CARRANZA'S

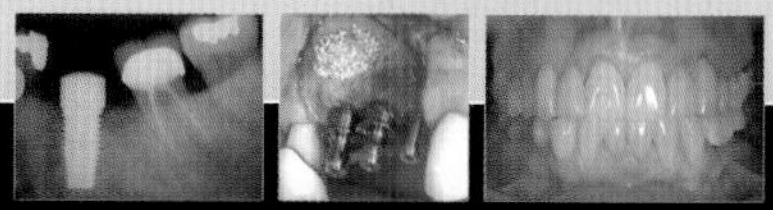

CLINICAL PERIODONTOLOGY

10

TENTH EDITION

MICHAEL G. NEWMAN, DDS

Adjunct Professor, Section of Periodontics
University of California, Los Angeles—School of Dentistry
Los Angeles, California

HENRY H. TAKEI, DDS, MS

Clinical Professor, Section of Periodontics
University of California, Los Angeles—School of Dentistry
Los Angeles, California

PERRY R. KLOKKEVOLD, DDS, MS

Associate Professor, Section of Periodontics
University of California, Los Angeles—School of Dentistry
Los Angeles, California

EDITOR EMERITUS

FERMIN A. CARRANZA, DR ODONT

Professor Emeritus, Section of Periodontics
University of California, Los Angeles—School of Dentistry
Los Angeles, California

SAUNDERS
ELSEVIER

SAUNDERS
ELSEVIER

An Imprint of Elsevier

11830 Westline Industrial Drive
St. Louis, Missouri 63146

CARRANZA'S CLINICAL PERIODONTOLOGY
Tenth Edition

ISBN 13 978-1-4160-2400-2
ISBN 10 1-4160-2400-X

NOTICE

Periodontology is an ever-changing field. Standard safety precautions must be followed, but as new research and clinical experience broaden our knowledge, changes in treatment and drug therapy may become necessary or appropriate. Readers are advised to check the most current product information provided by the manufacturer of each drug to be administered to verify the recommended dose, the method and duration of administration, and contraindications. It is the responsibility of the licensed health care provider, relying on experience and knowledge of the patient, to determine dosages and the best treatment for each individual patient. Neither the publisher nor the editors assume any liability for any injury and/or damage to persons or property arising from this publication.

The Publisher

International Standard Book Number 1-4160-2400-X

Publishing Director: Linda Duncan
Executive Editor: John Dolan
Developmental Editors: Jaime Pendill and John Dedeke
Publishing Services Manager: Patricia Tannian
Senior Project Manager: Anne Altepeter
Book Designer: Julia Dummitt

Printed in China

Last digit is the print number: 9 8 7 6 5 4 3 2 1

CARRANZA'S

CLINICAL PERIODONTOLOGY

EDITORS

ASSOCIATE EDITORS

David L. Cochran, DDS, PhD
Professor and Chairman, Department of Periodontics
Health Science Center at San Antonio
University of Texas
San Antonio, Texas

William V. Giannobile, DDS, DMSc
Najjar Professor of Dentistry and Director
Michigan Center for Oral Health Research
University of Michigan Clinical Research Center
Ann Arbor, Michigan

E. Barrie Kenney, BDSc, DDS, MS, FRACDS
Tarrson Family Professor of Periodontics and Chair
Section of Periodontics
University of California, Los Angeles—School of Dentistry
Los Angeles, California

M. John Novak, BDS, LDS, PhD
Professor of Periodontics and Associate Director
Center for Oral Health Research
University of Kentucky—College of Dentistry
Lexington, Kentucky

Section Editors

Jane L. Forrest, RDH, EdD
Division of Health Promotion, Disease Prevention, and Epidemiology
National Center for Dental Hygiene Research
University of Southern California—School of Dentistry
Los Angeles, California

Philippe P. Hujoel, PhD, DDS, MSD, MS
Department of Public Health Sciences
University of Washington—School of Dentistry
Seattle, Washington

Mark B. Lieberman, DDS
Clinical Lecturer
Section of Periodontics
University of California, Los Angeles—School of Dentistry
Los Angeles, California

CONTRIBUTORS

Elliot Abt, DDS, MS
Director
General Practice Residency Program
Advocate Illinois Masonic Medical Center
Chicago, Illinois

Alfredo Aguirre, DDS, MS
Professor and Program Director
Department of Oral Diagnostic Sciences
State University of New York at Buffalo—School of Dental Medicine
Buffalo, New York

William F. Ammons, Jr., DDS, MSD
Professor Emeritus
Department of Periodontics
University of Washington—School of Dentistry
Seattle, Washington

Maxwell H. Anderson, DDS, MS, MEd
Principal, Anderson Dental Consulting
Sequim, Washington

Akira Aoki, DDS, PhD
Instructor and Research Associate
Section of Periodontology
Department of Hard Tissue Engineering
Tokyo Medical and Dental University
Tokyo, Japan

Samuel J. Arbes, Jr., DDS, MPH, PhD
Clinical Research Coordinator
Division of Intramural Research
Environmental Diseases and Medicine Program
Laboratory of Respiratory Biology
National Institute of Environmental Health Sciences
Research Triangle Park, North Carolina

Robert R. Azzi, DDS
Assistant Clinical Professor
Department of Periodontics
University of Paris VII—School of Dentistry
Paris, France

Janet G. Bauer, DDS, MSEd, MSPH, MBA
Associate Professor
Section of Restorative Dentistry
University of California, Los Angeles—School of Dentistry
Los Angeles, California

James D. Beck, PhD
Distinguished Professor
Department of Dental Ecology
University of North Carolina
Chapel Hill, North Carolina

John Beumer, III, DDS, MS
Professor and Chair
Division of Advanced Prosthodontics, Biomaterials, and Hospital Dentistry
University of California, Los Angeles—School of Dentistry
Los Angeles, California

Carol A. Bibb, DDS, PhD
Assistant Dean, Adjunct Professor
Section of Oral Medicine
University of California, Los Angeles—School of Dentistry
Los Angeles, California

Jaime Bulkacz, PhD, DDS
Lecturer
Section of Periodontics
University of California, Los Angeles—School of Dentistry
Los Angeles, California

Paulo M. Camargo, DDS, MS
Associate Professor
Section of Periodontics
University of California, Los Angeles—School of Dentistry
Los Angeles, California

Fermin A. Carranza, Dr Odont
Professor Emeritus
Section of Periodontics
University of California, Los Angeles—School of Dentistry
Los Angeles, California

Ting-Ling Chang, DDS
Clinical Associate Professor
Division of Advanced Prosthodontics, Biomaterials, and Hospital Dentistry
University of California, Los Angeles—School of Dentistry
Los Angeles, California

Sebastian G. Ciancio, DDS, PhD
Distinguished Service Professor
Department of Periodontics and Endodontics
State University of New York at Buffalo—School of Dentistry
Buffalo, New York

David L. Cochran, DDS, PhD
Professor and Chair
Department of Periodontics
The University of Texas Health Science Center at San Antonio
San Antonio, Texas

Joseph P. Cooney, BDS, MS
Clinical Professor
Division of Advanced Prosthodontics, Biomaterials, and Hospital Dentistry
University of California, Los Angeles—School of Dentistry
Los Angeles, California

Raymond R. Derycke, DScD
Private Practice
Paris, France

Donald Duperon, DDS, MSc
Professor Emeritus
Section of Pediatric Dentistry
University of California, Los Angeles—School of Dentistry
Los Angeles, California

Daniel H. Etienne, DDS
Associate Professor
Department of Periodontology
University of Paris VII—School of Dentistry
Paris, France

Robert C. Fazio, DMD
Associate Clinical Professor in Surgery
Yale Medical School—College of Medicine
New Haven, Connecticut

Joseph P. Fiorellini, DSMc, DMD
Professor and Chair
Department of Oral Medicine, Infection, and Immunity
University of Pennsylvania
Philadelphia, Pennsylvania

Jane L. Forrest, RDH, EdD
Associate Professor and Chair
Division of Health Promotion, Disease Prevention, and Epidemiology
National Center for Dental Hygiene Research
University of Southern California—School of Dentistry
Los Angeles, California

Philippe C. Gault, DrOdont, CES, DUESC
Clinical Director
Natural Implant
Orleans, France

William V. Giannobile, DDS, DMSc
Najjar Professor of Dentistry and Director
Michigan Center for Oral Health Research
University of Michigan Clinical Research Center
Ann Arbor, Michigan

Stephen F. Goodman, DDS
Private Practice
New York, New York

Susan Kinder Haake, DMD, MDentSc, PhD
Associate Professor
Section of Periodontics
University of California, Los Angeles—School of Dentistry
Los Angeles, California

Thomas J. Han, DDS, MS
Associate Adjunct Professor
Section of Periodontics
University of California, Los Angeles—School of Dentistry
Los Angeles, California

Gerald W. Harrington, DDS, MSD
Professor Emeritus and Chair
Department of Endodontics
University of Washington—School of Dentistry
Seattle, Washington

James E. Hinrichs, DDS, MS
Professor and Director of Advanced Education in Periodontology
Department of Developmental/Surgical Sciences
University of Minnesota—School of Dentistry
Minneapolis, Minnesota

Eva L. Hogan, MD, DDS, MS
Lecturer
Section of Periodontics
University of California, Los Angeles—School of Dentistry
Los Angeles, California

Philippe P. Hujoel, PhD, DDS, MSD, MS
Professor
Department of Public Health Sciences
University of Washington—School of Dentistry
Seattle, Washington

Isao Ishikawa, DDS, PhD
Professor
Section of Periodontology
Department of Hard Tissue Engineering
Tokyo Medical and Dental University
Tokyo, Japan

Satoshi O. Ishikawa, DDS
Faculty Member
Section of Periodontology
Department of Hard Tissue Engineering
Tokyo Medical and Dental University
Tokyo, Japan

Carol A. Jahn, RDH, MS
Educational Programs Manager
Water-Pik Technologies
Warrenville, Illinois

David L. Jolkovsky, DMD, MS
Private Practice
Davis, California

Brian Kamel, Esq
Kamel and Maxwell, Attorneys At Law
Los Angeles, California

David M. Kim, DDS, DMSc
Instructor
Director of Predoctoral Periodontology
Department of Periodontology
Harvard University—School of Dental Medicine
Boston, Massachusetts

Keith L. Kirkwood, DDS, PhD
Assistant Professor
Department of Periodontics, Prevention, and Geriatrics
University of Michigan—School of Dentistry
Ann Arbor, Michigan

Perry R. Klokkevold, DDS, MS
Associate Professor
Section of Periodontics
University of California, Los Angeles—School of Dentistry
Los Angeles, California

Vincent G. Kokich, DDS, MS
Affiliate Professor
Department of Orthodontics
University of Washington—School of Dentistry
Seattle, Washington

Mark B. Lieberman, DDS
Clinical Lecturer
Section of Periodontics
University of California, Los Angeles—School of Dentistry
Los Angeles, California

Marina Maréchal, DDS, PhD
Associate Professor
Department of Periodontology
Catholic University, Leuven—School of Dentistry, Oral Pathology, and Maxillo-Facial Surgery
Leuven, Belgium

Phillip T. Marucha, DMD, PhD
Head
Department of Periodontics
University of Illinois at Chicago—College of Dentistry
Chicago, Illinois

Michael J. McDevitt, DDS
Private Practice
Atlanta, Georgia

Brian L. Mealey, DDS, MS
Clinical Associate Professor
Department of Periodontics
The University of Texas Health Science Center at San Antonio
San Antonio, Texas

Philip R. Melnick, DDS
Lecturer
Section of Periodontics
University of California, Los Angeles—School of Dentistry
Los Angeles, California

Robert L. Merin, DDS, MS
Private Practice
Woodland Hills, California

Bryan S. Michalowicz, DDS, MS
Director
Oral Health Clinical Research Center
University of Minnesota—School of Dentistry
Minneapolis, Minnesota

Syrene A. Miller, BA
Manager, National Center for Dental Hygiene Research
University of Southern California—School of Dentistry
Los Angeles, California

Kenneth T. Miyasaki, DDS, MS, PhD
Associate Professor
Section of Oral Biology
University of California, Los Angeles—School of Dentistry
Los Angeles, California

Richard J. Nagy, DDS
Private Practice
Santa Barbara, California

Ian Needleman, BDS, MSc, PhD, MRD
Senior Clinical Lecturer
Department of Periodontology
Eastman Dental Institute for Oral Health Care Sciences
University of London
London, England

Michael G. Newman, DDS
Adjunct Professor
Section of Periodontics
University of California, Los Angeles—School of Dentistry
Los Angeles, California

Russell J. Nisengard, DDS, PhD
Distinguished Teaching Professor
Associate Dean for Advanced Education and Research
State University of New York at Buffalo—School of Dentistry
Buffalo, New York

Karen F. Novak, DDS, MS, PhD
Associate Professor
Department of Periodontics
Center for Oral Health Research
University of Kentucky
Lexington, Kentucky

M. John Novak, BDS, LDS, PhD
Professor of Periodontics and Associate Director
Department of Periodontics
Center for Oral Health Research
University of Kentucky
Lexington, Kentucky

Joan Otomo-Corgel, DDS, MPH
Greater Los Angeles Veterans Administration Healthcare System
Adjunct Professor
Section of Periodontics
University of California, Los Angeles—School of Dentistry
Los Angeles, California

Kwang-Bum Park, DDS, MS, PhD
Visiting Assistant Researcher in Periodontics
University of California, Los Angeles—School of Dentistry
Los Angeles, California
Director, Perio-Line Institute of Clinical Periodontics and Implantology
Lecturer in Oral Anatomy and Histology
Kyung-Pook National University
Taegu, Korea

Anna M. Pattison, RDH, MS
Faculty Member
Department of Dental Hygiene
University of Southern California—School of Dentistry
Los Angeles, California

Gordon L. Pattison, DDS
Lecturer
Section of Periodontics
University of California, Los Angeles—School of Dentistry
Los Angeles, California

Dorothy A. Perry, RDH, PhD
Professor and Associate Dean for Education
Division of Dental Hygiene
University of California, San Francisco—School of Dentistry
San Francisco, California

Bruce L. Pihlstrom, DDS, MS
Acting Director, Center for Clinical Research
National Institute of Dental and Craniofacial Research
National Institutes of Health
Bethesda, Maryland

Philip M. Preshaw, BDS, FDS, RCSEd, PhD
Senior Lecturer in Periodontology
Department of Periodontology
University of Newcastle upon Tyne—School of Dental Sciences
Newcastle upon Tyne
England

Marc Quirynen, DDS, PhD
Professor
Department of Periodontology
Catholic University, Leuven—School of Dentistry, Oral Pathology, and Maxillo-Facial Surgery
Leuven, Belgium

Terry D. Rees, DDS, MSD
Professor
Department of Periodontics
Baylor College of Dentistry
Texas A&M Health Science Center
Dallas, Texas

Carlos Rossa, Jr., DDS, PhD
Professor
Diagnosis and Surgery Department
Universidade Estadual Paulista—Araraquara
Sao Paulo, Brazil

Eleni D. Roumanas, DDS
Associate Professor
Division of Advanced Prosthodontics, Biomaterials, and Hospital Dentistry
University of California, Los Angeles—School of Dentistry
Los Angeles, California

Maria Emanuel Ryan, DDS, PhD
Professor
Department of Oral Biology and Pathology
Stony Brook University—School of Dental Medicine
Stony Brook, New York

Mariano Sanz, MD, DDS
Dean and Professor
Department of Periodontics
Universidad Complutense de Madrid—Faculty of Dentistry
Madrid, Spain

Max O. Schmid, DMD
Private Practice
Aarau, Switzerland

Dennis A. Shanelec, DDS
Microsurgery Training Institute
Santa Barbara, California

Gerald Shklar, DDS, MS
Professor Emeritus
Charles A. Brackett Professor of Oral Pathology
Harvard University—School of Dental Medicine
Boston, Massachusetts

Thomas N. Sims, DDS
Lecturer
Section of Periodontics
University of California, Los Angeles—School of Dentistry
Los Angeles, California

Sue S. Spackman, DDS
Lecturer
Section of Restorative Dentistry
University of California, Los Angeles—School of Dentistry
Los Angeles, California

Frank M. Spear, DDS, MSD
Founder and Director
Seattle Institute for Advanced Dental Education
Seattle, Washington

Mario Taba, Jr., DDS, PhD
Professor
Department of Oral and Maxillofacial Surgery and Periodontics
University of São Paulo—School of Dentistry at Ribeirão Preto
Ribeirão Preto, SP, Brazil

Henry H. Takei, DDS, MS
Clinical Professor
Section of Periodontics
University of California, Los Angeles—School of Dentistry
Los Angeles, California

Sotirios Tetradis, PhD, DDS
Associate Professor
Section of Oral Radiology
University of California, Los Angeles—School of Dentistry
Los Angeles, California

Wim Teughels, DDS
Practical Assistant Professor
Department of Periodontology
Catholic University, Leuven—School of Dentistry, Oral Pathology, and Maxillo-Facial Surgery
Leuven, Belgium

Leonard S. Tibbetts, DDS, MSD
Private Practice
Arlington, Texas

Daniel van Steenberghe, MD, PhD
Professor
Department of Periodontology
Catholic University, Leuven—School of Dentistry, Oral Pathology, and Maxillo-Facial Surgery
Leuven, Belgium

Jose Luis Tapia Vazquez, DDS, MS
Assistant Professor
Department of Oral Diagnostic Sciences
State University of New York at Buffalo—School of Dental Medicine
Buffalo, New York

S. Jerome Zackin, DMD
Private Practice
Sarasota, Florida

ABOUT THE BOOK

Carranza's Clinical Periodontology is the definitive reference text on periodontics. Edited by Drs. Michael G. Newman, Henry H. Takei, new editor Perry R. Klokkevold, and editor emeritus Fermin A. Carranza, the tenth edition provides high-quality information for both students and practitioners. This outstanding resource has been completely updated to include the most current techniques and clinical aspects of modern periodontics while maintaining and upgrading detailed presentations of the fundamental basis of anatomy, physiology, etiology, and pathology. Major enhancements include a new full-color format, a detailed introduction to evidence-based decision making in dental practice, Science Transfer boxes in every chapter, and new chapters that address ethics, jurisprudence, and financial concerns of clinical practice. New contributors to the text provide fresh perspectives on key topics, and new information throughout the book ensures the most up-to-date coverage of the complete periodontal spectrum.

ABOUT THE E-DITION

With this tenth edition, *Carranza's Clinical Periodontology* is for the first time offered in an advanced electronic edition **(e-dition)** package, which combines the newly revised print textbook with a continuously updated companion website. Elsevier and the editors have put together a strong, comprehensive electronic component that combines the traditional printed textbook with additional features that are only possible electronically. The website offers many features such as a fully searchable text, text references with links to PubMed, regular content updates that enhance and refresh the information in the text, high-quality digital videos, case presentations, practice tests related to specific chapters, links to relevant websites, and much more. By offering continuous updates, the content of *Carranza's Clinical Periodontology* will remain in the forefront of periodontics throughout the lifetime of the tenth edition.

If you have purchased the print textbook without the e-dition, you may add Internet access at any time. Please go to www.elsevierhealth.com to order.

ABOUT THE AUTHORS

Michael G. Newman, DDS, FACD

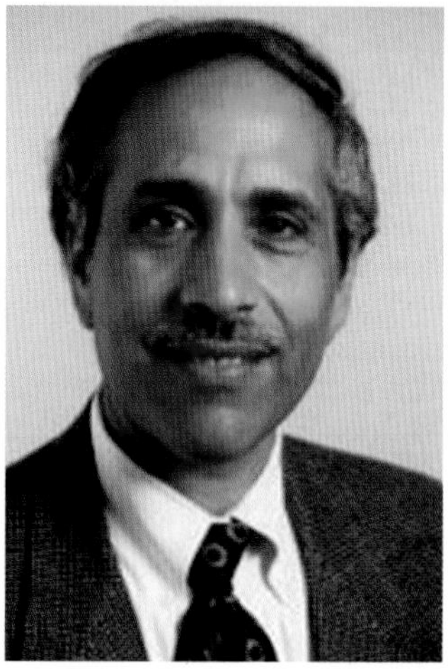

Dr. Michael G. Newman graduated from the University of California, Los Angeles (UCLA) College of Letters and Sciences with a degree in psychology. He completed his dental training at the UCLA School of Dentistry in 1972. Dr. Newman received a Certificate in Periodontics and Oral Medicine at the Harvard School of Dental Medicine and a Certificate in Oral Microbiology from the Forsyth Dental Institute under the mentorship of Dr. Sigmund Socransky. He is a diplomate of the American Board of Periodontology and an adjunct professor of periodontics at the UCLA School of Dentistry. Dr. Newman is a fellow and past president of the American Academy of Periodontology. In 1975, he won the Balint Orban Memorial Prize from the American Academy of Periodontology. He has been in private practice of periodontics for more than 25 years.

Dr. Newman has published more than 250 abstracts, journal articles, and book chapters and has co-edited eight textbooks. He has served as an ad hoc reviewer for the National Institute of Dental and Craniofacial Research, is a consultant to the Council on Scientific Affairs of the American Dental Association, and is a reviewer for numerous scientific and professional journals and governmental research organizations.

Dr. Newman has lectured throughout the world on microbiology, antimicrobials, evidence-based methodology, risk factors, and diagnostic strategies for periodontal disease. Dr. Newman has a strong interest in applied science and transfer of new technology for practical use. He has served as a consultant to many major dental and pharmaceutical companies throughout the world. Dr. Newman is the founding editor in chief of the *Journal of Evidence-Based Dental Practice* and was the associate editor of the *International Journal of Oral and Maxillofacial Implants.*

Henry H. Takei, DDS, MS, FACD

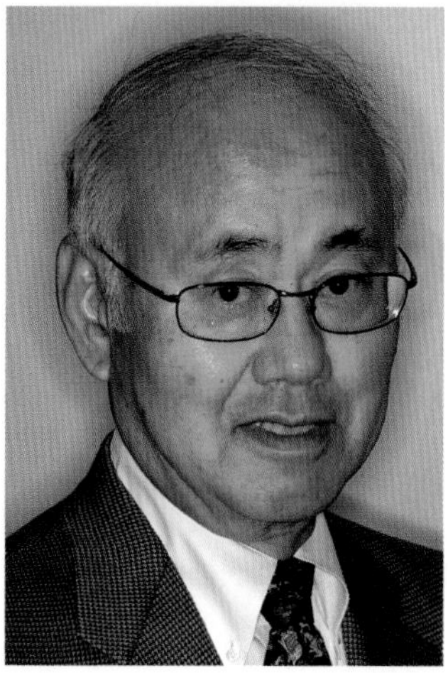

Dr. Henry H. Takei graduated in 1965 from the Marquette University School of Dentistry in Milwaukee, Wisconsin. He completed his Periodontics Certificate and Master of Science degree in 1967 at the Marquette University and the Veterans Administration Hospital in Wood, Wisconsin.

Dr. Takei is a clinical professor of periodontics at the UCLA School of Dentistry and a consultant in periodontics at the Veterans Administration Hospital in Los Angeles. He maintains a private practice limited to periodontics and implant surgery.

Dr. Takei has published numerous articles on periodontal surgery and has contributed chapters to five textbooks. He has been actively involved in continuing education and has lectured throughout the world on clinical periodontology and implant surgery. He has received many teaching awards from both universities and dental organizations nationally and internationally.

Dr. Takei has been honored by numerous periodontal organizations, universities, and study clubs for his contributions to education. He has received the Distinguished Alumnus Award by Marquette University and the Honorary Distinguished Alumnus Award by the University of California, Los Angeles.

ABOUT THE AUTHORS

Perry R. Klokkevold, DDS, MS

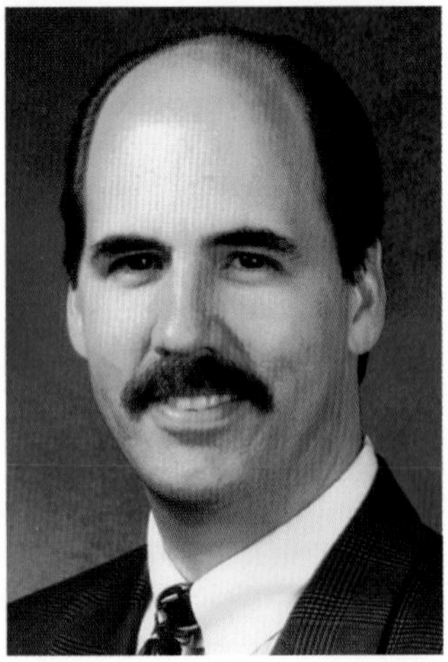

Dr. Perry R. Klokkevold graduated from the University of California, San Francisco School of Dentistry in 1986. His postdoctoral clinical training includes a general practice residency in hospital dentistry completed in 1987, a postgraduate periodontal residency completed in 1994, and a surgical implant fellowship completed in 1995. All of his postgraduate training was completed at the UCLA School of Dentistry. He completed a Master of Science degree program in oral biology at UCLA in 1995.

Dr. Klokkevold is a diplomate of the American Board of Periodontology. He is an associate professor in the Division of Associated Specialties, Section of Periodontics, at the UCLA School of Dentistry and director of the UCLA Postgraduate Periodontics Residency program. Dr. Klokkevold previously served as clinical director and director of the general practice residency program in hospital dentistry at UCLA School of Dentistry from 1987 to 1992. Dr. Klokkevold has maintained a faculty practice limited to the specialty of periodontics and dental implant surgery at UCLA for more than 10 years.

Dr. Klokkevold has published numerous articles for international journals and has written several book chapters on topics that include juvenile periodontitis, periodontal medicine, influence of systemic disease and risk factors on periodontitis, bone regeneration, and dental implants. He is a reviewer for several journals, including the *International Journal of Oral and Maxillofacial Implants,* and he is a special editor for the *Journal of Evidence-Based Dental Practice*. Dr. Klokkevold has lectured nationally and internationally on many periodontal and implant-related topics.

Fermin A. Carranza, Dr Odont, FACD

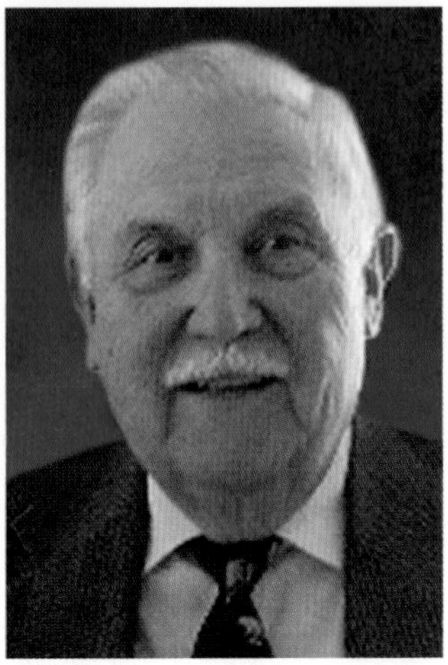

Dr. Fermin A. Carranza graduated from the University of Buenos Aires School of Dentistry in Argentina in 1948 and completed his postdoctoral training in periodontics at Tufts University School of Dental Medicine in 1952 under the mentorship of Dr. Irving Glickman.

Dr. Carranza is professor emeritus of periodontology at the UCLA School of Dentistry. He was head of the Department of Periodontics at the University of Buenos Aires from 1966 to 1974, and at UCLA from 1974 until his retirement in 1994.

Dr. Carranza has published more than 218 scientific papers and abstracts on basic and applied aspects of periodontics and 18 books, including the past five editions of *Clinical Periodontology*. He has received numerous awards and recognition for his work, including the IADR Science Award in Periodontal Disease and the Gies Award of the American Academy of Periodontology.

Dr. Carranza has lectured throughout the world on clinical periodontology, pathology, and therapy.

PREFACE

This tenth edition and companion e-dition is the most comprehensive textbook and information source about periodontology available anywhere. Utilizing Elsevier's advanced technology and high standards of quality, the editors and contributors have developed a major periodontal resource intended to be used by everyone with an interest in periodontology.

THE TEXT

Our goal in completely revising this classic textbook was to preserve the same tradition of comprehensiveness and organization that has made the book the number one choice among educators, students, clinicians, researchers, and policy makers. And, for the first time, the book is published in full color.

In addition to the book's all-color presentation, several new chapters and many revised chapters offer new content.

- A primer on evidence-based periodontology appears at the beginning of the text. We believe that the information contained in these chapters will greatly enhance understanding and incorporation of the information in the rest of the book.
- Each chapter throughout the book contains a new Science Transfer box, which provides expert interpretations of the content within the chapter. Sometimes these practical explanations describe the scientific basis for clinical procedures, bridging the gap between basic science and clinical practice. Other times the Science Transfer boxes contain state-of-the-art commentaries about the incorporation of techniques into clinical practice. The content of each Science Transfer box is unique and interesting and aims to convey a valued, expert perspective on the written material.
- The book concludes with an entirely new section and chapters devoted to ethics, jurisprudence, and financial aspects of clinical practice. A thorough understanding and application of the principles found in each of these chapters are crucial for dentists, hygienists, and periodontists who care for periodontal patients in clinical practice today.

THE E-DITION

Introduction of the *Clinical Periodontology E-dition* provides many new features and recognizes the ever-changing ways in which people learn and utilize information.

- The tenth edition's online counterpart contains all of the content of the printed book along with all of the illustrations, tables, and photographs.
- This web-based resource is fully searchable and contains many features that are designed to enhance learning and supplement the completely updated and revised content of the tenth edition.
- Important new information will be continually added to the site as updates to keep the content evergreen and useful to readers.

A complete description of *Carranza's Clinical Periodontology Online* can be found in the *Guide to Online Edition Resources*.

Since publication of the first edition of this book **53** years ago, periodontology has made tremendous progress. Analysis of periodontal tissues and elucidation of the mechanisms and causes of disease have extended far beyond histology and physiology and into the realm of cellular and molecular biological understanding. New therapeutic goals and clinical techniques, based on an improved understanding of disease, have facilitated better outcomes and brought us closer to achieving the ultimate goal of optimal periodontal health and function. Today, reconstruction of lost periodontal structures, replacement of compromised teeth with implants, and creation of esthetic results are integral parts of clinical practice.

This book is written for all individuals—from students to educators, clinicians to researchers, and specialists to generalists. It is our belief that periodontal care of the public is primarily the role of general dentists and dental hygienists. The responsibility to examine, diagnose, and either treat or refer *all* periodontal problems is unquestionable. Likewise, the role of periodontitis in systemic disease makes diagnosis essential and treatment imperative.

The multifaceted, complex task of producing the tenth edition and e-dition required the collaboration of numerous experts from various fields, and their contributions are invaluable. It is our hope that this new edition will continue to be as useful to dentists, hygienists, periodontists, students, educators, and researchers as the previous editions and that it will contribute to continuous progress of our profession.

Michael G. Newman
Henry H. Takei
Perry R. Klokkevold
Fermin A. Carranza

GUIDE TO ONLINE E-DITION RESOURCES

The study and practice of periodontology are ever changing, with new concepts, technology, and information emerging every day. The tenth edition of *Clinical Periodontology* is designed to evolve and grow continuously with each of these new developments in periodontics through the *Clinical Periodontology E-dition* website, a "living" online counterpart to this revised textbook. This resource is readily available to purchasers of the *Clinical Periodontology E-dition* or those who upgrade to web access. Resources of the *Clinical Periodontology E-dition* include the complete revised *Clinical Periodontology* text as well as a host of enhanced features not possible in a printed textbook.

Below is an introduction to each of the supplemental features found on the *Clinical Periodontology E-dition* website. These features form the core of the *Clinical Periodontology E-dition* but, just as periodontics continues to evolve, so does this interactive resource.

COMPLETE ONLINE, SEARCHABLE TEXT

The *Clinical Periodontology* online component allows the entire textbook to be searchable.

The accompanying search engine enables users to **instantly locate all content** related to a given topic.

CONTINUOUS CONTENT UPDATES

Changes in periodontology are addressed through regular amendments to the *Clinical Periodontology* text. These updates provide new information and multimedia on developments throughout the entire spectrum of periodontics and reflect the same quality coverage found in the textbook.

INTERACTIVE REFERENCES

All of the bibliographic material for *Clinical Periodontology* is presented in a searchable format that is directly linked, wherever possible, to the original full-text articles and abstracts referenced in the creation of the tenth edition.

CASE PRESENTATIONS

Online users can choose from a range of fully documented case studies that provide current, compelling information drawn from material in the text and other *Clinical Periodontology* online resources. The cases include histories, presenting symptoms, test results, diagnoses, and treatment options, as well as pertinent clinical photographs and radiographs.

VIDEO CLIPS

Important techniques, procedures, and concepts from *Clinical Periodontology* are supported by high-quality video clips accessible directly from the corresponding sections in the text.

TESTING CENTER

The *Clinical Periodontology* online Testing Center challenges users' knowledge of the text with online examinations accompanied by instant scoring and answer links to relevant text material.

ELECTRONIC IMAGE COLLECTION

Every image from the tenth edition of *Clinical Periodontology* is viewable in the electronic image collection. Students can review key points from the text, and instructors are able to customize lectures and lesson plans with supporting material taken directly from the tenth edition.

INSTANT ACCESS TO DENTAL DRUG DATABASE

Drug names throughout the online text are linked directly to corresponding monographs from *Mosby's Dental Drug Consult,* consistently updated with the most current data available for hundreds of dental drugs.

LEGAL CORNER

News alerts and articles on legal developments related to dentistry are presented as they occur, providing detailed information and commentary for a wide spectrum of topics.

To access the online content or for more information, visit www.clinicalperiodontology.com or contact Elsevier Customer Service at 1-800-545-2522.

ACKNOWLEDGMENTS

The originator of this book and author of its first four editions, published in 1953, 1958, 1964, and 1972, was Dr. Irving Glickman, professor and chairman of the Department of Periodontology at Tufts University School of Dental Medicine, in Boston, Massachusetts.

After Dr. Glickman's death in 1972 at age 58, responsibility for continuing this book moved to Dr. Fermin A. Carranza, once a student and collaborator of Dr. Glickman. At the time Dr. Carranza was professor and chairman of periodontics at the School of Dentistry, University of California, Los Angeles (UCLA). The following four editions were published in 1979, 1984, 1990, and 1996 under the guidance of Dr. Carranza, who is now professor emeritus at UCLA.

In 2002, the task of maintaining the book's tradition of almost half a century changed hands once again. Dr. Michael G. Newman and Dr. Henry H. Takei joined Dr. Carranza to take major responsibility for the ninth edition.

For this tenth edition, Dr. Perry R. Klokkevold from UCLA has joined as a co-editor, and Drs. E. Barrie Kenney, David Cochran, William V. Giannobile, and M. John Novak are associate editors.

Advances in basic science and clinical techniques have increased the knowledge base so dramatically that it is virtually impossible for a single individual to memorize and retain all of the information needed to practice excellently. It is also a certainty that the enormity of providing the information of a discipline must be borne by many experts willing to share their experience and knowledge.

The editors are indebted to everyone who has worked tirelessly to produce this milestone print and electronic edition of Carranza's Clinical Periodontology.

Many scientists and clinicians have shared their knowledge and expertise from previous editions of *Carranza's Clinical Periodontology,* but their names no longer appear as contributors to the present one. We express our deep gratitude to all of them for their many valuable concepts and ideas.

Our appreciation is given to Elsevier and particularly to Penny Rudolph, John Dolan, Jaime Pendill, John Dedeke, and Anne Altepeter. Their expertise and detailed attention to every word and every concept contributed greatly to producing a quality book and a truly useful website.

Very special thanks to Dominik Jacobs, whose hard work, steadfast determination, and superb organizational skills made production of this book possible.

We express gratitude to our parents, colleagues, friends, and mentors who have always been so tolerant, encouraging, and understanding, and who guided our first steps in our profession and helped us develop our ideas in the field.

Dr. Newman: my wife, *Susan;* my children *Andrea* and *Natalie;* my parents *Paul, Rose, John,* and *Inez. Sigmund S. Socransky, Stephen Stone, J.D. Murray, Fermin A. Carranza, Jr.,* and *Henry H. Takei.* Special thanks to *E. Barrie Kenney* for his support in providing me the opportunity to manage this large, complex, and time-consuming project. My gratitude to my co-editors and contributors whose expertise and willingness to participate in this work have made this book an excellent educational standard.

Dr. Takei: My wife, *June;* my children *Scott* and *Akemi;* their spouses, *Kozue* and *David;* my grandchildren, *Hana, Markus, Carter,* and *Arden.* My mentors, *Dr. Donald Van Scotter, Dr. Delbert Nachazel, Dr. John Pfeiffer,* and my co-editors, *Michael G. Newman, Fermin A. Carranza, Jr.,* and *Perry R. Klokkevold.* Special gratitude to *Laura Miyabe* for her professional support and *Rose Kitayama* for her technical support.

Dr. Klokkevold: my wife, *Angie;* my daughters *Ashley* and *Brianna;* my parents *Carl* and *Loretta Klokkevold;* my mentors *Henry H. Takei, John Beumer III, Bradley G. Seto, Charles N. Bertolami, Peter K. Moy,* and *E. Barrie Kenney.* I thank all of the residents with whom I have had the pleasure to work over the years, for the passion and inspiration they bring to me as an educator and clinician. Special thanks to my co-editors, *Michael G. Newman, Henry H. Takei,* and *Fermin A. Carranza, Jr.,* who have supported and encouraged me throughout the process of updating this classic textbook and creating the e-dition website.

Dr. Carranza: my wife, *Rita;* my children *Fermin, Patricia,* and *Laura;* and my grandchildren. *Irving Glickman, Fermin Carranza, Sr.,* and *Romulo L. Cabrini.* My gratitude also to my co-editors, who will continue the tradition of this book.

Michael G. Newman
Henry H. Takei
Perry R. Klokkevold
Fermin A. Carranza

CONTENTS

DETAILED CONTENTS

INTRODUCTION
The Historical Background of Periodontology

Gerald Shklar and Fermin A. Carranza

CHAPTER OUTLINE

Gingival and periodontal diseases, in their various forms, have afflicted humans since the dawn of history. Studies in paleopathology have indicated that destructive periodontal disease, as evidenced by bone loss, affected early humans in such diverse cultures as ancient Egypt and early pre-Columbian America. The earliest historical records dealing with medical topics reveal an awareness of periodontal disease and the need for treatment. Almost all the early writings that have been preserved have sections or chapters dealing with oral diseases, and periodontal problems comprise a significant amount of space in these writings. The relationship between calculus and periodontal disease often was considered, and underlying systemic disease was frequently postulated as a cause of periodontal disorders. However, methodic, carefully reasoned, therapeutic discussions did not exist until the Arabic surgical treatises of the Middle Ages, and modern treatment, with illustrated text and sophisticated instrumentation, did not develop until the time of Pierre Fauchard in the eighteenth century.

EARLY CIVILIZATIONS

Oral hygiene was practiced by the Sumerians of 3000 BC, and elaborately decorated gold toothpicks found in the excavations at Ur in Mesopotamia suggest an interest in cleanliness of the mouth. The Babylonians and Assyrians, like the earlier Sumerians, apparently suffered from periodontal problems, and a clay tablet of the period tells of treatment by gingival massage combined with various herbal medications.[25,33]

Periodontal disease was the most common of all diseases found in the embalmed bodies of the ancient Egyptians.[7,44] The Ebers papyrus contains many references to gingival disease and offers a number of prescriptions for strengthening the teeth and gums, applied in the form of a paste with honey, vegetable gum, or residue of beer as a vehicle.[14]

The medical works of ancient India devote significant space to oral and periodontal problems, including descriptions of severe periodontal disease with loose teeth and purulent discharge from the gingiva, stressing toothbrushing and oral hygiene.[47]

Ancient Chinese medical works also discussed periodontal disease. In the oldest book, about 2500 BC, a chapter is devoted to dental and gingival diseases. Gingival inflammations, periodontal abscesses, and gingival ulcerations are described. The Chinese used the "chewstick" as a toothpick and toothbrush to clean the teeth and massage the gingival tissues.[21]

The early Hebrews recognized the importance of oral hygiene. Many pathologic conditions of the teeth and surrounding structures are described in the Talmudic writings.

THE CLASSICAL WORLD

Among the ancient Greeks, Hippocrates of Cos (460–377 BC), the father of modern medicine, discussed the function and eruption of the teeth and the etiology of periodontal disease. He believed that inflammation of the gums could be caused by accumulations of "pituita" or calculus, with gingival hemorrhage occurring in cases of persistent splenic maladies.[10,27]

Among the Romans, Aulus Cornelius Celsus (25 BC–50 AD) referred to diseases that affect the soft parts of the mouth and their treatment, including oral hygiene. Paul of Aegina (625–690 AD) differentiated between "epulis," a fleshy excrescence of gums in the area of a tooth, and "parulis," which he described as an abscess of the gums. He wrote that tartar incrustations must be removed with either scrapers or a small file and that the teeth should be carefully cleaned after the last meal of the day.[41]

THE MIDDLE AGES

The decline and fall of the Roman Empire that plunged Europe into an age of darkness was accompanied by the rise of Islam and the golden age of Arabic science and medicine. Much of medieval and Renaissance "stomatology" and dentistry was derived directly from Arabic writings, particularly the treatises of Ibn Sina (Avicenna) and Abu'l-Qasim (Albucasis). The Arabic treatises derived their information from Greek medical treatises but added many refinements and novel approaches, particularly in surgical specialties.[45]

The contributions of Albucasis (936–1013) to dentistry and periodontology were outstanding achievements.[1] He had a clear understanding of the major etiologic role of calculus deposits and described the technique of scaling the teeth, using a set of instruments that he developed (Figure 1). He also wrote on the extraction of teeth, the splinting of loose teeth with gold wire, and the filing of gross occlusal abnormalities.

Born in Persia, Avicenna (980–1037) was possibly the greatest of the Arabic physicians. His *Canon,* a comprehensive treatise on medicine, was in continuous use for almost 600 years. Avicenna used an extensive "materia medica" for oral and periodontal diseases and rarely resorted to surgery.[3]

THE RENAISSANCE

During the Renaissance, with the rebirth of classical scholarship and the development of scientific thought and medical knowledge, in addition to the flowering of art, music, and literature, significant contributions were made to anatomy and surgery.

Paracelsus (1493–1541) developed an interesting and unusual theory of disease: the doctrine of calculus. He understood that pathologic calcification occurred in a variety of organs and considered it the result of metabolic disturbances whereby the body takes nourishment from food and discards the refuse as "tartarus," a material that cannot be broken down and is the ultimate matter, or *materia ultima.* Paracelsus recognized the extensive formation of tartar on the teeth and related this to toothache. Toothache was thus comparable to the pain produced by calculus in other organs, such as the kidneys.[39]

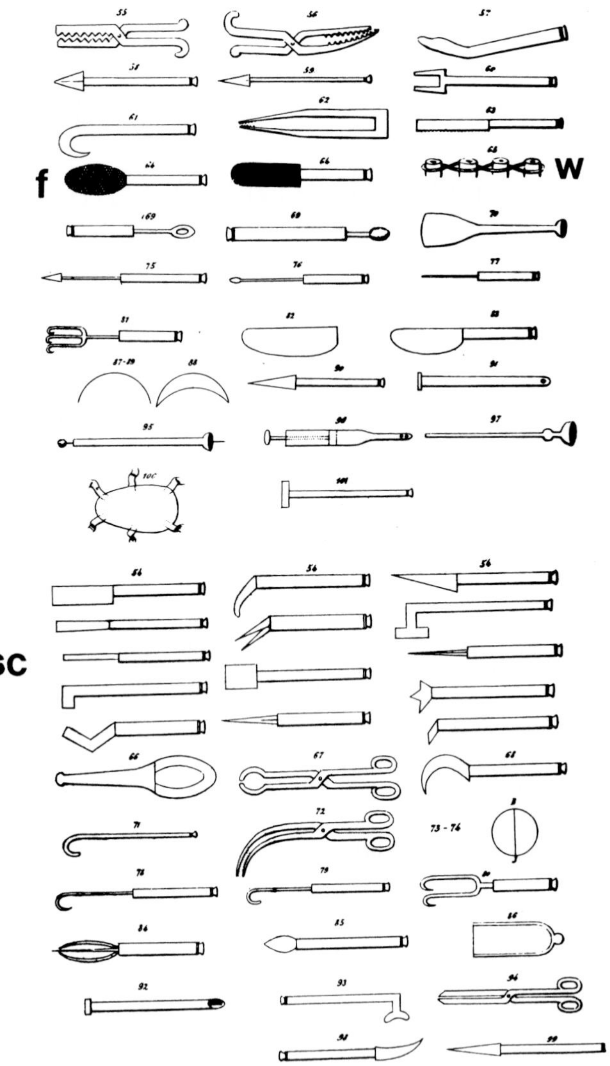

Figure 1 Illustration of Abu'l-Qasim's periodontal instruments, showing scalers *(sc),* files *(f),* and the wiring of loose teeth *(w).*

Andreas Vesalius (1514–1564), born in Brussels, taught at the University of Padua in the Venetian Republic, where he performed human dissections and wrote a magnificent book on anatomy with excellent illustrations throughout, which were drawn by Calcar, a student of Titian.[48]

Bartholomaeus Eustachius (1520–1574) of Rome was another outstanding anatomist and wrote a small book on dentistry, *Libellus de Dentibus* ("A Little Treatise on the Teeth"), in 30 chapters.[16] In many ways, his anatomic studies were more detailed and comprehensive than those of his more famous contemporary, Vesalius, but his major studies remained unknown until their publication in 1722. This was the first original book on the teeth and offered many new descriptions and concepts based on research and clinical studies, including a description of the periodontal tissues, diseases of the mouth, and their treatment modalities and rationale for treatment. For the treatment of periodontitis, Eustachius advised both scaling of calculus and curettage of granulation tissue so that actual reattachment of the gingival and periodontal tissues could take place.

Ambroise Paré (1509–1590), head surgeon at the Hôtel Dieu in Paris, was the outstanding surgeon of the Renaissance, and his contributions to dental surgery included gingivectomy for hyperplastic gingival tissues.[40] He also understood the etiologic significance of calculus and used a set of scalers to remove the hard deposits on the teeth.

The first book in a common language (German) and specifically devoted to dental practice, entitled *Artzney Buchlein* or *Zene Artzney* ("Medicine of the Teeth"), was published in Leipzig in 1530.[2] The book contains three chapters devoted to periodontal problems, including a crude concept of systemic and local factors in the etiology of periodontal disease. The presence of local infective agents, or "worms," also is mentioned. A variety of ointments, often astringent in nature, are suggested, and the binding of loose teeth to sound ones with silk or gold thread is recommended. Cauterizing the gingiva with a hot iron is mentioned.

The Italian physician, mathematician, and philosopher Girolamo Cardano (1501–1576) appears to have been the first to differentiate types of periodontal disease. In a publication dated 1562, he mentions one type of disease that occurs with advancing age and leads to progressive loosening and loss of teeth, as well as a second, very aggressive type that occurs in younger patients.[26] It was not until late in the twentieth century that this classification was rediscovered and became widely accepted.

Anton van Leeuwenhoek (1632–1723) of Delft, Holland, was a layman, but he had an inquisitive mind and a hobby of grinding lenses that allowed him to develop the microscope. He used it to discover microorganisms, cellular structure, blood cells, sperm, and various other microscopic structures, including the tubular structure of dentin.[9,13] Leeuwenhoek described his findings in letters written originally in Dutch to the Royal Society of London, which translated them into English and published them in its *Philosophical Transactions*. Using material from his own mouth, Leeuwenhoek first described oral bacterial flora, and his drawings offered a reasonably good presentation of oral spirochetes and bacilli (Figure 2). He even performed antiplaque experiments using strong vinegar in his own mouth and in vitro on bacteria in a dish.[13]

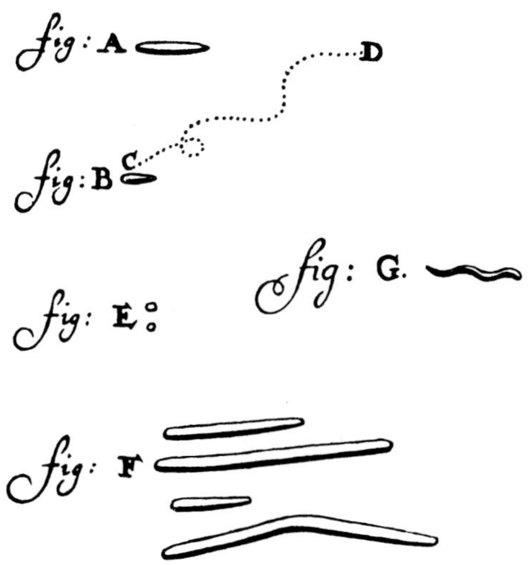

Figure 2 Leeuwenhoek's drawing of oral spirochetes, bacilli, and other microorganisms.

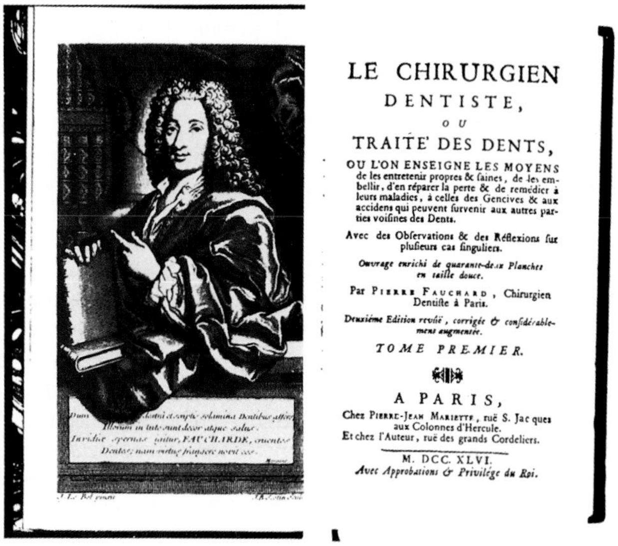

Figure 3 Frontispiece of Fauchard's book *The Surgeon Dentist* (1746 edition).

EIGHTEENTH CENTURY

Modern dentistry essentially developed in eighteenth-century Europe, particularly France and England. Pierre Fauchard, born in Brittany in 1678, is rightly regarded as the father of the dental profession as we know it. Self-educated in dentistry, he was able to develop a systematic approach to dental practice based on contemporary knowledge, and he significantly improved the instruments and technical skills required for dental treatment. His book *The Surgeon Dentist,* published in 1728, covered all aspects of dental practice, including restorative dentistry, prosthodontics, oral surgery, periodontics, and orthodontics[17] (Figure 3). Fauchard described in detail his periodontal instruments and the scaling technique to use them (Figure 4).

John Hunter (1728–1793), the most distinguished anatomist, surgeon, and pathologist of eighteenth-century England, wrote an excellent treatise on dentistry entitled *The Natural History of the Human Teeth.*[30] He offered remarkably clear illustrations of the anatomy of the teeth and their supporting structures. He also described the features of periodontal diseases and enunciated the concept of active and passive eruption of teeth.

A contemporary of Hunter, Thomas Berdmore (1740–1785), was considered the outstanding dentist in

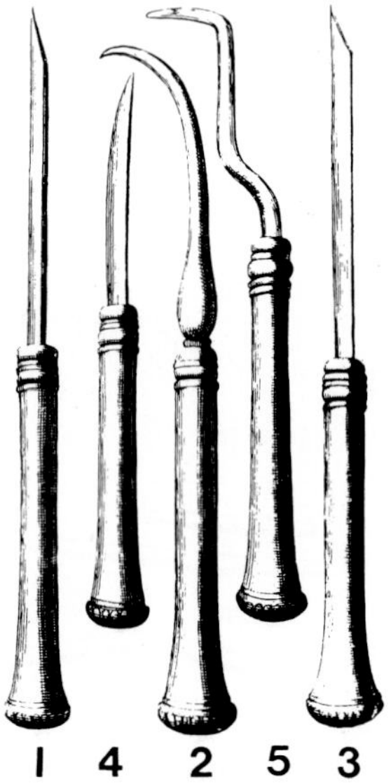

Figure 4 The five types of instruments used by Fauchard for detaching tartar from the teeth: *1,* chisel; *2,* parrot beak; *3,* graver; *4,* convex blade; and *5,* Z-shaped hook.

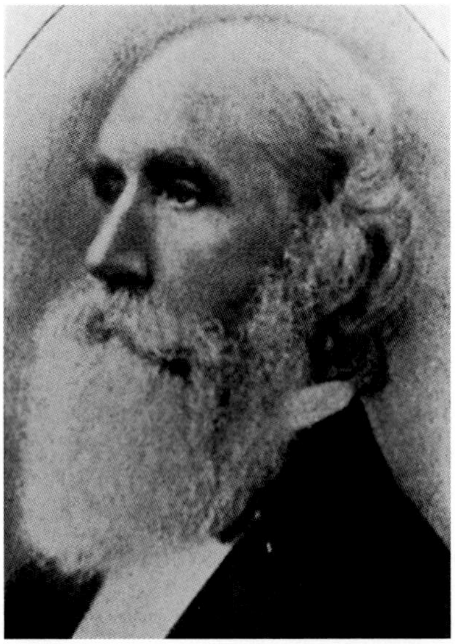

Figure 5 John W. Riggs (1811–1885). (From Hoffman-Axthelm W: *History of dentistry,* Chicago, 1981, Quintessence.)

England and published the *Treatise in the Disorders and Deformities of the Teeth and Gums* in 1770, with several chapters devoted to periodontal problems.[4]

NINETEENTH CENTURY

Leonard Koecker (1785–1850) was a German-born dentist who practiced in Baltimore. In a paper in 1821, he described inflammatory changes in the gingiva and calculus on teeth that led to their looseness and exfoliation. He mentioned the careful removal of tartar and the need for oral hygiene by the patient, recommending that it be performed in the morning and after every meal using an astringent powder and a toothbrush, placing "the bristles . . . into the spaces of the teeth." He also discouraged splinting because it loosened firm teeth, and he recommended that treatment of caries be postponed until after the gum treatment is completed and that placement of artificial teeth be avoided. Koecker was an early advocate of the "odontogenic focal infection" theory and recommended the extraction of all severely involved teeth and roots, including all unopposed molars, to prevent systemic infections.[35]

Levi Spear Parmly (1790–1859) was a New Orleans dentist who is considered the father of oral hygiene and the inventor of dental floss.[11,18]

In the mid-nineteenth century, John W. Riggs (1811–1885) was the leading authority on periodontal disease and its treatment in the United States, to the point that periodontitis was known as "Riggs' disease" (Figure 5). He was born in Seymour, Connecticut, and graduated from the Baltimore College of Dental Surgery in 1854. He practiced in Hartford, Connecticut, where he died on November 11, 1885. Riggs seems to have been the first individual to limit his practice to periodontics and therefore can be considered the first specialist in this field. Riggs' publications, however, are limited. In an 1876 paper, Riggs was a strong proponent of the so-called conservative approach to periodontal therapy, developing the concept of oral prophylaxis and prevention, advocating cleanliness of the mouth and opposing surgery, which at the time consisted of resection of the gums.[43]

Riggs and his disciples had great influence in the dental profession. Among Riggs followers were L. Taylor, D.D. Smith, R.B. Adair, and W.J. Younger. Many papers by followers and contemporaries of Riggs described clinical features and treatment of periodontal disease, the latter based mostly on hygienic measures.

William J. Younger (1838–1920) considered periodontal disease a local infection and was the first to discuss the possibility of "reattachment."[57] The instruments designed by Younger, and later modified by his student Robert Good, were used widely until well beyond the middle of the twentieth century.

Several major developments in medical science occurred in the second half of the nineteenth century, starting the era that can be called *modern medicine,* which includes dentistry.[9,36]

The first was the *discovery of anesthesia* by Horace Wells (1813–1848) of Hartford, Connecticut, in 1845 and by William Morton (1819–1868) of Boston in 1846, who discovered the general anesthetic effects of nitrous oxide and ether, respectively. *Local anestesia* was developed by the Vienna ophthalmologist Carl Köller (1857–1944), who produced anesthesia of the eye with drops of cocaine. Procaine (Novocaine) was developed in 1905 by the Munich chemists Alfred Einhorn and Richard Willstädter. Later, with the addition of adrenaline, discovered separately in the United States by Jokichi Takamine and Thomas Bell Aldrich, local anesthesia was born.[29]

The second scientific breakthrough was made by the French chemist Louis Pasteur (1822–1895), who finally proved that spontaneous generation of organisms does not exist and showed that one organism can cause disease in another, thus establishing the *germ theory of disease.* Subsequently, the German physician Robert Koch (1843–1910), in a series of brilliant investigations, discovered the microorganism that causes the cattle disease anthrax and the bacterial etiology of tuberculosis and cholera.

The concepts of Pasteur were transferred to clinical and surgical practice by Joseph Lister (1827–1912) of England, and thus the era of antisepsis (and later, asepsis) in surgery was born. Anesthesia and antisepsis made posible the extraordinary advances in surgical techniques.

Pasteur, Koch, and their collaborators and followers (Elie Metchnikoff, Emile Roux, Paul Ehrlich, Emil von Behring, Shibasaburo Kitasato, and many others) discovered the bacterial etiology of numerous diseases (e.g., pneumonia, puerperal fever, diphtheria, meningitis, plague, dysentery, syphilis) and gave birth to two sciences that became basic to periodontics: bacteriology and immunology.

A third scientific finding that changed the practice of dentistry in general and periodontics in particular was the *discovery of radiographs* by the German physicist Wilhelm Röntgen (1845–1923; also Roentgen). Röntgen's discovery was made in 1895 at the University of Würzburg and was purely a basic science finding, but it was immediately taken up by physicians and dentists and proved to be a crucial development in periodontics and many other areas of medicine and dentistry.

Also in the late nineteenth century, studies by Rudolph Virchow (1821–1902), Julius Cohnhein (1839–1884), Elie Metchnikoff (1845–1916), and others had started to reveal the microscopic changes occurring in inflammation.[8,9] This resulted in an understanding of the pathogenesis of periodontal disease based on histopathologic studies. The Russian N.N. Znamensky described the complex interaction of local and systemic factors in the etiology of periodontal disease. His observations and concepts were summarized in 1902 in a classic paper in which he described the presence in inflamed gingivae of a cellular infiltrate that extends deeper as the disease progresses, causing bone resorption associated to multinucleated cells (osteoclasts) and Howship's lacunae[58] (Figure 6).

The first individual to identify bacteria as the cause of periodontal disease appears to have been the German dentist Adolph Witzel (1847–1906).[23,56] The first true oral microbiologist, however, was the American Willoughby D. Miller (1853–1907), whose professional activities took place in Berlin, where he embarked on a research career that introduced modern bacteriology principles to dentistry. Although his greatest accomplishments were in caries research, in his classic book *The Microorganisms of the Human Mouth,* published in 1890, he described the features of periodontal disease and considered the role of predisposing factors, irritational factors, and bacteria in its etiology. He believed that the disease was not caused by a specific bacterium but by a complex array of various bacteria normally present in the oral cavity. This constitutes what was later known as the *nonspecific plaque hypothesis,* which went unchallenged for seven decades.[23,37]

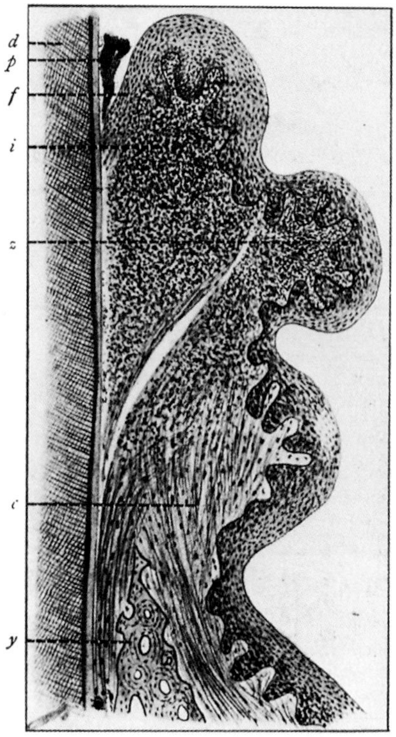

Figure 6 Microscopic features of periodontal disease as presented by Znamensky.

Bacterial plaque was described by J. Leon Williams (1852–1932), an American dentist who practiced in London and in 1897 described a gelatinous accumulation of bacteria adherent to the enamel surface in relation to caries.[55] In 1899, G.V. Black (1836–1915) coined the term "gelatinous microbic plaque."[5]

Salomon Robicsek (1845–1928) was born in Hungary and practiced dentistry in Vienna. He developed a surgical technique consisting of a scalloped, continuous gingivectomy excision, exposing the marginal bone for subsequent curettage and remodeling.[46]

The first description (1901) of a possible role of trauma from occlusion and bruxism in periodontal disease is generally attributed to the Austrian dentist Moritz Karolyi (1865–1945), who also recommended its correction by grinding occlusal surfaces and the preparation of bite plates.[34]

Necrotizing Ulcerative Gingivitis

Necrotizing ulcerative gingivitis (NUG) had been recognized in the fourth century BC by Xenophon, who mentioned that Greek soldiers were affected with "sore mouth and foul-smelling breath." In 1778, Hunter described the clinical features of this disease and differentiated it from scurvy and chronic periodontitis.

Hyacinthe Jean Vincent (1862–1950),[23,49] a French physician working at the Pasteur Institute in Paris, and Hugo Carl Plaut (1858–1928),[42] in Germany, described the spirillum and fusiform bacilli associated with what later became known as *Vincent's angina,* and in 1904 Vincent described these organisms in ulceronecrotic gingivitis.[50]

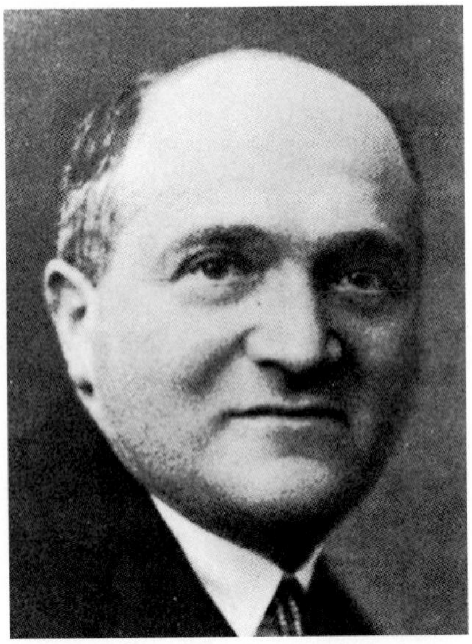

Figure 7 Bernhard Gottlieb (1885–1950). (From Gold SI: *J Clin Periodontol* 12:171, 1985.)

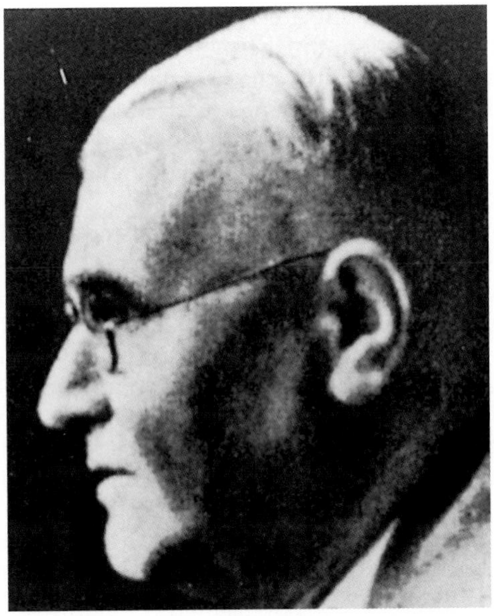

Figure 9 Oskar Weski (1879–1952). (From Hoffman-Axthelm W: *History of dentistry,* Chicago, 1981, Quintessence.)

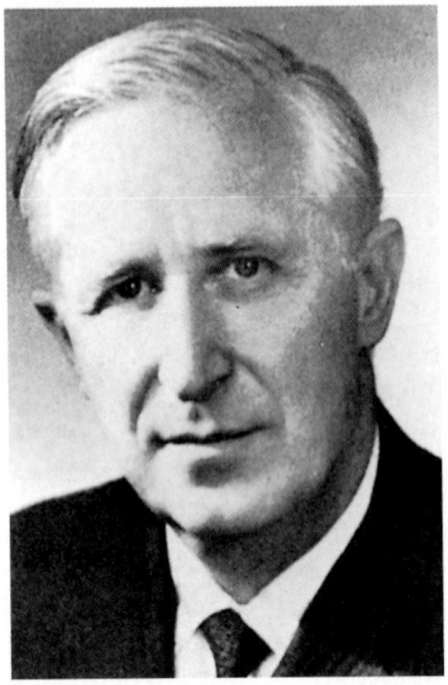

Figure 8 Balint J. Orban (1899–1960). (From *J Periodontol* 31:266, 1960.)

TWENTIETH CENTURY

In the first third of the twentieth century, periodontics flourished in central Europe, with two major centers of excellence: Vienna and Berlin.

Vienna

The Vienna school developed the basic histopathologic concepts on which modern periodontics was built. The major representative from this group was Bernhard Gottlieb (1885–1950), who published extensive microscopic studies of periodontal disease in human autopsy specimens (Figure 7). His major contributions appeared in the German literature in the 1920s and described the attachment of the gingival epithelium to the tooth, the histopathology of inflammatory and degenerative periodontal disease, the biology of the cementum, active and passive tooth eruption, and traumatic occlusion. A book published in 1938 by Gottlieb and Orban presented a complete review in English of the concepts developed by Gottlieb and his co-workers in Vienna.[24]

A younger contemporary of Gottlieb's in Vienna was Balint J. Orban (1899–1960) (Figure 8), who carried out extensive histologic studies on periodontal tissues that serve as the basis for much of current therapy. Other members of the Viennese school were Rudolph Kronfeld (1901–1940), Joseph P. Weinmann (1889–1960), and Harry Sicher (1889–1974). All these scientists emigrated to the United States in the 1930s and contributed greatly to the progress of American dentistry.

Berlin

The Berlin group consisted mostly of clinical scientists who developed and refined the surgical approach to periodontal therapy. Prominent in this group were Oskar Weski (Figure 9) and Robert Neumann (Figure 10).

Weski (1879–1952) carried out pioneering studies correlating radiographic and histopathologic changes in periodontal disease.[53] He also conceptualized the periodontium as formed by cementum, gingiva, periodontal ligament, and bone and gave it the name *paradentium,* which was later changed (for etymologic reasons) to *parodontium,* a term still used in Europe.

Neumann (1882–1958), in a book published in 1912[38] (with new editions in 1915, 1920, and 1924), described the principles of periodontal flap surgery, including osseous recontouring as it is currently known[20] (Figure 11). Other clinicians who described flap surgery at the beginning of the twentieth century were Leonard

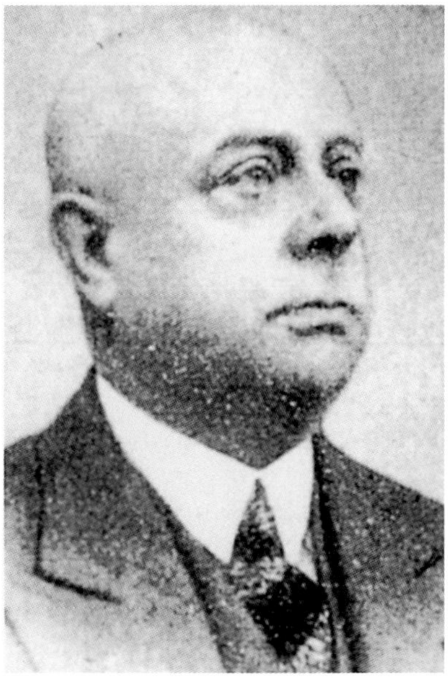

Figure 10 Robert Neumann (1882–1958). (Courtesy Dr. Steven I. Gold, New York, NY.)

Widman of Sweden (1871–1956)[54] and A. Cieszynski of Poland. A bitter controversy developed among Widman, Cieszynski, and Neumann in the 1920s over the priority in describing the periodontal flap.

United States and Other Countries

In the United States, before World War II, important contributions to periodontal surgery were made by A. Zentler, J. Zemsky, G.V. Black, O. Kirkland, A.W. Ward, A.B. Crane, H. Kaplan, and others. In 1923, Ward introduced the surgical pack under the trade name Wondr-Pak.[51]

The nonsurgical approach was championed by Isadore Hirschfeld (1882–1965) of New York, who wrote classic papers on oral hygiene,[28] local factors, and other topics. In 1913, Alfred Fones (1869–1938) opened the first school for dental hygienists in Bridgeport, Connecticut.[9]

In other countries, H.K. Box (Canada); M. Roy and R. Vincent (France); R. Jaccard and A.-J. Held (Switzerland); F.A. Carranza, Sr., and R. Erausquin (Argentina); W.W. James, A. Counsell, and E.W. Fish (Great Britain); and A. Leng (Chile) are well known for their important contributions. Probably the most comprehensive book on periodontics published in the first half of the twentieth century was *El Paradencio, Su Patologia y Tratamiento,* by the Uruguayan F.M. Pucci, which appeared in 1939.

Focal Infection

The concept of systemic diseases originating in dental and oral infections had been mentioned in the Assyrian clay tablets (seventh century BC), by Hippocrates (460–370 BC), in the Babylonian Talmud (third century AD), and by Girolamo Cardano and the German Walter Hermann Ryff in the sixteenth century.[29] In the nineteenth century, Benjamin Rush (famous physician and one of the signers of the American Declaration of Independence) in 1818 and Leonard Koecker in 1828 recognized the role of oral sepsis in rheumatic and other diseases. Later in the nineteenth century, W.D. Miller also mentioned oral infections as the cause of many diseases.[37]

In a paper published in 1900[31] and a decade later in a lecture at McGill University in Montreal,[32] William Hunter (1861–1937), a British physician, indicted dentistry as being the cause of oral sepsis, which in turn caused rheumatic and other chronic diseases. This idea was taken up by Billings, Rosenow, and many others, who advocated extractions of all teeth with periodontal or periapical infections to prevent systemic diseases. This led to wholesale extractions of teeth (and removal of tonsils).

The focal infection theory fell into disrepute when it was found that extractions failed to eliminate or reduce the systemic diseases to which the infected teeth were supposed to be linked.[15] However, the concept has been

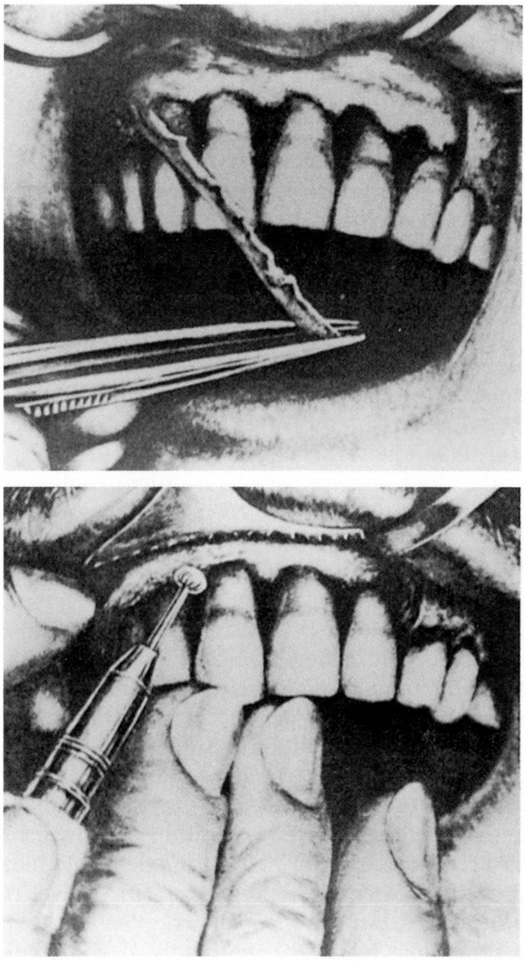

Figure 11 Surgical procedure advocated by Robert Neumann in the early part of the twentieth century. *Top,* After raising a mucoperiosteal flap, its edge is trimmed with scissors, leaving a scalloped outline. *Bottom,* Osseous recontouring with burs. (From Gold SI: *J Periodontol* 53:456, 1982.)

revisited in the 1990s, this time with a more solid research foundation.

Dental Implants

The replacement of human teeth by implants has been attempted for centuries. Skulls with metal or stone implants have been found in a Gallo-Roman necropolis in France from the second century AD and in a mandible of Mayan origin dated about 600 AD.[9]

In 1806 the Italian M. Maggiolo attempted to place solid-gold roots in human jaws, and later in the nineteenth century, several other investigators used porcelain and metallic implants. In the first half of the twentieth century, several attempts were made using elaborate surgical techniques and complicated constructs of gold and other precious metals, and microscopic investigations were begun on the tissue response to various metals.

In 1939, A.E. Strock of Harvard University started implanting cobalt-chromium (Vitallium) screws into tooth sockets. After World War II, numerous attempts were made with different materials and shapes of implants, including tantalum twisted spiral (Formiggini), Vitallium tree shaped (Lee), acrylic tooth root replica (Hodosh), Vitallium double helical spiral (Chércheve), tantalum tripodal pins (Scialom), tantalum vent-plant and titanium blade (Linkow), and vitreous carbon.[9]

In the 1950s the Swedish orthopedic surgeon Per-Ingvar Branemark developed a technique using titanium, screw-shaped intraosseous implants. This proved to be quite successful and was gradually adopted by the dental profession after the 1982 international conference in Toronto. The success and predictability of Branemark's technique are attributed to the achievement of direct contact between vital bone and the implant surface without intervening soft tissue, a phenomenon later termed "osseointegration."[6] Numerous variations of the Branemark concept were presented by A. Kirsch, G.A. Niznick, A. Schroeder, and others and are widely used at present.

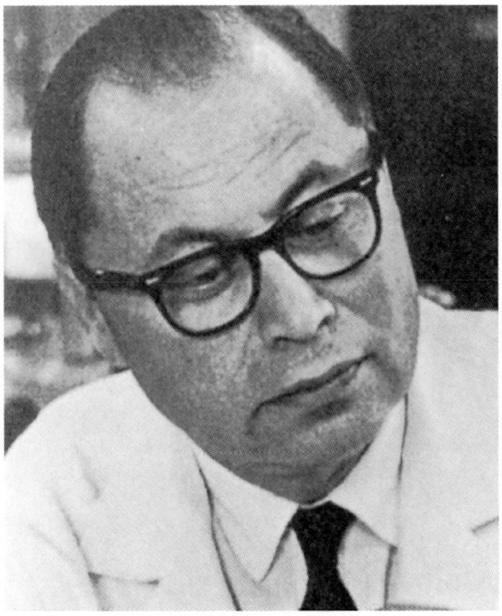

Figure 12 Irving Glickman (1914–1972).

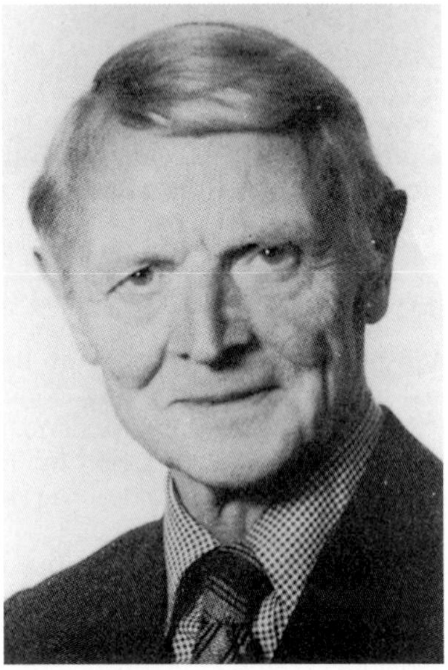

Figure 13 Jens Waerhaug (1907–1980). (From *J Clin Periodontol* 7:534, 1980.)

After World War II

The United States and Scandinavia took a leading role in basic and clinical periodontal research during and after the 1950s, with major advances in the fields of experimental pathology, microbiology, immunology, and therapy.

In the United States, five individuals led in the efforts to advance our understanding of the disease processes and the technical approaches to solve them: Irving Glickman (1914–1972) (Figure 12), Henry M. Goldman (1911–1991), Balint J. Orban (1899–1960) (see Figure 8), Sigurd P. Ramfjord (1911–1997), and Helmut A. Zander (1912–1991). In the clinical area, the influence of John Prichard (1907–1990) and Saul Schluger (1908–1990) led to new concepts and new directions in the pursuit of clinical success and excellence.

The leading figure of the Scandinavian group was Jens Waerhaug (1907–1980) of Oslo, whose dissertation, *The Gingival Pocket* (1952), opened a new era in the understanding of the biology of the periodontium (Figure 13).

The next generations centered their attention more on the role of microorganisms and the immunologic response. Their contributions, as well as those of their predecessors, are documented in this book.

Several workshops and international conferences have summarized the existing knowledge on the biologic and clinical aspects of periodontology. Worthy of mention are those that were conducted in 1951, 1966, 1977, 1989, and 1996 and cosponsored and published by the American Academy of Periodontology.

The American Academy of Periodontology (AAP), founded in 1914 by two female periodontists, Grace Rogers Spalding (1881–1953) and Gillette Hayden (1880–1929), has become the leader in organized periodontics. Its monthly scientific publication, *The Journal of Periodontology,* presents all the advances in this discipline. In Europe the periodontal societies have joined to form the European Federation of Periodontology, which meets regularly at the Europerio meeting. Their official publication is the *Journal of Clinical Periodontology*. Other scientific periodontal journals in English include *Journal of Periodontal Research, Periodontology 2000,* and *International Journal of Periodontics and Restorative Dentistry.* In other languages, *Journal de Parodontologie* (France), *Periodoncia* (Spain), and *Journal of the Japanese Association of Periodontology* deserve mention.

Periodontal education in the United States also has grown in the second half of the twentieth century, and most dental schools have separate and independent units for teaching and research in this discipline. Periodontics was recognized as a specialty of dentistry by the American Dental Association in 1947. The first university-based programs for the training of specialists in periodontics were begun in several universities (Columbia, Michigan, Tufts) in the late 1940s; these 1-year programs expanded to 2-year programs about 10 years later. In 1995 the AAP mandated that all postgraduate periodontal programs increase to a 3-year curriculum because of the increased knowledge in periodontics and the expansion of the scope of periodontics to include placement of dental implants and administration of conscious sedation. Currently, more than 50 periodontal graduate programs are based in universities and hospitals.

REFERENCES

1. Albucasis: *La Chirurgie,* Paris, Bailliére, 1861 (Translated by L LeClere).
2. *Artzney Buchlein,* Leipzig, 1530, Michael Blum (English translation in *Dent Cosmos* 29:1, 1887).
3. Avicenna: *Liber Canonis,* Venice, 1507 (Reprinted, Hildesheim, 1964, Georg Olms).
4. Berdmore T: *A treatise on the disorders and deformities of the teeth and gums,* London, 1786, B White.
5. Black GV: *Special dental pathology,* Chicago, 1915, Medico-Dental Publishers.
6. Branemark PI, Hansson BO, Adell R, et al: Osseointegrated implants in the treatment of the edentulous jaw: experience from a 10-year period, *Scand J Plast Reconstr Surg Suppl* 16:1, 1977.
7. Breasted JH: *The Edwin Smith surgical papyrus,* Chicago, 1930, University of Chicago Press.
8. Carranza FA: *Revolucionarios de la ciencia,* Buenos Aires, 1998, Vergara (editor).
9. Carranza F, Shklar G: *The history of periodontology,* Chicago, 2003, Quintessence.
10. Castiglione A: *History of medicine,* ed 2, New York, 1941, Knopf.
11. Chernin D, Shklar G: Levi Spear Parmly: father of dental hygiene and children's dentistry in America, *J Hist Dent* 51:15, 2003.
12. Dabry P: *La Medicine chez les Chinois,* Paris, 1863, Plon.
13. Dobell C: *Anton van Leeuwenhoek and his "little animals,"* New York, Harcourt, 1932 (Reprinted, New York, 1960, Dover Publications).
14. Ebbel B: *The Papyrus Ebers,* Copenhagen, 1937, Levin and Munksgaard.
15. Editorial, *JAMA* 150:490, 1952.
16. Eustachius B: *A little treatise on the teeth,* 1999, Science History Publishers/USA (Edited and introduced by DA Chernin and G Shklar; translated by JH Thomas).
17. Fauchard P: *Le Chirurgien Dentiste, ou Traite des Dents,* Paris, 1728, J Maruiette (Reprinted in facsimile, Paris, Prélat, 1961; English translation by L Lindsay, London, 1946, Butterworth & Co).
18. Fischman SL: The history of oral hygiene: how far have we come in 6000 years? *Periodontology 2000* 15:7, 1997.
19. Fleischmann L, Gottlieb B: Beitrage zur Histologie und Pathogenese der Alveolarpyorrhoe, *Z Stomatol* 2:44, 1920.
20. Gold SI: Robert Neumann: a pioneer in periodontal flap surgery, *J Periodontol* 53:456, 1982.
21. Gold SI: Periodontics: the past. Part I. Early sources, *J Clin Periodontol* 12:79, 1985.
22. Gold SI: Periodontics: the past. Part II. The development of modern periodontics, *J Clin Periodontol* 12:171, 1985.
23. Gold SI: Periodontics: the past. Part III. Microbiology, *J Clin Periodontol* 12:257, 1985.
24. Gottlieb B, Orban B: *Biology and pathology of the tooth and its supporting mechanism,* New York, 1938, Macmillan (Translated and edited by M Diamond).
25. Guerini V: *History of dentistry,* Philadelphia, 1909, Lea & Febiger.
26. Held A-J: *Periodontology—from its origins up to 1980: a survey,* Boston, 1989, Birkhauser.
27. Hippocrates: *Works,* London, 1923, 1931, Heinemann (Edited and translated by WHS Jones and ET Withington).
28. Hirschfeld I: *The toothbrush: its use and abuse,* New York, 1939, Dental Items of Interest Publishers.
29. Hoffman-Axthelm W: *History of dentistry,* Chicago, 1981, Quintessence.
30. Hunter J: *The natural history of the human teeth,* London, 1771, J Johnson (Reprinted as *Treatise in the natural history and diseases of the human teeth.* In Bell T, editor: *Collected works,* London, 1835, Longman Rees).
31. Hunter W: Oral sepsis as a cause of disease, *Br Med J* 1:215, 1900.
32. Hunter W: An address on the role of sepsis and antisepsis in nedicine, *Lancet* 1:79, 1911.
33. Jastrow N: The medicine of the Babylonians and Assyrians, *Proc Soc Med London* 7:109, 1914.
34. Karolyi M: Beobachtungen ber Pyorrhea Alveolaris, *Vjschr Zahnheilk* 17:279, 1901.
35. Koecker A: An essay on the devastation of the gums and the alveolar processes, *Philadelphia J Med Phys Sci* 2:282, 1821.
36. Major RHL: *A history of medicine,* Springfield, Ill, 1954, Charles C Thomas.
37. Miller WD: The human mouth as a focus of infection, *Dent Cosmos* 33:689, 789, 913, 1891.
38. Neumann R: *Die Alveolarpyorrhoe und ihre Behandlung,* Berlin, 1912, Meusser.
39. Paracelsus: *Sämtliche Werke* (Collected works in modern German), 14 volumes, Munich, 1922-1933, R Oldfenbourg (Edited by K Sudhoff).
40. Paré A: *Oeuvres Completes,* Paris, 1840, Bailliére (Edited by JF Malgaigne).
41. Paul of Aegina: *The Seven Books,* London, 1844, Sydenham Society (Translated by F Adams).
42. Plaut HC: Studien zur bakteriellen Diagnostik der Diphtherie und der Anginen, *Dtsch Med Wochenschr* 20:920, 1894.
43. Riggs JW: Suppurative inflammation of the gums and absorption of the gums and alveolar process, *Pa J Dent Sci* 3:99 1876 (Reprinted in *Arch Clin Oral Pathol* 2:423, 1938).
44. Ruffer MA: *Studies in the paleopathology of Egypt,* Chicago, 1921, University of Chicago Press.

45. Shklar G: Stomatology and dentistry in the golden age of Arabian medicine, *Bull Hist Dent* 17:17, 1969.
46. Stern IB, Everett FG, Robicsek K: S. Robicsek: a pioneer in the surgical treatment of periodontal disease, *J Periodontol* 36:265, 1965.
47. *Susruta Samhita,* Calcutta, 1907, KKL Bhishagratna.
48. Vesalius A: *De Humanis Corporis Fabrica,* Basle, 1542 (Reproduced in facsimile, Brussels, 1966, Culture et Civilisation).
49. Vincent HJ: Sur l'etiologie et sur les lesions anatomopathologiques de la pourriture d'hospital, *Ann de l'Inst Pasteur* 10:448, 1896.
50. Vincent HJ: Recherche sur l'etiologie de la stomatitis ulceromembraneuse primitive, *Arch Int Laryngol* 17:355, 1904.
51. Ward AW: Inharmonius cusp relation as a factor in periodontoclasia, *J Am Dent Assoc* 10:471, 1923.
52. Weinberger BW: *An introduction to the history of dentistry,* St Louis, 1948, Mosby.
53. Weski O: Roentgenographische-anatomische Studien auf dem Gebiete der Kieferpathologie, *Vjrsch Zahnh* 37:1, 1921.
54. Widman L: Surgical treatment of pyorrhea alveolaris, *J Periodontol* 42:571, 1971.
55. Williams JL: A contribution to the study of pathology of enamel, *Dent Cosmos* 39:169, 269, 353, 1897.
56. Witzel A: The treatment of pyorrhea alveolaris or infectious alveolitis, *Br J Dent Sci* 25:153, 209, 257, 1882.
57. Younger WJ: Pyorrhea alveolaris, *Schweiz Vierteljähresscrift Zahnheilk* 15:87, 1905.
58. Znamensky NN: Alveolar pyorrhoea: its pathological anatomy and its radical treatment, *J Br Dent Assoc* 23:585, 1902.

Evidence-Based Decision Making

Jane L. Forrest and Philippe P. Hujoel

PART

1

The principles of evidence-based methodologies provide a systematic framework for relying on scientific evidence in conjunction with clinical experience and judgment to answer questions and stay current with innovations in dentistry.

Learning and mastering the critical thinking skills associated with evidence-based methodologies is a key component in translating the discoveries of basic and clinical research found in this book into the realities of practice.

The three chapters in Part 1 provide an introduction to evidence-based decision making. Perspectives on the determination of clinical significance and examples of how to integrate the knowledge into practice are presented.

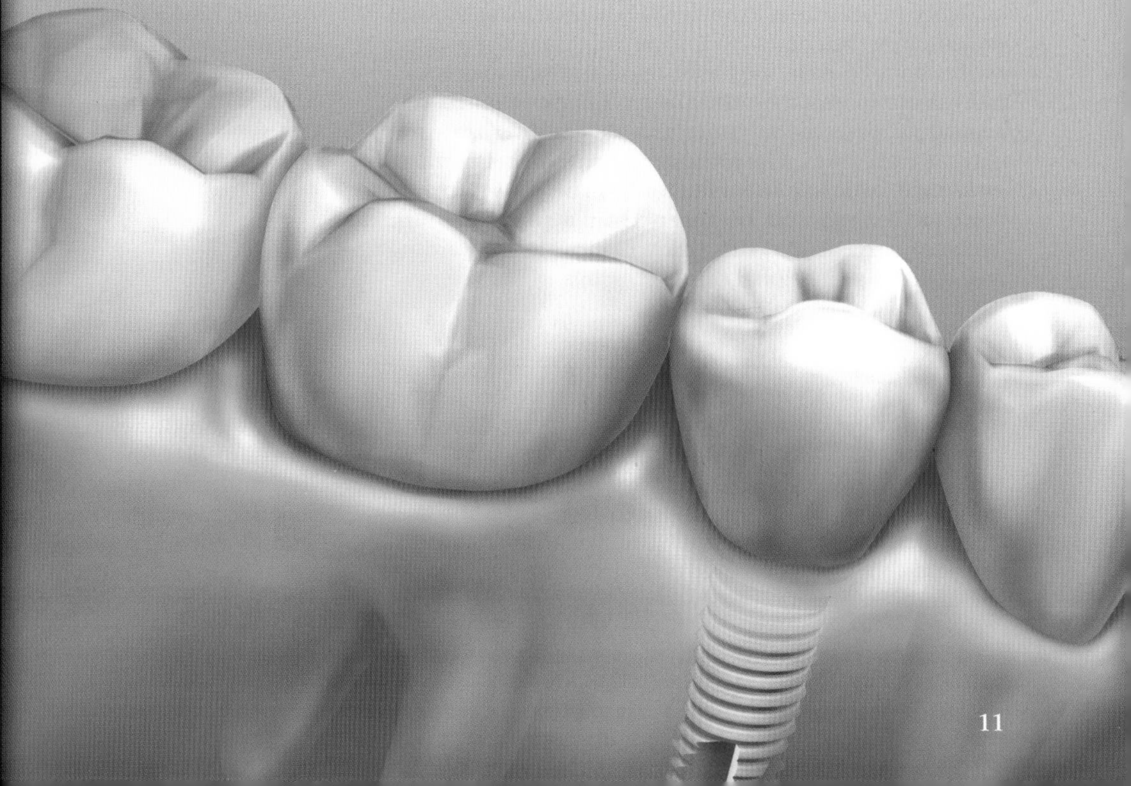

Introduction to Evidence-Based Decision Making

Jane L. Forrest, Syrene A. Miller, and Michael G. Newman

1

CHAPTER

■ ■ ■

CHAPTER OUTLINE

BACKGROUND AND DEFINITION
PRINCIPLES OF EVIDENCE-BASED DECISION MAKING
 Evidence-Based versus Traditional Decision Making
 Evidence-Based Dentistry
NEED FOR EVIDENCE-BASED DECISION MAKING
 Variations in Practice Patterns
 Assimilating Evidence into Practice

EVIDENCE-BASED DECISION-MAKING PROCESS
 AND SKILLS
 Asking Good Questions: the PICO Process
 Searching for and Acquiring the Evidence
 Appraising the Evidence
 Evaluating the Outcomes
CONCLUSION

Each day, dental care professionals make decisions about clinical care. It is important that these decisions incorporate the best available scientific evidence in order to maximize the potential for successful patient care outcomes. It is also important for readers of this book to have the background and skills necessary to evaluate information they read and hear about. These evaluative skills are as important as learning facts and clinical procedures. **The ability to find, discriminate, evaluate, and use information is the most important skill that can be learned as a professional.** Becoming excellent at this skill will provide a rewarding and fulfilled professional career.

BACKGROUND AND DEFINITION

Using evidence from the medical literature to answer questions, direct clinical action, and guide practice was pioneered at McMaster University, Ontario, Canada, in the 1980s. As clinical research and the publication of findings increased, so did the need to use the medical literature to guide practice. The traditional clinical problem-solving model based on individual experience or the use of information gained by consulting authorities (colleagues or textbooks) gave way to a new methodology for practice and restructured the way in which more

effective clinical problem solving should be conducted. This new methodology was termed *evidence-based medicine* (EBM).[17] EBM is defined as "the integration of the best research evidence with clinical expertise and patient values."[36]

The use of evidence to help guide clinical decisions is not new. However, the following aspects of EBM are new:

- The methods of generating high-quality evidence, such as randomized controlled trials and other well-designed methods.
- The statistical tools for synthesizing and analyzing the evidence (systematic reviews and meta-analysis).
- The ways for accessing the evidence (electronic databases) and applying it (evidence-based decision making and practice guidelines).[13,14]

Along with these changes has evolved the understanding of what constitutes the evidence and how to minimize sources of bias, quantify the magnitude of benefits and risks, and incorporate patient values.[18] "In other words, evidence-based practice is not just a new term for an old concept and as a result of advances, practitioners need 1) more efficient and effective online searching skills to find relevant evidence, and 2) critical appraisal skills to rapidly evaluate and sort out what is valid and useful, and what is not."[33]

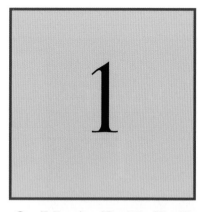

Evidence-based decision making (EBDM) is the formalized process and structure for learning these skills so that the best scientific evidence is considered when making patient care decisions.

PRINCIPLES OF EVIDENCE-BASED DECISION MAKING

Evidence-Based versus Traditional Decision Making

Initially, the focus of EBM emphasized using randomized clinical trials and other quantifiable methods. As EBM has evolved, however, so has the realization that the evidence from clinical research is only one key component of the decision-making process and does not tell a practitioner what to do.[20] In other words, *the use of current best evidence does not replace clinical expertise or input from the patient, but rather provides another dimension to the decision-making process,*[16,24,25] which is also placed in context with the patient's clinical circumstances (Figure 1-1). It is this decision-making process that we refer to as "evidence-based decision making." EBDM is not unique to medicine or any specific health discipline; it represents a concise way of referring to the application of evidence to clinical decision making.

EBDM focuses on solving clinical problems and involves two fundamental principles, as follows[18]:

1. Evidence alone is never sufficient to make a clinical decision.
2. Hierarchies of quality and applicability of evidence exist to guide clinical decision making.

EBDM is a structured process that incorporates a formal set of rules for interpreting the results of clinical research and places a lower value on authority or custom. In contrast to EBDM, traditional decision making relies more on intuition, unsystematic clinical experience, and pathophysiologic rationale.[18,31]

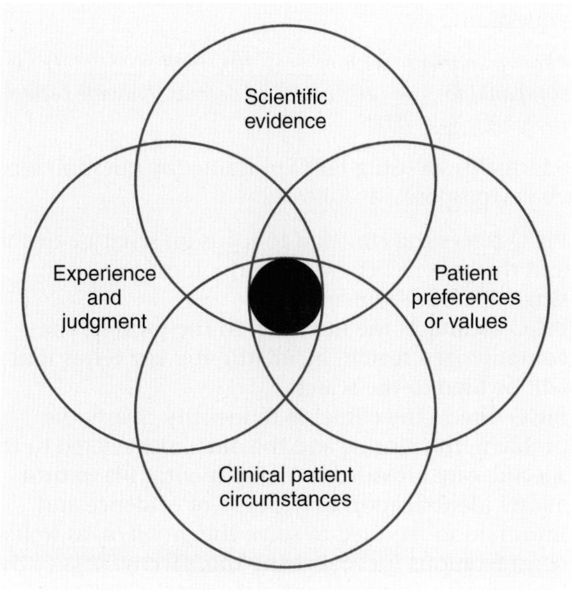

Figure 1-1 Evidence-based decision making.

Evidence-Based Dentistry

Since the 1990s, the evidence-based movement has continued to advance and is becoming widely accepted among the health care professions, with some refining the definition to make it more specific to their area of health care. The American Dental Association (ADA) has defined evidence-based dentistry (EBD) as "an approach to oral health care that requires the judicious integration of systematic assessments of clinically relevant scientific evidence, relating to the patient's oral and medical condition and history, with the dentist's clinical expertise and the patient's treatment needs and preferences."[3]

This definition is now incorporated in the ADA Accreditation Standards for Dental Education Programs.[2] Dental schools are expected to develop specific core competencies that focus on the need for graduates to become critical thinkers, problem solvers, and consumers of current research findings to enable them to become lifelong learners. These skills parallel those of evidence-based practice by teaching students to find, evaluate, and incorporate current evidence into their decision making.[2]

NEED FOR EVIDENCE-BASED DECISION MAKING

An evidence-based approach has emerged in response to the need to improve the quality of health care and to demonstrate the best use of limited resources.[16,25] Two forces driving the need to improve the quality of care are (1) the variations in practice patterns and (2) the difficulty that clinicians confront in assimilating scientific evidence into their practices.[9,33,36]

Variations in Practice Patterns

Studies of appropriateness in health care confirm that a wide range of variability exists between what is known and what is practiced.[7,8,15,22] Much too often, variations occur because of a gap between the time that current research knowledge becomes available and its application to care. Consequently, there is a delay in adopting useful procedures and in discontinuing ineffective or harmful ones.[5,12,19,23] This integration of new evidence has been slow partly because of the traditional approach to learning and practice, with its reliance on "authority" rather than on seeking out the most current empiric evidence. Coupled with the reliance on authority, clinicians tend to practice the same as they were taught in school. Consequently, trends indicate the longer clinicians are out of school, the greater the gap in their knowledge of up-to-date care.

Another explanation for the delay in integrating new evidence is the need for translating it into information that is useful for each decision maker, including the patient. Using a standard, unbiased method to evaluate information is considered better and necessary because the number of new scientific insights that emerge each year is overwhelming. Box 1-1 identifies why an evidence-based approach is better than using other methods of assessment.[30]

BOX 1-1

Advantages of Evidence-Based Approach Compared with Other Assessment Methods

The evidence-based approach:

- Is objective.
- Is scientifically sound.
- Is patient-focused.
- Incorporates clinical experience.
- Stresses good judgment.
- Is thorough and comprehensive.
- Uses transparent methodology.

Data from Newman M, Caton J, Gunsolly J: *Ann Periodontol* 8:1, 2003.

BOX 1-2

Skills and Abilities Needed to Apply Evidence-Based Decision-Making Process

1. Convert information needs and problems into clinical questions so that they can be answered.
2. Conduct a computerized search with maximum efficiency for finding the best external evidence with which to answer the question.
3. Critically appraise the evidence for its validity and usefulness (clinical applicability).
4. Apply the results of the appraisal, or evidence, in clinical practice.
5. Evaluate the process and your performance.

Data from Sackett DA, Strauss SE, Richardson WS, et al: *Evidence-based medicine: how to practice and teach EBM,* London, 2000, Churchill Livingstone.

Also contributing to variations in practice is the lack of, or weak scientific evidence for, answering specific clinical questions,[16] including those related to the most frequent treatments in dentistry and dental hygiene.[6,25] In these cases, an evidence-based approach serves another purpose by helping to inform the profession and investigators of needed research. The American Academy of Periodontology (AAP), the European Academy of Periodontology, the Academy of Osseointegration, and other organizations have responded to this need by using an evidence-based approach to plan and implement consensus conferences on periodontal and implant therapy. In a recent AAP consensus conference, 15 systematic reviews were prepared on topics relevant to contemporary periodontal practice, which then served as the basis for developing consensus reports, including implications for practice and additional research.[30]

Assimilating Evidence into Practice

Assimilating scientific evidence into practice requires keeping up-to-date through reading extensively, attending courses, and using the Internet and electronic databases, such as MEDLINE (PubMed) and the Cochrane Library, to search for published scientific articles. However, with the proliferation of clinical studies and journal publications, keeping current with relevant research is challenging. Consequently, substantial advances made in the knowledge of clinical dentistry and periodontics have not been translated into practice or fully applied to allow patients to receive the total benefit.

EVIDENCE-BASED DECISION-MAKING PROCESS AND SKILLS

The growth of evidence-based practice has been made possible through the development of online scientific databases such as MEDLINE (PubMed) and Web-based software, along with the use of desktop computers that enable users to quickly access relevant clinical evidence. This combination of *technology* and *good evidence* allows health care professionals to apply the benefits from clinical research to patient care.[35] EBDM recognizes that clinicians can never be completely current with all conditions, medications, materials, or available products, and it provides a mechanism for assimilating current research findings into everyday practice to answer questions and to stay current with innovations in dentistry. Translating the EBDM process into action is based on the abilities and skills identified in Box 1-2.[36]

Asking Good Questions: the PICO Process

Converting information needs and problems into clinical questions is a difficult skill to learn, but it is fundamental to evidence-based practice. The process almost always begins with a patient question or problem. A "well-built" question should include four parts that identify the patient problem or population *(P),* intervention *(I),* comparison *(C),* and outcome(s) *(O),* referred to as PICO.[36] Once these four components are clearly and succinctly identified, the following format can be used to structure the question:

> *"For a patient with _____ (P), will _____ (I) as compared to _____ (C) increase/ decrease/provide better/ in doing _____ (O)?"*

The formality of using PICO to frame the question serves three key purposes, as follows:

1. PICO forces the clinician to focus on what he or she and the patient believe to be the most important single issue and outcome.
2. PICO facilitates the next step in the process, the computerized search, by identifying key terms that will be used in the search.[36]
3. PICO directs the clinician to identify clearly the problem, the results, and the outcomes related to the specific care provided to that patient. This in turn allows identification of the type of evidence and information required to solve the problem, as well as considerations for measuring the effectiveness of the intervention and the application of the EBDM process.

BOX 1-3

Case Scenario Using PICO Process in Evidence-Based Decision Making

The health history of a new patient, Mr. Kramer, reveals that he is at risk for infective endocarditis and is allergic to penicillin. Typically, amoxicillin is used, but an alternative regimen is needed for individuals with a penicillin allergy.

Knowing that erythromycin and clindamycin may be possible alternatives, a search is conducted to determine the antibiotic and regimen most appropriate to prescribe before Mr. Kramer has periodontal scaling and root planing.

Based on this information, how should the question be structured so that the answer can be found quickly? Applying the PICO process, each key component is first identified:

P (problem)	=	Patient at risk for *infective endocarditis* and a penicillin allergy
I (intervention)	=	Clindamycin
C (comparison)	=	Erythromycin
O (outcome)	=	Provide effective antibiotic prophylaxis in terms of safety, better absorption, and more sustained serum levels

Next, the question is structured using the components:

> "For a patient at risk for infective endocarditis and a penicillin allergy, does clindamycin as compared to erythromycin provide more effective antibiotic prophylaxis in terms of safety, better absorption, and more sustained serum levels?"

From this question, key terms can be identified to use in conducting the search: "infective" or "endocarditis," which is indexed by the National Library of Medicine for the MEDLINE database as *bacterial endocarditis* (the medical subject heading [MeSH] term), "penicillin allergy," "clindamycin," "erythromycin," and "antibiotic prophylaxis."

SCIENCE TRANSFER

A significant problem in clinical medicine and dentistry is the delay between advances in research findings and their incorporation into daily clinical practice. One way to try to shorten this time is to perform evaluations of the findings and make them readily accessible to the clinician.

Current efforts focus on producing summaries of studies, and, appraising and incorporating the quality of the research. These rigorous analyses are called *systematic reviews*. If multiple similar studies have been performed, a statistical technique called a *meta-analysis* is used to combine the results. The clinician can then incorporate the findings of these more powerful tests into decision making.

Two points are important:

- Clinical experience and input from the patient must be incorporated in determining the final treatment plan no matter what evidence exists.
- Data about many advances are just beginning to become available suggesting that using evidence-based methods may shorten the time between research advances and their incorporation into practice. It is likely that multiple strategies will be required to accomplish this goal.

Periodontology has been the leader among dental specialties in embracing the concepts of evidence-based decision making (EBDM). Although this approach is superior to the concept of authoritative-centered decisions based solely on personal clinical experience, it is also superior practically speaking. EBDM, by design, incorporates clinical expertise to judge the evidence, and it requires that patients' preferences to be considered.

Currently in periodontics, there is a deficit of available clinical trials that truly meet the scientific criteria that allow multiple data sets to be evaluated together. Until the literature contains studies that incorporate evidence-based methodology, the clinician will need to balance clinical experience with the new process of EBDM. Each clinician should individually go through the process of EBDM and not rely on authoritative interpretation of the literature.

Thus, EBDM supports continuous quality improvements through measuring outcomes of care and self-reflection. Box 1-3 provides a case example showing the PICO process.

Searching for and Acquiring the Evidence

Evidence typically comes from studies related to questions about treatment/prevention, diagnosis, etiology/harm and prognosis of disease as well as from questions about the quality and economics of care. Evidence is considered the synthesis of all valid research that answers a specific question, which distinguishes it from a single research study.[21] Once synthesized, evidence can help inform decisions about whether a method of diagnosis or a treatment is effective relative to other methods of diagnoses or to other treatments, and under what circumstances. The challenge in using EBDM arises when there *is* only one research study available on a particular topic. In these cases individuals should be cautious in relying on the study because it can be contradicted by another study and it may only test efficacy and not effectiveness. This underscores the importance of staying current with the scientific literature, since the body of evidence evolves over time as more research is conducted.

Levels of Evidence

The highest level of evidence, or the "gold standard," is the *systematic review* (SR) and meta-analysis using two or more *randomized controlled trials* (RCTs) of human subjects. SRs and meta-analyses are considered the gold standard for evidence because of their strict protocols to reduce bias. These reviews provide a summary of multiple research studies that have investigated the same specific question. SRs use explicit criteria for retrieval, assessment, and synthesis of evidence from individual RCTs and other well-controlled methods.

Meta-analysis is a statistical process often used with SRs. It involves combining the statistical analyses of several individual studies into one analysis. When data from these studies are pooled, the sample size and power usually increase. As a result, the combined effect can increase the precision of estimates of treatment effects and exposure risks.[28]

Systematic reviews and meta-analyses are followed respectively by individual RCT studies, cohort studies, case-control studies, and then studies not involving human subjects.[32] In the absence of scientific evidence, the consensus opinion of experts in appropriate fields of research and clinical practice is used (Figure 1-2).

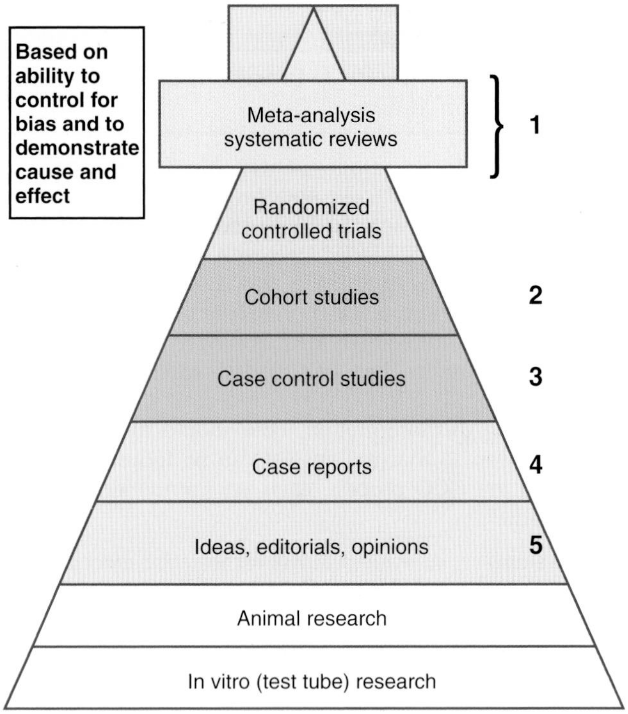

Figure 1-2 Levels of clinical evidence.

This hierarchy of evidence is based on the concept of causation and the need to control bias.[26,27] Although each level may contribute to the total body of knowledge, "not all levels are equally useful for making patient care decisions."[27] In progressing up the pyramid, the number of studies and correspondingly the amount of available literature decrease, while at the same time their relevance to answering clinical questions increases.

Evidence is judged on its rigor of methodology, and the level of evidence is directly related to the type of question asked, such as those derived from issues of therapy or prevention, diagnosis, etiology, and prognosis (Table 1-1). For example, the highest level of evidence associated with questions about therapy or prevention will be from SRs of RCT studies. However, the highest level of evidence associated with questions about prognosis will be from SRs of inception cohort studies.[34] Knowing which type of study will provide the best evidence for clinical decision making and how to retrieve this information quickly from the scientific literature is important to evidence-based practice.

Sources of Evidence

The two types of evidence-based sources are primary and secondary, as follows:

- *Primary sources* are original research publications that have not been filtered or synthesized.
- *Secondary sources* are synthesized publications of the primary literature. These include SRs and meta-analyses, evidence-based article reviews, and clinical practice guidelines and protocols.

Both primary and secondary sources can be found by conducting a search using such biomedical databases as MEDLINE (PubMed), EMBASE, HealthSTAR, and CINALH (Cumulative Index to Nursing and Allied Health). In addition, the Cochrane Collaboration Library provides access to systematic reviews. Many other secondary sources, such as evidence-based journals, are being developed by evidence-based groups to quickly inform the busy practitioner on important issues. However, it is also necessary to review the primary literature when secondary sources are not available.

Primary Sources of Evidence. PubMed is designed to provide access to both primary and secondary research from the biomedical literature. PubMed provides access to MEDLINE, the National Library of Medicine's premier bibliographic database covering the fields of medicine, nursing, dentistry, veterinary medicine, the health care system, and the preclinical sciences. MEDLINE contains bibliographic citations and author abstracts from more than 4800 biomedical journals published in the United States and 70 other countries. The database contains over 12 million citations dating back to 1966, and it adds more than 520,000 new citations each year.[29]

The PICO question provides the foundation for the search terms used in the database. By combining the patient problem or description with the intervention, comparison, and outcome being considered, one can quickly pinpoint a set of citations that will potentially provide an answer to the question being posed. Although online databases provide quicker access to the literature, knowing how databases filter information and having an understanding of how to use PICO and database features allows a more efficient search to be conducted.

These concepts are applied to the case scenario in the PubMed search illustrated in the History (Figure 1-3, *A*). By using the key terms identified in the PICO question and combining them using the Boolean operators "OR" and "AND," the number of relevant articles have been narrowed to a manageable 39.

TABLE 1-1
Type of Question Related to Type of Methodology and Levels of Evidence

Type of Question	Methodology of Choice[32]	Question Focus[27]
Therapy, prevention	Systematic Review (SR) of randomized controlled trials (RCTs) SR of cohort studies	Study effect of therapy or test on real patients; allows for comparison between intervention and control groups; largest volume of evidence-based literature.
Diagnosis	SR of controlled trials (Prospective cohort study) *Controlled trial* (Prospective: compare tests with a reference or "gold standard" test.)	Measures reliability of a particular diagnostic measure for a disease against the "gold standard" diagnostic measure for the same disease.
Etiology, causation, harm	SR of cohort studies *Cohort study* (Prospective data collection with formal control group.)	Compares a group exposed to a particular agent with an unexposed group; important for understanding prevention and control of disease.
Prognosis	SR of inception cohort studies *Inception cohort study* (All have disease but free of the outcome of interest.) *Retrospective cohort*	Follows progression of a group with a particular disease and compares with a group without the disease.

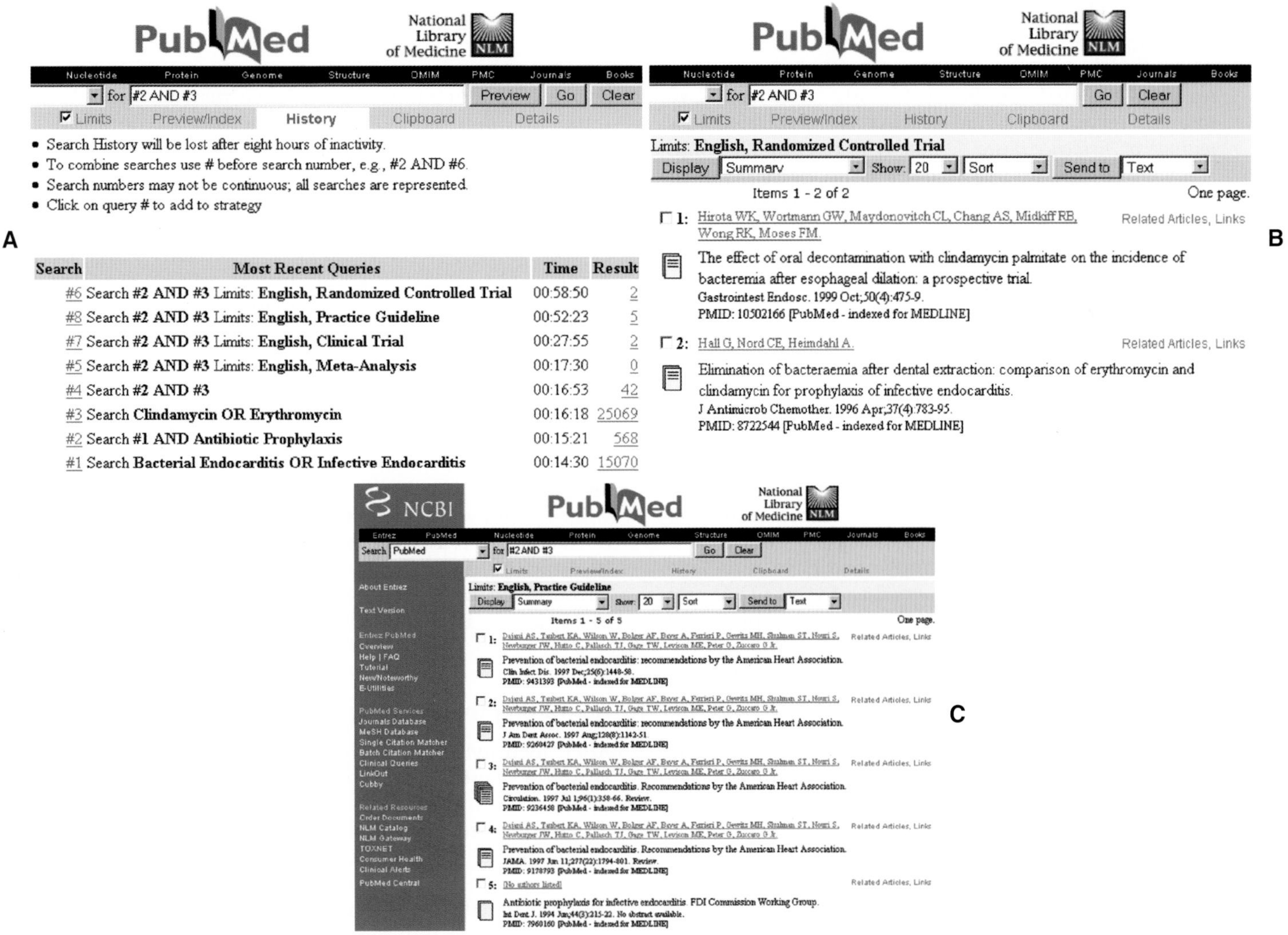

Figure 1-3 Case scenario PubMed search. **A,** Case search history. **B,** Case search results for randomized controlled trial. **C,** Case search results for practice guideline. (Courtesy the U.S. National Library of Medicine, Bethesda, MD.)

Knowing what constitutes the highest levels of evidence and knowing how to apply evidence-based limits and filters are necessary skills when searching the literature with maximum efficiency.[27] One can further refine the search using the "Limits" feature, allowing the user to search for publication types such as meta-analyses, RCTs, clinical trials, and practice guidelines. In the case shown here, the search results indicate there are no meta-analysis; two RCTs, one of which compares the effectiveness of clindamycin and erythromycin; and five citations related to the practice guidelines that outline the American Heart Associations recommendations for antibiotic prophylaxis for patients with infective (bacterial) endocarditis (Figure 1-3, *B* and *C*). Of the 39 citations, there are also two clinical trials, which happen to be the same as the RCTs.

Primary evidence is also available online through electronic journals. These are often peer reviewed, and they exist as electronic companions of print journals or stand-alone journals.

Secondary Sources of Evidence. Recognizing that finding relevant studies is difficult, evidence-based groups are developing many resources for easy access by busy practitioners. These resources include summaries of SRs and individual research articles, as well as clinical practice guidelines and protocols.

Summaries of Systematic Reviews and Research Articles. Evidence-based journals are an emerging resource designed specifically to assist clinicians. Two journals related to dental practice are published: the *Journal of Evidence-Based Dental Practice,* http://www.us.elsevierhealth.com/JEBDP/, and *Evidence-Based Dentistry,* http://www.naturesj.com/ebd. Depending on the journal, they provide concise and easy-to-read summaries of original research articles and of systematic reviews selected from the biomedical literature. A one- to two-page structured abstract, with an expert commentary highlighting the most relevant and practical information, is generally provided. In addition to summaries with commentary of SRs, selected abstracts of new SRs from the Cochrane Collaboration Library are provided.

The Cochrane Collaboration is an international, volunteer, nonprofit organization. There are approximately 50 specialist review groups in 13 countries, including an oral health group and a tobacco addiction group. All Cochrane groups provide peer-reviewed SRs that meet international standards[10] and have an obligation to update their reviews every 2 to 4 years to account for new evidence. The results of their work are stored in the Cochrane Library databases, one of which is the Cochrane Database of Systematic Reviews (COCH), a rapidly growing collection of SRs of the medical literature. There is no cost to access abstracts of the full SRs, which provide a concise summary of the background, objectives, search strategy, selection criteria, data collection and analysis, main results, and reviewer's conclusions.

Systematic reviews facilitate decision making by providing a clear summary of the current state of the existing evidence on a specific topic. SRs provide a way of *managing large quantities of information,*[28] making it easier to keep current with new research. SRs should not be confused with traditional literature reviews; Table 1-2 compares these two types of reviews.

Unfortunately, the already-appraised evidence does not cover many topics. In these cases, it is necessary to use the EBDM process to search for original studies in scientific databases, such as MEDLINE or PubMed.

Clinical Practice Guidelines and Protocols. Growing sources of synthesized information on a specific topic include practice guidelines and protocols. As defined by the Institute of Medicine, guidelines are "systematically developed statements to assist practitioner and patient decisions about appropriate health care for specific clinical circumstances."[11] The inclusion of scientific evidence in clinical practice guidelines has now become the standard, since guidelines should incorporate the best available scientific evidence. SRs support this process by putting together all that is known about a topic in an objective manner.

Although not identified as "guidelines," AAP *position papers, statements,* and *parameters of care* have been developed and updated on multiple aspects of periodontal practice. The AAP regularly monitors treatments, products, and concepts to ensure that even though these have been evaluated once, they are still the best available or as useful as originally envisioned.[1] Changing patterns of disease and improvements in treatments may render a previously accepted approach as inappropriate, whereas a test, device, drug, procedure or intervention for which there is new or mounting evidence may prove to be important only after thorough evaluation, continued development, and use in the field.[30] AAP position papers, statements, and parameters of care are posted on their website, http://www.perio.org/resources-products/posppr2.html.

The ADA posts information on a broader range of dental topics on their website, http://www.ada.org. The ADA Guidelines, Positions and Statements, can be accessed under the section *Professional Issues and Research.*[3] Practice guidelines related to treatment of specific medical conditions are found on other websites such as the American Heart Association.[4] The ADA also has evidence-based resources and information on its website.

When these papers, reports, guidelines, or protocols are published in a journal indexed by MEDLINE, they will be identified as a citation during the search, as found in the case with Mr. Kramer (see Box 1-3 and Figure 1-3). If difficulty identifying a guideline or protocol is encountered, or when it has not been formally published as an article in a journal, one can search the related website rather than assume that none exists.

Appraising the Evidence

After identifying the evidence gathered in order to answer a question, it is important to have the skills to understand the evidence found. In all cases, it is necessary to review the evidence, whether it is an SR or an original study, to determine if the methods were conducted rigorously and appropriately. International evidence-based groups have made this easier by developing appraisal forms and checklists that guide the user through a structured series of "YES/NO" questions

TABLE 1-2

Comparison of Characteristics of Systematic Reviews and Literature Reviews

Characteristic	Systematic Review	A Literature Review
Focus of review	Specific problem; narrow focus. *Example:* Effectiveness of Periostat as an adjunct to scaling and root planing for the treatment of adult periodontitis.	Range of issues on a topic; broad focus. *Example:* Effectiveness of adjunctive antimicrobial agents for treating periodontitis.
Who conducts	Multidisciplinary team	Individual
Selection of studies to include	Preestablished criteria based on validity of study design and specific problem. All studies that meet criteria are included. Bias minimized based on criteria.	Criteria not preestablished or reported in methods; search on range of issues. May include or exclude studies based on personal bias or support for the hypothesis, if one is stated. Inherent bias with lack of criteria.
Reported findings	Search strategy and databases searched. Number of studies that met and did not meet criteria; why studies were excluded. Description of study design, subjects, length of trial, state of health/disease, outcome measures.	Literature presentation format is crafted by individual author. Search strategy, databases, and total number of studies (pro and con) are rarely identified. Descriptive in nature, reporting the outcomes of studies rather than their study designs.
Synthesis of selected studies	Critical analysis of included studies. Determination if results could be statistically combined, and if so, how meta-analysis was conducted.	Reporting of studies that support a procedure or position and those that do not, rather than combining data or conducting a statistical analysis.
Main results	Summary of trials; total number of subjects. Definitive statements about findings in relation to objectives and outcome measures.	Summary of the findings by author in relation to purpose of literature review and specific objectives.
Conclusions or comments	Discussion of key findings with interpretation of the results, including potential biases and recommendations for future trials.	Discussion of key findings with interpretation of the results, including limitations and recommendations for future trials.

TABLE 1-3

Examples of Critical Analysis Guides

Guide	Purpose
CONSORT statement (Consolidated Standards of Reporting Trials)[2]	To improve the reporting and review of RCTs.
QUOROM (Quality of Reporting of Meta-Analyses)	To improve the reporting and review of SRs.
CASP (Critical Appraisal Skills Program)[13]	To review RCTs, SRs, and several other types of studies.

RCTs, Randomized controlled trials; *SRs,* systematic reviews.

to determine the validity of the individual study or systematic review. Table 1-3 provides examples of guides that can be used for critical analysis.

Common Ways Used to Report Results

Once the results are determined to be valid, the next step is to determine if the results; potential benefits (or harms) are important. Sackett and colleagues[36] identify the clinically useful measures for each type of study. For example, in determining the magnitude of therapy results, we would expect articles to report the control event rate (CER), the experimental event rate (EER), the absolute and relative risk reduction (ARR or RRR), and numbers needed to treat (NNT). NNT provides the number of patients (e.g., surfaces, periodontal pockets) that would need to be treated with the experimental treatment or intervention to achieve one additional patient (surfaces, periodontal pockets) who has a favorable response. These concepts are explained more fully in Chapter 2.

Evaluating the Outcomes

The final steps in the EBDM process are to evaluate the effectiveness of the intervention and clinical outcomes and to determine how effectively the EBDM process was applied. For example, one question to ask in evaluating the effectiveness of the intervention is, "Did the selected intervention or treatment achieve the desired result?" In the Mr. Kramer case scenario (see Box 1-3), the question is, "Did the antibiotic and regimen of choice provide adequate absorption and higher serum levels to maintain effective prophylaxis with no adverse effects?" Fortunately, looking up the regimens thought to provide prophylactic coverage (clindamycin and erythromycin) identified clindamycin as the antibiotic of choice given Mr. Kramer's health status and showed that erythromycin is not recommended by the American Heart Association as an alternative for an individual with a penicillin allergy.

Using an EBDM approach requires understanding new concepts and developing new skills. Questions that parallel each step in the EBDM process can be asked in evaluating self-performance. For example, "How well was the PICO question formulated so that key terms were easily identified for conducting the search?" As with most learning, time and practice are essential to mastering new techniques.

CONCLUSION

An EBDM approach closes the gap between clinical research and the realities of practice by providing dental practitioners with the skills to find, efficiently filter, interpret, and apply research findings so that what is known is reflected in the care provided. This approach assists clinicians in keeping current with conditions that a patient may have by providing a mechanism for addressing gaps in knowledge to provide the best care possible.

As EBDM becomes standard practice, individuals must be knowledgeable about what constitutes the evidence and how it is reported. Understanding evidence-based methodology and distinctions between different types of articles, such as systematic reviews and literature reviews, allows the clinician to judge better the validity and relevance of reported findings. To assist practitioners with this endeavor, systematic reviews are being conducted to answer specific clinical questions, and new journals devoted to evidence-based practice are being published to alert readers about important advances in a concise and user-friendly manner. By integrating good science with clinical judgment and patient preferences, clinicians enhance their decision-making ability and maximize the potential for successful patient care outcomes.

REFERENCES

1. American Academy of Periodontology (AAP): Index of AAP guidelines, position papers, statements and parameters of care, 2004, http://www.perio.org/resources-products/posppr2.html.
2. American Dental Association (ADA) Commission on Dental Accreditation: *Accreditation standards for dental education programs,* Chicago, 2002, ADA.
3. American Dental Association (ADA): ADA policy on evidence-based dentistry. professional issues and research, ADA guidelines, positions and statements, 2002, http://www.ada.org.
4. American Heart Association (AHA): Bacterial endocarditis guidelines, 2004, http://circ.ahajournals.org/cgi/content/full/96/1/358; *see also* Dajani AS, Taubert KA, Wilson W, et al: Prevention of bacterial endocarditis, *Circulation* 96:358, 1997.
5. Anderson G, Allison D: Intrapartum electronic fetal heart rate monitoring: a review of current status for the Task Force on the Periodic Health Examination. In *Preventing disease: beyond the rhetoric,* New York, 1990, Springer-Verlag, p 19.
6. Bader J, Ismail A: Survey of systematic reviews in dentistry, *J Am Dent Assoc* 135:464, 2004.
7. Bader JD, Shugars DA: Variation in dentists' clinical decisions, *J Public Health Dent* 55:181, 1995.
8. Bader J, Shugars D: Variation, treatment outcomes, and practice guidelines in dental practice, *J Dent Educ* 59:61, 1995.
9. Browman G, Levine M, Mohide E, et al: The practice guidelines development cycle: a conceptual tool for practice guidelines development and implementation, *J Clin Oncol* 13:502, 1995.
10. Cochrane Collaboration: What is the Cochrane Collaboration? 2004, http://www.cochrane.org/.
11. Committee on Quality of Health Care in America IOM: *Crossing the quality chasm: a new health system for the 21st century,* Washington, DC, 2000, National Academy of Sciences, p 151.
12. Crowley P, Chalmers I, Keirse M: The effects of corticosteroid administration before preterm delivery: an overview of the evidence from controlled trials, *Br J Obstet Gynecol* 97:11, 1990.
13. Davidoff F: In the teeth of the evidence: the curious case of evidence-based medicine, *Mt Sinai J Med* 66:75, 1999.
14. Davidoff F, Case K, Fried P, Cerra F: Evidence-based medicine: why all the fuss? *Ann Intern Med* 122:727, 1995.
15. Ecenbarger W: How honest are dentists? *Reader's Digest,* Feb, 1997, p 50.
16. Eisenberg J: Statement of health care quality before the House Subcommittee on Health and the Environment, Washington, DC, 1997, Agency for Health Care Policy and Research Archive.
17. Evidence-based Medicine Working Group: Evidence-based medicine: a new approach to teaching the practice of medicine, *JAMA* 268:2420, 1992.
18. Evidence-based Medicine Working Group: *Users' guides to the medical literature: a manual for EB clinical practice,* Chicago, 2002, American Medical Association.
19. Frazier P, Horowitz A: Prevention: a public health perspective. In *Oral health promotion and disease prevention,* Copenhagen, 1995, Munksgaard.
20. Greco P, Eisenberg J: Changing physicians' practices, *N Engl J Med* 329:1271, 1993.
21. Greenhalgh T: "Is my practice evidence-based?" Should be answered in qualitative, as well as quantitative terms, *BMJ* 313:957, 1996.
22. Grembowski D, Milgrom P, Fiset L: Dental decision-making and variation in dentist service rates, *Soc Sci Med* 32:287, 1991.
23. Grimes DA: Graduate education, *Evid Base Med* 86:451, 1995.
24. Haynes R: Some problems in applying evidence in clinical practice, *Ann NY Acad Sci* 703:210, 1999.
25. Institute of Medicine: *Dental education at the crossroads: challenges and change,* Washington, DC, 1995, National Academy Press.
26. Long A, Harrison S: The balance of evidence: evidence-based decision making, *Health Serv J* 6(suppl):1, 1995.
27. McKibbon A, Eady A, Marks S: *PDQ: evidence-based principles and practice,* Hamilton, Ontario, 1999, BC Decker.
28. Mulrow C: Rationale for systematic reviews, *BMJ* 309:597, 1994.
29. National Library of Medicine and NCBI, PubMed overview, 2004, National Library of Medicine, National Institutes of Health (NIH), http://pubmed.gov.
30. Newman M, Caton J, Gunsolly J: The use of the evidence-based approach in a periodontal therapy contemporary science workshop, *Ann Periodontol* 8:1, 2003.
31. NHS Centre for Reviews and Dissemination, University of York: Undertaking systematic reviews of research on effectiveness, 1997, http://www.york.ac.uk/inst/crd/report4.htm.

32. Oxford Centre for Evidence-Based Medicine: Levels of evidence and grades of recommendations, 1998, http://www.cebm.net/levels_of_evidence.asp.
33. Palmer J, Lusher A, Snowball R: Searching for the evidence, *Genitourinary Med* 73:70, 1997.
34. Phillips B, Ball C, Sackett DL, et al: Levels of evidence and grades of recommendations, Centre for Evidence-Based Medicine, 2001, http://www.cebm.net/levels_of_evidence.asp.
35. Rosenberg W, Donald A: Evidence based medicine: an approach to clinical problem-solving, *BMJ* 310:1122, 1995.
36. Sackett DA, Strauss SE, Richardson WS, et al: *Evidence-based medicine: how to practice and teach EBM,* London, 2000, Churchill Livingstone.

Assessing Evidence

Philippe P. Hujoel

CHAPTER

■ ■ ■

CHAPTER OUTLINE

TWELVE TOOLS FOR ASSESSING EVIDENCE
1. Be Skeptical.
2. Don't Trust Biologic Plausibility.
3. What Level of Controlled Evidence Is Available?
4. Did the Cause Precede the Effect?
5. No Betting on the Horse after the Race Is Over.
6. What Is a "Clinically Relevant Pretrial" Hypothesis?

7. Size Does Matter.
8. Is There "Even One Different Explanation That Works as Well or Better?"
9. Was the Study Properly Randomized?
10. When to Rely on Nonrandomized Evidence?
11. Placebo Effects: Real or Sham?
12. Was There Protection against Conflict of Interest?

CONCLUSION

Since 1965, there have been 1137 scientific articles on periodontal diseases and antibacterial agents. Which of these articles provide information that is clinically relevant? Are these 1137 articles accurately summarized in educational courses, textbooks, or systematic reviews? Relying on authority to provide answers to such questions is dangerous.[110]

Einstein purportedly said that "his own major scientific talent was his ability to look at an enormous number of experiments and journal articles, select the very few that were both correct and important, ignore the rest, and build a theory on the right ones."[13] Most evidence-based clinicians probably aspire toward the same goal in the evaluation of clinical evidence. In this search for good evidence, a "baloney detection kit"[57] is needed to separate salesmanship from science and suggestive hints from unequivocal evidence. This chapter discusses 12 tools that may be useful in assessing causality in clinical sciences.

TWELVE TOOLS FOR ASSESSING EVIDENCE

1. Be Skeptical.

Of all machines ours is the most complicated and inexplicable.

—Thomas Jefferson

By 1990, based on the results of a dozen studies, it was concluded that "available data thus strongly support the hypothesis that dietary carotenoids reduce the risk of lung cancer."[132] Beta carotene (β-carotene) was hypothesized to interfere passively with oxidative damage to deoxyribonucleic acid (DNA) and lipoproteins,[66] and these beliefs in part translated into $210 million sales of β-carotene in 1997 in the United States. Was this convincing evidence or should it be evaluated skeptically? Two large, randomized controlled trials were initiated, and both were stopped prematurely because they indicated that β-carotene increased lung cancer risk, cardiovascular disease risk, and overall mortality risk.[11,97] In 2005, the primary investigator of one of the trials reported that "beta-carotene should be regulated as a human carcinogen".[97]

Evidence on how to cure, manage, or prevent chronic diseases is notoriously contradictory, inconsistent, and unreliable. Mark Twain reminded people to be careful when reading health books because one may die of a misprint.[109] Three powerful forces, in addition to misprints, conspire to deliver a preponderance of misleading results:

1. Identifying a successful treatment for chronic diseases is challenging. It is estimated that less than 0.1% of all investigated treatments are effective. Because the

odds for identifying successful interventions for chronic diseases are so low, most so-called effective treatments identified in clinical trials turn out to be noneffective or even harmful.[116]

2. Most chronic diseases are complex[86] and include both environmental and genetic causes. Well-controlled studies on the etiology of chronic diseases can only do so much to elucidate the apparent infinite complexity of human disease causation. Incomplete and mistaken understandings of chronic disease etiology can lead to a cascade of wrong turns in the exploration of possible diagnosis, prognosis, and treatment.
3. Poor scientific methodology is a common problem permeating most of the evidence that surrounds us. Popular press headlines tell it all: "Lies, damned lies and medical statistics,"[108] "Undermined by an error of significance: a widespread misconception among scientists casts doubt on the reliability of a huge amount of research,"[85] and "Sloppy stats shame science."[114]

Several observations suggest that skepticism is required in the evaluation of periodontal evidence. First, the large number of "effective" periodontal treatments may be a telltale sign of a challenging chronic disease. Before 1917, there were 100 pneumonia treatments, none of which worked. Before the advent of antibiotics in the 1940s, none of the many tuberculosis treatments really worked. The current "therapeutic wealth" for periodontal diseases may well mean poverty and a suggestion we are dealing with a challenging chronic disease.[50] Second, periodontal diseases are by many no longer regarded as the simple, plaque-related diseases they were once thought to be, but rather as complex diseases with both environmental and genetic causes. Complex diseases are challenging to diagnose, treat, and investigate. Third, the scientific quality of periodontal studies has been rated as low.[8,9] Major landmark trials were analyzed using wrong statistics[60]; most randomized studies were not properly randomized[88]; and the primary drivers of the periodontitis epidemic may have been misunderstood because of the lack of properly controlled epidemiologic studies.[62,123] The chances that periodontal research somehow managed to escape the scientific challenges and hurdles that were present in research in other chronic diseases appears slim.

2. Don't Trust Biologic Plausibility.

Born but to die, and reasoning but to err.

—Alexander Pope

If an irregular heartbeat increases mortality risk, and if encainide can turn an irregular heartbeat into a normal heartbeat, then encainide should improve survival.[24] If high lipid levels increase myocardial infarction risk, and if clofibrate can successfully decrease lipid levels, clofibrate should improve survival.[105] Such "causal chain thinking" (A causes B, B causes C, therefore A causes C) is common and dangerous. These examples of treatment rationales, although seemingly reasonable and biologically plausible, turned out to harm patients. Causal chain thinking is sometimes referred to as "deductive inference," "deductive reasoning," or a "logical system."

In mathematics, "once the Greeks had developed the deductive method, they were correct in what they did, correct for all time."[10] In medicine or dentistry, decisions based on deductive reasoning have not been "correct for all time" and are certainly not universal. Because of an incomplete understanding of biology, the use of deductive reasoning for clinical decisions may be dangerous, and it largely failed for thousands of years to lead to medical breakthroughs. In evidence-based medicine, evidence that is based on deductive inference is classified as *level 5,* the lowest level of evidence available.

Unfortunately, much of our knowledge on how to prevent, manage, and cure chronic periodontitis depends largely on deductive reasoning. Small, short-term changes in pocket depth or attachment levels have been assumed to translate into tangible, long-term patient benefits, but minimal evidence to support this deductive inference leap is available. Plaque was related to experimental gingivitis in a small study,[77] and a "leap of faith" was made that plaque caused almost all periodontal diseases. Evidence that plaque control affects the most common forms of periodontal diseases is still weak[61] and largely based on "biologic plausibility" arguments. The use of antibiotics for painful periodontal abscesses[111] is similarly rationalized on deductive inference, a worrisome thought given the concerns about antibiotic resistance[92,124] and the increasing evidence that no antibiotics are needed for self-limiting infections.[2,37,52,101] A move toward a higher level of evidence (higher than biological plausibility) is needed to put periodontics on a firmer scientific footing.

3. What Level of Controlled Evidence Is Available?

Development of Western Science is based on two great achievements: the invention of a formal logical system (in Euclidean geometry) by the Greek philosophers, and the discovery of the possibility to find out causal relationships by systematic experiment (during the Renaissance).

—Albert Einstein

Rational thought requires reliance on either deductive reasoning (biologic plausibility) or on systematic experiments (sometimes referred to as inductive reasoning). Galileo is typically credited with the start of systematic experimentation in physics. Amazingly, it took until the latter half of the twentieth century before systematic experiments became part of clinical thinking. Three systematic experiments are now routine in clinical research: the case-control study, the cohort study, and the randomized controlled trial. In the following brief descriptions of these three systematic experimental designs, the term *exposure* refers to a suspected etiologic factor or an intervention, such as a treatment or a diagnostic test, and the term *endpoint* refers to the outcome of disease, quality-of-life measures, or any type of condition that may be of interest in clinical studies.

1. **Randomized controlled trial** (RCT). Individuals are randomly assigned to different exposures and monitored longitudinally for the endpoint of

interest. If the endpoint frequency differs between the exposure groups, an *association* between the exposure and the endpoint is present. The RCT is the "gold standard" design in clinical research. In evidence-based medicine, RCTs, when properly executed, are referred to as *level 1* evidence. Level 1 is the highest (best) level of evidence available.

2. **Cohort study.** Exposed individuals are compared to nonexposed individuals and monitored longitudinally for endpoint occurrence. If the endpoint frequency differs between exposed and nonexposed individuals, an *association* between exposure and endpoint is present. A cohort study is often considered the optimal study design in nonexperimental clinical research (i.e., for those study designs where no randomization is used). In evidence-based medicine, cohort studies, when properly executed, are referred to as *level 2* evidence.
3. **Case-control study.** *Cases* (individuals with the endpoint of interest) are compared with *controls* (individuals without the endpoint of interest) with respect to the prevalence of the exposure. If the prevalence of exposure differs between cases and controls, an *association* between the exposure and the endpoint is present. In a case-control study, it is challenging to select cases and controls in an unbiased manner and to obtain reliable information on possible causes of disease that occurred in the past. The case-control study is the most challenging study design to use for obtaining reliable evidence. As a result, in evidence-based medicine, case-control studies, when properly executed, are referred to as *level 3* evidence.

All three study designs permit us to study the association between the exposure and the endpoint. This association can be represented schematically as follows:

Exposure → Endpoint

An important challenge in the assessment of controlled evidence is determining whether the association identified (→) is causal. Criteria used to assess causality include factors such as the assessment of *temporality,* the presence of a *pretrial hypothesis,* and the size or strength of the reported *association.* Unlike deductive reasoning, where associations are either true or false, such absolute truths cannot be achieved with systematic experiments. Conclusions based on controlled study designs are always surrounded with a degree of uncertainty, a frustrating limitation to real-world clinicians who have to make yes/no decisions.

4. Did the Cause Precede the Effect?

You can't change the laws of physics, Captain.

—"Scotty" in Star Trek

In 2001 a study published in the *British Medical Journal* suggested that retroactive prayer shortened hospital stay in patients with bloodstream infection.[75] The only problem was that patients were already dismissed from the hospital when the nonspecified prayer to the nonspecified deity was made. To most scientists, findings in which the effect (shorter hospital stay) precedes the cause (the prayer) are impossible, and this provides an unequivocal example of a violation of correct temporality; the effect preceded the hypothesized cause. In chronic disease research, it is often challenging to disentangle temporality, and fundamental questions regarding temporality often remain disputed. For example, in Alzheimer's research the amyloid in the senile plaques in the brain is often considered to be the *cause* of Alzheimer's disease, but some researchers suggested that amyloid may be the *result* rather than the cause of Alzheimer's disease and that the amyloid actually may be protective.[74] Vigorous investigation of temporality is a key aspect in scientific investigation.

Temporality is the *only* criterion that needs to be satisfied for claiming causality; the cause needs to precede the effect. In periodontal research, many studies relating plaque or specific infections to periodontal diseases suffer from unclear temporality. Are observed microbial profiles the result or the cause of periodontitis? Do individuals with periodontitis have more plaque because they have more root surface areas to clean, or do they have poorer oral hygiene? Similarly, studies on the potential association between so-called chronic periodontitis and systemic diseases may not have adequately addressed the issue of temporality. Is chronic periodontitis preceding the systemic disease, or are chronic periodontitis and systemic disease comorbid conditions caused by a common causal factor, such as smoking? Unequivocal establishment of temporality is an essential element of causality and can

> **SCIENCE TRANSFER**
>
> Good science involves hypothesis testing and high-quality experimental design. If performed well, science yields the truth. For this reason, it is important to know what constitutes a good study and what the pitfalls and potential problems in experimental design may be. Learning to think in terms of hypothesis testing can be very beneficial to the clinician. The thrill of learning new information through hypothesis testing can stimulate career choices and become a passion.
>
> Each clinician needs to develop expertise in the scientific methodology of data evaluation. The 12 tools for assessing evidence presented in this chapter provide a basis to make decisions about patient care when reading published reports. These strict requirements for evidence are essential if true evidence-based decisions are to be incorporated into the daily practice of periodontics. Furthermore, the design of studies to solve periodontal questions must have a foundation based on these 12 tools, if they are to provide credible solutions. At present, much of what is accepted in periodontal therapy is scientifically flawed, and the future of periodontology must have a foundation of reliable scientific procedures; only then can evidence-based decisions become clear and reliable.

be difficult to establish for chronic diseases, including the epidemiology of periodontal diseases.

5. No Betting on the Horse after the Race Is Over.

Predictions are difficult, especially about the future.

—Niels Bohr

An acquired immunodeficiency syndrome (AIDS) researcher at an international AIDS conference was jeered when she claimed that AIDS therapy provided a significant benefit for a subgroup of trial participants.[94] A study published in the *New England Journal of Medicine*[79] was taken as a textbook example of poor science[40] when it claimed that coffee drinking was responsible for more than 50% of the pancreatic cancers in the United States. Results of a large collaborative study demonstrating that aspirin use after myocardial infarct increased mortality risk in patients born under Gemini or Libra provided a comical example of an important scientific concept; the unreliability of data-generated ideas.

An essence of science is that hypotheses or ideas predict observations, not that hypotheses or ideas can be fitted to observed data. This essential characteristic of scientific enterprise—prediction—is often lost in medical and dental research when poorly defined prestudy hypotheses result in convoluted data-generated ideas or hypotheses that fit the observed data. It has been reported that even for well-organized studies with carefully written protocols, investigators often do not remember which hypotheses were defined in advance, which hypotheses were data derived, which hypotheses were "a priori" considered plausible, and which were unlikely.[134] A wealth of data-generated ideas can be created by exploring patient subgroups, exposures, and endpoints, as shown by the following:

1. *Modifying study sample definition.* A common posttrial modification of a hypothesis is to evaluate proper or improper subgroups of the original study sample. *Improper subgroups* are based on patient characteristics that may have been influenced by the exposure. For example, one may evaluate tumor size only in those patients who survived or pocket depths only in those teeth that were not lost during the maintenance. Results of improper-subgroup analyses are almost always meaningless when establishing causality. *Proper subgroups* are based on patient characteristics that cannot be influenced by the exposure, such as gender, race, or patient's age. A review of trials in the area of cardiovascular disease suggested that even the results of proper-subgroup analyses turn out to be misleading in a majority of cases.[134] In the HIV area, one proper-subgroup analysis (based on racial characteristics) drew an investor lawsuit on the basis that company officials "deceived" investors with a "fraudulent scheme."[29]
2. *Modifying exposure definition.* After or during the conduct of a study, the exposure definition can be changed, or the number of exposures under study can be modified. In a controversial trial on the use of antibiotics for middle ear infections,[81] the placebo treatment was replaced with a boutique antibiotic,[33] causing a potentially misleading perception about the antibiotics' effectiveness. In another example of "betting on the horse after the race was over," a negative finding for cigarette smoking (the primary exposure) as a cause for pancreatic cancer led reportedly to the data-generated hypothesis that coffee drinking increased pancreatic cancer risk.[79] When this study was repeated in the same hospital, using the same protocol, but now with the pretrial hypothesis to evaluate coffee drinking, the results of the prior study could not be duplicated.[40]
3. *Modifying endpoint definition.* Almost all major trials specify one primary endpoint in the pretrial hypothesis. Any modification of this endpoint during or after the trial is cause for concern. In the initial investigation of the "clot buster" drug streptokinase, the primary endpoint was a measure of how well the heart pumped blood. When treatment had no effect on this endpoint, the endpoint definition was changed to reperfusion of the blocked artery.[21] In periodontal research the absence of a specific pretrial defined endpoint is common and permits effortless changing of the endpoint definition. The typical periodontal trial has six endpoints and does not specify which endpoint is primary,[59] and it is not always clear what is a good or a bad outcome.[104] Statistical trickery to reach desired conclusions under such circumstances may be child's play.

Deviating from the pretrial hypothesis is often compared to *data torturing*.[87] Detecting the presence of data torturing in a published article is often challenging; just as the talented torturer leaves no scars on the victim's body, the talented data torturer leaves no marks on the published study. Two types of torturing are recognized. *Opportunistic data torturing* refers to exploring data without the goal of "proving" a particular point of view. Opportunistic data torturing is an essential aspect of scientific activity and hypothesis generation. *Procrustean data torturing* refers to exploring data with the goal of proving a particular point of view. Just as the Greek mortal Procrusteus fitted guests perfectly to his guest bed either through bodily stretching or through chopping of the legs to ensure correspondence between body height and bed length, so can data be fitted to the pretrial hypothesis by Procrustean means.

6. What Is a Clinically Relevant Pretrial Hypothesis?

Far better an approximate answer to the right question, which is often vague, than the exact answer to the wrong question, which can always be made precise.

—John Tukey[127]

When alendronate was shown to lower fracture rates (a tangible benefit),[34] it became the leading worldwide treatment for postmenopausal osteoporosis, and its use is expected to continue to grow.[46] When a randomized trial showed that simvastatin saved lives of patients with prior heart disease (a tangible benefit),[73] sales increased by 80% in the first 9 months after the study's publication.

A pivotal trial on hormone replacement therapy[133] turned thriving drug sales into a major decline.[45] A pivotal trial found a routine eye surgery to be harmful, prompting the National Institutes of Health to send a clinical trial alert[64] to 25,000 ophthalmologists and neurologists.[6]

Clinically relevant questions are designed to have an impact on clinical practice and increasingly, trials on clinically relevant questions, succeed in exactly doing that; dramatically changing clinical practice. Usually, clinically relevant questions share four important characteristics of the pretrial hypothesis: (1) a clinically relevant endpoint (referred to as the **O**utcome in the PIC**O** question), (2) relevant exposure comparisons (referred to as the **I**ntervention and the **C**ontrol in the P**IC**O question, (3) a study sample representative of real-world clinical patients (should be representative of the **P**atient defined in the **P**ICO question), and (4) small error rates.

Clinically Relevant Endpoint

An *endpoint* is a measurement related to a disease process or a condition and used to assess the exposure effect. Two different types of endpoints are recognized. *True endpoints* are *tangible* outcomes that directly measure how a patient feels, functions, or survives[43]; examples include tooth loss, death, and pain. *Surrogate endpoints* are *intangible* outcomes used as a substitute for true endpoints[120]; examples include blood pressure and probing depths of periodontal pockets. Treatment effects on surrogates do not necessarily translate into real clinical benefit (Table 2-1). Use of surrogate endpoints has led to widespread use of deadly medications, and it has been suggested that such disasters should prompt policy changes in drug approval.[103] Analogously, most major causes of human disease (e.g., cigarette smoking) were identified through studies using true endpoints. A first requirement for a clinically relevant study is the pretrial specification of a true endpoint.

Common and Relevant Exposure Comparisons

The more prevalent a studied exposure, the more relevant is the clinical question. A clinically relevant exposure comparison implies (1) the absence of contrived control groups and (2) the use of a placebo control group when appropriate. Providing the control subjects with less than the standard dose of the standard treatment[80,98] or providing a control therapy that avoids the real clinical questions[33] are examples of clinically *irrelevant* research. In case-control or cohort studies the measurement and characterization of exposures (e.g., mercury, fluoride, chewing tobacco) can be difficult and imprecise, making answers imprecise. Moreover, a conclusion regarding the safety or efficacy of one particular type of exposure does not necessarily translate into safety or efficacy of apparently closely related exposures. This last consideration is important in the assessment of the "me-too" drugs or "me-too" implant systems.

Representative Study Sample

When cholesterol-lowering drugs provided a small benefit in middle-aged men with abnormally high cholesterol levels, it was concluded that those benefits "could and should be extended" to other age groups and women with "more modest elevations" of cholesterol levels.[76] Findings on lipids and heart disease derived mostly from Polish immigrants in the Framingham Study were generalized to a much more diverse population.[49] An antidepressant, which was approved for use in adults, was widely prescribed for children with unexpected, serious consequences.[1] Drugs primarily used by elderly individuals who take many drugs are often evaluated in younger individuals who take only one drug.[7] The larger the discrepancy between the study sample and the patient you seek to treat, the more questionable the applicability of the study's conclusions becomes.

Ideally, clinical trials should use simple entry criteria in which the enrolled patients reflect as closely as possible the real-world clinical practice situation.[48] Legislation has been enacted to reach this goal. In 1993, U.S. policy ensured the recruitment of women and minority groups in clinical trials.[19] A U.S. policy for the inclusion of children in clinical studies was then set into law in 1998. Similar efforts are currently being made for the inclusion of pregnant women into clinical studies.[27] Experiments with long lists of inclusion and exclusion criteria can be expensive recipes for failure because they can lead to study samples which are unrepresentative of most real-world clinical patients.

Small Type I and Type II Error Rates

The *type I error* rate is the likelihood of concluding there is an effect, when in truth there is no effect. The type I error rate is set by the investigator, and common values are 1% or 5%. The *type II error* rate is the likelihood of concluding there is no effect, when in truth there is an effect. The type II error rate is typically set by the investigator at 10% or 20%. The complement of the type II error rate (i.e., 1 – type II error rate) is referred to as the *power* of the study. The likelihood for a false-positive or false-negative result depends, in addition to the type I and II error rate, on the likelihood of finding an effect that is not under the investigator's control. For chronic diseases, in which the likelihood for identifying effective treatments or true causes is low, the false-positive rate can be high even when the type I error rate is low.[42] Clinically relevant studies require small type I and type II error rates to minimize false-positive and false-negative conclusions.

7. Size Does Matter.

Chronic hepatitis B infection increased the chances for liver cancer by more than 23,000%.[14] Proximity to electromagnetic radiation increased the chance for leukemia in children by 49%.[131] Periodontitis in populations with smokers increased the chance for coronary heart disease by 12%.[63] No one doubts the causality of the association between chronic hepatitis B infection and liver cancer, but the role of periodontitis in coronary heart disease or electromagnetic radiation in childhood leukemia remains controversial. Why? To a large extent, the size of the association drives the interpretation of causality.

The larger an association, the less likely it is caused by bias, and the more likely it is causal. One simple way to calculate the size of the association is to calculate an

TABLE 2-1

Examples of Potentially Misleading Surrogates*

Disease/ Conditions	Experimental Treatment	Control Treatment	Effect on Surrogate Endpoint	Effect on True Endpoint	Misleading Conclusion	Reference
AIDS	Immediate zidovudine	Delayed zidovudine	Significant increase of 30-35 CD4 cells/mm^3.	No change in incidence of AIDS, AIDS-related complex, or survival.	False-positive	3
Osteoporosis	Fluoride	Placebo	Significant increase of 16% in bone mineral density of lumbar spine.	Nonvertebral fracture rates increased by 85%.	False-positive	106
Lung cancer	ZD1839 (Iressa)	Placebo	Dramatic tumor shrinkage in 10% of patients.	No effect.	False-positive	32
Aphthous ulcers	Thalidomide	Placebo	Although thalidomide expected to decrease TNF-α production, significant increase of 4.4 pg/ml in TNF-α production occurred, suggesting harm.	Pain diminished and ability to eat improved.	False-negative	65
Edentulism dentures	Implant-supported	Conventional dentures	No impact on chewing cycles.	Improved oral health–related–quality of life	False-negative	12
Prostate cancer	Radical prostatectomy	Watchful waiting	Substantial elimination of tumor mass.	No effect on overall mortality risk.	False-positive	54
Advanced colorectal cancer	5-FU + LV	5-FU	23% of patients had 50% or greater reduction in tumor volume.	No effect on overall survival.	False-positive	4
Periodontitis	Surgery	Scaling	Mean pocket depth reduced by 0.5 mm.	Effect on tooth loss or quality of life unknown.	?	

AIDS, Acquired immunodeficiency syndrome; *TNF,* tumor necrosis factor; *FU,* fluorouracil; *LV,* leucovorin.

*For some examples, the experimental treatment led to improvements in surrogate endpoints while the true endpoint was either unaffected or worsened (a false-positive conclusion). For other examples, the experimental treatment had no impact or worsened the surrogate endpoint while the true endpoint improved (a false-negative conclusion).

TABLE 2-2

Two-by-Two Table Cross-Classifying Exposure and Endpoint*

		ENDPOINT	
		Failure	**Success**
Exposure	*Experimental*	A	B
	Control	C	D

*Note that the top left cell, by convention, tallies the number of failures for the experimental group.

TABLE 2-3

Two-by-Two Table on Association between Penciclovir and Oral Lesion Healing

		ENDPOINT	
		No Lesion Healing by Day 6	**Lesion Healing by Day 6**
Exposure	*1% Penciclovir*	376	878
	Placebo	526	757

TABLE 2-4

Two-by-Two Table on Association between Chronic Periodontitis and Fatal Myocardial Infarction (MI)

		ENDPOINT	
		Fatal MI	**No Fatal MI**
Exposure	*Chronic periodontitis (CP)*	2	257
	No gingivitis or CP	8	1241

odds ratio. The *odds* for an event is the probability that an event happens divided by the probability that an event does not happen. An *odds ratio* is a ratio of odds. To calculate an odds ratio, a two-by-two (2 × 2) table is constructed in which the outcome is cross-tabulated with the exposure (Table 2-2). Odds ratios can be calculated for data from RCTs, cohort studies, and case-control studies.

The odds ratio is the ratio of the cross-products (ad/bc). The odds ratio associated with penciclovir use for lesion healing is (376 × 757)/(526 × 878) = 0.62 (Table 2-3). The odds ratio associated with chronic periodontitis for a fatal myocardial infarction is (2 × 1241)/(8 × 257) = 1.21 (Table 2-4). The 95% confidence interval can be approximated by exp[*ln*(odds ratio) ±1.96 √(1/a + 1/b + 1/c + 1/d)]. The 95% confidence intervals of the odds ratio for lesion healing and fatal myocardial infarction are, respectively, exp(–0.48 ±1.96 √ 0.007), or 0.52 to 0.73, and exp(0.18 ±1.96 √ 0.63), or 0.25 to 5.72.

The *size* of the odds ratio ranges between 0 and infinity. An odds ratio of 1 indicates the absence of an association, and if the two-by-two table is set up with the reference cell (poor outcome-exposure of interest) in the left-hand side of the top data row, an odds ratio larger than 1 means a *harmful effect* (e.g., periodontitis increases the odds for a fatal myocardial infarction by 20%), and an odds ratio smaller than 1 means a *protective effect* (e.g., penciclovir decreases the odds for failed lesion healing by day 6 by 38%).

The *confidence interval* is the range of numbers between the upper confidence limit and the lower confidence limit. The confidence interval contains the true odds ratio with a certain predetermined probability (e.g., 95%). In a properly executed randomized trial, a conclusion of causality is typically made if the 95% confidence interval does not include the possibility of "no true association" (e.g., odds ratio = 1). For example, since the 95% confidence interval for the odds ratio associated with penciclovir use is 0.52 to 0.73 and does not include 1, the effect can be referred to as "statistically significant." For the chronic periodontitis–myocardial infarction example, the 95% confidence interval ranges from 0.25 to 5.72, includes 1, and is therefore referred to as "statistically insignificant."

In epidemiology, where there is no randomization of individuals to exposures, the interpretation of a confidence interval is challenging because no probabilistic basis (in the form of randomization) exists for making causal inference. A pessimist will claim that since no randomization was present, no statistical interpretations are allowed.[49] The emphasis should be on visual display of the identified associations and on sensitivity analyses where the results are interpreted under "what if" assumptions.[126] An optimist will argue that the absence of randomization does not preclude the making of statistical inferences, and that one always starts from the assumption that "assignments were random" (even when they were not).[135]

When individuals are *randomly* assigned to exposures, very small associations (i.e., associations very close to 1, such as 1.1) can reliably be identified. When individuals are *not* randomly assigned to exposures, as is the case in cohort studies and cases-control studies, the size of the reported association (e.g., the odds ratio) becomes key in the interpretation of the findings. Because of the inherent biases in epidemiologic research, *small* odds ratios *cannot* be reliably identified. But what is small? Leading epidemiologists provide some guidelines on how to interpret the size of an association with respect to possible causality. Richard Doll, one of the founders of epidemiology, said, "No single epidemiological study is persuasive by itself unless the lower limit of its 95% confidence level falls above a threefold (200%) increased risk." Trichopoulos, past chairperson of epidemiology at Harvard University, opts "for a fourfold (300%) increase at the lower limit (of the 95% confidence interval)." Marcia Angell, former editor of the *New England Journal of Medicine*, reported: "As a general rule of thumb we are looking for an odds ratio of 3 or more (≥200% increased odds) [before accepting a paper for publication]." Robert Temple, Director of the Food and Drug Administration, stated: "My basic rule is if the odds ratio isn't at least 3 or 4 (a 200% or 300% increased risk), forget it."[119] These opinions provide some guidelines on what size of odds ratio to look for when determining causality.

8. Is There "Even One Different Explanation That Works as Well or Better?"[58]

No amount of experimentation can ever prove me right; a single experiment can prove me wrong.

—Albert Einstein

When you have eliminated the impossible, whatever remains, however improbable, must be the truth.

—Sir Conan Doyle

Dozens of epidemiologic studies appeared to support the hypothesis that β-carotene intake lowered lung cancer risk. However, two RCTs provided unequivocal evidence to the contrary.[11,97] What went wrong? Different explanations that worked as well or better may have been inadequately explored. Possibly, smoking was not adequately considered as an alternative explanation and led to a misunderstanding on the health effects of β-carotene.[41,118] Similarly, epidemiology appeared to support the hypothesis that *Chlamydia pneumoniae* caused myocardial infarctions.[51] Again, however, a systematic review of RCTs suggested that the *C. pneumoniae* theory may be dead.[95] Why was epidemiology misleading? Again, different explanations may have been inadequately explored. Analyses restricted to "never-smokers" indicated that *C. pneumoniae* infection was not associated with an increased coronary heart disease risk,[121] a finding consistent with RCT results. The highest goal of a scientist is the attempt to refute, disprove, and vigorously explore factors and alternative hypotheses that may "explain away" the observed association.[22] Not vigorously exploring smoking as a potential confounder may have led to a significant waste of clinical research resources and a lost opportunity to explore more solid epidemiologic leads for lung cancer and coronary heart disease. Is it possible that similar mistakes are occuring in periodontics–systemic disease research?

For a factor to explain away an observed association, two criteria need to be fulfilled. First, the factor must be related to the exposure, but not necessarily in causal way. Second, the factor must be causally related to the outcome and must not be in the causal pathway. If both criteria are satisfied, the factor is referred to as a *confounder,* and *confounding* is said to be present. For example, smoking satisfied the criteria for a confounder in the β-carotene–lung cancer association because (1) cigarette smokers consumed less β-carotene than nonsmokers and (2) smoking caused lung cancer. Confounding is often represented schematically (Figure 2-1).

In randomized studies, confounding is not an issue because randomization balances known and unknown confounders across the compared groups with a high degree of certainty. In epidemiologic studies, in which no randomization is present, three questions related to

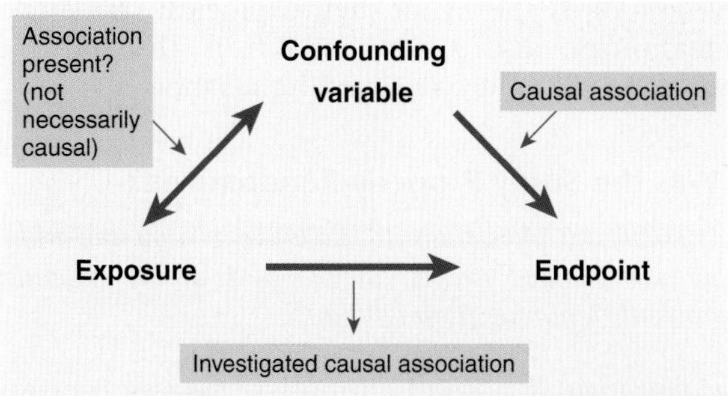

Figure 2-1 Schematic representation of the two necessary criteria for a variable to induce spurious associations (i.e., to be a confounding variable). The confounding variable (1) has to be associated with the exposure and (2) has to be causally linked to the outcome. When both criteria are satisfied, confounding is said to be present.

confounding need to be considered in the assessment of the causality, as addressed next.

First, were all important confounders identified? Complex diseases have multiple risk factors, which may act as confounders in the reported association. The multiple confounders need to be included in the statistical analyses. An association unadjusted for any potential confounders is sometimes referred to as the *crude association.* When this crude association is adjusted for potential confounders, it is referred to as an *adjusted association.* Typically, crude associations are adjusted for multiple confounders, and both crude and adjusted odds ratios are presented.

Second, how accurately were confounders measured? Some potential confounders, such as age, gender, and race, can be measured relatively accurately. Other potential confounders, such as smoking or lifestyle, are notoriously more difficult to measure. A discrepancy between what is measured and what is the truth will result in the incomplete removal of bias and lead to spurious associations. The remaining bias is sometimes referred to as *residual confounding.* Residual confounding is common in epidemiology and is one of the reasons why case-control and cohort studies are less effective research tools than randomized trials in identifying small effects. For instance, an accurate summary of smoking history over a person's lifetime may be impossible.[115]

Third, was the statistical modeling of the confounders appropriate? Any misspecification of the functional relationships causes bias. For example, assuming a linear relationship between a confounder and an endpoint, while in truth the relationship is quadratic, will cause bias.

Evaluating the impact of confounding is a complex challenge. The goal of an epidemiologist is to come up with the best possible defense why an identified association is spurious.[78] All possible efforts should be spent identifying known confounders, obtaining accurate measurements on the confounders, and exploring different analytic approaches to refute the observed association. Smoking, a potential confounder in many studies, has been found to be such a strong confounder that several leading epidemiologist have suggested that restriction to never-smokers is required to eliminate the potential for residual confounding by smoking.[99] Control for confounding is the major methodological challenge in epidemiology, and randomization is the only tool available to eliminate confounding reliably.

9. Was the Study Properly Randomized?

Attempts by physicians to circumvent randomization are not isolated events; they're part of an endemic problem stemming from ignorance.[94]

Randomization is a counterintuitive process because it (1) creates heterogeneity, (2) takes control over treatment assignment away from the physician, and (3) leads to apparently illogical situations in which patients randomly assigned to a treatment, but refusing it, still are analyzed as if they received the treatment. Although randomization was a radical innovation introduced for agriculture, it is doubtful whether it would have ever been introduced into medicine (and subsequently dentistry) were it not for a confluence of factors surrounding the end of World War II in Great Britain. Because of the revolutionary nature of randomization, fundamental misunderstandings of this process remain. About one third of the clinical trials published in elite medical journals apparently do *not* ensure that patients are assigned to different treatments by chance.[5] The majority of reported periodontal trials fail to convince reviewers that (1) the studies were properly randomized, (2) randomization was concealed, or (3) randomized patients were accounted for.[88] Tampering with the delicate process of randomization can quickly, using the words of Ronald Fisher, a statistician and geneticist, turn an "experiment into an experience."

Several studies have shown how an inadequate randomization process will bias study findings. In one review study, the ability to reject patients from the study *after* random treatment assignment tripled the likelihood of finding significant results and doubled the likelihood that confounders were unequally distributed among the compared groups.[25] Trials where clinicians can break the randomization code reported treatment effects that averaged 30% larger than effects in trials where the randomization could not be broken.[68] The common desire to eliminate noncompliant patients can similarly lead to biases, as shown by the following two examples. First, in one cardiovascular disease trial, patients compliant to a placebo pill had a 10% reduction in mortality risk compared with patients noncompliant to the placebo.[31] Second, in a caries trial, adolescents compliant to a placebo varnish had on average 2.2 fewer new caries lesions than adolescents noncompliant to a placebo varnish.[44] Clearly, factors related to compliance and unrelated to the treatments under investigation have a powerful influence on the outcome measured. Deleting such noncompliant patients may lead to biases.

Proper randomization ideally includes the following elements. First, subjects are enrolled into a study *prior to randomization:* important baseline disease characteristics are recorded and provided to an independent person or organization. This step ensures that baseline information is available for *every* patient who will be randomized. Without this step, randomized patients can be "lost," leading to biases. Subsequently, an independent person or organization *randomly* assigns subjects to treatments and informs the clinician regarding the treatment assignment. This randomization process needs to be auditable, making pseudorandom processes such as coin tosses unacceptable. The concealment of the randomization process ensures that clinicians cannot crack the code and that they will enroll only those patients they think are suited for the treatment that will be assigned. Finally, the outcome in the subject is evaluated regardless of follow-up time or compliance and according to the treatment assigned, *not* the treatment received. *Imputation* is used in sensitivity analyses to determine the extent that subjects with missing information can bias the conclusions. The whole process of randomization is complex and often deviated from leading to unreliable results.

10. When to Rely on Nonrandomized Evidence?

Randomize the first patient.

—*Thomas Chalmers*[26]

To tell the truth, all of the discussion today about the patient's informed consent still strikes me as absolute rubbish.

—*Sir Bradford Hill*

More than 50 epidemiologic studies reported evidence that hormone replacement therapy provided benefits to postmenopausal women.[39] Despite this "strong" evidence from "leading" researchers, and despite the opposition on ethical grounds to initiate a placebo-controlled trial, the Women's Health Initiative trial was initiated. The "miracle" of hormone replacement therapy was shown to lead to increases in breast cancer risk, dementia, myocardial infarction, and stroke. This example illustrates well the need for randomized studies and for questioning well-established and widely accepted beliefs based on numerous epidemiologic studies. Nonetheless, the initiation of randomized trials can become difficult because of ethical considerations and unaffordably large sample sizes.

Ethical principles dictate that proposed interventions do more good than harm, that the populations in whom the study will be conducted will benefit from the findings, that informed consent is obtained from enrolled subjects, and that a genuine uncertainty exists with respect to treatment efficacy. The interpretation of these ethical principles is largely determined by culture and era. Ethical principles also play an important role in determining which clinical questions are sufficiently important to warrant the conduct of a randomized controlled trial (RCT).

Sample size considerations may prevent the conduct of RCTs. The smaller the rate at which endpoints occur in an RCT, the larger the required sample size will be. For rare events such as bacterial endocarditis subsequent to a dental procedure or HIV conversion after exposure to an HIV-contaminated dental needle, RCTs may never be possible because the required sample sizes are in the 100,000s or millions of subjects.

In addition to both ethical and practical reasons, there can be powerful political issues surrounding the decision to initiate clinical trials. Nonetheless, unequivocal evidence requires the conduct of rigorously designed and executed RCTs. The smaller the beneficial effect identified in observational studies, the more prevalent is the exposure, and the larger the need for RCT evidence. Although certain important clinical questions may never have reliable answers, the absence of RCT evidence for important and answerable clinical questions can be frustrating to those who seek reliable evidence-based practice guidelines.

11. Placebo Effects: Real or Sham?

> *I never knew any advantage from electricity in (the treatment of) palsies that was permanent. And how far the apparent temporary advantage might arise from the exercise in the patient's journey, and coming daily to my house, or from the spirits given by the hope of success, enabling them to exert more strength in moving their limbs, I will not pretend to say.*
>
> **—Benjamin Franklin**[128]

Sham or *mock* surgeries have been used to evaluate whether implanting human fetal tissue in the brain decreases symptoms of Parkinson's disease,[96] whether surgical lavage and débridement decreases pain in arthritic knee joints,[89] whether mammary artery ligation improves heart disease outcomes,[28] and whether alveolar trephination relieves the pain of acute apical periodontitis.[55,93]

What motivates clinical investigators to subject patients to surgical risks, and yet knowingly provide no hypothesized benefits to these patients? A partial answer to this question lies in a phenomenon known as *placebo effects:* the beneficial effects some patients experience by simply participating in a study, by patient-physician interaction, by the patient's anticipation for improvement, or by the patient's desire to please the physician. A small, controlled study in 11 patients showed that placebo effects can cause changes in brain function,[18] providing plausibility to the argument that placebo effects may have biologic effects. Because of such placebo effects, without mock surgeries it would be impossible to tell whether the improvements observed in clinical trials are caused by the placebo effects associated with the surgical procedures or by the hypothesized active ingredient of the surgery itself.

Two studies have quantified the placebo effect. In the first study the magnitude of the placebo effect was estimated by evaluating patient responses to ineffective treatments.[107] Five treatments were identified as ineffective if the treatment had been abandoned by the medical profession and if at least one controlled study confirmed its ineffectiveness. With these ineffective treatments, good to excellent treatment responses were observed in 45% to 90% of the patients, a powerful placebo effect indeed. In the second study, placebo interventions (pharmacologic placebo, physical or psychologic intervention) were compared to true "no-treatment" interventions.[56] A significant placebo effect was observed for pain, the condition that was evaluated in the largest number of trials and that had the largest number of evaluated participants. No significant placebo effects were detected for other outcomes such as weight loss.

In dentistry, sound systematic reviews may provide some ability to evaluate placebo effects. One systematic review of 133 studies reported that the fluoride effect on caries was significantly larger when a no-treatment control group was used versus a placebo–control group.[82] One possible interpretation for these differences is a placebo effect: the placebo lowered caries rates. Other explanations, such as the scientific quality of the studies, may of course also be responsible for such observed differences, especially for pain. Overall, sufficient evidence is available to suggest that placebo effects can be real and measurable, and that the magnitude of the placebo effect may depend on the treatment under study and the type of outcome evaluated.

12. Was There Protection against Conflict of Interest?

> *Heartport Road Kill.*
>
> **—A phrase coined by cardiac surgeons to refer to patients who died or were injured using Heartport equipment**[72]

Can one trust clinical recommendations regarding a novel, noninvasive cardiac bypass surgery by a physician who has a $100 million stake in the procedure he is recommending? Is it possible that financial stakes are preventing physicians from disclosing a tenfold increased mortality risk?[72] Can one trust guidelines establishing sharply lowered lipid levels knowing that eight of the nine panel experts have financial connections to the manufacturers of lipid-lowering drugs?[67] Is it possible that science panelists are picked for ideology?[16] The answers to these questions are not straightforward and in general are discussed under the heading of "conflicts of interest."

Conflict of interest has been defined as "a set of conditions in which professional judgment concerning a primary interest (such as patient's welfare or validity of research) tends to be unduly influenced by a secondary interest."[122] A common secondary interest is financial but can include others, such as religious or scientific beliefs, ideologic or political beliefs, or academic interests (e.g., promotion). Some examples of how conflicts of interests can bias evidence are now given:

1. Evidence can be suppressed by lawsuits. For example, a company initiated a multimillion-dollar legal action[20] against the investigator who reported that their HIV vaccine was ineffective.[69] Also, two companies[84,129] suppressed submitted scientific articles that they perceived as incorrect.
2. Negative evidence can disappear into a "black hole."[53] If a drug is truly noneffective, and with a type I error rate of 5%, one can expect that 2 of 40 trials will provide positive results *by chance*. If the 38 negative trial reports go into a file drawer, and if the two positive reports are published in leading journals, a misleading perception of the drugs effectiveness will be given to the practicing community. Although a Food and Drug Administration (FDA) official indicated that such situations have never happened,[38] recent reports on nondisclosed negative trials on an antidepressant drug suggests such problems may exist.[71,130]

3. Conflicts of interest can lead to distortion of study designs and analyses to provide the desired results. Such distortions can range from data fabrication[47] and data falsification[83] to design and analysis "tweaks" such as contrived control groups,[80,98] unplanned subgroup analyses,[30] and only showing that time point in the analysis where the differences favor the investigated drug.[113]
4. Conflicts of interests related to loss of patents[23] or orphan drugs[125] can shunt available research resources to the conduct of clinical trials that are not necessarily in the best interest of public health.[7]

The potential for conflict of interest has increased over the past 20 years. The prevalence of industry-funded trials has increased from 32% to 62% between 1980 and 2000,[90,91] and two thirds of the universities hold stock in start-up companies that support clinical trials within that institution.[17] Such connections can be viewed with a skeptical eye: industry-sponsored studies are 3.6 times as likely to have pro-industry conclusions as non–industry-sponsored studies.[17] Even if industry-funded trials are executed with the highest degree of ethics and patient benefit in mind, the decrease of public trust caused by apparent conflict of interest can be damaging to the scientific reputation of journals, academic institutions, and science itself.[35]

Because of these issues, the proper handling of potential conflict-of-interest issues is an important aspect of clinical research. During the conduct of the research itself, independent data and safety monitoring boards provide protection against such biases. Policy regulations established by journals, academic institutions, and governments can further decrease the impact of perceived conflicts of interests. For instance, work is currently being done to eliminate the "file-drawer problem" by establishing a registry of RCTs where investigators need to deposit the RCT protocols before their initiation.[36,117]

Conflict-of-interest issues may be just as prevalent in dental research as in other medical areas dealing with chronic disease. In 2002 an article published in a leading dental journal ended up on the cover of the *New York Times*.[98] In part, the reason was a perceived conflict of interest; the article did not disclose that funding for the study came from an advertising company. Disclosure of conflict of interest is often poorly enforced, and some dental journals do not have regulations in place to reveal potential conflicts of interest of authors. Such situations (1) make it challenging for clinicians to recognize the potential for conflicts of interest, (2) may reduce trust in dental journals, and (3) may affect the scientific integrity of dental research.

CONCLUSION

Lessons learned from other chronic disease areas *do* apply to the evaluation of evidence in the periodontal disease research arena. Randomization or confounding is as important in periodontal research as it is in cancer research. Work remains to be done to integrate evidence-based thinking into clinical practice. The most challenging task may be to lessen the excessive reliance on biologic plausibility in determining both research priorities and patient management and to transition to clinical thinking that is based on controlled clinical observations, rather than biologic plausibility. Although the 12 proposed tools for assessing evidence do not cover all necessary tools, or even the most important tools, it is hoped that they provide a useful starting point for the further exploration of the issues and principles involved in the conduct of systematic experiments in periodontal disease research.

REFERENCES

1. Abbott A: British panel bans use of antidepressant to treat children, *Nature* 423:792, 2003.
2. Abbott AA, Koren LZ, Morse DR, et al: A prospective randomized trial on efficacy of antibiotic prophylaxis in asymptomatic teeth with pulpal necrosis and associated periapical pathosis, *Oral Surg Oral Med Oral Pathol* 66:722, 1988.
3. Aboulker JP, Swart AM: Preliminary analysis of the Concorde trial, Concorde Coordinating Committee (see comments), *Lancet* 341:889, 1993 (letter).
4. Advanced Colorectal Cancer Meta-Analysis Project: Modulation of fluorouracil by leucovorin in patients with advanced colorectal cancer: evidence in terms of response rate, *J Clin Oncol* 10:896, 1992.
5. Altman DG, Dore CJ: Randomisation and baseline comparisons in clinical trials, *Lancet* 335:149, 1990.
6. Altman LK: Study prompts call to halt a routine eye operation, *New York Times,* Feb 22, 1995, p C100.
7. Angell M: *The truth about the drug companies: how they deceive us and what to do about it,* New York, 2004, Random House.
8. Antczak AA, Tang J, Chalmers TC: Quality assessment of randomized control trials in dental research. I. Methods, *J Periodontal Res* 21:305, 1986.
9. Antczak AA, Tang J, Chalmers TC: Quality assessment of randomized control trials in dental research. II. Results: periodontal research, *J Periodontal Res* 21:315, 1986.
10. Asimov I: *A history of mathematics,* ed 2, New York, 1991, Wiley & Sons, p vii.
11. ATBC Cancer Prevention Study Group: The Alpha-Tocopherol, Beta-Carotene Lung Cancer Prevention Study: design, methods, participant characteristics, and compliance, *Ann Epidemiol* 4:1, 1994.
12. Awad MA, Locker D, Korner-Bitensky N, Feine JS: Measuring the effect of intra-oral implant rehabilitation on health-related quality of life in a randomized controlled clinical trial, *J Dent Res* 79:1659, 2000.
13. Barry JM, *The great influenza: the epic story of the deadliest plague in history,* New York, 2004, Viking, p 61.
14. Beasley RP, Hwang LY, Lin CC, Chien CS: Hepatocellular carcinoma and hepatitis B virus: a prospective study of 22,707 men in Taiwan, *Lancet* 2:1129, 1981.
15. Begley S: Seek and ye shall find, *Newsweek,* 1997.
16. Begley S: Now, science panelists are picked for ideology rather than expertise, *Wall Street Journal,* Dec 6, 2002, p B1.
17. Bekelman JE, Li Y, Gross CP: Scope and impact of financial conflicts of interest in biomedical research: a systematic review, *JAMA* 289:454, 2003.
18. Benedetti F, Colloca L, Torre E, Lanotte M, et al: Placebo-responsive Parkinson patients show decreased activity in single neurons of subthalamic nucleus, *Nat Neurosci* 7:587, 2004.
19. Bennett-J-C: Inclusion of women in clinical trials: policies for population subgroups (see comments), *N Engl J Med* 329:288, 1993.

20. Bodenheimer T, Collins R: The ethical dilemmas of drug, money, and medicine, *Seattle Times,* 2001.
21. Brody BA: *Ethical issues in drug testing, approval, and pricing: the clot dissolving drugs,* New York, 1995, Oxford University Press.
22. Buck C: Popper's philosophy for epidemiologists, *Int J Epidemiol* 4:159, 1975.
23. Burton TM: Why cheap drugs that appear to halt fatal sepsis go unused, *New York Times,* May 17, 2002, p A1.
24. Cardiac Arrhythmia Suppression Trial (CAST) investigators: Preliminary report: effect of encainide and flecainide on mortality in randomized trial of arrhythmia suppression after myocardial infarction, *N Engl J Med* 321:406, 1989.
25. Chalmers T, Celano P, Sacks H, Smith H: Bias in treatment assignment in controlled clinical trials, *New Engl J Med* 309:1358, 1983.
26. Chalmers TC: Randomization of the first patient, *Med Clin North Am* 59:1035, 1975.
27. Chauvenet M, Rimailho A, Hoog-Labouret N: Methodology for the evaluation of drugs in pregnant women, *Therapie* 58:247, 2003.
28. Cobb LA, Thomans GI, Dillard DH: An evaluation of internal mammary artery ligation by a double-blind technique, *N Engl J Med* 260:1115, 1959.
29. Cohen J: Clinical research: AIDS vaccine results draw investor lawsuits, *Science* 299:1965, 2003.
30. Cohen J: Public health: AIDS vaccine trial produces disappointment and confusion, *Science* 299:1290, 2003.
31. Coronary Drug Project Research Group: Influence of adherence to treatment and response of cholesterol on mortality in the Coronary Drug Project, *N Engl J Med* 303:1038, 1980.
32. Couzin J: Cancer drugs: smart weapons prove tough to design, *Science* 298:522, 2002.
33. Crossen C: The treatment: a medical researcher pays for challenging drug-industry funding, *Wall Street Journal,* Aug 6, 2001, p A1.
34. Cummings SR, Black DM, Thompson DE, et al: Effect of alendronate on risk of fracture in women with low bone density but without vertebral fractures: results from the Fracture Intervention Trial, *JAMA* 280:2077, 1998.
35. DeAngelis CD: Conflict of interest and the public trust, *JAMA* 284:2237, 2000.
36. DeAngelis CD, Drazen JM, Frizelle FA, et al: Clinical trial registration: a statement from the International Committee of Medical Journal Editors, *JAMA*, 2004.
37. Del Mar C, Glasziou P, Hayem M: Are antibiotics indicated as initial treatment for children with acute otitis media? A meta-analysis, *BMJ* 314:1526, 1997.
38. Ehrlich R: Can a sugar pill kill you? In *8 preposterous propositions,* Princeton, NJ, 2003, Princeton University Press.
39. Enserink M: Women's health: The vanishing promises of hormone replacement, *Science* 297:325, 2002.
40. Feinstein AR: Scientific standards in epidemiologic studies of the menace of daily life, *Science* 242:1257, 1988.
41. Feskanich D, Ziegler RG, Michaud DS, et al: Prospective study of fruit and vegetable consumption and risk of lung cancer among men and women, *J Natl Cancer Inst* 92:1812, 2000.
42. Fleming TR: Historical controls, data banks, and randomized trials in clinical research: a review, *Cancer Treat Rep* 66:1101, 1982.
43. Fleming TR, DeMets DL: Surrogate end points in clinical trials: are we being misled? *Ann Intern Med* 125:605, 1996.
44. Forgie AH, Paterson M, Pine CM, et al: A randomised controlled trial of the caries-preventive efficacy of a chlorhexidine-containing varnish in high-caries-risk adolescents, *Caries Res* 34:432, 2000.
45. Fuhrmans V: HRT worries give headaches to drug makers, *Wall Street Journal,* Oct 25, 2002, p B1.
46. Gilmartin RV: Chairman's report, Annual Meeting of Stockholders, 2002, Merck & Co.
47. Grady D: Breast cancer researcher admits falsifying data, *New York Times,* Feb 2000, p A7.
48. Gray R, Clarke M, Collins R, Peto R: Making randomised trials larger: a simple solution? *Eur J Surg Oncol* 21:137, 1995.
49. Greenland S: Randomization, statistics, and causal inference, *Epidemiology* 1: 21, 1990.
50. Guerini V: *History of dentistry,* New York, 1909, Lea & Febiger.
51. Gupta S, Camm AJ: *Chlamydia pneumoniae,* antimicrobial therapy and coronary heart disease: a critical overview, *Coron Artery Dis* 9:339, 1998.
52. Henry M, Reader A, Beck M: Effect of penicillin on postoperative endodontic pain and swelling in symptomatic necrotic teeth, *J Endod* 27:117, 2001.
53. Hensley S, Abboud L: Medical research has "black hole," *Wall Street Journal,* June 4, 2004, p B3.
54. Holmberg L, Bill-Axelson A, Helgesen F, et al: A randomized trial comparing radical prostatectomy with watchful waiting in early prostate cancer, *N Engl J Med* 347:781, 2002.
55. Houck V, Reader A, Beck M, Nist R, Weaver J: Effect of trephination on postoperative pain and swelling in symptomatic necrotic teeth, *Oral Surg Oral Med Oral Pathol Oral Radiol Endod* 90:507, 2000.
56. Hrobjartsson A and Gotzsche PC: Is the placebo powerless? An analysis of clinical trials comparing placebo with no treatment, *N Engl J Med* 344:1594, 2001.
57. http://www1.tpgi.com.au/users/tps-seti/baloney.html.
58. http://www.improbable.com/airchives/paperair/air-teachers-guide.html.
59. Hujoel PP, DeRouen TA: A survey of endpoint characteristics in periodontal clinical trials published 1988-1992, and implications for future studies, *J Clin Periodontol* 22:397, 1995.
60. Hujoel PP, Moulton LH: Evaluation of test statistics in split-mouth clinical trials, *J Periodontal Res* 23: 378, 1988.
61. Hujoel PP, Cunha-Cruz J, Loesche WJ, Robertson PR: Personal oral hygiene and chronic periodontitis: a systematic review, *Periodontology 2000* 37:29, 2005.
62. Hujoel PP, del Aguila MA, DeRouen TA, Bergstrom J: A hidden periodontitis epidemic during the 20th century? *Community Dent Oral Epidemiol* 31:1, 2003.
63. Hujoel PP, Drangsholt M, Spiekerman C, Derouen TA: Examining the link between coronary heart disease and the elimination of chronic dental infections, *J Am Dent Assoc* 132:883, 2001.
64. Ischemic Optic Neuropathy Decompression Trial Research Group: Optic nerve decompression surgery for nonarteritic anterior ischemic optic neuropathy (NAION) is not effective and may be harmful, *JAMA* 273:625, 1995.
65. Jacobson JM, Greenspan JS, Spritzler J, et al: Thalidomide for the treatment of oral aphthous ulcers in patients with human immunodeficiency virus infection, National Institute of Allergy and Infectious Diseases, AIDS Clinical Trials Group, *N Engl J Med* 336:1487, 1997.
66. Jha P, Flather M, Lonn E, et al: The antioxidant vitamins and cardiovascular disease: a critical review of epidemiologic and clinical trial data, *Ann Intern Med* 123:860, 1995.
67. Johnson LA: Group assails cholesterol advice over experts' ties to drugmakers, online, Associated Press, July 17.
68. Juni P, Altman DG, Egger M: Systematic reviews in health care: assessing the quality of controlled clinical trials, *BMJ* 323:42, 2001.

69. Kahn JO, Cherng DW, Mayer K, et al: Evaluation of HIV-1 immunogen, an immunologic modifier, administered to patients infected with HIV having 300 to 549 × 10^6/L CD4 cell counts: a randomized controlled trial, *JAMA* 284:2193, 2000.
70. Kennedy D: Drug discovery, *Science* 303:1729, 2004.
71. Kennedy D: The old file-drawer problem, *Science* 305:451, 2004.
72. King RJ: Keyhole heart surgery started fast: some say too fast, *Wall Street Journal,* May 5, 1999, p A1.
73. Kjekshus J, Pedersen TR: Reducing the risk of coronary events: evidence from the Scandinavian Simvastatin Survival Study (4S), *Am J Cardiol* 76:64C, 1995.
74. Lee HG, Casadesus G, Zhu X, et al: Perspectives on the amyloid-beta cascade hypothesis, *J Alzheimer Dis* 6:137, 2004.
75. Leibovici L: Effects of remote, retroactive intercessory prayer on outcomes in patients with bloodstream infection: randomised controlled trial, *BMJ* 323:1450, 2001.
76. Lipid Research Clinics Coronary Primary Prevention Trial: Results. I. Reduction in incidence of coronary heart disease, *JAMA* 251:351, 1984.
77. Löe H, Theilade E, Jensen SB: Experimental gingivitis in man, *J Periodontol* 36:177, 1965.
78. Maclure M: Multivariate refutation of aetiological hypotheses in non-experimental epidemiology, *Int J Epidemiol* 19:782, 1990.
79. MacMahon B, Yen S, Trichopoulos D, et al: Coffee and cancer of the pancreas, *N Engl J Med* 304:630, 1981.
80. Malakoff D: Human research: Nigerian families sue Pfizer, testing the reach of U.S. law, *Science* 293:1742, 2001.
81. Mandel EM, Rockette HE, Bluestone CD, et al: Efficacy of amoxicillin with and without decongestant-antihistamine for otitis media with effusion in children: results of a double-blind, randomized trial, *N Engl J Med* 316:432, 1987.
82. Marinho VC, Higgins JP, Logan S, Sheiham A: Topical fluoride (toothpastes, mouthrinses, gels or varnishes) for preventing dental caries in children and adolescents, *Cochrane Database Syst Rev*, CD002782, 2003.
83. Marshall E: Breast cancer: reanalysis confirms results of 'tainted' study, *Science* 270:1562, 1995.
84. Mathews A, Burton TM: Invasive procedure; After Medtronic lobbying push, the FDA had change of heart; Agency squelches an article raising doubts on safety of device to repair artery; Threat of 'criminal sanction,' *Wall Street Journal,* June 9, 2004, p A1.
85. Matthews R: *Statistics: Undermined by an error of significance, Financial Times,* 2004, p 9.
86. Merikangas KR, Risch N: Genomic priorities and public health, *Science* 302:599, 2003.
87. Mills JL: Data torturing, *N Engl J Med* 329:1196, 1993.
88. Montenegro R, Needleman I, Moles D, Tonetti M: Quality of RCTs in periodontology: a systematic review, *J Dent Res* 81:866, 2002.
89. Moseley JB, O'Malley K, Petersen NJ, et al: A controlled trial of arthroscopic surgery for osteoarthritis of the knee, *N Engl J Med* 347:81, 2002.
90. Moses H III, Martin JB: Academic relationships with industry: a new model for biomedical research, *JAMA* 285:933, 2001.
91. National Institutes of Health: Extramural data and trends, 2000, Bethesda, Md, NIH.
92. Neu HC: The crisis in antibiotic resistance, *Science* 257:1064, 1992.
93. Nist E, Reader A, Beck M: Effect of apical trephination on postoperative pain and swelling in symptomatic necrotic teeth, *J Endod* 27:415, 2001.
94. Nowak R: Problems in clinical trials go far beyond misconduct, *Science* 264:1538, 1994.
95. O'Connor CM, Dunne MW, Pfeffer MA, et al: Azithromycin for the secondary prevention of coronary heart disease events: the WIZARD study—a randomized controlled trial, *JAMA* 290:1459, 2003.
96. Olanow CW, Goetz CG, Kordower JH, et al: A double-blind controlled trial of bilateral fetal nigral transplantation in Parkinson's disease, *Ann Neurol* 54:403, 2003.
97. Omenn GS, Goodman GE, Thornquist MD, et al: Effects of a combination of beta carotene and vitamin A on lung cancer and cardiovascular disease, *N Engl J Med* 334:1150, 1996.
98. Peterson M: *Madison Ave. has growing role in the business of drug research, New York Times,* Nov 22, 2002, p A1.
99. Peto J: Cancer epidemiology in the last century and the next decade, *Nature* 411:390, 2001.
100. Peto R: Misleading subgroup analyses in GISSI, *Am J Cardiol* 66:771, 1990.
101. Pickenpaugh L, Reader A, Beck M, et al: Effect of prophylactic amoxicillin on endodontic flare-up in asymptomatic, necrotic teeth, *J Endod* 27:53, 2001.
102. Pilcher H: Starting to gel, *Nature* 430:138, 2004.
103. Psaty BM, Weiss NS, Furberg CD, et al: Surrogate end points, health outcomes, and the drug-approval process for the treatment of risk factors for cardiovascular disease, *JAMA* 282:786, 1999.
104. Ramfjord SP: Surgical periodontal pocket elimination: still a justifiable objective? *J Am Dent Assoc* 114:37, 1987.
105. Report of the Committee of Principal Investigators: WHO cooperative trial on primary prevention of ischaemic heart disease with clofibrate to lower serum cholesterol: final mortality follow-up, *Lancet* 2:600, 1984.
106. Riggs BL, Hodgson SF, O'Fallon WM, et al: Effect of fluoride treatment on the fracture rate in postmenopausal women with osteoporosis, *N Engl J Med* 322:802, 1990.
107. Roberts AH, Kewman DG, Mercier L, Hovell MF: The power of nonspecific effects in healing: implications for psychosocial and biological treatments, *Clin Psychol Rev* 13:375, 1993.
108. Ross PE: Lies, damned lies and medical statistics, *Forbes*, 1995, p 130.
109. Ryan M: *Who really said? The book that tests your "quote" IQ,* Hong Kong, 1967, Great Quotations Publishing Company.
110. Sagan C: *The demon-haunted world,* New York, 1996, Ballantine Books.
111. Schluger S, Yuodelis RA, Page RC: *Periodontal disease: basic phenomena, clinical management, and occlusal and restorative interrelationships,* Philadelphia, 1977, Lea & Febiger.
112. Second International Study of Infarct Survival (ISIS-2) Collaborative Group: Randomised trial of intravenous streptokinase, oral aspirin, both, or neither among 17,187 cases of suspected acute myocardial infarction, *Lancet* 2:349, 1988.
113. Silverstein FE, Faich G, Goldstein JL, et al: Gastrointestinal toxicity with celecoxib vs nonsteroidal anti-inflammatory drugs for osteoarthritis and rheumatoid arthritis: the CLASS study—a randomized controlled trial, Celecoxib Long-term Arthritis Safety Study, *JAMA* 284:1247, 2000.
114. Sloppy stats shame science, *Economist,* 2004.
115. Spiekerman CF, Hujoel PP, DeRouen TA: Bias induced by self-reported smoking on periodontitis–systemic disease associations, *J Dent Res* 82:345, 2003.
116. Staquet MJ, Rozencweig M, von Hoff DD, Muggia FM: The delta and epsilon errors in the assessment of cancer clinical trials, *Cancer Treat Rep* 63:1917, 1979.
117. Steinbrook R: Public registration of clinical trials, *N Engl J Med* 351:315, 2004.
118. Stram DO, Huberman M, Wu AH: Is residual confounding a reasonable explanation for the apparent protective effects

of beta-carotene found in epidemiologic studies of lung cancer in smokers? *Am J Epidemiol* 155:622, 2002.
119. Taubes G: News: Epidemiology faces its limits (see comments), *Science* 269:164, 1995.
120. Temple RJ: A regulatory authority's opinion about surrogate endpoints. In Tucker GT, editor: *Clinical measurement in drug evaluation,* New York, 1995, Wiley.
121. Thom DH, Grayston JT, Siscovick DS, et al: Association of prior infection with *Chlamydia pneumoniae* and angiographically demonstrated coronary artery disease, *JAMA* 268:68, 1992.
122. Thompson DF: Understanding financial conflicts of interest, *N Engl J Med* 329:573, 1993.
123. Tomar SL, Asma S: Smoking-attributable periodontitis in the United States: findings from NHANES III, National Health and Nutrition Examination Survey, *J Periodontol* 71:743, 2000.
124. Tomasz A: Multiple-antibiotic-resistant pathogenic bacteria: a report on the Rockefeller University Workshop, *N Engl J Med* 330:1247, 1994.
125. Tsintis P, La Mache E: CIOMS and ICH initiatives in pharmacovigilance and risk management: overview and implications, *Drug Saf* 27:509, 2004.
126. Tufte ER: *The visual display of quantitative information,* Cheshire, Conn, 1983, Graphics Press.
127. Tukey J: The future of data analysis, *Ann Math Stat* 33:1, 1962.
128. Van Doren C: *Benjamin Franklin,* New York, 1938, Viking.
129. Wadman M: Scientists cry foul as Elsevier axes paper on cancer mortality, *Nature* 429:687, 2004.
130. Wadman M: Spitzer sues drug giant for deceiving doctors, *Nature* 429:589, 2004.
131. Washburn EP, Orza MJ, Berlin JA, et al: Residential proximity to electricity transmission and distribution equipment and risk of childhood leukemia, childhood lymphoma, and childhood nervous system tumors: systematic review, evaluation, and meta-analysis, *Cancer Causes Control* 5:299, 1994.
132. Willett WC: Vitamin A and lung cancer, *Nutr Rev* 48:201, 1990.
133. Women's Health Initiative: Risks and benefits of estrogen plus progestin in healthy postmenopausal women: principal results from the Women's Health Initiative randomized controlled trial, *JAMA* 288:321, 2002.
134. Yusuf S, Wittes J, Probstfield J, Tyroler HA: Analyses and interpretation of treatment effects in subgroups of patients in randomized controlled trials, *JAMA* 266:93, 1991.
135. Zeger SL: RE: "Statistical reasoning in epidemiology," the author replies, *Epidemiology* 135:1187, 1992.

Implementing Evidence-Based Decisions in Clinical Practice

Elliot Abt

CHAPTER

3

■ ■ ■

CHAPTER OUTLINE

VARIATION IN CLINICAL DECISIONS
MANAGING UNCERTAINTY
INCORPORATING EVIDENCE INTO PRACTICE
LINKING OUTCOMES WITH DIAGNOSIS
 AND TREATMENT

Outcomes
Diagnosis
Treatment
IMPLEMENTING EVIDENCE-BASED DECISIONS
CHANGE MANAGEMENT

VARIATION IN CLINICAL DECISIONS

Clinical decision making has been the subject of much interest in the last decade. From papers examining dentists' treatment decisions[3] to the development of clinical practice guidelines, much has been written about the process of making clinical decisions. Interest in this discipline relates to variation in clinical practice among health professionals. **The dental literature supports the idea that there is significant variation in clinical decisions among dentists as a result of discrepancies in diagnosis, the need for and types of dental treatment recommended, and the outcomes of these interventions.[4]** Variations in clinical decisions, once defended as natural repercussions of the "art of dental practice," have come under closer scrutiny by educators, epidemiologists, and insurance companies. Many stakeholders are involved because the repercussions of clinical decisions affect patients, third-party payers, social and health policy, as well as the dental profession and its constituent societies.

Although it may seem routine to the seasoned practitioner, the process of making decisions can be complex. In its simplest form, reaching decisions involves taking a patient's chief complaint, performing a complete history and clinical examination, and using various diagnostic tests to obtain a diagnosis. The clinician must then decide if and which dental interventions are appropriate to optimize outcomes of therapy. Unfortunately, the road to

good decision making is filled with many pitfalls. Diagnosis and treatment planning are difficult skills based on assessing disease susceptibility and prognosis, which have historically been underemphasized in undergraduate dental education. Contemporary dental practice calls for decisions to be made efficiently while facing clinical uncertainty. Consequently, many of these decisions are made with an overreliance on past experience and input from colleagues or experts. The importance of making good decisions should not be discounted while facing these challenges.

Evidence-based practice has been defined as improving treatment outcomes by using research evidence, along with clinical experience and patient preferences, in making decisions about individual patients.[18] This chapter focuses on *qualitative* changes necessary to help align and improve clinical decisions using an evidence-based approach.

MANAGING UNCERTAINTY

Part of becoming a successful practitioner is making decisions in the face of clinical uncertainty. There will always be a lack of precision with diagnostic tests, diagnosis, and treatments and variability with outcomes of therapy.[13] This is especially true in the field of periodontics, where establishing a prognosis is an inherently imprecise skill. Additionally, the field of periodontics has experienced a significant increase in the number of diagnostic tests and therapeutic modalities in the past decade. These factors may further complicate the decision-making process.

There are psychologic issues in making decisions, especially while facing clinical uncertainty. Simply repeating old behavior patterns is generally much more comfortable than the insightfulness needed to question one's own actions and embrace change. Some individuals are more comfortable and skilled at making decisions, whereas others are inherently indecisive by nature. Contemporary dental practice often calls for treatment options and recommendations to be given quickly and confidently to patients, many of whom want to hear these options in quantitative terms.[13]

Unfortunately, many practitioners have actually been trained to be *indecisive*. Classic elementary education has trained us not to make decisions on our own, but to follow a prescribed set of rules. A simplified way of analyzing learning theory is to examine the way children and adults learn. The pedagogical learning theory states that children are "empty vessels" to be filled with knowledge; the "dominant" teacher disseminates known facts to the "submissive" student. The subject matter and logic dominate, motivation is external, and learning generally is not immediately applied. The *androgical theory* states that adults learn best by internal motivation and having an urgency to solve problems by drawing on existing knowledge. Adult learning is about discovering what is not known, accepting uncertainty, yet still being able to apply newfound knowledge immediately.

Traditional dental education has generally been pedagogical in nature. Students are given basic sciences but are then expected to adhere to "clinic rules" prescribed by the institution. Historically, these "rules" have consisted of a strict code of conduct and a series of *absolute* behavior patterns, as follows:

1. All cases must be mounted in centric relation.
2. All endodontically treated teeth require a post/core and crown.
3. Always replace missing teeth.
4. All oral surgery patients must receive antibiotics.
5. Never use cantilevers.
6. Always perform periodontal procedures before restorative procedures.

Students are given information from clinical instructors that may be scientific or anecdotal in nature; they generally are not given skills to discriminate which is which[1] or the latitude or training to make independent decisions. Training is limited in diagnosis, treatment planning, and assessing disease susceptibility. This results in a rather *linear* approach to clinical decision making. Instead of establishing a diagnosis, dental students and residents typically identify a presenting dental condition as needing a specific treatment to achieve or avoid a certain outcome (Figure 3-1). For example, dental residents generally view impacted wisdom teeth as requiring extraction to avoid future pathologic development and missing teeth as needing replacement to avoid arch collapse despite evidence to the contrary.[20]

This linear or "cookbook" approach to dental treatment could lead to successful outcomes, but it raises the question of overtreatment. This forms the basis for *traditional* decision making in dentistry: place a heavy emphasis on adherence to dental school principles when faced with clinical uncertainty. Many dental residents, when asked to make a clinical decision, simply state, "This is what we were told to do in dental school." Classic decision making overemphasizes past knowledge, input from experts, and previous clinical successes in an effort to obtain good outcomes.

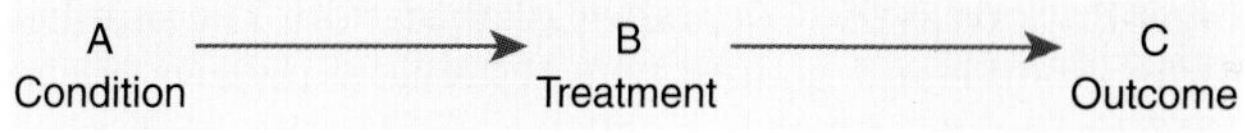

Figure 3-1 Linear, or traditional, method of making clinical decisions.

Implementing an *evidence-based approach* to clinical decision making has been advocated by the scientific literature.[5,14,15] This approach emphasizes decision making based on a clear understanding of accessing and appraising current best evidence. Use of research findings should be used *in conjunction with* clinical experience and patient values in determining optimal treatment recommendations. The literature has only begun to document better decisions and outcomes with an evidence-based rather than a traditional approach.[18] The purpose of clinical research is to provide valuable information for practitioners in helping care for their patients. Advances in dental practice include cosmetic bonding, osseointegration, and medical therapeutics for managing periodontal disease. Genetic research, once the domain of rare disorders, is now shedding new light on susceptibility to common dental diseases.[22] Ignoring research findings represents a significant barrier to the provision of optimal care. At a minimum, clinicians should attempt to base decisions on current evidence to help ensure more consistent, relevant treatment outcomes.

INCORPORATING EVIDENCE INTO PRACTICE

Before the existence of medical literature, practitioners had only their expertise and experience on which to base clinical decisions. Eventually, publication of research advances allowed practitioners to incorporate this evidence into clinical practice. This process, known as *science transfer,* has faced many challenges, such as the difficulty in accessing and evaluating evidence, practitioner resistance to changing behavior, and the high frequency of clinical success in dental practice.

One of the primary problems with evidence-based practice is practitioners' awareness of research findings. Although the lack of quality evidence in dentistry has been well documented,[5,15] there *is* quality research for *some* aspects of dental practice. It has been shown that dental residents and practitioners may not be aware of the current best evidence in dentistry.[2] This is understandable given the sheer number of dental journals, and the rate at which studies are being published make it difficult to stay current with the dental literature. This problem has been alleviated in part by the development of evidence-based journals as well as compilations of investigative findings *(systematic reviews)* by such organizations as the Cochrane Collaboration. The number of qualitative and quantitative systematic reviews *(meta-analyses)* in dentistry is small but is steadily increasing every year.

Searching for and critically appraising evidence are significant barriers facing dental practitioners. These two skills are difficult, generally develop over time, and require adequate training, which is just beginning to occur in dental schools. However, few opportunities exist for experienced practitioners to receive formal training in this area. Database-searching skills can be improved with online tutorials or help from medical librarians at hospitals or universities. The use of Boolean operators, medical subject headings (MeSH), truncations, and limits have made database searching more efficient.

When reading a scientific investigation, the dental professional should keep in mind the following three questions:

1. What are the results?
2. Are the results valid?
3. Are the findings relevant to my patient population?

These questions form the basis of *critical appraisal,* the ability to assess a study for clarity, validity, and generalizability. This skill has also been made easier by using critical appraisal worksheets that can be downloaded from various websites. These worksheets act as a guide to help readers in the decision to use or discard evidence. Once evidence has been obtained, evaluating it for quality and content can be difficult. Scientific investigations can be filled with many types of errors, bias, and confounders that can directly affect validity. Many studies have used incorrect designs, inappropriate sample sizes or statistical tests, and poor data analyses.

Practitioners have been hesitant to incorporate research findings into practicefor a variety of reasons, including one's ability to recognize the need for change and the ability to change behavior. Several investigations,[12,24] including qualitative studies,[10] have documented clinicians' hesitancy of incorporating known research into practice. Overdependence on clinical experience, the very nature of changing behavior, and concern with patients' reactions to treatment are among the reasons given for ignoring quality evidence.

There is a body of literature on the effectiveness of methods used for dissemination of evidence. It has been shown that passive diffusion of information and continuing education lectures are generally ineffective at getting research into practice and changing practitioner behavior.[6] Small, interactive group work, problem-based learning, and practice-specific interventions have been highly effective in facilitating these changes.[23]

Clinical success is a barrier to changing behavior and ultimately to evidence-based practice. Dental practice and procedures are highly successful, especially with short-term results. Failures do occur, but their impact often is not immediately experienced. Therefore, the impetus for change in dentistry may not be overwhelming. Conversely, the astute practitioner will base clinical practice on sound scientific research and continue to question the effectiveness of various interventions on long-term treatment outcomes. This inherent inquisitiveness can form the basis of lifelong learning in dentistry. As with medicine, the dental profession can experience significant gains by more effectively adopting quality evidence into clinical practice. Perhaps the difficulty with change is not so much accepting new practices, but in letting go of existing theories that have already determined practice. This inertia is what ultimately stalls the adoption of this paradigm shift in dentistry.

With the large number of articles published in the dental literature, the difficult nature of searching and critical appraisal, and practitioner resistance to change, it should become clearer why significant obstacles exist to the adoption of evidence in clinical practice.

LINKING OUTCOMES WITH DIAGNOSIS AND TREATMENT

Outcomes

Patients are treated with the understanding that certain therapies will have better long-term outcomes than others, and that these interventions are superior to "watchful waiting." However, dentistry is a treatment-oriented profession, and undergraduate dental education has traditionally supported treatment for outcomes with two overt themes: eliminate pathology and restore dental arches to an "ideal" occlusion. These two outcomes have been the hallmark of appropriate dental care. Dental students are trained to notate any pathologic entities or occlusal "conditions" with the understanding they will require some type of intervention to avoid poor outcomes.

However, these outcomes may be at odds with patient preferences. Other outcomes, not advocated by traditional dental education, should be strongly considered when making decisions about individual patients. Caries and periodontal disease are typical diagnoses but may have significant outcomes, including loss of tooth structure, pocket formation, mobility, abscess formation, and tooth loss. Other outcomes of significant relevance to patients include elimination of pain, difficulty with mastication, quality of life, and morbidity. The high costs of dental reconstructions can alter clinical decisions for some patients (Box 3-1). Additionally, dental education has traditionally recommended proactive treatment to avoid poor outcomes, such as crowning teeth with large amalgams, systematically removing impacted wisdom teeth, and replacing missing teeth. *The question for the dentist to consider is which of these outcomes is clinically relevant and how likely are these outcomes with or without intervention.* Making a prediction of outcome (prognosis) becomes an

BOX 3-1

Case Example: Interproximal Caries

The distal surface of tooth #4 was restored, whereas other incipient interproximal lesions were managed medically, by encouraging regular flossing and the application of fluoride gel.

important clinical skill (Figure 3-2). The astute clinician should recognize that decisions to intervene are crucial and in some cases may be *less* desirable to patients than watchful waiting.

Levels of intervention are linked to prognosis, which is based on susceptibility to disease. Patients who are highly susceptible to dental disease typically have poorer prognoses and require more urgent and often long-term interventions. That is, patients who are highly susceptible to dental disease are more likely to have tooth loss and quality-of-life issues than lower-risk patients. Underestimating disease susceptibility increases the risk of undertreatment. Perhaps more frequently, dental students and residents overestimate patient's risk of disease progression, which often leads to overtreatment.

Diagnosis

Although the number of strictly *dental* diagnoses is limited, establishing a diagnosis can be challenging for both new and experienced practitioners. Diagnosis is relatively simple when a patient presents with rampant caries. However, many dental students and residents have difficulty diagnosing both caries and periodontal disease in a surprisingly large percentage of cases. This difficulty manifests as both overdiagnosing and underdiagnosing disease. Deep occlusal fissures, with or without stain, can easily be diagnosed as pit and fissure caries with a sharp explorer. Interproximal caries tends to be underdiagnosed because of difficulties in radiographic interpretation (Box 3-1). Interproximal *root surface* carious lesions progress quickly, are often difficult to detect clinically, and are typically misdiagnosed or underdiagnosed (Box 3-2). Periodontal disease tends to be overdiagnosed by the novice practitioner, yet its subtleties allow it to be underdiagnosed by experienced practitioners. Emergencies present a host of diagnostic challenges as well. Distinguishing periapical abscess, periodontal abscess, and root fracture can be problematic for even the most experienced clinician.

Diagnosis has been facilitated by assessing a patient's susceptibility to dental disease. Scientific evidence has now identified risk factors for both caries and periodontal disease (Table 3-1). Assessment of susceptibility to dental disease facilitates both diagnosis and prognosis.

Good clinical decisions start with a complete history, clinical examination, and appropriate diagnostic tests. Treating before establishing a diagnosis or with a misdiagnosis usually leads to poor decisions and ultimately unfavorable outcomes (Box 3-2). Unfortunately, diagnosis has been underemphasized in favor of technical skill development at the undergraduate level.

Presenting condition → Assess disease susceptibility → Establish diagnosis

Establish prognosis → Evaluate need/level of intervention

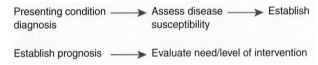

Figure 3-2 Relationship of prognosis to intervention.

BOX 3-2

Case Example: Root Surface Caries

A root surface carious lesion progressed extensively in 2 years. It was not visible clinically.

Treatment

Dental students and residents tend to be very treatment oriented, and they generally are skilled at rendering most types of dental treatment. This may be the result of (1) the nature of undergraduate dental education and (2) dentistry being a surgical discipline. First, dental schools have traditionally based fulfillment of graduation requirements on performing a certain number and type of clinical procedures. Thus, dental students monitor their clinical progress on rendered treatment rather than diagnostic, treatment-planning, or prognostic proficiency. Second, compared with other medical disciplines, dentistry is generally considered a surgical subspecialty in that most diseases are treated by surgical manipulation of diseased tissue. As in other surgical fields, dentistry is

TABLE 3-1

Risk Factors for Caries and Periodontal Disease in Adults

Disease	Risk Factors	Age when Susceptible
Pit and fissure caries	Anatomy of teeth	6-15 years (when teeth first erupt)
Smooth surface caries	Quality of saliva: buffering capacity and antibacterial potential; *Streptococcus mutans* levels	Age 15 into adulthood
Root surface caries	Quantity of saliva (xerostomia)	Adulthood; typically in sixth and seventh decades, depending on medications, history of radiation, etc.
Periodontal disease	Smoking; previous attachment loss; medical conditions (e.g., diabetes, AIDS); presence and amount of certain pathogenic bacteria; genetic risks	Fourth and fifth decades

BOX 3-3

Case Study: Diagnostic Error and Overtreatment

A healthy 65-year-old woman presents to the dental clinic complaining of moderate to severe dental pain for the past 2 months. Clinical examination reveals a missing lower left second molar (#18). Her dental history includes the diagnosis of acute pulpitis on the lower left second molar. Endodontic therapy had been completed on that tooth without any change in symptoms; the tooth was subsequently extracted. A clinical examination is performed, and after diagnostic tests, including radiographs, percussion, palpation, and pulp tests, it is determined that the lower left second bicuspid is the offending tooth. Endodontic therapy is initiated and provides immediate relief of symptoms.

This case is an unfortunate but rather common example of how errors in diagnosis often lead to overtreatment. Properly diagnosing this patient would have avoided unnecessary endodontic therapy and subsequent extraction of tooth #18.

SCIENCE TRANSFER

Clinical practice behavior is heavily influenced by what is learned in dental school. This usually involves a well-informed expert (teacher), knowledge from his or her past experiences, and previous successful behavior. Although this is effective for a number of years, new knowledge becomes available over time and should be incorporated into clinical decision making. Significant obstacles, however, impede such incorporation and include:

- A lack of dissemination of the new knowledge
- The ability to critically appraise the new knowledge
- A natural resistance to change

For example, advances in clinical decision making will occur as diagnostic testing and skills improve and when risk assessment is refined and incorporated into practice. Much excitement currently exists for incorporating evidence-based decision making versus a linear or traditional method of decision making; however, evaluation of the benefits of this approach are just beginning to be determined.

Clinicians need to be able to accept changes in the algorithms they currently use to treat periodontal disease. The excellent technical procedures that most dentists develop require a focus and dedication that can obscure other important skills such as diagnostic accuracy and careful documentation.

The intellectual embrace of evidence-based methods, coupled with clinical expertise and consideration of the patient's individual uniqueness and desires, is needed for all periodontal therapists if optimum care is the goal.

essentially a discipline where technical abilities are highly valued, unlike primary care medicine, where emphasis tends to be placed on diagnostic skills.

There is an expectation among many patients, especially those presenting with pain, that the dentist will render some form of treatment beyond the prescribing of medication. Patients and dentists usually view dentistry as a treatment-oriented profession that tends to discount the diagnostic phase of dental care. This can lead practitioners to treat without ruling in or ruling out a particular diagnosis. For example, if a patient presents with moderate to severe pain, the dentist may be unable to establish a diagnosis, but the patient wants treatment to relieve the pain. The novice practitioner should be cautious about rendering *irreversible* interventions at this point. Lacking a diagnosis, treatment should be limited to medical management and referral to a dental specialist in the hope of establishing a diagnosis. Unfortunately, many patients have undergone unnecessary endodontic and surgical procedures in the hope of elimination of pain caused by errors in diagnosis (Box 3-3).

Errors in *treatment planning* also lead to poor clinical decisions. Common examples are attempting to restore teeth that are too compromised by disease, saving teeth that serve as poor abutments for reconstructive cases, and using poor prosthesis design.

In private practice, certain aspects of rendering treatment can bias clinical decisions. One form of *bias* results from the comfort, familiarity, and pleasure derived from rendering a particular type of treatment. For example, a practitioner may enjoy the challenge of difficult endodontic procedures. Inherent bias may exist in the diagnosis of an endodontic problem, based on the clinician's desire to provide this type of service. Many practitioners have been hesitant to provide implant dentistry because of lack of training, comfort, or familiarity with the nuances of this discipline. However, research advances have shown implant-supported prostheses to be as good as, if not better than, conventional prostheses in terms of survival rates.[8,9,19] Another form of bias, financial bias, occurs when the compensation from more lucrative types of procedures unduly influences the decision-making process. In periodontics, surgical procedures are typically compensated at a higher rate than nonsurgical therapies, and clinicians have a built-in incentive to provide more costly services. The phrase "surgeons make their living by doing surgery" incorporates both types of bias. This vulnerability is inherent in all clinicians, and they must keep this in mind when making decisions about individual patients.

IMPLEMENTING EVIDENCE-BASED DECISIONS

The medical model of reaching clinical decisions is rather complex and uses combinations of algorithms, decision trees, chance trees, and clinical balance sheets. Some

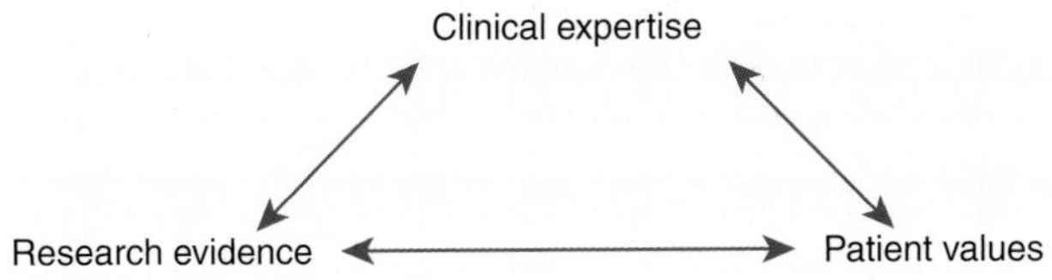

Figure 3-3 Basing clinical decisions on clinical experience and expertise, evidence, and patient values. (Modified from Sackett DA, Strauss SE, Richardson WS, et al: *Evidence-based medicine: how to practice and teach EBM,* London, 2000, Churchill Livingstone.

BOX 3-4

Case Study: Diagnosis and Patient Preference

A 45-year-old male presents to the dental clinic for a routine checkup. The patient has a 20–pack-year history of cigarette smoking and is not having any dental problems at this time. Clinical examination reveals mobility on the lower second bicuspid. There is 5-mm to 6-mm pocketing on this tooth, whereas there are no other pockets greater than 3 mm in all other areas. Radiographic analysis shows vertical bone defects in this area. The patient does not have periodontal disease, and a working diagnosis of root fracture has been established. Because this is a pathologic entity, extraction of this tooth was recommended to the patient. However, the patient has been aware of a problem on this tooth for several years, has never had any symptoms, and does not want the tooth extracted.

In this case a diagnosis has been established, and based on research evidence and clinical experience, extraction of the tooth would be warranted. This patient wanted no treatment, however, based on a lack of symptoms and the high costs associated with implants and bridgework.

of these methods are quantitative, in that success and failure rates are known, and are used mathematically in the decision-making process. Although this can be a difficult process, it is necessary when dealing with serious issues such as life span, morbidity, and quality of life. Although algorithms are used in the medical management of temporomandibular disorders, the use of these decision-making tools is less common in dental practice because of limited quantitative data on prognosis. However, it is still possible to implement evidence-based decisions by combining three key elements according to the definition of evidence-based practice of Sackett et al.[18]: clinical experience, research evidence, and patient preferences (Figure 3-3 and Box 3-4).

Research can be used to guide more appropriate decisions. For example, partial edentulism is not a pathologic entity, and current evidence suggests that failure to replace missing teeth does not result in loss of adjacent teeth or severe arch collapse.[21] The literature also suggests better long-term outcomes with implant versus conventional fixed prosthetics.[8,9,19] Using this evidence, patients

BOX 3-5

Elective Replacement of Missing Teeth

A 62-year-old healthy male presents to the dental clinic for routine examination. It is noted that the upper right first molar (tooth #3) is missing. History taking reveals the patient to be unconcerned about the missing tooth. He is not having difficulty chewing and is generally unaffected by its absence. Radiographically tracking this area shows the adjacent teeth to be in good health, and there is a lack of arch collapse or hypereruption associated with the loss of tooth #3 over a 13-year period.

should now be informed that replacement of missing teeth is elective, and that implants may offer better long-term success than fixed bridges (Box 3-5). This information becomes an important aspect of the decision-making process.

Good decisions begin by attempting to establish a diagnosis through a comprehensive medical and dental history. The medical profession has found that the *history of present illness* deserves the most attention to detail when performing a physical examination. Thoroughness during this phase of diagnosis will provide clues to the patient's experiences, needs, and fears, which helps to establish rapport, a vital ingredient to good dental practice. *Listening* to the patient is of the utmost importance, but studies have shown that clinicians often interrupt patients after only a few seconds of conversation, which can lead to bias in decision making.[7] The clinical examination should be deliberate and exhaustive because diagnosis is not an exact science.[13]

The next phase of providing quality care consists of using various tests to help establish a diagnosis. Radiographs, biopsy, electronic and thermal pulp tests, periodontal probing, and plaque indices are among the many diagnostic tests commonly available to clinicians.

At this point, the astute clinician should have an idea of the patient's susceptibility to dental disease, which helps to establish a diagnosis.

If a diagnosis has been reached, the question for the dentist to consider then is the *prognosis* for this patient. Of all the areas of patient management, prognosis is perhaps the least scientific. In medicine, prognostic difficulties arise with survival rates for patients with chronic illnesses. By examining age and risk factors, prognosis in dentistry can be simplified. For example, an elderly smoker with mild periodontitis may have a more favorable prognosis than the same condition in a young, nonsmoking patient. Unfortunately, even with bacteriologic and immunologic testing, challenges in periodontal prognosis persist. Prognostic proficiency facilitates good decisions because the clinician can make more accurate assessments of long-term outcomes. As such, the clinical picture should become clearer about which, if any, interventions are necessary to achieve good outcomes.

Dental students and residents are taught that decisions to intervene are critical and should be the third step in

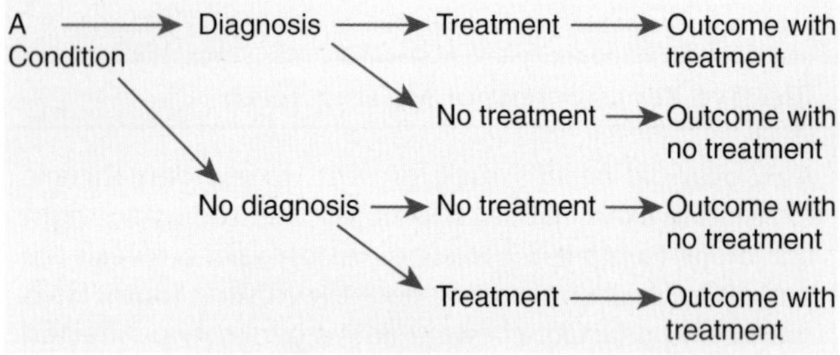

Figure 3-4 Four-step process of making decision to intervene, with or without a diagnosis.

a four-step process (Figure 3-4). Residents are encouraged to attempt to establish a diagnosis first before reaching decisions regarding intervention. If a diagnosis is reached, the resident *may* elect to intervene, depending on the evidence-based pattern of decision making illustrated in Figure 3-3. Occasionally, no diagnosis exists, but treatment may be initiated based on the patient's preferences; replacement of missing teeth and cosmetic bonding are common examples of this phenomenon. By delaying decisions on intervention, residents are taught to emphasize a diagnostic phase, which helps with familiarization of various pathologic conditions in dentistry. Residents are also encouraged to consider the long-term outcomes with or without intervention. What are the outcomes of not replacing missing teeth or not extracting wisdom teeth? In-depth discussions of this type tend to heighten the value of treatment decisions. This differs somewhat from Bader and Shugars' three-step model of clinical decision making in which decisions to intervene immediately follow the initial assessment phase.[4]

Evidence-based practice requires either knowledge of current evidence or the ability to access and evaluate it for content, validity, and relevance. Although the difficulties in evidence retrieval and appraisal have been acknowledged, several factors must be considered when searching the literature. *Randomized controlled trials* (RCTs) represent the appropriate methodology when looking for evidence on therapeutic interventions (see Chapter 1). *Systematic reviews* (SRs) are high-quality summaries of these trials that can provide quick, easy access to current evidence on these interventions. The Cochrane Collaboration provides many of these reviews on their library website. Evidence on diagnosis and prognosis, found in cross-sectional and cohort studies, respectively, may involve more complex database searching. Using various limits on search engines can quickly narrow a search to the appropriate publication type. Once the evidence has been evaluated for content, it should *not* be viewed as the ultimate authority in making decisions about individual patients. Again, evidence should be used in conjunction with clinical experience and patient preferences to make good decisions.

CHANGE MANAGEMENT

Three main challenges lie ahead with the implementation of evidence-based decisions: (1) individual changes and (2) organizational changes, both necessary to implement the evidence-based approach to patient care, and (3) allowing research findings to guide the decision-making process.

To implement evidence-based change, dental schools, dental societies, policies, and practices will need to evaluate their current belief systems. Change can occur only if administrators recognize the need for altering institutional policies and operating procedures. Much has been written about institutional and individual change management. There are no simple answers to effectuating lasting change, but several factors have been identified in the literature.[16] First, there must be the recognition of the need for change. This is a huge hurdle because the ability to recognize and admit the need for improvement is indeed rare. Second, an organizational analysis must be performed, followed by identification of all relevant stakeholders.[11] Third, all stakeholders need to be included early in the change process. Consensus building and teamwork are needed for change to occur, since hierarchical decisions tend to be ineffective.[17] Fourth, monitoring and evaluation are needed to ensure lasting change.

Implementing evidence-based change means providing training to current dental students.

Currently, most U.S. dental schools have only a minority of faculty members with adequate training in evidence-based principles. Thus, long-term change may need to replace ideas about immediate change in the workplace. For practitioners not trained in evidence-based principles, change may be even more difficult. The standard continuing-education seminar is generally representative of a pedagogical learning model, and research has shown that this type of educational intervention has been ineffective in changing practitioner behavior. Because adults typically do not learn best with this teaching method, it should become clearer that if evidence-based principles are to be disseminated to seasoned practitioners, the methods may need to change. The large lecture hall should be replaced by the small, interactive group work found at evidence-based seminars and conferences. Teachers should act as facilitators of knowledge transformation, that is, giving adults the tools needed to learn, rather than being active disseminators of known facts.

Change is typically a slow-moving process that can be influenced by several factors. Transforming our health care system from a traditional to an evidence-based model, with all its political, social, and economic repercussions, will depend on a clear need for change. Much of this change will be based on clinical research with clear patient benefits. It will also require data that support the idea that evidence-based teaching changes practitioner behavior and improves patient care. Currently, such data are lacking. However, a positive environment for evidence-based change exists. Many dental students, practitioners, administrators, and policy makers have expressed positive feelings about evidence-based principles and a desire to learn more about them. This positive environment, along with advancements in science, should help facilitate evidence-based change in the future.

REFERENCES

1. Abt E: A new perspective . . . two steps back: integration of the evidence-based method in a general practice residency program, *J Evid Base Dent Pract* 1(1):3, 2001.
2. Abt E: Evidence-based teaching and learning in a post-graduate dental education program, *J Evid Base Dent Pract* 4(1):100, 2004.
3. Bader JD, Shugars DA: Understanding dentist's restorative treatment decisions, *J Public Health Dent* 52(2):102, 1992.
4. Bader JD, Shugars DA: Variation, treatment outcomes, and practice guidelines in dental practice, *J Dent Educ* 59(1):61, 1995.
5. Bader J, Ismail A, Clarkson J: Evidence-based dentistry and the dental research community, *J Dent Res* 78(9):1480, 1999.
6. Bero LA, Grilli R, Grimshaw JM, et al: Closing the gap between research and practice: an overview of systematic reviews of interventions to promote the implementation of research findings, *BMJ* 317:465, 1998.
7. Chapman G, Sonnenberg F: *Decision making in health care,* New York, 2000, Cambridge University Press.
8. Creugers NH, Kayser AF, Van't Hot MA: A meta-analysis of durability data on conventional fixed bridges, *Community Dent Oral Epidemiol* 22:448, 1994.
9. Creugers NH, Kreulen CM, Snoek PA, de Kanter RJ: A systematic review of single-tooth restorations supported by implants, *J Dent* 28:209, 2000.
10. Freeman AC, Sweeney K: Why general practitioners do not implement evidence: qualitative study, *BMJ* 323:1, 2001.
11. Haines A, Donald A: Making better use of research findings, *BMJ* 317:72, 1998.
12. Haynes B, Haines A: Barriers and bridges to evidence based clinic practice, *BMJ* 317:273, 1998.
13. Hunink M, Glaziou P: *Decision making in health and medicine,* New York, 2001, Cambridge University Press.
14. Newman MG: Improved clinical decision making using the evidence-based approach, *Ann Periodontol* 1:i, 1996.
15. Niederman R, Badovinac R: Tradition-based dental care and evidence-based dental care, *Dent Res* 78(7):1288, 1999.
16. Oxman AD, Thomson MA, Davis DA, Haynes RB: No magic bullets: a systematic review of 102 trials of interventions to improve professional practice, *Can Med Assoc J* 153(10):1423, 1995.
17. Rycroft-Malone J, Kitson A, Harvey G, et al: Ingredients for change: revisiting a conceptual framework, *Qual Health Care* 11:117, 2002.
18. Sackett DA, Strauss SE, Richardson WS, et al: *Evidence-based medicine: how to practice and teach EBM,* London, 2000, Churchill Livingstone.
19. Scurria MS, Bader JD, Shugars DA: Meta-analysis of fixed partial denture survival: prostheses and abutments, *J Prosthet Dent* 79:459, 1998.
20. Shugars DA, Bader JD, Alexander B, et al: Survival rates of teeth adjacent to treated and untreated posterior bounded edentulous spaces, *J Am Dent Assoc* 129:1089, 1998.
21. Shugars DA, Bader JD, Phillips SW, et al: The consequences of not replacing a missing posterior tooth, *J Am Dent Assoc* 131:1317, 2000.
22. Slavkin HC: The human genome: implications for oral health and diseases, and dental education, *J Dent Educ* 65(5):463, 2001.
23. Thomson-O'Brien M, Freemantle N, Oxman AD, et al: Continuing education meetings and workshops: effects on professional practice and health care outcomes, *Cochrane Library* 1:1, 2003 (Cochrane Review).
24. University of York: Effective health care: getting evidence into practice, NHS Centre for Reviews and Dissemination, 5(1):1, 1999.

The Normal Periodontium

Michael G. Newman

PART 2

The periodontium consists of the investing and supporting tissues of the tooth: gingiva, periodontal ligament, cementum, and alveolar bone. It has been divided into two parts: the *gingiva,* the main function of which is protecting the underlying tissues, and the *attachment apparatus,* composed of the periodontal ligament, cementum, and alveolar bone. The cementum is considered a part of the periodontium because, with the bone, it serves as the support for the fibers of the periodontal ligament.

The periodontium is subject to morphologic and functional variations as well as changes associated with age. This section deals with the normal features of the tissues of the periodontium, since this knowledge is necessary for an understanding of periodontal diseases.

The soft and hard tissues surrounding dental implants have many similar features and some important differences with the periodontal tissues, as discussed in Chapter 73.

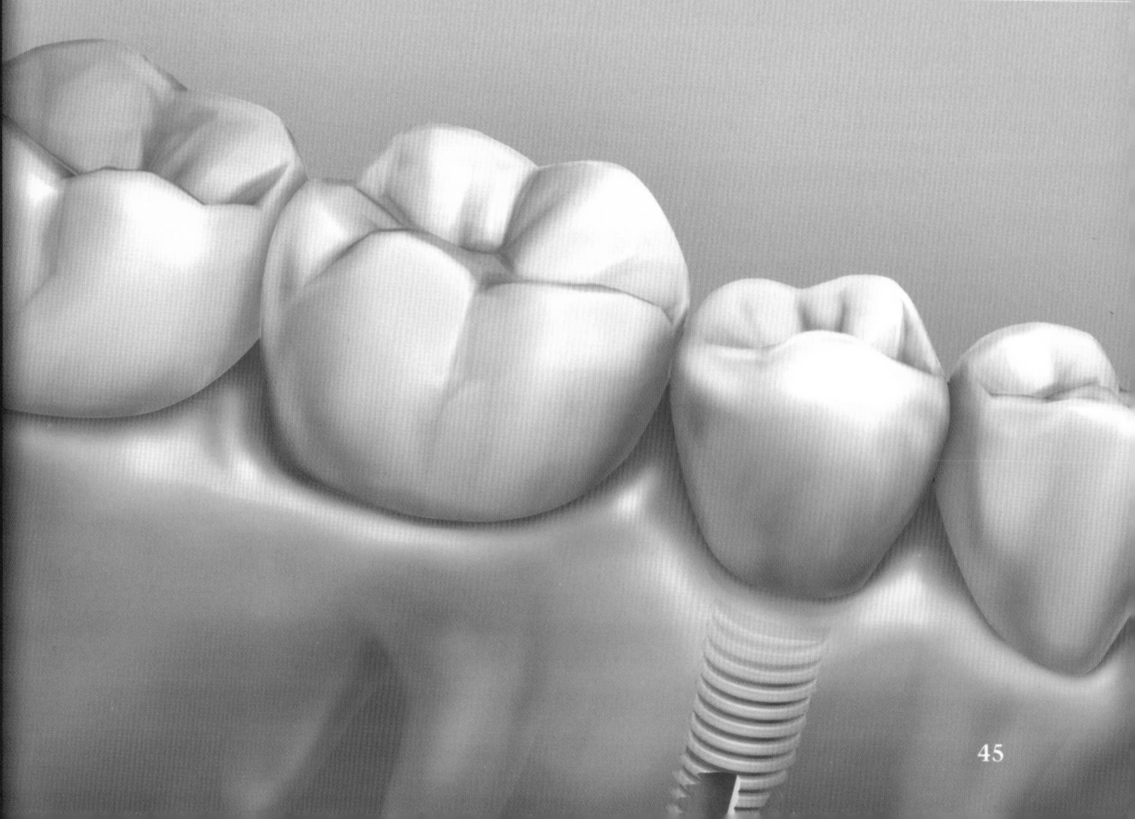

The Gingiva

Joseph P. Fiorellini, David M. Kim, and Satoshi O. Ishikawa

4

CHAPTER

CHAPTER OUTLINE

The *oral mucosa* consists of three zones:

1. The gingiva and the covering of the hard palate, termed the *masticatory mucosa*
2. The dorsum of the tongue, covered by *specialized mucosa*
3. The oral mucous membrane lining the remainder of the oral cavity. The *gingiva* is the part of the oral mucosa that covers the alveolar processes of the jaws and surrounds the necks of the teeth.

CLINICAL FEATURES

In an adult, normal gingiva covers the alveolar bone and tooth root to a level just coronal to the cementoenamel junction. The gingiva is divided anatomically into *marginal, attached,* and *interdental* areas. Although each type of gingiva exhibits considerable variation in differentiation, histology, and thickness according to its functional demands, all types are specifically structured to function appropriately against mechanical and microbial damage.[4] That is, the specific structure of different gingiva reflects its effectiveness as a barrier to the penetration by microbes and noxious agents into the deeper tissue.

Marginal Gingiva

The marginal, or *unattached,* gingiva is the terminal edge or border of the gingiva surrounding the teeth in collarlike fashion (Figures 4-1 and 4-2). In about 50% of cases, it is demarcated from the adjacent attached gingiva by a shallow linear depression, the *free gingival groove.*[3] Usually about 1 mm wide, the marginal gingiva forms the soft tissue wall of the gingival sulcus. It may be separated from the tooth surface with a periodontal probe.

Gingival Sulcus

The gingival sulcus is the shallow crevice or space around the tooth bounded by the surface of the tooth on one side and the epithelium lining the free margin of the gingiva on the other side. It is V shaped, and it barely permits the entrance of a periodontal probe. The clinical determination of the depth of the gingival sulcus is an important diagnostic parameter. Under absolutely normal or ideal conditions, the depth of the gingival sulcus is 0 mm or close to 0 mm.[49] These strict conditions of normalcy can be produced experimentally only in germ-free animals or after intense, prolonged plaque control.[8,23]

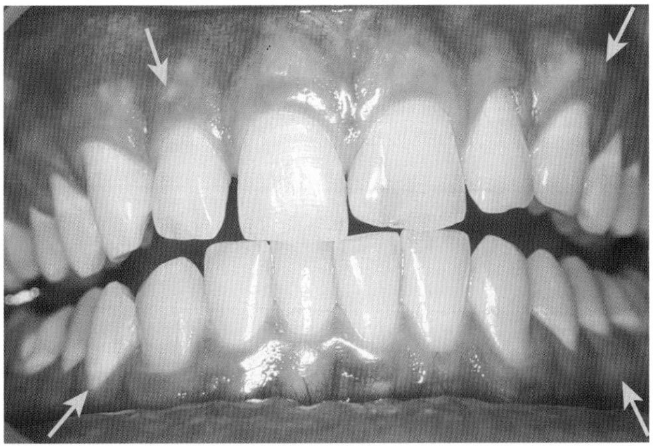

Figure 4-1 Normal gingiva in a young adult. Note the demarcation (mucogingival line) *(arrows)* between the attached gingiva and the darker alveolar mucosa.

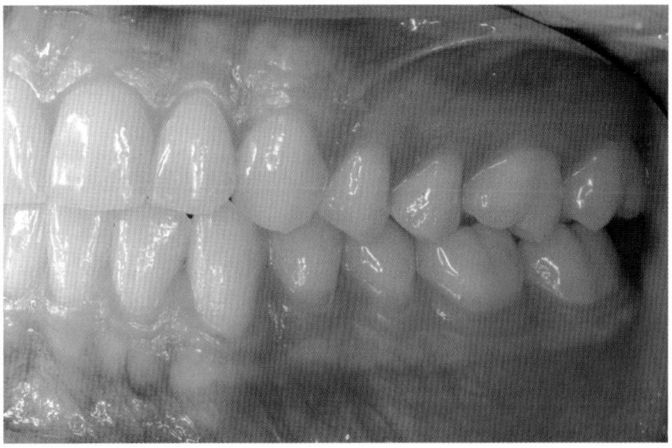

Figure 4-3 Mean width of attached gingiva in human permanent dentition.

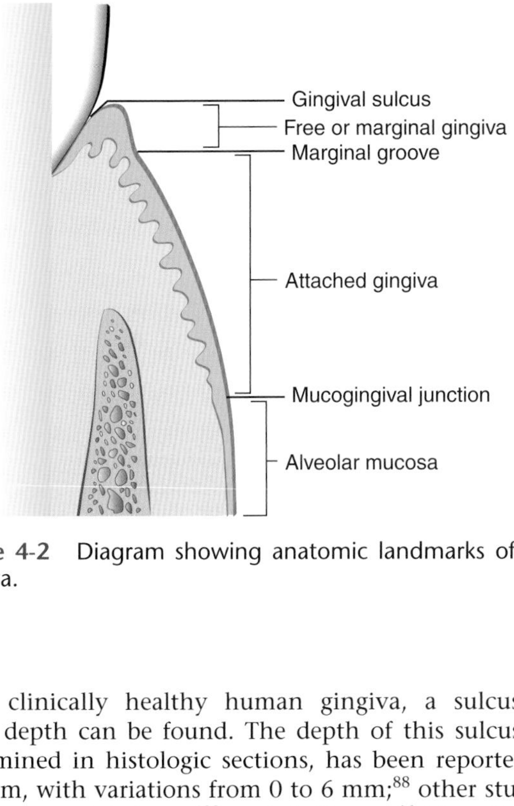

Figure 4-2 Diagram showing anatomic landmarks of the gingiva.

In clinically healthy human gingiva, a sulcus of some depth can be found. The depth of this sulcus, as determined in histologic sections, has been reported as 1.8 mm, with variations from 0 to 6 mm;[88] other studies have reported 1.5 mm[133] and 0.69 mm.[46] The clinical evaluation used to determine the depth of the sulcus involves the introduction of a metallic instrument, the periodontal probe, and the estimation of the distance it penetrates. The histologic depth of a sulcus does not need to be exactly equal to the depth of penetration of the probe. The so-called probing depth of a clinically normal gingival sulcus in humans is 2 to 3 mm (see Chapter 35).

Attached Gingiva

The attached gingiva is continuous with the marginal gingiva. It is firm, resilient, and tightly bound to the underlying periosteum of alveolar bone. The facial aspect of the attached gingiva extends to the relatively loose and movable alveolar mucosa and is demarcated by the *mucogingival junction* (see Figure 4-2).

The *width of the attached gingiva* is another important clinical parameter. It is the distance between the mucogingival junction and the projection on the external surface of the bottom of the gingival sulcus or the periodontal pocket. It should not be confused with the *width of the keratinized gingiva* because the latter also includes the marginal gingiva (see Figure 4-2).

The width of the attached gingiva on the facial aspect differs in different areas of the mouth.[16] It is generally greatest in the incisor region (3.5-4.5 mm in maxilla, 3.3-3.9 mm in mandible), and narrower in the posterior segments (1.9 mm in maxillary and 1.8 mm in mandibular first premolars)[3] (Figure 4-3).

Because the mucogingival junction remains stationary throughout adult life,[1] changes in the width of the attached gingiva are caused by modifications in the position of its coronal portion. The width of the attached gingiva increases with age[4] and in supraerupted teeth.[2] On the lingual aspect of the mandible, the attached gingiva terminates at the junction of the lingual alveolar mucosa, which is continuous with the mucous membrane lining the floor of the mouth. The palatal surface of the attached gingiva in the maxilla blends imperceptibly with the equally firm and resilient palatal mucosa.

Interdental Gingiva

The interdental gingiva occupies the gingival embrasure, which is the interproximal space beneath the area of tooth contact. The interdental gingiva can be pyramidal or can have a "col" shape. In the former the tip of one papilla is located immediately beneath the contact point; the latter presents a valleylike depression that connects a facial and lingual papilla and conforms to the shape of the interproximal contact[31] (Figures 4-4 and 4-5).

The shape of the gingiva in a given interdental space depends on the contact point between the two adjoining teeth and the presence or absence of some degree of

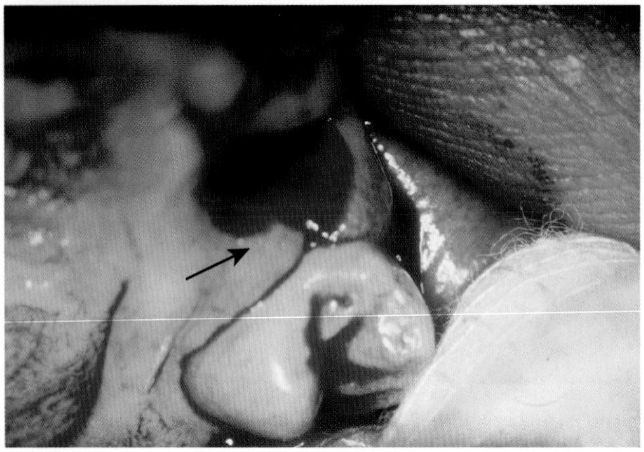

Figure 4-4 Site of extraction showing the facial and palatal interdental papillae and the intervening col *(arrow)*.

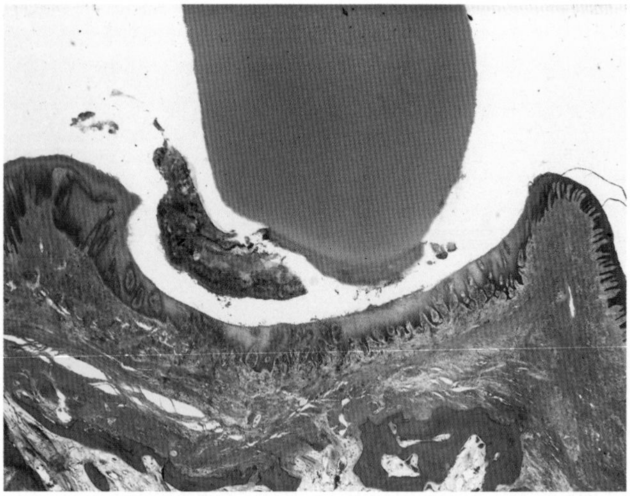

Figure 4-5 Faciolingual section (monkey) showing col between the facial and lingual interdental papillae. The col is covered with nonkeratinized stratified squamous epithelium.

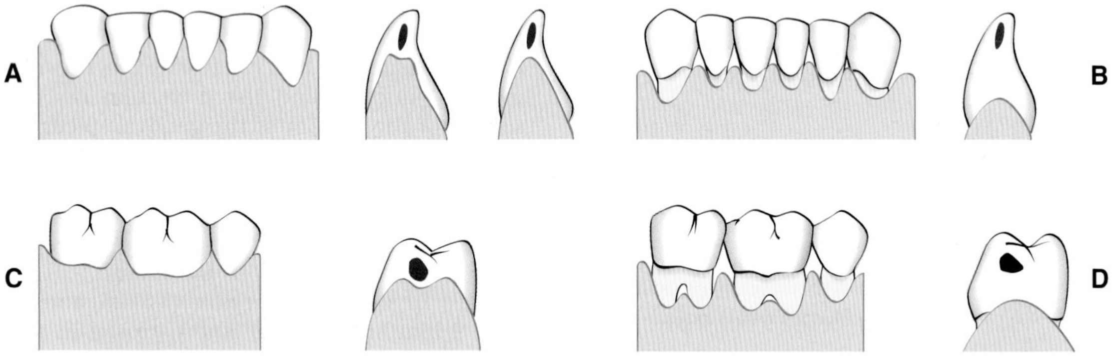

Figure 4-6 Diagram comparing anatomic variations of the interdental col in the normal gingiva *(left side)* and after gingival recession *(right side)*. **A** and **B,** Mandibular anterior segment, facial and buccolingual views, respectively. **C** and **D,** Mandibular posterior region, facial and buccolingual views, respectively. Tooth contact points are shown by black marks in lower individual teeth.

recession. Figure 4-6 depicts the variations in normal interdental gingiva.

The facial and lingual surfaces are tapered toward the interproximal contact area, whereas the mesial and distal surfaces are slightly concave. The lateral borders and tips of the interdental papillae are formed by the marginal gingiva of the adjoining teeth. The intervening portion consists of attached gingiva (Figure 4-7).

If a diastema is present, the gingiva is firmly bound over the interdental bone and forms a smooth, rounded surface without interdental papillae (Figure 4-8).

MICROSCOPIC FEATURES

Microscopic examination reveals that gingiva is composed of the overlying stratified squamous epithelium and the underlying central core of connective tissue. Although the epithelium is predominantly cellular in nature, the connective tissue is less cellular and composed primarily of collagen fibers and ground substance. These two tissues are considered separately.*

Gingival Epithelium

General Aspects of Gingival Epithelium Biology

Historically, the epithelial compartment was thought to provide only a physical barrier to infection and the underlying gingival attachment. However, we now believe that epithelial cells play an active role in innate host defense by responding to bacteria in an interactive manner.[33] That means the epithelium participates actively in responding to infection, in signaling further

*A detailed description of gingival histology can be found in Schroeder HE: *The periodontium,* New York, 1986, Springer-Verlag; and in Biological structure of the normal and diseased periodontium, *Periodontology 2000* 13, 1997.

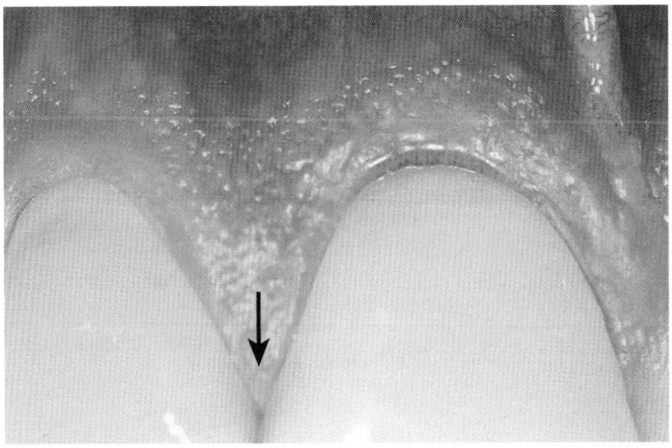

Figure 4-7 Interdental papillae *(arrow)* with central portion formed by attached gingiva. The shape of the papillae varies according to the dimension of the gingival embrasure. (Courtesy Dr. Osvaldo Costa.)

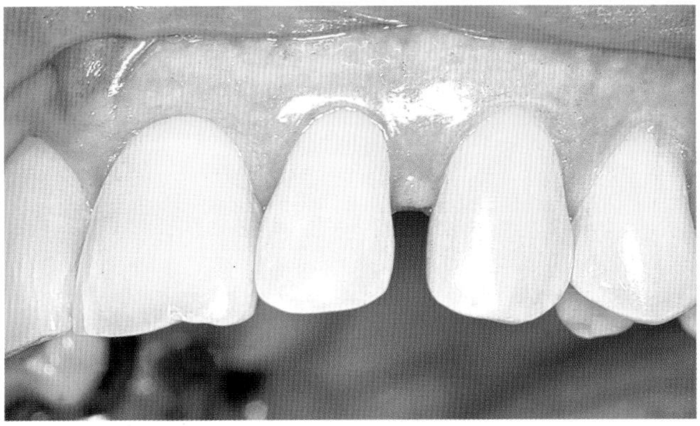

Figure 4-8 Absence of interdental papillae and col where proximal tooth contact is missing. (Courtesy Dr. Osvaldo Costa.)

host reactions, and in integrating innate and acquired immune responses. For example, epithelial cells may respond to bacteria by increased proliferation, alteration of cell-signaling events, changes in differentiation and cell death, and ultimately, alteration of tissue homeostasis.[33] To understand this new perspective of the epithelial innate defense responses and the role of epithelium in gingival health and disease, it is important to understand its basic structure and function (Box 4-1).

The gingival epithelium consists of a continuous lining of stratified squamous epithelium, and the three different areas can be defined from the morphologic and functional points of view: the oral or outer epithelium, sulcular epithelium, and junctional epithelium.

The principal cell type of the gingival epithelium, as well as of other stratified squamous epithelia, is the *keratinocyte*. Other cells found in the epithelium are the clear cells or nonkeratinocytes, which include the Langerhans cells, Merkel cells, and melanocytes.

The main function of the gingival epithelium is to protect the deep structures, while allowing a selective interchange with the oral environment. This is achieved by proliferation and differentiation of the keratinocytes.

BOX 4-1

Functions and Features of Gingival Epithelium

Functions
Mechanical, chemical, water, and microbial barrier
Signaling functions

Architectural Integrity
Cell-cell attachments
Basal lamina
Keratin cytoskeleton

Major Cell Type
Keratinocyte

Other Cell Types
Langerhans cells
Melanocytes, Merkel cells

Constant Renewal
Replacement of damaged cells

Cell-Cell Attachments
Desmosomes, adherens junctions
Tight junctions, gap junctions

Cell–Basal Lamina
Synthesis of basal lamina components
Hemidesmosome

Modified from Dale BA: *Periodontol 2000* 30:71, 2002.

Proliferation of keratinocytes takes place by mitosis in the basal layer and less frequently in the suprabasal layers, where a small proportion of cells remain as a proliferative compartment while a larger number begin to migrate to the surface.

Differentiation involves the process of keratinization, which consists of progressions of biochemical and morphologic events that occur in the cell as they migrate from the basal layer (Figure 4-9). The main morphologic changes are (1) progressive flattening of the cell with an increasing prevalence of tonofilaments, (2) intercellular junctions coupled to the production of keratohyaline granules, and (3) disappearance of the nucleus. (See Schroeder[103] for further details.)

A complete keratinization process leads to the production of an *orthokeratinized* superficial horny layer similar to that of the skin, with no nuclei in the stratum corneum and a well-defined stratum granulosum (Figure 4-10). Only some areas of the outer gingival epithelium are orthokeratinized; the other gingival areas are covered by parakeratinized or nonkeratinized epithelium,[20] considered to be at intermediate stages of keratinization. These areas can progress to maturity or dedifferentiate under different physiologic or pathologic conditions.

In *parakeratinized epithelia* the stratum corneum retains pyknotic nuclei, and the keratohyalin granules are dispersed, not giving rise to a stratum granulosum. The *nonkeratinized epithelium* (although cytokeratins

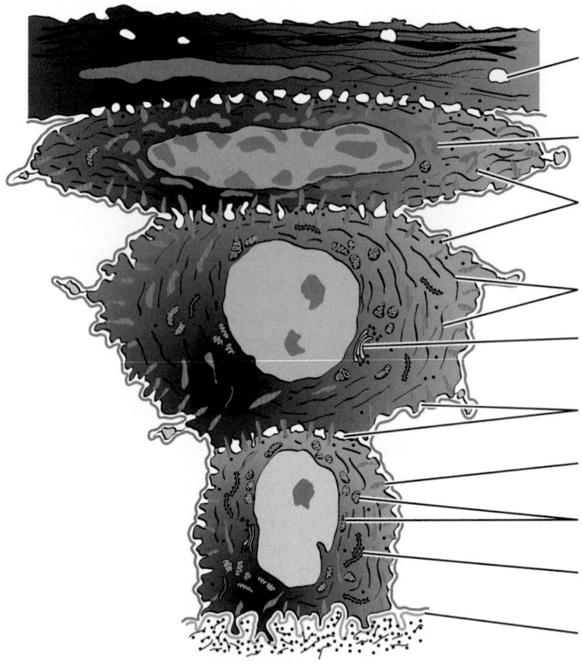

Figure 4-9 Diagram showing representative cells from the various layers of stratified squamous epithelium as seen by electron microscopy. (Modified from Weinstock A: In Ham AW: *Histology,* ed 7, Philadelphia, 1974, Lippincott.)

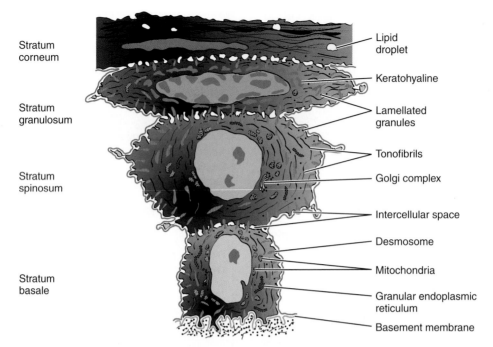

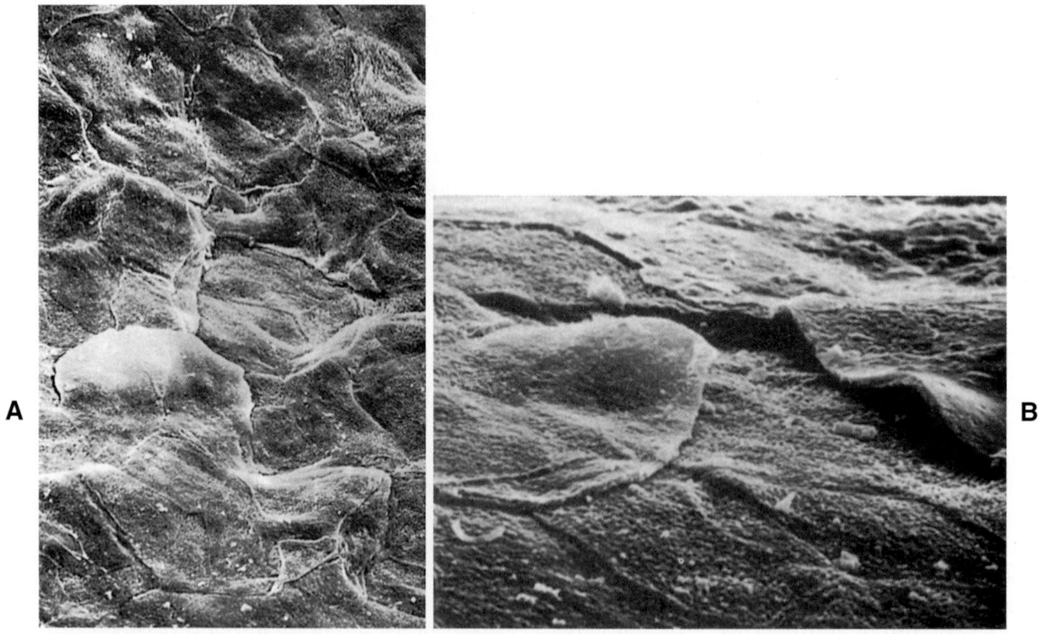

Figure 4-10 **A,** Scanning electron micrograph of keratinized gingiva showing the flattened keratinocytes and their boundaries on the surface of the gingiva (×1000). **B,** Scanning electron micrograph of gingival margin at edge of gingival sulcus showing several keratinocytes about to be exfoliated (×3000). (From Kaplan GB, Pameijer CH, Ruben MP: *J Periodontol* 48:446, 1977.)

are the major component, as in all epithelia) has neither granulosum nor corneum strata, whereas superficial cells have viable nuclei.

Immunohistochemistry, gel electrophoresis, and immunoblot techniques have made identification of the characteristic pattern of cytokeratins possible in each epithelial type. The keratin proteins are composed of different polypeptide subunits characterized by their isoelectric points and molecular weights. They are numbered in a sequence contrary to their molecular weight. Generally, basal cells begin synthesizing lower-molecular-weight keratins, such as K19 (40 kD), and express other higher-molecular-weight keratins as they migrate to the surface. K1 keratin polypeptide (68 kD) is the main component of the stratum corneum.[29]

Other proteins unrelated to keratins are synthesized during the maturation process. The most extensively studied are *keratolinin* and *involucrin,* which are precursors of a chemically resistant structure (the envelope) located below the cell membrane, and *filaggrin,* whose precursors are packed into the keratohyalin granules. In the sudden transition to the horny layer, the keratohyalin granules disappear and give rise to filaggrin, which forms the matrix of the most differentiated epithelial cell, the *corneocyte.*

Thus, in the fully differentiated state, the corneocytes are mainly formed by bundles of keratin tonofilaments embedded in an amorphous matrix of filaggrin and are surrounded by a resistant envelope under the cell membrane. The immunohistochemical patterns of the different keratin types, envelope proteins, and filaggrin change under normal or pathologic stimuli, modifying the keratinization process.[56-58]

Electron microscopy reveals that keratinocytes are interconnected by structures on the cell periphery called *desmosomes.*[69] These desmosomes have a typical structure consisting of two dense attachment plaques into which tonofibrils insert and an intermediate, electron-dense line in the extracellular compartment. Tonofilaments, which are the morphologic expression of the cytoskeleton of keratin proteins, radiate in brushlike fashion from the attachment plaques into the cytoplasm of the cells. The space between the cells shows cytoplasmic projections resembling microvilli that extend into the intercellular space and often interdigitate.

Less frequently observed forms of epithelial cell connections are tight junctions *(zonae occludens),* where the membranes of the adjoining cells are believed to be fused.[124,131] Evidence suggests that these structures allow ions and small molecules to pass from one cell to another.

Cytoplasmic organelle concentration varies among different epithelial strata. Mitochondria are more numerous in deeper strata and decrease toward the surface of the cell. Accordingly, histochemical demonstration of succinic dehydrogenase, nicotinamide-adenine dinucleotide, cytochrome oxidase, and other mitochondrial enzymes reveals a more active tricarboxylic cycle in basal and parabasal cells, where the proximity of the blood supply facilitates energy production through aerobic glycolysis.

Conversely, enzymes of the pentose shunt (an alternative pathway of glycolysis), such as glucose-6-phosphatase, increase their activity toward the surface. This pathway produces a larger amount of intermediate products for the production of ribonucleic acid (RNA), which in turn can be used for the synthesis of keratinization proteins. This histochemical pattern is in accordance with the increased volume and the amount of tonofilaments observed in cells reaching the surface; the intensity of the activity is proportional to the degree of differentiation.[35,42,55,91]

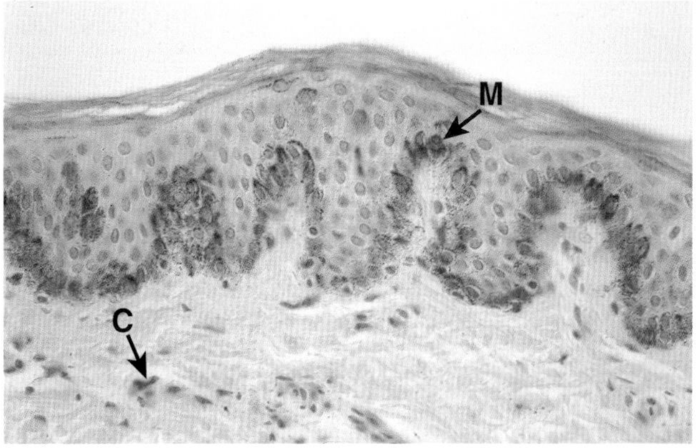

Figure 4-11 Pigmented gingiva of dog showing melanocytes *(M)* in the basal epithelial layer and melanophores *(C)* in the connective tissue (Glucksman technique).

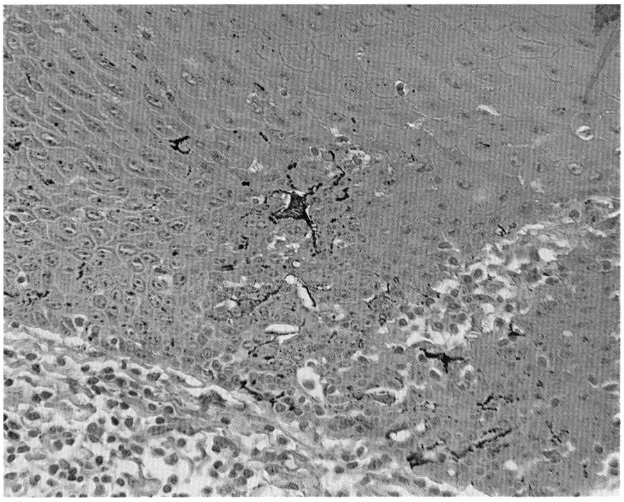

Figure 4-12 Human gingival epithelium, oral aspect. Immunoperoxidase technique showing Langerhans cells.

The uppermost cells of the stratum spinosum contain numerous dense granules, *keratinosomes* or *Odland bodies,* which are modified lysosomes. They contain a large amount of acid phosphatase, an enzyme involved in the destruction of organelle membranes, which occurs suddenly between the granulosum and corneum strata and during the intercellular cementation of cornified cells. Thus, acid phosphatase is another enzyme closely related to the degree of keratinization.[18,53,129]

Nonkeratinocyte cells are present in gingival epithelium as in other malpighian epithelia. *Melanocytes* are dendritic cells located in the basal and spinous layers of the gingival epithelium. They synthesize melanin in organelles called *premelanosomes* or *melanosomes*[30,100,117] (Figure 4-11). These contain tyrosinase, which hydroxylates tyrosine to dihydroxyphenylalanine (dopa), which in turn is progressively converted to melanin. Melanin granules are phagocytosed and contained within other cells of the epithelium and connective tissue called *melanophages* or *melanophores.*

Langerhans cells are dendritic cells located among keratinocytes at all suprabasal levels (Figure 4-12). They

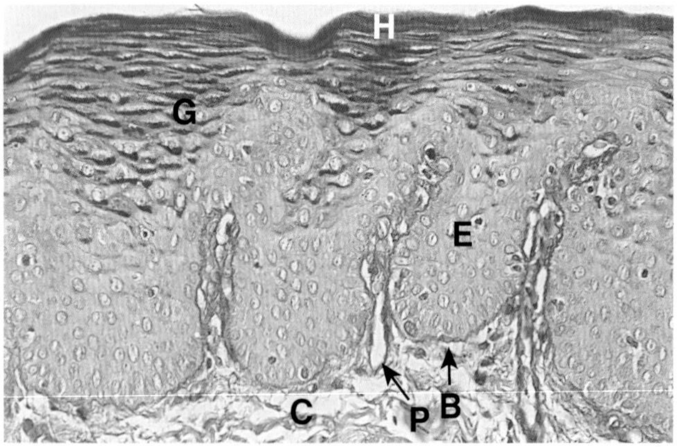

Figure 4-13 Normal human gingiva stained with the periodic acid–Schiff (PAS) histochemical method. The basement membrane *(B)* is seen between the epithelium *(E)* and the underlying connective tissue *(C)*. In the epithelium, glycoprotein material occurs in cells and cell membranes of the superficial hornified *(H)* and underlying granular layers *(G)*. The connective tissue presents a diffuse, amorphous ground substance and collagen fibers. The blood vessel walls stand out clearly in the papillary projections of the connective tissue *(P)*.

belong to the mononuclear phagocyte system (reticuloendothelial system) as modified monocytes derived from the bone marrow. They contain elongated granules and are considered macrophages with possible antigenic properties.[35] Langerhans cells have an important role in the immune reaction as antigen-presenting cells for lymphocytes. They contain g-specific granules (Birbeck's granules) and have marked adenosine triphosphatase activity. They are found in oral epithelium of normal gingiva and in smaller amounts in the sulcular epithelium; they are probably absent from the junctional epithelium of normal gingiva.

Merkel cells are located in the deeper layers of the epithelium, harbor nerve endings, and are connected to adjacent cells by desmosomes. They have been identified as tactile perceptors.[85]

The epithelium is joined to the underlying connective tissue by a *basal lamina* 300 to 400 Å thick, lying approximately 400 Å beneath the epithelial basal layer.[65,108,118] The basal lamina consists of lamina lucida and lamina densa. Hemidesmosomes of the basal epithelial cells abut the lamina lucida, which is mainly composed of the glycoprotein laminin. The lamina densa is composed of type IV collagen. The basal lamina, clearly distinguishable at the ultrastructural level, is connected to a reticular condensation of the underlying connective tissue fibrils (mainly collagen type IV) by the anchoring fibrils.[84,93,121] Anchoring fibrils have been measured at 750 nm in length from their epithelial end to their connective tissue end, where they appear to form loops around collagen fibers. The complex of basal lamina and fibrils is the periodic acid–Schiff (PAS)–positive and argyrophilic line observed at the optical level[110,122] (Figure 4-13). The basal lamina is permeable to fluids but acts as a barrier to particulate matter.

Structural and Metabolic Characteristics of Different Areas of Gingival Epithelium

The epithelial component of the gingiva shows regional morphologic variations that reflect tissue adaptation to the tooth and alveolar bone.[104] These variations include the oral epithelium, sulcular epithelium, and junctional epithelium. Whereas the oral epithelium and sulcular epithelium are largely protective in function, the junctional epithelium serves many more roles and is of considerable importance in regulating tissue health.[11] It is now recognized that epithelial cells are not "passive bystanders" in the gingival tissues; rather, they are metabolically active and capable of reacting to external stimuli by synthesizing a number of cytokines, adhesion molecules, growth factors, and enzymes.[11]

Oral (Outer) Epithelium. The oral, or outer, epithelium covers the crest and outer surface of the marginal gingiva and the surface of the attached gingiva. On average, the oral epithelium is 0.2 to 0.3 mm in thickness. It is keratinized or parakeratinized or presents various combinations of these conditions (Figure 4-14). The prevalent surface, however, is parakeratinized.[14,20,130]

The oral epithelium is composed of four layers: stratum basale (basal layer), stratum spinosum (prickle cell layer), stratum granulosum (granular layer), and stratum corneum (cornified layer).

The degree of gingival keratinization diminishes with age and the onset of menopause[90] but is not necessarily related to the different phases of the menstrual cycle.[59] Keratinization of the oral mucosa varies in different areas in the following order: palate (most keratinized), gingiva, ventral aspect of the tongue, and cheek (least keratinized).[82]

Keratins K1, K2, and K10 to K12, which are specific to epidermal-type differentiation, are immunohistochemically expressed with high intensity in orthokeratinized areas and with less intensity in parakeratinized areas. K6 and K16, characteristic of highly proliferative epithelia, and K5 and K14, stratification-specific cytokeratins, also are present. Parakeratinized areas express K19, which is usually absent from orthokeratinized normal epithelia.[15,98]

In keeping with the complete or almost-complete maturation, histoenzyme reactions for acid phosphatase and pentose-shunt enzymes are very strong.[19,55]

Glycogen can accumulate intracellularly when it is not completely degraded by any of the glycolytic pathways. Thus, its concentration in normal gingiva is inversely related to the degree of keratinization[109,130] and inflammation.[34,126,128]

Sulcular Epithelium. The sulcular epithelium lines the gingival sulcus (Figure 4-15). It is a thin, nonkeratinized stratified squamous epithelium without rete pegs, and it extends from the coronal limit of the junctional epithelium to the crest of the gingival margin (Figure 4-16). It usually shows many cells with hydropic degeneration.[14]

As with other nonkeratinized epithelia, the sulcular epithelium lacks granulosum and corneum strata and K1, K2, and K10 to K12 cytokeratins, but it contains K4 and K13, the so-called esophageal-type cytokeratins. It also expresses K19 and normally does not contain Merkel cells.

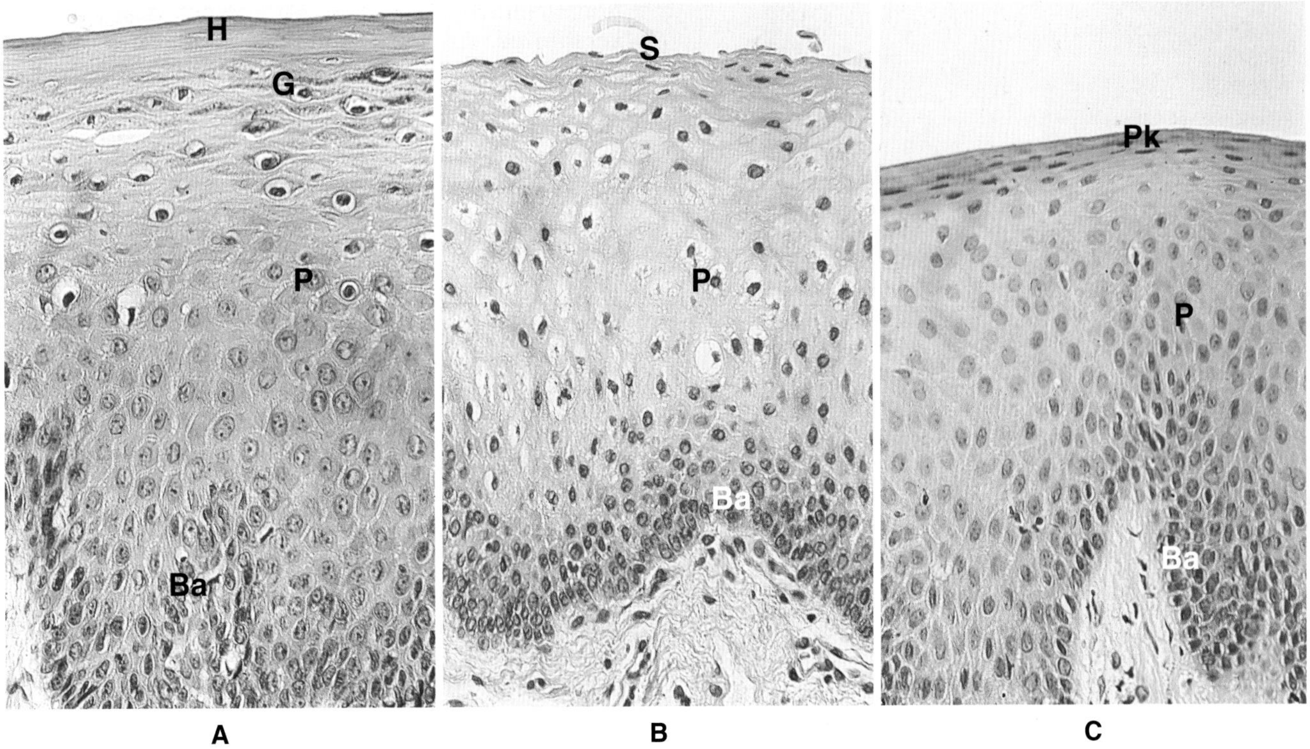

Figure 4-14 Variations in gingival epithelium. **A,** Keratinized. **B,** Nonkeratinized. **C,** Parakeratinized. Horny layer *(H)*, granular layer *(G)*, prickle cell layer *(P)*, basal cell layer *(Ba)*, flattened surface cells *(S)*, parakeratotic layer *(Pk)*.

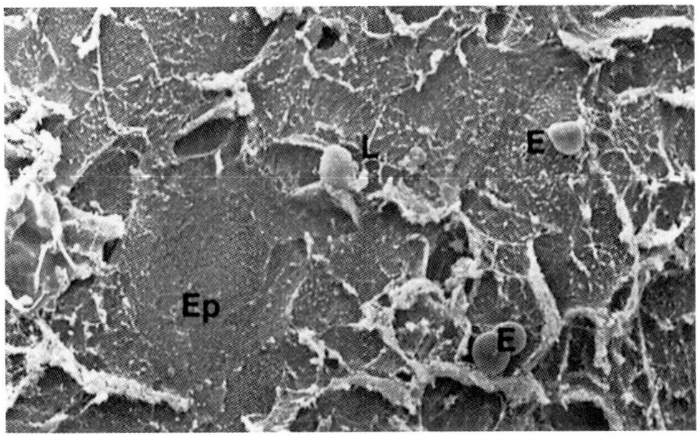

Figure 4-15 Scanning electron microscopic view of epithelial surface facing the tooth in a normal human gingival sulcus. The epithelium *(Ep)* shows desquamating cells, some scattered erythrocytes *(E)*, and a few emerging leukocytes *(L)*. (×1000.)

Histochemical studies of enzymes have consistently revealed a lower degree of activity in the sulcular than in the outer epithelium, particularly in the case of enzymes related to keratinization. Glucose-6-phosphate dehydrogenase expressed a faint and homogeneous reaction in all strata, unlike the increasing gradient toward the surface observed in cornified epithelia.[55] Acid phosphatase staining is negative,[18] although lysosomes have been described in exfoliated cells.[66]

Despite these morphologic and chemical characteristics, the sulcular epithelium has the potential to keratinize if (1) it is reflected and exposed to the oral cavity[17,21] or (2) the bacterial flora of the sulcus is totally eliminated.[22] Conversely, the outer epithelium loses its keratinization when it is placed in contact with the tooth.[22] These findings suggest that the local irritation of the sulcus prevents sulcular keratinization.

The sulcular epithelium is extremely important because it may act as a semipermeable membrane through which injurious bacterial products pass into the gingival and tissue fluid from the gingiva seeps into the sulcus.[123] Unlike the junctional epithelium, however, the sulcular epithelium is not heavily infiltrated by polymorphonuclear neutrophil leukocytes (PMNs), and it appears to be less permeable.[11]

Junctional Epithelium. The junctional epithelium consists of a collarlike band of stratified squamous nonkeratinizing epithelium. It is three to four layers thick in early life, but the number of layers increases with age to 10 or even 20 layers. Also, the junctional epithelium tapers from its coronal end, which may be 10 to 29 cells wide to one or two cells at its apical termination, located at the cementoenamel junction in healthy tissue. These cells can be grouped in two strata: the basal layer facing the connective tissue and the suprabasal layer extending to the tooth surface. The length of the junctional epithelium ranges from 0.25 to 1.35 mm.

The junctional epithelium is formed by the confluence of the oral epithelium and the reduced enamel epithelium

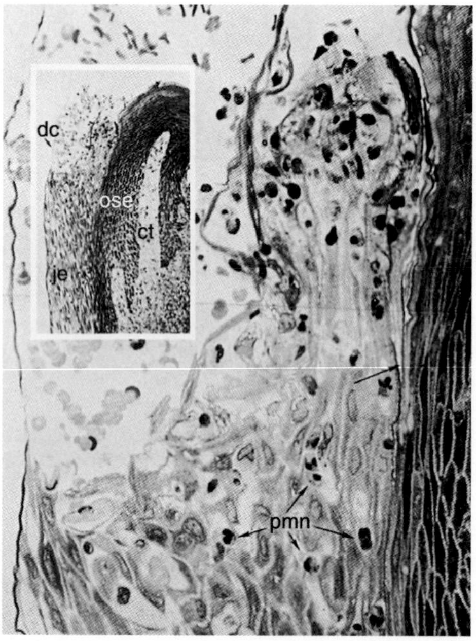

Figure 4-16 Epon-embedded human biopsy specimen showing a relatively normal gingival sulcus. The soft tissue wall of the gingival sulcus is made up of the oral sulcular epithelium *(ose)* and its underlying connective tissue *(ct)*, whereas the base of the gingival sulcus is formed by the sloughing surface of the junctional epithelium *(je)*. The enamel space is delineated by a dense cuticular structure *(dc)*. A relatively sharp line of demarcation exists between the junctional epithelium and the oral sulcular epithelium *(arrow)*, and several polymorphonuclear leukocytes *(pmn)* can be seen traversing the junctional epithelium. The sulcus contains red blood cells resulting from the hemorrhage occurring at the time of biopsy. (×391; inset ×55.) (From Schluger S, Youdelis R, Page RC: *Periodontal disease*, Philadelphia, 1977, Lea & Febiger.)

during tooth eruption (Figure 4-17). However, the reduced enamel epithelium is not essential for its formation; in fact, the junctional epithelium is completely restored after pocket instrumentation or surgery, and it forms around an implant.[68]

Cell layers not juxtaposed to the tooth exhibit numerous free ribosomes and prominent membrane-bound structures, such as Golgi complexes, and cytoplasmic vacuoles, presumably phagocytic. Lysosome-like bodies also are present, but the absence of keratinosomes (Odland bodies) and histochemically demonstrable acid phosphatase, correlated with the low degree of differentiation, may reflect a low defense power against microbial plaque accumulation in the gingival sulcus. Similar morphologic findings have been described in the gingiva of germ-free rats. PMNs are found routinely in the junctional epithelium of both conventional rats and germ-free rats.[134] Research has shown that although numerous migrating PMNs are evident and present around healthy junctional epithelium, a considerable increase in PMN numbers can be expected with the accumulation of dental plaque and gingival inflammation.[11]

The different keratin polypeptides of junctional epithelium have a particular histochemical pattern. Junctional epithelium expresses K19, which is absent from keratinized epithelia, and the stratification-specific cytokeratins K5 and K14.[98] Morgan et al.[83] reported that reactions to demonstrate K4 or K13 reveal a sudden change between sulcular and junctional epithelia, the junctional area being the only stratified nonkeratinized epithelium in the oral cavity that does not synthesize these specific polypeptides. Another particular behavior of junctional epithelium is the lack of expression of K6 and K16, which is usually linked to highly proliferative epithelia, although the turnover of the cells is very high.

Similar to sulcular epithelium, junctional epithelium exhibits lower glycolytic enzyme activity than outer epithelium, and it lacks acid phosphatase activity.[18,55]

The junctional epithelium is attached to the tooth surface (epithelial attachment) by means of an internal basal lamina. It is attached to the gingival connective tissue by an external basal lamina that has the same structure as other epithelial–connective tissue attachments elsewhere in the body.[70,75]

The internal basal lamina consists of a lamina densa (adjacent to the enamel) and a lamina lucida to which hemidesmosomes are attached. Hemidesmosomes have a decisive role in the firm attachment of the cells to the internal basal lamina on the tooth surface. Recent data suggest that the hemidesmosomes may also act as specific sites of signal transduction and thus may participate in regulation of gene expression, cell proliferation, and cell differentiation.[60] Organic strands from the enamel appear to extend into the lamina densa.[120] The junctional epithelium attaches to afibrillar cementum present on the crown (usually restricted to an area within 1 mm of the cementoenamel junction)[106] and root cementum in a similar manner.

Histochemical evidence for the presence of neutral polysaccharides in the zone of the epithelial attachment has been reported.[125] Data also have shown that the basal lamina of the junctional epithelium resembles that of endothelial and epithelial cells in its laminin content but differs in its internal basal lamina, which has no type IV collagen.[62,97] These findings indicate that the cells of the junctional epithelium are involved in the production of laminin and play a key role in the adhesion mechanism.

The attachment of the junctional epithelium to the tooth is reinforced by the gingival fibers, which brace the marginal gingiva against the tooth surface. For this reason, the junctional epithelium and the gingival fibers are considered a functional unit, referred to as the *dentogingival unit*.[72]

In conclusion, it is usually accepted that the junctional epithelium exhibits several unique structural and functional features that contribute to preventing pathogenic bacterial flora from colonizing the subgingival tooth surface.[92] First, junctional epithelium is firmly attached to the tooth surface, forming an epithelial barrier against plaque bacteria. Second, it allows access of gingival fluid, inflammatory cells, and components of the immunologic host defense to the gingival margin. Third, junctional epithelial cells exhibit rapid turnover, which contributes to the host-parasite equilibrium and rapid repair of damaged tissue. Also, some investigators indicate that the

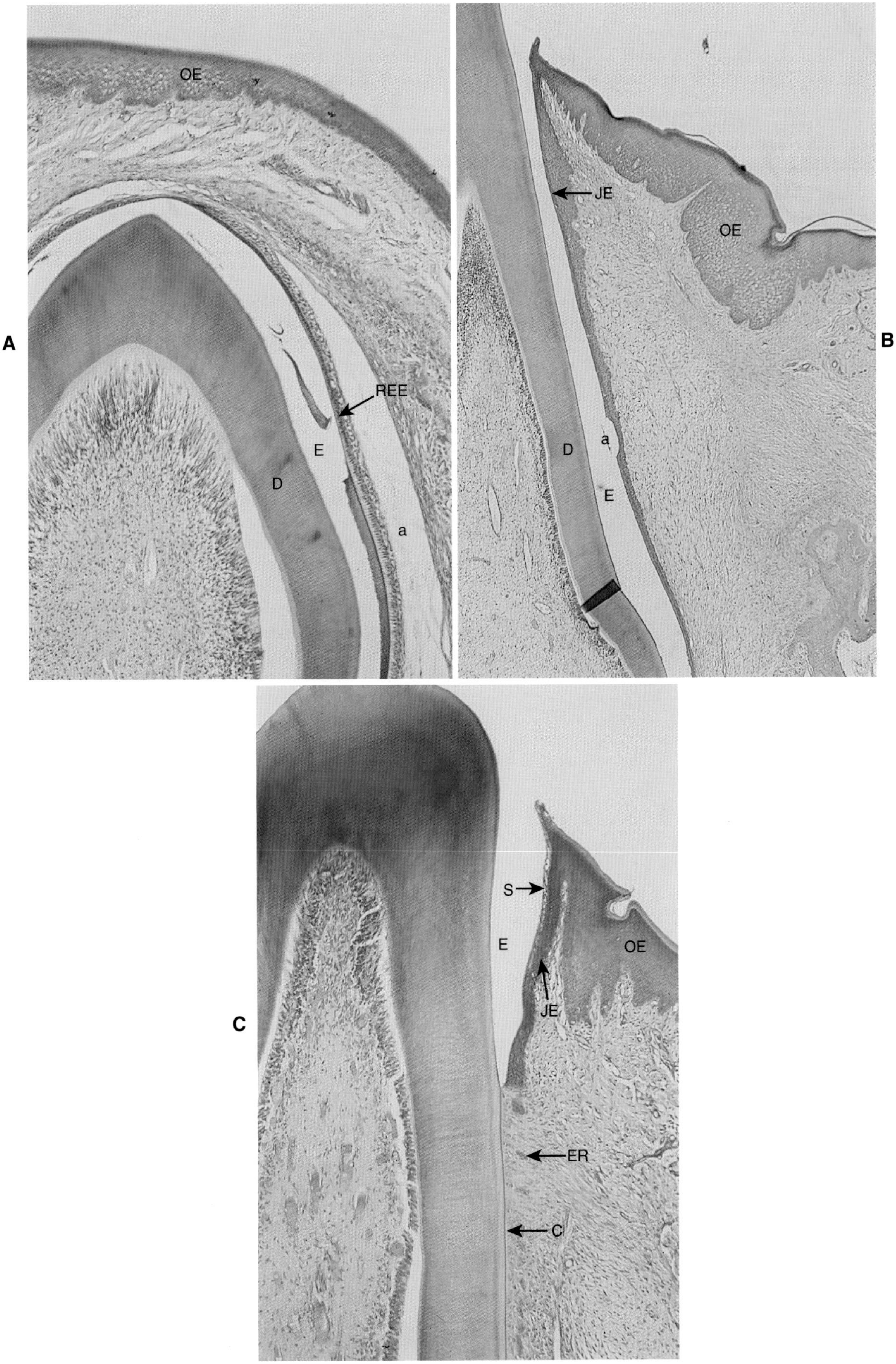

Figure 4-17 Eruption process in cat's tooth. **A,** Unerupted tooth. Dentin *(D)*, remnants of enamel matrix *(E)*, reduced enamel epithelium *(REE)*, oral epithelium *(OE)*, artifact *(a)*. **B,** Erupting tooth forming junctional epithelium *(JE)*. **C,** Completely erupted tooth. Sulcus with epithelial debris *(S)*, cementum *(C)*, and epithelial rests *(ER)*.

cells of the junctional epithelium have an endocytic capacity equal to that of macrophages and neutrophils, and that this activity might be protective in nature.[27]

Development of Gingival Sulcus

After enamel formation is complete, the enamel is covered with *reduced enamel epithelium* (REE), which is attached to the tooth by a basal lamina and hemidesmosomes.[71,119] When the tooth penetrates the oral mucosa, the REE unites with the oral epithelium and transforms into the junctional epithelium. As the tooth erupts, this united epithelium condenses along the crown, and the ameloblasts, which form the inner layer of the REE (see Figure 4-17), gradually become squamous epithelial cells. The transformation of the REE into a junctional epithelium proceeds in an apical direction without interrupting the attachment to the tooth. According to Schroeder and Listgarten,[106] this process takes between 1 and 2 years.

The junctional epithelium is a continually self-renewing structure, with mitotic activity occurring in all cell layers.[71,119] The regenerating epithelial cells move toward the tooth surface and along it in a coronal direction to the gingival sulcus, where they are shed[12] (Figure 4-18). The migrating daughter cells provide a continuous attachment to the tooth surface. The strength of the epithelial attachment to the tooth has not been measured.

The gingival sulcus is formed when the tooth erupts into the oral cavity. At that time, the junctional epithelium and REE form a broad band attached to the tooth surface from near the tip of the crown to the cementoenamel junction.

The gingival sulcus is the shallow, V-shaped space or groove between the tooth and gingiva that encircles the newly erupted tip of the crown. In the fully erupted tooth, only the junctional epithelium persists. *The sulcus consists of the shallow space that is coronal to the attachment of the junctional epithelium and bounded by the tooth on one side and the sulcular epithelium on the other. The coronal extent of the gingival sulcus is the gingival margin.*

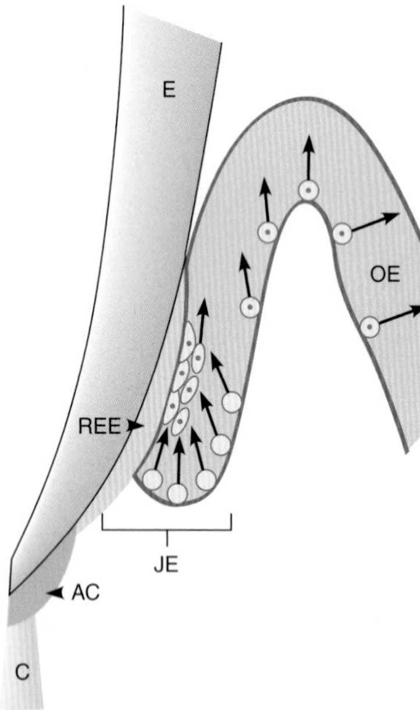

Figure 4-18 Junctional epithelium on an erupting tooth. The junctional epithelium *(JE)* is formed by the joining of the oral epithelium *(OE)* and the reduced enamel epithelium *(REE)*. *AC,* Afibrillar cementum, sometimes formed on enamel after degeneration of the REE. The arrows indicate the coronal movement of the regenerating epithelial cells, which multiply more rapidly in the JE than in the OE. *E,* Enamel; *C,* root cementum. A similar cell turnover pattern exists in the fully erupted tooth. (Modified from Listgarten MA: *J Can Dent Assoc* 36:70, 1970.)

Renewal of Gingival Epithelium

The oral epithelium undergoes continuous renewal. Its thickness is maintained by a balance between new cell formation in the basal and spinous layers and the shedding of old cells at the surface. The mitotic activity exhibits a 24-hour periodicity, with the highest and lowest rates occurring in the morning and evening, respectively.[120] The mitotic rate is higher in nonkeratinized areas and is increased in gingivitis, without significant gender differences. Opinions differ as to whether the mitotic rate is increased[74,75,81] or decreased[10] with age.

The mitotic rate in experimental animals varies among different areas of the oral epithelium in descending order: buccal mucosa, hard palate, sulcular epithelium, junctional epithelium, outer surface of the marginal gingiva, and attached gingiva.[6,51,74,127] The following have been reported as turnover times for different areas of the oral epithelium in experimental animals: palate, tongue, and cheek, 5 to 6 days; gingiva, 10 to 12 days, with the same or more time required with age; and junctional epithelium, 1 to 6 days.[12,116]

Regarding junctional epithelium, it was previously thought that only epithelial cells facing the external basal lamina were rapidly dividing. However, evidence indicates that a significant number of the cells, such as the basal cells along the connective tissue, are capable of synthesizing deoxyribonucleic acid (DNA), demonstrating their mitotic activity.[95,96] Rapid shedding of cells effectively removes bacteria adhering to the epithelial cells and therefore is an important part of the antimicrobial defense mechanisms at the dentogingival junction.[92]

Cuticular Structures on the Tooth

The term *cuticle* describes a thin, acellular structure with a homogeneous matrix, sometimes enclosed within clearly demarcated, linear borders.

Listgarten[73] has classified cuticular structures into coatings of developmental origin and acquired coatings. *Acquired coatings* include those of exogenous origin, such as saliva, bacteria, calculus, and surface stains (see Chapters 9 and 10). *Coatings of developmental origin* are those normally formed as part of tooth development. They include the REE, coronal cementum, and dental cuticle.

After enamel formation is completed, the ameloblastic epithelium is reduced to one or two layers of cells that remain attached to the enamel surface by hemidesmosomes and a basal lamina. This reduced enamel epithelium (REE) consists of postsecretory ameloblasts and cells from the stratum intermedium of the enamel organ.

In some animal species the REE disappears entirely and very rapidly, thereby placing the enamel surface in contact with the connective tissue. Connective tissue cells then deposit a thin layer of cementum known as *coronal cementum* on the enamel. In humans, thin patches of afibrillar cementum sometimes may be seen in the cervical half of the crown.

Electron microscopy has shown a *dental cuticle* consisting of a layer of homogeneous organic material of variable thickness (approximately 0.25 μm) overlying the enamel surface. It is nonmineralized and not always present. In some cases near the cementoenamel junction, it is deposited over a layer of afibrillar cementum, which in turn overlies enamel. The cuticle may be present between the junctional epithelium and the tooth. Ultrastructural histochemical studies have shown that the dental cuticle is proteinaceous,[63] and it may be an accumulation of tissue fluid components.[45,105]

Gingival Fluid (Sulcular Fluid)

The value of the gingival fluid is that it can be represented as either a transudate or an exudate. The gingival fluid contains a vast array of biochemical factors, offering potential use as a diagnostic or prognostic biomarker of the biologic state of the periodontium in health and disease.[41] The gingival fluid contains components of connective tissue, epithelium, inflammatory cells, serum, and microbial flora inhabiting the gingival margin or the sulcus (pocket).[40] In the healthy sulcus the amount of the gingival fluid is very small. During inflammation, however, the gingival fluid flow increases, and its composition start to resemble that of an inflammatory exudate.[28]

The main route of the gingival fluid diffusion is through the basement membrane, through the relatively wide intracellular spaces of the junctional epithelium, and then into the sulcus.[92]

The gingival fluid is believed to (1) cleanse material from the sulcus, (2) contain plasma proteins that may improve adhesion of the epithelium to the tooth, (3) possess antimicrobial properties, and (4) exert antibody activity to defend the gingiva (see Chapter 20).

Gingival Connective Tissue

The major components of the gingival connective tissue are collagen fibers (about 60% by volume), fibroblasts (5%), vessels, nerves, and matrix (about 35%).

The connective tissue of the gingiva is known as the *lamina propria* and consists of two layers: (1) a *papillary layer* subjacent to the epithelium, which consists of papillary projections between the epithelial rete pegs, and (2) a *reticular layer* contiguous with the periosteum of the alveolar bone. Connective tissue has a cellular and an extracellular compartment composed of fibers and ground substance. Thus the gingival connective tissue is largely a fibrous connective tissue that has elements originating directly from the oral mucosal connective tissue as well as some fibers (dentogingival) that originate from the developing dental follicle.[11]

The *ground substance* fills the space between fibers and cells, is amorphous, and has a high content of water. It is composed of proteoglycans, mainly hyaluronic acid and chondroitin sulfate, and glycoproteins, mainly fibronectin. Glycoproteins account for the faint PAS-positive reaction of the ground substance.[42] Fibronectin binds fibroblasts to the fibers and many other components of the intercellular matrix, helping mediate cell adhesion and migration. Laminin, another glycoprotein found in the basal lamina, serves to attach it to epithelial cells.

The three types of connective tissue fibers are collagen, reticular, and elastic. Collagen type I forms the bulk of the lamina propria and provides the tensile strength to the gingival tissue. Type IV collagen (argyrophilic reticulum fiber) branches between the collagen type I bundles and is continuous with fibers of the basement membrane and blood vessel walls.[75]

The elastic fiber system is composed of oxytalan, elaunin, and elastin fibers distributed among collagen fibers.[26]

Therefore, densely packed collagen bundles that are anchored into the acellular extrinsic fiber cementum just below the terminal point of the junctional epithelium form the connective tissue attachment. The stability of this attachment is a key factor in limiting the migration of junctional epithelium.[27]

Gingival Fibers

The connective tissue of the marginal gingiva is densely collagenous, containing a prominent system of collagen fiber bundles called the *gingival fibers.* They consist of type I collagen.[93] The gingival fibers have the following functions:

1. To brace the marginal gingiva firmly against the tooth.
2. To provide the rigidity necessary to withstand the forces of mastication without being deflected away from the tooth surface.
3. To unite the free marginal gingiva with the cementum of the root and the adjacent attached gingiva.

The gingival fibers are arranged in three groups: gingivodental, circular, and transseptal.[64]

Gingivodental Group. The gingivodental fibers are those on the facial, lingual, and interproximal surfaces. They are embedded in the cementum just beneath the epithelium at the base of the gingival sulcus. On the facial and lingual surfaces, they project from the cementum in fanlike conformation toward the crest and outer surface of the marginal gingiva, terminating short of the epithelium (Figures 4-19 and 4-20). They also extend externally to the periosteum of the facial and lingual alveolar bones, terminating in the attached gingiva or blending with the periosteum of the bone. Interproximally, the gingivodental fibers extend toward the crest of the interdental gingiva.

Circular Group. The circular fibers course through the connective tissue of the marginal and interdental gingivae and encircle the tooth in ringlike fashion.

Transseptal Group. Located interproximally, the transseptal fibers form horizontal bundles that extend between the cementum of approximating teeth into which they are embedded. They lie in the area between the epithelium at the base of the gingival sulcus and the

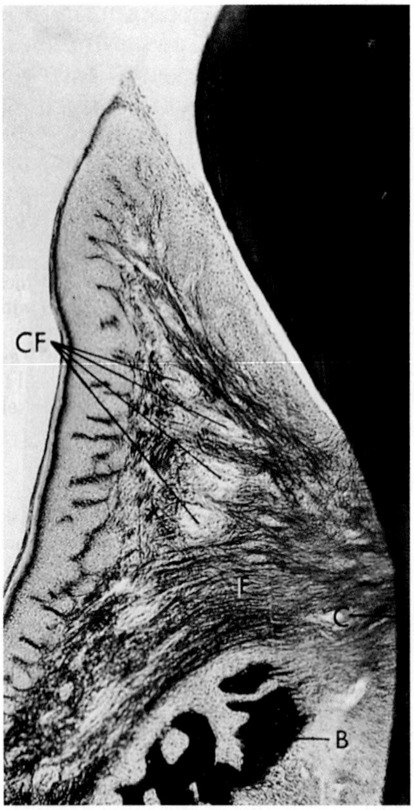

Figure 4-19 Faciolingual section of marginal gingiva showing gingival fibers *(F)* extending from the cementum *(C)* to the crest of the gingiva, to the outer gingival surface, and external to the periosteum of the bone *(B)*. Circular fibers *(CF)* are shown in cross section between the other groups. (Courtesy Sol Bernick.)

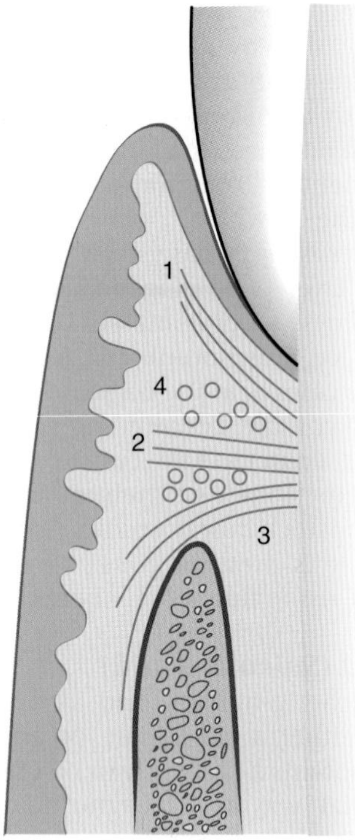

Figure 4-20 Diagram of the gingivodental fibers extending from the cementum *(1)* to the crest of the gingiva, *(2)* to the outer surface, and *(3)* external to the periosteum of the labial plate. Circular fibers *(4)* are shown in cross-section.

crest of the interdental bone and are sometimes classified with the principal fibers of the periodontal ligament.

Page et al.[89] also have described (1) a group of *semicircular fibers* that attach at the proximal surface of a tooth, immediately below the cementoenamel junction, go around the facial or lingual marginal gingiva of the tooth, and attach on the other proximal surface of the same tooth, and (2) a group of *transgingival fibers* that attach in the proximal surface of one tooth, traverse the interdental space diagonally, go around the facial or lingual surface of the adjacent tooth, again traverse diagonally the interdental space, and attach in the proximal surface of the next tooth.

Tractional forces in the extracellular matrix produced by fibroblasts are believed to be the forces responsible for generating tension in the collagen. This keeps the teeth tightly bound to each other and to the alveolar bone.

Cellular Elements

The preponderant cellular element in the gingival connective tissue is the *fibroblast.* Numerous fibroblasts are found between the fiber bundles. Fibroblasts are of mesenchymal origin and play a major role in the development, maintenance, and repair of gingival connective tissue. As with connective tissue elsewhere in the body, fibroblasts synthesize collagen and elastic fibers, as well as the glycoproteins and glycosaminoglycans of the amorphous intercellular substance. Fibroblasts also regulate collagen degradation through phagocytosis and secretion of collagenases.

Fibroblast heterogeneity is now a well-established feature of fibroblasts in the periodontium.[99] Although the biologic and clinical significance of such heterogeneity is not year clear, it seems that this is necessary for the normal functioning of tissues in health, disease, and repair.[11]

Mast cells, which are distributed throughout the body, are numerous in the connective tissue of the oral mucosa and the gingiva.[24,114,115,132] *Fixed macrophages* and *histiocytes* are present in the gingival connective tissue as components of the mononuclear phagocyte system (reticuloendothelial system) and are derived from blood monocytes. *Adipose cells* and *eosinophils,* although scarce, also are present in the lamina propria.

In clinically normal gingiva, small foci of plasma cells and lymphocytes are found in the connective tissue near the base of the sulcus (Figure 4-21). Neutrophils can be seen in relatively high numbers in both the gingival connective tissue and the sulcus. These inflammatory cells usually are present in small amounts in clinically normal gingiva.

Speculations about whether small amounts of leukocytes should be considered a normal component of the gingiva or an incipient inflammatory infiltrate without clinical expression are of theoretic rather than practical importance. Lymphocytes are absent when gingival normalcy is judged by strict clinical criteria or under

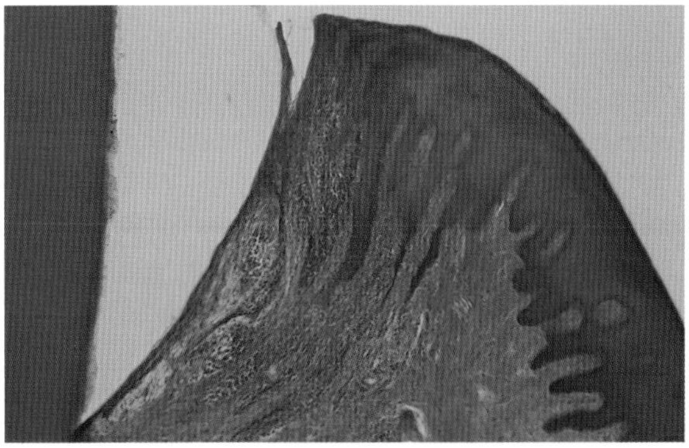

Figure 4-21 Section of clinically normal gingiva showing some degree of inflammation, which is almost always present near the base of the sulcus.

special experimental conditions,[8,87] but they are practically constant in healthy, normal gingiva, even before the complete tooth eruption.[67,77,102] Immunohistochemical studies using monoclonal antibodies have identified the different lymphocyte subpopulations. The infiltrate in the area below the junctional epithelium of healthy gingiva in newly erupted teeth in children is mainly composed of T lymphocytes (helper, cytotoxic, suppressor, and natural killer)[7,47,113] and thus could be interpreted as a normal lymphoid tissue involved in the early defense recognition system. As time elapses, B lymphocytes and plasma cells appear in greater proportions to elaborate specific antibodies against already-recognized antigens that are always present in the sulcus of clinically normal gingiva.[107]

Repair of Gingival Connective Tissue

Because of the high turnover rate, the connective tissue of the gingiva has remarkably good healing and regenerative capacity. Indeed, it may be one of the best healing tissues in the body and generally shows little evidence of scarring after surgical procedures. This is likely caused by rapid reconstruction of the fibrous architecture of the tissues.[80] However, the reparative capacity of gingival connective tissue is not as great as that of the periodontal ligament or the epithelial tissue.

Blood Supply, Lymphatics, and Nerves

Microcirculatory tracts, blood vessels, and lymphatic vessels play an important role in drainage of tissue fluid and in the spread of inflammation. In gingivitis and periodontitis, the microcirculation and vascular formation change greatly in the vascular network directly under the gingival sulcular epithelium and junctional epithelium.[79]

Blood vessels are easily evidenced in tissue sections by means of immunohistochemical reactions against proteins of endothelial cells (factor VIII and adhesion molecules). Before these techniques were developed, vascularization patterns of periodontal tissues had been described using histoenzymatic reactions for alkaline phosphatase and adenosine triphosphatase because of the great activity of these enzymes in endothelial cells.[25,135] In experimental animals the perfusion with India ink also was used to study vascular distribution. The injection and subsequent demonstration of peroxidase allow blood vessel identification and permeability studies.[112] The PAS reaction also outlines vascular walls by a positive line in their basal membrane.[110] Endothelial cells express 5-nucleotidase activity as well.[54] Scanning electron microscopy can be used after injection of plastic into the vessels through the carotid artery, followed by corrosion of the soft tissues.[43] In addition, laser Doppler

SCIENCE TRANSFER

The teeth are one of the few structures that penetrate the integument; that is, they go from inside the body to outside the body. As such, the gingival epithelium and connective tissue serve as a unique barrier to oral challenges. In addition, the shapes of the teeth are functionally adapted, and therefore the barrier morphology is adapted to correlate with the tooth shape. For example, the contact area varies between the teeth, as does the col shape of the interdental gingiva. Perhaps most important (and likely underestimated) are the functional qualities of the gingival barrier. The epithelium alone is a complex organ system with exquisite immune functions. Furthermore, the gingival fluid and connective tissues are complex and uniquely adaptive in the face of changes, such as those associated with aging, disease, and trauma. Superimposed on these unique barrier and functional qualities is the consistent and predominantly successful response against persistent microbial challenge. The last response in this area is a complicated, intertwined system of tissue changes and cellular responses of the immune system.

The integrity of the dentogingival complex depends on having an intact epithelial covering, with junctional epithelium forming a seal in the gingival sulcus. This seal operates because of the function of the dense type I collagen gingival fibers, which provide the mass and tensile strength to hold the tissues in tight apposition to the neck of the tooth.

Dental procedures such as root planing, subgingival restorative procedures, and crown and bridge gingival retraction techniques all damage both the epithelium and the gingival connective tissue.

The oral sulcular epithelium and junctional epithelium have a great ability to replenish themselves in a short turnover time of 1 to 6 days, and fibroblasts can also produce new collagen fibers. It is essential that dental procedures be as atraumatic as possible so that sufficient volume of gingival collagen fibers are maintained to hold the healing gingiva close to the roots. This allows a new, intact epithelial lining of the gingival sulcus to be quickly reconstituted and thus heal without any loss of attachment.

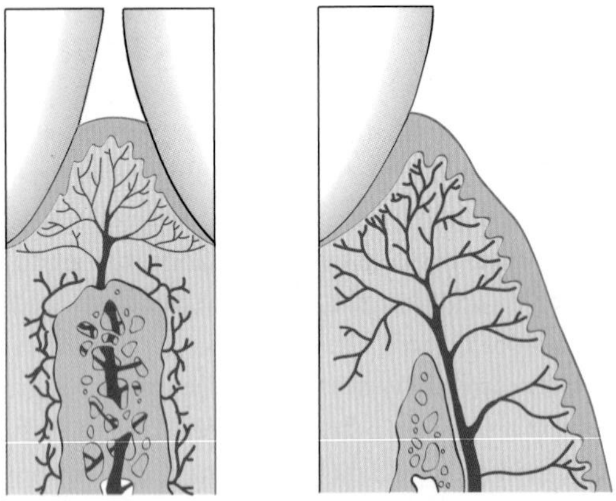

Figure 4-22 Diagram of arteriole penetrating the interdental alveolar bone to supply the interdental tissues *(left)* and a supraperiosteal arteriole overlying the facial alveolar bone, sending branches to the surrounding tissue *(right).*

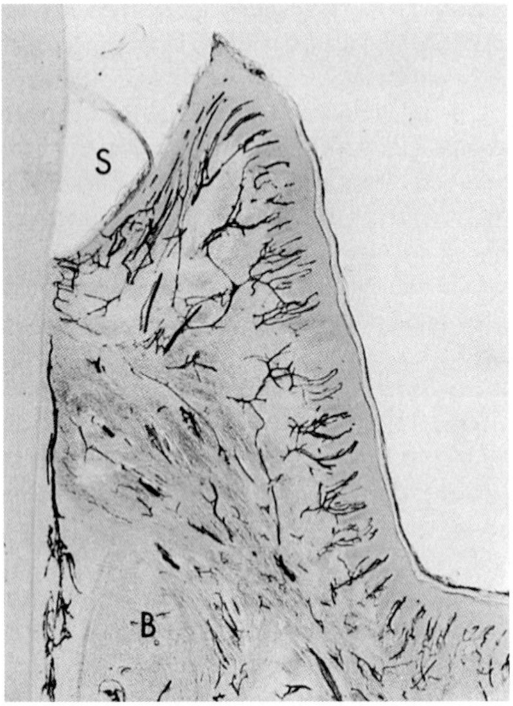

Figure 4-23 Blood supply and peripheral circulation of the gingiva. Tissues perfused with India ink. Note the capillary plexus parallel to the sulcus *(S)* and the capillary loops in the outer papillary layer. Note also the supraperiosteal vessels external to the bone *(B)*, which supply the gingiva, and a periodontal ligament vessel anastomosing with the sulcus plexus. (Courtesy Sol Bernick.)

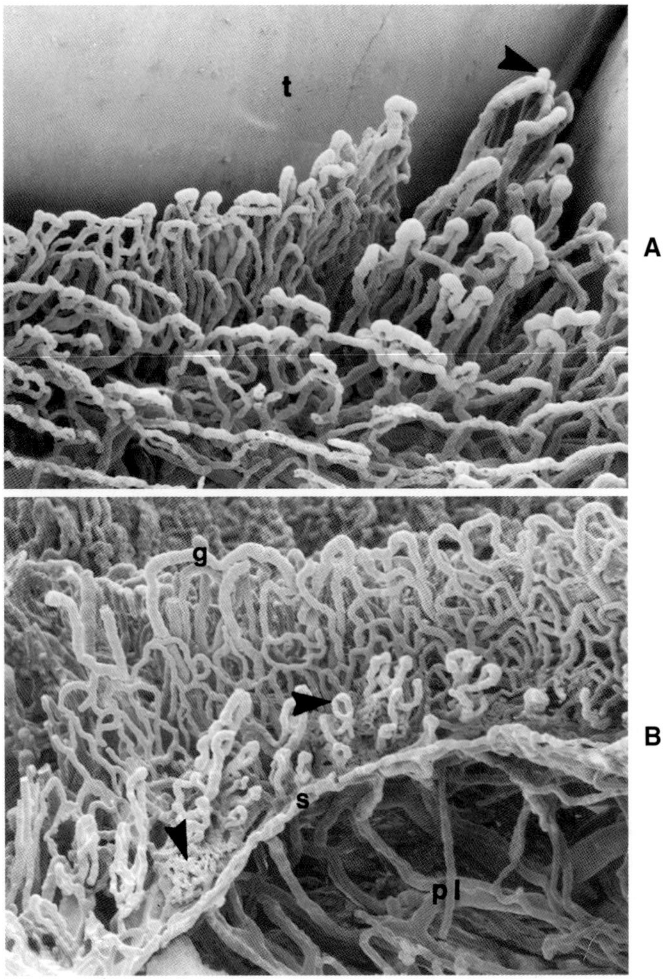

Figure 4-24 Scanning electron microscopic view of gingival tissues of rat molar palatal gingiva after vascular perfusion of plastic and corrosion of soft tissue. **A,** Oral view of gingival capillaries: *t,* tooth; interdental papilla *(arrowhead)* (×180). **B,** View from the tooth side. Note the vessels of the plexus next to the sulcular and junctional epithelium. The arrowheads point to vessels in sulcus area with mild inflammatory changes. *g,* Crest of marginal gingiva; *s,* bottom of gingival sulcus; *pl,* periodontal ligament vessels. (×150.) (Courtesy NJ Selliseth and K Selvig, University of Bergen, Norway.)

flow measurement provides a noninvasive means to observe blood flow modifications related to disease.[5]

Three sources of blood supply to the gingiva are as follows (Figures 4-22 and 4-23):

1. *Supraperiosteal arterioles* along the facial and lingual surfaces of the alveolar bone, from which capillaries extend along the sulcular epithelium and between the rete pegs of the external gingival surface.[38,52] Occasional branches of the arterioles pass through the alveolar bone to the periodontal ligament or run over the crest of the alveolar bone.
2. *Vessels of the periodontal ligament,* which extend into the gingiva and anastomose with capillaries in the sulcus area.
3. *Arterioles,* which emerge from the crest of the interdental septa[43] and extend parallel to the crest of the bone to anastomose with vessels of the periodontal ligament, with capillaries in the gingival crevicular areas and vessels that run over the alveolar crest.

Beneath the epithelium on the outer gingival surface, capillaries extend into the papillary connective tissue between the epithelial rete pegs in the form of terminal hairpin loops with efferent and afferent branches, spirals, and varices[25,52] (Figures 4-23 and 4-24). The loops are sometimes linked by cross-communications,[44] and flattened capillaries serve as reserve vessels when the circulation is increased in response to irritation.[48]

Along the sulcular epithelium, capillaries are arranged in a flat, anastomosing plexus that extends parallel to the enamel from the base of the sulcus to the gingival margin.[25] In the col area, a mixed pattern of anastomosing capillaries and loops occurs.

As mentioned, anatomic and histologic changes have been shown to occur in the gingival microcirculation with gingivitis. Prospective studies of the gingival vasculature in animals have demonstrated that in the absence of inflammation, the vascular network is arranged in a regular, repetitive, and layered pattern.[25,94] In contrast, the inflamed gingival vasculature exhibits an irregular vascular plexus pattern, with the microvessels exhibiting a looped, dilated, and convoluted appearance.[94]

The role of the lymphatic system in removing excess fluids, cellular and protein debris, microorganisms, and other elements is important in controlling diffusion and the resolution of inflammatory processes.[78] The *lymphatic drainage of the gingiva* brings in the lymphatics of the connective tissue papillae.[111] It progresses into the collecting network external to the periosteum of the alveolar process, then to the regional lymph nodes, particularly the submaxillary group. In addition, lymphatics just beneath the junctional epithelium extend into the periodontal ligament and accompany the blood vessels.

Neural elements are extensively distributed throughout the gingival tissues. Within the gingival connective tissues, most nerve fibers are myelinated and are closely associated with the blood vessels.[76] *Gingival innervation* is derived from fibers arising from nerves in the periodontal ligament and from the labial, buccal, and palatal nerves.[13] The following nerve structures are present in the connective tissue: a meshwork of terminal argyrophilic fibers, some of which extend into the epithelium; Meissner-type tactile corpuscles; Krause-type end bulbs, which are temperature receptors; and encapsulated spindles.[9]

CORRELATION OF CLINICAL AND MICROSCOPIC FEATURES

An understanding of the normal clinical features of the gingiva requires the ability to interpret them in terms of the microscopic structures they represent.

Color

The color of the attached and marginal gingiva is generally described as "coral pink" and is produced by the vascular supply, the thickness and degree of keratinization of the epithelium, and the presence of pigment-containing cells. The color varies among different persons and appears to be correlated with the cutaneous pigmentation. It is lighter in blond individuals with fair complexion than in swarthy, dark-haired individuals (Figure 4-25).

The attached gingiva is demarcated from the adjacent alveolar mucosa on the buccal aspect by a clearly defined mucogingival line. The alveolar mucosa is red, smooth, and shiny rather than pink and stippled. Comparison of the microscopic structure of the attached gingiva with that of the alveolar mucosa provides an explanation for the difference in appearance. The epithelium of the alveolar mucosa is thinner, is nonkeratinized, and contains no rete pegs (Figure 4-26). The connective tissue of the alveolar mucosa is loosely arranged, and the blood vessels are more numerous.

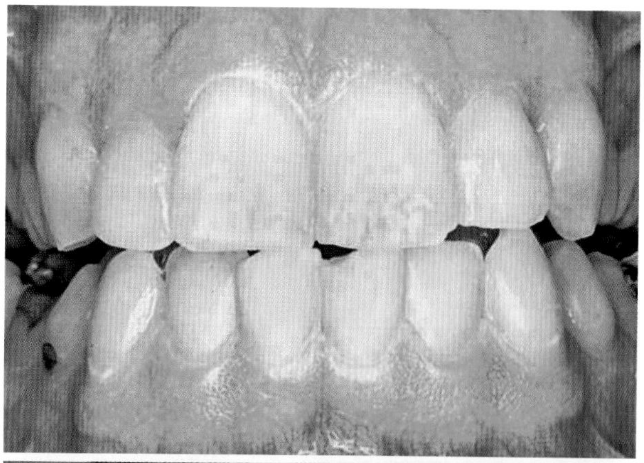
A

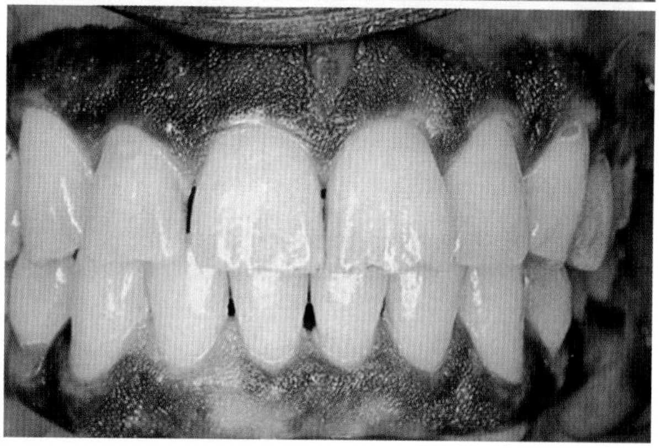
B

Figure 4-25 **A,** Clinically normal gingiva in a young adult. **B,** Heavily pigmented (melanotic) gingiva in a middle-aged adult. (From Glickman I, Smulow JB: *Periodontal disease: clinical, radiographic, and histopathologic features,* Philadelphia, 1974, Saunders.)

Physiologic Pigmentation (Melanin)

Melanin, a non–hemoglobin-derived brown pigment, is responsible for the normal pigmentation of the skin, gingiva, and remainder of the oral mucous membrane. It is present in all normal individuals, often not in sufficient quantities to be detected clinically, but is absent or severely diminished in albinos. Melanin pigmentation in the oral cavity is prominent in black individuals (see Figure 4-25).

According to Dummett,[36] the distribution of oral pigmentation in black individuals is as follows: gingiva, 60%; hard palate, 61%; mucous membrane, 22%; and tongue, 15%. Gingival pigmentation occurs as a diffuse, deep-purplish discoloration or as irregularly shaped, brown and light-brown patches. It may appear in the

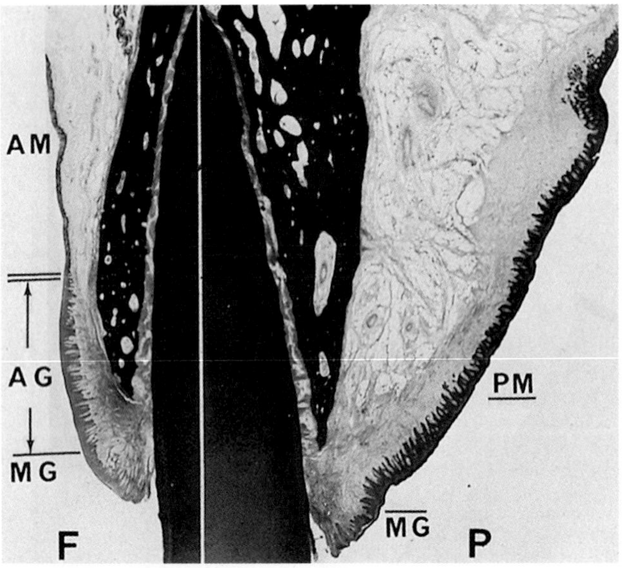

Figure 4-26 Oral mucosa, facial and palatal surfaces. The facial surface *(F)* shows the marginal gingiva *(MG)*, attached gingiva *(AG)*, and alveolar mucosa *(AM)*. The double line marks the mucogingival junction. Note the differences in the epithelium and connective tissue in the attached gingiva and alveolar mucosa. The palatal surface *(P)* shows the marginal gingiva *(MG)* and thick, keratinized palatal mucosa *(PM)*.

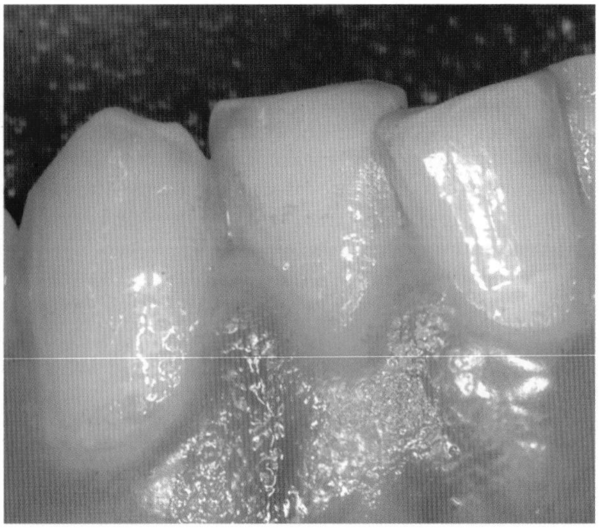

Figure 4-27 Thickened shelflike contour of gingiva on tooth in lingual version aggravated by local irritation caused by plaque accumulation.

gingiva as early as 3 hours after birth and often is the only evidence of pigmentation.[36]

Oral *repigmentation* refers to the clinical reappearance of melanin pigment after a period of clinical *depigmentation* of the oral mucosa resulting from chemical, thermal, surgical, pharmacologic, or idiopathic factors.[37] Information on the repigmentation of oral tissues after surgical procedures is extremely limited, and no definitive treatment is offered at this time.

Size

The size of the gingiva corresponds with the sum total of the bulk of cellular and intercellular elements and their vascular supply. Alteration in size is a common feature of gingival disease.

Contour

The contour or shape of the gingiva varies considerably and depends on the shape of the teeth and their alignment in the arch, the location and size of the area of proximal contact, and the dimensions of the facial and lingual gingival embrasures. The marginal gingiva envelops the teeth in collarlike fashion and follows a scalloped outline on the facial and lingual surfaces. It forms a straight line along teeth with relatively flat surfaces. On teeth with pronounced mesiodistal convexity (e.g., maxillary canines) or teeth in labial version, the normal arcuate contour is accentuated, and the gingiva is located farther apically. On teeth in lingual version, the gingiva is horizontal and thickened (Figure 4-27).

Shape

The shape of the interdental gingiva is governed by the contour of the proximal tooth surfaces and the location and shape of gingival embrasures. When the proximal surfaces of the crowns are relatively flat faciolingually, the roots are close together, the interdental bone is thin mesiodistally, and the gingival embrasures and interdental gingiva are narrow mesiodistally. Conversely, with proximal surfaces that flare away from the area of contact, the mesiodistal diameter of the interdental gingiva is broad (Figure 4-28). The height of the interdental gingiva varies with the location of the proximal contact. Thus, in the anterior region of the dentition, the interdental papilla is pyramidal in form, whereas the papilla is more flattened in a buccolingual direction in the molar region.

Consistency

The gingiva is firm and resilient and, with the exception of the movable free margin, tightly bound to the underlying bone. The collagenous nature of the lamina propria and its contiguity with the mucoperiosteum of the alveolar bone determine the firmness of the attached gingiva. The gingival fibers contribute to the firmness of the gingival margin.

Surface Texture

The gingiva presents a textured surface similar to an orange peel and is referred to as being *stippled* (see Figure 4-25). Stippling is best viewed by drying the gingiva. *The attached gingiva is stippled; the marginal gingiva is not.* The central portion of the interdental papillae is usually stippled, but the marginal borders are smooth. The pattern and extent of stippling vary among individuals and different areas of the same mouth.[50,94] Stippling is

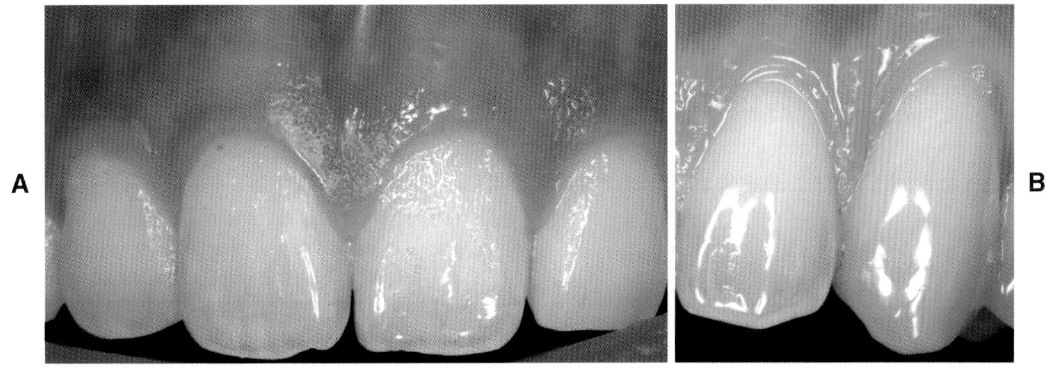

Figure 4-28 Shape of interdental gingival papillae correlated with shape of teeth and embrasures. **A,** Broad interdental papillae. **B,** Narrow interdental papillae.

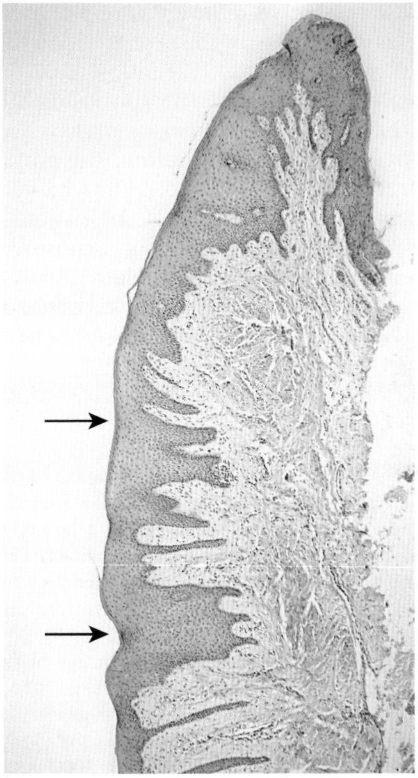

Figure 4-29 Gingival biopsy of patient shown in Figure 4-7, demonstrating alternate elevations and depressions *(arrows)* in the attached gingiva responsible for stippled appearance.

less prominent on lingual than facial surfaces and may be absent in some persons.

Stippling varies with age. It is absent in infancy, appears in some children at about 5 years of age, increases until adulthood, and frequently begins to disappear in old age.

Microscopically, stippling is produced by alternate rounded protuberances and depressions in the gingival surface. The papillary layer of the connective tissue projects into the elevations, and the elevated and depressed areas are covered by stratified squamous epithelium (Figure 4-29). The degree of keratinization and the prominence of stippling appear to be related.

Scanning electron microscopy has shown considerable variation in shape, but a relatively constant depth of stippling. At low magnification, a rippled surface is seen, interrupted by irregular depressions 50 μm in diameter. At higher magnification, cell micropits are seen.[30]

Stippling is a form of adaptive specialization or reinforcement for function. It is a feature of healthy gingiva, and reduction or loss of stippling is a common sign of gingival disease. When the gingiva is restored to health after treatment, the stippled appearance returns.

The surface texture of the gingiva is also related to the presence and degree of epithelial keratinization. Keratinization is considered a protective adaptation to function. It increases when the gingiva is stimulated by toothbrushing. However, research on free gingival grafts (see Chapter 69) has shown that when connective tissue is transplanted from a keratinized area to a nonkeratinized area, it becomes covered by a keratinized epithelium.[61] This finding suggests a connective tissue–based genetic determination of the type of epithelial surface.

Position

The *position* of the gingiva refers to the level at which the gingival margin is attached to the tooth. When the tooth erupts into the oral cavity, the margin and sulcus are at the tip of the crown; as eruption progresses, they are seen closer to the root. During this eruption process, as described earlier, the junctional epithelium, oral epithelium, and reduced enamel epithelium undergo extensive alterations and remodeling while maintaining the shallow physiologic depth of the sulcus. Without this remodeling of the epithelia, an abnormal anatomic relationship between the gingiva and the tooth would result.

Continuous Tooth Eruption

According to the concept of continuous eruption,[49] eruption does not cease when teeth meet their functional antagonists but continues throughout life. Eruption consists of an active and a passive phase. *Active eruption* is the movement of the teeth in the direction of the occlusal

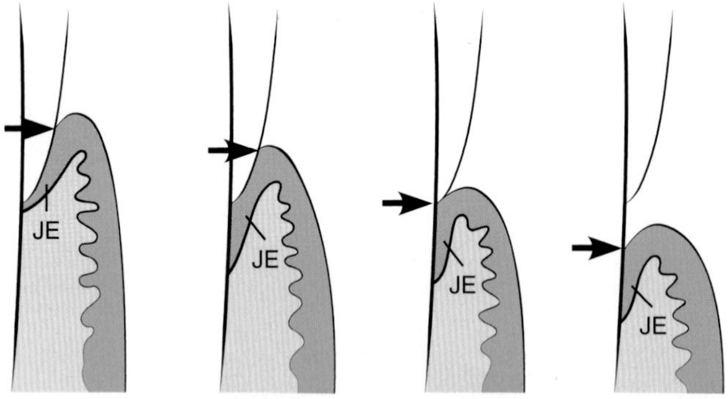

Figure 4-30 Diagrammatic representation of the four steps in passive eruption according to Gottlieb and Orban.[49] *1,* Base of the gingival sulcus *(arrow)* and the junctional epithelium *(JE)* are on the enamel. *2,* Base of the gingival sulcus *(arrow)* is on the enamel, and part of the junctional epithelium is on the root. *3,* Base of the gingival sulcus *(arrow)* is at the cementoenamel line, and the entire junctional epithelium is on the root. *4,* Base of the gingival sulcus *(arrow)* and the junctional epithelium are on the root.

plane, whereas *passive eruption* is the exposure of the teeth by apical migration of the gingiva.

This concept distinguishes between the *anatomic crown* (portion of the tooth covered by enamel) and the *anatomic root* (portion of the tooth covered by cementum) and between the *clinical crown* (part of the tooth that has been denuded of its gingiva and projects into the oral cavity) and *clinical root* (portion of the tooth covered by periodontal tissues). When the teeth reach their functional antagonists, the gingival sulcus and junctional epithelium are still on the enamel, and the clinical crown is approximately two thirds of the anatomic crown.

Gottlieb and Orban[49] believed that active and passive eruption proceed together. Active eruption is coordinated with attrition; the teeth erupt to compensate for tooth substance worn away by attrition. Attrition reduces the clinical crown and prevents it from becoming disproportionately long in relation to the clinical root, thus avoiding excessive leverage on the periodontal tissues. Ideally, the rate of active eruption keeps pace with tooth wear, preserving the vertical dimension of the dentition.

As teeth erupt, cementum is deposited at the apices and furcations of the roots, and bone is formed along the fundus of the alveolus and at the crest of the alveolar bone. In this way, part of the tooth substance lost by attrition is replaced by lengthening of the root, and socket depth is maintained to support the root.

Although originally thought to be a normal physiologic process, passive eruption is now considered a pathologic process. Passive eruption is divided into the following four stages (Figure 4-30):

Stage 1: The teeth reach the line of occlusion. The junctional epithelium and base of the gingival sulcus are on the enamel.

Stage 2: The junctional epithelium proliferates so that part is on the cementum and part is on the enamel. The base of the sulcus is still on the enamel.

Stage 3: The entire junctional epithelium is on the cementum, and the base of the sulcus is at the cementoenamel junction. As the junctional epithelium proliferates from the crown onto the root, it does not remain at the cementoenamel junction any longer than at any other area of the tooth.

Stage 4: The junctional epithelium has proliferated farther on the cementum. The base of the sulcus is on the cementum, a portion of which is exposed. Proliferation of the junctional epithelium onto the root is accompanied by degeneration of gingival and periodontal ligament fibers and their detachment from the tooth. The cause of this degeneration is not understood. At present, it is believed to be the result of chronic inflammation and therefore a pathologic process.

As noted, apposition of bone accompanies active eruption. The distance between the apical end of the junctional epithelium and the crest of the alveolus remains constant throughout continuous tooth eruption (1.07 mm).[46]

Exposure of the tooth by the apical migration of the gingiva is called *gingival recession,* or *atrophy.* According to the concept of continuous eruption, the gingival sulcus may be located on the crown, cementoenamel junction, or root, depending on the age of the patient and stage of eruption. Therefore, some root exposure with age would be considered normal and referred to as *physiologic recession.* Again, this concept is not accepted at present. Excessive exposure is termed *pathologic recession* (see Chapter 22).

REFERENCES

1. Ainamo A: Influence of age on the location of the maxillary mucogingival junction, *J Periodontal Res* 13:189, 1978.
2. Ainamo A, Ainamo J: The width of attached gingiva on supraerupted teeth, *J Periodontal Res* 13:194, 1978.
3. Ainamo J, Löe H: Anatomical characteristics of gingiva: a clinical and microscopic study of the free and attached gingiva, *J Periodontol* 37:5, 1966.
4. Ainamo J, Talari A: The increase with age of the width of attached gingiva, *J Periodontal Res* 11:182, 1976.
5. Ambrosini P, Cherene S, Miller N, et al: A laser Doppler study of gingiva blood flow variations following periosteal stimulation, *J Clin Periodontol* 29:103, 2002.
6. Anderson GS, Stern IB: The proliferation and migration of the attachment epithelium on the cemental surface of the rat incisor, *Periodontics* 4:15, 1966.
7. Armitt KL: Identification of T cell subsets in gingivitis in children, *Periodontology* 7:3, 1986.
8. Attstrom R, Graf-de Beer M, Schroeder HE: Clinical and histologic characteristics of normal gingiva in dogs, *J Periodontal Res* 10:115, 1975.
9. Avery JK, Rapp R: Pain conduction in human dental tissues, *Dent Clin North Am,* July 1959, p 489.
10. Barakat NJ, Toto PD, Choukas NC: Aging and cell renewal of oral epithelium, *J Periodontol* 40:599, 1969.
11. Bartold PM, Walsh LJ, Narayanan AS: Molecular and cell biology of the gingiva, *Periodontol 2000* 24:28, 2000.
12. Beagrie GS, Skougaard MR: Observations on the life cycle of the gingival epithelial cells of mice as revealed by autoradiography, *Acta Odontol Scand* 20:15, 1962.
13. Bernick S: Innervation of the teeth and periodontium, *Dent Clin North Am,* July 1959, p 503.

14. Biolcati EL, Carranza FA Jr, Cabrini RL: Variaciones y alteraciones de la queratinizacion en encias humanas clinicamente sanas, *Rev Asoc Odontol Argent* 41:446, 1953.
15. Bosch FX, Ouhayoun JP, Bader BL, et al: Extensive changes in cytokeratin expression patterns in pathologically affected human gingiva, *Virchows Arch B Cell Pathol* 58:59, 1989.
16. Bowers GM: A study of the width of the attached gingiva, *J Periodontol* 34:210, 1963.
17. Bral MM, Stahl SS: Keratinizing potential of human crevicular epithelium, *J Periodontol* 48:381, 1977.
18. Cabrini RL, Carranza FA Jr: Histochemical study on alkaline phosphatase in gingivae, varying the pH and the substrate, *J Dent Res* 30:28, 1951.
19. Cabrini RL, Carranza FA Jr: Histochemistry of periodontal tissues: a review of the literature, *Int Dent J* 16:466, 1966.
20. Cabrini R, Cabrini RL, Carranza FA Jr: Estudio histologico de la queratinizacion del epitelio gingival y de la adherencia epitelial, *Rev Asoc Odontol Argent* 41:212, 1953.
21. Caffesse RG, Karring T, Nasjleti CE: Keratinizing potential of sulcular epithelium, *J Periodontol* 48:140, 1977.
22. Caffesse RG, Nasjleti CE, Castelli WA: The role of sulcular environment in controlling epithelial keratinization, *J Periodontol* 50:1, 1979.
23. Caffesse RG, Kornman KS, Nasjleti CE: The effect of intensive antibacterial therapy on the sulcular environment in monkeys. Part II. Inflammation, mitotic activity and keratinization of the sulcular epithelium, *J Periodontol* 5:155, 1980.
24. Carranza FA Jr, Cabrini RL: Mast cells in human gingiva, *J Oral Surg* 8:1093, 1955.
25. Carranza FA Jr, Itoiz ME, Cabrini RL, et al: A study of periodontal vascularization in different laboratory animals, *J Periodontal Res* 1:120, 1966.
26. Chavier C: Elastic fibers of healthy human gingiva, *J Periodontol* 9:29, 1990.
27. Cho MI, Garant PR: Development and general structure of the periodontium, *Periodontol 2000* 24:9, 2000.
28. Cimasoni G: Crevicular fluid updated, *Monogr Oral Sci* 12:1, 1983.
29. Clausen H, Moe D, Buschard K, et al: Keratin proteins in human oral mucosa, *J Oral Pathol* 15:36, 1986.
30. Cleaton-Jones P, Buskin SA, Volchansky A: Surface ultrastructure of human gingiva, *J Periodontal Res* 13:367, 1978.
31. Cohen B: Morphological factors in the pathogenesis of periodontal disease, *Br Dent J* 107:31, 1959.
32. Cohen L: ATPase and DOPA oxidase activity in human gingival epithelium, *Arch Oral Biol* 12:1241, 1967.
33. Dale BA: Periodontal epithelium: a newly recognized role in health and disease, *Periodontol 2000* 30:70, 2002.
34. Dewar MR: Observations on the composition and metabolism of normal and inflamed gingivae, *J Periodontol* 26:29, 1955.
35. DiFranco CF, Toto PD, Rowden G, et al: Identification of Langerhans cells in human gingival epithelium, *J Periodontol* 56:48, 1985.
36. Dummett CO: Physiologic pigmentation of the oral and cutaneous tissues in the Negro, *J Dent Res* 25:421, 1946.
37. Dummett CO et al: Oral pigmentation: physiologic and pathologic, *NY State Dent J* 25:407, 1959.
38. Egelberg J: The topography and permeability of blood vessels at the dento-gingival junction in dogs, *J Periodontal Res* 1:1, 1967.
39. Eichel B, Shahrik HA, Lisanti VF: Cytochemical demonstration and metabolic significance of reduced diphosphopyridinenucleotide and triphospho-pyridinenucleotide reductases in human gingiva, *J Dent Res* 43:92, 1964.
40. Embery G, Waddington R: Gingival crevicular fluid: biomarkers of periodontal tissue activity, *Adv Dent Res* 8:329, 1994.
41. Embery G, Waddington RJ, Hall RC, et al: Connective tissue elements as diagnostic aids in periodontology, *Periodontol 2000* 24:193, 2000.
42. Engel MB: Water-soluble mucoproteins of the gingiva, *J Dent Res* 32:779, 1953.
43. Folke LE, Stallard RE: Periodontal microcirculation as revealed by plastic microspheres, *J Periodontal Res* 2:53, 1967.
44. Forsslund G: Structure and function of capillary system in the gingiva in man: development of stereophotogrammetric method and its application for study of the subepithelial blood vessels in vivo, *Acta Odontol Scand* 17:9, 1959.
45. Frank RM, Cimasoni G: On the ultrastructure of the normal human gingivo-dental junction, *Z Zellforsch Mikrosk Anat* 109:356, 1970.
46. Gargiulo AW, Wentz FM, Orban B: Dimensions and relations of the dentogingival junction in humans, *J Periodontol* 32:261, 1961.
47. Gillett R, Cruchley A, Johnson NW: The nature of the inflammatory infiltrates in childhood gingivitis, juvenile periodontitis and adult periodontitis: immunohistochemical studies using monoclonal antibody to HLADr, *J Clin Periodontol* 13:281, 1986.
48. Glickman I, Johannessen LB: Biomicroscopic (slit-lamp) evaluation of the normal gingiva of the albino rat, *J Am Dent Assoc* 41:521, 1950.
49. Gottlieb B, Orban B: Active and passive continuous eruption of teeth, *J Dent Res* 13:214, 1933.
50. Greene AH: A study of the characteristics of stippling and its relation to gingival health, *J Periodontol* 33:176, 1962.
51. Hansen ER: Mitotic activity of the gingival epithelium in colchicinized rats, *Odontol Tidskr* 74:229, 1966.
52. Hansson BO, Lindhe J, Branemark PI: Microvascular topography and function in clinically healthy and chronically inflamed dento-gingival tissues: a vital microscopic study in dogs, *Periodontics* 6:264, 1968.
53. Itoiz ME, Carranza FA Jr, Cabrini RL: Histotopographic distribution of alkaline and acid phosphatase in periodontal tissues of laboratory animals, *J Periodontol* 35:470, 1964.
54. Itoiz ME, Carranza FA Jr, Cabrini RL: Histotopographic study of esterase and 5-nucleotidase in periodontal tissues of laboratory animals, *J Periodontol* 38:130, 1967.
55. Itoiz ME, Carranza FA Jr, Gimenez IB, et al: Microspectrophotometric analysis of succinic dehydrogenase and glucose-6-phosphate dehydrogenase in human oral epithelium, *J Periodontal Res* 7:14, 1972.
56. Itoiz ME, Lanfranchi HE, Gimenez-Conti IB, et al: Immunohistochemical demonstration of keratins in oral mucosa lesions, *Acta Odontol Latinoam* 1:47, 1984.
57. Itoiz ME, Conti CJ, Lanfranchi HE, et al: Immunohistochemical detection of filaggrin in preneoplastic and neoplastic lesions of the human oral mucosa, *Am J Pathol* 119:456, 1985.
58. Itoiz ME, Conti CJ, Gimenez IB, et al: Immunodetection of involucrin in lesions of the oral mucosa, *J Oral Pathol* 15:205, 1986.
59. Iusem R: A cytology study of the cornification of the oral mucosa in women: a preliminary report, *J Oral Surg* 3:1516, 1950.
60. Jones JC, Hopkinson SB, Goldfinger LE: Structure and assembly of hemidesmosomes, *Bioessays* 20:488, 1998.
61. Karring T, Lang NP, Löe H: The role of gingival connective tissue in determining epithelial differentiation, *J Periodontal Res* 10:1, 1975.

62. Kobayashi K, Rose GG: Ultrastructural histochemistry of the dento-epithelial junction. II. Colloidal thorium and ruthenium red, *J Periodontal Res* 13:164, 1978.
63. Kobayashi K, Rose GG: Ultrastructural histochemistry of the dento-epithelial junction. III. Chloramine T–silver methenamine, *J Periodontal Res* 14:123, 1979.
64. Kronfeld R: *Histopathology of the teeth and their surrounding structures,* Philadelphia, 1939, Lea & Febiger.
65. Kurahashi Y, Takuma S: Electron microscopy of human gingival epithelium, *Bull Tokyo Dent Coll* 3:29, 1962.
66. Lange D, Camelleri GE: Cytochemical demonstration of lysosomes in exfoliated epithelial cells of the gingival cuff, *J Dent Res* 46:625, 1967.
67. Laurell L, Rylander H, Sundin Y: Histologic characteristics of clinically healthy gingiva in adolescents, *Scand J Dent Res* 95:456 1987.
68. Lavelle CLB: Mucosal seal around endosseous dental implants, *J Oral Implantol* 9:357, 1981.
69. Listgarten MA: The ultrastructure of human gingival epithelium, *Am J Anat* 114:49, 1964.
70. Listgarten MA: Electron microscopic study of the gingivo-dental junction of man, *Am J Anat* 119:147, 1966.
71. Listgarten MA: Phase-contrast and electron microscopic study of the junction between reduced enamel epithelium and enamel in unerupted human teeth, *Arch Oral Biol* 11:999, 1966.
72. Listgarten MA: Changing concepts about the dento-gingival junction, *J Can Dent Assoc* 36:70, 1970.
73. Listgarten MA: Structure of surface coatings on teeth: a review, *J Periodontol* 47:139, 1976.
74. Löe H, Karring T: Mitotic activity and renewal time of the gingival epithelium of young and old rats, *J Periodontal Res* 4:18, 1969.
75. Löe H, Karring T: A quantitative analysis of the epithelium–connective tissue interface in relation to assessments of the mitotic index, *J Dent Res* 48:634, 1969.
76. Luthman J, Johansson O, Ahlström U, et al: Immunohistochemical studies of the neurochemical markers CGRP, enkephalin, galanin, gamma-MSH, NPY, PHI, proctolin, PTH, somatostatin, SP, VIP, tyrosine hydroxylase and neurofilament in nerves and cells of the human attached gingiva, *Arch Oral Biol* 33:149, 1988.
77. Magnusson B: Mucosal changes in erupting molars in germ-free rats, *J Periodontal Res* 4:181, 1969.
78. Marchetti C, Poggi P: Lymphatic vessels in the oral cavity: different structures for the same function, *Microsc Res Tech* 56:42, 2002.
79. Matsuo M, Takahashi K: Scanning electron microscopic observation of microvasculature in periodontium, *Microsc Res Tech* 56:3, 2002.
80. Melcher AH: On the repair potential of periodontal tissues, *J Periodontol* 47:256, 1976.
81. Meyer J, Marwah AS, Weinmann JP: Mitotic rate of gingival epithelium in two age groups, *J Invest Dermatol* 27:237, 1956.
82. Miller SC, Soberman A, Stahl SS: A study of the cornification of the oral mucosa of young male adults, *J Dent Res* 30:4, 1951.
83. Morgan PR, Leigh IM, Purkis PE, et al: Site variation in keratin expression in human oral epithelia: an immunocytochemical study of individual keratins, *Epithelia* 1:31, 1987.
84. Moss ML: Phylogeny and comparative anatomy of oral ectodermal-ectomesenchymal inductive interactions, *J Dent Res* 48:732, 1969.
85. Ness KH, Morton TH, Dale BA: Identification of Merkel cells in oral epithelium using antikeratin and antineuroendocrine monoclonal antibodies, *J Dent Res* 66:1154, 1987.
86. Nuki K, Hock J: The organisation of the gingival vasculature, *J Periodontal Res* 9:305, 1974.
87. Oliver RC, Holm-Pederen P, Löe H: The correlation between clinical scoring, exudate measurements and microscopic evaluation of inflammation in the gingiva, *J Periodontol* 40:201, 1969.
88. Orban B, Kohler J: Die physiologische Zahn-fleischtasche, Epithelansatz und Epitheltiefenwucherung, *Z Stomatol* 22:353, 1924.
89. Page RC, Ammons WF, Schectman LR, et al: Collagen fibre bundles of the normal marginal gingiva in the marmoset, *Arch Oral Biol* 19:1039, 1972.
90. Papic M, Glickman I: Keratinization of the human gingiva in the menstrual cycle and menopause, *Oral Surg Oral Med Oral Pathol* 3:504, 1950.
91. Person P, Felton J, Fine A: Biochemical and histochemical studies of aerobic oxidative metabolism of oral tissues. 3. Specific metabolic activities of enzymatically separated gingival epithelium and connective tissue components, *J Dent Res* 44:91, 1965.
92. Pöllänen MT, Salonen JI, Uitto VJ: Structure and function of the tooth-epithelial interface in health and disease, *Periodontol 2000* 31:12, 2003.
93. Romanos GE, Bernimoulin JP: Collagen as a basic element of the periodontium: immunohistochemical aspects in the human and animal. 1. Gingiva and alveolar bone, *Parodontologie* 4:363, 1990.
94. Rosenberg HM, Massler M: Gingival stippling in young adult males, *J Periodontol* 38:473, 1967.
95. Salonen JI: Proliferative potential of the attached cells of human junctional epithelium, *J Periodontal Res* 29:41, 1994.
96. Salonen JI, Pöllänen MT: Junctional epithelial cells directly attached to the tooth, *Acta Med Dent Helv* 2:137, 1997.
97. Sawada T, Yamamoto T, Yanagisawa T, et al: Electron-immunocytochemistry of laminin and type-IV collagen in the junctional epithelium of rat molar gingiva, *J Periodontal Res* 25:372, 1990.
98. Sawaf MH, Ouhayoun JP, Forest N: Cytokeratin profiles in oral epithelial: a review and a new classification, *J Biol Buccale* 19:187, 1991.
99. Schor SL, Ellis I, Irwin CR, et al: Subpopulations of fetal-like gingival fibroblasts: characterisation and potential significance for wound healing and the progression of periodontal disease, *Oral Dis* 2:155, 1996.
100. Schroeder HE: Melanin containing organelles in cells of the human gingiva, *J Periodontal Res* 4:1, 1969.
101. Schroeder HE: Ultrastructure of the junctional epithelium of the human gingiva, *Helv Odontol Acta* 13:65, 1969.
102. Schroeder HE: Transmigration and infiltration of leucocytes in human junctional epithelium, *Helv Odontol Acta* 17:6, 1973.
103. Schroeder HE: *Differentiation of human oral stratified epithelia,* New York, 1981, Karger.
104. Schroeder HE: Gingiva. In Oksche A, Vollrath L, editors: *The periodontium handbook of microscopic anatomy,* vol. 5, Berlin, 1986, Springer-Verlag.
105. Schroeder HE: *The periodontium,* Berlin, 1986, Springer-Verlag.
106. Schroeder HE, Listgarten MA: Fine structure of the developing epithelial attachment of human teeth. In *Monographs in developmental biology,* vol 2, Basel, 1971, Karger.
107. Schroeder HE, Listgarten MA: The gingival tissues: the architecture of periodontal protection, *Periodontol 2000* 13:91, 1997.
108. Schroeder HE, Theilade J: Electron microscopy of normal human gingival epithelium, *J Periodontal Res* 1:95, 1966.
109. Schultz-Haudt SD, From S: Dynamics of periodontal tissues. I. The epithelium, *Odont T* 69:431, 1961.

110. Schultz-Haudt SD, Paus S, Assev S: Periodic acid–Schiff reactive components of human gingiva, *J Dent Res* 40:141, 1961.
111. Schweitzer G: Lymph vessels of the gingiva and teeth, *Arch Mik Anat Ent* 69:807, 1907.
112. Schwint AE, Itoiz ME, Cabrini RL: A quantitative histochemical technique for the study of vascularization in tissue sections using horseradish peroxidase, *Histochem J* 16:907, 1984.
113. Seymour GJ, Crouch MS, Powell RN, et al: The identification of lymphoid cell subpopulations in sections of human lymphoid tissue and gingivitis in children using monoclonal antibodies, *J Periodontal Res* 17:247, 1982.
114. Shapiro S, Ulmansky M, Scheuer M: Mast cell population in gingiva affected by chronic destructive periodontal disease, *J Periodontol* 40:276, 1969.
115. Shelton LE, Hall WB: Human gingival mast cells, *J Periodontal Res* 3:214, 1968.
116. Skougaard MR, Beagrie GS: The renewal of gingival epithelium in marmosets *(Callithrix jacchus)* as determined through autoradiography with thymidine-H3, *Acta Ondontol Scand* 20:467, 1962.
117. Squier CA, Waterhouse JP: The ultrastructure of the melanocyte in human gingival epithelium, *J Dent Res* 46:113, 1967.
118. Stern IB: Electron microscopic observations of oral epithelium. I. Basal cells and the basement membrane, *Periodontics* 3:224, 1965.
119. Stern IB: The fine structure of the ameloblast-enamel junction in rat incisors, epithelial attachment and cuticular membrane. Presented at 5th International Congress for Electron Microscopy, 1966, p 6.
120. Stern IB: Further electron microscopic observations of the epithelial attachment, International Association for Dental Research Abstracts, 45th general meeting, 1967, p 118.
121. Susi F: Histochemical, autoradiographic and electron microscopic studies of keratinization in oral mucosa, Tufts University, 1967 (PhD thesis).
122. Swift JA, Saxton CA: The ultrastructural location of the periodate-Schiff reactive basement membrane of the dermoepidermal junctions of human scalp and monkey gingiva, *J Ultrastruct Res* 17:23, 1967.
123. Thilander H: Permeability of the gingival pocket epithelium, *Int Dent J* 14:416, 1964.
124. Thilander H, Bloom GD: Cell contacts in oral epithelia, *J Periodontal Res* 3:96, 1968.
125. Thonard JC, Scherp HW: Histochemical demonstration of acid mucopolysaccharides in human gingival epithelial intercellular spaces, *Arch Oral Biol* 7:125, 1962.
126. Trott JR: An investigation into the glycogen content of the gingivae, *Dent Pract* 7:234, 1957.
127. Trott JR, Gorenstein SL: Mitotic rates in the oral and gingival epithelium of the rat, *Arch Oral Biol* 8:425, 1963.
128. Turesky S, Glickman I, Litwin T: A histochemical evaluation of normal and inflamed human gingivae, *J Dent Res* 30:792, 1951.
129. Waterhouse JP: The gingival part of the human periodontium, its ultrastructure and the distribution in it of acid phosphatase in relation to cell attachment and the lysosome concept, *Dent Pract Dent Rec* 15:409, 1965.
130. Weinmann JP, Meyer J: Types of keratinization in the human gingiva, *J Invest Dermatol* 32:87, 1959.
131. Weinstock A, Albright JT: Electron microscopic observations on specialized structures in the epithelium of the normal human palate, *J Dent Res* 45:79, 1966.
132. Weinstock A, Albright JT: The fine structure of mast cells in normal human gingiva, *J Ultrastruct Res* 17:245, 1967.
133. Weski O: Die chronische marginales Enzundungen des Alveolar-fortsatzes mit besonderer Berucksichtigung der Alveolarpyorrhoe, *Vierteljahrschr Zahnheilk* 38:1, 1922.
134. Yamasaki A, Nikai H, Niitani K, et al: Ultrastructure of the junctional epithelium of germ-free rat gingiva, *J Periodontol* 50:641, 1979.
135. Zander HA: The distribution of phosphatase in gingival tissue, *J Dent Res* 20:347, 1941.

The Tooth-Supporting Structures

Joseph P. Fiorellini, David M. Kim, and Satoshi O. Ishikawa

5

CHAPTER

CHAPTER OUTLINE

The normal periodontium provides the support necessary to maintain teeth in function. It consists of four principal components: gingiva, periodontal ligament, cementum, and alveolar bone. Each of these periodontal components is distinct in its location, tissue architecture, biochemical composition, and chemical composition, but all these components function together as a single unit. Recent research has revealed that the extracellular matrix components of one periodontal compartment can influence the cellular activities of adjacent structures. Therefore the pathologic changes occurring in one periodontal component may have significant ramifications for the maintenance, repair, or regeneration of other components of the periodontium.[9]

This chapter first discusses the structural components of the normal periodontium, then describes their development, vascularization, innervation, and functions.

PERIODONTAL LIGAMENT

The periodontal ligament is composed of a complex vascular and highly cellular connective tissue that surrounds the tooth root and connects it to the inner wall of the alveolar bone.[99] It is continuous with the connective tissue of the gingiva and communicates with the marrow spaces through vascular channels in the bone. Although the average width of the periodontal ligament space is documented to be about 0.2 mm, considerable variation exists. The periodontal space is diminished around teeth that are not in function and in unerupted teeth, but it is increased in teeth subjected to hyperfunction.

Periodontal Fibers

The most important elements of the periodontal ligament are the *principal fibers,* which are collagenous and arranged in bundles and follow a wavy course when viewed in longitudinal section (Figure 5-1). The terminal portions of the principal fibers that are inserted into cementum and bone are termed *Sharpey's fibers* (Figure 5-2). The principal fiber bundles consist of individual fibers that form a continuous anastomosing network between tooth and bone.[15,36] Once embedded in the wall of the alveolus or in the tooth, Sharpey's fibers calcify to a significant degree. They are associated with abundant noncollagenous proteins typically found in bone and also recently identified in tooth cementum.[22,79,100] Notable among these proteins are osteopontin and bone sialoprotein. These proteins are thought to contribute to the regulation of mineralization and to tissue cohesion at sites of increased biomechanical strain.[100]

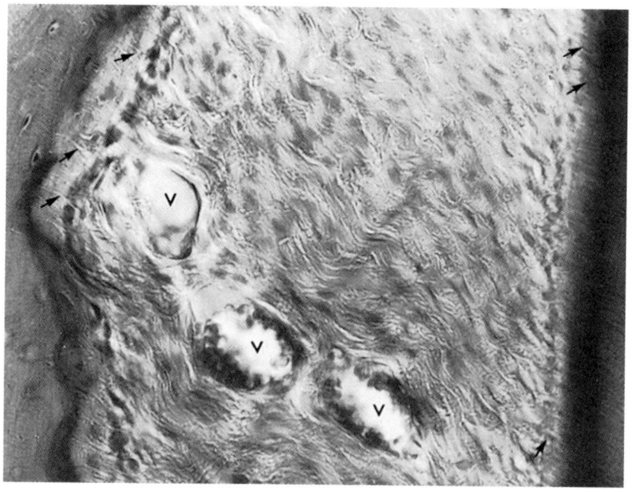

Figure 5-1 Principal fibers of the periodontal ligament follow a wavy course when sectioned longitudinally. The formative function of the periodontal ligament is illustrated by the newly formed osteoid and osteoblasts along a previously resorbed bone surface *(left)* and the cementoid and cementoblasts *(right)*. Note the fibers embedded in the forming calcified tissues *(arrows)*. *V,* Vascular channels.

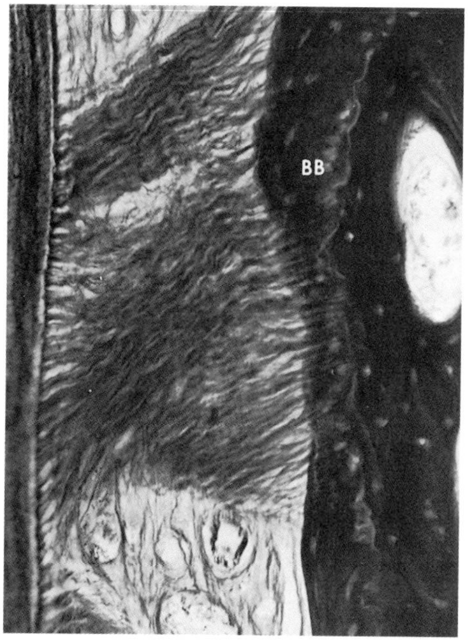

Figure 5-2 Collagen fibers embedded in the cementum *(left)* and bone *(right)* (silver stain). Note Sharpey's fibers within the bundle bone *(BB)* overlying lamellar bone.

Collagen is a protein composed of different amino acids, the most important of which are glycine, proline, hydroxylysine, and hydroxyproline.[32] The amount of collagen in a tissue can be determined by its hydroxyproline content. Collagen is responsible for maintenance of the framework and tone of tissue, and it exhibits a wide range of diversity.[45] There are at least 19 recognized collagen species encoded by at least 25 separate genes, dispersed among 12 chromosomes.[45]

Collagen biosynthesis occurs inside the fibroblasts to form tropocollagen molecules. These aggregate into microfibrils that are packed together to form fibrils. Collagen fibrils have a transverse striation with a characteristic periodicity of 64 nm; this striation is caused by the overlapping arrangement of the tropocollagen molecules. In collagen types I and III these fibrils associate to form fibers, and in collagen type I the fibers associate to form bundles (Figure 5-3).

Collagen is synthesized by fibroblasts, chondroblasts, osteoblasts, odontoblasts, and other cells. The several types of collagen are all distinguishable by their chemical composition, distribution, function, and morphology.[84] The principal fibers are composed mainly of collagen type I,[126] whereas reticular fibers are composed of collagen type III. Collagen type IV is found in the basal lamina.[127,128] The expression of type XII collagen during the tooth development is timed with the alignment and organization of periodontal fibers and is limited in tooth development to cells within the periodontal ligament.[94] Type VI collagen also has been immunolocalized in periodontal ligament and gingiva.[46]

The molecular configuration of collagen fibers provides them with a tensile strength greater than that of steel. Consequently, collagen imparts a unique combination of flexibility and strength to the tissues.[84]

The principal fibers of the periodontal ligament are arranged in six groups that develop sequentially in the developing root: the transseptal, alveolar crest, horizontal,

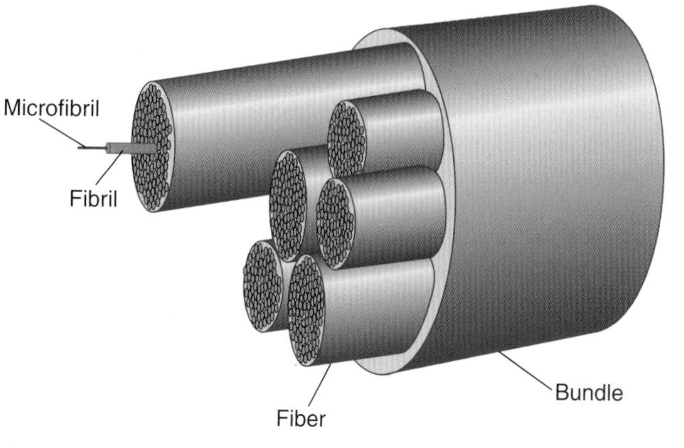

Figure 5-3 Collagen microfibrils, fibrils, fibers, and bundles.

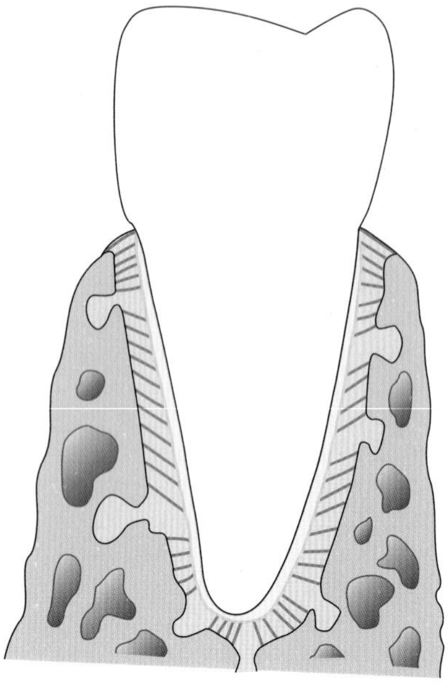

Figure 5-4 Diagram of principal fiber groups.

oblique, apical, and interradicular fibers (Figure 5-4), as follows:

Transseptal group. Transseptal fibers extend interproximally over the alveolar bone crest and are embedded in the cementum of adjacent teeth (Figure 5-5). They are reconstructed even after destruction of the alveolar bone resulting from periodontal disease. These fibers may be considered as belonging to the gingiva because they do not have osseous attachment.

Alveolar crest group. Alveolar crest fibers extend obliquely from the cementum just beneath the junctional epithelium to the alveolar crest (Figure 5-6). Fibers also run from the cementum over the alveolar crest and to the fibrous layer of the periosteum covering the alveolar bone. The alveolar crest fibers prevent the extrusion of the tooth[33] and resist lateral tooth movements. The incision of these fibers during periodontal surgery does not increase tooth mobility unless significant attachment loss has occurred.[57]

Horizontal group. Horizontal fibers extend at right angles to the long axis of the tooth from the cementum to the alveolar bone.

Oblique group. Oblique fibers, the largest group in the periodontal ligament, extend from the cementum in a coronal direction obliquely to the bone (see Figure 5-4). They bear the brunt of vertical masticatory stresses and transform them into tension on the alveolar bone.

Apical group. The apical fibers radiate in a rather irregular manner from the cementum to the bone at the apical region of the socket. They do not occur on incompletely formed roots.

Interradicular group. The interradicular fibers fan out from the cementum to the tooth in the furcation areas of multirooted teeth.

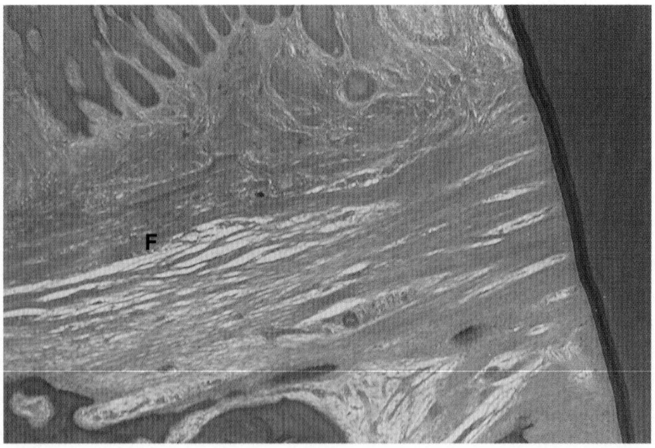

Figure 5-5 Transseptal fibers *(F)* at the crest of the interdental bone.

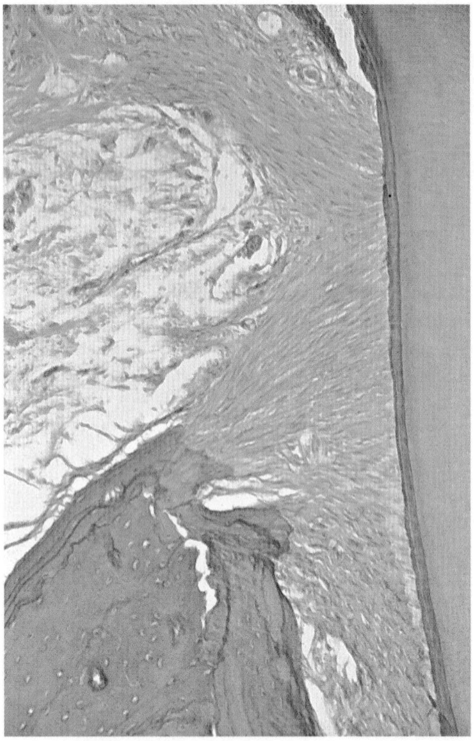

Figure 5-6 Rat molar section showing alveolar crest fibers radiating coronally.

Other well-formed fiber bundles interdigitate at right angles or splay around and between regularly arranged fiber bundles. Less regularly arranged collagen fibers are found in the interstitial connective tissue between the principal fiber groups; this tissue contains the blood vessels, lymphatics, and nerves.

Although the periodontal ligament does not contain mature elastin, two immature forms are found: oxytalan and eluanin. The so-called oxytalan fibers[50,61] run parallel to the root surface in a vertical direction and bend to attach to the cementum[50] in the cervical third of the root. They are thought to regulate vascular flow.[49] An elastic

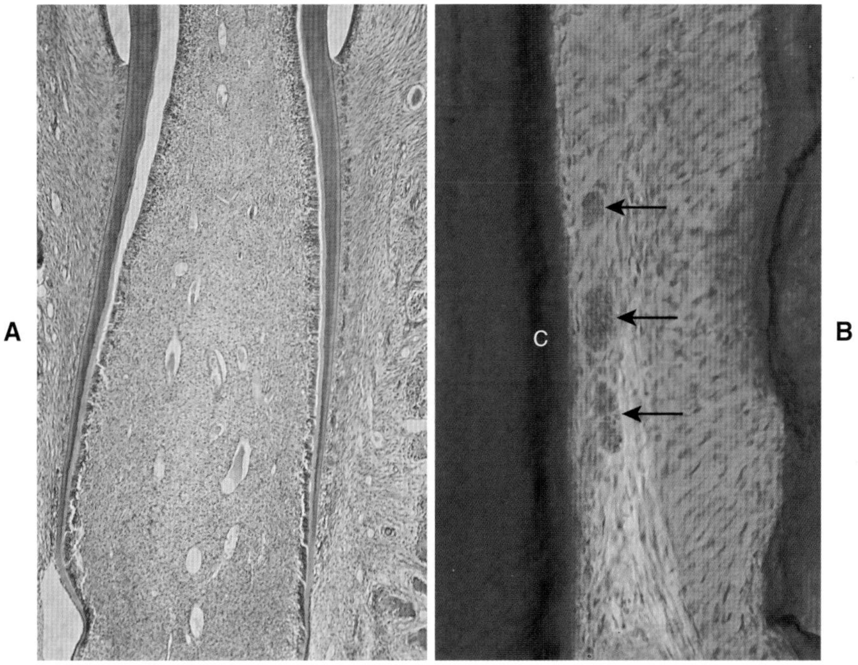

Figure 5-7 Epithelial rests of Malassez. **A,** Erupting tooth in a cat. Fragmentation of Hertwig's epithelial root sheath giving rise to epithelial rests located along, and close to, the root surface. **B,** Human periodontal ligament with rosette-shaped epithelial rests *(arrows)* lying close to the cementum *(C)*.

meshwork has been described in the periodontal ligament[80] as being composed of many elastin lamellae with peripheral oxytalan fibers and eluanin fibers. Oxytalan fibers have been shown to develop de novo in the regenerated periodontal ligament.[132]

The principal fibers are remodeled by the periodontal ligament cells to adapt to physiologic needs[150,167] and in response to different stimuli.[156]

In addition to these fiber types, small collagen fibers associated with the larger principal collagen fibers have been described. These fibers run in all directions, forming a plexus called the *indifferent fiber plexus*.[139]

Cellular Elements

Four types of cells have been identified in the periodontal ligament: connective tissue cells, epithelial rest cells, immune system cells, and cells associated with neurovascular elements.[16]

Connective tissue cells include fibroblasts, cementoblasts, and osteoblasts. Fibroblasts are the most common cells in the periodontal ligament and appear as ovoid or elongated cells oriented along the principal fibers, exhibiting pseudopodia-like processes.[125] These cells synthesize collagen and possess the capacity to phagocytose "old" collagen fibers and degrade them[150] by enzyme hydrolysis. Thus, collagen turnover appears to be regulated by fibroblasts in a process of intracellular degradation of collagen not involving the action of collagenase.[14]

Phenotypically distinct and functionally different subpopulations of fibroblasts exist in the adult periodontal ligament. They appear identical at both light and electron microscopic levels[69] but may have different functions, such as secretion of different collagen types and production of collagenase.

Osteoblasts and cementoblasts, as well as osteoclasts and odontoclasts, also are seen in the cemental and osseous surfaces of the periodontal ligament.

The *epithelial rests of Malassez* form a latticework in the periodontal ligament and appear as either isolated clusters of cells or interlacing strands (Figure 5-7), depending on the plane in which the microscopic section is cut. Continuity with the junctional epithelium has been suggested in experimental animals.[63] The epithelial rests are considered remnants of Hertwig's root sheath, which disintegrates during root development (Figure 5-7, *A*).

Epithelial rests are distributed close to the cementum throughout the periodontal ligament of most teeth and are most numerous in the apical area[122] and cervical area.[158,159] They diminish in number with age[141] by degenerating and disappearing or by undergoing calcification to become cementicles. The cells are surrounded by a distinct basal lamina, are interconnected by hemidesmosomes, and contain tonofilaments.[14]

Even though their functional properties are still considered to be unclear[145], the epithelial rests are reported to contain keratinocyte growth factors and have been shown to be positive for tyrosine kinase A neurotrophin receptor.[52,160,165] Also, epithelial rests proliferate when stimulated[146,151,155] and participate in the formation of periapical cysts and lateral root cysts.

The *defense cells* in the periodontal ligament include neutrophils, lymphocytes, macrophages, mast cells, and eosinophils. These cells, as well as those associated with neurovascular elements, are similar to the cells in other connective tissues.

Ground Substance

The periodontal ligament also contains a large proportion of ground substance, filling the spaces between fibers and cells. It consists of two main components: *glycosaminoglycans,* such as hyaluronic acid and proteoglycans, and *glycoproteins,* such as fibronectin and laminin. Ground substance also has a high water content (70%).

The cell surface proteoglycans participate in several biologic functions, including cell adhesion, cell-cell and cell-matrix interactions, binding to various growth factors as co-receptors, and cell repair.[166] For example, *fibromodulin,* a small proteoglycan rich in keratan sulfate and leucine, has recently been identified in bovine periodontal ligament.[162] The most comprehensive study of the proteoglycans in periodontal ligament was performed using fibroblast cultures of human ligament.[88]

The periodontal ligament may also contain calcified masses called *cementicles,* which are adherent to or detached from the root surfaces (Figure 5-8). Cementicles may develop from calcified epithelial rests; around small spicules of cementum or alveolar bone traumatically displaced into the periodontal ligament; from calcified Sharpey's fibers; and from calcified, thrombosed vessels within the periodontal ligament.[103]

Functions of Periodontal Ligament

The functions of the periodontal ligament are categorized into physical, formative and remodeling, nutritional, and sensory.

Physical Functions

The physical functions of the periodontal ligament entail the following:

1. Provision of a soft tissue "casing" to protect the vessels and nerves from injury by mechanical forces.
2. Transmission of occlusal forces to the bone.
3. Attachment of the teeth to the bone.
4. Maintenance of the gingival tissues in their proper relationship to the teeth.
5. Resistance to the impact of occlusal forces (shock absorption).

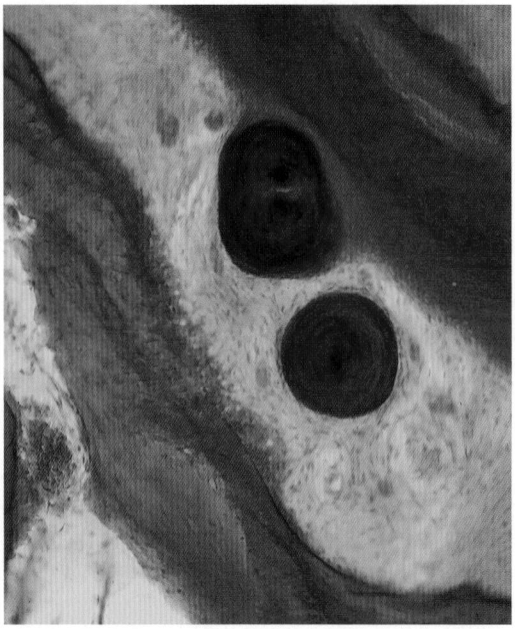

Figure 5-8 Cementicles in the periodontal ligament, one lying free and the other adherent to the tooth surface.

Resistance to Impact of Occlusal Forces (Shock Absorption). Two theories pertaining to the mechanism of tooth support have been considered: the tensional and viscoelastic system theories.

The *tensional theory* of tooth support states that the principal fibers of the periodontal ligament are the major factor in supporting the tooth and transmitting forces to the bone. When a force is applied to the crown, the principal fibers first unfold and straighten and then transmit forces to the alveolar bone, causing an elastic deformation of the bony socket. Finally, when the alveolar bone has reached its limit, the load is transmitted to the basal bone. Many investigators find this theory insufficient to explain available experimental evidence.

The *viscoelastic system theory* states that the displacement of the tooth is largely controlled by fluid movements, with fibers having only a secondary role.[21,31] When forces are transmitted to the tooth, the extracellular fluid passes from the periodontal ligament into the marrow spaces of bone through foramina in the cribriform plate. These perforations of the cribriform plate link the periodontal ligament with the cancellous portion of the alveolar bone and are more abundant in the cervical third than in the middle and apical thirds (Figure 5-9).

After depletion of tissue fluids, the fiber bundles absorb the slack and tighten. This leads to a blood vessel stenosis. Arterial back pressure causes ballooning of the vessels and passage of the blood ultrafiltrates into the tissues, thereby replenishing the tissue fluids.[21]

Transmission of Occlusal Forces to Bone. The arrangement of the principal fibers is similar to a suspension bridge or a hammock. When an axial force is applied to a tooth, a tendency toward displacement of the root into the alveolus occurs. The oblique fibers alter their wavy, untensed pattern; assume their full length; and sustain the major part of the axial force. When a horizontal

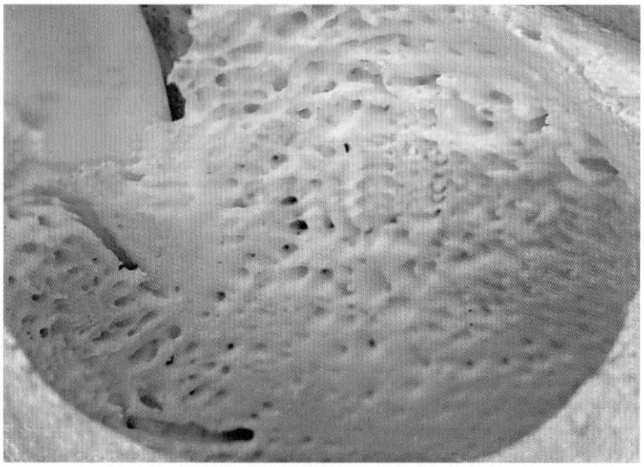

Figure 5-9 Foramina perforating the lamina dura (dog jaw).

or tipping force is applied, two phases of tooth movement occur. The first is within the confines of the periodontal ligament, and the second produces a displacement of the facial and lingual bony plates.[41] The tooth rotates about an axis that may change as the force is increased.

The apical portion of the root moves in a direction opposite to the coronal portion. In areas of tension, the principal fiber bundles are taut rather than wavy. In areas of pressure, the fibers are compressed, the tooth is displaced, and a corresponding distortion of bone exists in the direction of root movement.[118]

In single-rooted teeth the axis of rotation is located in the area between the apical third and the middle third of the root (Figure 5-10). The root apex[105] and the coronal half of the clinical root have been suggested as other locations of the axis of rotation. The periodontal ligament, which has an hourglass shape, is narrowest in the region of the axis of rotation[39,87] (Table 5-1). In multirooted teeth the axis of rotation is located in the bone between the roots (Figure 5-11). In compliance with the physiologic mesial migration of the teeth, the periodontal ligament is thinner on the mesial root surface than on the distal surface.

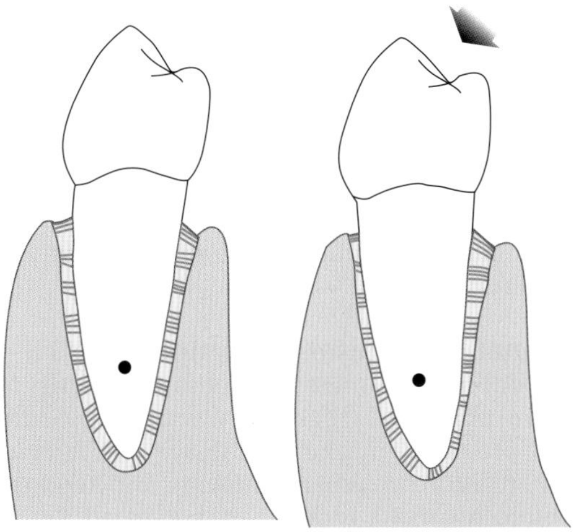

Figure 5-10 *Left,* Diagram of tooth (mandibular premolar) in a resting state. *Right,* When a force is exerted on the tooth, in this case in faciolingual direction *(arrow)* the tooth rotates around the fulcrum or axis of rotation *(black circle on root).* The periodontal ligament is compressed in areas of pressure and distended in areas of tension.

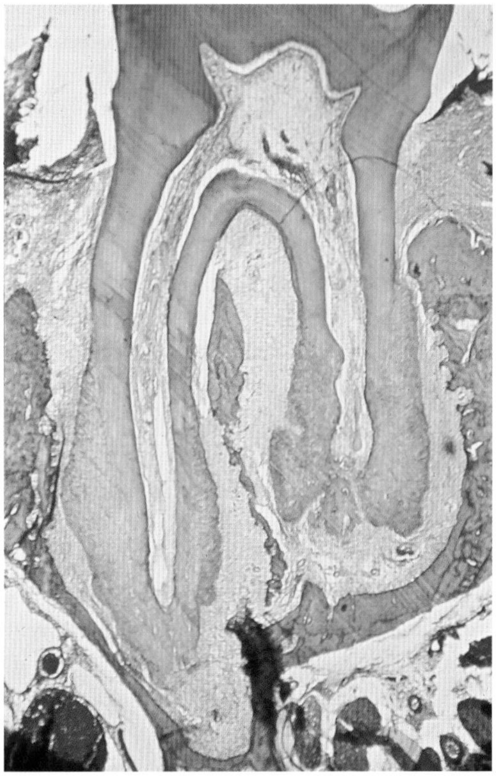

Figure 5-11 Microscopic view of rat molar subjected to occlusohorizontal forces. Note the alternating widened and narrowed areas of the periodontal ligament as the tooth rotates around its axis of rotation. The axis of rotation is in the interradicular space.

TABLE 5-1

Thickness of Periodontal Ligament of 172 Teeth from 15 Human Subjects

	Average of Alveolar Crest (mm)	Average of Midroot (mm)	Average of Apex (mm)	Average of Tooth (mm)
Ages 11-16 83 teeth from 4 jaws	0.23	0.17	0.24	0.21
Ages 32-50 36 teeth from 5 jaws	0.20	0.14	0.19	0.18
Ages 51-67 35 teeth from 5 jaws	0.17	0.12	0.16	0.15
Age 24 (1 case) 18 teeth from 1 jaw	0.16	0.09	0.15	0.13

Modified from Coolidge ED: *J Am Dent Assoc* 24:1260, 1937.

SCIENCE TRANSFER

The normal periodontium is a unique and complex dynamic structure. Each of its components (gingiva, periodontal ligament, cementum, and bone) has distinct functions that are capable of adaptation during the life of the structure. For example, as teeth respond to forces or migrate mesially with wear, the bone tissue is resorbed on the pressure side and added on the tension side. Cementum similarly adapts to wear on the occlusal surfaces of teeth by deposition in the apical area of the tooth root. The periodontal ligament itself is an area of high turnover, which allows the tooth not only to be suspended in the alveolar bone, but also to respond to the intermediate forces. Thus, although seemingly static, the structure of tooth support is made up from components of the periodontium that are highly specialized, adaptive, and dynamic structures.

The function of the periodontal ligament is most similar to a viscoelastic system that absorbs the first movement of loading, with collagen fibers then becoming important as a secondary phase of response to loading forces. This gives the periodontal ligament a shock-absorbing quality as well as a hydraulic-like tendency to respond to axial loading with an increased pressure that counteracts the apically directed tooth movement.

When a tooth is subjected to increased occlusal load, it will be slightly depressed, and when unloaded, it will have a rebound effect.

Therefore, correction of "high" restorations by grinding may require two or more checks over 2 to 5 minutes. Also, the use of heavy-bodied materials for crown and bridge impressions with sustained pressure can cause intrusion of a tooth, followed by a rebound extrusion after the impression is removed. The result will be a restoration that is high.

Being aware of these properties of the periodontal ligament can allow clinicians to modify their clinical procedures.

Formative and Remodeling Function

Periodontal ligament and alveolar bone cells are exposed to physical forces in response to mastication, parafunction, speech, and orthodontic tooth movement.[99] Cells of the periodontal ligament participate in the formation and resorption of cementum and bone, which occur in physiologic tooth movement; in the accommodation of the periodontium to occlusal forces; and in the repair of injuries. Variations in cellular enzyme activity are correlated with the remodeling process.[54-56] Although applied loads may induce vascular and inflammatory reactive changes in periodontal ligament cells, current evidence suggests that these cells have a mechanism to respond directly to mechanical forces by activation of various mechanosensory signaling systems, including adenylate cyclase, stretch-activated ion channels, and by changes in cytoskeletal organization.[99]

Cartilage formation in the periodontal ligament, although unusual, may represent a metaplastic phenomenon in the repair of this ligament after injury.[11]

The periodontal ligament is constantly undergoing remodeling. Old cells and fibers are broken down and replaced by new ones, and mitotic activity can be observed in the fibroblasts and endothelial cells.[106] Fibroblasts form the collagen fibers, and the residual mesenchymal cells develop into osteoblasts and cementoblasts. Therefore the rate of formation and the differentiation of osteoblasts, cementoblasts, and fibroblasts affect the rate of formation of collagen, cementum, and bone.

Radioautographic studies with radioactive thymidine, proline, and glycine indicate a high turnover rate of collagen in the periodontal ligament. The rate of collagen synthesis is twice as fast as that in the gingiva and four times as fast as that in the skin, as established in the rat molar.[142] A rapid turnover of sulfated glycosaminoglycans in the cells and amorphous ground substance of the periodontal ligament also occurs.[12]

It should be noted that most of these studies have been performed in rodents, and information on primates and humans is scarce.[136]

Nutritional and Sensory Functions

The periodontal ligament supplies nutrients to the cementum, bone, and gingiva by way of the blood vessels and also provides lymphatic drainage (see later discussion). In relation to other ligaments and tendons, the periodontal ligament is highly vascularized tissue, and almost 10% of its volume in the rodent molar is blood vessels.[24,98] This relatively high blood vessel content may provide hydrodynamic damping to applied forces, as well as high perfusion rates to the periodontal ligament.[99]

The periodontal ligament is abundantly supplied with sensory nerve fibers capable of transmitting tactile, pressure, and pain sensations by the trigeminal pathways.[6,20] Nerve bundles pass into the periodontal ligament from the periapical area and through channels from the alveolar bone that follow the course of the blood vessels. The bundles divide into single myelinated fibers, which ultimately lose their myelin sheaths and end in one of four types of neural termination: (1) free endings, which have a treelike configuration and carry pain sensation; (2) Ruffini-like mechanoreceptors, located primarily in the apical area; (3) coiled Meissner's corpuscles, also mechanoreceptors, found mainly in the midroot region; and (4) spindlelike pressure and vibration endings, which are surrounded by a fibrous capsule and located mainly in the apex.[49,95]

Regulation of Periodontal Ligament Width

Some of the most interesting features of the periodontal ligament in animals are its adaptability to rapidly changing applied force and its capacity to maintain its width at constant dimensions throughout its lifetime.[98]

These are important measures of periodontal ligament homeostasis, providing insight into the function of the biologic mechanisms that tightly regulate the metabolism and spatial locations of the cell populations involved in the formation of bone, cementum, and periodontal ligament fibers. Also, the ability of periodontal ligament cells to synthesize and secrete a wide range of regulatory molecules is an essential component of tissue remodeling and periodontal ligament homeostasis.[99]

CEMENTUM

Cementum is the calcified, avascular mesenchymal tissue that forms the outer covering of the anatomic root. The two main types of cementum are acellular *(primary)* and cellular *(secondary)* cementum.[62] Both consist of a calcified interfibrillar matrix and collagen fibrils.

The two main sources of collagen fibers in cementum are (1) Sharpey's fibers *(extrinsic)*, which are the embedded portion of the principal fibers of the periodontal ligament[127] and are formed by the fibroblasts, and (2) fibers that belong to the cementum matrix *(intrinsic)* and are produced by the cementoblasts.[137] Cementoblasts also form the noncollagenous components of the interfibrillar ground substance, such as proteoglycans, glycoproteins, and phosphoproteins. Proteoglycans are most likely to play a role in regulating cell-cell and cell-matrix interactions, both in normal development as well as in regeneration of the cementum.[8] In addition, immunohistochemical studies have shown that the distribution of proteoglycans is closely associated with the cementoblasts and cementocytes.[1,2]

The major proportion of the organic matrix of a cementum is composed of type I (90%) and type III (about 5%) collagens. Sharpey's fibers, which constitute a considerable proportion of the bulk of cementum, are composed of mainly collagen type I.[121] Type III collagen appears to coat the type I collagen of Sharpey's fibers.[7]

Acellular cementum is the first cementum formed, covers approximately the cervical third or half of the root, and does not contain cells (Figure 5-12). This cementum is formed before the tooth reaches the occlusal plane, and its thickness ranges from 30 to 230 µm.[141] Sharpey's fibers make up most of the structure of acellular cementum, which has a principal role in supporting the tooth. Most fibers are inserted at approximately right angles into the root surface and penetrate deep into the cementum, but others enter from several different directions. Their size, number, and distribution increase with function.[77] Sharpey's fibers are completely calcified, with the mineral crystals oriented parallel to the fibrils, as in dentin and bone, except in a 10- to 50-µm-wide zone near the cementodentinal junction, where they are only partially calcified. The peripheral portions of Sharpey's fibers in actively mineralizing cementum tend to be more calcified than the interior regions, according to evidence obtained by scanning electron microscopy.[83] Acellular cementum also contains intrinsic collagen fibrils that are calcified and irregularly arranged or parallel to the surface.[136]

Cellular cementum, formed after the tooth reaches the occlusal plane, is more irregular and contains cells (cementocytes) in individual spaces (lacunae) that communicate with each other through a system of anastomosing canaliculi (Figure 5-13). Cellular cementum is less calcified than the acellular type.[78] Sharpey's fibers occupy a smaller portion of cellular cementum and are separated by other fibers that are arranged either parallel to the root surface or at random. Sharpey's fibers may be completely or partially calcified or may have a central, uncalcified core surrounded by a calcified border.[81,137]

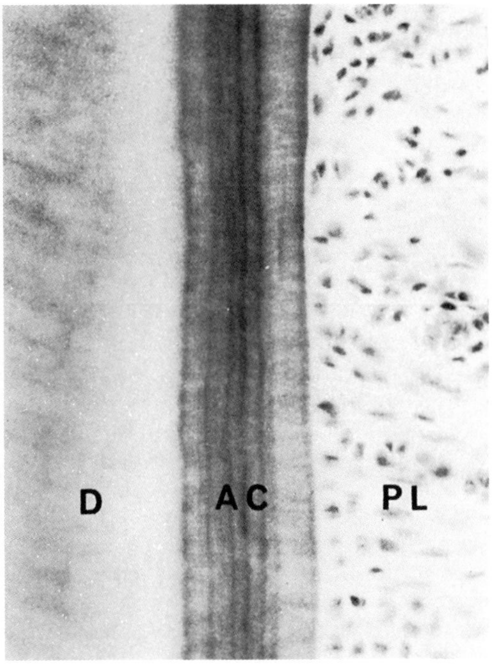

Figure 5-12 Acellular cementum *(AC)* showing incremental lines running parallel to the long axis of the tooth. These lines represent the appositional growth of cementum. Note the thin, light lines running into the cementum perpendicular to the surface; these represent Sharpey's fibers of the periodontal ligament *(PL)*. *D,* Dentin. (×300.)

Both acellular cementum and cellular cementum are arranged in lamellae separated by incremental lines parallel to the long axis of the root (see Figures 5-12 and 5-13). These lines represent "rest periods" in cementum formation and are more mineralized than the adjacent cementum.[129] In addition, loss of the cervical part of the reduced enamel epithelium at the time of tooth eruption may place portions of mature enamel in contact with the connective tissue, which then will deposit an acellular, afibrillar type of cementum over the enamel.[91]

Based on these findings, Schroeder[135,136] has classified cementum as follows:

Acellular afibrillar cementum (AAC) contains neither cells nor extrinsic or intrinsic collagen fibers, except for a mineralized ground substance. AAC is a product of cementoblasts and is found as coronal cementum in humans, with a thickness of 1 to 15 µm.

Acellular extrinsic fiber cementum (AEFC) is composed almost entirely of densely packed bundles of Sharpey's fibers and lacks cells. AEFC is a product of fibroblasts and cementoblasts and is found in

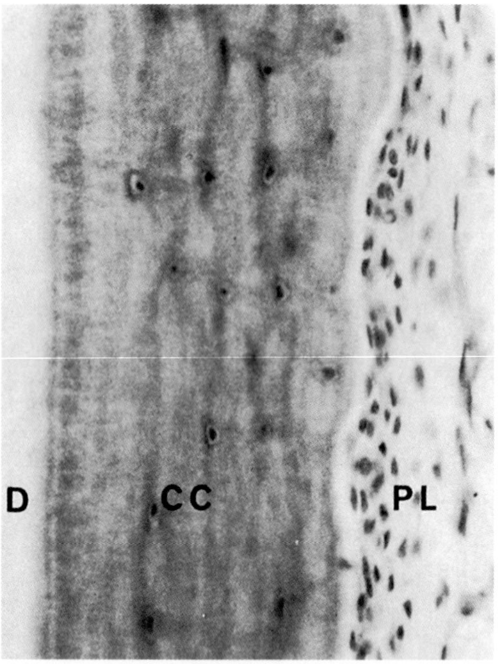

Figure 5-13 Cellular cementum *(CC)* showing cementocytes lying within lacunae. Cellular cementum is thicker than acellular cementum (see Figure 5-15). Evidence of incremental lines also exists, but they are less distinct than in acellular cementum. The cells adjacent to the surface of the cementum in the periodontal ligament *(PL)* space are cementoblasts. *D,* Dentin. (×300.)

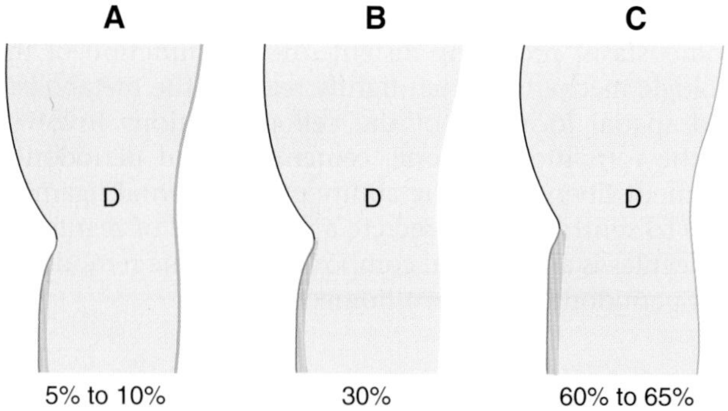

Figure 5-14 Normal variations in tooth morphology at the cementoenamel junction. **A,** Space between enamel and cementum with dentin *(D)* exposed. **B,** End-to-end relationship of enamel and cementum. **C,** Cementum overlapping the enamel.

the cervical third of roots in humans but may extend farther apically. Its thickness is between 30 and 230 μm.

Cellular mixed stratified cementum (CMSC) is composed of extrinsic (Sharpey's) and intrinsic fibers and may contain cells. CMSC is a co-product of fibroblasts and cementoblasts, and in humans it appears primarily in the apical third of the roots and apices and in furcation areas. Its thickness ranges from 100 to 1000 μm.

Cellular intrinsic fiber cementum (CIFC) contains cells, but no extrinsic collagen fibers. CIFC is formed by cementoblasts, and in humans it fills resorption lacunae.

Intermediate cementum is a poorly defined zone near the cementodentinal junction of certain teeth that appears to contain cellular remnants of Hertwig's sheath embedded in calcified ground substance.[43,90]

The inorganic content of cementum (hydroxyapatite; $Ca_{10}[Po_4]_6[OH]_2$) is 45% to 50%, which is less than that of bone (65%), enamel (97%), or dentin (70%).[171] Opinions differ about whether the microhardness increases[109] or decreases with age,[161] and no relationship has been established between aging and the mineral content of cementum.

It is well known that the protein extracts of mature cementum promote cell attachment and cell migration and stimulate protein synthesis of gingival fibroblasts and periodontal ligament cells.[134] Studies on cementum have identified adhesion proteins with RGD motifs (Arg-Gly-Asp sequences): bone sialoprotein, osteopontin, and osteonectin.[28,100] Bone sialoprotein and osteopontin are expressed during early tooth root development by cells along the root surface, and they are believed to play a major role in the differentiation of the cementoblast progenitor cells to the cementoblasts.[65,134]

Some of the molecules unique to the cementum have been described. Recent work has investigated the role of *cementum attachment protein* (CAP), a collagenous cementum-derived protein. CAP has been shown to promote the adhesion and spreading of mesenchymal cell types, with osteoblasts and periodontal ligament fibroblasts showing better adhesion than gingival fibroblasts and keratinocytes.[133] In addition, Ikezawa et al.[76] reported the characterization of *cementum-derived growth factor* (CGF), which is an insulin-like, growth factor I–like molecule. CGF has been shown to enhance proliferation of gingival fibroblasts and periodontal ligament cells.

Permeability of Cementum

In very young animals, acellular cementum and cellular cementum are very permeable and permit the diffusion of dyes from the pulp and external root surface. In cellular cementum the canaliculi in some areas are contiguous with the dentinal tubuli. The permeability of cementum diminishes with age.[25]

Cementoenamel Junction

The cementum at and immediately subjacent to the cementoenamel junction (CEJ) is of particular clinical importance in root-scaling procedures. Three types of relationships involving the cementum may exist at the CEJ.[110] In about 60% to 65% of cases, cementum overlaps the enamel (Figure 5-14); in about 30% an edge-to-edge butt joint exists; and in 5% to 10% the cementum and enamel fail to meet. In the last case, gingival recession may result in accentuated sensitivity because of exposed dentin.

Cementodentinal Junction

The terminal apical area of the cementum where it joins the internal root canal dentin is known as the cementodentinal junction (CDJ). When root canal treatment is performed, the obturating material should be at the CDJ. There appears to be no increase or decrease in the width of the CDJ with age; its width appears to remain relatively stable.[144] Scanning electron microscopy of the human teeth reveals that the CDJ is 2 to 3 μm wide. The fibril-poor layer contains a significant amount of proteoglycans, and fibrils intermingle between the cementum and dentin.[168,169]

Thickness of Cementum

Cementum deposition is a continuous process that proceeds at varying rates throughout life. Cementum formation is most rapid in the apical regions, where it compensates for tooth eruption, which itself compensates for attrition. The thickness of cementum on the coronal half of the root varies from 16 to 60 μm, or about the thickness of a hair. It attains its greatest thickness (up to 150-200 μm) in the apical third and in the furcation areas. It is thicker in distal surfaces than in mesial surfaces, probably because of functional stimulation from mesial drift over time.[40] Between 11 and 70 years of age, the average thickness of the cementum increases threefold, with the greatest increase in the apical region. Average thicknesses of 95 μm at age 20 and 215 μm at age 60 have been reported.[170]

Abnormalities in the thickness of cementum may range from an absence or paucity of cellular cementum (*cemental aplasia* or *hypoplasia*) to an excessive deposition of cementum (*cemental hyperplasia* or hypercementosis).[89]

The term *hypercementosis* refers to a prominent thickening of the cementum. It is largely an age-related phenomenon, and it may be localized to one tooth or affect the entire dentition. Because of considerable physiologic variation in the thickness of cementum among different teeth in the same person and also among different persons, distinguishing between hypercementosis and physiologic thickening of cementum is sometimes difficult. Nevertheless, excessive proliferation of cementum may occur in a broad spectrum of neoplastic and nonneoplastic conditions, including benign cementoblastoma, cementifying fibroma, periapical cemental dysplasia, florid cemento-osseous dysplasia, and other benign fibro-osseous lesions.[89]

Hypercementosis occurs as a generalized thickening of the cementum, with nodular enlargement of the apical third of the root. It also appears in the form of spikelike excrescences (cemental spikes) created by either the coalescence of cementicles that adhere to the root or the calcification of periodontal fibers at the sites of insertion into the cementum.[90]

Radiographically, the radiolucent shadow of the periodontal ligament and the radiopaque lamina dura are always seen on the outer border of an area of hypercementosis, enveloping it as it would in normal cementum.[89] On the other hand, from a diagnostic standpoint, periapical cemental dysplasia, condensing osteitis, and focal periapical osteopetrosis may be differentiated from hypercementosis because all these entities are located outside the shadow of the periodontal ligament and lamina dura.[164]

The etiology of hypercementosis varies and is not completely understood. The spikelike type of hypercementosis generally results from excessive tension from orthodontic appliances or occlusal forces. The generalized type occurs in a variety of circumstances. In teeth without antagonists, hypercementosis is interpreted as an effort to keep pace with excessive tooth eruption. In teeth subject to low-grade periapical irritation arising from pulp disease, it is considered compensation for the destroyed fibrous attachment to the tooth. The cementum is deposited adjacent to the inflamed periapical tissue. Hypercementosis of the entire dentition may occur in patients with Paget's disease.[131] Other systemic disturbances that may lead to or may be associated with hypercementosis include acromegaly, arthritis, calcinosis, rheumatic fever, and thyroid goiter.[89]

Hypercementosis itself does not require treatment. It could pose a problem if an affected tooth requires extraction. In multirooted tooth, sectioning of the tooth may be required before extraction.[10]

Cementum Resorption and Repair

Permanent teeth do not undergo physiologic resorption as do primary teeth. However, the cementum of erupted as well as unerupted teeth is subject to resorptive changes that may be of microscopic proportion, or sufficiently extensive to present a radiographically detectable alteration in the root contour. Microscopic cementum resorption is extremely common; in one study it occurred in 236 of 261 teeth (90.5%).[72] The average number of resorption areas per tooth was 3.5. Of the 922 areas of resorption, 708 (76.8%) were located in the apical third of the root, 177 (19.2%) in the middle third, and 37 (4.0%) in the gingival third. Approximately 70% of all resorption areas were confined to the cementum without involving the dentin.

Cementum resorption may be caused by local or systemic factors or may occur without apparent etiology (i.e., idiopathic). Local conditions causing cementum resorption include trauma from occlusion[113] (Figure 5-15); orthodontic movement[71,112,130]; pressure from malaligned erupting teeth, cysts, and tumors[86]; teeth without functional antagonists; embedded teeth; replanted and transplanted teeth[3,81]; periapical disease; and periodontal disease. Systemic conditions cited as predisposing to or inducing cemental resorption include calcium deficiency,[82] hypothyroidism,[13] hereditary fibrous osteodystrophy,[152] and Paget's disease.[131]

Cementum resorption appears microscopically as baylike concavities in the root surface. (Figure 5-16) Multinucleated giant cells and large mononuclear macrophages are generally found adjacent to cementum undergoing active resorption (Figure 5-17). Several sites of resorption may coalesce to form a large area of destruction. The resorptive process may extend into the underlying dentin and even into the pulp, but it is usually painless. Cementum resorption is not necessarily continuous and may alternate with periods of repair

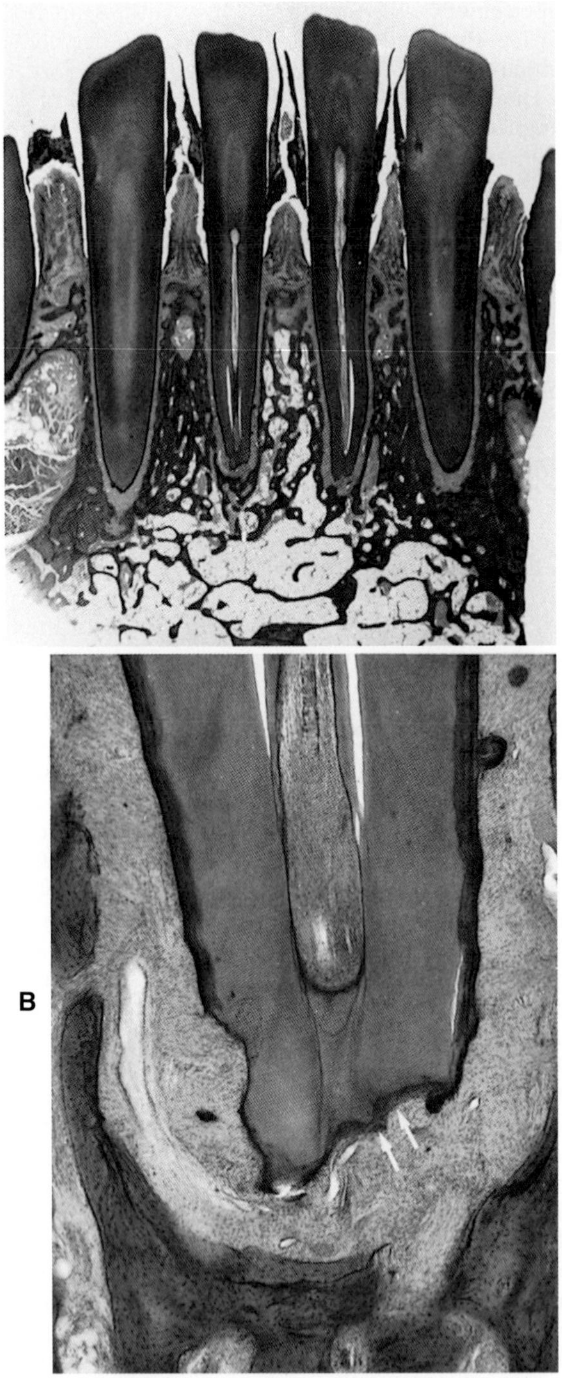

Figure 5-15 Cemental resorption associated with excessive occlusal forces. **A,** Low-power histologic section of mandibular anterior teeth. **B,** High-power micrograph of apex of left central incisor shortened by resorption of cementum and dentin. Note partial repair of the eroded areas *(arrows)* and cementicle at upper right.

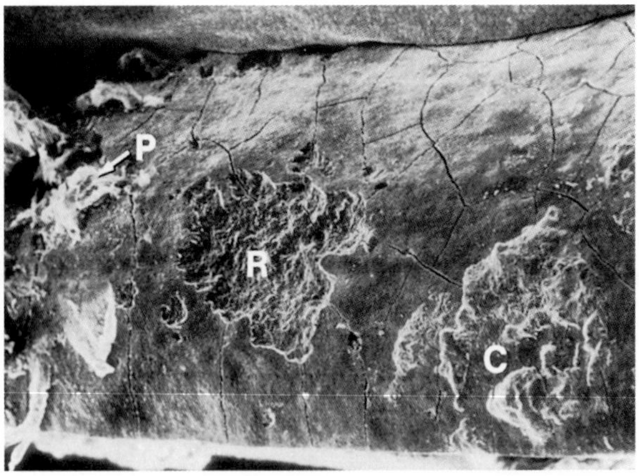

Figure 5-16 Scanning electron micrograph of root exposed by periodontal disease showing large resorption bay *(R)*. Remnants of the periodontal ligament *(P)* and calculus *(C)* are visible. Cracking of the tooth surface occurs as a result of the preparation technique. (×160.) (Courtesy Dr. John Sottosanti, La Jolla, Calif.)

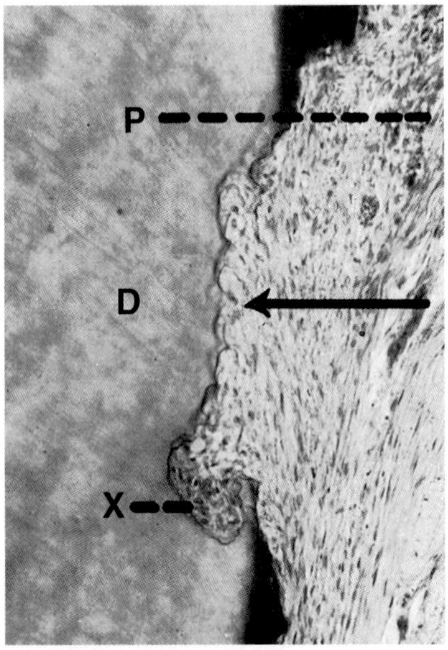

Figure 5-17 Resorption of cementum and dentin. A multinuclear osteoclast in seen at *X*. The direction of resorption is indicated by the arrow. Note the scalloped resorption front in the dentin *(D)*. The cementum is the darkly stained band at the upper and lower right. *P,* Periodontal ligament.

and the deposition of new cementum. The newly formed cementum is demarcated from the root by a deeply staining irregular line, termed a *reversal line,* which delineates the border of the previous resorption. A recent study showed that the reversal lines of human teeth contain a few collagen fibrils and highly accumulated proteoglycans with mucopolysaccharides (glycosaminoglycans), and that fibril intermingling occurs only in some places between reparative cementum and resorbed dentin or cementum.[168,169] Embedded fibers of the periodontal ligament reestablish a functional relationship in the new cementum.

Cementum repair requires the presence of viable connective tissue. If epithelium proliferates into an area of resorption, repair will not take place. Cementum repair can occur in devitalized as well as vital teeth.

Histologic evidence demonstrates that cementum formation is critical for appropriate maturation of the periodontium, both in development and in regeneration of lost periodontal tissues.[134] That is, a variety of macromolecules present in the extracellular matrix of the periodontium are likely to play a regulatory role in cementogenesis.[96] Regeneration of cementum requires cementoblasts, but the origin of the cementoblasts and the molecular factors regulating their recruitment and differentiation are not fully understood. Recent research, however, provides a better understanding; for example, the epithelial cell rests of Malassez are the only odontogenic epithelial cells that remain in the periodontium after the eruption of teeth, and they may have some function in cementum repair and regeneration under specific conditions.[68] The rests of Malassez may be related to cementum repair by activating their potential to secrete matrix proteins that have been expressed in tooth development, such as amelogenins, enamelins, and sheath proteins. Several growth factors have been shown to be effective in cementum regeneration, including members of the transforming growth factor superfamily (bone morphogenetic proteins), platelet-derived growth factor, insulin-like growth factor, and enamel matrix derivatives.[134]

Ankylosis

Fusion of the cementum and alveolar bone with obliteration of the periodontal ligament is termed *ankylosis.* Ankylosis occurs in teeth with cemental resorption, which suggests that it may represent a form of abnormal repair. Ankylosis also may develop after chronic periapical inflammation, tooth replantation, and occlusal trauma and around embedded teeth. This condition is relatively uncommon and occurs most frequently in the primary dentition.[101]

Ankylosis results in resorption of the root and its gradual replacement by bone tissue. For this reason, reimplanted teeth that ankylose will lose their roots after 4 to 5 years and will be exfoliated. Clinically, ankylosed teeth lack the physiologic mobility of normal teeth, which is one diagnostic sign for ankylotic resorption. In addition, these teeth usually have a special metallic percussion sound, and if the ankylotic process continues, they will be in infraocclusion.[51] However, clinical diagnosis of ankylosis by mobility and percussion tests alone is only reliable when at least 20% of the root surface is affected.[4]

As the periodontal ligament is replaced with bone in ankylosis, proprioception is lost because pressure receptors in the periodontal ligament are deleted or do not function correctly. Furthermore, the physiologic drifting and eruption of teeth can no longer occur, and thus the ability of the teeth and periodontium to adapt to altered force levels or directions of force is greatly reduced.[99] Radiographically, resorption lacunae are filled with bone, and the periodontal ligament space is missing.

Because no definitive causes can be found in ankylotic root resorption, no predictable treatment can be suggested. Treatment modalities range from a conservative approach, such as restorative intervention, to surgical extraction of the affected tooth.[107]

When titanium implants are placed in the jaw, healing results in bone that is formed in direct apposition to the implant without intervening connective tissue. This may be interpreted as a form of ankylosis. Because resorption of the metallic implant cannot occur, the implant remains indefinitely "ankylosed" to the bone. Also, a true periodontal pocket will not form because apical proliferation of the epithelium along the root, a key element of pocket formation, is not possible because of the ankylosis.

Exposure of Cementum to Oral Environment

Cementum becomes exposed to the oral environment in cases of gingival recession and as a result of loss of attachment in pocket formation. The cementum is sufficiently permeable to be penetrated in these cases by organic substances, inorganic ions, and bacteria. Bacterial invasion of the cementum occurs frequently in periodontal disease (see Chapter 27). Cementum caries can develop (see Chapter 35).

ALVEOLAR PROCESS

The alveolar process is the portion of the maxilla and mandible that forms and supports the tooth sockets (alveoli). It forms when the tooth erupts to provide the osseous attachment to the forming periodontal ligament; it disappears gradually after the tooth is lost.

Since the alveolar processes develop and undergo remodeling with the tooth formation and eruption, they are tooth-dependent bony structures.[135] Therefore the size, shape, location, and function of the teeth determine their morphology. Interestingly, although the growth and development of the bones of the jaw determine the position of the teeth, a certain degree of repositioning of teeth can be accomplished through occlusal forces and in response to orthodontic procedures that rely on the adaptability of the alveolar bone and associated periodontal tissues.[143]

The alveolar process consists of the following:

1. An external plate of cortical bone formed by haversian bone and compacted bone lamellae.
2. The inner socket wall of thin, compact bone called the *alveolar bone proper,* which is seen as the lamina dura in radiographs. Histologically, it contains a series of openings *(cribriform plate)* through which neurovascular bundles link the periodontal ligament with the central component of the alveolar bone, the cancellous bone.
3. Cancellous trabeculae, between these two compact layers, which act as supporting alveolar bone. The *interdental septum* consists of cancellous supporting bone enclosed within a compact border (Figure 5-18).

In addition, the bones of the jaw include the basal bone, which is the portion of the jaw located apically, but unrelated to the teeth (Figure 5-19).

The alveolar process is divisible into separate areas on an anatomic basis, but it functions as a unit, with all parts interrelated in the support of the teeth. Figures 5-20 and 5-21 show the relative proportions of cancellous bone and compact bone that form the alveolar process. Most of the facial and lingual portions of the sockets are formed by compact bone alone; cancellous bone

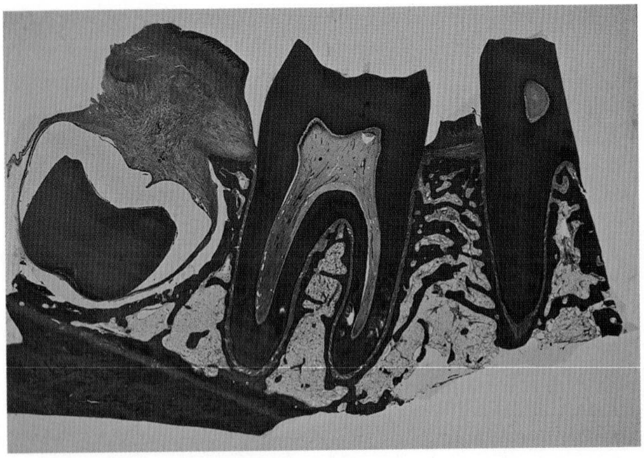

Figure 5-18 Mesiodistal section through mandibular molars of a 17-year-old female, obtained at autopsy. Note the interdental bony septa between first and second molar. The dense cortical bony plates represent the alveolar bone proper (cribriform plates) and are supported by cancellous bony trabeculae. The third molar is still in early stages of root formation and eruption.

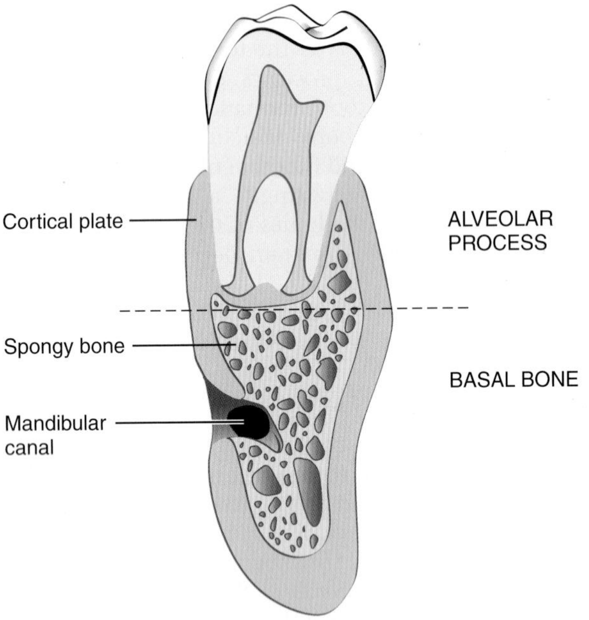

Figure 5-19 Section through human jaw with tooth in situ. The dotted line indicates the separation between basal bone and alveolar bone. (Redrawn from Ten Cate AR: *Oral histology: development, structure, and function,* ed 4, St Louis, 1994, Mosby.)

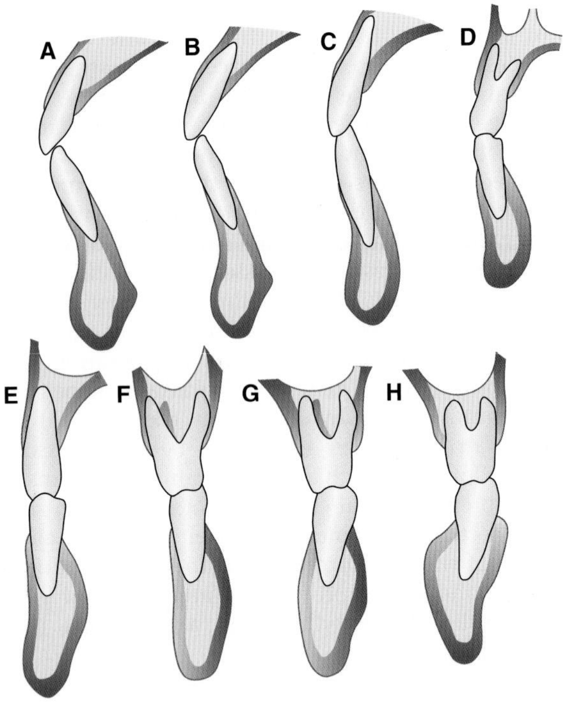

Figure 5-20 Relative proportions of cancellous bone and compact bone in a longitudinal faciolingual section of **A,** mandibular molars; **B,** lateral incisors; **C,** canines; **D,** first premolars; **E,** second premolars; **F,** first molars; **G,** second molars; and **H,** third molars.

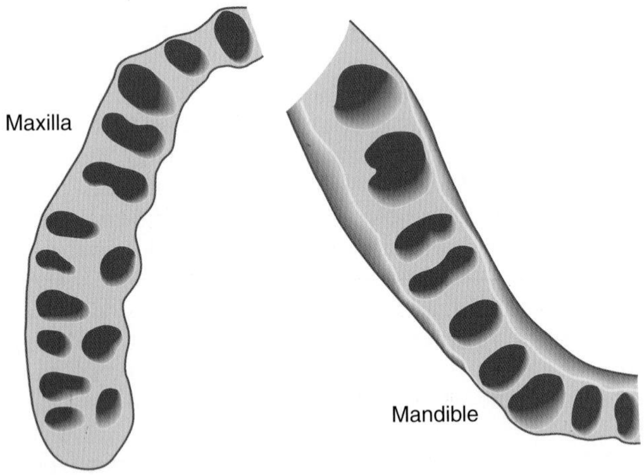

Figure 5-21 Shape of roots and surrounding bone distribution in a transverse section of maxilla and mandible at midroot level.

surrounds the lamina dura in apical, apicolingual, and interradicular areas.

Cells and Intercellular Matrix

Osteoblasts, the cells that produce the organic matrix of bone, are differentiated from pluripotent follicle cells. Alveolar bone is formed during fetal growth by intramembranous ossification and consists of a calcified matrix with osteocytes enclosed within spaces called *lacunae.* The osteocytes extend processes into *canaliculi* that radiate from the lacunae. The canaliculi form an anastomosing system through the intercellular matrix of the bone, which brings oxygen and nutrients to the osteocytes through the blood and removes metabolic waste products. Blood vessels branch extensively and travel through the periosteum. The endosteum lies adjacent to the marrow vasculature. Bone growth occurs by apposition of an organic matrix that is deposited by osteoblasts. Haversian systems *(osteons)* are the internal mechanisms that bring a vascular supply to bones too thick to be supplied only by surface vessels. These are found primarily in the outer cortical plates and the alveolar bone proper.

Bone consists of two-thirds inorganic matter and one-third organic matrix. The inorganic matter is composed principally of the minerals calcium and phosphate, along with hydroxyl, carbonate, citrate, and trace amounts of other ions,[59,60] such as sodium, magnesium, and fluorine. The mineral salts are in the form of hydroxyapatite crystals of ultramicroscopic size and constitute approximately two thirds of the bone structure.

The organic matrix[42] consists mainly of collagen type I (90%),[106] with small amounts of noncollagenous proteins such as osteocalcin, osteonectin, bone morphogenetic protein, phosphoproteins, and proteoglycans.[124] Osteopontin and bone sialoprotein are cell adhesion proteins that appear to be important for adhesion of both osteoclasts and osteoblasts.[92] In addition, paracrine factors, including cytokines, chemokines, and growth factors, have been implicated in the local control of mesenchymal condensations that occur at the onset of organogenesis. These factors probably play a prominent role in the development of the alveolar processes.[143]

Although the alveolar bone tissue is constantly changing in its internal organization, it retains approximately the same form from childhood through adult life. Bone deposition by osteoblasts is balanced by resorption by osteoclasts during tissue remodeling and renewal. It is well known that the number of osteoblasts decreases with aging; however, no remarkable change in the number of osteoclasts has ever been reported.[111]

Remodeling is the major pathway of bony changes in shape, resistance to forces, repair of wounds, and calcium and phosphate homeostasis in the body. Indeed, the coupling of bone resorption with bone formation constitutes one of the fundamental principles by which bone is necessarily remodeled throughout its life. Bone remodeling involves the coordination of activities of cells from two distinct lineages, the osteoblasts and the osteoclasts, which form and resorb the mineralized connective tissues of bone.[143]

Regulation of bone remodeling is a complex process involving hormones and local factors acting in an autocrine and a paracrine manner on the generation and activity of differentiated bone cells.[143] Bone contains 99% of the body's calcium ions and therefore is the major source for calcium release when the calcium blood levels decrease; this is monitored by the parathyroid gland. A decrease in blood calcium is mediated by receptors on the chief cells of the parathyroid glands, which then release parathyroid hormone (PTH). PTH stimulates osteoblasts to release interleukin-1 and interleukin-6, which stimulate monocytes to migrate into the bone area. Leukemia-inhibiting factor (LIF), secreted by osteoblasts, coalesces monocytes into multinucleated osteoclasts, which then resorb bone, releasing calcium ions from hydroxyapatite into the blood. This release normalizes the blood level of calcium. A feedback mechanism of normal blood levels of calcium turns off the secretion of PTH. Meanwhile, osteoclasts have resorbed organic matrix along with hydroxyapatite. The breakdown of collagen from the organic matrix releases various osteogenic substrates, which are covalently bound to collagen, and this in turn stimulates the differentiation of osteoblasts, which ultimately deposit bone. This interdependency of osteoblasts and osteoclasts in remodeling is called *coupling*.

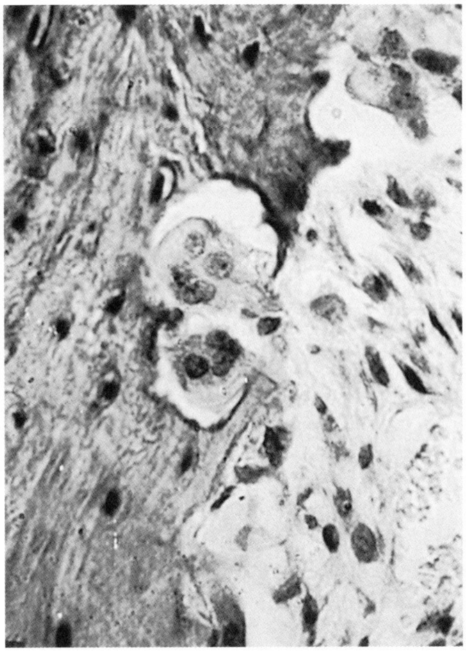

Figure 5-22 Rat alveolar bone. Histologic view of two multinucleated osteoclasts in Howship's lacuna.

The bone matrix that is laid down by osteoblasts is nonmineralized *osteoid*. While new osteoid is being deposited, the older osteoid located below the surface becomes mineralized as the mineralization front advances.

Bone resorption is a complex process morphologically related to the appearance of eroded bone surfaces (Howship's lacunae) and large, multinucleated cells (osteoclasts) (Figure 5-22). Osteoclasts originate from hematopoietic tissue[35,66,115] and are formed by the fusion of mononuclear cells of asynchronous populations.[17,85,117,149] When osteoclasts are active rather than resting, they possess an elaborately developed ruffled border from which hydrolytic enzymes are believed to be secreted.[157] These enzymes digest the organic portion of bone. The activity of osteoclasts and morphology of the ruffled border can be modified and regulated by hormones such as PTH (indirectly) and calcitonin, which has receptors on the osteoclast membrane.

Another mechanism of bone resorption involves the creation of an acidic environment on the bone surface, leading to the dissolution of the mineral component of bone. This event can be produced by different conditions, including a proton pump through the cell membrane of the osteoclast,[23] bone tumors, and local pressure,[115] translated through the secretory activity of the osteoclast.

Ten Cate[149] described the sequence of events in the resorptive process as follows:

1. Attachment of osteoclasts to the mineralized surface of bone.

2. Creation of a sealed acidic environment through action of the proton pump, which demineralizes bone and exposes the organic matrix.
3. Degradation of the exposed organic matrix to its constituent amino acids by the action of released enzymes, such as acid phosphatase and cathepsin.
4. Sequestering of mineral ions and amino acids within the osteoclast.

Notably, the cellular and molecular events involved in bone remodeling have a strong similarity to many aspects of inflammation and repair. The relationship between matrix molecules, such as osteopontin, bone sialoprotein, SPARC (secreted protein, acidic, rich in cysteine), and osteocalcin, and blood clotting and wound healing are clearly evident.[143]

Socket Wall

The socket wall consists of dense, lamellated bone, some of which is arranged in haversian systems and bundle bone. *Bundle bone* is the term given to bone adjacent to the periodontal ligament that contains a great number of Sharpey's fibers[163] (Figure 5-23). It is characterized by thin lamellae arranged in layers parallel to the root, with intervening appositional lines (Figure 5-24). Bundle bone is localized within the alveolar bone proper. Some Sharpey's fibers are completely calcified, but most contain an uncalcified central core within a calcified outer layer.[137] Bundle bone is not unique to the jaws; it occurs throughout the skeletal system wherever ligaments and muscles are attached.

The cancellous portion of the alveolar bone consists of trabeculae that enclose irregularly shaped marrow spaces lined with a layer of thin, flattened endosteal cells. Wide variation occurs in the trabecular pattern of cancellous bone,[116] which is affected by occlusal forces. The matrix of the cancellous trabeculae consists of irregularly arranged lamellae separated by deeply staining incremental and resorption lines indicative of previous bone activity, with an occasional haversian system.

Cancellous bone is found predominantly in the interradicular and interdental spaces and in limited amounts facially or lingually, except in the palate. In the adult human, more cancellous bone exists in the maxilla than in the mandible.

Bone Marrow

In the embryo and newborn the cavities of all bones are occupied by red hematopoietic marrow. The red marrow gradually undergoes a physiologic change to the fatty or yellow inactive type of marrow. In the adult the marrow of the jaw is normally of the latter type, and red marrow is found only in the ribs, sternum, vertebrae, skull, and humerus. However, foci of red bone marrow are occasionally seen in the jaws, often accompanied by resorption of bony trabeculae.[29] Common locations are the maxillary tuberosity, the maxillary and mandibular molar and premolar areas, and the mandibular symphysis and ramus angle, which may be visible radiographically as zones of radiolucency.

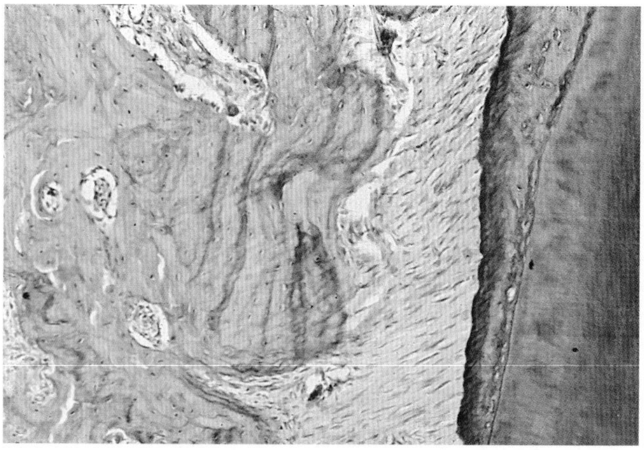

Figure 5-23 Deep penetration of Sharpey's fibers into bundle bone (rat molar).

Periosteum and Endosteum

Layers of differentiated osteogenic connective tissue cover all the bone surfaces. The tissue covering the outer surface of bone is termed *periosteum,* whereas the tissue lining the internal bone cavities is called *endosteum.*

The periosteum consists of an *inner layer* composed of osteoblasts surrounded by osteoprogenitor cells, which have the potential to differentiate into osteoblasts, and an *outer layer* rich in blood vessels and nerves and composed of collagen fibers and fibroblasts. Bundles of periosteal collagen fibers penetrate the bone, binding the periosteum to the bone. The endosteum is composed of a single layer of osteoblasts and sometimes a small amount of connective tissue. The inner layer is the osteogenic layer, and the outer layer is the fibrous layer.

Cellular events at the periosteum modulate bone size throughout an individual's life span, and change in bone size is probably the result of the balance between periosteal osteoblastic and osteoclastic activities. Currently, little is known about the control of periosteal osteoblastic activity or the clinical importance of variations in periosteal bone formation.[114] Moreover, the nature and impact of periosteal bone resorption are virtually unexplored.

Interdental Septum

The interdental septum consists of cancellous bone bordered by the socket wall cribriform plates (lamina dura or alveolar bone proper) of approximating teeth and the facial and lingual cortical plates (Figure 5-25). If the interdental space is narrow, the septum may consist of only the cribriform plate. In one study, for example, the space between mandibular second premolars and first molars consisted of cribriform plate and cancellous bone in 85% of the cases and only cribriform plate in the remaining 15%.[70] If roots are too close together, an irregular "window" can appear in the bone between adjacent roots (Figure 5-26). Between maxillary molars, the septum consisted of cribriform plate and cancellous

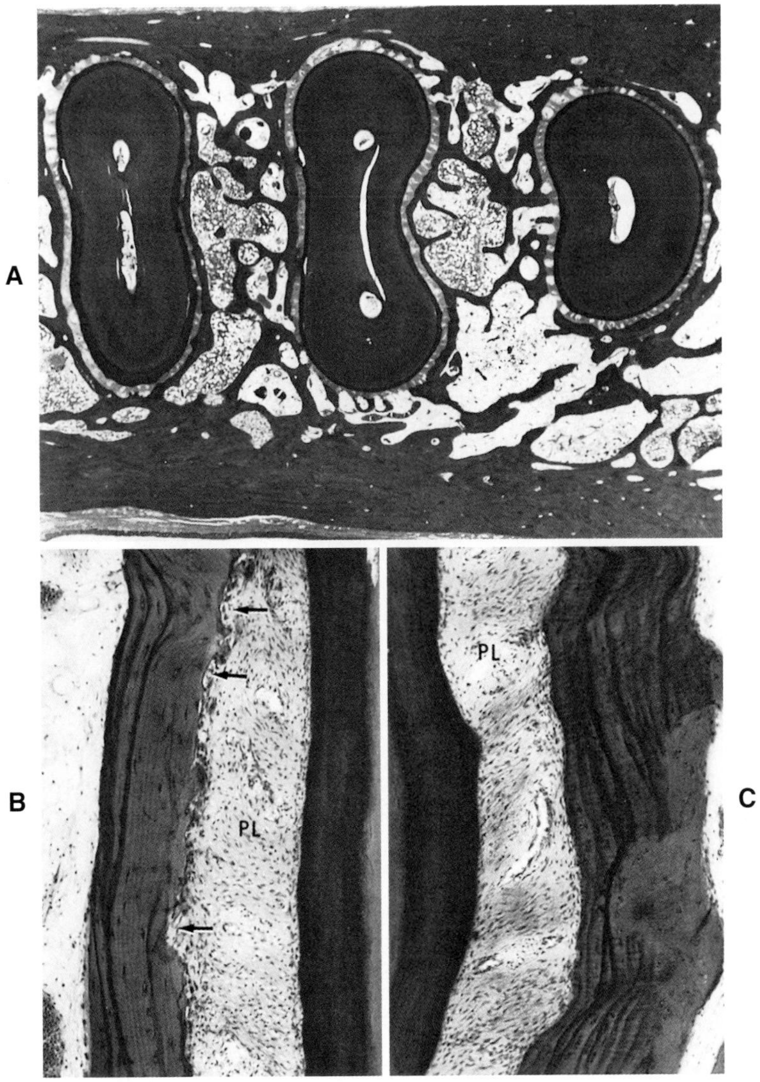

Figure 5-24 Bundle bone associated with physiologic mesial migration of the teeth. **A,** Horizontal section through molar roots in the process of mesial migration (*left,* mesial; *right,* distal). **B,** Mesial root surface showing osteoclasis of bone *(arrows).* **C,** Distal root surface showing bundle bone that has been partially replaced with dense bone on the marrow side. *PL,* Periodontal ligament.

bone in 66.6% of cases, was composed of only cribriform plate in 20.8%, and had a fenestration in 12.5%.[70]

Determining root proximity radiographically is important (see Chapter 36). The mesiodistal angulation of the crest of the interdental septum usually parallels a line drawn between the cementoenamel junctions of the approximating teeth.[124] The distance between the crest of the alveolar bone and the cementoenamel junction in young adults varies between 0.75 and 1.49 mm (average, 1.08 mm). This distance increases with age to an average of 2.81 mm.[53] However, this phenomenon may not be as much a function of age as of periodontal disease.

The mesiodistal and faciolingual dimensions and shape of the interdental septum are governed by the size and convexity of the crowns of the two approximating teeth, as well as by the position of the teeth in the jaw and their degree of eruption.[124]

Osseous Topography

The bone contour normally conforms to the prominence of the roots, with intervening vertical depressions that taper toward the margin (Figure 5-27). Alveolar bone anatomy varies among patients and has important clinical implications. The height and thickness of the facial and lingual bony plates are affected by the alignment of the teeth, angulation of the root to the bone, and occlusal forces.

On teeth in labial version, the margin of the labial bone is located farther apically than on teeth in proper alignment. The bone margin is thinned to a knife-edge and presents an accentuated arc in the direction of the apex. On teeth in lingual version, the facial bony plate is thicker than normal. The margin is blunt, rounded, and horizontal rather than arcuate. The effect of the root-to-bone angulation on the height of alveolar bone is

A
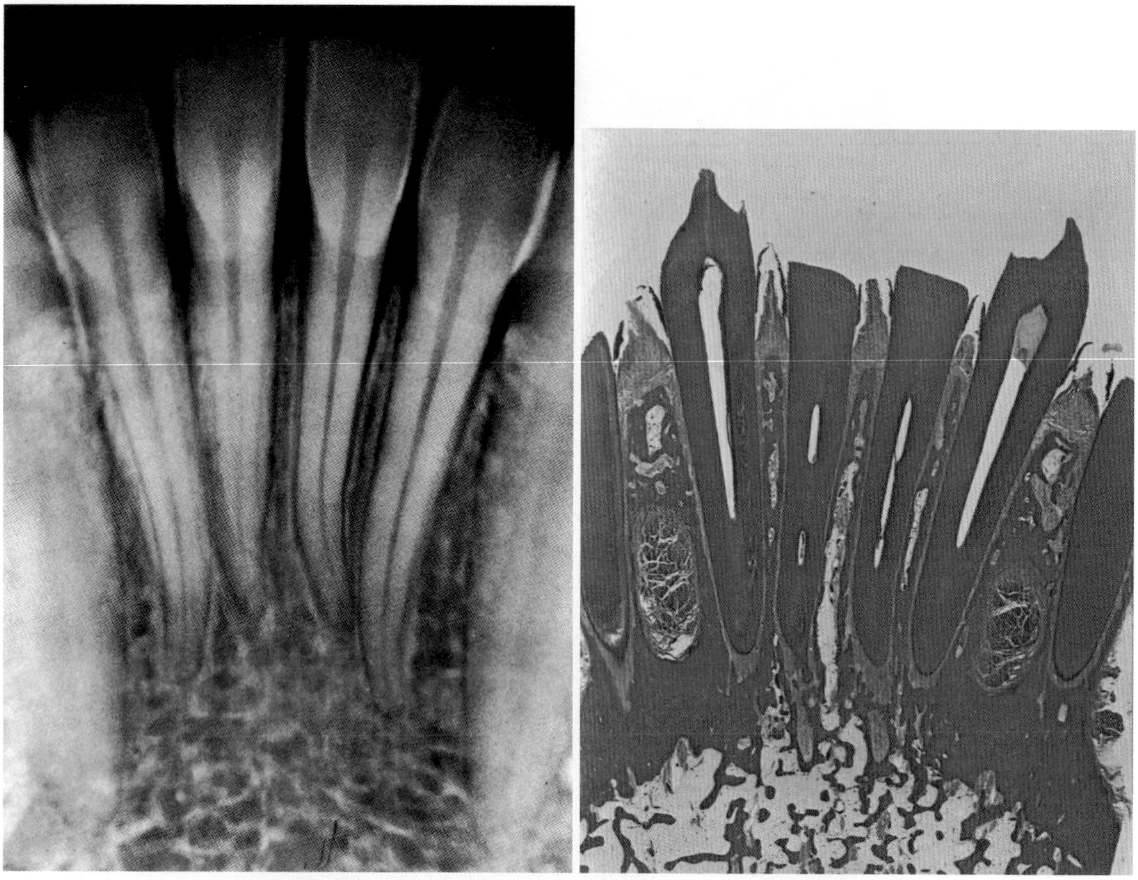
B

Figure 5-25 Interdental septa. **A,** Radiograph of mandibular incisor area. Note the prominent lamina dura. **B,** Interdental septa between the mandibular anterior teeth shown in *A*. There is a slight reduction in bone height with widening of the periodontal ligament in the coronal areas. The central cancellous portion is bordered by the dense bony cribriform plates of the socket, which form the lamina dura around the teeth in the radiograph. Attachments for the mentalis muscle are seen between the canine and lateral incisors. (From Glickman I, Smulow J: *Periodontal disease: clinical, radiographic, and histopathologic features,* Philadelphia, 1974, Saunders.)

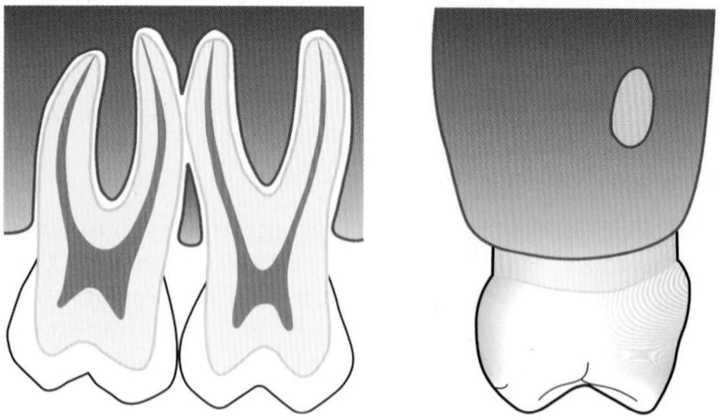

Figure 5-26 Boneless "window" between adjoining close roots of molars.

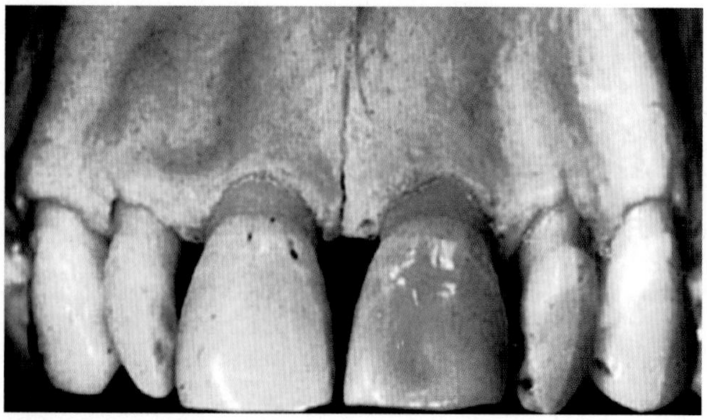

Figure 5-27 Normal bone contour conforms to the prominence of the roots.

most noticeable on the palatal roots of maxillary molars. The bone margin is located farther apically on the roots, which forms relatively acute angles with the palatal bone.[74] The cervical portion of the alveolar plate is sometimes considerably thickened on the facial surface, apparently as reinforcement against occlusal forces (Figure 5-28).

Fenestration and Dehiscence

Isolated areas in which the root is denuded of bone and the root surface is covered only by periosteum and overlying gingiva are termed *fenestrations*. In these areas the marginal bone is intact. When the denuded areas extend through the marginal bone, the defect is called a

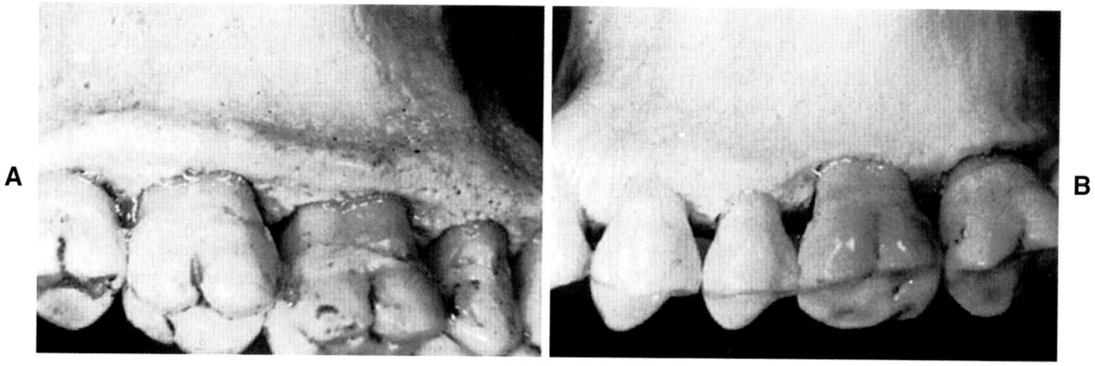

Figure 5-28 Variation in the cervical portion of the buccal alveolar plate. **A,** Shelflike conformation. **B,** Comparatively thin buccal plate.

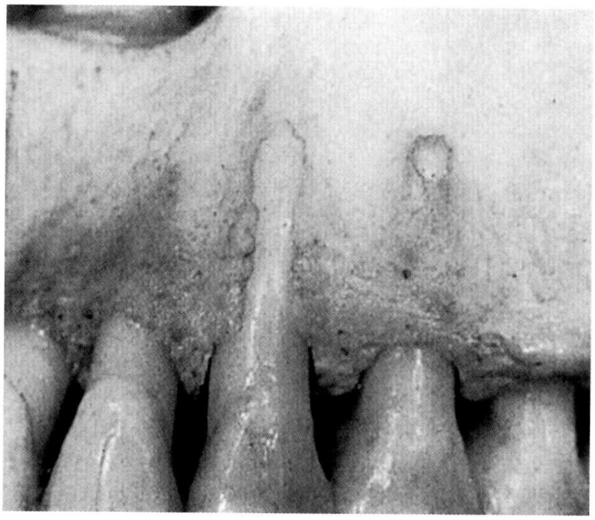

Figure 5-29 Dehiscence on the canine and fenestration of the first premolar.

dehiscence (Figure 5-29). Such defects occur on approximately 20% of the teeth; they occur more often on the facial bone than on the lingual bone, are more common on anterior teeth than on posterior teeth, and are frequently bilateral. Microscopic evidence of lacunar resorption may be present at the margins. The cause of these defects is not clear. Prominent root contours, malposition, and labial protrusion of the root combined with a thin bony plate are predisposing factors.[44] Fenestration and dehiscence are important because they may complicate the outcome of periodontal surgery.

Remodeling of Alveolar Bone

In contrast to its apparent rigidity, alveolar bone is the least stable of the periodontal tissues because its structure is in a constant state of flux. A considerable amount of internal remodeling takes place by means of resorption and formation, which is regulated by local and systemic influences. Local influences include functional requirements on the tooth and age-related changes in bone cells. Systemic influences are probably hormonal (e.g., parathyroid hormone, calcitonin, or vitamin D_3).

The remodeling of the alveolar bone affects its height, contour, and density, and this is manifested in the following three areas: adjacent to the periodontal ligament, in relation to the periosteum of the facial and lingual plates, and along the endosteal surface of the marrow spaces.

DEVELOPMENT OF THE ATTACHMENT APPARATUS

After the crown has formed, the stratum intermedium and the stellate reticulum of the enamel organ disappear. The outer and inner epithelia of the enamel organ remain and form *reduced enamel epithelium.* The apical portion of this constitutes *Hertwig's epithelial root sheath,* which will continue to grow apically and determines the shape of the root. Before the beginning of root formation, the root sheath bends horizontally at the future cementoenamel junction, narrowing the cervical opening and forming the *epithelial diaphragm.* The epithelial diaphragm separates the dental follicle from the dental papilla.

After root dentin formation starts, Hertwig's root sheath breaks up and partially disappears; the remaining cells form the epithelial clusters or strands known as *epithelial rests of Malassez* (see Figure 5-7, *A*). In multirooted teeth the epithelial diaphragm grows in such a way that tonguelike extensions develop horizontally, leaving spaces for each of the future roots to form.

The role of Hertwig's epithelial root sheath in root development, especially as it relates to the initiation of cementogenesis, has become a focus of research.[154] Based on various studies, it is now generally accepted that there is a transient period of secretion of proteins, including bone sialoprotein, osteopontin, and amelin, by the cells of Hertwig's epithelial root sheath.[26,48] In addition, research shows that growth and differentiation factors may play roles in the development of the attachment apparatus of periodontal tissues. Pluripotent dental follicle cells have been shown to differentiate into osteoblasts, cementoblasts, or periodontal fibroblasts.[138]

Cementum

The rupture of Hertwig's root sheath allows the mesenchymal cells of the dental follicle to contact the dentin, where they start forming a continuous layer of cementoblasts. Based on immunochemical and ultrastructural studies, Thomas[153] and others[24,93] have speculated that cementoblasts also can be of epithelial origin (Hertwig's root sheath), which would undergo an epithelial mesenchymal transformation.

Cementum formation begins by deposition of a meshwork of irregularly arranged collagen fibrils sparsely distributed in a ground substance or matrix called *precementum* or *cementoid.* This is followed by a phase of matrix maturation, which subsequently mineralizes to form cementum. Cementoblasts, which are initially separated from the cementum by uncalcified cementoid, sometimes become enclosed within the matrix and are trapped. Once they are enclosed, they are referred to as *cementocytes* and will remain viable in a manner similar to that of osteocytes.

A layer of connective tissue known as the *dental sac* surrounds the enamel organ, including the epithelial root sheath as it develops. The zone immediately in contact with the dental organ and continuous with the ectomesenchyme of the dental papilla is called the *dental follicle*[147,148,151] and consists of undifferentiated fibroblasts.

Periodontal Ligament

As the crown approaches the oral mucosa during tooth eruption, these fibroblasts become active and start producing collagen fibrils. They initially lack orientation, but they soon acquire an orientation oblique to the tooth. The first collagen bundles then appear in the region immediately apical to the cementoenamel junction and give rise to the gingivodental fiber groups. As tooth eruption progresses, additional oblique fibers appear and become attached to the newly formed cementum and bone. The transseptal and alveolar crest fibers develop when the tooth merges into the oral cavity. Alveolar bone deposition occurs simultaneously with periodontal ligament organization.[142]

Studies of the squirrel monkey have shown that during eruption, cemental Sharpey's fibers appear first, followed by Sharpey's fibers emerging from bone.[64] Sharpey's fibers are fewer in number and more widely spaced than those emerging from the cementum. At a later stage, alveolar fibers extend into the middle zone to join the lengthening cemental fibers and attain their classic orientation, thickness, and strength when occlusal function is established.

Early investigators had suggested that the individual fibers, rather than being continuous, consisted of two separate parts spliced together midway between the cementum and the bone in a zone that is called the *intermediate plexus*. The plexus has been reported in the periodontal ligament of continuously growing incisors, but not in the posterior teeth of rodents[73,102,172] or in actively erupting human and monkey teeth,[64] and not after teeth reach occlusal contact. Rearrangement of the fiber ends in the plexus is supposed to accommodate tooth eruption without necessitating the embedding of new fibers into the tooth and the bone.[102] The existence of such a plexus, however, has not been confirmed by radioautographic data and other studies, and it is considered a microscopic artifact.[136]

The developing periodontal ligament, as well as the mature periodontal ligament, contains undifferentiated stem cells that retain the potential to differentiate into osteoblasts, cementoblasts, and fibroblasts.[97]

Alveolar Bone

Just before mineralization, osteoblasts start producing matrix vesicles. These vesicles contain enzymes, such as alkaline phosphatase, that help jump-start the nucleation of hydroxyapatite crystals. As these crystals grow and develop, they form coalescing bone nodules, which, with fast-growing nonoriented collagen fibers, are the substructure of woven bone and the first bone formed in the alveolus. Later, through bone deposition, remodeling, and secretion of oriented collagen fibers in sheets, mature lamellar bone is formed.[18,19]

The hydroxyapatite crystals are generally aligned with their long axes parallel to the collagen fibers and appear to be deposited on and within the collagen fibers in mature lamellar bone. In this way, bone matrix is able to withstand the heavy mechanical stresses applied to it during function.

The alveolar bone develops around each tooth follicle during odontogenesis. When a deciduous tooth is shed, its alveolar bone is resorbed. The succedaneous permanent tooth moves into place, developing its own alveolar bone from its own dental follicle. As the tooth root forms and the surrounding tissues develop and mature, alveolar bone merges with the separately developing basal bone, and the two become one continuous structure. Although alveolar bone and basal bone have different intermediate origins, both are ultimately derived from neural crest ectomesenchyme.

Mandibular basal bone begins mineralization at the exit of the mental nerve from the mental foramen, whereas the maxillary basal bone begins at the exit of the infraorbital nerve from the infraorbital foramen.

Physiologic Migration of the Teeth

Tooth movement does not end when active eruption is completed and the tooth is in functional occlusion. With time and wear, the proximal contact areas of the teeth are flattened, and the teeth tend to move mesially. This is referred to as *physiologic mesial migration*. By age 40, it results in a reduction of about 0.5 cm in the length of the dental arch from the midline to the third molars. Alveolar bone is reconstructed in compliance with the physiologic mesial migration of the teeth. Bone resorption is increased in areas of pressure along the mesial surfaces of the teeth, and new layers of bundle bone are formed in areas of tension on the distal surfaces (see Figure 5-24).

EXTERNAL FORCES AND THE PERIODONTIUM

The periodontium exists for the purpose of supporting teeth during function and depends on the stimulation it receives from function for the preservation of its structure. Therefore a constant and sensitive balance is present between external forces and the periodontal structures.

TABLE 5-2

Comparison of Periodontal Width of Functioning and Functionless Teeth in a 38-Year-Old Man

	AVERAGE WIDTH OF PERIODONTAL SPACE (mm)		
	Entrance of Alveolus	**Middle of Alveolus**	**Fundus of Alveolus**
Heavy function: Left upper second bicuspid	0.35	0.28	0.30
Light function: Left lower first bicuspid	0.14	0.10	0.12
Functionless: Left upper third molar	0.10	0.06	0.06

Modified from Kronfeld R: *J Am Dent Assoc* 18:1242, 1931.

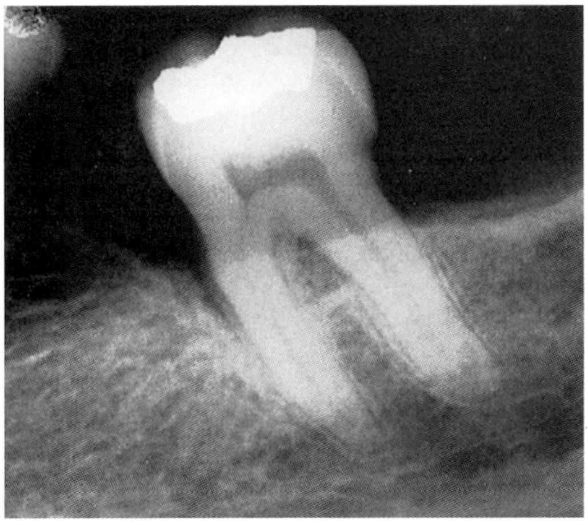

Figure 5-30 Bony trabeculae realigned perpendicular to the mesial root of tilted molar.

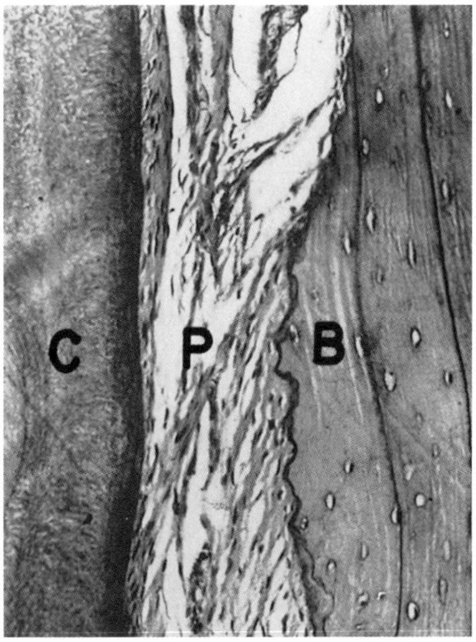

Figure 5-31 Atrophic periodontal ligament *(P)* of a tooth devoid of function. Note the scalloped edge of the alveolar bone *(B)*, indicating that resorption has occurred. *C*, Cementum.

Alveolar bone undergoes constant physiologic remodeling in response to external forces, particularly occlusal forces. Bone is removed from areas where it is no longer needed and added to areas where it is presently needed. The socket wall reflects the responsiveness of alveolar bone to external forces. Osteoblasts and newly formed osteoid line the socket in areas of tension; osteoclasts and bone resorption occur in areas of pressure. Forces exerted on the tooth also influence the number, density, and alignment of cancellous trabeculae. The bony trabeculae are aligned in the path of the tensile and compressive stresses to provide maximal resistance to the occlusal force with a minimum of bone substance[58,140] (Figure 5-30). When forces are increased, the cancellous bony trabeculae increase in number and thickness, and bone may be added to the external surface of the labial and lingual plates.

The periodontal ligament also depends on stimulation provided by function to preserve its structure. Within physiologic limits, the periodontal ligament can accommodate increased function with an increase in width (Table 5-2), a thickening of its fiber bundles, and an increase in diameter and number of Sharpey's fibers. Forces that exceed the adaptive capacity of the periodontium produce injury called *trauma from occlusion*. Since trauma from occlusion can only be confirmed histologically, the clinician is challenged to use clinical and radiographic surrogate indicators in an attempt to facilitate and assist in its diagnosis[67] (see Chapter 29).

When occlusal forces are reduced, the number and thickness of the trabeculae are reduced.[38] The periodontal ligament also atrophies, appearing thinned, and the fibers are reduced in number and density, disoriented,[5,123] and ultimately arranged parallel to the root surface (Figure 5-31). This phenomenon is termed *disuse atrophy* or *afunctional atrophy*. In this condition the cementum is either unaffected[38] or thickened, and the distance from the cementoenamel junction to the alveolar crest is increased.[119]

Decreased occlusal function causes changes in the periodontal microvasculature, such as occlusion of blood vessels and a decrease in the number of blood vessels.[75]

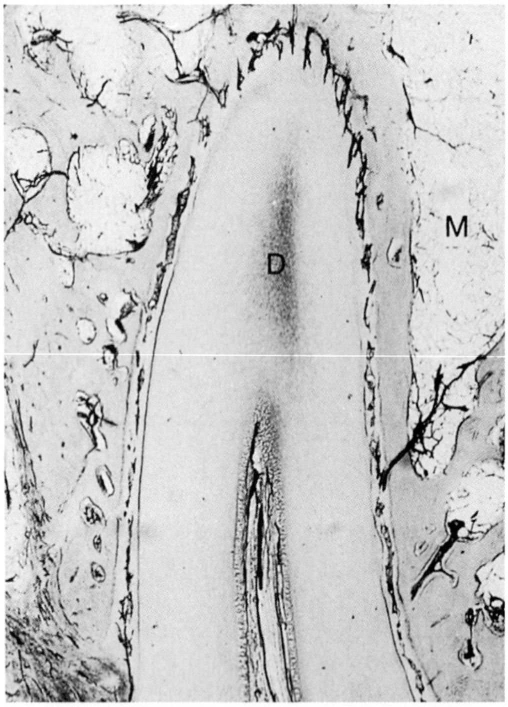

Figure 5-32 Vascular supply of monkey periodontium (perfused with India ink). Note the longitudinal vessels in the periodontal ligament and alveolar arteries passing through channels between the bone marrow *(M)* and periodontal ligament. *D,* Dentin. (Courtesy Dr. Sol Bernick, Los Angeles.)

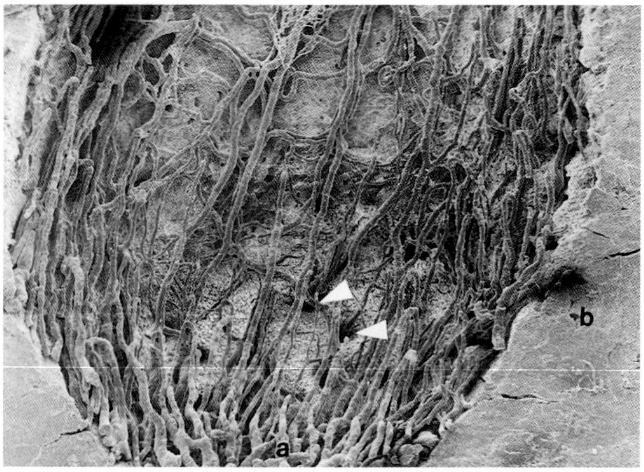

Figure 5-33 Vascular supply to the periodontal ligament in rat molar, as viewed by scanning electron microscopy after perfusion with plastic and tissue corrosion. Middle and apical areas of the periodontal ligament are shown with longitudinal blood vessels from apex *(below)* to gingiva *(above)*, perforating vessels entering the bone *(b)*, and many transverse connections *(arrowheads)*. Apical vessels *(a)* form a cap that connects with the pulpal vessels. (Courtesy NJ Selliseth and K Selvig, University of Bergen, Norway.)

For example, Murrell et al.[108] reported that the application and removal of orthodontic force produced significant changes in blood vessel number and density. However, no evidence-based explanation exists for why the force stimulated such changes in blood vessel number.

Orthodontic tooth movement is believed to result from site-specific bone remodeling in the absence of inflammation. It is well recognized that tensional forces will stimulate the formation and activity of osteoblastic cells, whereas compressive forces promote osteoclastic activity.[143]

VASCULARIZATION OF THE SUPPORTING STRUCTURES

The blood supply to the supporting structures of the tooth is derived from the inferior and superior alveolar arteries to the mandible and maxilla, and it reaches the periodontal ligament from three sources: apical vessels, penetrating vessels from the alveolar bone, and anastomosing vessels from the gingiva.[37] The branches of the apical vessels supply the apical region of the periodontal ligament before the vessels enter the dental pulp. The transalveolar vessels are branches of the intraseptal vessels that perforate the lamina dura and enter the ligament. The intraseptal vessels continue to vascularize the gingiva; these gingival vessels in turn anastomose with the periodontal ligament vessels of the cervical region.[47]

The vessels within the periodontal ligament are contained in interstitial spaces of loose connective tissue between the principal fibers and are connected in a netlike plexus that runs longitudinally and closer to the bone than the cementum[34] (Figures 5-32 and 5-33). The blood supply increases from the incisors to the molars; is greatest in the gingival third of single-rooted teeth, less in the apical third, and least in the middle; is equal in the apical and middle thirds of multirooted teeth; is slightly greater on the mesial and distal surfaces than on the facial and lingual surfaces; and is greater on the mesial surfaces of mandibular molars than on the distal surfaces.[22]

The vascular supply to the bone enters the interdental septa through nutrient canals together with veins, nerves, and lymphatics. Dental arterioles, which also branch off the alveolar arteries, send tributaries through the periodontal ligament, and some small branches enter the marrow spaces of the bone through the perforations in the cribriform plate. Small vessels emanating from the facial and lingual compact bone also enter the marrow and spongy bone.

The **venous drainage** of the periodontal ligament accompanies the arterial supply. Venules receive the blood through the abundant capillary network. Also, arteriovenous anastomoses bypass the capillaries; these are seen more frequently in apical and interradicular regions, and their significance is unknown.

Lymphatics supplement the venous drainage system. Lymphatic channels draining the region just beneath the junctional epithelium pass into the periodontal ligament and accompany the blood vessels into the periapical region.[30] From there, they pass through the alveolar bone to the inferior dental canal in the mandible or the infraorbital canal in the maxilla, then to the submaxillary lymph nodes.

REFERENCES

1. Ababneh KT, Hall RC, Embery G: Immunolocalization of glycosaminoglycans in ageing, healthy and periodontally diseased human cementum, *Arch Oral Biol* 43:235, 1998.
2. Ababneh KT, Hall RC, Embery G: The proteoglycans of human cementum: immunohistochemical localization in healthy, periodontally involved and ageing teeth, *J Periodontal Res* 34:87, 1999.
3. Agnew RG, Fong CC: Histologic studies on experimental transplantation of teeth, *J Oral Surg* 9:18, 1956.
4. Andersson L, Blomlof L, Lindskog S, et al: Tooth ankylosis: clinical, radiographic and histological assessments, *Int J Oral Surg* 13:423, 1984.
5. Anneroth G, Ericsson SG: An experimental histological study of monkey teeth without antagonist, *Odontol Rev* 18:345, 1967.
6. Avery JK, Rapp R: Pain conduction in human dental tissues, *Dent Clin North Am,* July 1959, p 489.
7. Bartold PM: Turnover in periodontal connective tissues: dynamic homeostasis of cells, collagen and ground substances, *Oral Dis* 1:238, 1995.
8. Bartold PM, Narayanan AS: *Biology of the periodontal connective tissues,* Chicago, 1998, Quintessence.
9. Bartold PM, Walsh LJ, Narayanan AS: Molecular and cell biology of the gingiva, *Periodontol 2000* 24:28, 2000.
10. Basdra EK, Stellzig A, Komposch G: Generalized hypercementosis in a young female patient, *Oral Surg Oral Med Oral Pathol Oral Radiol Endod* 83:418, 1997.
11. Bauer WH: Effect of a faultily constructed partial denture on a tooth and its supporting tissue, with special reference to formation of fibrocartilage in the periodontal membrane as a result of disturbed healing caused by abnormal stresses, *Am J Orthod Oral Surg* 27:640, 1941.
12. Baumhammers A, Stallard RE: S35-sulfate utilization and turnover by connective tissues of the periodontium, *J Periodontal Res* 3:187, 1968.
13. Becks H: Root resorptions and their relation to pathologic bone formation, *Int J Orthod Oral Surg* 22:445, 1936.
14. Beertsen W, McCullough CAG, Sodek J: The periodontal ligament: a unique, multifunctional connective tissue, *Periodontol 2000* 13:20, 1997.
15. Berkovitz BK: The structure of the periodontal ligament: an update, *Eur J Orthod* 12:51, 1990.
16. Berkovitz BK, Shore RC: Cells of the periodontal ligament. In: Berkovitz BK, Moxham BJ, Newman HE, editors: *The periodontal ligament in health and disease,* London, 1982, Pergamon.
17. Bernard GW, Ko JS: Osteoclast formation in vitro from bone marrow mononuclear cells in osteoclast-free bone, *Am J Anat* 161:415, 1981.
18. Bernard GW, Marvaso V: Matrix vesicles as an assay for primary tissue calcification *in vivo* and *in vitro.* In Ascenzi A, Bonucci B, DeBernard B, editors: *Matrix vesicles: Proceedings of the 3rd International Conference on Matrix Vesicles,* Milano, 1981, Wichtig.
19. Bernard GW, Pease DC: An electron microscopic study of initial intramembranous osteogenesis, *Am J Anat* 125:271, 1969.
20. Bernick S: Innervation of teeth and periodontium, *Dent Clin North Am* July 1959, p 503.
21. Bien SM: Hydrodynamic damping of tooth movement, *J Dent Res* 45:907, 1966.
22. Birn H: The vascular supply of the periodontal membrane: an investigation of the number and size of perforations in the alveolar wall, *J Periodontal Res* 1:51, 1966.
23. Blair HC, Teitelbaum SL, Ghiselli R, et al: Osteoclastic bone resorption by a polarized vacuolar proton pump, *Science* 245:855, 1989.
24. Blaushild N, Michaeli Y, Steigman S: Histomorphometric study of the periodontal vasculature of the rat incisor, *J Dent Res* 71:1908, 1992.
25. Blayney JR, Wassermann F, Groetzinger G, et al: Further studies in mineral metabolism of human teeth by the use of radioactive phosphorus, *J Dent Res* 29:559, 1941.
26. Bosshardt DD, Nanci A: Immunolocalization of epithelial and mesenchymal matrix constituents in association with inner enamel epithelial cells, *J Histochem Cytochem* 46:135, 1998.
27. Bosshardt DD, Schroeder HE: Cementogenesis reviewed: a comparison between human premolars and rodent molars, *Anat Rec* 245:267, 1996.
28. Bosshardt DD, Zalzal S, McKee MD, et al: Developmental appearance and distribution of bone sialoprotein and osteopontin in human and rat cementum, *Anat Rec* 250:13, 1998.
29. Box HK: Bone resorption in red marrow hyperplasia in human jaws, *Can Dent Res Found,* Bulletin 21, 1936.
30. Box KF: Evidence of lymphatics in the periodontium, *J Can Dent Assoc* 15:8, 1949.
31. Boyle PE: Tooth suspension: a comparative study of the paradental tissues of man and of the guinea pig, *J Dent Res* 17:37, 1938.
32. Carneiro J, Fava de Moraes F: Radioautographic visualization of collagen metabolism in the periodontal tissues of the mouse, *Arch Oral Biol* 10:833, 1955.
33. Carranza FA, Carranza FA Jr: The management of the alveolar bone in the treatment of the periodontal pocket, *J Periodontol* 27:29, 1956.
34. Carranza FA Jr, Itoiz ME, Cabrini RL, et al: A study of periodontal vascularization in different laboratory animals, *J Periodontal Res* 1:120, 1966.
35. Chambers TJ: The cellular basis of bone resorption, *Clin Orthop,* September 1980, p 283.
36. Ciancio SC, Neiders ME, Hazen SP: The principal fibers of the periodontal ligament, *Periodontics* 5:76, 1967.
37. Cohen L: Further studies into the vascular architecture of the mandible, *J Dent Res* 39:936, 1960.
38. Cohn SA: Disuse atrophy of the periodontium in mice, *Arch Oral Biol* 10:909, 1965.
39. Coolidge ED: The thickness of the human periodontal membrane, *J Am Dent Assoc* 24:1260, 1937.
40. Dastmalchi R, Polson A, Bouwsma O, et al: Cementum thickness and mesial drift, *J Clin Periodontol* 17:709, 1990.
41. Davies WR, Picton DC: Dimensional changes in the periodontal membrane of monkeys' teeth with horizontal thrusts, *J Dent Res* 46:114, 1967.
42. Eastoe JE: The organic matrix of bone. In Bourne GH, editor: *The biochemistry and physiology of bone,* New York, 1956, Academic Press.
43. El Mostehy MR, Stallard RE: Intermediate cementum, *J Periodontal Res* 3:24, 1968.
44. Elliot JR, Bowers GM: Alveolar dehiscence and fenestration, *Periodontics* 1:245, 1963.
45. Embery G, Waddington RJ, Hall RC, et al: Connective tissue elements as diagnostic aids in periodontology, *Periodontol 2000* 24:193, 2000.
46. Everts V, Niehof A, Jansen D, et al: Type VI collagen is associated with microfibrils and oxytalan fibers in the extracellular matrix of periodontium, mesenterium and periosteum, *J Periodontal Res* 33:118, 1998.
47. Folke LE, Stallard RE: Periodontal microcirculation as revealed by plastic microspheres, *J Periodontal Res* 2:53, 1967.
48. Fong CD, Slaby I, Hammarström L, et al: Amelin: an enamel-related protein, transcribed in the cells of epithelial root sheath, *J Bone Miner Res* 11:892, 1996.

49. Freeman E: The periodontium. In Ten Cate R, editor: *Oral histology,* ed 4, St Louis, 1994, Mosby.
50. Fullmer HM, Sheetz JH, Narkates AJ: Oxytalan connective tissue fibers: a review, *J Oral Pathol* 3:291, 1974.
51. Fuss Z, Tsesis I, Lin S: Root resorption: diagnosis, classification and treatment choices based on stimulation factors, *Dent Trauma* 19:175, 2003.
52. Gao Z, Flaitz CM, Mackenzie IC: Expression of keratinocyte growth factor in periapical lesions, *J Dent Res* 75:1658, 1996.
53. Gargiulo AW, Wentz FM, Orban B: Dimensions and relations of the dentogingival junction in humans, *J Periodontol* 32:261, 1961.
54. Gibson WA, Fullmer HM: Histochemistry of the periodontal ligament. I. The dehydrogenases, *Periodontics* 4:63, 1966.
55. Gibson WA, Fullmer HM: Histochemistry of the periodontal ligament. 2. The phosphatases, *Periodontics* 5:226, 1967.
56. Gibson WA, Fullmer HM: Histochemistry of the periodontal ligament. 3. The esterases, *Periodontics* 6:71, 1968.
57. Gillespie BR, Chasens AI, Brownstein CN, et al: The relationship between the mobility of human teeth and their supracrestal fiber support, *J Periodontol* 50:120, 1979.
58. Glickman I, Roeber FW, Brion M, et al: Photoelastic analysis of internal stresses in the periodontium created by occlusal forces, *J Periodontol* 41:30, 1970.
59. Glimcher MJ, Friberg UA, Levine PT: The identification and characterization of a calcified layer of coronal cementum in erupted bovine teeth, *J Ultrastruct Res* 10:76, 1964.
60. Glimcher MJ: The nature of the mineral component of bone and the mechanism of calcification. In Avioli LV, Krane SM, editors: *Metabolic bone disease and clinical related disorders,* Philadelphia, 1990, Saunders.
61. Goggins JF: The distribution of oxytalan connective tissue fibers in periodontal ligaments of deciduous teeth, *Periodontics* 4:182, 1966.
62. Gottlieb B: Biology of the cementum, *J Periodontol* 13:13, 1942.
63. Grant D, Bernick S: A possible continuity between epithelial rests and epithelial attachment in miniature swine, *J Periodontol* 40:87, 1969.
64. Grant D, Bernick S: Formation of the periodontal ligament, *J Periodontol* 43:17, 1972.
65. Grzesik WJ, Narayanan AS: Cementum and periodontal wound healing and regeneration, *Crit Rev Oral Biol Med* 13:474, 2002.
66. Hagel-Bradway S, Dziak R: Regulation of bone cell metabolism, *J Oral Pathol Med* 18:344, 1989.
67. Hallmon WW, Harrel SK: Occlusal analysis, diagnosis and management in the practice of periodontics, *Periodontol 2000* 34:151, 2004.
68. Hasegawa N, Kawaguchi H, Ogawa T, et al: Immunohistochemical characteristics of epithelial cell rests of Malassez during cementum repair, *J Periodontal Res* 38:51, 2003.
69. Hassell TM, Stanek EJ 3rd: Evidence that healthy human gingiva contains functionally heterogenous fibroblast subpopulations, *Arch Oral Biol* 28:617, 1983.
70. Heins PJ, Wieder SM: A histologic study of the width and nature of inter-radicular spaces in human adult premolars and molars, *J Dent Res* 65:948, 1986.
71. Hemley S: The incidence of root resorption of vital permanent teeth, *J Dent Res* 20:133, 1941.
72. Henry JL, Weinmann JP: The pattern of resorption and repair of human cementum, *J Am Dent Assoc* 42:270, 1951.
73. Hindle MC: Quantitative differences in periodontal membrane fibers, *J Dent Res* 43:953, 1964.
74. Hirschfeld I: A study of skulls in the American Museum of Natural History in relation to periodontal disease, *J Dent Res* 5:241, 1923.
75. Howard PS, Kucich U, Taliwal R, et al: Mechanical forces alter extracellular matrix synthesis by human periodontal ligament fibroblasts, *J Periodontal Res* 33:500, 1998.
76. Ikezawa K, Hart CE, Williams DC, et al: Characterization of cementum derived growth factor as an insulin-like growth factor-I like molecule, *Connect Tissue Res* 36:309, 1997.
77. Inoue M, Akiyoshi M: Histological investigation on Sharpey's fibers in cementum of teeth in abnormal function, *J Dent Res* 41:503, 1962.
78. Ishikawa G, Yamamoto H, Ito K, et al: Microradiographic study of cementum and alveolar bone, *J Dent Res* 43:936, 1964.
79. Johnson RB: A new look at the mineralized and unmineralized components of intraosseous fibers of the interdental bone of the mouse, *Anat Rec* 206:1, 1983.
80. Johnson RB, Pylypas SP: A re-evaluation of the distribution of the elastic meshwork within the periodontal ligament of the mouse, *J Periodontal Res* 27:239, 1992.
81. Jones ML, Aldred MJ, Hardy P: Tooth resorption in the two-stage transplantation technique: a case report, *Br J Orthod* 10:157, 1983.
82. Jones MR, Simonton FV: Mineral metabolism in relation to alveolar atrophy in dogs, *J Am Dent Assoc* 15:881, 1928.
83. Jones SJ, Boyde A: A study of human root cementum surfaces as prepared for and examined in the scanning electron microscope, *Z Zellforsch Mikrosk Anat* 130:318, 1972.
84. Junqueira LC, Carneiro J, Kelley RO: *Basic histology,* ed 6, Norwalk, Conn, 1989, Appleton & Lange.
85. Ko JS, Bernard GW: Osteoclast formation in vitro from bone marrow mononuclear cells in osteoclast-free bone, *Am J Anat* 161:415, 1981.
86. Kronfeld R: Histologic study of the influence of function on the human periodontal membrane, *J Am Dent Assoc* 18:1242, 1931.
87. Kronfeld R: The biology of cementum, *J Am Dent Assoc* 25:1451, 1938.
88. Larjava H, Häkkinen L, Rahemtulla F: A biochemical analysis of human periodontal tissue proteoglycans, *Biochem J* 284:267, 1992.
89. Leider AS, Garbarino VE: Generalized hypercementosis, *Oral Surg Oral Med Oral Pathol* 63:375, 1987.
90. Lester KS: The incorporation of epithelial cells by cementum, *J Ultrastruct Res* 27:63, 1969.
91. Listgarten MA: A light and electron microscopic study of coronal cementogenesis, *Arch Oral Biol* 13:93, 1968.
92. Mackie EJ: Osteoblasts: novel roles in orchestration of skeletal architecture, *Int J Biochem Cell Biol* 35:1301, 2003.
93. MacNeil RL, Thomas HF: Development of the murine periodontium. II. Role of the epithelial root sheath in formation of the periodontal attachment, *J Periodontol* 64:285, 1993.
94. MacNeil RL, Berry JE, Strayhorn CL, et al: Expression of type I and XII collagen during development of the periodontal ligament in the mouse, *Arch Oral Biol* 43:779, 1998.
95. Maeda T, Kannari K, Sato O, et al: Nerve terminals in human periodontal ligament as demonstrated by immunohistochemistry for neurofilament protein (NFP) and S-100 protein, *Arch Histol Cytol* 53:259, 1990.
96. Matias MA, Li H, Young WG, et al: Immunohistochemical localization of fibromodulin in the periodontium during cementogenesis and root formation in the rat molar, *J Periodontal Res* 38:502, 2003.
97. McCulloch CA: Basic considerations in periodontal wound healing to achieve regeneration, *Periodontol 2000* 1:16, 1993.

98. McCulloch CA, Melcher AH: Cell density and cell generation in the periodontal ligament of mice, *Am J Anat* 167:43, 1983.
99. McCulloch CA, Lekic P, McKee MD: Role of physical forces in regulating the form and function of the periodontal ligament, *Periodontol 2000* 24:56, 2000.
100. McKee MD, Zalzal S, Nanci A: Extracellular matrix in tooth cementum and mantle dentin: localization of osteopontin and other noncollagenous proteins, plasma proteins, and glycoconjugates by electron microscopy, *Anat Rec* 245:293, 1996.
101. McNamara TG, O'Shea D, McNamara CM, et al: The management of traumatic ankylosis during orthodontics: a case report, *J Clin Pediatr Dent* 24:265, 2000.
102. Melcher AH: Remodeling of the periodontal ligament during eruption of the rat incisor, *Arch Oral Biol* 12:1649, 1967.
103. Mikola OJ, Bauer WH: "Cementicles" and fragments of cementum in the periodontal membrane, *Oral Surg Oral Med Oral Pathol* 2:1063, 1949.
104. Miller EJ: A review of biochemical studies on the genetically distinct collagens of the skeletal system, *Clin Orthop* 92:260, 1973.
105. Mühlemann HR: The determination of tooth rotation centers, *Oral Surg* 7:392, 1954.
106. Mühlemann HR, Zander HA, Halberg F: Mitotic activity in the periodontal tissues of the rat molar, *J Dent Res* 33:459, 1954.
107. Mullally BH, Blakely D, Burden DJ: Ankylosis: an orthodontic problem with a restorative solution, *Br Dent J* 179:426, 1995.
108. Murrell EF, Yen EH, Johnson RB: Vascular changes in the periodontal ligament after removal of orthodontic forces, *Am J Orthod Dentofac Orthop* 110:280, 1996.
109. Nihei I: A study on the hardness of human teeth, *J Osaka Univ Dent Soc* 4:1, 1959.
110. Noyes FB, Schour I, Noyes HJ: *A textbook of dental histology and embryology,* ed 5, Philadelphia, 1938, Lea & Febiger.
111. Ogasawara T, Yoshimine Y, Kiyoshima T, et al: In situ expression of RANKL, RANK, osteoprotegerin and cytokines in osteoclasts of rat periodontal tissue, *J Periodontal Res* 39:42, 2004.
112. Oppenheim A: Human tissue response to orthodontic intervention of short and long duration, *Am J Orthodont Oral Surg* 28:263, 1942.
113. Orban B: Tissue changes in traumatic occlusion, *J Am Dent Assoc* 15:2090, 1928.
114. Orwoll ES: Toward an expanded understanding of the role of the periosteum in skeletal health, *J Bone Miner Res* 18:949, 2003.
115. Otero RL, Parodi RJ, Ubios AM, et al: Histologic and histometric study of bone resorption after tooth movement in rats, *J Periodontal Res* 8:327, 1973.
116. Parfitt GJ: An investigation of the normal variations in alveolar bone trabeculation, *Oral Surg Oral Med Oral Pathol* 15:1453, 1962.
117. Parodi RJ, Ubios AM, Mayo J, et al: Total body irradiation effects on the bone resorption mechanism in rats subjected to orthodontic movement, *J Oral Pathol* 2:1, 1973.
118. Picton DC, Davies WI: Dimensional changes in the periodontal membrane of monkeys *(Macaca irus)* due to horizontal thrusts applied to the teeth, *Arch Oral Biol* 12:1635, 1967.
119. Pihlstrom BL, Ramfjord SP: Periodontal effect of nonfunction in monkeys, *J Periodontol* 42:748, 1971.
120. Raisz LG, Rodan GA: Cellular basis for bone turnover. In Avioli LV, Krane SM, editors: *Metabolic bone disease and clinical related disorders,* Philadelphia, 1990, Saunders.
121. Rao LG, Wang HM, Kalliecharan R, et al: Specific immunohistochemical localization of type I collagen in porcine periodontal tissues using the peroxidase-labelled antibody technique, *Histochem J* 11:73, 1979.
122. Reeve CM, Wentz FM: The prevalence, morphology and distribution of epithelial rests in the human periodontal ligament, *Oral Surg Oral Med Oral Pathol* 15:785, 1962.
123. Rippin JW: Collagen turnover in the periodontal ligament under normal and altered functional forces. II. Adult rat molars, *J Periodontal Res* 13:149, 1978.
124. Ritchey B, Orban B: The crests of the interdental alveolar septa, *J Periodontol* 24:75, 1953.
125. Roberts WE, Chamberlain JG: Scanning electron microscopy of the cellular elements of rat periodontal ligament, *Arch Oral Biol* 23:587, 1978.
126. Romaniuk K: Some observations of the fine structure of human cementum, *J Dent Res* 46:152, 1967.
127. Romanos GE, Schroter-Kermani C, Bernimoulin J-P: Das Kollagen als Basis-element des Parodonts: Immunohistochemische Aspekte bein Menschen und bei Tieren, *Parodontologie* 1:47, 1991.
128. Romanos G, Schroter-Kermani C, Hinz N, et al: Immunohistochemical distribution of the collagen types IV, V and VI and glycoprotein laminin in the healthy rat, marmoset *(Callithrix jacchus)* and human gingivae, *Matrix* 11:125, 1991.
129. Romanos GE, Schroter-Kermani C, Hinz N, et al: Immunohistochemical localization of collagenous components in healthy periodontal tissues of the rat and marmoset *(Callithrix jacchus)*. I. Distribution of collagens type I and III, *J Periodontal Res* 27:101, 1992.
130. Rudolph CE: An evaluation of root resorption occurring during orthodontic treatment, *J Dent Res* 19:367, 1940.
131. Rushton MA: The dental tissues in osteitis deformans, *Guy's Hosp Rep* 88:163, 1938.
132. Saffar JL, Lasfargues JJ, Cherruau M: Alveolar bone and the alveolar process: the socket that is never stable, *Periodontol 2000* 13:76, 1997.
133. Saito M, Narayana AS: Signaling reactions induced in human fibroblasts during adhesion to cementum-derived attachment protein, *J Bone Miner Res* 14:65, 1999.
134. Saygin NE, Giannobile WV, Somerman MJ: Molecular and cell biology of cementum, *Periodontol 2000* 24:73, 2000.
135. Schroeder H: *Oral structural biology,* New York, 1991, Time Medical Publishers.
136. Schroeder HE: *The periodontium,* Berlin, 1986, Springer-Verlag.
137. Selvig KA: The fine structure of human cementum, *Acta Odontol Scand* 23:423, 1965.
138. Sena K, Morotome Y, Baba O, et al: Gene expression of growth differentiation factors in the developing periodontium of rat molars, *J Dent Res* 82:166, 2003.
139. Shackleford JM: The indifferent fiber plexus and its relationship to principal fibers of the periodontium, *Am J Anat* 131:427, 1971.
140. Sicher H, DuBrul EL: *Oral anatomy,* ed 6, St Louis, 1975, Mosby.
141. Simpson HE: The degeneration of the rest of Malassez with age as observed by the apoxestic technique, *J Periodontol* 36:288, 1965.
142. Sodek J: A comparison of the rates of synthesis and turnover of collagen and non-collagen proteins in adult rat periodontal tissues and skin using a microassay, *Arch Oral Biol* 22:655, 1977.
143. Sodek J, McKee MD: Molecular and cellular biology of alveolar bone, *Periodontol 2000* 24:99, 2000.
144. Stein TJ, Corcoran JF: Anatomy of the root apex and its histologic changes with age, *Oral Surg, Oral Med Oral Pathol* 69:238, 1990.

145. Tadokoro O, Maeda T, Heyeraas KJ, et al: Merkel-like cells in Malassez epithelium in the periodontal ligament of cats: an immunohistochemical, confocal-laser scanning and immuno electron-microscopic investigation, *J Periodontal Res* 37:456, 2002.
146. Ten Cate AR: The histochemical demonstration of specific oxidative enzymes and glycogen in the epithelial cell rests of Malassez, *Arch Oral Biol* 10:207, 1965.
147. Ten Cate AR: The development of the periodontium. In Melcher AH, Bowen WH, editors: *Biology of the periodontium,* New York, 1969, Academic Press.
148. Ten Cate AR: Formation of supporting bone in association with periodontal ligament organization in the mouse, *Arch Oral Biol* 20:137, 1975.
149. Ten Cate AR: Hard tissue formation and destruction. In Ten Cate AR, editor: *Oral histology: development, structure, and function,* ed 4, St Louis, 1994, Mosby.
150. Ten Cate AR, Deporter DA: The degradative role of the fibroblast in the remodeling and turnover of collagen in soft connective tissue, *Anat Rec* 182:1, 1975.
151. Ten Cate AR, Mills C, Solomon G: The development of the periodontium: a transplantation and autoradiographic study, *Anat Rec* 170:365, 1971.
152. Thoma KH, Sosman MC, Bennett GA: An unusual case of hereditary fibrous osteodystrophy (fragilitas ossium) with replacement of dentine by osteocementum, *Am J Orthodont Oral Surg* 29:1, 1943.
153. Thomas HF: Root formation, *Int J Dev Biol* 39:231, 1995.
154. Thomas HF, Kollar EJ: Tissue interactions in normal murine root development. In Davidovitch Z, editor: *The biological mechanisms of tooth eruption and root resorption,* Birmingham, 1988, EBSCO Media.
155. Trowbridge HO, Shibata F: Mitotic activity in epithelial rests of Malassez, *Periodontics* 5:109, 1967.
156. Ubios AM, Cabrini RL: Tritiated thymidine uptake in periodontal tissue subject to orthodontic movement, *J Dent Res* 50:1160, 1971.
157. Vaes G: Cellular biology and biochemical mechanism of bone resorption: a review of recent developments on the formation, activation, and mode of action of osteoclasts, *Clin Orthop* 231:239, 1988.
158. Valderhaug JP, Nylen MU: Function of epithelial rests as suggested by their ultrastructure, *J Periodontal Res* 1:69, 1966.
159. Valderhaug JP, Zander H: Relationship of "epithelial rests of Malassez" to other periodontal structures, *Periodontics* 5:254, 1967.
160. Vandevska-Radunovic V, Kvinnsland IH, Kvinnsland S, et al: Immunocompetent cells in rat periodontal ligament and their recruitment incident to experimental orthodontic tooth movement, *Eur J Oral Sci* 105:36, 1997.
161. Warren EB, Hansen NM, Swartz ML, et al: Effects of periodontal disease and of calculus solvents on microhardness of cementum, *J Periodontol* 35:505, 1964.
162. Watanabe T, Kubota T: Characterization of fibromodulin isolated from bovine periodontal ligament, *J Periodontal Res* 33:1, 1998.
163. Weinmann JP, Sicher H: *Bone and bones: fundamentals of bone biology,* ed 2, St Louis, 1955, Mosby.
164. Wood NK, Goaz PW: *Differential diagnosis of oral lesions,* ed 2, St Louis, 1984, Mosby.
165. Woodnutt DA, Wager-Miller J, O'Neill PC, et al: Neurotrophin receptors and nerve growth factor are differentially expressed in adjacent nonneuronal cells of normal and injured tooth pulp, *Cell Tissue Res* 299:225, 2000.
166. Worapamorn W, Li H, Pujic Z, et al: Expression and distribution of cell-surface proteoglycans in the normal Lewis rat molar periodontium, *J Periodontal Res* 35:214, 2000.
167. Yamamoto T, Wakita M: Bundle formation of principal fibers in rat molars, *J Periodontal Res* 27:20, 1992.
168. Yamamoto T, Domon T, Takahashi S, et al: The fibrillar structure of cement lines on resorbed root surfaces of human teeth, *J Periodontal Res* 35:208, 2000.
169. Yamamoto T, Domon T, Takahashi S, et al: The fibrous structure of the cemento-dentinal junction in human molars shown by scanning electron microscopy combined with NaOH-maceration, *J Periodontal Res* 35:59, 2000.
170. Zander HA, Hurzeler B: Continuous cementum apposition, *J Dent Res* 37:1035, 1958.
171. Zipkin J: The inorganic composition of bones and teeth. In Schraer H, editor: *Biological calcification,* New York, 1970, Appleton-Century-Crofts.
172. Zwarych PD, Quigley MB: The international plexus of the periodontal ligament history and further observations, *J Dent Res* 44:383, 1965.

Aging and the Periodontium

Ian Needleman

CHAPTER

6

■ ■ ■

CHAPTER OUTLINE

EFFECTS OF AGING ON THE PERIODONTIUM
 Gingival Epithelium
 Gingival Connective Tissue
 Periodontal Ligament
 Cementum
 Alveolar Bone

Bacterial Plaque
Immune Responses
EFFECTS OF AGING ON PROGRESSION OF
 PERIODONTAL DISEASE
AGING AND RESPONSE TO TREATMENT OF THE
 PERIODONTIUM

*I*ncreased health awareness and improvements in preventive dentistry have led to decreasing tooth loss for all age groups. The effects of this shift in tooth retention need to be considered carefully. In particular, increased life expectancy and greater health expectations may lead to changes in demand from older individuals for periodontal treatment. Therefore, an understanding of the impact of aging on the periodontium is critical. This chapter first reviews the literature concerning the fundamental aspects of aging on the periodontal tissues, then examines broader aspects of aging and the possible effects on treatment outcomes.

The evidence base is not without problems, many of which make it difficult to draw conclusions on the effects of aging. Some of these problems include inconsistency in the definition of a true "older" group, inadequate exclusion of adults with systemic diseases that can modify study findings, and attempts to extrapolate results from animal research. For the purposes of this chapter, the effects of aging are limited to a narrow review of possible biologic and microbiologic changes.* The reader should

be fully aware that this excludes many important age-associated phenomena, including the reduction in an individual's cognitive or motor function skills, which may have a direct impact on periodontal management. Chapter 45 discusses these issues in more detail.

Since this chapter was first written 5 years ago, little new research has been generated that investigates the impact of aging. However, much effort and many resources have been employed in researching questions partially related to this topic. These include the effect of periodontal infection on general health (see Chapter 18) and the impact of osteoporosis on periodontal status (see Chapter 43).

EFFECTS OF AGING ON THE PERIODONTIUM

Gingival Epithelium

Thinning and decreased keratinization of the gingival epithelium have been reported with age.[35] The significance of these findings could mean an increase in epithelial permeability to bacterial antigens, a decreased resistance to functional trauma, or both. If so, such changes might influence long-term periodontal outcomes. However, other studies have found no age-related differences in the gingival epithelium of humans or dogs.[7,16] Other reported changes with aging include the flattening of rete

*For further reading on the effects of aging on the dental and periodontal patient, the reader should consult Holm-Pederson P, editor: *Textbook of geriatric dentistry,* ed 2, Copenhagen, 1996, Munksgaard; and Ellen RP, editor: Periodontal disease among older adults, *Periodontol 2000* 16, 1998.

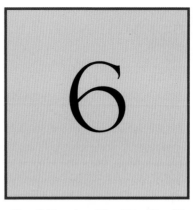

SCIENCE TRANSFER

From a purely physiologic perspective, the effect of aging is clinically insignificant with regard to increased risk of loss of periodontal support. However, other aspects such as cognitive and behavioral factors may be highly influential to oral health and may be affected by ageing. Similarly and importantly, this holds true for the alveolar bone and for bony healing. Thus the extraction of teeth at virtually any age in healthy patients results in healing of the extraction site by means of osseous filling. Likewise, endosseous dental implants can be placed in older patients with the same success rate as in younger patients. These examples reinforce that the oral cavity, as in other areas of the body, responds in physiologic terms and is therefore somewhat predictable based on physiology. Plaque will stimulate inflammation in all patients, and removal of plaque decreases this physiologic response. As with tooth extraction, periodontal surgery results in a wound that heals in a predicable sequence of events. *Thus, understanding physiologic responses is the basis for understanding many of the events that occur in the oral cavity.*

Older patients have an equal ability to resist the progression of the plaque-induced attachment loss as younger patients, and thus, in this respect, they can be managed in the same manner. There may be less bone regeneration capacity with increasing age, although this needs to be confirmed in clinical studies before recommendations can be made for treatment planning.

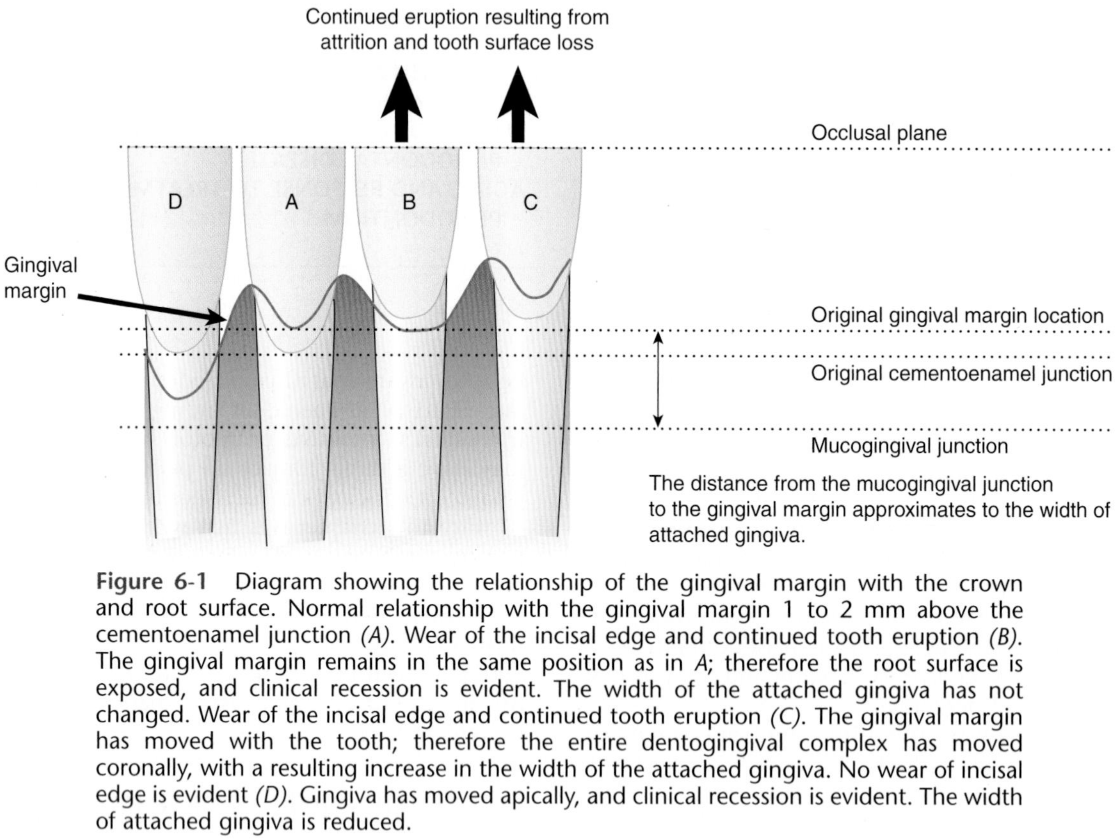

Figure 6-1 Diagram showing the relationship of the gingival margin with the crown and root surface. Normal relationship with the gingival margin 1 to 2 mm above the cementoenamel junction *(A)*. Wear of the incisal edge and continued tooth eruption *(B)*. The gingival margin remains in the same position as in *A*; therefore the root surface is exposed, and clinical recession is evident. The width of the attached gingiva has not changed. Wear of the incisal edge and continued tooth eruption *(C)*. The gingival margin has moved with the tooth; therefore the entire dentogingival complex has moved coronally, with a resulting increase in the width of the attached gingiva. No wear of incisal edge is evident *(D)*. Gingiva has moved apically, and clinical recession is evident. The width of attached gingiva is reduced.

pegs and altered cell density. Conflicting data regarding surgical regeneration times for gingival epithelium have been ascribed to problems in research methodology.[38]

The effect of aging on the location of the junctional epithelium has been the subject of much speculation. Some reports show migration of the junctional epithelium from its position in healthy individuals (i.e., on enamel) to a more apical position on the root surface, with accompanying gingival recession.[7] In other animal studies, however, no apical migration has been noted.[19] With continuing gingival recession, the width of the attached gingiva would be expected to decrease with age, but the opposite appears to be true.[2,3] Alternatively, the migration of the junctional epithelium to the root surface could be caused by the tooth erupting through the gingiva in an attempt to maintain occlusal contact with its opposing tooth (passive eruption) as a result of tooth surface loss from attrition (Figure 6-1). The consensus is

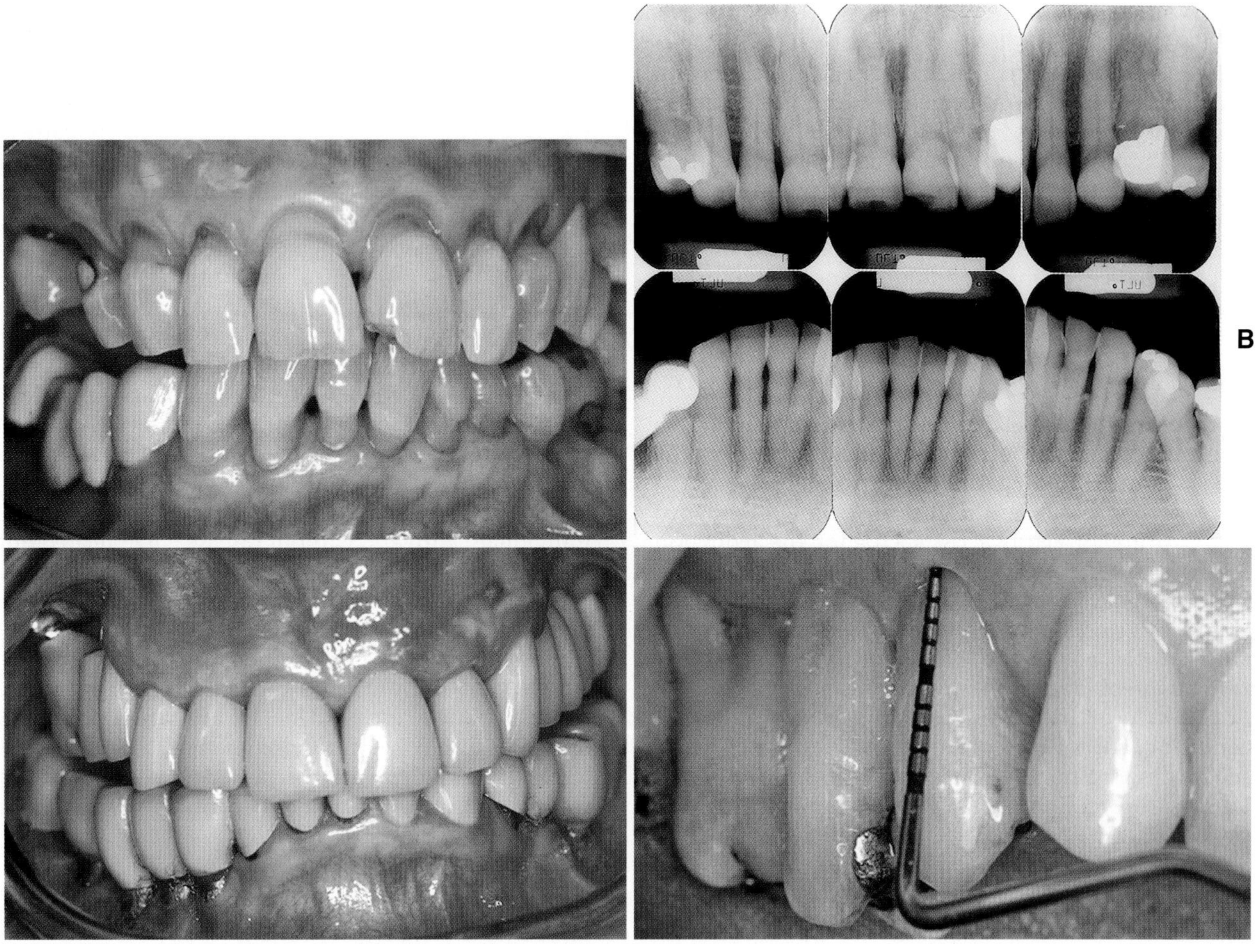

Figure 6-2 Three scenarios illustrating the variation in the position of the gingival margin with age. **A,** Overeruption with recession in older individual (68-year-old woman) with generalized recession and history of periodontitis (treated). Note some overeruption of lower anterior teeth and wear of teeth related to oral hygiene measures. **B,** Radiographs of the patient in *A.* **C,** Overeruption without recession in an older individual (72-year-old woman) with no periodontitis but marked wear of lower incisors and overeruption. Note how the gingival margin has migrated coronally with the erupting teeth. **D,** Extensive recession in young individual (32-year-old man) with marked recession and no history of periodontitis. The recession has resulted from a combination of anatomically thin tissues and toothbrush-related trauma.

that gingival recession is not an inevitable physiologic process of aging but is explained by cumulative effects of inflammation or trauma on the periodontium[6,7] (see later discussion) (Figure 6-2).

Gingival Connective Tissue

Increasing age results in coarser and denser gingival connective tissues.[41] Qualitative and quantitative changes to collagen include an increased rate of conversion of soluble to insoluble collagen, increased mechanical strength, and increased denaturing temperature. These results indicate increased collagen stabilization caused by changes in the macromolecular conformation.[23] Not surprisingly, a greater collagen content has been found in the gingivae of older animals despite a lower rate of collagen synthesis with age.[7,23,38]

Periodontal Ligament

Changes in the periodontal ligament reported with aging include decreased numbers of fibroblasts and a more irregular structure, paralleling the changes in the gingival connective tissues.[7,23,38] Other findings include decreased organic matrix production and epithelial cell rests and increased amounts of elastic fiber.[38] Conflicting results have been reported for changes in the width of the periodontal ligament in human and animal models. Although true variation might exist, this finding probably reflects the functional status of the teeth in the studies, because the width of the space will decrease if the tooth is unopposed (hypofunction) or will increase with excessive occlusal loading.[23,38] Both scenarios might be anticipated as a result of tooth loss in this population. These effects also might explain the variability in studies reporting qualitative changes within the periodontal ligament.

Cementum

Some consensus exists regarding aging effects on cementum. An increase in cemental width is a common finding; this increase may be 5 to 10 times with increasing age.[7] This finding is not surprising because deposition continues after tooth eruption. The increase in width is greater apically and lingually.[38] Although cementum has limited capacity for remodeling, an accumulation of resorption bays explains the finding of increasing surface irregularity.[13]

Alveolar Bone

Reports of morphologic changes in alveolar bone mirror age-related changes in other bony sites. Specific to the periodontium are findings of a more irregular periodontal surface of bone and less regular insertion of collagen fibers.[38] Although age is a risk factor for the reduction of bone mass in osteoporosis, it is not causative and therefore should be distinguished from physiologic aging processes.[15] Overriding the diverse observations of bony changes with age is the important finding that the healing rate of bone in extraction sockets appears to be unaffected by increasing age.[4] Indeed, the success of osseointegrated dental implants, which rely on intact bone-healing responses, does not appear to be age related.[8] However, balancing this view is the observation that bone graft preparations (decalcified freeze-dried bone) from donors more than 50 years old possessed significantly less osteogenic potential than graft material from younger donors.[34] The possible significance of this phenomenon on normal healing responses needs to be investigated.

Bacterial Plaque

Dentogingival plaque accumulation has been suggested to increase with age.[14] This might be explained by the increase in hard tissue surface area resulting from gingival recession and the surface characteristics of the exposed root surface as a substrate for plaque formation compared with enamel. Other studies have shown no difference in plaque quantity with age. This contradiction might reflect the different age ranges of experimental groups with variable degrees of gingival recession and root surface exposure. For supragingival plaque, no real qualitative differences have been shown for plaque composition.[14] For subgingival plaque, one study has shown similar subgingival flora to a normal flora, whereas another study reported increased numbers of enteric rods and pseudomonads in older adults.[27,37] Mombelli[26] suggests caution in the interpretation of this finding because of increased oral carriage of these species among older adults. It has been speculated that a shift occurs in the importance of certain periodontal pathogens with age, specifically including an increased role for *Porphyromonas gingivalis* and a decreased role for *Actinobacillus actinomycetemcomitans*. However, differentiating true age effects from the changes in ecologic determinants for periodontal bacteria will be difficult.[26]

Immune Responses

Recent advances in the study of the effects of aging on the immune response *(immunosenescence)* have altered the understanding of this phenomenon. In particular, more recent studies have set tighter controls on excluding individuals with systemic conditions known to affect the immune response. As a result, age has been recognized as having much less effect in altering the host response than previously thought.[17,24] Differences between young and older individuals can be demonstrated for T and B cells, cytokines, and natural killer cells, but not for polymorphonuclear cells and macrophage activity. McArthur[24] concludes, "Measurement of indicators of immune and inflammatory competency suggested that, within the parameters tested, there was no evidence for age-related changes in host defenses correlating with periodontitis in an elderly (65 to 75 years) group of individuals, with and without disease." Age-related differences in the inflammatory response in gingivitis have been clearly demonstrated and are discussed later in this textbook.

In summary, although many contradictions exist, a survey of the literature demonstrates that some age related changes are evident in the periodontium and host response. Whether these changes are significant in altering the progression of periodontal diseases or the response of an older adult to periodontal treatment is examined next.

EFFECTS OF AGING ON PROGRESSION OF PERIODONTAL DISEASE

In a classic experimental gingivitis study, subjects were rendered plaque and inflammation free through frequent professional cleaning. Once this was achieved, the subjects abstained from oral hygiene measures for periods of 3 weeks to allow gingivitis to develop.[22] In this experimental model, a comparison of developing gingivitis between young and older individuals demonstrated a greater inflammatory response in older subjects, both in humans and dogs.[7,11,12,14] In the older age group (65-80 years), the findings included a greater size of infiltrated connective tissue, increased gingival crevicular fluid flow, and increased gingival index.[11,12] Other studies have not demonstrated differences between subjects; this may be related to smaller differences between the ages of the younger and older experimental groups.[42] Intriguingly, even at the baseline level of excellent gingival health before commencing plaque accumulation, differences may exist between groups, with older individuals demonstrating more inflammation.[11,12]

The phrase "getting long in the tooth" expresses a widespread belief that age is inevitably associated with an increased loss of connective tissue attachment. However, this observation might equally well reflect a cumulative exposure to a number of potentially destructive processes. These exposures might include plaque-associated periodontitis, chronic mechanical trauma from toothbrushing, and iatrogenic damage from unfavorable restorative dentistry or repeated scaling and root planing. The effects of these exposures act in one direction only (i.e., increased loss of attachment).[39]

In an attempt to differentiate the effects of age from these other processes, several studies have been designed to eliminate confounding issues and address more clearly the question of age as a risk factor for periodontitis. A *risk factor* is defined as an exposure or factor that increases the probability that the disease (periodontitis) will occur.[31] The conclusions from these studies are strikingly consistent and show that the effect of age either is nonexistent or provides a small and clinically insignificant increased risk of loss of periodontal support.[9,21,28,31,32] Indeed, in comparison with the odds ratio of 20.52 for poor oral hygiene status and periodontitis, the odds ratio for age was only 1.24,[1] and smoking is much more influential than age.[28] Therefore, age has been suggested as being not a true risk factor but a background or an associated factor for periodontitis.[31] In addition, the recent reports of a genetic basis for susceptibility to severe forms of periodontitis underline the overriding importance of plaque, smoking, and susceptibility in explaining most of the variation in periodontal disease severity between individuals.[18,25] A longitudinal study of essentially untreated periodontitis in an elderly Japanese population (at least 70 years of age) indicated that 296 of 394 individuals (75%) had a least one site with loss of attachment of 3 mm or more over a 2-year period.[29] Smoking and baseline attachment level of 6 mm or more were significantly associated with the disease progression.

AGING AND RESPONSE TO TREATMENT OF THE PERIODONTIUM

The successful treatment of periodontitis requires both meticulous plaque control by the patient at home and meticulous supragingival and subgingival débridement by the therapist.[10] Unfortunately, only a few studies have directly compared such an approach among patients of different age groups. These few studies clearly demonstrate that despite the histologic changes in the periodontium with aging, no differences in response to nonsurgical or surgical treatment have been shown for periodontitis.[5,20,40] If plaque control is not ideal, however, continued loss of attachment is inevitable. Attempts to aid plaque control by chemical means have also been reported.[36]

A purely biologic or physiologic review indicates that the effects of aging on the structure of the periodontium, the function of the immune response, and the nature of either supragingival or subgingival plaque have a negligible impact on an individual's experience with periodontal disease. Aging might affect other aspects of managing periodontal health, such as the risk of root caries[33] (see Chapter 45), and the resulting difficulties should not be underestimated. Interestingly, a recent study has identified greater compliance with supportive maintenance among older individuals than younger patients.[30]

REFERENCES

1. Abdellatif HM, Burt BA: An epidemiological investigation into the relative importance of age and oral hygiene status as determinants of periodontitis, *J Dent Res* 66:13, 1987.
2. Ainamo A, Ainamo J, Poikkeus R: Continuous widening of the band of attached gingiva from 23 to 65 years of age, *J Periodontal Res* 16:595, 1981.
3. Ainamo J, Talari A: The increase with age of the width of attached gingiva, *J Periodontal Res* 11:182, 1976.
4. Amler MH: Age factor in human alveolar bone repair, *J Oral Impl* 19:138, 1993.
5. Axelsson P, Lindhe J, Nystrom B: On the prevention of caries and periodontal disease: results of a 15-year longitudinal study in adults, *J Clin Periodontol* 18:182, 1991.
6. Baker DL, Seymour GJ: The possible pathogenesis of gingival recession: a histological study of induced recession in the rat, *J Clin Periodontol* 3:208, 1976.
7. Berglundh T: Clinical and structural characteristics of periodontal tissues in young and old dogs, *J Clin Periodontol* 18:616, 1991.
8. Bryant SR, Zarb GA: Osseointegration of oral implants in older and younger adults, *Int J Maxillofac Impl* 13:492, 1998.
9. Burt BA: Periodontitis and aging: reviewing recent evidence, *J Am Dent Assoc* 125:273, 1994.
10. Cobb CM: Nonsurgical pocket therapy: mechanical, *Ann Periodontol* 1:443, 1996.
11. Fransson C, Berglundh T, Lindhe J: The effect of age on the development of gingivitis, *J Clin Periodontol* 23:379, 1996.
12. Fransson C, Mooney J, Kinane DF, et al: Differences in the inflammatory response in young and old human subjects during the course of experimental gingivitis, *J Clin Periodontol* 26:453, 1999.
13. Grant D, Bernick S: The periodontium of aging humans, *J Periodontol* 43:660, 1972.
14. Holm-Pedersen P, Agerbaek N, Theilade E: Experimental gingivitis in young and elderly individuals, *J Clin Periodontol* 2:14, 1975.
15. Jeffcoat MK: Osteoporosis: a possible modifying factor in oral bone loss, *Ann Periodontol* 3:312, 1998.
16. Karring T, Löe H: A computerized method for quantitative estimation of the epithelium–connective tissue interface applied to the gingiva of various age groups, *Acta Odontol Scand* 31:241, 1973.
17. Kay MM: Immunology and aging. In Holm-Pedersen P, editor: *Textbook of geriatric dentistry,* ed 2, Copenhagen, 1996, Munksgaard.
18. Kornman KS, Crane A, Wang HY, et al: The interleukin-1 genotype as a severity factor in adult periodontal disease, *J Clin Periodontol* 24:72, 1997.
19. Lindhe J, Hamp SE, Löe H: Plaque-induced periodontal disease in beagle dogs: a 4-year clinical, roentgenographical and histometrical study, *J Periodontal Res* 10:243, 1975.
20. Lindhe J, Socransky S, Nyman S, et al: Effect of age on healing following periodontal therapy, *J Clin Periodontol* 12:774, 1985.
21. Locker D, Slade GD, Murray H: Epidemiology of periodontal disease among older adults: a review, *Periodontol 2000* 16:16, 1999.
22. Löe H, Theilade E, Jensen SB: Experimental gingivitis in man, *J Periodontol* 36:177, 1965.
23. Mackenzie IC, Holm-Pedersen P, Karring T: Age changes in the oral mucous membranes and periodontium. In Holm-Pedersen P, editor: *Textbook of geriatric dentistry,* ed 2, Copenhagen, 1996, Munksgaard.
24. McArthur WP: Effect of aging on immunocompetent and inflammatory cells, *Periodontol 2000* 16:53, 1999.
25. McGuire MK, Nunn ME: Prognosis versus actual outcome. IV. The effectiveness of clinical parameters and IL-1 genotype in accurately predicting prognoses and tooth survival, *J Periodontol* 70:49, 1999.

26. Mombelli A: Aging and the periodontal and periimplant microbiota, *Periodontol 2000* 16:44, 1999.
27. Newman MG, Grinenco V, Weiner M, et al: Predominant microbiota associated with periodontal health in the aged, *J Periodontol* 49:553, 1978.
28. Norderyd O, Hugoson A, Grusovin G: Risk of severe periodontal disease in a Swedish adult population: a longitudinal study, *J Clin Periodontol* 26:608, 1999.
29. Ogawa H, Yoshihara A, Hirotomi T, et al: Risk factors for periodontal disease progression among elderly people, *J Clin Periodontol* 29:592, 2002.
30. Ojima M, Hanioka T, Shizukuishi S: Survival analysis for degree of compliance with supportive periodontal therapy, *J Clin Periodontol* 28:1091, 2001.
31. Page RC, Beck JD: Risk assessment for periodontal diseases, *Int Dent J* 47:61, 1997.
32. Papapanou PN, Lindhe J, Sterrett JD, et al: Considerations on the contribution of ageing to loss of periodontal tissue support, *J Clin Periodontol* 18:611, 1991.
33. Reiker J, van der Velden U, Barendregt DS, Loos B: A cross-sectional study into the prevalence of root caries in periodontal maintenance patients, *J Clin Periodontol* 26:26, 1999.
34. Schwartz Z, Somers A, Mellonig JT, et al: Ability of commercial demineralized freeze-dried bone allograft to induce new bone formation is dependent on donor age but not gender, *J Periodontol* 69:470, 1998.
35. Shklar G: The effects of aging upon oral mucosa, *J Invest Dermatol* 47:115, 1966.
36. Simons D, Brailsford S, Kidd E, Beighton D: The effect of chlorhexidine acetate/xylitol chewing gum on the plaque and gingival indices of elderly occupants in residential homes: a 1-year clinical trial, *J Clin Periodontol* 28:1010, 2001.
37. Slots J, Feik D, Rams TE: Age and sex relationships of superinfecting microorganisms in periodontitis patients, *Oral Microbiol Immunol* 5:305, 1990.
38. Van der Velden U: Effect of age on the periodontium, *J Clin Periodontol* 11:81, 1984.
39. Waerhaug J: Epidemiology of periodontal disease: review of the literature. In Ramfjord SP, Kerr DA, Ash MM, editors: *World workshop in periodontics,* Ann Arbor, Mich, 1966, American Academy of Periodontology.
40. Wennstrom JL, Serino G, Lindhe J, et al: Periodontal conditions of adult regular dental care attendants: a 12-year longitudinal study, *J Clin Periodontol* 20:714, 1993.
41. Wentz FM, Maier AW, Orban B: Age changes and sex differences in the clinically "normal" gingiva, *J Periodontol* 23:13, 1952.
42. Winkel EG, Abbas F, der Van V, et al: Experimental gingivitis in relation to age in individuals not susceptible to periodontal destruction, *J Clin Periodontol* 14:499, 1987.

PART

3

Classification and Epidemiology of Periodontal Diseases

Michael G. Newman

Periodontal disease classifications are useful to help establish diagnosis, determine prognosis, and facilitate treatment planning. Different classifications of periodontal diseases have been used over the years and have been replaced as new knowledge has improved our understanding of the etiology and pathology of the diseases of the periodontium, as discussed in Chapter 7.

Also, as covered in Chapter 8, Part 3 includes information about the epidemiology of periodontal diseases that will help the student and clinician analyze a disease and base their diagnostic and therapeutic decisions on its prevalence, incidence, and distribution in large populations or groups. Knowledge of the epidemiology of a disease improves our understanding and sharpens our decisions in individual cases.

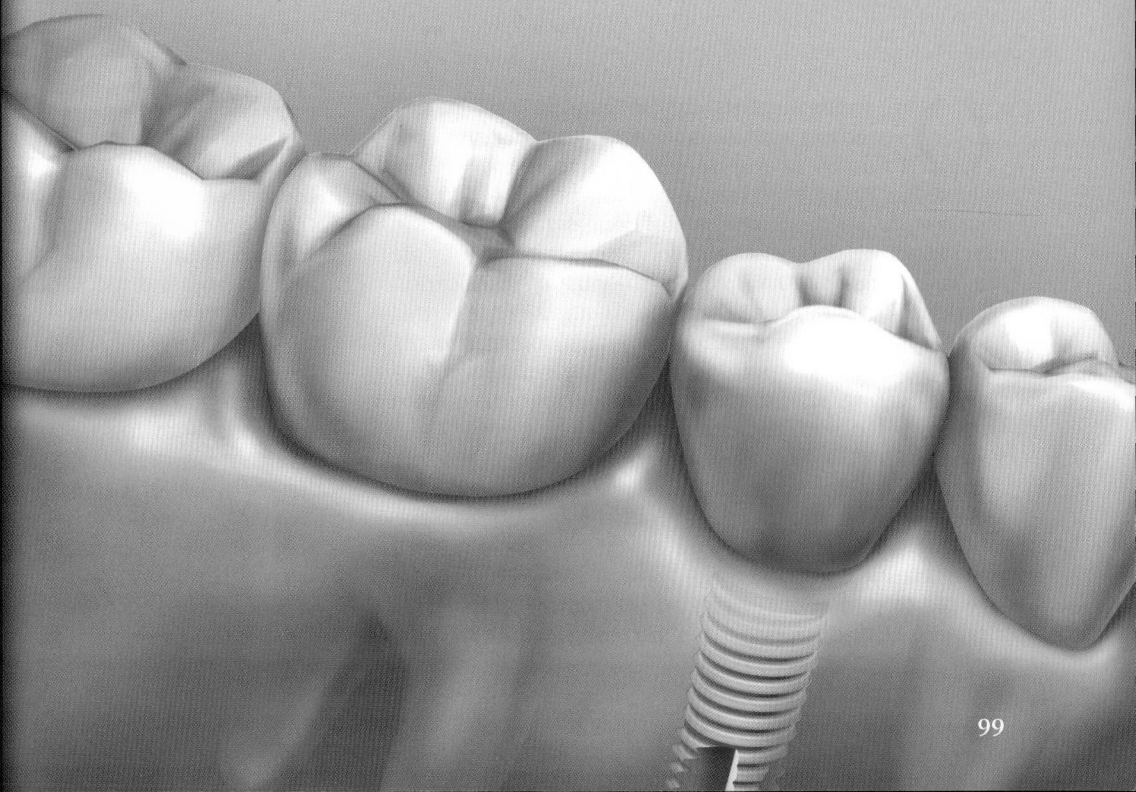

Classification of Diseases and Conditions Affecting the Periodontium

M. John Novak

7 CHAPTER

Chapter Outline

Our understanding of the etiology and pathogenesis of oral diseases and conditions is continually changing with increased scientific knowledge. In light of this, a classification can be most consistently defined by the differences in the clinical manifestations of diseases and conditions because they are clinically consistent and require little, if any, clarification by scientific laboratory testing. The classification presented in this chapter is based on the most recent, internationally accepted, consensus opinion of the diseases and conditions affecting the tissues of the periodontium and was presented and discussed at the 1999 International Workshop for the Classification of the Periodontal Diseases organized by the American Academy of Periodontology (AAP).[2] Box 7-1 presents the overall classification system, and each of the diseases or conditions are discussed where clarification is needed. In each case, the reader is referred to pertinent reviews on the subject and specific chapters within this book that discuss the topics in more detail.

GINGIVAL DISEASES

Dental Plaque–Induced Gingival Diseases

Gingivitis that is associated with dental plaque formation is the most common form of gingival disease[1] (Box 7-2), and its epidemiology (Chapter 8), its etiology (Chapters 9 through 16), and its clinical characteristics (Chapters 20 through 26) are discussed elsewhere in this textbook and in other sources.[8,10,12,19,20] Gingivitis has been previously characterized by the presence of clinical signs of inflammation that are confined to the gingiva and associated with teeth showing no attachment loss. Gingivitis also has been observed to affect the gingiva of periodontitis-affected teeth that have previously lost attachment but have received periodontal therapy to stabilize any further attachment loss. In these treated cases, plaque-induced gingival inflammation may recur, but without any evidence of further attachment loss.

From this evidence it has been concluded that plaque-induced gingivitis may occur on a periodontium with

BOX 7-1

Classification of Periodontal Diseases and Conditions

Gingival Diseases
Plaque-induced gingival diseases*
Non–plaque-induced gingival lesions

Chronic Periodontitis†
Localized
Generalized

Aggressive Periodontitis
Localized
Generalized

Periodontitis as a Manifestation of Systemic Diseases

Necrotizing Periodontal Diseases
Necrotizing ulcerative gingivitis (NUG)
Necrotizing ulcerative periodontitis (NUP)

Abscesses of the Periodontium
Gingival abscess
Periodontal abscess
Pericoronal abscess

Periodontitis Associated with Endodontic Lesions
Endodontic–periodontal lesion
Periodontal–endodontic lesion
Combined lesion

Developmental or Acquired Deformities and Conditions
Localized tooth-related factors that predispose to plaque-induced gingival diseases or periodontitis
Mucogingival deformities and conditions around teeth
Mucogingival deformities and conditions on edentulous ridges
Occlusal trauma

*These diseases may occur on a periodontium with no attachment loss or on a periodontium with attachment loss that is stable and not progressing.
†Chronic periodontitis can be further classified based on extent and severity. As a general guide, extent can be characterized as *localized* (<30% of sites involved) or *generalized* (>30% of sites involved). Severity can be characterized based on the amount of *clinical attachment loss* (CAL) as follows: *slight* = 1 or 2 mm CAL; *moderate* = 3 or 4 mm CAL; and *severe* ≥5 mm CAL. Data from Armitage GC: *Ann Periodontol* 4:1, 1999.

SCIENCE TRANSFER

Disease classification is helpful to distinguish the various conditions affecting the periodontium and to facilitate treatment planning. In periodontics, several classifications have been used, predominantly based on clinical manifestations, including location, degree of tissue change or loss, and rate of destruction. Because of a lack of understanding about specific etiology and pathogenic mechanisms, arbitrary designations have been used, such as "age" and separate "early" versus "adult" forms of disease. More recent work has suggested classification based on less subjective criteria. Additionally, despite limited microbiologic and biochemical differences, the classification of the periodontal diseases has facilitated treatment alternatives and therapeutic outcomes. Better understanding of the host response and the inflammation stimulated by microbial plaque should enhance the ability to distinguish periodontal diseases even more clearly.

The most widely accepted classification of periodontal diseases is that developed and presented at the 1994 International Workshop for the Classification of Periodontal Diseases. This is the basis for clinicians to diagnose lesions of the gingival and periodontal tissues and to clarify the disease status of patients. Periodontitis has been subdivided into three categories: *chronic periodontitis, aggressive periodontitis,* and *periodontitis as a manifestation of systemic disease.* Gingivitis now has the subcategories of *dental plaque–induced gingival disease* and *non–plaque-induced gingival disease.*

no attachment loss or on a periodontium with previous attachment loss that is stable and not progressing. This implies that gingivitis may be the diagnosis for inflamed gingival tissues associated with a tooth with no previous attachment loss or with a tooth that has previously undergone attachment and bone loss (reduced periodontal support) but is not currently losing attachment or bone, even though gingival inflammation is present. For this diagnosis to be made, longitudinal records of periodontal status, including clinical attachment levels, should be available.

Gingivitis Associated with Dental Plaque Only

Plaque-induced gingival disease is the result of an interaction between the microorganisms found in the dental plaque biofilm and the tissues and inflammatory cells of the host. The plaque-host interaction can be altered by the effects of local factors, systemic factors, medications, and malnutrition, all of which can influence the severity and duration of the response. Local factors that may contribute to gingivitis, in addition to plaque-retentive calculus formation on crown and root surfaces, are discussed later (see Developmental or Acquired Deformities and Conditions). These factors are contributory because of their ability to retain plaque microorganisms and inhibit their removal by patient-initiated plaque control techniques.

BOX 7-2

Gingival Diseases

Dental Plaque–Induced Gingival Diseases

These diseases may occur on a periodontium with no attachment loss or on a periodontium with attachment loss that is stable and not progressing.

- I. Gingivitis associated with dental plaque only
  - A. Without local contributing factors
  - B. With local contributing factors (see Box 7-4)
- II. Gingival diseases modified by systemic factors
  - A. Associated with endocrine system
    - 1. Puberty-associated gingivitis
    - 2. Menstrual cycle–associated gingivitis
    - 3. Pregnancy associated
      - a. Gingivitis
      - b. Pyogenic granuloma
    - 4. Diabetes mellitus–associated gingivitis
  - B. Associated with blood dyscrasias
    - 1. Leukemia-associated gingivitis
    - 2. Other
- III. Gingival diseases modified by medications
  - A. Drug-influenced gingival diseases
    - 1. Drug-influenced gingival enlargements
    - 2. Drug-influenced gingivitis
      - a. Oral contraceptive–associated gingivitis
      - b. Other
- IV. Gingival diseases modified by malnutrition
  - A. Ascorbic acid deficiency gingivitis
  - B. Other

Non–Plaque-Induced Gingival Lesions

- I. Gingival diseases of specific bacterial origin
  - A. *Neisseria gonorrhoeae*
  - B. *Treponema pallidum*
  - C. *Streptococcus* species
  - D. Other
- II. Gingival diseases of viral origin
  - A. Herpesvirus infections
    - 1. Primary herpetic gingivostomatitis
    - 2. Recurrent oral herpes
    - 3. Varicella zoster
  - B. Other
- III. Gingival diseases of fungal origin
  - A. *Candida* species infections: generalized gingival candidiasis
  - B. Linear gingival erythema
  - C. Histoplasmosis
  - D. Other
- IV. Gingival lesions of genetic origin
  - A. Hereditary gingival fibromatosis
  - B. Other
- V. Gingival manifestations of systemic conditions
  - A. Mucocutaneous lesions
    - 1. Lichen planus
    - 2. Pemphigoid
    - 3. Pemphigus vulgaris
    - 4. Erythema multiforme
    - 5. Lupus erythematosus
    - 6. Drug induced
    - 7. Other
  - B. Allergic reactions
    - 1. Dental restorative materials
      - a. Mercury
      - b. Nickel
      - c. Acrylic
      - d. Other
    - 2. Reactions attributable to:
      - a. Toothpastes or dentifrices
      - b. Mouth rinses or mouthwashes
      - c. Chewing gum additives
      - d. Foods and additives
    - 3. Other
- VI. Traumatic lesions (factitious, iatrogenic, or accidental)
  - A. Chemical injury
  - B. Physical injury
  - C. Thermal injury
- VII. Foreign body reactions
- VIII. Not otherwise specified

Data from Holmstrup P: *Ann Periodontol* 4:20, 1999; and Mariotti A: *Ann Periodontol* 4:7, 1999.

Gingival Diseases Modified by Systemic Factors

Systemic factors contributing to gingivitis, such as the endocrine changes associated with puberty, the menstrual cycle, pregnancy, and diabetes, may be exacerbated because of alterations in the gingival inflammatory response to plaque.[10,12,19] This altered response appears to result from the effects of systemic conditions on the host's cellular and immunologic functions. These changes are most apparent during pregnancy, when the prevalence and severity of gingival inflammation may increase even in the presence of low levels of plaque. Blood dyscrasias such as leukemia may alter immune function by disturbing the normal balance of immunologically competent white blood cells supplying the periodontium. Gingival enlargement and bleeding are common findings and may be associated with swollen, spongy gingival tissues caused by excessive infiltration of blood cells.

Gingival Diseases Modified by Medications

Gingival diseases modified by medications are increasingly prevalent because of the increased use of anticonvulsant drugs known to induce gingival enlargement, such as phenytoin, immunosuppressive drugs such as cyclosporine (cyclosporin A), and calcium channel blockers such as nifedipine, verapamil, diltiazem, and sodium valproate.[8,12,20] The development and severity of gingival enlargement in response to medications are patient specific and may be influenced by uncontrolled plaque accumulation. The increased use of oral contraceptives by premenopausal women has been associated with a higher incidence of gingival inflammation and development of gingival enlargement, which may be reversed by discontinuation of the oral contraceptive.

Gingival Diseases Modified by Malnutrition

Gingival diseases modified by malnutrition have received attention because of clinical descriptions of bright-red, swollen, and bleeding gingiva associated with severe ascorbic acid (vitamin C) deficiency or scurvy.[12] Nutritional deficiencies are known to affect immune function and may affect the host's ability to protect itself against some of the detrimental effects of cellular products, such as oxygen radicals. Unfortunately, little scientific evidence is available to support a role for specific nutritional deficiencies in the development or severity of gingival inflammation or periodontitis in humans.

Non–Plaque-Induced Gingival Lesions

Oral manifestations of systemic conditions that produce lesions in the tissues of the periodontium are rare. These effects are observed in lower socioeconomic groups, developing countries, and immunocompromised individuals.[9]

Gingival Diseases of Specific Bacterial Origin

Gingival diseases of specific bacterial origin are increasing in prevalence, especially as a result of sexually transmitted diseases such as gonorrhea *(Neisseria gonorrhoeae)* and to a lesser degree, syphilis *(Treponema pallidum)*.[21,24] Oral lesions may be secondary to systemic infection or may occur through direct infection. Streptococcal gingivitis or gingivostomatitis is a rare condition that may present as an acute condition with fever, malaise, and pain associated with acutely inflamed, diffuse, red, and swollen gingiva with increased bleeding and occasional gingival abscess formation. The gingival infections usually are preceded by tonsillitis and have been associated with group A β-hemolytic streptococcal infections.

Gingival Diseases of Viral Origin

Gingival diseases of viral origin may be caused by a variety of deoxyribonucleic acid (DNA) and ribonucleic acid (RNA) viruses, the most common being the herpesviruses. Lesions are frequently related to reactivation of latent viruses, especially as a result of reduced immune function. The oral manifestations of viral infection have been comprehensively reviewed.[9,21,24]

Gingival Diseases of Fungal Origin

Gingival diseases of fungal origin are relatively uncommon in immunocompetent individuals but occur more frequently in immunocompromised individuals and those with normal oral flora disturbed by the long-term use of broad-spectrum antibiotics.[9,24,25] The most common oral fungal infection is candidiasis, caused by infection with *Candida albicans,* which also can be seen under prosthetic devices, in individuals using topical steroids, and in individuals with decreased salivary flow, increased salivary glucose, or decreased salivary pH. A generalized candidal infection may manifest as white patches on the gingiva, tongue, or oral mucous membrane that can be removed with gauze, leaving a red, bleeding surface. In individuals infected with human immunodeficiency virus (HIV), candidal infection may present as erythema of the attached gingiva and has been referred to as *linear gingival erythema* or *HIV-associated gingivitis* (see Chapter 34).

Diagnosis of candidal infection can be made by culture, smear, and biopsy. Less common fungal infections have also been described.[24,25]

Gingival Diseases of Genetic Origin

Gingival diseases of genetic origin may involve the tissues of the periodontium and have been described in detail.[1] One of the most clinically evident conditions is *hereditary gingival fibromatosis,* which exhibits autosomal dominant or (rarely) autosomal recessive modes of inheritance. The gingival enlargement may completely cover the teeth, delay eruption, and present as an isolated finding or may be associated with several more generalized syndromes.

Gingival Manifestations of Systemic Conditions

Gingival manifestations of systemic conditions may appear as desquamative lesions, ulceration of the gingiva, or both.[9,18,23] Allergic reactions that manifest with gingival changes are uncommon but have been observed in association with several restorative materials, toothpastes, mouthwashes, chewing gum, and foods (see Box 7-2). The diagnosis of these conditions may prove difficult and may require an extensive history and selective elimination of potential culprits.

Traumatic Lesions

Traumatic lesions may be *factitious* (produced by artificial means; unintentionally produced), as in the case of toothbrush trauma resulting in gingival ulceration, recession, or both; *iatrogenic* (trauma to the gingiva induced by the dentist or health professional), as in the case of preventive or restorative care that may lead to traumatic injury of the gingiva; or *accidental,* as in the case of damage to the gingiva through minor burns from hot foods and drinks.[9]

Foreign Body Reactions

Foreign body reactions lead to localized inflammatory conditions of the gingiva and are caused by the introduction of foreign material into the gingival connective tissues through breaks in the epithelium.[9] Common examples are the introduction of amalgam into the gingiva during the placement of a restoration or extraction of a tooth, leaving an amalgam tattoo, or the introduction of abrasives during polishing procedures.

PERIODONTITIS

Periodontitis is defined as "an inflammatory disease of the supporting tissues of the teeth caused by specific microorganisms or groups of specific microorganisms, resulting in progressive destruction of the periodontal ligament and alveolar bone with pocket formation, recession, or both." The clinical feature that distinguishes periodontitis from gingivitis is the presence of clinically detectable attachment loss. This often is accompanied by periodontal pocket formation and changes in the density and height of subjacent alveolar bone. In some cases, recession of the marginal gingiva may accompany attachment loss, thus masking ongoing disease progression if pocket depth measurements are taken without measurements of clinical attachment levels. Clinical signs of inflammation, such as changes in color, contour, and consistency and bleeding on probing, may not always be positive indicators of ongoing attachment loss. However, the presence of continued bleeding on probing at sequential visits has proved to be a reliable indicator of the presence of inflammation and the potential for subsequent attachment loss at the bleeding site. The attachment loss associated with periodontitis has been shown to progress either continuously or in episodic bursts of disease activity.

Although many classifications of the different clinical manifestations of periodontitis have been presented over the past 20 years, consensus workshops in North America in 1989[5] and Europe in 1993[3] identified that periodontitis may present in early-onset, adult-onset, and necrotizing forms (Table 7-1). In addition, the AAP consensus concluded that periodontitis may be associated with systemic conditions such as diabetes and HIV infection and that some forms of periodontitis may be refractory to conventional therapy. Early-onset disease was distinguished from adult-onset disease by the age of onset (35 years of age was set as an arbitrary separation of diseases), the rate of disease progression, and the presence of alterations in host defenses. The early-onset diseases were more aggressive, occurred in individuals younger than 35 years old, and were associated with defects in host defenses, whereas adult forms of disease were slowly progressive, began in the fourth decade of life, and were not associated with defects in host defenses. In addition, early-onset periodontitis was subclassified into prepubertal, juvenile, and rapidly progressive forms with localized or generalized disease distributions.

TABLE 7-1

Classification of the Various Forms of Periodontitis

Classification	Forms of Periodontitis	Disease Characteristics
AAP World Workshop in Clinical Periodontics, 1989[5]	Adult periodontitis	Age of onset >35 years Slow rate of disease progression No defects in host defenses
	Early-onset periodontitis (may be prepubertal, juvenile, or rapidly progressive)	Age of onset <35 years Rapid rate of disease progression Defects in host defenses Associated with specific microflora
	Periodontitis associated with systemic disease	Systemic diseases that predispose to rapid rates of periodontitis Diseases: diabetes, Down syndrome, HIV infection, Papillon-Lefèvre syndrome
	Necrotizing ulcerative periodontitis	Similar to acute necrotizing ulcerative gingivitis but with associated clinical attachment loss
	Refractory periodontitis	Recurrent periodontitis that does not respond to treatment
European Workshop in Periodontology, 1993[3]	Adult periodontitis	Age of onset: fourth decade of life Slow rate of disease progression No defects in host response
	Early-onset periodontitis	Age of onset: before fourth decade of life Rapid rate of disease progression Defects in host defense
	Necrotizing periodontitis	Tissue necrosis with attachment and bone loss
AAP International Workshop for Classification of Periodontal Diseases, 1999[2]	Chronic periodontitis Aggressive periodontitis Periodontitis as a manifestation of systemic diseases	See Box 7-3.

AAP, American Academy of Periodontology; *HIV,* human immunodeficiency virus.

Extensive clinical and basic scientific research of these disease entities has been performed in many countries, and some disease characteristics outlined 10 years ago no longer stand up to rigid scientific scrutiny.[6,11,26] In particular, supporting evidence was lacking for the distinct classifications of adult periodontitis, refractory periodontitis, and the various different forms of early-onset periodontitis as outlined by the AAP Workshop for the International Classification of Periodontal Diseases in 1999[2] (see Table 7-1). It has been observed that chronic periodontal destruction, caused by the accumulation of local factors such as plaque and calculus, can occur before age 35 years and that the aggressive disease seen in young patients may be independent of age but has a familial (genetic) association. With respect to refractory periodontitis, little evidence supports that this is indeed a distinct clinical entity because the causes of continued loss of clinical attachment and alveolar bone after periodontal therapy are currently poorly defined and apply to many disease entities. In addition, the clinical and etiologic manifestations of the different diseases outlined in North America in 1989 and in Europe in 1993 were not consistently observed in different countries around the world and did not always fit the models presented. As a result, the AAP held an International Workshop for the Classification of Periodontal Diseases in 1999 to clarify further a classification system based on current clinical and scientific data.[2] The resulting classification of the different forms of periodontitis was simplified to describe three general clinical manifestations of periodontitis: chronic periodontitis, aggressive periodontitis, and periodontitis as a manifestation of systemic diseases (see Table 7-1 and Box 7-3).

Chronic Periodontitis

Chronic periodontitis is the most common form of periodontitis[6]; Box 7-3 outlines the characteristics of this form of periodontitis. Chronic periodontitis is most prevalent in adults but can be observed in children; therefore the age range of older than 35 years previously designated for the classification of this disease has been discarded. Chronic periodontitis is associated with the accumulation of plaque and calculus and generally has a slow to moderate rate of disease progression, but periods of more rapid destruction may be observed. Increases in the rate of disease progression may be caused by the impact of local, systemic, or environmental factors that may influence the normal host-bacteria interaction. Local factors may influence plaque accumulation (see Box 7-4); systemic diseases such as diabetes mellitus and HIV infection may influence the host defenses, and environmental factors such as cigarette smoking and stress also may influence the response of the host to plaque accumulation. Chronic periodontitis may occur as a localized disease in which less than 30% of evaluated sites demonstrate attachment and bone loss, or it may occur as a more generalized disease in which greater than 30% of sites are affected. The disease also may be described by the severity of disease as slight, moderate, or severe based on the amount of clinical attachment loss (see Box 7-3).

Aggressive Periodontitis

Aggressive periodontitis differs from the chronic form primarily by (1) the rapid rate of disease progression seen in an otherwise healthy individual, (2) an absence of large accumulations of plaque and calculus, and (3) a family history of aggressive disease suggestive of a genetic trait[16,26] (see Box 7-3). This form of periodontitis was previously classified as early-onset periodontitis (see Table 7-1) and therefore still includes many of the characteristics previously identified with the localized and generalized forms of early-onset periodontitis. Although the clinical presentation of aggressive disease appears to be universal, the etiologic factors involved are not always consistent; Box 7-3 outlines additional clinical, microbiologic, and immunologic characteristics of aggressive disease that may be present. As was previously described for early-onset disease, aggressive forms of periodontitis usually affect young individuals at or after puberty and may be observed during the second and third decade of life (i.e., 10 to 30 years of age). The disease may be localized as previously described for localized juvenile periodontitis (LJP) or generalized as previously described for generalized juvenile periodontitis (GJP) and rapidly progressive periodontitis (RPP) (see Table 7-1). Box 7-3 provides the common features of the localized and generalized forms of aggressive periodontitis.

Periodontitis as a Manifestation of Systemic Diseases

Several hematologic and genetic disorders have been associated with the development of periodontitis in affected individuals[10,11] (see Box 7-3). The majority of these observations of effects on the periodontium are the result of case reports, and few research studies have been performed to investigate the exact nature of the effect of the specific condition on the tissues of the periodontium. It is speculated that the major effect of these disorders is through alterations in host defense mechanisms that have been clearly described for disorders such as neutropenia and leukocyte adhesion deficiencies but are less well understood for multifaceted syndromes. The clinical manifestation of many of these disorders appears at an early age and may be confused with aggressive forms of periodontitis with rapid attachment loss and the potential for early tooth loss. With the introduction of this form of periodontitis in this and previous classification systems (see Table 7-1), the potential exists for overlap and confusion between periodontitis as a manifestation of systemic disease and both the aggressive and the chronic form of disease when a systemic component is suspected. At present, "periodontitis as a manifestation of systemic disease" is the diagnosis to be used when the systemic condition is the major predisposing factor and local factors such as large quantities of plaque and calculus are not clearly evident. In the case where periodontal destruction is clearly the result of local factors but has been exacerbated by the onset of such conditions as diabetes mellitus or HIV infection, the diagnosis should be "chronic periodontitis modified by" the systemic condition.

BOX 7-3

Periodontitis

The disease periodontitis can be subclassified into the following three major types based on clinical, radiographic, historical, and laboratory characteristics.

Chronic Periodontitis
The following characteristics are common to patients with chronic periodontitis:

- Prevalent in adults but can occur in children.
- Amount of destruction consistent with local factors.
- Associated with a variable microbial pattern.
- Subgingival calculus frequently found.
- Slow to moderate rate of progression with possible periods of rapid progression.
- Possibly modified by or associated with the following:
  - — Systemic diseases such as diabetes mellitus and HIV infection.
  - — Local factors predisposing to periodontitis.
  - — Environmental factors such as cigarette smoking and emotional stress.

Chronic periodontitis may be further subclassified into *localized* and *generalized* forms and characterized as *slight, moderate,* or *severe* based on the common features described above and the following specific features:

- Localized form: <30% of sites involved.
- Generalized form: >30% of sites involved.
- Slight: 1 to 2 mm of clinical attachment loss.
- Moderate: 3 to 4 mm of clinical attachment loss.
- Severe: ≥5 mm of clinical attachment loss.

Aggressive Periodontitis
The following characteristics are common to patients with aggressive periodontitis:

- Otherwise clinically healthy patient.
- Rapid attachment loss and bone destruction.
- Amount of microbial deposits inconsistent with disease severity.
- Familial aggregation of diseased individuals.

The following characteristics are common but not universal:

- Diseased sites infected with *Actinobacillus actinomycetemcomitans.*
- Abnormalities in phagocyte function.
- Hyperresponsive macrophages, producing increased prostaglandin E_2 (PGE_2) and interleukin-1β.
- In some cases, self-arresting disease progression.

Aggressive periodontitis may be further classified into *localized* and *generalized* forms based on the common features described here and the following specific features:

Localized form

- Circumpubertal onset of disease.
- Localized first molar or incisor disease with proximal attachment loss on at least two permanent teeth, one of which is a first molar.
- Robust serum antibody response to infecting agents.

Generalized form

- Usually affecting persons under 30 years of age (however, may be older).
- Generalized proximal attachment loss affecting at least three teeth other than first molars and incisors.
- Pronounced episodic nature of periodontal destruction.
- Poor serum antibody response to infecting agents.

Periodontitis as a Manifestation of Systemic Diseases
Periodontitis may be observed as a manifestation of the following systemic diseases:

1. Hematologic disorders
   a. Acquired neutropenia
   b. Leukemias
   c. Other
2. Genetic disorders
   a. Familial and cyclic neutropenia
   b. Down syndrome
   c. Leukocyte adhesion deficiency syndromes
   d. Papillon-Lefèvre syndrome
   e. Chédiak-Higashi syndrome
   f. Histiocytosis syndromes
   g. Glycogen storage disease
   h. Infantile genetic agranulocytosis
   i. Cohen syndrome
   j. Ehlers-Danlos syndrome (types IV and VIII AD)
   k. Hypophosphatasia
   l. Other
3. Not otherwise specified

Data from Flemmig TF: *Ann Periodontol* 4:32, 1999; Kinane DF: *Ann Periodontol* 4:54, 1999; and Tonetti MS, Mombelli A: *Ann Periodontol* 4:39, 1999.

NECROTIZING PERIODONTAL DISEASES

The clinical characteristics of necrotizing periodontal diseases may include but are not limited to ulcerated and necrotic papillary and marginal gingiva covered by a yellowish white or grayish slough or pseudomembrane, blunting and cratering of papillae, bleeding on provocation or spontaneous bleeding, pain, and fetid breath. These diseases may be accompanied by fever, malaise, and lymphadenopathy, although these characteristics are not consistent. Two forms of necrotizing periodontal disease have been described: *necrotizing ulcerative gingivitis* (NUG) and *necrotizing ulcerative periodontitis* (NUP). NUG has been previously classified under "gingival diseases" or "gingivitis" because clinical attachment loss is not a consistent feature, whereas NUP has been classified as a form of "periodontitis" because attachment loss is present. Recent reviews of the etiologic and clinical characteristics of NUG and NUP have suggested that the two diseases represent clinical manifestations of the same disease, except that distinct features of NUP are clinical attachment and bone loss. As a result, both NUG and NUP have been determined as a separate group of diseases that have *tissue necrosis* as a primary clinical feature (see Box 7-1).

Necrotizing Ulcerative Gingivitis

The clinical and etiologic characteristics of NUG[22] are described in detail in Chapter 26. The defining characteristics of NUG are its bacterial etiology, its necrotic lesion, and predisposing factors such as psychologic stress, smoking, and immunosuppression. In addition, malnutrition may be a contributing factor in developing countries. NUG is usually seen as an acute lesion that responds well to antimicrobial therapy combined with professional plaque and calculus removal and improved oral hygiene.

Necrotizing Ulcerative Periodontitis

NUP differs from NUG in that loss of clinical attachment and alveolar bone is a consistent feature.[15] All other characteristics appear to be the same between the two forms of necrotizing disease. The characteristics of NUP are described in detail in Chapter 32. NUP may be observed among patients with HIV infection and manifests as local ulceration and necrosis of gingival tissue with exposure and rapid destruction of underlying bone, spontaneous bleeding, and severe pain. HIV-infected patients with NUP are 20.8 times more likely to have CD4+ cell counts below 200 cells/mm^3 of peripheral blood than HIV-infected patients without NUP, suggesting that immunosuppression is a major contributing factor. In addition, the predictive value of NUP for HIV-infected patients with CD4+ cell counts below 200 cells/mm^3 was 95.1%, and the cumulative probability of death within 24 months of a NUP diagnosis in HIV-infected individuals was 72.9%. In developing countries, NUP also has been associated with severe malnutrition, which may lead to immunosuppression in some patients.

ABSCESSES OF THE PERIODONTIUM

A periodontal abscess is a localized purulent infection of periodontal tissues and is classified by its tissue of origin.[13] The clinical, microbiologic, immunologic, and predisposing characteristics are discussed in Chapters 8 and 9.

PERIODONTITIS ASSOCIATED WITH ENDODONTIC LESIONS

Classification of lesions affecting the periodontium and pulp is based on the disease process sequence.[4]

Endodontic–Periodontal Lesions

In endodontic–periodontal lesions, pulpal necrosis precedes periodontal changes. A periapical lesion originating in pulpal infection and necrosis may drain to the oral cavity through the periodontal ligament, resulting in destruction of the periodontal ligament and adjacent alveolar bone. This may present clinically as a localized, deep, periodontal pocket extending to the apex of the tooth. Pulpal infection also may drain through accessory canals, especially in the area of the furcation, and may lead to furcal involvement through loss of clinical attachment and alveolar bone.

Periodontal–Endodontic Lesions

In periodontal–endodontic lesions, bacterial infection from a periodontal pocket associated with loss of attachment and root exposure may spread through accessory canals to the pulp, resulting in pulpal necrosis. In the case of advanced periodontal disease, the infection may reach the pulp through the apical foramen. Scaling and root planing removes cementum and underlying dentin and may lead to chronic pulpitis through bacterial penetration of dentinal tubules. However, many periodontitis-affected teeth that have been scaled and root-planed show no evidence of pulpal involvement.

Combined Lesions

Combined lesions occur when pulpal necrosis and a periapical lesion occur on a tooth that also is periodontally involved. A radiographically evident intrabony defect is seen when infection of pulpal origin merges with infection of periodontal origin.

In all cases of periodontitis associated with endodontic lesions, the endodontic infection should be controlled before beginning definitive management of the periodontal lesion, especially when regenerative or bone-grafting techniques are planned.

DEVELOPMENTAL OR ACQUIRED DEFORMITIES AND CONDITIONS

Localized Tooth-Related Factors That Modify or Predispose to Plaque-Induced Gingival Diseases or Periodontitis

In general, these factors are considered to be those local factors that contribute to the initiation and progression of periodontal disease through an enhancement of plaque accumulation or the prevention of effective plaque removal by normal oral hygiene measures.[4] These factors fall into four subgroups (Box 7-4).

Tooth Anatomic Factors

These factors are associated with malformations of tooth development or tooth location. Anatomic factors such as cervical enamel projections and enamel pearls have been associated with clinical attachment loss, especially in furcation areas. Cervical enamel projections are found on 15% to 24% of mandibular molars and 9% to 25% of maxillary molars, and strong associations have been

BOX 7-4

Developmental or Acquired Deformities and Conditions

Localized Tooth-Related Factors That Modify or Predispose to Plaque-Induced Gingival Diseases or Periodontitis

1. Tooth anatomic factors
2. Dental restorations or appliances
3. Root fractures
4. Cervical root resorption and cemental tears

Mucogingival Deformities and Conditions around Teeth

1. Gingival or soft tissue recession
   a. Facial or lingual surfaces
   b. Interproximal (papillary)
2. Lack of keratinized gingiva
3. Decreased vestibular depth
4. Aberrant frenum or muscle position
5. Gingival excess
   a. Pseudopocket
   b. Inconsistent gingival margin
   c. Excessive gingival display
   d. Gingival enlargement (see Box 7-2)
   e. Abnormal color

Mucogingival Deformities and Conditions on Edentulous Edges

1. Vertical and/or horizontal ridge deficiency
2. Lack of gingiva or keratinized tissue
3. Gingival or soft tissue enlargements
4. Aberrant frenum or muscle position
5. Decreased vestibular depth
6. Abnormal color

Occlusal Trauma

1. Primary occlusal trauma
2. Secondary occlusal trauma

Data from Blieden TM: *Ann Periodontol* 4:91, 1999; Halmon WW: *Ann Periodontol* 4:102, 1999; and Pini Prato GP: *Ann Periodontol* 4:98, 1999.

observed with furcation involvement. Palatogingival grooves, found primarily on maxillary incisors, are observed in 8.5% of individuals and are associated with increased plaque accumulation, clinical attachment, and bone loss. Proximal root grooves on incisors and maxillary premolars also predispose to plaque accumulation, inflammation, and loss of clinical attachment and bone.

Tooth location is considered important in the initiation and development of disease. Tooth malalignment predisposes to plaque accumulation and inflammation in children and may predispose to clinical attachment loss in adults, especially when associated with poor oral hygiene. In addition, open contacts have been associated with increased loss of alveolar bone, most probably through food impaction.

Dental Restorations or Appliances

Dental restorations or appliances are frequently associated with the development of gingival inflammation, especially when they are located subgingivally. This may apply to subgingivally placed onlays, crowns, fillings, and orthodontic bands. Restorations may impinge on the biologic width by being placed deep in the sulcus or within the junctional epithelium. This may promote inflammation and loss of clinical attachment and bone, with apical migration of the junctional epithelium and reestablishment of the attachment apparatus at a more apical level.

Root Fractures

Root fractures caused by traumatic forces or restorative or endodontic procedures may lead to periodontal involvement through an apical migration of plaque along the fracture when the fracture originates coronal to the clinical attachment and is exposed to the oral environment.

Cervical Root Resorption and Cemental Tears

Cervical root resorption and cemental tears may lead to periodontal destruction when the lesion communicates with the oral cavity and allows bacteria to migrate subgingivally.

Mucogingival Deformities and Conditions around Teeth

Mucogingival is defined as "a generic term used to describe the mucogingival junction and its relationship to the gingiva, alveolar mucosa, frenula, muscle attachments, vestibular fornices, and the floor of the mouth." A *mucogingival deformity* may be defined as "a significant departure from the normal shape of gingiva and alveolar mucosa" and may involve the underlying alveolar bone. *Mucogingival surgery* is defined as "periodontal surgical procedures designed to correct defects in the morphology, position, and/or amount of gingiva" and is described in detail in Chapter 69. The surgical correction of mucogingival deformities may be performed for esthetic reasons, to enhance function, or to facilitate oral hygiene.[17]

Mucogingival Deformities and Conditions on Edentulous Ridges

Mucogingival deformities and conditions on edentulous ridges usually require corrective surgery to restore form and function before the prosthetic replacement of missing teeth or implant placement.[17]

Occlusal Trauma

The etiology of trauma from occlusion and its effects on the periodontium[8] is discussed in detail in Chapters 29, 30, and 56.

REFERENCES

1. Aldred MJ, Bartold PM: Genetic disorders of the gingivae and periodontium, *Periodontol 2000* 18:7, 1998.
2. Armitage GC: Development of a classification system for periodontal diseases and conditions, *Ann Periodontol* 4:1, 1999.
3. Attstrom R, Vander Velden U: Summary of session 1. In Lang N, Karring T, editors: *Proceedings of the 1st European Workshop in Periodontology,* Berlin, 1993, Quintessence.
4. Blieden TM: Tooth-related issues, *Ann Periodontol* 4:91, 1999.
5. Caton J: Periodontal diagnosis and diagnostic aids: consensus report. In *Proceedings of the World Workshop in Clinical Periodontics,* 1989, American Academy of Periodontology.
6. Flemmig TF: Periodontitis, *Ann Periodontol* 4:32, 1999.
7. Hallmon WW: Occlusal trauma: effect and impact on the periodontium, *Ann Periodontol* 4:102, 1999.
8. Hallmon WW, Rossmann JA: The role of drugs in the pathogenesis of gingival overgrowth, *Periodontol 2000* 21:176, 1999.
9. Holmstrup P: Non–plaque-induced gingival lesions, *Ann Periodontol* 4:20, 1999.
10. Kinane DF: Blood and lymphoreticular disorders, *Periodontol 2000* 21:84, 1999.
11. Kinane DF: Periodontitis modified by systemic factors, *Ann Periodontol* 4:54, 1999.
12. Mariotti A: Dental plaque-induced gingival diseases, *Ann Periodontol* 4:7, 1999.
13. Meng HX: Periodontal abscess, *Ann Periodontol* 4:79, 1999.
14. Meng HX: Periodontic-endodontic lesions, *Ann Periodontol* 4:84, 1999.
15. Novak MJ: Necrotizing ulcerative periodontitis, *Ann Periodontol* 4:74, 1999.
16. Novak MJ, Novak KF: Early-onset periodontitis, *Curr Opin Periodontol* 3:45, 1996.
17. Pini Prato GP: Mucogingival deformities, *Ann Periodontol* 4:98, 1999.
18. Plemons JM, Gonzalez TS, Burkhart NW: Vesiculobullous diseases of the oral cavity, *Periodontol 2000* 21:158, 1999.
19. Porter SR: Gingival and periodontal aspects of diseases of the blood and blood-forming organs and malignancy, *Periodontol 2000* 18:102, 1998.
20. Rees TD: Drugs and oral disorders, *Periodontol 2000* 18:21, 1998.
21. Rivera Hidalgo F, Stanford TW: Oral mucosal lesions caused by infective microorganisms. I. Viruses and bacteria, *Periodontol 2000* 21:106, 1999.
22. Rowland RW: Necrotizing ulcerative gingivitis, *Ann Periodontol* 4:65, 1999.
23. Scully C, Laskaris G: Mucocutaneous disorders, *Periodontol 2000* 18:81, 1998.
24. Scully C, Monteil R, Sposto MR: Infectious and tropical diseases affecting the human mouth, *Periodontol 2000* 18:47, 1998.
25. Stanford TW, Rivera-Hidalgo F: Oral mucosal lesions caused by infective microorganisms. II. Fungi and parasites, *Periodontol 2000* 21:125, 1999.
26. Tonetti MS, Mombelli A: Early-onset periodontitis, *Ann Periodontol* 4:39, 1999.

CHAPTER 8

Epidemiology of Gingival and Periodontal Diseases

James D. Beck and Samuel J. Arbes, Jr.

CHAPTER OUTLINE

Although information about the epidemiology of a disease is based on groups of people, whereas clinicians are primarily interested in the individual patient being treated, thoughtful clinicians understand the value of epidemiologic information for the decisions they must make about the philosophy of their practice and the treatment of each patient. Questions that frame the diagnosis of an individual patient include the following:

- Is this a rare or common condition?
- Does my patient fit the profile of people likely to have this disease?
- Where on the continuum of normality to disease are the signs and symptoms I see in my patient?

Epidemiologic studies identifying risk factors for diseases provide guidance for primary prevention recommendations, and newer molecular epidemiology studies help identify where to intervene in the disease process. Treatment-related questions such as, "What is the natural history of the disease that I am treating?" lead to decisions about whether to treat now or continue to evaluate the condition. Similarly, much of our knowledge about the prognosis for an individual patient receiving a specific treatment comes from epidemiologic studies of treatment outcomes.

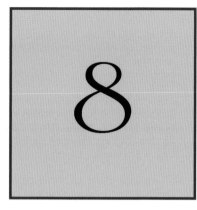

The focus of this chapter is on the clinician; therefore, many of the topic headings address clinical issues, such as abnormality, definition of a case, diagnosis, and risk for new disease and disease progression. A short review of epidemiology and study designs used in epidemiologic and clinical studies precedes discussion of these clinical issues. (For those who are well versed in these areas, the authors recommend skipping the next section and using it as a reference for the remainder of the chapter.)

WHAT IS EPIDEMIOLOGY?

Epidemiology is "the study of the distribution and determinants of health-related states or events in specified populations, and the application of this study to control health problems."[43] Epidemiology traditionally has been considered a basic science of public health. What distinguishes public health practice from clinical practice is that *public health* practice emphasizes the health of population groups, whereas *clinical* practice is concerned with the health of individual patients. The determinants of disease in an individual patient may be quite different from the determinants of disease in a population. For example, a periodontist may attribute a patient's periodontal disease to the accumulation of plaque and calculus (factors that can be addressed in a practice), whereas a public health practitioner may attribute the high prevalence of periodontal disease in a given population to low socioeconomic status or the lack of access to preventive dental services.

As the definition implies, epidemiology has three purposes: (1) to determine the amount and distribution of a disease in a population, (2) to investigate causes for the disease, and (3) to apply this knowledge to the control of the disease. Perhaps the most basic question in public health and clinical practice is, "How much disease is present?" Descriptive studies are used to measure the amount of disease in a population. Disease often is described in terms of the percentage of persons affected and its distribution among subgroups (defined by age, gender, ethnicity, education levels, or other characteristics) in the population. The underlying assumption in epidemiology is that the distribution of disease among members of a population is not random.[33] Some members or subgroups of the population have characteristics that make them more susceptible to disease. These characteristics include the physical, biologic, behavioral, cultural, and social factors that determine health.[43] Epidemiologists use analytic study designs such as case-control or cohort studies to investigate factors associated with a disease.

The final purpose of epidemiology is to apply the knowledge gained from studies to "promote, protect, and restore health."[43] Epidemiologic data are the foundation for much of our public health policy. One of the most successful public health interventions has been the fluoridation of public drinking water to prevent dental caries. Epidemiologic data also have been the foundation for much of clinical practice.[33] Diagnostic tests, prognoses, and selection of appropriate therapies are based on studies of groups of people. The practice of evidence-based dentistry requires clinical practitioners to use the best available scientific information in making decisions about the care of individual patients. Much of this scientific information comes from epidemiologic studies and randomized clinical trials in particular.

Epidemiologic Measures of Disease

Prevalence

Prevalence is the proportion of persons in a population who have the disease of interest at a given point in or period of time.[34] It is calculated by dividing the number of persons in the population who have the disease by the number of persons in the population.

Prevalence, which can be reported as a proportion or percentage, is a measure of the burden of disease in a population. Information about prevalence can be useful for estimating the need for health care resources. For example, prevalence data on dental disease are used for estimating the number of new general dentists and specialists that dental schools should train.

Several factors influence the prevalence of disease. The prevalence of a disease at a given point in time is the result of the dynamic situation between the addition of new cases (incidence), which increases prevalence, and the removal of cases through death or cure, which decreases prevalence.[33] Ironically, the introduction of more sensitive diagnostic tests or new treatments that enhance survival increases prevalence. Also, the prevalence of a nonfatal chronic disease, such as chronic adult periodontitis, tends to increase with increasing age. This increase in prevalence with age, which is simply caused by the accumulation of cases, often is misinterpreted as meaning that older adults are at higher risk for the disease.

Incidence

Incidence, also referred to as *risk* or *cumulative incidence,* is the average percentage of unaffected persons who will develop the disease of interest during a given period of time.[3] Incidence can be viewed as the risk or probability that a person will become a case. It is calculated by dividing the number of new cases of disease by the number of persons in the population who are at risk for the disease.

Whereas prevalence is a measure of the amount of disease existing in a population, incidence is a measure of the occurrence of new disease. The numerator of the incidence equation is the number of persons who transition from a nondiseased state to a diseased state during the period of observation. The denominator in the equation must contain only those persons in the population who are at risk for but do not have the disease at the start of observation. For example, in a study of oral cancer, only individuals who are free of oral cancer at the beginning of the study would be included in the population at risk. In the expression of incidence, specifying the period of observation is necessary. Without a specified time period, such as per month or per year, incidence has little meaning.

In the study of periodontal disease, rarely, if ever, does *incident periodontal disease* refer strictly to the onset of disease in previously periodontitis-free adults. Instead, it usually refers to the development of new periodontal lesions in people who may have had other periodontal lesions at baseline and to the progression of existing lesions (see later discussion). Incident periodontal disease is typically measured as a change in attachment level over time, and studies rarely differentiate between the development of new lesions and the progression of existing lesions.

Epidemiologic Study Designs

To investigate the prevalence and incidence of disease, risk factors associated with disease, and the effectiveness and efficacy of interventions, researchers conduct epidemiologic studies. Most epidemiologic studies are observational. In these studies the researchers observe natural occurrences in the population. The most common observation studies are cross-sectional, cohort, and case-control studies. In addition to observational studies, epidemiologists also conduct experimental studies in which they manipulate exposures, such as in drug trials when one group of subjects receives the study drug and another group receives a placebo (or delayed treatment, or the current standard treatment). Experimental studies are useful in studying the efficacy of preventive interventions, treatments, and drugs. Community intervention trials and randomized clinical trials are two types of experimental studies. Because researchers can control the exposures, these studies provide the strongest evidence for cause and effect. For more information on community intervention and clinical trials, the interested reader is referred to texts by Hulley et al.,[39] Lilienfeld et al.,[44] and Friedman et al.[31] Features of the most common observational study designs are reviewed here.

Cross-Sectional Studies

In cross-sectional studies the presence or absence of disease and the characteristics of the members of a population are measured at a point in time. These studies are useful for providing prevalence data on a disease, comparing the characteristics of persons with and without disease, and generating hypotheses regarding the etiology of a disease. Whereas cohort and case-control studies are considered *analytic* study designs, cross-sectional studies are considered *descriptive*. Cross-sectional studies also are referred to as *disease frequency surveys* or *prevalence studies*. Depending on the size of the population and the resources available to the researchers, the entire population or a representative sample of the population can be studied. Cross-sectional studies repeated at regular intervals can provide information on trends in disease over time or the effectiveness of prevention or treatment programs.

Cross-sectional studies have two major limitations. First, cross-sectional studies can only identify prevalent cases of disease. Because these studies do not follow a population at risk of the disease over time, incidence cannot be determined. Second, although cross-sectional studies may show that a certain characteristic is associated with having the disease, determining whether the characteristic preceded the disease is not always possible. For example, a cross-sectional study may reveal that people with periodontal disease are more likely to be smokers; however, it cannot always be determined whether the smoking or the disease occurred first. Establishing the temporal relationship between a particular characteristic and the onset of disease is an important criterion for determining whether the characteristic is a cause of the disease. Cohort studies that observe people over time are required to calculate incidence and establish temporality.

The advantages of cross-sectional studies are that they are generally less expensive than longitudinal studies and can be conducted more quickly.

Cohort Studies

Unlike cross-sectional studies, cohort studies follow subjects over time. The purpose of a cohort study is to determine whether an exposure or characteristic is associated with the development of a disease or condition. At the beginning of the study, all subjects must be free of the disease of interest. Subjects are classified into "exposed" and "unexposed" groups and then followed over time and monitored for the development of the disease. Incidence can be calculated because new cases of disease are assessed. If the incidence of disease is greater in the exposed group than in the unexposed group, the study provides evidence that the exposure is a risk factor for the disease. Because a cohort study can demonstrate that an exposure preceded a disease, it provides strong support for an association. The disadvantages of cohort studies are that they can require long periods of follow-up and can be expensive to conduct. Also, if the disease of interest is rare, large numbers of subjects will need to be followed. The preferred study design for investigating rare diseases is the case-control study.

Case-Control Studies

Case-control studies provide an efficient way to investigate the association between an exposure and a disease, especially a rare disease. In a case-control study, persons with the disease *(cases)* and persons without the disease *(controls)* are recruited into the study and assessed for the exposure of interest. If an association exists between the exposure and the disease, the proportion of exposed persons would be expected to be greater among the cases than the controls.

Because case-control studies do not follow subjects over time, they require fewer resources and can be conducted more quickly than cohort studies. For rare diseases such as oral cancer, recruiting existing cases is much more efficient than enrolling a large, cancer-free cohort and observing the subjects over time. The major disadvantage of the case-control study is that the temporal relationship between the exposure and the onset of disease cannot always be determined because the exposure is usually assessed when the disease status is established. Also, the prevalence or incidence of a disease cannot be determined from a case-control study because the subjects are recruited into the study based on their disease status.

More information on the basics of epidemiology can be found in texts by Gordis[33] and Greenberg.[34]

DIAGNOSIS

Normal versus Abnormal; Health versus Disease

For epidemiologists to study disease in populations or for clinicians to care for individual patients, they must be able to identify individuals with disease. For some conditions, the distinction between health and disease is apparent. For example, if a teenager has extensive bone loss around the first molars and lower incisors, the clinical diagnosis of "localized, aggressive periodontitis" (formerly localized juvenile periodontitis) is obvious. For many conditions, however, a gray area exists between health and disease. Does a patient with a diastolic blood pressure of 90 mm Hg have hypertension? If the tip of a dental explorer "sticks" on the occlusal surface of a molar with no obvious cavitation, is dental caries present? Does a patient with 3 mm of periodontal attachment loss on only one tooth have periodontitis? The consequences of making the wrong decision could be significant. In clinical practice, misdiagnosing diseased and disease-free patients could mean that persons without disease would face the costs and risks of unnecessary treatment while persons with disease go untreated. In epidemiologic studies the misclassification of subjects would result in the underestimation or overestimation of the prevalence of disease. It also could lead to invalid conclusions about the association between a disease and some exposure or characteristic.

When making diagnoses, clinicians assimilate information from a variety of sources, such as patient interviews, clinical examinations, radiographs, and laboratory data. From this information, the clinician needs to distinguish between normal and abnormal findings. One approach for making this distinction is to consider abnormal as "unusual."[29] In clinical practice, this refers to the unexpected or infrequent finding or test result. What is unexpected or infrequent is sometimes based on statistically defined *thresholds,* such as two standard deviations from the mean or the 95th percentile (those in the upper 5%). However, thresholds based on statistical considerations are not adequate for all diseases. As Fletcher et al.[29] point out, if the same statistical threshold was chosen for all clinical tests, the prevalence of all diseases would be the same. Another approach is to establish the threshold using observations associated with an increased risk of disease. For example, 90 mm Hg is chosen as the threshold for hypertension because observations that are above that value are associated with greater risk for developing cardiovascular disease.

Principles of Diagnostic Testing

Practitioners use diagnostic tests to increase the probability of making correct diagnoses. In dentistry the diagnosis of periodontal disease is made by the assimilation of clinical and radiographic information, such as bleeding on probing, pocket depth, attachment loss, and bone loss. However, progress is being made in the development of diagnostic tests for periodontal disease. Because periodontal disease is a chronic, infectious disease, microbiologic tests have been developed to detect the presence of specific periodontal pathogens in the gingival sulcus or pockets. These tests are useful for planning treatment for new patients, selecting appropriate recall intervals, monitoring periodontal therapy, determining appropriate antibiotic therapy for patients who do not respond to conventional therapy, and screening patients before extensive restorative or implant therapy.[85] Also, immunologic and biochemical tests to measure the individual's response to periodontal pathogens are being developed. As more of these tests become available, it will become increasingly important for dental practitioners to understand the principles of diagnostic testing.

Sensitivity and Specificity

When a diagnostic test for a disease or condition gives a positive result, the result can be correct *(true positive)* or incorrect *(false positive).* When a test gives a negative result, the result can be true *(true negative)* or false *(false negative)* (Table 8-1). The ability of a test to give a correct answer is indicated by its sensitivity and specificity.

The *sensitivity* of a test is the proportion of subjects with the disease who test positive.

A highly sensitive test is unlikely to be negative when someone has the disease (false negative). A clinician should choose a highly sensitive test when the consequences of not identifying a person with a disease could be severe, such as during testing for human immunodeficiency virus (HIV) infection. Another example would be a microbiologic test for active periodontal disease. Although the consequences would not be as potentially severe as in the HIV example, a false-negative result for active periodontal disease could mean that appropriate therapy would not be prescribed. Sensitive tests also are useful when a clinician wants to rule out possible diseases during the early stages of diagnostic workups or to screen for diseases during routine physical examinations. Because sensitive tests rarely give false-negative results, sensitive tests are most informative when the results are negative.[29] That is, if the results are negative, the clinician can be reasonably sure the person does not have the disease.

The *specificity* of a test is the proportion of subjects without the disease who test negative.

A highly specific test is unlikely to be positive when a person does not have the disease (false positive). Specific tests are especially indicated when the misdiagnosis of disease in the absence of disease could harm a person emotionally, physically, or financially.[29] For example, a false-positive screening test for HIV could cause significant

TABLE 8-1

Comparison of Diagnostic Test Results with True Disease Status

	TRUE DISEASE STATUS	
Test Result	**Disease**	**No Disease**
Positive	A (True positive)	B (False positive)
Negative	C (False negative)	D (True negative)
Sensitivity	A ÷ (A + C)	
Specificity	D ÷ (B + D)	
Positive predictive value	A ÷ (A + B)	
Negative predictive value	D ÷ (C + D)	

emotional stress until more definitive testing could be performed. Although a false-positive microbiologic test for active periodontal disease could mean unnecessary treatment and expense, it also could mean that a person who desires extensive restorative treatment or dental implants would inappropriately be considered as too "high–risk" for such care. Because highly specific tests rarely give false-positive results, specific tests are most informative to clinicians when the results are positive.[29]

Ideally, a diagnostic test would be highly sensitive and specific; however, for most tests, sensitivity comes at the expense of specificity, and vice versa. This is because most diagnostic test results take on values distributed over a range of values. In such cases, a threshold, or cutoff point, must be established to distinguish between positive and negative results. As the threshold is moved higher or lower, the sensitivity and the specificity change in opposite directions. Currently, the threshold for hypertension is a diastolic blood pressure of 90 mm Hg. However, if the threshold for hypertension were increased to 100 mm Hg, the number of false positives would decrease (increased specificity) while the number of false negatives would increase (decreased sensitivity). The decision of where to place a threshold for a test depends on the penalty for making the wrong decision. If the penalty for a false-negative result is higher than the penalty for a false-positive result, a threshold that makes the test more sensitive should be selected. If the penalty for a false-positive result is higher, however, a threshold that makes the test more specific should be selected. Because diagnostic tests are rarely both sensitive and specific, a highly sensitive test is sometimes administered first to rule out people who do not have the disease. Then the people who test positive are given a highly specific test to rule in people who have the disease.

Predictive Value

Sensitivity and specificity are characteristics of a diagnostic test that are useful in choosing an appropriate test. However, once a clinician has received the test result, the most relevant question becomes, "Given this test result, what is the probability that it is right?" The answer to this question is the *predictive value* of the test. The probability that a person with a positive test has the disease is called the *positive predictive value* of the test (A ÷ [A + B], as shown in Table 8-1). The probability that a person with a negative test does not have the disease is referred to as the *negative predictive value* (D ÷ [C + D]). For a given diagnostic test, the predictive values are influenced by the prevalence of the disease in the population tested.[29] As the prevalence of disease in the population decreases, a higher proportion of the positive tests are false. As the prevalence of disease increases, a higher proportion of negative tests are false. This situation is better explained by looking at the extremes of prevalence.

Consider a population in which no one has the disease. In such a group, all positive results, even for a very specific test, will be false positives. Therefore, as the prevalence of disease in a population approaches zero, the positive predictive value of a test also approaches zero. Conversely, if everyone in a population tested has the disease, all negative results will be false negatives, even for a very sensitive test. As prevalence approaches 100%, negative predictive value approaches zero.[29] Because of the influence of prevalence on the predictive values of tests, clinicians need to be aware of the patient's probability of having disease.

RISK VERSUS PROGNOSIS

Risk, Risk Factors, and Risk Assessment

In addition to determining who has a disease at a given point in time, clinicians and epidemiologists are also interested in predicting *who* will get the disease. The likelihood that a person will get a disease in a specified time period is called *risk*. For any given disease, the risk of developing the disease differs among individuals. The characteristics of individuals that place them at increased risk for getting a disease are called *risk factors*. As the definition implies, exposure to a risk factor must occur before the onset of disease. Exposure to a risk factor may have been at a single point in time, episodic, or continuous. Removal of a risk factor or a reduction in exposure should reduce an individual's risk of getting the disease, but once a person has the disease, removal of the risk factor may not make the disease disappear. Also, rarely does a single risk factor explain a person's entire risk for a disease. The identification and importance of risk factors for a disease are based on current knowledge, and as knowledge about relationships between factors and disease changes, new factors may become important while previously identified factors become less important or irrelevant.

The process of predicting an individual's probability of disease is called *risk assessment*. Clinicians use risk assessment in several ways. One way is to predict which patients are at risk for disease. For example, people who smoke cigarettes or have diabetes are at a higher risk of developing periodontal disease than nonsmokers or nondiabetic persons. This information may be important for scheduling the frequency of hygiene appointments. Another way clinicians use risk assessment is to aid in the diagnosis of disease. In adolescent patients with localized bone loss on the lower first molars, the detection of significant numbers of *Actinobacillus actinomycetemcomitans* can help in the diagnosis of early-onset periodontitis. Finally, clinicians often use risk assessment to prevent disease by identifying and modifying risk factors. For example, dental providers typically identify cigarette smokers within their practices and offer smoking cessation services. The amount of disease prevented depends on the success of the intervention in reducing the risk and the number of risk factors associated with the disease.

Prognosis, Prognostic Factors, and Prognosis Assessment

Once disease is identified, the patient and clinician usually turn their attention to the course of disease. Unlike risk, which deals with the prediction of new disease, *prognosis* is the prediction of the course or outcome of the disease. Depending on the disease, important outcomes may include death, survival, or quality-of-life issues, such as pain and disability. For periodontal disease, important outcomes include tooth loss, recurrent disease, and loss of function. The characteristics or factors that predict the outcome of a disease once disease is present are known as *prognostic factors,* and the process of using prognostic factors to predict the course of a disease is called *prognosis assessment.* In periodontics, factors often considered in the generation of a prognosis include, but are not limited to, tooth type, furcation involvement, bone loss, pocket depth, tooth mobility, occlusal force, patient's home dental care, presence of systemic disease, and cigarette smoking (see Chapter 38).

As discussed earlier, measures of disease incidence usually include new periodontal lesions in sites without previous disease and progression of disease in already-diseased sites. In reality, the latter event is actually disease *progression,* not disease incidence. Although this distinction may not be extremely important when considering the incidence of disease, the difference between risk factors and prognostic factors should be remembered. Some factors (e.g., smoking) may be both risk factors and prognostic factors, whereas others are either risk factors or prognostic factors. Thus, once a person has the disease, two processes must be considered: reducing the risk in healthy sites and increasing the risk for a positive prognosis in the sites with disease.

GINGIVAL DISEASE

A gingivitis case clearly involves a person with gingivitis. The more difficult part involves deciding when a person has gingivitis. An early definition of gingivitis simply stated that gingivitis was inflammation of the gingiva.[52] Another definition in the literature states that gingivitis is inflammation of the gingiva in which the junctional epithelium remains attached to the tooth at its original level.[32] This definition implies that gingivitis does not exist if the tooth has periodontitis. In other words, if the inflammatory process involves the gingiva and the periodontium and loss of periodontal attachment has occurred, then according to this definition, the condition should be called *periodontitis,* not gingivitis. The presence of plaque-induced gingivitis in a patient with existing but nonprogressing attachment loss has recently been classified (see Box 7-2). Whether the presence or absence of gingivitis is conditional on the presence of attachment loss has important implications for the estimation of the prevalence of gingivitis.

Although the clinical signs of gingivitis are easy to detect, it is not clear how much inflammation a person must have to be considered a gingivitis case. A universally accepted threshold for the amount or severity of gingival inflammation that must be present in an individual does not exist. In studies of gingivitis, a variety of indices have been used. Because different indices have different clinical criteria for establishing the presence or absence of gingivitis, the definition of a gingivitis case varies across studies. In general, however, a gingivitis case is a person with at least mild inflammation in at least one of the gingival units that are assessed. Depending on the study, a "gingival unit" may be an anatomic structure of the gingiva, such as the interdental papilla, marginal gingiva, or attached gingiva, or it may be a gingival site defined in relation to a tooth, such as the facial, lingual, mesial, or distal gingiva.

How Is Gingivitis Measured?

Gingivitis is measured by gingival indices. *Indices* are methods for quantifying the amount and severity of diseases or conditions in individuals or populations. Indices are used in clinical practice to assess the gingival status of patients and follow any changes in gingival status over time. Gingival indices are used in epidemiologic studies to compare the prevalence of gingivitis in population groups. In clinical studies, gingival indices are used to test the efficacy of therapeutic agents or devices. The ideal index is simple and quick to use, accurate, reproducible, and quantitative. All gingival indices measure one or more of the following: gingival color, gingival contour, gingival bleeding, extent of gingival involvement, and gingival crevicular fluid flow.[25] Most indices assign numbers on an ordinal scale (0, 1, 2, 3, and so on) to represent the extent and severity of the gingival condition. These numbers usually can be summarized to represent the gingival status in an individual or a population. The first quantitative methods for assessing gingivitis appeared around the end of World War II. Many gingival indices have been introduced since that time, and no single index has universal application or acceptance.[46]

Gingival Index

The gingival index (GI) was proposed in 1963 as a method for assessing the severity and quantity of gingival inflammation in individual patients or among subjects in large population groups (Box 8-1).[48,50] Only gingival tissues are assessed with the GI. According to this method, each of the four gingival areas of the tooth (facial, mesial, distal, and lingual) is assessed for inflammation and given a score from 0 to 3. Box 8-1 identifies the criteria for quantifying the severity of gingival inflammation. Bleeding is assessed by running a periodontal probe along the soft tissue wall of the gingival crevice. The scores for the four areas of the tooth can be totaled and divided by four to give a tooth score. By adding the tooth scores together and dividing by the number of teeth examined, an individual's GI score can be obtained. The gingival areas of all teeth or selected teeth can be assessed. A GI

BOX 8-1

Scores and Criteria for Gingival Index (GI)

0 = Normal gingiva.
1 = Mild inflammation: slight change in color and slight edema; *no bleeding on probing.*
2 = Moderate inflammation: redness, edema, and glazing; *bleeding on probing.*
3 = Severe inflammation: marked redness and edema; ulceration; *tendency to spontaneous bleeding.*

Data from Löe H: *J Periodontol* 38(suppl):610, 1967.

BOX 8-2

Scores and Criteria for Modified Gingival Index (MGI)

0 = Absence of inflammation.
1 = Mild inflammation: slight change in color; little change in texture of any portion of, but not the entire, marginal or papillary gingival unit.
2 = Mild inflammation: criteria as above, but involving the entire marginal or papillary gingival unit.
3 = Moderate inflammation: glazing, redness, edema, and/or hypertrophy of the marginal or papillary gingival unit.
4 = Severe inflammation: marked redness, edema, and/or hypertrophy of the marginal or papillary gingival unit; spontaneous bleeding, congestion, or ulceration.

Modified from Lobene RR, Weatherford T, Ross NM, et al: *Clin Prev Dent* 8:3, 1986.

score of 0.1 to 1.0 indicates *mild* inflammation, 1.1 to 2.0 indicates *moderate* inflammation, and 2.1 to 3.0 indicates *severe* inflammation.[48]

Modified Gingival Index

The modified gingival index (MGI) introduced two important changes to the GI: (1) elimination of gingival probing to assess the presence or absence of bleeding and (2) redefinition of the scoring system for mild and moderate inflammation (Box 8-2).[47] The developers of the MGI decided to eliminate probing, which could disturb plaque and irritate the gingiva. A noninvasive index would allow for repeated evaluations and permit intracalibration and intercalibration of examiners. Also, the developers wanted an index that would be more sensitive to earlier, more subtle changes in gingival inflammation.[47] To achieve this, they assigned a score of 1 to mild inflammation that involved only a portion of the marginal or papillary gingival unit and a score of 2 to mild inflammation that involved the entire marginal or papillary gingival unit. Scores of 3 and 4 correspond with the original scores of 2 and 3, respectively, of the GI. Box 8-2 provides the scoring criteria for the MGI. As with the GI, four gingival units per tooth (two marginal, two papillary) are assessed. Either a full or a partial mouth assessment can be performed. A mean score for an individual can be calculated by summing the gingival unit scores and dividing by the number of gingival units examined.

The MGI is perhaps the most widely used index in clinical trials of therapeutic agents.[25] As with its predecessors, the MGI does not assess the presence of periodontal pockets or attachment loss. Thus, these indices cannot identify gingivitis in the absence of periodontitis.

Gingival Bleeding Indices

Whereas the clinical assessment of gingival color, form, and texture is subjective in nature, gingival bleeding is an *objective* diagnostic sign of inflammation. Research suggests that bleeding on gentle probing of the gingival sulcus may occur before changes in color, form, or texture are apparent.[35,38,54] Since 1974, numerous indices that measure bleeding only, such as the gingival bleeding index and the Eastman interdental bleeding index, have been published and reviewed elsewhere.[22,23,56] Periodontal probes are used with most indices; however, toothpicks and dental floss are used to elicit bleeding with some indices.[56] Among the indices that require the use of periodontal probes, the type of probe and the angulation, depth, and force of probing vary. Even though gingival bleeding is a sign of inflammation, the bleeding from the gingival sulcus may be associated with other forms of periodontal disease, not just gingivitis. For indices that require insertion of the periodontal probe to the bottom of the gingival sulcus, bleeding may be a sign of periodontitis rather than gingivitis. Gingival bleeding indices are used in clinical practice, surveys of population groups, and clinical trials of antiplaque and antigingivitis agents.

Nidcr Protocol for Assessment of Gingival Bleeding. In several of its national surveys, such as the NIDR National Survey of Oral Health in U.S. Employed Adults and Seniors (1985–1986) and the Third National Health and Nutrition Examination Survey (1988–1994), the National Institute of Dental and Craniofacial Research (NIDCR) has used the presence or absence of gingival bleeding as an indication of gingival health. The gingival assessment is just one of several components of the NIDCR protocol for the assessment of periodontal disease. For this approach, the facial and mesiofacial sites of teeth in two randomly selected quadrants, one maxillary and one mandibular, are assessed for bleeding. A special probe known as the *NIDR probe* is used in these assessments. The NIDR probe is color-coded and is graduated at 2, 4, 6, 8, 10, and 12 mm. To begin the assessment, the examiner dries a quadrant of teeth with air. Then, starting with the most posterior tooth in the quadrant (excluding the third molar), the examiner places a periodontal probe 2 mm into the gingival sulcus at the facial site and carefully sweeps the probe from the mesiofacial to the mesial interproximal area. After probing the sites in the quadrant, the examiner assesses the presence or absence of bleeding at each probed site. The same procedure is repeated for the remaining quadrant. For an individual, the number or percentage of teeth or sites with bleeding can be calculated. For population groups, the prevalence of gingival bleeding, usually defined as bleeding at one or more sites, can be determined.

How Much Gingivitis Is Present?

Data on the dental health of the U.S. population come from the third National Health and Nutrition Examination Survey (NHANES III), conducted from 1988 to 1994. The survey was the seventh in a series of national surveys designed to provide estimates of the health status of the U.S. population. This survey used the NIDCR protocol for gingival bleeding, as just described. According to data from NHANES III, 54% of the noninstitutionalized civilian U.S. population age 13 years and older had gingival bleeding in at least one gingival site.[79] Gingival bleeding

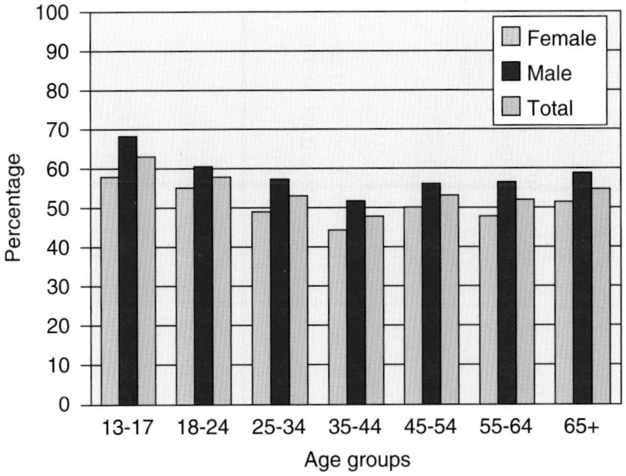

Figure 8-1 Percentage of persons in the United States with one or more sites of gingival bleeding. (Data from US Department of Health and Human Services, National Center for Health Statistics: *Third National Health and Nutrition Examination Survey, 1988–1994,* NHANES III Examination Data File (CD-ROM), Public Use Data File Documentation Number 76200, Hyattsville, Md, 1996, Centers for Disease Control and Prevention.)

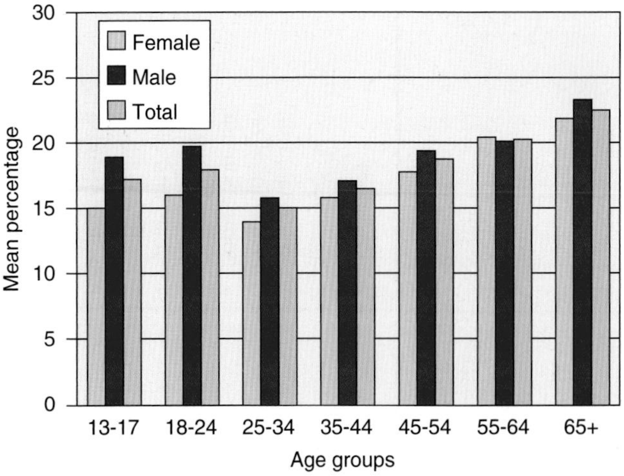

Figure 8-2 Mean percentage of sites per person with gingival bleeding among persons in the United States with gingival bleeding. (Data from US Department of Health and Human Services, National Center for Health Statistics: *Third National Health and Nutrition Examination Survey, 1988–1994,* NHANES III Examination Data File (CD-ROM), Public Use Data File Documentation Number 76200, Hyattsville, Md, 1996, Centers for Disease Control and Prevention.)

was most prevalent in the 13- to 17-year-old group (63%) and declined gradually through the 35- to 44-year-old group (Figure 8-1). The prevalence increased again at the 45- to 54-year-old group but remained fairly constant in older groups. On average per person, 10% of all sites had gingival bleeding; however, among persons with gingival bleeding, an average of 18% of sites had gingival bleeding. The extent of gingival bleeding among persons with gingival bleeding was higher in the younger and older groups than in the middle age groups (Figure 8-2).

A study of U.S. schoolchildren age 14 to 17 years reported that the prevalence of gingival bleeding was 61.5%, essentially identical to the prevalence reported among those age 13 to 17 years in the NHANES III study.[14] Both surveys used the NIDCR gingival sweep method for eliciting gingival bleeding. The prevalence decreased with age from a high of 65% in 14-year-olds to a low of 57% in 17-year-olds. On average per child, 6% of sites measured had gingival bleeding with probing.

In NHANES III, gingival bleeding was assessed at periodontal sites without regard to the periodontal status of the tooth. According to a definition cited earlier, gingivitis is inflammation of the gingiva in which the junctional epithelium remains attached to the tooth at its original level.[32] If the prevalence of gingival bleeding from NHANES III data is recalculated using only periodontal sites without attachment loss (<1 mm), the prevalence of one or more sites per person with gingival bleeding decreases slightly from 54% to 47%. This indicates that about 7% of the people had bleeding only in sites with attachment loss. The remainder of individuals either did not have any bleeding in sites with attachment loss or had bleeding in sites with and without attachment loss.

Is More or Less Gingivitis Present Now than Previously?

Although it is generally believed that the prevalence of gingivitis is declining in the United States, the epidemiologic data needed to make that claim do not exist.[8] Since 1960, several national health surveys have assessed periodontal health: the Health Examination Survey (HES) (1960–1962), NHANES I (1971–1974), the Health Resources and Services Administration (HRSA) survey of households (1981), the National Institute of Dental Research (NIDR) study of employed adults (1985–1986), and NHANES III (1988–1994). However, because of differences in populations, sampling methods, and periodontal measurement methods, comparisons of results between these surveys are difficult, if not impossible, to make. Table 8-2 summarizes periodontal findings from studies based on data from these surveys. Even if results from these studies could be compared, they do not support the view that the prevalence of gingivitis is declining.

Does My Patient with Gingivitis Fit the Typical Profile?

Gingivitis is so common that any patient presenting with gingivitis could be considered typical; however, gingivitis is more prevalent among certain groups. Adolescents have a higher prevalence of gingivitis than prepubertal children or adults. The rise of sex hormones during adolescence is suspected to be the cause of the increased prevalence. Studies suggest that the increase in sex hormones during puberty affects the composition of the subgingival microflora.[36,53,55] One study found that increased serum levels of testosterone in boys and estradiol

TABLE 8-2

U.S. Population-Based Prevalence Studies* of Periodontal Disease

	HES[79]	HANES I[80]	HRSA Survey[16]	NIDR Survey[17]	NHANES III[74]
Year(s) conducted	1960–1962	1971–1974	1981	1985–1986	1988–1994
Population sampled	Total civilian, non-institutionalized population age 18-79 years	Total civilian, non-institutionalized population age 1-74 years	Households (including military personnel and their families)	Employed persons age 18-64	Total civilian, non-institutionalized population age 2 months and older
Age at periodontal assessment	18-79 years	6-74 years	19 years and older	18-64 years	13 years and older
Method of periodontal assessment	Periodontal index (PI) No probing	Periodontal index No probing	Periodontal index (with modifications) Pocket depth measured in millimeters (mm) at mesial of every permanent erupted tooth	Bleeding on probing Ramfjord probing technique Measured mesiofacial and midfacial sites in one upper and one lower quadrant (maximum of 28 sites in 14 teeth)	Bleeding on probing Ramfjord probing technique Measured mesiofacial and midfacial sites in one upper and one lower quadrant (maximum of 28 sites in 14 teeth)
Prevalence of gingivitis	48.5%	25%	50% had gingivitis any pockets ≥4 mm	44% had one or more sites without with bleeding	54% had one or more sites with bleeding
Prevalence of periodontal pockets person: 1.13	25.4% had pockets Average PI per Average PI per person: 0.83	4.5% had 1-3 pockets 12.1% had ≥4 pockets 8% had 1 or more teeth with pocket ≥6 mm	28% had 1 or more teeth with pocket 4-6 mm 0.6% had one or more sites with pocket ≥7 mm	13.4% had one or more sites with pocket 4-6 mm ≥4 mm	21.0% had one or more sites with pocket
Prevalence of attachment loss	Not assessed	Not assessed	Not assessed	43.8% had one or more sites with attachment loss ≥3 mm	38.1% had one or more sites with attachment loss ≥3 mm

*References refer to published studies that analyzed data from these surveys. Periodontal findings in any given column are from the study referenced in the top cell.

HES, Health Examination Survey; *HANES I,* First Health and Nutrition Examination Survey; *HRSA,* Health Resources and Services Administration; *NIDR,* National Institute of Dental Research; *NHANES III,* Third National Health and Nutrition Survey.

SCIENCE TRANSFER

There is a widespread tendency to misinterpret epidemiologic data on periodontal disease by assuming that a statistically significant relationship between two variables proves cause and effect. Even if the increase in one variable precedes in time the increases in another, this type of data can only suggest, not prove, a causal relationship. Another confounding process is that both variables may change because of the effect of a third variable or groups of variables, further complicating the true connection between them (see Chapter 2). These relationships have importance, however, since they can be the basis for planning inductive research to establish cause and effect.

Different techniques for measuring gingival bleeding on probing are used in epidemiologic estimations of gingivitis and are described as specific procedures for different indices. Clinically, the bleeding seen with routine probing of pockets on individual patients during periodontal charting is comparable to Bleeding on Probing (BOP) used in epidemiologic research. The deeper penetration of the probe with charting will most likely increase the chance of bleeding compared with the epidemiologic indices of gingivitis that use superficial probing with sweeping techniques. All bleeding on probing is caused by gingival inflammation coupled with ulceration of the epithelial lining of the gingival sulcus. This can occur as early as 2 days after gingivitis begins in healthy gingiva and frequently persists throughout the development of gingivitis and periodontitis. In many cases, if plaque and calculus are removed, the epithelial ulceration will heal, and gingival bleeding on probing is eliminated. This healing of the ulceration can take 7 to 10 days. If plaque then reaccumulates in the region (e.g., because of inadequate oral hygiene), ulceration and bleeding can return in 2 days. Thus, for individual patients, bleeding on probing is a good indicator of current inflammatory disease activity at all stages of periodontal disease.

Factors such as smoking appear to be related to the incidence of periodontal disease, but these confirmed etiologic relationships do not necessarily have the same degree of effect on the patient's response to treatment. Response to treatment is a separate issue that clinicians need to focus on in order to give a basis for scientifically based treatment planning. Surgical procedures in which blood supply is of paramount importance (e.g., mucogingival surgery for root coverage) may be more affected by smoking than regenerative bone-grafting procedures in which osteoprogenitor cell activation is pivotal.

and progesterone in girls were associated with increased levels of the periodontal pathogens *Prevotella intermedia* and *Prevotella nigrescens*.[55] Hormonal effects also may be responsible for the increased prevalence during pregnancy and among women.[30]

As shown in Figure 8-1, males in all age groups are more likely to have gingivitis than females. The prevalence of gingivitis is especially high for males age 13 to 17 years. Also, males with gingivitis have more involved sites than females (see Figure 8-2), especially in the younger groups. Although the reason for the existence of these gender differences is not known, poorer plaque control among males could likely explain much of their higher prevalence and extent of disease.

Why Do Patients Have Gingivitis, and What Puts Them at Risk?

It is clear from experimental and epidemiologic studies that microbial plaque is the direct cause of gingivitis.[45,51,59,65] The cause-and-effect relationship between plaque and gingival inflammation was demonstrated in a classic study by Löe et al.[51] in which 12 individuals (9 dental students, 1 instructor, and 2 laboratory technicians) were asked to abstain from all measures of oral hygiene. Dental plaque began to form quickly, and the amount of plaque increased with time. All subjects developed gingivitis within 10 to 21 days. The mean GI score increased from 0.27 at baseline to 1.05 at the end of the "no-brushing" period. Gingival inflammation resolved in all subjects within 1 week of resuming hygiene measures. The authors concluded that bacterial plaque was essential in the production of gingival inflammation.

Because bacterial plaque is the cause of the most common form of gingivitis, factors that influence the oral hygiene status of individuals would likely influence the prevalence of gingivitis. The generally poorer oral hygiene status of males may explain the higher prevalence and extent among males.[3] Poorer oral hygiene also may explain the higher prevalence of gingivitis among adolescents. Even though the increased levels of circulating sex hormones have been implicated in the higher prevalence, the influence of plaque control on gingivitis may be more important than the rising levels of hormones.[77] The conversion of bleeding gingival sites to nonbleeding sites with oral hygiene interventions alone provide strong evidence for the role of poor oral hygiene in the etiology of gingivitis.[7,15,24]

Few population-based studies of the association between oral hygiene status and gingivitis have been published. In NHANES I, information on toothbrushing frequency and oral hygiene status was collected. A study that investigated the associations between these factors and the periodontal index (PI) reported that increased toothbrushing frequency and better oral hygiene scores were associated with lower PI scores.[76] These associations remained statistically significant after controlling for age, race, socioeconomic status, alcohol consumption, smoking habits, and dental visits. Although this study was based on the PI, an index of periodontal disease, gingivitis is a component of all but the most severe category. In NHANES III, information on the presence or absence of calculus was collected. However, this study has not reported any association between calculus and gingival health.

Although smoking is one of the most important risk factors for adult periodontitis, its role in gingivitis is unclear. Several studies have indicated that gingival bleeding is reduced among smokers.[13,66] Plaque levels in the smokers were either similar to or greater than plaque levels in nonsmokers. This reduction in gingival bleeding among smokers may be the result of the vasoconstrictive effects of nicotine in cigarette smoke. In clinical practice the smoking status of patients should be considered when gingival bleeding is assessed.

CHRONIC PERIODONTITIS

Periodontitis is inflammation of the periodontium that extends beyond the gingiva and produces destruction of the connective tissue attachment of the teeth.[68] No longer considered a single disease, periodontitis is now considered to exist in three primary forms: chronic, aggressive, and as a manifestation of systemic diseases (see Box 7-3). Chronic periodontitis is the most common form. Chronic periodontitis progresses slowly and generally becomes clinically significant in adults but may be observed in children. For epidemiologic purposes, a case of chronic periodontitis is a person with the disease. As with gingivitis, methods to measure periodontitis and the amount of disease necessary to consider a person a case vary widely across studies.

How Is Periodontitis Measured?

Periodontal Index

In the early 1950s, gingivitis indices were gaining in popularity; however, no index was available to measure more advanced stages of periodontal disease. Motivated by the lack of valid indices for measuring the prevalence of periodontal disease in population groups, Russell[69] developed the *periodontal index* (Box 8-3). Use of the PI requires a minimum of equipment: a light source, a mouth mirror, and an explorer. The supporting tissues for each tooth in the mouth are scored according to a progressive scale that gives little weight to gingival inflammation and relatively great weight to advanced periodontal disease.[69] Box 8-3 identifies the scoring criteria for the PI. An *individual's score* is the sum of the tooth scores divided by the number of teeth examined. The *population score* is the sum of the individual scores divided by the number of persons examined. Periodontal probing was not recommended because, according to Russell, it "added little and proved to be a troublesome focus of examiner disagreement."[69]

BOX 8-3

Scores and Criteria* for Periodontal Index (PI)

0 = *Negative.* There is neither overt inflammation in the investing tissues nor loss of function caused by destruction of supporting tissues.
1 = *Mild gingivitis.* There is an overt area of inflammation in the free gingiva, but this area does not circumscribe the tooth.
2 = *Gingivitis.* Inflammation completely circumscribes the tooth, but there is no apparent break in the epithelial attachment.
6 = *Gingivitis with pocket formation.* The epithelial attachment has been broken, and there is a pocket (not merely a deepened gingival crevice caused by swelling in the free gingiva). There is no interference with normal masticatory function; the tooth is firm in its socket and has not drifted.
8 = *Advanced destruction with loss of masticatory function.* The tooth may be loose, may have drifted, may sound dull on percussion with a metallic instrument, and may be depressible in its socket.

*Criteria and scoring for field studies.
Modified from Russell AL: *J Dent Res* 35:350, 1956.

The PI is fast and easy to use. However, one important criticism of the index is that it underestimates the prevalence of disease.[67]

Periodontal Disease Index

As a consultant to the World Health Organization for a 1957 study of periodontal disease in India, Ramfjord[67] was faced with the inadequacies of the available indices for measuring periodontal disease. Taking the most valuable features of existing indices and adding new features to compensate for their shortcomings, Ramfjord developed his own system for measuring periodontal disease.[67] This system became known as the *periodontal disease index* (PDI). One unique aspect of the PDI was the examination of six preselected teeth in the mouth: the maxillary right first molar, maxillary left central incisor, maxillary left first premolar, mandibular left first molar, mandibular right central incisor, and mandibular right first premolar. This selection of teeth became known as the *Ramfjord teeth.* Another unique aspect of the PDI was the use of the *cementoenamel junction* (CEJ) as a fixed landmark for measuring periodontal attachment loss.

To begin an assessment using the PDI, the examiner dries the areas around the six teeth. Next, the examiner assesses the severity of gingival inflammation around the six teeth. Gingival scores for a tooth range from G0 for "absence of inflammation" to G3 for "severe gingivitis." At the mesial, facial, distal, and lingual side of each of the six teeth, the distance from the free gingival margin to the CEJ and the distance from the free gingival margin to the bottom of the gingival sulcus are measured in millimeters with a periodontal probe. If the free gingival margin is on the cementum, its distance from the CEJ is

BOX 8-4

Scores and Criteria for Periodontal Disease Index (PDI)

Perform Gingival Assessment

G0 = Absence of inflammation.
G1 = Mild to moderate inflammatory gingival changes not extending all around the tooth.
G2 = Mild to moderate severe gingivitis extending all around the tooth.
G3 = Severe gingivitis characterized by marked redness, tendency to bleed, and ulceration.

Record Pockets

The distance from the free gingival margin to the cementoenamel junction (CEJ) and the distance from the free gingival margin to the bottom of the gingival crevice or pocket should be recorded for the mesial, the facial, the distal, and the lingual aspects of each tooth examined. The interproximal recording should be secured at the buccal aspect of the interproximal contact areas with the probe pointing in the direction of the long axis of the tooth.

If the gingival margin is on enamel:

1. Measure from gum margin to the CEJ, and record the measurement on the crown of the schematic tooth. If the epithelial attachment is on the crown and the CEJ cannot be felt by the probe, record the depth of the gingival crevice on the crown.
2. Measure from the gingival margin to the bottom of the pocket when the crevice extends apically to the CEJ, and record the measurement on the root of the schematic tooth. (The distance from the CEJ to the bottom of the pocket can then be found by subtracting measurement number 1 from measurement number 2.)

If the gingival margin is on cementum:

1. Measure from the CEJ to the gingival margin. Record as a minus value on the root of the schematic tooth.
2. Measure from the CEJ to the bottom of the gingival crevice. Record value on the root.

Modified from Ramfjord SP: *J Periodontol* 30:51, 1959.

recorded as a negative number. The distance from the CEJ to the bottom of the gingival sulcus is the difference between these two measurements. The distance from the CEJ to the bottom of the gingival sulcus is a measurement of periodontal attachment loss. Ramfjord's method for measuring this distance is often referred to as the *indirect method for measuring periodontal attachment loss.* The PDI score for each tooth is based on the assessment of gingival inflammation and the depth of the gingival sulcus in relation to the CEJ (Box 8-4). If the gingival sulcus does not extend apically to the CEJ in any of the measured areas, the PDI score for the tooth is the gingival score. If the gingival sulcus extends below the CEJ in any of the measured areas by 3 mm or less, the PDI score is 4. Teeth with sulcus measurements of 3 to 6 mm and greater than 6 mm are given scores of 5 and 6, respectively. The PDI for the individual is the sum of the tooth scores divided by the number of teeth examined. If any of the six preselected teeth are missing, another tooth is not substituted in its place. In addition to the PDI score for periodontal disease, the PDI provides a method for calculating tooth scores for calculus, occlusal attrition, mobility, and proximal contacts.

Although the PDI is rarely used today, two aspects of the index are often used: selection of the six Ramfjord teeth and the method for measuring pocket depth and loss of periodontal attachment. Ramfjord's technique for measuring pocket depth and periodontal attachment loss has been used in national surveys (e.g., NHANES).

Extent and Severity Index

The PI and the PDI yield scores that represent the severity of periodontal disease in individuals or populations, but these scores do not provide information on the extent of disease. The *extent and severity index* (ESI) of periodontal disease was developed to provide separate estimates of the extent and severity of periodontal disease in individuals and populations.[21] Unlike the PI and PDI, the ESI does not assess gingival inflammation. Instead, it estimates the loss of periodontal attachment using the periodontal probing method developed by Ramfjord for the PDI.[67] A threshold of disease must be established to calculate the extent score for an individual. In their initial study of the ESI, Carlos et al.[21] considered a site to be diseased when attachment loss exceeded 1 mm. (Because the measurements in epidemiology studies are rounded down to the next lowest millimeter, "greater than 1 mm" means 2 mm or greater, or ≥2 mm.) For an individual, the *extent score* is the percentage of sites examined that have attachment loss greater than 1 mm. The *severity score* for an individual is the average loss of attachment per site among the disease sites. The ESI is expressed as a bivariate statistic: ESI = (Extent, Severity). For example, an individual's ESI of (20, 3.0) would be interpreted as 20% of sites examined had disease, and of the diseased sites, the average loss of attachment was 3.0 mm. The ESI for a population would be the average extent and severity scores for the individuals examined.

When ESI scores from two sites per tooth in the whole mouth were compared with an assessment of one upper and one lower quadrant, the developers of the ESI found that little information was lost from the half-mouth assessment.[21] However, the ESI has been used for full-mouth examinations on as many as six sites per tooth.

NIDCR Protocol for Periodontal Disease Assessment

The NIDCR periodontal disease assessment, as used in NHANES III, contains three parts: a periodontal destruction assessment, gingival assessment, and calculus assessment.[79] The gingival assessment is described in the previous section on gingivitis. The "periodontal destruction" examination involves an assessment of loss of periodontal attachment and furcation involvement.

Loss of periodontal attachment is the distance (in millimeters) from the CEJ to the bottom of the gingival sulcus. This distance is measured at the facial and mesiofacial sites of teeth in two randomly selected quadrants, one maxillary and one mandibular, using the indirect measurement method developed by Ramfjord.[67] Probing is carried out with the use of the NIDCR probe, which is color-coded and has markings at 2, 4, 6, 8, 10, and 12 mm. In NHANES III, loss of attachment was reported in millimeters for each site measured. Periodontal pocket depth, or the distance from the free gingival margin to the bottom of the sulcus, also was reported in millimeters for each site.

Furcation involvement is assessed on eight teeth: the maxillary first and second molars, the maxillary first premolars, and the mandibular first and second molars. The assessment requires the use of a #17 dental explorer for the maxillary teeth and a #3 cowhorn explorer for the mandibular teeth. The extent of furcation involvement is assessed at the mesial, facial, and distal surfaces of the maxillary molars; the mesial and distal sides of the premolars; and the facial and lingual surfaces of the mandibular molars. If furcation involvement does not exist, the site is scored as 0. If partial involvement exists but the probe cannot pass through the furcation, the site is scored as 1. If the explorer can pass between the roots (through involvement), the site is scored as 2.

At each site assessed for loss of attachment, the presence or absence of supragingival and subgingival calculus is assessed. Subgingival calculus is detected using the NIDCR probe. A score of 0 is recorded for the site if no calculus is present; a score of 1 is recorded if only supragingival calculus is present; and a score of 2 is recorded if supragingival and subgingival calculus are present.

Beginning in 1999, NHANES became a continuous, annual survey (e.g., NHANES 1999, 2000, 2001) rather than a periodic survey. All other aspects of the examination were the same as for NHANES III. The survey data are released every 2 years. Thus the data-release cycle for the ongoing (and continuous) NHANES is described as NHANES 1999–2000, NHANES 2001–2002, NHANES 2003–2004, and so on. To produce estimates with greater statistical reliability, combining two or more 2-year cycles of the continuous NHANES is encouraged and strongly recommended. The NIDCR periodontal protocol was slightly modified for the NHANES 1999–2000 studies by adding a mesiofacial site to the examination, resulting in three sites examined per tooth.

Radiographic Assessment of Bone Loss

The radiographic assessment of bone loss is an important part of the clinical diagnosis of periodontal disease. However, for the purposes of estimating the prevalence or incidence of periodontitis in population groups, radiographs are rarely used because of ethical and practical considerations. In studies in which radiographic bone loss is used as a measure of periodontitis, bone loss is usually measured from bite-wing radiographs as the distance from the CEJ to the alveolar crest. Bone loss can be expressed as this distance in millimeters or as a percentage of the root length. Various studies have used

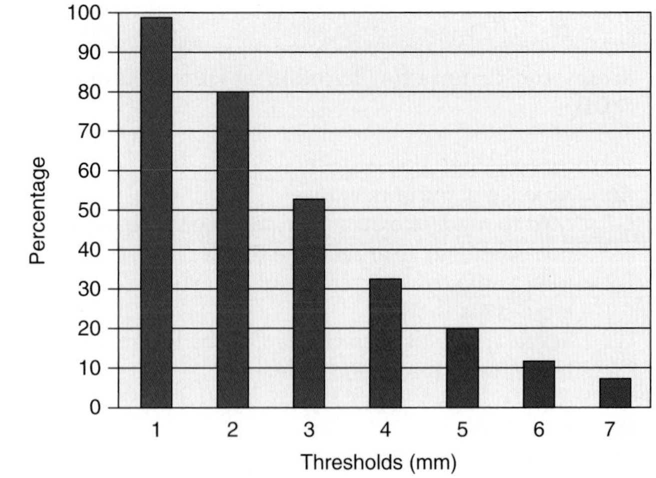

Figure 8-3 Percentage of persons in the United States with periodontal attachment loss according to different thresholds of attachment loss. (Data from Albandar JM, Brunelle JA, Kingman A: Destructive periodontal disease in adults 30 years of age and older in the United States, 1988–1994, *J Periodontol* 70:13, 1999.)

bone loss thresholds ranging from greater than 1 mm to greater than 3 mm.[9] Bone loss measurements from radiographs are highly correlated with measurements of attachment loss taken with periodontal probes.[9] The three main sources of error in the assessment of bone loss are (1) variations in projection geometry, (2) variations in film contrast and density, and (3) obstruction of the view by other anatomic structures.[9] Computerized programs can detect bone changes as small as 0.5 mm when measuring bone loss from sequential radiographs.[41] Also, advanced image-processing techniques, such as digital subtraction radiography and computer-assisted densitometric image analysis, can enhance the ability to detect bone loss over time.[41]

How Much Chronic Periodontitis Is Present?

The most recent data for the prevalence of periodontal disease in the United States come from NHANES III (1988–1994). Because the assessment of periodontitis in a cross-sectional survey such as NHANES III is a cumulative measure of periodontal destruction, separating chronic periodontitis in adults from other forms is not possible. However, an analysis of NHANES III data for adults age 30 years and older was reported.[4] The prevalence of periodontal attachment loss depends greatly on the threshold chosen, ranging from a high of 99% for a threshold of greater than 1 mm to a low of 7% for a threshold of greater than 7 mm (Figure 8-3). At a threshold of greater than 3 mm, the prevalence of attachment loss in at least one site in the mouth was 53.1%. The prevalence of attachment loss increased steadily with age, from a low of 35.7% for the 30- to 39-year-old group to a high of 89.2% for the 80- to 90-year-old group (Figure 8-4). On average per person, 19.6% of the teeth had attachment loss greater than 3 mm. Among people with at least one site of attachment loss greater than 3 mm, an average of 36.6% of the teeth per person was affected. The mean

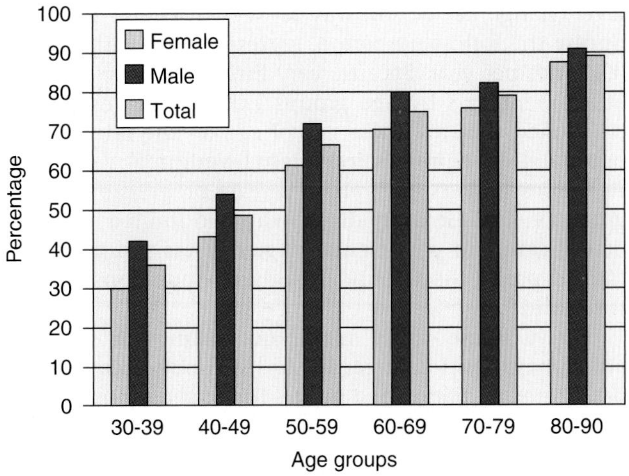

Figure 8-4 Percentage of persons in the United States with periodontal attachment loss of greater than 3 mm. (Data from Albandar JM, Brunelle JA, Kingman A: *J Periodontol* 70:13, 1999.)

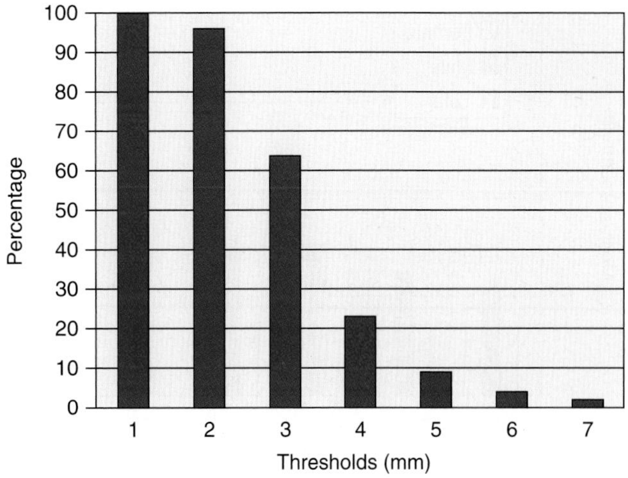

Figure 8-6 Percentage of persons in the United States with periodontal pockets according to different thresholds of pocket depth. (Data from Albandar JM, Brunelle JA, Kingman A: *J Periodontol* 70:13, 1999.)

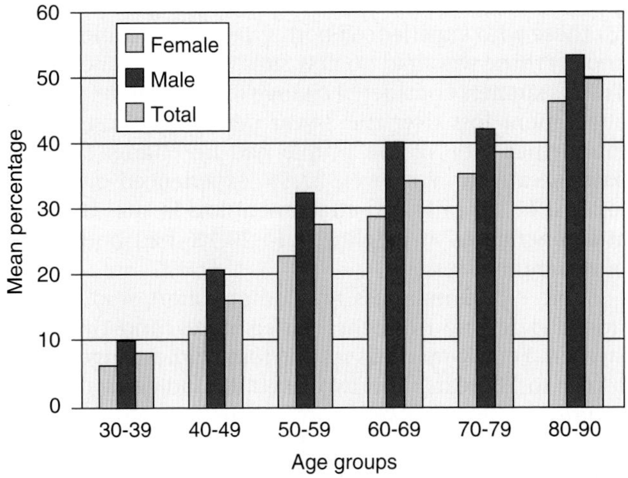

Figure 8-5 Mean percentage of teeth per person in the United States with attachment loss of greater than 3 mm. (Data from Albandar JM, Brunelle JA, Kingman A: *J Periodontol* 70:13, 1999.)

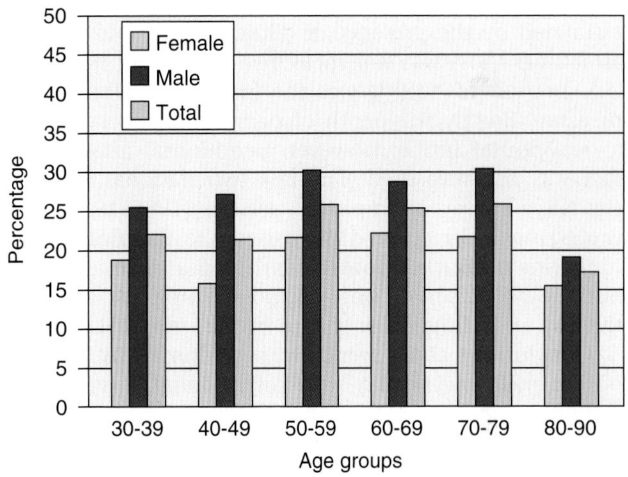

Figure 8-7 Percentage of persons in the United States with periodontal pockets of greater than 4 mm. (Data from Albandar JM, Brunelle JA, Kingman A: *J Periodontol* 70:13, 1999.)

percentage of teeth affected also increased with age (Figure 8-5). Maxillary molars and mandibular incisors were more likely than other teeth to have attachment loss greater than 3 mm, whereas maxillary central incisors were the least likely.

As with attachment loss, the prevalence of periodontal pockets depends greatly on the threshold chosen (Figure 8-6). Generally, pockets greater than 3 mm are considered to reflect disease. The prevalence of periodontal pockets greater than 4 mm was 23.1%. The increase in the prevalence of attachment loss with increasing age is not seen with pocket depth (Figure 8-7). The average extent of pockets greater than 4 mm was 5.2% of teeth per person, and the extent varied little with age (Figure 8-8).

The answer to the question, "How much adult periodontitis is out there?" must be, "It depends on the case definition used."

Is More or Less Chronic Periodontitis Present Now than Previously?

It is frequently stated that the prevalence of periodontal disease has decreased in the United States over the past 30 years. Again, however, because of methodologic differences in the national surveys conducted, it is difficult to draw any conclusions about changes in the prevalence of periodontal disease. Drawing any conclusions about trends in the chronic form of periodontitis is even more difficult. Table 8-2 provides a comparison of the methodologies and results from five national surveys conducted in the United States. The first two surveys, the HES (1960–1962) and HANES I (1971–1974), used the PI to measure periodontal disease. The PI relies only on visible signs of inflammation to determine the severity of periodontal disease. The presence of periodontal pockets was

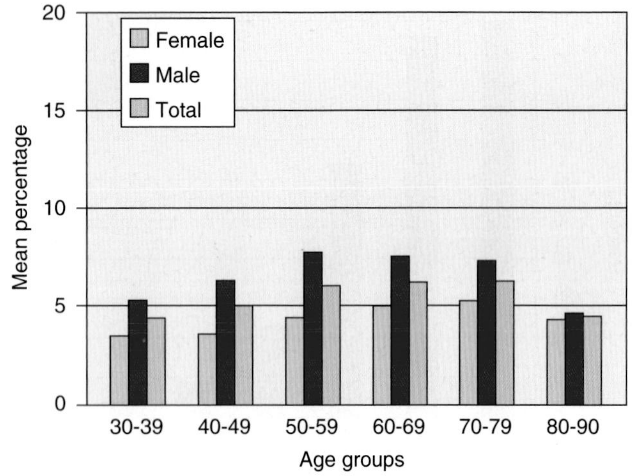

Figure 8-8 Mean percentage of teeth per person in the United States with pocket depths of greater than 4 mm. (Data from Albandar JM, Brunelle JA, Kingman A: *J Periodontol* 70:13, 1999.)

estimated by the presence of clinical signs, and clinical attachment loss was not measured. The HRSA survey of U.S. households (1981) was the first national survey to measure directly the depth of periodontal pockets with a periodontal probe; however, periodontal attachment loss was not measured. The last two national surveys, the NIDR survey of employed persons (1985–1986) and the NHANES III (1988–1994), used the Ramfjord technique for measuring pocket depth and attachment loss, but the NIDR survey only included employed persons, thereby excluding major groups in the United States.

Conclusions about trends in periodontal disease will not be available until a series of national surveys that similarly measure periodontal disease are conducted. However, as Douglas and Fox[27] concluded in their study of trends in periodontal disease, "Even if the prevalence and severity of periodontal disease are seen as declining over the next 30 years, it would seem that a substantial proportion of this decline will be counterbalanced by the sizable increase in number of persons and number of teeth per person at risk of disease." In fact, the authors estimated that for U.S. adults over age 25 years, the number of adults with some manifestation of periodontal disease would increase at least through the year 2010.[27]

How Much New or Progressing Chronic Periodontitis Is Present?

In contrast to prevalence data, no nationally representative longitudinal studies are available in the United States. The incidence rates must be taken from studies representative of local or regional groups in the United States and other countries.

A 10-year follow-up study among Chinese individuals age 20 to 80 years found that 79.8% of all sites measured (4 sites per tooth) experienced attachment loss.[10] Approximately 48% of the sites measured lost more than 2 mm, 21.8% of the sites lost greater than 3 mm, and 9% of the sites lost more than 4 mm. The average attachment level change per person was between 1.45 and 1.86 mm during the follow-up period, corresponding with 0.15 to 0.19 mm per year. Because very little difference in mean attachment loss by age groups existed, the researchers concluded that the influence of age on the rate of periodontal disease progression might be minimal. According to the researchers, the rate of disease progression in this group of Chinese individuals, who had limited access to dental care and poor dental hygiene, was similar to the rate of progression found in other populations around the world.

The Chinese study made no distinction between attachment level changes in sites without disease at the baseline examination and in sites that had existing disease. One study that made a distinction between disease onset and disease progression was a study of community-dwelling older adults (age 65 years and older) living in five contiguous North Carolina counties.[12] The subjects, who were followed for 36 months, were categorized into four groups according to their type of periodontal attachment loss: (1) those who only had attachment loss in previously nondiseased sites, (2) those with only progression of attachment loss in previously diseased sites, (3) those who experienced both types of attachment loss, and (4) those who had no new sites with attachment loss. The researchers considered change to be 3 mm or more of attachment loss over the 3-year period. The researchers found that 40% of the people had no change in their baseline attachment level, 27.5% experienced only new lesions, 11.1% only had attachment loss in sites that had attachment loss at baseline, and 20.1% had both types of attachment loss.

Table 8-3 summarizes four other cohort studies: one from Japan, one from the United States, and two from Sweden. Follow-up times for the four studies ranged from 1 year to 28 years. The two Swedish studies used radiographs to assess changes in alveolar bone height, whereas the studies from the United States and Japan used periodontal probing to assess changes in clinical attachment levels. Mean annual loss of bone or attachment loss per person, ranging from approximately 0.03 to 0.14 mm, was fairly consistent across the three studies that reported this information. Each study shows that attachment loss or alveolar bone loss progressed in only a small percentage of periodontal sites and subjects. Ismail et al.[27] reported that 59.3% of the periodontal sites present at baseline showed no change in attachment loss over the 28 years of follow-up. Only 13.3% of the subjects had a mean change in attachment loss of 2 mm or greater. Approximately 90% of the sites followed in the study by Albandar and Kingman[5] showed no change in bone height in the 6 years that passed between baseline and reexamination. In that study, 70% of the subjects had few or no sites with additional bone loss. From the results in these studies, adult periodontitis appears to progress fairly slowly and in only a minority of the adult population.

Does My Patient with Chronic Periodontitis Fit the Typical Profile?

Chronic periodontitis generally becomes clinically significant after age 30.[68] The disease is characterized by

TABLE 8-3

Other Studies of Periodontal Disease Progression among Adults

Study	Length	Subjects	Methodology	Results
Haffajee et al.[37]	1 year	Random sample of 271 residents of Ushiku, Japan, age 20-79 years.	Clinical attachment loss measured at six sites on all teeth. Change defined as attachment loss of ≥3 mm in 1 year.	27.3% of persons had attachment loss at one or more sites. Older subjects had greater risk of disease progression than younger subjects. Persons with attachment loss at baseline were more likely to have progression.
Ismail et al.[40]	28 years	526 residents of Tecumseh, Mich, age 5-60, examined at baseline in 1959. 167 reexamined in 1987.	Clinical attachment loss measured at four sites per tooth on all teeth present. Calculated mean attachment loss per person over the 28 years.	13.3% of persons had mean loss ≥2 mm. 3.0% of persons had mean loss ≥3 mm. 1.2% of persons had mean loss ≥4 mm. 59.3% of all sites did not change. Mean annual attachment loss per person was 0.04 mm. Only 10.9% of teeth lost during follow-up.
Albandar[4]	6 years	293 employees of industrial plant in Oslo, Sweden, age 18-67, examined at baseline. 142 reexamined at 2 and 6 years.	Radiographic alveolar bone height measured from periapical films. Change defined as ≥1 mm of bone loss during two consecutive exams.	70 % of subjects had few or no sites with bone loss. 25% of subjects had moderate progression. 5% had high rates of progression. 90% of all sites did not change. Mean annual bone loss per person ranged by age from 0.03-0.05 mm.
Papapanou et al.[64]	10 years	531 Swedes examined at baseline in 1974–1976. 201, age 25-70 at baseline, reexamined in 1985–1986.	Radiographic alveolar bone height measured at mesial and distal of each tooth. Reported mean bone loss per person over 10 years.	17% of persons had mean loss of ≥2 mm. Mean annual bone loss per person was 0.07-0.14 mm in those age 25-65 (at baseline), 0.28 mm in those age 70.

a slow progression of attachment loss over time. With 53% of U.S. adults having at least one periodontal site with attachment loss of 3 mm or more, periodontitis is a common disease. Among adults, the prevalence of attachment loss and periodontal pockets are higher in males than females (see Figures 8-4 and 8-7). Males also are more likely than females to have more teeth with attachment loss and more teeth with pockets (see Figures 8-5 and 8-8). Typically, the prevalence and extent of periodontal attachment loss increases with age (see Figures 8-4 and 8-5). This increased prevalence with age more likely reflects the cumulative effect of attachment loss over time rather than an increased susceptibility to periodontitis. Unlike attachment loss, the prevalence or extent of periodontal pocketing does not show much variation with age (see Figures 8-7 and 8-8). The increase in attachment loss with age without a corresponding increase in pocket depth may result from the increasing prevalence of gingival recession with age. In the United States the prevalence of greater than 1 mm of gingival recession increases from 38% in the 30- to 39-year-old group to 90% in the 80- to 90-year-old group.[5]

Why Do Patients Have Chronic Periodontitis, and What Puts Them at Risk?

Periodontitis is an infectious disease associated with a group of mainly gram-negative bacteria.[84] The scientific literature on the pathogenesis of periodontal disease and the role of microbial factors was extensively reviewed at the 1996 World Workshop in Periodontics.[57,84] The section members concluded by consensus that sufficient evidence exists to consider three microorganisms as etiologic agents: *Actinobacillus actinomycetemcomitans, Porphyromonas gingivalis,* and *Tannerella forsythia* (formally *Bacteriodes forsythus*). Of these bacteria, *P. gingivalis* and

T. forsythia often are found in chronic periodontitis, whereas *A. actinomycetemcomitans* often is found in cases of aggressive periodontitis. Evidence suggests that other microorganisms also may be involved in the development of periodontitis.

Although these pathogens are necessary to cause periodontitis, their presence is not sufficient to cause disease. Epidemiologic studies have shown that the presence of microorganisms in the subgingival plaque explains only a small portion of the cases of periodontitis. To explain these findings, periodontal researchers recently have begun to talk about a "new paradigm" for the etiology of adult periodontitis.[61] This paradigm indicates that microorganisms are the cause of periodontitis, but that the clinical expression of the disease (extent and severity) depends on how the host responds to the extent and virulence of the microbial burden. In response to periodontal pathogens and their endotoxins, immune cells in the periodontium, particularly monocytes, secrete proinflammatory mediators such as prostaglandin E, interleukin-1, and tumor necrosis factor. The body's inflammatory response is an attempt to protect itself from the pathogens, but at the same time the inflammation can lead to periodontal connective tissue destruction and bone degeneration as the body attempts to rid itself of the infectious tooth. Further understanding of the role of differences in immune response should help in understanding an individual's susceptibility to periodontal disease.

Much epidemiologic research has focused on the identification of environmental and host factors involved in the initiation and progression of periodontal disease. Of all the environmental factors known to be associated with periodontitis, *cigarette smoking* may be the most important. Evidence for the role of smoking in periodontitis includes (1) a higher prevalence of disease among smokers in cross-sectional studies, (2) a higher incidence of periodontitis among smokers in longitudinal studies, (3) a statistically significant association even after controlling for other risk factors, (4) increased prevalence and incidence of disease with increased amounts of smoking, and (5) biologically plausible mechanisms that can explain how smoking is involved in the destruction of periodontal tissues.[63] Cigarette smokers are up to five times more likely than nonsmokers to develop severe periodontitis, and the risk of the disease increases with the amount of cigarettes smoked.[60]

Diabetes mellitus is another factor that enhances an individual's susceptibility to periodontitis. The prevalence and severity of periodontitis are significantly higher in type 1 (formally called *insulin-dependent* but now called *immune-mediated*) and type 2 (formally called *non–insulin-dependent*) diabetic patients than in nondiabetic persons.[28,76] Type 1 diabetes mellitus typically occurs during childhood or adolescence, whereas type 2 usually occurs after age 45. Approximately 9 of 10 individuals with diabetes have type 2 diabetes mellitus. Much of clinicians' understanding of the epidemiologic association between diabetes and periodontitis comes from studies of the Pima Indians of the Gila River Indian Community in Arizona. The Pimas have the highest incidence of type 2 diabetes ever recorded.[42] Among the Pimas, diabetic individuals have a threefold risk of developing periodontitis.[28] The effects of diabetes appear to be similar among individuals with type 1 and type 2 diabetes as long as the duration of their disease is similar. However, type 1 diabetic patients often have had diabetes longer than those with type 2 and therefore may be at risk of developing more periodontitis.[58] In addition to the duration of diabetes, the long-term metabolic control of diabetes is an important factor in periodontitis. Compared with well-controlled and moderately controlled diabetic patients, the prevalence, severity, and extent of periodontitis are increased among poorly controlled diabetic patients.[75] The encouraging news is that well-controlled diabetic patients have similar levels of periodontal disease as nondiabetic persons, and diabetic patients treated for moderate to advanced adult periodontitis are able to maintain a healthy periodontium.[58,82]

Although numerous cross-sectional studies indicate that the prevalence and severity of periodontitis increase with age, the current opinion is that *aging* does not cause periodontitis. In cross-sectional studies, indicators of periodontitis such as attachment loss and bone loss are cumulative measures of disease over an individual's lifetime. The greater prevalence and severity of periodontitis among older persons in these studies results from the cumulative effects of the disease over time rather than a greater susceptibility of older people.[19] In fact, studies support the view that if a person is susceptible to severe periodontal destruction, the tendency will be seen early.[20] Longitudinal studies examining the association between age and periodontitis have been inconclusive.[11] One longitudinal study indicated that when good oral hygiene is maintained throughout a lifetime, periodontal disease progression is negligible.[2] In that study, oral hygiene was shown to be the most important predictor for periodontitis, and in all age groups, more than 95% of individuals with good oral hygiene did not have periodontitis. The authors concluded, "The effect of age on the progression of periodontitis could therefore be considered negligible when good oral hygiene is maintained."[2] Finally, the benefit of continuing the debate on whether age is a risk factor is unclear, because the question of whether the risk for periodontal disease is reduced by intervention cannot be tested (i.e., people cannot become younger).

Several other characteristics have been investigated as possible risk factors for adult periodontitis. The following list, adapted from Page and Beck,[60] summarizes many of those characteristics in terms of current evidence to support their candidacy as risk factors.

- *Nutrition.* Most information regarding nutrition and periodontal diseases is dated and primarily based on animal studies that involved severe nutritional deficiencies. Minor nutritional deficiencies or imbalances failed to demonstrate an effect on periodontal disease in these animal models. Longitudinal studies that control for possible confounders meeting our stated criteria for evaluation of nutrition as a risk factor are lacking.
- *Low socioeconomic and educational status.* Periodontal disease is more severe in individuals of lower

socioeconomic status and poorer education. However, when periodontal status is adjusted for oral hygiene and smoking, the associations between lower socioeconomic and educational status and severe periodontal disease are not seen. Thus, socioeconomic and educational status does not appear to affect the pathogenesis directly.

- *Osteoporosis*. Longitudinal data are scarce, and multivariate analyses produce inconsistent results.
- *HIV infection and AIDS*. Longitudinal data are scarce. Multivariable analyses generally are lacking. HIV infection and acquired immunodeficiency syndrome (AIDS) appear to elevate risk for severe periodontitis.
- *Infrequent dental visits*. Longitudinal data are available. However, multivariate analyses are inconsistent, and risk assessments and intervention studies have not been completed.
- *Bacteria*. Longitudinal data are available. Multivariate analyses implicate certain bacteria, and assessments and some interventions have been completed. Bacteria are generally considered to be causal. However, whether the presence of putative pathogenic species can be used as a strong indicator for future clinical attachment loss remains controversial. Although some reports claim that the presence of these species is a good predictor, others observed an association with disease progression but found that the presence of putative pathogenic species was unreliable as a predictor for future clinical attachment loss in individual patients and at specific sites. Subject prediction usually is more accurate than site prediction. The absence of any of the group of five to seven putative periodontal pathogens is a reliable indicator for the absence of future clinical attachment loss for most patients.
- *Bleeding on probing*. Longitudinal data are available. Multivariate analyses implicate bleeding on probing in combination with increasing pocket depth. Because bleeding on probing is an indicator of active inflammation, it is likely to be predictor of attachment loss rather than causal. At present, bleeding on probing is widely used as an indication for needed treatment. However, bleeding on probing alone is not a predictor of elevated risk for future loss of clinical attachment. On the other hand, a lack of bleeding on probing, especially on two or more occasions, is an excellent indicator of periodontal health, with a predictive value of 0.972.
- *Previous periodontal disease*. Longitudinal data are available. Multivariate analyses implicate past disease. The risk for future periodontal deterioration in a given individual is strongly associated with the presence and severity of existing periodontitis. In other words, individuals with the most advanced existing periodontitis are at greatest risk for future clinical attachment loss. Individuals who are currently free of periodontitis are less likely to experience future clinical attachment loss than those with periodontitis. However, past disease is only a good clinical predictor. It is not likely to be causal, and it is unclear whether past disease is predictive of both incidental attachment loss and progression of current disease.
- *Genetic factors*. Longitudinal data are available. Multivariate analyses implicate genetic factors. Genetic factors are strongly associated with the aggressive forms and, to a lesser extent, with chronic periodontitis.
- *Stress*. Most studies involve necrotizing ulcerative gingivitis (NUG). Case control and a few short-term longitudinal studies indicate associations. Multivariate and intervention studies are needed. Biologic mechanisms are known.

In addition, *obesity* has been implicated as a risk factor for several chronic health conditions, such as diabetes and hypertension, and an increasing prevalence of overweight and obese individuals in the United States has generated concern. Recent studies have focused on the relationship between obesity and periodontal disease. Studies in Japan[70,71] and the United States[6,83] found that obese individuals were more likely to have periodontal disease after adjusting for traditional risk factors for periodontitis. For example, a Japanese study found that the risk of periodontitis for each 5% increase in body fat was 1.3 ($p = 0.02$) after adjusting for age, gender, oral hygiene status, and smoking history.[70] In addition, neither the subjects' glycosylated hemoglobin values nor their fasting blood glucose concentrations were correlated with the incidence of periodontitis, indicating that any association between obesity and periodontal status was independent of measures often associated with obesity. If we evaluate the status of obesity as a risk factor for periodontal disease in a manner similar to the factors previously listed, we find that even though the association exists after multivariable analyses and there are some supportive animal studies, only a few studies report this association in humans, and those studies are cross-sectional in nature. At this time, more research is needed before obesity can be classified as a risk factor for periodontitis.

AGGRESSIVE PERIODONTITIS

Aggressive periodontitis (formerly known as *early-onset periodontitis*) is periodontal destruction that becomes clinically significant during adolescence or early adulthood. The disease has been classified into two types: localized and generalized.[68] Other terms found in the literature that have been used to describe aggressive forms of periodontitis include juvenile, localized juvenile, generalized juvenile, rapidly progressive, severe, and prepubertal periodontitis[68] (see Box 7-3). The distinction between the localized and generalized forms is based on the distribution of the periodontal destruction in the mouth. *Localized* aggressive periodontitis is characterized by bone loss around the first molars and incisors. As the name implies, *generalized* aggressive periodontitis is characterized by a more widespread pattern of periodontal destruction.

Although aggressive periodontitis is characterized by age at onset and pattern of periodontal destruction, case definitions for early-onset disease or its subtypes have varied across epidemiologic studies. In a national survey of the oral health of U.S. schoolchildren, three case definitions were used for aggressive periodontitis, as follows[49]:

- *Localized aggressive periodontitis:* At least one first molar and at least one incisor or second molar and two or fewer canines or premolars had greater than 3 mm of attachment loss.
- *Generalized aggressive periodontitis:* Criteria for localized disease were not met; four or more teeth had greater than 3 mm of attachment loss; and at least two affected teeth were second molars, canines, or premolars.
- *Incidental loss of periodontal attachment:* Criteria for localized or generalized were not met, and one or more teeth had greater than 3 mm of attachment loss.

Other studies have based case definitions on various combinations of disease patterns and the extent and severity of pocket depth, attachment loss, and bone loss. Papapanou[62] provides a thorough review of studies that have investigated aggressive forms of periodontitis in childhood and adolescence. As our understanding of aggressive periodontitis changes, the nomenclature for the disease and case definitions will likely continue to evolve.

How Much Aggressive Periodontitis Is Present?

Most studies from the United States and other countries that have examined localized aggressive periodontitis in adolescents have reported prevalence estimates below 1%.[62] In the United States the prevalence of localized and generalized aggressive periodontitis was estimated at 0.53% and 0.13%, respectively.[49] Another 1.61% of the adolescents had incidental attachment loss—attachment loss that did not fit the study's case definitions for localized or generalized disease.[76] Although these prevalence estimates are small, together they represented almost 300,000 U.S. adolescents at the time of the study (1986–87).[49]

How Much New Aggressive Periodontitis Is Present?

Very few longitudinal studies of aggressive periodontitis have been conducted. One longitudinal study conducted in the United Kingdom followed 167 subjects from ages 14 to 19 years.[26] Periodontal attachment loss was measured on the mesiofacial surfaces of the first molars, first premolars, and central incisors. During the 5 years of follow-up, the percentage of subjects with attachment loss on one or more of the examined teeth increased dramatically: from 3% to 77% for attachment loss of greater than 1 mm and from 0% to 14% for attachment loss of greater than 2 mm. By age 19 years, 31% of the sites examined had attachment loss greater than 1 mm, and 3.1% had attachment loss greater than 2 mm. The teeth most often affected were the maxillary first molars and the mandibular central incisors. In the 19-year-old subjects, 9% of the maxillary molars had attachment loss of more than 2 mm. The presence of subgingival calculus and plaque at baseline was a significant predictor of loss of attachment at 5 years. Although this study provides useful information on the change in prevalence of aggressive periodontitis, the authors noted that the cohort was not a randomly selected group of 14-year-olds, and therefore the results cannot be generalized to the population at large.

Another study that followed a cohort of 14-year-old subjects was conducted among Norwegians.[1] Of the 2767 subjects examined at baseline (14 years old) in 1984, 215 were reexamined in 1992 (they were also examined in 1986 and 1988). At each examination, the prevalence of radiographic alveolar bone loss was assessed on sets of bite-wing radiographs. Bone loss was measured on the mesial and distal surfaces of fully erupted teeth (distal of canines to mesial of second molars) and was defined as the distance from the cementoenamel junction to the alveolar crest. The distance had to exceed 2 mm for bone loss to be present. At baseline, the prevalence of subjects with one or more lesions was approximately 3.5%. By 1992, the prevalence of subjects with bone loss had doubled. The percentage of subjects with three or more sites with bone loss also increased during that time, from 2.5% to 33.3%.

A review of the available longitudinal studies of periodontitis in childhood and adolescence concluded that subjects with signs of periodontal disease at a young age are likely to have further periodontal deterioration. Progression is more extensive at initially infected sites and among subjects of low socioeconomic status.[62]

Does My Patient with Aggressive Periodontitis Fit the Typical Profile?

The prevalence of aggressive periodontitis is higher in African Americans than in whites. In a study of aggressive periodontitis among U.S. adolescents, it was estimated that 2.05% of African Americans had localized periodontitis compared with 0.14% of whites.[49] For generalized disease, the prevalence was 0.59% for African Americans and 0.03% for whites. The prevalence of incidental attachment loss was much higher among African Americans than whites: 4.63% versus 0.91%.

Whether or not the prevalence of aggressive periodontitis differs by gender is unclear. Early case reports and small studies often found the condition to be more prevalent among women; however, findings from larger studies have suggested the distribution of the disease is fairly equal between the genders.[72] The 1986–1987 survey of U.S. schoolchildren indicated that males had slightly higher but statistically insignificant prevalence of localized and generalized aggressive periodontitis and incidental attachment loss.[49] However, when the distribution of the disease by gender was examined among race groups, differences by gender became much more evident. Among African Americans, males were 2.9 times more likely than females to have localized disease. Among whites, the association was reversed. White females were 2.5 times more likely than white males to have localized disease.

Why Do Patients Have Aggressive Periodontitis, and What Puts Them at Risk?

The bacterium *A. actinomycetemcomitans* is found in high numbers in localized aggressive periodontal lesions and is the primary pathogen associated with the disease.[84] Elimination of the pathogen is associated with clinical improvement. The bacterium produces a strong leukotoxin that kills neutrophils, which provide an important defense against periodontal infections. Different strains of *A. actinomycetemcomitans* produce different levels of leukotoxin. Highly toxic strains produce 10 to 20 times the levels of leukotoxin as do minimally toxic strains.[86] Patients with localized aggressive periodontitis are more likely to harbor the highly leukotoxic strains than periodontally healthy persons or persons with chronic periodontitis.[86] In a study of 21 families with at least one family member who had localized disease, children infected with the highly leukotoxic strains of *A. actinomycetemcomitans* were more likely to develop localized aggressive periodontitis.[18] Persons with African backgrounds have been found more likely to be infected with the more virulent strains of *A. actinomycetemcomitans,* which may explain the elevated risk of localized juvenile periodontitis among African Americans.[73] Although infection with *A. actinomycetemcomitans* is strongly associated with cases of localized disease, not all individuals infected with this organism develop localized aggressive periodontitis, and not all individuals with localized disease have detectable levels of *A. actinomycetemcomitans.*

Another factor believed to be involved in the pathogenesis of aggressive periodontitis is *defective neutrophil function.* "Depressed neutrophil chemotaxis" is a consistent finding among patients with localized or generalized forms of the disease. Studies have shown that 70% to 75% of patients with localized disease have depressed neutrophil chemotaxis.[81] Localized aggressive periodontitis tends to occur in families, and this neutrophil chemotactic abnormality is genetic in origin and may predispose individuals to localized disease. However, not all individuals with localized disease have depressed neutrophil chemotaxis, and not all individuals with depressed neutrophil chemotaxis develop localized disease. Other, currently unidentified host factors are likely involved in the pathogenesis of aggressive periodontitis.

REFERENCES

1. Aass AM, Tollefsen T, Gjermo P: A cohort study of radiographic alveolar bone loss during adolescence, *J Clin Periodontol* 21:133, 1994.
2. Abdellatif HM, Burt BA: An epidemiological investigation into the relative importance of age and oral hygiene status as determinants of periodontitis, *J Dent Res* 66:13, 1987.
3. Addy M, Hunter ML, Kingdon A, et al: An 8-year study of changes in oral hygiene and periodontal health during adolescence, *Int J Paediatr Dent* 4:75, 1994.
4. Albandar JM: A 6-year study on the pattern of periodontal disease progression, *J Clin Periodontol* 17:467, 1990.
5. Albandar JM, Kingman A: Gingival recession, gingival bleeding, and dental calculus in adults 30 years of age and older in the United States, 1988–1994, *J Periodontol* 70:30, 1999.
6. Al-Zahrani MS, Bissada NF, Borawskit EA: Obesity and periodontal disease in young, middle-aged, and older adults, *J Periodontol* 74:610, 2003.
7. Amato R, Caton J, Polson A, Espeland M: Interproximal gingival inflammation related to the conversion of a bleeding to a nonbleeding state, *J Periodontol* 57:63, 1986.
8. Anonymous: Consensus report. Periodontal diseases: pathogenesis and microbial factors, *Ann Periodontol* 1:926, 1996.
9. Armitage GC: Periodontal diseases: diagnosis, *Ann Periodontol* 1:37, 1996.
10. Baelum V, Luan WM, Chen X, Fejerskov O: A 10-year study of the progression of destructive periodontal disease in adult and elderly Chinese, *J Periodontol* 68:1033, 1997.
11. Beck JD: Periodontal implications: older adults, *Ann Periodontol* 1:322, 1996.
12. Beck JD, Koch GG, Offenbacher S: Incidence of attachment loss over 3 years in older adults: new and progressing lesions, *Community Dent Oral Epidemiol* 23:291, 1995.
13. Bergstrom J: Oral hygiene compliance and gingivitis expression in cigarette smokers, *Scand J Dent Res* 98:497, 1990.
14. Bhat M: Periodontal health of 14-17–year-old US schoolchildren, *J Public Health Dent* 51:5, 1991.
15. Bouwsma O, Caton J, Polson A, Espeland M: Effect of personal oral hygiene on bleeding interdental gingiva: histologic changes, *J Periodontol* 59:80, 1988.
16. Brown LJ, Oliver RC, Löe H: Periodontal diseases in the U.S. in 1981: prevalence, severity, extent, and role in tooth mortality, *J Periodontol* 60:363, 1989.
17. Brown LJ, Oliver RC, Löe H: Evaluating periodontal status of US employed adults, *J Am Dent Assoc* 121:226, 1990.
18. Bueno LC, Mayer MP, DiRienzo JM: Relationship between conversion of localized juvenile periodontitis-susceptible children from health to disease and *Actinobacillus actinomycetemcomitans* leukotoxin promoter structure (see comments), *J Periodontol* 69:998, 1998.
19. Burt BA: Periodontitis and aging: reviewing recent evidence, *J Am Dent Assoc* 125:273, 1994.
20. Burt BA, Eklund SA: Dentistry, dental practice, and the community, Philadelphia, 1999, Saunders.
21. Carlos JP, Wolf MD, Kingman A: The extent and severity index: a simple method for use in epidemiologic studies of periodontal disease, *J Clin Periodontol* 13:500, 1986.
22. Carter HG, Barnes GP: The gingival bleeding index, *J Periodontol* 45:801, 1974.
23. Caton JG, Polson AM: The interdental bleeding index: a simplified procedure for monitoring gingival health, *Compend Contin Educ Dent* 6:88, 1985.
24. Caton J, Bouwsma O, Polson A, Espeland M: Effects of personal oral hygiene and subgingival scaling on bleeding interdental gingiva, *J Periodontol* 60:84, 1989.
25. Ciancio S: Current status of indices of gingivitis, *J Clin Periodontol* 13:375, 1986.
26. Clerehugh V, Lennon MA, Worthington HV: 5-year results of a longitudinal study of early periodontitis in 14- to 19-year-old adolescents, *J Clin Periodontol* 17:702, 1990.
27. Douglas CW, Fox CH: Cross-sectional studies in periodontal disease: current status and implications for dental practice, *Adv Dent Res* 7:25, 1993.
28. Emrich LJ, Shlossman M, Genco RJ: Periodontal disease in non-insulin-dependent diabetes mellitus (see comments), *J Periodontol* 62:123, 1991.
29. Fletcher RH, Fletcher SW, Wagner EH: *Clinical epidemiology: the essentials,* Baltimore, 1988, Williams & Wilkins, p 246.
30. Folkers SA, Weine FS, Wissman DP: Periodontal disease in the life stages of women, *Compendium* 13:852, 1992.
31. Friedman LM, Furberg CD, DeMets DL: *Fundamentals of clinical trials,* St Louis, 1996, Mosby, p 361.
32. Genco RJ: Classification and clinical and radiographic features of periodontal disease. In Genco RJ, Goldman HM, Cohen DW: *Contemporary periodontics,* St Louis, 1990, Mosby.
33. Gordis L: *Epidemiology,* Philadelphia, 1996, Saunders.

34. Greenberg RS: *Medical epidemiology,* Norwalk, Conn, 1996, Appleton & Lange, p 196.
35. Greenstein G: The role of bleeding upon probing in the diagnosis of periodontal disease: a literature review, *J Periodontol* 55:684, 1984.
36. Gusberti FA, Mombelli A, Lang NP, Minder CE: Changes in subgingival microbiota during puberty: a 4-year longitudinal study, *J Clin Periodontol* 17:685, 1990.
37. Haffajee AD, Socransky SS, Lindhe J, et al: Clinical risk indicators for periodontal attachment loss, *J Clin Periodontol* 18:117, 1991.
38. Hirsch RS, Clarke NG, Townsend GC: The effect of locally released oxygen on the development of plaque and gingivitis in man, *J Clin Periodontol* 8:21, 1981.
39. Hulley SB, Cummings SR, Browner WS: *Designing clinical research: an epidemiologic approach,* Baltimore, 1988, Williams & Wilkins, p 247.
40. Ismail AI, Morrison EC, Burt BA, et al: Natural history of periodontal disease in adults: findings from the Tecumseh Periodontal Disease Study, 1959–87, *J Dent Res* 69:430, 1990.
41. Jeffcoat MK, Wang IC, Reddy MS: Radiographic diagnosis in periodontics, *Periodontol 2000* 7:54, 1995.
42. Knowler WC, Pettitt DJ, Savage PJ, Bennett PH: Diabetes incidence in Pima Indians: contributions of obesity and parental diabetes, *Am J Epidemiol* 113:144, 1981.
43. Last JM, Abramson JH, International Epidemiological Association: *A dictionary of epidemiology,* New York, 1995, Oxford University Press.
44. Lilienfeld DE, Stolley PD, Lilienfeld AM: *Foundations of epidemiology,* New York, 1994, Oxford University Press, p 371.
45. Lindhe J, Hamp S, Löe H: Experimental periodontitis in the beagle dog, *J Periodontal Res* 8:1, 1973.
46. Lobene RR: Discussion: clinical status of indices for measuring gingivitis, *J Clin Periodontol* 13:381, 1986.
47. Lobene RR, Weatherford T, Ross NM, et al: A modified gingival index for use in clinical trials, *Clin Prev Dent* 8:3, 1986.
48. Löe H: The gingival index, the plaque index and the retention index systems, *J Periodontol* 38(suppl):610, 1967.
49. Löe H, Brown LJ: Early onset periodontitis in the United States of America, *J Periodontol* 62:608, 1991.
50. Löe H, Silness J: Periodontal disease in pregnancy. I. Prevalence and severity, *Acta Odontol Scand* 21:533, 1963.
51. Löe H, Theilade E, Jensen SB: Experimental gingivitis in man, *J Periodontol* 36:177, 1965.
52. Lyons H, Kerr DM, Hine MK: Report from the 1949 Nomenclature Committee of the American Association of Periodontology, *J Periodontol* 21:40, 1950.
53. Mombelli A, Lang NP, Burgin WB, Gusberti FA: Microbial changes associated with the development of puberty gingivitis, *J Periodontal Res* 25:331, 1990.
54. Muhlemann HR, Son S: Gingival sulcus bleeding: a leading symptom in initial gingivitis, *Helv Odontol Acta* 15:107, 1971.
55. Nakagawa S, Fujii H, Machida Y, Okuda K: A longitudinal study from prepuberty to puberty of gingivitis: correlation between the occurrence of *Prevotella intermedia* and sex hormones, *J Clin Periodontol* 21:658, 1994.
56. Newbrun E: Indices to measure gingival bleeding, *J Periodontol* 67:555, 1996.
57. Offenbacher S: Periodontal diseases: pathogenesis, *Ann Periodontol* 1:821, 1996.
58. Oliver RC, Tervonen T: Diabetes: a risk factor for periodontitis in adults? *J Periodontol* 65:530, 1994.
59. Page RC: Gingivitis, *J Clin Periodontol* 13:345, 1986.
60. Page RC, Beck JD: Risk assessment for periodontal diseases, *Int Dent J* 47:61, 1997.
61. Page RC, Offenbacher S, Schroeder HE, et al: Advances in the pathogenesis of periodontitis: summary of developments, clinical implications and future directions, *Periodontol 2000* 14:216, 1997.
62. Papapanou PN: Periodontal diseases: epidemiology, *Ann Periodontol* 1:1, 1996.
63. Papapanou PN: Risk assessments in the diagnosis and treatment of periodontal diseases, *J Dent Educ* 62:822, 1998.
64. Papapanou PN, Wennstrom JL, Grondahl K: A 10-year retrospective study of periodontal disease progression, *J Clin Periodontol* 16:403, 1989.
65. Payne WA, Page RC, Ogilvie AL, Hall WB: Histopathologic features of the initial and early stages of experimental gingivitis in man, *J Periodontal Res* 10:51, 1975.
66. Preber H, Bergstrom J: Occurrence of gingival bleeding in smoker and non-smoker patients, *Acta Odontol Scand* 43:315, 1985.
67. Ramfjord SP: Indices for prevalence and incidence of periodontal disease, *J Periodontol* 30:51, 1959.
68. Ranney R: Classification of periodontal diseases, *Periodontol 2000* 2:13, 1993.
69. Russell AL: A system of classification and scoring for prevalence surveys of periodontal disease, *J Dent Res* 35:350, 1956.
70. Saito T, Shimazaki Y, Sakamoto M: Obesity and periodontitis, *N Engl J Med* 339:482, 1998.
71. Saito T, Shimazaki Y, Koga T, et al: Relationship between upper body obesity and periodontitis, *J Dent Res* 80:1631, 2001.
72. Saxby MS: Sex ratio in juvenile periodontitis: the value of epidemiological studies, *Community Dent Health* 1:29, 1984.
73. Schenkein HA: Etiology of localized juvenile periodontitis, *J Periodontol* 69:1068, 1998 (editorial; comment).
74. Slade G, Beck J: Plausibility of periodontal disease estimates from NHANES III, *J Public Health Dent* 59:67, 1999.
75. Tervonen T, Oliver RC: Long-term control of diabetes mellitus and periodontitis, *J Clin Periodontol* 20:431, 1993.
76. Thorstensson H, Hugoson A: Periodontal disease experience in adult long-duration insulin-dependent diabetics, *J Clin Periodontol* 20:352, 1993.
77. Tiainen L, Asikainen S, Saxen L: Puberty-associated gingivitis, *Community Dent Oral Epidemiol* 20:87, 1992.
78. US Department of Health and Human Services (DHHS), National Center for Health Statistics: *Third National Health and Nutrition Examination Survey, 1988–1994,* NHANES III Examination Data File (CD-ROM), Public Use Data File Documentation Number 76200, Hyattsville, Md, 1996, Centers for Disease Control and Prevention.
79. US Public Health Service, National Center for Health Statistics: *Periodontal disease in adults, United States, 1960–62,* DHEW Pub No (PHS) 1000, Vital and Health Statistics, Series 11, No 12, Washington, DC, 1965, US Government Printing Office.
80. US Public Health Service, National Center for Health Statistics: *Basic data on dental examination findings of persons 1-74 years, United States, 1971–74,* DHEW Pub No (PHS) 79-1662, Vital and Health Statistics, Series 11, No 214. Washington, DC, 1979, US Government Printing Office.
81. Van Dyke TE, Schweinebraten M, Cianciola LJ, et al: Neutrophil chemotaxis in families with localized juvenile periodontitis, *J Periodontal Res* 20:503, 1985.
82. Westfelt E, Rylander H, Blohme G, et al: The effect of periodontal therapy in diabetics: results after 5 years, *J Clin Periodontol* 23:92, 1996.
83. Wood N, Johnson RB, Streckfus CF: Comparison of body composition and periodontal disease using nutritional assessment techniques, Third National Health and Nutrition Examination Survey (NHANES III), *J Clin Periodontol* 30:321, 2003.

84. Zambon JJ: Periodontal diseases: microbial factors, *Ann Periodontol* 1:879, 1996.
85. Zambon JJ, Haraszthy VI: The laboratory diagnosis of periodontal infections, *Periodontol 2000* 7:69, 1995.
86. Zambon JJ, Haraszthy VI, Hariharan G, et al: The microbiology of early-onset periodontitis: association of highly toxic *Actinobacillus actinomycetemcomitans* strains with localized juvenile periodontitis, *J Periodontol* 67(suppl):282, 1996.

Etiology of Periodontal Diseases

William V. Giannobile

PART 4

As many as 600 different species of bacteria that colonize the oral cavity can affect the delicate balance of host-bacterial interactions leading to health or disease. Periodontal infection is initiated by specific invasive oral pathogens that colonize dental plaque biofilms on the tooth root surface. Local and systemic factors can also modulate an individual's susceptibility to periodontitis. This chronic challenge of virulent microorganisms leads to destruction of tooth-supporting soft and hard tissues of the periodontium, including alveolar bone, tooth root cementum, and periodontal ligament (PDL).

Although periodontitis is initiated by the subgingival microbiota, it is generally accepted that mediators of connective tissue breakdown are generated to a large extent by the host's response to the pathogenic infection. In a susceptible host, microbial virulence factors trigger the release of host-derived enzymes and proinflammatory cytokines that can lead to periodontal tissue destruction. The implications of periodontal microbiota-associated by-products such as endotoxin on induction of the innate immune response, toll-like receptor (TLR) signaling, generation of pathogen-associated molecular patterns (PAMPs), and their role in periodontal disease pathogenesis are crucial to the extent of disease severity.

Elevated levels of tissue-destructive enzymes such as collagenases and other host-derived proinflammatory cytokines initiated by periodontal pathogens have been detected in inflamed gingiva and in oral fluids such as gingival crevicular fluid and saliva. In addition to antimicrobials traditionally used to manage bacterial infections in periodontitis, alternative adjunctive approaches to manage the disease target the blockade of host response modifiers such as inhibitors of proteases or proinflammatory cytokines such as tumor necrosis factor alpha and interleukin-1 beta.

The role of host genes in the etiology and pathogenesis of the periodontal diseases is critically important to the determination of patient risk for periodontal tissue breakdown. Genetic tests may prove useful for identifying patients who are most likely to develop disease, suffer from recurrent disease, or experience tooth loss as a result of disease. Given the complex etiology of the periodontal diseases, it is likely that any genetic test will be useful in only a subset of patients or populations. Knowledge of specific genetic risk factors or inflammatory biomarkers could enable clinicians to direct environmentally based prevention and treatments to individuals who are most susceptible to disease.

Furthermore, associations between periodontal infection and systemic diseases such as cardiovascular disease, osteoporosis, or other diseases highlight the view that periodontitis represents a polygenic disease with multiple etiologies with interactions with other chronic inflammatory illnesses.

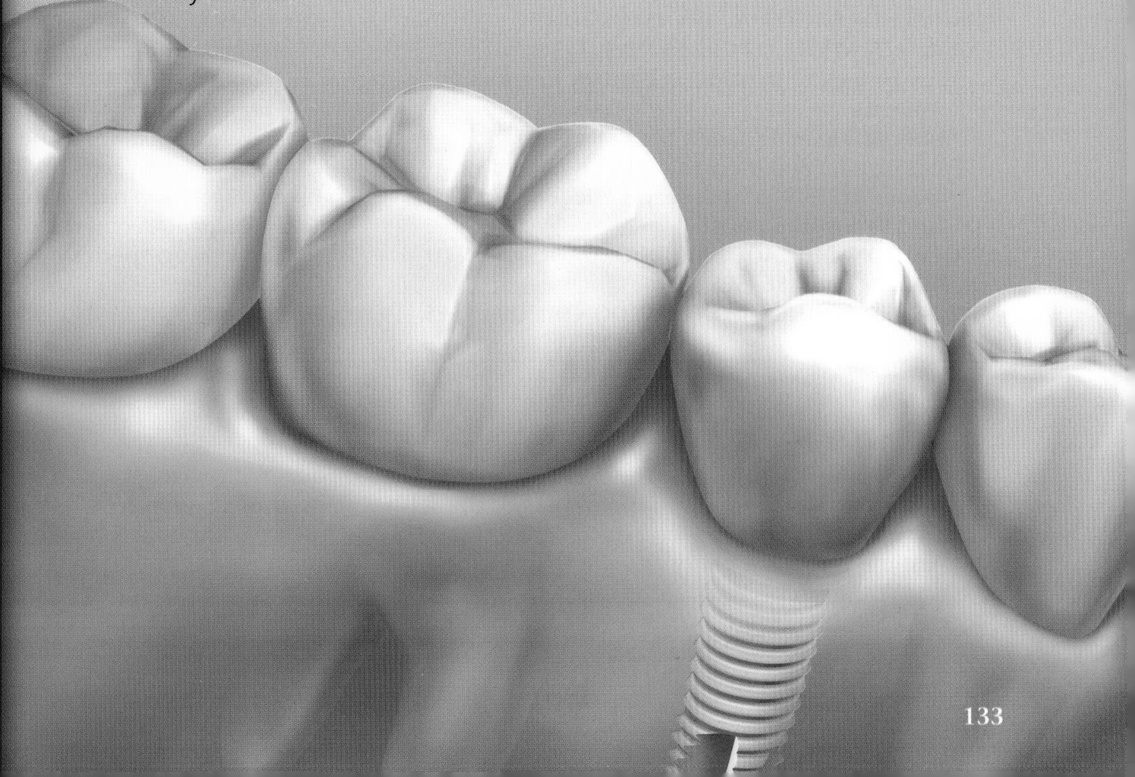

Microbiology of Periodontal Diseases

Marc Quirynen, Wim Teughels, Susan Kinder Haake, and Michael G. Newman

9

CHAPTER

CHAPTER OUTLINE

The human fetus inside the uterus is sterile, but after passing through the birth canal, the fetus acquires vaginal and fecal microorganisms.[70] The colonization of the oral cavity also starts about the time of birth. Within hours after birth, the sterile oral cavity becomes colonized by low numbers of mainly facultative and aerobic bacteria.[235] Beginning the second day, anaerobic bacteria can be detected in the infant's edentulous mouth.[60,204] Within 2 weeks, a nearly mature *microbiota* is established in the gut of the newborn. After weaning (>2 years), the entire human microbial flora is formed by a complex collection of approximately 10^{14} microorganisms consisting of more than 400 different types of bacteria.[158] From this moment on, the body contains *10 times more bacteria* than human cells. In general, this microbiota lives in harmony with the host, but under special conditions (increased mass or pathogenicity, reduced host response), disease may occur. Often, bacteria and host cells form a commensal relationship, which is beneficial for both parties. The host vaginal epithelial cells, for example, supply glucose for the colonized lactobacilli, which in turn produce acid. A lowering of the pH prevents the growth of many other species that have deleterious effects on the vaginal environment.[201] These endogenous bacteria and their products can thus be considered a necessary and beneficial component of a healthy body.

After tooth eruption, a more complex oral flora becomes established. It is estimated that *more than 500 different species* are capable of colonizing the adult mouth, and that any individual may typically harbor 150 or more different species.[159,234] Most of the oral bacteria are commensal and beneficial. The latter is clearly illustrated by the development of yeast infections when this normal oral flora is reduced, such as after long-term use of systemic antibiotics.[257]

From an ecologic viewpoint, the oral cavity, which communicates with the pharynx (the *oropharynx*), should be considered as an "open growth system" with uninterrupted ingestion and removal of microorganisms and their nutrients. In this system a dynamic equilibrium exists between the adhesion forces of microorganisms and a variety of removal forces originating from (1) swallowing, mastication, and blowing the nose; (2) tongue and oral hygiene implements; (3) washout effect of the salivary, nasal, and crevicular fluid outflow; and (4) active motion of the ciliae (nasal and sinus walls). Most organisms can survive in the oropharynx only when they adhere to either the soft tissues (short term) or the hard surfaces (teeth, dentures, and implants) where a biofilm is formed.

DIVERSITY OF INTRAORAL SURFACES FOR BACTERIAL ADHESION

On the basis of physical and morphologic criteria, the oral cavity can be divided into the following *five major ecosystems* (also called *niches*), each with distinct ecologic determinants:

1. Intraoral, supragingival, hard surfaces (teeth, implants, restorations, and prostheses)
2. Periodontal/periimplant pocket (with its crevicular fluid, the root cementum or implant surface, and the pocket epithelium)
3. Buccal epithelium, palatal epithelium, and epithelium of the floor of the mouth
4. Dorsum of the tongue
5. Tonsils

Table 9-1 summarizes several studies on the detection frequency of periodontal pathogens in these different niches. Most species (with the exception of spirochetes) are able to colonize all of them. Some periodontal pathogens (*Fusobacterium nucleatum* and *Prevotella intermedia*) have been involved in the etiology of tonsillitis, and most pathogens are able to colonize the maxillary sinus.[23,255]

Bacterial adhesion to epithelial cells generally shows large intersubject variability. Several studies clearly illustrate a positive correlation between the adhesion rate of pathogenic bacteria to different epithelia and the susceptibility of that patient to certain infections (for review, see Ofek and Doyle[169]). Females prone to urinary tract infections, for example, harbor five times more bacteria per cell in adhesion assays of *Escherichia coli* to different epithelial cells of their urogenital tract (periurethral, vaginal, uroepithelial cells). The same is true for the adhesion of *Streptococcus pneumoniae* to nasopharyngeal epithelial cells of children prone to recurrent otitis media infections, as well as for the adhesion of *Haemophilus influenzae* to buccal cells of subjects prone to acute bronchitis.[47,246] Some studies indicate that the same may be true for periodontal infections. Isogai et al.[97] reported a significantly lower adherence rate of *Porphyromonas gingivalis* and *Prevotella intermedia* strains to gingival epithelial cells in rats that were resistant to gingivitis compared with susceptible rats. A recent in vitro study on cultured human pocket epithelial cells showed a same tendency when patients resistant to periodontitis were compared to patients with severe periodontal breakdown[189] (Figure 9-1). Fortunately, the high turnover rate of the intraoral epithelial cells, especially of the gingiva, prevents the permanent accumulation of large masses of microorganisms on these surfaces. In essence, this is a natural cleansing mechanism.

From a microbiologic viewpoint, teeth and implants are unique for two reasons: they provide a hard, nonshedding surface that allows the development of extensive structured bacterial deposits, and they form a unique ectodermal interruption. A special seal of epithelium and connective tissue exists between the external environment and the internal parts of the body. The accumulation and metabolism of bacteria on these hard surfaces are considered the primary cause of caries, gingivitis, periodontitis, periimplantitis, and often, bad breath.

Teeth are the primary habitat for periopathogens. Indeed, soon after full-mouth tooth extraction in patients with severe periodontitis, key pathogens such as *Actinobacillus actinomycetemcomitans* and *P. gingivalis* will disappear from all their natural intraoral habitats.[49] *P. intermedia* and other black-pigmented *Prevotella* species can remain, but at lower frequencies and numbers (see Table 9-1). Therefore, teeth can even be considered as a "port of entry" for periopathogens. Recent studies using newer microbial technologies, however, indicate that *A. actinomycetemcomitans* and *P. gingivalis* are not entirely eradicated after full-mouth extraction; they may remain at very low concentrations.[192] The same applies to edentulous infants or full-denture wearers, in whom significant proportions of periodontal pathogens, again except for *A. actinomycetemcomitans* and *P. gingivalis,* have been recorded.[48,112]

Cariogenic species, however, seem relatively restricted to solid surfaces (see Table 9-1). For this reason, *Streptococcus mutans* is often called an "obligate periphyte."[245] In infants this species can only be detected from the time the deciduous teeth erupt in the oral cavity.[35] In a longitudinal observation of adults with severe dental caries, the cariogenic species fell below detection level after

TABLE 9-1

Intraoral Habitats (Periodontal Pocket, Buccal Mucosa, Tongue, Saliva, Tonsils, and Supragingival [Supra] Plaque) for Periodontopathogenic and Cariogenic Species

Study	Infection	Age Group (*number*)	Species	Number Positive Patients*	DIFFERENT INTRAORAL NICHES: Pocket	Mucosa	Tongue	Saliva	Tonsils	Supra
Asikainen et al. (1991)	Periodontitis	Adult	*Aa*	—	100%[a]	—	56%	72%	—	—
Petit et al. (1994)	—	Child (*n* = 45)	*Aa*	5	4[b]	3	1	3	2	—
			Pg	1	0	1	0	1	1	—
			Pi	34	23	18	25	31	22	—
			Spi	13	6	0	7	3	1	—
Petit et al. (1994)	Periodontitis	Adult (*n* = 24)	*Aa*	13	13[b]	11	11	11	5	—
			Pg	18	18	14	7	10	11	—
			Pi	24	24	22	23	23	23	—
			Spi	22	22	0	2	5	1	—
Von Troil-Lindén et al. (1995)	Periodontitis	Adult (*n* = 10)	*Aa*	—	6[c]	—	—	6	—	—
			Pg	—	7	—	—	4	—	—
			Pi	—	10	—	—	9	—	—
Danser et al. (1994)	Perio/E[†]	Adult (*n* = 8)	*Aa*	2	2/–[d]	2/0	2/0	2/0	2/0	1/0
			Pg	6	6/–	2/0	4/0	4/0	3/0	2/0
			Pi	8	8/–	4/1	6/3	6/4	5/3	6/1
			Prev	8	3/–	4/5	7/6	7/5	4/6	5/4
Danser et al. (1996)	Perio/R[‡]	Adult (*n* = 15)	*Aa*	11	9/4[e]	10/9	—	5/2	—	2/0
			Pg	10	6/5	9/7	—	4/1	—	6/0
			Pi	15	11/1	15/15	—	14/13	—	11/1
Gibbons and van Houte	—[f]	—[f]	*Sm*	—	?	<1[f]	<1	<1	—	0-50
			L		?	<0.1	<0.1	<1	—	0-1

*Number of patients positive for specific species: Pg, *Porphyromonas gingivalis;* Pi, *Prevotella intermedia;* Aa, *Actinobacillus actinomycetemcomitans; Spi,* spirochetes; Prev, *Prevotella* species (e.g., *P. melaninogenica, P. denticola, P. loeschii, P. veroralis*); Sm, *Streptococcus mutans;* L, *Lactobacillus* spp.).
[†]Perio/Early onset.
[‡]Perio/Refractory.
[a]Percentage of "specific" positive sites in positive patients.
[b]Number of "specific" positive sites in positive patients.
[c]Number of "specific" positive sites in patients with advanced periodontitis.
[d]Number of "specific" positive sites in positive patients before/after full-mouth extraction.
[e]Number of "specific" positive sites in positive patients before/after periodontal therapy, including surgery.
[f]Percentage of total flora cultivable in anaerobically incubated agar in nonspecific patients, as estimated from several studies.

A

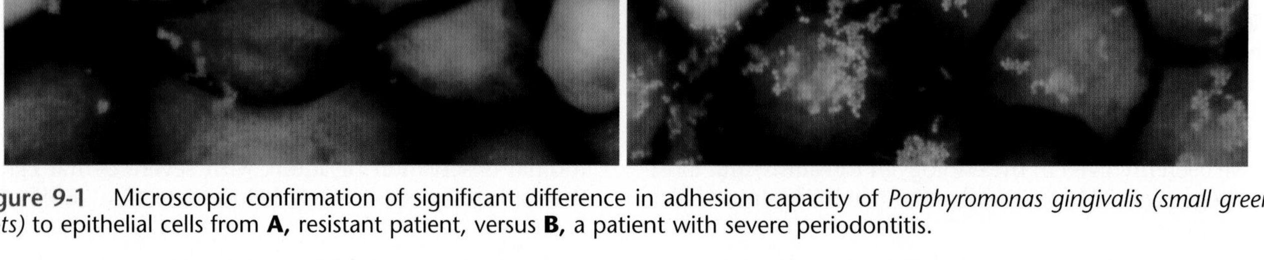

B

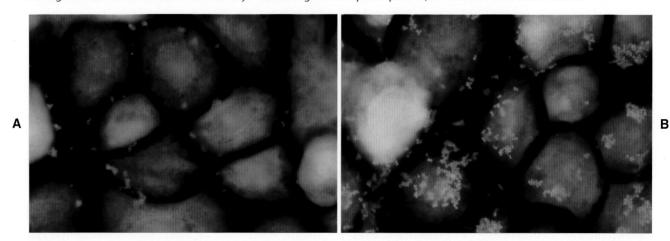

Figure 9-1 Microscopic confirmation of significant difference in adhesion capacity of *Porphyromonas gingivalis (small green dots)* to epithelial cells from **A,** resistant patient, versus **B,** a patient with severe periodontitis.

full-mouth extraction but reappeared in a few days after denture insertion.[34] Based on these reports and on their own observations, Caufield and Gibbons[37] assumed that most of the *S. mutans* cells in the saliva or on the tongue are derived from the biofilm present on the teeth, and that the mucosae could not act as a reservoir for the infection of teeth by those organisms.

STRUCTURE AND COMPOSITION OF DENTAL PLAQUE

Dental plaque is defined clinically as a structured, resilient, yellow-grayish substance that adheres tenaciously to the intraoral hard surfaces, including removable and fixed restorations[18] (Figure 9-2). Plaque is primarily composed of bacteria in a matrix of salivary glycoproteins and extracellular polysaccharides. This matrix makes it impossible to remove the plaque by rinsing or the use of sprays. Plaque can thus be differentiated from other deposits that may be found on the tooth surface, such as materia alba and calculus. *Materia alba* refers to soft accumulations of bacteria and tissue cells that lack the organized structure of dental plaque, and it is easily displaced with a water spray. *Calculus* is a hard deposit that forms by mineralization of dental plaque, and it is generally covered by a layer of unmineralized plaque.

Dental plaque is composed primarily of microorganisms. One gram of plaque (wet weight) contains approximately 10^{11} bacteria.[221,237] The number of bacteria in supragingival plaque on a single tooth surface can exceed 10^9. In a periodontal pocket, counts can range from 10^3 bacteria in a healthy crevice to greater than 10^8 bacteria in a deep pocket. More than 500 distinct microbial species are found in dental plaque.[159] New molecular approaches for bacterial identification, which rely on analysis of ribosomal deoxyribonucleic acid (DNA) sequences, suggest that as much as 30% of the microorganisms associated with gingivitis may represent uncultivated species.[117] Thus it is apparent that substantial numbers of plaque microorganisms have yet to be identified. One individual may harbor 150 or more different species. Nonbacterial microorganisms that are found in plaque include *Mycoplasma* species, yeasts, protozoa, and viruses.[43] The microorganisms exist within an intercellular matrix that also contains a few host cells, such as epithelial cells, macrophages, and leukocytes.

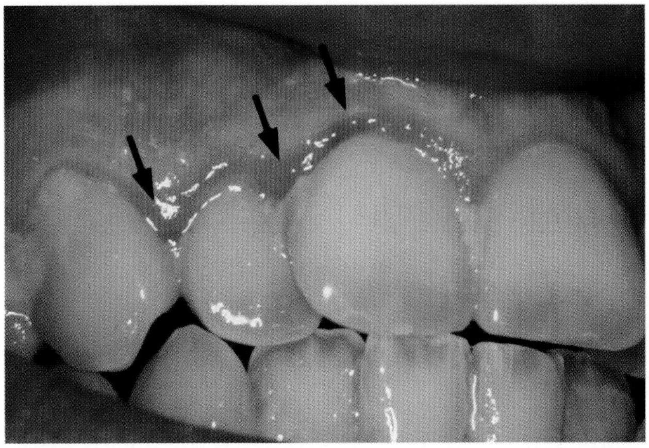

Figure 9-2 Clinical photo of 10-day-old supragingival plaque. The first symptoms of gingival inflammation *(arrows)* are becoming visible.

Dental plaque is broadly classified as supragingival or subgingival based on its position on the tooth surface toward the gingival margin, as follows:

- *Supragingival plaque* is found at or above the gingival margin; when in direct contact with the gingival margin, it is referred to as *marginal plaque*.
- *Subgingival plaque* is found below the gingival margin, between the tooth and the gingival pocket epithelium.

Supragingival plaque typically demonstrates a stratified organization of a multilayered accumulation of bacterial morphotypes (Figure 9-3). Gram-positive cocci and short rods predominate at the tooth surface, whereas gram-negative rods and filaments, as well as spirochetes, predominate in the outer surface of the mature plaque mass.

In general, the subgingival microbiota differs in composition from the supragingival plaque, primarily because of the local availability of blood products and a low oxidation-reduction (redox) potential, which characterizes the anaerobic environment. One can even question whether the presence of some specific microorganisms in the periodontal pocket is the cause or the consequence of the disease.[239] Many periodontal pathogens are indeed fastidious, strict anaerobes and as such may contribute little to the initiation of disease in shallow gingival pockets. In deep periodontal pockets, however, they find their preferred habitat.

The environmental parameters of the subgingival region differ from those of the supragingival region. The gingival crevice or pocket is bathed by the flow of crevicular fluid, which contains many substances that bacteria may use as nutrients (see later discussion). Host inflammatory cells and mediators are likely to have considerable influence on the establishment and growth of bacteria in the subgingival region. Both morphologic and microbiologic studies of subgingival plaque reveal distinctions between the tooth-associated and tissue-associated regions of subgingival plaque[130,163] (Figure 9-4, *A, B,* and *C*).

The tooth-associated cervical plaque, adhering to the root cementum, does not greatly differ from that observed in gingivitis. At this location, filamentous microorganisms dominate, but cocci and rods also occur. This plaque is dominated by gram-positive rods and cocci, including *Streptococcus mitis, S. sanguis, Actinomyces viscosus, A. naeslundii,* and *Eubacterium* species. In the deeper parts of the pocket, however, the filamentous organisms become fewer in numbers, and in the apical portion, they seem to be virtually absent. Instead, the microbiota is dominated by smaller organisms without a particular orientation.[130] *The apical border of the plaque mass is separated from the junctional epithelium by a layer of host leukocytes, and the bacteria of this apical tooth-associated region show an increased concentration of gram-negative rods* (Figure 9-4, *D*).

The layers of microorganisms facing the soft tissue lack a definite intermicrobial matrix and contain primarily

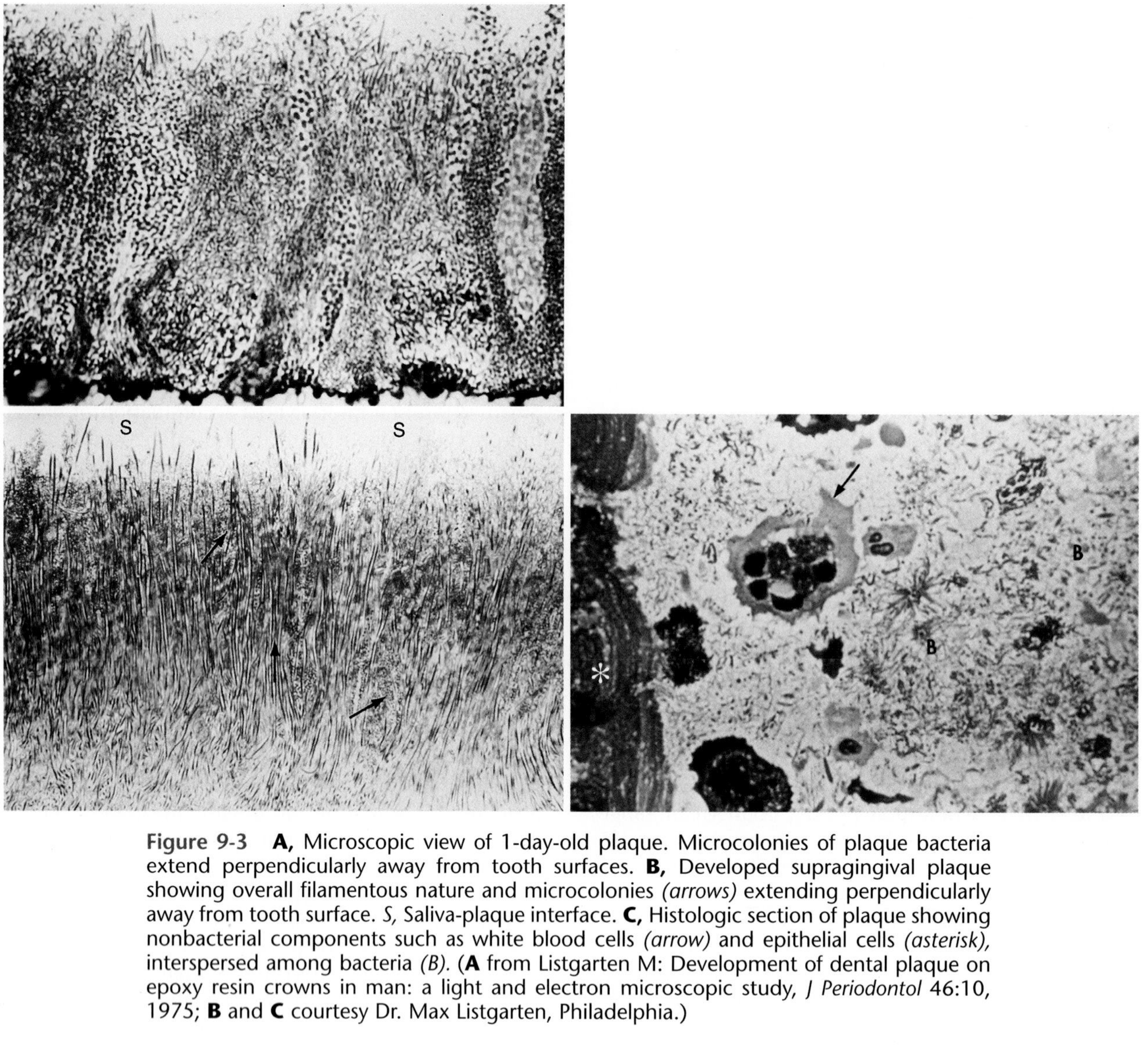

Figure 9-3 **A,** Microscopic view of 1-day-old plaque. Microcolonies of plaque bacteria extend perpendicularly away from tooth surfaces. **B,** Developed supragingival plaque showing overall filamentous nature and microcolonies *(arrows)* extending perpendicularly away from tooth surface. *S,* Saliva-plaque interface. **C,** Histologic section of plaque showing nonbacterial components such as white blood cells *(arrow)* and epithelial cells *(asterisk),* interspersed among bacteria *(B).* (**A** from Listgarten M: Development of dental plaque on epoxy resin crowns in man: a light and electron microscopic study, *J Periodontol* 46:10, 1975; **B** and **C** courtesy Dr. Max Listgarten, Philadelphia.)

gram-negative rods and cocci, as well as large numbers of filaments, flagellated rods, and spirochetes. Studies on tissue-associated plaque indicate a predominance of species such as *Streptococcus oralis, Streptococcus intermedius, Peptostreptococcus micros, Porphyromonas gingivalis, Prevotella intermedia, Tannerella forsythia,* and *Fusobacterium nucleatum.*[53,57] Host tissue cells (e.g., white blood cells and epithelial cells) may also be found in this region. Sometimes, bacteria are found within the host tissues (in the soft tissues as well as in the dentinal tubules).[210,211]

The composition of the subgingival plaque thus depends on the pocket depth. The apical part is dominated by spirochetes, cocci, and rods, whereas in the coronal part, more filaments are observed.

The site specificity of plaque is significantly associated with diseases of the periodontium. Marginal plaque, for example, is of prime importance in the initiation and development of gingivitis. Supragingival plaque and tooth-associated subgingival plaque are critical in calculus formation and root caries, whereas tissue-associated subgingival plaque is important in the tissue destruction that characterizes different forms of periodontitis.

Biofilms also form on artificial surfaces exposed to the oral environment, such as prostheses and implants. A large series of studies compared the microbiota in pockets around teeth with those around implants of partially edentulous patients; the similarities were striking.*

PLAQUE AS A BIOFILM

Biofilms, in general, have an organized structure. They are composed of microcolonies of bacterial cells non-randomly distributed in a shaped matrix or glycocalyx. In the lower plaque layers, which are dense, microbes are bound together in a polysaccharide matrix with other organic and inorganic materials. On top of the lower

*References 11, 94, 95, 103, 105, 121, 125, 148, 156, 172, 180, 213.

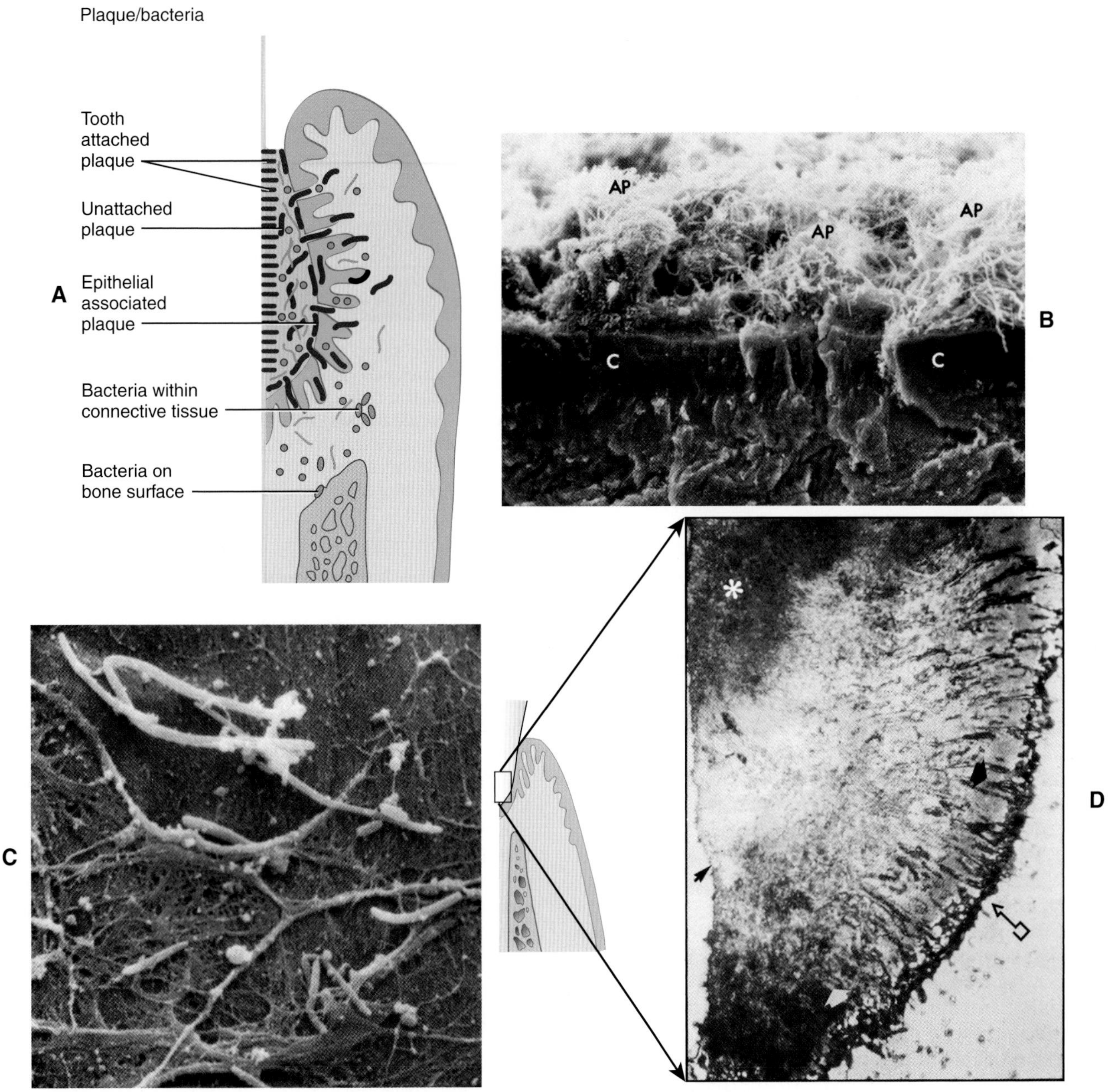

Figure 9-4 **A,** Diagram depicting the plaque-bacteria association with tooth surface and periodontal tissues. **B,** Scanning electron photomicrograph of cross section of cementum *(C)* with attached subgingival plaque *(AP).* Area shown is within a periodontal pocket. **C,** Scanning electron micrograph of cocci and filaments associated with surface of pocket epithelium in a case of marginal gingivitis (×3000). **D,** *Left,* Diagrammatic representation of the histologic structure of subgingival plaque. *Right,* Histologic section of subgingival plaque. *Arrow with box,* Sulcular epithelium. *White arrow,* Predominantly gram-negative unattached zone. *Black arrow,* Tooth surface. *Asterisk,* Predominantly gram-positive attached zone. (**B** courtesy Dr. J. Sottosanti, La Jolla, Calif; **D** from Listgarten M: *J Periodontol* 46:10, 1975.)

layer, a looser layer appears that is often irregular in appearance; it can extend into the surrounding medium (for teeth, the saliva). The fluid layer bordering the biofilm has a rather stationary sublayer and a fluid layer in motion. Nutrient components penetrate this fluid medium by molecular diffusion. Steep diffusion gradients, especially for oxygen, exist in the more compact lower regions of biofilm, which further explains changes in microbial composition.

The dental plaque biofilm has a similar structure. It is heterogeneous in structure, with clear evidence of open fluid-filled *channels* running through the plaque mass[44,45,268] (Figure 9-5). These water channels permit the passage of nutrients and other agents throughout

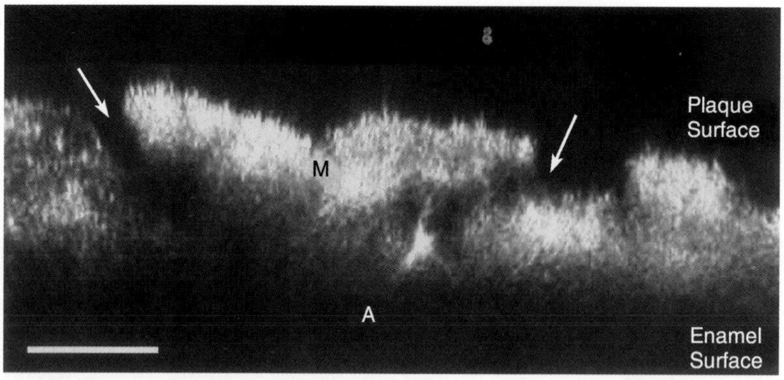

Figure 9-5 Vertical section through a 4-day human plaque sample. An intraoral device designed for in vivo generation of plaque biofilms on enamel was used. Confocal microscopy enabled visualization of the section of plaque without the dehydration steps used in conventional histologic preparations. Note the channels *(white arrows)* that traverse from the plaque surface through the bacterial mass (*M*; gray-white areas) to the enamel surface. An area in which the bacterial mass appears to attach to the enamel surface *(A)* is indicated. Scale bar = 25 μm. (From Wood SR, Kirkham J, Marsh PD, et al: *J Dent Res* 79:21, 2000.)

the biofilm, acting as a primitive "circulatory" system. Nutrients make contact with the sessile (attached) microcolonies by diffusion from the water channels to the microcolony, rather than from the matrix. The bacteria exist and proliferate within the intercellular matrix through which the channels run. The matrix confers a specialized environment, which distinguishes bacteria that exist within the biofilm from those that are free floating, the so-called planktonic state in solutions such as saliva or crevicular fluid. The biofilm matrix functions as a barrier. Substances produced by bacteria within the biofilm are retained and essentially concentrated, which fosters metabolic interactions among the different bacteria, as discussed later.

The intercellular matrix consists of organic and inorganic materials derived from saliva, gingival crevicular fluid, and bacterial products.

Organic constituents of the matrix include polysaccharides, proteins, glycoproteins, and lipid material. Albumin, probably originating from crevicular fluid, has been identified as a component of the plaque matrix. The lipid material consists of debris from the membranes of disrupted bacterial and host cells and possibly food debris. Glycoproteins from saliva are an important component of the pellicle, which initially coats a clean tooth surface (see next section), but they also become incorporated into the developing plaque biofilm. Polysaccharides produced by bacteria, of which dextran is the predominant form, also contribute to the organic portion of the matrix. They play a major role in maintaining the integrity of the biofilm.

The inorganic components of plaque are predominantly calcium and phosphorus, with trace amounts of other minerals, including sodium, potassium, and fluoride. The source of inorganic constituents of supragingival plaque is primarily saliva. As the mineral content increases, the plaque mass becomes calcified to form calculus. Calculus is frequently found in areas of the dentition adjacent to salivary ducts (e.g., lingual surface of mandibular incisors and canines, buccal surface of maxillary first molars), reflecting the high concentration of minerals available from saliva in those regions. The inorganic components of subgingival plaque are derived from crevicular fluid (a serum transudate). Calcification of subgingival plaque also results in calculus formation. Subgingival calculus is typically dark green or dark brown, probably reflecting the presence of blood products associated with subgingival hemorrhage.

The fluoride component of plaque is largely derived from external sources such as fluoridated toothpastes, rinses, and fluoridated drinking water. Fluoride is used therapeutically to aid in remineralization of tooth structures, prevention of demineralization of tooth structures, and inhibition of the growth of many plaque microorganisms.[202]

PLAQUE FORMATION AT THE ULTRASTRUCTURAL LEVEL

The process of plaque formation can be divided into three major phases: (1) the formation of the pellicle on the tooth surface, (2) initial adhesion and attachment of bacteria, and (3) and colonization and plaque maturation.

Formation of the Pellicle

All surfaces of the oral cavity (both hard and soft tissues) are coated with a pellicle (initial phase of plaque development). Within nanoseconds after a vigorously polishing the teeth, a thin, saliva-derived layer, called the *acquired pellicle,* covers the tooth surface. This pellicle consists of numerous components, including glycoproteins (mucins), proline-rich proteins, phosphoproteins (e.g., statherin), histidine-rich proteins, enzymes (e.g., α-amylase), and other molecules that can function as adhesion sites for bacteria (receptors). Currently the term "acquired pellicle" is less frequently used because it is misleading. Indeed, it may imply that bacteria can colonize the tooth surface only when this pellicle is in place for some hours. However, it has been proved that bacteria can be part of the very early deposit, within seconds after prophylaxis.[203] Studies of early (2-hour) enamel pellicle reveal that its amino acid composition differs from that of saliva, indicating that the pellicle forms by selective adsorption of the environmental macromolecules.[214] The mechanisms involved in enamel pellicle formation include electrostatic, van der Waals, and hydrophobic forces. The specific components of a pellicle also depend on the underlying surface. The physical and chemical nature of the solid substratum significantly affects several physicochemical surface properties of the pellicle, including its composition, packing, density, and its configuration.[15,62,120,205,209] Thus the characteristics of the underlying hard surface are transferred through the pellicle layers and can still influence initial bacterial adhesion.[175,176] Absolom et al.[1] even observed a clear relationship between the type of proteins adsorbed in the pellicle and the free energy of the substratum surface. In an in vitro study, Busscher et al.[29] observed that the detachment of adhering bacteria might occur through a cohesive failure in the conditioning film between bacteria and surface (i.e., the pellicle).

Initial Adhesion and Attachment of Bacteria

Although, according to the present state of the art, no completely satisfactory picture of the bacterial adhesion to hard surfaces exists, the following concept helps to understand most aspects of this adhesion process.[161] It would be impossible and erroneous to conclude that a single mechanism dictates the adhesive tendency of micro-organisms, since the situation is too complex.[91] This concept approaches the microbial adhesion to surfaces in an aquatic environment as a four-stage sequence[30,31,220,251,252] (Figure 9-6, *A*). Similar principles are applicable in the marine environment, pipelines, cardiovascular prostheses, and airplane wings. This diagram of events can also clarify the importance of hard-surface characteristics in plaque formation.

Phase 1: Transport to the surface. The first stage involves the initial transport of the bacterium to the tooth surface. Random contacts may occur, for example, through brownian motion (average displacement of 40 µm/hour), through sedimentation of microorganisms, through liquid flow (several orders of magnitude faster than diffusion), or through active bacterial movement (chemotactic activity).

Phase 2: Initial adhesion. The second stage results in an initial, *reversible* adhesion of the bacterium, initiated by the interaction between the bacterium and the surface, from a certain distance (50 nm), through long-range and short-range forces, including van der Waals attractive forces and electrostatic repulsive forces (see Figure 9-6). Derjaguin, Landau, Verwey, and Overbeek (DLVO) have postulated that, above a separation distance of 1 nm, the summation of the previous two forces describes the total long-range interaction.[208] Figure 9-6, *B,* shows the total interaction energy, also called the *total Gibbs energy* (G_{TOT}). The result of this summation ($G_{TOT} = G_A + G_E$), is a function of the separation distance between a negatively charged particle and a negatively charged surface in a medium ionic strength suspension medium (e.g., saliva). For most bacteria, G_{TOT} consists of a *secondary minimum* (where a reversible binding takes place: 5-20 nm from the surface), a *positive maximum* (an energy barrier *B*) to adhesion, and a steep *primary minimum* (located at <2 nm away from the surface), where an irreversible adhesion is established. For bacteria in the mouth, the secondary minimum does not often reach large negative values, which means a "weak" reversible adhesion. If a particle reaches the primary minimum (<1 nm from the surface), a group of short-range forces (e.g., hydrogen bonding, ion pair formation, steric interaction) dominates the adhesive interaction and determines the strength of adhesion (see Figure 9-6, *A*).

Phase 3: Attachment. After initial adhesion, a *firm anchorage* between bacterium and surface will be established by specific interactions (covalent, ionic, or hydrogen bonding). This follows direct contact or bridging true extracellular filamentous appendages (with length up to 10 nm). *On a rough surface, bacteria are better protected against shear forces so that a change from reversible to irreversible bonding occurs more easily and more frequently. The substratum surface free energy becomes important when the water film between the interacting surfaces has to be removed before short-range forces can be involved.* The bonding between bacteria and pellicle is mediated by specific extracellular proteinaceous components (adhesions) of the organism and complementary receptors (i.e., proteins, glycoproteins, or polysaccharides) on the surface (e.g., pellicle) and is species specific. Each *Streptococcus* and *Actinomyces* strain binds specific salivary molecules.[61,63,149] Streptococci (especially *S. sanguis*), the principal early colonizers, bind to acidic proline-rich-proteins and other receptors in the pellicle, such as α-amylase and sialic acid.[93,218] *Actinomyces* species can also function as primary colonizers; for example, *A. viscosus* possesses *fimbriae* that contain *adhesins* that specifically bind to proline-rich proteins of the dental pellicle.[69,149] Some molecules from the pellicle (e.g., proline-rich-proteins) evidently undergo a conformational change when they adsorb to the tooth surface so that new receptors become available. Indeed, *A. viscosus* recognizes cryptic segments of the proline-rich-proteins, which are only available in adsorbed molecules.[68,69] This provides a microorganism with a mechanism for efficiently attaching to teeth and also offers a molecular explanation for their sharp tropisms. It is convenient to refer to such hidden receptors for bacterial adhesins as *cryptitopes* (*cryptic,* hidden; *topo,* place).

Phase 4: Colonization of the surface and biofilm formation. See following discussion.

Colonization and Plaque Maturation

When the firmly attached microorganisms start growing and the newly formed bacterial clusters remain attached, microcolonies or a biofilm can develop (Figure 9-7). From this stage forward, new mechanisms are involved because now intrabacterial connections may occur. At least 18 genera from the oral cavity have shown some form of *coaggregation* (cell-to-cell recognition of genetically distinct partner cell types).[110] Essentially all oral bacteria possess surface molecules that foster some type of cell-to-cell interaction[108] (Figure 9-8). This process occurs primarily through the highly specific stereochemical

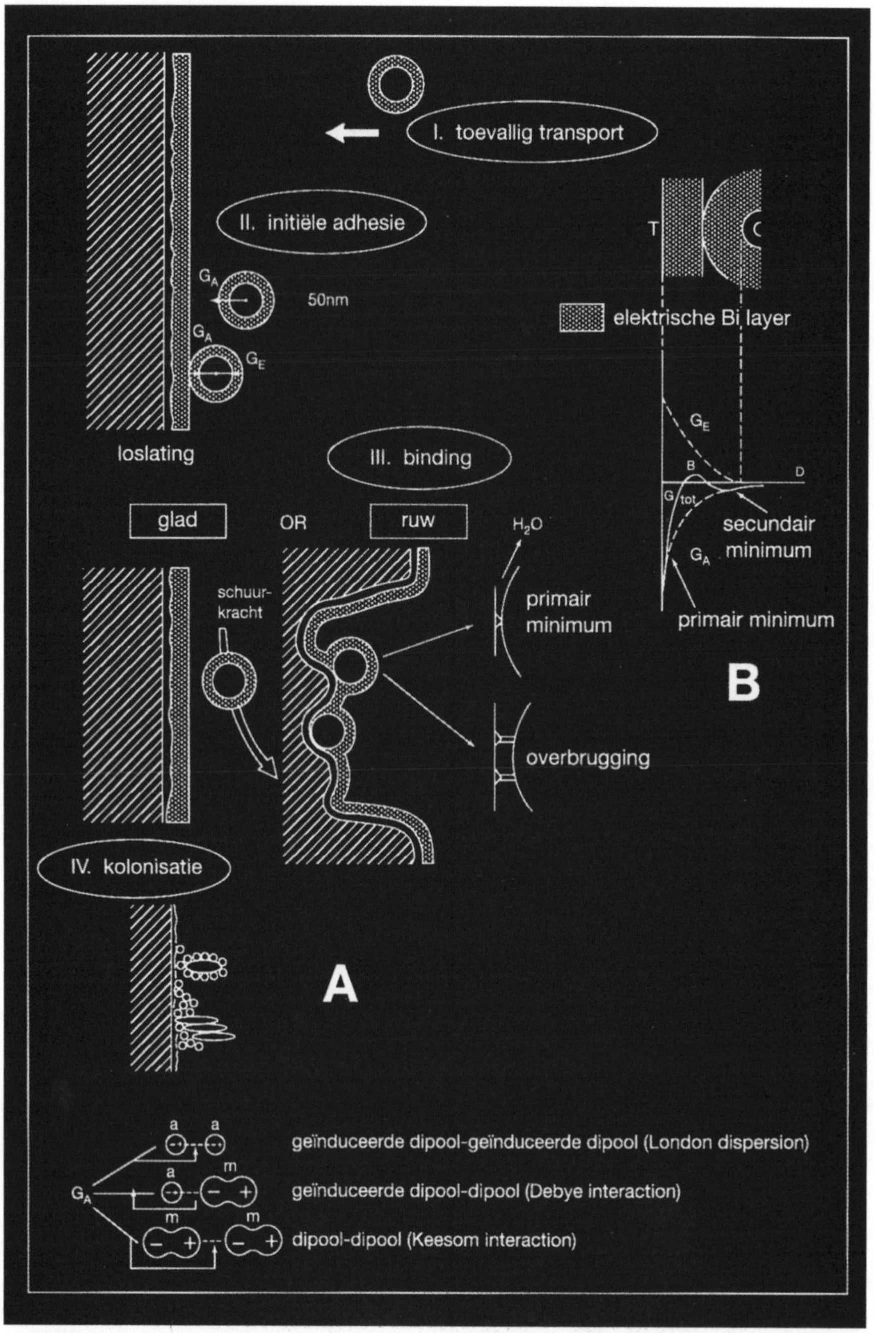

Figure 9-6 **A,** Schematic representation of the dynamic plaque formation process as a four-stage sequence. *1,* Random transport of bacterium to the surface. 2, Initial adhesion at secondary minimum (which often does not reach large negative values so that the adhesion is reversible: R) or directly at the primary minimum (with an irreversible binding: IR), depending on the result of the van der Waals attractive force *(G_A)* and the electrostatic repulsive force *(G_E)*. *3,* Attachment of bacterium to the surface by specific interactions after bridging the separation gap or after passing the energy barrier. *4,* Colonization of the surface and biofilm formation (primarily by cell dividing and by bacterial intrageneric and/or intergeneric coaggregation). **B,** Long-range interaction between a negatively charged bacterium and a negatively charged surface according to the DLVO theory.[208] The Gibbs energy of interaction (G_{TOT}) is calculated in relation to the separation gap *(D),* as the summation of the van der Waals force (G_A) and the electrostatic interaction (G_E). Electrostatic interactions start when the electrical double layers overlap each other (see upper part of figure with *S,* solid surface; *C,* bacterial cell; *t,* thickness of the electrical double layer or Stern layer). Note that the size of the bacterium is too small in relation to the separation gap. (Modified and data from van Loosdrecht MC, Norde W, Zehnder AJ, et al: *J Biomater Appl* 5:91, 1990; Busscher HJ, Sjollema J, van der Mei HC: Relative importance of surface free energy as a measure of hydrophobicity in bacterial adhesion to solid surfaces. In Doyle RJ, Rosenberg M, editors: *Microbial cell surface hydrophobicity,* Washington, DC, 1990, American Society for Microbiology, p 335; and Quirynen M, Bollen CM: *J Clin Periodontol* 22:1, 1995.)

A

B

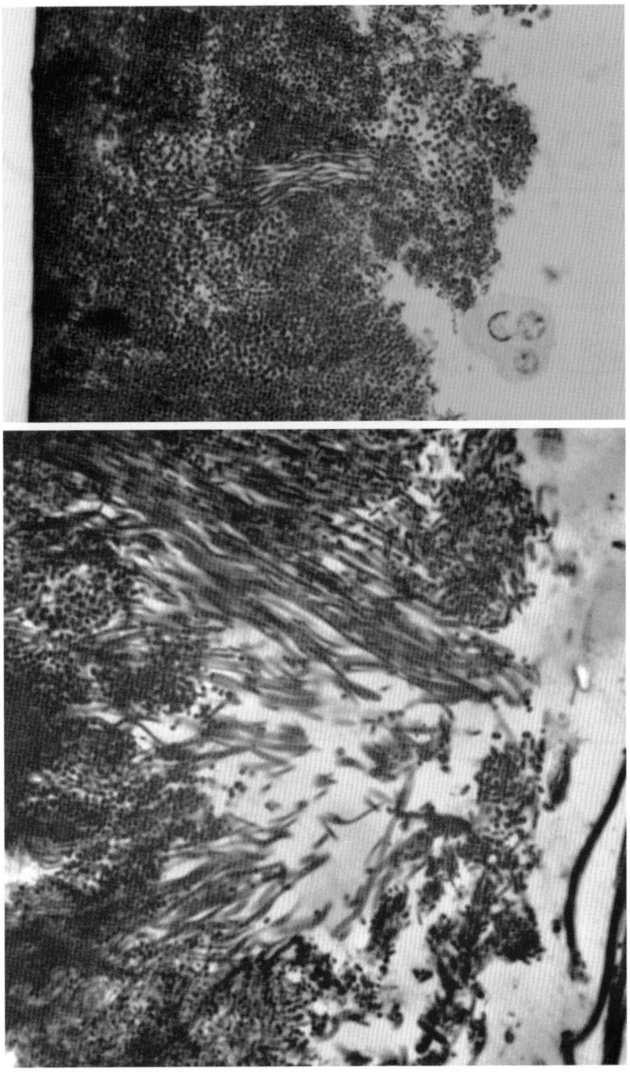

Figure 9-7 When a single microorganism enables to adhere to the tooth surface **(A),** it can start to multiply and slowly forms a microcolony of daughter cells **(B).** These views were taken after plaque formation on a strip glued to a tooth surface (e.g., see Figure 9-10).

interaction of protein and carbohydrate molecules located on the bacterial cell surfaces, in addition to the less specific interactions resulting from hydrophobic, electrostatic, and van der Waals forces.[55,64,106,108] Fusobacteria coaggregate with all other human oral bacteria, whereas veillonellae, capnocytophagae, and prevotellae bind to streptococci and actinomycetes.[108,111,264] Each newly accreted cell becomes itself a nascent surface and therefore may act as a coaggregation bridge to the next potentially accreting cell type that passes. Most coaggregations among strains of different genera are mediated by lectinlike adhesins and can be inhibited by lactose and other galactosides.

The significance of coaggregation in oral colonization has been documented in studies on biofilm formation in vitro as well as in animal model studies.[20] Well-characterized interactions of secondary colonizers with early colonizers include the coaggregation of *Fusobacterium nucleatum* with *Streptococcus sanguis, Prevotella loescheii* with *Actinomyces viscosus,* and *Capnocytophaga ochraceus* with *A. viscosus.*[100,259-261] Most studies of coaggregation have focused on interactions among different gram-positive species and between gram-positive and gram-negative species. Streptococci show intrageneric coaggregation, allowing them to bind to the nascent monolayer of already-bound streptococci.[93,109,168,226]

Each strain of early colonizer is coated with distinct molecules. Identical cells coated with a specific salivary molecule may agglutinate, which would lead to a microconcentration and juxtapositioning of a particular strain. Alternatively, growth of a particular accreted strain can lead to a microcolony coated with specific salivary molecules (see Figure 9-7).

Both streptococci and actinomycetes are facultative anaerobes, and doubling times for microbial populations during the first 4 hours of development are less than 1 hour.[258] Consequently, these two groups of primary colonizers are taught to prepare a favorable environment for later (secondary) colonizers, which have more fastidious growth requirements. Secondary colonizers (e.g., *P. intermedia, P. loescheii, Capnocytophaga* spp., *F. nucleatum, Porphyromonas gingivalis*) do not initially colonize clean tooth surfaces but adhere to bacteria already in the plaque mass.[108] In the latter stages of plaque formation, coaggregation between different gram-negative species is likely to predominate. Examples of these types of interactions are the coaggregation of *F. nucleatum* with *P. gingivalis* or *Treponema denticola.*[102,107,111]

This coaggregation concept opens new perspectives, especially for the use of probiotics. Special examples of coaggregations are the "corncob" formation (Figure 9-9), in which, for example, streptococci adhere to filaments of *Bacterionema matruchotii* or *Actinomyces* species, and the "test tube brush," composed of filamentous bacteria to which gram-negative rods adhere.[42,130,162]

Recent analyses of more than 13,000 plaque samples, looking for 40 subgingival microorganisms using a DNA hybridization methodology, defined "complexes" of periodontal microorganisms. The composition of the different complexes was based on the frequency with which different clusters of microorganisms were recovered.[238] Interestingly, the early colonizers are either independent of defined complexes *(Actinomyces naeslundii, A. viscosus)* or members of the yellow (*Streptococcus* spp.) or purple complexes *(Actinomyces odontolyticus).* The microorganisms primarily considered secondary colonizers fell into the green, orange, or red complexes. The green complex includes *Eikenella corrodens, Actinobacillus actinomycetemcomitans* serotype a, and *Capnocytophaga* species. The orange complex includes *Fusobacterium, Prevotella,* and *Campylobacter* species. The green and orange complexes include species recognized as pathogens in periodontal and nonperiodontal infections. The red complex consists of *P. gingivalis, Tannerella forsythia,* and *Treponema denticola.* This complex is of particular interest because it is associated with bleeding on probing, which is an important clinical parameter of destructive periodontal diseases.[238] The existence of complexes of species in plaque is another reflection of bacterial interdependency in the biofilm environment.

GROWTH DYNAMICS OF DENTAL PLAQUE

Ultrastructural Aspects

Important changes in the plaque growth rate can be detected within the first 24 hours.[129] During the first 2 to 8 hours, the adherent pioneering streptococci saturate the salivary pellicular binding sites and thus cover 3% to 30% of the enamel surface.[128] Instead of the expected steady growth during the next 20 hours (Loesche[138] suggested a 4- to 6-hour generation time), a short period of rapid growth is observed. After 1 day, the term *biofilm* is fully deserved because organization takes place within it.

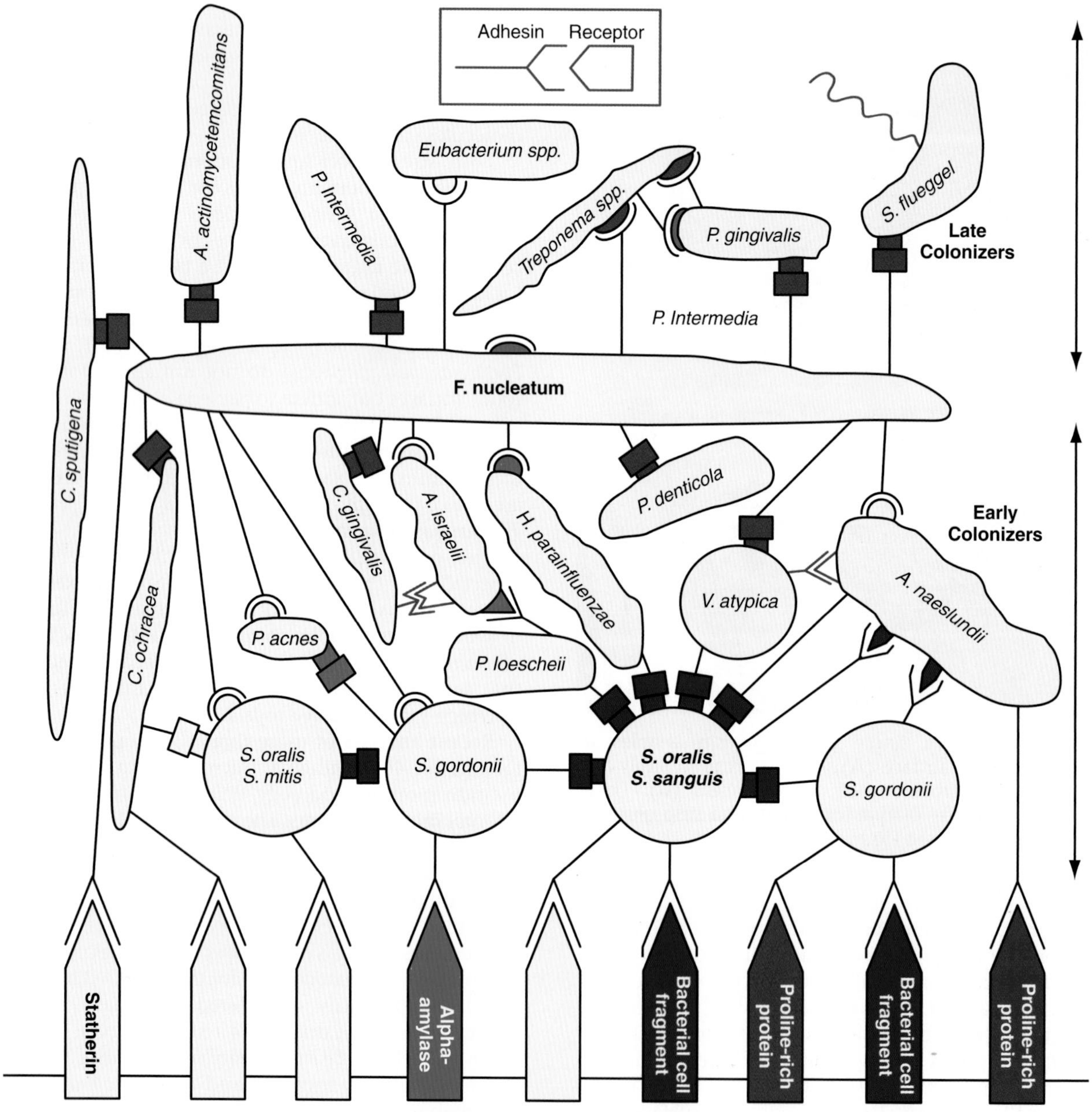

Figure 9-8 Diagrammatic representation of initial plaque formation. Early colonizers bind to receptors in the pellicle. Each adherent cell becomes in turn the nascent surface and bridge for additional species (secondary colonizers). The complementary sets of adhesin receptor symbols (example in box) represent the various types of coaggregations as well as the interactions with molecules in the pellicle. The symbol with a stem (adhesin) represents a cellular component that is heat inactivated (cell suspension heated to 85° C for 30 minutes) and sensitive to protease treatment. The cell type exhibiting the complementary symbol (receptor) is insensitive to either treatment. The symbols with a rectangular shape represent lactose-inhibitable coaggregations; others are lactose-noninhibitable coaggregations. (Modified from Kolenbrander PE, London J: *J Bacteriol* 175:3247, 1993.)

Microorganisms, packed closely together, form a palisade, whereas others start to develop a pleomorphism. Each crack is filled with one type of microorganism (Figure 9-10). As the bacterial densities approach approximately 2 to 6 million bacteria/mm^2 on the enamel surface, a marked increase in growth rate (about three or four doublings) can be observed to 32 million bacteria/mm^2. This further growth of the plaque mass occurs preferably by the multiplication of already-adhering microorganisms rather than by new colonizers.[22] This growth period is independent of subject, surface, tooth, or timebut appears to be dependent on cell density. The thickness of the plaque increases slowly with time, increasing to 20 to 30 μm after 3 days.

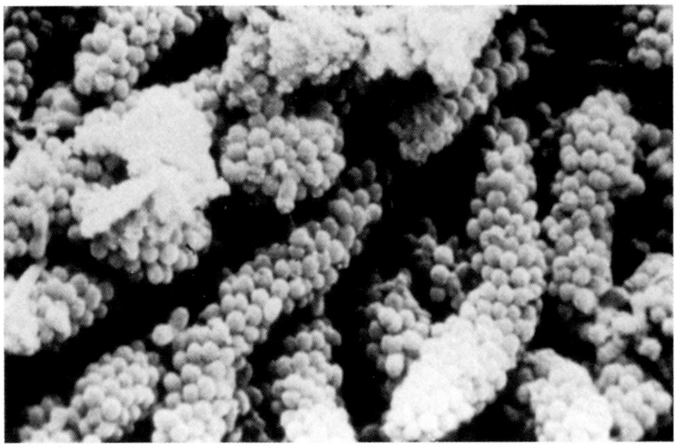

Figure 9-9 Long-standing supragingival plaque near the gingival margin demonstrates "corncob" arrangement. A central gram-negative filamentous core supports the outer coccal cells, which are firmly attached by interbacterial adherence or coaggregation.

De Novo Supragingival Plaque Formation: Clinical Aspects

Clinically, early undisturbed plaque formation on teeth follows an exponential growth curve when measured planimetrically.[188] During the first 24 hours, starting from a clean tooth surface, plaque growth is negligible from a clinical viewpoint (<3% coverage of the vestibular tooth surface, an amount that is clinically almost undetectable). During the following 3 days, plaque growth increases at a rapid rate, then slows down from that point onward. After 4 days, on average, 30% of the total tooth crown area will be covered with plaque. Although plaque does not seem to increase substantially with time after the fourth day, several reports have proved that its composition will change further, with a shift toward more

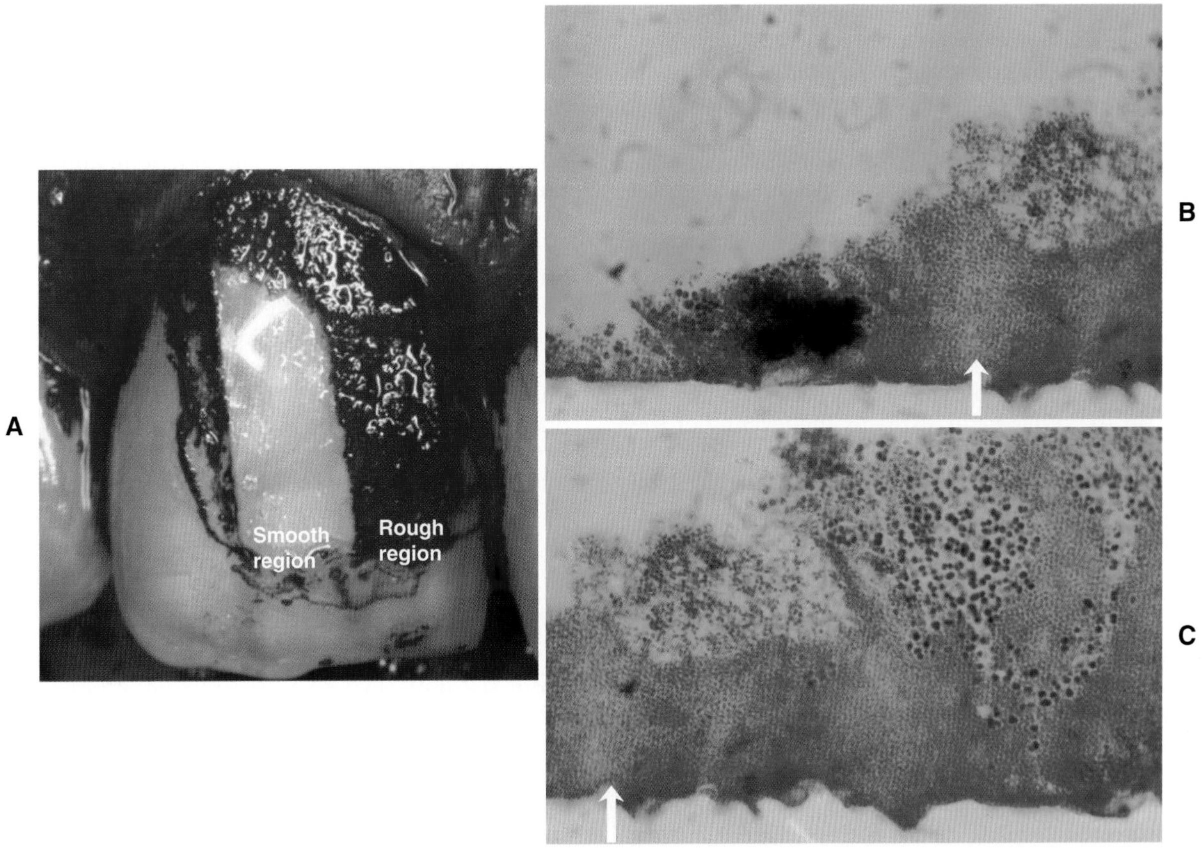

Figure 9-10 **A,** Small plastic strip divided in half (a rough region, average roughness [R_a] 2.0 μm, located mesially, and a smooth region, R_a 0.1 μm, distally located) was glued to the central upper incisors of a patient who refrained from oral hygiene for 3 days. **B** and **C,** After removal, the strip was cut in small slices for microscopic evaluation. The rough part **(C)** contains a thicker plaque layer than the smooth part **(B).** Arrow shows border between rough and smooth surface.

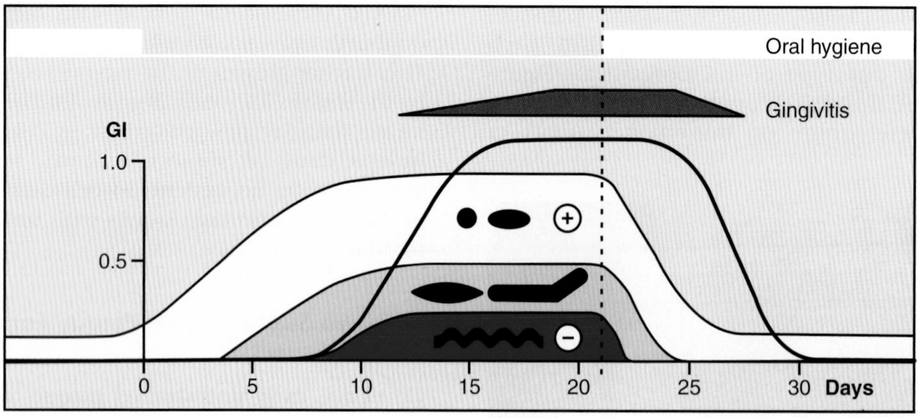

Figure 9-11 Experimental gingivitis model. From day 0 on, when mechanical plaque control was stopped, plaque will slowly form on the teeth. With time the plaque composition changes, with a shift to more gram-negative species (see color) and more rods, filaments, and from day 7 on, spiriles and spirochetes (see morphotypes in black). From day 3 on, the first symptoms of gingival inflammation become visible. When proper plaque control is reestablished, the plaque composition returns to the initial situation. and the symptoms of gingivitis disappear.

anaerobic and gram-negative flora, including an influx of fusobacteria, filaments, spiral forms, and spirochetes (Figure 9-11), as illustrated in several experimental gingivitis studies.[243,248] *In this ecologic shift within of the biofilm, there is a transition from the early aerobic environment characterized by gram-positive facultative species to a highly oxygen-deprived environment in which gram-negative anaerobic microorganisms predominate.*

The slow start of the plaque growth curve can be partly explained by a colony of bacteria needing to reach a certain size before it can be clinically detected. The observations that the early increase in plaque mass originates largely from the proliferation of bacteria already present, and only to a limited extent from new adhering species, fit with the observed exponential growth.[22] The lengthening of the microbial generation time (1 hour for initial plaque to 12 hours for 3-day-old plaque), on the other hand, explains the leveling of the slope from day 4 onward.[258]

During the night, plaque growth rate is reduced by about 50%.[181] This seems surprising because one would expect that reduced plaque removal and the decreased salivary flow at night would enhance plaque growth. The fact that the supragingival plaque obtains its nutrients mainly from the saliva seems to be of greater significance than the antibacterial activity of saliva.[34]

Topography of Supragingival Plaque

Early plaque formation on teeth follows a typical topographic pattern (Figure 9-12), with initial growth along the gingival margin and from the interdental space (areas protected against shear forces). Later, further extension in the coronal direction can be observed.[152,181] This pattern may fundamentally change when the tooth surface contains irregularities that offer a favorable growth path (Figure 9-13). Plaque formation can also start from grooves, cracks, perikymata, or pits. Scanning electron microscopy studies clearly reveal that the early colonization of the enamel surface starts from surface irregularities, where bacteria escape shear forces, allowing the time needed to change from reversible to irreversible binding.[126,127,167,179] By multiplication, the bacteria subsequently spread out from these initial areas as a relatively even monolayer. Surface irregularities are also responsible for the "individualized" plaque growth pattern (see Figure 9-13), which is reproduced in the absence of optimal oral hygiene.[152,153] This phenomenon illustrates the importance of surface roughness in plaque growth, which should lead to proper clinical treatment options.

Surface Microroughness

Rough intraoral surfaces (e.g. crowns, implant abutments, denture bases) accumulate and retain more plaque and calculus in terms of thickness, area, and colony-forming units (for review, see Quirynen and Bollen[179]). Ample plaque also reveals an increased maturity and pathogenicity of its bacterial components, characterized by an increased proportion of motile organisms and spirochetes, or a denser packing of bacteria (Figure 9-14). Smoothing an intraoral surface decreases the rate of plaque formation. Below a certain surface roughness (average roughness [R_a] <0.2 µm), however, further smoothing does not result in additional reduction in plaque formation.[17,184] There seems to be a threshold level for surface roughness (R_a about 0.2 µm), above which bacterial adhesion will be facilitated.[16] Although surface free energy and surface roughness are two factors influencing plaque growth, the latter predominates (see Figure 9-14).

Individual Variables Influencing Plaque Formation

The rate of plaque formation differs significantly between subjects, and these differences might overrule surface characteristics. A distinction is often made between "heavy" (fast) and "light" (slow) plaque formers. From 133 individuals, Simonsson et al.[224] selected one group

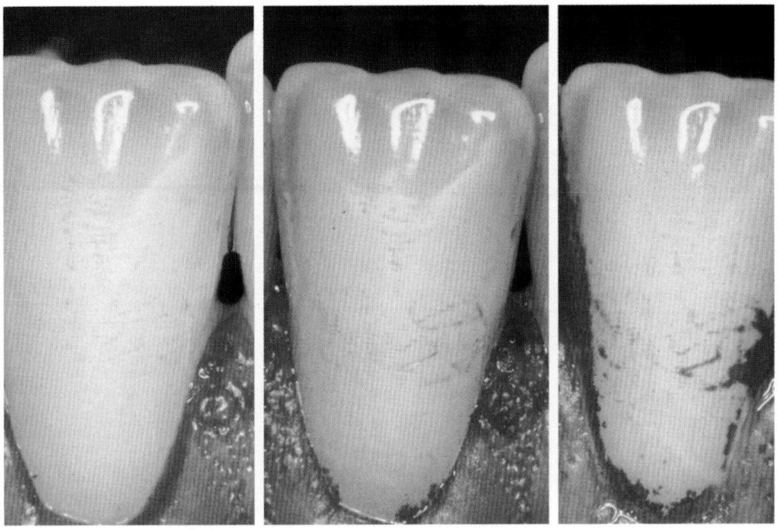

Figure 9-12 Clinical photos of the typical topography of plaque growth. Initial growth starts along the gingival margin and from the interdental space (areas protected against shear forces), to extend farther in a coronal direction. This pattern may fundamentally change when the tooth surface contains presents irregularities (midbuccal area).

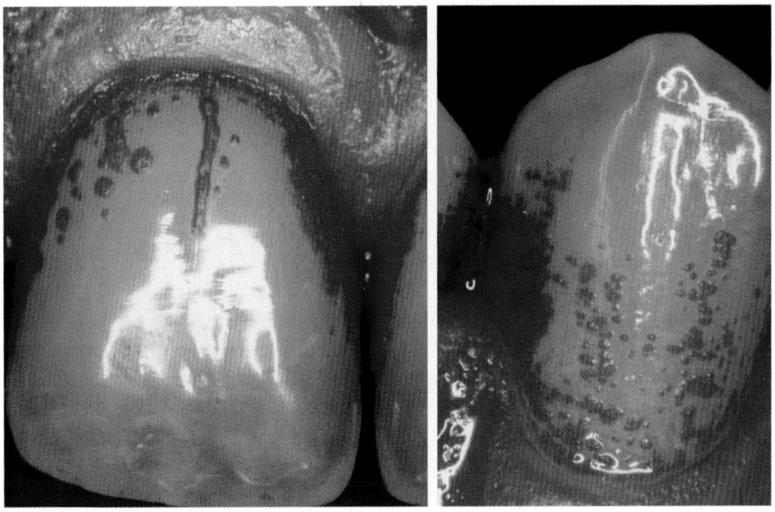

Figure 9-13 Important surface irregularities (*left,* crack on central upper incisor; *right,* several small pits on canine) are also responsible for the "individualized" plaque growth pattern.

of heavy and one group of light plaque formers. Both groups were investigated for clinical, biochemical, biophysical, and microbiologic variables. In a comparative analysis, there were only minor differences between the groups, and no single variable was considered as the only explanation for the great differences in the rate of plaque formation. A multiple regression analysis showed that the clinical wettability of the tooth surfaces, the saliva-induced aggregation of oral bacteria, and the relative salivary flow conditions around the sampled teeth explained 90% of the variation. Moreover, the saliva from light plaque formers reduced the colloidal stability of bacterial suspensions of, for example, *Streptococcus sanguis.*[223]

Zee et al.[273] followed de novo plaque formation on small enamel blocks that were bonded onto the teeth of slow and heavy plaque formers. After 1 day, the heavy plaque formers showed more plaque with a more complex supragingival structure. From days 3 to 14, however, there were no discernible differences between both groups, except for a more prominent intermicrobial matrix in the group of fast growers. In another study, Zee et al.[272] detected qualitative differences in the composition of the plaque between slow and rapid plaque formers. Rapid plaque formers demonstrated higher proportions of gram-negative rods (35% vs. 17%) in 14-day-old plaque.

The intersubject variation in plaque formation can also be explained by factors such as diet, chewing fibrous

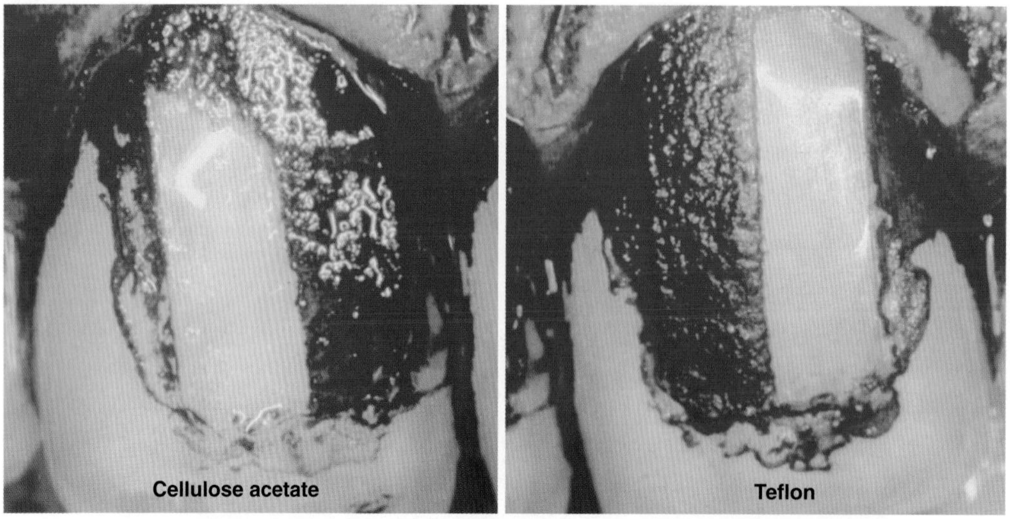

Figure 9-14 Photographs showing the clinical impact of surface roughness and surface free energy on de novo plaque formation. Two small strips were glued to the central upper incisors of a patient who refrained from oral hygiene for 3 days. Each strip was divided in half: a rough region (R_a 2.0 μm), located mesially, and a smooth region (R_a 0.1 μm), located distally. **A,** Strip of cellulose acetate (medium surface free energy (sfe): 58 erg/cm^{-2}); **B,** strip of Teflon (low sfe: 20 erg/cm^{-2}). Plaque was disclosed with 0.5% neutral red solution. The smooth regions show the decrease in biofilm formation caused by the low surface free energy; the rough regions demonstrate the predominance of surface roughness, that is, more plaque with no difference between the two surfaces, even with different surface free energies. (From Quirynen M, Listgarten MA: *Clin Oral Implants Res* 1:8, 1990.)

food, smoking, the presence of copper amalgam, tongue and palate brushing, the colloid stability of bacteria in the saliva, antimicrobial factors present in the saliva, the chemical composition of the pellicle, and the retention depth of the dentogingival area.*

Variation within the Dentition

Within a dental arch, large differences in plaque growth rate can be detected. In general, early plaque formation occurs faster (1) in the lower jaw compared to the upper jaw, (2) in molar areas, (3) on the buccal tooth surfaces compared to oral sites (especially in the upper jaw), and (4) in the interdental regions compared to the strict buccal or oral surfaces.[66,119,178]

Impact of Gingival Inflammation

Several studies clearly indicate that early in vivo plaque formation is more rapid on tooth surfaces facing inflamed gingival margins than on those adjacent to healthy gingivae.[182,193,194] These studies suggest that the increase in crevicular fluid production enhances plaque formation. Most likely, some substance from this exudate (e.g. mineral, protein, carbohydrate) favors both the initial adhesion and the growth of the early colonizing bacteria.

Impact of Patient's Age

Although past studies were contradictory, recent papers clearly indicate that the subject's age does not influence de novo plaque formation. Fransson et al.[65] could detect no differences in de novo plaque formation, either in amount or in composition, between a group of young (20-25 years) and older (65-80 years) subjects who withheld mechanical tooth-cleaning measures for 21 days. This observation largely confirms data by Holm-Pedersen et al.[92] and Winkel et al.[266] The developed plaque in the older patient group, however, resulted in more severe gingival inflammation, which seems to indicate an increased susceptibility to gingivitis with aging.

Spontaneous Tooth Cleaning

Many clinicians still believe that plaque is removed spontaneously from the teeth, such as during eating. However, based on the firm attachment between bacteria and surface, as previously discussed, this seems unlikely. Even in the occlusal part of the molars, plaque remains, even after chewing fibrous food (e.g., carrots, apples, chips). The inefficiency of spontaneous plaque removal is well illustrated by the clinical photos in Figure 9-15, taken before and after dinner, starting from 4 days of undisturbed plaque formation. Only negligible differences in plaque extension could be observed.

De Novo Subgingival Plaque Formation

It is technically impossible to record the dynamics of subgingival plaque formation in an established dentition for the simple reason that one cannot sterilize a periodontal pocket at present. Some early studies, using culturing techniques, examined the changes within the subgingival microbiota during the first week after mechanical debridement and reported only partial

*References 2, 5, 13, 96, 98, 222-224.

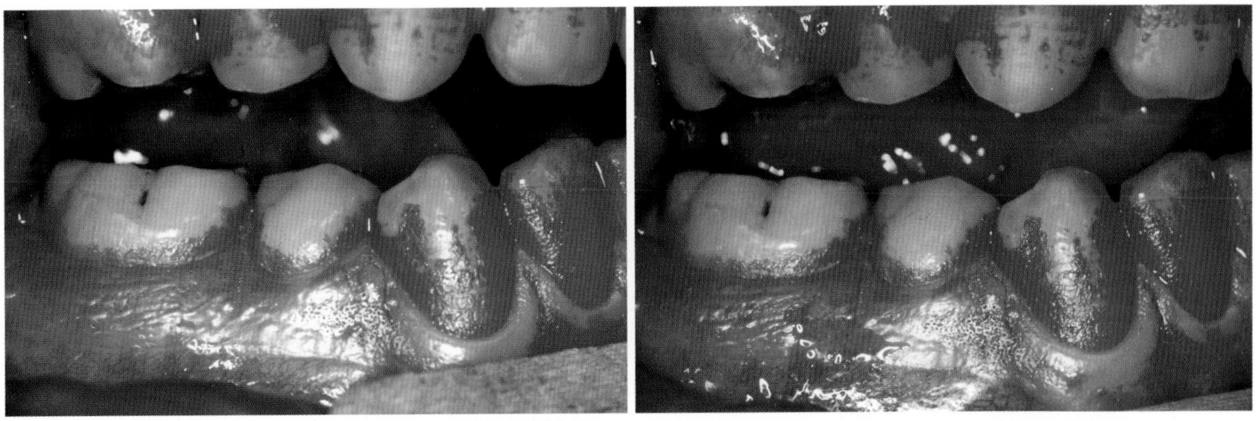

Figure 9-15 Lower premolars and molars from a dental student who refrained from oral hygiene for 100 hours so that undisturbed plaque formation could be evaluated. **A,** Before dinner, and **B,** after diner, eating fibrous food. Almost no reduction in plaque extension could be observed, illustrating the absence of spontaneous plaque removal.

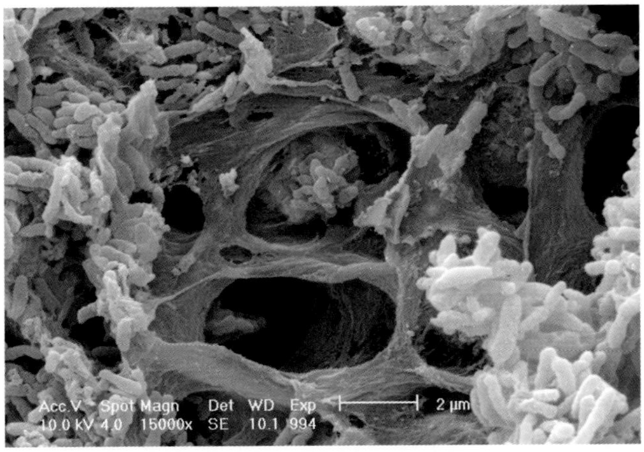

Figure 9-16 Scanning electron micrograph of bacteria invading the dentinal tubules.

reduction of about 3 logs (from 10^8 to 10^5), followed by a fast regrowth to almost pretreatment levels (–0.5 log) within 7 days.[73,86,144] The rapid recolonization was explained by several factors. A critical review of the effectiveness of subgingival debridement, for example, revealed that a high proportion of treated tooth surfaces (5%-80%) still harbored plaque and calculus after scaling. These remaining bacteria were considered the primary source for the subgingival recolonization.[174] Some pathogens penetrate the soft tissues or the dentinal tubules and eventually escape instrumentation[4,72,206] (Figure 9-16).

The introduction of oral implants (see Chapter 73), especially of the two-stage type, provides a new experimental setup. Indeed, when the transmucosal part of the implant (the abutment) is inserted on top of the osseointegrated endosseous part, a new "pristine" surface is created on which the intraoral translocation of bacteria can be investigated.[184] Recent studies demonstrate that a complex subgingival microbiota, including most periopathogens, is established within 1 week after abutment insertion. This is followed by a slow increase of especially the number of pathogenic species.[191,192] This microbiota appears at periimplant sites independent of shallow or intermediate depth. Since the supragingival environment (saliva, tongue, and dental plaque) served as the only sources of colonization of the "pristine" periimplant pockets, the importance of cross-infection is once more highlighted (see later discussion).

Oral implants have been used as a model to study the impact of surface roughness on the subgingival plaque formation.* Smooth abutments (R_a <0.2 µm) were found to harbor 25 times less bacteria than rough ones, with a slightly higher density of coccoid (i.e., nonpathogenic) cells. The subgingival flora was also largely dependent on the remaining presence of teeth and the degree of periodontitis in the remaining natural dentition (for review, see Quirynen et al.[186]). These aspects again point to the importance of the intraoral bacterial translocation or cross-infection.

In a beagle dog study, Leknes et al.[124] studied the extent of subgingival colonization in 6-mm pockets with smooth or rough root surfaces. The authors also observed that smooth surfaces harbored significantly less plaque and concluded that subgingival irregularities shelter submerged microorganisms by impeding the cleaning action of the gingival crevicular fluid. Moreover, biopsies of the soft tissues showed a higher proportion of inflammatory cells in the junctional epithelium (and the underlying connective tissue) facing the rough surfaces.[123] Finally, the same group reported higher rates of attachment loss around teeth with grooves in the root surface.[122]

PHYSIOLOGIC PROPERTIES OF DENTAL PLAQUE

The transition from gram-positive to gram-negative microorganisms observed in the structural development of dental plaque is paralleled by a physiologic transition

*References 17, 28, 81, 184, 190, 200.

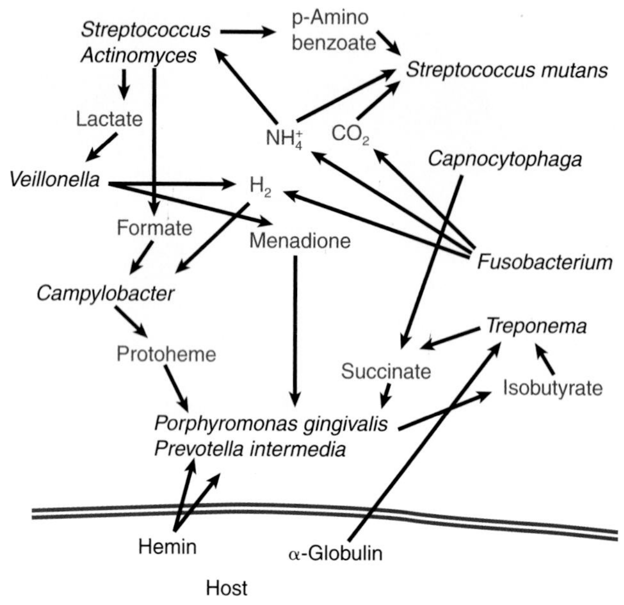

Figure 9-17 Schematic illustration of metabolic interactions among different bacterial species found in plaque and between the host and plaque bacteria. These interactions are likely to be important to the survival of bacteria in the periodontal environment.

in the developing plaque. The early colonizers (e.g., streptococci, *Actinomyces* species) use oxygen and lower the redox potential of the environment, which then favors the growth of anaerobic species.[52,256] Gram-positive species use sugars as an energy source and saliva as a carbon source. The bacteria that predominate in mature plaque are anaerobic and asaccharolytic and use amino acids and small peptides as energy sources.[136] Laboratory studies have demonstrated many physiologic interactions among the different bacteria found in dental plaque (Figure 9-17). Lactate and formate are byproducts of the metabolism of streptococci and actinomycetes and may be used in the metabolism of other plaque microorganisms. The growth of *Porphyromonas gingivalis* is enhanced by metabolic byproducts produced by other microorganisms, such as succinate from *Capnocytophaga ochraceus* and protoheme from *Campylobacter rectus*.[75,76,147]

The host also functions as an important source of nutrients. For example, the bacterial enzymes that degrade host proteins result in the release of ammonia, which may be used by bacteria as a nitrogen source.[33] Hemin iron from the breakdown of host hemoglobin may be important in the metabolism of *P. gingivalis*.[21] Increases in steroid hormones are associated with significant increases in the proportions of *Prevotella intermedia* found in subgingival plaque.[114] Physiologic interactions occur both between different microorganisms in plaque and between the host and plaque microorganisms. These nutritional interdependencies are probably critical to the growth and survival of microorganisms in dental plaque and may partly explain the evolution of highly specific structural interactions observed among bacteria in plaque.

Some researchers even consider the pathologic flora as a result of environmental perturbations to the habitat, the "ecological plaque hypothesis."[145,146] A change in the nutrient status of a pocket or chemical and physical changes to the habitat are thus considered the primary cause for the overgrowth by pathogens. For example, laboratory studies indicated that an increased flow of gingival crevicular fluid leads to the enrichment of proteolytic species (e.g., periopathogens) by providing essential nutrients, including heme-containing molecules.[247] This hypothesis, if correct, could lead to new treatment concepts. For periodontitis, attempts could be made to alter the local environment by reducing the crevicular flow rate, or the site could be made less anaerobic by the use of redox agents.[146]

SPECIAL BACTERIAL BEHAVIOR IN BIOFILMS

Bacteria growing in microbial communities adherent to a surface do not "behave" the same as bacteria growing suspended in a liquid environment ("planktonic" or unattached state). For example, the resistance of bacteria to antimicrobial agents is dramatically increased in the biofilm.[8,44,87,177] Almost without exception, organisms in a biofilm are 1000 to 1500 times more resistant to antibiotics than in their planktonic state. The mechanisms of this increased resistance differ from species to species, from antibiotic to antibiotic, and for biofilm growing in different habitats.

It is generally accepted that the resistance of bacteria to antibiotics is affected by their nutritional status, growth rate, temperature, pH, and prior exposure to subeffective concentrations of antimicrobial agents.[26,27,265] Variations in any of these parameters will thus lead to a varied response to antibiotics within a biofilm. Another important mechanism of resistance appears to be the slower rate of growth of bacterial species in a biofilm, which makes them less susceptible to many, but not all, antibiotics.[14,24,44,269] The biofilm matrix, although not a significant barrier in itself to the diffusion of antibiotics, does have certain properties that can resist diffusion. For example, strongly charged or chemically highly reactive agents can fail to reach the deeper zones of the biofilm because the biofilm acts as an ion-exchange resin, removing such molecules from solution.[71] In addition, extracellular enzymes such as β-lactamase, formaldehyde lyase, and formaldehyde dehydrogenase may become trapped and concentrated in the extracellular matrix, thus inactivating some antibiotics (especially positively charged hydrophilic antibiotics). Some antibiotics, such as the macrolides, which are positively charged but hydrophobic, are unaffected by this process. Recently, "super-resistant" bacteria were identified within a biofilm; these cells have multidrug-resistance pumps that can extrude antimicrobial agents from the cell.[24] Because these pumps place the antibiotics outside the outer membrane, the process offers protection against antibiotics that target, for example, cell wall synthesis. All these observations are critical to the use of antimicrobials in the treatment of periodontal infections.

In a biofilm, bacteria have the capacity to communicate with each other *(quorum sensing)*. This involves the regulation of expression of specific genes through the accumulation of signaling compounds that mediate inter-cellular communication. When these signaling compounds reach a threshold level (quorum cell density), gene expression can be activated. The latter can occur more easily in microcolonies because the signaling compounds do not dissolve in the surroundings and thus remain concentrated. Such quorum sensing seems to play a role in expressing genes for antibiotic resistance and in encouraging the growth of beneficial species to the biofilm and discouraging the growth of competitors.

The high density of bacterial cells in a biofilm also facilitates the exchange of genetic information among cells of the same species and across species and even genera. *Conjugation* (exchange of genes through a direct interbacterial connection formed by a sex pilus), *transformation* (movement of small pieces of DNA from the environment into the bacterial chromosome), plasmid transfer, and transposon transfer have all been shown to occur more easily in a biofilm.

PRINCIPLE OF BACTERIAL TRANSMISSION, TRANSLOCATION, OR CROSS-INFECTION

Bacterial "fingerprinting" clearly illustrates that periodontal pathogens are transmissible within members of a families.[270] This bacterial *transmission* between subjects (and even between animals and humans) should not be confused with *contagion* ("contagious" refers to the likelihood of a microorganism causing disease, after being transmitted from an infected to an uninfected host). Similar observations were made for the transmission of cariogenic species from mother to child.[104]

The existence of an "intraoral" transmission of bacteria (from one niche to another, also called *translocation* or *cross-infection*) has recently been thoroughly investigated. Such a transmission of pathogens, from one *locus* to another, could jeopardize the outcome of periodontal therapy. The significance of such an intraoral translocation is difficult to prove or quantify. The existence of intraoral transmission of bacteria was first examined in cariology. Loesche et al.[139] showed that streptomycin-resistant strains of *Streptococcus mutans*, grown on a dental inlay, were spontaneously transmitted to the neighboring teeth (probably through saliva) and could even reach the contralateral quadrant after transmission with a dental explorer. Earlier, Edman et al.[59] had been successful in implanting *S. mutans* in two volunteers by means of inoculated dental flosses.

Comparable observations have been made for periodontal pathogens. Christersson et al.[41] demonstrated translocation of *A. actinomycetemcomitans* by periodontal probes in patients with localized aggressive periodontitis. The authors were able to inoculate noninfected pockets with *A. actinomycetemcomitans* by a single course of probing with a probe previously inserted in an infected pocket of the same patient. Although the inoculation was only temporary, the question remained whether the inoculation could have become permanent if the site had offered more suitable growth conditions (e.g., a deep pocket, as frequently encountered immediately after initial periodontal therapy).

Microbiology of Implants in Partially Edentulous Patients

A large series of studies compared the microbiota in pockets around teeth with that in periimplant pockets in partially edentulous patients and reported a striking similarity.* Based on this similarity, it has been suggested that, at least in partially edentulous patients, teeth might act as a reservoir for the (re)colonization of the subgingival area around implants. This hypothesis was supported by Sumida et al.,[242] who detected similar intrasubject pulsed-field gel-electrophoresis patterns for periopathogens from teeth and implants compared with large intersubject variations.

Translocation and Guided Tissue Regeneration

Nowzari et al.[166] evaluated the amount of guided tissue regeneration and membrane contamination after treatment of mandibular bony defects in either a group of patients with a healthy periodontium in the remaining dentition or a group of patients with multiple deep pockets and numerous pathogens. The healthy group showed significantly less membrane contamination both immediately after insertion as well as at removal after 6 weeks. The healthy group also showed significantly more clinical gain in attachment than the disease group (3.4 vs. 1.4 mm). Mombelli et al.[155] compared the clinical and microbial changes when tetracycline fibers (local application of antibiotics) were applied only to the two deepest pockets in the mouth (without further treatment to the remaining pockets) with those changes obtained when all teeth were cleaned and pockets with a depth greater than 3 mm were treated. After 6 months, significant "additional" improvements (clinical as well as microbiologic) were recorded in the group of patients with the more global approach. Their pockets showed a probing depth reduction (1.7 mm) and attachment gain (0.7 mm) that were significantly higher than in the patients with some remaining pockets (0.9 and 0.3 mm, respectively). The authors concluded that pathogens most likely were transferred through saliva from infected untreated periodontal lesions or other niches to the treated sites.

Translocation and Mechanical Debridement

To reduce the chance for an intraoral translocation, a treatment strategy called *one-stage, full-mouth disinfection* was introduced by the Leuven group in the 1990s.[185] This strategy attempts to eradicate, or at least suppress, periodontal pathogens in a short time not only from the periodontal pockets, but also from all their intraoral habitats (mucous membranes, tongue, and saliva). The one-stage, full-mouth disinfection concept consists of a combination of the following therapeutic efforts[185]:

- Full-mouth scaling and root planing within 24 hours to reduce the number of subgingival pathogenic organisms.

*References 11, 94, 95, 103, 105, 121, 125, 148, 156, 172, 180, 213.

- Subgingival irrigation of all pockets with a 1% chlorhexidine gel to kill remaining bacteria.
- Tongue brushing with an antiseptic to suppress the bacteria in the niche.
- Mouth rinsing with an antiseptic to reduce the bacteria in the saliva and on the tonsils.

Several studies comparing this approach with the standard therapy (root planing per quadrant at 2-week intervals) from the Leuven group clearly illustrate the benefits of the one-stage, full-mouth approach in relation to (1) gain in attachment, (2) pocket depth reduction, and (3) microbiologic shifts (for review, see Quirynen et al.[186]). A study by Apatzidou and Kinane[10] was less convincing but still reported benefits for the one-stage, full-mouth approach (0.8-mm gain in attachment) for deep pockets.

Intraoral Equilibrium between Cariogenic Species and Periopathogens

Several clinical studies followed the detection frequency and relative proportion of cariogenic species after periodontal therapy. All suggest a relative increase in the number as well as the detection frequency of *S. mutans* up to 8 months after mechanical debridement.[51,187] In a cross-sectional study, subgingival plaque samples from adult periodontitis patients were tested for the presence and levels of mutans streptococci and putative periodontal pathogens.[250] Patients were divided into four groups based on the stage of their periodontal treatment: (1) untreated, (2) after initial periodontal therapy, (3) maintenance phase without periodontal surgery, and (4) after periodontal surgery. The prevalence of mutans streptococci in the four groups was equivalent. The shift toward a more cariogenic flora observed after initial therapy and after surgical periodontal therapy could be explained by:

(1) subgingival outgrowth by *S. mutans* occupying spots that became available after periodontal therapy (e.g., increased number of free adhesion/receptor sites),
(2) creation of a new ecosystem in the subgingival area which is characterized by being more anaerobic, and having a lower redox potential, lower pH and a protein concentrated nutritional environment This niche allows or facilitates the growth of *S. mutans* species, and
(3) "down growth" of *S. mutans* from the supragingival area, where the species could survive in the saliva.

SCIENCE TRANSFER

The oral cavity has the potential to harbor at least 600 different bacterial species, and in any given patient, more than 150 species may be present. One surface of a tooth can have as many as a billion bacteria in its attached bacterial plaque.

A number of gram-negative rods and spirochetes are putative periodontal pathogens, but these organisms may also be present, although in smaller concentrations, in healthy patients. In addition, the bacteria in periodontal pockets exist in a biofilm that gives them more than a thousandfold increased resistance to antibiotics. These complexities, together with variations in patients' host response, mean that in general, periodontal disease cannot be treated by antibiotic therapies restricted to specific bacteria.

A recent, innovative approach to treating periodontal pockets involves complete mouth debridement and the use of antiseptic rinses and gels within 24 hours to reduce the potential for bacteria from untreated sites to colonize treated areas. This may result in additional improvements in attachment gain and pocket reduction, compared to the conventional four-appointment initial therapy.

ASSOCIATION OF PLAQUE MICROORGANISMS WITH PERIODONTAL DISEASES

The current concept on the etiology of periodontitis considers three groups of factors that determine whether active periodontitis will occur in a subject: (1) a susceptible host, (2) the presence of pathogenic species, and (3) the absence, or a small proportion, of "beneficial bacteria."[9,231,233,236,267] The clinical manifestations of periodontal destruction thus result from a complex interplay between the etiologic agents, in this case specific pathogens in dental plaque, and the host tissues. In general, small amounts of bacterial plaque can be controlled by the body's defense mechanisms without destruction, but when the balance between bacterial load and host response is disturbed, periodontal destruction may occur. This may result when the subject is extremely susceptible to periodontal infections or when the patient is infected by a large amount of bacteria or by an extremely pathogenic microbiota.

The **susceptibility** of the host is partially hereditary but can be influenced by environmental and behavioral factors, such as smoking, stress, and diabetes. Recently, genetic variations or mutations have been identified that modulate the individual's response to the intraoral bacterial insult (e.g., inadequate or unregulated immunologic response) and that are associated with severe forms of periodontal disease. Several studies demonstrated a significant link between specific genetic markers (associated with increased interleukin-1 production) and periodontitis susceptibility (for review, see Albandar and Rams[6]). Especially for patients with early-onset periodontitis (high susceptibility), the hereditary aspect seems to play a key role.[67,150] Grossi et al.[79,80] found a direct and linear dose response between destructive periodontitis and the level of smoking (odds ratio of 2.0 to 5.0 when attachment loss was considered). Smokers were also found to heal less satisfactorily after periodontal therapy than nonsmokers.[84,101,271] Patients with diabetes are also at higher risk for periodontal destruction.[78,241] Severe stress conditions (e.g., divorce, financial strain), especially in combination with inadequate coping behavior, seem to aggravate the periodontal destruction, probably by influencing the environmental factors (e.g., smoking, oral hygiene) and modifying the immune response. More recently, viruses (e.g., cytomegalovirus, Epstein-Barr virus, papillomavirus, herpesvirus) were suspected to play a role in causing periodontal diseases, possibly by changing the host response to the local subgingival microbiota.[43,229]

The second essential factor for disease initiation and progression is the presence of one or more **pathogens,** of the susceptible clonal type and in sufficient numbers. Despite the difficulties inherent in characterizing the microbiology of periodontal diseases (see later discussion), a small group of pathogens is recognized because of their close association with disease. There are obvious data to consider *Actinobacillus actinomycetemcomitans, Tannerella forsythia,* and *Porphyromonas gingivalis* as key pathogens because they are strongly associated with periodontal disease status, disease progression, and unsuccessful therapy. For the following bacteria, however, moderate evidence for etiology has been reported, at least if their concentration passes a certain threshold level: *Prevotella intermedia, Prevotella nigrescens, Campylobacter rectus, Peptostreptococcus micros, Fusobacterium nucleatum, Eubacterium nodatum,* and various spirochetes.[9,231,233,236,267] The significance for the role of these key pathogens is largely based on epidemiologic data, the ability of these microorganisms to produce disease when inoculated in animals, and their capacity to produce virulence factors. However, the mere presence of putative periodontal pathogens in the gingival crevice is *not* sufficient to initiate or cause periodontal inflammation. An elevation in the relative proportion or number of these pathogens to reach a critical mass seems more crucial to mount an effective tissue-damaging process. Indeed, even in health, periodontal pathogens may be present in the gingival crevice, although in low numbers, as members of the normal resident flora.[141]

The role of "**beneficial** species" of the host is less obvious in the progression of disease.[233] Such bacteria can affect disease progression in different ways: (1) by passively occupying a niche that may otherwise be colonized by pathogens, (2) by actively limiting a pathogen's ability to adhere to appropriate tissue surfaces, (3) by adversely affecting the vitality or growth of a pathogen, (4) by affecting the ability of a pathogen to produce virulence factors, or (5) by degrading virulence factors produced by the pathogen. One well-documented example of such a beneficial action is the effect of *Streptococcus sanguis* on *A. actinomycetemcomitans. S. sanguis* produces hydrogen peroxide (H_2O_2), which either directly or by host-enzyme amplification can kill *A. actinomycetemcomitans.*[90]

Since it is impossible at present to alter the susceptibility of the host, periodontal therapy is necessarily focused on the reduction or elimination of periodontal pathogens in combination with the reestablishment, often by surgical pocket elimination, of a more suitable environment (less anaerobic) for a more beneficial microbiota. Several studies have indicated that the presence of the previously mentioned periodontal pathogens (persisting or reestablished after treatment) is associated with a negative clinical outcome of periodontal treatment.[46,84,196,197,238]

Recent studies demonstrate a potential association between periodontitis and nosocomial pneumonia as well as between periodontitis and an adverse pregnancy outcome.[216,217] Moreover, a more modest association is observed between periodontal disease and the occurrence of atherosclerosis, cardiovascular disease, and stroke.[215] Thus, host factors act locally in reducing resistance to periodontal tissue destruction as a result of bacterial challenge, and the bacterial challenge may produce local or systemic responses that contribute to a systemic disease.

MICROBIAL SPECIFICITY OF PERIODONTAL DISEASES

Nonspecific Plaque Hypothesis

In the mid-1900s, periodontal diseases were believed to result from an accumulation of plaque over time, eventually in conjunction with a diminished host response and increased host susceptibility with age. This thinking, termed the *nonspecific plaque theory,* was supported by epidemiologic studies that correlated both the patient's age and the amount of plaque with evidence of periodontitis.[142,207,219]

The nonspecific plaque hypothesis maintains that periodontal disease results from the "elaboration of noxious products by the entire plaque flora."[137] According to this theory, when only small amounts of plaque are present, the noxious products are neutralized by the host. Similarly, large amounts of plaque would produce large amounts of noxious products, which would essentially overwhelm the host's defenses. Inherent in the nonspecific plaque hypothesis is the concept that control of periodontal disease depends on control of the amount of plaque accumulation. The current standard treatment of periodontitis by debridement (nonsurgical or surgical) and oral hygiene measures still focuses on the removal of plaque and its products and is founded in the nonspecific plaque hypothesis. Thus, although the nonspecific plaque hypothesis has been discarded in favor of the specific plaque hypothesis, much clinical treatment is still based on the nonspecific theory.

Several observations contradicted the conclusions of the nonspecific plaque hypothesis. First, some individuals with considerable amounts of plaque and calculus, as well as gingivitis, never developed destructive periodontitis. Furthermore, individuals who did present with periodontitis demonstrated considerable site specificity in the pattern of disease. Some sites were unaffected, whereas advanced disease was found in adjacent sites. In the presence of a uniform host response, these findings were inconsistent with the concept that all plaque was equally pathogenic. Recognition of the differences in plaque at sites of different clinical status (i.e., disease vs. health) led to a renewed search for *specific* pathogens in periodontal diseases and a conceptual transition from the nonspecific to the specific plaque hypothesis.[135,228,237]

Specific Plaque Hypothesis

The specific plaque hypothesis states that only certain plaque is pathogenic, and its pathogenicity depends on the presence of or increase in specific microorganisms.[137] This concept predicts that plaque harboring specific bacterial pathogens results in a periodontal disease because these organisms produce substances that mediate the destruction of host tissues.

The association of specific bacterial species with disease originated in the early 1960s, when microscopic examination of plaque revealed that different bacterial morphotypes were found in healthy versus periodontally diseased sites. At about the same time, major advances were made in techniques used to isolate and identify periodontal microorganisms. These included improvements in procedures to sample subgingival plaque, handling of samples to prevent killing the bacteria, and media used to grow the bacteria in the laboratory.[233] The result was a tremendous increase in the ability to isolate periodontal microorganisms and considerable refinement in bacterial taxonomy.[117] Acceptance of the specific plaque hypothesis was spurred by the recognition of *A. actinomycetemcomitans* as a pathogen in localized aggressive periodontitis.[164,228] These advances led to a series of association studies that focused on identifying specific periodontal pathogens by examining the microbiota associated with states of health and disease in cross-sectional and longitudinal studies.

Complicating Factors

The identification of bacterial pathogens in periodontal diseases has been difficult because of a number of factors.[233] The periodontal microbiota is a complex community of microorganisms, many of which are still difficult or impossible to isolate in the laboratory. The chronic nature of periodontal disease has complicated the search for bacterial pathogens. It was previously thought that periodontal diseases progressed at a slow but steady rate. However, epidemiologic studies established that disease progresses at different rates, with alternating episodes of rapid tissue destruction and periods of remission (Figure 9-18). Identification of the microorganisms found during the different phases of the disease progression is technically challenging. Furthermore, the interpretation of microbiologic data is greatly influenced by the clinical classification of disease status, an area that has undergone a number of recent revisions.[12] Previous and perhaps current classifications involve the grouping of potentially different disease states because of the difficulties in accurately distinguishing them clinically. It is important to recognize that these types of groupings may obscure microbiologic associations.

Currently, periodontitis is considered a mixed infection, which has a significant impact on both its diagnosis and its treatment. For the diagnosis the clinician must evaluate the presence of up to 10 species, and it is still unclear whether some combinations of species are more pathogenic than others. The treatment is directed to the eradication or reduction of the number of all key periopathogens. Because several species might be involved, the use of antimicrobials (especially antibiotics) is extremely difficult, because not all expected periopathogens are susceptible to the same antibiotic. Therefore, several studies analyzed the success of combinations of several

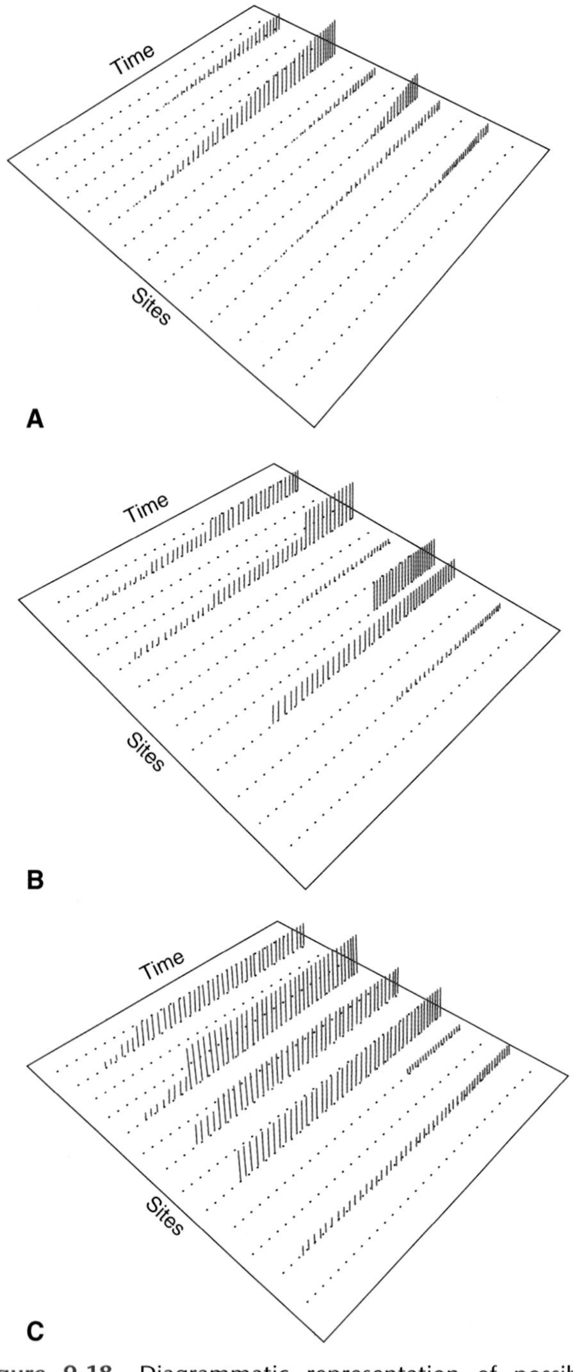

Figure 9-18 Diagrammatic representation of possible modes of progression of chronic destructive periodontal diseases. Sites on the *x* axis are plotted against time on the *y* axis, and activity is shown on the *z* axis. **A,** Some sites show progressive loss of attachment over time, whereas others show no destruction. The time of onset and the extent of destruction vary among sites. **B,** Random burst model. Activity occurs at random at any site. Some sites show no activity, whereas others show one or several bursts of activity. The cumulative extent of destruction varies among sites. **C,** Asynchronous multiple-burst model. Several sites show bursts of activity over a finite period, followed by prolonged periods of inactivity. Occasional bursts may occur infrequently at certain sites at later periods. Other sites show no periodontal disease activity at any time. The difference from the model shown in **B** is that in **C** the majority of destructive disease activity takes place within a few years of the individual's life. (Courtesy Drs. S. Socransky, A. Haffajee, M. Goodson, and J. Lindhe, Boston and Göteborg, Sweden.)

antibiotics, although this approach increased the chance of severe side effects.

Recent microbiologic tests clearly indicate that the presence of periodontal pathogens by itself is not sufficient for the development of periodontitis. Because of the high sensitivity of these tests, several pathogens have been detected in periodontitis-free patients. Thus, rather than their presence, the *amount* of pathogens plays the key role in relation to disease. Again, these observations have major clinical implications, as follows:

1. This approach dramatically reduces the specificity of microbial examinations (*specificity* = presence of pathogen means periodontitis). In other words, even though a microbiologic analysis is positive, the patient may not have disease. This undermines the reliability and usefulness of these tests.
2. The understanding of the etiology becomes more complicated because the threshold level for periopathogens between health and disease is unknown and subject dependent.
3. For several species, large intrastrain variations in genetic information have been detected (different genotypes), so information on the genotype level is needed before the pathogenicity of the strain can be estimated.[38,50,77,173] Besides the bacteria, the quality of the host response also plays an essential role but still cannot be correctly estimated.
4. One can question whether periopathogens are endogenous species or exogenous, since the newer techniques have reported high detection frequencies of all pathogens in healthy subjects as well. This again has significant impact on the treatment strategies. For *endogenous* species, the endpoint of a therapy is reduction of the species, whereas for *exogenous* species, the endpoint is eradication and prevention of reinfection.

These observations emphasize that several key questions remain unanswered. Some researchers still question whether the presence of specific microorganisms in the periodontal pocket is the cause or the consequence of the disease.[239] Because periodontopathogens are fastidious strict anaerobes, they may contribute little to the initiation of disease in shallow gingival pockets, only finding their preferred habitat in deep periodontal pockets.

Criteria for Identification of Periodontal Pathogens

In the 1870s, Robert Koch developed the classic criteria by which a microorganism can be judged to be a causative agent in human infections. These criteria, known as *Koch's postulates,* stipulate the following for the causative agent:

1. Must be routinely isolated from diseased individuals.
2. Must be grown in pure culture in the laboratory.
3. Must produce a similar disease when inoculated into susceptible laboratory animals.
4. Must be recovered from lesions in a diseased laboratory animal.

Streptococcus mutans, for example, has been shown to fulfill Koch's postulates as an etiologic agent of dental caries. However, difficulties exist in the application of these criteria to other types of diseases, and the applicability of Koch's postulates has been increasingly challenged in recent years. In the case of periodontitis, three primary problems are (1) the inability to culture all the organisms that have been associated with disease (e.g., many of the oral spirochetes), (2) the difficulties inherent in defining and culturing sites of active disease, and (3) the lack of a good animal model system for the study of periodontitis.[233]

Sigmund Socransky, a researcher at the Forsyth Dental Center in Boston, proposed criteria by which periodontal microorganisms may be judged to be potential pathogens.[233] These criteria stipulate the following for a potential pathogen:

1. Must be associated with disease, as evident by increases in the number of organisms at diseased sites.
2. Must be eliminated or decreased in sites that demonstrate clinical resolution of disease with treatment.
3. Must demonstrate a host response, in the form of an alteration in the host cellular or humoral immune response.
4. Must be capable of causing disease in experimental animal models.
5. Must demonstrate virulence factors responsible for enabling the microorganism to cause destruction of the periodontal tissues.

As presented earlier, data support the role of *A. actinomycetemcomitans* and *P. gingivalis* as periodontal pathogens, based on these criteria. The association and elimination criteria are discussed in the preceding sections. The latter three criteria focus on the host-parasite interaction, which is discussed in Chapter 13.

MICROORGANISMS ASSOCIATED WITH SPECIFIC PERIODONTAL DISEASES

Early studies with appropriate microscopy clearly demonstrated that the number and proportion of different subgingival bacterial groups varied in periodontal health compared with the disease state.[131,228,237] The total number of bacteria, determined by microscopic counts per gram of plaque, was twice as high in periodontally diseased sites than in healthy sites.[237] Because considerably more plaque is found at diseased sites, this suggests that the total bacterial load seems greater than that at healthy sites.

The differences between periodontal health and disease also are evident when the morphotypes of the bacteria from healthy and diseased sites are examined (Figure 9-19). Fewer coccal cells and more motile rods and spirochetes are found in diseased sites than in healthy sites by means of phase-contrast or dark-field microscopy.[131] One should remember that almost all key periodontal pathogens except *Campylobacter rectus* are immobile rods, which adds to the confusion when bacterial etiologies are overlooked. On culturing, it appears that bacteria from periodontally healthy sites consist predominantly of gram-positive facultative rods and cocci (approximately 75%).[228] The recovery of this group of microorganisms is decreased proportionally in gingivitis

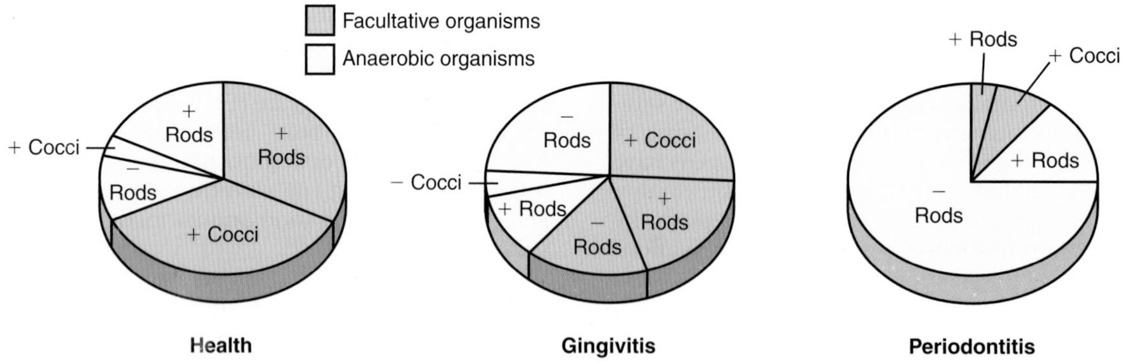

Figure 9-19 Pie charts based on culturing studies, representing the relative proportion of different morphotypes in subgingival samples in cases of periodontal health, gingivitis, and periodontitis. A clear distinction is made between facultative species and obligate anaerobic species. Spirochetes are not included.

(44%) and periodontitis (10%-13%). These decreases are accompanied by increases in the proportions of gram-negative rods, from 13% in health to 40% in gingivitis and 74% in advanced periodontitis (see Figure 9-15).

Periodontal Health

The recovery of microorganisms from periodontally healthy sites is meager compared with that from diseased sites. The bacteria associated with periodontal health are primarily gram-positive facultative species and members of the genera *Streptococcus* and *Actinomyces* (e.g., *S. sanguis, S. mitis, A. viscosus, A. naeslundii*). Small proportions of gram-negative species are also found, most frequently *P. intermedia, F. nucleatum,* and *Capnocytophaga, Neisseria,* and *Veillonella* species. Microscopic studies indicate that a few spirochetes and motile rods also may be found.

Certain bacterial species have been proposed to be protective or beneficial to the host, including *S. sanguis, Veillonella parvula,* and *C. ochraceus.* They are typically found in high numbers at periodontal sites that do not demonstrate attachment loss (inactive sites), but in low numbers at sites where active periodontal destruction occurs.[58,233] These species probably function in preventing the colonization or proliferation of pathogenic microorganisms. As noted earlier, a mechanism by which this may occur is the production of H_2O_2 by *S. sanguis;* H_2O_2 is known to be lethal to cells of *A. actinomycetemcomitans.* Clinical studies have shown that sites with high levels of *C. ochraceus* and *S. sanguis* are associated with a greater gain in attachment after therapy, further supporting this concept.[233] A better understanding of plaque ecology and the interactions between bacteria and their products in plaque will undoubtedly reveal many other examples.

Gingivitis

The development of gingivitis has been extensively studied in a model system referred to as *experimental gingivitis* and initially described by Löe et al.[135] and Theilade et al.[248] Periodontal health is first established in human subjects by cleaning and rigorous oral hygiene measures, followed by abstinence from oral hygiene for 21 days. After 8 hours without oral hygiene, bacteria may be found at concentrations of 10^3 to $10^4/mm^2$ of tooth surface and will increase in number by a factor of 100 to 1000 in the next 24-hour period.[240] After 36 hours the plaque becomes clinically visible. The initial microbiota of experimental gingivitis consists of gram-positive rods, gram-positive cocci, and gram-negative cocci (see Figure 9-11). The transition to gingivitis is evident by inflammatory changes and is accompanied first by the appearance of gram-negative rods and filaments, then by spirochetal and motile microorganisms.[248]

The microbiota of *dental plaque-induced gingivitis (chronic gingivitis)* consist of approximately equal proportions of gram-positive (56%) and gram-negative (44%) species, as well as facultative (59%) and anaerobic (41%) microorganisms.[228] Predominant gram-positive species include *S. sanguis, S. mitis, S. intermedius, S. oralis, A. viscosus, A. naeslundii,* and *P. micros.* The gram-negative microorganisms are predominantly *F. nucleatum, P. intermedia,* and *V. parvula,* as well as *Haemophilus, Capnocytophaga,* and *Campylobacter* species.[154,159,228]

Pregnancy-associated gingivitis is an acute inflammation of the gingival tissues associated with pregnancy. This condition is accompanied by increases in steroid hormones in crevicular fluid and dramatic increases in the levels of *P. intermedia,* which uses the steroids as growth factors.[114]

Studies of gingivitis support the conclusion that disease development is associated with selected alterations in the microbial composition of dental plaque and is not simply the result of an accumulation of plaque. Gingivitis was generally believed to precede the development of chronic periodontitis; however, many individuals demonstrate long-standing gingivitis that never advances to destruction of the periodontal attachment.[25,134]

Chronic Periodontitis

Numerous forms of periodontal disease are found in adult populations, characterized by different rates of progression (see Figure 9-18) and different responses to therapy.[12]

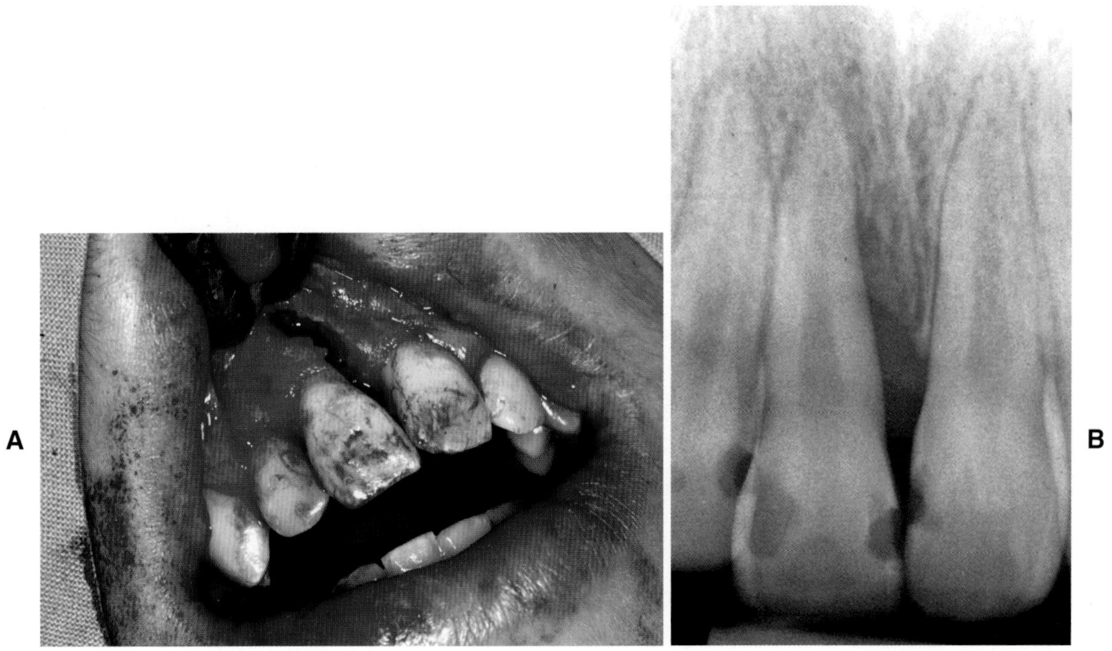

Figure 9-20 **A,** Clinical photo, and **B,** intraoral radiograph, showing dramatic bone destruction in adolescent with localized aggressive periodontitis.

Studies in which untreated populations were examined over long intervals indicate disease progression at mean rates ranging from 0.05 to 0.3 mm of attachment loss per year (i.e., the *gradual model*).[25] When populations are examined over short intervals, individual sites demonstrated short phases of attachment destruction interposed by periods of no disease activity (i.e., the *burst model*).[74] It is unclear from recent studies whether the gradual or burst model of disease progression, or some other model, is correct.[12]

Microbiologic examinations of chronic periodontitis have been carried out in both cross-sectional and longitudinal studies; the latter have been conducted with and without treatment. These studies support the concept that chronic periodontitis is associated with specific bacterial agents. Microscopic examination of plaque from sites with chronic periodontitis has consistently revealed elevated proportions of spirochetes.[131,140] Cultivation of plaque microorganisms from sites of chronic periodontitis reveals high percentages of anaerobic (90%) and gram-negative (75%) bacterial species[227,228] (see Figure 9-19).

In chronic periodontitis the bacteria most often cultivated at high levels include *P. gingivalis, T. forsythia, P. intermedia, C. rectus, E. corrodens, F. nucleatum, A. actinomycetemcomitans, P. micros,* and *Treponema* and *Eubacterium* species.* When periodontally active sites (i.e., with recent attachment loss) were examined in comparison with inactive sites (i.e., with no recent attachment loss), *C. rectus, P. gingivalis, P. intermedia, F. nucleatum,* and *T. forsythia* were found to be elevated in the active sites.[56] Furthermore, detectable levels of *P. gingivalis, P. intermedia, T. forsythia, C. rectus,* and *A. actinomycetemcomitans* are associated with disease progression, and their elimination by therapy is associated with an improved clinical response.[39,56,83,230,262] Both *P. gingivalis* and *A. actinomycetemcomitans* are known to invade host tissue cells, which may be significant in aggressive forms of adult periodontitis. [36,40,210]

Recent studies have documented an association between chronic periodontitis and viral microorganisms of the herpesvirus group, most notably Epstein-Barr virus-1 (EBV-1) and human cytomegalovirus (HCMV).[43] Further, the presence of subgingival EBV-1 and HCMV are associated with high levels of putative bacterial pathogens, including *P. gingivalis, T. forsythia, P. intermedia,* and *T. denticola.* These data support the hypothesis that viral infection may contribute to periodontal pathogenesis, but the potential role of viral agents remains to be determined.

Microbial Shift During Disease

Comparing the microbiota in health, gingivitis, and periodontitis, the following microbial shifts can be identified:

- From gram positive to gram negative.
- From cocci to rods (and at a later stage to spirochetes).
- From nonmotile to motile organisms.
- From facultative anaerobes to obligate anaerobes.
- From fermenting to proteolytic species.

Localized Aggressive Periodontitis

Several forms of periodontitis are characterized by rapid and severe attachment loss occurring in individuals during or before puberty. Localized aggressive periodontitis (previously referred to as "localized juvenile periodontitis")

*References 116, 118, 136, 159, 228, 232, 233, 244.

develops around the time of puberty, is observed in females more often than in males, and typically affects the permanent first molars and incisors (Figure 9-20). This condition is almost uniformly seen in individuals who demonstrate some systemic defect in immune regulation, and affected individuals often demonstrate defective neutrophil function. Without treatment, the local form often extends to a more generalized form with severe attachment loss around many teeth. The first symptoms of localized aggressive periodontitis are already detectable in the deciduous dentition, especially by periodontal destruction around the canines and second molars.[225]

The microbiota associated with localized aggressive periodontitis is predominantly composed of gram-negative, capnophilic, and anaerobic rods.[164,165,228] Microbiologic studies indicate that almost all disease sites harbor *A. actinomycetemcomitans,* which may compose as much as 90% of the total cultivable microbiota.[115,157] Other organisms found in significant levels include *P. gingivalis, E. corrodens, C. rectus, F. nucleatum, B. capillus, Eubacterium brachy, Capnocytophaga* species, and spirochetes.[115,151,157,160] Herpesviruses, including EBV-1 and HCMV, also have been associated with localized aggressive periodontitis.[43,151,249]

A. actinomycetemcomitans is generally accepted as the primary etiologic agent in most, but not all, cases of localized aggressive periodontitis.[113,233] Studies of therapy indicate that mechanical debridement in combination with systemic antibiotic treatment is necessary to control the levels of *A. actinomycetemcomitans* in this disease.[115,198,199] The failure of mechanical therapy alone may relate to the ability of this organism to invade host tissues.[36,40,210]

Necrotizing Periodontal Diseases

Necrotizing periodontal diseases present as an acute inflammation of the gingival and periodontal tissues characterized by necrosis of the marginal gingival tissue and interdental papillae (Figure 9-21). Clinically, these conditions often are associated with stress or human immunodeficiency virus (HIV) infection. Necrotizing diseases may be accompanied by malodor, pain, and possibly systemic symptoms, including lymphadenopathy, fever, and malaise. Microbiologic studies indicate that high levels of *P. intermedia,* and especially of spirochetes, are found in necrotizing ulcerative gingivitis lesions. Spirochetes are found to penetrate necrotic tissue and apparently unaffected connective tissue.[132,133]

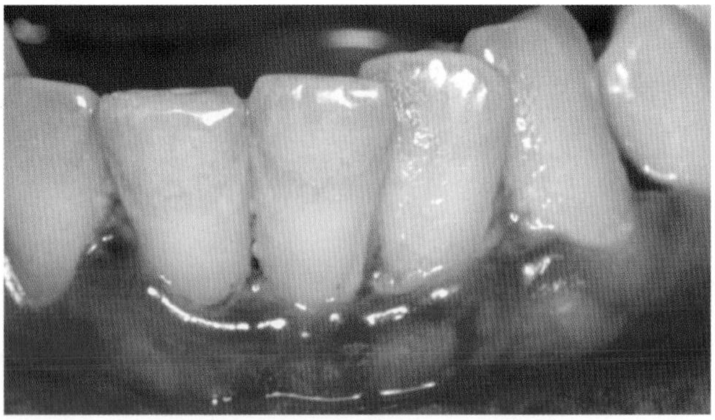

Figure 9-21 Clinical photo of lower front teeth with necrotizing gingivitis.

Abscesses of the Periodontium

Periodontal abscesses are acute lesions that may result in very rapid destruction of the periodontal tissues (Figure 9-22). They often occur in patients with untreated periodontitis but also may be found in patients during maintenance or after scaling and root planing of deep pockets. Periodontal abscesses also may occur in the absence of periodontitis; for example, associated with impaction of a foreign object (e.g., popcorn kernel, dental floss) or with endodontic problems.[88] Typical clinical symptoms of periodontal abscesses include pain, swelling, suppuration, bleeding on probing, and mobility of the involved tooth. Signs of systemic involvement may be present, including cervical lymphadenopathy and an elevated white blood cell count.[89] Investigations reveal that bacteria recognized as periodontal pathogens are typically found in significant numbers in periodontal abscesses. These microorganisms include *F. nucleatum, P. intermedia, P. gingivalis, P. micros,* and *T. forsythia.*[85,89,164]

Periodontitis as Manifestation of Systemic Disease

Previous classification schemes delineated "prepubertal periodontitis" as a rare form of periodontitis found to affect the primary dentition. This group has now been reclassified under the heading of *periodontitis as a manifestation of systemic disease* because most children with severe periodontal destruction also demonstrate profound immunologic abnormalities. The underlying immune deficiency may vary and includes neutrophil defects and leukocyte adhesion defects.[54,99] Recent studies have demonstrated that some cases of severe periodontal destruction are associated with a mutation in the cathepsin C gene in affected children (see Chapter 11). Studies of patients with "prepubertal periodontitis" indicate that subgingival bacteria associated with other forms of periodontal disease also are found in these patients.[159,171] This is consistent with the concept that the occurrence of severe destruction at an early age is a reflection of increased host susceptibility, in this case resulting from systemic disease. Identification of severe periodontal destruction in a child may be one of the first signs of systemic disease.

Microbial Specificity in Periodontitis

Table 9-2 provides an overview of the detection frequency for most key pathogens in different forms of periodontal infections. It is immediately obvious that there is no "black-or-white" situation; most pathogens *might* be present, but do not necessarily *have* to be present, for specific forms of periodontitis. This overview also illustrates that one cannot use the microbial composition to differentiate between different forms of periodontal infections.

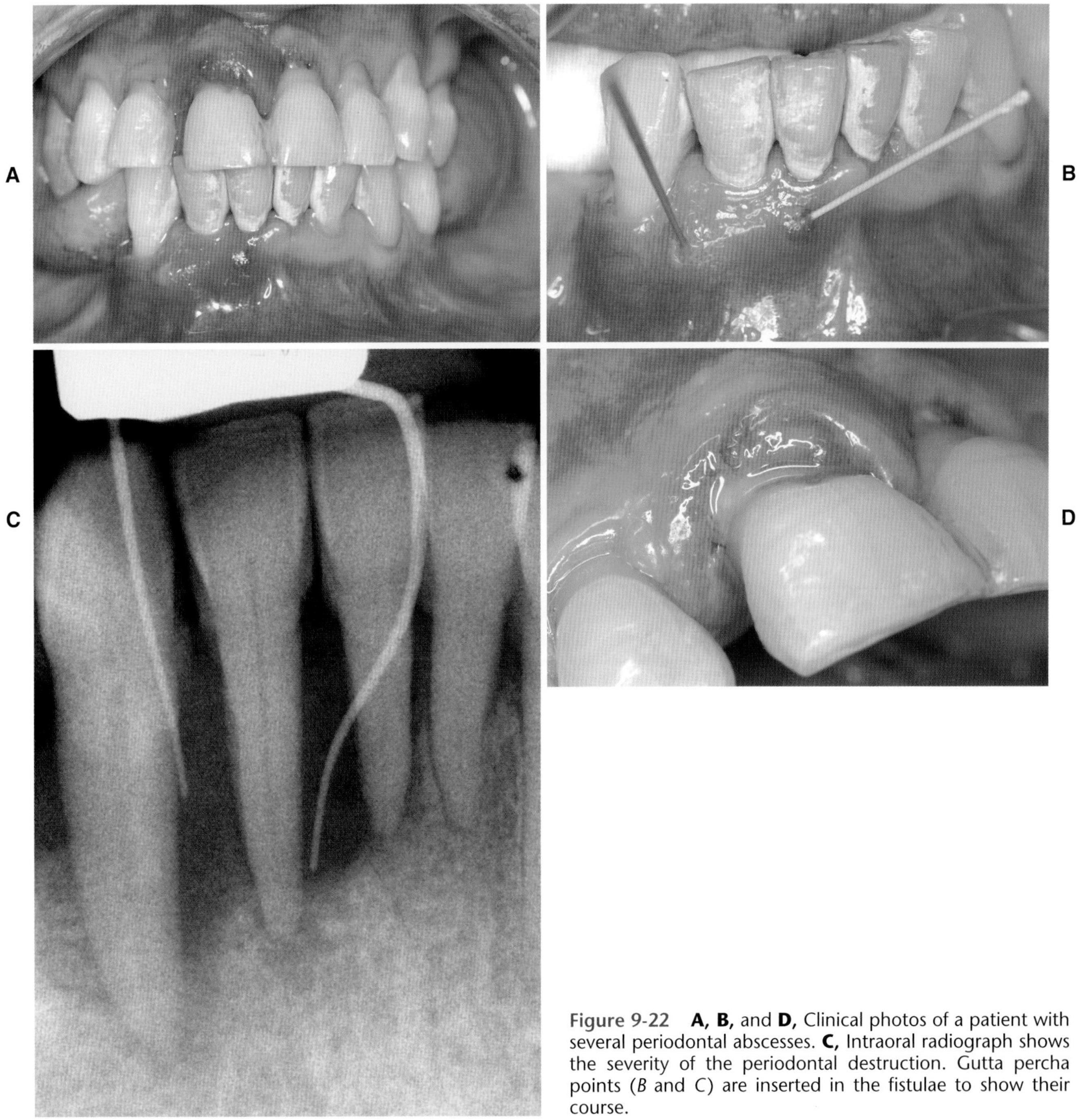

Figure 9-22 **A, B,** and **D,** Clinical photos of a patient with several periodontal abscesses. **C,** Intraoral radiograph shows the severity of the periodontal destruction. Gutta percha points (*B* and *C*) are inserted in the fistulae to show their course.

Table 9-3 shows the prevalence of key pathogens, further highlighting the complexity of the microbiology of periodontitis. Most periopathogens can also be detected in healthy subjects with frequencies ranging from 10% to 85%. This automatically reduces the specificity of microbiologic testing in periodontology.

Periimplantitis

The term *periimplantitis* refers to an "inflammatory process" affecting the tissues around an already-osseointegrated implant and resulting in loss of supporting bone[12] (see Chapter 81). In animal studies and in cross-sectional and longitudinal observations in humans, this inflammatory process has been associated with a microbiota comparable to that of periodontitis (high proportion of anaerobic gram-negative rods, motile organisms, and spirochetes), but this association does not necessarily prove a causal relationship (for review, see Quirynen et al.[183]). Healthy periimplant pockets are characterized by high proportions of coccoid cells, a low ratio anaerobic/aerobic species, a low number of gram-anaerobic species, and low detection frequencies for periodontal pathogens.[3,19,121,170]

Implants with periimplantitis reveal a complex microbiota encompassing conventional periodontal pathogens.

TABLE 9-2

Microbial Species Associated with Various Clinical Forms of Periodontitis

	FORMS OF PERIODONTITIS			
Species	**Adult**	**Refractory**	**Localized Aggressive**	**Early onset**
Actinobacillus actinomycetemcomitans	++	++	+++	++
Porphyromonas gingivalis	+++	++	O	+++
Prevotella intermedia/nigrescens	+++	+++	++	+++
Tannerella forsythia	+++	++	O	++
Fusobacterium species	+++	++	+	++
Peptostreptococcus micros	+++	++	O	++
Eubacterium species	++	+	NE	+
Campylobacter rectus	++	+	+	++
Treponema species	+++	++	++	+++
Enteric rods and pseudomonads	O	+	NE	NE
Candida species	NE	0	NE	NE

Modified from Haffajee AD, Socransky SS: *Periodontol 2000* 5:78, 1994.

NE, Not elevated in comparison to health; *O,* occasionally isolated; +, less than 10% of patients positive; ++, less than 50% of patients positive; +++, more than 50% of patients positive.

TABLE 9-3

Prevalence of Key-Pathogens in Healthy Subjects and Patients with Periodontitis

	PREVALENCE		SIGNIFICANCE OF DIFFERENCE	
Species	**Health**	**Periodontitis**	***p* value**	**Odds ratio***
Actinobacillus actinomycetemcomitans	12.8	31.0	0.002	3.1
Porphyromonas gingivalis	10.6	59.5	<0.001	12.3
Prevotella intermedia/nigrescens	69.1	87.9	0.001	3.3
Tannerella forsythia	47.9	90.5	<0.001	10.4
Fusobacterium nucleatum	85.1	95.7	0.014	3.9
Peptostreptococcus micros	67	94	<0.001	7.7
Campylobacter rectus	13.8	20.7	ns	1.6

Modified from van Winkelhoff AJ, Loos BG, van der Reijden WA, et al: *J Clin Periodontol* 29:1023, 2002.

*Ratio of the probability of developing the disease to the probability of the disease not occurring; thus "3" means three times times more chance that the disease will develop.

ns, Not significant.

Species such as *A. actinomycetemcomitans, P. gingivalis, T. forsythia, P. micros, C. rectus, Fusobacterium,* and *Capnocytophaga* are often isolated from failing sites but can also be detected around healthy periimplant sites. Other species, such as *Pseudomonas aeruginosa,* enterobacteriaceae, *Candida albicans,* and staphylococci, are also frequently detected around implants.[7] These organisms are uncommon in the subgingival area but have been associated with refractory periodontitis.[231] High proportions of *Staphylococcus aureus* and *S. epidermidis* on oral implants have also been reported.[195] The relative resistance of these organisms to common antibiotics suggests that their presence might represent an opportunistic colonization secondary to systemic antibiotic therapy.[230]

Some large-scale clinical follow-up studies seem to indicate that implant failures cluster within patients, with increased odd ratios for a second implant failure in patients who already lost one implant.[253,263] These observations indicate that "within-patient" factors, or systemic factors, are important in the characterization of implant losses.

KEY CHARACTERISTICS OF SPECIFIC PERIOPATHOGENS

Actinobacillus actinomycetemcomitans

A. actinomycetemcomitans is a small, short (0.4-1 μm), straight or curved rod with rounded ends. It is nonmotile and gram negative.

Forms: From this species, multiple biotypes and five serotypes (*a* to *e*) have been described based on differences

A

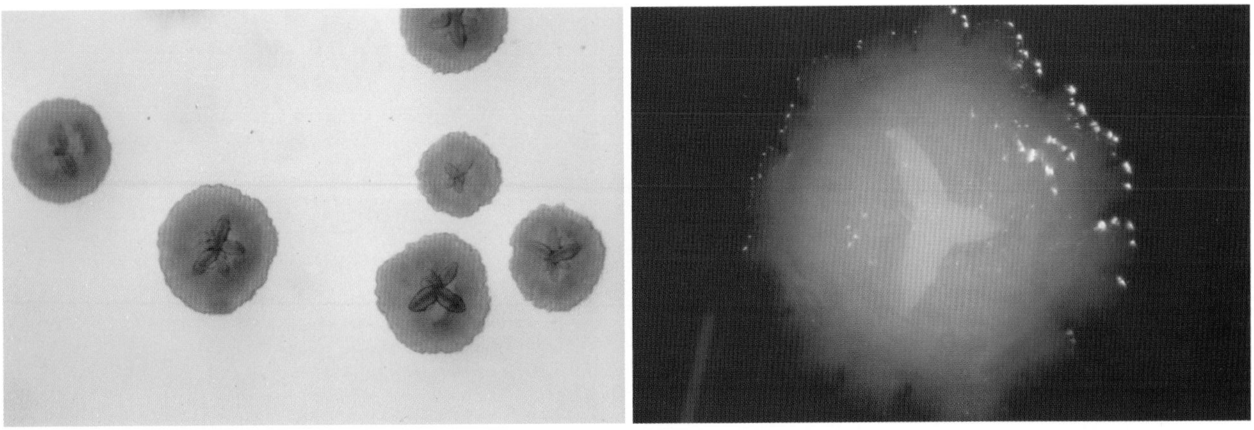

B

Figure 9-23 Colony morphology of an *Actinobacillus actinomycetemcomitans* strain on **A,** a specific medium, and **B,** a nonspecific medium. The internal star is easily seen.

in polysaccharide composition. Recently, differences between strains from different geographic areas have been noted. Strains from patients in Africa, for example, seem to have an increased leukotoxin production.

Culture conditions and identification: It grows as a white, translucent, smooth, nonhemolytic colony on blood agar; because of its low density, *A. actinomycetemcomitans* is preferably identified on a specific growth medium (with vancomycin and bacitracin as antibiotics to suppress other species) under 5% to 10% carbon dioxide, where it appears as a white, translucent colony with a star-shaped internal structure (Figure 9-23).

Special pathogenic characteristics: It possesses a number of virulence factors, including lipopolysaccharide (endotoxin), a leukotoxin (forms pores in neutrophil granulocytes, monocytes, and some lymphocytes, which consequently die because of osmotic pressure), collagenase (destruction of connective tissue), and a protease (able to cleave IgG). The leukotoxin especially plays a significant role in the pathogenicity of *A. actinomycetemcomitans.*

Tannerella forsythia

T. forsythia is a nonmotile, spindle-shaped, highly pleomorphic rod and a gram-negative obligate anaerobe.

Culture conditions and identification: It grows slowly (14 days for minute colonies) only under anaerobic conditions and needs several growth factors (e.g., *N*-acetylmuramic acid) from other species (e.g., *F. nucleatum*).

Pathogenicity: This species produces several proteolytic enzymes that are able to destroy immunoglobulins and factors of the complement system. *T. forsythia* also induces apoptotic cell death.

Porphyromonas gingivalis

P. gingivalis is a nonmotile, pleomorphic (coccal to short) rod and gram-negative obligate anaerobe.

Forms: From this species, different genotypes have been described, based on the capsule type.

Culture conditions and identification: It grows anaerobically (anaerobic chamber or special jars), with dark

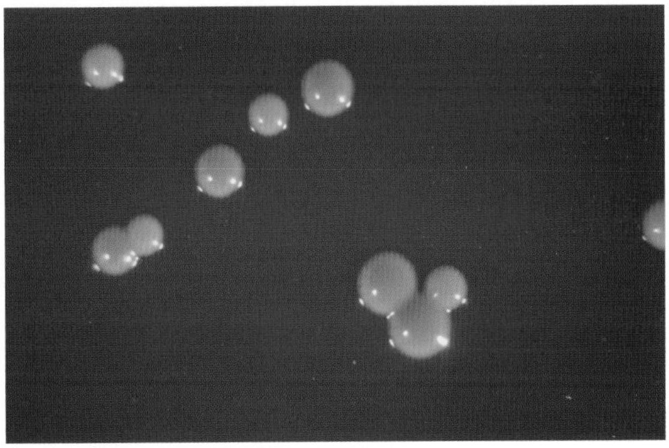

Figure 9-24 Colony morphology of a pure culture of *Porphyromonas gingivalis* strain on a nonspecific blood-agar Petri dish.

pigmentation (brown, dark green, or black) on blood agar because of a metabolic end product from blood (hemin). *P. gingivalis* has a strong proteolytic activity (degradation of proteins) (Figure 9-24).

Special pathogenic characteristics: It is an aggressive periodontal pathogen. Its fimbriae mediate adhesion, and its capsule defends against phagocytosis. This species produces a series of virulence factors, including many proteases (e.g., for the destruction of immunoglobulins, complement factors, and heme-sequestering proteins; degradation of host cell collagenase inhibitors), a hemolysin, and a collagenase. This species can inhibit migration of polymorphonuclear leukocytes (PMNs) across an epithelial barrier and affects the production or degradation of cytokines by mammalian cells.[143,212] *P. gingivalis* also has the capacity to invade soft tissues.

Prevotella intermedia and *Prevotella nigrescens*

Species from the *Prevotella* group are short, round-ended, nonmotile, gram-negative rods.

Forms: In this group, *P. intermedia* and *P. nigrescens* are the most pathogenic of the several species classified.

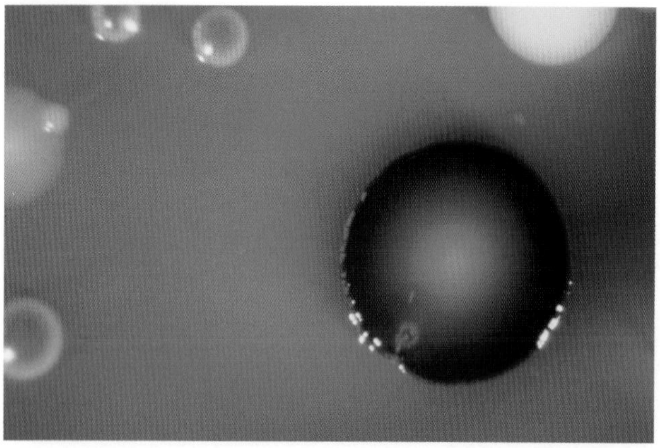

Figure 9-25 Colony morphology of a *Prevotella intermedia* strain (large black colony) on a nonspecific blood-agar Petri dish. The green colonies are *Porphyromonas gingivalis.*

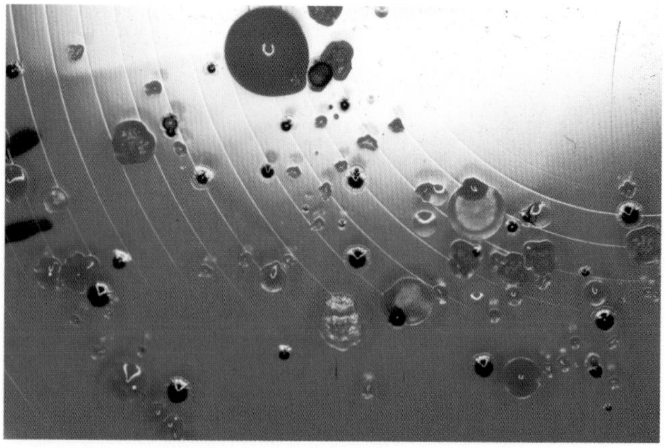

Figure 9-26 Colony morphology of a *Campylobacter rectus* strain (gray-black colonies) on a specific medium.

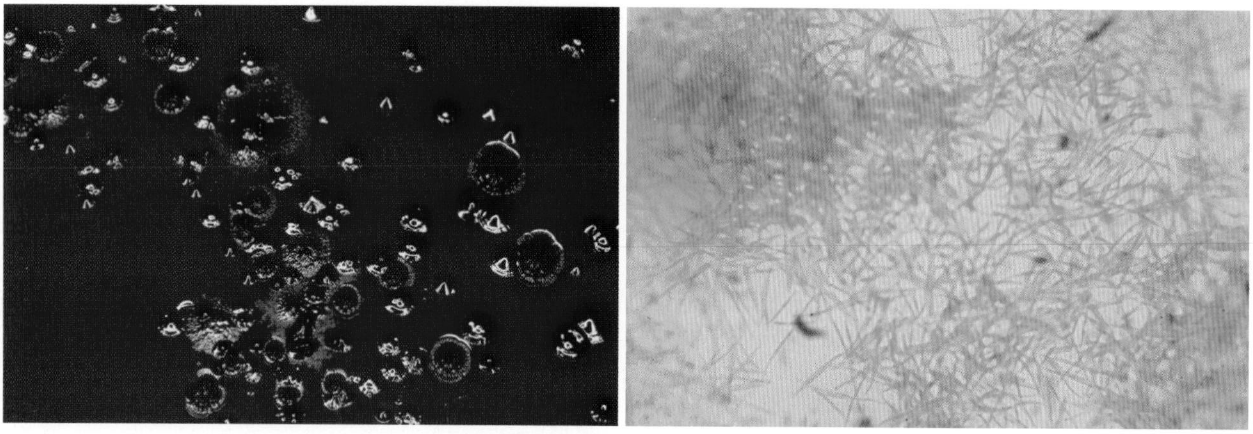

Figure 9-27 Colony morphology of a *Fusobacterium nucleatum* strain on **A,** a specific medium (purple colonies), and **B,** with Gram stain.

Culture conditions and identification: These species grow anaerobically, with dark pigmentation (brown-black colonies) on blood agar. (Figure 9-25).

Special pathogenic characteristics: The *Prevotella* species are less virulent and less proteolytic than *P. gingivalis.*

Campylobacter rectus

C. rectus is one of the rare motile organisms involved in periodontitis. It is a gram-negative, short rod, curved (vibrio) or helical. The motility results from the polar flagellum.

Culture conditions and identification: It grows anaerobically (anaerobic chamber or special jars), with dark pigmentation when sulfide is added to the medium, which is transformed to FeS, giving a gray stain (Figure 9-26).

Special pathogenic characteristics: This species, as with *A. actinomycetemcomitans,* produces a leukotoxin. *C. rectus* is less virulent and less proteolytic than *P. gingivalis.*

Fusobacterium nucleatum

F. nucleatum is a gram-negative, cigar-shaped bacillus with pointed ends.

Forms: In this group, several subspecies (ss) are classified, including *F. nucleatum* ss *nucleatum, F. nucleatum* ss *polymorphum, F. nucleatum* ss *vincentii,* and *F. periodonticum.*

Culture conditions and identification: It grows anaerobically on blood agar and can easily be identified on a specific medium (Figure 9-27).

Special pathogenic characteristics: This organism can induce apoptotic cell death in mononuclear and polymorphonuclear cells and can trigger the release of cytokines, elastase, and oxygen radicals from leukocytes. Because fusobacteria coaggregate with most oral microorganisms, they are believed to be important bridging organisms between the primary (early) and secondary (late) colonizers during colonization.

Peptostreptococcus micros

P. micros is one of the rare cocci in periodontitis. This species is gram positive and grows obligate anaerobically.

Eubacterium species

Eubacterium is a gram-positive, obligate anaerobic, small, pleomorphic rod.

Forms: Several species of *Eubacterium* are classified, including: *E. nodatum, E. brachy,* and *E. timidum.*

Culture conditions and identification: These species grow anaerobically, but with difficulty on standard blood agar.

Spirochetes

Spirochetes represent a diverse group of spiral, motile organisms. They are helical rods 5 to 15 μm long with a diameter of 0.5 μm. They have three to eight irregular spirals. Their cell wall is gram negative, but they stain poorly.

Forms: Classified species of spirochetes include *Treponema denticola, Treponema vincentii, Treponema socranskii* (often associated with periodontitis), and *Treponema pallidum* (associated with secondary syphilis).

Culture conditions and identification: Oral spirochetes are extremely difficult to grow and need strict anaerobic conditions and a specific medium.

Special pathogenic characteristics: The ability of these species to travel trough viscous environments enables them to migrate within the gingival crevicular fluid and to penetrate both the epithelium and the connective tissue. Some spirochetes have the capacity to degrade collagen and even dentin. *T. denticola* produces proteolytic enzymes that can destroy immunoglobulins (IgA, IgM, IgG) or complement factors.

FUTURE ADVANCES IN PERIODONTAL MICROBIOLOGY

Scientific progress at the end of the twentieth century, particularly in the field of molecular biology, has led to advances in periodontal microbiology. DNA-based methodology for the identification and detection of specific bacteria and viruses offers remarkable advantages in time and cost savings compared with culturing techniques. The number of samples that can be examined and the number of microorganisms enumerated have increased dramatically. Perhaps even more relevant is the present ability to detect microorganisms that cannot be cultivated thus far, which has underscored the limitations of our knowledge of this complex ecologic niche. Becoming aware that the host response is also of major significance will further improve our understanding of the severity and therapy of periodontal infections. Finally, the recognition of the beneficial activity of several groups of commensal species, such as probiotics, might open new strategies for periodontal therapy.

REFERENCES

1. Absolom DR, Zingg W, Neumann AW: Protein adsorption to polymer particles: role of surface properties, *J Biomed Mater Res* 21:161, 1987.
2. Adamson M, Carlsson J: Lactoperoxidase and thiocyanate protect bacteria from hydrogen peroxide, *Infect Immun* 35:20, 1982.
3. Adell R, Lekholm U, Rockler B, et al: Marginal tissue reactions at osseointegrated titanium fixtures (I): a 3-year longitudinal prospective study, *Int J Oral Maxillofac Surg* 15:39, 1986.
4. Adriaens PA, De Boever JA, Loesche WJ: Bacterial invasion in root cementum and radicular dentin of periodontally diseased teeth in humans: a reservoir of periodontopathic bacteria, *J Periodontol* 59:222, 1988.
5. Ainamo J, Asikainen S, Ainamo A, et al: Plaque growth while chewing sorbitol and xylitol simultaneously with sucrose flavored gum, *J Clin Periodontol* 6:397, 1979.
6. Albandar JM, Rams TE: Global epidemiology of periodontal diseases: an overview, *Periodontol 2000* 29:7, 2002.
7. Alcoforado GA, Slots J: *Actinobacillus actinomycetemcomitans* and black-pigmented bacteroides in advanced periodontitis in man: theoretical and practical considerations, *Rev Port Estomatol Cir Maxilofac* 31:89, 1990.
8. Allison DG, Gilbert P: Modification by surface association of antimicrobial susceptibility of bacterial populations, *J Ind Microbiol* 15:311, 1995.
9. American Academy of Periodontology: *Proceedings of the 1996 World Workshop in Periodontics,* 1996, p 926.
10. Apatzidou DA, Kinane DF: Quadrant root planing versus same-day full-mouth root planing, *J Clin Periodontol* 31:152, 2004.
11. Apse P, Ellen RP, Overall CM, et al: Microbiota and crevicular fluid collagenase activity in the osseointegrated dental implant sulcus: a comparison of sites in edentulous and partially edentulous patients, *J Periodontal Res* 24:96, 1989.
12. Armitage GC: Development of a classification system for periodontal diseases and conditions, *Ann Periodontol* 4:1, 1999.
13. Arnim SS: The use of disclosing agents for measuring tooth cleanliness, *J Periodontol* 34:217, 1963.
14. Ashby MJ, Neale JE, Knott SJ, et al: Effect of antibiotics on non-growing planktonic cells and biofilms of *Escherichia coli, J Antimicrob Chemother* 33:443, 1994.
15. Baier RE, Glantz PO, Characterization of oral in vivo films formed on different types of solid surfaces, *Acta Odontol Scand* 36:289, 1978.
16. Bollen CM, Mongardini C, Papaioannou W, et al: The effect of a one-stage full-mouth disinfection on different intraoral niches: clinical and microbiological observations, *J Clin Periodontol* 25:56, 1998.
17. Bollen CM, Papaioanno W, van Eldere J, et al: The influence of abutment surface roughness on plaque accumulation and peri-implant mucositis, *Clin Oral Implants Res* 7:201, 1996.
18. Bowen WH: Nature of plaque, *Oral Sci Rev* 9:3, 1976.
19. Bower RC, Radny NR, Wall CD, et al: Clinical and microscopic findings in edentulous patients 3 years after incorporation of osseointegrated implant-supported bridgework, *J Clin Periodontol* 16:580, 1989.
20. Bradshaw DJ, Marsh PD, Watson GK, et al: Role of *Fusobacterium nucleatum* and coaggregation in anaerobe survival in planktonic and biofilm oral microbial communities during aeration, *Infect Immun* 66:4729, 1998.
21. Bramanti TE, Holt SC: Roles of porphyrins and host iron transport proteins in regulation of growth of *Porphyromonas gingivalis* W50, *J Bacteriol* 173:7330, 1991.
22. Brecx M, Theilade J, Attstrom R: An ultrastructural quantitative study of the significance of microbial multiplication during early dental plaque growth, *J Periodontal Res* 18:177, 1983.
23. Brook I, Foote PA, Slots J: Immune response to *Fusobacterium nucleatum, Prevotella intermedia* and other anaerobes in children with acute tonsillitis, *J Antimicrob Chemother* 39:763, 1997.
24. Brooun A, Liu S, Lewis K: A dose-response study of antibiotic resistance in *Pseudomonas aeruginosa* biofilms, *Antimicrob Agents Chemother* 44:640, 2000.
25. Brown LJ, Löe H: Prevalence, extent, severity and progression of periodontal disease, *Periodontol 2000* 2:57, 1993.

26. Brown MR, Williams P: The influence of environment on envelope properties affecting survival of bacteria in infections, *Annu Rev Microbiol* 39:527, 1985;
27. Brown MR, Collier PJ, Gilbert P: Influence of growth rate on susceptibility to antimicrobial agents: modification of the cell envelope and batch and continuous culture studies, *Antimicrob Agents Chemother* 34:1623, 1990.
28. Brunette DM, Chehroudi B, Gould TRL: Electron microscopic observations on the effects of surface topography on the behaviour of cells attached to percutaneous and subcutaneous implants. In Laney WR, Tonato M, editors: *Tissue integration in oral, orthopedic & maxillofacial reconstruction,* Chicago, 1982, Quintessence Books, p 21.
29. Busscher HJ, Bos R, van der Mei HC: Initial microbial adhesion is a determinant for the strength of biofilm adhesion, *FEMS Microbiol Lett* 128:229, 1995.
30. Busscher HJ, Retief DH, Arends J: Relationship between surface-free energies of dental resins and bond strengths to etched enamel, *Dent Mater* 3:60, 1987.
31. Busscher HJ, Sjollema J, van der Mei HC: Relative importance of surface free energy as a measure of hydrophobicity in bacterial adhesion to solid surfaces. In Doyle RJ, Rosenberg M, editors: *Microbial cell surface hydrophobicity,* Washington, DC, 1990, American Society for Microbiology, p 335.
32. Carlsson J: Symbiosis between host and microorganisms in the oral cavity, *Scand J Infect Dis Suppl* 24:74, 1980.
33. Carlsson J: Microbiology of plaque associated periodontal disease. In Lindhe J, editor: *Textbook of clinical periodontology,* Munksgaard, 1983; Munksgaard International Publishers.
34. Carlsson J, Soderholm G, Almfeldt I: Prevalence of *Streptococcus sanguis* and *Streptococcus mutans* in the mouth of persons wearing full-dentures, *Arch Oral Biol* 14:243, 1969.
35. Carlsson J, Grahnen H, Jonsson G, et al: Establishment of *Streptococcus sanguis* in the mouths of infants, *Arch Oral Biol* 15:1143, 1970.
36. Carranza FA Jr, Saglie R, Newman MG, et al: Scanning and transmission electron microscopic study of tissue-invading microorganisms in localized juvenile periodontitis, *J Periodontol* 54:598, 1983.
37. Caufield PW, Gibbons RJ: Suppression of *Streptococcus mutans* in the mouths of humans by a dental prophylaxis and topically-applied iodine, *J Dent Res* 58:1317, 1979.
38. Chen C, Slots J: Clonal analysis of *Porphyromonas gingivalis* by the arbitrarily primed polymerase chain reaction, *Oral Microbiol Immunol* 9:99, 1994.
39. Christersson LA, Zambon JJ, Genco RJ: Dental bacterial plaques: nature and role in periodontal disease, *J Clin Periodontol* 18:441, 1991.
40. Christersson LA, Albini B, Zambon JJ, et al: Tissue localization of *Actinobacillus actinomycetemcomitans* in human periodontitis. I. Light, immunofluorescence and electron microscopic studies, *J Periodontol* 58:529, 1987.
41. Christersson LA, Slots J, Zambon JJ, et al: Transmission and colonization of *Actinobacillus actinomycetemcomitans* in localized juvenile periodontitis patients, *J Periodontol* 56:127, 1985.
42. Cisar JO: Coaggregation reactions between oral bacteria: studies of specific cell-to-cell adherence mediated by microbial lectins. In Genco RJ, Mergenhagen S, editors: *Host parasite interactions in periodontal diseases,* Washington, DC, 1982, American Society for Microbiology, p 121.
43. Contreras A, Slots J: Herpesviruses in human periodontal disease, *J Periodontal Res* 35:3, 2000.
44. Costerton JW, Stewart PS, Greenberg EP: Bacterial biofilms: a common cause of persistent infections, *Science* 284:1318, 1999.
45. Costerton JW, Lewandowski Z, Caldwell DE, et al: Microbial biofilms, *Annu Rev Microbiol* 49:711, 1995.
46. Cugini MA, Haffajee AD, Smith C, et al: The effect of scaling and root planing on the clinical and microbiological parameters of periodontal diseases: 12-month results, *J Clin Periodontol* 27:30, 2000.
47. Danino J, Joachims HZ, Barak M: Predictive value of an adherence test for acute otitis media, *Otolaryngol Head Neck Surg* 118:400, 1998.
48. Danser MM, Timmerman MF, van Winkelhoff AJ, et al: The effect of periodontal treatment on periodontal bacteria on the oral mucous membranes, *J Periodontol* 67:478, 1996.
49. Danser MM, van Winkelhoff AJ, de Graaff J, et al: Short-term effect of full-mouth extraction on periodontal pathogens colonizing the oral mucous membranes, *J Clin Periodontol* 21:484, 1994.
50. Darveau RP, Tanner A, Page RC: The microbial challenge in periodontitis, *Periodontol 2000* 14:12, 1997.
51. De Soete M, De Keyser C, Pauwels M, et al: Outgrowth of cariogenic bacteria after initial periodontal therapy, *J Dent Res* 84:48, 2005.
52. Diaz PI, Zilm PS, Rogers AH: The response to oxidative stress of *Fusobacterium nucleatum* grown in continuous culture, *FEMS Microbiol Lett* 187:31, 2000.
53. Dibart S, Skobe Z, Snapp KR, et al: Identification of bacterial species on or in crevicular epithelial cells from healthy and periodontally diseased patients using DNA-DNA hybridization, *Oral Microbiol Immunol* 13:30, 1998.
54. Dougherty N, Gataletto MA: Oral sequelae of chronic neutrophil defects: case report of a child with glycogen storage disease type 1b, *Pediatr Dent* 17:224, 1995.
55. Doyle RJ, Rosenberg M, Drake D: Hydrophobicity of oral bacteria. In Doyle RJ, Rosenberg M, editors: *Microbial cell surface hydrophobicity,* Washington, DC, 1990, American Society for Microbiology.
56. Dzink JL, Socransky SS, Haffajee AD: The predominant cultivable microbiota of active and inactive lesions of destructive periodontal diseases, *J Clin Periodontol* 15:316, 1988.
57. Dzink JL, Gibbons RJ, Childs WC III, et al: The predominant cultivable microbiota of crevicular epithelial cells, *Oral Microbiol Immunol* 4:1, 1989.
58. Dzink JL, Tanner AC, Haffajee AD, et al: Gram negative species associated with active destructive periodontal lesions, *J Clin Periodontol* 12:648, 1985.
59. Edman DC, Keene HJ, Shklair IL, et al: Dental floss for implantation and sampling of Streptococcus mutans from approximal surfaces of human teeth, *Arch Oral Biol* 20:145, 1975.
60. Evaldson G, Heimdahl A, Kager L, et al: The normal human anaerobic microflora, *Scand J Infect Dis Suppl* 35:9, 1982.
61. Fachon-Kalweit S, Elder BL, Fives-Taylor P: Antibodies that bind to fimbriae block adhesion of *Streptococcus sanguis* to saliva-coated hydroxyapatite, *Infect Immun* 48:617, 1985.
62. Fine DH, Wilton JM, Caravana C: In vitro sorption of albumin, immunoglobulin G, and lysozyme to enamel and cementum from human teeth, *Infect Immun* 44:332, 1984.
63. Fives-Taylor PM, Thompson DW: Surface properties of *Streptococcus sanguis* FW213 mutants nonadherent to saliva-coated hydroxyapatite, *Infect Immun* 47:752, 1985.
64. Fletcher M: The physiological activity of bacteria attached to solid surfaces, *Adv Microb Physiol* 32:53, 1991.
65. Fransson C, Berglundh T, Lindhe J: The effect of age on the development of gingivitis: clinical, microbiological and histological findings, *J Clin Periodontol* 23:379, 1996.
66. Furuichi Y, Lindhe J, Ramberg P, et al: Patterns of de novo plaque formation in the human dentition, *J Clin Periodontol* 19:423, 1992.

67. Genco RJ, Löe H: The role of systemic conditions and disorders in periodontal disease, *Periodontol 2000* 2:98, 1993.
68. Gibbons RJ, Hay DI: Human salivary acidic proline-rich proteins and statherin promote the attachment of *Actinomyces viscosus* LY7 to apatitic surfaces, *Infect Immun* 56:439, 1988.
69. Gibbons RJ, Hay DI, Cisar JO, et al: Adsorbed salivary proline-rich protein 1 and statherin: receptors for type 1 fimbriae of *Actinomyces viscosus* T14V-J1 on apatitic surfaces, *Infect Immun* 56:2990, 1988.
70. Gibson GR, Roberfroid MB: Dietary modulation of the human colonic microbiota: introducing the concept of prebiotics, *J Nutr* 125:1401, 1995.
71. Gilbert P, Allison DG: Biofilms and their resistance towards antimicrobial agents. In Newman HN, Wilson M, editors: *Dental plaque revisited,* New York, 1999, Cambridge University Press, p 125.
72. Giuliana G, Pizzo G, Milici ME, et al: In vitro antifungal properties of mouthrinses containing antimicrobial agents, *J Periodontol* 68:729, 1997.
73. Goodson JM, Tanner A, McArdle S, et al: Multicenter evaluation of tetracycline fiber therapy. III. Microbiological response, *J Periodontal Res* 26:440, 1991.
74. Goodson JM, Tanner AC, Haffajee AD, et al: Patterns of progression and regression of advanced destructive periodontal disease, *J Clin Periodontol* 9:472, 1982.
75. Grenier D, Nutritional interactions between two suspected periodontopathogens, *Treponema denticola* and *Porphyromonas gingivalis, Infect Immun* 60:5298, 1992.
76. Grenier D, Mayrand D: [Studies of mixed anaerobic infections involving *Bacteroides gingivalis*], *Can J Microbiol* 29:612, 1983.
77. Griffen AL, Leys EJ, Fuerst PA: Strain identification of *Actinobacillus actinomycetemcomitans* using the polymerase chain reaction, *Oral Microbiol Immunol* 7:240, 1992.
78. Grossi SG, Genco RJ: Periodontal disease and diabetes mellitus: a two-way relationship, *Ann Periodontol* 3:51, 1998.
79. Grossi SG, Genco RJ, Machtei EE, et al: Assessment of risk for periodontal disease. II. Risk indicators for alveolar bone loss, *J Periodontol* 66:23, 1995.
80. Grossi SG, Zambon JJ, Ho AW, et al: Assessment of risk for periodontal disease. I. Risk indicators for attachment loss, *J Periodontol* 65:260, 1994.
81. Guy SC, McQuade MJ, Scheidt MJ, et al: In vitro attachment of human gingival fibroblasts to endosseous implant materials, *J Periodontol* 64:542, 1993.
82. Haffajee AD, Socransky SS: Microbial etiological agents of destructive periodontal diseases, *Periodontol 2000* 5:78, 1994.
83. Haffajee AD, Cugini MA, Dibart S, et al: Clinical and microbiological features of subjects with adult periodontitis who responded poorly to scaling and root planing, *J Clin Periodontol* 24:767, 1997.
84. Haffajee AD, Cugini MA, Dibart S, et al: The effect of SRP on the clinical and microbiological parameters of periodontal diseases, *J Clin Periodontol* 24:324, 1997.
85. Hafstrom CA, Wikstrom MB, Renvert SN, et al: Effect of treatment on some periodontopathogens and their antibody levels in periodontal abscesses, *J Periodontol* 65:1022, 1994.
86. Harper DS, Robinson PJ: Correlation of histometric, microbial, and clinical indicators of periodontal disease status before and after root planing, *J Clin Periodontol* 14:190, 1987.
87. Helmerhorst EJ, Hodgson R, van 't Hof W, et al: The effects of histatin-derived basic antimicrobial peptides on oral biofilms, *J Dent Res* 78:1245, 1999.
88. Herrera D, Roldan S, Sanz M: The periodontal abscess: a review, *J Clin Periodontol* 27:377, 2000.
89. Herrera D, Roldan S, Gonzalez I, et al: The periodontal abscess. I. Clinical and microbiological findings, *J Clin Periodontol* 27:387, 2000.
90. Hillman JD, Socransky SS, Shivers M: The relationships between streptococcal species and periodontopathic bacteria in human dental plaque, *Arch Oral Biol* 30:791, 1985.
91. Ho CS: An understanding of the forces in the adhesion of micro-organisms to surfaces, *Process Biochemistry*, 1986, p 148.
92. Holm-Pedersen P, Agerbaek N, Theilade E: Experimental gingivitis in young and elderly individuals, *J Clin Periodontol* 2:14, 1975.
93. Hsu SD, Cisar JO, Sandberg AL, et al: Adhesive properties of viridans streptococcal species, *Microb Ecol Health Dis*, 1994, p 125.
94. Hultin M, Gustafsson A, Klinge B: Long-term evaluation of osseointegrated dental implants in the treatment of partly edentulous patients, *J Clin Periodontol* 27:128, 2000.
95. Hultin M, Gustafsson A, Hallstrom H, et al: Microbiological findings and host response in patients with peri-implantitis, *Clin Oral Implants Res* 13:349, 2002.
96. Hyyppä T, Paunio K: The plaque-inhibiting effects of copper amalgam, *J Clin Periodontol* 4:231, 1977.
97. Isogai E, Isogai H, Sawada H, et al: Bacterial adherence to gingival epithelial cells of rats with naturally occurring gingivitis, *J Periodontol* 57:225, 1986.
98. Jacobson SE, Crawford JJ, McFall WR Jr: Oral physiotherapy of the tongue and palate: relationship to plaque control, *J Am Dent Assoc* 87:134, 1973.
99. Kamma JJ, Lygidakis NA, Nakou M: Subgingival microflora and treatment in prepubertal periodontitis associated with chronic idiopathic neutropenia, *J Clin Periodontol* 25:759, 1998.
100. Kaufman J, DiRienzo JM: Isolation of a corncob (coaggregation) receptor polypeptide from *Fusobacterium nucleatum, Infect Immun* 57:331, 1989.
101. Kinane DF, Radvar M: The effect of smoking on mechanical and antimicrobial periodontal therapy, *J Periodontol* 68:467, 1997.
102. Kinder SA, Holt SC: Characterization of coaggregation between *Bacteroides gingivalis* T22 and *Fusobacterium nucleatum* T18, *Infect Immun* 57:3425, 1989.
103. Kohavi D, Greenberg RS, Raviv E, et al: Subgingival and supragingival microbial flora around healthy osseo-integrated implants in partially edentulous patients, *Int J Oral Maxillofac Implants*, 1994, p 673.
104. Kohler B, Krasse B, Carlen A: Adherence and *Streptococcus mutans* infections: in vitro study with saliva from non-infected and infected preschool children, *Infect Immun* 34:633, 1981.
105. Koka S, Razzoog ME, Bloem TJ, et al: Microbial colonization of dental implants in partially edentulous subjects, *J Prosthet Dent* 70:141, 1993.
106. Kolenbrander PE: Surface recognition among oral bacteria: multigeneric coaggregations and their mediators, *Crit Rev Microbiol* 17:137, 1989.
107. Kolenbrander PE, Andersen RN: Inhibition of coaggregation between *Fusobacterium nucleatum* and *Porphyromonas (Bacteroides) gingivalis* by lactose and related sugars, *Infect Immun* 57:3204, 1989.
108. Kolenbrander PE, London J: Adhere today, here tomorrow: oral bacterial adherence, *J Bacteriol* 175:3247, 1993.
109. Kolenbrander PE, Andersen RN, Moore LV: Intrageneric coaggregation among strains of human oral bacteria: potential role in primary colonization of the tooth surface, *Appl Environ Microbiol* 56:3890, 1990.

110. Kolenbrander PE, Ganeshkumar N, Cassels FJ, et al: Coaggregation: specific adherence among human oral plaque bacteria, *FASEB J* 7:406, 1993.
111. Kolenbrander PE, Parrish KD, Andersen RN, et al: Intergeneric coaggregation of oral *Treponema* spp. with *Fusobacterium* spp. and intrageneric coaggregation among *Fusobacterium* spp, *Infect Immun* 63:4584, 1995.
112. Kononen E, Asikainen S, Jousimies-Somer H: The early colonization of gram-negative anaerobic bacteria in edentulous infants, *Oral Microbiol Immunol* 7:28, 1992.
113. Kornman KS, Löe H: The role of local factors in the etiology of periodontal diseases, *Periodontol 2000* 2:83, 1993.
114. Kornman KS, Loesche WJ: Effects of estradiol and progesterone on *Bacteroides melaninogenicus* and *Bacteroides gingivalis, Infect Immun* 35:256, 1982;.
115. Kornman KS, Robertson PB: Clinical and microbiological evaluation of therapy for juvenile periodontitis, *J Periodontol* 56:443, 1985.
116. Kremer BH, Loos BG, van der Velden U, et al: *Peptostreptococcus micros* smooth and rough genotypes in periodontitis and gingivitis, *J Periodontol* 71:209, 2000.
117. Kroes I, Lepp PW, Relman DA: Bacterial diversity within the human subgingival crevice, *Proc Natl Acad Sci USA* 96:14547, 1999.
118. Lai CH, Listgarten MA, Shirakawa M, et al: *Bacteroides forsythus* in adult gingivitis and periodontitis, *Oral Microbiol Immunol* 2:152, 1987.
119. Lang NP, Cumming BR, Löe H: Toothbrushing frequency as it relates to plaque development and gingival health, *J Periodontol* 44:396, 1973.
120. Lee RG, Adamson C, Kim SW: Competitive adsorption of plasma proteins onto polymer surfaces, *Thromb Res* 4:485, 1974.
121. Lekholm U, Ericsson I, Adell R, et al: The condition of the soft tissues at tooth and fixture abutments supporting fixed bridges: a microbiological and histological study, *J Clin Periodontol* 13:558, 1986.
122. Leknes KN, Lie T, Selvig KA: Root grooves: a risk factor in periodontal attachment loss, *J Periodontol* 65:859, 1994.
123. Leknes KN, Lie T, Wikesjo UM, et al: Influence of tooth instrumentation roughness on gingival tissue reactions, *J Periodontol* 67:197, 1996.
124. Leknes KN, Lie T, Wikesjo UM, et al: Influence of tooth instrumentation roughness on subgingival microbial colonization, *J Periodontol* 65:303, 1994.
125. Leonhardt A, Renvert S, Dahlen G: Microbial findings at failing implants, *Clin Oral Implants Res* 10:339, 1999.
126. Lie T: Morphologic studies on dental plaque formation, *Acta Odontol Scand* 37:73, 1979.
127. Lie T, Gusberti F: Replica study of plaque formation on human tooth surfaces, *Acta Odontol Scand* 37:65, 1979.
128. Liljemark WF, Bloomquist C: Human oral microbial ecology and dental caries and periodontal diseases, *Crit Rev Oral Biol Med* 7:180, 1996.
129. Liljemark WF, Bloomquist CG, Reilly BE, et al: Growth dynamics in a natural biofilm and its impact on oral disease management, *Adv Dent Res* 11:14, 1997.
130. Listgarten MA: Structure of the microbial flora associated with periodontal health and disease in man: a light and electron microscopic study, *J Periodontol* 47:1, 1976.
131. Listgarten MA, Hellden L: Relative distribution of bacteria at clinically healthy and periodontally diseased sites in humans, *J Clin Periodontol* 5:115, 1978.
132. Listgarten MA, Socransky SS: Ultrastructural characteristics of a spirochete in the lesion of acute necrotizing ulcerative gingivostomatitis (Vincent's infection), *Arch Oral Biol* 16:95, 1964.
133. Listgarten MA, Socransky SS: Electron microscopy as an aid in the taxonomic differentiation of oral spirochetes, *Arch Oral Biol* 10:127, 1965.
134. Löe H: Periodontal diseases: a brief historical perspective, *Periodontol 2000* 2:7, 1993.
135. Löe H, Theilade E, Jensen SB: Experimental gingivitis in man, *J Periodontol* 36:177, 1965.
136. Loesche WJ: Importance of nutrition in gingival crevice microbial ecology, *Periodontics* 6:245, 1968.
137. Loesche WJ: Chemotherapy of dental plaque infections, *Oral Sci Rev* 9:65, 1976.
138. Loesche WJ: Ecology of the oral flora. In Nisengard RJ, Newman MG, editors: *Oral microbiology and immunology,* Philadelphia, 1988, Saunders, p 307.
139. Loesche WJ, Svanberg ML, Pape HR: Intraoral transmission of *Streptococcus mutans* by a dental explorer, *J Dent Res* 58:1765, 1979.
140. Loesche WJ, Syed SA, Schmidt E, et al: Bacterial profiles of subgingival plaques in periodontitis, *J Periodontol* 56:447, 1985.
141. Loomer PM: Microbiological diagnostic testing in the treatment of periodontal diseases, *Periodontol 2000* 34:49, 2004.
142. Lovdal A, Arno A, Waerhaug J: Incidence of clinical manifestations of periodontal disease in light of oral hygiene and calculus formation, *J Am Dent Assoc* 56:21, 1958.
143. Madianos PN, Papapanou PN, Sandros J: *Porphyromonas gingivalis* infection of oral epithelium inhibits neutrophil transepithelial migration, *Infect Immun* 65:3983, 1997.
144. Maiden MF, Tanner A, McArdle S, et al: Tetracycline fiber therapy monitored by DNA probe and cultural methods, *J Periodontal Res* 26:452, 1991.
145. Marsh PD: Oral ecology and its impact on oral microbial diversity. In Kuramitsu HK, Ellen RP, editors: *Oral bacterial ecology: the molecular basis,* Norfolk, Va, 2000, Horizon Scientific Press, p 12.
146. Marsh PD, Bradshaw DJ: Physiological approaches to the control of oral biofilms, *Adv Dent Res* 11:176, 1997.
147. Mayrand D, McBride BC: Exological relationships of bacteria involved in a simple, mixed anaerobic infection, *Infect Immun* 27:44, 1980.
148. Mengel R, Stelzel M, Hasse C, et al: Osseointegrated implants in patients treated for generalized severe adult periodontitis: an interim report, *J Periodontol* 67:782, 1996.
149. Mergenhagen SE, Sandberg AL, Chassy BM, et al: Molecular basis of bacterial adhesion in the oral cavity, *Rev Infect Dis* 9(suppl 5):S467, 1987.
150. Michalowicz BS: Genetic and heritable risk factors in periodontal disease, *J Periodontol* 65:479, 1994.
151. Michalowicz BS, Ronderos M, Camara-Silva R, et al: Human herpesviruses and *Porphyromonas gingivalis* are associated with juvenile periodontitis, *J Periodontol* 71:981, 2000.
152. Mierau HD: [Relations between plaque formation, tooth surface roughness and self-cleaning], *Dtsch Zahnarztl Z* 39:691, 1984.
153. Mierau HD, Singer D, [Reproducibility of plaque formation in the dento-gingival region (3)], *Dtsch Zahnarztl Z* 33:566, 1978.
154. Mombelli A, Lang NP, Burgin WB, et al: Microbial changes associated with the development of puberty gingivitis, *J Periodontal Res* 25:331, 1990.
155. Mombelli A, Lehmann B, Tonetti M, et al: Clinical response to local delivery of tetracycline in relation to overall and local periodontal conditions, *J Clin Periodontol* 24:470, 1997.
156. Mombelli A, Marxer M, Gaberthuel T, et al: The microbiota of osseointegrated implants in patients with a history of periodontal disease, *J Clin Periodontol* 22:124, 1995.

157. Moore WE: Microbiology of periodontal disease, *J Periodontal Res* 22:335, 1987.
158. Moore WE, Holdeman LV: Special problems associated with the isolation and identification of intestinal bacteria in fecal flora studies, *Am J Clin Nutr* 27:1450, 1974.
159. Moore WE, Moore LV: The bacteria of periodontal diseases, *Periodontol 2000* 5:66, 1994.
160. Moore WE, Holdeman LV, Cato EP, et al: Comparative bacteriology of juvenile periodontitis, *Infect Immun* 48:507, 1985.
161. Morra M, Cassinelli C: Bacterial adhesion to polymer surfaces: a critical review of surface thermodynamic approaches, *J Biomater Sci Polym Ed* 9:55, 1997.
162. Mouton C, Reynolds HS, Genco RJ: Characterization of tufted streptococci isolated from the "corn cob" configuration of human dental plaque, *Infect Immun* 27:235, 1980.
163. Newman HN: The approximal apical border of plaque on children's teeth. 1. Morphology, structure and cell content, *J Periodontol* 50:561, 1979.
164. Newman MG, Socransky SS: Predominant cultivable microbiota in periodontosis, *J Periodontal Res* 12:120, 1977.
165. Newman MG, Socransky SS, Savitt ED, et al: Studies of the microbiology of periodontosis, *J Periodontol* 47:373, 1976.
166. Nowzari H, MacDonald ES, Flynn J, et al: The dynamics of microbial colonization of barrier membranes for guided tissue regeneration, *J Periodontol* 67:694, 1996.
167. Nyvad B, Fejerskov O: Scanning electron microscopy of early microbial colonization of human enamel and root surfaces in vivo, *Scand J Dent Res* 95:287, 1987.
168. Nyvad B, Kilian M: Microflora associated with experimental root surface caries in humans, *Infect Immun* 58:1628, 1990.
169. Ofek I, Doyle RJ, editors: *Bacterial adhesion to cells and tissues*, London, 1994, Chapman & Hall.
170. Ong ES, Newman HN, Wilson M, et al: The occurrence of periodontitis-related microorganisms in relation to titanium implants, *J Periodontol* 63:200, 1992.
171. Page RC, Schroeder HE, editors: *Periodontitis in man and other animals*, Basel, 1982, Karger.
172. Papaioannou W, Quirynen M, van Steenberghe D: The influence of periodontitis on the subgingival flora around implants in partially edentulous patients, *Clin Oral Implants Res* 7:405, 1996.
173. Pearce MA, Devine DA, Dixon RA, et al: Genetic heterogeneity in *Prevotella intermedia, Prevotella nigrescens, Prevotella corporis* and related species isolated from oral and nonoral sites, *Oral Microbiol Immunol* 15:89, 2000.
174. Petersilka GJ, Ehmke B, Flemmig TF: Antimicrobial effects of mechanical debridement, *Periodontol 2000* 28:56, 2002.
175. Pratt-Terpstra IH, Weerkamp AH, Busscher HJ: The effects of pellicle formation on streptococcal adhesion to human enamel and artificial substrata with various surface free-energies, *J Dent Res* 68:463, 1989.
176. Pratt-Terpstra IH, Mulder J, Weerkamp AH, et al: Secretory IgA adsorption and oral streptococcal adhesion to human enamel and artificial solid substrata with various surface free energies, *J Biomater Sci Polym Ed* 2:239, 1991.
177. Pratten J, Barnett P, Wilson M: Composition and susceptibility to chlorhexidine of multispecies biofilms of oral bacteria, *Appl Environ Microbiol* 64:3515, 1998.
178. Quirynen M: Anatomical and inflammatory factors influence bacterial plaque growth and retention in man, 1986.
179. Quirynen M, Bollen CM: The influence of surface roughness and surface-free energy on supra- and subgingival plaque formation in man: a review of the literature, *J Clin Periodontol* 22:1, 1995.
180. Quirynen M, Listgarten MA: Distribution of bacterial morphotypes around natural teeth and titanium implants ad modum Branemark, *Clin Oral Implants Res* 1:8, 1990.
181. Quirynen M, van Steenberghe D: Is early plaque growth rate constant with time? *J Clin Periodontol* 16:278, 1989.
182. Quirynen M, Dekeyser C, van Steenberghe D: The influence of gingival inflammation, tooth type, and timing on the rate of plaque formation, *J Periodontol* 62:219, 1991.
183. Quirynen M, Gijbels F, Jacobs R: An infected jawbone site compromising successful osseointegration, *Periodontol 2000* 33:129, 2003.
184. Quirynen M, Bollen CM, Papaioannou W, et al: The influence of titanium abutment surface roughness on plaque accumulation and gingivitis: short-term observations, *Int J Oral Maxillofac Implants* 11:169, 1996.
185. Quirynen M, Bollen CM, Vandekerckhove BN, et al: Full- vs. partial-mouth disinfection in the treatment of periodontal infections: short-term clinical and microbiological observations, *J Dent Res* 74:1459, 1995.
186. Quirynen M, De Soete M, Dierickx K, et al: The intra-oral translocation of periodontopathogens jeopardises the outcome of periodontal therapy: a review of the literature, *J Clin Periodontol* 28:499, 2001.
187. Quirynen M, Gizani S, Mongardini C, et al: The effect of periodontal therapy on the number of cariogenic bacteria in different intra-oral niches, *J Clin Periodontol* 26:322, 1999.
188. Quirynen M, Marechal M, Busscher HJ, et al: The influence of surface free-energy on planimetric plaque growth in man, *J Dent Res* 68:796, 1989.
189. Quirynen M, Papaioannou W, van Steenbergen TJ, et al: Adhesion of *Porphyromonas gingivalis* strains to cultured epithelial cells from patients with a history of chronic adult periodontitis or from patients less susceptible to periodontitis, *J Periodontol* 72:626, 2001.
190. Quirynen M, van der Mei HC, Bollen CM, et al: An in vivo study of the influence of the surface roughness of implants on the microbiology of supra- and subgingival plaque, *J Dent Res* 72:1304, 1993.
191. Quirynen M, Vogels R, Pauwels M, et al: Initial subgingival colonization of pristine pockets in an established environment, *J Dent Res* 84:340, 2005.
192. Quirynen M, Vogels R, Peeters W, et al: Dynamics of initial subgingival colonization of peri-implant pockets, *Clin Oral Implants Res* 2005.
193. Ramberg P, Axelsson P, Lindhe J: Plaque formation at healthy and inflamed gingival sites in young individuals, *J Clin Periodontol* 22:85, 1995.
194. Ramberg P, Lindhe J, Dahlen G, et al: The influence of gingival inflammation on de novo plaque formation, *J Clin Periodontol* 21:51, 1994.
195. Rams TE, Feik D, Slots J: Staphylococci in human periodontal diseases, *Oral Microbiol Immunol* 5:29, 1990.
196. Renvert S, Dahlen G, Wikstrom M: Treatment of periodontal disease based on microbiological diagnosis: relation between microbiological and clinical parameters during 5 years, *J Periodontol* 67:562, 1996.
197. Renvert S, Dahlen G, Wikstrom M: The clinical and microbiological effects of non-surgical periodontal therapy in smokers and non-smokers, *J Clin Periodontol* 25:153, 1998.
198. Renvert S, Wikstrom M, Dahlen G, et al: Effect of root debridement on the elimination of *Actinobacillus actinomycetemcomitans* and *Bacteroides gingivalis* from periodontal pockets, *J Clin Periodontol* 17:345, 1990.
199. Renvert S, Wikstrom M, Dahlen G, et al: On the inability of root debridement and periodontal surgery to eliminate *Actinobacillus actinomycetemcomitans* from periodontal pockets, *J Clin Periodontol* 17:351, 1990.

200. Rimondini L, Fare S, Brambilla E, et al: The effect of surface roughness on early in vivo plaque colonization on titanium, *J Periodontol* 68:556, 1997.
201. Roberts FA, Darveau RP: Beneficial bacteria of the periodontium, *Periodontol 2000* 30:40, 2002.
202. Rolla G, Ogaard B, Cruz RA: Topical application of fluorides on teeth: new concepts of mechanisms of interaction, *J Clin Periodontol* 20:105, 1993.
203. Ronstrom A, Edwardsson S, Atistrom R: *Streptococcus sanguis* and *Streptococcus salivarius* in early plaque formation on plastic films, *J Periodontal Res* 12:331, 1977.
204. Rotimi VO, Duerden BI: The development of the bacterial flora in normal neonates, *J Med Microbiol* 14:51, 1981.
205. Ruan MS, Di Paola C, Mandel ID: Quantitative immunochemistry of salivary proteins adsorbed in vitro to enamel and cementum from caries-resistant and caries-susceptible human adults, *Arch Oral Biol* 31:597, 1986.
206. Rudney JD, Chen R, Sedgewick GJ: Intracellular *Actinobacillus actinomycetemcomitans* and *Porphyromonas gingivalis* in buccal epithelial cells collected from human subjects, *Infect Immun* 69:2700, 2001.
207. Russel AL: Epidemiology of periodontal disease, *Int Dent J* 17:282, 1967.
208. Rutter PR, Vincent B: Physicochemical interactions of the substratum, microorganisms and the fluid phase. In Marshall KC, editors: *Microbial adhesion and aggregation,* Berlin, 1984, Springer Verlag, p 21.
209. Rykke M, Sonju T: Amino acid composition of acquired enamel pellicle collected in vivo after 2 hours and after 24 hours, *Scand J Dent Res* 99:463, 1991.
210. Saglie FR, Marfany A, Camargo P: Intragingival occurrence of *Actinobacillus actinomycetemcomitans* and *Bacteroides gingivalis* in active destructive periodontal lesions, *J Periodontol* 59:259, 1988.
211. Saglie FR, Carranza FA Jr, Newman MG, et al: Identification of tissue-invading bacteria in human periodontal disease, *J Periodontal Res* 17:452, 1982.
212. Sandros J, Karlsson C, Lappin DF, et al: Cytokine responses of oral epithelial cells to *Porphyromonas gingivalis* infection, *J Dent Res* 79:1808, 2000.
213. Sbordone L, Barone A, Ciaglia RN, et al: Longitudinal study of dental implants in a periodontally compromised population, *J Periodontol* 70:1322, 1999.
214. Scannapieco FA, Levine MJ: Saliva and dental pellicles. In Genco RJ, Goldman HM, Cohen DW, editors: *Contemporary periodontics,* St Louis, 1990, Mosby.
215. Scannapieco FA, Bush RB, Paju S: Associations between periodontal disease and risk for atherosclerosis, cardiovascular disease, and stroke: a systematic review, *Ann Periodontol* 8:38, 2003.
216. Scannapieco FA, Bush RB, Paju S: Periodontal disease as a risk factor for adverse pregnancy outcomes: a systematic review, *Ann Periodontol* 8:70, 2003.
217. Scannapieco FA, Bush RB, Paju S: Associations between periodontal disease and risk for nosocomial bacterial pneumonia and chronic obstructive pulmonary disease: a systematic review, *Ann Periodontol* 8:54, 2003.
218. Scannapieco FA, Torres GI, Levine MJ: Salivary amylase promotes adhesion of oral streptococci to hydroxyapatite, *J Dent Res* 74:1360, 1995.
219. Schei O, Waerhaug J, Loval A: Alveolar bone loss as related to oral hygiene and age, *J Periodontol* 30:7, 1959.
220. Scheie AA: Mechanisms of dental plaque formation, *Adv Dent Res* 8:246, 1994.
221. Schroeder HE, De Boever J: The structure of microbial dental plaque. In McHugh WD, editors: *Dental plaque,* Edinburgh, 1970, Livingstone, p 49.
222. Sheiham A: Periodontal disease and oral cleanliness in tobacco smokers, *J Periodontol* 42:259, 1971.
223. Simonsson T: Aspects of dental plaque formation with special reference to colloid-chemical phenomena, *Swed Dent J Suppl* 58:1, 1989.
224. Simonsson T, Ronstrom A, Rundegren J, et al: Rate of plaque formation: some clinical and biochemical characteristics of "heavy" and "light" plaque formers, *Scand J Dent Res* 95:97, 1987.
225. Sjodin B, Crossner CG, Unell L, et al: A retrospective radiographic study of alveolar bone loss in the primary dentition in patients with localized juvenile periodontitis, *J Clin Periodontol* 16:124, 1989.
226. Skopek RJ, Liljemark WF, Bloomquist CG, et al: Dental plaque development on defined streptococcal surfaces, *Oral Microbiol Immunol* 8:16, 1993.
227. Slots J: The predominant cultivable microflora of advanced periodontitis, *Scand J Dent Res* 85:114, 1977.
228. Slots J: Subgingival microflora and periodontal disease, *J Clin Periodontol* 6:351, 1979.
229. Slots J: Update on human cytomegalovirus in destructive periodontal disease, *Oral Microbiol Immunol* 19:217, 2004.
230. Slots J, Listgarten MA: *Bacteroides gingivalis, Bacteroides intermedius* and *Actinobacillus actinomycetemcomitans* in human periodontal diseases, *J Clin Periodontol* 15:85, 1988.
231. Slots J, Rams TE: New views on periodontal microbiota in special patient categories, *J Clin Periodontol* 18:411, 1991.
232. Socransky SS, Haffajee AD: Microbial mechanisms in the pathogenesis of destructive periodontal diseases: a critical assessment, *J Periodontal Res* 26:195, 1991.
233. Socransky SS, Haffajee AD: The bacterial etiology of destructive periodontal disease: current concepts, *J Periodontol* 63:322, 1992.
234. Socransky SS, Haffajee AD: The nature of periodontal diseases, *Ann Periodontol* 2:3, 1997.
235. Socransky SS, Manganiello SD: The oral microbiota of man from birth to senility, *J Periodontol* 42:485, 1971.
236. Socransky SS, Smith C, Haffajee AD: Subgingival microbial profiles in refractory periodontal disease, *J Clin Periodontol* 29:260, 2002.
237. Socransky SS, Gibbons RJ, Dale AC, et al: The microbiota of the gingival crevice area of man. I. Total microscopic and viable counts of specific microorganisms, *Arch Oral Biol* 8:275, 1953.
238. Socransky SS, Haffajee AD, Cugini MA, et al: Microbial complexes in subgingival plaque, *J Clin Periodontol* 25:134, 1998.
239. Socransky SS, Haffajee AD, Smith GL, et al: Difficulties encountered in the search for the etiologic agents of destructive periodontal diseases, *J Clin Periodontol* 14:588, 1987.
240. Socransky SS, Manganiello AD, Propas D, et al: Bacteriological studies of developing supragingival dental plaque, *J Periodontal Res* 12:90, 1977.
241. Soskolne WA, Klinger A: The relationship between periodontal diseases and diabetes: an overview, *Ann Periodontol* 6:91, 2001.
242. Sumida S, Ishihara K, Kishi M, et al: Transmission of periodontal disease-associated bacteria from teeth to osseointegrated implant regions, *Int J Oral Maxillofac Implants* 17:696, 2002.
243. Syed SA, Loesche WJ: Bacteriology of human experimental gingivitis: effect of plaque age, *Infect Immun* 21:821, 1978.
244. Tanner AC, Haffer C, Bratthall GT, et al: A study of the bacteria associated with advancing periodontitis in man, *J Clin Periodontol* 6:278, 1979.

245. Tappuni AR, Challacombe SJ: Distribution and isolation frequency of eight streptococcal species in saliva from predentate and dentate children and adults, *J Dent Res* 72:31, 1993.
246. Taylor DC, Clancy RL, Cripps AW, et al: An alteration in the host-parasite relationship in subjects with chronic bronchitis prone to recurrent episodes of acute bronchitis, *Immunol Cell Biol* 72:143, 1994.
247. Ter Steeg PF, van der Hoeven JS, de Jong MH, et al: Enrichment of subgingival microflora on human serum leading to accumulation of *Bacteroides* species, peptostreptococci and fusobacteria, *Antonie Van Leeuwenhoek* 53:261, 1987.
248. Theilade E, Wright WH, Jensen SB, et al: Experimental gingivitis in man. II. A longitudinal clinical and bacteriological investigation, *J Periodontal Res* 1:1, 1966.
249. Ting M, Contreras A, Slots J: Herpesvirus in localized juvenile periodontitis, *J Periodontal Res* 35:17, 2000.
250. Van der Reijden WA, Dellemijn-Kippuw N, Stijne-van Nes AM, et al: Mutans streptococci in subgingival plaque of treated and untreated patients with periodontitis, *J Clin Periodontol* 28:686, 2001.
251. Van Loosdrecht MC, Lyklema J, Norde W, et al: Influence of interfaces on microbial activity, *Microbiol Rev* 54:75, 1990.
252. Van Loosdrecht MC, Norde W, Zehnder AJ: Physical chemical description of bacterial adhesion, *J Biomater Appl* 5:91, 1990.
253. Van Steenberghe D, Jacobs R, Desnyder M, et al: The relative impact of local and endogenous patient-related factors on implant failure up to the abutment stage, *Clin Oral Implants Res* 13:617, 2002.
254. Van Winkelhoff AJ, Loos BG, van der Reijden WA, et al: *Porphyromonas gingivalis, Bacteroides forsythus* and other putative periodontal pathogens in subjects with and without periodontal destruction, *J Clin Periodontol* 29:1023, 2002.
255. Wade WG, Addy M: In vitro activity of a chlorhexidine-containing mouthwash against subgingival bacteria, *J Periodontol* 60:521, 1989.
256. Walden WC, Hentges DJ: Differential effects of oxygen and oxidation-reduction potential on the multiplication of three species of anaerobic intestinal bacteria, *Appl Microbiol* 30:781, 1975.
257. Walker CB: Selected antimicrobial agents: mechanisms of action, side effects and drug interactions, *Periodontol 2000* 10:12, 1996.
258. Weiger R, Netuschil L, von Ohle C, et al: Microbial generation time during the early phases of supragingival dental plaque formation, *Oral Microbiol Immunol* 10:93, 1995.
259. Weiss EI, Eli I, Shenitzki B, et al: Identification of the rhamnose-sensitive adhesin of Capnocytophaga ochracea ATCC 33596, *Arch Oral Biol* 35(suppl):127S, 1990.
260. Weiss EI, London J, Kolenbrander PE, et al: Characterization of monoclonal antibodies to fimbria-associated adhesins of *Bacteroides loescheii* PK1295, *Infect Immun* 56:219, 1988.
261. Weiss EI, London J, Kolenbrander PE, et al: Localization and enumeration of fimbria-associated adhesins of *Bacteroides loescheii, J Bacteriol* 170:1123, 1988.
262. Wennstrom JL, Heijl L, Dahlen G, et al: Periodic subgingival antimicrobial irrigation of periodontal pockets. I. Clinical observations, *J Clin Periodontol* 14:541, 1987.
263. Weyant RJ, Burt BA: An assessment of survival rates and within-patient clustering of failures for endosseous oral implants, *J Dent Res* 72:2, 1993.
264. Whittaker CJ, Clemans DL, Kolenbrander PE: Insertional inactivation of an intrageneric coaggregation-relevant adhesin locus from *Streptococcus gordonii* DL1 (Challis), *Infect Immun* 64:4137, 1996.
265. Williams P: Role of the cell envelope in bacterial adaptation to growth in vivo in infections, *Biochimie* 70:987, 1988.
266. Winkel EG, Abbas F, van der Velden U, et al: Experimental gingivitis in relation to age in individuals not susceptible to periodontal destruction, *J Clin Periodontol* 14:499, 1987.
267. Wolff L, Dahlen G, Aeppli D: Bacteria as risk markers for periodontitis, *J Periodontol* 65:498, 1994.
268. Wood SR, Kirkham J, Marsh PD, et al: Architecture of intact natural human plaque biofilms studied by confocal laser scanning microscopy, *J Dent Res* 79:21, 2000.
269. Xu KD, McFeters GA, Stewart PS: Biofilm resistance to antimicrobial agents, *Microbiology* 146(pt 3):547, 2000.
270. Zambon JJ: Periodontal diseases: microbial factors, *Ann Periodontol* 1:879, 1996.
271. Zambon JJ, Grossi SG, Machtei EE, et al: Cigarette smoking increases the risk for subgingival infection with periodontal pathogens, *J Periodontol* 67:1050, 1996.
272. Zee KY, Samaranayake LP, Attstrom R: Predominant cultivable supragingival plaque in Chinese "rapid" and "slow" plaque formers, *J Clin Periodontol* 23:1025, 1996.
273. Zee KY, Samaranayake LP, Attstrom R: Scanning electron microscopy of microbial colonization of 'rapid' and 'slow' dental-plaque formers in vivo, *Arch Oral Biol* 42:735, 1997.

The Role of Dental Calculus and Other Predisposing Factors

James E. Hinrichs

10

CHAPTER

■ ■ ■

CHAPTER OUTLINE

CALCULUS
 Supragingival and Subgingival Calculus
 Prevalence
 Composition
 Attachment to the Tooth Surface
 Formation
 Etiologic Significance
 Materia Alba, Food Debris, and Dental Stains

OTHER PREDISPOSING FACTORS
 Iatrogenic Factors
 Malocclusion
 Periodontal Complications Associated with
 Orthodontic Therapy
 Extraction of Impacted Third Molars
 Habits and Self-Inflicted Injuries
 Tobacco Use
 Radiation Therapy

*T*he primary cause of gingival inflammation is bacterial plaque (see Chapters 9, 12, and 13), along with other predisposing factors. These predisposing factors include calculus, malocclusion, faulty restorations, complications associated with orthodontic therapy, self-inflicted injuries, use of tobacco, and radiation therapy.

CALCULUS

Calculus consists of mineralized bacterial plaque that forms on the surfaces of natural teeth and dental prostheses. Calculus is classified as supragingival or subgingival, according to its relation to the gingival margin.

Supragingival and Subgingival Calculus

Supragingival calculus is located coronal to the gingival margin and therefore is visible in the oral cavity. It is usually white or whitish yellow in color, hard with claylike consistency, and easily detached from the tooth surface. After removal, it may rapidly recur, especially in the lingual area of the mandibular incisors. The color is influenced by contact with such substances as tobacco and food pigments. It may localize on a single tooth or group of teeth, or it may be generalized throughout the mouth.

The two most common locations for supragingival calculus to develop are the buccal surfaces of the maxillary molars (Figure 10-1) and the lingual surfaces of the mandibular anterior teeth (Figure 10-2).[51] Saliva from the parotid gland flows over the facial surfaces of upper molars through Stensen's duct, whereas the orifices of Wharton's duct and Bartholin's duct empty onto the lingual surfaces of the lower incisors from the submaxillary and sublingual glands, respectively. In extreme cases, calculus may form a bridgelike structure over the interdental papilla of adjacent teeth or cover the occlusal surface of teeth without functional antagonists.

Subgingival calculus is located below the crest of the marginal gingiva and therefore is not visible on routine clinical examination. The location and extent of subgingival calculus may be evaluated by careful tactile perception with a delicate dental instrument such as an explorer. Clerehugh et al.[46] used a World Health Organization #621 probe to detect and score subgingival calculus. Subsequently, these teeth were extracted and visually scored for subgingival calculus. An agreement of 80% was

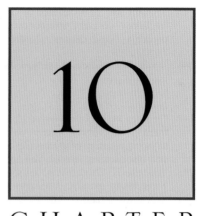

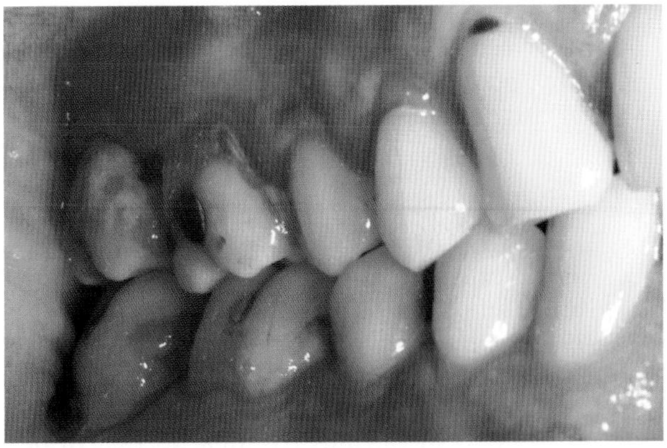

Figure 10-1 Supragingival calculus is depicted on the buccal surfaces of maxillary molars adjacent to orifice for Stensen's duct.

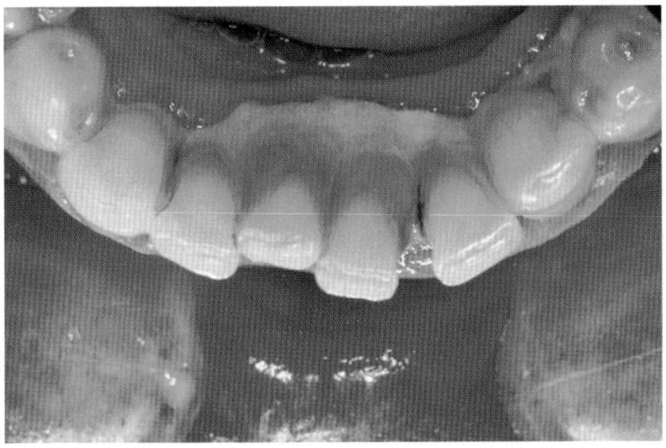

Figure 10-2 Extensive supragingival calculus is present on the lingual surfaces of lower anterior teeth.

found between these two scoring methods. Subgingival calculus is typically hard and dense and frequently appears dark brown or greenish black while being firmly attached to the tooth surface (Figure 10-3). Supragingival calculus and subgingival calculus generally occur together, but one may be present without the other. Microscopic studies demonstrate that deposits of subgingival calculus usually extend nearly to the base of periodontal pockets in chronic periodontitis but do not reach the junctional epithelium.

When the gingival tissues recede, subgingival calculus becomes exposed and is therefore reclassified as supragingival (Figure 10-4). Thus, supragingival calculus can be composed of both supragingival calculus and previous subgingival calculus. A reduction in gingival inflammation and probing depths with a gain in clinical attachment can be observed after the removal of subgingival plaque and calculus (Figure 10-5) (see Chapter 51).

Prevalence

Anerud et al.[6] observed the periodontal status of a group of Sri Lankan tea laborers and a group of Norwegian academicians for a 15-year period. The Norwegian population had ready access to preventive dental care throughout their lives, whereas the Sri Lankan tea laborers did not. The formation of supragingival calculus was observed early in life in the Sri Lankan individuals, probably shortly after the teeth erupted. The first areas to exhibit calculus deposits were the facial aspects of

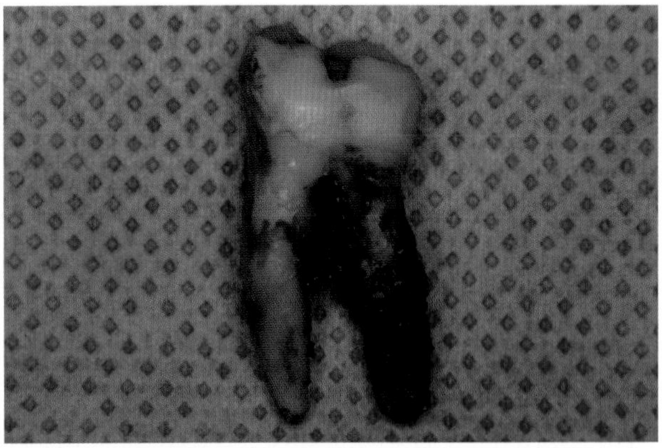

Figure 10-3 Dark-pigmented deposits of subgingival calculus are shown on the distal root of an extracted lower molar.

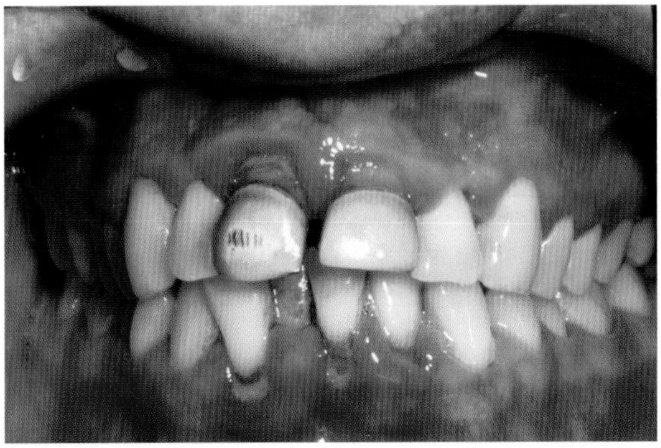

Figure 10-4 A 31-year-old Caucasian male is shown with extensive supragingival and subgingival calculus deposits throughout his dentition.

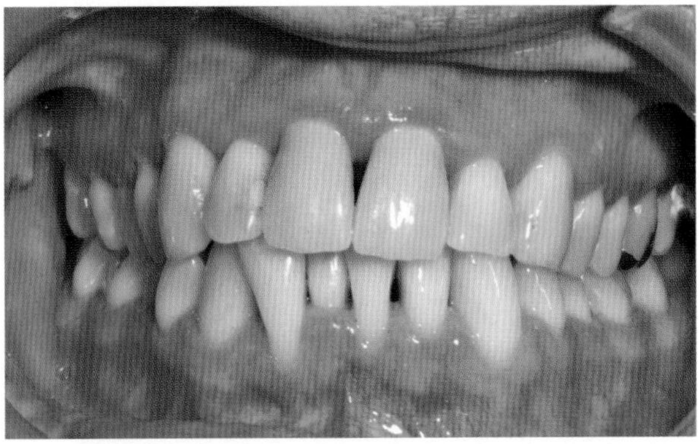

Figure 10-5 Same patient shown in Figure 10-4, 1 year after receiving thorough scaling and root planing to remove supragingival and subgingival calculus deposits, followed by restorative care. Note the substantial reduction in gingival inflammation.

maxillary molars and the lingual surfaces of mandibular incisors. Deposition of supragingival calculus continued as individuals aged, reaching a maximal calculus score around 25 to 30 years of age. At this time, most of the teeth were covered by calculus, although the facial surfaces had less calculus than the lingual or palatal surfaces. Calculus accumulation appeared to be symmetric, and by age 45 only a few teeth, typically the premolars, were without calculus. Subgingival calculus appeared first either independently or on the interproximal aspects of areas where supragingival calculus already existed. By age 30, all surfaces of all teeth had subgingival calculus without any pattern of predilection.

The Norwegian academicians received oral hygiene instructions and frequent preventive dental care throughout their lives. The Norwegians exhibited a marked reduction in the accumulation of calculus compared with the Sri Lankan group. However, despite that 80% of teenagers formed supragingival calculus on the facial surfaces of the upper molars and the lingual surfaces of lower incisors, no additional calculus formation occurred on other teeth, and calculus did not increase with age.[6]

More recently, the third National Health and Nutrition Examination Survey (NHANES III) evaluated 9689 adults in the United States between 1988 and 1994.[4] This survey revealed that 91.8% of the subjects had detectable calculus and 55.1% had subgingival calculus.

Both supragingival calculus and subgingival calculus may be seen on radiographs (see Chapter 36). Highly calcified interproximal calculus deposits are readily detectable as radiopaque projections that protrude into the interdental space (Figure 10-6). However, the sensitivity level of calculus detection by radiographs is low.[36] The location of calculus does not indicate the bottom of the periodontal pocket because the most apical plaque is not sufficiently calcified to be visible on radiographs.

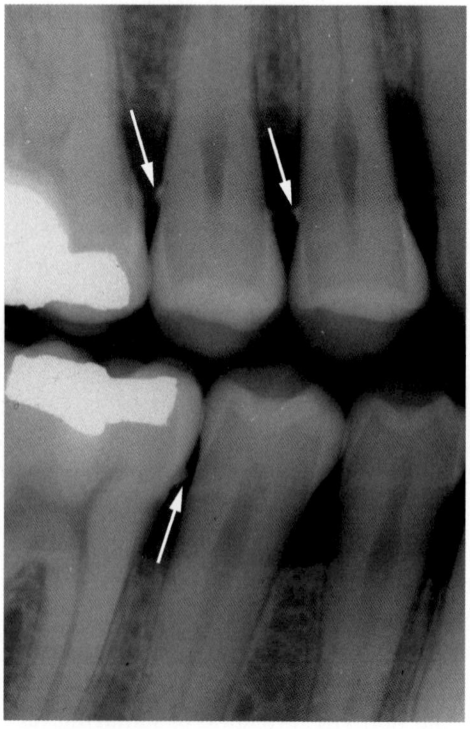

Figure 10-6 Bite-wing radiograph illustrating extensive subgingival calculus deposits, appearing as interproximal spurs *(arrows).*

Composition

Inorganic Content

Supragingival calculus consists of inorganic (70%-90%)[69] and organic components. The inorganic portion consists of 75.9% calcium phosphate, $Ca_3(PO_4)_2$; 3.1% calcium carbonate, $CaCO_3$; and traces of magnesium phosphate, $Mg_3(PO_4)_2$, and other metals.[215] The percentage of inorganic constituents in calculus is similar to that in other calcified tissues of the body. The principal inorganic components are calcium, 39%; phosphorus, 19%; carbon dioxide, 1.9%; magnesium, 0.8%; and trace amounts of sodium, zinc, strontium, bromine, copper, manganese, tungsten, gold, aluminum, silicon, iron, and fluorine.[141]

At least two thirds of the inorganic component is crystalline in structure.[111] The four main crystal forms and their percentages are as follows:

Hydroxyapatite, approximately 58%
Magnesium whitlockite, approximately 21%
Octacalcium phosphate, approximately 12%
Brushite, approximately 9%

Generally, two or more crystal forms are typically found in a sample of calculus. Hydroxyapatite and octacalcium phosphate are detected most frequently (in 97% to 100% of all supragingival calculus) and constitute the bulk of the specimen. Brushite is more common in the mandibular anterior region and magnesium whitlockite in the posterior areas. The incidence of the four crystal forms varies with the age of the deposit.[26]

Organic Content

The organic component of calculus consists of a mixture of protein-polysaccharide complexes, desquamated epithelial cells, leukocytes, and various types of microorganisms.[126] Between 1.9% and 9.1% of the organic component is carbohydrate, which consists of galactose, glucose, rhamnose, mannose, glucuronic acid, galactosamine, and sometimes arabinose, galacturonic acid, and glucosamine.[117,125,196] All these organic components are present in salivary glycoprotein, with the exception of arabinose and rhamnose. Salivary proteins account for 5.9% to 8.2% of the organic component of calculus and include most amino acids. Lipids account for 0.2% of the organic content in the form of neutral fats, free fatty acids, cholesterol, cholesterol esters, and phospholipids.[116]

The composition of subgingival calculus is similar to that of supragingival calculus, with some differences. Subgingival calculus has the same hydroxyapatite content, more magnesium whitlockite, and less brushite and octacalcium phosphate than supragingival calculus.[178,202] The ratio of calcium to phosphate is higher subgingivally, and the sodium content increases with the depth of periodontal pockets.[115] Salivary proteins present in supragingival calculus are not found subgingivally.[16] Dental calculus, salivary duct calculus, and calcified dental tissues are similar in inorganic composition.

Attachment to the Tooth Surface

Differences in the manner in which calculus is attached to the tooth surface affect the relative ease or difficulty encountered in its removal. The following four modes of attachment have been described[107,180,222]:

1. Attachment by means of an organic pellicle on enamel (Figures 10-7 and 10-8).
2. Mechanical locking into surface irregularities, such as resorption lacunae (Figure 10-9).
3. Close adaptation of calculus undersurface depressions to the gently sloping mounds of the unaltered cementum surface[196] (Figure 10-10).
4. Penetration of calculus bacteria into cementum.

However, not all investigators acknowledge the fourth mode of attachment[107] (Figure 10-11). Calculus embedded deeply in cementum may appear morphologically similar to cementum and thus has been termed *calculocementum*.[187]

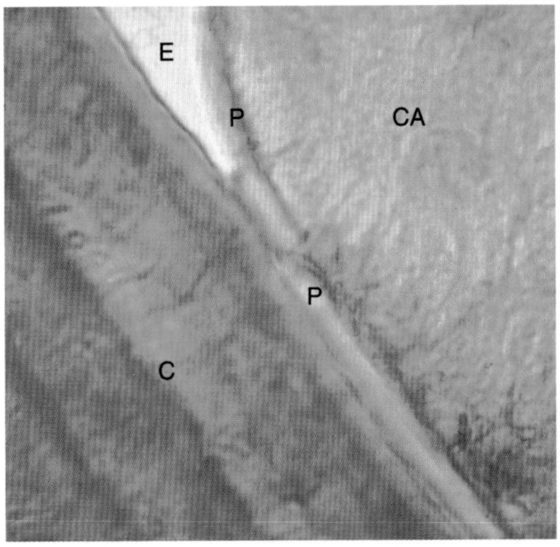

Figure 10-7 Calculus attached to pellicle on enamel surface and cementum. An enamel void *(E)* has been created in the preparation of the specimen. *CA,* Calculus; *P,* pellicle; *C,* cementum.

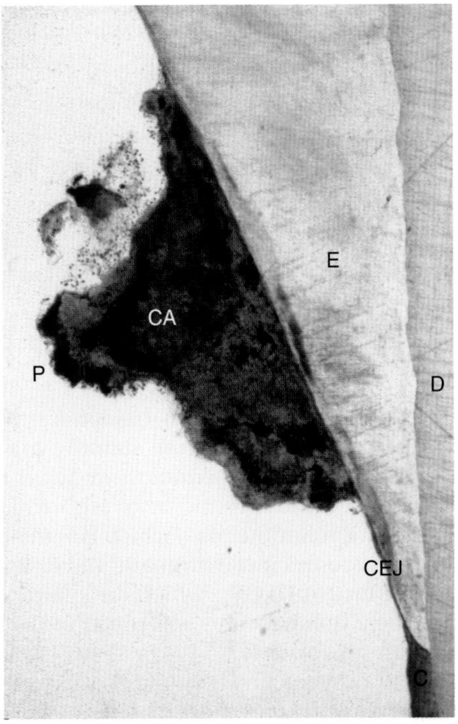

Figure 10-8 Nondecalcified specimen with calculus *(CA)* attached to enamel *(E)* surface just coronal to cementoenamel junction *(CEJ)*. Note plaque *(P)* on the surface of the calculus while dentin (D) and cementum (C) are identified. (Courtesy Dr. Michael Rohrer, Minneapolis.)

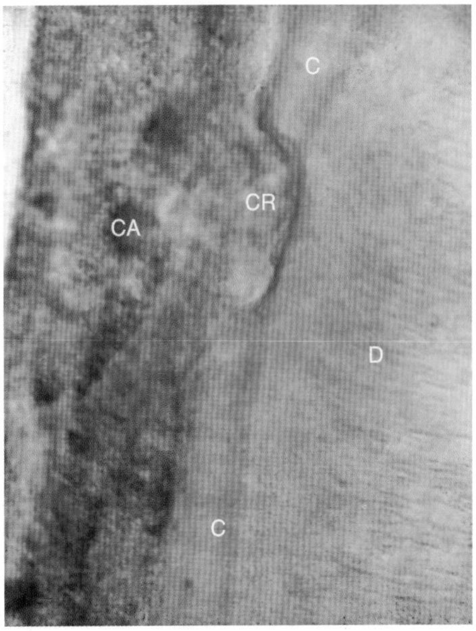

Figure 10-9 Calculus *(CA)* attached in a cemental resorption area *(CR)* with cementum *(C)* adjacent to dentin *(D)*.

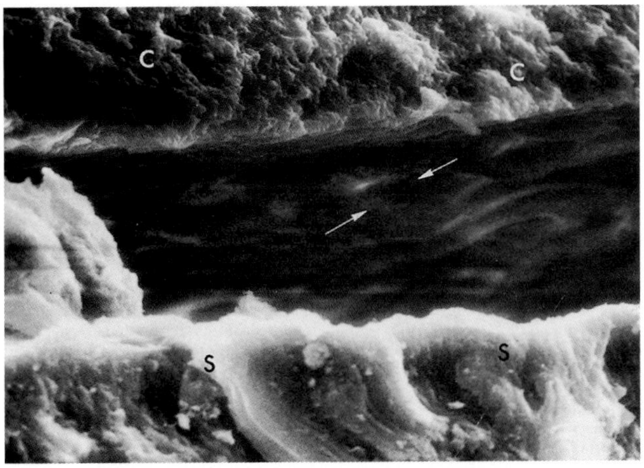

Figure 10-10 Undersurface of subgingival calculus *(C)* previously attached to the cementum surface *(S)*. Note impression of cementum mounds in calculus *(arrows)*. (Courtesy Dr. John Sottosanti, La Jolla, Calif.)

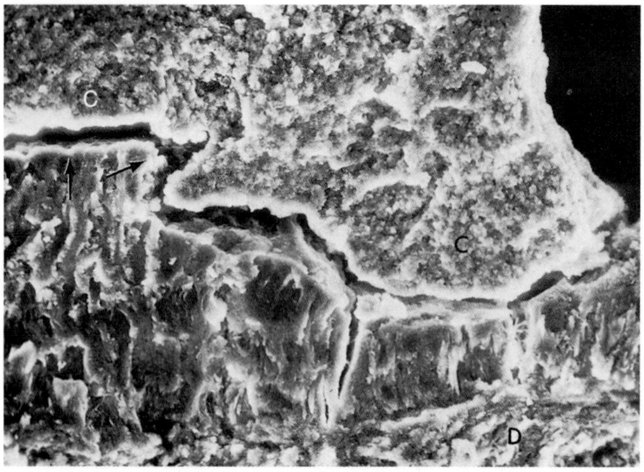

Figure 10-11 Subgingival calculus *(C)* embedded beneath the cementum surface *(arrows)* and penetrating to the dentin *(D)*, making removal difficult. (Courtesy Dr. John Sottosanti, La Jolla, Calif.)

> **SCIENCE TRANSFER**
>
> Investigators have shown calculus can attach to tooth surfaces in four modes. Simple attachment to enamel via an organic pellicle means that clinicians can easily remove the calculus with conventional scalers and curettes. However, attachment interlocks between calculus and the cementoenamel junction (CEJ) or to root surface irregularities makes calculus removal more challenging. Penetration of calculus into the cementum results in a dramatic change in techniques of calculus removal. Root planing to produce a smooth, noncalculus surface is required to remove surface cementum. This technique is one of the most difficult clinical skills to master because it requires the ability to control curettes to produce a glasslike surface as well as the tactile ability to detect the end point of the procedure. Clinicians need to understand how calculus is attached to each tooth surface so that appropriate techniques and time are used.
>
> A major etiologic factor in periodontal disease is bacterial plaque. A sequelae of plaque accumulation is the resulting mineralization process, which results in calculus. The calculus provides another site for further plaque accumulation. Calculus accumulation provides an environment that makes plaque removal difficult. Other conditions also make plaque removal difficult and as such are referred to as *predisposing factors.* In all these cases, the significance of these conditions lies in the fact that microbial accumulation is facilitated and the body responds predictably with an inflammatory response. This inflammatory response can be physiologic, but under certain conditions, becomes pathologic and results in tissue loss or periodontitis. Thus, a predominant tenant of periodontal treatment is the control of inflammation, accomplished in part by plaque and calculus removal and control of predisposing factors.

Formation

Calculus *is dental plaque that has undergone mineralization.* The soft plaque is hardened by the precipitation of mineral salts, which usually starts between the first and fourteenth days of plaque formation. However, calcification has been reported to occur as soon as 4 to 8 hours.[203] Calcifying plaques may become 50% mineralized in 2 days and 60% to 90% mineralized in 12 days.[140,181,191] All plaque does not necessarily undergo calcification. Early plaque contains a small amount of inorganic material, which increases as the plaque develops into calculus. Plaque that does not develop into calculus reaches a plateau of maximal mineral content within 2 days.[182] Microorganisms are not always essential in calculus formation because calculus occurs readily in germ-free rodents.[79]

Saliva is the source of mineralization for supragingival calculus, whereas the serum transudate called *gingival crevicular fluid* furnishes the minerals for subgingival calculus.[94,198] Plaque has the ability to concentrate calcium at 2 to 20 times its level in saliva.[26] Early plaque of patients who are heavy calculus formers contains more calcium, three times more phosphorus, and less potassium than that of non–calculus formers, suggesting that phosphorus may be more critical than calcium in plaque mineralization.[126] Calcification entails the binding of calcium ions to the carbohydrate-protein complexes of the organic matrix and the precipitation of crystalline calcium phosphate salts.[124] Crystals form initially in the intercellular matrix and on the bacterial surfaces and finally within the bacteria.[70,223]

Calcification begins along the inner surface of the supragingival plaque and in the attached component of subgingival plaque adjacent to the tooth. Separate foci of calcification increase in size and coalesce to form solid masses of calculus (Figure 10-12). Calcification may be accompanied by alterations in the bacterial content and staining qualities of the plaque. As calcification progresses, the number of filamentous bacteria increases, and foci of calcification change from basophilic to eosinophilic. There is a reduction in the staining intensity of groups exhibiting a positive periodic acid–Schiff reaction. Sulfhydryl and amino groups also are reduced and instead stain with toluidine blue, which is initially orthochromatic but becomes metachromatic and disappears.[211] Calculus is formed in layers, which are often separated by a thin cuticle that becomes embedded in the calculus as calcification progresses.[128]

The initiation of calcification and the rate of calculus accumulation vary from person to person, for different teeth, and at different times in the same person.[141,207] On the basis of these differences, persons may be classified as *heavy, moderate,* or *slight* calculus formers or as non–calculus formers. The average daily increment in calculus formers is from 0.10% to 0.15% of dry weight.[191,207]

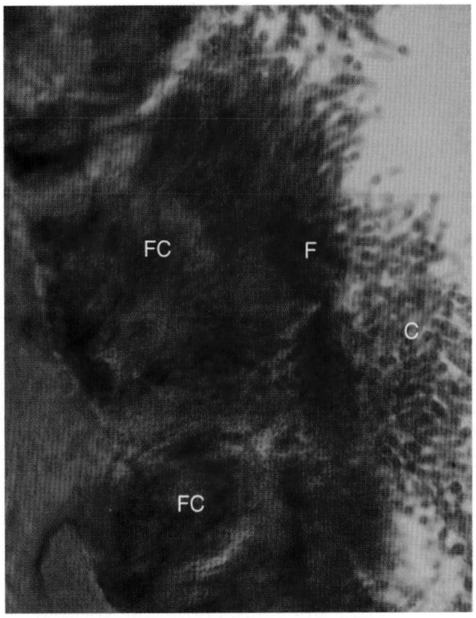

Figure 10-12 Plaque and calculus on tooth surface. Note the spherical areas of focal calcification *(FC)* and the perpendicular alignment of the filamentous *(F)* organisms along the inner surface of plaque and cocci *(C)* on the outer surface.

Calculus formation continues until it reaches a maximum, after which it may be reduced in amount. The time required to reach the maximal level has been reported as 10 weeks[47] and 6 months.[209] The decline from maximal calculus accumulation, referred to as *reversal phenomenon,* may be explained by the vulnerability of bulky calculus to mechanical wear from food and from the cheeks, lips, and tongue.

Anticalculus (antitartar) dentifrices claim to reduce the quantity and quality of calculus formed, making it easier for removal by the clinician. These products appear to be helpful for some patients.

Theories on Mineralization of Calculus

The theoretic mechanisms by which plaque becomes mineralized can be stratified into two principal categories, as follows[142]:

1. Mineral precipitation results from a local rise in the degree of saturation of calcium and phosphate ions, which may occur through the following mechanisms:
   - An *increase in the pH* of the saliva causes precipitation of calcium phosphate salts by lowering the precipitation constant. The pH may be elevated by the loss of carbon dioxide and the formation of ammonia by dental plaque bacteria or by protein degradation during stagnation.[25,89]
   - *Colloidal proteins* in saliva bind calcium and phosphate ions and maintain a supersaturated solution with respect to calcium phosphate salts. With stagnation of saliva, colloids settle out, and the supersaturated state is no longer maintained, leading to precipitation of calcium phosphate salts.[165,184]
   - *Phosphatase* liberated from dental plaque, desquamated epithelial cells, or bacteria precipitates calcium phosphate by hydrolyzing organic phosphates in saliva, thus increasing the concentration of free phosphate ions.[213] *Esterase* is another enzyme that is present in the cocci and filamentous organisms, leukocytes, macrophages, and desquamated epithelial cells of dental plaque.[10] Esterase may initiate calcification by hydrolyzing fatty esters into free fatty acids. The fatty acids form soaps with calcium and magnesium that are later converted into the less-soluble calcium phosphate salts.
2. Seeding agents induce small foci of calcification that enlarge and coalesce to form a calcified mass.[144] This concept has been referred to as the *epitactic concept*, or more appropriately, *heterogeneous nucleation*. The seeding agents in calculus formation are not known, but it is suspected that the intercellular matrix of plaque plays an active role.[127,140,223] The carbohydrate-protein complexes may initiate calcification by removing calcium from the saliva (chelation) and binding with it to form nuclei that induce subsequent deposition of minerals.[124,210]

Role of Microorganisms in Mineralization of Calculus

Mineralization of plaque starts extracellularly around both gram-positive organisms and gram-negative organisms;[109] it may also start intracellularly. filamentous organisms, diphtheroids, and *Bacterionema* and *Veillonella* species have the ability to form intracellular apatite crystals (Figure 10-13). Calculus formation spreads until the matrix and bacteria are calcified.[70,223]

Bacterial plaque may actively participate in the mineralization of calculus by forming phosphatases, which changes the pH of the plaque and induces mineralization,[56,124] but the prevalent opinion is that these bacteria are only passively involved[70,174,213] and are simply calcified with other plaque components. The occurrence of calculus-like deposits in germ-free animals supports this opinion.[79] However, other experiments suggest that transmissible factors are involved in calculus formation and that penicillin in the diets of some of these animals reduces calculus formation.[11]

Etiologic Significance

Distinguishing between the effects of calculus and plaque on the gingiva is difficult because calculus is always covered with a nonmineralized layer of plaque.[182] A positive correlation between the presence of calculus and the prevalence of gingivitis exists,[168] but this correlation is not as great as that between plaque and gingivitis.[73] In young persons, periodontal conditions are more closely related to plaque accumulation than to calculus, but the situation is reversed with age.[73,112] The incidence of calculus, gingivitis, and periodontal disease increases with age. It is extremely rare to find periodontal pockets in adults without subgingival calculus, although subgingival calculus may be of microscopic proportion in some cases.

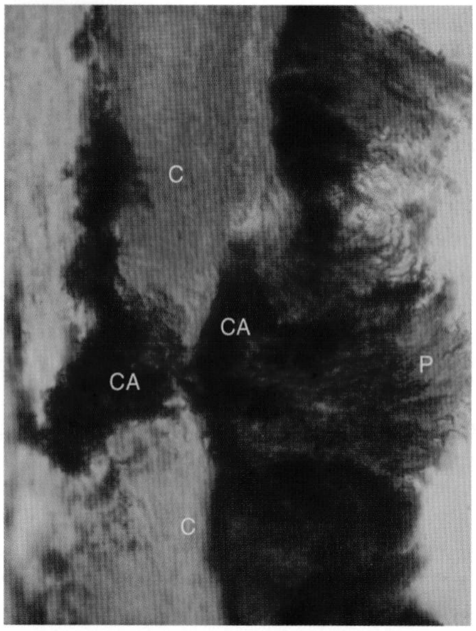

Figure 10-13 Calculus *(CA)* penetrates the tooth surface and is embedded within the cementum *(C)*. Note plaque *(P)* attached to the calculus.

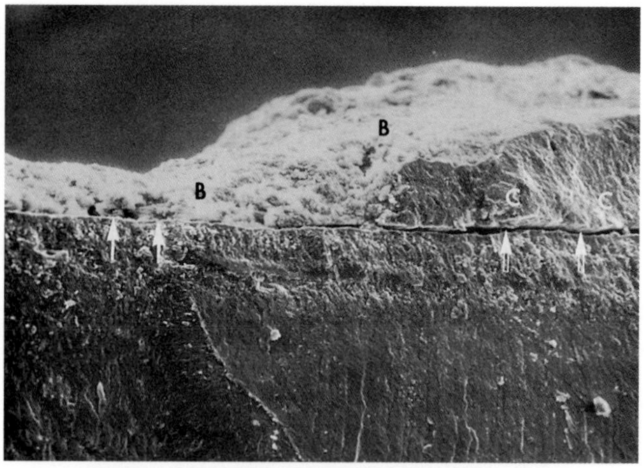

Figure 10-14 Scanning electron microscope view of an extracted human tooth, fracture experimentally, showing a cross section of subgingival calculus *(C)* that is not firmly attached to the cemental surface *(arrows)*. Note bacteria *(B)* attached to calculus and cemental surface. (Courtesy Dr. John Sottosanti, La Jolla, Calif.)

The nonmineralized plaque on the calculus surface is the principal irritant, but the underlying calcified portion may be a significant contributing factor (Figure 10-14). It does not irritate the gingiva directly but provides a fixed nidus for the continued accumulation of plaque and retains it close to the gingiva. Subgingival calculus may be the *product* rather than the cause of periodontal pockets. Plaque initiates gingival inflammation, which starts pocket formation, and the pocket in turn provides a sheltered area for plaque and bacterial accumulation. The increased flow of gingival fluid associated with gingival inflammation provides the minerals that convert the continually accumulating plaque into subgingival calculus. Over a 6-year period, Albander et al.[4] observed 156 teenagers with histories of aggressive periodontitis. The authors noted that areas with detectable subgingival calculus at the initiation of the study were much more likely to experience loss of periodontal attachment than sites that did not initially exhibit subgingival calculus.

Although the bacterial plaque that coats the teeth is the main etiologic factor in the development of periodontal disease, the removal of subgingival plaque and calculus constitutes the cornerstone of periodontal therapy. Calculus plays an important role in maintaining and accentuating periodontal disease by keeping plaque in close contact with the gingival tissue and creating areas where plaque removal is impossible. Therefore the clinician must not only possess the clinical skill to remove the calculus and other irritants that attach to the teeth, but also must be conscientious about performing this task.

Materia Alba, Food Debris, and Dental Stains

Materia alba is a concentration of microorganisms, desquamated epithelial cells, leukocytes, and a mixture of salivary proteins and lipids, with few or no food particles, and it lacks the regular internal pattern observed in plaque.[183] It is a yellow or grayish white, soft, sticky deposit and is somewhat less adherent than dental plaque. The irritating effect of materia alba on the gingiva is caused by bacteria and their products.

Most food debris is rapidly liquefied by bacterial enzymes and cleared from the oral cavity by salivary flow and the mechanical action of the tongue, cheeks, and lips. The rate of clearance from the oral cavity varies with the type of food and the individual. Aqueous solutions are typically cleared within 15 minutes, whereas sticky foods may adhere for more than 1 hour.[100,208] Dental plaque is not a derivative of food debris, and food debris is not an important cause of gingivitis.[55] Although oral microflora is the main determinant of gingival status, short-chain carboxylic acids found in retained food particles may also affect periodontal status.[100]

Pigmented deposits on the tooth surface are called *dental stains*. Stains are primarily an aesthetic problem and do not cause inflammation of the gingiva. The use of tobacco products (Figure 10-15), coffee, tea, certain mouth rinses, and pigments in foods can contribute to stain formation.[118]

OTHER PREDISPOSING FACTORS

Iatrogenic Factors

Deficiencies in the quality of dental restorations or prostheses are contributing factors to gingival inflammation and periodontal destruction. Inadequate dental procedures that contribute to the deterioration of the periodontal tissues are referred to as *iatrogenic factors*. Characteristics of dental restorations and removable partial dentures that are important to the maintenance of periodontal health include (1) the location of the gingival margin

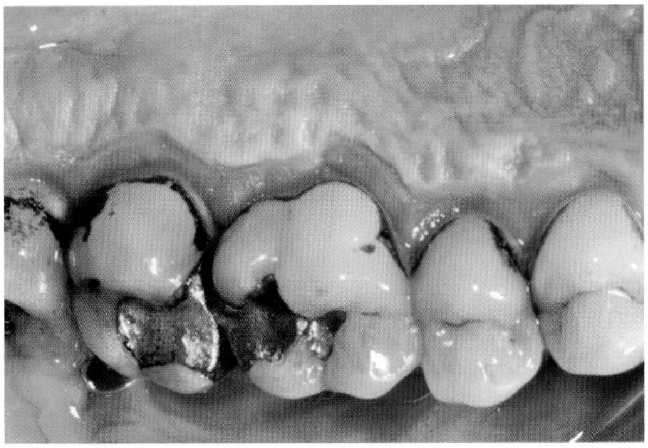

Figure 10-15 Tobacco stains on the apical third of the clinical crown caused by cigarette smoking.

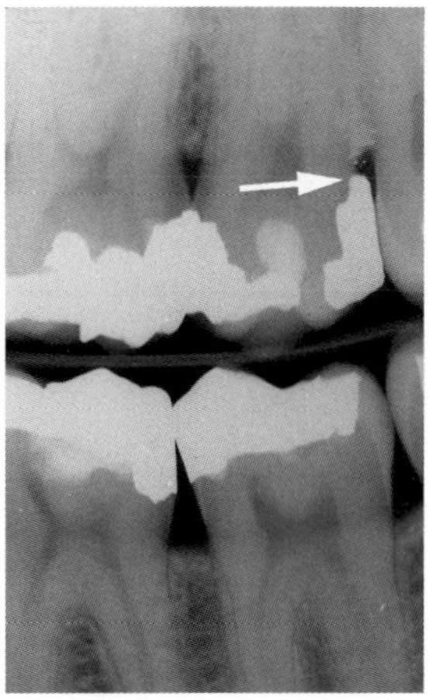

Figure 10-16 Radiograph of amalgam overhang on the distal surface of maxillary second molar that is a contributing source of plaque retention and gingival inflammation.

for the restoration, (2) the space between the margin of the restoration and the unprepared tooth, (3) the contour of restorations, (4) the occlusion, (5) materials used in the restoration, (6) the restorative procedure itself, and (7) the design of the removable partial denture. These characteristics are described in this chapter as they relate to the etiology of periodontal disease. A more comprehensive review, with special emphasis on the interrelationship between restorative procedures and periodontal status, is presented in Chapters 71 and 72.

Margins of Restorations

Overhanging margins of dental restorations contribute to the development of periodontal disease by (1) changing the ecologic balance of the gingival sulcus to an area that favors the growth of disease-associated organisms (predominantly gram-negative anaerobic species) at the expense of the health-associated organisms (predominantly gram-positive facultative species)[110] and (2) inhibiting the patient's access to remove accumulated plaque.

The frequency of overhanging margins of proximal restorations varies from 16.5% to 75% in different studies.[28,67,93,150] A highly significant statistical relationship has been reported between marginal defects and reduced bone height.[28,84,93] Removal of overhangs permits more effective control of plaque, resulting in a reduction of gingival inflammation and a small increase in radiographic alveolar bone support[72,86,193] (Figures 10-16 and 10-17).

The location of the gingival margin for a restoration is directly related to the health status of adjacent periodontal tissues.[192] Numerous studies have shown a positive correlation between margins located apical to the marginal gingiva and the presence of gingival inflammation.[67,90,99,170,193] Subgingival margins are associated with large amounts of plaque, more severe gingivitis, and deeper pockets. Even high-quality restorations, if placed subgingivally, will increase plaque accumulation, gingival inflammation,[108,110,139,171] and the rate of gingival fluid flow.[19,75] Margins placed at the level of the gingival crest induce less severe inflammation, whereas supragingival margins are associated with a degree of periodontal health

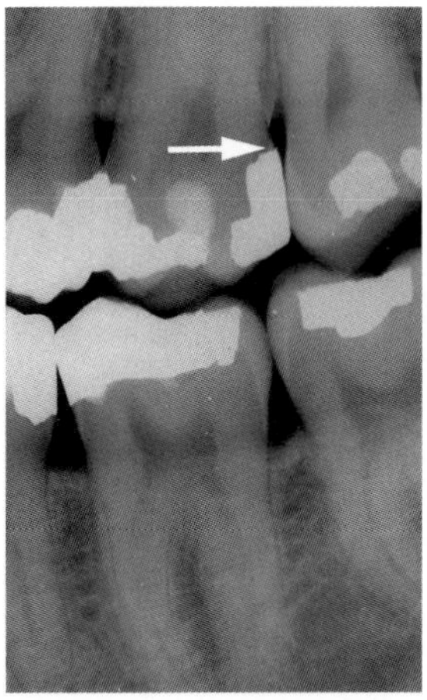

Figure 10-17 Radiograph of same patient shown in Figure 10-16 after the excessive amalgam has been removed.

similar to that seen with nonrestored interproximal surfaces.[63,192]

Roughness in the subgingival area is considered to be a major contributing factor to plaque buildup and subsequent gingival inflammation.[192] The subgingival zone is composed of the margin of the restoration, the luting material, and the prepared as well as the unprepared tooth surface. Sources of marginal roughness include the following:

- Grooves and scratches in the surface of carefully polished acrylic resin, porcelain, or gold restorations (Figure 10-18).
- Separation of the restoration margin and luting material from the cervical finish line, thereby exposing the rough surface of the prepared tooth (Figure 10-19).
- Dissolution and disintegration of the luting material between the preparation and the restoration, leaving a space (Figure 10-20).
- Inadequate marginal fit of the restoration.

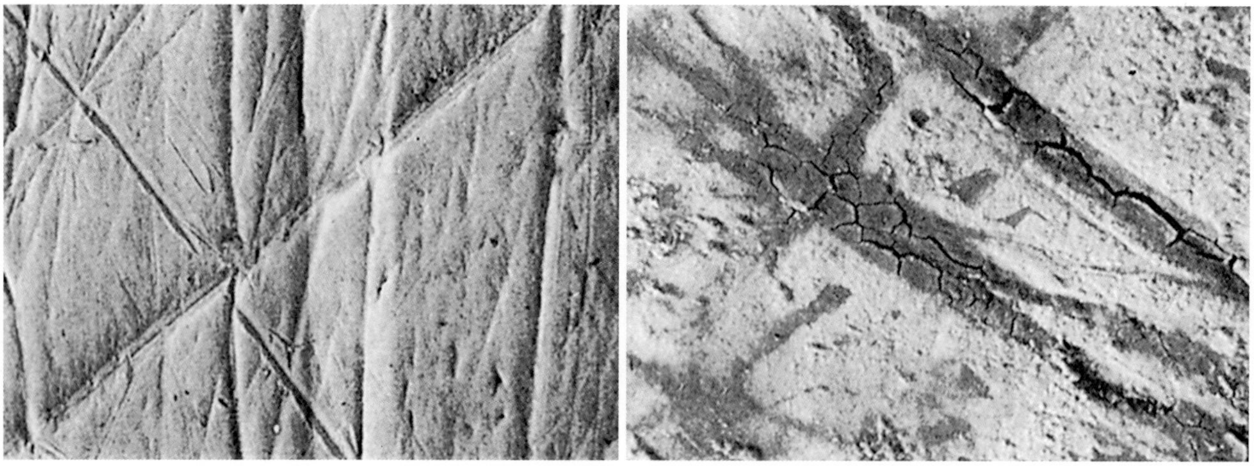

Figure 10-18 **A,** Polished gold alloy crown demonstrates surface scratches. **B,** Gold alloy crown that had been in the mouth for several years has scratches filled with deposits. (From Silness J: *Dental Clin North Am* 24:317, 1980.)

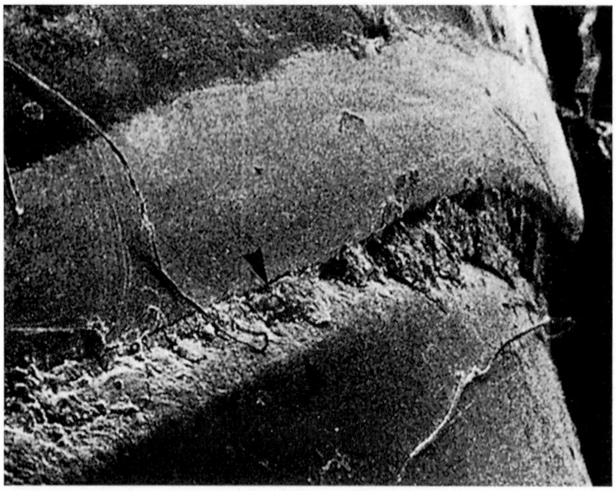

Figure 10-19 After cementation, luting material prevents approximation of the crown margin and the finishing line, leaving part of the prepared tooth uncovered (area between *arrowheads*). (From Silness J: *Dent Clin North Am* 24:317, 1980.)

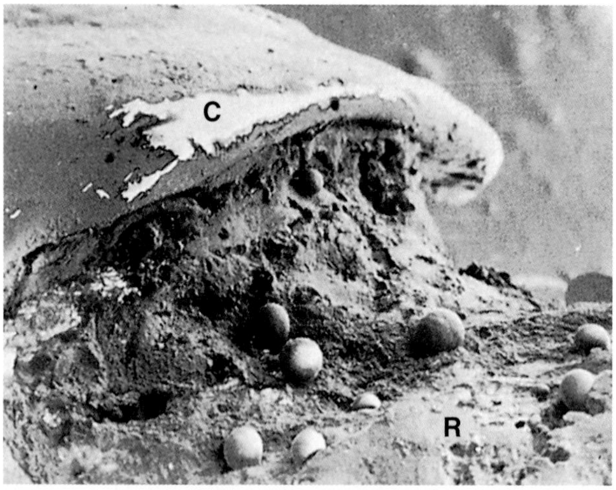

Figure 10-20 Craters have formed after dissolution and disintegration of the luting material. Spherical bodies are not identified. *C,* Crown; *R,* root. (From Silness J: *Dent Clin North Am* 24:317, 1980.)

Subgingival margins typically have a gap of 20 to 40 μm between the margin of the restoration and the unprepared tooth.[190] Colonization of this gap by bacterial plaque undoubtedly contributes to the detrimental effect of margins placed in a subgingival environment.

Contours and Open Contacts

Overcontoured crowns and restorations tend to accumulate plaque and possibly prevent the self-cleaning mechanisms of the adjacent cheek, lips, and tongue[7,105,137,220] (Figures 10-21 and 10-22). Restorations that fail to reestablish adequate interproximal embrasure spaces are associated with papillary inflammation. Undercontoured crowns that lack a protective height of contour may not be as detrimental during mastication as once thought.[220]

The contour of the occlusal surface, as established by the marginal ridges and related developmental grooves, normally serves to deflect food away from the interproximal spaces. The optimal cervico-occlusal location for a posterior contact is at the longest mesiodistal diameter of the tooth, which is generally just apical to the crest of the marginal ridge. The integrity and location of the proximal contacts along with the contour of the marginal ridges and developmental grooves typically prevent interproximal food impaction. *Food impaction* is the forceful wedging of food into the periodontium by occlusal forces. As the teeth wear down, their originally convex proximal surfaces become flattened, and the wedging effect of the opposing cusp is exaggerated. Cusps that tend to wedge food forcibly into interproximal embrasures are known as *plunger cusps*. The interproximal plunger cusp effect may also be observed when missing teeth are not replaced and the relationship between proximal contacts of adjacent teeth is altered. An intact,

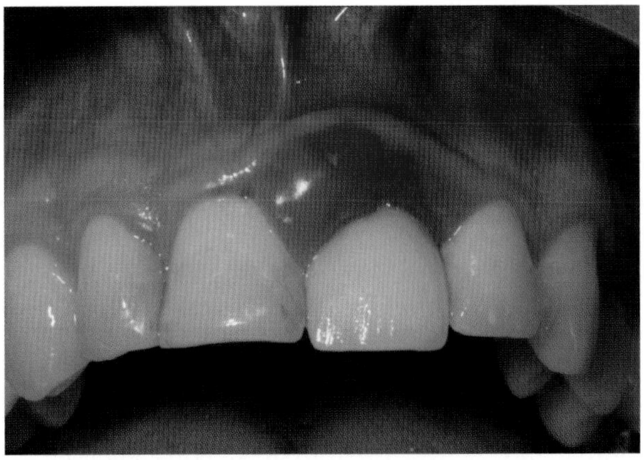

Figure 10-21 Inflamed marginal and papillary gingiva adjacent to overcontoured porcelain-fused-to-metal crown on the maxillary left central incisor.

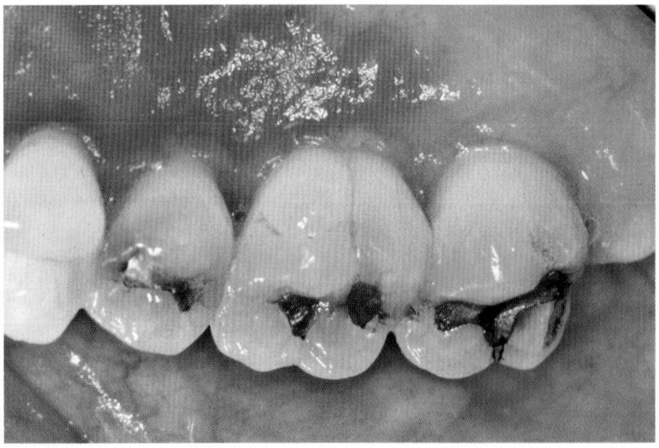

Figure 10-23 Inflamed palatal gingiva associated with a maxillary provisional acrylic partial denture. Note the substantial difference in color of the inflamed gingiva adjacent to the premolars and first molar compared with the gingiva adjacent to the second molar.

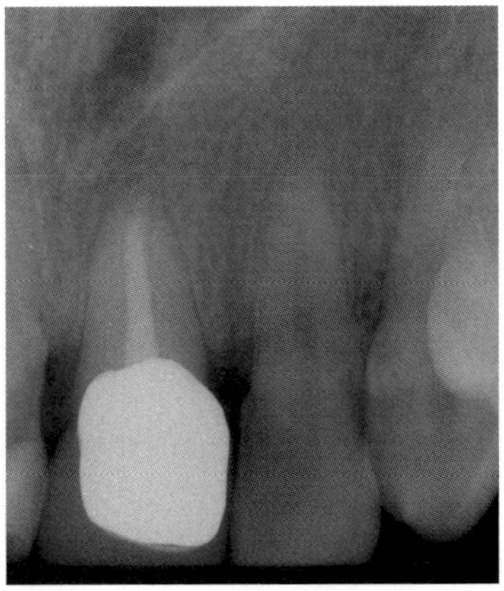

Figure 10-22 Radiograph of poorly fitting porcelain-fused-to-metal crown shown in Figure 10-21.

firm proximal contact precludes the forceful wedging of food into the interproximal embrasure space, whereas a light or open contact is conducive to impaction.

The classic analysis of the factors leading to food impaction was made by Hirschfeld,[88] who recognized the following factors: uneven occlusal wear, opening of the contact point as a result of loss of proximal support or from extrusion, congenital morphologic abnormalities, and improperly constructed restorations.

The presence of abnormalities does not necessarily lead to food impaction and periodontal disease. A study of interproximal contacts and marginal ridge relationships[110] in three groups of periodontally healthy males revealed that 0.7% to 76% of the proximal contacts were defective and 33.5% of adjacent marginal ridges were uneven.[149] However, greater probing depth and loss of clinical attachment have been reported for sites that exhibited both an open contact and food impaction compared with contralateral control sites without open contacts or food impaction.[95] Excessive anterior overbite is a common cause of food impaction on the lingual surfaces of the maxillary anterior teeth and the facial surfaces of the opposing mandibular teeth. These areas may be exemplified by attachment loss with gingival recession.

Materials

In general, restorative materials are not inherently injurious to the periodontal tissues.[7,101] One exception to this may be self-curing acrylics[212] (Figure 10-23).

Plaque that forms at the margins of restorations is similar to that founded on adjacent nonrestored tooth surfaces. The composition of plaque formed on all types of restorative materials is similar, with the exception of that formed on silicate.[145] Although surface textures of restorative materials differ in their capacity to retain plaque,[212,217] all can be adequately cleaned if they are polished[146,179] and accessible to methods of oral hygiene. The undersurface of pontics in fixed bridges should barely touch the mucosa. Access for oral hygiene is impeded by excessive pontic-to-tissue contact, thereby contributing to plaque accumulation, which will cause gingival inflammation and possibly formation of pseudopockets.[61,194]

Design of Removable Partial Dentures

After the insertion of partial dentures, the mobility of the abutment teeth, gingival inflammation, and periodontal pocket formation increase,[27,38,186] because partial dentures favor the accumulation of plaque, particularly if they cover the gingival tissue. Partial dentures that are worn during both night and day induce more plaque formation than those worn only during the day.[27] These observations emphasize the need for careful and personalized oral hygiene instruction to avoid harmful effects of partial dentures on the remaining teeth and periodontium.[19] The presence of removable partial dentures induces not only quantitative changes in dental plaque[65] but also qualitative changes, promoting the emergence of spirochetal microorganisms.[66]

Restorative Dentistry Procedures

The use of rubber dam clamps, matrix bands, and burs in such a manner as to lacerate the gingiva results in varying degrees of mechanical trauma and inflammation. Although such transient injuries generally heal, they are needless sources of discomfort to the patient. Forceful packing of a gingival retraction cord into the sulcus to prepare subgingival margins on a tooth or for the purpose of obtaining an impression may mechanically injure the periodontium and leave behind impacted debris capable of causing a foreign body reaction. (See Chapter 72 for a more detailed explanation.)

Malocclusion

Irregular alignment of teeth as found in cases of malocclusion may make plaque control more difficult. Several authors have found a positive correlation between crowding and periodontal disease,[37,152,200] whereas others have not.[64] Uneven marginal ridges of contiguous posterior teeth have a low correlation with pocket depth, loss of attachment, plaque, calculus, and gingival inflammation.[104] Roots of teeth that are prominent in the arch (Figures 10-24 and 10-25), such as in buccal or lingual version, or that are associated with a high frenal attachment and small quantities of attached gingiva, frequently exhibit recession.[2,134]

Failure to replace missing posterior teeth may have adverse consequences on the periodontal support for the remaining teeth.[43] The following scenario illustrates the possible ramifications of not replacing a missing posterior tooth. When the mandibular first molar is extracted, the initial change is a mesial drifting and tilting of the mandibular second and third molars with extrusion of the maxillary first molar. As the mandibular second molar tips mesially, its distal cusps extrude and act as plungers. The distal cusps of the mandibular second molar wedge between the maxillary first and second molars and open the contact by deflecting the maxillary second molar distally. Subsequently, food impaction may occur and may be accompanied by gingival inflammation, with eventual loss of the interproximal bone between the maxillary first and second molars.

The preceding example does not occur in all patients in whom mandibular first molars are not replaced. However, drifting and tilting of the remaining teeth with an accompanying alteration of the proximal contacts are generally a consequence of not replacing posterior teeth that have been extracted.

Tongue thrusting exerts excessive lateral pressure on the anterior teeth, which may result in spreading and tilting of the anterior teeth (Figures 10-26 and 10-27). Tongue thrusting is an important contributing factor in pathologic tooth migration and the development of an

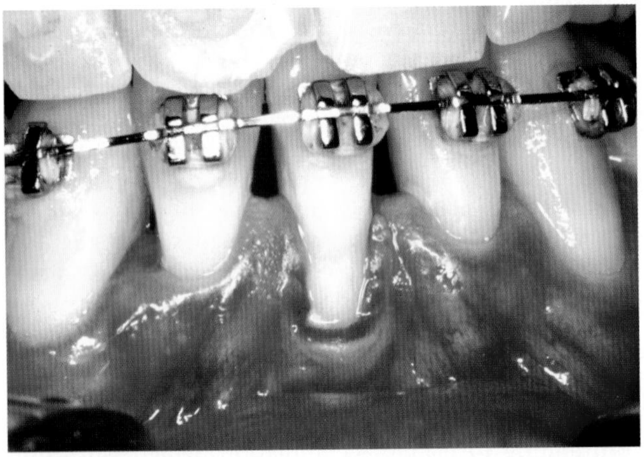

Figure 10-24 Lower incisor showing prominent root with gingival recession and lacking attached gingiva.

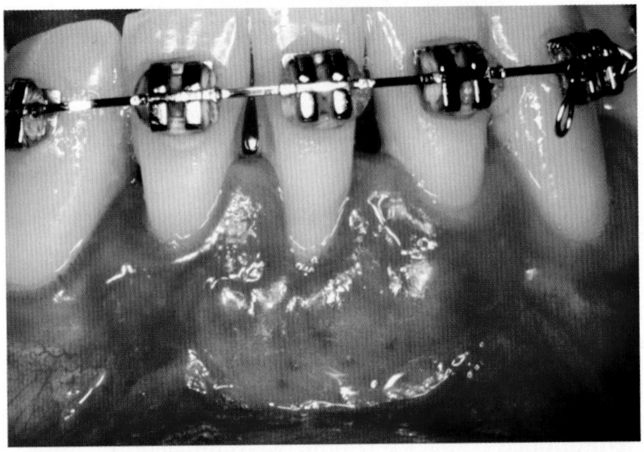

Figure 10-25 Same patient shown in Figure 10-24 after placement of a soft tissue graft to gain attached gingiva and treat gingival recession.

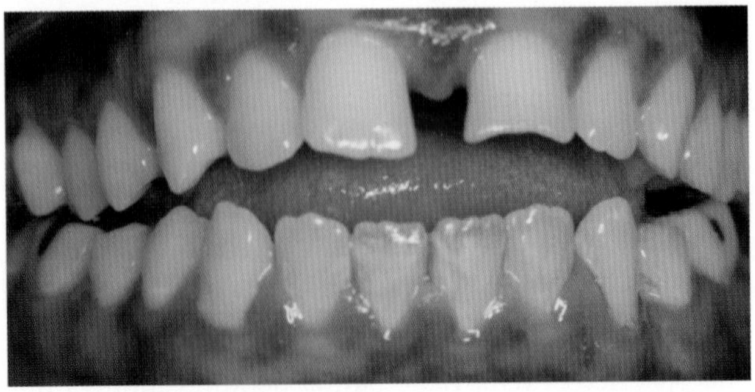

Figure 10-26 Anterior open bite with flared incisors, as observed in association with a habit of tongue thrusting.

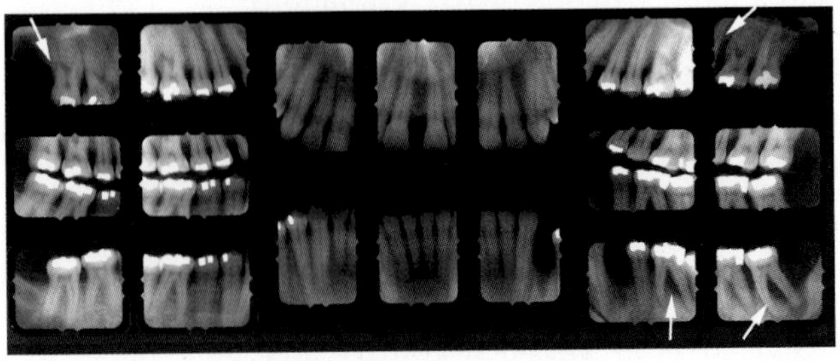

Figure 10-27 Radiographs of same patient shown in Figure 10-26 depicting anterior open bite. Note severe periodontal destruction *(arrows)* on molar regions.

anterior open bite.[40] Mouth breathing may be observed in association with a habit of tongue thrusting and an anterior open bite. Marginal and papillary gingivitis is frequently encountered in the maxillary anterior sextant in cases involving an anterior open bite with mouth breathing. However, the role of mouth breathing as a local etiologic factor is unclear because of the following conflicting evidence:

1. Mouth breathing has no effect on the prevalence or extent of gingivitis, except when considerable amounts of calculus are present.[5]
2. Mouth breathers have more severe gingivitis than non–mouth breathers with similar plaque scores.[91]
3. No relationship exists between mouth breathing and prevalence of gingivitis, except a slight increase in severity.[200]
4. Crowding of teeth is associated with gingivitis only in mouth breathers.[92]

Restorations that do not conform to the occlusal pattern of the mouth result in occlusal disharmonies that may cause injury to the supporting periodontal tissues. Histologic features of the periodontium for a tooth subjected to traumatic occlusion include a widened subcrestal periodontal ligament space, a reduction in collagen content of the oblique and horizontal fibers, an increase in vascularity and leukocyte infiltration, and an increase in the number of osteoclasts on bordering alveolar bone.[24] However, these observations are generally apical and separate from the bacterial-induced inflammation that occurs at the base of the sulcus. On the basis of current human trials, it is still impossible to answer definitively the question, "Does occlusal trauma modify the progression of periodontal attachment loss associated with sulcular inflammation?"[188] (See Chapter 29 for a more detailed explanation of periodontal trauma from occlusion and the periodontal response to external forces.)

Periodontal Complications Associated with Orthodontic Therapy

Orthodontic therapy may affect the periodontium by favoring plaque retention, by directly injuring the gingiva as a result of overextended bands, and by creating excessive forces, unfavorable forces, or both on the tooth and supporting structures.

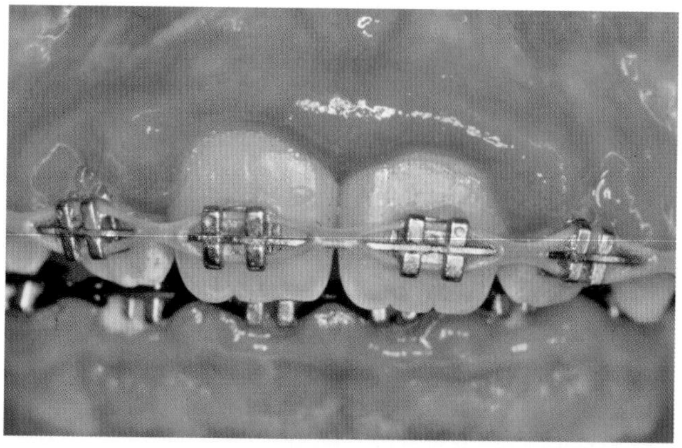

Figure 10-28 Gingival inflammation and enlargement associated with orthodontic appliance and poor oral hygiene.

Plaque Retention and Composition

Orthodontic appliances not only tend to retain bacterial plaque and food debris, resulting in gingivitis (Figure 10-28), but also are capable of modifying the gingival ecosystem. An increase in *Prevotella melaninogenica, Prevotella intermedia,* and *Actinomyces odontolyticus* and a decrease in the proportion of facultative microorganisms were detected in the gingival sulcus after placement of orthodontic bands.[53] *Actinobacillus actinomycetemcomitans* was found in at least one site in 85% of children wearing orthodontic appliances, compared with only 15% of the control subjects.[151]

Gingival Trauma and Alveolar Bone Height

Orthodontic treatment is often started soon after eruption of the permanent teeth, when the junctional epithelium is still adherent to the enamel surface. Orthodontic bands should not be forcefully placed beyond the level of attachment because this will detach the gingiva from the tooth and result in apical proliferation of the junctional epithelium, with an increased incidence of gingival recession.[153]

The mean alveolar bone loss per patient for adolescents who underwent 2 years of orthodontic care during a 5-year observation period ranged between 0.1 and 0.5 mm.[31] This small magnitude of alveolar bone loss was also noted in the control group and therefore was considered to be of little clinical significance. However, the degree of bone loss during adult orthodontic care may be higher than that observed in adolescents,[120] especially if the periodontal condition is not treated before initiating orthodontic therapy.

Tissue Response to Orthodontic Forces

Orthodontic tooth movement is possible because the periodontal tissues are responsive to externally applied forces.[169,185] Alveolar bone is remodeled by osteoclasts inducing bone resorption in areas of pressure and osteoblasts forming bone in areas of tension. Although moderate orthodontic forces usually result in bone remodeling and repair, excessive force may produce necrosis of the periodontal ligament and adjacent alveolar bone.[157-159] Excessive orthodontic forces also increase the risk of apical root resorption.[34,35] The prevalence of severe root resorption, as indicated by resorption of more than one third of the root length, during orthodontic therapy in adolescents has been reported at 3%.[98] The incidence of moderate to severe root resorption for incisors among adults age 20 to 45 years has been reported as 2% before treatment and 24.5% after treatment[120] (Figures 10-29, 10-30, and 10-31). *It is important to avoid excessive force and too-rapid tooth movement in orthodontic treatment.*

The use of elastics to close a diastema may result in severe attachment loss with possible tooth loss as the elastics migrate apically along the root (Figures 10-32 and 10-33). Surgical exposure of impacted teeth and orthodontic-assisted eruption may compromise the periodontal attachment on adjacent teeth (Figures 10-34

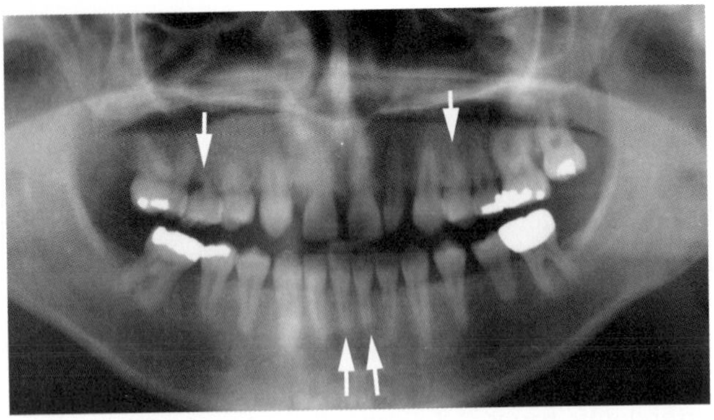

Figure 10-29 Panoramic radiograph illustrating that a limited degree of pretreatment root resorption *(arrows)* existed before orthodontic care was initiated.

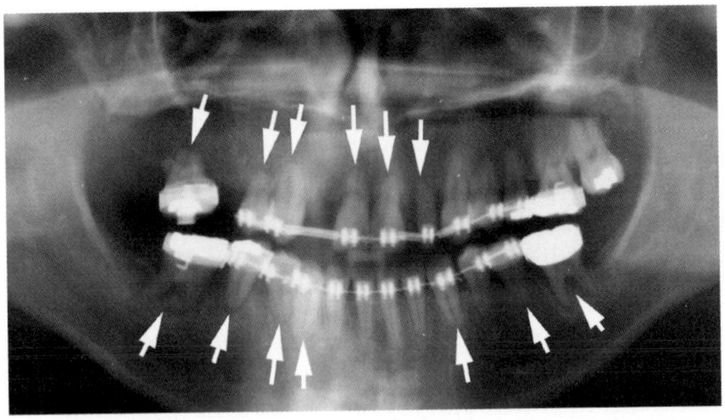

Figure 10-30 Panoramic radiograph of same patient depicted in Figure 10-29 after 4 years of intermittent orthodontic treatment. Note that several roots have undergone severe resorption *(arrows)* during orthodontic care.

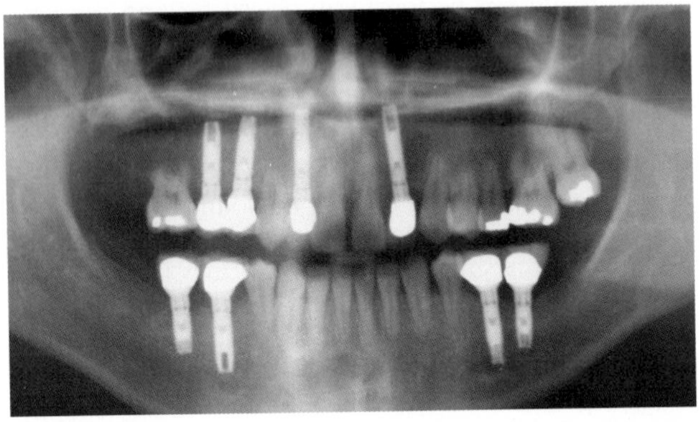

Figure 10-31 Panoramic radiograph of same patient depicted in Figure 10-30. Note the teeth that had developed extensive root resorption with accompanying hypermobility have been extracted and replaced by implant-supported bridgework.

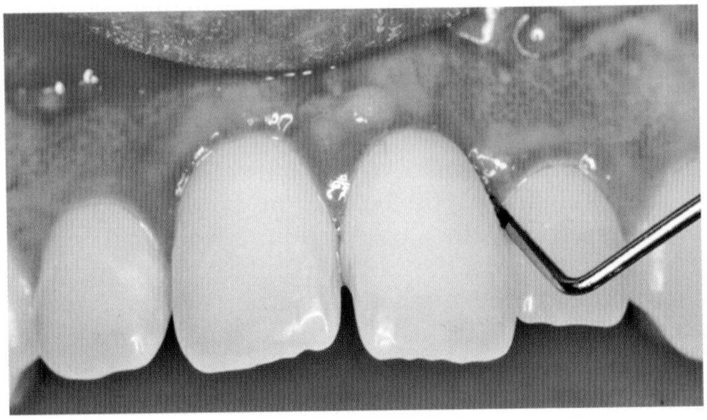

Figure 10-32 Maxillary central incisors in which an elastic ligature was used to close a midline diastema. Note inflamed gingiva and deep probing depths.

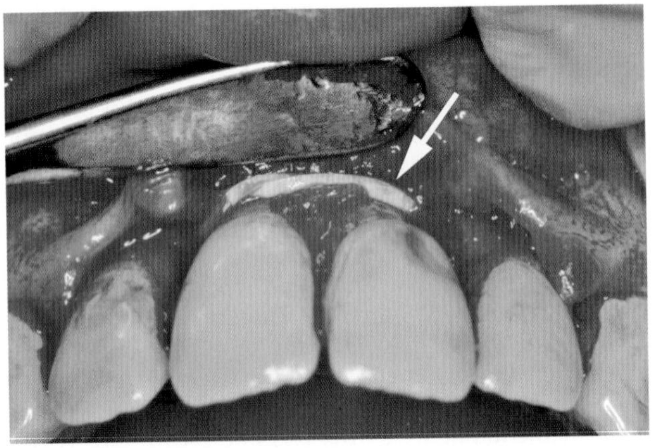

Figure 10-33 Same patient shown in Figure 10-32. A full-thickness mucoperiosteal flap has been reflected to expose the elastic ligature and angular intrabony defects around the central incisors.

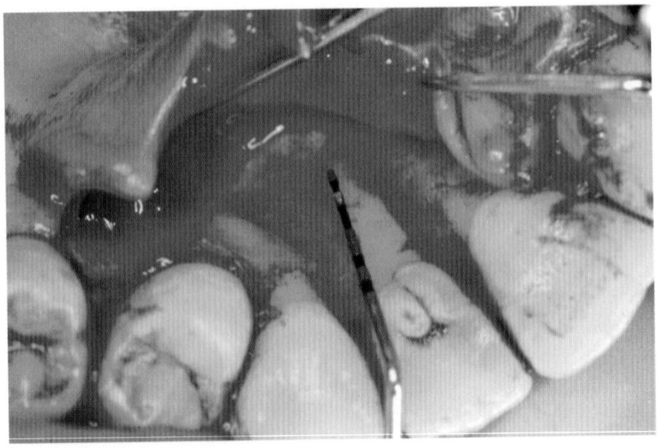

Figure 10-34 Radiograph of impacted maxillary canine that required surgical exposure and orthodontic assistance to erupt.

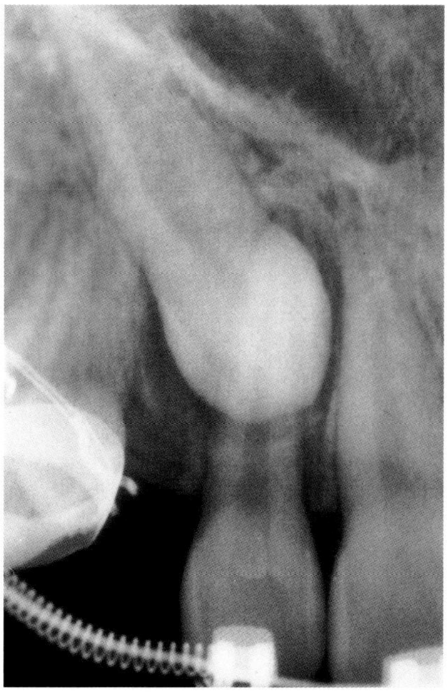

Figure 10-35 Palatal flap reflected to reveal bony dehiscence on the maxillary lateral incisor shown on radiograph in Figure 10-34.

and 10-35). However, the majority of impacted teeth surgically exposed and assisted in their eruption by orthodontic treatment subsequently exhibited 90% or more of their attachment as being intact.[87]

It has been reported that the dentoalveolar gingival fibers located within the marginal and attached gingiva are stretched when teeth are rotated during orthodontic therapy.[54] Surgical severing or removal of these gingival fibers in combination with a brief period of retention may reduce the incidence of relapse after orthodontic treatment intended to realign rotated teeth.[33,136]

Extraction of Impacted Third Molars

Numerous clinical studies have reported that the extraction of impacted third molars often results in the creation of vertical defects distal to the second molars.[8] This iatrogenic effect is unrelated to flap design[44] and appears to occur more often when third molars are extracted in individuals older than 25 years.[8,106,131] Other factors that appear to play a role in the development of lesions on the distal surface of second molars, particularly in those older than 25 years, include the presence of visible plaque, bleeding on probing, root resorption in the contact area between second and third molars, presence of a pathologically widened follicle, inclination of the third molar, and proximity of the third molar to the second molar[106] (Figure 10-36).

Habits and Self-Inflicted Injuries

Patients might not be aware of their self-inflicted injurious habits that may be important to the initiation and progression of their periodontal disease. Mechanical

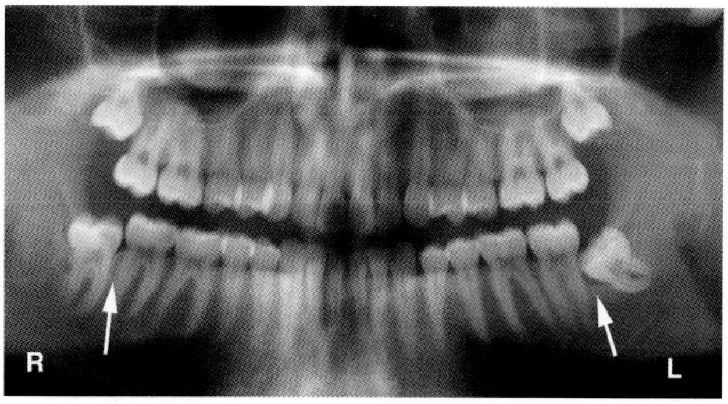

Figure 10-36 Panoramic radiograph illustrating a mesially impacted lower-left third molar with a widened follicle and no apparent bone on the distal interproximal surface of the second molar. Alternatively, the lower-right third molar is vertically impacted and exhibits interproximal bone distal to the second molar and the mesial surface of the third molar.

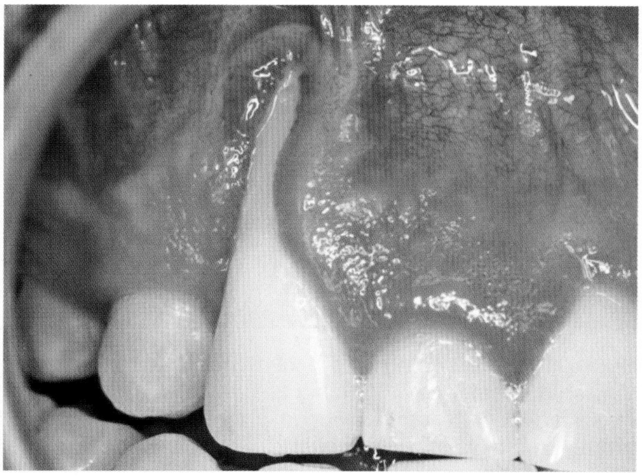

Figure 10-37 Gingival recession on a maxillary canine caused by self-inflicted trauma from the patient's fingernail.

forms of trauma can result from improper use of a toothbrush, wedging of toothpicks between the teeth, application of fingernail pressure against the gingiva, and other causes (e.g., burns from pizza)[29] (Figure 10-37). Sources of chemical irritation include topical application of caustic medications (e.g., aspirin, cocaine), allergic reactions to toothpaste and chewing gum, and use of chewing tobacco or concentrated mouth rinses.[189]

Trauma Associated with Oral Jewelry

The use of piercing jewelry in the lip or tongue has become more common recently among teenagers and young adults (Figure 10-38). Whittle and Lamden[216] surveyed 62 dentists and found that 97% had seen patients with either lip- or tongue-piercing jewelry within the previous 12 months. The incidence of lingual recession with pocket formation (Figure 10-39) and radiographic evidence of bone loss (Figure 10-40) was 50% among subjects with a mean age of 22 years who wore lingual "barbells" for 2 or more years.[38] Chipped lower anterior teeth were noted in 47% of the patients who wore tongue-piercing jewelry for 4 years or more. Patients need to be informed

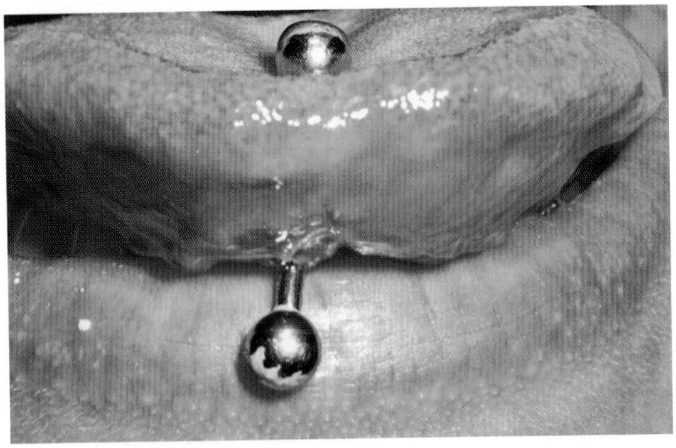

Figure 10-38 Pierced tongue with oral jewelry.

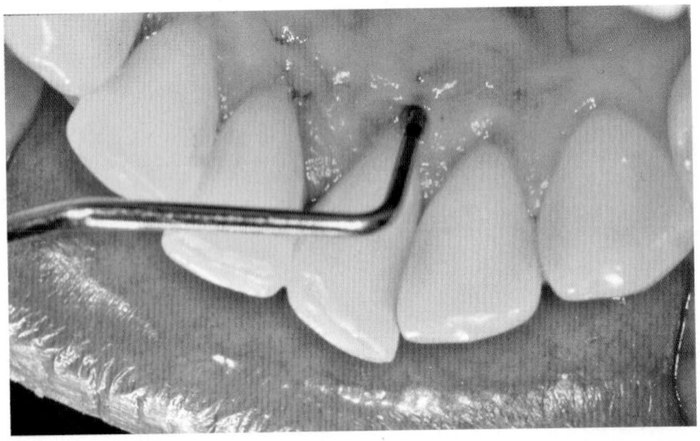

Figure 10-39 Probing depth of 8 mm with 10 mm of clinical attachment loss on lingual surface of lower central incisor adjacent to oral jewelry in pierced tongue. Pulp for central incisor was found to be vital on both ice and electrical stimulation. (Courtesy Dr. Leonidas Batas, Minneapolis.)

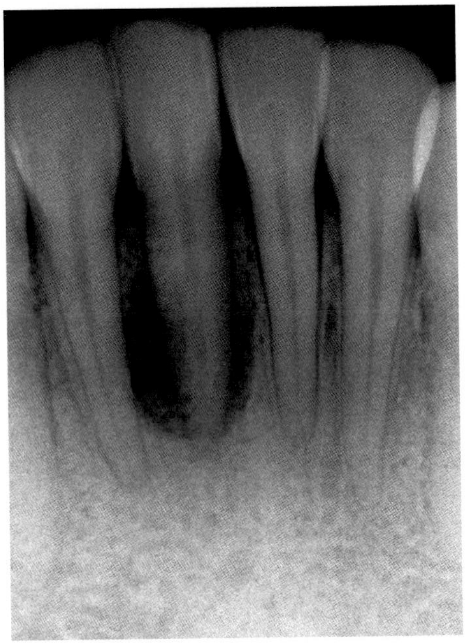

Figure 10-40 Radiograph of lower incisor shown in Figure 10-39, depicting bone loss associated with pierced tongue and oral jewelry.

of the risks of wearing oral jewelry and cautioned against such practices.

Toothbrush Trauma

Abrasions of the gingiva as well as alterations in tooth structure may result from aggressive brushing in a horizontal or rotary fashion. The deleterious effect of abusive brushing is accentuated when highly abrasive dentifrices are used. The gingival changes attributable to toothbrush trauma may be acute or chronic. The acute changes vary in their appearance and duration, from scuffing of the epithelial surface to denudation of the underlying connective tissue with the formation of a painful gingival ulcer (Figure 10-41). Diffuse erythema and denudation of the attached gingiva throughout the mouth may be striking sequelae of overzealous brushing. Signs of acute gingival abrasion are frequently noted when the patient first uses a new brush. Puncture lesions may be produced when heavy pressure is applied to firm bristles that are aligned perpendicular to the surface of the gingiva. A forcibly embedded toothbrush bristle may be retained in the gingiva and cause an acute gingival abscess (see Chapter 24).

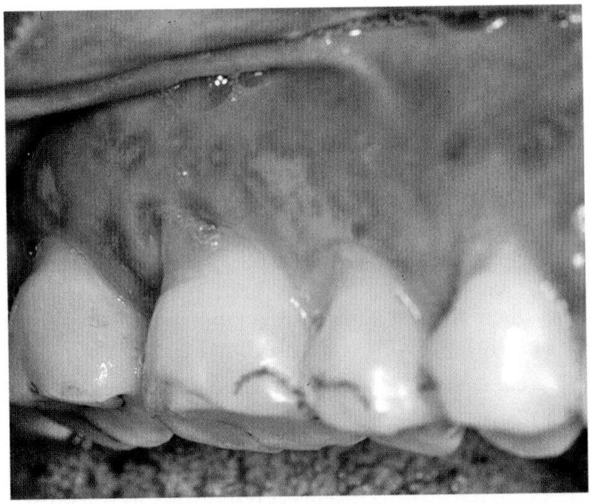

Figure 10-41 Overzealous use of a toothbrush may denude the gingival epithelial surface and expose the underlying connective tissue as a painful ulcer.

Chronic toothbrush trauma results in gingival recession with denudation of the root surface. Interproximal attachment loss is generally a consequence of bacteria-induced periodontitis, whereas buccal and lingual attachment loss is frequently the result of toothbrush abrasion.[195] Improper use of dental floss may result in lacerations of the interdental papilla.

Chemical Irritation

Acute gingival inflammation may be caused by chemical irritation resulting from either sensitivity or nonspecific tissue injury. In allergic inflammatory states, the gingival changes range from simple erythema to painful vesicle

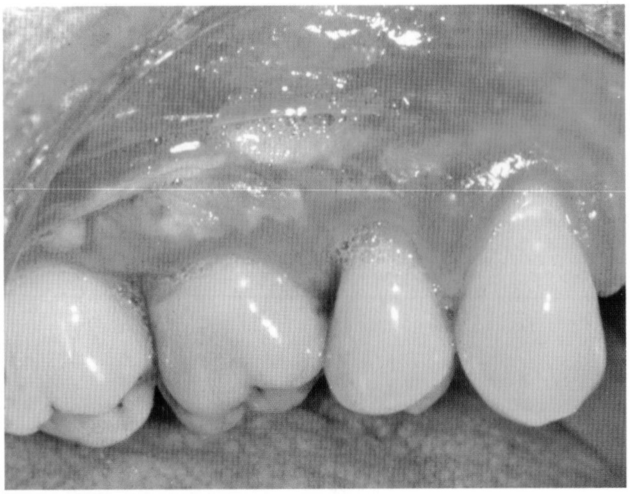

Figure 10-42 Chemical burn caused by aspirin, with sloughing of gingival tissue and accompanying recession.

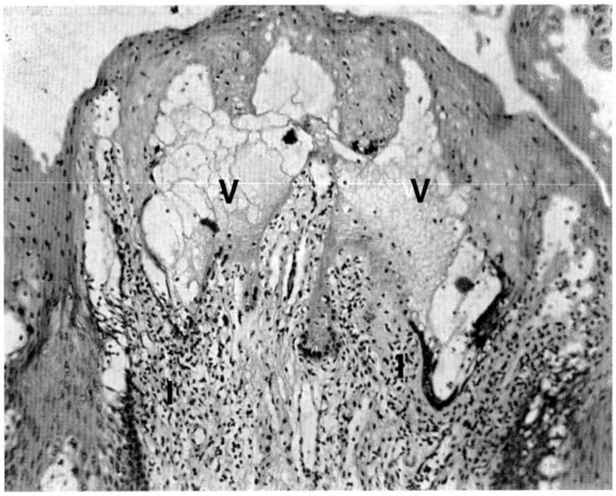

Figure 10-43 Biopsy of aspirin-induced chemical burn. Note intraepithelial vesicles *(V)* and inflammatory infiltrate *(I)* within the underlying connective tissue.

formation and ulceration. This chemical irritation often explains the severe reactions to ordinarily innocuous mouthwashes, dentifrices, and denture materials.

Acute inflammation with ulceration may be produced by the nonspecific injurious effect of chemicals on the gingival tissues. The indiscriminate use of strong mouthwashes, topical application of corrosive drugs such as aspirin (Figure 10-42) or cocaine, and accidental contact with drugs such as phenol or silver nitrate are common examples of chemicals that cause irritation of the gingiva. A histologic view of an aspirin-induced chemical burn depicts vacuoles with serous exudates and inflammatory infiltrates in the connective tissue (Figure 10-43).

Tobacco Use

Approximately 25% of the U.S. population smokes cigarettes,[41] and in other areas of the world, the percentage of smokers is even higher.[15,122] Smoking was associated with the prevalence of necrotizing ulcerative gingivitis (NUG) as early as 1947.[155,156] In investigations in which plaque levels were kept to a minimum for both smoking and nonsmoking groups or the data were adjusted for this difference, smokers had more sites with deeper pockets[22,23,113] and greater attachment loss.[9,17,78,113] The prevalence of furcation involvement among smokers was higher,[9,143] as was the degree of alveolar bone loss.[21,75,218] It can be concluded that smokers have greater attachment loss and bone loss, an increased number of deep pockets, and an increased amount of calculus formation. However, smokers demonstrate varied levels of plaque and inflammation, with a tendency toward decreased inflammation.

Depending on which clinical parameters are used to assess periodontal disease, smokers are 2.6 to 6 times more likely to develop periodontal disease than nonsmokers.[18,23,78,81,199] The odds ratio for a moderate smoker (15-30 pack-years) to have periodontal disease is 2.77 times that of a nonsmoker, and a heavy smoker (≥30 pack-years) is 4.75 times more likely to have periodontal disease than a nonsmoker.[22] *Pack-years* can be defined as the number of cigarettes (packs) smoked per day multiplied by the number of years that an individual smoked. Smoking also appears to be a contributing factor for periodontitis.[1,121,123] MacFarlane et al.[121] reported that greater than 90% of their refractory periodontitis patients were smokers, compared with approximately 30% of the general population being smokers. Periodontal maintenance patients who smoke are reported to be twice as likely to lose teeth over a 5-year period compared with periodontal maintenance patients who do not smoke.[133] Smoking is one of the most significant risk factors currently available to predict the development and progression of periodontitis.[17,18,78]

Two possible explanations for smokers experiencing more prevalent and severe periodontal disease are (1) they harbor more pathogenic subgingival microflora and (2) their flora might be more virulent. However, several investigations failed to find any significant difference in the percentage of periodontal pathogens recovered from deep pockets in smokers and nonsmokers.[163,164,199] The analysis of subgingival plaque samples collected from a large cross-sectional population in Erie County, New York, revealed that smokers were more likely to be infected with *A. actinomycetemcomitans, Porphyromonas gingivalis,* and *Bacteroides forsythus* (now *Tannerella forsythia*) than nonsmokers.[221] However, the elevated values for these putative pathogens were not statistically higher than those found in nonsmokers. A diminished response to nonsurgical therapy has been reported for smokers. Recent research has indicated that it is more difficult to suppress certain bacteria such as *A. actinomycetemcomitans,*[172] *P. gingivalis,*[77,83] and *B. forsythus*[77] in smokers than in nonsmokers, which may partially explain a diminished response.

Although bacteria are the primary etiologic factors of periodontal disease, a patient's diminished host response may contribute to increased disease susceptibility. Smokers exhibit depressed numbers of helper T lymphocytes, which are important to stimulate B-cell function for antibody production,[14,49,68] thereby reducing serum levels of immunoglobulin G (IgG).[14] Smoking has been shown to decrease serum IgG2 levels in adult Caucasian subjects[166] and correlate with a dramatic reduction in levels of serum IgG2, anti–*A. actinomycetemcomitans* in African-American smokers with generalized, aggressive periodontitis.[201] Smokers have also been reported to exhibit reduced serum IgG antibodies to *Prevotella intermedia* and *Fusobacterium nucleatum*.[80] Neutrophils from smokers with refractory periodontitis exhibit impaired phagocytosis.[121] Neutrophils with diminished chemotaxis, phagocytosis, or both[103] may be a consequence of a lower antibody titer, which curtails opsonization. Nicotine has been shown to decrease gingival blood flow.[45] Periodontal wound healing may be adversely affected by exposure to tobacco or nicotine, which may impair revascularization in soft tissues[138] and hard tissues.[173]

Smoking has been identified as a significant variable to predict the response to periodontal treatment.[133,145] Most investigations that evaluated the effect of smoking on nonsurgical therapy have demonstrated less reduction in probing depth* and smaller gains in attachment levels in smokers compared with nonsmokers.[3,83] Smokers who were treated with surgical periodontal therapy and subsequently followed with maintenance care exhibited less probing depth reduction,[3,97,162] smaller gains in clinical attachment levels[3,97] and less gain in bone height[32] than nonsmokers. Heavy cigarette smoking decreases the amount of root coverage obtainable with thick, free gingival grafts,[134] whereas the effect of smoking on subepithelial connective tissue grafts is not conclusive.[85,224] Gains in clinical attachment were less in smokers than nonsmokers when guided tissue regenerative procedures were employed.[48,119,176,205,206] Several studies have found implant success rates to be lower in smokers.[13,52,71,96] Implant success rates greater than 95% have been reported among nonsmokers versus less than 89% in smokers during a 6-year period.[13] Patients who quit smoking 1 week before surgery and abstained for 8 weeks after surgical placement of their implants had only one-third as many failures compared with those individuals who continued to smoke.[12] Implant failure rates in these subjects were similar to rates in nonsmokers. However, other retrospective implant studies have failed to identify smoking as a variable associated with failure.[135,214] A 15-year longitudinal study detected a slightly greater amount of marginal bone loss around implants supporting mandibular fixed prosthesis in smokers compared with nonsmokers.[114]

In summary, smoking has a negative effect on periodontal therapy. However, periodontal therapy did result in an improvement in the periodontal condition of both smokers and nonsmokers when compared with their pretreatment status.

The prevalence and severity of periodontal disease in former smokers are between those of nonsmokers and current smokers.[30,81,82] This implies that once the patients stop smoking, additional adverse effects attributed to smoking may be minimized. However, previous damage is not reversed. Both nonsmokers and former smokers respond more favorably to periodontal therapy than current smokers, whereas no significant difference in response was noted between former smokers and nonsmokers.[77,97] The benefits of terminating smoking on periodontal treatment do not appear to be related to the number of years since smoking was halted.[77] Therefore a past history of smoking does not appear to be deleterious to the response of current periodontal treatment.

*References 3, 76, 77, 83, 97, 161, 172.

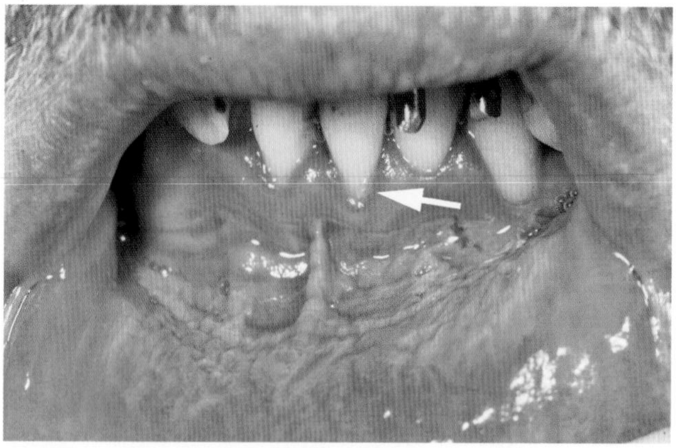

Figure 10-44 Gingival recession and hyperkeratosis of the vestibular mucosa that developed following the use of chewing tobacco.

Feldman et al.[60] reported that plaque, calculus, probing depth, and bone loss measurements for cigar smokers were intermediate to those for nonsmokers and cigarette smokers while tending to be closer to nonsmoker values.

Approximately 9% of the U.S. high school population currently uses smokeless tobacco products such as snuff and chewing tobacco.[42] The relationship between the use of smokeless tobacco and squamous cell carcinoma in the oral cavity is well established.[219] A strong relationship has been established between white oral mucosal lesions and the use of smokeless tobacco by athletes[58,175] and adolescents.[50,148,204] These white mucosal lesions occur in approximately 50% to 60% of smokeless tobacco users, whereas 25% to 30% exhibit localized attachment loss in the form of gingival recession on the facial surfaces of mandibular anterior teeth[74,160,175] (Figure 10-44). One study demonstrated that 97.5% of these leukoplakia lesions are clinically resolved after abstaining from smokeless tobacco for 6 weeks.[132]

Radiation Therapy

Radiation therapy has cytotoxic effects on both normal cells and malignant cells. A typical total dose of radiation for head and neck tumors is in the range of 5000 to 8000 centigrays (cGy = 1 rad).[154] The total dose of radiation is generally given in partial incremental doses referred to as *fractionation*. Fractionation helps minimize the adverse effects of the radiation while maximizing the death rate for the tumor cells.[62] Fractionated doses are typically administered in the range of 100 to 1000 cGy per week.

Radiation treatment induces an obliterative endarteritis that results in soft tissue ischemia and fibrosis while irradiated bone becomes hypovascular and hypoxic.[129] Adverse affects of head and neck radiation therapy include dermatitis and mucositis of the irradiated area as well as muscle fibrosis and trismus, which may restrict access to the oral cavity.[177] The mucositis typically develops 5 to 7 days after radiation therapy is initiated. The severity of the mucositis can be reduced by asking the patient to avoid secondary sources of irritation to the mucous membrane, such as smoking, alcohol, and spicy foods. Use of a chlorhexidine digluconate mouth rinse may help reduce the mucositis.[167] However, all chlorhexidine mouth rinses currently available in the United States have a high alcohol content that may act as an astringent, which dehydrates the mucosa, thereby intensifying the pain. Saliva production is permanently impaired when salivary glands located within the portal of radiation receive 6000 cGy or more.[130] Xerostomia results in greater plaque accumulation and a reduced buffering capacity from the remaining saliva. The use of effective oral hygiene, professional dental prophylactic cleaning, fluoride application, and frequent dental examinations are essential to control caries and periodontal disease. The use of customized trays appears to be a more effective method of fluoride application than using the toothbrush.[102]

Periodontal attachment loss and tooth loss were greater on the radiated side in cancer patients treated with high-dose unilateral radiation compared with the nonradiated control side of the dentition.[57] Irradiated patients should receive prophylactic antibiotic coverage before receiving appropriate nonsurgical periodontal therapy after the patient's initial recovery from radiation therapy.[59] Dental and periodontal infections can pose a severe risk to a patient who has been treated with head and neck radiation. Therefore the dental therapist may choose to consult with the patient's oncologist before initiating therapy. The risk of osteoradionecrosis must be evaluated before extracting a tooth or performing periodontal surgery in an irradiated site. Precautions must be taken regarding prophylactic antibiotics, atraumatic surgical technique, microbiologic culture and sensitivity, restricted use of local anesthetic with vasoconstrictor, and the need for hyperbaric oxygen therapy. (Refer to Chapter 44 for more detail on the periodontal management of medically compromised patients.)

REFERENCES

1. Adams D: Diagnosis and treatment of refractory periodontitis, *Curr Opin Dent* 2:33, 1992.
2. Addy M, Dummer P, Hunter M, et al: A study of the association of fraenal attachment, lip coverage and vestibular depth with plaque and gingivitis, *J Periodontol* 58:752, 1987.
3. Ah M, Johnson G, Kaldahl W, et al: The effect of smoking on the response to periodontal therapy, *J Clin Periodontol* 21:91, 1994.
4. Albandar J, Kingman A, Brown L, et al: Gingival inflammation and subgingival calculus as determinants of disease progression in early-onset periodontitis, *J Clin Periodontol* 25:231, 1998.
5. Alexander A: Habitual mouth breathing and its effect on gingival health, *Parodontologie* 24:49, 1970.
6. Anerud A, Löe H, Boysen H: The natural history and clinical course of calculus formation in man, *J Clin Periodontol* 18:160, 1991.
7. App G: Effect of silicate, amalgam and cast gold on the gingiva, *J Prosthet Dent* 11:522, 1961.
8. Ash M, Costich E, Hayward J: A study of periodontal hazards of third molars, *J Periodontol* 33:209, 1962.
9. Axelsson P, Paulander J, Lindhe J: Relationship between smoking and dental status in 35-, 50-, 65-, and 75-year old individuals, *J Clin Periodontol* 25:297, 1998.
10. Baer P, Burstone M: Esterase activity associated with formation of deposits on teeth, *Oral Surg* 12:1147, 1959.
11. Baer P, Keyes P, White C: Studies on experimental calculus formation in the rat. XII. On the transmissibility of factors affecting dental calculus, *J Periodontol* 39:86, 1968.
12. Bain C: Smoking and implant failure: benefits of a smoking cessation protocol, *Int J Oral Maxillofac Implants* 11:756, 1996.
13. Bain C, Moy P: The association between the failure of dental implants and cigarette smoking, *Int J Oral Maxillofac Implants* 8:609, 1993.
14. Barbour S, Nakashim K, Zhang J, et al: Tobacco and smoking: environmental factors that modify the host response (immune system) and have an impact on periodontal health, *Crit Rev Oral Biol Med* 8:437, 1997.
15. Bartecchi C, MacKenzie T, Schrier R: The human costs of tobacco use. I, *N Engl J Med* 331:907, 1994.
16. Baumhammers A, Stallard R: A method for the labeling of certain constituents in the organic matrix of dental calculus, *J Dent Res* 45:1568, 1966.
17. Beck J, Koch C, Offenbacher S: Incidence of attachment loss over 3 years in older adults: new and progressing lesions, *Community Dent Oral Epidemiol* 23:291, 1995.
18. Beck J, Koch G, Rozier R, et al: Prevalence and risk indicators for periodontal attachment loss in a population of older community-dwelling blacks and whites, *J Periodontol* 61:521, 1990.
19. Bergman B, Hugoson A, Olsson C: Periodontal and prosthetic conditions in patients treated with removable partial dentures and artificial crowns, *Acta Odontol Scand* 29:621, 1971.
20. Bergström J: Cigarette smoking as risk factor in chronic periodontal disease, *Community Dent Oral Epidemiol* 17:245, 1989.
21. Bergström J, Eliasson S: Cigarette smoking and alveolar bone height in subjects with high standard of oral hygiene, *J Clin Periodontol* 14:466, 1987.
22. Bergström J, Eliasson S: Noxious effect of cigarette smoking on periodontal health, *J Periodont Res* 22:513, 1987.
23. Bergström J, Preber H: Tobacco use as a risk factor, *J Periodontol* 65:545, 1994.
24. Biancu S, Ericsson I, Lindhe J: Periodontal ligament tissue reactions to trauma and gingival inflammation: an experimental study in beagle dogs, *J Clin Periodontol* 22:772, 1995.
25. Bibby B: The formation of salivary calculus, *Dent Cosmos* 77:668, 1935.
26. Birkeland J, Jorkjend L: The effect of chewing apples on dental plaque and food debris, *Community Dent Oral Epidemiol* 2:161, 1974.
27. Bissada N, Ibrahim S, Barsoum W: Gingival response to various types of removable partial dentures, *J Periodontol* 45:651, 1974.
28. Bjorn AL, Bjorn H, Grcovic B: Marginal fit of restorations and its relation to periodontal bone level, *Odont Rev* 20:311, 1969.
29. Blanton P, Hurt W, Largent M: Oral factitious injuries, *J Periodontol* 48:33, 1977.

30. Bolin A, Eklund G, Frithiof L, et al: The effect of changed smoking habits on marginal alveolar bone loss, *Swed Dent J* 17:211, 1993.
31. Bondemark L: Interdental bone changes after orthodontic treatment: a 5-year longitudinal study, *Am J Orthod Dentofac Orthop* 114:25, 1998.
32. Bostrom L, Linder L, Bergström J: Influence of smoking on the outcome of periodontal surgery: a 5-year follow-up, *J Clin Periodontol* 25:194, 1998.
33. Brain W: The effect of surgical transsection of free gingival fibers on the regression of orthodontically rotated teeth in the dog, *Am J Orthod* 55:50, 1969.
34. Brezniak N, Wasserstein A: Root resorption after orthodontic treatment. Part 1. Literature review, *Am J Orthod Dentofac Orthop* 103:62, 1993.
35. Brezniak N, Wasserstein A: Root resorption after orthodontic treatment. Part 2. Literature review, *Am J Orthod Dentofac Orthop* 103:138, 1993.
36. Buchanan S, Jenderseck R, Granet M, et al: Radiographic detection of dental calculus, *J Periodontol* 58:747, 1987.
37. Buckley L: The relationship between malocclusion and periodontal disease, *J Periodontol* 43:415, 1972.
38. Campbell A, Moore A, Williams E, et al: Tongue piercing: impact of time and barbell stem length on lingual gingival recession and tooth chipping, *J Periodontol* 73:289, 2002.
39. Carlsson G, Hedegard B, Koivumaa K: Studies in partial dental prosthesis. IV. Final results of a four-year longitudinal investigation of dentogingivally supported partial dentures, *Acta Odontol Scand* 23:443, 1965.
40. Carranza F Sr, Carraro J: El empuje lingual como factor traumatizante en periodoncia, *Rev Asoc Odontol Argent* 47:105, 1959.
41. Centers for Disease Control and Prevention: Cigarette smoking among adults, *MMWR* 48:1217, 1997.
42. Centers for Disease Control and Prevention: Tobacco use among high school students—United States, *MMWR* 47:229, 1998.
43. Chaikin B: Anterior periodontal destruction due to the loss of one or more unreplaced molars, *Dent Items Int* 61:17, 1939.
44. Chin Quee T, Gosselin D, Millar E, et al: Surgical removal of the fully impacted mandibular third molar: the influence of flap design and alveolar bone height, *J Periodontol* 56:625, 1985.
45. Clarke N, Shephard B, Hirsch R: The effects of intra-arterial epinephrine and nicotine on gingival circulation, *Oral Surg Oral Med Oral Pathol* 52:577, 1981.
46. Clerehugh V, Abdeia R, Hull P: The effect of subgingival calculus on the validity of clinical probing measurements, *J Dent* 24:329, 1996.
47. Conroy C, Sturzenberger O: The rate of calculus formation in adults, *J Periodontol* 39:142, 1968.
48. Cortellini P, Pini Prato G, Tonetti M: Long-term stability of clinical attachment following guided tissue regeneration and conventional therapy, *J Clin Periodontol* 23:106, 1996.
49. Costabel U, Bross K, Reuter C, et al: Alterations in immunoregulatory T-cell subsets in cigarette smokers: a phenotypic analysis of bronchoalveolar and blood lymphocytes, *Chest* 90:39, 1986.
50. Creath C, Cutter G, Bradley D, et al: Oral leukoplakia and adolescent smokeless tobacco use, *Oral Surg Oral Med Oral Pathol* 72:35, 1991.
51. Dawes C: Recent research on calculus, *NZ Dent J* 94:60, 1998.
52. De Bruyn H, Collaert B: The effect of smoking on early implant failure, *Clin Oral Implant Res* 5:260, 1994.
53. Diamanti-Kipioti A, Gusberti F, Lang N: Clinical and microbiological effects of fixed orthodontic appliances, *J Clin Periodontol* 14:326, 1987.
54. Edwards J: A study of the periodontium during orthodontic rotation of teeth, *Am J Orthod* 54:441, 1968.
55. Egelberg J: Local effect of diet on plaque formation and development of gingivitis in dogs. III. Effect of frequency of meals and tube feeding, *Odontol Rev* 16:50, 1965.
56. Ennever J: Microbiologic mineralization: a calcifiable cell-free extract from a calcifiable microorganism, *J Dent Res* 41:1383, 1983.
57. Epstein J, Lunn R, Le N, et al: Periodontal attachment loss in patients after head and neck radiation therapy, *Oral Surg Oral Med Oral Pathol* 86:673, 1998.
58. Ernster V, Grady DG, Greene JC, et al: Smokeless tobacco use and health effects among baseball players, *JAMA* 264:218, 1990.
59. Fattore L, Strauss R, Bruno J: The management of periodontal disease in patients who have received radiation therapy for head and neck cancer, *Spec Care Dentist* 7:120, 1987.
60. Feldman R, Alman J, Chauncey H: Periodontal disease indexes and tobacco smoking in healthy aging men, *Gerodontics* 3:43, 1987.
61. Flemmig T, Sorensen J, Newman M, et al: Gingival enhancement in fixed prosthodontics. Part II. Microbiologic findings, *J Prosthet Dent* 65:365, 1991.
62. Fletcher G: The role of irradiation in the management of squamous-cell carcinomas of the mouth and throat, *Head Neck Surg* 1:441, 1979.
63. Flores-de-Jacoby L, Zafiropoulos G, Ciancio S: The effect of crown margin location on plaque and periodontal health, *Int J Periodont Restor Dent* 9:197, 1989.
64. Geiger A, Wasserman B, Turgeon L: Relationship of occlusion and periodontal disease. VIII. Relationship of crowding and spacing to periodontal destruction and gingival inflammation, *J Periodontol* 45:43, 1974.
65. Ghamrawy E: Quantitative changes in dental plaque formation related to removable partial dentures, *J Oral Rehabil* 3:115, 1976.
66. Ghamrawy E: Qualitative changes in dental plaque formation related to removable partial dentures, *J Oral Rehabil* 6:183, 1979.
67. Gilmore N, Sheiham A: Overhanging dental restorations and periodontal disease, *J Periodontol* 42:8, 1971.
68. Ginns L, Goldenheim P, Miller L: T-lymphocyte subsets in smoking and lung cancer: analyses of monoclonal antibodies and flow cytometry, *Am Rev Res Dis* 126:265, 1982.
69. Glock G, Murray M: Chemical investigation of salivary calculus, *J Dent Res* 17:257, 1938.
70. Gonzales F, Sognnaes R: Electromicroscopy of dental calculus, *Science* 131:156, 1960.
71. Gorman L, Lambert P, Morris H, et al: The effect of smoking on implant survival at second stage surgery: DICRG Interim Report No 5, Dental Implant Clinical Research Group, *Implant Dent* 3:165, 1994.
72. Gorzo I, Newman H, Strahan J: Amalgam restoration, plaque removal and periodontal health, *J Clin Periodontol* 6:98, 1979.
73. Greene J: Oral hygiene and periodontal disease, *Am J Public Health* 53:913, 1963.
74. Greer R, Poulson T: Oral tissue alterations associated with the use of smokeless tobacco by teen-agers. Part I. Clinical findings, *Oral Surg Oral Med Oral Pathol* 56:275, 1983.
75. Grossi S, Genco R, Machtei E, et al: Assessment of risk for periodontal disease. II. Risk indicators for alveolar bone loss, *J Periodontol* 66:23, 1995.

76. Grossi S, Skrepcinski F, DeCaro T, et al: Response to periodontal therapy in diabetics and smokers, *J Periodontol* 67:1094, 1996.
77. Grossi S, Zambon J, Machtei E, et al: Effects of smoking and smoking cessation on healing after mechanical therapy, *J Am Dent Assoc* 128:599, 1997.
78. Grossi S, Zambon J, Ho A, et al: Assessment of risk for periodontal disease. I. Risk indicators for attachment loss, *J Periodontol* 65:260, 1994.
79. Gustafsson B, Krasse B: Dental calculus in germ free rats, *Acta Odontol Scand* 20:135, 1962.
80. Haber J: Cigarette smoking: a major risk factor for periodontitis, *Compend Contin Educ Dent* 15:1002, 1994.
81. Haber J, Kent RL: Cigarette smoking in periodontal practice, *J Periodontol* 63:100, 1992.
82. Haber J, Wattles J, Crowley M, et al: Evidence for cigarette smoking as a major risk factor for periodontitis, *J Periodontol* 64:16, 1993.
83. Haffajee A, Cugini M, Dibart S, et al: The effect of SRP on the clinical and microbiological parameters of periodontal diseases, *J Clin Periodontol* 24:324, 1997.
84. Hakkarainen K, Ainamo J: Influence of overhanging posterior tooth restorations of alveolar bone height in adults, *J Clin Periodontol* 7:114, 1980.
85. Harris R: The connective tissue with partial thickness double pedicle graft: the results of 100 consecutively treated defects, *J Periodontol* 65:448, 1994.
86. Highfield J, Powell R: Effects of removal of posterior overhanging metallic margins of restorations upon the periodontal tissues, *J Clin Periodontol* 5:169, 1978.
87. Hinrichs J, El Deeb M, Waite D, et al: Periodontal evaluation of canines erupted through grafted alveolar cleft defects, *J Oral Maxillofac Surg* 42:717, 1984.
88. Hirschfeld I: Food impaction, *J Am Dent Assoc* 17:1504, 1930.
89. Hodge H, Leung S: Calculus formation, *J Periodontol* 21:211, 1950.
90. Huttner G: Follow-up study of crowns and abutments with regard to the crown edge and the marginal periodontium, *Dtsch Zahnarztl Z* 26:724, 1971.
91. Jacobson L: Mouth breathing and gingivitis, *J Periodontal Res* 8:269, 1973.
92. Jacobson L, Linder-Aronson S: Crowding and gingivitis: a comparison between mouth breathers and non-mouth breathers, *Scand J Dent Res* 80:500, 1972.
93. Jeffcoat M, Howell T: Alveolar bone destruction due to overhanging amalgam in periodontal disease, *J Periodontol* 51:599, 1980.
94. Jenkins G: *The physiology of the mouth,* Oxford, 1966, Blackwell Scientific Publications.
95. Jernberg G, Bakdash B, Keenan K: Relationship between proximal tooth open contact and periodontal disease, *J Periodontol* 54:529, 1983.
96. Jones J, Triplett R: The relationship of cigarette smoking to impaired intraoral wound healing: a review of evidence and implications for patient care, *J Oral Maxillofac Surg* 50:237, 1992.
97. Kaldahl W, Johnson G, Patil K, et al: Levels of cigarette consumption and response to periodontal therapy, *J Periodontol* 67:675, 1996.
98. Kaley J, Phillips C: Factors related to root resorption in edgewise practice, *Angle Orthod* 61:125, 1991.
99. Karlsen K: Gingival reactions to dental restorations, *Acta Odontol Scand* 28:895, 1970.
100. Kashket S, Zhang J, Niederman R: Gingival inflammation induced by food and short-chain carboxylic acids, *J Dent Res* 77:412, 1998.
101. Kawakara H, Yamagani A, Nakamura M Jr: Biological testing of dental materials by means of tissue culture, *Int Dent J* 18:443, 1968.
102. Keene H, Fleming T, Toth B: Cariogenic microflora in patients with Hodgkin's disease before and after mantle field radiotherapy, *Oral Surg Oral Med Oral Pathol* 78:577, 1994.
103. Kenney EG, Kraal JH, Saxe SR, et al: The effect of cigarette smoke on human oral polymorphonuclear leukocytes, *J Periodontal Res* 12:227, 1977.
104. Kepic T, O'Leary T: Role of marginal ridge relationships as an etiologic factor in periodontal disease, *J Periodontol* 49:570, 1978.
105. Koivumaa K, Wennstrom A: A histological investigation of the changes in gingival margins adjacent to gold crowns, *Odont T* 68:373, 1960.
106. Kugelberg C: Third molar surgery, *Curr Opin Dent* 2:9, 1992.
107. Kupczyk L, Conroy M: The attachment of calculus to root planed surfaces, *Periodontics* 6:78, 1968.
108. Lang N, Kiel R, Anderhalden K: Clinical and microbiological effect of subgingival restorations with overhanging or clinically perfect margins, *J Clin Periodontol* 10:563, 1983.
109. Leach S, Saxton C: An electron microscopic study of the acquired pellicle and plaque formed on the enamel of human incisors, *Arch Oral Biol* 11:1081, 1966.
110. Leon A: Amalgam restorations and periodontal disease, *Br Dent J* 140:377, 1976.
111. Leung S, Jensen A: Factors controlling the deposition of calculus, *Int Dent J* 8:613, 1958.
112. Lilienthal B, Amerena V, Gregory G: An epidemiological study of chronic periodontal disease, *Arch Oral Biol* 10:553, 1965.
113. Linden G, Mullally B: Cigarette smoking and periodontal destruction in young adults, *J Periodontol* 65:718, 1994.
114. Lindquist L, Carlsson G, Jemt T: A prospective 15-year follow-up study of mandibular fixed prosthesis supported by osseointegrated implants: clinical results and marginal bone loss, *Clin Oral Implant Res* 7:329, 1996.
115. Little M, Hazen S: Dental calculus composition. 2. Subgingival calculus: ash, calcium, phosphorus, and sodium, *J Dent Res* 43:645, 1964.
116. Little M, Bowman L, Dirksen T: The lipids of supragingival calculus, *J Dent Res* 43:836, 1964.
117. Little M, Bowman L, Casciani C, et al: The composition of dental calculus. III. Supragingival calculus: the amino acid and saccharide component, *Arch Oral Biol* 11:385, 1966.
118. Löe H, Schiott C: The effect of mouth rinses and topical application of chlorhexidine on the development of dental plaque and gingivitis in man, *J Periodontal Res* 5:79, 1970.
119. Luepke P, Mellonig J, Brunvold M: A clinical evaluation of a bioresorbable barrier with and without decalcified freeze-dried bone allograft in the treatment of molar furcations, *J Clin Periodontol* 24:440, 1998.
120. Lupi J, Handelman C, Sadowsky C: Prevalence and severity of apical root resorption and alveolar bone loss in orthodontically treated adults, *Am J Orthod Dentofac Orthop* 109:28, 1996.
121. MacFarlane G, Herzberg M, Wolff L, et al: Refractory periodontitis associated with abnormal polymorphonuclear leukocyte phagocytosis and cigarette smoking, *J Periodontol* 63:908, 1992.
122. MacKenzie T, Bartecchi C, Schrier R: The human costs of tobacco use. II, *N Engl J Med* 331:975, 1994.
123. Magnusson I, Walker C: Refractory periodontitis or recurrence of disease, *J Clin Periodontol* 23:289, 1996.
124. Mandel I: Calculus formation: the role of bacteria and mucoprotein, *Dent Clin North Am* 4:731, 1960.

125. Mandel I: Histochemical and biochemical aspects of calculus formation, *Periodontics* 1:43, 1963.
126. Mandel I: Biochemical aspects of calculus formation, *J Periodontal Res* 4(suppl):7, 1969.
127. Mandel I, Levy B, Wasserman B: Histochemistry of calculus formation, *J Periodontol* 28:132, 1957.
128. Manly R: A structureless recurrent deposit on teeth, *J Dent Res* 22:479, 1973.
129. Marciani R, Ownby H: Osteoradionecrosis of the jaw, *J Oral Maxillofac Surg* 44:218, 1986.
130. Markitziu A, Zafiropoulos G, Tsalkis L, et al: Gingival health and salivary function in head and neck–irradiated patients: a five-year follow-up, *Oral Surg Oral Med Oral Pathol* 73:427, 1992.
131. Marmary Y, Brayer L, Tzukert A, et al: Alveolar bone repair following extraction of impacted mandibular third molars, *Oral Surg Oral Med Oral Pathol* 61:324, 1986.
132. Martin G, Brown J, Eifler C, et al: Oral leukoplakia status six weeks after cessation of smokeless tobacco use, *J Am Dent Assoc* 130:945, 1999.
133. McGuire M, Nunn M: Prognosis versus actual outcome. III. The effectiveness of clinical parameters in accurately predicting tooth survival, *J Periodontol* 67:666, 1996.
134. Miller P: Root coverage with the free gingival graft: factors associated with incomplete coverage, *J Periodontol* 58:674, 1987.
135. Minsk L, Polson A, Weisgold A, et al: Outcome failures of endosseous implants from a clinical training center, *Compend Contin Educ Dent* 17:849, 1996.
136. Moffett B: Remodeling changes of the facial sutures, periodontal and temporomandibular joints produced by orthodontic forces in rhesus monkeys, *Bull Pac Coast Soc Orthod* 44:46, 1969.
137. Morris M: Artificial crown contours and gingival health, *J Prosthet Dent* 12:1146, 1962.
138. Mosely L, Finseth F, Goody M: Nicotine and its effects on wound healing, *Plast Reconstr Surg* 61:570, 1978.
139. Mueller H: The effect of artificial crown margins on the periodontal conditions in a group of periodontally supervised patients treated with fixed bridges, *J Clin Periodontol* 13:97, 1986.
140. Mühlemann H, Schroeder H: Dynamics of supragingival calculus formation, *Adv Oral Biol* 1:175, 1964.
141. Mühler J, Ennever J: Occurrence of calculus through several successive periods in a selected group of subjects, *J Periodontol* 33:22, 1962.
142. Mukherjee S: Formation and prevention of supragingival calculus, *J Periodontal Res* 3(suppl 2):1, 1968.
143. Mullally B, Linden G: Molar furcation involvement associated with cigarette smoking in periodontal referrals, *J Clin Periodontol* 23:658, 1996.
144. Neuman W, Neuman M: *The chemical dynamics of bone mineral*, Chicago, 1958, University of Chicago Press.
145. Newman M, Kornman K, Holtzman S: Association of clinical risk factors with treatment outcomes, *J Periodontol* 65:489, 1994.
146. Norman R, Mehia R, Swartz M, et al: Effect of restorative materials on plaque composition, *J Dent Res* 51:1596, 1972.
147. Normann W, Regolati B, Renggli H: Gingival reaction to well-fitted subgingival proximal gold inlays, *J Clin Periodontol* 1:120, 1974.
148. Offenbacher S, Weathers D: Effects of smokeless tobacco on the periodontal, mucosal and caries status of adolescent males, *J Oral Pathol* 14:169, 1985.
149. O'Leary T, Badell M, Bloomer R: Interproximal contact and marginal ridge relationships in periodontally healthy young males classified as to orthodontic status, *J Periodontol* 46:6, 1975.
150. Pack A, Coxhead L, McDonald B: The prevalence of overhanging margins in posterior amalgam restorations and periodontal consequences, *J Clin Periodontol* 17:145, 1990.
151. Paolantonio M, Girolamo G, Pedrazzoli V, et al: Occurrence of *Actinobacillus actinomycetemcomitans* in patients wearing orthodontic appliances: a cross-sectional study, *J Clin Periodontol* 23:112, 1996.
152. Paunio K: The role of malocclusion and crowding in the development of periodontal disease, *Int Dent J* 23:420, 1973.
153. Pearson L: Gingival height of lower central incisors, orthodontically treated and untreated, *Angle Orthod* 38:337, 1968.
154. Peterson D, D'Ambrosio J: Nonsurgical management of head and neck cancer patients, *Dent Clin North Am* 38:425, 1994.
155. Pindborg J: Tobacco and gingivitis. I. Statistical examination of the significance of tobacco in the development of ulceromembranous gingivitis and in the formation of calculus, *J Dent Res* 26:261, 1947.
156. Pindborg J: Tobacco and gingivitis. II. Correlation between consumption of tobacco, ulceromembranous gingivitis and calculus, *J Dent Res* 28:460, 1949.
157. Polson A: The relative importance of plaque and occlusion in periodontal disease, *J Clin Periodontol* 13:923, 1986.
158. Polson A, Reed BE: Long-term effect of orthodontic treatment on crestal alveolar bone levels, *J Periodontol* 55:28, 1984.
159. Polson A, Adams R, Zander H: Osseous repair in the presence of active tooth hypermobility, *J Clin Periodontol* 10:370, 1983.
160. Poulson T, Lindenmuth J, Greer R: A comparison of the use of smokeless tobacco in rural and urban teenagers, *CA Cancer J Clin* 34:248, 1984.
161. Preber H, Bergström J: The effect of non-surgical treatment on periodontal pockets in smokers and non-smokers, *J Clin Periodontol* 13:319, 1986.
162. Preber H, Bergström J: Effect of cigarette smoking on periodontal healing following surgical therapy, *J Clin Periodontol* 17:324, 1990.
163. Preber H, Bergström J, Linder L: Occurrence of periopathogens in smoker and non-smoker patients, *J Clin Periodontol* 19:667, 1992.
164. Preber H, Linder L, Bergström J: Periodontal healing and periopathogenic microflora in smokers and non-smokers, *J Clin Periodontol* 22:946, 1995.
165. Prinz H: The origin of salivary calculus, *Dent Cosmos* 63:231, 1921.
166. Quinn S, Zhang J, Gunsolley J, et al: The influence of smoking and race on adult periodontitis and serum IgG2 levels, *J Periodontol* 69:171, 1998.
167. Raether D, Walker P, Bostrum B, et al: Effectiveness of oral chlorhexidine for reducing stomatitis in a pediatric bone marrow transplant population, *Pediatr Dent* 11:37, 1989.
168. Ramfjord S: The periodontal status of boys 11 to 17 years old in Bombay, India, *J Periodontol* 32:237, 1961.
169. Reitan K: Tissue changes following experimental tooth movement as related to the time factor, *Dent Rec* 73:559, 1953.
170. Renggli H: The influence of subgingival proximal filling borders on the degree of inflammation of the adjacent gingiva: a clinical study, *Schweiz Monatsschr Zahnheilkd* 84:181, 1974.
171. Renggli H, Regolati B: Gingival inflammation and plaque accumulation by well-adapted supragingival and subgingival proximal restorations, *Helv Odontol Acta* 16:99, 1972.
172. Renvert S, Dahlen G, Widstrom M: The clinical and microbiological effects of non-surgical periodontal therapy

in smokers and non-smokers, *J Clin Periodontol* 25:153, 1998.
173. Riebel G, Boden S, Whitesides T, et al: The effect of nicotine on incorporation of cancellous bone graft in an animal model, *Spine* 20:2198, 1995.
174. Rizzo A, Martin G, Scott D, et al: Mineralization of bacteria, *Science* 135:439, 1962.
175. Robertson P, Walsh M, Greene J, et al: Periodontal effects associated with the use of smokeless tobacco, *J Periodontol* 61:438, 1990.
176. Rosen P, Marks M, Reynolds M: Influence of smoking on long-term clinical results of intrabony defects treated with regenerative therapy, *J Periodontol* 67:1159, 1996.
177. Rothwell B: Prevention and treatment of the orofacial complications of radiotherapy, *J Am Dent Assoc* 114:316, 1987.
178. Rowles S: The inorganic composition of dental calculus. In Blackwood HJ, editor: *Bone and tooth,* Oxford, 1964, Pergamon Press.
179. Sanchez-Sotres L, van Huysen G, Gilmore H: A histologic study of gingival tissue response to amalgam, silicate and resin restorations, *J Periodontol* 42:8, 1969.
180. Schoff F: Periodontia: an observation on the attachment of calculus, *Oral Surg* 8:154, 1955.
181. Schroeder H: Inorganic content and histology of early dental calculus in man, *Helv Odontol Acta* 7:17, 1963.
182. Schroeder H: Crystal morphology and gross structures of mineralizing plaque and of calculus, *Helv Odontol Acta* 9:73, 1965.
183. Schroeder H: Formation and inhibition of dental calculus, Berne, 1969, Hans Huber.
184. Schroeder H, Bambauer H: Stages of calcium phosphate crystallization during calculus formation, *Arch Oral Biol* 11:1, 1966.
185. Schwartz A: Tissue changes incidental to orthodontic tooth movement, *Orthod Oral Surg Rad Int J* 18:331, 1932.
186. Scoman S: Study of the relationship between periodontal disease and the wearing of partial dentures, *Aust Dent J* 8:206, 1963.
187. Selvig J: Attachment of plaque and calculus to tooth surfaces, *J Periodontal Res* 5:8, 1970.
188. Serio F, Hawley C: Periodontal trauma and mobility: diagnosis and treatment planning, *Dent Clin North Am* 43:37, 1999.
189. Serio F, Siegel M, Slade B: Plasma cell gingivitis of unusual origin, *J Periodontol* 62:390, 1991.
190. Setz J, Diehl J: Gingival reaction on crowns with cast and sintered metal margins: a progressive study, *J Prosthet Dent* 71:442, 1994.
191. Sharawy A, Sabharwal K, Socransky S, et al: A quantitative study of plaque and calculus formation in normal and periodontally involved mouths, *J Periodontol* 37:495, 1966.
192. Silness J: Fixed prosthodontics and periodontal health, *Dent Clin North Am* 24:317, 1980.
193. Sorensen J, Larsen I, Jorgensen K: Gingival and alveolar bone response to marginal fit of subgingival crown margins, *Scand J Dent Res* 94:109, 1986.
194. Sorensen J, Doherty F, Newman M, et al: Gingival enhancement in fixed prosthodontics. Part I. Clinical findings, *J Prosthet Dent* 65:100, 1991.
195. Spieler E: Preventing toothbrush abrasion and the efficacy of the Alert toothbrush, *Compend Contin Educ Dent* 17:478, 1996.
196. Standford J: Analysis of the organic portion of dental calculus, *J Dent Res* 45:128, 1966.
197. Stanton G: The relation of diet to salivary calculus formation, *J Periodontol* 40:167, 1969.
198. Stewart R, Ratcliff P: The source of components of subgingival plaque and calculus, *Periodont Abstr* 14:102, 1966.
199. Stoltenberg J, Osborn J, Pihlstrom B, et al: Association between cigarette smoking, bacterial pathogens, and periodontal status, *J Periodontol* 64:1225, 1993.
200. Sutcliffe P: Chronic anterior gingivitis: an epidemiological study in school children, *Br Dent J* 125:47, 1968.
201. Tangada S, Califano J, Nakashima K, et al: The effect of smoking on serum IgG2 reactive with *Actinobacillus actinomycetemcomitans* in early-onset periodontitis patients, *J Periodontol* 68:842, 1997.
202. Theilade J, Schroeder H: Recent results in dental calculus research, *Int Dent J* 16:205, 1966.
203. Tibbetts L, Kashiwa H: A histochemical study of early plaque mineralization, Abstract No 616, *J Dent Res* 19:202, 1970.
204. Tomar S, Winn D, Swango P, et al: Oral mucosal smokeless tobacco lesions among adolescents in the United States, *J Dent Res* 76:1277, 1997.
205. Tonetti M, Pini-Prato G, Cortellini P: Effect of cigarette smoking on periodontal healing following GTR in infrabony defects: a preliminary retrospective study, *J Clin Periodontol* 22:229, 1995.
206. Trombelli L, Kim C, Zimmerman G, et al: Retrospective analysis of factors related to clinical outcome of guided tissue regeneration procedures in intrabony defects, *J Clin Periodontol* 24:366, 1997.
207. Turesky S, Renstrup G, Glickman I: Effects of changing the salivary environment on progress of calculus formation, *J Periodontol* 33:45, 1962.
208. Volker J, Pinkerton D: Acid production in saliva carbohydrates, *J Dent Res* 26:229, 1947.
209. Volpe A, Kupczak L, King W, et al: In vivo calculus assessment. Part IV. Parameters of human clinical studies, *J Periodontol* 40:76, 1969.
210. Von der Fehr F, Brudevold F: In vitro calculus formation, *J Dent Res* 39:1041, 1960.
211. Waerhaug J: The source of mineral salts in subgingival calculus, *J Dent Res* 34:563, 1955.
212. Waerhaug J, Zander H: Reaction of gingival tissue to self-curing acrylic restorations, *J Am Dent Assoc* 54:760, 1957.
213. Wasserman B, Mandel J, Levy BM: In vitro calcification of calculus, *J Periodontol* 29:145, 1958.
214. Weyant R: Characteristics associated with the loss and peri-implant tissue health of endosseous dental implants, *Int J Oral Maxillofac Implants* 9:95, 1994.
215. White D: Dental calculus: recent insights into occurrence, formation, prevention, removal and oral health effects of supragingival and subgingival deposits, *Eur J Oral Sci* 105:508, 1997.
216. Whittle JG, Lamden KH: Lip and tongue piercing: experiences and views of general dental practitioners in South Lancashire, *Prim Dent Care* 11:92, 2004.
217. Wise M, Dykema R: The plaque retaining capacity of four dental materials, *J Prosthet Dent* 33:178, 1975.
218. Wouters F, Salonen L, Frithiof L, et al: Significance of some variables on interproximal alveolar bone height based on cross-sectional epidemiologic data, *J Clin Periodontol* 20:199, 1993.
219. Wray A, McGuirt F: Smokeless tobacco usage associated with oral carcinoma: incidence, treatment, outcome, *Arch Otolaryngol Head Neck Surg* 119:929, 1993.
220. Yuodelis R, Weaver J, Sapkos S: Facial and lingual contours of artificial complete crowns and their effect on the periodontium, *J Prosthet Dent* 29:61, 1973.
221. Zambon J, Grossi S, Machtei E, et al: Cigarette smoking increases the risk for subgingival infection with periodontal pathogens, *J Periodontol* 67:1050, 1996.

222. Zander H: The attachment of calculus to root surfaces, *J Periodontol* 24:16, 1953.
223. Zander H, Hazen S, Scott D: Mineralization of dental calculus, *Proc Soc Exp Biol Med* 103:257, 1960.
224. Zucchelli G, Clauser C, De Sanctis M, et al: Mucogingival versus guided tissue regeneration procedures in the treatment of deep recession type defects, *J Periodontol* 69:138, 1998.

Genetic Factors Associated with Periodontal Disease

Bryan S. Michalowicz and Bruce L. Pihlstrom

11

CHAPTER

■ ■ ■

CHAPTER OUTLINE

GENETIC STUDY DESIGNS
 Segregation Analyses
 Twin Studies
 Linkage and Association Studies
AGGRESSIVE PERIODONTAL DISEASES
 Associations with Genetic and Inherited Conditions
 Segregation Analyses

Linkage Studies
Association Studies
CHRONIC PERIODONTITIS
 Twin Studies
 Association Studies
CLINICAL IMPLICATIONS OF GENETIC STUDIES
FUTURE OF GENETIC STUDIES IN PERIODONTOLOGY

Traditionally, periodontitis was thought to be strictly environmental in origin. Despite this belief, it was recognized that only a portion of the variability of disease in the population could be explained by environmental factors alone. In a classic study of the natural history of periodontitis, Löe et al.[53] found that among individuals with poor oral hygiene and no access to dental care, some developed disease at a rapid rate, whereas others experienced little or no disease. This variation must have been attributable to either unrecognized environmental factors or to individual differences in susceptibility to disease. Because host susceptibility may be defined in terms of genetic variation, a relatively recent focus in periodontology has been to quantify genetic risk and identify specific gene variants that determine disease susceptibility. At present, the specific role that genes play in defining susceptibility remains largely unknown.

The purpose of this chapter is to provide the reader with a brief overview of some approaches used to ascertain genetic risk and to discuss genetic risk factors for the various forms of periodontal disease.

Portions of this chapter were adapted from Pihlstrom BL, Michalowicz BS: Genetic risk for periodontal diseases: a clinical perspective, *J Paradontol Implantol Orale* 17:123, 1998.

In 1999, the American Academy of Periodontology established a new diagnostic scheme for the periodontal diseases.[4] Diagnoses, which had been based on the age of onset, are now based primarily on the rate of disease progression. Previously, the "early-onset diseases," which included "juvenile periodontitis," occurred by definition only in children, adolescents, and young adults. The terms "localized juvenile periodontitis" and "generalized juvenile periodontitis" have been replaced with *localized aggressive periodontitis* and *generalized aggressive periodontitis,* respectively. The term *chronic periodontitis* is now used to describe any slow or moderately progressing disease. Previously, "adult periodontitis" referred to slowly progressing disease in patients 35 years of age and older. Most studies discussed in this chapter used diagnostic schemes that included these former age restrictions.

GENETIC STUDY DESIGNS

A person's unique genetic code is contained in the sequences of nucleotide bases (adenine, thymine, cytosine, and guanine), which make up deoxyribonucleic acid (DNA). The human genome consists of more than 3 billion pairs of bases contained in 22 pairs of chromosomes, termed *autosomes,* and two sex chromosomes (Figure 11-1).

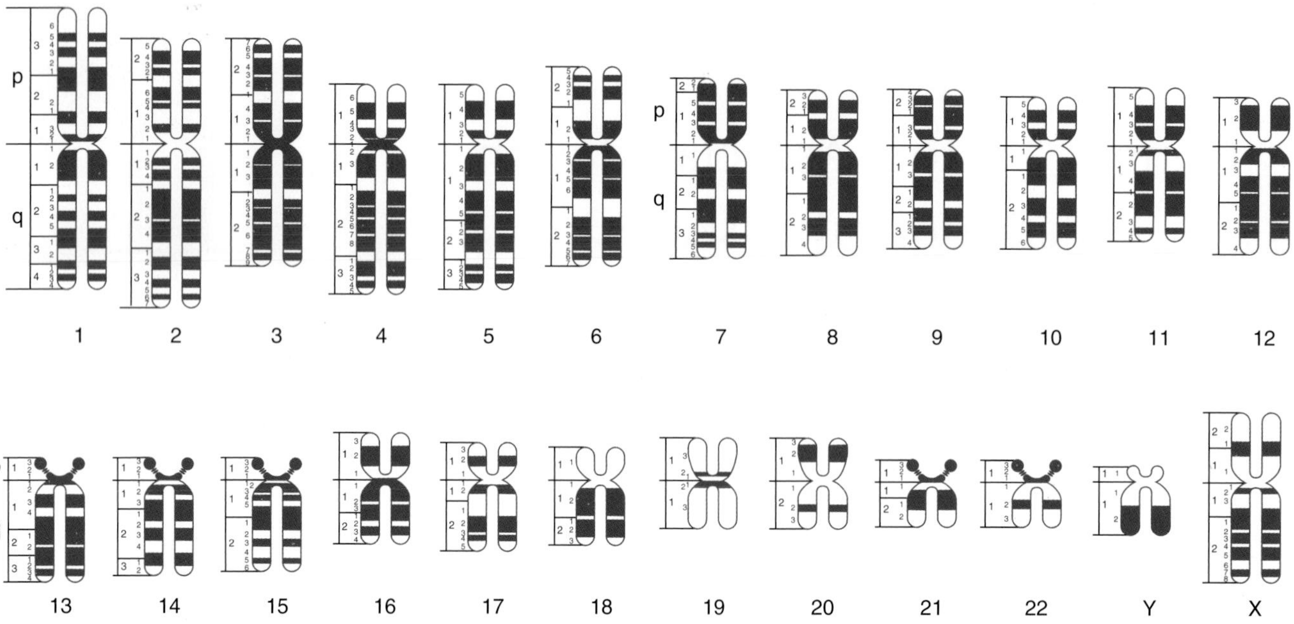

Figure 11-1 The nomenclature used to locate positions along chromosomes is based on the physical appearance and staining patterns of chromosomes viewed during prophase or early metaphase. Each chromosome contains a short arm (*p,* or petite) and long arm *(q).* In this schematic, termed an *ideogram,* the chromosomes are depicted as they appear after Giemsa staining (thus the term *G banding patterns*). Genes are located based on their positions within these bands. For example, 11q23 denotes a position in the third band of the second region on the long arm of chromosome 11. Sub-bands are designated by decimal points (e.g., 11q23.2). (From Jorde LB, Carey JC, White RL, editors: *Medical genetics,* St Louis, 1995, Mosby.)

Genes are sequences of nucleotide bases contained in noncontiguous segments called *exons.* The exons provide the DNA template for the subsequent synthesis of polypeptides that regulate all developmental, physiologic, and immunologic processes in the body. The human genome contains about 25,000 to 35,000 genes.[101]

The genetic composition of an organism is termed the *genotype,* and the collection of traits or characteristics is termed the *phenotype.* The phenotype is determined by the interaction of genes and the environment.[51] Traits and diseases might be caused by a single gene *(monogenic),* several genes *(oligogenic),* or many genes *(polygenic).* Diseases with etiologies that include both genetic and environmental factors are referred to as *multifactorial.* Most common diseases are multifactorial.

Specific locations on chromosomes are referred to as *loci,* and variations in the nucleotide sequence at a locus are termed *alleles.* At a given locus, an individual is considered homozygous if the alleles are identical on homologous chromosomes or heterozygous if the alleles are different. Some alleles are associated with profound changes in the phenotype, whereas others have no measurable effects. Phenotypic differences in the population may be caused by the effects of alleles in the coding region of a gene or in flanking noncoding regions that control gene transcription or expression.

The term *genetic marker* refers to any gene or nucleotide sequence that can be mapped to a specific location or region on a chromosome. Any marker that is sufficiently polymorphic, or variable, in the population can be used to map or locate disease alleles. There is an important distinction between the role of genes in monogenic disorders such as Huntington's disease and their role in complex multifactorial diseases such as periodontitis. In monogenic disorders, genes are referred to as *causative* because almost everyone with the mutation develops the condition. Environmental factors generally play a minor role in determining the phenotype. In contrast, genes involved in complex multifactorial diseases are often referred to as *susceptibility genes* (or more correctly, *susceptibility alleles*). For these diseases, individuals who inherit susceptibility alleles will not develop disease unless they are exposed to deleterious environments. For the periodontal diseases, important environmental risk factors include gram-negative anaerobic microorganisms, cigarette smoking, and poor oral hygiene.

The theory that genes influence susceptibility to common diseases such as periodontitis is not new or revolutionary. Given the complex etiology and pathogenesis of periodontitis, variations in any number or combination of genes that control the development of the periodontal tissues or the competency of the cellular and humoral immune systems could affect an individual's risk for disease. Critics might even argue that every trait or disease likely has some genetic variation and that merely confirming this fact has little or no practical value. Once the genetic basis for a disease has been established, it is equally important to determine (1) which alleles have a measurable effect on the phenotype and (2) whether the prevention, diagnosis, or treatment of the disease can be improved once disease alleles are identified. The first issue can be addressed in a systematic but nontrivial manner. The second issue is more complex and involves debate on scientific, ethical, and public health grounds.

Segregation Analyses

Inherited diseases "run" in families. The pattern of transmission through generations depends on (1) whether the disease alleles are contained in autosomes or sex chromosomes, (2) whether they are dominant or recessive, and (3) whether they are fully or partially penetrant. Generally, a *dominant* allele determines the phenotype in a heterozygote with another recessive allele. A *recessive* allele determines the phenotype only when present at both loci on homologous chromosomes. *Penetrance* refers to the probability that a particular phenotype will result from a genotype. *Partially penetrant* means that only a fraction of individuals who inherit the disease alleles will be affected.

In segregation analyses, the observed pattern of disease is compared with those expected under various models of inheritance to select the best-fitting model. The statistical power of this design depends on the number and composition of the families and the heterogeneity of the disease. *Heterogeneity* means that there are different causes of disease. Generally, segregation analyses have low power to resolve heterogeneity. Segregation analyses cannot distinguish between genetic effects and unmeasured environmental causes of disease, such as the transmission of pathogenic organisms within families.[22]

Twin Studies

The relative influence of genetic and environmental factors on complex diseases can be estimated using twin data. In the classic twin study, reared-together monozygotic and dizygotic twins are compared to estimate the effects of shared genes. *Monozygotic* (MZ) twins are genetically identical, whereas *dizygotic* (DZ) or fraternal twins share on average 50% of their genes by descent. For binary traits (present or absent), a genetic effect is inferred if the positive *concordance rate,* or percentage of twin pairs in which both twins are affected, is greater for MZ than DZ twins. For continuous measures, such as periodontal probing depth or attachment loss, twin-pair similarities are assessed using intraclass correlations. These correlations reflect the variation between twin pairs relative to the variation within pairs. Typically, twin data are used to estimate *heritability,* which is the proportion of phenotypic variation attributed to genetic variation. A heritability estimate of 50% means that half of the variance in the population is attributed to genetic variance; it does not mean that a child of an affected parent has a 50% chance of being similarly affected. Very large samples of reared-together twins are needed to estimate heritability with precision.

Heritability also can be estimated from MZ twins who are separated at birth and raised apart. Because they do not share a common family environment, any similarities in these twins may be attributed to the effects of shared genes. (Raised-apart twins share an in utero environment and often a common culture. To the extent that these environments affect the phenotype, heritability estimates from MZ twins raised apart may be artificially inflated.) Although more powerful than the classic twin design, few such studies have been conducted because of the scarcity of such twins. Regardless of the method of estimation, heritability pertains to populations and not individuals. Such estimates describe the impact of genes on specific populations exposed to a particular range of environments.

Linkage and Association Studies

Linkage and association studies are used to map disease alleles to specific regions on chromosomes. These studies exploit a unique feature of how alleles segregate during meiosis. During gametogenesis, diploid cells (containing 2N copies of each allele) divide to become haploid (containing one copy of each parental allele). The probability that two alleles at different loci will recombine (termed a *recombination* or *crossover event*) is generally proportional to the distance between them. Two alleles selected at random from the genome will likely recombine, and the chance that any two maternal or paternal alleles will be transmitted together to an offspring is 50%. Alleles at nearby loci, however, tend to segregate together; that is, they are linked. By identifying genetic markers that segregate with a disease, researchers can infer the location of putative disease alleles. It is not necessary for the same marker allele to be transmitted with the disease allele in all affected families, and a marker that is linked to the disease allele within a family may not be associated with disease in the population. Allelic associations *(linkage disequilibrium)* occur when the *same* marker allele is linked to disease in multiple families (Figure 11-2).

Linkage studies use sets of families, or *pedigrees,* containing multiple affected individuals. Genotypes are determined for affected and unaffected family members, and complex statistical models are used to determine whether the marker allele(s) and disease cosegregate in the families under a given inheritance model. Parameters that must be specified in the model include the mode of inheritance, frequency of the marker allele in the population, and disease penetrance. The summary statistic used to assess linkage is the *logarithm of the odds* (LOD) *score,* which is a measure of the likelihood that the marker and disease alleles are linked versus not linked at a given recombination rate, or θ. Although linkage analyses are typically conducted for qualitative traits or diseases, methods to evaluate linkage for quantitative traits or measures have been developed. Once linkage to a particular region has been established, the task of identifying the actual disease allele or mutation is far from trivial. Linkage can be detected if the marker and disease alleles are within 20 to 30 centimorgans (cM) of one another. In humans, 1 cM represents approximately 1 million nucleotide bases. Because sequencing 20 million to 30 million base pairs in search of mutations remains a daunting task at present, fine marker mapping is used to further refine the regions of interest. Fortunately, given the rapid advances in human genomics, it will soon be possible to identify all nearby candidate genes for study once linkage is established.

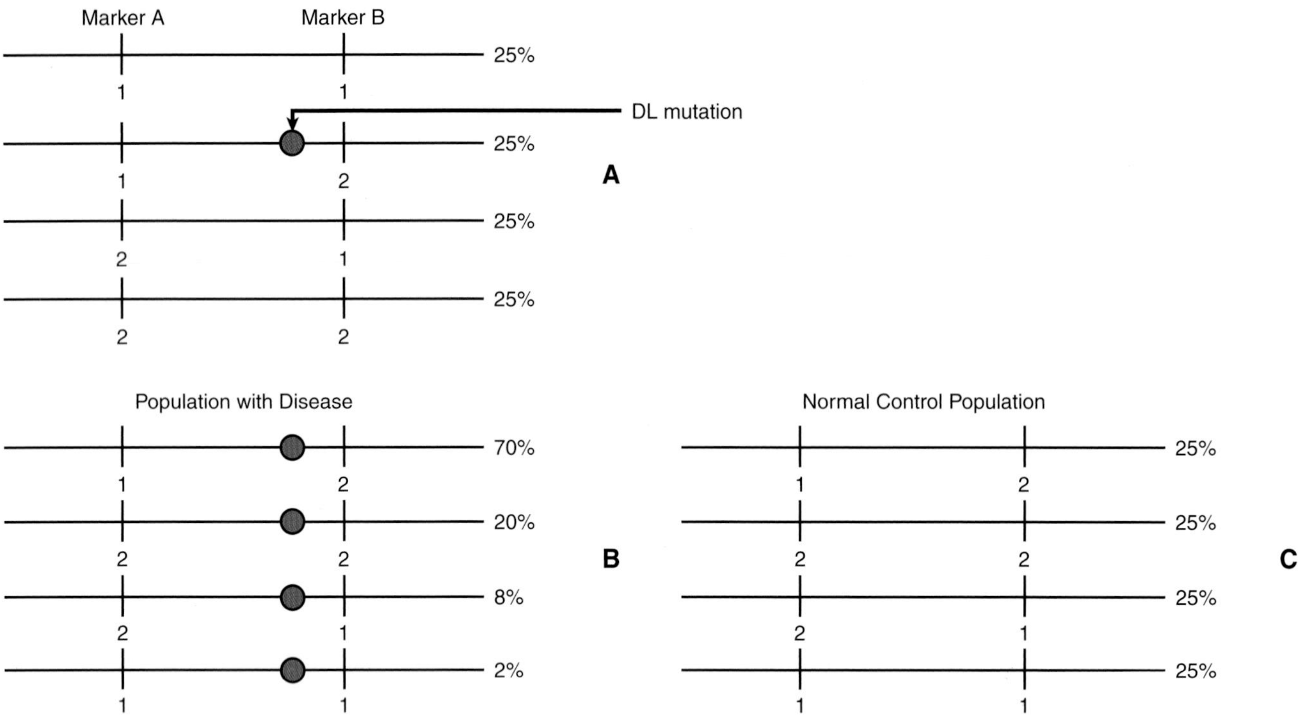

Figure 11-2 Linkage disequilibrium between a disease locus *(DL)* and two linked loci, **A** and **B.** The DL mutation first arises on the chromosome with the A_1B_2 haplotype. After a number of generations, most chromosomes carrying the DL mutation still have the A_1B_2 haplotype, but as a result of recombination, the DL mutation is also found on other haplotypes. Because the A_1B_2 haplotype is seen in 70% of DL chromosomes but only 25% of normal chromosomes, there is linkage disequilibrium between the DL and loci *A* and *B.* Because locus *B* is closer to DL, it is in greater linkage disequilibrium with DL than is locus *A.* **C,** Normal control population. (Modified from Jorde LB, Carey JC, White RL, editors: *Medical genetics,* St Louis, 1995, Mosby.)

To test for associations (linkage disequilibrium), the frequency of alleles at a given locus is compared between subjects with disease (cases) and healthy controls sampled from the same population. Although often used in genetic epidemiology, results from case-control studies should be interpreted with caution. An association does not necessarily imply a biologic link between the disease and an allele. The association may result from some environmental component causing both the marker and the disease to increase in the population, from an unrecognized difference in the racial or ethnic makeup of the cases and controls, or from chance alone.[16] True linkage disequilibrium in an outbred and random mating population implies that the disease and marker alleles lie very close to one another on a chromosome.

Associations (linkage disequilibrium) suggest that the presence of an allele confers risk for disease within a defined environment. This is an important qualifier when discussing common multifactorial diseases such as periodontitis. Alleles that can be used to predict disease in one population may not be useful in other populations or even in the same population when exposed to extremely different environments. For example, suppose the humoral response to a particular class of bacterial antigens varies in the population because of genetic variation. Suppose also that individuals who fail to mount a robust immunologic response cannot suppress the growth of pathogens expressing these antigens. In the presence of the pathogens, individuals with the low-response allele develop disease. On the other hand, no relationship may exist between the disease and this allele in populations where the particular bacteria are either never or only rarely present. Thus the notion of "high-risk" alleles may be specific to an environment.

AGGRESSIVE PERIODONTAL DISEASES

The search for periodontitis-susceptibility alleles is complicated because (1) multiple causes (both genetic and nongenetic) may exist for the same disease *(etiologic heterogeneity)* and (2) different genetic mechanisms may lead to the same clinical endpoint *(genetic heterogeneity)*.[45] Most studies of the aggressive periodontal (AP) diseases to date have had inadequate statistical power to resolve substantial genetic heterogeneity. In addition, the periodontal disease diagnoses are based on clinical and radiographic criteria, but the immunologic and microbiologic characteristics can vary substantially within diagnostic categories. The variability in the clinical presentation of these diseases and the limited criteria used to establish disease diagnoses also have made the search for susceptibility genes more difficult. Nonetheless, evidence from a variety of sources suggests that the risk for AP disease may be substantially heritable.[87]

TABLE 11-1

Genetic and Inherited Disorders Associated with Aggressive Periodontitis

Disorder	Protein or Tissue Defect
Leukocyte adhesion deficiency type I	CD18 (β-2 integrin chain of LFA molecule)
Leukocyte adhesion deficiency type II	CD15 (neutrophil ligand for E and P selectins); inborn error in fucose metabolism
Acatalasia	Catalase enzyme
Chronic and cyclic neutropenias	Unknown
Chédiak-Higashi syndrome	Abnormal transport of vesicles to and from neutrophil lysosomes caused by mutations in lysosomal trafficking regulator gene
Ehler-Danlos syndrome (EDS types IV and VIII)	Type III collagen for EDS type IV, unknown for EDS type VIII
Papillion-Lefèvre syndrome	Cathepsin C (dipeptidyl aminopeptidase I)
Hypophosphatasia	Tissue-nonspecific alkaline phosphatase
Trisomy 21	Multiple; critical trisomic region at least 5 Mb long
Prepubertal periodontitis (nonsyndromic)	Cathepsin C
Kindler syndrome	Defect in actin–extracellular matrix linkage caused by loss of function mutations in KIND-1

LFA, Leukocyte function–associated antigen; *Mb,* megabase; *KIND-1,* gene associated with Kindler syndrome.

Associations with Genetic and Inherited Conditions

Early and aggressive periodontitis is a consistent feature in several inherited or genetic disorders (Table 11-1), which demonstrates the variety of ways in which gene mutations can affect risk for AP disease. The disorders have been grouped according to the resultant protein or biochemical defect(s); the mutant alleles may affect the function of phagocytic immune cells or the structure of epithelia, connective tissue, or the teeth themselves. The specific gene or tissue defect responsible for the condition has been identified for some but not all disorders.

Hypophosphatasia is a rare disorder caused by mutations in the tissue-nonspecific alkaline phosphatase gene (1p36.1-p34).[81] Mutations leading to deficiency in alkaline phosphatase activity result in abnormal bone mineralization, skeletal anomalies, and cementum hypoplasia. Both autosomal dominant forms and recessive forms have been reported. Although the infantile form is usually fatal, milder forms can occur in children and adults. The condition leads to the premature loss of the primary teeth and occasionally the permanent teeth.[17]

Papillon-Lefèvre syndrome (PLS) is a rare autosomal recessive disorder characterized by palmoplantar hyperkeratosis and aggressive periodontitis[28,38] (Figure 11-3). Both the primary dentitions and secondary dentitions can be affected. PLS is caused by mutations in the cathepsin C gene, which is located on chromosome 11 (11q14-q21).[34,99] *Cathepsin C* is a cysteine protease normally expressed at high levels in various cells, including epithelium and polymorphonuclear leukocytes (PMNs).[79] Cathepsin C appears to play a role in degrading proteins and activating proenzymes in immune and inflammatory cells.

PLS patients, who lack virtually all cathepsin C activity,[79] are either mutant homozygotes (i.e., they have inherited the same mutation from both parents) or compound heterozygotes (i.e., they have inherited a different mutation from each parent).[32] A late-onset PLS patient with no loss of function mutation in the cathepsin C gene has recently been reported.[74] This suggests there might be other genetic causes for this form of PLS.

In some PLS patients, AP disease is associated with the virulent microorganism *Actinobacillus actinomycetemcomitans.* The periodontal destruction in PLS patients can be arrested by eliminating *A. actinomycetemcomitans,*[77] which suggests that AP disease is not a direct result of a gene mutation, but rather the consequence of a specific bacterial infection in a highly susceptible host.

Inherited disorders such as acatalasia, leukocyte adhesion deficiency, and Chédiak-Higashi syndrome highlight the importance of competent phagocytes in the defense against periodontal infections. Many, but not all, patients with prepubertal periodontitis also have some inherited or congenital defect in phagocytic cell function. The immunologic defects associated with these syndromes can be profound, and patients generally have systemic infections in addition to periodontitis. Although the mutant alleles responsible for these syndromes may be uncommon, other, more common alleles at the same loci may serve as candidate markers for nonsyndromic forms of AP disease. Recently, nonsyndromic prepubertal periodontitis-affected individuals in a Jordanian family were found to be homozygous for a cathepsin C gene mutation (Figure 11-4).[35] Others have argued that prepubertal periodontitis is heterogeneous and in some families simply is a partially penetrant form of PLS.[40]

To reach the periodontal tissues, blood-borne phagocytes must adhere to and then traverse the blood vessel wall. Surface molecules present on both the phagocyte and the endothelium mediate this adhesion. Three adhesion molecules expressed on leukocytes are composed of a unique α subunit (CD11a, b, or c) and a common β subunit (CD18). When too few of these molecules are present, cells cannot adhere to endothelium, and an important component of the cellular immune response is compromised. Patients with inherited deficiencies in leukocyte adhesion molecules are at high risk for AP disease, and prepubertal periodontitis in particular. Two inherited forms of leukocyte adhesion deficiency have been described, each of which affects a different adhesion molecule. Homozygotes carrying two copies of the mutant allele experience a dramatic reduction in the number of leukocyte adhesion molecules and develop

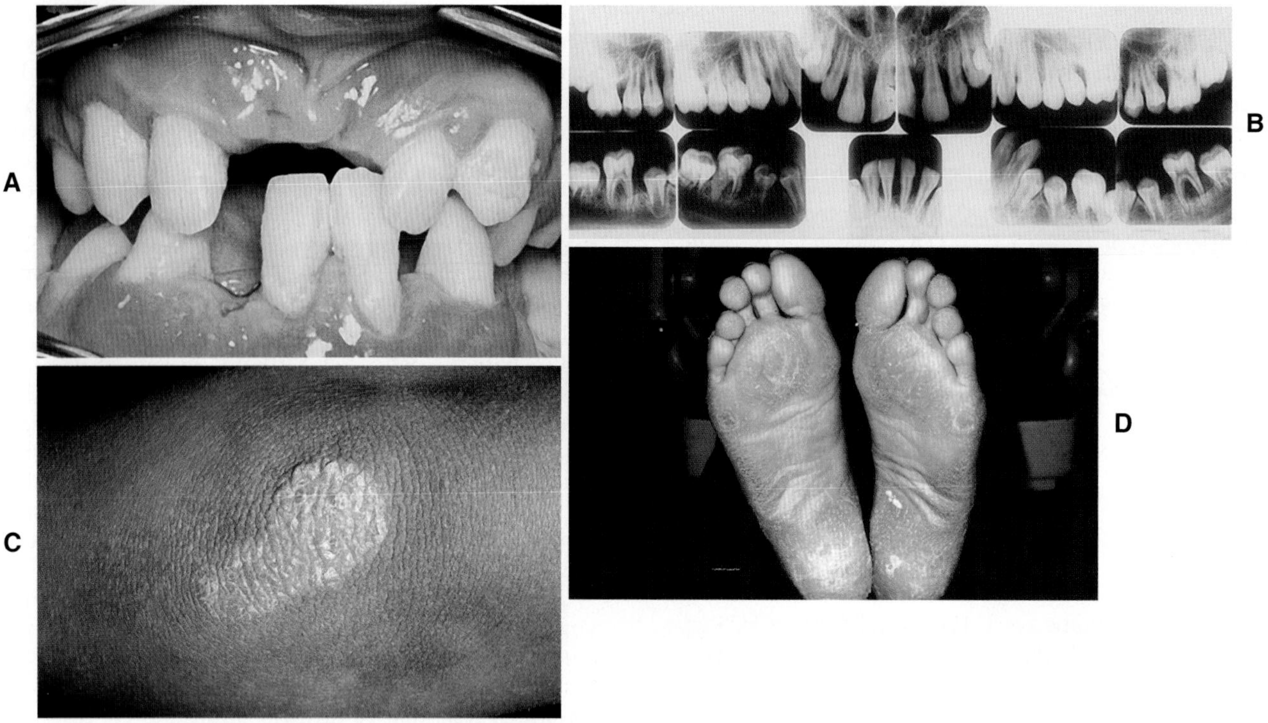

Figure 11-3 Oral **(A)**, radiographic **(B)**, and dermatologic (**C** and **D**) findings in the Papillon-Lefèvre syndrome (PLS). Pocketing and bone loss usually affect the primary and secondary teeth shortly after eruption. Although numerous palmoplantar keratodermas have been described, the hyperkeratotic lesions of PLS can affect the elbows **(C)** and knees and the palms and plantar surfaces of the feet **(D)**. (Courtesy Dr. Robert J. Gorlin, Minneapolis.)

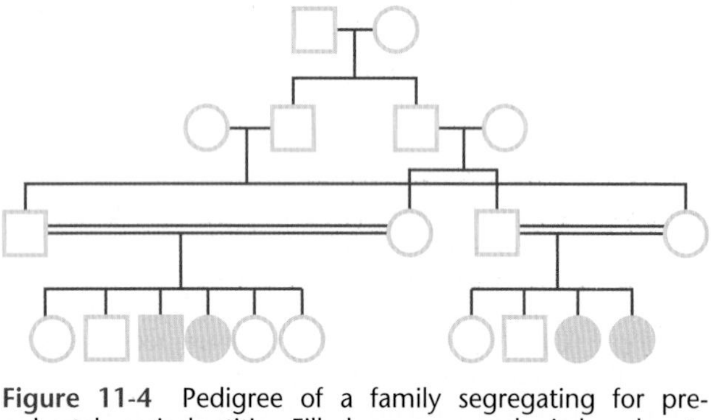

Figure 11-4 Pedigree of a family segregating for prepubertal periodontitis. Filled squares and circles denote affected males and females, respectively. The double lines between the parents of affected individuals indicate they are blood relatives (in this case, first cousins), which is a frequent finding in rare autosomal recessive disorders. Affected individuals were homozygous by descent for a mutation in the cathepsin C gene. The four parents of the affected individuals were heterozygous for the mutation, as were the two unaffected siblings. None of these heterozygotes had clinical evidence of the disease. (From Hart TC, Hart PS, Michalec MD, et al: *J Med Genet* 37:95, 2000.)

recurrent infections, including periodontitis (Figure 11-5). Expression is about half of normal in heterozygotes, who carry only one mutant allele. Although cell adherence is usually normal in heterozygotes, they may be at increased risk for adult-onset disease.[102]

Segregation Analyses

Aggressive periodontitis aggregates in families.[11,15] Such clustering suggests but does not prove the disease has a genetic basis because family members can share deleterious components of their environment as well. Several research groups have used segregation analyses to determine the likely mode of inheritance for AP disease.

In most such studies, the localized and generalized forms of AP disease have been considered variants of the same disorder. This theory is supported by the observation that both forms frequently occur in the same family;[54,57] the probability of two rare diseases occurring in the same family is exceedingly small. Various forms of aggressive periodontitis (e.g., prepubertal and juvenile periodontitis) have been observed in the same family[92] and found to occur sequentially in the same individual.[90] These findings suggest there are common genetic risk factors for the subforms of AP disease.

There are many reports in the literature describing families with multiple affected individuals. The patterns of disease in these families have led investigators to postulate both dominant and recessive modes of inheritance for AP diseases. However, few formal segregation analyses have been conducted. and even these have yielded disparate results (Table 11-2). Melnick et al.[61] proposed X-linked inheritance because of the preponderance of female probands (the initially identified disease-afflicted individual in the family) and affected family members. The preponderance of affected females in these

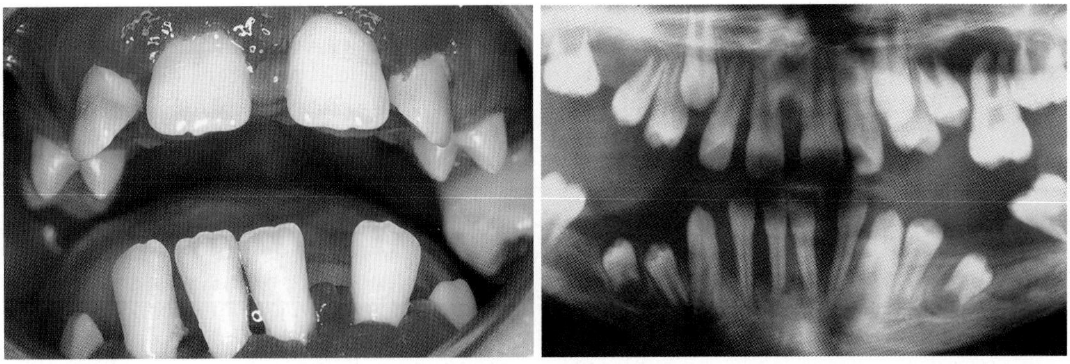

Figure 11-5 Oral **(A)** and radiographic **(B)** appearance of a patient with leukocyte adhesion deficiency (LAD). The child was deficient in CD18 (i.e., LAD type I), which results in absent or severely reduced levels of the β-2 integrin molecule. The patient suffered from recurrent infections of the middle ear, tongue, and perirectal areas as well as the periodontium. (From Majorana A, Notarangelo LD, Savoldi E, et al: Leukocyte adhesion deficiency in a child with severe oral involvement, *Oral Surg Oral Med Oral Pathol Oral Radiol Endod* 87:691, 1999.)

TABLE 11-2

Segregation Analyses of Aggressive Periodontitis

Racial/Ethnic Groups	No. Families (individuals)	Favored Model	Comments	Ref.
Caucasian and African American	19 (88)	X-linked dominant	Reviewed cases in the literature plus 2 new ones. Recognized paucity of males in families. Penetrance estimated at 75%.	61
Finnish	31 (158)	Autosomal recessive	Genetic ratio 0.26 for complete and 0.17 for very incomplete ascertainment. No affected parents observed.	84
	30 (142)	Autosomal recessive	Genetic ratios highly consistent with AR mode. No affected parents observed.	85
Triracial isolate	1 (50)	Autosomal dominant	One five-generation family. JP cosegregated with dentinogenesis imperfecta. Disease allele linked to chromosome 4.	14
African American, Caucasian, Asian	32 (199)	Autosomal recessive	Tested AR, XD and sporadic models. XD mode favored in 8 of 33 kindreds.	54
Not specified, U.S. sample	28 (157)	Autosomal recessive	High type II error realized for mistakenly accepting AR over AD model. Tested AR, XD, and sporadic models.	8
African American, Caucasian	100 (631)	Autosomal dominant	Evidence of racial heterogeneity. Disease allele more frequent in blacks than whites.	57

AR, Autosomal recessive; *JP,* juvenile (aggressive) periodontitis; *XD,* X-linked dominant; *AD,* autosomal dominant.

reports has been attributed to ascertainment bias because women are more likely than men to seek dental care and participate in family studies.[37] Also, father-to-son transmissions, which were not seen in earlier studies (the lack of such transmissions suggests X-linked inheritance), were subsequently reported. An autosomal recessive mode of inheritance was clearly favored in Finnish populations where parents of probands were not consistently unaffected.[83,85] In contrast, in the largest U.S. study conducted to date, the autosomal dominant mode was favored in African-American and Caucasian families.[57] The estimated frequency of the disease allele, however, was significantly higher in African Americans and reflects the higher prevalence of AP disease in this group.

Despite inconsistent conclusions regarding their mode of inheritance, segregation analyses consistently have supported the role of a major gene in the etiology of the AP diseases. Multifactorial or polygenic models alone cannot adequately account for the patterns of disease observed in families. Results from these studies, however, are prone to error because of the difficulty in correctly diagnosing older individuals, the variable clinical appearance of disease, and the likely etiologic and genetic heterogeneity of these diseases.[13,76] Beaty et al.[8] recognized that the narrow age range in which AP diseases can reliably be diagnosed increases the chance that an incorrect model of inheritance is favored over the true one.

Schenkein[86] proposed a model of inheritance that distinguishes between the etiologies of localized and generalized aggressive periodontitis and allows for family clustering. He theorized that AP disease and immunoglobulin G2 (IgG2) responsiveness to bacterial lipopolysaccharide (LPS) segregate independently as dominant and codominant traits, respectively. Under this model, subjects with one AP disease allele and two copies of the high-IgG2-response allele would develop only localized disease. In contrast, subjects who carry the AP disease allele and only one copy of the IgG2 allele would develop more widespread disease because their IgG2 response to LPS would be less robust. This model, although appealing, requires more rigorous testing, and the work needed to resolve the confounding effects of race and smoking on IgG2 levels and disease is far from trivial.

Linkage Studies

To date, few linkage studies of AP diseases have been performed. Boughman et al.[14] were the first to report linkage between aggressive periodontitis and a specific chromosomal region. They studied an extended family in which an autosomal dominant form of AP disease was found to cosegregate with *dentinogenesis imperfecta* (DGI). Using polymorphic protein markers, the putative AP disease gene was localized to the long arm of chromosome 4 (4q11-13) near the gene for DGI. Aggressive periodontitis does not typically cosegregate with DGI, however, and it is highly unlikely an important AP disease gene resides within this chromosomal region in the more general population.[36]

Saxen and Koskimies[84] typed a small number of multiplex Finnish families for the HLA antigens and concluded it was unlikely that AP disease was linked to this region. Recently, AP disease has been linked in four families with localized aggressive periodontitis (LAP) to a marker on chromosome 1 (1q25) with a LOD score of 3.48 and theta of 0.0.[52] The region containing the putative LAP locus spans over 25 million base pairs, and denser marker sets or extensive sequencing will be needed to narrow the region of interest.

Association Studies

Because of their role in regulating immune responses, the *human leukocyte antigens* (HLA) have long been considered as candidate genetic risk markers for AP disease. More than 40 diseases, most of which are autoimmune in nature, have been associated with various HLA antigens.[98] Genes for the class I and II antigens are located on chromosome 6 in humans. Nearby genes encode for complement fragments and the proinflammatory cytokine, tumor necrosis factor alpha (TNF-α). Currently, more than 150 HLA antigens have been defined serologically. Dissection of the coding sequences has revealed even more impressive variation at the genotypic level. More than 220 alleles have been identified in the gene that encodes the β-1 molecule of the dimeric class II DR antigen (DRB1 alleles). Although this variation is desirable for linkage studies (because most individuals will be heterozygotic for a given marker), it can hinder the search for allelic associations. With so many antigens and alleles, the chance of obtaining an adequate number of subjects with any particular HLA type is small except in large, homogeneous samples. The possibility that an association will be caused by chance alone also increases with the number of statistical tests conducted. For example, consider a study that tests for associations between periodontal disease and all known HLA antigens. At a standard significance level of 5%, approximately 7 antigens (150 antigens multiplied by 0.05) would be expected to be associated with the disease by chance alone. Although statistical methods to adjust for multiple hypotheses testing are available, such corrections have not always been made.

Despite the many case-control studies of HLA antigens, few consistent findings have been reported (Table 11-3). This inconsistency may be caused by false-positive findings, differences in the racial or ethnic makeup of the study groups, differences in the clinical criteria used to define patient groups, or true genetic heterogeneity. *Two antigens that appear to be consistently associated with AP diseases are HLA-A9 and B15.* The risk of disease in subjects with HLA-A9 or B15 is about 1.5 to 3.5 times greater than in those lacking these antigens.[91] In contrast, the HLA-A2 antigen appears to be less prevalent in patients with aggressive periodontitis than in controls, suggesting that this antigen somehow may be protective.[42,43,97]

The class II DR4 antigen has been of particular interest in periodontology because of its association with type 1 (insulin-dependent) diabetes mellitus (DM). Type 1 DM patients with the DR4 antigen are at increased risk for diabetes-related complications,[82] including periodontitis. It has been suggested that the HLA-D antigens may mediate the association between periodontal disease and type 1 DM.[23] Although the number of cases was small, Katz et al.[44] found the DR4 antigen to be more prevalent in patients with AP disease than in controls. Others, however, have found no association with this antigen (see Table 11-3).

In early genetic epidemiologic studies of periodontitis, investigators often compared the distribution of inherited tissue markers (e.g., HLA antigens or blood types) between patients and healthy controls. More recent studies have examined variation at the gene rather than the protein level. Although it may soon be feasible to conduct systematic, genome-wide searches for allelic associations, to date researchers have focused on candidate gene regions. These regions lie within or near genes that code for enzymes or regulatory molecules that are likely to be involved in the pathogenesis of disease. The number and variety of candidates for AP diseases are vast. Polymorphisms in genes that encode the immunoglobulin receptors, LPS-binding proteins, prostaglandins, and cytokines are all suitable markers for study.[33,104]

TABLE 11-3

HLA Antigens and Alleles in the Periodontal Diseases: Summary of Association Studies

Disease	Ages of Cases (years)	Racial/Ethnic Group	No. Cases	No. Controls	Associations with Disease	Comments	Ref.
AP and non-AP	13-30	Caucasians	19 AP, 28 non-AP	41* 267†	↓A2, A5 in non-AP	Trend for ↓A2 in AP. No associations with ANUG.	42, 97
AP (RPP)	23-39, median 31	Caucasians	44	2041†	↑A9 (A24)	Subjects had no evidence of past AP. No significant ↑ in B15 or DR antigens although trend for DR5.	46
AP and non-AP	13-30	Caucasians	33 AP, 41 non-AP	53	↓A2 in non-AP	Similar trend for AP. No difference in A9, A28, Bw15. Also tested ABO blood groups	43
AP	11-29 Mode 21	Caucasians	39	1967†	↑A9, A28, Bw15	No significant associations with CP. Trend for ↓A2 in AP group.	80
AP	≤25	Caucasians and African–Americans	30	341	↑Bw15 in blacks (Class I only)	Trend for ↑B12 in whites. Small samples. No evidence of linkage to HLA region in collection of 8 families.	21
AP	Mean 26.5	Japanese	24	47	None (Class II only)	Trend for ↑DRB1 ×1401, ×1501 and DQB1 ×0503, ×0602. DR association thought to result from linkage disequilibrium with DQ alleles.	71
AP	15-25	African Caribbeans	38	42	↑A1, B22, A28, DR7 ↓A68(28), B5, DR2	None remained significant after corrections for multiple comparisons.	68
AP (RPP)	21-35	Ashkenazi and non-Ashkenazi Jews	10	120	↑DR4	Small sample size. Borderline and uncorrected *p* value.	44
AP	Puberty to 35	Non-Ashkenazi Jews	26	113†	↑A9, B15	Associations in GAP, not LAP, group. No association with DR antigens.	89
AP (RPP)	20-35	6 ethno-geographic groups	12	55	↑DRB1 ×0401, ×0404, ×0405, or ×0408	Small sample of AP. No significant association for all patients ($n = 48$) or for all DR alleles combined.	12
AP (LAP, RPP)	LAP: puberty-24; RPP: puberty-35	Turkish citizens	30 LAP, 30 RPP	3731†	↑A9 (A24), DR4	↑DR4 in both patient groups.	25

*Resistant group.

†Population-based controls, disease status not determined.

HLA, Human leukocyte antigen; *AP,* aggressive periodontitis; *ANUG,* acute necrotizing ulcerative gingivitis; *RPP,* rapidly progressive periodontitis; GAP, generalized AP; LAP, localized AP; *CP,* chronic periodontitis.

Continued

TABLE 11-3

HLA Antigens and Alleles in the Periodontal Diseases: Summary of Association Studies—cont'd

Disease	Ages of Cases (years)	Racial/Ethnic Group	No. Cases	No. Controls	Associations with Disease	Comments	Ref.
AP and CP (?)	25-40, Mean 33.0	Not specified	49	70* 600[2]	↑A9; ↓A10	↑A9 in patients vs. resistant group. ↓A10 in resistant group vs. undiagnosed controls.	2
AP and CP	Mean 34.9	Japanese	55	26	None (Class II only)	Atypical enzyme restriction site in DQB1 gene detected in a subgroup of patients.	95
GAP	Not reported	European Caucasians	90	88	None (DQB1 gene only)	Tested for association with restriction site described in ref. 96.	41
Not specified	Mean 35.9	Caucasians	30[3]	30‡	↑DR4, DR53, DQ3 (Class II only)	Association between diabetes and periodontitis may be mediated by D antigens.	1, 23
AP and CP	20-49	Not specified	50	257†	↑A9, B44(12), Bw35, Cw4	Cw4 and Bw35 in strong disequilibrium (gametic association).	58
CP	40-73, Mean 49.9	Caucasians and African Americans	25	25* 22,000†	↓A28, B5	Significant ↓ in A28 in blacks and B5 in whites compared with undiagnosed controls.	29
CP	38-73	Caucasians	102	102 157†	↑↑B14, –Cw ×08 ↓↓A3	Differences reported later in haplotypes and homozygotic and heterozygotic states.	56
AP	19-43	Caucasians	50	102 157†	↑DRB1 ×13(6) ↓Non-DRB3/4/5		56

‡Fifteen subjects with insulin-dependent (type 1) diabetes mellitus.

Polymorphisms in the *interleukin-1* (IL-1 gene have been studied extensively because of the prominent role IL-1 plays in the initiation and progression of the periodontal lesion. Produced primarily by activated monocytes, its actions are pleiotropic; IL-1 stimulates bone resorption, inhibits collagen synthesis, and upregulates matrix metalloproteinase activity and prostaglandin synthesis.[49,96] IL-1 exists in two forms, IL-1α and IL-1β. An IL-1 antagonist blocks the activity of IL-1 by competitively binding to its receptor.

In humans, genes encoding IL-1 and its receptor antagonist are clustered on the long arm of chromosome 2.[69] Although several polymorphisms have been identified in this region, few appear to be functional. One variant, a single-nucleotide base-pair substitution in the IL-1β coding region, designated IL-1β^{+3954}, has been associated with a fourfold increase in IL-1β production.[33]

The more common allele at the IL-1β^{+3954} site was reported in linkage disequilibrium with generalized aggressive periodontitis,[22] suggesting that at least one disease allele is at or very close to the +3954 site. In this study, linkage disequilibrium was detected using the *transmission disequilibrium test,* which contrasts the number of marker alleles transmitted versus not transmitted from heterozygous parents to affected offspring. The probability that an unlinked marker allele will be transmitted is 50%. If the marker and disease allele are in linkage disequilibrium, however, the marker will be transmitted more than 50% of the time. The number of nuclear families in this report was small, however, and sibling pair analyses of the same population provided little if any evidence of linkage to this region.[33] This "high-risk" IL-1β allele, however, may be too common in African Americans—who are at higher risk than Caucasians for AP disease—to be of diagnostic value.[103]

Polymorphisms in the vitamin D receptor[39,93] and IL-1 receptor antagonist genes[94] and mutations in the *N*-formyl-1-methionyl-1-leucyl-1-phenylalanine (FMLP) receptor gene[30] have been associated with AP disease. Few of these associations, however, have been verified in independent study. Interestingly, the IL-1 composite, which has been associated with chronic disease (see below), does not appear to increase one's risk for aggressive periodontitis.

CHRONIC PERIODONTITIS

Clinicians have long known that susceptibility to periodontitis differs among racial and ethnic groups. In the United States, African Americans have more severe disease than Caucasians.[10,72] Elsewhere, Sri Lankans and South Pacific islanders appear to be more prone to disease than other groups with similar environments.[7] Although these differences may be caused by unrecognized environmental factors, they also may be the result of race-based or ethnic-based differences in genetic makeup.

Measures of periodontitis and gingivitis are correlated within families.[9,100] The basis of this similarity, whether it be shared environments or genes or both, has been investigated in several large family studies. Initially, studies of Japanese and Hawaiian children suggested that gingivitis was caused by recessive genes.[88] Later, correlations within families (e.g., sibling, parent-offspring) were used to estimate genetic and environmental variances for periodontitis among various racial groups in Hawaii. It was concluded that similarities within families were caused by shared cultures and family environments, but not shared genes.[18,78] Beaty et al.[9] reported similar results in a sample comprised mostly of African Americans. The correlations in clinical periodontal measures were greater between mothers and offspring than between fathers and offspring. Sibling correlations in this study were generally low, and the null hypothesis of "no familial correlation" (and thus no genetic effect) could not be rejected.

Twin Studies

As early as 1940, Noack[70] recognized that the periodontal conditions of identical twins were often similar. Independent twin studies in Minnesota and Virginia concluded that a significant heritable component to chronic periodontitis exists. The Minnesota group[62-64,66] studied both reared-together and reared-apart adult twins (Figures 11-6 and 11-7). Between 38% and 82% of the population variance for gingivitis, probing depth, and clinical attachment loss could be attributed to genetic variation. A significant heritable influence on radiographic crestal alveolar bone height was found in these same twins. Moreover, reared-apart MZ twins were no less similar than reared-together MZ twins, indicating that the family environment had no significant influence on clinical measures of disease. The latter finding was surprising because it is within this environment that oral hygiene behaviors are learned and pathogenic bacteria may be acquired from other family members.

Despite the usefulness of the twin study design, very large sample sizes are needed to estimate heritability precisely. For example, heritability for clinical attachment loss in the preceding study was estimated to be 48%.[64] The 90% confidence interval for this estimate was quite large, ranging from 21% to 71%.

A questionnaire survey of several thousand adult twin pairs provided further evidence of the heritable component to periodontitis.[20] The concordance rate for disease was significantly greater in MZ twins (23%) than DZ twins (8%). Although the assessment method is questionable—twins may not be aware of their own or their twin's periodontal condition—the findings were confirmed in a clinical study from the same population.[65] Heritability estimates for the extent and severity of disease were approximately 50%, which were consistent with previous estimates. The heritable component for periodontitis was not associated with behaviors such as smoking, utilization of dental care, and oral hygiene habits. This implies that genes controlling biologic mechanisms, and not behaviors, mediate the genetic influence on disease.

The twin design also has been used to study whether host genes affect the composition of the oral microbiota. Oral bacteria can be transmitted within families,[6] which could partly explain why periodontitis clusters in families. Although the introduction of a bacterium into the oral cavity is an environmental event, long-term colonization of the host may be determined by both host genetic factors and environmental factors. Adolescent

A

B

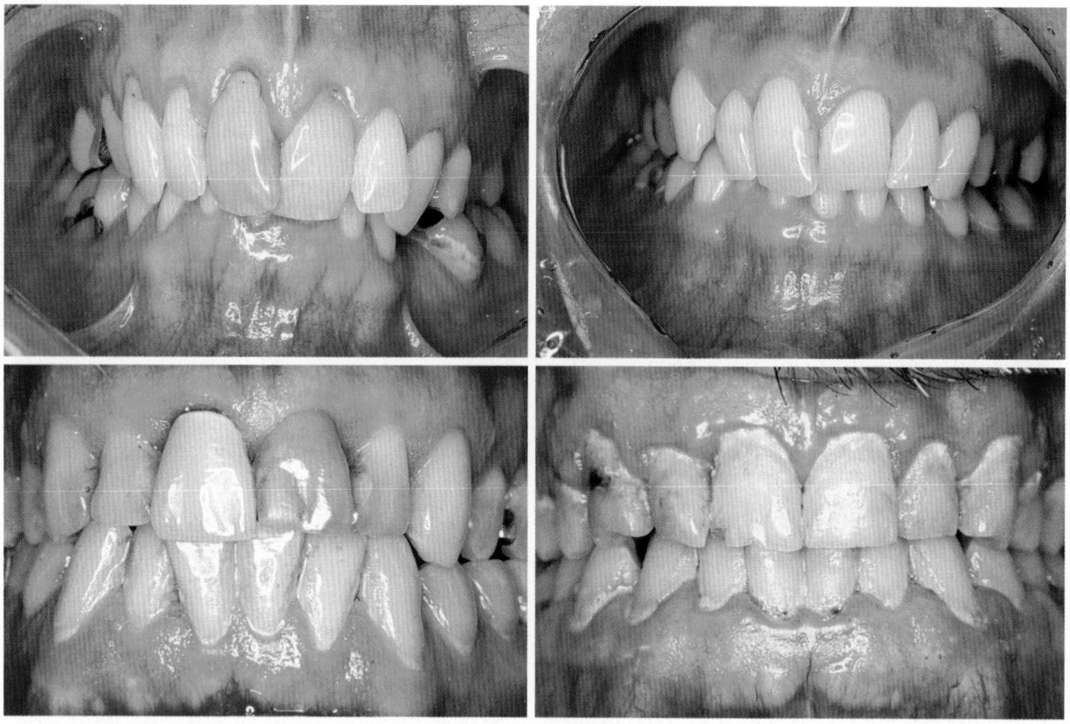

Figure 11-6 Reared-apart twin pairs. **A,** 37-year-old female identical twins. Note the similarity in tooth and arch forms in the twins. **B,** 40-year-old male fraternal twins. (From Philstrom B, Michalowicz B: *J Paradontol Implantol Orale* 17:123, 1998.)

A

B

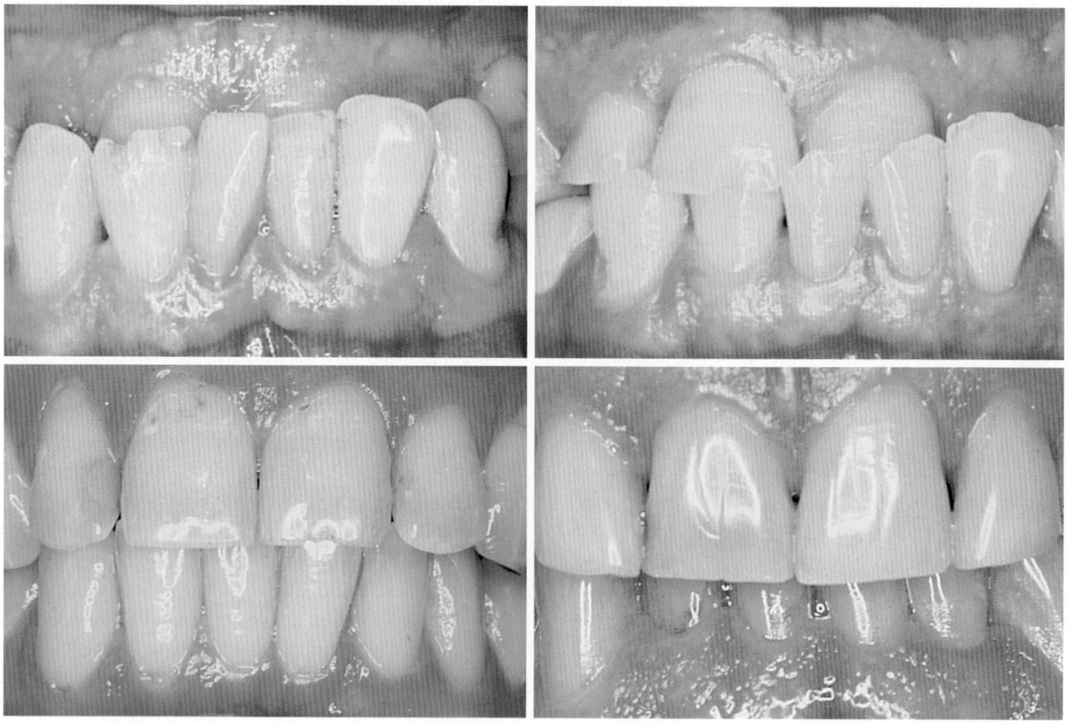

Figure 11-7 Reared-together twin pairs. **A,** 70-year-old male identical twins. **B,** 67-year-old male fraternal twins. (From Philstrom B, Michalowicz B: *J Paradontol Implantol Orale* 17:123, 1998.)

twins have been found to be more similar in their oral microbiota than pairs of unrelated individuals.[67] In adults, however, neither host genes nor early family environments appear to have a significant influence on the presence of periodontal bacteria in subgingival plaque.[66] Together, these findings suggest that although host genes may influence initial bacterial colonization of the oral cavity, the effect does not persist into adulthood.

Association Studies

Many of the same gene polymorphisms considered as candidates for aggressive periodontitis are suitable for study in chronic periodontitis (CP). As with AP disease, the role of the HLA antigens in determining risk for CP is poorly understood (see Table 11-3). One study found the HLA-B5 antigen to be more prevalent in adults resistant to disease.[29]

Kornman et al.[49] reported that a "composite" IL-1 genotype, consisting of at least one copy of the more rare allele at both an IL-1α and IL-1β loci, was associated with severe periodontitis in Northern European adults. Genotype "positive" nonsmokers were 6.8 times more likely to have severe (as opposed to mild) periodontal disease. In contrast, Gore et al.[27] found the more rare IL-1β allele, but not the composite genotype, to be more prevalent in patients with advanced CP. The IL-1α and IL-1β sites were in linkage disequilibrium, which meant that the apparent role of the IL-1α allele could be caused by its association with the IL-1β allele and not with the disease itself. There is similar evidence that risk for CP is conferred more by the IL-1β than IL-1α allele.[22] Importantly, it appears that the IL-1 composite genotype occurs too infrequently in Asian populations to be of value as a diagnostic or prognostic test.[3,5]

Galbraith et al.[26] found no association between CP and TNF-α polymorphisms, although one genotype was correlated with elevated TNF-α production by oral PMNs in patients with advanced disease. Similarly, Engebretson et al.[24] reported a difference in the amount of IL-1 in the gingival crevicular fluid of patients with periodontitis who were positive for the composite IL-1 genotype. The TNF-α and IL-1 variants are examples of functional polymorphisms. In other words, they are variations in coding sequences that affect either the structure (and thus function) or the production of the final protein product. The identification of additional functional polymorphisms, especially within genes that regulate immune responsiveness, should facilitate the discovery of alleles that determine host susceptibility to periodontitis.

Patients who continue to lose clinical attachment and bone support after treatment are said to have "refractory periodontitis." Both aggressive and chronic periodontitis can be refractory to treatment. Neutrophils from refractory disease patients usually display some functional defect.[55] Kobayashi et al.[47] tested the association between neutrophil IgG receptor (FcγR) polymorphisms and CP in a Japanese population. These polymorphisms, which reside in genes that encode receptors for the IgG isotypes, help determine how efficiently PMNs phagocytose opsonized antigens. Although the distribution of FcγR genotypes did not differ between patients and controls, the FcγRIIIb-NA2 allele was found to be more prevalent in those with recurrent disease. Others, however, have not found this same association in refractory patients.[19]

Few investigators have examined how genetic polymorphisms interact with the environment to affect risk for periodontitis. Smoking is one factor that may affect the expression of disease alleles. Large sample sizes are needed to test for gene-by-environment interactions, and most studies have been inadequately powered to detect such interactions. In the seminal report on IL-1 polymorphisms and periodontal disease, Kornman, et al.[49] found the IL-1 "composite" genotype was associated with severe disease only in nonsmokers, which supports the theory that some harmful environments may overwhelm any genetically determined susceptibility or resistance to disease. Tooth loss in periodontal maintenance patients was subsequently shown to be greatest in smokers who were genotype "positive."[59] A more recent population-based study found the IL-1 genotype was associated with disease in smokers but not nonsmokers,[60] which is in stark contrast to the findings of Kornman et al.[49] Thus, although smoking and the IL-1 genotype appear to interact to affect risk for periodontitis, the nature and direction of this interaction are poorly understood. As with all epidemiologic findings, it is critical that such interactions be verified in independent samples.

> **SCIENCE TRANSFER**
>
> Evidence indicates that aggressive periodontitis is more common in some families and may be caused by a genetic susceptibility. Chronic periodontitis in Caucasians (but not in all Asians) is more likely to occur in patients who have a composite genotype that affects interleukin-1 (IL-1) expression, which can result in a fourfold increase in IL-1 production. Also, specific syndromes that include periodontal disease are associated with the parents' genetic profile, such as Papillon-Lefèvre syndrome, hypophosphatasia, and leukocyte function abnormalities. *Clinicians need to be aware of these connections and, where necessary, extend periodontal evaluations to family members of affected individuals.* Genetic makeup also can affect response to periodontal therapy, and a susceptible patient's maintenance care and retreatment need to be increased.

CLINICAL IMPLICATIONS OF GENETIC STUDIES

The role of host genes in the etiology and pathogenesis of the periodontal diseases is just beginning to be understood. Genetic tests may prove useful for identifying patients who are most likely to develop disease, suffer from recurrent disease, or suffer tooth loss as a result of disease. The utility of any screening tool, however, must be evaluated in diverse populations. Given the complex etiology of the periodontal diseases, it is likely that any genetic test will be useful in only a subset of patients or populations. Genetic testing to determine risk for complex diseases (e.g., cancer) is becoming increasingly more common. With the availability of such tests, practitioners have the responsibility to inform the demanding public fully about what genetic tests can do, to act on the results, and to advise and support individuals before and after testing.[75]

Knowledge of specific genetic risk factors could enable clinicians to direct environmentally based prevention and treatments to individuals who are most susceptible to disease. For example, early and aggressive efforts to prevent pathogenic microorganisms from colonizing the oral cavity may be effective in preventing disease in highly susceptible individuals. At present, however, the efficacy of specific preventive and treatment strategies in susceptible patients has yet to be clearly established.

Genetic information also may prove to be useful in predicting treatment outcomes. A retrospective cohort study of periodontal maintenance patients suggests that a patient's periodontal prognosis may depend in part on his or her IL-1 genotype.[59] In this study, the composite genotype described earlier was found to increase an individual's risk of tooth loss 2.7 times. The combined effect of a positive genotype and heavy smoking increased the risk of tooth loss nearly eightfold. Although prospective studies are needed to control for other known risk factors, this study demonstrated that a patient's IL-1 genotype might be an important factor for predicting future disease.

The identification of genetic risk factors for periodontitis in no way mitigates the importance of recognizing and controlling important environmental risk factors. For example, tobacco use is a major risk factor in chronic periodontitis. The risk of disease attributed to smoking appears to override any genetic susceptibility or resistance to disease.[48] For patients who smoke, preventive strategies must address the overwhelming environmental factor: tobacco use. It also is possible that new treatment strategies will be developed to directly counter the deleterious effects of certain risk allele(s). A simple theoretic example is the use of select antiinflammatory drugs in patients who are genetically programmed to be hyperresponders to bacterial antigens.

FUTURE OF GENETIC STUDIES IN PERIODONTOLOGY

Genome-wide searches for risk alleles are not yet feasible because of the large number of markers required in this approach.[50] At present, therefore, the search for risk alleles must focus on candidate gene regions. *Single-nucleotide polymorphisms* (SNPs) are likely to be valuable tools in this search. SNPs are single-nucleotide base-pair substitutions that occur frequently (i.e., about every 1000 base pairs) throughout the genome. Few SNPs alter the amino acid sequences of proteins or even reside in exons. From an epidemiologic viewpoint, however, SNPs are useful because they represent variation in the population.

Given the completion of the human genome project, it should be feasible in the near future to identify all alleles that confer even a moderate risk for disease. Even today, more than 800 SNPs have been identified within the 75 genes thought to be candidates for hypertension.[31] A similar number of candidate SNPs probably exists for the periodontal diseases, especially in genes whose products regulate humoral or cellular immune responses.

Since 1997, dozens of studies exploring the relationship between periodontal disease and genetic polymorphisms have been reported in the literature. To date, however, few polymorphisms have been consistently associated with a periodontal disease. Furthermore, the number of subjects or families studied has been relatively small, and the risk attributable to any one allele or genotype has not been estimated precisely. Before any nucleotide sequence variant is touted as a risk marker for periodontitis, the gene it affects should have some established or biologically plausible role in the pathogenesis of the disease, and its association with periodontitis should be confirmed in independent populations. Given the vast number of annotated variants in the human genome, the potentially large number of false-positive results could lead to clinicians and researchers alike to become disillusioned with the potential clinical utility of such tests.

Periodontitis is clearly multifactorial, and researchers need to design studies that examine the role of important environmental and genetic factors simultaneously. Given the large numbers of genes in the human genome and bacteria in the oral cavity, it is likely that genes and the environment interact in important but as-yet unrecognized ways to alter disease risk. Most importantly, identifying specific genetic risk factors may be academically appealing but is of little use unless it leads to improvements in the prevention or treatment of disease.

REFERENCES

1. Alley CS, Reinhardt RA, Maze CA, et al: HLA-D and T lymphocyte reactivity to specific periodontal pathogens in type 1 diabetic periodontitis, *J Periodontol* 64:974, 1993.
2. Amer A, Singh G, Darke C, et al: Association between HLA antigens and periodontal disease, *Tissue Antigens* 31:53, 1988.
3. Anusaksathien O, Sukboon A, Sitthiphong P, Teanpaisan R: Distribution of interleukin-1beta(+3954) and IL-1alpha(-889) genetic variations in a Thai population group, *J Periodontol* 74:1796, 2003.
4. Armitage GC: Development of a classification system for periodontal diseases and conditions, *Ann Periodontol* 4:1, 1999.
5. Armitage GC, Wu Y, Wang HY, et al: Low prevalence of a periodontitis-associated interleukin-1 composite genotype in individuals of Chinese heritage, *J Periodontol* 71:164, 2000.
6. Asikainen S, Chen C, Alaluusua S, et al: Can one acquire periodontal bacteria and periodontitis from a family member? *J Am Dent Assoc* 128:1263, 1997.
7. Baelum V, Chen X, Manji F, et al: Profiles of destructive periodontal disease in different populations, *J Periodontal Res* 31:17, 1996.
8. Beaty TH, Boughman JA, Yang P, et al: Genetic analysis of juvenile periodontitis in families ascertained through an affected proband, *Am J Hum Genet* 40:443, 1987.
9. Beaty TH, Colyer CR, Chang YC, et al: Familial aggregation of periodontal indices, *J Dent Res* 72:544, 1993.
10. Beck JD, Koch GG, Rozier RG, et al: Prevalence and risk indicators for periodontal attachment loss in a population of older community dwelling blacks and whites, *J Periodontol* 61:521, 1990.
11. Benjamin SD, Baer PN: Familial patterns of advanced alveolar bone loss in adolescence (periodontosis), *Periodontics* 5:82, 1967.
12. Bonfil JJ, Dillier FL, Mercier P, et al: A "case control" study on the role of HLA DR4 in severe periodontitis rapidly progressive periodontitis: identification of types and subtypes using molecular biology (PCR.SSO), *J Clin Periodontol* 26:77, 1999.
13. Boughman JA, Beaty TH, Yang P, et al: Problems of genetic model testing in early onset periodontitis, *J Periodontol* 59:332, 1988.
14. Boughman JA, Halloran SL, Roulston D, et al: An autosomal-dominant form of juvenile periodontitis: its

localization to chromosome 4 and linkage to dentinogenesis imperfecta and Gc, *J Craniofac Genet Dev Biol* 6:341, 1986.
15. Butler JH: A familial pattern of juvenile periodontitis (periodontosis), *J Periodontol* 40:115, 1969.
16. Cantor RM, Rotter JI: Analysis of genetic data: methods and interpretation. In King RA, Rotter JI, Motulsky AG, editors: *The genetic basis of common diseases,* New York, 1992, Oxford University Press.
17. Chapple IL: Hypophosphatasia: dental aspects and mode of inheritance, *J Clin Periodontol* 20:615, 1993.
18. Chung CS, Kau MCW, Chung SSC, et al: A genetic and epidemiologic study of periodontal disease in Hawaii. II. Genetic and environmental influence, *Am J Hum Genet* 29:76, 1977.
19. Colombo AP, Eftimiadi C, Haffajee AD, et al: Serum IgG2 level, Gm(23) allotype and Fc gamma RIIa and Fc gamma RIIIb receptors in refractory periodontal disease, *J Clin Periodontol* 25:465, 1998.
20. Corey LA, Nance WE, Hofstede P, et al: Self-reported periodontal disease in a Virginia twin population, *J Periodontol* 64:1205, 1993.
21. Cullinan MP, Sachs J, Wolf E, et al: The distribution of HLA-A and -B antigens in patients and their families with periodontosis, *J Periodontal Res* 15:177, 1980.
22. Diehl SR, Wang YF, Brooks CN, et al: Linkage disequilibrium of interleukin-1 genetic polymorphisms with early onset periodontitis, *J Periodontol* 70:418, 1999.
23. Dyer JK, Peck MA, Reinhardt RA, et al: HLA-D types and serum IgG responses to *Capnocytophaga* in diabetes and periodontitis, *J Dent Res* 76:1825, 1997.
24. Engebretson SP, Lamster IB, Herra-Abreu M, et al: The influence of interleukin polymorphisms on expression of interleukin-1 and tumor necrosis factor-α in periodontal tissue and gingival crevicular fluid, *J Periodontol* 70:567, 1999.
25. Firatli E, Kantarci A, Cebeci I, et al: Association between HLA antigens and early onset periodontitis, *J Clin Periodontol* 23:563, 1996.
26. Galbraith GM, Steed RB, Sanders JJ, et al: Tumor necrosis factor alpha production by oral leukocytes: influence of tumor necrosis factor genotype, *J Periodontol* 69:428, 1998.
27. Gore EA, Sanders JJ, Pandey JP, et al: Interleukin-1 beta+3953 allele 2: association with disease status in adult periodontitis, *J Clin Periodontol* 25:781, 1998.
28. Gorlin RJ, Sedano H, Anderson VF: The syndrome of palmar-plantar hyperkeratosis and premature periodontal destruction of the teeth, *J Pediatr* 65:985, 1964.
29. Goteiner D, Goldman MJ: Human lymphocyte antigen haplotype and resistance to periodontitis, *J Periodontol* 55:155, 1984.
30. Gwinn MR, Sharma A, De Nardin E: Single nucleotide polymorphisms of the N-formyl peptide receptor in localized juvenile periodontitis, *J Periodontol* 70:1194, 1999.
31. Halushka MK, Fan JB, Bentley K, et al: Patterns of single-nucleotide polymorphisms in candidate genes for blood-pressure homeostasis, *Nat Genet* 22:239, 1999.
32. Hart PS, Zhang Y, Firatli E, et al: Identification of cathepsin C mutations in ethnically diverse Papillon-Lefèvre syndrome patients, *J Med Genet* 37:927, 2000.
33. Hart TC, Kornman KS: Genetic factors in the pathogenesis of periodontitis, *Periodontol 2000* 14:202, 1997.
34. Hart TC, Hart PS, Bowden DW, et al: Mutations of the cathepsin C gene are responsible for Papillon-Lefèvre syndrome, *J Med Genet* 36:881, 1999.
35. Hart TC, Hart PS, Michalec MD, et al: Localisation of a gene for prepubertal periodontitis to chromosome 11q14 and identification of a cathepsin C gene mutation, *J Med Genet* 37:95, 2000.
36. Hart TC, Marazita ML, McCanna KM, et al: Reevaluation of the chromosome 4q candidate region for early onset periodontitis, *Hum Genet* 91:416, 1993.
37. Hart TC, Marazita ML, Schenkein HA, et al: No female preponderance in juvenile periodontitis after correction for ascertainment bias, *J Periodontol* 62:745, 1991.
38. Hart TC, Stabholz A, Meyle J, et al: Genetic studies of syndromes with severe periodontitis and palmoplantar hyperkeratosis, *J Periodontal Res* 32(pt 2):81, 1997.
39. Hennig BJ, Parkhill JM, Chapple IL, et al: Association of a vitamin D receptor gene polymorphism with localized early onset periodontal diseases, *J Periodontol* 70:1032, 1999.
40. Hewitt C, McCormick D, Linden G, et al: The role of cathepsin C in Papillon-Lefèvre syndrome, prepubertal periodontitis, and aggressive periodontitis, *Hum Mutat* 23:222, 2004.
41. Hodge PJ, Riggio MP, Kinane DF: No association with HLA-DQB1 in European Caucasians with early onset periodontitis, *Tissue Antigens* 54:205, 1999.
42. Kaslick RS, West TL, Chasens AI, et al: Association between HL-A2 antigen and various periodontal diseases in young adults, *J Dent Res* 54:424, 1975.
43. Kaslick RS, West TL, Chasens AI: Association between ABO blood groups, HL-A antigens and periodontal diseases in young adults: a follow-up study, *J Periodontol* 51:339, 1980.
44. Katz J, Goultschin J, Benoliel R, et al: Human leukocyte antigen (HLA) DR4: positive association with rapidly progressing periodontitis, *J Periodontol* 58:607, 1987.
45. King RA, Rotter JI, Motulsky AG: The approach to genetic bases of common diseases. In King RA, Rotter JI, Motulsky AG, editors: *The genetic basis of common diseases,* New York, 1992, Oxford University Press.
46. Klouda PT, Porter SR, Scully C, et al: Association between HLA-A9 and rapidly progressive periodontitis, *Tissue Antigens* 28:146, 1986.
47. Kobayashi T, Westerdaal NA, Miyazaki A, et al: Relevance of immunoglobulin G Fc receptor polymorphism to recurrence of adult periodontitis in Japanese patients, *Infect Immun* 65:3556, 1997.
48. Kornman KS, di Giovine FS: Genetic variations in cytokine expression: a risk factor for severity of adult periodontitis, *Ann Periodontol* 3:327, 1998.
49. Kornman KS, Crane A, Wang HY, et al: The interleukin-1 genotype as a severity factor in adult periodontal disease, *J Clin Periodontol* 24:72, 1997.
50. Kruglyak L: Prospects for whole-genome linkage disequilibrium mapping of common disease genes, *Nat Genet* 22:139, 1999.
51. Lewin B: *Genes,* ed 4, New York, 1994, Oxford University Press.
52. Li Y, Xu L, Hasturk H, et al: Localized aggressive periodontitis is linked to human chromosome 1q25, *Hum Genet*114:291, 2004.
53. Löe H, Anerud A, Boysen H, et al: Natural history of periodontal disease in man: rapid moderate, and no loss of attachment in Sri Lankan laborers 14 to 46 years of age, *J Clin Periodontol* 13:431, 1986.
54. Long JC, Nance WE, Waring P, et al: Early onset periodontitis: a comparison and evaluation of two proposed modes of inheritance, *Genet Epidemiol* 4:13, 1987.
55. MacFarlane GD, Herzberg MC, Wolff LF, et al: Refractory periodontitis associated with abnormal polymorphonuclear leukocyte phagocytosis and cigarette smoking, *J Periodontol* 63:908, 1992.
56. Machulla HK, Stein J, Gautsch A, et al: HLA-A, B, Cw, DRB1, DRB3/4/5, DQB1 in German patients suffering from rapidly progressive periodontitis (RPP) and adult periodontitis (AP), *J Clin Periodontol* 29:573, 2002.

57. Marazita ML, Burmeister JA, Gunsolley JC, et al: Evidence for autosomal dominant inheritance and race-specific heterogeneity in early onset periodontitis, *J Periodontol* 65:623, 1994.
58. Marggraf E, von Keyserlingk-Eberius HJ, Komischke B, et al: [Association of histocompatibility antigens (HLA antigens) with deep periodontopathies], *Dtsch Zahnarztl Z* 38:585, 1983.
59. McGuire MK, Nunn ME: Prognosis versus actual outcome. IV. The effectiveness of clinical parameters and IL-1 genotype in accurately predicting prognoses and tooth survival, *J Periodontol* 70:49, 1999.
60. Meisel P, Siegemund A, Grimm R, et al: The interleukin-1 polymorphism, smoking, and the risk of periodontal disease in the population-based SHIP study, *J Dent Res* 82:189, 2003.
61. Melnick M, Shields ED, Bixler D: Periodontosis: a phenotypic and genetic analysis, *Oral Surg Oral Med Oral Pathol* 42:32, 1976.
62. Michalowicz BS: Genetic and heritable risk factors in periodontal disease, *J Periodontol* 65(5 suppl):479, 1994.
63. Michalowicz BS, Aeppli DM, Kuba RK, et al: A twin study of genetic variation in proportional radiographic alveolar bone height, *J Dent Res* 70:1431, 1991.
64. Michalowicz BS, Aeppli D, Virag JG, et al: Periodontal findings in adult twins, *J Periodontol* 62:293, 1991.
65. Michalowicz BS, Diehl SR, Gunsolley JC, et al: Evidence of a substantial genetic basis for risk of adult periodontitis, *J Periodontol* 71:1699, 2000.
66. Michalowicz BS, Wolff LF, Klump, D, et al: Periodontal bacteria in adult twins, *J Periodontol* 70:263, 1999.
67. Moore WE, Burmeister JA, Brooks CN, et al: Investigation of the influences of puberty, genetics, and environment on the composition of subgingival periodontal floras, *Infect Immun* 61:2891, 1993.
68. Moses JH, Tsichti H, Donaldson P, et al: HLA and susceptibility to juvenile periodontitis in Afro-Caribbeans, *Tissue Antigens* 43:316, 1994.
69. Nicklin MJ, Weith A, Duff GW: A physical map of the region encompassing the human interleukin-1 alpha, interleukin-1 beta, and interleukin-1 receptor antagonist genes. Genomics 1994; 19:382.
70. Noack B: Die Parodontoseätiologie im Lichte der Vererbung. Untersuchungen an erbverschiedenen und erbgleichen Zwillingspaaren, *Osterr Zschr Stomat* 38:267, 1940.
71. Ohyama H, Takashiba S, Oyaizu K, et al: HLA Class II genotypes associated with early onset periodontitis: DQB1 molecule primarily confers susceptibility to the disease, *J Periodontol* 67:888, 1996.
72. Oliver RC, Brown LJ, Löe H: Variations in the prevalence and extent of periodontitis, *J Amer Dent Assoc* 122:43, 1991.
73. Pihlstrom BL, Michalowicz BS: Genetic risk for periodontal diseases: a clinical perspective, *J Paradontol Implantol Orale* 17:123, 1998.
74. Pilger U, Hennies HC, Truschnegg A, Aberer E: Late-onset Papillon-Lefèvre syndrome without alteration of the cathepsin C gene, *J Am Acad Dermatol* 49(5 suppl):S240, 2003.
75. Ponder BA: Costs, benefits and limitations of genetic testing for cancer risk, *Br J Cancer* 80(suppl 1):46, 1999.
76. Potter RH: Etiology of periodontitis: the heterogeneity paradigm, *J Periodontol* 60:593, 1989 (guest editorial).
77. Preus HR: Treatment of rapidly destructive periodontitis in Papillon-Lefèvre syndrome: laboratory and clinical observations, *J Clin Periodontol* 15:639, 1988.
78. Rao DC, Chung CS, Morton NE: Genetic and environmental determinants of periodontal disease, *Am J Med Genet* 4:39, 1979.
79. Rao NV, Rao GV, Hoidal JR: Human dipeptidyl-peptidase I: gene characterization, localization, and expression, *J Biol Chem* 272:10260, 1997.
80. Reinholdt J, Bay I, Svejgaard A: Association between HLA-antigens and periodontal disease, *J Dent Res* 56:1261, 1977.
81. Root AW: Recent advances in the genetics of disorders of calcium homeostasis, *Adv Pediatr* 43:77, 1996.
82. Rotter JR, Vadheim CM, Rimoin DL: Diabetes mellitus. In King RA, Rotter JI, Motulsky AG, editors: *The genetic basis of common diseases,* New York, 1992, Oxford University Press.
83. Saxen L: Heredity of juvenile periodontitis, *J Clin Periodontol* 7:276, 1980.
84. Saxen L, Koskimies S: Juvenile periodontitis—no linkage with HLA-antigens, *J Periodontal Res* 19:441, 1984.
85. Saxen L, Nevanlinna HR: Autosomal recessive inheritance of juvenile periodontitis: test of a hypothesis, *Clin Genet* 25:332, 1984.
86. Schenkein HA: Genetics of early onset periodontal diseases. In Genco R et al, editors: *Molecular pathogenesis of periodontal disease,* Washington, DC, 1994, American Society for Microbiology.
87. Schenkein HA: Inheritance as a determinant of susceptibility for periodontitis, *J Dent Educ* 62:840, 1998.
88. Schull WJ, Neel JV: Effects of inbreeding on Japanese children, New York, 1965, Harper & Row.
89. Shapira L, Eizenburg S, Sela MN, et al: HLA A9 and B15 are associated with generalized form, but not the localized form, of early onset periodontal diseases, *J Periodontol* 65:219, 1994.
90. Shapira L, Smidt A, Van Dyke TE, et al: Sequential manifestation of different forms of early onset periodontitis: a case report, *J Periodontol* 65:631, 1994.
91. Sofaer JA: Genetic approaches in the study of periodontal diseases, *J Clin Periodontol* 17:401, 1990.
92. Spektor MD, Vandesteen GE, Page RC: Clinical studies of one family manifesting rapidly progressive, juvenile and prepubertal periodontitis, *J Periodontol* 56:93, 1985.
93. Tachi Y, Shimpuku H, Nosaka Y, et al: Association of vitamin D receptor gene polymorphism with periodontal diseases in Japanese and Chinese, *Nucleic Acids Res Suppl* 1:111, 2001.
94. Tai H, Endo M, Shimada Y, et al: Association of interleukin-1 receptor antagonist gene polymorphisms with early onset periodontitis in Japanese, *J Clin Periodontol* 29:882, 2002.
95. Takashiba S, Noji S, Nishimura F, et al: Unique intronic variations of HLA-DQ beta gene in early onset periodontitis, *J Periodontol* 65:379, 1994.
96. Tatakis DN: Interleukin-1 and bone metabolism: a review, *J Periodontol* 64(5 suppl):416, 1993.
97. Terasaki PI, Kaslick RS, West TL, et al: Low HL-A2 frequency and periodontitis, *Tissue Antigens* 5:286, 1975.
98. Thomson G: HLA disease associations: models for the study of complex human genetic disorders, *Crit Rev Clin Lab Sci* 32:183, 1995.
99. Toomes C, James J, Wood AJ, et al: Loss-of-function mutations in the cathepsin C gene result in periodontal disease and palmoplantar keratosis, *Nat Genet* 23:421, 1999.
100. van der Velden U, Abbas F, Armand S, et al: The effect of sibling relationship on the periodontal condition, *J Clin Periodontol* 20:683, 1993.
101. Venter JC, Adams MD, Myers EW, et al: The sequence of the human genome, *Science* 291:1304, 2001.
102. Waldrop TC, Anderson DC, Hallmon WW, et al: Periodontal manifestations of the heritable Mac-1, LFA-1, deficiency syndrome: clinical, histopathologic and molecular characteristics, *J Periodontol* 58:400, 1987.
103. Walker SJ, van Dyke TE, Rich S, et al: Genetic polymorphisms of the IL-1alpha and IL-1beta genes in African-American LJP patients and an African-American control population, *J Periodontol* 71:723, 2000.
104. Wilson ME, Kalmar JR: Fc-gamma-RIIA (CD32)—a potential marker defining host susceptibility to localized juvenile periodontitis, *J Periodontol* 67:323, 1996.

Immunity and Inflammation: Basic Concepts

Keith L. Kirkwood, Russell J. Nisengard, Susan Kinder Haake, and Kenneth T. Miyasaki

12

CHAPTER

■ ■ ■

CHAPTER OUTLINE

CELLS OF IMMUNITY AND INFLAMMATION
 Mast Cells
 Dermal Dendrocytes
 Peripheral Dendritic Cells
 Neutrophils and Monocytes/Macrophages
 Lymphocytes
 T Cells
 B Cells
 Natural Killer (NK) Cells
COMPLEMENT

TRANSENDOTHELIAL MIGRATION
LEUKOCYTE FUNCTIONS
 Chemotaxis
 Phagocytosis
 Antigen Processing and Presentation
SPECIFIC IMMUNE RESPONSES
T-CELL RESPONSES
B-CELL RESPONSES AND ANTIBODIES
SUMMARY

*T*he common periodontal diseases found in humans are gingivitis and periodontitis. These are inflammatory responses in the periodontal tissues induced by microorganisms in dental plaque, which contribute to tissue destruction, bone loss, and eventually tooth loss. This chapter focuses on the role of the immune system in inflammation. The immune system is a network designed for the homeostasis of large molecules *(oligomers)* and cells based on specific recognition processes. Recognition of the structural features of an oligomer by receptors on immune cells is an important component of the *specificity* of the immune system.

Immune responses are categorized as either innate or adaptive. *Innate immune responses* may adapt with exposure to the same pathogen but subside once the threat has been eliminated. An example of innate immunity is phagocytic cells (i.e., monocytes, macrophages, neutrophils), which possess a number of inherently antimicrobial peptides and proteins that kill many different pathogens rather than one specific pathogen. In contrast, the specific immune responses will increase after exposure to a pathogen and usually maintain higher levels for years. Lymphocytes (e.g., T cells, B cells) are important in the fundamental form of specific

adaptive immunity referred to as the *specific immune response.* The ability of T cells and B cells to recognize specific oligomeric structures on a pathogen and generate progeny that also recognize the structure enables the immune system to respond more rapidly and effectively when reexposed to that same pathogen.

Inflammation is an observable alteration in tissues associated with changes in vascular permeability and dilation, often with the infiltration of leukocytes into affected tissues. These changes result in the erythema, edema, heat, pain, and loss of function that are the "cardinal signs" of inflammation. Typically, inflammation can progress through three stages: immediate, acute, and chronic. *Leukocytes,* the white blood cells, control all three stages of inflammation (Table 12-1 and Figure 12-1).

Leukocytes originate in the bone marrow and exit from the blood by *transendothelial migration* under normal conditions, accounting for the *resident leukocytes* (or nonelicited leukocytes) found in tissues. Among the most important resident leukocytes are mast cells, peripheral dendritic cells, and monocyte derivatives such as dermal dendrocytes (histiocytes). These resident leukocytes transmit information that initiates the processes of *immediate inflammation* (Figure 12-2). Immediate

TABLE 12-1

Cells of the Immune System

Leukocytes	Normal Blood Levels (per mm^2)	Notable Properties (Cell Diameter in Blood)	Key Receptors in Interactions with Antigens*	Important Functions in Inflammation
Myeloid Cells				
Neutrophil	4000 to 8000	Terminally differentiated in blood, granular cytoplasm (9-10 μm)	CR1, CR3 (Mac-1) CR4 FcγRII C5aR(CD88)	Phagocytic killing of microorganisms
Monocyte	200 to 800	Immature in blood (9-10 μm)	CR1, CR3 (Mac-1) CR4, CD1 FcγRI, FcγRII MHC class II C5aR (CD88)	Can differentiate to macrophages with diameters >20 μm Functions in phagocytosis and antigen processing and presentation
Peripheral dendritic cell	N/A	Immature in blood (9-10 μm)	IAM-1, LFA-1 MHC Class II CD1	Resident in parabasilar epithelium Functions in processing and presentation of antigen
Eosinophil	50 to 300	Terminally differentiated in blood, granular cytoplasm (9-10 μm)	FCεRII (low affinity) FcγRII C5aR (CD88) CR1, CR3 (Mac-1) CR4	Antiparasitic and antihelminthic activity, mediated by IgE
Basophil	0 to 100	Terminally differentiated in blood, granular cytoplasm (9-10 μm)	FCεRII (high affinity) CR1, CR3, CR4 C5aR (CD88)	Receptor profile suggests that cells may respond to bacterial and parasitic infections.
Mast cell	N/A	N/A	FCεRII (high affinity) C3aR C5aR (CD88) CR4, no CR3	Resident of perivascular connective tissue Anaphylactic effects in response to C3a and C5a Antigen recognized by IgE
Lymphoid Cells				
CD4+ cells	400-1600	(8-10 μm)	TCR, CD4	Scanning antigen presented by professional antigen-presenting cells; in inflammation, this may result in clonal expansion of B cells or T cells.
CD8+ cells	200 to 800	(8-10 μm)	TCR, CD8	Scanning antigen presented by all cells; in inflammation, this may result in clonal expansion and filling of the cell presenting antigen.
B cell	200 to 800	(8-10 μm)	BCR, MHC class II	Binding soluble antigen, antigen processing and presentation; in inflammation, this may result in clonal expansion and antibody secretion.
Natural killer – (NK) cell	100 to 500	(8-15 μm)	KIR, KAR	Scanning cell antigens, target cell killing if KAR scans antigen, no killing if KIR scans antigen

*All cells present self-derived antigens using major histocompatibility complex (MHC) class I molecules. See text for explanation of receptor designations.

N/A, Not applicable.

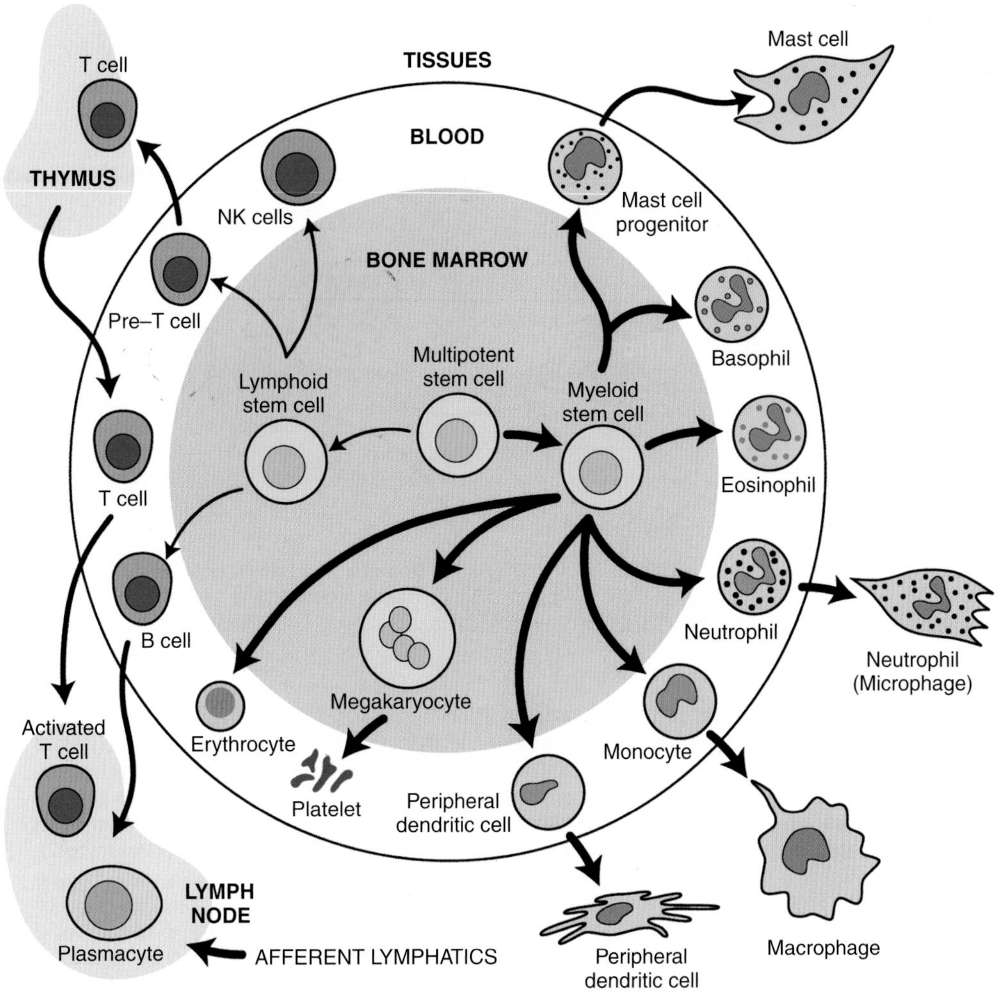

Figure 12-1 The main cells of the immune system are derived from the lymphoid and myeloid arms of the hematopoietic system. In the bone marrow, the myeloid arm gives rise to peripheral dendritic cells (DCs), phagocytes (neutrophils and monocytes), mast cell precursors, basophils, eosinophils, platelets, and erythrocytes. In the tissues, peripheral DCs, monocytes, and mast cell precursors further differentiate. The monocyte can become a macrophage. In the bone marrow, the lymphoid arm gives rise to natural killer (NK) cells, B cells, and pre–T cells. The pre–T cells differentiate to T cells in the thymus. Secondary lymphoid organs, including lymph nodes and the spleen, are areas where antigen-presenting cells, B cells, and DCs present antigen to T cells. Terminal differentiation of B and T cells also occurs in these organs.

inflammation is followed within minutes by a short-lived period (up to several hours) of *acute inflammation* that is characterized by an influx of neutrophils to the area after they exit the blood. If the problem is not resolved, acute inflammation gives way to a potentially unending period of *chronic inflammation* dominated by the migration of lymphocytes and macrophages to the local tissues. The leukocytes recruited into tissues in acute and chronic inflammation are termed *inflammatory leukocytes.*

CELLS OF IMMUNITY AND INFLAMMATION

Cells of the immune system that are important in inflammation and host defenses include mast cells, dermal dendrocytes (histiocytes), peripheral dendritic cells, neutrophils, monocytes/macrophages, T cells, B cells, and natural killer (NK) cells (see Table 12-1 and Figure 12-1). Other hematopoietic leukocytes, including basophils, eosinophils, erythrocytes, and platelets, also participate in certain forms of inflammation or immune function but are not described here.

Cells possess *receptors,* which are molecules on the cell surfaces that enable the cell to interact with other molecules or cells. Receptors reflect and dictate the function of cells. Historically, the names given to receptors often related to function. In addition to these common names, a systematic nomenclature known as the *CD* (cluster of differentiation) *system* has been developed. Under this system, receptors are identified as CD1, CD2, and so on. In this chapter, multiple designations are provided for specific receptors when the different designations have been commonly used.

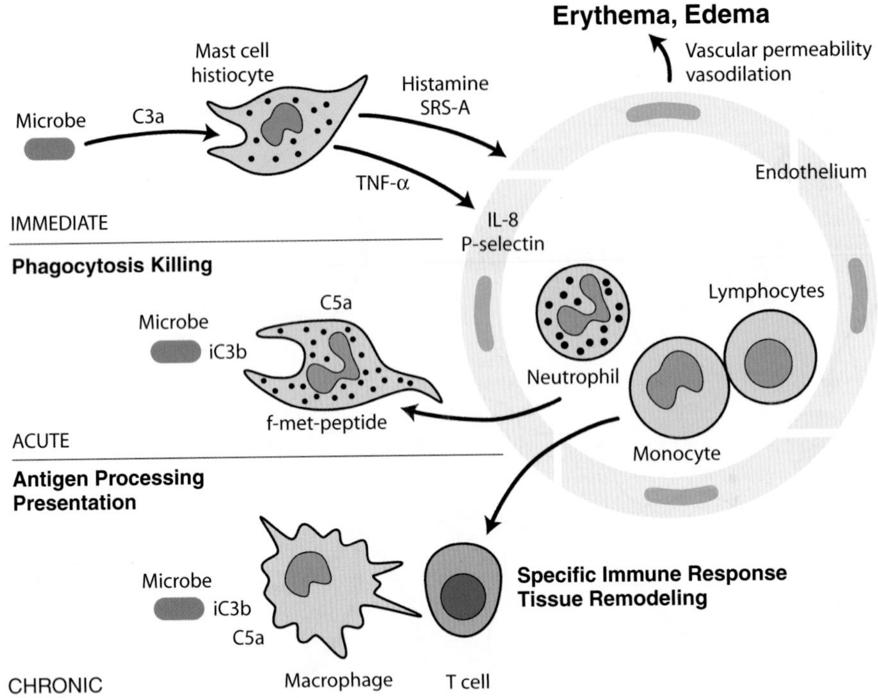

Figure 12-2 The natural history of inflammation actually starts before an irritant exists, with the transendothelial migration of resident leukocytes, especially the mast cell. Mast cells are among the most effective cells in alerting the endothelium of a local problem. Mast cell interaction with the vascular system leads to erythema and edema, which are two of the five cardinal signs of inflammation. Mast cells also signal the endothelial cells to recruit inflammatory leukocytes. The inflammatory leukocytes are active in phagocytosis, killing, antigen processing and presentation, specific immune responses, and tissue remodeling. They cause the infiltrated area to lose function (the fifth cardinal sign of inflammation) as a side effect of their intense focus on resolving the problem and remodeling the tissue. Also depicted are the complement metabolites, iC3b, C3a, and C5a. These molecules are important in allowing the immune system to "see" substances for which they do not possess receptors. *TNF-α,* Tumor necrosis factor alpha; *IL-8,* interleukin-8; *SRS-A,* slow-reacting substance of anaphylaxis.

SCIENCE TRANSFER

In periodontal disease the inflammatory response causes tissue resistance to bacterial invasion but also provides mechanisms that contribute to tissue damage. The acute inflammatory cells, such as mast cells, macrophages, dermal dendrocytes, Langerhans cells, and polymorphonuclear leukocytes (PMNs), all combine to form a potent antibacterial defense mechanism, but the initial signs of gingival inflammation (e.g., swelling, redness, bleeding on probing) represent the tissue-destructive aspects of these cells. In established periodontal disease, there is also chronic inflammatory change, with B cells and T cells adding to the antibacterial spectrum. These lymphocytic cells also have the capacity to release cytokines, which may induce the synthesis of arachidonate metabolites (especially PGE_2), and to stimulate macrophages and osteoclasts to release hydrolases and collagenases, which are responsible for loss of collagen and bone. Each patient with dental plaque has a complex balance between these protective and damaging scenarios that results either in a slowly progressive loss of attachment (periodontitis) or in a restriction of tissue inflammation to the peripheral tissues (gingivitis).

Mast Cells

Mast cells are important in immediate inflammation (see Table 12-1 and Figure 12-1). They possess receptors for complement components (C3a and C5a) as well as receptors for the Fc portion of the antibody molecules immunoglobulin E (IgE) and immunoglobulin G (IgG): FcεR and FcγR, respectively.[4] More recently, mast cells have been shown to express toll-like receptors.[20] These receptors allow the innate immune system to adapt (e.g., express the major histocompatibility complex [MHC; see later discussion] class II molecules, produce nitric oxide and so on). This adaptation is transitory. The stimulation of these receptors can result in activation and secretion of vasoactive substances that increase vascular permeability and dilation, two important signs of *anaphylaxis*. Anaphylaxis can be life threatening if it is widespread (systemic), but it is usually localized and is important in initiating inflammatory responses against local microbial invasion.[17] Mast cells feature prominent cytoplasmic granules, termed *lysosomes,* which store inflammatory mediators such as histamine, eosinophil chemotactic factor, neutrophil chemotactic factor, and heparin. Mast cells can synthesize, de novo, other inflammatory mediators, such as the slow-reacting substances of anaphylaxis (SRS-A), tumor necrosis factor alpha (TNF-α), interleukin-6 (IL-6), and leukotriene C4.

Dermal Dendrocytes

Dermal dendrocytes *(histiocytes)* are widely distributed and form a large system of collagen-associated dendritic cells of myeloid origin. These cells are distributed near blood vessels and possess receptors for the complement component C3a, by which they participate in immediate inflammation. They express the MHC class II molecules.[27] More recently, it has been found that histiocytes can express matrix metalloproteinases (MMPs) in response to bacterial challenge and thus potentially contribute directly to periodontal tissue destruction.[18]

Peripheral Dendritic Cells

Peripheral dendritic cells (DCs) are leukocytes with cytoplasmic projections, or *dendrites* (see Table 12-1).[32] *Langerhans cells* are DCs that reside in the suprabasilar portions of squamous epithelium. DCs ingest antigen locally and transport the antigen to the lymph nodes through the afferent lymphatics. DCs express high levels of MHC class II molecules and CD1, as well as cell adhesion molecules (e.g., intercellular adhesion molecule-1 [ICAM-1], leukocyte function–associated antigen-3 [LFA-3]) and co-stimulatory factors (e.g., B7-1, B7-2; discussed later).

Neutrophils and Monocytes/Macrophages

Neutrophils and monocytes are closely related phagocytic leukocytes. The fundamental difference between these two cells is that neutrophils differentiate almost completely within the bone marrow (14 days), whereas monocytes exit the bone marrow after 2 days in a relatively immature state and may differentiate in the tissues. Neutrophils and monocytes are almost the same size (10-μm diameter) in the blood.

Neutrophils, also known as *polymorphonuclear leukocytes* (PMNs), are the predominant leukocyte in blood, accounting for about two thirds of all blood leukocytes (4000-8000 cells/mm^3; see Table 12-1). They possess many lysosomes within their cytoplasm. Because neutrophils do not need to differentiate substantially to function, they are suited for rapid responses. Neutrophils possess receptors for metabolites of the complement molecule C3, designated complement receptors 1, 3, and 4 (CR1, CR3, CR4) and C5 (C5aR). They also possess receptors for IgG antibody (FcγR). These receptors enable neutrophils to (1) be recruited from the blood, (2) locate offending agents, and (3) ingest (phagocytose) and kill the offending agents.

By convention, monocytes are referred to as *macrophages* when they leave the blood. They complete their differentiation in the local tissues and may become greater than 22 μm in diameter; thus the *macro*phage designation. Because macrophages differentiate and live in the local tissues, they are suited for communicating with lymphocytes and other surrounding cells. Macrophages live long enough to present antigen to T cells. Together, macrophages and lymphocytes orchestrate the chronic immune response. Monocytes/macrophages possess CR1, CR3, CR4, C5aR receptors, several classes of Fcγ receptors (FcγRI, FcγRII, FcγRIII), and molecules important in antigen presentation (MHC class II receptor, CD1).

Lymphocytes

The three main types of lymphocytes are distinguished on the basis of their receptors for antigens: T lymphocytes, B –lymphocytes, and natural killer (NK) cells. In the blood, B cells and T cells are inactive and fairly small (8-10 μm). NK cells may differentiate extensively in the bone marrow and appear in blood as large, granular lymphocytes. With a diameter of 15 μm or greater, NK cells are larger than any other leukocytes in the blood.

T Cells

T cells recognize diverse antigens using a low-affinity transmembranous complex, the *T-cell antigen receptor* (TCR). Antigens are recognized by T cells in association with either MHC class I or class II molecules on the surface of the antigen-presenting cell. T cells are subdivided based on whether they possess the co-receptors CD4 or CD8. The CD4 co-receptor reversibly binds (scans for) MHC class II molecules (HLA-DR, HLA-DP, HLA-DQ) that are found on DCs, macrophages, and B cells. CD4+ T cells initiate and help with immune responses by providing proliferation and differentiation signals. The CD8 co-receptor scans for MHC class I molecules, which are found on all cells. The CD8+ T cells are predominantly cytotoxic T cells involved in controlling intracellular antigens (e.g., certain bacteria, hyphal fungi, viruses).

B Cells

B cells help control extracellular antigens such as bacteria, fungal yeast, and virions. B cells recognize diverse antigens using the *B-cell antigen receptor* (BCR), which is a high-affinity antigen receptor. The high-affinity interaction between BCR and antigen enables the B cell to bind and ingest the antigen without antigen presentation. The antigen is tightly bound, not scanned. Ingested antigen is degraded and presented to T cells.

Before antigen exposure, B cells express immunoglobulin M (IgM) as part of the BCR. After antigen exposure, some B cells differentiate to form *plasma cells* dedicated to the production and secretion of antibodies of the IgM isotype. Others in the presence of T cells may differentiate along the memory pathway, forming *memory B cells.* Memory B cells give rise to plasma cells on secondary exposure to antigen and produce high-affinity antibodies of the appropriate isotype.

Natural Killer (NK) Cells

NK cells recognize and kill certain tumor and virally infected cells. The NK cells possess several classes of antigen receptors, including *killer inhibitory receptor* (KIR) and *killer activating receptor* (KAR). These receptors will recognize antigens associated with MHC class I molecules, MHC class I molecules themselves, and certain other surface glycoproteins. Normal cells possess MHC class I molecules that present antigens recognized as "self"; these interact with KIRs and protect the cells from NK cell–mediated killing. Alterations in antigens presented by the MHC class I molecules, occurring in tumor-infected and virally infected cells, may result in NK-cell activation because the KIRs do not detect sufficient self-antigens. Additionally, cells can present self-antigens in response to stress or other alteration, which are recognized by the KARs. KAR activation can override KIR inhibition and cause the NK cell to kill the target cell.

COMPLEMENT

Complement (C) is an interacting network of about 30 membrane-associated cell receptors and soluble serum glycoproteins (Table 12-2). Soluble components of this system account for about 5% (3-4 mg/ml) of the total serum protein. Most soluble components are synthesized in the liver, but many also may be produced by macrophages (C1, C2, C3, C4, C5, factor B, C1–INA, factor D, and factor H). The soluble components of the complement system were first observed to cause bacteriolysis and cytolysis in association with antibody (a "complement" of antibody), and later in the absence of antibody. These lytic effects are famous but represent only one function of complement.

The complement system is a central component of inflammation that enables endothelium and leukocytes to recognize and bind foreign substances for which they lack receptors. Complement promotes inflammation by generating the following:

- A vasoactive substance, termed *kinin-like,* C2a, which induces pain and increases vascular permeability and dilation.
- Molecules, termed *anaphylatoxins,* C3a and C5a, which produce anaphylaxis by inducing mast cell secretion.
- A chemotaxin, C5a, which attracts leukocytes and stimulates phagocyte secretion.
- An opsonin, iC3b, covalently bound to molecular aggregates, particles, or cells, which enables phagocytes to ingest them.

C3 is the most important component of complement (Figure 12-3, *A*). It also is the predominant component, accounting for about one third of the total complement (1.6 mg/ml). A sequestered, internal thioester bond is the essential feature of C3, and it shares this feature with the related molecule, C4. Splitting of C3 forms C3a and C3b and exposes the internal thioester bond residing within the C3b fragment. Two main pathways result in the splitting of C3: the *alternative* and *classical* pathways (Figure 12-3, *B*). The outcome of C3b generation is dictated by the presence or absence of the regulators of complement activation (see following discussion).

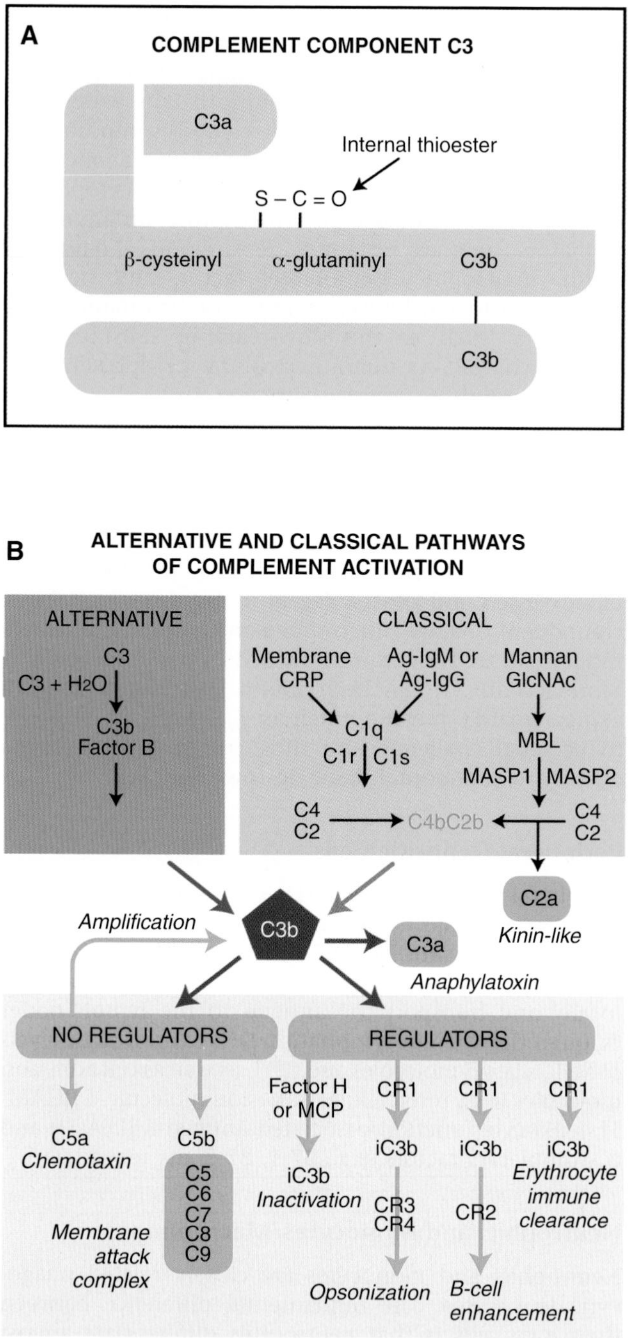

Figure 12-3 **A,** The central component of complement is C3. (See text for details of the importance and function of C3.) **B,** The central goal of the complement system is the formation of C3b. Both the alternative and classical pathways lead to formation of C3 convertase enzymes (C3bBb, C4bC2b) and the generation of C3b. The biologic consequences of C3b formation depend on the presence or absence of regulators. (See text for details of the complement pathways.)

TABLE 12-2

Complement Components

Component/Serum	Molecular Weight (kD)	Concentration (μg/ml)*
Classical Pathway Initiators		
C1q†	410	150 to 180
C1r	85	50
C1s	85	100
Mannose-binding lectin (MBL)	400	1.5 to 1.8
MASP1	93 (proform)	1.5 to 12
MASP2	90 (proform)	Undetermined
C3 Convertase and C3/C5 Convertase Formation		
C2	110	30
C3	195	1200 to 1300
C4	210	400 to 450
Factor B	93	200 to 225
Factor D	25	1.5
Membrane Attach Complex Formation		
C5	205	80
C6	128	75
C7	121	55
C8	155	80
C9	79	200
C1-INA	109	180
Factor I	88 to 93	25 to 35
Anaphylatoxin inactivator	310	30
Soluble Regulators of Complement Activation		
Factor H	150	500 to 520
C4BP	570	200
Membrane Regulators of Complement Activation		**Location**
MCP (CD46)	45 to 70	All cells
DAF (CD55)	75 to 80	All cells
CR1 (CD35)	250	Phagocytes, B cells, erythrocytes
CR2 (CD21)	140	B cells
Opsonic Receptors of iC3b		
CR3 (Mac-1; CD11b/CD18)	165/95‡	Phagocytes, dendritic cells
CR4 (p150/95; CD11c/CD18)	150/95‡	Phagocytes

*Normal serum protein concentration range is 60 to 78 mg/ml.

†See text for explanation of abbreviations.

‡Molecular weights of individual subunits of the receptors are provided.

Both the alternative pathway and the classical pathway lead to inflammation and phagocytosis through an enzyme that is designated a *bound C3 convertase.* The alternative pathway is initiated without provocation by a spontaneous hydrolysis of the internal thioester bond of C3 by water. This pathway leads to the hydrolysis of C3b by larger structures (designated *R*), including the hydroxyls and amines on macromolecules and bacterial cell surfaces. The resulting covalent structure, C3b-R, leads to the bound C3 convertase (R-C3bBb).

The classical pathway is initiated in response to the presence of some irritant. Irritants include antibody-antigen complexes, certain membranes, or suspicious polymers (e.g., mannans). This pathway involves the activation of a serine protease (e.g., C1qrs) that has attached to an irritant. The protease serves as a C4/C2 convertase and leads to formation of a C3 convertase covalently bound to R (R-C4bC2b), with release of the vasoactive kinin-like substance C2a. The classical pathway also may be activated in the absence of such irritants, but this is controlled by an inactivator, C1 inactivator (C1-INA). A deficiency of C1-INA (often occurring secondary to infection) can result in swollen lips or eyelids (angioedema) because of such spontaneous activation of the classical pathway.

Two main processes can occur with the formation of bound C3 convertase in the absence of regulators, such as in the presence of bacterial cells (Figure 12-3, *B*). First, amplification occurs, and second, the membrane attack complex is formed. *Amplification* is an exponential increase in the formation of C3b. This results because the bound C3 convertase (either R-C3bBb or R-C4bC2b) forms more C3b, and the resultant C3b may form more C3 convertases (R-C3bBb). Formation of C3b also is associated with the production of the anaphylatoxin C3a.

Formation of the *membrane attack complex* is initiated after approximately 100 molecules of C3b are formed, when the thioester of one C3b is hydrolyzed by the C3 convertase (R-C3bBb or R-C4bC2b) itself at a specific site on the C3b (or C4b) subunit of the convertase.[8] This results in the formation of the structure R-C3b-C3bBb or R-C3b-C4bC2b. These new complexes can bind and cleave both C3 and C5; thus they are called *C3/C5 convertases*. The C5 convertase activity is monumentally slow (one of the slowest enzymatic activities known); at best, one C5 is converted every 4 minutes by one C5 convertase. Nonetheless, the cleavage of C5 produces two important fragments, C5a and C5b. The C5a fragment is the main leukocyte chemoattractant derived from complement and is an important anaphylatoxin. The C5b component associates with C6, C7, C8, and C9, forming a membrane attack complex that can lyse certain bacteria and cells by forming a large pore in the target cell membrane.

The six *regulators of complement activation* are encoded in a tight cluster on chromosome 1: *factor H, membrane cofactor protein* (MCP), *complement receptor 1* (CR1), *complement receptor 2* (CR2), *decay-accelerating factor* (DAF), and *C4-binding protein* (C4BP). Four of these regulators are cofactors working with the proteolytic soluble enzyme *factor I:* factor H, MCP, CR1, and C4BP.

Factor H and C4BP are serum cofactors that are most important in the inactivation of fluid phase C3b and C4b, respectively. Factor H enables factor I to inactivate C3b by clipping out a small piece, forming inactivated C3b (iC3b). The iC3b is inactive because it no longer can bind factor G and thus can no longer generate C3 convertases. MCP and DAF are widely distributed on host cells and are mainly designed to protect the host cell against C3b and C3 convertase, respectively, which have bound to the same host cell. MCP binds to R-C3b and enables factor I to convert the R-C3b to R-iC3b. This halts further amplification. Eventually, iC3b is further metabolized and destroyed.

CR1 is a transmembrane molecule expressed by phagocytes (neutrophils and macrophages), B cells, and red blood cells. CR1 binds C3b that is attached covalently to the surface of another particle, and it attracts factor I, leading to the inactivation of amplification by the formation of iC3b. Phagocytes possess receptors for iC3b and will efficiently ingest the iC3b-bound cell or particle in a process known as *opsonic phagocytosis* (see later), with subsequent destruction of the ingested material. Thus, whereas MCP protects host cells, CR1 targets foreign or altered cells or molecules in the area for destruction.

In summary, the complement system is essential for identifying and neutralizing substances for which the host does not possess specific receptors. Local expression of complement components (e.g. C2a, C3a, and C5a) enhances the inflammatory response and enables the endothelium and leukocytes to respond to eliminate the antigen. The complement system also facilitates phagocytosis and destruction of foreign substances as well as direct destruction of cells or microorganisms through the membrane attack complex.

TRANSENDOTHELIAL MIGRATION

The directed movement of leukocytes from the blood into the local tissues is central to inflammation. Transendothelial migration is a selective interaction between leukocytes and endothelium that results in the leukocyte pushing its way between endothelial cells to exit the blood and enter the tissues. Defects in transendothelial migration are associated with aggressive periodontitis, reflecting the importance of this process in periodontal diseases.

Neutrophils and monocytes spend less than 12 hours in circulation. B cells and T cells stay in the blood for only about 30 minutes at a time. B cells and T cells require the additional influence of lymphoid organs (lymph nodes, spleen, tonsils, Peyer's patches, adenoids) to function properly. Thus they constantly exit the blood, pass through lymphatics and secondary lymphoid organs, and reenter the blood in a perpetual process known as *lymphocyte recirculation.* The blood contains only 2% of all lymphocytes at any given time, and lymphocytes are estimated to recirculate as much as 50 times a day.[26]

In a local inflammatory response, transendothelial migration occurs in the following sequential phases (Figure 12-4): rolling (step 1), an insult to local tissue (step 2), signaling the endothelium (step 3), increased rolling (step 4), signal for rolling arrest (step 5), strong adhesion (arrested rolling) (step 6), and the zipper phase (step 7).

Leukocytes use the lectin (a nonenzymatic carbohydrate-binding protein) designated *L-selectin* to interact with carbohydrate molecules known as *vascular addressins* (e.g., sialomucin CD34)[16] on the luminal surface of endothelial cells (step 1, Figure 12-4). This brief interaction manifests itself as the *rolling* of the leukocyte along the luminal surface of the endothelium, a process whereby the leukocyte essentially pauses to inspect the endothelium.

A local insult (step 2, Figure 12-4) triggers the release of a variety of inflammatory signals (e.g., interleukin-1β [IL-1β], tumor necrosis factor alpha [TNF-α]) from cells in the tissue, especially from resident leukocytes such as mast cells.[30] Mast cells are crucial in initiating neutrophil recruitment against bacteria and responding to anaphylatoxins such as C3a and C5a (step 3, Figure 12-4).

IL-1β, TNF-α, C5a, and lipopolysaccharides can stimulate endothelial cells to express *P-selectin* and *E-selectin* on their luminal surfaces.[19] Either of these selectins can bind carbohydrate molecules found on the leukocyte, resulting in an increase in the time the leukocyte remains associated with the endothelium. This appears microscopically as an increase in number of leukocytes attached to the luminal surface of the endothelium, or *increased rolling.* Note that endothelial cells, not inflammatory

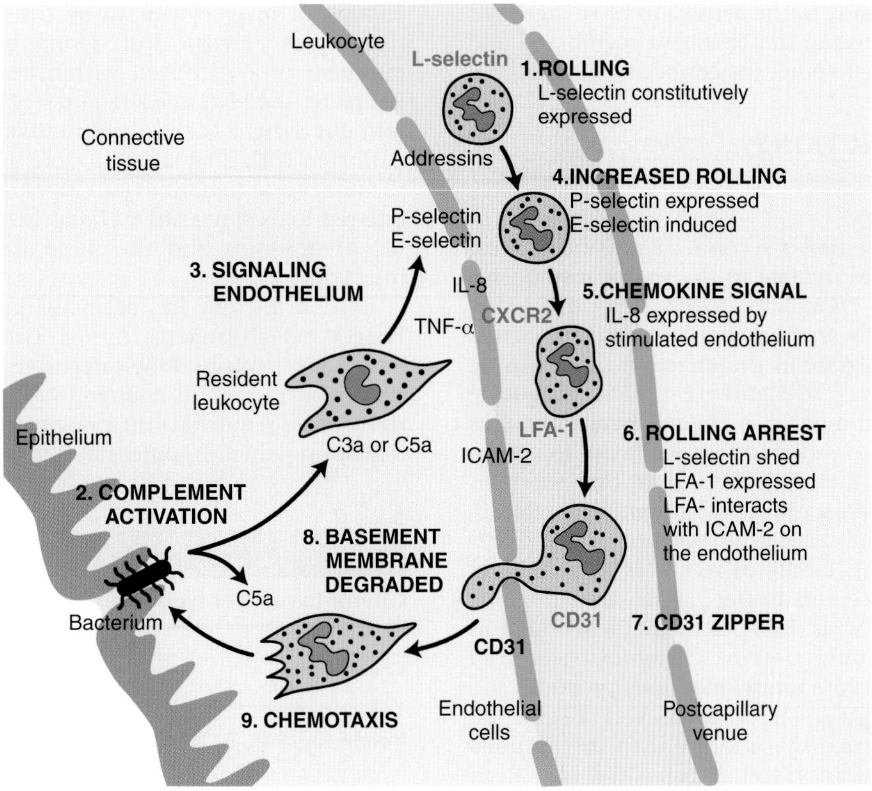

Figure 12-4 Inflammation is a result of the interaction between complement, resident leukocytes, endothelium, and the recruited inflammatory leukocytes. Endothelial components are indicated in gray type; leukocyte components are indicated in red type. (See text for the events involved in transendothelial migration.)

leukocytes, initially respond to local inflammatory signals from the resident leukocytes.

The stimulated endothelium also releases chemokines. *Chemokines* are small peptide cytokines, first recognized for their chemoattractant activities, which play a fundamental role as selective signals for leukocytes to exit the blood (step 5, Figure 12-4). Chemokines function as a *signal for rolling arrest.* The interaction of a chemokine, interleukin-8 (IL-8), with the leukocyte receptor CXCR2 causes the leukocyte to shed L-selectin and upregulate the integrin *leukocyte function–associated antigen-1* (LFA-1).[12,28] Integrins are transmembrane adhesins, some of which have been adapted for use by the immune system. LFA-1 binds *intercellular adhesion molecule-2* (ICAM-2), which is expressed constitutively by endothelium (step 6, Figure 12-4). This results in *rolling arrest* because the phagocyte becomes firmly associated with the endothelium. Prolonged or severe disturbances of the endothelium can upregulate ICAM-1, which is a more efficient ligand for LFA-1.

Because leukocytes differ with respect to their chemokine receptors, the chemokines dictate which leukocytes (e.g., neutrophils, macrophages, lymphocytes, eosinophils, basophils) dominate the leukocyte infiltrate. Different stimuli (e.g., cytokines, tissue injury, viral or microbial insults) can lead to expression of different chemokines.[13,14,19] For example, hypoxia, a condition in which only neutrophils can function successfully, favors endothelial release of IL-8, a chemokine to which neutrophils are responsive. The integrin phase of transendothelial migration (i.e., the interaction of LFA-1 with ICAM-2) also can be somewhat selective. Thus, chronic inflammatory leukocytes (monocytes and lymphocytes) possess integrins that are not expressed by neutrophils. One such integrin, *very late antigen-4* (VLA-4), binds endothelial *vascular cell adhesion molecule-1* (VCAM-1). Endothelium expresses VCAM-1 after prolonged inflammation, thus providing a mechanism for the selection of chronic inflammatory cells.

CD31 (platelet–endothelial cell adhesion molecule-1) is a 130-kD transmembrane glycoprotein present at the intercellular borders of endothelial cells facing into lumen and on all leukocytes. CD31 is a homophilic adhesion molecule because CD31 molecules bind to one another. The binding of CD31 on endothelium with CD31 on leukocytes guides leukocytes to the boundaries between endothelial cells (step 7, Figure 12-4). Once the leukocyte locates the interendothelial junction, it uses its own CD31 as a zipper *(CD31 zipper)* with the CD31 of the endothelial cells. This zipper effect has been proposed as a mechanism of minimizing the leakage of fluid. As the endothelium unzips its CD31, the leukocyte rapidly "zips" between the endothelial cells.

Leukocytes accumulate briefly between the basement membrane and the endothelial cell. This pause may reflect a period of secretion of proteases to degrade the basement membrane (step 8, Figure 12-4). Leukocytes possess several proteases, including *urokinase plasminogen activator receptor* (uPAR). The uPAR leads to the activation of collagenase, which then may degrade the basement membrane and enable the leukocyte to enter the connective tissues.[10]

LEUKOCYTE FUNCTIONS

Chemotaxis

Once the leukocyte enters the connective tissue, it must be able to locate and migrate to the site of insult. This is accomplished by *chemotaxis,* which depends on the leukocyte's ability to sense a chemical gradient across its cell body and migrate in the direction of increasing concentration[19,29] (step 9, Figure 12-4). The phagocyte senses only a limited number of chemicals: chemotaxins for which it has receptors and chemotaxin receptors. Table 12-3 lists some molecules that can serve as chemotaxins and their sources. The receptors for chemotaxis belong to a family called the *G-protein coupled family* (Figure 12-5, *A*). This family of receptors also includes the various light receptors in our retinas; thus in some ways, leukocytes "see" a chemotactic gradient much as we see light. The only class of chemotaxins derived directly from bacteria are formyl-methionyl peptides.

To migrate toward a target, leukocytes assume an asymmetric or polarized shape rather than the rounded morphology evident in blood (Figure 12-5, *B*). Even under ideal experimental conditions, neutrophil migration has been observed to be primarily random until the neutrophil is one to two body lengths (10-20 μm) away from a recognizable target particle.

Phagocytosis

Phagocytosis is the process by which cells ingest particles of a size visible to light microscopy. Neutrophils and monocytes/macrophages are the only cells efficient enough at phagocytosis to be considered "professional phagocytes." Phagocytosis results in the eventual containment of a pathogen within a membrane-delimited structure, the *phagosome* (Figures 12-6 and 12-7, *A*). The immune system has evolved mechanisms of coating the pathogen with a few recognizable ligands, which enable the phagocyte to bind to and ingest the pathogen. This is referred to as *opsonization.* Table 12-4 provides a selected list of opsonins and the molecules with which they interact.

Once a microbe has been ingested, it may be killed. Phagocytes kill bacteria through two broad categories of killing mechanisms. One category is based on the reduction of oxygen and is referred to as "oxidative." *Oxidative mechanisms* require (1) the presence of oxygen and (2) an oxidation-reduction potential, Eh, at or above –160 mV.

TABLE 12-3

Chemotaxins for Neutrophils

Chemotaxin	Source
Tumor necrosis factor (TNF)	Macrophages/monocytes
Interleukin-8 (IL-8)	Neutrophils (PMNs), endothelium
Platelet-activating factor	Many cells
Leukotriene B4	
C5a	Serum/plasma
Neutrophil chemotactic factor	Mast cells
Interleukin-1 (IL-1)	B cells, macrophage
Interferon-γ (IFN-γ)	Activated T cells
N-formyl-methionyl peptides	Bacteria

PMNs, Polymorphonuclear leukocytes.

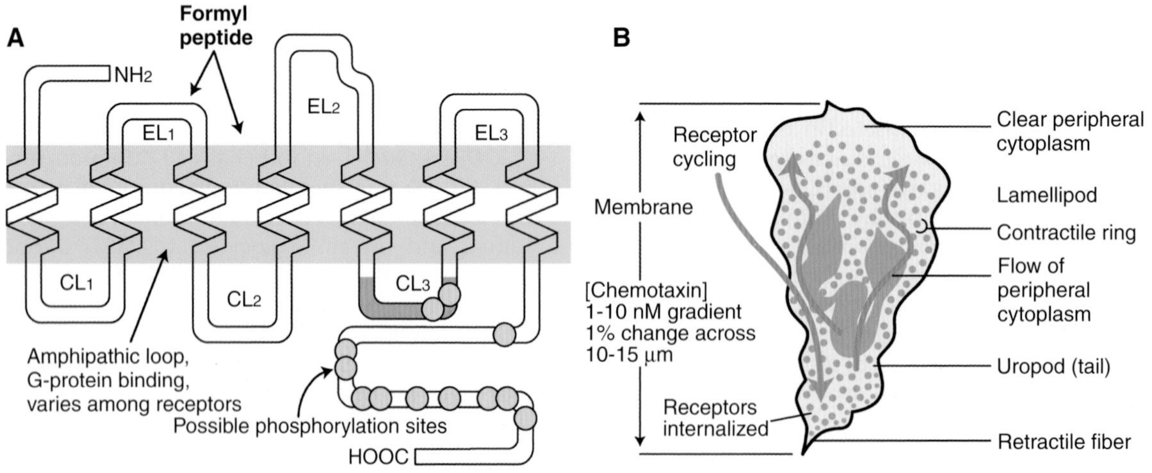

Figure 12-5 Leukocytes can "hone in" on various irritants, such as a microorganism, by chemotaxis. This requires a chemotaxin receptor **(A).** The chemotaxin receptors are members of the G-protein coupled family. Seven transmembranous domains, three extracellular loops *(EL1-EL3),* and three cytosolic loops *(CL1-CL3)* characterize this family of molecules. **B,** Neutrophils polarize, forming an anterior lamellipod and a posterior uropod. Cytoplasm appears to squirt through a contractile ring. Neutrophils exhibit strikingly sensitive chemotaxis and can detect a 1% gradient over the length of its cell body at nanomolar concentrations.

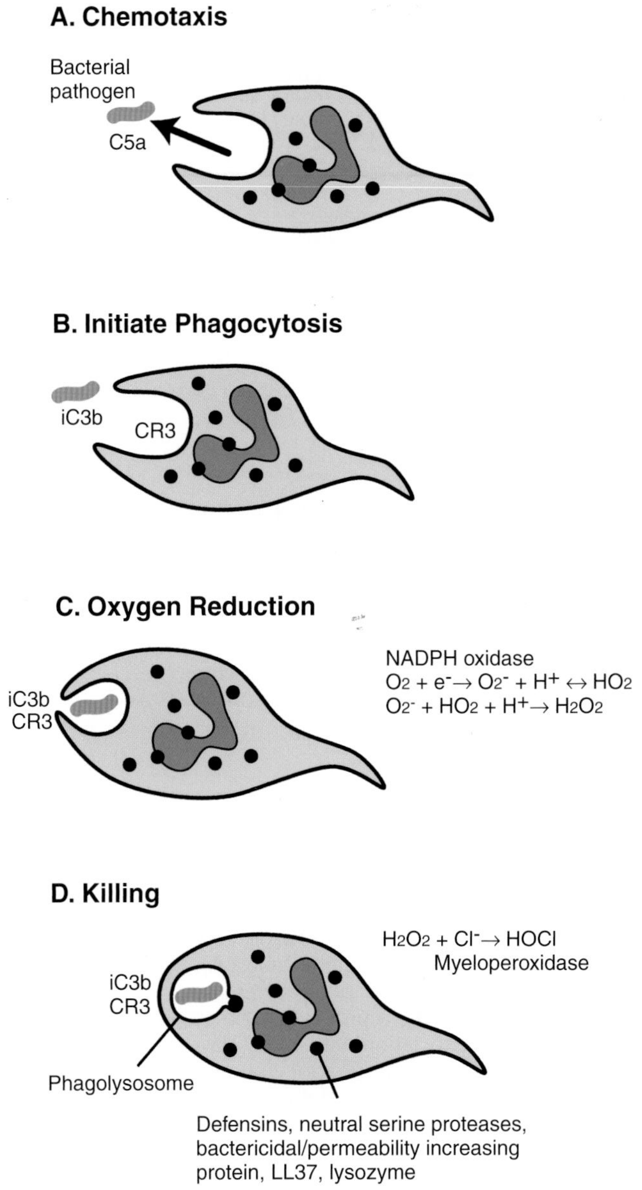

Figure 12-6 After neutrophils exit the blood, they must kill the offending pathogens. This process consists of overlapping steps, which are illustrated in this diagram. **A,** *Chemotaxis* refers to directed motility that enables the leukocyte to locate its target. C5a is a chemotaxin, which may be generated by any target that activates complement. **B,** *Phagocytosis* also requires the interaction of receptors with a few ligands. The diagram illustrates the important interaction between the opsonin iC3b, which will coat an offending particle or cell, and the opsonic receptor CR3. **C,** *Oxygen reduction* requires the presence of oxygen and a certain oxidation-reduction (redox) potential, both of which can vary in the gingival crevice. The formation of several oxygen metabolites can kill some bacteria. **D,** *Killing* involves several processes. First, phagocytosis traps the microorganism in the stringent environment of the phagosome. Second, the phagosome and lysosomes (granules) fuse to form the phagolysosome. In this step, all the toxic compounds of the lysosome (e.g., defensins, neutral serine proteases) are dumped into the phagolysosome. Third, myeloperoxidase in the phagolysosome can convert hydrogen peroxide *(H_2O_2)* to hypochlorous acid *(HOCl)*.

Both variables may be suboptimal within the gingival crevice. Neutrophils do not require oxygen for energy and can function under anaerobic conditions. Thus, phagocytes also must possess capabilities for the second category of killing mechanisms, the *nonoxidative mechanisms*.

Nonoxidative killing requires *phagosome-lysosome fusion*. This process involves the movement toward and subsequent membrane fusion of the lysosome with the phagosome, which forms a *phagolysosome*. This results in the secretion of lysosomal components into the phagolysosome. Each neutrophil possesses two main types of lysosomes, or granules: *specific granules*, designed for both extracellular and intraphagolysosomal secretion, and *azurophil granules*, designed mainly for intraphagolysosomal secretion. Less than 30 seconds after phagocytosis, neutrophils secrete specific granule components into the phagolysosome. Specific granules contain several microbiocidal components, including lysozyme and lactoferrin. *Lysozyme* is an enzyme that possesses enzyme-dependent bactericidal activity and enzyme-independent bactericidal and fungicidal activity. *Lactoferrin* is a bacteriostatic compound that contains a bactericidal peptide domain, lactoferricin. Neutrophils secrete azurophil granule components into the phagolysosome minutes after the secretion of the specific granules. Among the microbicidal compounds are small antimicrobial peptides known as *α-defensins* (e.g., HNP-1, HNP-2, HNP-3, and HNP-4), *serprocidins* (elastase, proteinase 3, azurocidin), cathepsin G, and lysozyme. These nonoxidative mechanisms of neutrophil killing may be of particular importance in periodontal diseases because of the highly anaerobic conditions in the subgingival environment.

In the presence of oxygen, phagocytes additionally possess mechanisms of *oxidative killing*. In particular, neutrophils exert intense microbicidal activity by forming toxic, reduced-oxygen metabolites such as superoxide anion (O_2^-) using the *NADPH oxidase system*. The superoxide anion also contributes to the formation of hydrogen peroxide (H_2O_2), which is capable of diffusing across membranes. Inside a target cell, H_2O_2 may be further reduced to the hydroxyl radical, which can cause DNA damage. More importantly, H_2O_2 is a substrate for *myeloperoxidase* (MPO). In the presence of H_2O_2 and chloride, MPO catalyzes the formation of hypochlorous acid (HOCl). This molecule is the acidic form of the laundry bleach salt, sodium hypochlorite (NaOCl), which also is used as an antimicrobial cleansing irrigant in endodontics. Deficiencies in the NADPH oxidase system result in *chronic granulomatous disease*, a severe, recurrent, focal infection by organisms that do not release H_2O_2 on their own. Chronic granulomatous disease has been associated inconsistently with aggressive periodontal disease, suggesting that oxidative microbicidal mechanisms are of some importance in periodontal infections.

In summary, phagocytosis is of primary importance in the ability of a host to resist or combat infection. Once a pathogenic microorganism is ingested, several mechanisms of killing are possible. Because of the highly anaerobic conditions in the periodontal environment, nonoxidative mechanisms of killing are of particular importance.

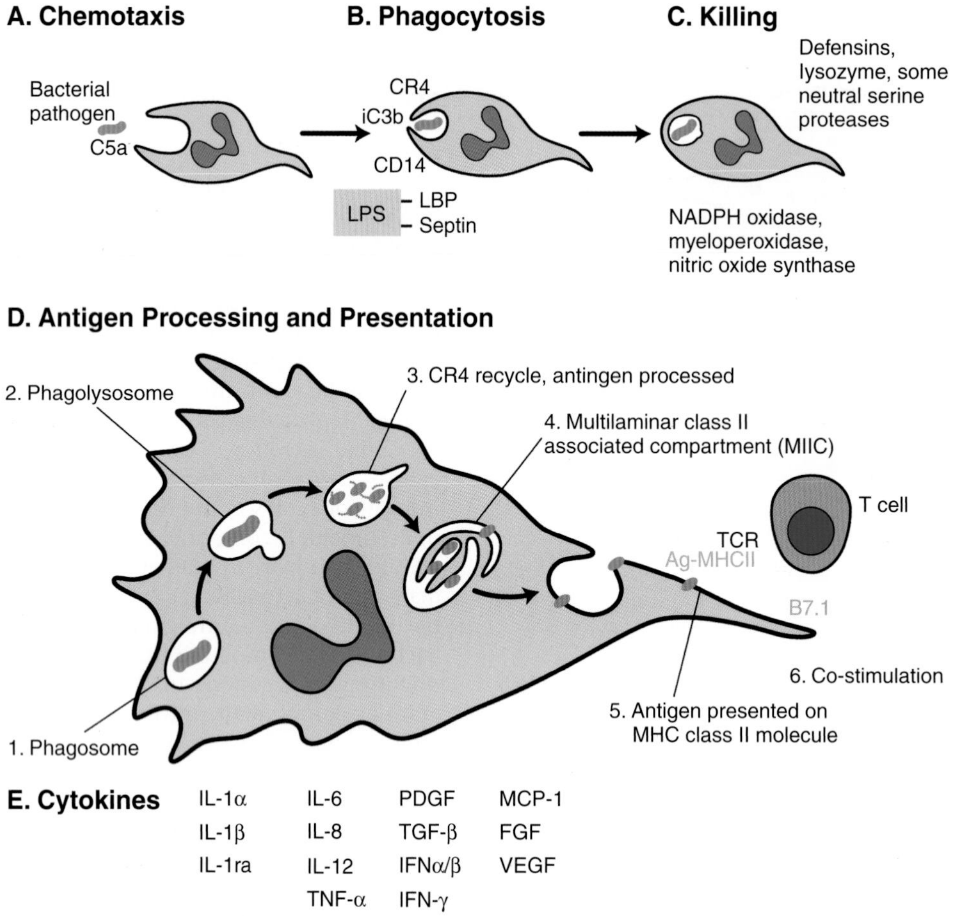

Figure 12-7 Mononuclear phagocytes (monocytes in blood, macrophages in tissues) are closely related to neutrophils. Their activities are similar, and they exhibit chemotaxis **(A)**, phagocytosis **(B)**, and killing **(C)**, similar to neutrophils. Mononuclear phagocytes are particularly adept at processing and presenting antigen to T cells **(D)**, a process that may require more than 20 hours. Note that antigen is presented in association with MHC class II molecules along with a co-stimulatory signal *(B7.1)*. Mononuclear phagocytes also release cytokines **(E)** that direct lymphocyte differentiation. (See text for details of the interactions illustrated.)

Antigen Processing and Presentation

The *major histocompatibility complex* (MHC) is a locus on the short arm of chromosome 6 (6p21.3) that encodes a number of molecules, including MHC classes I, II, and III molecules, which are involved with antigen uptake, processing, and presentation. All cells process and present self-derived antigens (intracellular antigens) in association with MHC class I molecules. MHC class I molecules are used to present intracellular antigens to CD8+ T cells and NK cells. MHC class III molecules include complement factors B, C2, and C4.

Antigens derived from extracellular sources are presented by professional *antigen-presenting cells* (APCs) in association with MHC class II molecules. The three main professional APCs are peripheral DCs, monocyte derivatives, and B cells. These cells are specialized to present antigen to CD4+ T cells, which recognize antigen in association with the MHC class II molecule. This is important because CD4+ T cells control the proliferation of other T and B cells.

The professional APC expresses MHC class II molecules (i.e., HLA-DP, HLA-DQ, HLA-DR) constitutively. Externally derived antigens are processed by phagocytosis, and the resulting peptide molecules associate with the MHC class II molecules on the cell surface. As shown in Figure 12-7, *D,* antigen associates with the MHC class II molecule within the multilaminar class II–associated compartment (MIIC). Oligomeric peptide fragments derived from extracellular polymers are bound by as many as four specificity pockets found in the MHC class II molecule. Because the binding specificity is not for the entire peptide sequence, MHC class II molecules are somewhat "promiscuous" and may bind to many different peptides.

Molecules of MHC classes I, II, and III are among the most pleomorphic molecules in humans. *Pleomorphism* refers to stable variations among individuals within a species, based on the occurrence of variants of certain genes. Pleomorphism in the MHC is particularly high near the specificity pockets. This means that the antigens bound by one person's MHC class I or II molecules may

TABLE 12-4

Opsonins and Opsonic Receptors

Target	Opsonin	Opsonic Receptor	Cell Possessing Opsonic Receptor
Gram-negative bacteria	LPS-binding protein (LBP) or septin	CD14	Macrophages Neutrophils (if primed with TNF-α)
Any particle or cell	iC3b	CR3 (Mac1)	Neutrophils
		CR4	Macrophages Macrophages
Any particle or cell	IgG1, IgG2, IgG3	FcγRI	Macrophages
		FcγRII	Macrophages Neutrophils

LPS, Lipopolysaccharide; TNF-α, tumor necrosis factor alpha; IgG, immunoglobulin G.

TABLE 12-5

Selected TNF Superfamily Molecules Involved in Co-Stimulation

Stimulating Cell (Antigen Presentor)	Co-Stimulatory Factor	Stimulated Cell	Co-Stimulatory Receptor on Stimulated Cell
APC	B7-2 (CD86)	CD4+ and CD8+ T –cells	CD28
APC	B7-2 (CD80)	Activated T cells	CD28
Nonprofessional APC	B7-3	T cells	CD28
Stimulated B cells	CD70 (TNF-SF7)	CD4+ T cells	CD27

TNF, Tumor necrosis factor; *APC,* antigen-presenting cell.

not bind exactly the same peptides as those from a different individual. The existence of such pleomorphism may be important in species survival (as opposed to individual survival) and has become a significant consideration in transplantation (thus the term *histocompatibility*). If the donor tissue is not well matched in the MHC, it will present a multitude of new antigens, and the donor tissue will be rejected by the resulting immune response.

The interaction between two cells permits a high level of sophistication unattainable by the simple interaction of two molecules, enabling the APC to present antigen to the T cell with a second signal. The most important second signal is called *co-stimulation.* Co-stimulation reaffirms to the T cell that it has recognized an undesirable antigen. In the absence of co-stimulation, T cells may become unresponsive or apoptotic and die. Co-stimulation is mediated by a variety of transmembrane molecules of the tumor necrosis factor (TNF) superfamily (Table 12-5), a family of molecules that deals with issues of cellular life and death. Co-stimulation performs three functions: (1) makes the T cell resistant to *apoptosis* (a programmed cell death); (2) upregulates growth factor receptors on the T cell, thereby stimulating its proliferation; and (3) decreases the amount of time needed to trigger the T cell (also referred to as *amplification*).[6,15]

Increases in the expression of co-stimulatory molecules occur in the presence of certain environmental stimuli. Macrophages increase the expression of co-stimulatory molecules if they are exposed to bacterial lipoplysaccharide (LPS),[3] as well as particulate and occasionally soluble antigen. B cells exposed to antigen to which they are specific, to selected bacterial membrane components (e.g., specific proteins, LPS), or to a B-cell activator molecule produced by T cells (Gp39) respond by increasing the expression of the co-stimulatory molecules B7-1, B7-2, or both.[9] In addition, viral infection or certain chemical irritants can upregulate B7-1 or B7-3 on nonprofessional APCs.[11] A receptor molecule named "toll," first identified in fruit flies (*Drosophila* spp.), was shown to be important in certain responses to injury or infection. The human *toll-like receptors* (TLRs) are stimulated by highly conserved bacterial components such as LPS and are important in dictating the adaptations found in the innate immune system.[23] TLRs cause APCs to upregulate the co-stimulatory B7 molecules.[21,24] Although T cells may constantly interact with antigen, co-stimulation enables this interaction to progress to T-cell proliferation. (TLR activation and cell-signaling events in periodontal tissues are extensively reviewed in Chapter 15 and the Chapter 15 supplemental material found on *Carranza's Clinical Periodontology Online.*)

SPECIFIC IMMUNE RESPONSES

Chronic inflammation, if protracted, can result in an adaptation called the *specific immune response.* The specific immune response requires lymphocytes, which use two types of receptors, to generate specific immune

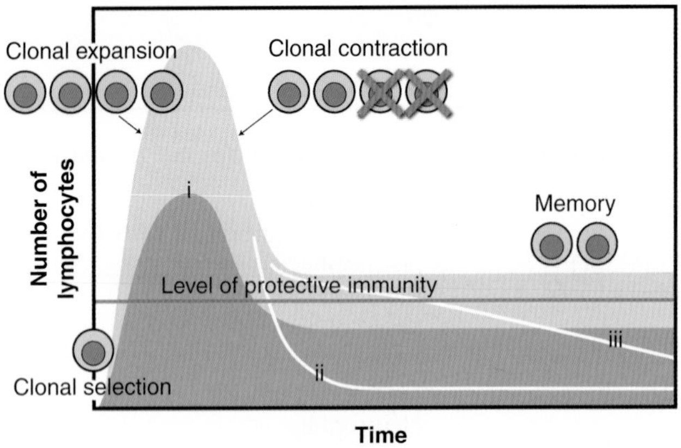

Figure 12-8 Schematic illustration of the four phases of the specific immune response in relation to the occurrence of protective immunity. See the text for details of the four phases: clonal selection, clonal expansion, clonal contraction, and memory. Protective immunity is achieved if an adequate number of the lymphocytes are maintained in the memory phase, and the individual is said to be "immune." However, this does not always occur because an individual (1) may not undergo sufficient clonal expansion, (2) may undergo excessive clonal contraction, or (3) may be unable to maintain memory. (Modified from Ahmed R, Gray D: *Science* 272(5258):54, 1996.)

responses, the B-cell antigen receptor (BCR) and the T-cell antigen receptor (TCR). Four phases are involved in the generation of specific immunity: (1) *clonal selection,* the selection of lymphocytes that bear receptors (BCRs or TCRs) recognizing the specific antigen; (2) *clonal expansion,* the proliferation of those lymphocytes; (3) *clonal contraction,* the death of "effector" lymphocytes; and (4) *memory,* the maintenance of an expanded clone of cells that bears the specific receptors (BCRs or TCRs) recognizing the antigen (Figure 12-8). As long as a sufficient number of lymphocytes are maintained to provide protection against a specific antigen, the individual is said to be "immune."

T cells are selected when their TCR interacts with antigen presented by MHC class I or II molecules. B-cell clonal selection requires only the multivalent binding of antigen by the BCR. A proliferation of the antigen-specific cells occurs after clonal selection. This process of clonal expansion results in a 100- to 5000-fold increase in these cells.[1] In B-cell responses, some antigen-specific receptors are produced as soluble *antibodies.* The increase in antibody concentration and the strength of antibody binding is referred to as an "increase in titer." *Titer* is operationally defined as the reciprocal dilution of antibody required to detect a standardized amount of antigen. Clonal contraction occurs by apoptosis at a rate equal to that of clonal expansion. More than 95% of antigen-specific T cells are lost during the contraction phase,[1] usually occurring over several weeks. After clonal contraction, an increased population of memory T cells or B cells is maintained; this is the essence of the specific immune response.

The increase in antibody titer or antigen-specific T cells resulting from the exposure of a host to an antigen for the first time is referred to as the *primary response.* The *secondary response* develops after a subsequent exposure to that same antigen. Because of the generation of memory (i.e., the expanded pool of cells recognizing antigen), the secondary response (1) is more rapid in onset, (2) is longer in duration, (3) is greater in strength because of higher titers, and (4) for Bcells, may have greater specificity against the antigen compared with the primary response. The expanded pool of memory cells provides a reservoir of cells that is sustained for years by constant stimulation of antigen maintained by follicular DCs (nonhematopoetic cells found in the lymphoid tissues). The primary response takes slightly more than 1 week (8-14 days) to become measurable and biologically or clinically useful. Secondary responses are measurable within 1 to 3 days and are so effective that an individual may not be aware of the infection. *Vaccination* is the development of immunity, or resistance to infection, after a secondary response (the booster) that is adequate to consider the individual *immune* to a subsequent infection.

T-CELL RESPONSES

To obtain a specific immune response, the T cell must interact with the APC. This is a complex process requiring that the T cell recognize the antigen on the APC, receive co-stimulation, activate growth cytokine receptors, and produce cytokines. These processes signal and support growth and differentiation. Once activated, the T cell undergoes proliferation and differentiation, leading to one of several possible mature T-cell phenotypes.

T-cell antigen recognition is a function of the TCR, a low-affinity receptor of the immunoglobulin superfamily. T cells may express 3000 to 50,000 TCRs on their surface. Antigens are presented to the TCR by MHC class I or II molecules on the APC. CD1 is a related antigen-presenting molecule that presents specific antigens to NK T cells, a unique subpopulation of CD4– and CD8—T cells. The TCR recognizes and binds the MHC-peptide complex.[25] Antigen (Ag) is contacted by the TCR using variable domains found at the *N*-terminus of the TCR α and β subunits. TCR-peptide binding is more specific than that of the MHC-peptide complex, which is based on recognition of a smaller number of discontinuous amino acids. Thus the T cell may recognize fewer antigens than those presented by the MHC.

The TCR consists of a number of components in addition to those that bind antigen. These include components that form the *CD3 transductory apparatus* (TCR-CD3), which is important in the activation of the TCR and the eventual transmission or transduction of the signal into the cell. *CD8* and *CD4* are *T-cell co-receptors,* whose recognition of MHC class I and II molecules, respectively, on APCs is essential for T-cell function and subsequent TCR activation. Activation of these co-receptors increases the excitability of the TCR and increases the binding between the T cell and the APC.

The low affinity of the TCR enables the T cell to bind APCs in a reversible manner, which occurs between multiple TCRs and one or a few antigens over time. This time-dependent interaction of many TCRs with a few

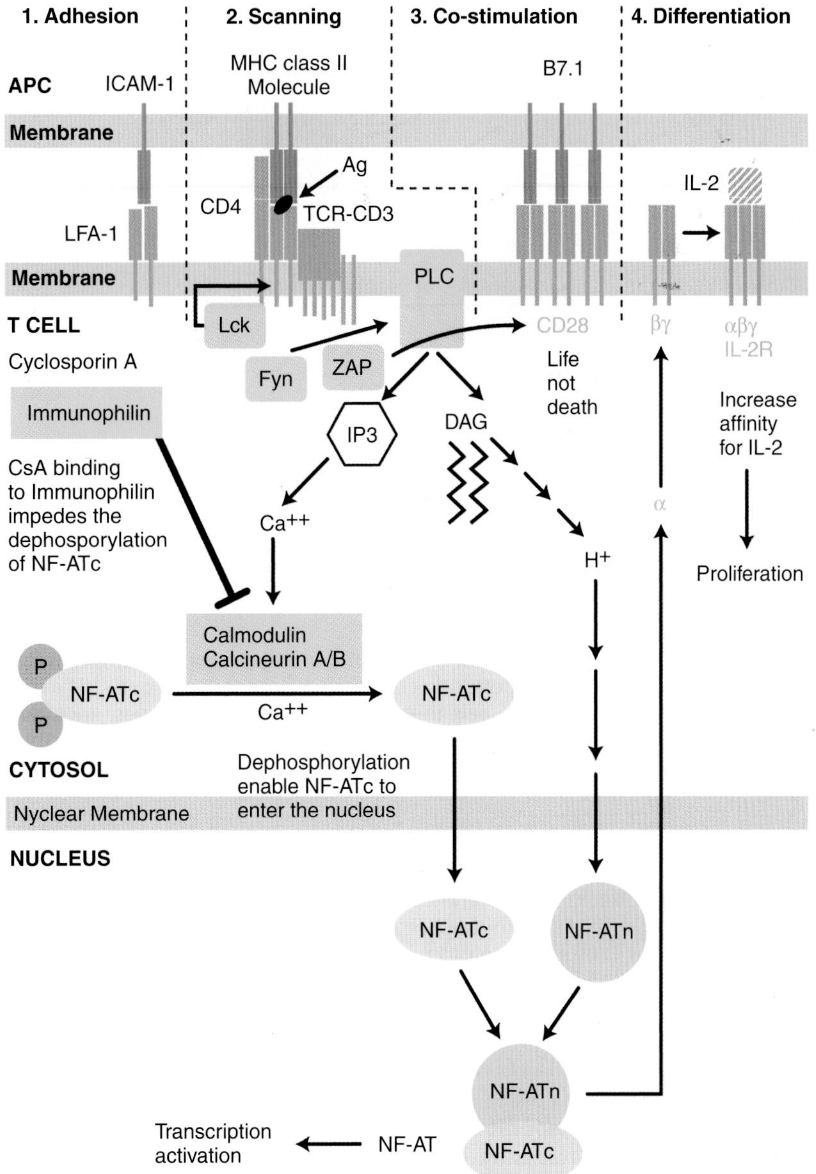

Figure 12-9 Schematic illustration of receptor-mediated events leading to T-cell activation. *1,* Adhesion between the T cell and the antigen-presenting cell *(APC)* is mediated by adhesins such as leukocyte function–associated antigen-1 *(LFA-1)* and intercellular adhesion molecule-1 *(ICAM-1). 2,* Scanning of the APC by the T-cell co-receptors, CD4 or CD8, helps activate the TCR using the kinase *Lck.* Recognition of antigen by the TCR results in activation of phospholipase C *(PLC)* and CD28 by *Fyn* and *ZAP,* respectively. *3,* Activated CD28 binds co-stimulatory factors such as B7-1. The co-stimulatory factors are upregulated by environmental cues and reinforce the activation signal. *4,* The scanning of antigen results in transcription of an important growth hormone receptor subunit, the IL-2 receptor α subunit. This increases the affinity of the interleukin-2 *(IL-2)* receptor. Later, the T cell produces IL-2, which interacts with the IL-2 receptor to stimulate its own proliferation.

antigens is referred to as *scanning.* Scanning that leads to T-cell activation is called *serial triggering.* To fully activate T-cells, multiple TCR engagement must be sustained for 2 to 20 hours.

Activation of T cells leads to proliferative differentiation. This process begins with activation of the protein tyrosine kinases *lck, fyn,* and *ZAP,* which activate the TCR, phospholipase C (PLC), and CD28, respectively (Figure 12-9). Activation of CD28 prepares the T cell to receive the co-stimulatory signals, which are important in T-cell survival and function. Activation of PLC results in the generation of diacylglycerol (DAG) and 1,4,5-inositol triphosphate (IP3). DAG signals the activation of a transcription-activating cofactor, NF-ATn. IP3 stimulates the release of Ca^{++}, which results in the activation of a calmodulin-calcineurin A/B phosphatase. This phosphatase dephosphorylates NF-ATc and enables it to enter the nucleus, where it combines with NF-ATn to form active

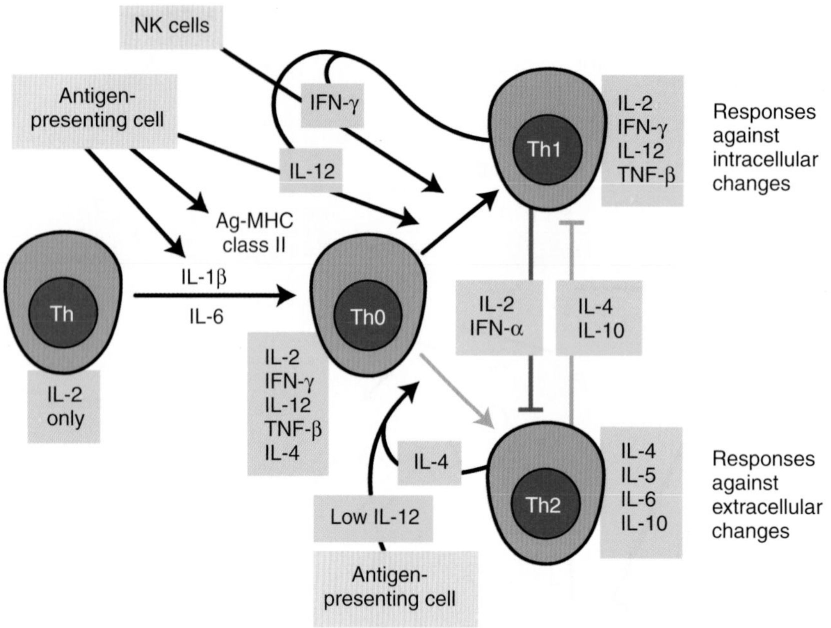

Figure 12-10 Schematic illustration of T-cell differentiation. Early inflammatory signals from macrophages and peripheral dendritic cells such as interleukin-1β *(IL-1β)* activate the CD4+ T-helper *(Th)* T cell. The Th cell then produces many cytokines, including IL-2, interferon-γ *(IFN-γ)* and IL-4, and is referred to as a *Th0 T cell.* The Th0 T cell further differentiates to form Th1 or Th2 T cells, which regulate immune responses against intracellular and extracellular antigens, respectively. A key signal determining which pathway the T cell follows is the level of IL-12 provided by the antigen-presenting cell. High levels of IL-12 favor the Th1 pathway, and low levels of IL-12 favor the Th2 pathway. Subsequently, the Th1 phenotype is favored in the presence of Th1 cytokines such as IFN-γ, which stimulates Th1 differentiation and blocks Th2 differentiation. Similarly, the Th2 cytokines such as IL-4 block Th1 differentiation while promoting Th2 differentiation. The Th3 T cell, which produces IgA and functions in mucosal defense, is not illustrated here. *Ag-MHC,* Antigen major histocompatibility complex; *NK,* natural killer; *TNF-β,* tumor necrosis factor beta.

nuclear factor of activated T cells (NF-AT). NF-AT then upregulates transcription of genes, such as those for interleukin-2 (IL-2) and the IL-2 receptor α subunit (IL-2Rα), which support T-cell growth and differentiation. The latent cytoplasmic transcription factor NF-κβ also is activated and is important in delaying apoptosis. One of the most important proliferative differentiation signals is by the cytokine IL-2. The activated transcription factors are required for the T cell to express one of the subunits of the heterotrimeric receptor for IL-2 (IL-2R) and the IL-2Rα and also to produce IL-2.[7] Thus, IL-2 produced by the activated T cell interacts with the IL-2R on the same cell to stimulate proliferative differentiation.

Clinically important immunosuppressants block the intracellular processes of T-cell activation. *Immunophilins* are regulatory factors that diminish the action of calcineurin. Immunosuppressants such as *cyclosporin A* and *tacrolimus* bind and activate immunophilins, resulting in their immunosuppressive effects.

CD4+ T cells mature to form phenotypic subpopulations that are distinguishable on the basis of their cytokine production[22] (Figure 12-10). In addition to antigen and co-stimulation, professional APCs provide immature *T-helper* (Th) *T cells* with the maturational signal interleukin-1 (IL-1β), which induces T-cell maturation to a multifaceted *Th0 T-cell* phenotype. Th0 T cells produce cytokines, which can stimulate both B cells and CD8+ T cells. Other cells in the area, especially macrophages, DCs, other T cells, and NK cells, provide further differentiation signals. High or low concentrations of interleukin-12 (IL-12) or cytokines such as interferon-γ (IFN-γ), IL-2, IL-4, IL-10, and tumor growth factor beta (TGF-β) then can induce T cells to mature to the Th1, Th2, or Th3 phenotypes. The *Th1* phenoytpe is important in controlling altered cells and intracellular molecules; the *Th2* phenotype is important in proinflammatory responses against extracellular antigens; and the *Th3* phenotype is important in antiinflammatory responses against extracellular antigens. These later T-cell maturational subpopulations are important in B-cell development.

B-CELL RESPONSES AND ANTIBODIES

B cells produce immunoglobulin. An immunoglobulin that binds a known antigen is an *antibody.* Once antigen is bound, a number of consequences can occur, as dictated by the type (isotype) of immunoglobulin involved (Table 12-6). Immunoglobulin accounts for about 20% to 25% (15 mg/ml) of the total serum protein (60-70 mg/ml). Humans possess nine genetically distinct isotypes of immunoglobulins: IgM, IgD, IgG1, IgG2, IgG3, IgG4, IgA1, IgA2, and IgE. When B cells exit the bone marrow,

TABLE 12-6

Selected Properties of Immunoglobulin Isotypes

Immunoglobulin Isotype	IgG1	IgG2	IgG3	IgG4	IgM	IgA1	IgA2	IgD	IgE
Concentration in serum (mg/ml)	9	3	1	0.5	1.5	3	0.5	0.03	0.00005
Molecular weight (kilodaltons)	146	146	170	146	970	160	160	184	188
Present on naive B cells	–	–	–	–	+	–	–	+	–
Activation of complement (classical pathway)	++	+	+++	–	+++	–	–	–	–
Functions as opsonin without complement	+	–	+	+	–	–	–	–	–
With antigen, stimulates mast cells	–	–	–	–	–	–	–	–	++++
With antigen, stimulates eosinophils	–	–	–	–	–	–	–	–	++
Functions in mucosal immunity	–	–	–	–	–	+	+	–	–

they possess receptors bearing only IgM, and the cells are capable of producing soluble IgM. IgM functions in the primitive agglutination reactions that facilitate antigen clearance.

Secondary immunoglobulin response classes permit a more discriminating response. To form secondary response isotypes, B cells must enter a pathway of differentiation. In this memory pathway, B cells undergo the process of isotype switching. One example of the significance of this process to periodontal diseases is that certain pathogens, such as *Actinobacillus actinomycetemcomitans,* can only be controlled by neutrophils when opsonized by antibody of the IgG isotype. Complement, LPS-binding protein (LBP), and any other immunoglobulin isotypes are not effective.

The ability of B cells to respond to antigen depends on the B-cell antigen receptor (BCR). The BCR is formed partly by immunoglobulin molecules on the B-cell surface, which serve as highly specific antigen receptors, and partly by transductory elements of the immunoglobulin superfamily. The BCR binds antigen with a high affinity and is designed for binding. This contrasts with the low-affinity binding of the TCR, which is ideal for scanning. B cells are capable of responding to certain antigens in the absence of T cells. This is referred to as *T-independent B-cell antibody response.* However, these B-cell responses do not mature (i.e., they do not enter the memory pathway). The cells maintain an IgM isotype, and their antibody products retain a relatively low affinity for antigen binding. B cells must interact with T cells to enter the memory pathway, and thus the memory pathway is considered to be T cell dependent.

B cells bind soluble antigens using the BCR. If enough antigen is bound, they then are ingested and processed, and parts of the antigen are presented to specific CD4+ T cells using MHC class II molecules. After antigen presentation, the T cells provide an *activation* signal to the B cell. T-cell activators are transmembranous molecules, analogous to the co-stimulatory factors for T cells discussed previously. Activators include T-cell-derived Gp39 and Gp34, which interact with the B-cell receptors, CD40 or OX40, respectively. Mutations in the gene for Gp39 lead to a condition called *X-linked hyper-immunoglubulinemia M syndrome,* characterized by a deficiency in most immunoglobulin isotypes.[5] A compensatory increase in IgM T-cell Gp39 enables B-cell entry into the memory pathway, whereas the absence of Gp39 leads to terminal differentiation of the B cells toward IgM, producing plasma cells.[2] B cells upregulate B7-1 and B7-2 if activated by Gp39. These co-stimulatory factors enable the T cells to differentiate, both with respect to proliferation and in the production of cytokines. Some T-cell cytokines are *switch factors;* these cytokines fall into three classes: Th1 (IL-2, IFN-γ), Th2 (IL-4, IL-10), and Th3 (TGF-β). Th1 and Th2 switch signals generally promote switching to inflammatory immunoglobulins (IgG or IgE). The Th3 signal promotes a switch to an antiinflammatory isotype (IgA).[31] Unlike the activators, switch factors are usually soluble rather than membrane associated. Figure 12-11 shows effects of various combinations of activators and switch factors.

B cells that differentiate to become plasma cells no longer express surface immunoglobulin and CD40; however, they do express secreted immunoglobulin. IgM is a primordial, all-purpose, *primary-response immunoglobulin.* IgM is capable of complement activation but not direct opsonization (i.e., no Fc receptors exist for IgM). IgD is often co-expressed on B cells with IgM and is believed to help increase B-cell responses to antigen. The memory B cells give rise to the *secondary-response immunoglobulins.* These B cells produce immunoglobulin isotypes that can be divided into the IgE- or IgG-mediated inflammatory isotype responses and the IgA-mediated antiinflammatory isotype responses. IgA is considered antiinflammatory because it does not stimulate complement activation, tends to antagonize IgE and IgG, and does not serve as a direct opsonin. Daily, humans produce about three times more IgA than all other immunoglobulin isotypes combined. IgA protects mucosal surfaces above and below the epithelium and is an important molecule in mucosal immunity.

SUMMARY

This chapter focuses on the role of the immune system in inflammation, which is the host response to injury or insult and plays a central in the pathogenesis of periodontal diseases. Innate immunity provides critical early-phase defenses against invading microorganisms.

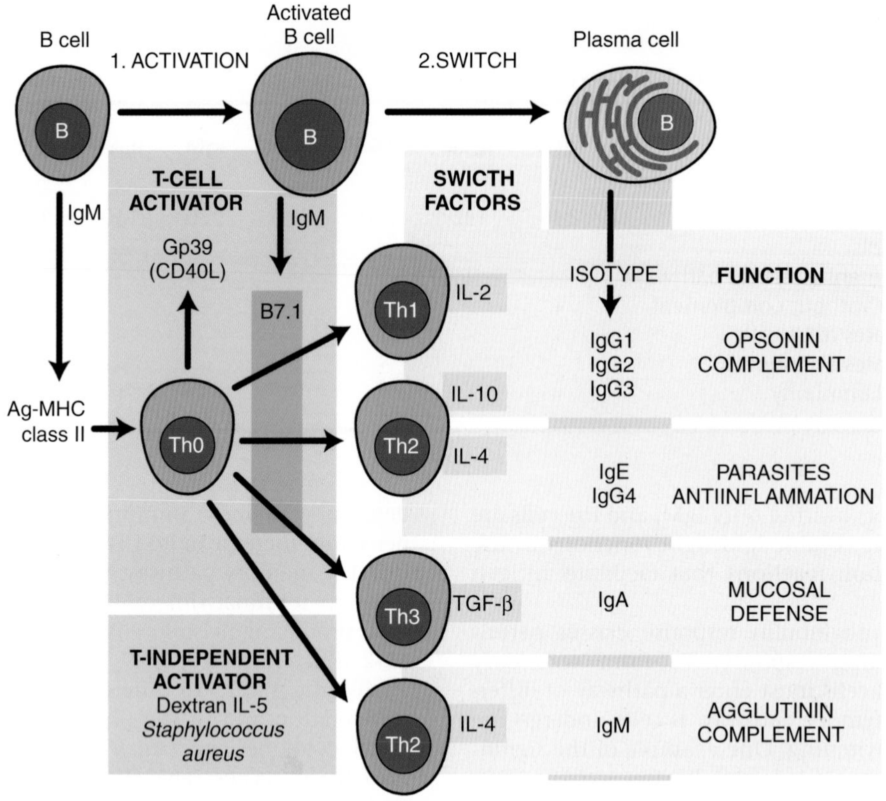

Figure 12-11 Schematic illustration of B-cell differentiation. The essential signals in B-cell differentiation are activator and switch factors. *1,* The activator signal often requires cell contact because T-cell activators (Gp37, Gp34) are transmembranous. T cells express Gp39 after antigen has been scanned. In the absence of T-cell switch signals, T-independent activation can result in an immunoglobulin M *(IgM)* response. Once the B cell is activated, it can provide co-stimulation to the T cells, which allows them to respond to differentiation signals (see Figure 12-10). *2,* Switch signals also are derived from T cells, and T cells are required for isotype switching. Notice that IgG1, IgG2, and IgG3 can function in responses against both extracellular (Th2) and intracellular (Th2) pathogens. In contrast, Th1 responses are not that important for generation of IgA and IgE, which function in mucosal defenses.

Adaptive immunity, including the development of the specific immune response, provides mechanisms by which the host can become more efficient in protecting against specific pathogens. Chapter 15 discusses the interaction of the immune system with microbial pathogens involved in periodontal diseases.

REFERENCES

1. Ahmed R, Gray D: Immunological memory and protective immunity: understanding their relation, *Science* 272(5258): 54, 1996.
2. Arpin C, Dechanet J, Van Kooten C, et al: Generation of memory B cells and plasma cells in vitro, *Science* 268(5211): 720, 1995.
3. Banchereau J, Briere F, Caux C, et al: Immunobiology of dendritic cells, *Annu Rev Immunol* 18:767, 2000.
4. Boyce JA: Mast cells: beyond IgE, *J Allergy Clin Immunol* 111:24, 2003.
5. Callard RE, Smith SH, Matthews DJ: Regulation of human B cell growth and differentiation: lessons from the primary immunodeficiencies, *Chem Immunol* 67:114, 1997.
6. Carroll RG, Riley JL, Levine BL, et al: Differential regulation of HIV-1 fusion cofactor expression by CD28 costimulation of CD4+ T cells, *Science* 276(5310):273, 1997.
7. Cerdan C, Martin Y, Courcoul M, et al: CD28 costimulation up-regulates long-term IL-2R beta expression in human T cells through combined transcriptional and post-transcriptional regulation, *J Immunol* 154:1007, 1995.
8. Cole DS, Morgan BP: Beyond lysis: how complement influences cell fate, *Clin Sci (Lond)* 104:455, 2003.
9. Constant S, Schweitzer N, West J, et al: B lymphocytes can be competent antigen-presenting cells for priming CD4+ T cells to protein antigens in vivo, *J Immunol* 155:3734, 1995.
10. Cook-Mills JM, Deem TL: Active participation of endothelial cells in inflammation, *J Leukoc Biol* 77:487, 2005.
11. Dezzutti CS, Rudolph DL, Lal RB: Infection with human T-lymphotropic virus types I and II results in alterations of cellular receptors, including the up-modulation of T-cell counterreceptors CD40, CD54, and CD80 (B7-1), *Clin Diagn Lab Immunol* 2:349, 1995.
12. Diacovo TG, Roth SJ, Buccola JM, et al: Neutrophil rolling, arrest, and transmigration across activated, surface-adherent platelets via sequential action of P-selectin and the beta 2-integrin CD11b/CD18, *Blood* 88:146, 1996.

13. Hoffmann E, Dittrich-Breiholz O, Holtmann H, Kracht M: Multiple control of interleukin-8 gene expression, *J Leukoc Biol* 72:847, 2002.
14. Huang D, Han Y, Rani MR, et al: Chemokines and chemokine receptors in inflammation of the nervous system: manifold roles and exquisite regulation, *Immunol Rev* 177:52, 2000.
15. Huber AR, Kunkel SL, Todd RF III, Weiss SJ: Regulation of transendothelial neutrophil migration by endogenous interleukin-8, *Science* 254(5028):99, 1991.
16. Lepique AP, Palencia S, Irjala H, Petrie HT: Characterization of vascular adhesion molecules that may facilitate progenitor homing in the post-natal mouse thymus, *Clin Dev Immunol* 10:27, 2003.
17. Malaviya R, Georges A: Regulation of mast cell–mediated innate immunity during early response to bacterial infection, *Clin Rev Allergy Immunol* 22:189, 2002.
18. Maldonado A, He L, Game BA, et al: Pre-exposure to high glucose augments lipopolysaccharide-stimulated matrix metalloproteinase-1 expression by human U937 histiocytes, *J Periodontal Res* 39:415, 2004.
19. Marshall D, Haskard DO: Clinical overview of leukocyte adhesion and migration: where are we now? *Semin Immunol* 14:133, 2002.
20. Marshall JS, McCurdy JD, Olynych T: Toll-like receptor–mediated activation of mast cells: implications for allergic disease? *Int Arch Allergy Immunol* 132:87, 2003.
21. Medzhitov R, Preston-Hurlburt P, Kopp E, et al: MyD88 is an adaptor protein in the hToll/IL-1 receptor family signaling pathways, *Mol Cell* 2:253, 1998.
22. Mosmann TR, Schumacher JH, Street NF, et al: Diversity of cytokine synthesis and function of mouse CD4+ T cells, *Immunol Rev* 123:209, 1991.
23. O'Neill LA, Greene C: Signal transduction pathways activated by the IL-1 receptor family: ancient signaling machinery in mammals, insects, and plants, *J Leukoc Biol* 63:650, 1998.
24. Pasare C, Medzhitov R: Toll-like receptors: linking innate and adaptive immunity, *Microbes Infect* 6:1382, 2004.
25. Reinherz EL, Tan K, Tang L, et al: The crystal structure of a T cell receptor in complex with peptide and MHC class II, *Science* 286(5446):1913, 1999.
26. Rosenberg YJ, Anderson AO, Pabst R: HIV-induced decline in blood CD4/CD8 ratios: viral killing or altered lymphocyte trafficking? *Immunol Today* 19:10, 1998.
27. Sontheimer RD, Matsubara T, Seelig LL Jr: A macrophage phenotype for a constitutive, class II antigen-expressing, human dermal perivascular dendritic cell, *J Invest Dermatol* 93:154, 1989.
28. Tangemann K, Gunn MD, Giblin P, Rosen SD: A high endothelial cell–derived chemokine induces rapid, efficient, and subset-selective arrest of rolling T lymphocytes on a reconstituted endothelial substrate, *J Immunol* 161:6330, 1998.
29. Van Haastert PJ, Devreotes PN: Chemotaxis: signalling the way forward, *Nat Rev Mol Cell Biol* 5:626-634, 2004.
30. Walsh LJ: Mast cells and oral inflammation, *Crit Rev Oral Biol Med* 14:188, 2003.
31. Zhang K: Immunoglobulin class switch recombination machinery: progress and challenges, *Clin Immunol* 95(Pt 1):1, 2000;
32. Ziegler-Heitbrock HW: Definition of human blood monocytes, *J Leukoc Biol* 67:603, 2000.

CHAPTER 13

Microbial Interactions with the Host in Periodontal Diseases

Russell J. Nisengard, Susan Kinder Haake, Michael G. Newman, and Kenneth T. Miyasaki

CHAPTER OUTLINE

Gingivitis and periodontitis, as well as other less common periodontal diseases, are chronic infectious diseases. The interaction of the microorganism with the host determines the course and extent of the resulting disease. Microorganisms may exert pathogenic effects directly by causing tissue destruction or indirectly by stimulating and modulating host responses. The host response is mediated by the microbial interaction and inherent characteristics of the host, including genetic factors that vary among individuals. In general, the host response functions in a protective capacity by preventing the local infection from progressing to a systemic, life-threatening infection. However, local alteration and destruction of host tissues as a result of the microbial-host interactions may manifest as periodontal disease. The varying balance between locally harmful and beneficial effects of the pathogenic microorganisms and the host accounts for the wide variety of patterns of tissue changes observed among patients.

MICROBIOLOGIC ASPECTS OF THE MICROBIAL-HOST INTERACTION

The specific microorganisms found to be associated with differing states of health and disease are discussed in Chapter 9. In general, gram-negative facultative or anaerobic bacteria appear to represent the predominant microorganisms associated with disease. Predominant bacterial species that have been implicated in the disease processes include *Porphyromonas gingivalis, Actinobacillus actinomycetemcomitans, Tannerella forsythia, Fusobacterium nucleatum, Prevotella intermedia, Campylobacter rectus, Peptostreptococcus micros*, and *Eikenella corrodens*. This chapter focuses on how the interaction of bacterial pathogens with host tissues results in disease. These issues relate to three of the criteria established by Socransky to identify periodontal pathogens (see Chapter 9). Studies of microbial interactions with the host involve analysis of the host response as well as the ability of a microorganism to cause disease in an animal model system.

SCIENCE TRANSFER

The central role of dental plaque bacteria in the etiology of gingivitis, periodontitis, aggressive periodontitis, necrotizing periodontal diseases, and periodontal abscesses involves direct tissue destruction by bacterially expressed toxins; bacterial interactions with the immune response–related, tissue-destructive processes also play a role. Each type of gingival and periodontal disease has been associated with specific plaque-bacterial cohorts made up of gram-negative anaerobic rods and spirochetes. Clinicians are able to treat each patient with appropriate surgical and nonsurgical therapy directed at removal of plaque bacteria and the establishment of shallow gingival crevices that become an inhospitable milieu for large numbers of anaerobic organisms. Recent advances in microbiology and host defense studies allow clinicians to couple conventional mechanical therapy with locally and systemically delivered antimicrobial and host modulation agents.

The properties of a microorganism that enable it to cause disease are referred to as *virulence factors.*

Considerable research is currently focused on defining the virulence factors of periodontal pathogens. From a simplistic viewpoint, to function as a pathogen, a bacterium must colonize the appropriate host tissue site and then cause destruction of the host tissues. In periodontitis, the initial step in the disease process is the colonization of the periodontal tissues by pathogenic species. Entry of the bacterium itself (invasion) or of bacterial products into the periodontal tissues may be important in the disease process. Furthermore, inherent in successful colonization of host tissues is the ability of the bacterium to evade host defense mechanisms aimed at eliminating the bacterium from the periodontal environment. The process of tissue destruction results from the interaction of bacteria or bacterial substances with host cells, which directly or indirectly lead to degradation of the periodontal tissues. Thus, virulence properties can be broadly categorized into two groups: (1) factors that enable a bacterial species to colonize and invade host tissues and (2) factors that enable a bacterial species to cause host tissue damage directly or indirectly.

Bacterial Colonization and Survival in the Periodontal Region

Bacterial Adherence in the Periodontal Environment

The gingival sulcus and periodontal pocket are bathed in gingival crevicular fluid, which flows outward from the base of the pocket. Bacterial species that colonize this region must attach to available surfaces to avoid displacement by the fluid flow. Therefore, adherence represents a virulence factor for periodontal pathogens.

The surfaces available for attachment include the tooth or root, tissues, and preexisting plaque mass. Numerous interactions between periodontal bacteria and these surfaces have been characterized, and in some cases the molecules responsible for mediating these highly specific interactions have been determined (Table 13-1). Bacteria that initially colonize the periodontal environment most likely attach to the pellicle- or saliva-coated tooth surface. A relevant example is the adherence of *Actinomyces viscosus* and *Porphyromonas gingivalis* through fimbriae on the bacterial surface to proline-rich proteins found on saliva-coated tooth surfaces.[3,120] Through its fimbriae, *P. gingivalis* also binds to epithelial cells and fibroblasts.[3]

Bacterial attachment to preexisting plaque is studied by examining the adherence between different bacterial strains *(coaggregation).* One of the best-characterized interactions is the adherence of *A. viscosus* through surface fimbriae to a polysaccharide receptor on cells of *Streptococcus sanguis.*[118] These types of interactions are thought to be of primary importance in the colonization of the periodontal environment. In addition, the adherence of bacteria to host tissues likely plays a role in colonization and may be a critical step in the process of bacterial invasion. Thus the ability of *P. gingivalis* to attach to other bacteria,[86-88] epithelial cells,[30] and the connective tissue components fibrinogen and fibronectin[97,98] are all likely to be important in the virulence of this microorganism.

Host Tissue Invasion

The presence of bacteria in host tissues in patients with necrotizing ulcerative gingivitis (NUG) has been recognized for years, based on histologic studies.[101] Investigations carried out largely in the 1980s demonstrated the presence of bacteria in periodontal tissues in gingivitis,[44] advanced chronic adult periodontitis,[47,153] and juvenile periodontitis.[20,24] Both gram-positive and gram-negative bacteria, including cocci, rods, filaments, and spirochetes, have been observed in gingival connective tissue and in proximity to alveolar bone. Bacteria may enter host tissues through ulcerations in the epithelium of the gingival sulcus or pocket and have been observed in intercellular spaces of the gingival tissues (Figures 13-1 to 13-4). Another means of tissue invasion may involve the direct penetration of bacteria into host epithelial or connective tissue cells. Laboratory investigations have demonstrated the ability of *A. actinomycetemcomitans,*[166] *P. gingivalis*[154] (Figure 13-5), *F. nucleatum,*[62] and *Treponema denticola*[184] to invade host tissue cells directly.

The clinical significance of bacterial invasion is not clear. Bacterial species that have been identified as capable of tissue invasion are strongly associated with disease, and the ability to invade has been proposed as a key factor that distinguishes pathogenic from nonpathogenic gram-negative species or strains.[105] Certainly, localization of bacteria to the tissues provides an ideal position from which the organism can effectively deliver toxic molecules and enzymes to the host tissue cells, and this may be the significance of invasion as a virulence factor. Indeed, some investigators have speculated that the "bursts of

TABLE 13-1

Select Bacterial Adhesins and Target Substrates

Probable Attachment Surface	Substrate	Bacterial Species	Bacterial Adhesion	Substrate Receptor
Tooth	Saliva-coated mineralized surfaces	*A. viscosus*	Fimbriae	Saliva-treated hydroxyapatite
		A. viscosus	Fimbriae	Proline-rich proteins
	Saliva-coated surfaces	*S. mitis*	70- to 90-kD protein	Sialic acid residues
		F. nucleatum	300- to 330-kD outer membrane protein	Galactosyl residues
Tissue	Epithelial cells	*P. gingivalis*	Fimbriae	Galactosyl residues
		A. viscosus	Fimbriae	Galactosyl residues
		A. naeslundii		
	Fibroblasts	*T. denticola*	Surface protein	Galactosyl or mannose residues
	Polymorphonuclear leukocytes	*A. viscosus*	Fimbriae	Galactosyl residues
		A. naeslundii		
		F. nucleatum	Protein	Galactosyl residues
	Connective tissue components	*P. gingivalis*	Membrane protein	Fibrinogen, fibronectin
		P. intermedia	Membrane protein	Fibrinogen
Preexisting plaque mass	*S. sanguis*	*A. viscosus*	Fimbriae	Repeating heptasaccharide on polysaccharide
	S. sanguis	*C. ochraceus*	Heat-sensitive protein	Rhamnose, fucose, *N*-acetylneuraminic acid residue
	A. naeslundii			
	A. israelii			
	S. sanguis	*P. loescheii*	75- to 45-kD fimbrial proteins	Galactosyl residues
	A. israelii			
	P. gingivalis	*F. nucleatum*	Heat- and protease-sensitive protein	Galactosyl residues
	T. denticola			
	P. micros			

Data from Socransky SS, Haffajee AD: *J Periodontal Res* 26:195, 1991; Lantz MS, Allen RD, Bounelis P, et al: *J Bacteriol* 172:716, 1990; Lantz MS, Allen RD, Duck LW, et al: *J Bacteriol* 173:4263, 1991; Bas HA, van Steenbergen M: *FEMS Microbiol Lett* 182:57, 2000; and Kolenbrander PE, Parrish KD, Andersen RN, et al: *Infect Immun* 63:4584, 1995.

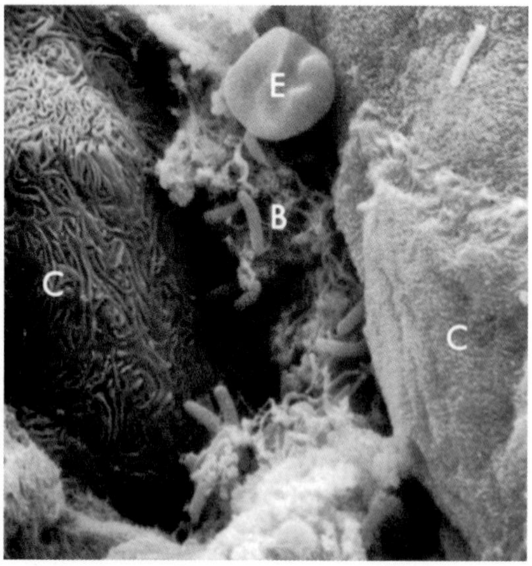

Figure 13-1 Scanning electron micrograph of epithelial intercellular spaces containing bacterial plaque *(B)* enmeshed in a fibrinlike material. *C,* Epithelial cells; *E,* erythrocyte. The cells to the left show signs of necrosis. (×4000.)

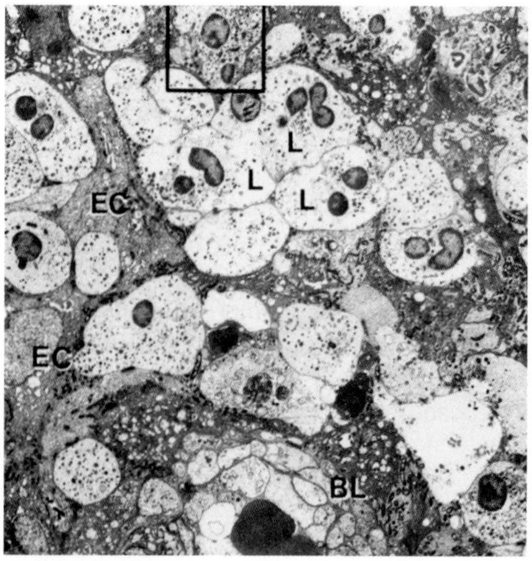

Figure 13-2 Interface between pocket epithelium and connective tissue separated by the basement lamina *(BL).* Abundant bacteria can be seen in the intercellular spaces. Numerous infiltrating polymorphonuclear leukocytes *(L)* are seen between epithelial cells *(EC).* Some leukocytes show engulfed bacteria. (×3908.)

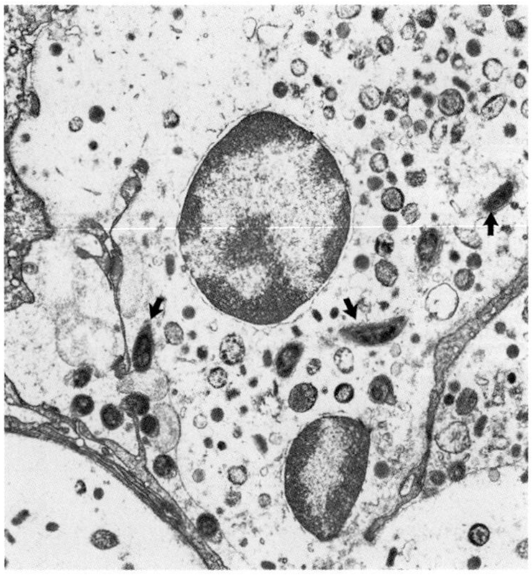

Figure 13-3 Higher magnification of the polymorphonuclear leukocyte in square in Figure 13-2 with engulfed bacteria *(arrows)* (×15,000).

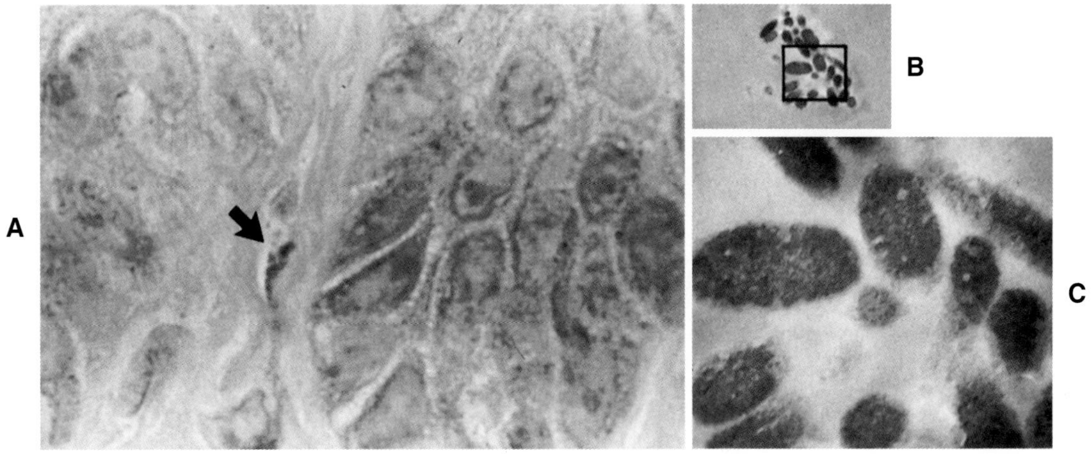

Figure 13-4 **A,** Gingival tissue of a patient with localized juvenile periodontitis showing granular-positive *(dark gray)* staining in the connective tissue for *Actinobacillus actinomycetemcomitans (arrow);* formalin paraffin section, peroxidase antiperoxidase method, anti–*A. actinomycetemcomitans,* counterstained with hematoxylin (×1200). **B,** Electron micrograph of the same paraffin section showing the area indicated by the arrow in *A,* which was reembedded in plastic (modified "pop-off" technique) (×40,000). **C,** Higher magnification of the rectangle in *B* showing the short coccobacillary rod with approximately the size and shape of *A. actinomycetemcomitans* (×80,000).

disease activity" observed in periodontitis may be related to phases of bacterial invasion of the tissues.[152] An additional possibility is that bacteria in the tissues may enable persistence of that species in the periodontal pocket by providing a reservoir for recolonization. Consistent with this hypothesis is the observation that mechanical debridement alone is insufficient, and that systemic antibiotics in combination with surgical therapy is required, to eliminate *A. actinomycetemcomitans* from lesions in patients with localized aggressive periodontitis (LAP).[23,91]

Bacterial Evasion of Host Defense Mechanisms

To survive in the periodontal environment, bacteria must neutralize or evade the host mechanisms involved in bacterial clearance and killing. Bacterial adherence and invasion are representative strategies by which microorganisms accomplish this task. The ability to adhere allows bacteria to avoid displacement by host secretions, and eukaryotic cell invasion disrupts the natural barriers formed by host tissue cells. Periodontal bacteria neutralize or evade host defenses through numerous other mechanisms (Table 13-2). For example, immunoglobulins might function to facilitate phagocytosis of bacteria by opsonization or may block adherence by binding to the bacterial cell surface and restricting access to bacterial adhesins. The production of immunoglobulin-degrading proteases by specific microorganisms may counteract these host defenses. Similarly, bacteria produce substances that suppress the activity of or kill polymorphonuclear leukocytes (PMNs) and lymphocytes normally involved

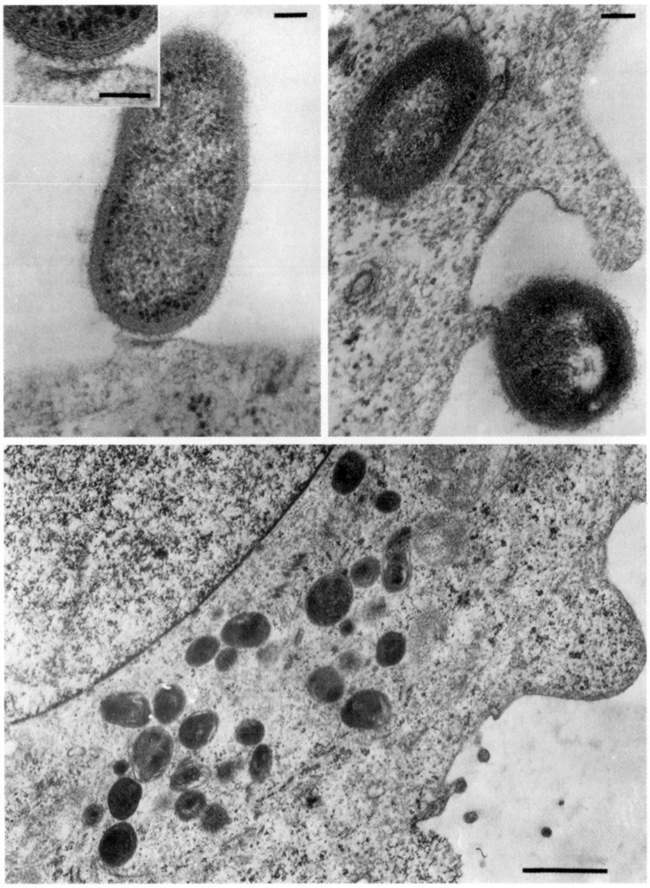

Figure 13-5 High-magnification electron photomicrographs of the interaction of *Porphyromonas gingivalis* strain W50 with the epithelial cell HEp-2. **A,** *P. gingivalis* is attached to the HEp-2 plasma membrane by its tip. *Inset,* Note the electron-dense region juxtaposed to the site of interaction, possibly an early stage of clatherin pit formation. **B,** *P. gingivalis* is seen in transverse section attached to a microvillus extension. An internalized *P. gingivalis* also is apparent in the cell section. **C,** Numerous *P. gingivalis* W50 cells are seen in the HEp-2 cytoplasm. (Courtesy Dr. Stanley C. Holt, Boston.)

in host defenses. An example of this is the production by *A. actinomycetemcomitans* of two toxins (a leukotoxin and cytolethal distending toxin) that may be important in the virulence of this microorganism in aggressive periodontitis and possibly in chronic periodontitis. Similarly, *T. forsythia*[2] and *F. nucleatum*[73] have been shown to induce apoptosis, a form of cellular "suicide," in lymphocytes. Many periodontal pathogens stimulate the production of interleukin-8 (IL-8), a proinflammatory chemokine that provides a signal for the recruitment of neutrophils (PMNs) to a local site (see later discussion). *P. gingivalis* is able to inhibit the production of IL-8 by epithelial cells, which may provide the microorganism with an advantage in evading PMN-mediated killing (see Chapter 15).

Microbial Mechanisms of Host Tissue Damage

Research on virulence factors has focused on the properties of bacteria related to the destruction of host tissues. These bacterial properties can be broadly categorized as those resulting directly in degradation of host tissues and those causing the release of biologic mediators from host tissue cells that lead to host tissue destruction.

Some bacterial products inhibit the growth or alter the metabolism of host tissue cells; these include a number of metabolic byproducts such as ammonia; volatile sulfur compounds; and fatty acids, peptides, and indoles.[159,181] An important class of molecules in tissue destruction is the variety of enzymes produced by periodontal microorganisms (Table 13-3). These enzymes appear to be capable of degrading essentially all host tissue and intercellular matrix molecules.[26,94] In particular, a wide range of proteolytic enzymes have been identified from *P. gingivalis* (see Chapter 15), including a trypsinlike enzyme and those that degrade collagen, fibronectin, and immunoglobulins. Bacterial enzymes may facilitate tissue destruction and invasion of bacteria into host tissues. However, the exact role of bacterially derived proteases in the disease process has not been determined because similar enzymes (e.g., collagenases) in the periodontal environment originate from host tissue cells. Indeed, one mechanism by which bacteria may indirectly cause tissue damage is by induction of host tissue proteinases such as elastase and matrix metalloproteinases (MMPs)[31,32] (see later discussion and Chapters 16 and 53).

The host immune system involves a complex network of interactions among cells and regulatory molecules.

TABLE 13-2

Select Bacterial Properties Involved in Evasion of Host Defense Mechanisms

Host Defense Mechanism	Bacterial Species	Bacterial Property	Biologic Effect
Specific antibody	*P. gingivalis* *P. intermedia* *P. melaninogenica* *Capnocytophaga* spp.	IgA- and IgG-degrading proteases	Degradation of specific antibody
Polymorphonuclear leukocytes (PMNs)	*A. actinomycetem-comitans*	Leukotoxin	Inhibition of PMN function
	F. nucleatum	Heat-sensitive surface protein	Apoptosis (programmed cell death) of PMN
	P. gingivalis	Capsule	Inhibition of phagocytosis
	T. denticola	Inhibition of superoxide production	Decreased bacterial killing
Lymphocytes	*A. actinomycetem-comitans*	Leukotoxin	Killing of mature B and T cells; nonlethal suppression of activity
		Cytolethal distending toxin	Impairment of function by arresting of lymphocyte cell cycle
	F. nucleatum	Heat-sensitive surface protein	Apoptosis of mononuclear cells
	T. forsythia	Cytotoxin	Apoptosis of lymphocytes
	P. intermedia	Suppression	Decreased response to antigens and mitogens
	T. denticola *A. actinomycetem-comitans*		
Release of interleukin-8 (IL-8)	*P. gingivalis*	Inhibition of IL-8 production by epithelial cells	Impairment of PMN response to bacteria

Data from Socransky SS, Haffajee AD: *J Periodontal Res* 26:195, 1991; Jewett A, Hume WR, Le H, et al: *Infect Immun* 68:1893, 2000; Shenker BJ, McKay T, Datar S, et al: *J Immunol* 162:4773, 1999; Arakawa S, Nakajima T, Ishikura H, et al: *Infect Immun* 68:4611, 2000; Darveau RP, Belton CM, Reife RA, et al: *Infect Immun* 66:1660, 1998; and Huang GT, Haake SK, Kim JW, et al: *Oral Microbiol Immunol* 13:1301, 1998.

TABLE 13-3

Bacterial Enzymes Capable of Degrading Host Tissues

Bacterial Enzyme	Species
Collagenase	*P. gingivalis* *A. actinomycetemcomitans*
Trypsinlike enzyme	*P. gingivalis* *A. actinomycetemcomitans* *T. denticola*
Arysulfatase	*C. rectus*
Neuraminidase	*P. ginivalis* *T. forsythia* *P. melaninogenica*
Fibronectin-degrading enzyme	*P. gingivalis* *P. intermedia*
Phospholipase A	*P. intermedia* *P. melaninogenica*

Bacterial products may perturb the system, resulting in tissue destruction (Table 13-4). Well-characterized interactions involve the release of interleukin-1 (IL-1), tumor necrosis factor (TNF), and prostaglandins from monocytes, macrophages, and PMNs exposed to bacterial endotoxin (lipopolysaccharide).[146,192] These host-derived mediators have the potential to stimulate bone resorption and activate or inhibit other host immune cells. Many additional examples of this type of interaction exist, and the mechanisms underlying their manipulation of the host response are the focus of the next section.

IMMUNOLOGIC ASPECTS OF THE MICROBIAL-HOST INTERACTION

Periodontal disease is dependent on bacteria, as discussed previously, and bacteria may directly interact with the host tissues in mediating tissue destruction. In addition, many tissue changes associated with periodontal diseases appear to be well-orchestrated responses, suggesting the influence of host regulation. Among the orchestrated responses are the antimicrobial activities by acute inflammatory cells (neutrophils) and the adaptive activities brought about by monocytes/macrophages and lymphocytes. Adaptive responses include the epithelial alterations, angiogenesis, episodic remodeling of the underlying hard and soft connective tissues, and antigen-specific immune responses. Remodeling of the connective tissues appears to be episodic and occurs in cycles of destruction and reconstruction. Excessive destruction or inadequate reconstruction can result in periodontal disease.

TABLE 13-4

Examples of Effects of Bacteria and Their Products on Production of Biologically Active Molecules by Host Tissues

Effect on Cytokine Levels	Bacterial Species	Bacterial Component	Target Host Tissue
Increased release of interleukin-1	*A. actinomycetemcomitans*	LPS	PMNs
	F. nucleatum		
	A. actinomycetemcomitans	37-kD protein	Macrophages
	P. gingivalis	LPS	Monocytes
Increased release of interleukin-6	*A. actinomycetemcomitans*	37-kD protein	Macrophages
	A. actinomycetemcomitans	Whole cells	Gingival fibroblasts
	C. rectus		
	E. corrodens	Whole cells	Epithelial cells
Increased release of interleukin-8	*A. actinomycetemcomitans*	Whole cells	Epithelial cells
	E. corrodens		
	F. nucleatum		
	A. actinomycetemcomitans	Whole cells	Gingival fibroblasts
	C. rectus		
	A. actinomycetemcomitans	LPS	PMNs
	F. nucleatum		
Increased release of tumor necrosis factor	*A. actinomycetemcomitans*	LPS	PMNs
	F. nucleatum		
	A. actinomycetemcomitans	37-kD protein	Macrophages
Stimulated release of prostaglandin E_2	*C. rectus*	LPS	Monocytes
	A. actinomycetemcomitans		
	P. intermedia		
	P. gingivalis		

Modified from Socransky SS, Haffajee AD: *J Periodontal Res* 26:195, 1991; data from references 28, 33, 50, 62, 69, 70, 146, 171, 192, and 193.
LPS, Lipopolysaccharide; *PMNs,* polymorphonuclear leukocytes; *kD,* kilodalton.

This section presents a paradigm for the role of the immune system in periodontal pathogenesis. The paradigm is consistent with the specific plaque hypothesis, current concepts in immunology, and the classic clinical and histologic observations (see Chapters 20 and 26) regarding periodontal diseases. The paradigm involves the following in response to bacterial infection:

1. Innate factors such as complement, resident leukocytes, and especially mast cells play an important role in signaling endothelium, thus initiating inflammation.
2. Acute inflammatory cells (i.e., neutrophils) protect local tissues by controlling the periodontal microbiota within the gingival crevice and junctional epithelium.
3. Chronic inflammatory cells, macrophages, and lymphocytes protect the entire host from within the subjacent connective tissues and do all that is necessary to prevent a local infection from becoming systemic and life threatening, including the sacrifice of local tissues.

In this paradigm, periodontal disease represents a well-regulated response to protracted bacterial infection directed by the inflammatory cells of the host immune system (Figure 13-6). Neutrophils function primarily as antimicrobial cells, and chronic inflammatory cells orchestrate adaptive responses. Neutrophils function to contain the microbial challenge through phagocytosis and killing and may contribute to local tissue changes by the release of tissue-degrading enzymes. The chronic inflammatory cells, the lymphocytes and monocytes, orchestrate connective tissue changes associated with both periodontal infection and periodontal repair and healing. They also function to assist the neutrophils in controlling bacterial infection by forming specific opsonic antibodies. The host response in the connective tissues may result in local destruction of the tissue, which is evident as periodontal disease. In recent years the potential systemic impact of periodontal disease has been increasingly recognized (see Chapters 17 and 18). However, the end result of the periodontal host response is largely successful in preventing progressive spread of the infection despite local tissue destruction.

Innate Factors and Initiation of Inflammation

The onset of inflammation involves the development of edema and erythema, which are signs of vascular changes. Complement activation in response to bacterial infection results in generation of the complement-derived anaphylatoxins C3a and C5a. *Anaphylatoxins* are substances that stimulate vascular changes indirectly by causing degranulation of the resident leukocytes, the mast cells. Degranulated mast cells increase within the gingival connective tissue as gingival inflammation increases.

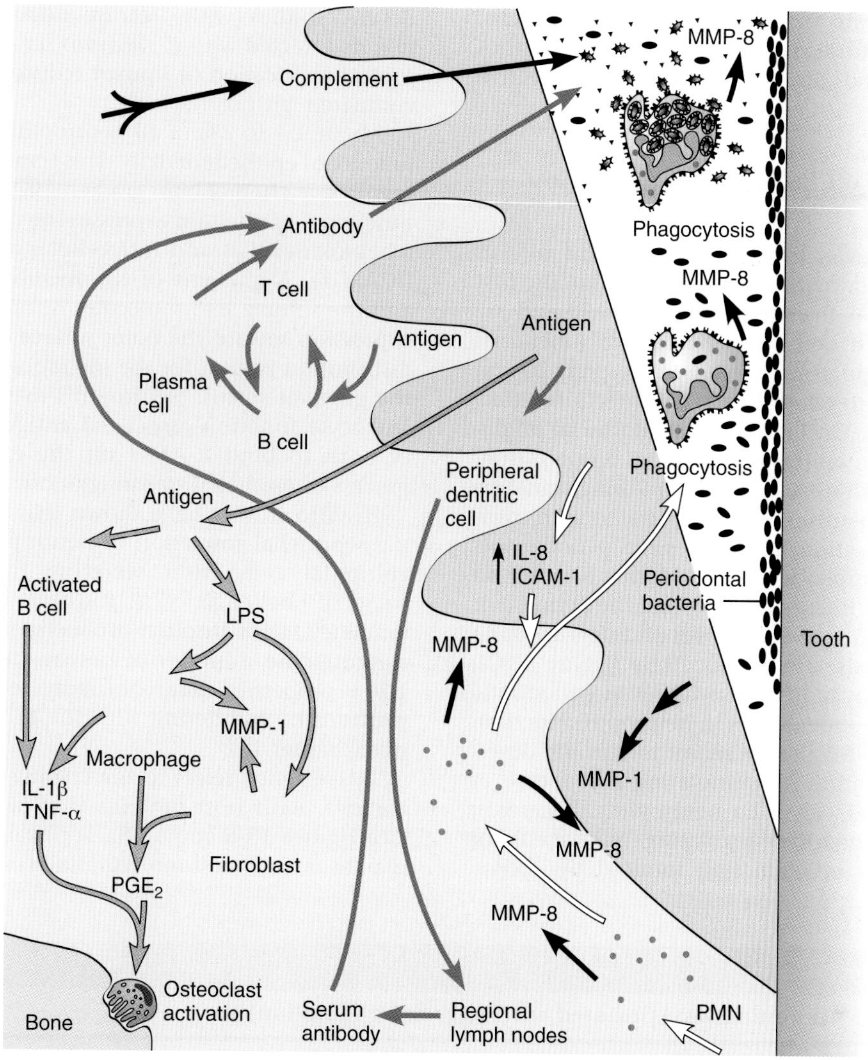

Figure 13-6 Schematic illustration of key processes of the host bacterial interaction in periodontal diseases. Interactions of the bacteria or bacterial antigen with host tissues leads to neutrophil recruitment *(white arrows)*, antibody production *(gray arrows)*, and bone resorption *(light-gray arrows with black outline)*. Interleukin-8 *(IL-8)* and intercellular adhesion molecule-1 *(ICAM-1)* production in the epithelial cells in response to periodontal bacteria provides a chemotactic signal for neutrophils *(PMN)*. Neutrophils function to control the bacterial assault by phagocytosis but also secrete matrix metalloproteinases *(MMP-8)*, which may contribute to tissue destruction. The interaction of bacterial antigens with peripheral dendritic cells leads to the generation of systemic antibody, whereas interaction with local B cells leads to production of local antibody. Antibody specific to many of the periodontal microorganisms is essential for phagocytosis. Complement components also may contribute to efficient bacterial phagocytosis. The production of interleukin-1β *(IL-1β)*, tumor necrosis factor alpha *(TNF-α)*, and prostaglandin E_2 *(PGE_2)* in response to bacterial lipopolysaccharides *(LPS)* leads to bone resorption through osteoclast activation, proliferation, and differentiation.

Mast cells constitutively transcribe tumor necrosis factor alpha (TNF-α), transforming growth factor beta (TGF-β), interleukin-4 (IL-4), and interleukin-6 (IL-6); when stimulated, they induce transcription of proinflammatory cytokines such as IL-1, IL-6, interferon-γ (IFN-γ), and others.[121] The stimulation of endothelial cells by C5a, IL-1β, TNF-α, and bacterial lipopolysaccharide (LPS) results in the expression of selectins on the luminal surface of the endothelial cells and release of chemokines from the endothelial cells. These processes are central in transendothelial migration of leukocytes (see Figure 12-4), which results in the movement of leukocytes into the local tissues.

In healthy individuals, complement levels in gingival crevicular fluid (GCF) are about 3% of that in serum. As periodontal inflammation increases, a concomitant increase in the levels of complement components occurs. The levels of C3 and C4, for example, can increase to 25% and 85% of that in serum.[155] The levels of complement components in GCF are more than adequate to support the recruitment of acute and chronic inflammatory cells, opsonization and neutralization of pathogens or pathogenic substances, and local regulation of connective tissue changes.

Controlling Bacterial Challenge: Primary Role for Neutrophils

Neutrophils are believed to play an important role in controlling the periodontal microbiota. They are the first leukocytes to arrive at the site of inflammation and are always the dominant cell type within the junctional epithelium and the gingival crevice (see Chapters 20 and 26.) For neutrophils to control bacterial infections effectively, their functions, including transendothelial migration, chemotaxis, transepithelial migration, opsonization, phagocytosis, and intraphagolysosomal killing, must be intact. Disorders of neutrophils are associated with invasive periodontal infection and aggressive periodontitis (Table 13-5). For example, severe periodontal destruction involving both the primary dentition and the permanent dentition is evident in individuals with disorders affecting neutrophil chemotaxis and phagocytosis (Figure 13-7). Also, otherwise-healthy individuals with severe periodontal problems may have subtle defects in neutrophil function, as discussed later. TNF-α plays a major role in the development of inflammation by stimulating the release of cytokines, including IL-1β, from neutrophils.[144] Lipoxin A_4 is an important cytokine-regulating lipid mediator that can reduce the inflammation induced by TNF-α. Recent studies with ligature-induced periodontitis in rabbits infected with *P. gingivalis* have demonstrated that topical application of lipoxin reduced alveolar bone loss compared with controls.[181]

About 1% to 2% of all neutrophils migrate across the junctional epithelium daily. This transepithelial migration requires a chemotaxin gradient (see Figure 13-6). The junctional epithelium expresses the chemotactic cytokine (chemokine) IL-8 and intercellular adhesion molecule-1 (ICAM-1). A gradient of the membrane-bound ICAM-1 and the soluble IL-8 molecules is formed, with increased expression toward the outer surface of the tissue.[122] This distribution is ideal for the migration of neutrophils into the gingival sulcus. Neutrophils may use their adhesins leukocyte function–associated antigen-1 (LFA-1), Mac-1, or both to bind ICAM-1 on the epithelial cell in the process of epithelial transmigration.

In vitro studies have shown that *P. gingivalis* impedes transepithelial migration of neutrophils[111] and prevents epithelial cells from secreting IL-8 in response to bacterial challenge.[28,70] *P. gingivalis* also has a potential virulence factor through production of periodontain, an α_1-proteinase inhibitor of human neutrophil elastase.[129] These properties may contribute to the virulence of *P. gingivalis* by interfering with the host immune response (see Chapter 15).

Opsonization refers to the coating of particles, such as bacteria, with host proteins that facilitate phagocytosis (see Figures 13-6 and 13-8). For example, a bacterial cell may be coated with molecules derived from complement

TABLE 13-5

Systemic Neutrophil Abnormalities Associated with Aggressive Periodontitis

Condition	Neutrophil Abnormality	Periodontal Manifestations
Neutropenia, agranulocytosis	Decreased number of neutrophils.	Severe aggressive periodontitis.
Chédiak-Higashi syndrome	Decreased neutrophil chemotaxis and secretion. Neutrophil granules fuse to form characteristic giant granules called *megabodies*.	Aggressive periodontitis and oral ulceration. Syndrome caused by mutation in the vesicle trafficking regulator gene, LYST.
Papillon-Lefèvre syndrome	Multiple functional neutrophil defects, including myeloperoxidase deficiency, defective chemotaxis, and phagocytosis.	Severe aggressive periodontal destruction at an early age, which may involve primary and permanent dentition. Recently associated with mutation in cathepsin C gene (see Chapter 11).
Leukocyte adhesion deficiency type 1 (LAD-1)	Defects in leukocyte function caused by lack of integrin β-2 subunit (CD18). Neutrophil defects include impaired migration and phagocytosis. Histologically, almost no extravascular neutrophils are evident in periodontal lesions.	Aggressive periodontitis at an early age and affecting primary and permanent dentition, in individuals who are homozygous for the defective gene.
Leukocyte adhesion deficiency type 2 (LAD-2)	Neutrophils fail to express the ligand (CD15) for P- and E-selectins, resulting in impaired transendothelial migration in response to inflammation.	Aggressive periodontitis at a young age.

Data from references 12, 29, 52, 63, 64, 127, 144, 158, 182.

components (e.g., iC3b) for which the neutrophil has receptors (CR3). Similarly, bacterial cells may be coated with specific antibody that fixes complement and results in surface deposition of C3b that is recognized by the CR3 neutrophil receptor when converted to iC3b. Specific antibody of the immunoglobulin G (IgG) isotype also facilitates phagocytosis directly by binding with the neutrophil Fc receptor and appears to be essential for phagocytosis of certain periodontal pathogens (see later discussion).

Patients with periodontitis often exhibit very high serum titers of IgG to specific periodontal pathogens. Although B cells are directly responsible for antibody production, T cells are required to regulate the isotype switch from immunoglobulin M (IgM) to IgG. Antigen-presenting cells (APCs) such as the peripheral dendritic cells (e.g., Langerhans cells, macrophages, B cells) are abundant within the gingival tissues[135] and can transport antigen to regional lymph nodes, thus promoting the production of serum IgG antibody. Local immunoglobulin production also has been documented within the gingiva, and the gingival tissues are impregnated with very high levels of immunoglobulins.

Scaling and root planing stimulates antibody production against microorganisms such as *P. gingivalis* and *A. actinomycetemcomitans*.[22,160] Variability in the levels, types, and strength of binding of the antibody is evident in different patients, and the significance of the antibody depends on its functional capabilities.[85] The antibody may function to facilitate host clearance of periodontal pathogens. For example, the antibody appears to be essential for opsonization and phagocytosis of *A. actinomycetemcomitans*[11] and virulent strains of *P. gingivalis*.[27] The antibody also may function to neutralize bacterial components important in colonization or host cell interactions. A monoclonal antibody preparation specific for a hemagglutinin of *P. gingivalis* has been shown to prevent recolonization of deep periodontal pockets in vivo in periodontitis patients.[15,78] More information is needed to clarify the role of antibodies to specific bacterial epitopes in disease progression and resolution. It is noteworthy that in LAP, the absence of a host antibody response has been postulated to contribute to disease progression (see following discussion).

Once the bacterial cell is bound to the neutrophil, ingestion (phagocytosis) results in entrapment of the

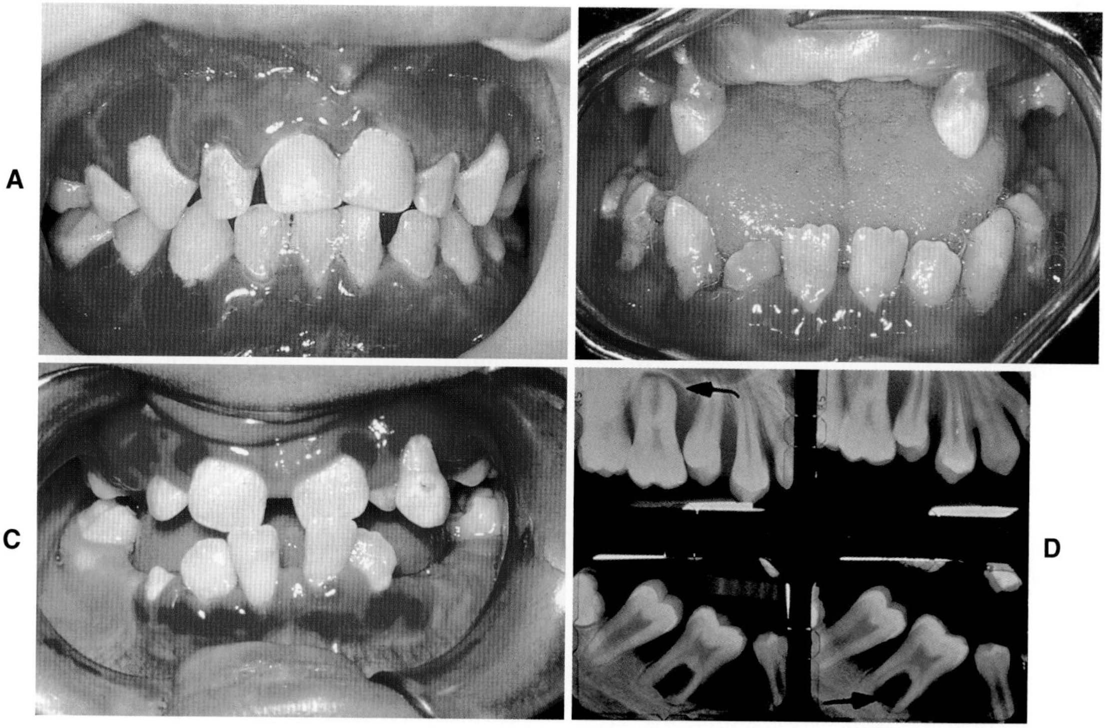

Figure 13-7 Periodontal manifestations of disorders affecting neutrophil function. **A** and **B,** Clinical appearance of patients with *cyclic neutropenia,* a condition that involves reduction in the number of circulating neutrophils (blood neutrophil levels <1500/mm^4). **A,** Five-year-old boy with cyclic neutropenia. Note the aggressive and extensive inflammation in the gingival tissues. **B,** Seven-year-old boy with cyclic neutropenia demonstrating acute and extensive gingival inflammation and advanced attachment loss with recession evident. **C** and **D,** Clinical and radiographic appearance of patients with *leukocyte adhesion deficiency* (LAD type 1). This disorder involves defects in neutrophil transendothelial migration, resulting in a lack of extravascular neutrophils in periodontal lesions. However, dense infiltrates of mononuclear leukocytes are found in the periodontal lesions. Note the tissue inflammation evident clinically **(C)** and the extensive bone loss seen in these patients (**D,** arrows).[181] (For additional information, see text and Table 13-5.) (**A** and **B** courtesy Dr. Max Listgarten; **C** and **D** courtesy Dr. D.C. Anderson.)

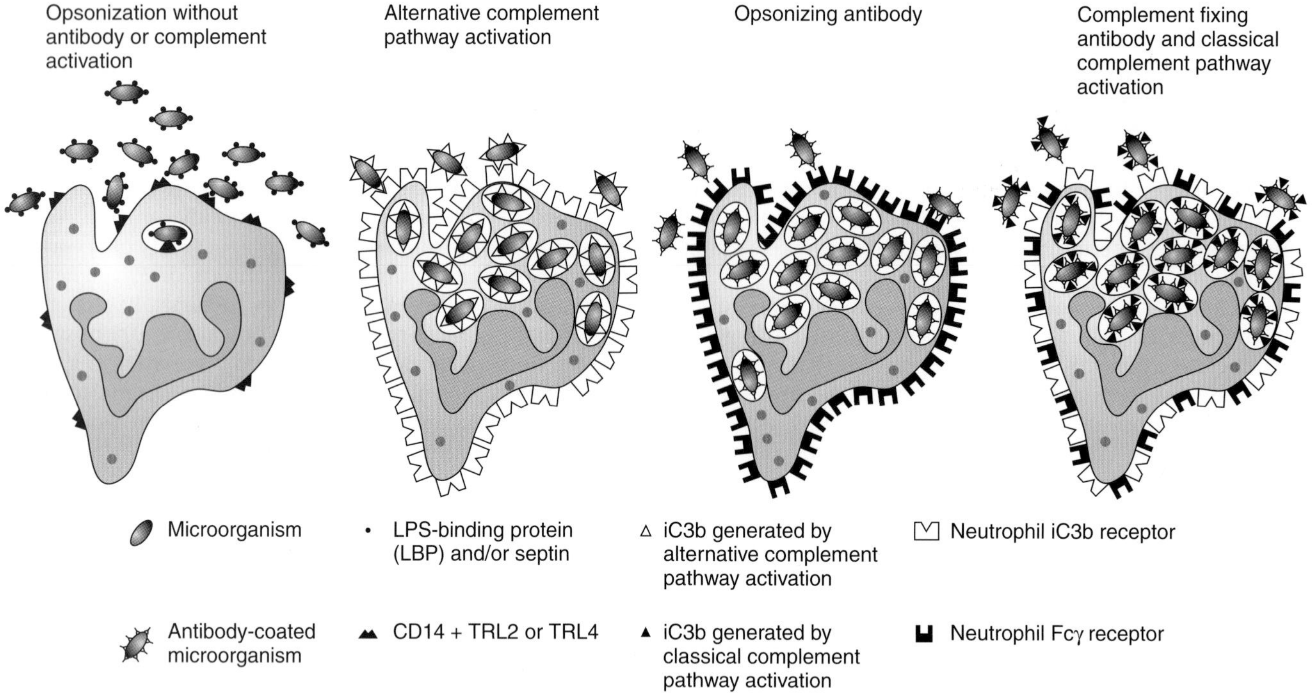

Figure 13-8 Schematic illustration of some routes of opsonization and phagocytosis. Bacterial control in the periodontal environment is achieved largely by opsonization, phagocytosis, and killing of the bacteria by neutrophils. *Opsonization* refers to the coating of the bacterial cell with host-derived proteins such as LPS-binding protein (LBP), specific antibody, or the complement component iC3b (*LPS,* lipopolysaccharide). Opsonization with specific antibody of the IgG subclass is required for phagocytosis of certain bacteria, such as *Actinobacillus actinomycetemcomitans.* (See text for further details.)

bacterial cell into the membrane-delimited structure known as the *phagosome.* Bacteria within the phagosome and phagolysosome may be killed by oxidative or nonoxidative mechanisms. The gingival sulcus is characteized by a diminished level of oxygen, and the oxidation-reduction (redox) potential of the periodontal pocket is more reduced than the gingival sulcus. This is indicated by measurements of crevicular oxygen levels and redox potential[79] and reflected by the growth of strictly anaerobic bacteria such as *P. gingivalis* and the oral spirochetes. The oxidative killing mechanisms of crevicular neutrophils may be intact in a healthy sulcus but impaired in the periodontal pocket. A shutdown of oxidative killing may be an important factor in the progression to periodontitis. Nonoxidative mechanisms of killing involve phagosome-lysosome fusion, resulting in secretion of bactericidal substances such as lysozyme, cathepsin G, and α-defensins into the phagolysosome containing the ingested bacterium. Some periodontal pathogens evade phagocytic cells as a virulence mechanism. For example, the leukotoxin of *A. actinomycetemcomitans* kills phagocytes by binding to the LFA-1 adhesin and subsequently lysing the eukaryotic cell.[96] Recently it was demonstrated in vitro that specific antibodies to *A. actinomycetemcomitans* or antileukotoxin serum protects neutrophils from leukotoxin-mediated injury and enables phagocytosis to proceed.[74]

Connective Tissue Alterations: Tissue Destruction in Periodontitis

A central feature of periodontitis is the remodeling of connective tissues that leads to a net loss of local soft tissues, bone, and the periodontal attachment apparatus. The fundamental event in the transition from gingivitis to periodontitis is the loss of the soft tissue attachment to the tooth and the subsequent loss of alveolar bone. Bacterial components that contribute directly or indirectly to tissue destruction have been discussed previously. Mediators produced as a part of the host response that contribute to tissue destruction include proteinases, cytokines, and prostaglandins.

Proteinases

Matrix metalloproteinases (MMPs) are considered to be primary proteinases involved in periodontal tissue destruction by degradation of extracellular matrix molecules. MMPs are a family of proteolytic enzymes found in neutrophils, macrophages, fibroblasts, epithelial cells, osteoblasts, and osteoclasts[150] that degrade extracellular matrix molecules, such as collagen, gelatin, and elastin. MMP-8 and MMP-1 are both collagenases; MMP-8 is released by infiltrating neutrophils, whereas MMP-1 is expressed by resident cells, including fibroblasts, monocytes/macrophages, and epithelial cells (see Figure 13-6). MMPs are also produced by the periodontal pathogens

P. gingivalis and *A. actinomycetemcomitans,* although this is not considered a major factor in disease progression.[122] Collagenase is elevated in tissues and GCF associated with periodontitis compared with gingivitis or healthy controls.[72,147]

MMPs are secreted in an inactive (latent) form. Enzyme activity in the tissues is partly controlled by activation of the latent enzyme and the level of enzyme inhibitors present. One mechanism of MMP activation involves the proteolytic cleavage of a portion of the latent enzyme. Proteases capable of activating MMPs include bacterial enzymes such as the chymotrypsin-like protease produced by *Treponema denticola,* as well as host cell enzymes such as the neutrophil cathepsin G. MMPs are inactivated by α-macroglobulins found in serum and GCF and by tissue inhibitors of MMPs (TIMPs) produced by many cell types and common in host tissues and fluids.[14] Tetracyclines appear to inactivate neutrophil MMP and to have some therapeutic potential[54,57] (see Chapter 16).

Other proteinases associated with periodontitis include the neutrophil serine proteinases, elastase and cathepsin G. *Elastase* is capable of degrading a wide range of molecules, including elastin, collagen, and fibronectin. *Cathepsin G* is a bactericidal proteinase that also may function in the activation of MMP-8. Endogenous inhibitors of elastase and cathepsin G (e.g., α_1-proteinase inhibitor, α_1-antichymotrypsin, α_2-macroglobulin) are found in plasma and GCF.[66] The role of these enzymes in pathogenesis probably depends on the balance of enzyme and enzyme inhibitor in the local tissue. Cathepsin G is elevated in the gingival tissues and GCF in adult (chronic) periodontitis.[173] Elevated levels of elastase in GCF are associated with active periodontal attachment loss,[3] and elastase may provide a convenient clinical marker of disease progression.

Cytokines

Three proinflammatory cytokines, interleukin-1 (IL-1), IL-6, and tumor necrosis factor (TNF), appear to have a central role in periodontal tissue destruction[57,138] (see Figure 13-6). IL-1 is found in two active forms, IL-1α and IL-1β, encoded by separate genes. Both are potent proinflammatory molecules and are the main constituents of what was once called "osteoclast-activating factor." The IL-1 family also includes the IL-1 receptor antagonist (IL-1ra), which will bind the IL-1 receptor without stimulation of the host cell. IL-6, another inflammatory cytokine, leads to bone remodeling.[112] TNF also is found in two forms, TNF-α and TNF-β. TNF-α shares many of the same biologic activities as IL-1, including the stimulation of bone resorption.

IL-1 is produced primarily by activated macrophages or lymphocytes but also may be released by other cells, including mast cells, fibroblasts, keratinocytes, and endothelial cells. Bacterial LPS is a potent activator of macrophage IL-1 production, whereas TNF-α and IL-1 itself also can activate macrophage IL-1 production. The ability of IL-1 to upregulate its own production may provide a significant amplification mechanism. TNF-α also is produced by activated macrophages, particularly in response to bacterial LPS. TNF-β is primarily produced by the Th1 subset of CD4+ T cells that have been activated by antigen or mitogen. The proinflammatory effects of IL-1 and TNF-α include (1) stimulation of endothelial cells to express selectins that facilitate recruitment of leukocytes, (2) activation of macrophage IL-1 production, and (3) induction of prostaglandin E_2 (PGE_2) by macrophages and gingival fibroblasts.[138]

The properties of these cytokines that relate to tissue destruction involve stimulation of bone resorption and induction of tissue-degrading proteinases. IL-1 is a potent stimulant of osteoclast proliferation, differentiation, and activation. TNF-α has similar effects on osteoclasts but is much less potent than IL-1. Both IL-1 and TNF-α induce production of proteinases in mesenchymal cells, including MMPs, which may contribute to connective tissue destruction.[57,138]

Substantial data from in vivo studies support the concept that IL-1 and TNF-α are key molecules in the pathogenesis of periodontitis. IL-1, IL-6, and TNF-α are found in significant concentrations in GCF from periodontally diseased sites. Reductions in IL-1 concentration are associated with successful treatment,[110,158] and elevated levels of IL-6 in GCF are associated with sites that do not respond well in initial nonsurgical phases of therapy.[115] Increasing severity of periodontitis is associated with increased concentrations of IL-1 and decreasing concentrations of IL-1ra.[145] In a primate model of experimental periodontitis, application of antagonists to IL-1 and TNF resulted in an 80% reduction in recruitment of inflammatory cells in proximity to the alveolar bone and a 60% reduction in bone loss.[9]

Prostaglandins

Prostaglandins are arachidonic acid metabolites generated by cyclooxygenases (COX-1, COX-2). Arachidonic acid is a 20-carbon polyunsaturated fatty acid found in the plasma membrane of most cells. COX-2 is upregulated by IL-1β, TNF-α, and bacterial LPS and appears to be responsible for generating the prostaglandin (PGE_2) that is associated with inflammation. The primary cells responsible for PGE_2 production in the periodontium are macrophages and fibroblasts. PGE_2 is increased in periodontal sites demonstrating inflammation and attachment loss.[90,136] Induction of MMPs and osteoclastic bone resorption is induced by PGE_2 (see Figure 13-6).

PGE_2 appears to be partly responsible for the bone loss associated with periodontitis. PGE_2 is elevated in gingivitis and periodontitis, particularly in active disease. Assays in GCF may eventually be considered as a diagnostic marker for future bone loss.[115] Studies in vitro demonstrated that bone loss associated with several periodontal pathogens was inhibited in part by inhibitors of prostaglandin synthesis.[196] In addition, use of a nonsteroidal antiinflammatory drug (NSAID) as an inhibitor of prostaglandin synthesis in human subjects with advanced periodontitis resulted in significantly less bone loss compared with placebo.[185] PGE_2 release from monocytes of patients with severe or aggressive periodontitis is greater than that from patients with little to no periodontal destruction.[49,136] It has been postulated that high-risk periodontal patients have a "monocyte hypersecretory trait" that results in an exaggerated response both locally and systemically to bacterial LPS.[136]

Summary

The production of proteinases and mediators as well as their inhibitors by host tissue cells are influenced by bacteria and regulatory molecules produced by host cells that are resident within, or recruited to, the periodontal tissues. In normal tissue turnover, a balance exists such that no net loss of tissue occurs. In disease, tissue loss occurs, suggesting that this balance is disrupted. In addition, although bacterial proteinases do not appear predominant in this environment, their effects locally within the periodontal "econiche" may be significant. Loss of bone in periodontal diseases appears to occur in part through the action of regulatory molecules, including IL-1, IL-6, TNF-α, and PGE_2.

Connective Tissue Alterations: Healing Processes in Periodontitis

The chronic immune system plays an important role in healing processes, which consist of regeneration and repair. *Regeneration* involves the replacement of tissues with new, identical tissues that function the same as the original tissues. Periodontal tissues are limited in their regenerative capacity, and considerable research is being devoted to developing techniques and materials to augment host processes that facilitate regeneration (see Chapters 67 and 77).

Repair involves replacement of one tissue with another tissue, such as fibrous connective tissue, which may not function the same as the tissue replaced. After traumatic or surgical injury, healing is initiated as part of the immediate and acute inflammatory responses. A clot that usually provides hemostasis almost immediately after injury also forms a matrix rich in platelet-derived cytokines that stimulates and facilitates healing. In contrast, periodontal infections do not normally produce the massive, platelet-rich clot observed in traumatic injury. Thus the periodontal "healing" cycle during the pathogenesis of periodontal disease is primarily postinflammatory, and cellular elements other than platelets provide important signals in this process. Periodontal repair occurs in overlapping phases of inflammation shutdown, angiogenesis, and fibrogenesis.

In the postinflammatory healing process, the shutdown of inflammatory processes and initiation of postinflammatory healing is orchestrated by leukocytes. Some of the important antiinflammatory signals generated by leukocytes include *IL-1 receptor antagonist* (IL-1ra) and *transforming growth factor beta* (TGF-β).[51] Other cytokines that depress an inflammatory response include IL-4, IL-10, and IL-11.[112] In inflamed periodontal tissues, macrophages are a source of IL-1ra,[75] whereas neutrophils, macrophages, and mast cells and lymphocytes produce TGF-β.[168]

Angiogenesis and fibrogenesis, as well as cytokines such as IL-1β and TNF-β that help to induce these processes, participate in both inflammation and healing. IL-1β and IL-1α are indirectly involved in inducing fibroblast proliferation and collagen synthesis by stimulating the production of PGE_2 or the release of "secondary" cytokines such as *platelet-derived growth factor* (PDGF) and TGF-β. PDGF is a protein complex formed by different combinations of A, B, C, and D chains, resulting in five isoforms: PDGF-AA, PDGF-AB, PDGF-BB, PDGF-CC, and PDGF-DD. It is produced by numerous cells and tissues, including endothelium, vascular smooth muscle, and macrophages. PDGF activates fibroblasts and osteoblasts, resulting in the induction of protein synthesis.[53] The PDGFs are related structurally and functionally to *vascular endothelial growth factor* (VEGF), an important factor in endothelial proliferation. VEGF is a glycoprotein produced by many cells, including monocytes/macrophages, and it is induced by antiinflammatory factors such as TGF-β.

TGF-β is a multifunctional peptide that stimulates osteoblasts and fibroblasts and inhibits osteoclasts, epithelial cells, and most immune cells. Receptors for TGF-β are found in almost all cells. TGF-β is produced as a propeptide, and activation requires acidic conditions. TGF-β is known for its ability to promote the elaboration of fibroblast extracellular matrix adhesion.

Other fibrogenic cytokines that may play a role include *basic fibroblast growth factor* (bFGF), TGF-α, and TNF-α. TGF-α and TNF-α are produced mainly by cells of the monocyte lineage, and within the periodontium, bFGF is produced primarily by periodontal ligament (PDL) cells and endothelium.[48]

In the healing of alveolar bone, regeneration of bone within a defect clearly can occur. The immune system can induce regenerative bone healing by preventing osteoclast formation and activation and by activating osteoblasts. By blocking osteoclast formation or increasing osteoclast death, it is possible to cause a marked decrease in osteoclastic activity. TGF-β is a potent inhibitor of osteoclast formation. Bone matrix itself contains TGF-β, which is released by osteoclastic resorption,[126] and osteoclasts may provide the acidic conditions necessary for TGF-β activation. Osteoclast differentiation and activation are inhibited by interferon-γ (IFN-γ), which is secreted by natural killer (NK) cells, Th1 T cells, and macrophages. The main effect of IFN-γ appears to be inhibition of IL-1 and TNF-α–induced osteoclast activation. IL-1ra also is effective in blocking IL-1 and TNF-α–induced osteoclast activation.

Much research in bone healing has focused on activation of osteoblasts and PDL cells as a means of promoting regenerative healing. Two substances, *insulin-like growth factor-I* (IGF-I) and PDGF, have been shown to induce or augment periodontal tissue repair.[68,108,141] The insulin-like growth factors induce osteoblast growth, differentiation, and synthesis of collagen. Several studies in nonhuman primates indicate that the combination of IGF-I and PDGF effectively and significantly enhances regeneration of periodontal structures, including new bone and cementum.[53,149]

MICROBIOLOGY AND IMMUNOLOGY IN GINGIVAL HEALTH

The gingival crevice harbors bacteria in both health and disease. In a clinically healthy periodontium, the microbial flora is largely composed of gram-positive facultative microorganisms, predominantly species of genera such as *Actinomyces* and *Streptococcus*. Gram-negative species and spirochetal forms also may be found, but they are considerably less prevalent and occur in much smaller numbers. Serum antibodies to microorganisms are usually in low titers, suggesting the minimal systemic antigenic stimulation by plaque during gingival health. The gingival tissues typically demonstrate some evidence of inflammation. Tissues are usually infiltrated with chronic inflammatory cells, generally lymphocytes. Neutrophils also are common within the junctional epithelium and in the gingival crevice. The infiltration of inflammatory cells is thought to be a response to bacterial plaque, and host defense mechanisms in a healthy individual are effective in managing the bacterial challenge. Physical mechanisms of host defense include the integrity of the epithelial cell layer, as well as the shedding of epithelial cells and the flow of crevicular fluid, which may function to clear bacteria and their products from the subgingival environment. It is likely that the complement, neutrophils, and antibody production contribute to controlling the sulcular microbiota.

MICROBIOLOGY AND IMMUNOLOGY IN PERIODONTAL DISEASES

Gingivitis

The most common form of gingivitis is *plaque-induced gingivitis.*[112] Common clinical findings in gingivitis include erythema, edema, tissue enlargement, and bleeding. Two forms of plaque-induced gingivitis have been investigated: a naturally occurring gingivitis and experimental gingivitis. Experimental gingivitis is a longitudinal clinical model that has been widely used in human and animal studies.[103] In humans, experimental gingivitis is induced through abstinence from oral hygiene measures; in animal studies a soft diet favoring plaque accumulation is instituted. The studies of experimental gingivitis have clearly demonstrated that plaque accumulation invariably causes gingivitis and that gingivitis is reversible with removal of the plaque deposits.

Page and Schroeder[139] reviewed the histopathology of human and animal experimental gingivitis in a classic article that delineated three temporal stages of gingivitis: the initial, early, and established lesions (see Chapter 20). Central to the histopathologic changes are the vascular inflammation and infiltration of neutrophils and then lymphocytes in the early stages. The early lymphocytic infiltrate is dominated by T cells, but eventually B cells become dominant. The established lesion is characterized by a predominance of B cells that have transformed into plasma cells in the connective tissues. Neutrophils continue to dominate the junctional epithelium and gingival crevice with a marked increase in GCF flow. It is noteworthy that collagen loss in the involved tissues is evident in the earliest stages of gingivitis. Page and Schroeder[139] report a predominance of plasma cells in the established lesion. Although several studies of human experimental gingivitis have failed to demonstrate plasma cell dominance,[16,17,156] increases in the proportions of plasma cells are evident with long-standing gingivitis.[16]

The development of experimental gingivitis occurs in parallel with a tremendous increase in the number of bacteria present in plaque. A distinct shift in the bacterial composition of the plaque also occurs, with increasing proportions of gram-negative anaerobes.[169] Studies on the microbiology of naturally occurring gingivitis indicate relatively equal proportions of gram-positive facultative and gram-negative anaerobic bacteria,[161] with evidence of a greater shift toward more gram-negative organisms when compared with experimental gingivitis. The host response to plaque bacteria is fundamentally an inflammatory response involving the processes described previously. Although gingivitis is not associated with loss of connective tissue attachment, it is evident histologically that some loss of collagen occurs within the connective tissues.

Specialized forms of gingivitis include those associated with hormonal changes, with medications, and with systemic disease.[113] In these cases, evidence exists of an altered host environment that appears to contribute to an increase in host susceptibility to gingivitis. For example, the inflammatory response to plaque during pregnancy appears to be exaggerated, with an increased prevalence and severity of gingivitis beyond that expected for the level of plaque accumulation.[111] Alterations in the subgingival microbiota and the host immune response to bacterial antigens during pregnancy have been reported.[89,107]For example, increases in hormone levels appear to correlate with increases in the subgingival proportions of *Prevotella intermedia*, a microorganism that can substitute progesterone or estradiol[8] for vitamin K as an essential bacterial growth factor.[89] These alterations, as well as the increased clinical susceptibility to gingivitis, resolve postpartum.

Chronic Periodontitis

Gingivitis and periodontitis share the clinical feature of inflammation. In contrast, periodontitis involves clinically detectable levels of host tissue destruction that are not found in gingivitis. These include clinical attachment loss, periodontal pocketing, and alveolar bone loss. In the common form of periodontitis, chronic periodontitis, the amount of tissue destruction is consistent with the local etiologic factors of plaque and calculus[46] and is associated with a variable microbial pattern. The clinical course of disease follows a slow to moderate rate of progression, but periods of rapid progression may occur.[56]

Bacterial Etiology

Despite a remarkable diversity of bacteria found in the periodontal microbiota, only a few species have been associated with periodontitis (see Chapter 9). These include *Porphyromonas gingivalis, Tannerella forsythia, Prevotella intermedia, Campylobacter rectus, Eikenella corrodens, Fusobacterium nucleatum, Actinobacillus actinomycetemcomitans, Peptostreptococcus micros,* and *Treponema denticola.** Studies of the microbiologic responses to periodontal therapy support a role for these species in the disease process. Decreases in the prevalence and numbers of *P. gingivalis, T. forsythia,* and *T. denticola* are associated

*References 93, 95, 104, 110, 123, 161, 163, 164, 172.

with successful clinical treatment of disease.[25,61,106] When diseased sites with recent attachment loss are compared with inactive sites, increases in the recovery of *P. gingivalis, F. nucleatum, P. intermedia, T. forsythia, E. corrodens, A. actinomycetemcomitans,* and *C. rectus* are evident in the active sites.[34,35,39] In addition, when treatment results are compared with microorganisms detected before treatment, poorly responding sites demonstrate higher levels of *F. nucleatum* and *P. micros.*[59]

Alterations in the host response associated with specific periodontal pathogens are clearly evident. Increases in serum and GCF antibody specific to putative pathogens,[38,39,85,133] including *P. gingivalis, A. actinomycetemcomitans, P. intermedia, E. corrodens, F. nucleatum,* and *C. rectus,* are evident in patients with periodontitis. Therapy itself is associated with initial increases in serum antibody levels, which return to pretreatment levels by 8 to 12 months after treatment.[10,37]

Studies in animal models have been used to demonstrate the pathologic potential of periodontal microorganisms in vivo. A common animal model involves abscess formation in mice driven by *P. gingivalis, C. rectus, P. micros, P. intermedia, Prevotella nigrescens, A. actinomycetemcomitans, F. nucleatum,* and *T. denticola.*[40,81,82,128,177] Differences in the virulence of distinct strains of the same species also are evident in the abscess model.[128] Furthermore, *P. gingivalis, C. rectus,* and *A. actinomycetemcomitans* demonstrate increased virulence in mice that are depleted of neutrophils, indicating an important role for neutrophils in responding to the bacterial challenge.[40]

Synergistic interactions between microbial pathogens appear to be important in bacterial virulence. In the mouse model, simultaneous infection with *P. gingivalis* and *F. nucleatum* enhanced virulence when compared to infection with *P. gingivalis* alone.[43] In a rabbit abscess model, *T. forsythia* in combination with either *P. gingivalis* or *F. nucleatum* produced abscesses, whereas none of the microorganism alone caused abscess formation.[170] Evidence of synergy in virulence, exemplified by these data, is an important consideration in infections that are polymicrobial.

Another area that has been addressed using animal model systems is the generation of immunity to infection. Inoculation with a specific microorganism or specific bacterial component that results in protective immunity suggests that the microorganism or molecule may be important in the disease process. Studies in which *P. gingivalis* outer membrane or fimbriae were used as immunogens have demonstrated a protective effect in a rodent model.[13,42] Using a nonhuman primate model of periodontal disease, immunization with whole cells of *P. gingivalis* or the cysteine protease of *P. gingivalis* has resulted in decreased periodontal destruction.[125,142] Although these investigations are useful in assessing microbial interactions in the disease process, much more investigation is needed for consideration of vaccine therapy in humans, particularly with regard to the polymicrobial nature of periodontitis.

Immunologic Considerations

Considerable information is available regarding components of the host immune response that are not specific to a given microbial pathogen but occur in response to the infection and are likely to contribute to pathogenesis. Chronic periodontitis is characterized primarily as involving alternative pathway activation of complement, with C3 and C3B cleavage in gingival fluids observed. This suggests that even though pathogen-specific antibodies are formed in chronic periodontitis, activation of the classical complement pathway by processes involving antibody-antigen binding does not predominate. It also is possible that specific cleavage products in GCF result from the action of bacterial enzymes. *P. gingivalis,* for example, produces an enzyme that can cleave C5 to its active metabolite, C5a.[190]

Collagenase activity is associated with active periodontal destruction.[100] MMP-8 is elevated in chronic periodontitis, whereas the levels of TIMP (TIMP-1) are not.[72] The ability of the chymotrypsin-like enzyme of *T. denticola* to activate MMPs may contribute to MMP-mediated tissue destruction at periodontitis sites with high levels of this microorganism.[165] In addition, studies of GCF in chronic periodontitis reveal that collagenase activity is as much as sixfold greater than that of gingivitis. Most of the collagenase activity associated with chronic periodontitis is caused by the neutrophil collagenase MMP-8.[147] Some microorganisms may modulate neutrophil secretion of collagenase. For example, the phagocytosis of *F. nucleatum* and *T. denticola* is associated with the release of high levels of elastase and MMP-8 from neutrophils.[31,32]

Clear evidence of variation exists among individuals in their susceptibility to periodontitis. Despite considerable accumulation of bacterial plaque, including the presence of putative pathogens, some individuals appear to be resistant to the disease process, whereas others develop disease. These differences relate primarily to variability in the host immunoinflammatory response to the infectious challenge, but the underlying basis for varying susceptibility may be genetic or environmental in nature.

Systemic factors that modify susceptibility to periodontitis include conditions such as diabetes and human immunodeficiency virus (HIV) infection and environmental influences such as smoking and stress.[84] Epidemiologic studies indicate that the prevalence and severity of periodontitis are increased in patients with *diabetes,* and poorly controlled diabetic patients appear to be particularly susceptible.[150] Periodontitis has been recently recognized as one of six primary complications of diabetes.[102] *HIV infection* is associated with alterations in the CD4+ T cells and monocytes/macrophages. HIV patients may exhibit acute necrotizing periodontal conditions, particularly when CD4+ T-cell levels are very low.[84,134] *Smoking* is strongly associated with periodontitis in epidemiologic studies. Smoking affects the vasculature, immune system, and inflammatory processes and is an important risk factor for development of periodontitis.[84] *Stress* is associated with necrotizing ulcerative gingivitis (NUG) and an increased prevalence of periodontitis. The effects of stress may be mediated by alterations in the immune response and inflammatory processes.[84] Diminished wound healing is associated with stress, and thus diminished reparative processes may play a role in periodontal pathogenesis.[114,183] Although the specific mechanisms behind the association of these conditions with periodontitis are not clear (see discussions in Chapter 18), a central role of alterations in the host inflammatory processes appears to be a consistent theme.

A *genetic* basis for variations in periodontal disease susceptibility is indicated by recent studies demonstrating an association between a composite genotype involving the IL-1 genes and the occurrence of chronic periodontitis. The composite genotype consists of a variant of the IL-1β gene with a single base-pair alteration in the DNA sequence at the +3953 position, in combination with similar alterations at the −889 and the +4845 positions of the IL-1α gene.[41,92] Studies indicate that individuals, primarily those of Caucasian European decent, carrying the composite genotype are at significantly increased risk (odds ratio of approximately 5 to 7) of having moderate to severe periodontitis.[92,116] The occurrence of these alleles in the IL-1 genes are considerably lower in individuals of Chinese and African-American heritage.[6,183] Thus these genetic polymorphisms may not contribute to variations in susceptibility and may be less useful as markers in these populations. The IL-1β allele (+3953) of the composite genotype is known to be associated with a twofold to fourfold increase in IL-1β production. Individuals negative for the composite genotype undergoing periodontal treatment demonstrate decreases in GCF levels of IL-1β, whereas those with the composite genotype do not demonstrate this response to treatment.[41] These data provide some information as to the molecular basis for variations in host susceptibility, and it is likely that additional genetic loci will be identified that also influence these processes (see Chapter 11).

Refractory Periodontitis

The majority of patients with chronic periodontitis are successfully managed with conventional treatment regimens. However, a small proportion of patients do not respond to treatment and demonstrate continued clinical periodontal destruction. These individuals are referred to as "refractory periodontitis patients." Prominent periodontal pathogens such as *P. gingivalis, T. forsythia, F. nucleatum, P. micros, E. corrodens,* and *Streptococcus intermedius* have been found to be elevated in patients who do not respond to treatment.[59,60] Often, patients identified as refractory to treatment have other factors, particularly smoking, that may contribute to the disease process.[76,77] The impact of smoking on the response to treatment may relate to alterations in neutrophil chemotaxis and phagocytosis, as well as altered levels of cytokines (e.g., IL-1, IL-6) at the local sites.[65,80,99,109]

Aggressive Periodontitis

A primary characteristic of aggressive periodontitis that differentiates it from chronic periodontitis is the rapid progression of attachment and bone loss that is evident.[176] Other consistent features of patients with aggressive periodontitis are that they are otherwise healthy and that the disease demonstrates a familial pattern of occurrence. A number of features are generally, but not universally, associated with aggressive periodontitis. These include inconsistencies between the amount of microbial deposits and the severity of periodontal destruction; the presence of elevated levels of *A. actinomycetemcomitans;* and evidence of phagocyte abnormalities and hyperresponsive monocytes/macrophages, leading to elevations in PGE_2 and IL-1β. Furthermore, the disease process is self-limiting in some cases of aggressive periodontitis.

Aggressive periodontitis may be localized or generalized. The classic form of localized aggressive periodontitis was initially referred to as "periodontosis"[129] and then as "localized juvenile periodontitis" (LJP). Classic LJP was defined by several distinguishing characteristics: onset around the time of puberty, aggressive periodontal destruction localized almost exclusively to the incisors and first molars, and a familial pattern of occurrence. The incidence of LJP is low, ranging from 0.1% to 2.3% of juveniles and adolescents. [45] However, studies of this distinctive disease process have provided a window into the processes underlying periodontal pathogenesis. *Localized aggressive periodontitis* (LAP) is the new classification designated to replace LJP. Thus, in the following discussions, LAP will be used synonymously with LJP. *Generalized aggressive periodontitis* (GAP) is differentiated from the localized form by the extent of involvement of the permanent teeth, and it is considered to include some of the individuals previously categorized as having rapidly progressive periodontitis. Patients with GAP frequently have subgingival gram-negative rods, including *P. gingivalis,* and exhibit suppressed neutrophil chemotaxis.[189]

Localized Aggressive Periodontitis

Bacterial Etiology. Early microbiologic studies of LAP provided clear evidence of a strong association between disease and a unique bacterial microbiota dominated by a microorganism later identified as *A. actinomycetemcomitans*.[129-132] Other microorganisms that have been associated with LAP include *P. gingivalis, E. corrodens, C. rectus, F. nucleatum, Bacillus capillus,* and *Capnocytophaga* species and spirochetes.[91,124,129,131,132] However, subsequent research has continued to provide support for a primary etiologic role of *A. actinomycetemcomitans* in LAP. These findings are summarized as follows:

1. The prevalence of a humoral immune response to this organism is elevated in patients with LAP. *A. actinomycetemcomitans* has been isolated in up to 97% of LAP patients, compared with 21% of adult periodontitis patients and 17% of healthy subjects.[195] Not only is the prevalence of *A. actinomycetemcomitans* six times greater in LAP than in healthy patients, but its proportion of the cultivable subgingival flora also is elevated. Among the three serotypes, serotype B is the most common, followed by serotype A.
2. The incidence of *A. actinomycetemcomitans* is greater in younger than in older LAP patients.[7] If age is considered relative to the duration of the disease, younger patients have more destructive disease developing within a shorter period. This suggests that the presence of this organism correlates with disease activity.
3. A large number of *A. actinomycetemcomitans* organisms occur in lesions in LAP patients, but such

organisms are absent or occur in low numbers in healthy sites.[45]

4. *A. actinomycetemcomitans* can be identified by electron microscopy, immunofluorescence, and culture from LAP lesions within the gingival connective tissues.[194]
5. *A. actinomycetemcomitans* is quite virulent, producing a leukotoxin, collagenase, phosphatases, and bone-resorbing factors, as well as other factors important in invasion of host tissue cells, evasion of host defenses, immunosuppression, and destruction of periodontal tissues.[45,74]
6. A positive correlation exists between the elimination of this organism from the subgingival flora and successful clinical treatment of LAP.[23,162]

A primary focus of studies on the virulence properties of *A. actinomycetemcomitans* has been on the leukotoxin produced by this bacterium. The ability of this molecule to bind to and lyse phagocytes is considered to be an important mechanism of host defense.[74,96] Early studies revealed that the levels of leukotoxin produced by different strains varied considerably. More recent investigations have linked the strains producing high levels of leukotoxin with a deletion in the promoter region of the leukotoxin gene[18] and further linked the onset of LAP in a high-risk population with the presence of these high–leukotoxin-producing strains.[19] The molecular basis of leukotoxin expression is discussed further in Chapter 15. Another potentially important virulence determinant is the production of an immunosuppressive factor[157] capable of inhibiting lymphocyte functions.

The familial occurrence of LAP raises the question as to whether transmission of specific strains of *A. actinomycetemcomitans* between family members could contribute to the disease process. Recognition of variations in virulence between different strains further suggests that this could be important. Genetic analyses of *A. actinomycetemcomitans* strains isolated from family members suggest that transmission of a strain between spouses or from parent to child occurred in approximately one third of the families investigated.[8]

Therapeutic approaches to infections involving *A. actinomycetemcomitans* must take into account the host-parasite interaction. Mechanical methods alone do not predictably control this microorganism. The ability of *A. actinomycetemcomitans* to invade and reside within the gingival tissues appears to provide a reservoir by which the bacterium can rapidly repopulate the pocket. Periodontal sites that continue to deteriorate after treatment harbor substantial levels of *A. actinomycetemcomitans.* Clinical studies suggest that surgery and antibiotic therapy may be required to control *A. actinomycetemcomitans* infection.[23,91,162]

Immunologic Considerations. Numerous mechanisms of serum-mediated bacterial killing are available, including lysis by the membrane attack complex of complement and antimicrobial substances such as lysozyme. However, some bacteria, including all known strains of *A. actinomycetemcomitans* as well as some strains of most putative periodontal pathogens, are resistant to serum-mediated killing mechanisms.[11] For serum-resistant bacteria, the neutrophil is the primary host response mechanism of bacterial control. Studies of LAP have revealed a number of aspects of neutrophil function that may result in compromised bacterial killing and have been key in demonstrating the importance of neutrophil function in periodontal health and disease.

Approximately 75% of patients with LAP have dysfunctional neutrophils, involving a decreased expression of G-protein coupled receptors. The defect is evident as a decrease in the chemotactic response to several chemotactic agents, including the complement component C5a, *N*-formyl-methionyl leucyl phenylalanine (FMLP), and leukotriene B4.[137] The defect is associated with a 40% deficiency in a 110-kilodalton membrane glycoprotein, GP110, on the neutrophil surface.[180] The function of GP110 is unknown, but diminished GP110 expression is associated with diminished surface expression of all G-protein coupled receptors. For this reason, this neutrophil defect has been called a *global membrane receptor defect.* The precise dysfunction caused by the G-protein coupled receptor deficiency responsible for disease has not been identified. However, neutrophil transendothelial migration, transepithelial migration, chemotaxis, secretion, and priming can be affected. The molecular basis for the receptor defect is postulated to be inherited as an intrinsic cellular defect or a modulation of neutrophil receptor expression by elevated levels of proinflammatory cytokines, including IL-1 and TNF-α.[1,179] LAP patients (25%) who do not show G-protein coupled receptor deficiency have the same clinical picture as those with this neutrophil defect. This suggests that the G-protein coupled receptor deficiency is sufficient but not essential for LAP, and other alterations of the host-bacterial interaction may yield a similar clinical outcome.

In LAP the predominant collagenase found in tissues and crevicular fluid is MMP-1, and elevated levels of TIMP-1 are present.[72] This contrasts with the situation in chronic periodontitis, in which the collagenous activity is caused by MMP-8 from neutrophils. The differences in MMPs may relate to altered neutrophil functions and further underscore the evidence that varying mechanisms of tissue destruction occur in these different forms of periodontal destruction.

Patients with LAP demonstrate elevated antibodies to *A. actinomycetemcomitans,*[36] and antibody as well as complement are essential for opsonization and efficient phagocytosis.[11] In LAP the dominant serum antibody isotype IgG2 is specific for surface antigens of *A. actinomycetemcomitans,* including LPS and at least one major outer membrane protein.[187,188] Some individuals possess a variant of the Fc receptor on neutrophils (R131 allele of FcγRII-α) that does not efficiently bind IgG2, and this is one possible basis for disease susceptibility.[186] It has been hypothesized that because this binding is less efficient, an antibody response more vigorous than normal is necessary to control the *A. actinomycetemcomitans* infection in LAP, and that the progression in LAP is limited by the development of a strong antibody response. This is further supported by the observation that patients with an elevated antibody response have significantly less loss of attachment.[20] In comparison, individuals with generalized early-onset periodontitis do not develop a strong antibody response,[58,174] which supports the hypothesis that antibodies function to limit the disease process.

Summary. The evidence indicates that LAP is a form of periodontitis that is clearly distinct from chronic periodontitis. The pathogenesis of LAP is characterized by a highly specific infection involving predominantly *A. actinomycetemcomitans*. This bacterium is capable of tissue destruction and inhibition of host defenses through the production of a leukotoxin and an immunosuppressive factor. The host response is characterized by the high prevalence of neutrophil chemotaxis defects in affected individuals as well as a selective antibody response dominated by high titers of IgG2. This antibody response may necessitate particularly high levels of antibody for efficient opsonization and phagocytosis of *A. actinomycetemcomitans*.

Generalized Aggressive Periodontitis

The recent reclassifications limit the information available pertinent to this group of patients. Some but not all of the individuals previously classified as having rapidly progressive periodontitis (RPP) would likely be considered to have GAP. Studies of RPP indicate a diverse microbial pattern that includes microorganisms associated with chronic periodontitis and a host response often characterized by defects in either neutrophils or monocytes.[140]

Necrotizing Periodontal Diseases

Two forms of necrotizing ulcerative periodontal diseases are *necrotizing ulcerative gingivitis* (NUG) and *necrotizing ulcerative periodontitis* (NUP). These conditions represent acute forms of periodontal destruction typically associated with some form of host compromise.

The essential components of NUG are interdental gingival necrosis, pain, and bleeding; variable features include lymphadenopathy, fever, and malaise.[148] The tissue necrosis results in an appearance often described as "punched-out" papillae. Microbiologic studies indicate that predominant organisms associated with NUG include *P. intermedia, Fusobacterium* species, and spirochetal microorganisms. Electron microscopic studies of NUG reveal a zone of tissue infiltration of spirochetal microorganisms in advance of the region of tissue necrosis.[101] NUG is normally associated with predisposing host factors, including stress, immunosuppression, and malnutrition.[148]

NUP is distinguished from NUG by the loss of clinical attachment and bone in affected sites, but the clinical presentation and etiologic factors are similar to that of NUG in the absence of systemic disease.[134] In the presence of systemic immunosuppression, exemplified by HIV infection, NUP may result in rapid and extensive necrosis to the tissues and underlying alveolar bone.[191]

Periodontal Abscesses

Periodontal abscesses are purulent infections localized to the gingival, periodontal, or pericoronal regions. In the presence of periodontitis, a periodontal abscess represents an acute infectious process with active tissue and bone destruction. Microorganisms that are prevalent in periodontal abscesses are *P. intermedia, F. nucleatum,* and *P. gingivalis*; other periodontal pathogens that are found include *T. forsythensis, P. micros, Prevotella melaninogenica,* and *C. rectus*.[62,125] Histologic studies indicate the presence of neutrophils and macrophages surrounding an internal region of dead leukocytes and tissue debris. In the absence of periodontitis, abscesses are typically associated with impaction of foreign objects, such as dental floss or a popcorn kernel.

SUMMARY

The pathogenesis of periodontal destruction involves a complex interplay between bacterial pathogens and the host tissues. For some time it has been recognized that "not all dental plaque is equal" and that specific bacterial pathogens appear to be responsible for the changes resulting in disease. It also has been recognized that in the process of effectively limiting the bacterial assault of the periodontal tissues, host defense mechanisms contribute to the destruction of tissues locally.

Recent investigations have revealed that not all strains of a specific microbial species are equal in their capacity to cause disease, and not all hosts are equal in their susceptibility to disease. The challenge for the future is to be able to better identify the more virulent bacterial strains and the more susceptible hosts. In this manner it may be possible to predict accurately the individuals at risk for future disease and to develop more effective strategies to prevent the onset and progression of periodontitis.

REFERENCES

1. Agarwal S, Suzuki JB, Riccelli AE: Role of cytokines in the modulation of neutrophil chemotaxis in localized juvenile periodontitis, *J Periodontal Res* 29:127, 1994.
2. Arakawa S, Nakajima T, Ishikura H, et al: Novel apoptosis-inducing activity in *Bacteroides forsythus:* a comparative study with three serotypes of *Actinobacillus actinomycetemcomitans, Infect Immun* 68:4611, 2000.
3. Amano A: Molecular interaction of *Porphyromonas gingivalis* with host cells: implication for the microbial pathogenesis of periodontal disease, *J Periodontol* 74:90, 2003.
4. Armitage GC: Development of a classification system for periodontal diseases and conditions, *Ann Periodontol* 4:1, 1999.
5. Armitage GC, Jeffcoat MK, Chadwick DE, et al: Longitudinal evaluation of elastase as a marker for the progression of periodontitis, *J Periodontol* 65:120, 1994.
6. Armitage GC, Wu Y, Wang HY, et al: Low prevalence of a periodontitis-associated interleukin-1 composite genotype in individuals of Chinese heritage, *J Periodontol* 71:164, 2000.
7. Asikainen S: Occurrence of *Actinobacillus actinomycetemcomitans* and spirochetes in relation to age in localized juvenile periodontitis, *J Periodontol* 57:537, 1986.
8. Asikainen S, Chen C, Slots J: Likelihood of transmitting *Actinobacillus actinomycetemcomitans* and *Porphyromonas gingivalis* in families with periodontitis, *Oral Microbiol Immunol* 11:387, 1996.
9. Assuma R, Oates T, Cochran D, et al: IL-1 and TNF antagonists inhibit the inflammatory response and bone loss in experimental periodontitis, *J Immunol* 160:403, 1998.

10. Aukhil I, Lopatin DE, Syed SA, et al: The effects of periodontal therapy on serum antibody (IgG) levels to plaque microorganisms, *J Clin Periodontol* 15:544, 1988.
11. Baker PJ, Wilson ME: Opsonic IgG antibody against *Actinobacillus actinomycetemcomitans* in localized juvenile periodontitis, *Oral Microbiol Immunol* 4:98, 1989.
12. Barbosa MD, Nguyen QA, Tchernev VT, et al: Identification of the homologous beige and Chédiak-Higashi syndrome genes, *Nature* 382:262, 1996.
13. Bird PS, Gemmell E, Polak B, et al: Protective immunity to *Porphyromonas gingivalis* infection in a murine model, *J Periodontol* 66:351, 1995.
14. Birkedal-Hansen H: Role of matrix metalloproteinases in human periodontal diseases, *J Periodontol* 64:474, 1993.
15. Booth V, Ashley FP, Lehner T: Passive immunization with monoclonal antibodies against *Porphyromonas gingivalis* in patients with periodontitis, *Infect Immun* 64:422, 1996.
16. Brecx MC, Frohlicher I, Gehr P, et al: Stereological observations on long-term experimental gingivitis in man, *J Clin Periodontol* 15:621, 1988.
17. Brecx MC, Lehmann B, Siegwart CM, et al: Observations on the initial stages of healing following human experimental gingivitis: a clinical and morphometric study, *J Clin Periodontol* 15:123, 1988.
18. Brogan JM, Lally ET, Poulsen K, et al: Regulation of *Actinobacillus actinomycetemcomitans* leukotoxin expression: analysis of the promoter regions of leukotoxic and minimally leukotoxic strains, *Infect Immun* 62:501, 1994.
19. Bueno LC, Mayer MP, DiRienzo JM: Relationship between conversion of localized juvenile periodontitis–susceptible children from health to disease and *Actinobacillus actinomycetemcomitans* leukotoxin promoter structure, *J Periodontol* 69:998, 1998.
20. Califano JV, Pace BE, Gunsolley JC, et al: Antibody reactive with *Actinobacillus actinomycetemcomitans* leukotoxin in early-onset periodontitis, *Oral Microbiol Immunol* 12:20, 1997.
21. Carranza FA Jr, Saglie R, Newman MG, et al: Scanning and transmission electron microscopic study of tissue-invading microorganisms in localized juvenile periodontitis, *J Periodontol* 54:598, 1983.
22. Chen HA, Johnson BD, Sims TJ, et al: Humoral immune responses to *Porphyromonas gingivalis* before and following therapy in rapidly progressive periodontitis patients, *J Periodontol* 62:781, 1991.
23. Christersson LA, Slots J, Rosling BG, et al: Microbiological and clinical effects of surgical treatment of localized juvenile periodontitis, *J Clin Periodontol* 12:465, 1985.
24. Christersson LA, Albini B, Zambon JJ, et al: Tissue localization of *Actinobacillus actinomycetemcomitans* in human periodontitis. I. Light, immunofluorescence and electron microscopic studies, *J Periodontol* 58:529, 1987.
25. Cugini MA, Haffajee AD, Smith C, et al: The effect of scaling and root planing on the clinical and microbiological parameters of periodontal diseases: 12-month results, *J Clin Periodontol* 27:30, 2000.
26. Curtis MA, Kuramitsu HK, Lantz M, et al: Molecular genetics and nomenclature of proteases of *Porphyromonas gingivalis*, *J Periodontal Res* 34:464, 1999.
27. Cutler CW, Kalmar JR, Arnold RR: Phagocytosis of virulent *Porphyromonas gingivalis* by human polymorphonuclear leukocytes requires specific immunoglobulin G, *Infect Immun* 59:2097, 1991.
28. Darveau RP, Belton CM, Reife RA, et al: Local chemokine paralysis, a novel pathogenic mechanism for *Porphyromonas gingivalis*, *Infect Immun* 66:1660, 1998.
29. Delcourt-Debruyne EM, Boutigny HR, Hildebrand HF: Features of severe periodontal disease in a teenager with Chédiak-Higashi syndrome, *J Periodontol* 71:816, 2000.
30. Dickinson DP, Kubiniec MA, Yoshimura F, et al: Molecular cloning and sequencing of the gene encoding the fimbrial subunit protein of *Bacteroides gingivalis*, *J Bacteriol* 170:1658, 1988.
31. Ding Y, Uitto VJ, Haapasalo M, et al: Membrane components of *Treponema denticola* trigger proteinase release from human polymorphonuclear leukocytes, *J Dent Res* 75:1986, 1996.
32. Ding Y, Haapasalo M, Kerosuo E, et al: Release and activation of human neutrophil matrix metallo- and serine proteinases during phagocytosis of *Fusobacterium nucleatum*, *Porphyromonas gingivalis*, and *Treponema denticola*, *J Clin Periodontol* 24:237, 1997.
33. Dongari-Bagtzoglou AI, Ebersole JL: Production of inflammatory mediators and cytokines by human gingival fibroblasts following bacterial challenge, *J Periodontal Res* 31:90, 1996.
34. Dzink JL, Socransky SS, Haffajee AD: The predominant cultivable microbiota of active and inactive lesions of destructive periodontal diseases, *J Clin Periodontol* 15:316, 1988.
35. Dzink JL, Tanner AC, Haffajee AD, et al: Gram negative species associated with active destructive periodontal lesions, *J Clin Periodontol* 12:648, 1985.
36. Ebersole JL, Taubman MA: The protective nature of host responses in periodontal diseases, *Periodontology 2000* 5:112, 1994.
37. Ebersole JL, Taubman MA, Smith DJ, et al: Effect of subgingival scaling on systemic antibody responses to oral microorganisms, *Infect Immun* 48:534, 1985.
38. Ebersole JL, Taubman MA, Smith DJ, et al: Human immune responses to oral microorganisms: patterns of systemic antibody levels to *Bacteroides* species, 51:507, 1986.
39. Ebersole JL, Taubman MA, Smith DJ, et al: Human serum antibody responses to oral microorganisms. IV. Correlation with homologous infection, *Oral Microbiol Immunol* 2:53, 1987.
40. Ebersole JL, Kesavalu L, Schneider SL, et al: Comparative virulence of periodontopathogens in a mouse abscess model, *Oral Dis* 1:115, 1995.
41. Engebretson SP, Lamster IB, Herrera-Abreu M, et al: The influence of interleukin gene polymorphism on expression of interleukin-1β and tumor necrosis factor-α in periodontal tissue and gingival crevicular fluid, *J Periodontol* 70:567, 1999.
42. Evans RT, Klausen B, Sojar HT, et al: Immunization with *Porphyromonas (Bacteroides) gingivalis* fimbriae protects against periodontal destruction, *Infect Immun* 60:2926, 1992.
43. Feuille F, Ebersole JL, Kesavalu L, et al: Mixed infection with *Porphyromonas gingivalis* and *Fusobacterium nucleatum* in a murine lesion model: potential synergistic effects on virulence, *Infect Immun* 64:2095, 1996.
44. Fillery ED, Pekovic DD: Identification of microorganisms in immunopathological mechanisms on human gingivitis, *J Dent Res* 61:253, 1982.
45. Fives-Taylor PM, Meyer DH, Mintz KP, et al: Virulence factors of *Actinobacillus actinomycetemcomitans*, *Periodontol 2000* 20:136, 1999.
46. Flemmig TF: Periodontitis, *Ann Periodontol* 4:32, 1999.
47. Frank RM: Bacterial penetration in the apical wall of advanced human periodontitis, *J Periodontal Res* 15:563, 1980.
48. Gao J, Jordan TW, Cutress TW: Immunolocalization of basic fibroblast growth factor (bFGF) in human periodontal ligament (PDL) tissue, *J Periodontal Res* 31:260, 1996.
49. Garrison SW, Nichols FC: LPS-elicited secretory responses in monocytes: altered release of PGE_2 but not IL-1β in patients with adult periodontitis, *J Periodontal Res* 24:88, 1989.

50. Garrison SW, Holt SC, Nichols FC: Lipopolysaccharide-stimulated PGE_2 release from human monocytes: comparison of lipopolysaccharides prepared from suspected periodontal pathogens, *J Periodontol* 59:684, 1988.
51. Genco RJ: Host responses in periodontal diseases: current concepts, *J Periodontol* 63:338, 1992.
52. Genco RJ, Wilson ME, De Nardin E: Periodontal complications and neutrophil abnormalities. In Genco RJ, Goldman HM, Cohen DW, editors: *Contemporary periodontics*, St Louis, 1990, Mosby.
53. Giannobile WV, Hernandez RA, Finkelman RD, et al: Comparative effects of platelet-derived growth factor-BB and insulin-like growth factor-I, individually and in combination, on periodontal regeneration in *Macaca fascicularis, J Periodontal Res* 31:301, 1996.
54. Golub L, Sorsa T, Lee HM, et al: Doxycycline inhibits neutrophil (PMN)-type matrix metalloproteinases in human adult periodontitis gingiva, *J Clin Periodontol* 21:1, 1995.
55. Golub L, Lee H, Greenwald R, et al: A matrix metalloproteinase inhibitor reduces bone-type collagenase in gingival crevicular fluid during adult periodontitis, *Inflamm Res* 4:310, 1997.
56. Goodson JM, Tanner AC, Haffajee AD, et al: Patterns of progression and regression of advanced destructive periodontal disease, *J Clin Periodontol* 9:472, 1982.
57. Graves DT: The potential role of chemokines and inflammatory cytokines in periodontal disease progression, *Clin Infect Dis* 28:482, 1999.
58. Gunsolley JC, Burmeister JA, Tew JG, et al: Relationship of serum antibody to attachment level patterns in young adults with juvenile periodontitis or generalized severe periodontitis, *J Periodontol* 58:314, 1987.
59. Haffajee AD, Socransky SS, Ebersole JL: Survival analysis of periodontal sites before and after periodontal therapy, *J Clin Periodontol* 12:553, 1985.
60. Haffajee AD, Socransky SS, Dzink JL, et al: Clinical, microbiological and immunological features of subjects with refractory periodontal diseases, *J Clin Periodontol* 15:390, 1988.
61. Haffajee AD, Cugini MA, Dibart S, et al: Clinical and microbiological features of subjects with adult periodontitis who responded poorly to scaling and root planing, *J Clin Periodontol* 24:767, 1997.
62. Han YW, Shi W, Huang GT, et al: Interactions between periodontal bacteria and human oral epithelial cells: *Fusobacterium nucleatum* adheres to and invades epithelial cells, *Infect Immun* 68:3140, 2000.
63. Hart TC, Stabholz A, Meyle J, et al: Genetic studies of syndromes with severe periodontitis and palmoplantar hyperkeratosis, *J Periodontal Res* 32:81, 1997.
64. Hart TC, Hart PS, Bowden DW, et al: Mutations of the cathepsin C gene are responsible for Papillon-Lefèvre syndrome, *J Med Genet* 36:881, 1999.
65. Hernichel-Gorbach E, Kornman KS, Holt SC, et al: Host responses in patients with generalized refractory periodontitis, *J Periodontol* 65:8, 1994.
66. Herrera D, Roldan S, Sanz M: The periodontal abscess: a review, *J Clin Periodontol* 27:377, 2000.
67. Herrera D, Roldan S, Gonzalez I, et al: The periodontal abscess. I. Clinical and microbiological findings, *J Clin Periodontol* 27:387, 2000.
68. Howell TH, Fiorellini JP, Paquette DW, et al: A phase I/II clinical trial to evaluate a combination of recombinant human platelet-derived growth factor-BB and recombinant human insulin-like growth factor-I in patients with periodontal disease, *J Periodontol* 68:1186, 1997.
69. Huang GT-J, Kinder Haake S, Park N-H: Gingival epithelial cells increase interleukin-8 secretion in response to *Actinobacillus actinomycetemcomitans* challenge, *J Periodontol* 69:1105, 1998.
70. Huang GT-J, Kinder Haake S, Kim J-W, et al: Differential expression of interleukin-8 and intercellular adhesion molecule-1 by human gingival epithelial cells in response to *Actinobacillus actinomycetemcomitans* or *Porphyromonas gingivalis* infection, *Oral Microbiol Immunol* 13:301, 1998.
71. Ingman T, Sorsa T, Kangaspunta P, et al: Elastase and α1–proteinase inhibitor in gingival crevicular fluid and gingival tissue in adult and juvenile periodontitis, *J Periodontol* 65:702, 1994.
72. Ingman T, Tervahartiala T, Ding Y, et al: Matrix metalloproteinases and their inhibitors in gingival crevicular fluid and saliva of periodontitis patients, *J Clin Periodontol* 23:1127, 1996.
73. Jewett A, Hume WR, Le H, et al: Induction of apoptotic cell death in peripheral blood mononuclear and polymorphonuclear cells by an oral bacterium, *Fusobacterium nucleatum, Infect Immun* 68:1893, 2000.
74. Johansson A, Sandstrom G, Claesson R, et al: Anaerobic neutrophil-dependent killing of *Actinobacillus actinomycetemcomitans* in relation to the bacterial leukotoxicity, *Eur J Oral Sci* 108:136, 2000.
75. Kabashima H, Nagata K, Hashiguchi I, et al: Interleukin-1 receptor antagonist and interleukin-4 in gingival crevicular fluid of patients with inflammatory periodontal disease, *J Oral Pathol Med* 25:449, 1996.
76. Kaldahl WB, Johnson GK, Patil KD, et al: Levels of cigarette consumption and response to periodontal therapy, *J Periodontol* 67:675, 1996.
77. Kaldahl WB, Kalkwarf KL, Patil KD, et al: Long-term evaluation of periodontal therapy: II. Incidence of sites breaking down, *J Periodontol* 67:103, 1996.
78. Kelly CG, Booth V, Kendal H, et al: The relationship between colonization and haemagglutination inhibiting and B cell epitopes of *Porphyromonas gingivalis, Clin Exp Immunol* 110:285, 1997.
79. Kenney EB, Ash MM, Jr: Oxidation reduction potential of developing plaque, periodontal pockets and gingival sulci, *J Periodontol* 40:630, 1969.
80. Kenney EB, Kraal JH, Saxe SR, et al: The effect of cigarette smoke on human oral polymorphonuclear leukocytes, *J Periodontal Res* 12:227, 1977.
81. Kesavalu L, Holt SC, Crawley RR, et al: Virulence of *Wolinella recta* in a murine abscess model, *Infect Immun* 59:2806, 1991.
82. Kesavalu L, Ebersole JL, Machen RL, et al: *Porphyromonas gingivalis* virulence in mice: induction of immunity to bacterial components, *Infect Immun* 60:1455, 1992.
83. Kiecolt-Glaser JK, Marucha PT, Malarkey WB, et al: Slowing of wound healing by psychological stress, *Lancet* 346:1194, 1995.
84. Kinane DF: Periodontitis modified by systemic factors, *Ann Periodontol* 4:54, 1999.
85. Kinane DF, Mooney J, Ebersole JL: Humoral immune response to *Actinobacillus actinomycetemcomitans* and *Porphyromonas gingivalis* in periodontal disease, *Periodontol 2000* 20:289, 1999.
86. Kinder SA, Holt SC: Characterization of coaggregation between *Bacteroides gingivalis* T22 and *Fusobacterium nucleatum* T18, *Infect Immun* 57:3425, 1989.
87. Kinder SA, Holt SC: Carbohydrate receptor on *Porphyromonas gingivalis* T22 mediating coaggregation with *Fusobacterium nucleatum* T18, *J Dent Res* 70:275, 1991.
88. Kolenbrander PE, Andersen RN: Inhibition of coaggregation between *Fusobacterium nucleatum* and *Porphyromonas (Bacteroides) gingivalis* by lactose and related sugars, *Infect Immun* 57:3204, 1989.

89. Kornman KS, Loesche WJ: Effects of estradiol and progesterone on *Bacteroides melaninogenicus* and *Bacteroides gingivalis*, *Infect Immun* 35:256, 1982.
90. Kornman KS: Host modulation as a therapeutic strategy in the treatment of periodontal disease, *Clin Infect Dis* 28:520, 1999.
91. Kornman KS, Robertson PB: Clinical and microbiological evaluation of therapy for juvenile periodontitis, *J Periodontol* 56:443, 1985.
92. Kornman KS, Crane A, Wang HY, et al: The interleukin-1 genotype as a severity factor in adult periodontal disease, *J Clin Periodontol* 24:72, 1997.
93. Kremer BH, Loos BG, van der Velden U, et al: *Peptostreptococcus micros* smooth and rough genotypes in periodontitis and gingivitis, *J Periodontol* 71:209, 2000.
94. Kuramitsu HK: Proteases of *Porphyromonas gingivalis:* what don't they do? *Oral Microbiol Immunol* 13:263, 1998.
95. Lai CH, Listgarten MA, Shirakawa M, et al: *Bacteroides forsythus* in adult gingivitis and periodontitis, *Oral Microbiol Immunol* 2:152, 1987.
96. Lally ET, Kieba IR, Sato A, et al: RTX toxins recognize a β-2 integrin on the surface of human target cells, *J Biol Chem* 272:30463, 1997.
97. Lantz MS, Rowland RW, Switalski LM, et al: Interactions of *Bacteroides gingivalis* with fibrinogen, *Infect Immun* 54:654, 1986.
98. Lantz MS, Allen RD, Duck LW, et al: Identification of *Porphyromonas gingivalis* components that mediate its interactions with fibronectin, *J Bacteriol* 173:4263, 1991.
99. Lee HJ, Kang IK, Chung CP, et al: The subgingival microflora and gingival crevicular fluid cytokines in refractory periodontitis, *J Clin Periodontol* 22:885, 1995.
100. Lee W, Aitken S, Sodek J, et al: Evidence of a direct relationship between neutrophil collagenase activity and periodontal tissue destruction in vivo: role of active enzyme in human periodontitis, *J Periodontal Res* 30:23, 1995.
101. Listgarten MA: Electron microscopic observations on the bacterial flora of acute necrotizing ulcerative gingivitis, *J Periodontol* 36:328, 1965.
102. Löe H: Periodontal disease: the sixth complication of diabetes mellitus, *Diabetes Care* 16:329, 1993.
103. Löe H, Theilade E, Jensen SB: Experimental gingivitis in man, *J Periodontol* 36:177, 1965.
104. Loesche WJ: Importance of nutrition in gingival crevice microbial ecology, *Periodontics* 6:245, 1968.
105. Loesche WJ: Bacterial mediators in periodontal disease, *Clin Infect Dis* 16(suppl 4):S203, 1993.
106. Loesche WJ, Syed SA, Schmidt E, et al: Bacterial profiles of subgingival plaques in periodontitis, *J Periodontol* 56:447, 1985.
107. Lopatin DE, Kornman KS, Loesche WJ: Modulation of immunoreactivity to periodontal disease–associated microorganisms during pregnancy, *Infect Immun* 28:713, 1980.
108. Lynch SE, Nixon JC, Colvin RB, et al: Role of platelet-derived growth factor in wound healing: synergistic effects with other growth factors, *Proc Natl Acad Sci USA* 84:7696, 1987.
109. MacFarlane GD, Herzberg MC, Wolff LF, et al: Refractory periodontitis associated with abnormal polymorphonuclear leukocyte phagocytosis and cigarette smoking, *J Periodontol* 63:908, 1992.
110. Macuch PJ, Tanner AC: *Campylobacter* species in health, gingivitis, and periodontitis, *J Dent Res* 79:785, 2000.
111. Madianos PN, Papapanou PN, Sandros J: *Porphyromonas gingivalis* infection of oral epithelium inhibits neutrophil transepithelial migration, *Infect Immun* 65:3983, 1997.
112. Manolagas SC: Birth and death of bone cells: basic regulatory mechanisms and implications for the pathogenesis and treatment of osteoporosis, *Endocr Rev* 21:115, 2000.
113. Mariotti A: Dental plaque-induced gingival diseases, *Ann Periodontol* 4:7, 1999.
114. Marucha PT, Kiecolt-Glaser JK, Favagehi M: Mucosal wound healing is impaired by examination stress, *Psychosom Med* 60:362, 1998.
115. Masada MP, Persson R, Kenney JS, et al: Measurement of interleukin-1α and -1β in gingival crevicular fluid: implications for the pathogenesis of periodontal disease, *J Periodontal Res* 25:156, 1990.
116. McCauley LK, Nohutcu RM: Mediators of periodontal osseous destruction and remodeling: principles and implications for diagnosis and therapy, *J Periodontol* 73:1377, 2002.
117. McDevitt MJ, Wang HY, Knobelman C, et al: Interleukin-1 genetic association with periodontitis in clinical practice, *J Periodontol* 71:156, 2000.
118. McIntire FC, Bush CA, Wu SS, et al: Structure of a new hexasaccharide from the coaggregation polysaccharide of *Streptococcus sanguis* 34, *Carbohydr Res* 166:133, 1987.
119. Meng HX: Periodontal abscess, *Ann Periodontol* 4:79, 1999.
120. Mergenhagen SE, Sandberg AL, Chassy BM, et al: Molecular basis of bacterial adhesion in the oral cavity, *Rev Infect Dis* 9:S467, 1987.
121. Metcalfe DD, Costa JJ, Burd PR: Mast cells and basophils. In Gallin JI, Goldstein IM, Snyderman R, editors: *Inflammation: basic principles and clinical correlates,* ed 2, New York, 1992, Raven Press.
122. Modulation of the host response in periodontology, American Academy of Periodontology, *J Periodontol* 73:460, 2002.
123. Moore WE, Moore LV: The bacteria of periodontal diseases, *Periodontol 2000* 5:66, 1994.
124. Moore WE, Holdeman LV, Cato EP, et al: Comparative bacteriology of juvenile periodontitis, *Infect Immun* 48:507, 1985.
125. Moritz AJ, Cappelli D, Lantz MS, et al: Immunization with *Porphyromonas gingivalis* cysteine protease: effects on experimental gingivitis and ligature-induced periodontitis in *Macaca fascicularis, J Periodontol* 69:686, 1998.
126. Mundy GR: Inflammatory mediators and the destruction of bone, *J Periodontal Res* 26:213, 1991.
127. Nagle DL, Karim MA, Woolf EA, et al: Identification and mutation analysis of the complete gene for Chédiak-Higashi syndrome, *Nat Genet* 14:307, 1996.
128. Neiders ME, Chen PB, Suido H, et al: Heterogeneity of virulence among strains of *Bacteroides gingivalis*, *J Periodontal Res* 24:192, 1989.
129. Nelson D, Potempa J, Kordula T, Travis J: Purification and characterization of a novel cysteine proteinase (periodontain) from *Porphyromonas gingivalis, J Biol Chem* 274:12245, 1999.
130. Newman MG, Sims TN: The predominant cultivable microbiota of the periodontal abscess, *J Periodontol* 50:350, 1979.
131. Newman MG, Socransky SS: Predominant cultivable microbiota in periodontosis, *J Periodontal Res* 14:120, 1977.
132. Newman MG, Socransky SS, Savitt ED, et al: Studies of the microbiology of periodontosis, *J Periodontol* 47:373, 1976.
133. Nisengard RJ: The role of immunology in periodontal disease, *J Periodontol* 48:505, 1977.
134. Novak MJ: Necrotizing ulcerative periodontitis, *Ann Periodontol* 4:74, 1999.
135. Nunes IP, Johannessen AC, Matre R, et al: Epithelial expression of HLA class II antigens and Fc gamma receptors in

patients with adult periodontitis, *J Clin Periodontol* 21:526, 1994.
136. Offenbacher S, Salvi GE: Induction of prostaglandin release from macrophages by bacterial endotoxin, *Clin Infect Dis* 28:505, 1999.
137. Offenbacher S, Scott SS, Odle BM, et al: Depressed leukotriene B4 chemotactic response of neutrophils from localized juvenile periodontitis patients, *J Periodontol* 58:602, 1987.
138. Page RC: The role of inflammatory mediators in the pathogenesis of periodontal disease, *J Periodontal Res* 26:230, 1991.
139. Page RC, Schroeder HE: Pathogenesis of inflammatory periodontal disease: a summary of current work, *Lab Invest* 34:235, 1976.
140. Page RC, Altman LC, Ebersole JL, et al: Rapidly progressive periodontitis: a distinct clinical condition, *J Periodontol* 54:197, 1983.
141. Park JB, Matsuura M, Han KY, et al: Periodontal regeneration in class III furcation defects of beagle dogs using guided tissue regenerative therapy with platelet-derived growth factor, *J Periodontol* 66:462, 1995.
142. Persson GR, Engel D, Whitney C, et al: Immunization against *Porphyromonas gingivalis* inhibits progression of experimental periodontitis in nonhuman primates, *Infect Immun* 62:1026, 1994.
143. Pouliot M, Serhan CN: Lipoxin A_4 and aspirin-triggered 15-epi-LXA_4 inhibit tumor necrosis factor-α–initiated neutrophil responses and trafficking: novel regulators of a cytokine-chemokine axis relevant to periodontal diseases, *J Periodontal Res* 34:370, 1999.
144. Price TH, Ochs HD, Gershoni-Baruch R, et al: In vivo neutrophil and lymphocyte function studies in a patient with leukocyte adhesion deficiency type II, *Blood* 84:1635, 1994.
145. Rawlinson A, Dalati MH, Rahman S, et al: Interleukin-1 and IL-1 receptor antagonist in gingival crevicular fluid, *J Clin Periodontol* 27:738, 2000.
146. Roberts FA, Richardson GJ, Michalek SM: Effects of *Porphyromonas gingivalis* and *Escherichia coli* lipopolysaccharides on mononuclear phagocytes, *Infect Immun* 65:3248, 1997.
147. Romanelli R, Mancini S, Laschinger C, et al: Activation of neutrophil collagenase in periodontitis, *Infect Immun* 67:2319, 1999.
148. Rowland RW: Necrotizing ulcerative gingivitis, *Ann Periodontol* 4:65, 1999.
149. Rutherford RB, Niekrash CE, Kennedy JE, et al: Platelet-derived and insulin-like growth factors stimulate regeneration of periodontal attachment in monkeys, *J Periodontal Res* 27:285, 1992.
150. Ryan ME Golub LM: Modulation of matrix metalloproteinase activities in periodontitis as a treatment strategy, *Periodontol 2000* 24:226, 2000.
151. Safkan-Seppala B, Ainamo J: Periodontal conditions in insulin-dependent diabetes mellitus, *J Clin Periodontol* 19:24, 1992.
152. Saglie FR, Marfany A, Camargo P: Intragingival occurrence of *Actinobacillus actinomycetemcomitans* and *Bacteroides gingivalis* in active destructive periodontal lesions, *J Periodontol* 59:259, 1988.
153. Saglie R, Newman MG, Carranza FA Jr, et al: Bacterial invasion of gingiva in advanced periodontitis in humans, *J Periodontol* 53:217, 1982.
154. Sandros J, Papapanou P, Dahlen G: *Porphyromonas gingivalis* invades oral epithelial cells in vitro, *J Periodontal Res* 28:219, 1993.
155. Schenkein HA: The role of complement in periodontal diseases, *Crit Rev Oral Biol Med* 2:65, 1991.
156. Seymour GJ, Powell RN, Aitken JF: Experimental gingivitis in humans: a clinical and histologic investigation, *J Periodontol* 54:522, 1983.
157. Shenker BJ, Hoffmaster RH, McKay TL, et al: Expression of the cytolethal distending toxin (Cdt) operon in *Actinobacillus actinomycetemcomitans:* evidence that the CdtB protein is responsible for G2 arrest of the cell cycle in human T cells, *J Immunol* 165:2612, 2000.
158. Shibutani T, Gen K, Shibata M, et al: Long-term follow-up of periodontitis in a patient with Chédiak-Higashi syndrome: a case report, *J Periodontol* 71:1024, 2000.
159. Singer RE, Buckner BA: Butyrate and propionate: important components of toxic dental plaque extracts, *Infect Immun* 32:458, 1981.
160. Sjostrom K, Ou J, Whitney C, et al: Effect of treatment on titer, function, and antigen recognition of serum antibodies to *Actinobacillus actinomycetemcomitans* in patients with rapidly progressive periodontitis, *Infect Immun* 62:145, 1994.
161. Slots J: Subgingival microflora and periodontal disease, *J Clin Periodontol* 6:351, 1979.
162. Slots J, Rosling BG: Suppression of the periodontopathic microflora in localized juvenile periodontitis by systemic tetracycline, *J Clin Periodontol* 10:465, 1983.
163. Socransky SS, Haffajee AD: Microbial mechanisms in the pathogenesis of destructive periodontal diseases: a critical assessment, *J Periodontal Res* 26:195, 1991.
164. Socransky SS, Haffajee AD: The bacterial etiology of destructive periodontal disease: current concepts, *J Periodontol* 63:322, 1992.
165. Sorsa T, Ding YL, Ingman T, et al: Cellular source, activation and inhibition of dental plaque collagenase, *J Clin Periodontol* 22:709, 1995.
166. Sreenivasan PK, Meyer DH, Fives-Taylor PM: Requirements for invasion of epithelial cells by *Actinobacillus actinomycetemcomitans, Infect Immun* 61:1239, 1993.
167. Stashenko P, Jandinski JJ, Fujiyoshi P, et al: Tissue levels of bone resorptive cytokines in periodontal disease, *J Periodontol* 62:504, 1991.
168. Steinsvoll S, Halstensen TS, Schenck K: Extensive expression of TGF-beta1 in chronically inflamed periodontal tissue, *J Clin Periodontol* 26:366, 1999.
169. Syed SA, Loesche WJ: Bacteriology of human experimental gingivitis: effect of plaque age, *Infect Immun* 21:821, 1978.
170. Takemoto T, Kurihara H, Dahlen G: Characterization of *Bacteroides forsythus* isolates, *J Clin Microbiol* 35:1378, 1997.
171. Tani Y, Tani M, Kato I: Extracellular 37–kDa antigenic protein from *Actinobacillus actinomycetemcomitans* induces TNF-alpha, IL-1 beta, and IL-6 in murine macrophages, *J Dent Res* 76:1538, 1997.
172. Tanner AC, Haffer C, Bratthall GT, et al: A study of the bacteria associated with advancing periodontitis in man, *J Clin Periodontol* 6:278, 1979.
173. Tervahartiala T, Konttinen YT, Ingman T, et al: Cathepsin G in gingival tissue and crevicular fluid in adult periodontitis, *J Clin Periodontol* 23:68, 1996.
174. Tew JG, Zhang JB, Quinn S, et al: Antibody of the IgG2 subclass, *Actinobacillus actinomycetemcomitans,* and early-onset periodontitis, *J Periodontol* 67:317, 1996.
175. Tonetti MS, Mombelli A: Early-onset periodontitis, *Ann Periodontol* 4:39, 1999.
176. Tonetti MS, Imboden MA, Lang NP: Neutrophil migration into the gingival sulcus is associated with transepithelial gradients of interleukin-8 and ICAM-1, *J Periodontol* 69:1139, 1998.
177. Van Dalen PJ, van Deutekom-Mulder EC, de Graaff J, et al: Pathogenicity of *Peptostreptococcus micros* morphotypes and *Prevotella* species in pure and mixed culture, *J Med Microbiol* 47:135, 1998.

178. Van Dyke TE, Serhan CN: Resolution of inflammation: a new paradigm for the pathogenesis of periodontal disease, *J Dent Res* 82:82, 2003.
179. Van Dyke TE, Schweinebraten M, Cianciola LJ, et al: Neutrophil chemotaxis in families with localized juvenile periodontitis, *J Periodontal Res* 20:503, 1985.
180. Van Dyke TE, Wilson-Burrows C, Offenbacher S, et al: Association of an abnormality of neutrophil chemotaxis in human periodontal disease with a cell surface protein, *Infect Immun* 55:2262, 1987.
181. Van Steenbergen TJ, van der Mispel LM, de Graaff J: Effects of ammonia and volatile fatty acids produced by oral bacteria on tissue culture cells, *J Dent Res* 65:909, 1986.
182. Waldrop TC, Anderson DC, Hallmon WW, et al: Periodontal manifestations of the heritable Mac-1, LFA-1, deficiency syndrome: clinical, histopathologic and molecular characteristics, *J Periodontol* 58:400, 1987.
183. Walker SJ, van Dyke TE, Rich S, et al: Genetic polymorphisms of the IL-1alpha and IL-1beta genes in African-American LJP patients and an African-American control population, *J Periodontol* 71:723, 2000.
184. Wang B, Holt SC: Interaction of *Treponema denticola* with HEp-2 cells, *J Dent Res* 72:324, 1993.
185. Williams RC, Jeffcoat MK, Howell TH, et al: Altering the progression of human alveolar bone loss with the nonsteroidal anti-inflammatory drug flurbiprofen, *J Periodontol* 60:485, 1989.
186. Wilson M, Kalmar JR: FcγRIIa (CD32): a potential marker defining susceptibility to localized juvenile periodontitis, *J Periodontol* 67:323, 1996.
187. Wilson ME, Hamilton RG: Immunoglobulin G subclass response of localized juvenile periodontitis patients to *Actinobacillus actinomycetemcomitans* Y4 lipopolysaccharide, *Infect Immun* 60:1806, 1992.
188. Wilson ME, Hamilton RG: Immunoglobulin G subclass response of juvenile periodontitis subjects to principal outer membrane proteins of *Actinobacillus actinomycetemcomitans, Infect Immun* 63:1062, 1995.
189. Wilson ME, Zambon JJ, Suzuki JP, Genco RJ: Generalized juvenile periodontitis, defective neutrophil chemotaxis and *Bacteroides gingivalis* in a 13-year-old female, *J Periodontol* 56:457, 1985.
190. Wingrove JA, DiScipio RG, Chen Z, et al: Activation of complement components C3 and C5 by a cysteine proteinase (gingipain-1) from *Porphyromonas (Bacteroides) gingivalis, J Biol Chem* 267:18902, 1992.
191. Winkler JR, Robertson PB: Periodontal disease associated with HIV infection, *Oral Surg Oral Med Oral Pathol* 73:145, 1992.
192. Yoshimura A, Hara Y, Kaneko T, et al: Secretion of IL-1 beta, TNF-alpha, IL-8 and IL-1ra by human polymorphonuclear leukocytes in response to lipopolysaccharides from periodontopathic bacteria, *J Periodontal Res* 32:279, 1997.
193. Yumoto H, Nakae H, Fujinaka K, et al: Interleukin-6 (IL-6) and IL-8 are induced in human oral epithelial cells in response to exposure to periodontopathic *Eikenella corrodens, Infect Immun* 67:384, 1999.
194. Zambon JJ: *Actinobacillus actinomycetemcomitans* in human periodontal disease, *J Clin Periodontol* 12:1, 1985.
195. Zambon JJ, Christersson LA, Slots J: *Actinobacillus actinomycetemcomitans* in human periodontal disease: prevalence in patient groups and distribution of biotypes and serotypes within families, *J Periodontol* 54:707, 1983.
196. Zubery Y, Dunstan CR, Story BM, et al: Bone resorption caused by three periodontal pathogens in vivo in mice is mediated in part by prostaglandin, *Infect Immun* 66:4158, 1998.

Smoking and Periodontal Disease

M. John Novak and Karen F. Novak

CHAPTER

■ ■ ■

CHAPTER OUTLINE

EFFECTS OF SMOKING ON PREVALENCE AND SEVERITY
OF PERIODONTAL DISEASE
 Gingivitis
 Periodontitis
EFFECTS OF SMOKING ON ETIOLOGY AND
PATHOGENESIS OF PERIODONTAL DISEASE
 Microbiology
 Immunology
 Physiology

EFFECTS OF SMOKING ON RESPONSE TO
PERIODONTAL THERAPY
 Nonsurgical Therapy
 Surgical Therapy and Implants
 Maintenance Therapy
 Recurrent (Refractory) Disease

*A*n estimated 27.9% of dentate U.S. adults are current smokers, and 23.3% are former smokers. The prevalence of smoking is higher in individuals older than 34 years of age compared with with older age groups and in males (30.9%) compared with females (25.1%), with the highest prevalence seen in non-Hispanic black men (38.6%). Current smoking is more common among low-income adults (37.1%) compared with medium- or high-income earners and increases with decreasing years of education.[69]

Increasing evidence points to smoking as a major risk factor for periodontitis, affecting the prevalence, extent, and severity of disease. In addition, smoking may influence the clinical outcome of nonsurgical and surgical therapy as well as the long-term success of implant placement. With 41.9% of periodontitis cases in the United States associated with smoking, it has become increasingly important to understand its impact on the initiation, progression, and management of the disease in patients who smoke. This chapter discusses the effects of smoking on the prevalence, severity, etiology, and pathogenesis of periodontal disease as well as the impact on treatment. The reader is referred to several excellent reviews on the topic for the detailed results of studies.[34,49,50,53,70]

EFFECTS OF SMOKING ON PREVALENCE AND SEVERITY OF PERIODONTAL DISEASE

Gingivitis

Controlled clinical studies have demonstrated that in human models of experimental gingivitis, the development of inflammation in response to plaque accumulation is reduced in smokers compared with nonsmokers[8,16] (Table 14-1). In addition, cross-sectional studies have consistently demonstrated that smokers present with less gingival inflammation than nonsmokers.[5-7,54,55] These data suggest that smokers have a decreased expression of clinical inflammation in the presence of plaque accumulation compared with nonsmokers. The microbiologic, immunologic, and physiologic factors that might account for this observation are discussed in detail later.

Periodontitis

Although gingival inflammation in smokers appears to be reduced in response to plaque accumulation compared with nonsmokers, an overwhelming body of data points to smoking as a major risk factor for increasing the

TABLE 14-1

Effects of Smoking on Prevalence and Severity of Periodontal Disease

Periodontal Disease	Impact of Smoking
Gingivitis	↓Gingival inflammation and bleeding on probing
Periodontitis	↑Prevalence and severity of periodontal destruction ↑Pocket depth, attachment loss, and bone loss ↑Rate of periodontal destruction ↑Prevalence of severe periodontitis ↑Tooth loss ↑Prevalence with increased number of cigarettes smoked per day ↓Prevalence and severity with smoking cessation

↓, Decreased; ↑, increased.

prevalence and severity of periodontal destruction. Multiple cross-sectional and longitudinal studies have demonstrated that pocket depth, attachment loss, and alveolar bone loss are more prevalent and severe in patients who smoke compared with nonsmokers.[34,49,50,53,70]

An assessment of the relationship between cigarette smoking and periodontitis was performed in more than 12,000 dentate individuals over age 18 years as part of the third National Health and Nutrition Examination Survey (NHANES III).[69] Periodontitis was defined as one or more sites with clinical attachment loss of 4 mm or greater and pocket depth of 4 mm or greater. Using criteria established by the Centers for Disease Control and Prevention (CDC), "current smokers" were defined as those who had smoked 100 or more cigarettes over their lifetime and smoked at the time of the interview; "former smokers" had smoked 100 or more cigarettes in their lifetime but were not currently smoking; and "nonsmokers" had not smoked 100 or more cigarettes in their lifetime. Of the 12,000 individuals studied, 9.2% had periodontitis. This represented approximately 15 million cases of periodontitis in the United States. On average, smokers were four times as likely to have periodontitis as persons who had never smoked after adjusting for age, gender, race/ethnicity, education, and income/poverty ratio. Former smokers were 1.68 times more likely to have periodontitis than persons who had never smoked. This study also demonstrated a dose-response relationship between cigarettes smoked per day and the odds of having periodontitis. In subjects smoking nine or fewer cigarettes per day, the odds for having periodontitis was 2.79, whereas subjects smoking 31 or more cigarettes per day were almost six times more likely to have periodontitis. With former smokers, the odds of having periodontitis declined with the number of years since quitting. These data indicated that approximately 42% of periodontitis cases (6.4 million cases) in the U.S. adult population were attributable to current smoking, and approximately 11% (1.7 million cases) were attributable to former smoking.

These data are consistent with the findings of other cross-sectional studies performed in the United States and Europe. The odds ratio for periodontitis in current smokers has been estimated to range from as low as 1.5 to as high as 7.3, depending on the observed severity of periodontitis.[50] A meta-analysis of data from six such studies involving 2361 subjects indicated that current smokers were almost three times more likely to have severe periodontitis than nonsmokers.[49] The detrimental impact of long-term smoking on the periodontal and dentate status of older adults has been clearly demonstrated. Older-adult smokers are approximately three times more likely to have severe periodontal disease,[4,44] and the number of years of tobacco use is a significant factor in tooth loss, coronal root caries, and periodontal disease.[32,33] Smoking also has been shown to affect periodontal disease severity in younger individuals. Cigarette smoking is associated with increased severity of generalized aggressive periodontitis (formerly termed "early-onset periodontitis") in young adults,[64] and those age 19 to 30 years who smoke are 3.8 times more likely to have periodontitis than nonsmokers.[26] Longitudinal studies have demonstrated that young individuals smoking more than 15 cigarettes per day showed the highest risk for tooth loss.[30] Also, smokers are more than six times as likely as nonsmokers to demonstrate continued attachment loss.[31] Over a 10-year period, bone loss has been reported to be twice as rapid in smokers as in nonsmokers[11] and proceeds more rapidly even in the presence of excellent plaque control.[9]

Less information is available on the effects of cigar and pipe smoking, but it appears that effects similar to cigarette smoking may be observed with these forms of tobacco use.[2,20,21,42] The prevalence of moderate and severe periodontitis and the percentage of teeth with 5 mm or more of attachment loss was most severe in current cigarette smokers, but cigar and pipe smokers showed a severity of disease intermediate between the current cigarette smokers and nonsmokers.[2] Tooth loss is also increased in cigar and pipe smokers compared with nonsmokers.[42]

Smokeless tobacco use has been associated with oral leukoplakia and carcinoma.[15,75] However, no generalized effects on periodontal disease progression seem to occur, other than localized attachment loss and recession at the site of tobacco product placement.[60]

Interestingly, former smokers have less risk for periodontitis than current smokers but more risk than nonsmokers, and the risk for periodontitis decreases with the increasing number of years since quitting smoking.[69] This suggests that (1) the effects of smoking on the host are reversible with smoking cessation and (2) smoking cessation programs should be an integral component of periodontal education and therapy. Several tobacco intervention approaches can be used in helping the patient deal with the nicotine withdrawal symptoms and psychologic factors associated with smoking cessation. An appropriate approach for the dental office is the five-step program recommended by the Agency for Health

TABLE 14-2

Effects of Smoking on Etiology and Pathogenesis of Periodontal Disease

Etiologic Factor	Impact of Smoking
Microbiology	No effect on rate of plaque accumulation ↑Colonization of shallow periodontal pockets by periodontal pathogens ↑Levels of periodontal pathogens in deep periodontal pockets
Immunology	Altered neutrophil chemotaxis, phagocytosis, and oxidative burst ↑TNF-α and PGE_2 in gingival crevicular fluid (GCF) ↑Neutrophil collagenase and elastase in GCF ↑Production of PGE_2 by monocytes in response to LPS
Physiology	↓Gingival blood vessels with ↑ inflammation ↓GCF flow and bleeding on probing with ↑ inflammation ↓Subgingival temperature ↑Time needed to recover from local anesthesia

↑, Increased; ↓, decreased; *TNF-α,* tumor necrosis factor alpha, *PGE_2,* prostaglandin E_2; *LPS,* lipopolysaccharide.

Care Research and Quality.[34] This program uses the "five As" approach for smoking cessation: (1) *ask* (identify patient's tobacco use status), (2) *advise* (on associations between oral disease and smoking and the benefits of cessation), (3) *assess* (patient's interest and readiness to participate in tobacco cessation programs), (4) *assist* (use appropriate techniques to assist patient in tobacco cessation), and (5) *arrange* (follow-up contacts with the patient).[34] In addition, pharmacotherapeutic treatments such as nicotine replacement therapy and sustained bupropion administration have proved effective.

EFFECTS OF SMOKING ON ETIOLOGY AND PATHOGENESIS OF PERIODONTAL DISEASE

The increased prevalence and severity of periodontal destruction associated with smoking suggests that the host-bacterial interactions normally seen in chronic periodontitis are altered, resulting in more aggressive periodontal breakdown (Table 14-2) (see Chapters 9, 12, and 13). This imbalance between bacterial challenge and host response may be caused by changes in the composition of the subgingival plaque, with increases in the numbers and virulence of pathogenic organisms, changes in the host response to the bacterial challenge, or a combination of both. This section discusses recent evidence on the effects of smoking on the microbiology, immunology, and physiology of periodontitis.

Microbiology

Studies have failed to demonstrate a difference in the rate of plaque accumulation of smokers compared with nonsmokers, suggesting that if an alteration in the microbial challenge in smokers exists, it results from a *qualitative* rather than quantitative alteration in the plaque.[5] Several studies have explored the possible changes in subgingival plaque caused by smoking, with conflicting and inconclusive results. In a study of 142 patients with chronic periodontitis, plaque samples from deep pockets (≥6 mm) showed no differences in the counts of *Actinobacillus actinomycetemcomitans, Porphyromonas gingivalis,* and *Prevotella intermedia.*[57] In a similar study of 615 patients using immunoassay, the prevalence of *A. actinomycetemcomitans, P. gingivalis, P. intermedia,* and *Eikenella corrodens* was not found to be significantly different between smokers and nonsmokers.[67] In contrast, other studies have shown differences in the microbial composition of subgingival plaque between smokers and nonsmokers.

In a study of 798 subjects with different smoking histories, it was found that smokers had significantly higher levels of *Bacteroides forsythus* (now *Tannerella forsythia*) and that smokers were 2.3 times more likely to harbor *T. forsythia* than nonsmokers and former smokers.[76] Of particular interest was the observation that smokers do not respond to mechanical therapy as well as nonsmokers; this is associated with increased levels of *T. forsythia, A. actinomycetemcomitans,* and *P. gingivalis* remaining in the pockets after therapy in the smoking group when compared with nonsmokers.[23,24,28,59]

Many discrepancies between the findings of microbiologic studies are a function of the methodology involved, including bacterial counts versus proportions or prevalence of bacteria, number of sites sampled and the pocket depths selected, the sampling technique, the disease status of the subject, and the methods of bacterial enumeration and data analysis. In an attempt to overcome some of these problems, a recent study sampled subgingival plaque from all teeth with the exception of third molars in 272 adult subjects, including 50 current smokers, 98 past smokers, and 124 nonsmokers.[27] Using checkerboard DNA-DNA hybridization technology to screen for 29 different subgingival species, it was found that members of the orange and red complexes (see Chapter 9), including *Eikenella nodatum, Fusobacterium nucleatum* ss. *vincentii, P. intermedia, Peptostreptococcus micros, Prevotella nigrescens, T. forsythia, P. gingivalis, and Treponema denticola* were significantly more prevalent in current smokers than in nonsmokers and former smokers. The increased prevalence of these periodontal pathogens was caused by an increased colonization of shallow sites (pocket depth ≤4 mm), with no differences among smokers, former smokers, and nonsmokers in pockets 4 mm or greater. In addition, these pathogenic bacteria were more prevalent in the maxilla than the mandible. These data suggest that smokers have a greater extent of colonization by periodontal pathogens than nonsmokers or former smokers and that this colonization may lead to an increased prevalence of periodontal breakdown.

Immunology

The immune response of the host to plaque accumulation is essentially protective. In periodontal health and gingivitis, a balance exists between the bacterial challenge of plaque and the immune response from within the gingival tissues, with no resulting loss of periodontal support. In contrast, periodontitis appears to be associated with an alteration in the host-bacterial balance that may be initiated by changes in the bacterial composition of subgingival plaque, changes in the immune response, or a combination of both elements (see Chapters 9, 12, and 13).

Smoking exerts a major effect on the protective elements of the immune response, resulting in an increase in the extent and severity of periodontal destruction. The deleterious effects of smoking appear to result in part from a downregulation of the immune response to bacterial challenge. The neutrophil is an important component of the host response to bacterial infection, and alterations in neutrophil number or function may result in localized and systemic infections. Critical functions of neutrophils include *chemotaxis* (directed locomotion from the bloodstream to the site of infection), *phagocytosis* (internalization of foreign particles such as bacteria), and *killing* using oxidative and nonoxidative mechanisms. Neutrophils obtained from the peripheral blood, oral cavity, or saliva of smokers or exposed in vitro to whole tobacco smoke or nicotine have been shown to demonstrate functional alterations in chemotaxis, phagocytosis, and the oxidative burst.[19,38] In vitro studies of the effects of tobacco products on neutrophils have shown detrimental effects on cell movement as well as the oxidative burst.[14,37,43,62,65] In addition, the production of antibody essential for phagocytosis and killing of bacteria, specifically, immunoglobulin G2 (IgG2) levels to periodontal pathogens, has been reported to be reduced in smokers versus nonsmokers with periodontitis,[13,25,58,68] suggesting that smokers may have reduced protection against periodontal infection. In contrast, elevated levels of tumor necrosis factor alpha (TNF-α) have been demonstrated in the gingival crevicular fluid (GCF) of smokers,[12] as well as elevated levels of prostaglandin E_2 (PGE_2), neutrophil elastase, and matrix metalloproteinase-8 (MMP-8).[66] In vitro studies also have shown that exposure to nicotine increases the secretion of PGE_2 by monocytes in response to lipopolysaccharide (LPS).[51]

These data suggest that smoking may impair the response of neutrophils to periodontal infection but may also increase the release of tissue-destructive enzymes. The exact changes in the immunologic mechanisms involved in the rapid tissue destruction seen in smokers are currently unclear. Further studies are needed to define the effects of tobacco use on the immune response and tissue destruction in periodontitis.

Physiology

Previous studies have shown that the clinical signs of inflammation are less pronounced in smokers than in nonsmokers.[6,16] This may result from alterations in the inflammatory response in smokers, as outlined previously, or from alterations in the vascular response of the gingival tissues. Although no significant differences in the vascular density of healthy gingiva have been observed between smokers and nonsmokers,[52] the response of the microcirculation to plaque accumulation appears to be altered in smokers compared with nonsmokers. With developing inflammation, increases in GCF flow, bleeding on probing,[8] and gingival blood vessels[10] were less in smokers than nonsmokers. In addition, the oxygen concentration in healthy gingival tissues appears to be less in smokers than nonsmokers, although this condition is reversed in the presence of moderate inflammation.[29] Subgingival temperatures are lower in smokers than nonsmokers,[18] and recovery from the vasoconstriction caused by local anaesthetic administration takes longer in smokers.[39,72]

SCIENCE TRANSFER

Smoking has detrimental effects on the periodontium, which can be observed particularly in regard to periodontal therapy. Although the exact mechanisms are not known, it appears that the host response to bacterial plaque and the ability of the wound healing response in the host are significantly affected. Much of the impairment centers on *vascularity* and the functions of vascularity, such as the ability to provide oxygen, nutrients, cells, and growth stimulants to the tissues. Even slight alteration in the vascularity can have significant and profound effects on tissues and may account for the diminished response of periodontal therapy in smokers. Importantly, cessation of smoking appears to allow the host to respond more like nonsmokers, and therefore the effects on the vascularity appear reversible. This provides the basis for smoking cessation therapies and attests to the resiliency of the host.

A reduced gingival vascular response to dental plaque has been documented in smokers compared with nonsmokers. This is associated with an increased severity of periodontal disease directly related to quantitative assessments of cigarette utilization. *Clinicians must be focused in their assessment of periodontal disease in smokers because the appearance of healthy-appearing, nonbleeding gingiva often is accompanied by deep pockets and advanced bone loss.*

Cigarette smoking reduces the favorable outcomes of periodontal therapy. This is most dramatic in mucogingival root coverage surgical procedures and regenerative surgical procedures such as guided tissue regeneration and bone grafts. *It is recommended that smoking patients should be following a successful smoking cessation program before these surgical procedures are implemented.*

These cumulative data suggest that significant alterations are present in the gingival microvasculature of smokers compared with nonsmokers, and that these changes lead to decreased blood flow and decreased clinical signs of inflammation.

EFFECTS OF SMOKING ON RESPONSE TO PERIODONTAL THERAPY

Nonsurgical Therapy

Numerous studies have indicated that current smokers do not respond as well to periodontal therapy as nonsmokers or former smokers (Table 14-3). The majority of clinical research supports the observation that pocket depth reduction is more effective in nonsmokers than in smokers after nonsurgical periodontal therapy (Phase I therapy), including oral hygiene instruction, scaling, and root planing.*

*References 1, 23, 24, 28, 36, 56, 59.

TABLE 14-3

Effects of Smoking on Response to Periodontal Therapy

Therapy	Effects of Smoking
Nonsurgical	↓Clinical response to scaling and root planing
	↓Reduction in pocket depth
	↓Gain in clinical attachment levels
	↓Negative impact of smoking with ↑ level of plaque control
Surgery and implants	↓Pocket depth reduction after surgery
	↑Deterioration of furcations after surgery
	↓Gain in clinical attachment levels, ↓ bone fill, ↑ recession, and ↑ membrane exposure after GTR
	↓Pocket depth reduction after DFDBA
	↓Pocket depth reduction and gain in clinical attachment levels after open flap debridement
	Conflicting data on the impact of smoking on implant success.
	Smoking cessation should be recommended before implants.
Maintenance	↑Pocket depth during maintenance therapy
	↓Gain in clinical attachment levels
Recurrent (refractory) disease	↑Recurrent/refractory disease in smokers
	↑Need for re-treatment in smokers
	↑Need for antibiotics in smokers to control the negative effects of periodontal infection on surgical outcomes
	↑Tooth loss in smokers after surgical therapy

↓, Decreased; ↑, increased; *GTR,* guided tissue regeneration, *DFDBA,* decalcified freeze-dried bone allograft.

In addition, gains in clinical attachment as a result of scaling and root planing are less pronounced in smokers than in nonsmokers. In a study of patients with previously untreated advanced periodontal disease, scaling and root planing plus oral hygiene resulted in significantly greater average reductions in pocket depth and bleeding on probing in nonsmokers than in smokers when evaluated 6 months after completion of therapy.[59] Average pocket reductions of 2.5 mm for nonsmokers and 1.9 mm for smokers were observed in pockets that averaged 7 mm before treatment, even though plaque scores were less than favorable. In another study, the nonsurgical management of pockets 5 mm or greater showed that smokers had less pocket depth reduction than nonsmokers after 3 months (1.29 vs. 1.76 mm) as well as fewer gains in clinical attachment levels.[23] When a higher level of plaque control can be achieved as part of nonsurgical care, the differences in the resolution of 4-mm to 6-mm pockets between nonsmokers and smokers become clinically less significant.[56] When pockets persist in smokers and nonsmokers after therapy, adjunctive topical antimicrobial therapy can be used to try to resolve the remaining pocket depths (see Chapter 52). When scaling and root planing are used in combination with topical subgingivally placed tetracycline fibers, subgingival minocycline gel, or subgingival metronidazole gel, smokers continue to show less pocket reduction than nonsmokers.[40]

It can be concluded that smokers respond less well to nonsurgical therapy than nonsmokers. With excellent plaque control, however, these differences may be minimized. When comparing current smokers with former smokers and nonsmokers, the former and nonsmoking subjects appear to respond equally well to nonsurgical care,[23] reinforcing the need for patients to be informed of the benefits of smoking cessation.

Surgical Therapy and Implants

The less favorable response of the periodontal tissues to nonsurgical therapy that is observed in current smokers also appears to apply to surgical therapy. In a longitudinal comparative study of the effects of four different treatment modalities, including coronal scaling, root planing, modified Widman flap surgery, and osseous resection surgery, smokers ("heavy" defined as ≥20 cigarettes/day; "light" defined as ≤19 cigarettes/day) consistently showed less pocket reduction and less gain in clinical attachment levels than nonsmokers or former smokers.[36] These differences began immediately after the completion of therapy and continued throughout 7 years of supportive periodontal therapy. During the 7 years, deterioration of furcation areas was greater in heavy and light smokers than in former smokers and nonsmokers.

Smoking also has been shown to have a negative impact on the outcomes of guided tissue regeneration (GTR)[71,73] and the treatment of intrabony defects by bone allografts.[61] By 12 months after GTR therapy for deep intrabony defects, smokers gained less than half as much clinical attachment as nonsmokers (2.1 vs. 5.2 mm).[71] In a second study, 73 smokers also showed less gain in clinical attachment (1.2 vs. 3.2 mm), more gingival

TABLE 14-4

Postsurgical Changes in Clinical Parameters of Healing Response in Smoker and Nonsmoker Patients

	Smokers	Nonsmokers	p Value
CAL gain	1.2 ± 1.3 mm	3.2 ± 2.0 mm	<0.007
GR increase	2.8 ± 1.2 mm	1.3 ± 1.3 mm	<0.008
PBL gain	0.5 ± 1.5 mm	3.7 ± 2.2 mm	<0.000
ME	10/10	15/28	<0.008

Modified from Trombelli M, Kim CK, Zimmerman GJ, et al: *J Clin Periodontol* 24:366, 1997.

CAL, Clinical attachment level; *GR,* gingival recession; *PBL,* probing bone level; *ME,* prevalence of membrane exposure at removal.

recession, and less gain in bone fill of the defect. In addition, the GTR membranes were exposed in all the smokers and approximately half the nonsmokers (Table 14-4).

Similarly, after the use of decalcified freeze-dried bone allograft (DFDBA) for the treatment of intrabony defects, smokers showed less percentage of reduction in presurgical pocket depth than nonsmokers (41.9% vs. 48.3%).[61]

Open flap debridement surgery without regenerative or grafting procedures is the most common surgical procedure used for accessing the root and osseous surfaces. By 6 months after this procedure, smokers showed significantly less reduction of deep pockets (≥7 mm) than nonsmokers (3 mm for smokers vs. 4 mm for nonsmokers) and significantly less gain in clinical attachment (1.8 vs. 2.8 mm), even though the patients received supportive periodontal therapy every month for 6 months.[63] Of increased significance was the observation that only 16% of deep pockets in smokers returned to 3 mm or less at 6 months after surgery, whereas 47% of the deep pockets in nonsmokers were 3 mm or less after completion of therapy.

The impact of smoking on implant success is unclear at present. Several studies have shown that implant success rates are reduced in smokers,[3,17,22,35] whereas other studies have shown no effect.[48,74] Since numerous factors can influence implant success (see Chapters 73-81), further controlled clinical trials are needed to address the role of smoking as an independent variable in implant failure. However, with existing evidence supporting a negative effect of smoking on long-term implant success, patients should be informed and advised of the benefits of smoking cessation and the potential risks of smoking for implant failure.

Maintenance Therapy

The detrimental effects of smoking on treatment outcomes appears to be long-lasting and independent of the frequency of maintenance therapy. After four different modalities of therapy, including scaling, scaling and root planing, modified Widman flap surgery, and osseous surgery, maintenance therapy was performed by an hygienist every 3 months for 7 years.[36] Smokers consistently had deeper pockets than nonsmokers and less gain in attachment when evaluated each year for the 7-year period. Heavy smokers (≥20 cigarettes/day) had more plaque than light smokers, former smokers, and nonsmokers. Even with more intensive maintenance therapy given every month for 6 months after flap surgery,[63] smokers had deeper and more residual pockets than nonsmokers, even though no significant differences in plaque or bleeding on probing scores were found.

These data suggest that the effects of smoking on the quality of subgingival plaque, the host response, and the healing characteristics of the periodontal tissues may have a long-term effect on pocket resolution in smokers that may not be managed by conventional periodontal therapy. More studies are needed to examine the effects of antimicrobial agents combined with host-modulating agents in an attempt to control periodontal disease in smokers.

Recurrent (Refractory) Disease

Because of the difficulty in controlling periodontal disease in smokers, many smokers become refractory to traditional periodontal treatment and tend to show more periodontal breakdown than nonsmokers after therapy.[45,46] The question has been raised as to whether patients are truly refractive to therapy or whether the therapy administered was insufficient to control the disease process.[41,46] It is now thought that patients formerly considered refractive to therapy actually undergo continuous or recurrent disease; for this reason, the diagnosis of "refractory periodontitis" has been removed as a distinct classification (see Chapter 7).

The complex effects of smoking on the subgingival microflora and host response provide a model for studying new modalities of therapy for controlling periodontitis. In studies of patients who failed to respond to conventional therapy, including different combinations of oral hygiene instruction, scaling and root planing, surgery, and antibiotics, approximately 90% of these "refractory" patients were smokers.[45,47] In one study the mean age of the refractory patients was 42 years, and 28 of the 31 refractory patients were smokers.[45] Of the 31 patients, 19% had been retreated once surgically for pocket elimination, 10% had been re-treated twice surgically, and the patients had received an average of four episodes of adjunctive antibiotics. During the course of treatment, 36% of patients had lost an average of three teeth (range, 1-10).

It is clear from these studies that smokers (1) may present with periodontal disease at an early age, (2) may be difficult to treat with conventional therapy, and (3) may continue to have progressive or recurrent periodontitis leading to tooth loss. Further studies are needed to determine the level and type of therapy required to provide long-term maintenance of periodontal health in individuals who choose to continue smoking.

REFERENCES

1. Ah MK, Johnson GK, Kaldahl WB, et al: The effect of smoking on the response to periodontal therapy, *J Clin Periodontol* 21:91, 1994.

2. Albandar JM, Streckfus CF, Adesanya MR, et al: Cigar, pipe, and cigarette smoking as risk factors for periodontal disease and tooth loss, *J Periodontol* 71:1874, 2000.
3. Bain CA, Moy PK: The association between the failure of dental implants and cigarette smoking, *Int J Oral Maxillofac Implants* 8:609, 1993.
4. Beck JD, Koch GG, Rozier RG, et al: Prevalence and risk indicators for periodontal attachment loss in a population of older community-dwelling blacks and whites, *J Periodontol* 61:521, 1990.
5. Bergstrom J: Cigarette smoking as a risk factor in chronic periodontal disease, *Community Dent Oral Epidemiol* 17:245, 1989.
6. Bergstrom J: Oral hygiene compliance and gingivitis expression in cigarette smokers, *Scand J Dent Res* 98:497, 1990.
7. Bergstrom J, Floderus-Myrhed B: Co-twin control study of the relationship between smoking and some periodontal disease factors, *Community Dent Oral Epidemiol* 11:113, 1983.
8. Bergstrom J, Preber H: The influence of cigarette smoking on the development of experimental gingivitis, *J Periodont Res* 21:668, 1986.
9. Bergstrom J, Eliasson S, Dock J: A 10-year prospective study of tobacco smoking and periodontal health, *J Periodontol* 71:1338, 2000.
10. Bergstrom J, Persson L, Preber H: Influence of cigarette smoking on vascular reaction during experimental gingivitis, *Scand J Dent Res* 96:34, 1988.
11. Bolin A, Eklund G, Frithiof L, et al: The effect of changed smoking habits on marginal alveolar bone loss: a longitudinal study, *Swed Dent J* 17:211, 1993.
12. Bostrum L, Linder LE, Bergstrom J: Clinical expression of TNF-α in smoking-associated periodontal disease, *J Clin Periodontol* 25:767, 1998.
13. Califano JV, Schifferle RE, Gunsolley JC, et al: Antibody reactive with *Porphyromonas gingivalis* serotypes K1–6 in adult and generalized early-onset periodontitis, *J Periodontol* 70:730, 1999.
14. Codd EE, Swim AT, Bridges RB: Tobacco smokers' neutrophils are desensitized to chemotactic peptide-stimulated oxygen uptake, *J Lab Clin Med* 110:648, 1987;.
15. Creath CJ, Cutter G, Bradley DH, et al: Oral leukoplakia and adolescent smokeless tobacco use, *Oral Surg Oral Med Oral Pathol* 72:35, 1991.
16. Danielsen B, Manji F, Nagelkerke N, et al: Effect of cigarette smoking on the transition dynamics in experimental gingivitis, *J Clin Periodontol* 17:159, 1990.
17. De Bruyn H, Collaert B: The effect of smoking on early implant failure, *Clin Oral Implants Res* 5:260, 1994.
18. Dinsdale CR, Rawlinson A, Walsh TF: Subgingival temperature in smokers and nonsmokers with periodontal disease, *J Clin Periodontol* 24:761, 1997.
19. Eichel B, Sharik HA: Tobacco smoke toxicity: loss of human oral leukocyte function and fluid cell metabolism, *Science* 166:1424, 1969.
20. Feldman RS, Alman JE, Chauncey HH: Periodontal disease indexes and tobacco smoking in healthy aging men, *Gerodontics* 3:43, 1987.
21. Feldman RS, Bravacos JS, Close CL: Associations between smoking different tobacco products and periodontal disease indexes, *J Periodontol* 54:481, 1983.
22. Gorman LM, Lambert PM, Morris HF, et al: The effect of smoking on implant survival at second stage surgery: DICRG Interim Report No. 5, Dental Implant Clinical Research Group, *Implant Dent* 3:165, 1994.
23. Grossi SG, Skrepcinski FB, DeCaro T, et al: Response to periodontal therapy in diabetics and smokers, *J Periodontol* 67:1094, 1996.
24. Grossi SG, Zambon J, Machtei EE, et al: Effects of smoking and smoking cessation on healing after mechanical therapy, *J Am Dent Assoc* 128:599, 1997.
25. Gunsolley JC, Pandey JP, Quinn SM, et al: The effect of race, smoking and immunoglobulin allotypes on IgG subclass concentrations, *J Periodontal Res* 32:380, 1997.
26. Haber J, Wattles J, Crowley M, et al: Evidence for cigarette smoking as a major risk factor for periodontitis, *J Periodontol* 64:16, 1993.
27. Haffajee AD, Socransky SS: Relationship of cigarette smoking to the subgingival microbiota, *J Clin Periodontol* 28:377, 2001.
28. Haffajee AD, Cugini MA, Dibart S, et al: The effects of scaling and root planing on the clinical and microbiologic parameters of periodontal diseases, *J Clin Periodontol* 24:324, 1997.
29. Hanioka T, Tanaka M, Ojima M, et al: Oxygen sufficiency in the gingiva of smokers and nonsmokers with periodontal disease, *J Periodontol* 71:1846, 2000.
30. Holm G: Smoking as an additional risk for tooth loss, *J Periodontol* 65:996, 1994.
31. Ismail AI, Morrison EC, Burt BA, et al: Natural history of periodontal disease in adults: findings from the Tecumseh Periodontal Disease Study, *J Dent Res* 69:430, 1990.
32. Jette AM, Feldman HA, Douglass C: Oral disease and physical disability in community dwelling older persons, *J Am Geriatr Soc* 41:1102, 1993.
33. Jette AM, Feldman HA, Tennstedt SL: Tobacco use: a modifiable risk factor for dental disease among the elderly, *Am J Public Health* 83:1271, 1993.
34. Johnson GK, Hill M: Cigarette smoking and the periodontal patient, *J Periodontol* 75:196, 2004.
35. Jones JK, Triplett RG: The relationship of cigarette smoking to impaired intraoral wound healing: a review of evidence and implications for patient care, *J Oral Maxillofac Surg* 50:237, 1992.
36. Kaldahl WB, Johnson GK, Patil KD, et al: Levels of cigarette consumption and response to periodontal therapy, *J Periodontol* 67:675, 1996.
37. Kalra J, Chandhary AK, Prasad K: Increased production of oxygen free radicals in cigarette smokers, *Int J Exp Pathol* 72:1, 1991.
38. Kenney EB, Kraal JH, Saxe SR, et al: The effect of cigarette smoke on human oral polymorphonuclear leukocytes, *J Periodontal Res* 12:227, 1977.
39. Ketabi M, Hirsch RS: The effects of local anesthetic containing adrenaline on gingival blood flow in smokers and nonsmokers, *J Clin Periodontol* 24:888, 1997.
40. Kinane DF, Radvar M: The effect of smoking on mechanical and antimicrobial periodontal therapy, *J Periodontol* 68:467, 1997.
41. Kornman KS: Refractory periodontitis: critical questions in clinical management, *J Clin Periodontol* 23:293, 1996.
42. Krall EA, Garvey AJ, Garcia RI: Alveolar bone loss and tooth loss in male cigar and pipe smokers, *J Am Dent Assoc* 130:57, 1999.
43. Lannan S, McLean A, Drost E, et al: Changes in neutrophil morphology and morphometry following exposure to cigarette smoke, *Int J Exp Pathol* 73:183, 1992.
44. Locker D, Leake JL: Risk indicators and risk markers for periodontal disease experience in older adults living independently in Ontario, Canada, *J Dent Res* 72:9, 1993.
45. MacFarlane GD, Herzberg MC, Wolff LF, et al: Refractory periodontitis associated with abnormal polymorphonuclear leukocyte phagocytosis and cigarette smoking, *J Periodontol* 63:908, 1992.
46. Magnussen I, Walker CB: Refractory periodontitis or recurrent disease, *J Clin Periodontol* 23:289, 1996.

47. Magnussen I, Low S, McArthur WP, et al: Treatment of subjects with refractory periodontal disease, *J Clin Periodontol* 21:628, 1994.
48. Minsk L, Polson AM, Weisgold A, et al: Outcome failures of endosseous implants from a clinical training center, *Compend Contin Educ Dent* 17:848, 1996.
49. Papapanou PN: Periodontal diseases: epidemiology, *Ann Periodontol* 1:1, 1996.
50. Papapanou PN: Risk assessments in the diagnosis and treatment of periodontal diseases, *J Dent Educ* 62:822, 1998.
51. Payne JB, Johnson GK, Reinhardt RA, et al: Nicotine effects on PGE2 and IL-1β release by LPS-treated human monocytes, *J Periodontal Res* 31:99, 1996.
52. Persson L, Bergstrom J: Smoking and vascular density of healthy marginal gingival, *Eur J Oral Sci* 106:953, 1998.
53. Position paper: Tobacco use and the periodontal patient, *J Periodontol* 70:1419, 1999.
54. Preber H, Bergstrom J: Occurrence of gingival bleeding in smoker and nonsmoker patients, *Acta Odontol Scand* 43:315, 1985.
55. Preber H, Bergstrom J: Cigarette smoking in patients referred for periodontal treatment, *Scand J Dent Res* 94:102, 1986.
56. Preber H, Bergstrom J: The effect of non-surgical treatment on periodontal pockets in smokers and nonsmokers, *J Clin Periodontol* 13:319, 1986.
57. Preber H, Bergstrom J, Linder LE: Occurrence of periopathogens in smoker and nonsmoker patients, *J Clin Periodontol* 19:667, 1992.
58. Quinn SM, Zhang JB, Gunsolley JC, et al: The influence of smoking and race on adult periodontitis and serum IgG_2 levels, *J Periodontol* 69:171, 1998.
59. Renvert S, Dahlen G, Wikstrom M: The clinical and microbiologic effects of non-surgical periodontal therapy in smokers and nonsmokers, *J Clin Periodontol* 25:153, 1998.
60. Robertson PB, Walsh M, Greene J, et al: Periodontal effects associated with the use of smokeless tobacco, *J Periodontol* 61:438, 1990.
61. Rosen PS, Marks MH, Reynolds MA: Influence of smoking on long-term clinical results of intrabony defects treated with regenerative therapy, *J Periodontol* 67:1159, 1996.
62. Ryder MI, Fujitaki R, Johnson G, et al: Alterations of neutrophil oxidative burst by in vitro smoke exposure: implications for oral and systemic diseases, *Ann Periodontol* 3:76, 1998.
63. Scabbia A, Cho K-S, Sigurdsson TJ, et al: Cigarette smoking negatively affects healing response following flap debridement surgery, *J Periodontol* 72:43, 2001.
64. Schenkein HA, Gunsolley JC, Koertge TE, et al: Smoking and its effects on early-onset periodontitis, *J Am Dent Assoc* 126:1107, 1995.
65. Selby C, Drost E, Brown D, et al: Inhibition of neutrophil adherence and movement by acute cigarette smoke exposure, *Exp Lung Res* 18:813, 1992.
66. Soder B: Neutrophil elastase activity, levels of prostaglandin E2, and matrix metalloproteinase-8 in refractory periodontitis sites in smokers and nonsmokers, *Acta Odont Scand* 57:77, 1999.
67. Stoltenberg JL, Osborn JB, Pihlstrom BL, et al: Association between cigarette smoking, bacterial pathogens and periodontal status, *J Periodontol* 64:1225, 1993.
68. Tangada SD, Califano JV, Nakashima K, et al: The effect of smoking on serum IgG_2 reactive with *Actinobacillus actinomycetemcomitans* in early-onset periodontitis, *J Periodontol* 68:842, 1997.
69. Tomar SL, Asma S: Smoking-attributable periodontitis in the United States: findings from NHANES III, *J Periodontol* 71:743, 2000.
70. Tonetti MS: Cigarette smoking and periodontal diseases: etiology and management of disease, *Ann Periodontol* 3:88, 1998.
71. Tonetti MS, Pino-Prato G, Cortellini P: Effect of cigarette smoking on periodontal healing following GTR in infrabony defects, *J Clin Periodontol* 22:229, 1995.
72. Trikilis N, Rawlinson A, Walsh TF: Periodontal probing depth and subgingival temperature in smokers and non-smokers, *J Clin Periodontol* 26:38, 1999.
73. Trombelli M, Kim CK, Zimmerman GJ, et al: Retrospective analysis of factors related to clinical outcome of guided tissue regeneration procedures in intrabony defects, *J Clin Periodontol* 24:366, 1997.
74. Weyant RJ: Characteristics associated with the loss and peri-implant tissue health of endosseous dental implants, *Int J Oral Maxillofac Implants* 9:95, 1994.
75. Wray A, McGuirt WF: Smokeless tobacco usage associated with oral carcinoma: incidence, treatment, outcome, *Arch Otolaryngol Head Neck Surg* 119:929, 1993.
76. Zambon JJ, Grossi SG, Machtei EE, et al: Cigarette smoking increases the risk for subgingival infection with periodontal pathogens, *J Periodontol* 67:1050, 1996.

Molecular Biology of the Host-Microbe Interaction in Periodontal Diseases: Selected Topics: Molecular Signaling Aspects of Pathogen-Mediated Bone Destruction in Periodontal Diseases

15

CHAPTER

Keith L. Kirkwood; Mario Taba, Jr.; Carlos Rossa, Jr.; Philip M. Preshaw; and William V. Giannobile

CHAPTER OUTLINE

This chapter provides an overview on the molecular biology of the host-parasite relationship from a cellular signaling perspective specific to the pathogen-associated lipopolysaccharide (LPS). Specific topics reviewed include the implications of periodontal microbiota-associated LPS on the induction of the innate immune response, toll-like receptor signaling, and the generation of pathogen-associated molecular patterns and their role in the pathogenesis of periodontal disease. The second half of the chapter highlights the pathobiology of periodontal disease and the induction of disease by proinflammatory cytokines that generate host tissue destruction and alveolar bone loss. The chapter concludes with ramifications for the development of therapeutic strategies that perturb LPS signal transduction for the treatment of periodontitis.

INNATE-IMMUNE RESPONSE AND TOLL-LIKE RECEPTORS

The host defense against periodontopathic bacteria comprises innate and acquired immunity. These two distinct sets of responses are sequentially activated during periodontal disease and ultimately target the elimination of the microbial pathogen. Whereas the *innate* immune system is activated quickly (within minutes) after the invasion of the host and is responsible for the defense during the initial hours and days of the infection, *acquired* immunity requires at least 7 to 10 days before an adequate cellular or humoral response occurs. Although the innate immune system, consisting of cellular and humoral components, is very effective in dealing with the vast majority of infections, it is believed to be nonspecific to invading pathogens. Any lapse in host protection presumably will be overcome by secondary activation of specific acquired immunity mediated by T and B lymphocytes to eliminate the organism.

One of the primary challenges of the innate immune system is to discriminate among a large number of periodontal pathogens from the host with a limited number of cell surface receptors. This challenge is compounded because microbial pathogens have the ability to mutate as a mechanism to escape host recognition. The innate immune system has met this challenge through recognition of evolutionary conserved structures on pathogens that are not present in higher eukaryotes, called *pattern recognition receptors* (PRRs). These molecular motifs, known as *pathogen-associated molecular patterns* (PAMPs), have essential roles in the pathogen's ability to evade host defense and thus are not subject to high mutation rates.[105] PAMPs are shared among pathogens but not expressed by the host.[104] Although many PRRs have been known for years, it was not clear how the innate immune system functioned until the discovery of the *toll-like receptors* (TLRs), which have proved to be critical for recognition of microbes by the innate immune system and for bridging the innate and acquired immune responses.

Toll was first described initially as the gene for a type I transmembrane receptor, with an important role in the dorsoventral development of the *Drosophila* (fruit fly) embryo.[165] In addition, it had become apparent that the absence of *toll* in genetically deficient *Drosophila* also resulted in a severely impaired defense against fungi and gram-positive bacteria.[89] These initial data suggested that *toll* is an important component of *Drosophila* antimicrobial defense and that mammalian homologs might have similar functions. Indeed, 10 different mammalian TLRs have been identified in humans to date.

Despite the alleged nonspecificity of the innate immune response, it has long been known that cytokine release on stimulation with gram-positive or gram-negative bacteria showed important quantitative and qualitative differences. During the last few years, research in this field has identified TLRs as a major class of signaling receptors, recognizing conserved bacterial structures. The specificity of TLR recognition for several important PAMPs has been identified, including recognition of *peptidoglycan* (PGN), bacterial lipoproteins, atypical LPS, and zymosan by TLR-2; double-stranded ribonucleic acid (RNA) by TLR-3; LPS and heat-shock proteins (HSPs) by TLR-4; flagellin by TLR-5; and CpG motifs of bacterial deoxyribonucleic acid (DNA) by TLR-9.[73] Table 15-1 lists periopathogenic PAMPs and the TLR use for each particular PAMP. Most studies have focused on TLR-2 and TLR-4 because these recognize gram-positive and gram-negative bacterial PAMPs, respectively. Of particular note is *Porphyromonas gingivalis* LPS, which preferentially utilizes TLR-2 and not TLR-4.[11,65] Earlier data indicated that *P. gingivalis* LPS bound TLR-4 in gingival fibroblasts.[168,169] TLRs are expressed by myleomonocytic cells as well as by endothelial, epithelial, and various other cells, including gingival fibroblasts.[168] Within periodontal tissues, TLR-2 and TLR-4 expression appears to be increased in severe disease states.[109]

TLRs all contain a common extracellular leucine-rich domain and a conserved intracellular domain.[3] The intracellular tail of the receptor was shown to be homologous with the intracellular domain of the *interleukin-1 receptor* (IL-1R) type I, currently being designated as the *toll/IL-1R* (TIR) *domain*. The TLR-PAMP interaction results in the recruitment of specific adapter molecules such as MyD88 and Mal, which then bind the *IL-1R–associated kinase* (IRAK). The signal is thereafter transmitted through a chain of signaling molecules, which is apparently common to all TLRs, involving *tumor necrosis factor* (TNF) *receptor–associated factor-6* (TRAF6) and *mitogen-activated protein kinases* (MAPKs). Thereafter, activation of *nuclear factor kappa B* (NF-κB) and *activated protein-1* (AP-1) leads to transcription of genes involved in the activation of the innate host defense, notably proinflammatory cytokines[2] (Figure 15-1).

TOLL-LIKE RECEPTOR EXPRESSION AND MICROBIAL RECOGNITION IN PERIODONTAL TISSUES

Human gingival fibroblasts and human periodontal ligament fibroblasts are representative constituents of periodontal tissues and produce various inflammatory cytokines, such as interleukin-1 (IL-1), IL-6, and IL-8 when stimulated by oral bacterial LPS fractions, such as those from *P. gingivalis, Prevotella intermedia,* or *Actinobacillus actinomycetemcomitans*. Fibroblasts are generally devoid of membrane CD14 (cluster of differentiation, *CD*), which is responsible for pattern recognition of common bacterial cell surface components such as LPS and PGN.[164] There appears to be controversy in the literature regarding CD14 expression in gingival fibroblasts. It has been reported that human gingival fibroblasts lacking both membrane CD14 and messenger RNA (mRNA) expression were activated by *Escherichia coli* LPS in a soluble CD14–dependent

TABLE 15-1

Toll-Like Receptors (TLRs) and Ligands in Periodontal Disease

PRR	PAMP	Periodontal Pathogen	References
TLR-2	Lipoproteins	*Bacteroides forsythus**	57
	Atypical LPS	*P. gingivalis, C. ochracea*	50, 65, 98, 174
	Outer membrane proteins	Oral treponemes	8, 58
	Fimbriae	*P. gingivalis*	9, 49, 51, 52, 64
	Nonendotoxic glycoprotein	*P. intermedia*	153
TLR-4	HSP-60 (GroEL)	*P. gingivalis*	163
	LPS	*A. actinomycetemcomitans, F. nucleatum*	174
TLR-9	CpG-containing DNA	*A. actinomycetemcomitans, P. gingivalis, P. micros*	116

**Tannerella forsythia.*

PRR, Pattern recognition receptor; *PAMP,* pathogen-associated molecular pattern; *LPS,* lipopolysaccharide; *HSP,* heat-shock protein.

manner.[62] In contrast, others reported that human gingival fibroblasts expressed membrane CD14 and responded to *P. gingivalis* LPS in a membrane CD14–dependent manner.[171] Part of this disparity in the literature may be caused by heterogeneity of membrane CD14 expression in human gingival fibroblasts, as indicated in studies where CD14 expression is directly correlated with chemokine production.[152] This variation has been also recently observed in PDL fibroblasts, ranging from 5% to 22.9% of CD14+ cells.[60]

Besides membrane-bound CD14, both gingival fibroblasts[156] and *periodontal ligament* (PDL) fibroblasts[60] constitutively express TLR-2 and TLR-4. Consistent with the concept of significant differences between gingival fibroblasts and PDL cells, the latter expressed higher levels of TLR-2, whereas TLR-4 was expressed at similar levels. More recent data have shown that cementoblasts also express TLR-2 and TLR-4 as well as CD-14.[115] It has been suggested that TLR-4 mediates the response to LPS, whereas TLR-2 is involved in the response to other bacterial cell wall components and antigens, such as PGN and lipoprotein.[168] Whether there is such specificity of TLRs, however, remains a controversial issue, because both TLR-2 and TLR-4 can be involved in response to LPS stimulation in gingival fibroblasts cells,[156] using different signaling pathways.

Collectively, these data provide evidence that gingival fibroblasts and PDL cells are equipped to respond to LPS stimulation. Nevertheless, the signaling pathways involved in LPS stimulation are only partially understood, especially in these cell types. Despite the similarity of the intracellular domain of TLRs and IL-1R, which is supported by activation of some common "upstream" kinases (e.g., IRAK–IL-1R–associated kinase, TRAF6–TNF receptor–associated kinase) as well as activation of a common "downstream" transcription factor (NF-κB), there is a great complexity in terms of the adapter proteins involved in signaling by TLRs.[3] Some of these adapter proteins may be common to all known TLRs (MyD88), whereas others may be specific to only one (e.g., MD-2

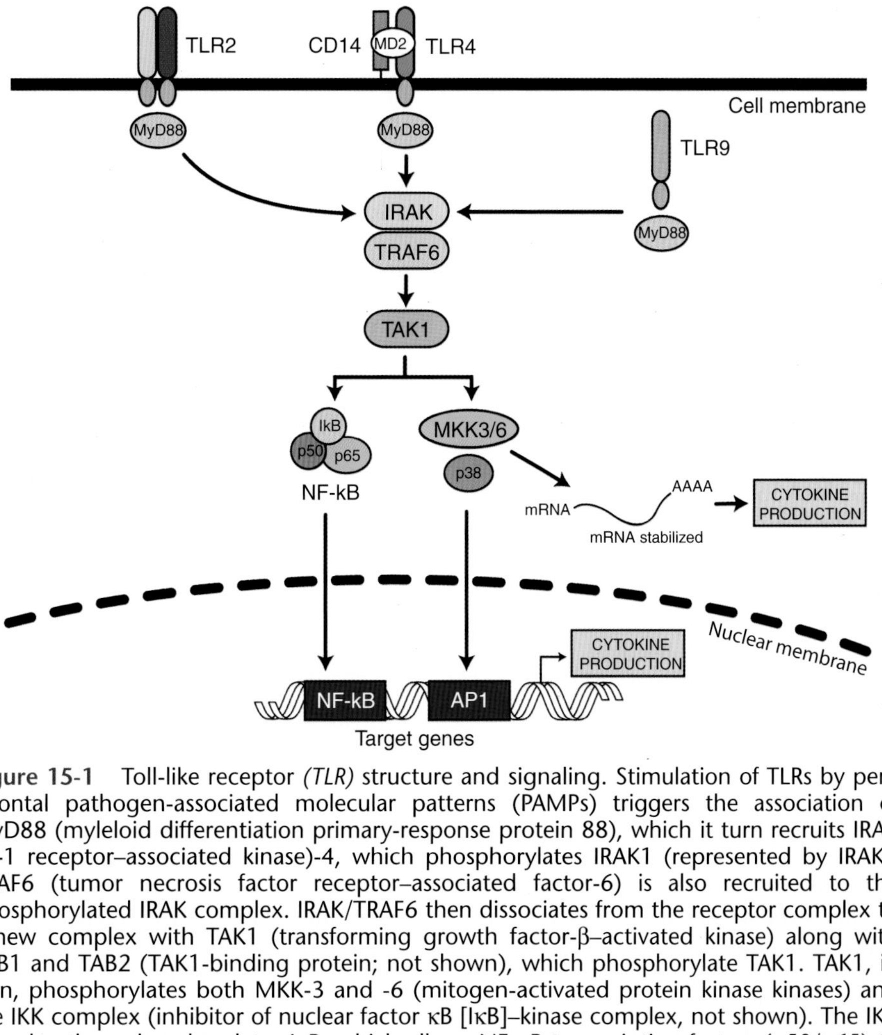

Figure 15-1 Toll-like receptor *(TLR)* structure and signaling. Stimulation of TLRs by periodontal pathogen-associated molecular patterns (PAMPs) triggers the association of MyD88 (myleloid differentiation primary-response protein 88), which it turn recruits IRAK (IL-1 receptor–associated kinase)-4, which phosphorylates IRAK1 (represented by IRAK). TRAF6 (tumor necrosis factor receptor–associated factor-6) is also recruited to the phosphorylated IRAK complex. IRAK/TRAF6 then dissociates from the receptor complex to a new complex with TAK1 (transforming growth factor-β–activated kinase) along with TAB1 and TAB2 (TAK1-binding protein; not shown), which phosphorylate TAK1. TAK1, in turn, phosphorylates both MKK-3 and -6 (mitogen-activated protein kinase kinases) and the IKK complex (inhibitor of nuclear factor κB [IκB]–kinase complex, not shown). The IKK complex then phosphorylates IκB, which allows NF-κB transcription factors (p50/p65) to translocate to the nucleus to induce expression of cytokine genes. Similarly, MKK3/6 can phosphorylate p38 MAPK to activate AP-1 (activated protein-1) transcription factors and initiate gene expression. In addition, p38 can phosphorylate RNA-binding proteins, which can stabilize cytokine mRNA and thus amplify cytokine production.

for TLR-4) or a few types of TLRs (e.g., TIRAP, also known as Mal for TLR-2 and TLR-4).[91]

The current signaling pathways models for TLR-2 and TLR-4 are summarized in Figure 15-1, but various other pathways may be implicated downstream of the binding of periodontal pathogen components to these receptors. The pathways involved include recruitment of different adapter proteins and activation of various MAPK cascades, such as ERK-1 and ERK-2,[5] JNK, and p38.[141] In general, the ERKs are activated by growth factors and hormones, whereas both JNKs and p38 MAPKs are activated by environmental stress and inflammatory cytokines.[22,129] One of the main bifurcation points in LPS signaling through TLRs is proximal to the cytoplasmic domain of the toll/IL-1R where, on dimerization of the receptor, an adapter protein is recruited called *MyD88*. The MyD88-dependent pathway leads to subsequent activation of IRAK, TRAF6, and ultimately NF-κB, and it is essential for cytokine induction. On the other hand, the MyD88-independent pathway does not activate IRAK and leads to activation of NF-κB with delayed kinetics. This pathway requires different adapter proteins, such as TIRAP, TRIF, and TRAM, and probably does not lead to cytokine induction. Rather, it is related to interferon-β (IFN-β) secretion and indirect upregulation of IFN-dependent genes.[110,113,155] The second bifurcation point is represented by *MAP kinase-kinase-kinase* (MAPKKK), also known as TAK-1, and is located downstream to MAPK. It can lead to activation of either AP-1, through MAPK pathways, or NF-κB, through the *inhibitor of nuclear factor kappa B* (IKK) pathway. The significance of the activation of various pathways by the same receptor is not completely understood and may be related to compensatory mechanisms or to the specificity of cell response in terms of modulation of biologic cell response by the production of proinflammatory or antiinflammatory cytokines.[113,168]

ROLE OF PATHOGEN-ASSOCIATED MOLECULAR PATTERNS IN PERIODONTAL DISEASE

Host-pathogen interactions in destructive periodontal diseases are very complex because diverse PAMPs can stimulate many cell types, including resident cells normally present in the periodontal tissues in the absence of disease, as well as nonresident or inflammatory cells attracted to the periodontal tissues as a result of the pathogenic process. Cell death by necrosis or apoptosis may result from the exposure to those PAMPs[39,55]; however, this section focuses on the host-derived substances produced after that exposure. Activated host cells can produce biologically active substances that will affect other cells, forming an intricate network of proinflammatory cytokines and chemokines with the main purpose of preventing sepsis. However, some PAMPs have the opposite effect of inhibiting the host response, which is regarded as a mechanism of enhancing the infectiveness for some microbial species by evading the host immune system. For example, proteinases from *P. gingivalis* degrade tumor necrosis factor alpha (TNF-α), which may be induced by other PAMPs in different cells.[15]

Great progress has been made toward understanding this network of inflammatory cytokines during the past few years, and this knowledge can provide the rationale for new preventive and therapeutic approaches to the management of periodontal diseases.

Effects on Resident Cells

Cells normally present in the periodontal tissues are the first to be exposed to PAMPs as the disease initiates. These cells remain exposed and stimulated by these factors as the disease progresses, so they have important roles in both establishment and modulation of the host response (Figure 15-2).

When disease is initiated at a previously healthy periodontium, the first cell type to be stimulated by PAMPs is the **epithelial cell.** These cells express TLR-2 and TLR-9,[106] and in addition to the biologic mediators listed in Table 15-2, LPS from *A. actinomycetemcomitans* increases the expression of *intercellular adhesion molecule-1* (ICAM-1), the ligand for *lymphocyte function–associated antigen-1* (LFA-1). The binding between these molecules can direct the attachment and migration of leukocytes toward the antigen on the lumen of the pocket. These cells have also been shown to produce interleukin-8 (IL-8), a neutrophil chemoattractant and activator, in response to LPS from various periodontal pathogens,[53,67] whereas expression of both ICAM-1 and IL-8 are down-regulated by *P. gingivalis* LPS.[68] Besides activating other host cells, such as endothelial cells, macrophages, dendritic cells, and neutrophils, these cells produce *matrix metalloproteinases* (MMPs)[170] after stimulation with PAMPs, suggesting a direct mechanism of tissue damage.

Dendritic cells (DCs, or *Langerhan cells*) are resident cells present in the epithelium and connective tissue that function as sentinels of the innate immune system, continually surveying their surroundings for antigens. These cells are also exposed to PAMPs as soon as the subgingival area becomes colonized by putative periodontal pathogens. When DCs express TLR-9, they are able to recognize antigens, including PAMPs, which initiates a maturation process. Mature DCs not only can present antigens in a major histocompatibilty complex (MHC) class II–peptide complex, but also can produce cytokines and costimulatory molecules (CD40, CD54, CD80, CD86) that induce activation of T lymphocytes, resulting in either Th1-type or Th2-type immune responses.[83] DCs provide an important link for the generation and modulation of the immune response to PAMPs; when invaded by fimbriated *P. gingivalis* and co-cultured with T lymphocytes, these cells stimulate a Th1 type of response. However, stimulation of DCs from *P. gingivalis* LPS may have the opposite effect, resulting in a shift on the pattern of immune response from Th1 to Th2.[77] This differential activation by distinct PAMPs is related to the type of TLR/signaling pathway activated by those stimuli, since *P. gingivalis* LPS activates TLR-2 and not TLR-9.[29]

As periodontitis progresses and PAMPs gain access to connective tissues, **macrophages,** which are usually found in low numbers in the clinically healthy situation, are also directly activated. The macrophages are highly efficient resident *antigen-presenting cells* (APCs) derived

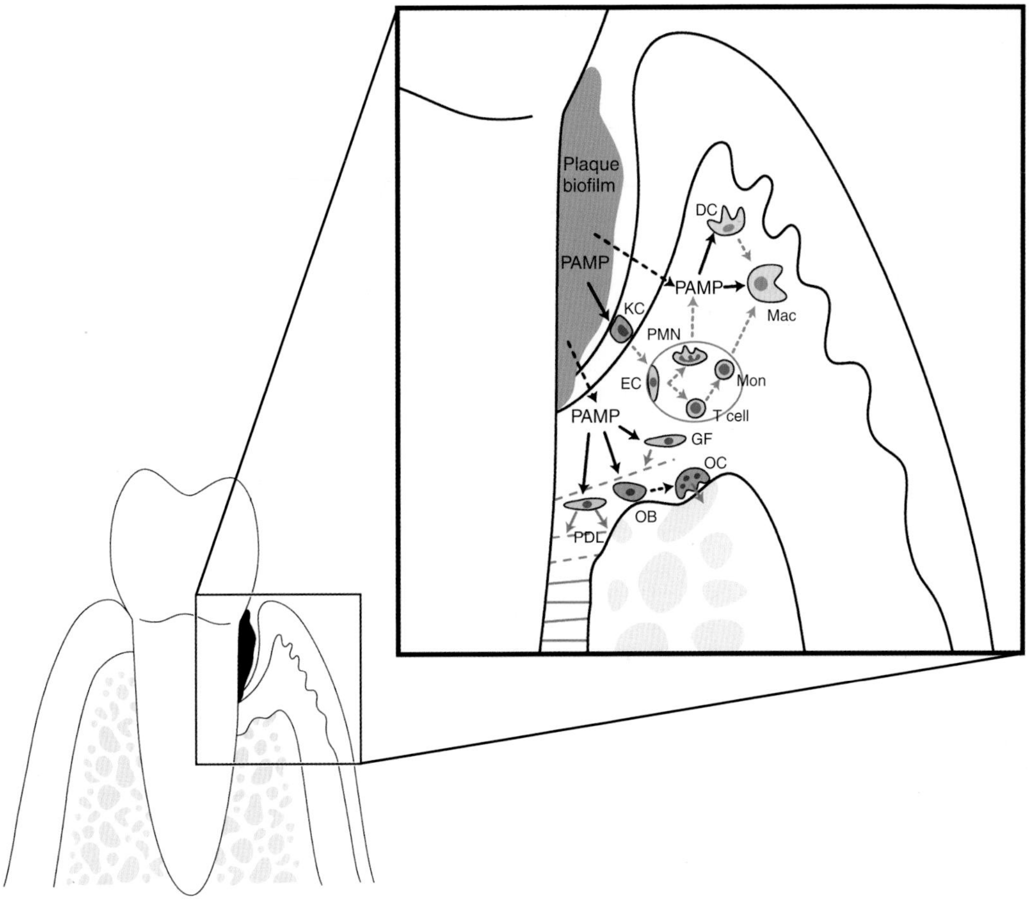

Figure 15-2 Effects of PAMPs on cells. PAMPs from microorganisms in the dental biofilm can directly activate various cell types *(black arrows)*, which will produce a number of biologic mediators. These mediators, in turn, will either affect other cells *(blue-dashed arrows)*, by inducing the expression of other mediators (RANKL expression by osteoblasts) or by triggering chemotaxis *(green-dashed arrows)*. Examples of these effects include the expression of RANKL by osteoblasts and secretion of IL-8 by epithelial cells, respectively. Direct damage to periodontal tissues may also result after PAMP stimulation *(red arrows)*, such as metalloproteinase secretion by gingival and periodontal ligament fibroblasts. See text for more details on the network of events initiated by PAMP stimulation. *PAMP,* Pathogen-associated molecular pattern; *RANKL,* receptor activator of nuclear factor kappa B ligand; *IL-8,* interleukin-8; *KC,* keratinocyte; *DC,* dendritic cell; *Mac,* macrophage; *GF,* gingival fibroblast; *PDL,* periodontal ligament fibroblast; *OB,* osteoblast; *OC,* osteoclast; *EC,* endothelial cell; *PMN,* polymorphonuclear neutrophil; *Mon,* monocyte; *T cell,* T lymphocyte.

from peripheral blood monocytes and can produce various cytokines as well as other biologic mediators (e.g., MMP-1, nitric oxide) when stimulated by CpG and LPS from different periodontal pathogens.[103,116,173]

The **fibroblast** is the most abundant cell of the periodontium and has a central role in homeostasis, pathogenesis, and healing.[59] Gingival fibroblasts and PDL fibroblasts possess distinct phenotypes;[60,146] the PDL fibroblast population presents alkaline phosphatase activity similar to osteoblasts. Gingival fibroblasts can produce a number of proinflammatory cytokines and also express adhesion molecules in response to diverse PAMPs, including LPS, PGN, and CpG DNA from various periodontal pathogens.[60-62,116,122,123,171] However, different PAMPs can have opposing effects, which explains the mechanism used by some microorganisms to evade host immune responses. For example, the capsular polysaccharide from *A. actinomycetemcomitans* strain Y4 can inhibit expression of IL-6 and IL-8 induction in gingival fibroblasts by LPS from the same microorganism. This inhibition of IL-6 and IL-8 can modulate the immune response toward a blocking of bone resorption, which is supported by the increased expression of *osteoprotegerin* (OPG) by LPS-stimulated gingival fibroblasts.[111]

PDL fibroblasts are reported to lack expression of CD14 receptors, which may account for the lower levels of IL-8 produced after LPS stimulation compared with gingival fibroblasts. On stimulation with PGN, however, PDL cells express higher levels of IL-8 than gingival fibroblasts, which may be related to the higher levels of TLR-2 expression.[60] These cells are also able to secrete proteinases, which can result in direct degradation of

TABLE 15-2

Biologic Mediators Elicited by PAMPs in Resident and Nonresident Cells Involved in Pathogenesis of Destructive Periodontal Disease

Cell Type	PAMPs*	Biologic Mediator*	References
Epithelial cells	LPS, fimbriae, glycoprotein, whole bacteria, cell wall extracts	IL-8, G-CSF, GM-CSF, β-defensin-2, MMP-3, MMP-9	21, 26, 53, 66, 68, 140, 154, 170
Dendritic cells	Fimbriae, LPS, CpG DNA, DNA	IFN-α, IL-6, IL-8, IL-10, IL-12, TNF-α, GM-CSF	72, 77, 78, 128, 147
Endothelial cells	LPS, heat-shock proteins	IL-6, GM-CSF, ICAM-1	27, 35, 76, 97
Gingival fibroblasts	LPS, peptidoglycan, CpG DNA	IL1β, IL-6, IL-8, TNF-α, PGE_2, MCP-1	31, 60, 116, 122, 123, 130, 131, 157, 170, 171
Periodontal ligament fibroblasts	LPS	IL-6, IL-8, MMP-13	60, 133, 172
Cementoblasts	LPS	OPN, OCN, RANKL	115
Macrophages	LPS, CpG DNA	IL-1α, IL-1β, IL-6, IL-12, TNF-α, MMP-1, NO	103, 116, 122, 132, 159
Osteoblasts	LPS	IL-1β, IL-6, TNF-α, RANKL, PGE_2, NO, MMP-2, MMP-9	79, 125, 150, 176
Neutrophils	DNA	IL-8, chemotaxis, shedding of L-selectin	161, 162
Monocytes	LPS, CpG DNA, fimbriae	IFN-γ, IL-1β, IL-6, IL-8, IL-12, TNF-α, RANKL, PGE_2	12, 27, 30, 35, 52, 56, 74, 85, 95, 111, 131, 132
B lymphocytes	CpG DNA, heat-stress proteins, cell sonicate extracts	IL-6, IL-10, IL-12, TNF-α, proliferation, antibody production	18, 120, 166, 175
T lymphocytes	LPS, CpG DNA, peptidoglycan	IFN-β, IL-4, IL-10, IL-13, inhibition of apoptosis	40, 100, 101, 128, 175

*See text for clarification of PAMPs and mediators.

both soft and mineralized tissues. Also present in the periodontal ligament (PDL) region, **cementoblasts** stimulated by LPS exhibit decreased levels of expression of the *receptor activator of NF-κB ligand* (RANKL) and, similar to gingival fibroblasts, increased expression of both OPG as well as *osteopontin* (OPN). Moreover, these effects were mediated by TLR-4 in one study, and possibly by TLR-2, and may be a protective mechanism against bone and root resorption.[115]

Endothelial cells lining blood vessels may be stimulated by IL-8 secreted by other host cells and also directly by LPS through TLR-4 and the p38 MAPK pathway,[34] ultimately leading to activation and increased adhesion of monocytes.[30] This effect is related to the induction of cytokine production and increased expression of adhesion molecules E-selectin, ICAM-1, and VCAM-1 induced by PAMPs.[35,76] These cells can also function as APCs, expressing both MHC class I and MHC class II. In fact, activated endothelial cells may induce the production of IL-2, IL-4, and IFN-β by both naive and memory T cells in the presence of a co-stimulatory factor (LFA-3), even though this effect is insufficient to promote differentiation of naive T cells into T helper type 1 (Th1) effector cells.[93]

Osteoblasts are also sensitive to PAMPs; in particular, LPS can induce production of multiple proinflammatory cytokines and biologic mediators involved in bone resorption, as well as inhibit expression of the bone-protecting factor OPG.[125,150] *P. intermedia* LPS also inhibits osteoblast differentiation and mineralization, resulting in a shift in bone homeostasis.[125] Moreover, LPS from different periodontal pathogens, CpG DNA, and capsular polysaccharide from *A. actinomycetemcomitans* promote osteoclast differentiation of bone marrow cells.[70,114,176-178] In the absence of stromal cells and osteoblasts, however, LPS inhibits RANKL-induced differentiation of osteoclast precursors (bone marrow–derived monocytes) as a result of decreased levels of both macrophage colony-stimulating factor (M-CSF) receptor and RANK (see later discussion). Interestingly, if these osteoclast precursor cells are primed with RANKL, LPS synergistically increases differentiation, and this effect is influenced by autocrine stimulation with LPS-induced TNF-α and prostaglandin E_2 (PGE_2).[114,176]

Effects on Nonresident Cells

Neutrophils respond to cytokines secreted by activated host cells, such as IL-8 released by epithelial cells, and to the adhesion molecules expressed by stimulated endothelial cells. PAMPs may also directly stimulate these cells, inducing chemotaxis, shedding of the adhesion molecule L-selectin, and cytokine production, effects mediated by TLR-2 expression.[161]

Monocytes stimulated by PAMPs produce inflammatory cytokines[12,56,95,120-122,132] and also increase proliferation[132] and adhesion to endothelial cells.[30] Importantly, LPS induces differentiation of monocytes into osteoclasts even in the absence of osteoblasts, and the induction RANKL expression is thought to play a central role on this effect.[74] However, some of these effects of PAMPs on monocytes are hypothesized to be either dependent or at least enhanced by the presence of co-stimulatory factors, such as granulocyte-macrophage colony-stimulating factor (GM-CSF). Secretion of IL-12 plays an important role in the activation of T cells to produce IFN-γ, which leads to the development of a Th1 T-cell response, characterized by cell-mediated immunity. In the presence of IL-12, *P. gingivalis* LPS significantly increases IFN-γ production by T cells and also augments production of IL-12 by monocytes, suggesting a positive-feedback mechanism enhancing the Th1 immune response.[175] On the other hand, without co-stimulatory factors, *P. gingivalis* LPS fails to induce proinflammatory cytokines on monocytes; on the contrary, it induces expression of antiinflammatory IL-10 that can downregulate IL-12 levels and shift the immune response toward a Th2 pattern. These effects are counteracted by inhibition of MEK1 (ERK1/2) and phosphatidylinositol-3 kinase (PI3K) pathways, resulting in an increase of IL-12 and a decrease in IL-10 expression.[99] Differential regulation by distinct signaling pathways is also shown for LPS-induced MMP expression. Although MMP-1 is positively regulated by p38 MAPK, one study showed that ERK 1/2 MAPK regulated both MMP-1 and MMP-9 expression induced by LPS.[85] On the other hand, interleukin-1 receptor antagonist (IL-1ra) production is potently induced by *P. gingivalis* LPS, which may result in inhibition of inflammatory destructive processes.[132]

B lymphocytes are also directly stimulated by PAMPs, specifically CpG DNA, because they lack expression of TLR-4 while also expressing TLR-9.[166] This leads to proliferation, antibody production in plasmocytes, expression of co-stimulatory factors (e.g., MHC class II, CD80, CD86), and production of inflammatory cytokines,[179] including IL-12, in the presence of co-stimulatory factors.[166]

T lymphocytes usually are activated through interaction with other cells and their biologic mediators, resulting in differentiation of either a Th1 or a Th2 type of immune response. However, LPS can also directly induce proliferation and secretion of cytokines, but this effect depends on the microorganism species and probably is also influenced by the strain within the same species. LPS from *E. coli* was demonstrated to induce both CD4+ and CD8+ T cells to produce IFN-γ, whereas *P. gingivalis* LPS resulted in higher levels of Th2 cytokines.[128] These effects of LPS on T cells are thought to be dependent on the presence of viable monocytes and soluble co-stimulatory factors.[100,101] Interestingly, no difference was observed for the proliferative effects of LPS between naive and memory CD4+ T lymphocytes.[100] Besides activating and inducing differentiation of T cells, CpG DNA, which is a ligand for TLR-3 and TLR-9, was shown to inhibit CD4+ apoptosis; however, PGN and LPS, ligands for TLR-2 and TLR-4, respectively, did not have the same effect,[40] demonstrating that the activation of different receptors by PAMPs may trigger diverse signaling pathways, resulting in the modulation of a cell response.

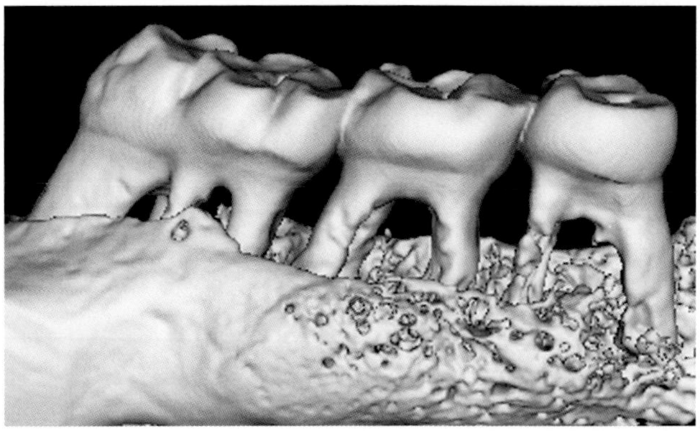

Figure 15-3 Lipopolysaccharide (LPS)-mediated experimental bone destruction. MicroCT three-dimensional reconstruction of rat maxilla after 8 weeks of *P. gingivalis* LPS injection at the interproximal area three times a week. This palatal view shows severe horizontal and vertical bone destruction and generalized furcation lesions around the first, second, and third molar teeth.

PATHOBIOLOGY OF LIPOPOLYSACCHARIDE-MEDIATED BONE DESTRUCTION

P. gingivalis LPS is considered a key factor in the development of periodontitis; Figure 15-3 shows an example of *P. gingivalis* LPS-mediated experimental periodontitis. LPS induction of disease leads to the initiation of a local host response in gingival tissues that involves recruitment of inflammatory cells, generation of prostanoids and cytokines, elaboration of lytic enzymes, and activation of osteoclasts.[41,92] Specifically, LPS increases osteoblastic expression of RANKL, IL-1, PGE_2, and TNF-α, each known to induce osteoclast activity, viability, and differentiation.[176] Figure 15-4 provides an overview of bone resorption/formation and remodeling.

SIMILARITIES OF PERIODONTAL DISEASES TO OTHER CHRONIC INFLAMMATORY DISEASES: RHEUMATOID ARTHRITIS

A variety of immune-associated cell populations are responsible for the pathogenesis of periodontal diseases, including specific CD+ T cells. The pathogenic process is most likely a response to exogenous periodontal pathogens such as *P. gingivalis* associated with plaque biofilms.[25] Consequently, recruited monocytes, macrophages, and fibroblasts produce cytokines (e.g., TNF-α, IL-1β) within periodontal lesions. These cytokines may be localized in periodontal tissues as well as in gingival crevicular fluid

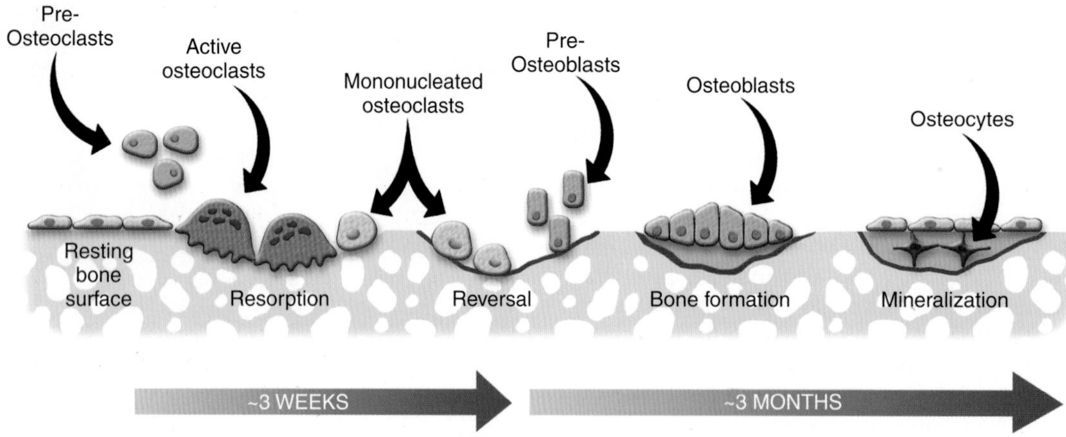

Figure 15-4 Bone-remodeling cycle. Pre-osteoclasts are recruited to sites of resorption, induced to differentiate into active osteoclasts, and form resorption pits. After their period of active resorption, they are replaced by transient mononuclear cells. Through the process of coupling, pre-osteoblasts are recruited, differentiate into active matrix-secreting cells, and form bone. Some osteoblasts become entrapped in the matrix and become osteocytes. (Modified from McCauley LK, Koh-Paige AJ, Chen H, et al: *Endocrinology* 142:1975, 2001.)

TABLE 15-3

Comparison of Pathobiology: Periodontal Disease and Rheumatoid Arthritis

	Periodontal Disease	Rheumatoid Arthritis
Proinflammatory cytokines: IL-1, IL-6, TNF-α	High levels	High levels
MMPs	High levels	High levels
TIMPs (MMP inhibitors)	Low levels	Low levels
PGE_2	Present	Present
Inflammatory infiltrate on lesion site	Present	Present
Active osteoclast	Present	Present
C-reactive protein	Elevated level	Elevated level
NSAID effect	Reported	Reported

Modified from Mercado FB, Marshall RI, Klestov AC, et al: *J Periodontol* 72:779, 2001; and Mercado FB, Marshall RI, Bartold PM: *J Clin Periodontol* 30:761, 2003.

IL-1, -6, Interleukin-1, -6; *TNF-α,* tumor necrosis factor alpha; *MMPs,* matrix metalloproteinases; *TIMP,* tissue inhibitors of metalloproteinase; *PGE_2,* prostaglandin E_2; *NSAID,* nonsteroidal antiinflammatory drug.

(GCF) associated with the lesion. These cytokines are central to the damaging cascade, ultimately triggering the production of MMPs, prostaglandins, and osteoclasts. The end result of this cascade is an irreversible damage to tooth-supporting soft tissues and alveolar bone.[47,48] Although the disease is initiated by specific oral pathogens that colonize and invade the oral tissues, the host inflammatory response is a major factor in the progression of disease.

Chronic periodontal disease also demonstrates a high degree of similarity in terms of pathogenesis to rheumatoid arthritis (RA), a bone-destructive disease that displays periods of remission and exacerbation[107,108] (Table 15-3).

Targets for Inflammatory Periodontal Diseases

Inflammatory reactions involve a number of biochemical and cellular alterations. An inappropriate inflammatory response is the cause of many common diseases, including periodontitis and RA. The local inflammatory reaction, in response to plaque bacteria, is characterized by an initial increase in blood flow, enhanced vascular permeability, and the influx of cells from the peripheral blood to the gingival crevice. Polymorphonuclear leukocytes (PMNs), or neutrophils, migrate through the epithelial lining of the gingival pocket to be the first line of defense against invading plaque bacteria and their byproducts.[94] These cells are nonspecific phagocytes responsible for an acute and rapid defense. Subsequently, monocytes/macrophages, T cells, and B cells appear at the site of injury or infection.[37] These cells are antigen specific and modulate the immune responses.[87,42] Once activated, they produce inflammatory mediators such as anaphylatoxins of the complement cascade, kinins of the coagulation system, leukotrienes, prostaglandins, and neuropeptides. Cytokines responsible for early responses include IL-1α, IL-1β, IL-6, and TNF-α.[86] Other proinflammatory mediators include leukemia-inhibiting factor (LIF); IFN-γ; oncostatin M (OSM); ciliary neurotrophic factor (CNTF); transforming growth factor beta (TGF-β); GM-CSF; IL-11, IL-12, IL-17, IL-18, IL-8, and a variety of other chemokines that attract inflammatory cells; and various neuromodulatory factors.[17,119,135-139] The net effect of an inflammatory response is determined by the balance between proinflammatory cytokines and antiinflammatory cytokines such as IL-4, IL-10, IL-13, IL-16, IFN-α, TGF-β, IL-1ra, GM-CSF, and soluble receptors for TNF or IL-6.[48,88] Table 15-4 lists bone resorptive cytokines.

TABLE 15-4

Mediators of Bone Resorption

Stimulators	Inhibitors
Interleukin-1 (IL-1)	Interferon-γ (IFN-γ)
Interleukin-6 (IL-6)	Osteoprotegerin (OPG)
Tumor necrosis factor (TNF)	Estrogens
Parathyroid hormone (PTH)	Androgens
PTH-related protein (PTHrP)	Calcitonin (CT)
Prostaglandin E_2 (PGE_2)	Cyclosporin
Macrophage colony-stimulating factor (M-CSF)	
Receptor activator of NF-κB (RANK)	
RANK ligand (RANKL)	
1,25-Dihydroxyvitamin D_3 (vitamin D)	

Modified from McCauley LK, Koh-Paige AJ, Chen H, et al: *Endocrinology* 142:1975, 2001.

Cytokines and Inflammatory Diseases

Macrophages are exquisitely sensitive to the LPS produced by specific pathogens. They respond by producing cytokines, notably TNF-α, but also IL-1 and IL-6. These mediators induce the *acute-phase response,* which is a rapid systemic response that potently increases the concentration of many key serum proteins to aid the host defense response, such as *C-reactive protein* (CRP) and mannose-binding protein, natural activators of the complement system.[144,145] CRP levels in subjects with either periodontal or cardiovascular disease display twofold increases above subjects with neither disease, whereas a threefold increase in CRP is noted in subjects with both diseases.[43] On the other hand, resolution of the inflammation has been shown to ameliorate the associated elevated inflammatory markers. CRP and IL-6 levels are positively influenced by conventional periodontal treatment and may significantly improve the systemic condition.[24]

TNF-α, an inflammatory cytokine that is released by activated monocytes/macrophages and T lymphocytes, promotes inflammatory responses that are important in the pathogenesis of RA and periodontal diseases. TNF-α binds to two receptors that are expressed by a variety of cells, the *type 1 TNF receptor* (p55) and the *type 2 TNF receptor* (p75).[14] Activation of TNF-R1 upregulates the inflammatory response, whereas TNF-R2 appears to dampen the response.[126] TNF-R1 is expressed on multiple cell types, whereas TNF-R2 is more restricted to expression on endothelial cells and cells of hematopoietic lineage.[69] Blocking TNF-α effectively inhibits osteoclast formation.[20] Indeed, the blockade of TNF can be used as a probe to understand the molecular basis of osteoclastogenesis and also as a target to therapeutic agent development.

Patients with RA and periodontal disease have high concentrations of TNF in the synovial fluid and GCF, respectively. Studies of experimental models of RA and periodontal diseases have shown a strong association of active bone resorption coincident with high local levels of TNF at the disease sites. Both IL-1 and TNF-α have been found to be significantly elevated in diseased periodontal sites compared with healthy or inactive sites.[33,36,45,149] IL-1 has also been positively correlated to increased probing depth and attachment loss.[28] In addition, IL-1β has synergistic activity with TNF-α or lymphotoxin in stimulating bone resorption. Incubation of IL-1 with TNF or lymphotoxin in an in vitro model resulted in a twofold increase in the bone-resorbing activity of IL-1 and a 100-fold increase in activity of TNF or lymphotoxin.[148] Reduction of the bacteria and associated metabolic byproducts through periodontal therapy also results in a decrease in both IL-1β[4,124] and TNF-α.[36,71]

Although periodontal treatment can successfully reduce inflammation, some individuals have demonstrated aggressive bone destruction and high levels of proinflammatory cytokines that cannot be completely explained by bacteria alone. Based on susceptibility analysis, cells from individuals with immune-mediated diseases exhibit different cytokine secretion profiles, which may be explained by genetic differences between individuals causing the hyperresponsiveness.[63] These variances, termed *single-nucleotide polymorphisms* (SNPs), elicit exuberant inflammation in certain individuals and vary significantly in different racial and ethnic populations[7,127,167] (see Chapter 11).

PATHOBIOLOGY OF PERIODONTAL DISEASE PROGRESSION

The pathogenic processes of periodontal diseases are largely the result of the host response to microbial-induced tissue destruction. As previously discussed, these destructive processes are initiated by bacteria, mainly LPS, but are propagated by the host. Periodontal pathogens produce harmful products and enzymes (e.g., hyaluronidases, collagenases, proteases) that break down extracellular matrices such as collagen and even host cell membranes in order to produce nutrients for their growth[13] for subsequent tissue invasion. Arg- and Lys-gingipain cysteine proteinases produced by *P. gingivalis* are key virulence factors and are believed to be essential for significant tissue component degradation, leading to host tissue invasion.[6] Many of the microbial surface protein molecules are actually capable of eliciting an immune response in the host and are also effective in creating local tissue inflammation.[25] *P. gingivalis* possesses multiple virulence factors, such as cytoplasmic membranes, peptidoglycans (PGNs), outer membrane proteins, LPS, capsules, and fimbriae, on the cell surface.[118] All these virulence factors are competent to activate the host response.

Once the immune and inflammatory processes are initiated, various inflammatory molecules, including proteases, MMPs, cytokines, prostaglandins, and host enzymes, are released from leukocytes and fibroblasts or structural cells of the tissues.[81] Proteases tend to break up the collagen structure of the tissues and thus create inroads for further leukocyte infiltration.[6] Mature collagen cross-links *hydroxylysylpyridinoline* (HP) and its deoxy analog, *lysylpyridinoline* (LP), also referred to as

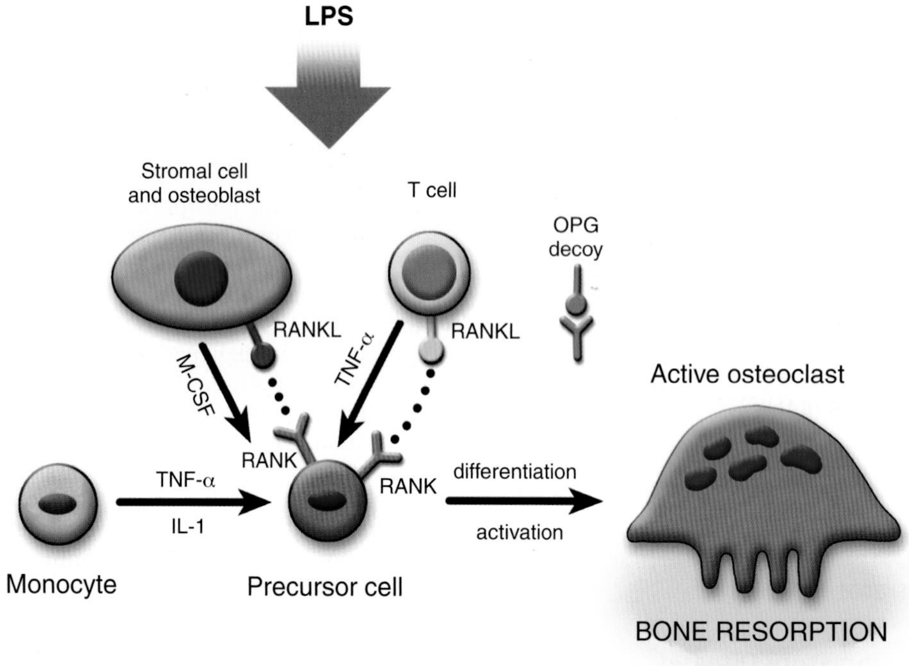

Figure 15-5 Stimuli factors regulating osteoclast formation and function: Cytokines such as interleukin-1 *(IL-1)*, tumor necrosis factor alpha *(TNF-α)*, and macrophage colony-stimulating factor *(M-CSF)*, produced by bone marrow stromal cells, osteoblasts, monocytes, and T cells are key regulators on this process. Osteoprotegerin *(OPG)* acts as a decoy receptor that prevents RANKL from binding to its receptor RANK on precursor cells and downregulate the osteoclastogenesis.

pyridinoline (Pyr) and deoxypyridinoline, respectively, are widely distributed in vertebrate connective tissues, whereas LP, although widely distributed, features most prominently in bone and dentin.[54] Both HP and LP are elevated in tissue with increased collagen resorption, and the pyridinoline residues from collagenase digestion can be used as markers.[42] Although the production of collagenase from infiltrating neutrophils is part of the natural host response to infection, an imbalance exists between the level of activated tissue-destroying MMPs and their endogenous inhibitors in periodontal disease and other inflammatory diseases.[44]

As periodontal disease progresses, the collagen fibers and connective tissue attachment to the tooth are destroyed, the epithelial cells proliferate apically along the root surface, and periodontal pockets deepen. As the junctional epithelium migrates apically, so too does the extent of the tissue inflammatory infiltrate. Moreover, activated osteoclasts initiate bone destruction. The activation signaling is modulated by RANKL, RANK, and OPG, three novel members of the TNF ligand and receptor superfamilies[90] (Figure 15-5). Briefly, a number of hormones and cytokines modulate osteoclastogenesis by enhancing osteoclast differentiation, activation, life span, and function. These include parathyroid hormone (PTH), calcitriol, PTH-related protein, PGE_2, thyroxine, and IL-11.[32,102,151] The formation of active osteoclasts requires M-CSF[96,158] and involves cell-to-cell contact between precursors of the monocyte/macrophage lineage and osteoblasts, marrow stromal cells, and T and B cells.

SCIENCE TRANSFER

Many signaling pathways result in periodontal inflammation and bone loss, and multiple cells are involved in significant interactions between inflammatory mediators and their antagonists. Elucidation of the molecular bases for periodontal breakdown offers the opportunity for therapeutic manipulation of advancing periodontal destruction. Matrix metalloproteinase (MMP) inhibitors such as doxycycline already are being used to treat periodontal disease. In addition, soluble antagonists of the destructive cytokines interleukin-1 (IL-1) and tumor necrosis factor (TNF), together with cytokine inhibitors that interrupt cell-signaling NF-κB and p38 mitogen-activated protein kinase (MAPK) pathways, are potential local agents for future use in patient care.

These cells express the receptor activator of NF-κB ligand *(RANKL)*, a member of the TNF ligand family, which is essential for this process. RANKL attaches to *RANK*, a receptor on the cell surface of osteoclasts and osteoclast precursors, to stimulate proliferation and differentiation of cells to form the osteoclast phenotype and inhibit apoptosis.[23] Osteoprotegerin (OPG), a soluble decoy

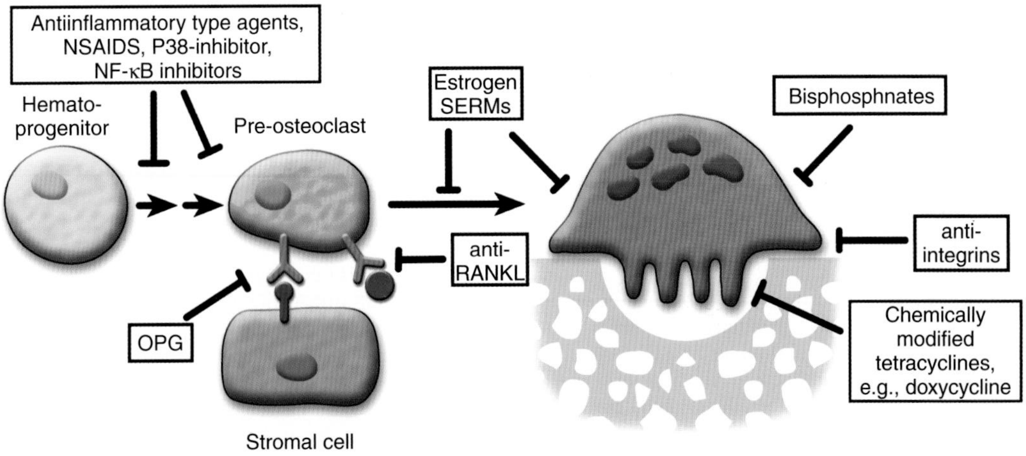

Figure 15-6 Potential therapeutic strategies to treat bone resorption. Agents that block the differentiation or activity of osteoclasts are potential therapeutic agents. Osteoprotegerin *(OPG)* inhibits the differentiation of osteoclasts through its action as a decoy receptor that blocks RANKL and RANK juxtacrine interaction. Nonsteroidal antiinflammatory drugs *(NSAIDs)* and other antiinflammatory molecules can inhibit the formation of hematoprogenitor cells to pre-osteoclasts. Antibodies to RANKL can also block this interaction. Estrogen and selective estrogen receptor modulators (*SERMs)* may inhibit the activity of osteoclasts but also may promote apoptosis of osteoclasts, thus reducing their active life span. Bisphosphonates also promote osteoclast apoptosis. Chemically modified tetracyclines reduce the protease degradation of the organic matrix, and antiintegrins block the initial osteoclast adhesion to the matrix. (Modified from McCauley LK, Koh-Paige AJ, Chen H, et al: *Endocrinology* 142:1975, 2001.)

receptor produced by osteoblasts, marrow stromal cells, and other cells, profoundly modifies the effects of RANKL by inhibiting RANKL/RANK interaction;[143] OPG has shown promising results for the treatment of bone-related diseases.[82] In the presence of periodontal pathogens (e.g., *A. actinomycetemcomitans*), CD4+ T cells present increased expression of RANKL, triggering the activation of osteoclasts and causing bone loss.[160] Similar mechanisms leading to bone loss are caused by excessive osteoclastic activity in RA[46] and osteoporosis.[112] Once the destructive pattern continues, the accumulation of subgingival plaque increases, with subsequent increase in microbial density to propagate further the destructive periodontal lesion. As the pocket deepens, the flora becomes more anaerobic, and the host response becomes more destructive and chronic. Eventually, the periodontitis lesion progresses to such an extent that the tooth is lost.[80,88]

THERAPEUTIC STRATEGIES DISRUPTING HOST-CELL SIGNALING FOR TREATMENT OF PERIODONTAL DISEASES

A variety of treatment strategies have been developed to target the host response to LPS-mediated tissue destruction (Figure 15-6). Chapters 16 and 53 provide mechanistic overviews and clinical applications on the use of host modulatory therapeutic regimens for periodontal disease management. MMP inhibitors, such as low-dose formulations of doxycycline, have been used in combination with scaling and root planing[16] or surgical therapy.[38] In addition, high-risk patient populations, such as diabetic patients or those with refractory periodontal disease, have benefited from systemic MMP administration.[19,117,134] Encouraging results have been shown using soluble antagonists of TNF and IL-1 delivered locally to periodontal tissues in nonhuman primates,[10] as well as more recent evidence using gene therapy vectors to provide a longer-term delivery of TNF receptor antagonists at the periodontium (Taba and Giannobile, personal communication).

Other therapeutic strategies being explored are aimed at inhibiting signal transduction pathways involved in inflammation. Pharmacologic inhibitors of NF-κB and p38 MAPK pathways are actively being developed to manage RA and inflammatory bone diseases[1,75,84] (see Figures 15-1 and 15-6). Using this novel strategy, inflammatory mediators, including proinflammatory cytokines (IL-1, TNF, IL-6) and MMPs, would be inhibited at the level of cell-signaling pathways required for transcription factor activation necessary for inflammatory gene expression or mRNA stability. These therapies may provide the next wave of adjuvant chemotherapeutic agents, which may be used to manage chronic periodontitis.

REFERENCES

1. Adams JL, Badger AM, Kumar S, et al: p38 MAP kinase: molecular target for the inhibition of pro-inflammatory cytokines, *Prog Med Chem* 38:1, 2001.
2. Akira S: Toll-like receptors and innate immunity, *Adv Immunol* 78:1, 2001.
3. Akira S: Toll-like receptor signaling, *J Biol Chem* 278:38105, 2003.
4. Al-Shammari KF, Giannobile WV, Aldredge WA, et al: Effect of non-surgical periodontal therapy on C-telopeptide pyridinoline cross-links (ICTP) and interleukin-1 levels, *J Periodontol* 72:1045, 2001.

5. An H, Yu Y, Zhang M, et al: Involvement of ERK, p38 and NF-κB signal transduction in regulation of TLR2, TLR4 and TLR9 gene expression induced by lipopolysaccharide in mouse dendritic cells, *Immunology* 106:38, 2002.
6. Andrian E, Grenier D, Rouabhia M: In vitro models of tissue penetration and destruction by *Porphyromonas gingivalis, Infect Immun* 72:4689, 2004.
7. Armitage GC, Wu Y, Wang HY, et al: Low prevalence of a periodontitis-associated interleukin-1 composite genotype in individuals of Chinese heritage, *J Periodontol* 71:164, 2000.
8. Asai Y, Jinno T, Ogawa T: Oral treponemes and their outer membrane extracts activate human gingival epithelial cells through toll-like receptor 2, *Infect Immun* 71:717, 2003.
9. Asai Y, Ohyama Y, Gen K, et al: Bacterial fimbriae and their peptides activate human gingival epithelial cells through toll-like receptor 2, *Infect Immun* 69:7387, 2001.
10. Assuma R, Oates T, Cochran D, et al: IL-1 and TNF antagonists inhibit the inflammatory response and bone loss in experimental periodontitis, *J Immunol* 160:403, 1998.
11. Bainbridge BW, Darveau RP: *Porphyromonas gingivalis* lipopolysaccharide: an unusual pattern recognition receptor ligand for the innate host defense system, *Acta Odontol Scand* 59:131, 2001.
12. Baqui AA, Meiller TF, Chon JJ, et al: Granulocyte-macrophage colony-stimulating factor amplification of interleukin-1beta and tumor necrosis factor alpha production in THP-1 human monocytic cells stimulated with lipopolysaccharide of oral microorganisms, *Clin Diagn Lab Immunol* 5:341, 1998.
13. Bartold PM, Page RC: The effect of chronic inflammation on gingival connective tissue proteoglycans and hyaluronic acid, *J Oral Pathol* 15:367, 1986.
14. Bouwmeester T, Bauch A, Ruffner H, et al: A physical and functional map of the human TNF-α/NF-κB signal transduction pathway, *Nat Cell Biol* 6:97, 2004.
15. Calkins CC, Platt K, Potempa J, et al: Inactivation of tumor necrosis factor-alpha by proteinases (gingipains) from the periodontal pathogen, *Porphyromonas gingivalis:* implications of immune evasion, *J Biol Chem* 273:6611, 1998.
16. Caton JG, Ciancio SG, Blieden TM, et al: Subantimicrobial dose doxycycline as an adjunct to scaling and root planing: post-treatment effects, *J Clin Periodontol* 28:782, 2001.
17. Cavaillon JM: Cytokines and macrophages, *Biomed Pharmacother* 48:445, 1994.
18. Champaiboon C, Yongvanitchit K, Pichyangkul S, et al: The immune modulation of B-cell responses by *Porphyromonas ginginvalis* and interleukin-10, *J Periodontol* 71:468, 2000.
19. Chang KM, Ryan ME, Golub LM, et al: Local and systemic factors in periodontal disease increase matrix-degrading enzyme activities in rat gingiva: effect of micocycline therapy, *Res Commun Mol Pathol Pharmacol* 91:303, 1996.
20. Cheng X., Kinosaki M, Murali R, et al: The TNF receptor superfamily: role in immune inflammation and bone formation, *Immunol Res* 27:287, 2003.
21. Chung WO, Dale BA: Innate immune response of oral and foreskin keratinocytes: utilization of different signaling pathways by various bacterial species, *Infect Immun* 72:352, 2004.
22. Cobb MH, Goldsmith EJ: How MAP kinases are regulated, *J Biol Chem* 270:14843, 1995.
23. Crotti TN, Ahern MJ, Lange K, et al: Variability of RANKL and osteoprotegerin staining in synovial tissue from patients with active rheumatoid arthritis: quantification using color video image analysis, *J Rheumatol* 30:2319, 2003.
24. D'Aiuto F, Parkar M, Andreou G, et al: Periodontitis and systemic inflammation: control of the local infection is associated with a reduction in serum inflammatory markers, *J Dent Res* 83:156, 2004.
25. Darveau RP, Tanner A, Page RC: The microbial challenge in periodontitis, *Periodontol 2000* 14:12, 1997.
26. Darveau RP, Belton CM, Reife RA, et al: Local chemokine paralysis, a novel pathogenic mechanism for *Porphyromonas gingivalis, Infect Immun* 66:1660, 1998.
27. Darveau RP, Arbabi S, Garcia I, et al: *Porphyromonas gingivalis* lipopolysaccharide is both agonist and antagonist for p38 mitogen-activated protein kinase activation, *Infect Immun* 70:1867, 2002.
28. Delima AJ, Karatzas S, Amar S, et al: Inflammation and tissue loss caused by periodontal pathogens is reduced by interleukin-1 antagonists, *J Infect Dis* 186:511, 2002.
29. Dillon S, Agrawal A, van Dyke T, et al: A toll-like receptor 2 ligand stimulates Th2 responses in vivo, via induction of extracellular signal–regulated kinase mitogen-activated protein kinase and c-Fos in dendritic cells, *J Immunol* 172:4733, 2004.
30. Doherty DE, Zagarella L, Henson PM, et al: Lipopolysaccharide stimulates monocyte adherence by effects on both the monocyte and the endothelial cell, *J Immunol* 143:3673, 1989.
31. Dongari-Bagtzoglou AI, Ebersole JL: Production of inflammatory mediators and cytokines by human gingival fibroblasts following bacterial challenge, *J Periodontal Res* 31:90, 1996.
32. Duong LT, Rodan GA: Regulation of osteoclast formation and function, *Rev Endocr Metab Disord* 2:95, 2001.
33. Ejeil AL, Gaultier F, Igondjo-Tchen S, et al: Are cytokines linked to collagen breakdown during periodontal disease progression? *J Periodontol* 74:196, 2003.
34. Faure E, Equils O, Sieling PA, et al: Bacterial lipopolysaccharide activates NF-κB through toll-like receptor 4 (TLR-4) in cultured human dermal endothelial cells: differential expression of TLR-4 and TLR-2 in endothelial cells, *J Biol Chem* 275:11058, 2000.
35. Galdiero M, de l'Ero GC, Marcatili A: Cytokine and adhesion molecule expression in human monocytes and endothelial cells stimulated with bacterial heat shock proteins, *Infect Immun* 65:699, 1997.
36. Gamonal J, Acevedo A, Bascones A, et al: Levels of interleukin-1 beta, -8, and -10 and RANTES in gingival crevicular fluid and cell populations in adult periodontitis patients and the effect of periodontal treatment, *J Periodontol* 71:1535, 2000.
37. Gamonal J, Acevedo A, Bascones A, et al: Characterization of cellular infiltrate, detection of chemokine receptor CCR5 and interleukin-8 and RANTES chemokines in adult periodontitis, *J Periodontal Res* 36:194, 2001.
38. Gapski R, Barr JL, Sarment DP, et al: Effect of systemic matrix metalloproteinase inhibition on periodontal wound repair: a proof of concept trial, *J Periodontol* 75:441, 2004.
39. Geatch DR, Harris JI, Heasman PA, et al: In vitro studies of lymphocyte apoptosis induced by the periodontal pathogen *Porphyromonas gingivalis, J Periodontal Res* 34:70, 1999.
40. Gelman AE, Zhang J, Choi Y, et al: Toll-like receptor ligands directly promote activated CD4+ T cell survival, *J Immunol* 172:6065, 2004.
41. Genco CA, van Dyke T, Amar S: Animal models for *Porphyromonas gingivalis*–mediated periodontal disease, *Trends Microbiol* 6:444, 1998.
42. Giannobile WV, Lynch SE, Denmark RG, et al: Crevicular fluid osteocalcin and pyridinoline cross-linked carboxy-terminal telopeptide of type I collagen (ICTP) as markers

of rapid bone turnover in periodontitis: a pilot study in beagle dogs, *J Clin Periodontol* 22:903, 1995.
43. Glurich I, Grossi S, Albini B, et al: Systemic inflammation in cardiovascular and periodontal disease: comparative study, *Clin Diagn Lab Immunol* 9:425, 2002.
44. Golub LM, Lee HM, Greenwald RA, et al: A matrix metalloproteinase inhibitor reduces bone-type collagen degradation fragments and specific collagenases in gingival crevicular fluid during adult periodontitis, *Inflamm Res* 46:310, 1997.
45. Gorska R, Gregorek H, Kowalski J, et al: Relationship between clinical parameters and cytokine profiles in inflamed gingival tissue and serum samples from patients with chronic periodontitis, *J Clin Periodontol* 30:1046, 2003.
46. Gravallese EM, Goldring SR: Cellular mechanisms and the role of cytokines in bone erosions in rheumatoid arthritis, *Arthritis Rheum* 43:2143, 2000.
47. Graves DT: The potential role of chemokines and inflammatory cytokines in periodontal disease progression, *Clin Infect Dis* 28:482, 1999.
48. Graves DT, Delima AJ, Assuma R, et al: Interleukin-1 and tumor necrosis factor antagonists inhibit the progression of inflammatory cell infiltration toward alveolar bone in experimental periodontitis, *J Periodontol* 69:1419, 1998.
49. Hajishengallis G, Genco RJ: Downregulation of the DNA-binding activity of nuclear factor-kappaB p65 subunit in *Porphyromonas gingivalis* fimbria-induced tolerance, *Infect Immun* 72:1188, 2004.
50. Hajishengallis G, Martin M, Schifferle RE, et al: Counteracting interactions between lipopolysaccharide molecules with differential activation of toll-like receptors, *Infect Immun* 70:6658, 2002.
51. Hajishengallis G, Martin M, Sojar HT, et al: Dependence of bacterial protein adhesins on toll-like receptors for proinflammatory cytokine induction, *Clin Diagn Lab Immunol* 9:403, 2002.
52. Hajishengallis G, Sojar H, Genco RJ, et al: Intracellular signaling and cytokine induction upon interactions of *Porphyromonas gingivalis* fimbriae with pattern-recognition receptors, *Immunol Invest* 33:157, 2004.
53. Han YW, Shi W, Huang GT, et al: Interactions between periodontal bacteria and human oral epithelial cells: *Fusobacterium nucleatum* adheres to and invades epithelial cells, *Infect Immun* 68:3140, 2000.
54. Hanson DA, Eyre DR: Molecular site specificity of pyridinoline and pyrrole cross-links in type I collagen of human bone, *J Biol Chem* 271:26508, 1996.
55. Harris JI, Russell RR, Curtis MA, et al: Molecular mediators of *Porphyromonas gingivalis*–induced T-cell apoptosis, *Oral Microbiol Immunol* 17:224, 2002.
56. Hartmann G, Krieg AM: CpG DNA and LPS induce distinct patterns of activation in human monocytes, *Gene Ther* 6:893, 1999.
57. Hasebe A, Yoshimura A, Into T, et al: Biological activities of *Bacteroides forsythus* lipoproteins and their possible pathological roles in periodontal disease, *Infect Immun* 72:1318, 2004.
58. Hashimoto M, Asai Y, Ogawa T: Treponemal phospholipids inhibit innate immune responses induced by pathogen-associated molecular patterns, *J Biol Chem* 278:44205, 2003.
59. Hassell TM: Tissues and cells of the periodontium, *Periodontol 2000* 3:9, 1993.
60. Hatakeyama J, Tamai R, Sugiyama A, et al: Contrasting responses of human gingival and periodontal ligament fibroblasts to bacterial cell-surface components through the CD14/toll-like receptor system, *Oral Microbiol Immunol* 18:14, 2003.
61. Hayashi F, Means TK, Luster AD: Toll-like receptors stimulate human neutrophil function, *Blood* 102:2660, 2003.
62. Hayashi J, Masaka T, Saito I, et al: Soluble CD14 mediates lipopolysaccharide-induced intercellular adhesion molecule 1 expression in cultured human gingival fibroblasts, *Infect Immun* 64:4946, 1996.
63. Hill AV: Immunogenetics: defence by diversity, *Nature* 398(6729):668, 1999.
64. Hiramine H, Watanabe K, Hamada N, et al: *Porphyromonas gingivalis* 67-kDa fimbriae induced cytokine production and osteoclast differentiation utilizing TLR2, *FEMS Microbiol Lett* 229:49, 2003.
65. Hirschfeld M, Weis JJ, Toshchakov V, et al: Signaling by toll-like receptor 2 and 4 agonists results in differential gene expression in murine macrophages, *Infect Immun* 69:1477, 2001.
66. Huang GT, Haake SK, Park NH: Gingival epithelial cells increase interleukin-8 secretion in response to *Actinobacillus actinomycetemcomitans* challenge, *J Periodontol* 69:1105, 1998.
67. Huang GT, Haake SK, Kim JW, et al: Differential expression of interleukin-8 and intercellular adhesion molecule-1 by human gingival epithelial cells in response to *Actinobacillus actinomycetemcomitans* or *Porphyromonas gingivalis* infection, *Oral Microbiol Immunol* 13:301, 1998.
68. Huang GT, Kim D, Lee JK, et al: Interleukin-8 and intercellular adhesion molecule 1 regulation in oral epithelial cells by selected periodontal bacteria: multiple effects of *Porphyromonas gingivalis* via antagonistic mechanisms, *Infect Immun* 69:1364, 2001.
69. Idriss HT, Naismith JH: TNF alpha and the TNF receptor superfamily: structure-function relationship(s), *Microsc Res Tech* 50:184, 2000.
70. Ito HO, Shuto T, Takada H, et al: Lipopolysaccharides from *Porphyromonas gingivalis, Prevotella intermedia* and *Actinobacillus actinomycetemcomitans* promote osteoclastic differentiation in vitro, *Arch Oral Biol* 41:439, 1996.
71. Iwamoto Y, Nishimura F, Soga Y, et al: Antimicrobial periodontal treatment decreases serum C-reactive protein, tumor necrosis factor-alpha, but not adiponectin levels in patients with chronic periodontitis, *J Periodontol* 74:1231, 2003.
72. Jakob T, Walker PS, Krieg AM, et al: Activation of cutaneous dendritic cells by CpG-containing oligodeoxynucleotides: a role for dendritic cells in the augmentation of Th1 responses by immunostimulatory DNA, *J Immunol* 161:3042, 1998.
73. Janeway CA Jr, Medzhitov R: Innate immune recognition, *Annu Rev Immunol* 20:197, 2002.
74. Jiang Y, Mehta CK, Hsu TY, et al: Bacteria induce osteoclastogenesis via an osteoblast-independent pathway, *Infect Immun* 70:3143, 2002.
75. Jimi E, Aoki K, Saito H, et al: Selective inhibition of NF-κB blocks osteoclastogenesis and prevents inflammatory bone destruction in vivo, *Nat Med* 10:617, 2004.
76. Jirik FR, Podor TJ, Hirano T, et al: Bacterial lipopolysaccharide and inflammatory mediators augment IL-6 secretion by human endothelial cells, *J Immunol* 142:144, 1989.
77. Jotwani R, Cutler CW: Fimbriated *Porphyromonas gingivalis* is more efficient than fimbria-deficient *P. gingivalis* in entering human dendritic cells in vitro and induces an inflammatory Th1 effector response, *Infect Immun* 72:1725, 2004.
78. Jotwani R, Pulendran B, Agrawal S, et al: Human dendritic cells respond to *Porphyromonas gingivalis* LPS by promoting a Th2 effector response in vitro, *Eur J Immunol* 33:2980, 2003.
79. Kikuchi T, Matsuguchi T, Tsuboi N, et al: Gene expression of osteoclast differentiation factor is induced by lipopolysaccharide in mouse osteoblasts via toll-like receptors, *J Immunol* 166:3574, 2001.

80. Kinane DF, Lappin DF: Clinical, pathological and immunological aspects of periodontal disease, *Acta Odontol Scand* 59:154, 2001.
81. Kornman KS, Page RC, Tonetti MS: The host response to the microbial challenge in periodontitis: assembling the players, *Periodontol 2000* 14:33, 1997.
82. Kostenuik PJ, Bolon B, Morony S, et al: Gene therapy with human recombinant osteoprotegerin reverses established osteopenia in ovariectomized mice, *Bone* 34:656, 2004.
83. Krieg AM: CpG motifs in bacterial DNA and their immune effects, *Annu Rev Immunol* 20:709, 2002.
84. Kumar S, Votta BJ, Rieman DJ, et al: IL-1- and TNF-induced bone resorption is mediated by p38 mitogen activated protein kinase, *J Cell Physiol* 187:294, 2001.
85. Lai WC, Zhou M, Shankavaram U, et al: Differential regulation of lipopolysaccharide-induced monocyte matrix metalloproteinase (MMP)-1 and MMP-9 by p38 and extracellular signal–regulated kinase 1/2 mitogen-activated protein kinases, *J Immunol* 170:6244, 2003.
86. Lamster IB, Novak MJ: Host mediators in gingival crevicular fluid: implications for the pathogenesis of periodontal disease, *Crit Rev Oral Biol Med* 3:31, 1992.
87. Lappin DF, Koulouri O, Radvar M, et al: Relative proportions of mononuclear cell types in periodontal lesions analyzed by immunohistochemistry, *J Clin Periodontol* 26:183, 1999.
88. Lappin DF, MacLeod CP, Kerr A, et al: Anti-inflammatory cytokine IL-10 and T cell cytokine profile in periodontitis granulation tissue, *Clin Exp Immunol* 123:294, 2001.
89. Lemaitre B, Nicolas E, Michaut L, et al: The dorsoventral regulatory gene cassette spatzle/toll/cactus controls the potent antifungal response in *Drosophila* adults, *Cell* 86:973, 1996.
90. Lerner UH: New molecules in the tumor necrosis factor ligand and receptor superfamilies with importance for physiological and pathological bone resorption, *Crit Rev Oral Biol Med* 15:64, 2004.
91. Lien E, Golenbock DT: Adjuvants and their signaling pathways: beyond TLRs, *Nat Immunol* 4:1162, 2003.
92. Listgarten MA, Wong MY, Lai CH: Detection of *Actinobacillus actinomycetemcomitans, Porphyromonas gingivalis,* and *Bacteroides forsythus* in an *A. actinomycetemcomitans*–positive patient population, *J Periodontol* 66:158, 1995.
93. Ma W, Pober JS: Human endothelial cells effectively costimulate cytokine production by, but not differentiation of, naive CD4+ T cells, *J Immunol* 161:2158, 1998.
94. Madianos PN, Papapanou PN, Sandros J: *Porphyromonas gingivalis* infection of oral epithelium inhibits neutrophil transepithelial migration, *Infect Immun* 65:3983, 1997.
95. Mahanonda R, Sa-Ard-Iam N, Charatkulangkun O, et al: Monocyte activation by *Porphyromonas gingivalis* LPS in aggressive periodontitis with the use of whole-blood cultures, *J Dent Res* 83:540, 2004.
96. Manolagas SC: Birth and death of bone cells: basic regulatory mechanisms and implications for the pathogenesis and treatment of osteoporosis, *Endocr Rev* 21:115, 2000.
97. Mao S, Maeno N, Matayoshi S, et al: The induction of intercellular adhesion molecule-1 on human umbilical vein endothelial cells by a heat-stable component of *Porphyromonas gingivalis, Curr Microbiol* 48:108, 2004.
98. Martin M, Katz J, Vogel SN, et al: Differential induction of endotoxin tolerance by lipopolysaccharides derived from *Porphyromonas gingivalis* and *Escherichia coli, J Immunol* 167:5278, 2001.
99. Martin M, Schifferle RE, Cuesta N, et al: Role of the phosphatidylinositol 3 kinase-Akt pathway in the regulation of IL-10 and IL-12 by *Porphyromonas gingivalis* lipopolysaccharide, *J Immunol* 171:717, 2003.
100. Mattern T, Thanhauser A, Reiling N, et al: Endotoxin and lipid A stimulate proliferation of human T cells in the presence of autologous monocytes, *J Immunol* 153:2996, 1994.
101. Mattern T, Flad HD, Brade L, et al: Stimulation of human T lymphocytes by LPS is MHC unrestricted, but strongly dependent on B7 interactions, *J Immunol* 160:3412, 1998.
102. McCauley LK, Koh-Paige AJ, Chen H, et al: Parathyroid hormone stimulates fra-2 expression in osteoblastic cells in vitro and in vivo, *Endocrinology* 142:1975, 2001.
103. McCoy SL, Kurtz SE, Hausman FA, et al: Activation of RAW264.7 macrophages by bacterial DNA and lipopolysaccharide increases cell surface DNA binding and internalization, *J Biol Chem* 279:17217, 2004.
104. Medzhitov R: Toll-like receptors and innate immunity, *Nat Rev Immunol* 1:135, 2001.
105. Medzhitov R, Janeway C Jr: The toll receptor family and microbial recognition, *Trends Microbiol* 8:452, 2000.
106. Mempel M, Voelcker V, Kollisch G, et al: Toll-like receptor expression in human keratinocytes: nuclear factor kappaB controlled gene activation by *Staphylococcus aureus* is toll-like receptor 2 but not toll-like receptor 4 or platelet activating factor receptor dependent, *J Invest Dermatol* 121:1389, 2003.
107. Mercado FB, Marshall RI, Bartold PM: Inter-relationships between rheumatoid arthritis and periodontal disease: a review, *J Clin Periodontol* 30:761, 2003.
108. Mercado FB, Marshall RI, Klestov AC, et al: Relationship between rheumatoid arthritis and periodontitis, *J Periodontol* 72:779, 2001.
109. Mori Y, Yoshimura A, Ukai T, et al: Immunohistochemical localization of toll-like receptors 2 and 4 in gingival tissue from patients with periodontitis, *Oral Microbiol Immunol* 18:54, 2003..
110. Muzio M, Mantovani A: Toll-like receptors (TLRs) signalling and expression pattern, *J Endotoxin Res* 7:297, 2001.
111. Nagasawa T, Kobayashi H, Kiji M, et al: LPS-stimulated human gingival fibroblasts inhibit the differentiation of monocytes into osteoclasts through the production of osteoprotegerin, *Clin Exp Immunol* 130:338, 2002.
112. Nanes MS: Tumor necrosis factor-alpha: molecular and cellular mechanisms in skeletal pathology, *Gene* 321:1, 2003.
113. Netea MG, van der Graaf C, van der Meer JW, et al: Toll-like receptors and the host defense against microbial pathogens: bringing specificity to the innate-immune system, *J Leukoc Biol* 75:749, 2004.
114. Nishihara T, Ueda N, Amano K, et al: *Actinobacillus actinomycetemcomitans* Y4 capsular-polysaccharide-like polysaccharide promotes osteoclast-like cell formation by interleukin-1 alpha production in mouse marrow cultures, *Infect Immun* 63:1893, 1995.
115. Nociti FH Jr, Foster BL, Barros SP, et al: Cementoblast gene expression is regulated by *Porphyromonas gingivalis* lipopolysaccharide partially via toll-like receptor-4/MD-2, *J Dent Res* 83:602, 2004.
116. Nonnenmacher C, Dalpke A, Zimmermann S, et al: DNA from periodontopathogenic bacteria is immunostimulatory for mouse and human immune cells, *Infect Immun* 71:850, 2003.
117. Novak MJ, Johns LP, Miller RC, et al: Adjunctive benefits of subantimicrobial dose doxycycline in the management of severe, generalized, chronic periodontitis, *J Periodontol* 73:762, 2002.
118. Offenbacher S: Periodontal diseases: pathogenesis, *Ann Periodontol* 1:821, 1996.
119. Offenbacher S, Salvi GE: Induction of prostaglandin release from macrophages by bacterial endotoxin, *Clin Infect Dis* 28:505, 1999.

120. Ogawa T: Immunobiological properties of chemically defined lipid A from lipopolysaccharide of *Porphyromonas (Bacteroides) gingivalis, Eur J Biochem* 219:737, 1994.
121. Ogawa T, Uchida H: Differential induction of IL-1β and IL-6 production by the nontoxic lipid A from *Porphyromonas gingivalis* in comparison with synthetic *Escherichia coli* lipid A in human peripheral blood mononuclear cells, *FEMS Immunol Med Microbiol* 14:1, 1996.
122. Ogawa T, Asai Y, Yamamoto H, et al: Immunobiological activities of a chemically synthesized lipid A of *Porphyromonas gingivalis, FEMS Immunol Med Microbiol* 28:273, 2000.
123. Ohguchi Y, Ishihara Y, Ohguchi M, et al: Capsular polysaccharide from *Actinobacillus actinomycetemcomitans* inhibits IL-6 and IL-8 production in human gingival fibroblast, *J Periodontal Res* 38:191, 2003.
124. Oringer RJ, Al-Shammari KF, Aldredge WA, et al: Effect of locally delivered minocycline microspheres on markers of bone resorption, *J Periodontol* 73:835, 2002.
125. Pelt P, Zimmermann B, Ulbrich N, et al: Effects of lipopolysaccharide extracted from *Prevotella intermedia* on bone formation and on the release of osteolytic mediators by fetal mouse osteoblasts in vitro, *Arch Oral Biol* 47:859, 2002.
126. Peschon JJ, Torrance DS, Stocking KL, et al: TNF receptor–deficient mice reveal divergent roles for p55 and p75 in several models of inflammation, *J Immunol* 160:943, 1998.
127. Pontes CC, Gonzales JR, Novaes AB Jr, et al: Interleukin-4 gene polymorphism and its relation to periodontal disease in a Brazilian population of African heritage, *J Dent* 32:241, 2004.
128. Pulendran B, Kumar P, Cutler CW, et al: Lipopolysaccharides from distinct pathogens induce different classes of immune responses in vivo, *J Immunol* 167:5067, 2001.
129. Raingeaud J, Gupta S, Rogers JS, et al: Pro-inflammatory cytokines and environmental stress cause p38 mitogen-activated protein kinase activation by dual phosphorylation on tyrosine and threonine, *J Biol Chem* 270:7420, 1995.
130. Reddi K, Henderson B, Meghji S, et al: Interleukin 6 production by lipopolysaccharide-stimulated human fibroblasts is potently inhibited by naphthoquinone (vitamin K) compounds, *Cytokine* 7:287, 1995.
131. Reddi K, Poole S, Nair S, et al: Lipid A–associated proteins from periodontopathogenic bacteria induce interleukin-6 production by human gingival fibroblasts and monocytes, *FEMS Immunol Med Microbiol* 11:137, 1995.
132. Roberts FA, Richardson GJ, Michalek SM: Effects of *Porphyromonas gingivalis* and *Escherichia coli* lipopolysaccharides on mononuclear phagocytes, *Infect Immun* 65:3248, 1997.
133. Rossa C Jr, Patil C, Ehmann K, et al: p38 MAPK mediates cytokine-induced MMP13 expression in PDL cells, *J Dent Res* 83(A):3765, 2004.
134. Ryan ME, Usman A, Ramamurthy NS, et al: Excessive matrix metalloproteinase activity in diabetes: inhibition by tetracycline analogues with zinc reactivity, *Curr Med Chem* 8:305, 2001.
135. Salvi GE, Beck JD, Offenbacher S: PGE_2, IL-1β, and TNF-α responses in diabetics as modifiers of periodontal disease expression, *Ann Periodontol* 3:40, 1998.
136. Salvi GE, Williams RC, Offenbacher S: Nonsteroidal anti-inflammatory drugs as adjuncts in the management of periodontal diseases and peri-implantitis, *Curr Opin Periodontol* 4:51, 1997.
137. Salvi GE, Brown CE, Fujihashi K, et al: Inflammatory mediators of the terminal dentition in adult and early onset periodontitis, *J Periodontal Res* 33:212, 1998.
138. Salvi GE, Collins JG, Yalda B, et al: Monocytic TNF-α secretion patterns in IDDM patients with periodontal diseases, *J Clin Periodontol* 24:8, 1997.
139. Salvi GE, Yalda B, Collins JG, et al: Inflammatory mediator response as a potential risk marker for periodontal diseases in insulin-dependent diabetes mellitus patients, *J Periodontol* 68:127, 1997.
140. Sandros J, Karlsson C, Lappin DF, et al: Cytokine responses of oral epithelial cells to *Porphyromonas gingivalis* infection, *J Dent Res* 79:1808, 2000.
141. Schumann RR, Pfeil D, Lamping N, et al: Lipopolysaccharide induces the rapid tyrosine phosphorylation of the mitogen-activated protein kinases erk-1 and p38 in cultured human vascular endothelial cells requiring the presence of soluble CD14, *Blood* 87:2805, 1996.
142. Seymour GJ, Gemmell E, Kjeldsen M, et al: Cellular immunity and hypersensitivity as components of periodontal destruction, *Oral Dis* 2:96, 1996.
143. Simonet WS, Lacey DL, Dunstan CR, et al: Osteoprotegerin: a novel secreted protein involved in the regulation of bone density, *Cell* 89:309, 1997.
144. Slade GD, Offenbacher S, Beck JD, et al: Acute-phase inflammatory response to periodontal disease in the US population, *J Dent Res* 79:49, 2000.
145. Slade GD, Ghezzi EM, Heiss G, et al: Relationship between periodontal disease and C-reactive protein among adults in the Atherosclerosis Risk in Communities study, *Arch Intern Med* 163:1172, 2003.
146. Somerman MJ, Foster RA, Imm GM, et al: Periodontal ligament cells and gingival fibroblasts respond differently to attachment factors in vitro, *J Periodontol* 60:73, 1989.
147. Sparwasser T, Koch ES, Vabulas RM, et al: Bacterial DNA and immunostimulatory CpG oligonucleotides trigger maturation and activation of murine dendritic cells, *Eur J Immunol* 28:2045, 1998.
148. Stashenko P, Dewhirst FE, Peros WJ, et al: Synergistic interactions between interleukin 1, tumor necrosis factor, and lymphotoxin in bone resorption, *J Immunol* 138:1464, 1987.
149. Stashenko P, Jandinski JJ, Fujiyoshi P, et al: Tissue levels of bone resorptive cytokines in periodontal disease, *J Periodontol* 62:504, 1991.
150. Suda K, Udagawa N, Sato N, et al: Suppression of osteoprotegerin expression by prostaglandin E2 is crucially involved in lipopolysaccharide-induced osteoclast formation, *J Immunol* 172:2504, 2004.
151. Suda T, Takahashi N, Udagawa N, et al: Modulation of osteoclast differentiation and function by the new members of the tumor necrosis factor receptor and ligand families, *Endocr Rev* 20:345, 1999.
152. Sugawara S, Sugiyama A, Nemoto E, et al: Heterogeneous expression and release of CD14 by human gingival fibroblasts: characterization and CD14-mediated interleukin-8 secretion in response to lipopolysaccharide, *Infect Immun* 66:3043, 1998.
153. Sugawara S, Yang S, Iki K, et al: Monocytic cell activation by nonendotoxic glycoprotein from *Prevotella intermedia* ATCC 25611 is mediated by toll-like receptor 2, *Infect Immun* 69:4951, 2001.
154. Sugiyama A, Uehara A, Iki K, et al: Activation of human gingival epithelial cells by cell-surface components of black-pigmented bacteria: augmentation of production of interleukin-8, granulocyte colony-stimulating factor and granulocyte-macrophage colony-stimulating factor and expression of intercellular adhesion molecule 1, *J Med Microbiol* 51:27, 2002.
155. Swantek JL, Tsen MF, Cobb MH, et al: IL-1 receptor–associated kinase modulates host responsiveness to endotoxin, *J Immunol* 164:4301, 2000.

156. Tabeta K, Yamazaki K, Akashi S, et al: Toll-like receptors confer responsiveness to lipopolysaccharide from *Porphyromonas gingivalis* in human gingival fibroblasts, *Infect Immun* 68:3731, 2000.
157. Takeshita A, Imai K, Hanazawa S: CpG motifs in *Porphyromonas gingivalis* DNA stimulate interleukin-6 expression in human gingival fibroblasts, *Infect Immun* 67:4340, 1999.
158. Tanaka S, Takahashi N, Udagawa N, et al: Macrophage colony-stimulating factor is indispensable for both proliferation and differentiation of osteoclast progenitors, *J Clin Invest* 91:257, 1993.
159. Tani Y, Tani M, Kato I: Extracellular 37-kDa antigenic protein from *Actinobacillus actinomycetemcomitans* induces TNF-α, IL-1β, and IL-6 in murine macrophages, *J Dent Res* 76:1538, 1997.
160. Teng YT, Nguyen H, Gao X, et al: Functional human T-cell immunity and osteoprotegerin ligand control alveolar bone destruction in periodontal infection, *J Clin Invest* 106:R59, 2000.
161. Trevani AS, Chorny A, Salamone G, et al: Bacterial DNA activates human neutrophils by a CpG-independent pathway, *Eur J Immunol* 33:3164, 2003.
162. Tsukahara Y, Lian Z, Zhang X, et al: Gene expression in human neutrophils during activation and priming by bacterial lipopolysaccharide, *J Cell Biochem* 89:848, 2003.
163. Ueki K, Tabeta K, Yoshie H, et al: Self-heat shock protein 60 induces tumour necrosis factor-alpha in monocyte-derived macrophage: possible role in chronic inflammatory periodontal disease, *Clin Exp Immunol* 127:72, 2002.
164. Ulevitch RJ: Regulation of receptor-dependent activation of the innate immune response, *J Infect Dis* 187(suppl 2):S351, 2003.
165. Underhill DM, Ozinsky A: Toll-like receptors: key mediators of microbe detection, *Curr Opin Immunol* 14:103, 2002.
166. Wagner M, Poeck H, Jahrsdoerfer B, et al: IL-12p70-dependent Th1 induction by human B cells requires combined activation with CD40 ligand and CpG DNA, *J Immunol* 172:954, 2004.
167. Walker SJ, van Dyke TE, Rich S, et al: Genetic polymorphisms of the IL-1α and IL-1β genes in African-American LJP patients and an African-American control population, *J Periodontol* 71:723, 2000.
168. Wang PL, Ohura K: *Porphyromonas gingivalis* lipopolysaccharide signaling in gingival fibroblasts-CD14 and toll-like receptors, *Crit Rev Oral Biol Med* 13:132, 2002.
169. Wang PL, Azuma Y, Shinohara M, et al: Toll-like receptor 4–mediated signal pathway induced by *Porphyromonas gingivalis* lipopolysaccharide in human gingival fibroblasts, *Biochem Biophys Res Commun* 273:1161, 2000.
170. Warner RL, Bhagavathula N, Nerusu KC, et al: Matrix metalloproteinases in acute inflammation: induction of MMP-3 and MMP-9 in fibroblasts and epithelial cells following exposure to pro-inflammatory mediators in vitro, *Exp Mol Pathol* 76:189, 2004.
171. Watanabe A, Takeshita A, Kitano S, et al: CD14-mediated signal pathway of *Porphyromonas gingivalis* lipopolysaccharide in human gingival fibroblasts, *Infect Immun* 64:4488, 1996.
172. Yamaji Y, Kubota T, Sasaguri K, et al: Inflammatory cytokine gene expression in human periodontal ligament fibroblasts stimulated with bacterial lipopolysaccharides, *Infect Immun* 63:3576, 1995.
173. Yeo SJ, Yoon JG, Hong SC, et al: CpG DNA induces self and cross-hyporesponsiveness of RAW264.7 cells in response to CpG DNA and lipopolysaccharide: alterations in IL-1 receptor–associated kinase expression, *J Immunol* 170:1052, 2003.
174. Yoshimura A, Kaneko T, Kato Y, et al: Lipopolysaccharides from periodontopathic bacteria *Porphyromonas gingivalis* and *Capnocytophaga ochracea* are antagonists for human toll-like receptor 4, *Infect Immun* 70:218, 2002.
175. Yun PL, DeCarlo AA, Collyer C, et al: Modulation of an interleukin-12 and gamma interferon synergistic feedback regulatory cycle of T-cell and monocyte cocultures by *Porphyromonas gingivalis* lipopolysaccharide in the absence or presence of cysteine proteinases, *Infect Immun* 70:5695, 2002.
176. Zou W, Bar-Shavit Z: Dual modulation of osteoclast differentiation by lipopolysaccharide, *J Bone Miner Res* 17:1211, 2002.
177. Zou W, Amcheslavsky A, Bar-Shavit Z: CpG oligodeoxynucleotides modulate the osteoclastogenic activity of osteoblasts via toll-like receptor 9, *J Biol Chem* 278:16732, 2003.
178. Zou W, Schwartz H, Endres S, et al: CpG oligonucleotides: novel regulators of osteoclast differentiation, *FASEB J* 16:274, 2002.
179. Zugel U, Kaufmann SH: Immune response against heat shock proteins in infectious diseases, *Immunobiology* 201:22, 1999.

Host Modulation

Maria Emanuel Ryan and Philip M. Preshaw

16

CHAPTER

Chapter Outline

Host modulation is a new term that has been incorporated into our dental vocabulary, but it has not been well defined. *Host* can be defined as "the organism from which a parasite obtains its nourishment," or in the transplantation of tissue, "the individual who receives the graft." *Modulation* is defined as "the alteration of function or status of something in response to a stimulus or an altered chemical or physical environment" (*Taber's Medical Dictionary,* 2004). In diseases of the periodontium that are initiated by bacteria, the "host" clearly is the individual who harbors these pathogens; however, it was not clear for many years whether it was possible to modulate the host response to these pathogens. Host modulation with chemotherapeutic therapy or drugs is a promising new adjunctive therapeutic option for the management of periodontal diseases.

The concept of host modulation is fairly new to the field of dentistry but is universally understood by most physicians who routinely apply the principles of host modulation to the management of a number of chronic progressive disorders, such as arthritis and osteoporosis. The concept of host modulation was first introduced to dentistry by Williams[27] and Golub et al.[10] and then expanded on by many other scholars in the dental profession. In 1990, Williams concluded, "There are compelling data from studies in animals and human trials indicating that pharmacologic agents that modulate the host responses believed to be involved in the pathogenesis of periodontal destruction may be efficacious in slowing the progression of periodontitis."[27] In 1992, Golub and colleagues discussed "host modulation with tetracyclines and their chemically modified analogues."[10] The future that these authors described has arrived, and to better understand this new era in disease management, we must first look to the past to see how this new concept of host modulation has evolved.

HISTORICAL PERSPECTIVE

From the earliest times, the human race has been plagued by a variety of dental problems and has attempted to alleviate these conditions, which were often painful if left untreated. The first dental healers were physicians, with Hippocrates describing a malady of loose teeth and bleeding gums.[1] In Rome, Celsus (30 BC) recommended vinegar as a remedy for gingival disorders,[6] perhaps the first documented attempt at managing the disease with chemotherapeutics. From these early times, periodontal disease had been regarded as incurable, and teeth attacked by it doomed to extraction, until Riggs introduced his techniques for the treatment of periodontal disease at the 1881 International Medical Congress in London, which led to the term "Riggs' disease."[4]

Based on the work of Riggs, Younger and later Hutchinson advocated surgical treatment of periodontal inflammation by pocket obliteration, which was undertaken by numerous dentists in the early part of the twentieth century. At the same time, C.M. Carr developed "scalers" for the removal of subgingival deposits and for the planing of root surfaces, from which most aspects of modern periodontics actually started. About 1910, encouraged by initial treatment successes, several dentists began to limit their practices to periodontal treatment or, as it was then known, "pyorrhoea" treatment. At the same time a British physician, William Hunter, introduced the concept that chronic infection is the cause of certain systemic diseases, directing remarks on etiology largely to mouth infections, with special emphasis on periodontal infections.[23] Occasionally, medical rather than surgical treatment was attempted, including attempts to develop suitable vaccines for "pyorrhoea."

A major step forward was taken in 1948 when the National Institute of Dental Research, now the National Institute of Dental and Craniofacial Research, was established by the United States Public Health Service, which was ultimately incorporated into the National Institutes of Health (NIH). Through this act, Congress recognized the importance of dental health,[22] providing a means for investigation into the epidemiology of periodontal disease, as well as its pathogenesis. By the 1960s it was also recognized that systemic disorders often play an important role in the etiology of certain periodontal diseases. Thus it became clear that periodontal disease, in some of its phases, constituted a medicodental problem. It was also recognized that the mouth was part of the body and could not be separated from it, although the vital connection seemed at times to be rather tenuous. In a report to the World Health Organization (WHO) in 1961, A.L. Russell of the U.S. Public Health Service and J. Kostlan of the Czechoslovakian Institute of Dental Research stated that periodontitis is a "spectacular disease affecting the majority of the world's population."[23] They emphasized the importance of periodontal disease as a world health threat in view of its deleterious systemic effects and its worldwide distribution.

Theories about the pathogenesis of periodontitis have evolved from a purely plaque-associated disease to the more recent hypotheses, placing considerable emphasis on the host's response to the bacteria.[5] The first Surgeon General's report on "Oral Health in America," published in 2000, has recognized the importance of dental health in the overall general health and well-being of a patient.[26] Recent research findings indicate possible associations between chronic oral infections, such as periodontitis, and systemic disorders, such as diabetes, heart and lung diseases, stroke, and adverse pregnancy outcomes. These findings are addressed in the Surgeon General's report, which assesses these emerging associations and explores factors that may underlie these oral-systemic disease connections.

Along with these findings and the emergence of the discipline of periodontal medicine, there have been many developments in therapeutic approaches to the management of periodontitis. The development of the chemo-therapeutic approach known as "host modulation" required a thorough understanding of the host response.

THE HOST RESPONSE AND POTENTIAL TARGETS FOR HOST MODULATION

Many individuals harbor the putative pathogens associated with periodontal disease, but they do not develop the disease. Periodontal disease does not appear to act as a classic infection, but more as an *opportunistic* infection. There is no way to eliminate bacteria from the oral cavity, so bacteria are always present in the periodontal milieu. When certain, more virulent species exist in an environment that allows for their presence in greater proportion, there is the opportunity for periodontal destruction to occur. However, although plaque appears to be essential for the development of periodontal disease, the severity and pattern of disease are not explained solely by the amount of plaque present.

In 1985, research began to focus on bacterial-host interactions.[15] It had been recognized that although bacterial pathogens initiate the periodontal inflammation, the host response to these pathogens is equally, if not more, important in mediating connective tissue breakdown, including bone loss. It has become clear that the host-derived enzymes known as the *matrix metalloproteinases* (MMPs), as well as changes in osteoclast activity driven by cytokines and prostanoids, cause most of the tissue destruction in the periodontium.[18] This shift in paradigms, with a focus on the host response, led to the development of *host modulatory therapies* to improve therapeutic outcomes, slow the progression of disease, and allow for more predictable management of patients. This therapeutic strategy not only may be relevant to individuals at greater risk for periodontal disease, but also may be important in the management of those at risk for a number of related systemic diseases.

To better understand the host factors that clinicians are attempting to modulate, we need a more detailed assessment of the role of the host response in periodontal pathogenesis (Figure 16-1). After the accumulation of subgingival plaque bacteria, a variety of microbial substances, including chemotactic factors such as *lipopolysaccharide* (LPS), microbial peptides, and other bacterial antigens, diffuse across the junctional epithelium into the gingival connective tissues. The periodontium is anatomically unique in that the junctional epithelium ends on the tooth surface, which is nonliving tissue; there is no other such discontinuous lining over the entire surface of the body. The dentogingival junction indicates *a priori* vulnerability to bacterial attack. Epithelial and connective tissue cells are thus stimulated to produce inflammatory mediators that result in an inflammatory response in the tissues. The gingival vasculature dilates (vasodilation) and becomes increasingly permeable to fluid and cells. Fluid accumulates in the tissues, and defense cells migrate from the circulation toward the source of the chemotactic stimulus (bacteria and their products) in the gingival crevice. Neutrophils, or polymorphonuclear leukocytes (PMNs), predominate in the early stages of gingival inflammation, and these cells phagocytose and kill plaque bacteria. Bacterial killing by PMNs involves both intracellular mechanisms (after phagocytosis of bacteria within membrane-bound structures inside the cell) and extracellular mechanisms (by release of PMN enzymes and oxygen radicals outside the cell). As bacterial products

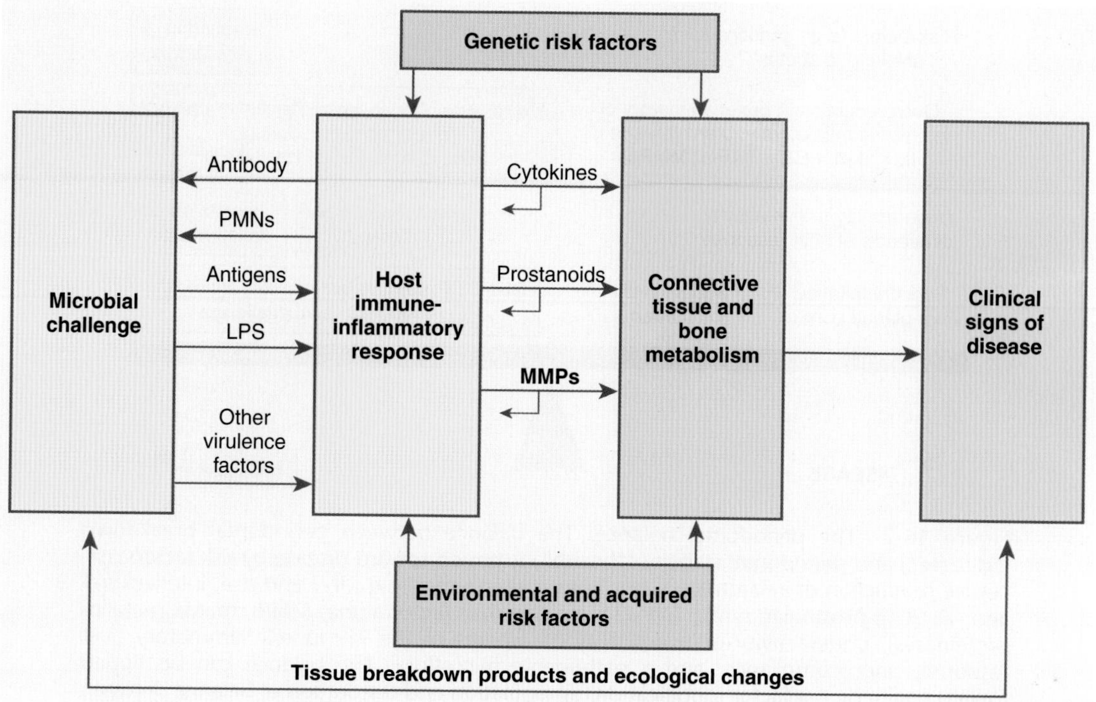

Figure 16-1 Schematic illustration of the pathogenesis of periodontitis. The microbial challenge presented by subgingival plaque bacteria results in an upregulated host immune-inflammatory response in the periodontal tissues that is characterized by the excessive production of inflammatory cytokines (e.g., interleukins, tumor necrosis factor), prostanoids (e.g., prostaglandin E_2) and enzymes, including the matrix metalloproteinases *(MMPs)*. These proinflammatory mediators are responsible for the majority of periodontal breakdown that occurs, leading to the clinical signs and symptoms of periodontitis. The process is modified by environmental (e.g., tobacco use) and acquired risk factors (e.g., systemic diseases) and genetic susceptibility. *PMNs,* Polymorphonuclear leukocytes; *LPS,* lipopolysaccharide. (Modified from Kornman KS: *Clin Infect Dis* 28:520, 1999.)

enter the circulation, committed lymphocytes return to the site of infection, and B lymphocytes are transformed to plasma cells, which produce antibodies against specific bacterial antigens. Antibodies are released in the gingival tissues and, in the presence of complement, facilitate and enhance PMN phagocytosis and bacterial killing.

Thus, a host immune-inflammatory response is established in the gingival tissues, and the clinical signs of gingivitis develop. This response is essentially protective in intent, to combat the bacterial infection and prevent ingress of bacteria into the tissues. In persons who are not susceptible to periodontitis *(disease resistant),* these primary defense mechanisms control the infection, and chronic inflammation (i.e., chronic gingivitis) may persist indefinitely. In *disease-susceptible* individuals, however, inflammatory events extend apically and laterally to involve deeper connective tissues and alveolar bone. There is proliferation of the junctional epithelium, which becomes increasingly permeable and ulcerated, thus accelerating the ingress of bacterial products, and the inflammation worsens. Further defense cells are recruited to the area, including macrophages and lymphocytes. Large numbers of PMNs migrate into the tissues, secreting excessive quantities of destructive enzymes and inflammatory mediators. These enzymes include the MMPs, such as collagenases, which break down collagen fibers in the gingival and periodontal tissues. The infiltrating inflammatory and immune cells are accommodated by the breakdown of structural components of the periodontium. MMPs are a primary target for host modulation. Pharmacologic agents or chemotherapeutics can be administered to suppress excessive levels of MMPs.

Macrophages are recruited to the area and are activated (by binding to LPS) to produce prostaglandins (e.g., prostaglandin E_2, PGE_2), interleukins (e.g., IL-1α, IL-1β, IL-6), tumor necrosis factor alpha (TNF-α), and MMPs. The cytokines (interleukins and TNF-α) and prostanoids are additional targets for host modulatory therapeutics. Interleukins and TNF-α bind to fibroblasts, which are stimulated to produce additional quantities of PGE_2, interleukins, TNF-α, and MMPs in positive-feedback cycles. The concentration of these enzymes and inflammatory mediators becomes pathologically high in the periodontal tissues. Host modulatory therapy can be used to interrupt these positive-feedback loops and ultimately reduce the excessive levels of cytokines, prostanoids, and enzymes resulting in tissue destruction. MMPs break down collagen fibers, disrupting the normal anatomy of the gingival tissues and resulting in destruction of the periodontal ligament. The inflammation extends apically, and osteoclasts are stimulated to resorb alveolar bone by the high levels of prostaglandins, interleukins, and TNF-α in the

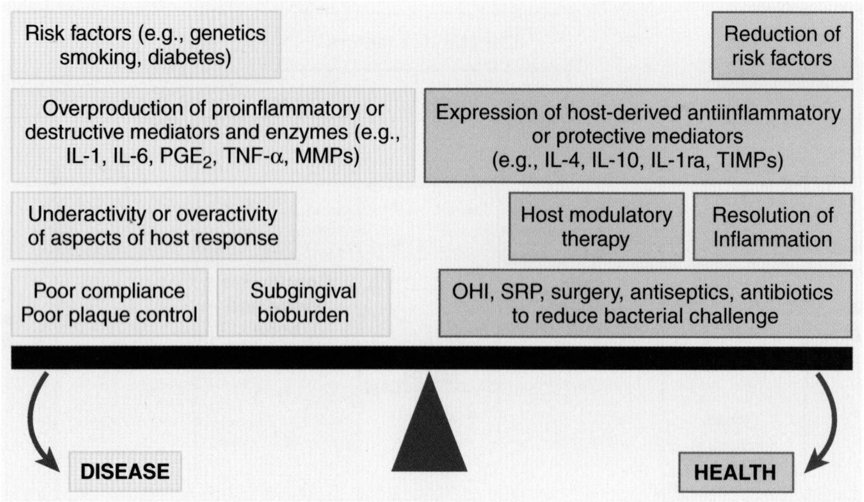

Figure 16-2 The periodontal balance. The balance between periodontal breakdown ("disease") and periodontal stability ("health") is tipped toward disease by risk factors, excessive production of inflammatory cytokines and enzymes (e.g., *IL-1* and *IL-6,* interleukin-1 and –6; *PGE$_2$,* prostaglandin E_2; *TNF-α,* tumor necrosis factor alpha; *MMPs,* matrix metalloproteinases), underactivity or overactivity of aspects of the immune-inflammatory host response, poor compliance, and a pathogenic microflora. The balance can be tipped toward health by risk factor modification, upregulation and restoration of balance between naturally occurring inhibitors of inflammation (e.g., *IL-4* and *IL-10,* interleukins 4 and 10; *IL-1ra,* interleukin-1 receptor antagonist; *TIMPs,* tissue inhibitors of metalloproteinases), *HMT* (host modulatory therapy), and antibacterial treatments such as *OHI* (oral hygiene instructions), *SRP* (scaling and root planning), surgery, antiseptics, and antibiotics.

tissues. The osteoclasts themselves are targets for host modulation. Drugs can be administered to downregulate osteoclastic activity and ultimately to inhibit bone resorption by these cells.

The elevations in the proinflammatory or destructive mediators in response to bacterial challenge are counterbalanced by elevations in antiinflammatory or protective mediators such as the cytokines IL-4 and IL-10, as well as other mediators such as IL-1ra (receptor antagonist) and tissue inhibitors of matrix metalloproteinases (TIMPs) (Figure 16-2). Under conditions of health, the antiinflammatory or protective mediators serve to control tissue destruction. If there are adequate levels of these antiinflammatory or protective mediators to keep the host response to the bacterial challenge in check, the individual will be disease resistant. If an imbalance occurs, with excessive levels of the proinflammatory or destructive mediators present in the host tissues, tissue destruction will ensue in the susceptible host. Another potential target for host modulation could entail the use of pharmacologic agents, which either mimic or result in elevations of endogenous antiinflammatory or protective mediators.

Thus, plaque bacteria initiate the disease, and bacterial antigens that cross the junctional epithelium drive the inflammatory process. Therefore, bacteria are essential for periodontitis to occur, but they are insufficient to cause disease alone. For periodontitis to develop, a susceptible host is also required. The majority of periodontal breakdown (bone loss, attachment loss) is caused by host-derived destructive enzymes (MMPs) and inflammatory mediators (prostaglandins, interleukins) that are released during the cascade of destructive events that occur as part of the inflammatory response[21] (see Figure 16-1). Paradoxically, the inflammatory response, which is essentially protective in design, is responsible for much of the breakdown of the soft and hard periodontal tissues. Periodontal disease is characterized by high concentrations of MMPs, cytokines, and prostanoids in the periodontal tissues, whereas periodontal health is characterized by the opposite situation.[20] The purpose of host modulation therapy is to restore the balance of proinflammatory or destructive mediators and antiinflammatory or protective mediators to that seen in healthy individuals. Pocket formation occurs as coronal junctional epithelium is broken down and restored at a more apical location. Plaque bacteria then migrate apically along the root surface deeper into the pocket, where the physical conditions favor the proliferation of gram-negative anaerobic species. Bacterial products continue to challenge the host, and the host continues its frustrated response against these products. Inflammation extends further and further apically, more bone is resorbed, and periodontal ligament (PDL) is broken down. The pocket deepens, and the associated attachment and bone loss result in clinical and radiographic signs of periodontitis. Intervention is required to prevent eventual tooth loss and other sequelae of the disease.

HOST MODULATORY THERAPY

Intervention in periodontal disease can now include host modulatory therapy (HMT) as one of the available adjunctive treatment options. The term *adjunctive* is meant to imply "in addition to conventional therapies" or "in

BOX 16-1

Risk Factors for Periodontal Disease

- Heredity: family history, PST test
- Smoking: frequency, current history, past history
- Diabetes: duration, control
- Stress: reported by patient
- Medications: calcium channel blockers, dilantin, cyclosporin, drugs known to cause dry mouth
- Nutrition
- Poor oral hygiene: plaque and calculus
- Faulty dentistry: overhangs, subgingival margins
- Hormonal variations: *pregnancy* (increased estradiol and progesterone), *menopause* (decreased estrogen, osteoporosis)
- Immunocompromise: HIV, neutropenia
- Connective tissue diseases
- Previous history of periodontitis

PST, Periodontal screening test; *HIV,* human immunodeficiency virus.

BOX 16-2

Risk Assessment and Therapy for Periodontitis*

- Heredity: chemotherapeutics
- Smoking: cessation, chemotherapeutics
- Diabetes: improved control, work with physician; chemotherapeutics
- Stress: management, chemotherapeutics
- Medications: change medications, work with physician; chemotherapeutics
- Nutrition: supplements
- Poor oral hygiene: improved oral hygiene, chemotherapeutics
- Faulty dentistry: corrective dentistry
- Hormonal variations: consult with physician, chemotherapeutics
- Immunocompromise: consult with physician, chemotherapeutics
- Connective tissue diseases: consult with physician, chemotherapeutics

*In addition to more frequent dental visits (treatment/maintenance).

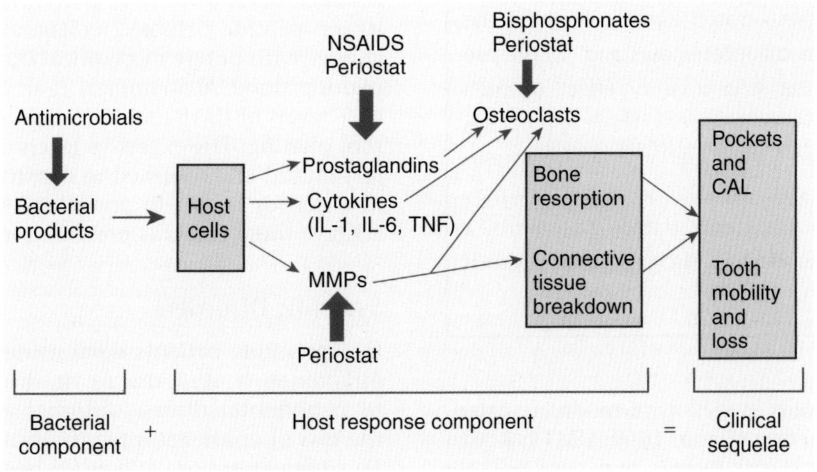

Figure 16-3 Potential adjunctive therapeutic approaches. Possible adjunctive therapies and points of intervention in the treatment of periodontitis are presented related to the pathologic cascade of events. *CAL,* Clinical attachment loss.

addition to other established therapies." For the management of periodontal diseases, conventional approaches were initially mechanical in nature, as reviewed in the historical section, that is, surgery as well as scaling and root planing. Initially, adjunctive therapies were solely antimicrobial, such as the use of antiseptics and antibiotics. New adjunctive approaches involve modulation of the host response.

When considering factors that increase an individual's risk for developing periodontitis, it has been recognized that genetic, environmental (e.g., tobacco use), and acquired risk factors (e.g., systemic disease) can increase a patient's susceptibility to developing this disease. These risk factors may lead to the imbalance between the proinflammatory and antiinflammatory mediators seen in susceptible individuals (see Figure 16-2). Risk factors can affect onset, rate of progression, and severity of periodontal disease, as well as response to therapy[7,12,25] (Box 16-1). Some of these risk factors can be modified to reduce a patient's susceptibility. Risk assessment and therapy may include smoking cessation, improved control of diabetes, nutritional supplementation, improved oral hygiene, changes in medication, stress management, and more frequent dental visits (Box 16-2). The use of chemotherapeutic agents or drugs specifically designed to treat periodontal diseases is emerging to aid in this risk assessment and reduction strategy. Chemotherapeutic agents can include adjuncts such as locally applied and systemically delivered antimicrobials and host modulatory therapies. HMT can be used to reduce excessive levels of enzymes,

SCIENCE TRANSFER

In the past, an understanding of the etiology and pathogenesis of the periodontal disease focused on the microbial aspect of the diseases. More recent investigations recognize the importance of the host response and the critical role the host response plays in the protection and, in fact, the destruction of the periodontal tissues. Therapeutic efforts in the past therefore focused on the mechanical or chemotherapeutic removal of the bacterial flora. More recent therapeutic efforts focus on altering (modulating) the host response. Ironically, without realizing it, past efforts removing the bacterial flora indirectly modulated the host because when the bacterial insult was minimized, the host response could be more effective. Therefore, periodontists have long been doing host modulation therapy (HMT) indirectly. At present, new strategies incorporate more direct HMT in addition to the indirect approaches.

The modulation of host responses to bacterially initiated periodontal disease focuses on two approaches: (1) the use of tetracycline-related agents to inhibit the production of matrix metalloproteinases and (2) the use of agents that limit the inflammatory effect of such mediators as prostanoids and cytokines. These approaches are adjunctive to conventional periodontal treatment, and because most are systemic in application, they may be part of an overall treatment strategy to control a variety of other chronic diseases such as atherosclerosis and osteoporosis.

cytokines, and prostanoids as well as to modulate osteoclast and osteoblast function (Figure 16-3). HMT is key to addressing many of these risk factors that have adverse effects on the host response, which are either not easily managed (e.g., smoking, diabetes) or cannot be changed (e.g., genetic susceptibility). A program of risk assessment and reduction is critical to optimal periodontal therapy in the same way that it is key to the successful medical care of diabetic or cardiac patients (see Chapter 38).

Clearly, when considering the imbalance in destructive or proinflammatory mediators versus protective or antiinflammatory mediators in the diseased state, physicians should contemplate the use of pharmacologic agents or HMT. HMT may be used systemically and locally to restore the balance that is present in health and to prevent further progression of disease and improve therapeutic outcomes. As with current approaches, future host modulatory therapies for the management of periodontal diseases will primarily target the excessive levels of proinflammatory mediators (see Chapter 53). In addition, host modulatory agents might be used to increase the levels of a person's own protective or antiinflammatory mediators. Use of systemic HMTs for treatment of a patient's periodontal condition may also provide benefits for other inflammatory disorders, such as arthritis, cardiovascular disease, dermatologic conditions, diabetes, and osteoporosis. Also, patients who are currently taking host modulatory agents, such as nonsteroidal antiinflammatory drugs (NSAIDS), bisphosphonates, or tetracyclines, as well as newer agents targeting specific cytokines for the management of medical conditions, may be experiencing periodontal benefits from these systemic medications.

HOST MODULATION FACTORS

Periodontitis

When considering the pathogenesis of periodontitis, it becomes clear that host modulation should play a role in the management of this multifactorial disease, along with an antimicrobial approach and risk reduction. As discussed, the excessive host response in susceptible patients leads to an imbalance in destructive proinflammatory mediators versus protective or antiinflammatory mediators. Indeed, studies have demonstrated that markers of disease located in the gingival crevicular fluid (GCF) of pockets in patients with periodontitis, including IL-1, MMPs, and bone and connective tissue breakdown products such as ICTP (a pyrodinoline-containing cross-linked peptide of type I collagen), undergo little to no change with purely mechanical therapy, scaling, and root planing alone. Al Shammari et al[2] reported no changes in GCF levels of IL-1β and ICTP before and after scaling and root planing. The excessive levels of these factors need to be reduced and returned to constitutive or normal levels in order for health to prevail. HMT can help physicians achieve these goals, as presented in Chapter 53.

Systemic Disorders

In susceptible patients demonstrating an excessive local inflammatory response to the bacterial stimuli leading to periodontal disease, another consideration involves the loss of epithelial integrity in the periodontal pocket. This tissue response allows for bacterial penetration into the inflamed tissues and eventual entry of the bacteria into the systemic circulation. Patients with untreated periodontitis have an increased risk for transient bacteremias. Bacteremia and associated endotoxemia may incite the overproduction of destructive proinflammatory mediators at distant sites in the periodontitis patient. Therefore, patients with periodontitis may be at greater risk for developing a number of systemic conditions associated with a similar overactive host response to external stimuli, such as cardiovascular disease, adverse pregnancy outcomes, and diabetic complications. Elevated levels of cytokines, prostanoids, and enzymes are evident in all these conditions.

In the era of periodontal medicine, systemic host modulatory approaches need to be considered (see Chapter 18). As mentioned, host modulators used to manage periodontal disease, such as an MMP, cytokine, and prostanoid inhibitors, may have additional beneficial effects on systemic diseases that have been linked to periodontal disease, such as cardiovascular disease, diabetes, and premature birth. In cardiovascular disease, preliminary studies have indicated that individuals with periodontal disease are almost twice as likely to have a fatal heart attack and three times as likely to have a stroke.[3] MMPs and cytokines have been found to play a major role in weakening the plaques formed with cardiovascular disease, leading to rupture and eventual thrombosis and infarction.[8] In fact, Golub et al.[9] suggested that tetracyclines could reduce the incidence of acute myocardial infarction[17] by blocking collagenase and stabilizing the collagen cap on the atherosclеromatous arterial plaques.

In diabetes, the same MMPs and cytokines involved in the development of periodontitis as the sixth long-term complication of diabetes[16] also play a role in the development of other well-known complications of diabetes, such as nephropathy, angiopathy, retinopathy, and wound-healing problems.[24] Modulation of these proinflammatory mediators in diabetic patients may impede the development of multiple long-term complications.

Finally, periodontal disease has been found to put pregnant women at an increased risk of giving birth to preterm, low-weight babies, because endotoxins drive up the levels of prostanoids involved in contraction.[19] In addition, MMPs have been found to play a role in the cervical effacement and dilation that precede labor. MMPs also may serve as biochemical markers of risk for preterm delivery[14] because they are involved in preterm premature rupture of the membranes, playing a role in preterm parturition.[11]

An inhibitor of MMPs, cytokines, and prostanoids used in the treatment of periodontitis may have an indirect effect on these disease processes if a patient's risk for developing these disorders is increased by the presence of untreated periodontitis. HMT may also directly aid in the treatment and prevention of cardiovascular disease, diabetic complications, and premature birth.

SUMMARY

The executive summary of the Surgeon General's report on oral health reveals that most adults show signs of periodontal or gingival disease, with severe periodontitis affecting about 14% of adults age 45 to 54 and 23% of adults age 54 to 74 years.[26] Adding the population of underdeveloped countries to this statistic could increase the prevalence of disease to above 33%. It is also known that 17% to 28% of the treated periodontal patients develop refractory or recurrent periodontitis. Clearly there is a need for improved diagnosis and cost-effective means of managing this chronic progressive disease, which has been linked to other systemic diseases.

Periodontal pathogens and destructive host responses are involved in the initiation and progression of periodontitis. Therefore the successful long-term management of this disease may require a treatment strategy that integrates therapies that address both etiologic components. Evidence for the role of MMPs, cytokines, and other mediators in the pathogenesis of periodontal disease distinguishes them as viable targets for a chemotherapeutic approach. The introduction of novel, adjunctive therapies such as host modulation to enhance the efficacy of existing mechanical procedures can contribute favorably to an integrated approach for the long-term, clinical management of periodontitis. The use of HMT as an adjunct may be particularly useful in susceptible, high-risk patients in whom a prolonged and excessive host response to the presence of bacteria promotes the activity of MMPs and osteoclasts.

The Surgeon General's report recognizes "the mouth as a mirror of health or disease, as a sentinel or early warning system, as an accessible model for the study of other tissues and organs, and as a potential source of pathology affecting other systems and organs."[26] The findings discussed in this chapter with regard to the use of host modulation to better manage chronic periodontal disease may have applications to other chronic progressive tissue-destructive diseases such as arthritis. The effects of host modulation on periodontitis in diabetic patients may have implications on other long-term complications of diabetes, such as cardiovascular disease, retinopathy, nephropathy, neuropathy, and wound healing. Future studies may demonstrate that host modulation for the management of periodontal disease can have profound positive effects on the cardiovascular status of patients. The future holds much promise for host modulation as an important tool not only for the management of periodontitis, but also for the clinical practice of periodontal medicine.

REFERENCES

1. Adams FR: *The genuine works of Hippocrates,* Charlottesville, Va, 1891, Unbound Medicine.
2. Al Shammari KF, Giannobile WV, Aldredge WA, et al: Effect of non-surgical periodontal therapy on C-telopeptide pyridinoline cross-links (ICTP) and interleukin-1 levels, *J Periodontol* 72:1045, 2001.
3. Beck JD, Offenbacher S, Williams R, et al: Periodontitis: a risk factor for coronary heart disease? *Ann Periodontol* 3:127, 1998.
4. Bremner M: *The story of dentistry from the dawn of civilization,* New York, 1939, Dental Items of Interest.
5. Carranza FA, editor: *Clinical periodontology,* ed 8, Philadelphia, 1996, Saunders.
6. Elliot JS: *Outlines of Greek and Roman medicine,* Boston, 1972, Milford House.
7. Genco RJ:. Host responses in periodontal diseases: current concepts, *J Periodontol* 63:338, 1992.
8. Genco RJ, Offenbacher S, Beck J, Rees T: Cardiovascular disease and oral infections. In Rose LF, editor: *Periodontal medicine,* Ontario, 1999, BC Decker.
9. Golub LM, Greenwald RA, Thompson RW: Tetracyclines and risk of subsequent first-time acute mycoardial infarction, *JAMA* 282:1997, 1999 (letter to the editor).
10. Golub LM, Suomalainen K, Sorsa T:. Host modulation with tetracyclines and their chemically modified analogues, *Curr Opin Dent* 2:80, 1992.
11. Gomez R, Romero R, Edwin SS, David C: Pathogenesis of preterm labor and preterm premature rupture of membranes associated with intraamniotic infection, *Infect Dis Clin North Am* 11:135, 1997.
12. Grossi SG, Zambon JJ, Ho AW, et al: Assessment of risk for periodontal disease. I. Risk indicators for attachment loss, *J Periodontol* 65:260, 1994.
13. Kornman KS: Host modulation as a therapeutic strategy in the treatment of periodontal disease, *Clin Infect Dis* 28:520, 1999.
14. Lockwood CJ, Kuczynski E: Markers of risk for preterm delivery, *J Perinat Med* 27:5, 1999.

15. Maynard J: Eras in periodontics. Periodontal Disease Management: a Conference for the Dental Team, Boston, 1993, American Academy of Periodontology.
16. Mealy B: *Diabetes mellitus in periodontal medicine,* Ontario, 1999, BC Decker.
17. Meier CR, Derby LE, Jick SS, et al: Antibiotics and risk of subsequent first-time acute myocardial infarction, *JAMA* 281:427, 1999.
18. Offenbacher S: Periodontal diseases: pathogenesis, *Ann Periodontol* 1:821, 1996.
19. Offenbacher S, Jared HL, O'Reilly PG, et al: Potential pathogenic mechanisms of periodontitis-associated pregnancy complications, *Ann Periodontol* 3:233, 1998.
20. Page RC: Milestones in periodontal research and the remaining critical issues, *J Periodontal Res* 34:331, 1999.
21. Page RC, Kornman KS: The pathogenesis of human periodontitis: an introduction, *Periodontol 2000* 14:9, 1997.
22. Prinz H: *Dental chronology: a record of the more important historic events in the evolution of dentistry,* Philadelphia, 1945, Lea & Febiger.
23. Russell S, Kostlan J: Spectacular report from World Health Organization, *NY J Dent* 31:98, 1961.
24. Ryan ME: Host response in diabetes-associated periodontitis: effects of tetracycline analogues, Stony Brook, 1998, State University of New York (PhD thesis).
25. Salvi GE, Lawrence HP, Offenbacher S, Beck JD: Influence of risk factors on the pathogenesis of periodontitis, *Periodontol 2000* 14:173, 1997.
26. US Department of Health and Human Services (DHHS): *Oral health in America: a Report of the Surgeon General,* Executive Summary, Rockville, Md, 2000, DHHS, NIDCR, National Institutes of Health.
27. Williams RC: Periodontal disease, *N Engl J Med* 322:373, 1990.

Relationship between Periodontal Disease and Systemic Health

Perry R. Klokkevold

PART 5

An interrelationship between periodontal disease and systemic health has been suspected for centuries, but evidence to explain the connection has only been elucidated in the past few decades.

Inflammation is the primary pathologic feature of periodontal disease, and bacterial plaque is the essential etiologic factor responsible for inducing the host inflammatory process. However, it is host susceptibility and ability of the host defense to respond appropriately to the bacterial challenge that results in differences in the severity of periodontal disease from one individual to another. Thus, individual susceptibility to periodontitis is influenced by a number of factors, including systemic diseases and conditions. Conversely, recent evidence indicates that the presence of chronic inflammatory periodontal disease may significantly affect systemic health conditions such as coronary heart disease, stroke, or adverse pregnancy outcomes.

Consequently, the relationship between periodontal disease and systemic health is a two-way road, with systemic host factors acting locally to reduce resistance to periodontal destruction and the local bacterial challenge generating widespread effects with the potential to induce adverse systemic outcomes. This part describes the influence of systemic disease and conditions on the periodontium and the role of inflammatory periodontal disease on systemic conditions. The relationship of oral malodor to oral, periodontal, and systemic disease is also described.

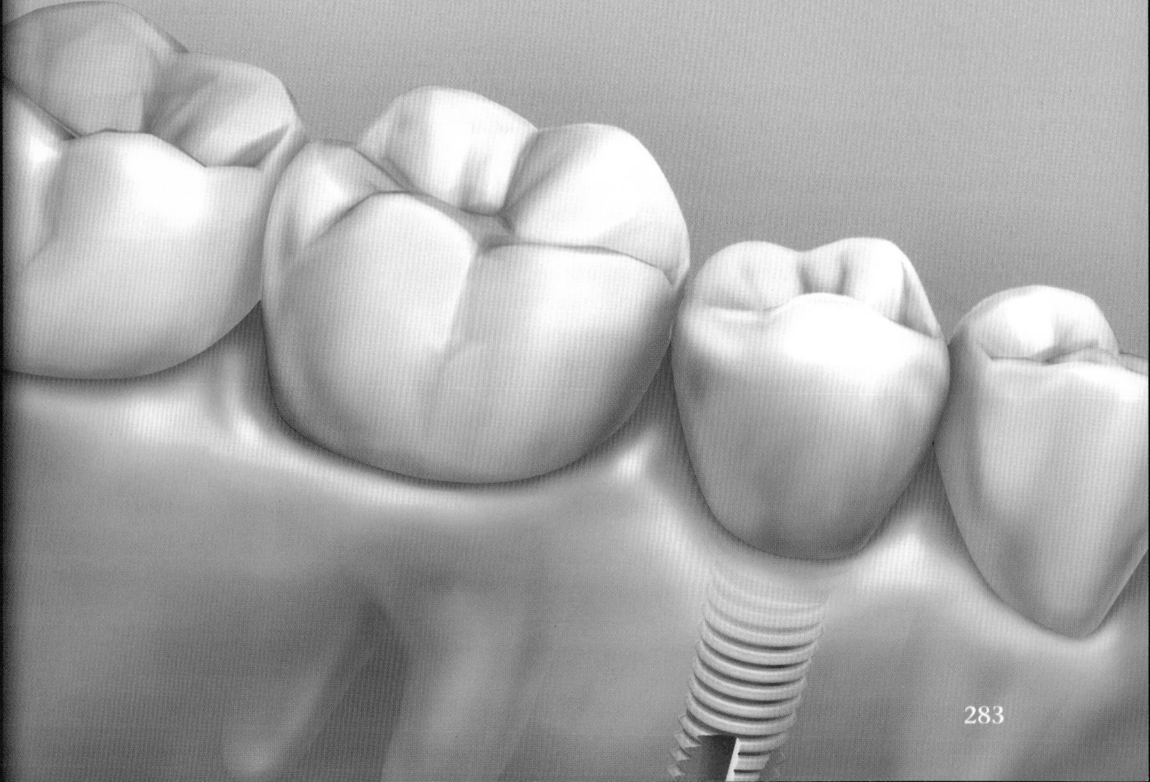

Influence of Systemic Disorders and Stress on the Periodontium

Perry R. Klokkevold and Brian L. Mealey

17

CHAPTER

CHAPTER OUTLINE

Many systemic diseases and disorders have been implicated as risk indicators or risk factors in periodontal disease. Clinical and basic science research over the past several decades has led to an improved understanding and appreciation for the complexity and pathogenesis of periodontal diseases.[140] Clearly, there is an *essential* bacterial etiology, and there are *specific* bacteria (periodontal pathogens) associated with destructive periodontal diseases. However, these pathogens do not invariably cause disease simply by their presence alone. Their absence, on the other hand, appears to be consistent with periodontal health. The role of bacteria in disease etiology and pathogenesis are discussed in Chapters 9 and 13.

Perhaps the most significant change in our understanding of the pathogenesis of periodontitis is that the host response varies between individuals and that an insufficient host immune response or an exaggerated host immune response to bacterial pathogens may lead to more severe forms of the disease. In other words, the individual host immune response to periodontal pathogens is very important and likely explains much of the differences in disease severity observed from one individual to another. Furthermore, certain systemic disorders and conditions alter host tissues and physiology, which may impair host barrier integrity and host defense to periodontal infection, resulting in more destructive disease.

Recent evidence also suggests that periodontal infections can adversely affect systemic health with manifestations such as coronary heart disease, stroke, diabetes, preterm labor, low-birth-weight delivery, and respiratory disease.[126] The potential role of periodontal infections on these systemic health conditions is discussed in Chapter 18.

The interrelationships between periodontal infections and host defense are complex. A number of environmental, physical, and psychosocial factors have the potential to alter periodontal tissues and the host immune response, resulting in more severe periodontal disease expression. It is important to appreciate that these disorders and conditions do not initiate periodontitis, but they may predispose, accelerate, or otherwise increase its progression. This chapter discusses the influence of systemic disorders and stress on the periodontium.

ENDOCRINE DISORDERS AND HORMONAL CHANGES

Endocrine diseases such as diabetes and hormonal fluctuations that are associated with puberty and pregnancy are well-known examples of systemic conditions that adversely affect the condition of the periodontium. Endocrine disturbances and hormone fluctuations affect the periodontal tissues directly, modify the tissue response to local factors, and produce anatomic changes in the gingiva that may favor plaque accumulation and disease progression. This section describes the evidence supporting the relationship among endocrine disorders, hormonal changes, and periodontal disease.

Diabetes Mellitus

Diabetes mellitus is an extremely important disease from a periodontal standpoint. It is a complex metabolic disorder characterized by chronic hyperglycemia. Diminished insulin production, impaired insulin action, or a combination of both result in the inability of glucose to be transported from the bloodstream into the tissues, which in turn results in high blood glucose levels and excretion of sugar in the urine. Lipid and protein metabolism is altered in diabetes as well. Uncontrolled diabetes (chronic hyperglycemia) is associated with several long-term complications, including microvascular diseases (retinopathy, nephropathy, neuropathy), macrovascular diseases (cardiovascular, cerebrovascular), an increased susceptibility to infections, and poor wound healing. An estimated 15.7 million individuals, or 5.9% of the U.S. population, have diabetes.[132] Almost half of these individuals are unaware that they have the disease.

There are two major types of diabetes, type 1 and type 2, with several less common secondary types. *Type 1* diabetes mellitus, formerly insulin-dependent diabetes mellitus (IDDM), is caused by a cell-mediated autoimmune destruction of the insulin-producing beta cells of the islets of Langerhans in the pancreas, which results in insulin deficiency. Type 1 diabetes accounts for 5% to 10% of all cases of diabetes and most often occurs in children and young adults. This type of diabetes results from a lack of insulin production and is very unstable and difficult to control. It has a marked tendency toward ketosis and coma, is not preceded by obesity, and requires injected insulin to be controlled. Patients with type 1 diabetes mellitus present with the symptoms traditionally associated with diabetes, including polyphagia, polydipsia, polyuria, and predisposition to infections.

Type 2 diabetes mellitus, formerly non–insulin-dependent diabetes mellitus (NIDDM), is caused by peripheral resistance to insulin action, impaired insulin secretion, and increased glucose production in the liver. The insulin-producing beta cells in the pancreas are not destroyed by cell-mediated autoimmune reaction. Type 2 diabetes is the most common form of diabetes, accounting for 90% to 95% of all cases, and usually has an adult onset. Individuals often are not aware they have the disease until severe symptoms or complications occur. Type 2 generally occurs in obese individuals and can often be controlled by diet and oral hypoglycemic agents. Ketosis and coma are uncommon. Type 2 diabetes can present with the same symptoms as type 1 diabetes, but typically in a less severe form.

An additional category of diabetes is *hyperglycemia* secondary to other diseases or conditions. A prime example of this type of hyperglycemia is *gestational diabetes* associated with pregnancy. Gestational diabetes develops in 2% to 5% of all pregnancies but disappears after delivery. Women who have had gestational diabetes are at increased risk of developing type 2 diabetes later in life. Other secondary types of diabetes are those associated with diseases that involve the pancreas and destruction of the insulin-producing cells. Endocrine diseases such as acromegaly and Cushing's syndrome, tumors, pancreatectomy, and drugs or chemicals that cause altered insulin levels are included in this group. Experimentally induced types of diabetes generally belong in this category rather than in type 1 or 2 diabetes mellitus.

Oral Manifestations

Numerous oral changes have been described in diabetic patients, including cheilosis, mucosal drying and cracking, burning mouth and tongue, diminished salivary flow, and alterations in the flora of the oral cavity, with greater predominance of *Candida albicans,* hemolytic streptococci, and staphylococci.[1,16,76,121] An increased rate of dental caries has also been observed in poorly controlled diabetes.[54,63] Importantly, however, these changes are not always present, are not specific, and are not pathognomonic for diabetes.[124] Furthermore, these changes are less likely to be observed in well-controlled diabetic patients. Individuals with controlled diabetes have a normal tissue response, a normally developed dentition, a normal defense against infections, and no increase in the incidence of caries.[178]

The influence of diabetes on the periodontium has been thoroughly investigated. Although it is difficult to make definitive conclusions about the specific effects of diabetes on periodontium, a variety of changes have been described, including a tendency toward enlarged gingiva, sessile or pedunculated gingival polyps, polypoid gingival proliferations, abscess formation, periodontitis, and loosened teeth[84] (Figure 17-1). Perhaps the most striking changes in uncontrolled diabetes are the reduction in defense mechanisms and the increased susceptibility to infections, leading to destructive periodontal disease. In fact, periodontal disease is considered to be the sixth complication of diabetes.[110]

Periodontitis in type 1 diabetic patients appears to start after age 12 years.[35] The prevalence of periodontitis has been reported as 9.8% in 13- to 18-year-old patients, increasing to 39% in those 19 years and older.

The extensive literature on this subject and the overall impression of clinicians indicate that *periodontal disease in diabetic patients follows no consistent or distinct pattern.* Severe gingival inflammation, deep periodontal pockets, rapid bone loss, and frequent periodontal abscesses often

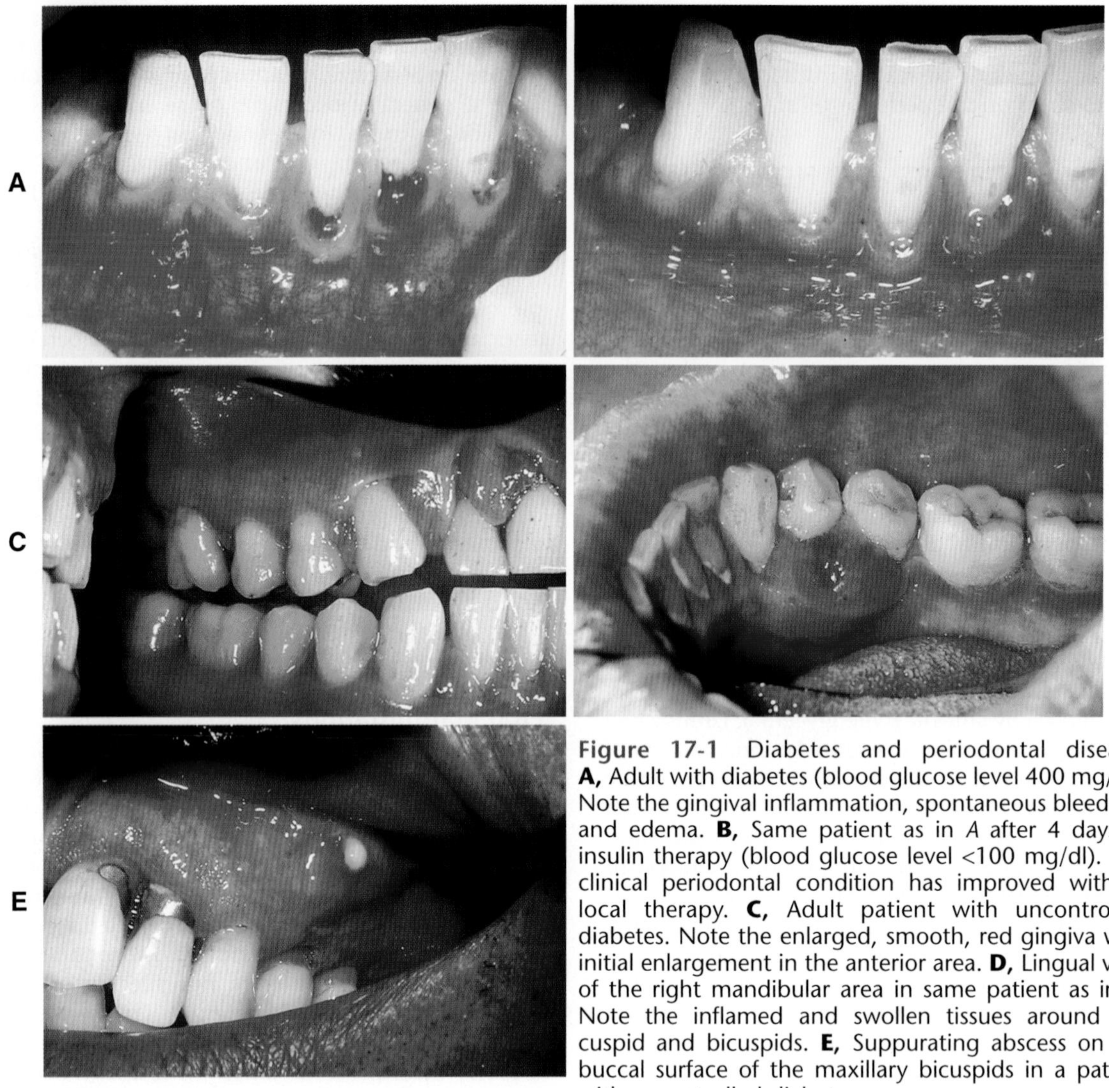

Figure 17-1 Diabetes and periodontal disease. **A,** Adult with diabetes (blood glucose level 400 mg/dl). Note the gingival inflammation, spontaneous bleeding, and edema. **B,** Same patient as in *A* after 4 days of insulin therapy (blood glucose level <100 mg/dl). The clinical periodontal condition has improved without local therapy. **C,** Adult patient with uncontrolled diabetes. Note the enlarged, smooth, red gingiva with initial enlargement in the anterior area. **D,** Lingual view of the right mandibular area in same patient as in *C*. Note the inflamed and swollen tissues around the cuspid and bicuspids. **E,** Suppurating abscess on the buccal surface of the maxillary bicuspids in a patient with uncontrolled diabetes.

occur in diabetic patients with poor oral hygiene[2] (Figure 17-2). Children with type 1 diabetes tend to have more destruction around the first molars and incisors than elsewhere, but this destruction becomes more generalized at older ages.[35] In juvenile diabetic patients, extensive periodontal destruction often occurs because of their age.

Other investigators have reported that the rate of periodontal destruction appears to be similar for those with diabetes and those without diabetes, up to age 30 years.[67,175] After age 30, diabetic patients have a greater degree of periodontal destruction, possibly related to disease destruction over time. Patients showing overt diabetes over more than 10 years have greater loss of periodontal structures than those with a diabetic history of less than 10 years.[67] This destruction may also be related to the diminished tissue integrity that continues to deteriorate over time. (See later description of altered collagen metabolism for an explanation of this observation.)

Despite that some studies have not found a correlation between the diabetic state and the periodontal condition, the majority of well-controlled studies show a higher prevalence and severity of periodontal disease in individuals with diabetes than in nondiabetic persons with similar local factors.* Findings include a greater loss of attachment, increased bleeding on probing, and increased tooth mobility. The lack of consistency is most likely related to the different degrees of diabetic involvement and control of the disease in patients examined and the diversity of indices and patient sampling.

Recent studies suggest that uncontrolled or poorly controlled diabetes is associated with an increased susceptibility and severity of infections, including periodontitis.[11,157] As with other systemic conditions associated with periodontitis, diabetes mellitus does not cause gingivitis or periodontitis, but evidence indicates that it alters the response of the periodontal tissues to local factors, hastening bone loss and delaying postsurgical healing of the periodontal tissues. Frequent periodontal abscesses appear to be an important feature of periodontal

*References 9, 16, 27, 38, 81, 133, 135, 136, 176.

A

B

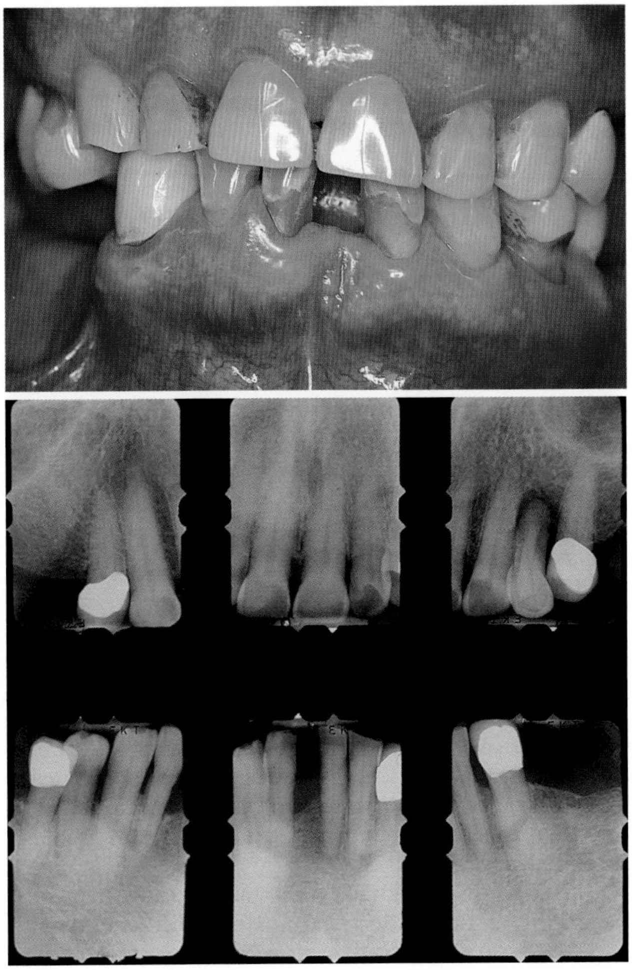

Figure 17-2 Diabetic patient. **A,** Gingival inflammation and periodontal pockets in 34-year-old patient with diabetes of long duration. **B,** Extensive, generalized bone loss in the patient shown in *A.* Failure to replace posterior teeth adds to the occlusal burden of the remaining dentition.

disease in diabetic patients. A study of risk indicators for a group of 1426 patients, ages 25 to 74, revealed that individuals with diabetes are twice as likely to exhibit attachment loss as nondiabetic individuals.[79]

Approximately 40% of adult Pima Indians in Arizona have type 2 diabetes. A comparison of individuals with or without diabetes in this Native American tribe has shown a clear increase in prevalence of destructive periodontitis, as well as a 15% increase in edentulousness, in diabetic patients.[46] The risk of developing destructive periodontitis increases threefold in these individuals.[52]

Bacterial Pathogens

The glucose content of gingival fluid and blood is higher in individuals with diabetes than in those without diabetes, with similar plaque and gingival index scores.[57] The increased glucose in the gingival fluid and blood of diabetic patients could change the environment of the microflora, inducing qualitative changes in bacteria that could contribute to the severity of periodontal disease observed in those with poorly controlled diabetes.

Patients with type 1 diabetes mellitus and periodontitis have been reported to have a subgingival flora composed mainly of *Capnocytophaga,* anaerobic vibrios, and *Actinomyces* species. *Porphyromonas gingivalis, Prevotella intermedia,* and *Actinobacillus actinomycetemcomitans,* which are common in periodontal lesions of individuals without diabetes, are present in low numbers in those with the disease.[80,122] Other studies, however, found scarce *Capnocytophaga* and abundant *A. actinomycetemcomitans* and black-pigmented *Bacteroides,* as well as *P. intermedia, P. melaninogenica,* and *Campylobacter rectus.*[121,160] Black-pigmented species, especially *P. gingivalis, P. intermedia,* and *C. rectus,* are prominent in severe periodontal lesions of Pima Indians with type 2 diabetes.[65,199] Although these results suggest an altered flora in the periodontal pockets of patients with diabetes, the exact role of these microorganisms has not been determined.

Polymorphonuclear Leukocyte Function

The increased susceptibility of diabetic patients to infection has been hypothesized as being caused by polymorphonuclear leukocyte deficiencies resulting in impaired chemotaxis, defective phagocytosis, or impaired adherence.[125,146] In patients with poorly controlled diabetes, the function of polymorphonuclear leukocytes (PMNs) and monocytes/macrophages is impaired.[88] As a result, the primary defense (PMNs) against periodontal pathogens is diminished, and bacterial proliferation is unchecked. No alteration of immunoglobulin A (IgA), G (IgG), or M (IgM) has been found in diabetic patients.[154]

Altered Collagen Metabolism

Increased collagenase activity and decreased collagen synthesis is found in individuals with poorly controlled diabetes who have chronic hyperglycemia. Decreased collagen synthesis, osteoporosis, and reduction in the height of alveolar bone occur in diabetic animals, with comparable osteoporosis in other bones.[68,162] Chronic hyperglycemia adversely affects the synthesis, maturation, and maintenance of collagen and extracellular matrix. In the hyperglycemic state, numerous proteins and matrix molecules undergo a nonenzymatic glycosylation, resulting in *accumulated glycation end products* (AGEs). The formation of AGEs occurs at normal glucose levels as well, but in hyperglycemic environments, AGE formation is excessive. Many types of molecules are affected, including proteins, lipids, and carbohydrates. Collagen is cross-linked by AGE formation, making it less soluble and less likely to be normally repaired or replaced. Cellular migration through cross-linked collagen is impeded, and perhaps more importantly, tissue integrity is impaired as a result of damaged collagen remaining in the tissues for longer periods (i.e., collagen is not renewed at a normal rate).[79] As a result, collagen in the tissues of patients with poorly controlled diabetes is aged and more susceptible to breakdown (i.e., less resistant to destruction by periodontal infections).

AGEs play a central role in the classic complications of diabetes[23] and may play a significant role in the progression of periodontal disease as well. Poor glycemic control, with the associated increase in AGEs, renders the periodontal tissues more susceptible to destruction.[161]

The cumulative effects of altered cellular response to local factors, impaired tissue integrity, and altered collagen metabolism undoubtedly play a significant role in the susceptibility of diabetic patients to infections and destructive periodontal disease.

Female Sex Hormones

There are several types of gingival disease in which modification of the female sex hormones is considered to be either the initiating or the complicating factor. Gingival alterations such as pubertal gingivitis, pregnancy gingivitis, and menopausal gingivostomatitis are associated with physiologic hormonal changes and are characterized by nonspecific inflammatory reactions with a predominant vascular component, leading clinically to a marked hemorrhagic tendency. These conditions are briefly described here; Chapter 43 provides a detailed discussion of issues related to the female patient.

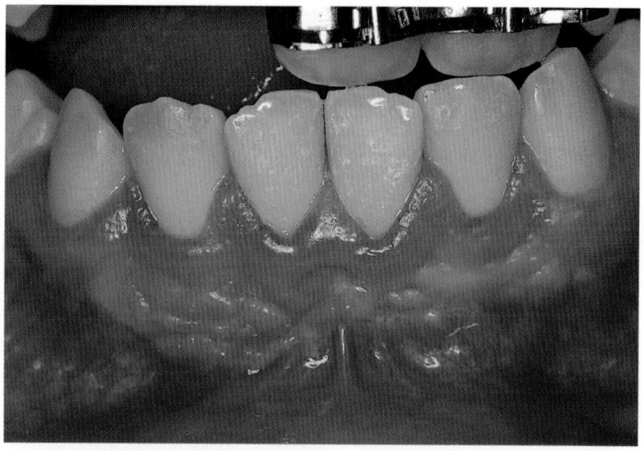

Figure 17-3 Gingivitis in puberty, with edema, discoloration, and enlargement.

The Gingiva in Puberty

Puberty is often accompanied by an exaggerated response of the gingiva to plaque.[172] Pronounced inflammation, bluish red discoloration, edema, and gingival enlargement result from local factors that would ordinarily elicit a comparatively mild gingival response (Figure 17-3).

As adulthood approaches, the severity of the gingival reaction diminishes, even when local factors persist. However, complete return to normal health requires removal of these factors. Although the prevalence and severity of gingival disease are increased in puberty, gingivitis is not a universal occurrence during this period; with good oral hygiene, it can be prevented (see Chapter 25).

Gingival Changes Associated with Menstrual Cycle

As a general rule, *the menstrual cycle is not accompanied by notable gingival changes,* but occasional problems do occur. Gingival changes associated with menstruation have been attributed to hormonal imbalances and in some patients may be accompanied by a history of ovarian dysfunction.

During the menstrual period, the prevalence of gingivitis increases. Some patients may complain of bleeding gums or a bloated, tense feeling in the gums in the days preceding menstrual flow. The exudate from inflamed gingiva is increased during menstruation, suggesting that existing gingivitis is aggravated by menstruation, but the crevicular fluid of normal gingiva is unaffected.[86] Tooth mobility does not change significantly during the menstrual cycle.[62] The salivary bacterial count is increased during menstruation and at ovulation up to 14 days earlier.[147]

Gingival Disease in Pregnancy

Gingival changes in pregnancy were described as early as 1898, even before any knowledge about hormonal changes in pregnancy was available.[18] *Pregnancy itself does not cause gingivitis.* Gingivitis in pregnancy is caused by bacterial plaque, just as it is in nonpregnant women. Pregnancy accentuates the gingival response to plaque and modifies the resultant clinical picture (Figure 17-4). *No notable changes occur in the gingiva during pregnancy in the absence of local factors.*

The reported incidence of gingivitis in pregnancy in well-conducted studies varies from about 50% to 100%.[109,116] Pregnancy affects the severity of previously inflamed areas; it does not alter healthy gingiva. Impressions of increased incidence may be created by the aggravation of previously inflamed but unnoticed areas. Tooth mobility, pocket depth, and gingival fluid are also increased in pregnancy.[87,106,150]

The severity of gingivitis is increased during pregnancy beginning in the second or third month. Patients with slight chronic gingivitis that attracted no particular attention before the pregnancy become aware of the gingiva because previously inflamed areas become enlarged, edematous, and more notably discolored. Patients with little or no noticeable gingival bleeding before pregnancy become concerned about an increased tendency to bleed (Figure 17-4, *A*).

Gingivitis becomes more severe by the eighth month and decreases during the ninth month of pregnancy; plaque accumulation follows a similar pattern.[109] Some investigators report that the greatest severity is between the second and third trimesters.[39] The correlation between gingivitis and the quantity of plaque is greater after parturition than during pregnancy, which suggests that pregnancy introduces other factors that aggravate the gingival response to local factors.[100]

Partial reduction in the severity of gingivitis occurs by 2 months postpartum, and after 1 year the condition of the gingiva is comparable to that of patients who have not been pregnant.[39] However, the gingiva does not return to normal as long as local factors are present. Tooth mobility, pocket depth, and gingival fluid are also reduced after pregnancy. In a longitudinal investigation of the periodontal changes during pregnancy and for 15 months postpartum, no significant loss of attachment was observed.[39]

Pronounced ease of bleeding is the most striking clinical feature. The gingiva is inflamed and varies in color from a bright red to bluish red.[200,201] The marginal and interdental gingivae are edematous, pit on pressure, appear

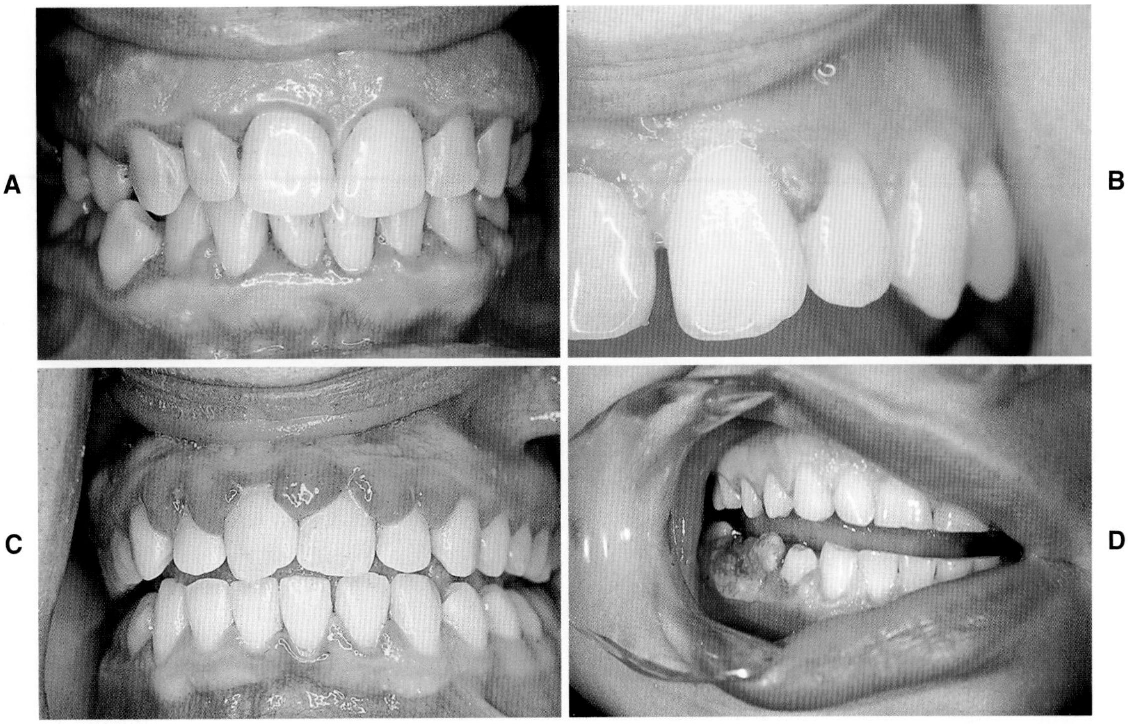

Figure 17-4 **A,** Marginal erythema and easily bleeding gingiva in a woman 5 months pregnant. **B,** Localized, incipient gingival enlargement between the maxillary central and lateral incisors in a woman 4 months pregnant. **C,** Generalized gingival enlargement of the papilla and gingival margins on the facial surface of the maxillary incisors in a pregnant woman. **D,** Extensive gingival enlargement localized on the buccal surface of teeth #28 to #30 in a pregnant woman. These lesions are often referred to as "pregnancy tumors."

smooth and shiny, are soft and pliable, and sometimes present a raspberry-like appearance. The extreme redness results from marked vascularity, and there is an increased tendency to bleed (see Figure 17-4, *A*). The gingival changes are usually painless unless complicated by acute infection. In some cases the inflamed gingiva forms discrete "tumorlike" masses, referred to as *pregnancy tumors* (Figure 17-4, *D*).

Microscopically, gingival disease in pregnancy appears as nonspecific, vascularizing, proliferative inflammation.[116,201] Marked inflammatory cellular infiltration occurs, with edema and degeneration of the gingival epithelium and connective tissue. The epithelium is hyperplastic, with accentuated rete pegs, reduced surface keratinization, and various degrees of intracellular and extracellular edema and infiltration by leukocytes.[181] Newly formed engorged capillaries are present in abundance.

The possibility that bacterial-hormonal interactions may change the composition of plaque and lead to gingival inflammation has not been extensively explored. Kornman and Loesche[101] reported that the subgingival flora changes to a more anaerobic flora as pregnancy progresses; the only microorganism that increases significantly during pregnancy is *P. intermedia*. This increase appears to be associated with elevations in systemic levels of estradiol and progesterone and to coincide with the peak in gingival bleeding. It has also been suggested that during pregnancy, a depression of the maternal T-lymphocyte response may be a factor in the altered tissue response to plaque.[137]

The aggravation of gingivitis in pregnancy has been attributed principally to the increased levels of progesterone, which produce dilation and tortuosity of the gingival microvasculature, circulatory stasis, and increased susceptibility to mechanical irritation, all of which favor leakage of fluid into the perivascular tissues.[129,136] A marked increase in estrogen and progesterone occurs during pregnancy, with a reduction after parturition. Animal studies with radioactive estradiol have demonstrated that the gingiva is a target organ for female sex hormones.[59] The severity of gingivitis varies with the hormonal levels in pregnancy.[87]

It has also been suggested that the accentuation of gingivitis in pregnancy occurs in two peaks: during the first trimester, when there is overproduction of gonadotropins, and during the third trimester, when estrogen and progesterone levels are highest.[109] Destruction of gingival mast cells by the increased sex hormones and the resultant release of histamine and proteolytic enzymes may also contribute to the exaggerated inflammatory response to local factors.[108]

Hormonal Contraceptives and the Gingiva

Hormonal contraceptives aggravate the gingival response to local factors in a manner similar to that seen in pregnancy and, when taken for more than $1^1/_2$ years, increase periodontal destruction.[50,99,107]

Although some brands of oral contraceptives produce more dramatic changes than others, no correlation has been found to exist on the basis of differences in progesterone or estrogen content in various brands.[116,145] Cumulative exposure to oral contraceptives apparently has no effect on gingival inflammation or oral debris index scores.[93]

Menopausal Gingivostomatitis (Senile Atrophic Gingivitis)

During menopause the usual rhythmic hormonal fluctuations of the female cycle are ended as estradiol ceases to be the major circulating estrogen.[127] As a result, females can develop a gingivostomatitis. This condition occurs during menopause or in the postmenopausal period. Mild signs and symptoms sometimes appear, associated with the earliest menopausal changes. Menopausal gingivostomatitis is not a common condition. The term used for its designation has led to the erroneous impression that it invariably occurs associated with menopause, whereas the opposite is true. Oral disturbances are not a common feature of menopause.[193]

The gingiva and remaining oral mucosa are dry and shiny, vary in color from abnormal paleness to redness, and bleed easily. Fissuring occurs in the mucobuccal fold in some women, and comparable changes may occur in the vaginal mucosa.[152] Microscopically, the gingiva exhibits atrophy of the germinal and prickle cell layers of the epithelium and, in some patients, areas of ulceration. The patient complains of a dry, burning sensation throughout the oral cavity, associated with extreme sensitivity to thermal changes; abnormal taste sensations described as "salty," "peppery," or "sour"; and difficulty with removable partial prostheses.[123]

The signs and symptoms of menopausal gingivostomatitis are somewhat comparable to those of chronic desquamative gingivitis (see Chapters 26 and 45). Signs and symptoms similar to those of menopausal gingivostomatitis occasionally occur after ovariectomy or sterilization by radiation in the treatment of malignant neoplasms.

Corticosteroid Hormones

In humans, systemic administration of cortisone and adrenocorticotropic hormone (ACTH) appears to have no effect on the incidence and severity of gingival and periodontal disease.[103] However, renal transplant patients who are receiving immunosuppressive therapy (prednisone or methylprednisone, azathioprine or cyclophosphamide) have significantly less gingival inflammation than control subjects with similar amounts of plaque.[14,95,138,179]

Exogenous cortisone may have an adverse effect on bone quality and physiology. The systemic administration of cortisone in experimental animals results in osteoporosis of alveolar bone; capillary dilation and engorgement, with hemorrhage in the periodontal ligament and gingival connective tissue; degeneration and reduction in the number of collagen fibers of the periodontal ligament; and increased destruction of the periodontal tissues, associated with inflammation.[72]

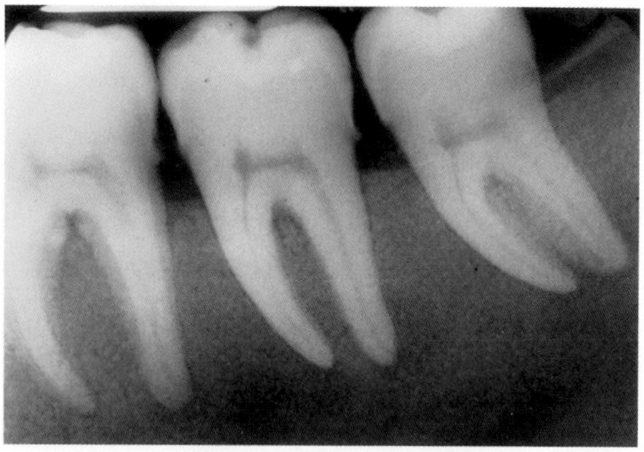

Figure 17-5 Secondary hyperparathyroidism in 35-year-old woman with advanced kidney disease. This periapical radiograph shows ground-glass appearance of bone and loss of lamina dura. (Courtesy Dr. L. Roy Eversole, San Francisco.)

Stress increases circulating cortisol levels through stimulation of the adrenal glands (hypothalamic-pituitary-adrenal axis). This increased exposure to endogenous cortisol may have adverse effects on the periodontium by diminishing the immune response to periodontal bacteria (see later discussion of psychosocial stress).

Hyperparathyroidism

Parathyroid hypersecretion produces generalized demineralization of the skeleton, increased osteoclasis with proliferation of the connective tissue in the enlarged marrow spaces, and formation of bone cysts and giant cell tumors.[190] The disease is called *osteitis fibrosa cystica,* or von Recklinghausen's bone disease.

Oral changes include malocclusion and tooth mobility, radiographic evidence of alveolar osteoporosis with closely meshed trabeculae, widening of the periodontal ligament space, absence of the lamina dura, and radiolucent cystlike spaces (Figures 17-5 and 17-6). Bone cysts become filled with fibrous tissue with abundant hemosiderin-laden macrophages and giant cells. These cysts have been called *brown tumors,* although they are not really tumors but reparative giant cell granulomas. In some cases these lesions appear in the periapical region of teeth and can lead to a misdiagnosis of a lesion of endodontic origin.[112]

Loss of the lamina dura and giant cell tumors in the jaws are late signs of hyperparathyroid bone disease, which in itself is uncommon. Complete loss of the lamina dura does not occur often, and clinicians may attach too much diagnostic significance to it. Loss of lamina dura may also occur in Paget's disease, fibrous dysplasia, and osteomalacia.

Different investigators report that 25%, 45%, and 50% of patients with hyperparathyroidism have associated oral changes.[155,168,171] A relationship has been suggested between periodontal disease in dogs and hyperparathyroidism secondary to calcium deficiency in the diet,[82] but this has not been confirmed by other studies.[173]

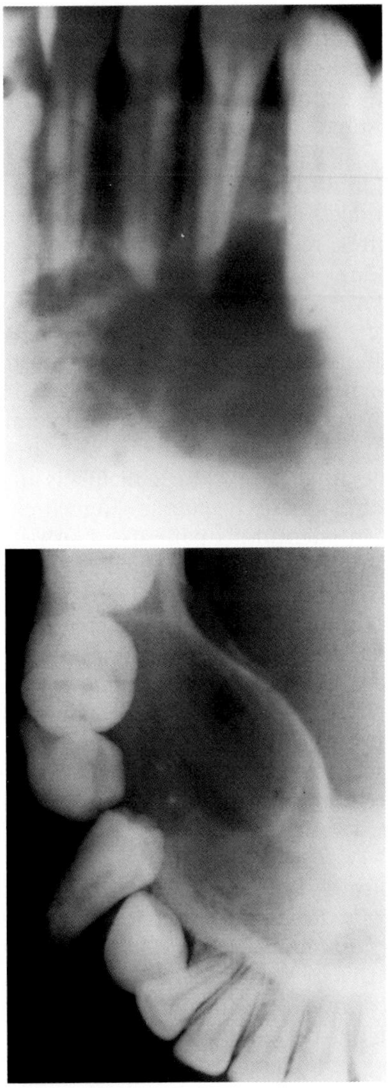

A

B

Figure 17-6 **A,** Periapical, and **B,** occlusal, radiographic views of brown tumors in patient with hyperparathyroidism. (Courtesy Dr. L. Roy Eversole, San Francisco.)

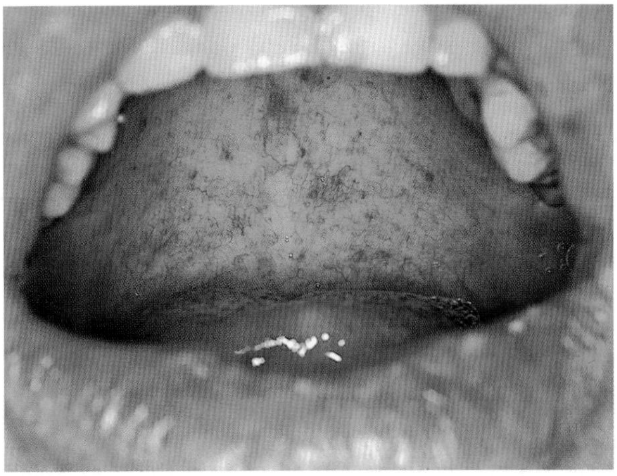

Figure 17-7 Petechiae evident on the soft palate of patient with underlying bleeding disorder.

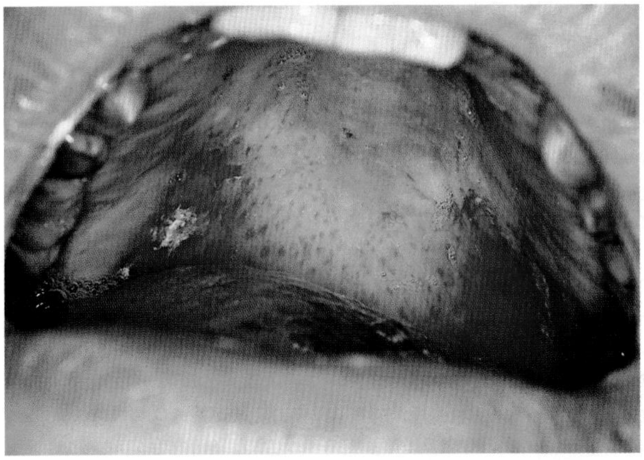

Figure 17-8 Ecchymosis evident on the lateral aspects of the soft palate and tonsillar pillars of patient with chemotherapy-induced thrombocytopenia.

HEMATOLOGIC DISORDERS AND IMMUNE DEFICIENCIES

All blood cells play an essential role in the maintenance of a healthy periodontium. White blood cells (WBCs) are involved in inflammatory reactions and are responsible for cellular defense against microorganisms as well as for proinflammatory cytokine release. Red blood cells (RBCs) are responsible for gas exchange and nutrient supply to the periodontal tissues and platelets and are necessary for normal hemostasis as well as recruitment of cells during inflammation and wound healing. Disorders of any blood cells or blood-forming organs can have a profound effect on the periodontium.

Certain oral changes such as hemorrhage may suggest the existence of a blood dyscrasia. However, a specific diagnosis requires a complete physical examination and a thorough hematologic study. Comparable oral changes occur in more than one form of blood dyscrasia, and secondary inflammatory changes produce a wide range of variation in the oral signs.

Gingival and periodontal disturbances associated with blood dyscrasias must be viewed in terms of fundamental interrelationships between the oral tissues and the blood cells and blood-forming organs rather than in terms of a simple association of dramatic oral changes with hematologic disease. Hemorrhagic tendencies occur when the normal hemostatic mechanisms are disturbed. Abnormal bleeding from the gingiva or other areas of the oral mucosa that is difficult to control is an important clinical sign suggesting a hematologic disorder. Petechiae and ecchymosis observed most often in the soft palate area are signs of an underlying bleeding disorder (Figures 17-7 and 17-8). It is essential to diagnose the specific etiology in order to address any bleeding or immunologic disorder appropriately.

Deficiencies in the host immune response may lead to severely destructive periodontal lesions. These deficiencies may be primary (inherited) secondary, caused by immunosuppressive drug therapy or pathologic destruction of the lymphoid system. Leukemia, Hodgkin's disease, lymphomas, and multiple myeloma all may result in secondary immunodeficiency disorders. This section discusses common hematologic and certain immunodeficiency disorders (see Chapter 34 for a detailed discussion of the HIV-infected patient).

Leukemia

The leukemias are malignant neoplasias of WBC precursors characterized by (1) diffuse replacement of the bone marrow with proliferating leukemic cells, (2) abnormal numbers and forms of immature WBCs in the circulating blood, and (3) widespread infiltrates in the liver, spleen, lymph nodes, and other body sites.[153]

According to the lineage of WBC involved, leukemias are classified as *lymphocytic* or *myelocytic;* a subgroup of the myelocytic leukemias is *monocytic* leukemia. According to their evolution, leukemias can be *acute,* which is rapidly fatal; *subacute;* or *chronic.* In acute leukemia the primitive "blast" cells are released into the peripheral circulation, whereas in chronic leukemia the abnormal cells tend to be more mature with normal morphologic characteristics and function when released into the circulation.

All leukemias tend to displace normal components of the bone marrow elements with leukemic cells, resulting in reduced production of RBCs, WBCs, and platelets and leading to anemia, *leukopenia* (reduction in number of *nonmalignant* WBSs) and thrombocytopenia. *Anemia* results in poor tissue oxygenation, making tissues more friable and susceptible to breakdown. A reduction of normal WBCs in the circulation leads to an increased susceptibility to infections. *Thrombocytopenia* leads to bleeding tendency, which can occur in any tissue but in particular affects the oral cavity, especially the gingival sulcus (Figure 17-9). Some patients may have normal blood counts while leukemic cells reside primarily in the bone marrow; this type of disease is called *aleukemic leukemia.*[74]

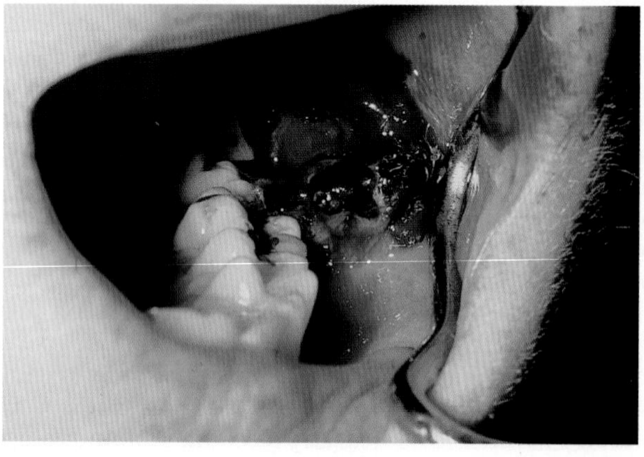

Figure 17-9 Spontaneous bleeding from the gingival sulcus in patient with thrombocytopenia. Normal coagulation is evident by the large clot that forms in the mouth. However, platelets are inadequate to establish hemostasis.

The Periodontium in Leukemic Patients

Oral and periodontal manifestations of leukemia consist of leukemic infiltration, bleeding, oral ulcerations, and infections. The expression of these signs is more common in acute and subacute forms of leukemia than in chronic forms.

Leukemic Infiltration. Leukemic cells can infiltrate the gingiva and less frequently the alveolar bone. Gingival infiltration often results in *leukemic gingival enlargement* (see Chapter 23).

A study of 1076 adult patients with leukemia showed that 3.6% of the patients with teeth had leukemic gingival proliferative lesions, with the highest incidence in patients with acute monocytic leukemia (66.7%), followed by acute myelocytic-monocytic leukemia (18.7%) and acute myelocytic leukemia (3.7%).[49] It should be noted, however, that monocytic leukemia is an extremely rare form of the disease. Leukemic gingival enlargement is not found in edentulous patients or in patients with chronic leukemia. Leukemic gingival enlargement consists of a basic infiltration of the gingival corium by leukemic cells that increases the gingival thickness and creates gingival pockets where bacterial plaque accumulates, initiating a secondary inflammatory lesion that contributes to the enlargement of the gingiva. Clinically, the gingiva appears initially bluish red and cyanotic, with a rounding and tenseness of the gingival margin; then it increases in size, most often in the interdental papilla and partially covering the crowns of the teeth (Figures 17-10 and 17-11).

Microscopically, the gingiva exhibits a dense, diffuse infiltration of predominantly immature leukocytes in the attached and marginal gingiva. Occasionally, mitotic figures indicative of ectopic hematopoiesis may be seen. The normal connective tissue components of the gingiva are displaced by the leukemic cells (Figure 17-12). The nature of the cells depends on the type of leukemia. The cellular accumulation is denser in the entire reticular connective tissue layer. In almost all cases the papillary layer contains comparatively few leukocytes. The blood vessels are distended and contain predominantly leukemic cells, and the RBCs are reduced in number. The epithelium presents a variety of changes and may be thinned or hyperplastic. Common findings include degeneration associated with intercellular and intracellular

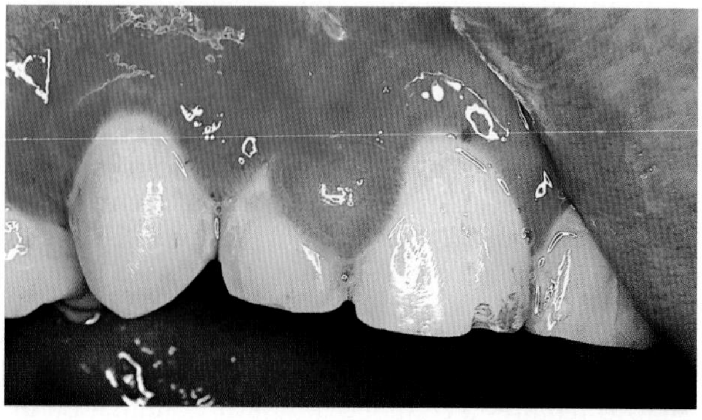

Figure 17-10 Leukemic infiltration causing localized gingival swelling of the interdental papillae.

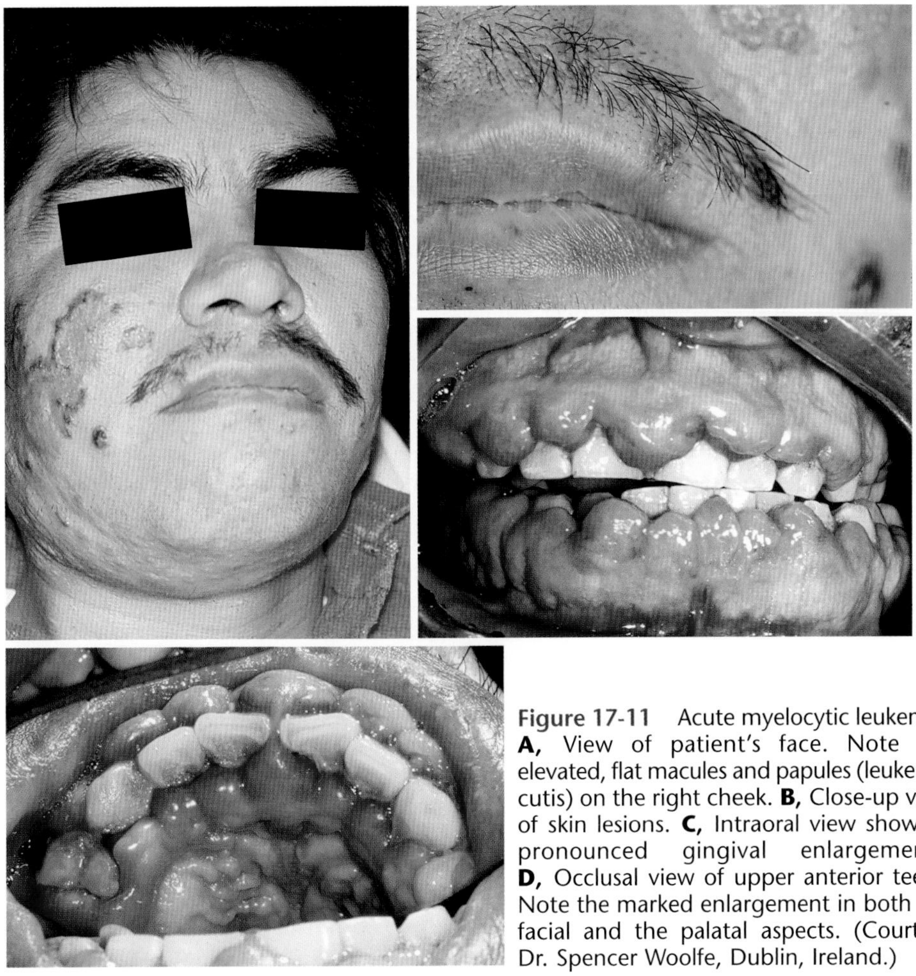

Figure 17-11 Acute myelocytic leukemia. **A,** View of patient's face. Note the elevated, flat macules and papules (leukemia cutis) on the right cheek. **B,** Close-up view of skin lesions. **C,** Intraoral view showing pronounced gingival enlargements. **D,** Occlusal view of upper anterior teeth. Note the marked enlargement in both the facial and the palatal aspects. (Courtesy Dr. Spencer Woolfe, Dublin, Ireland.)

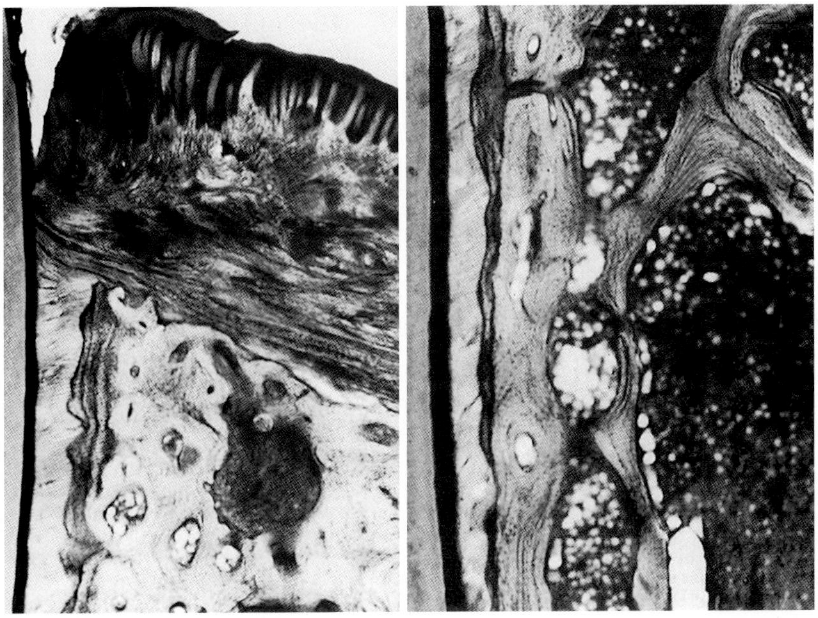

Figure 17-12 **A,** Leukemic infiltrate in gingiva and bone in human autopsy specimen. **B,** Same case as in *A.* Note the dense infiltrate in marrow spaces and the lack of extension to the periodontal ligament.

edema and leukocytic infiltration with diminished surface keratinization.

The microscopic picture of the marginal gingiva differs from that of other gingival locations in that it usually exhibits a notable inflammatory component, in addition to the leukemic cells. Scattered foci of plasma cells and lymphocytes with edema and degeneration are common findings. The inner aspect of the marginal gingiva is usually ulcerated, and marginal necrosis with pseudomembrane formation may also be seen.

The periodontal ligament and alveolar bone may also be involved in acute and subacute leukemia. The periodontal ligament may be infiltrated with mature and immature leukocytes. The marrow of the alveolar bone exhibits a variety of changes, such as localized areas of necrosis, thrombosis of the blood vessels, infiltration with mature and immature leukocytes, occasional RBCs, and replacement of the fatty marrow by fibrous tissue.

In leukemic mice the presence of infiltrate in marrow spaces and the periodontal ligament results in osteoporosis of the alveolar bone with destruction of the supporting bone and disappearance of the periodontal fibers[21,28] (Figure 17-13).

The abnormal accumulation of leukemic cells in the dermal and subcutaneous connective tissue is called *leukemia cutis* and forms elevated and flat macules and papules[49,153] (see Figure 17-11, A).

Bleeding. Gingival hemorrhage is a common finding in leukemic patients (see Figure 17-9), even in the absence of clinically detectable gingivitis. Bleeding gingiva can be an early sign of leukemia. It is caused by the thrombocytopenia resulting from replacement of the bone marrow cells by leukemic cells and from the inhibition of normal stem cell function by leukemic cells or their products.[153] This bleeding tendency can also manifest in the skin and throughout the oral mucosa, where petechiae are often found, with or without leukemic infiltrates. A more diffuse submucosal bleeding manifests as ecchymosis (see Figure 17-8). Oral bleeding has been reported as a presenting sign in 17.7% of patients with acute leukemia and in 4.4% of patients with chronic leukemia.[114] Bleeding may also be a side effect of the chemotherapeutic agents used to treat leukemia.

Oral Ulceration and Infection. In leukemia the response to bacterial plaque or other local irritation is altered; the cellular component of the inflammatory exudate differs both quantitatively and qualitatively from that in nonleukemic individuals. There is pronounced infiltration of immature leukemic cells in addition to the usual inflammatory cells. As a result, the normal inflammatory response may be diminished.

Granulocytopenia (diminished WBC count) results from the displacement of normal bone marrow cells by leukemic cells, which increases the host susceptibility to opportunistic microorganisms and leads to ulcerations and infections. Discrete, punched-out ulcers penetrating deeply into the submucosa and covered by a firmly attached white slough can be found on the oral mucosa.[10] These lesions occur in sites of trauma such as the buccal mucosa in relation to the line of occlusion or on the palate. Patients with past history of herpes infection may develop recurrent herpetic oral ulcers, often in multiple sites, and large atypical forms, especially after chemotherapy is instituted[78] (Figure 17-14).

A gingival (bacterial) infection in leukemic patients can be the result of an exogenous bacterial infection or an existing bacterial infection (e.g., gingival or periodontal disease). Acute gingivitis and lesions resembling necrotizing ulcerative gingivitis are more frequent and severe in terminal cases of acute leukemia[15] (Figures 17-15 and 17-16).

The inflamed gingiva in patients with leukemia differs clinically from that in nonleukemic individuals. Gingiva is a peculiar bluish red, is spongelike and friable,

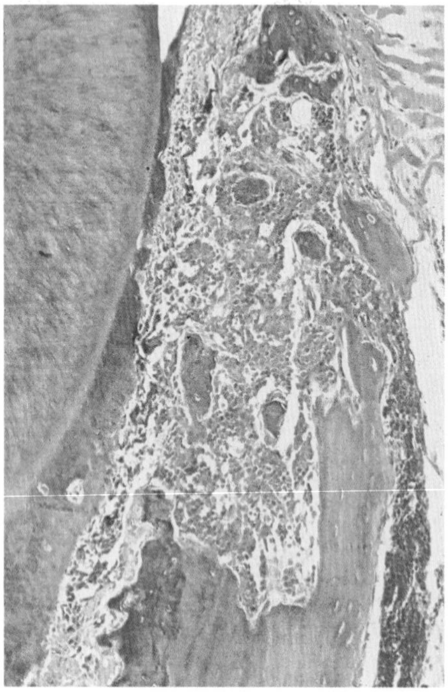

Figure 17-13 Leukemic infiltrate in alveolar bone in leukemic mouse. Note the leukemic infiltrate causing destruction of bone and loss of periodontal ligament.

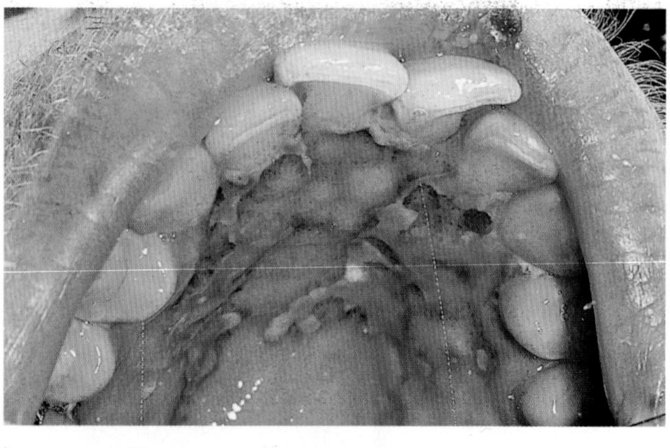

Figure 17-14 Large ulcerations on the palate of patient with granulocytopenia secondary to leukemia. These atypical ulcerations are caused by herpesvirus opportunistic infection. Notice the smaller, discrete, round ulcerations that have coalesced into the larger lesion.

A 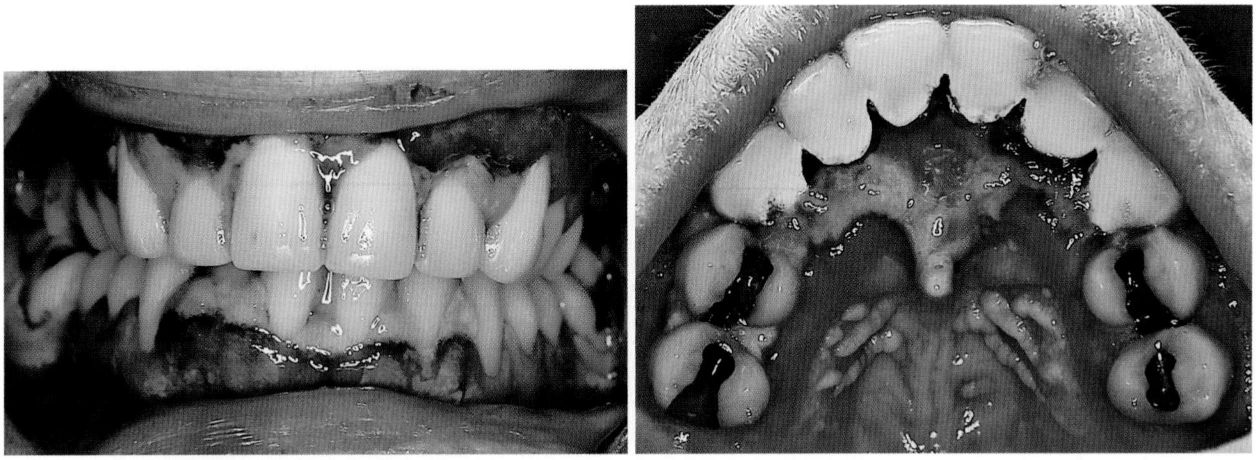 B

Figure 17-15 **A,** Anterior view of patient with acute myelocytic leukemia. Interdental papillae are necrotic with a highly inflamed and swollen base. **B,** Palatal view demonstrating extensive necrosis of interdental and palatal tissue.

A 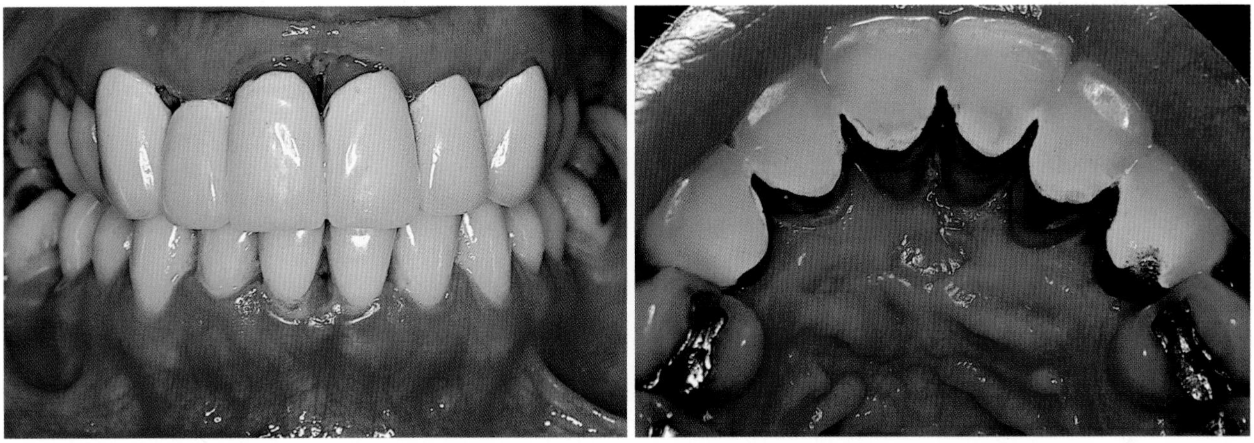 B

Figure 17-16 Same patient as in Figure 17-16 after chemotherapy and initial induction of remission. **A,** Anterior view reveals that although tissue health has dramatically improved, the interdental papillae have been lost. **B,** Palatal view shows extensive loss of gingival tissue around maxillary incisors.

and bleeds persistently on the slightest provocation or even spontaneously in leukemic patients. This greatly altered and degenerated tissue is extremely susceptible to bacterial infection, which can be so severe as to cause acute gingival necrosis and pseudomembrane formation (Figures 17-17 and 17-18). These are secondary oral changes superimposed on the oral tissues altered by the blood dyscrasia. They produce associated disturbances that may be a source of considerable difficulty to the patient, such as systemic toxic effects, loss of appetite, nausea, blood loss from persistent gingival bleeding, and constant gnawing pain. Eliminating or reducing local factors (e.g., bacterial plaque) can minimize severe oral changes in leukemia. In some patients with severe acute leukemia, symptoms may only be relieved by treatment that leads to remission of the disease.

In chronic leukemia, clinical oral changes suggesting a hematologic disturbance are rare. The microscopic

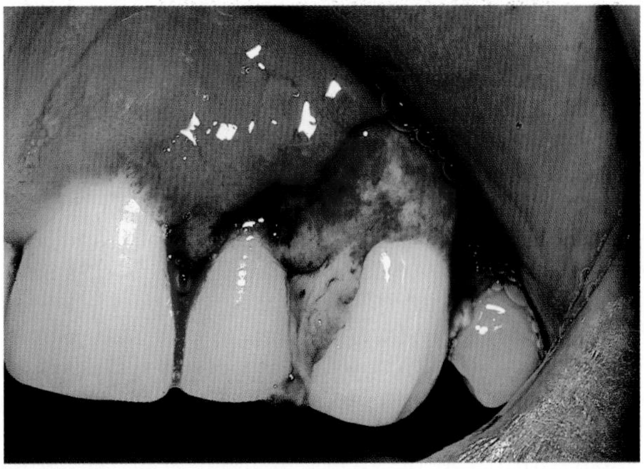

Figure 17-17 Opportunistic bacterial infection of gingiva in patient with leukemia. Gingival tissue is highly inflamed, bleeding, and necrotic with pseudomembrane formation.

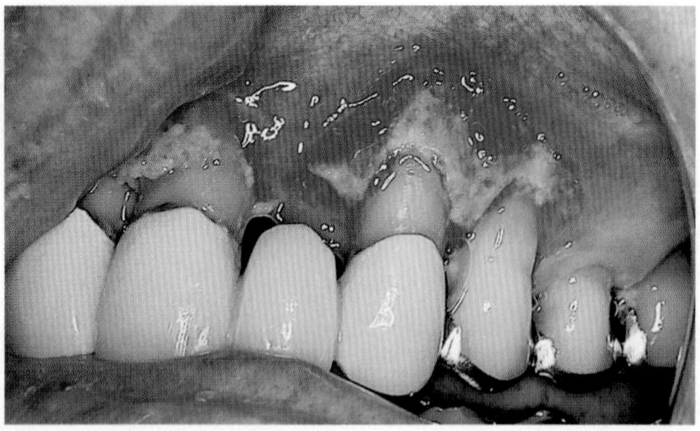

Figure 17-18 Opportunistic bacterial infection in immunosuppressed patient caused complete destruction of gingiva, exposing underlying alveolar bone.

changes in chronic leukemia may consist of replacing the normal fatty marrow of the jaws with islands of mature lymphocytes, or lymphocytic infiltration of the marginal gingiva without dramatic clinical manifestations.

The existence of leukemia is sometimes revealed by a gingival biopsy performed to clarify the nature of a troublesome gingival condition. In such cases the gingival findings must be corroborated by medical examination and hematologic study. In patients with recognized leukemia, gingival biopsy may indicate the extent to which leukemic infiltration is responsible for the altered clinical appearance of the gingiva. *Although such findings are of interest, their benefit to the patient is insufficient to warrant routine gingival biopsy studies in patients with leukemia.* Furthermore, it is important to note that the absence of leukemic involvement in a gingival biopsy specimen does not rule out the possibility of leukemia. A gingival biopsy in a patient with chronic leukemia may reveal typical gingival inflammation without any suggestion of a hematologic disturbance.

Anemia

Anemia is a deficiency in the quantity or quality of the blood, as manifested by a reduction in the number of erythrocytes and in the amount of hemoglobin. Anemia may be the result of blood loss, defective blood formation, or increased RBC destruction. Anemias are classified according to cellular morphology and hemoglobin content as (1) macrocytic hyperchromic anemia (pernicious anemia), (2) microcytic hypochromic anemia (iron deficiency anemia), (3) sickle cell anemia, or (4) normocytic-normochromic anemia (hemolytic or aplastic anemia).

Pernicious anemia results in tongue changes in 75% of patients. The tongue appears red, smooth, and shiny because of atrophy of the papillae (Figure 17-19). There is also marked pallor of the gingiva (Figure 17-20). *Iron deficiency anemia* induces similar tongue and gingival changes. A syndrome consisting of glossitis and ulceration of the oral mucosa and oropharynx, inducing dysphagia (Plummer-Vinson syndrome) has been described in patients with iron deficiency anemia. *Sickle cell anemia* is a hereditary form of chronic hemolytic anemia that occurs almost exclusively in blacks. It is characterized by pallor, jaundice, weakness, rheumatoid manifestations, and leg ulcers. Oral changes include generalized osteoporosis of the jaws, with a peculiar stepladder alignment of the trabeculae of the interdental septa, along with pallor and yellowish discoloration of the oral mucosa. Periodontal infections may precipitate sickle cell crisis.[149] *Aplastic anemia* result from a failure of the bone marrow to produce erythrocytes. The etiology is usually the effect of toxic drugs on the marrow or displacement of RBCs by leukemic cells. Oral changes include pale discoloration of the oral mucosa and increased susceptibility to infection because of the concomitant neutropenia.

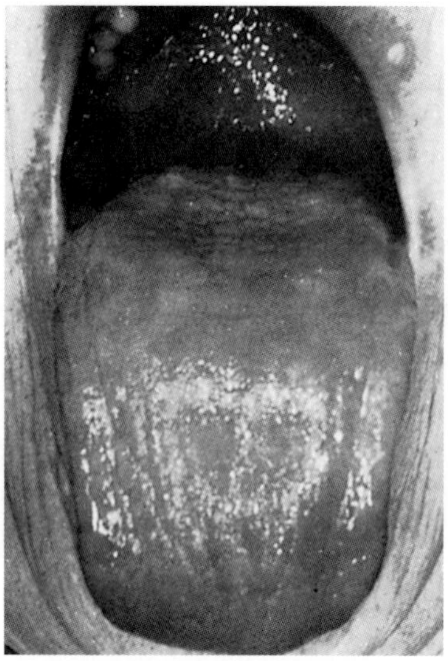

Figure 17-19 Smooth tongue in patient with pernicious anemia.

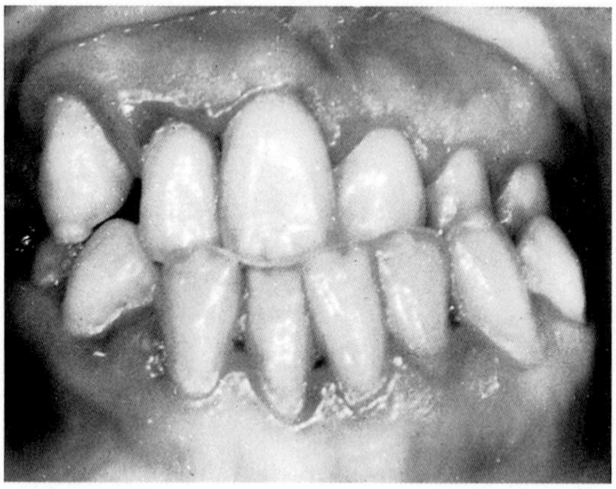

Figure 17-20 Diffuse pallor of gingiva in patient with anemia. The discolored, inflamed gingival margin stands out in sharp contrast to the adjacent pale, attached gingiva.

Thrombocytopenia

Thrombocytopenia is a term used to describe the condition of reduced platelet count resulting from either lack of platelet production or increased loss of platelets. *Purpura* refers to the purplish appearance of the skin or mucous membranes where bleeding has occurred as a result of decreased platelets. *Thrombocytopenic purpura* may be

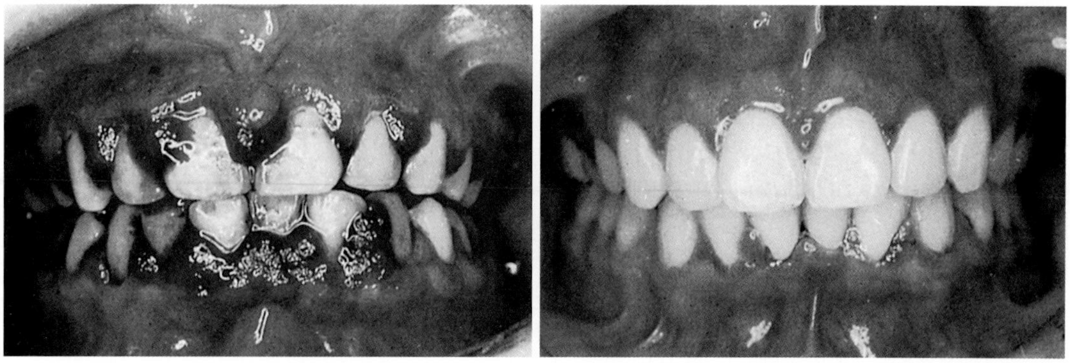

Figure 17-21 Thrombocytopenic purpura. **A,** Hemorrhagic gingivitis in patient with thrombocytopenic purpura. **B,** Marked reduction in severity of gingival disease after removal of surface debris and careful scaling.

idiopathic (i.e., of unknown etiology, as in Werlhof's disease) or may occur secondary to some known etiologic factor responsible for a reduced amount of functioning marrow and a resultant reduction in the number of circulating platelets. Such etiologic factors include aplasia of the marrow; displacement of the megakaryocytes in the marrow, as in leukemia; replacement of the marrow by tumor; and destruction of the marrow by irradiation or radium or by drugs, such as benzene, aminopyrine, and arsenical agents.

Thrombocytopenic purpura is characterized by a low platelet count, a prolonged clot retraction and bleeding time, and a normal or slightly prolonged clotting time. There is spontaneous bleeding into the skin or from mucous membranes. Petechiae and hemorrhagic vesicles occur in the oral cavity, particularly in the palate, tonsillar pillars, and the buccal mucosa (see Figures 17-7 and 17-8). The gingivae are swollen, soft, and friable. Bleeding occurs spontaneously or on the slightest provocation and is difficult to control. *Gingival changes represent an abnormal response to local irritation;* the severity of the gingival condition is dramatically alleviated by removal of the local factors (Figure 17-21).

Leukocyte (Neutrophil) Disorders

Disorders that affect production or function of leukocytes may result in severe periodontal destruction. The polymorphonuclear leukocyte (neutrophil, PMN) in particular plays a critical role in bacterial infections because PMNs are the first line of defense (see Chapter 13). Many systemic conditions associated with or predisposing to periodontal destruction include genetic disorders that result in an inadequate number or function of circulating neutrophils. This underscores the importance of the neutrophil in the protection of the periodontium against infection.

Severe periodontitis has been observed in individuals with *primary* neutrophil disorders such as neutropenia, agranulocytosis, Chédiak-Higashi syndrome, and lazy leukocyte syndrome. In addition, severe periodontitis has also been observed in individuals who exhibit *secondary* neutrophil impairment, as seen in Down syndrome, Papillon-Lefèvre syndrome, and inflammatory bowel disease. This section discusses conditions with primary and secondary leukocyte disorders.

Neutropenia

Neutropenia is a blood disorder that results in low levels of circulating neutrophils. An individual with an *absolute neutrophil count* (ANC) of less than 1500 cells per microliter is considered to be neutropenic. Neutropenia has numerous causes; it can be genetic or drug induced or may result from a viral infection. It may be chronic or cyclic, severe or benign. It affects as many as one in three patients receiving chemotherapy for cancer. Neutropenia is a serious condition. Infections are sometimes difficult to manage and may be life threatening, particularly when the ANC is less than 500 cells per microliter.

Agranulocytosis

Agranulocytosis is characterized by a reduction in the number of circulating granulocytes and results in severe infections, including ulcerative necrotizing lesions of the oral mucosa, skin, and gastrointestinal and genitourinary tracts. Less severe forms of the disease are called neutropenia or granulocytopenia.

Drug idiosyncrasy is the most common cause of agranulocytosis, but in some cases, its cause cannot be explained. Agranulocytosis has been reported after the administration of drugs such as aminopyrine, barbiturates and their derivatives, benzene ring derivatives, sulfonamides, gold salts, or arsenical agents.[102,115,128,149] It generally occurs as an acute disease. It may be chronic or periodic with recurring neutropenic cycles (e.g., cyclic neutropenia).[177]

The onset of disease is accompanied by fever, malaise, general weakness, and sore throat. Ulceration in the oral cavity, oropharynx, and throat is characteristic. The mucosa exhibits isolated necrotic patches that are black and gray and are sharply demarcated from the adjacent uninvolved areas.[96,119] *The absence of a notable inflammatory reaction caused by lack of granulocytes is a striking feature.* The gingival margin may or may not be involved. Gingival hemorrhage, necrosis, increased salivation, and fetid odor are accompanying clinical features. In cyclic neutropenia the gingival changes recur with recurrent exacerbation of the disease.[37] The occurrence of aggressive

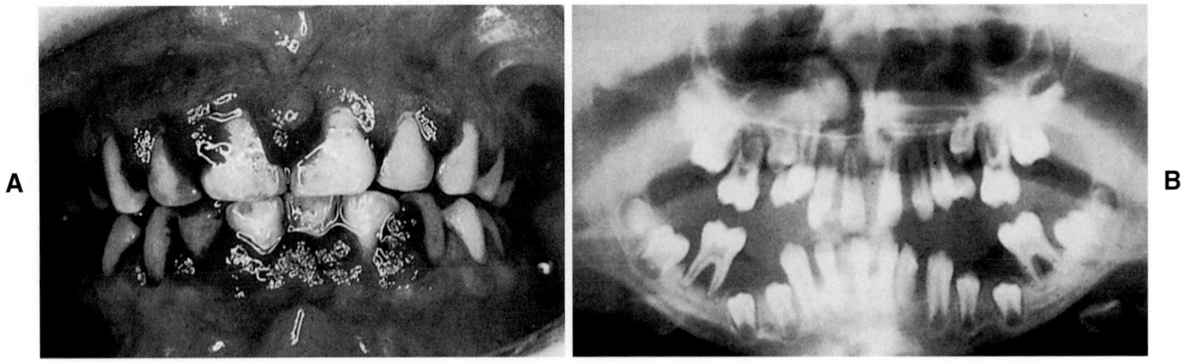

Figure 17-22 Prepubertal periodontitis **A,** Clinical presentation of 10-year-old male with cyclic neutropenia and agammaglobulinemia. Note the severe erythema and migration of teeth caused by loss of bone support. **B,** Panoramic radiograph demonstrating severe bone loss around all permanent teeth that have erupted into the oral cavity.

(formerly termed "rapidly progressive") periodontitis has been described in cyclic neutropenia[165] (Figure 17-22).

Because infection is a common feature of agranulocytosis, differential diagnosis involves consideration of such conditions as acute necrotizing ulcerative gingivitis, diphtheria, noma, and acute necrotizing inflammation of the tonsils. Definitive diagnosis depends on the hematologic findings of pronounced leukopenia and almost complete absence of neutrophils.

Chédiak-Higashi Syndrome

Chédiak-Higashi syndrome is a rare disease that affects the production of organelles found in almost every cell. It affects mostly the melanocytes, platelets, and phagocytes. It causes partial albinism, mild bleeding disorders, and recurrent bacterial infections. Neutrophils contain abnormal, giant lysosomes that can fuse with the phagosome, but their ability to release their contents is impaired. As a result, killing of ingested microorganisms is delayed. Aggressive (formerly termed "rapidly destructive") periodontitis has been described in these patients. Chédiak-Higashi syndrome has been described as a genetically transmitted disease in ranch-raised mink[8,142] (see Chapter 11).

Lazy Leukocyte Syndrome

Lazy leukocyte syndrome is characterized by susceptibility to severe microbial infections, neutropenia, defective chemotactic response by neutrophils, and an abnormal inflammatory response.[144] Individuals diagnosed with lazy leukocyte syndrome are susceptible to aggressive periodontitis with destruction of bone and early tooth loss.

Leukocyte Adhesion Deficiency

Leukocyte adhesion deficiency (LAD) is a very rare genetic disorder. Only a few hundred cases have been diagnosed. Because LAD is an inherited disease, it is categorized as a primary immunodeficiency most often diagnosed at birth. Many children do not survive.

LAD results from the inability to produce or failure to express normally an important cell surface integrin (CD18), which is necessary for leukocytes to adhere to the vessel wall at the site of infection. When leukocytes cannot effectively adhere to the vessel wall near the site of infection, they cannot migrate to the infection. As a result, bacterial infections are able to continue to destroy host tissues unimpeded by the normal host immune response. Infections act similarly to those observed in neutropenic patients because phagocytes are unable to reach the site of infection.

Cases of periodontal disease attributed to LAD are rare. They begin during or immediately after eruption of the primary teeth. Extremely acute inflammation and proliferation of the gingival tissues with rapid destruction of bone are found. Profound defects in peripheral blood neutrophils and monocytes and an absence of neutrophils in the gingival tissues have been noted in patients with LAD.[141,142] These patients also have frequent respiratory tract infections and sometimes otitis media. Both primary and permanent teeth are affected, often resulting in early tooth loss.[189]

Papillon-Lefèvre Syndrome

Papillon-Lefèvre syndrome is inherited and appears to follow an autosomal recessive pattern. Parents are not affected, and both must carry the autosomal genes for the syndrome to appear in the offspring. It may occur in siblings; males and females are equally affected. The estimated frequency is 1 to 4 cases per 1 million individuals. Rare cases of adult onset of this syndrome, although with mild periodontal lesions, have also been described.[24]

The syndrome is characterized by hyperkeratotic skin lesions, severe destruction of the periodontium, and in some cases, calcification of the dura.[30,55] The cutaneous and periodontal changes usually appear together before the age of 4 years. The skin lesions consist of hyperkeratosis and ichthyosis of localized areas on palms, soles, knees, and elbows (Figures 17-23 and 17-24).

Periodontal involvement consists of early inflammatory changes that lead to bone loss and exfoliation of teeth. Primary teeth are lost by 5 or 6 years of age. The permanent dentition then erupts normally, but within a few years the permanent teeth are lost because of destructive periodontal disease. By age 15 years, patients are usually edentulous except for the third molars. These

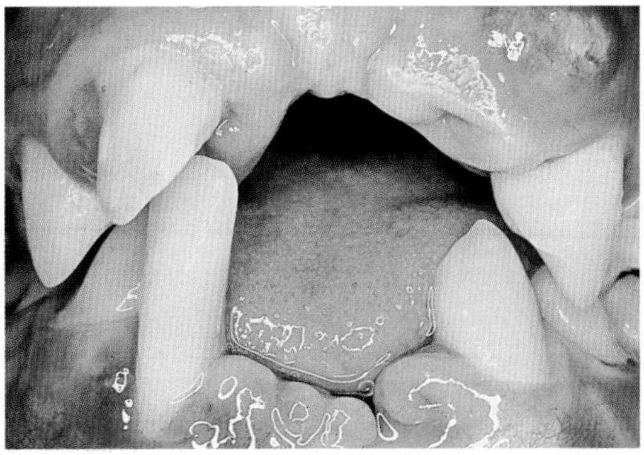

Figure 17-23 Dentition of 17-year-old boy with Papillon-Lefèvre syndrome. The missing teeth were exfoliated.

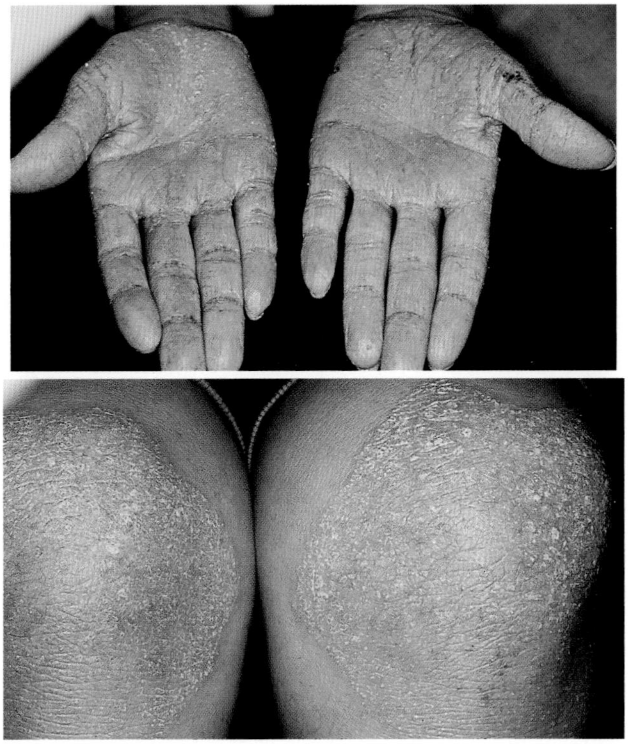
A

B

Figure 17-24 **A,** Palms, and **B,** knees, of the patient in Figure 17-24. Note the hyperkeratotic, scaly lesions.

also are lost a few years after they erupt. Tooth extraction sites heal uneventfully.[56] The microscopic changes reported include marked chronic inflammation of the lateral wall of the pocket with a predominantly plasma cell infiltrate, considerable osteoclastic activity and apparent lack of osteoblastic activity, and an extremely thin cementum.[120] Bacterial flora studies of plaque in a patient with Papillon-Lefèvre syndrome revealed a similarity to bacterial flora in chronic periodontitis.[113] Spirochete-rich zones in the apical portion of the pockets, as well as spirochete adherence to the cementum and microcolony formation of *Mycoplasma* species, have been reported in Papillon-Lefèvre syndrome.[92] Gram-negative cocci and rods appear at the apical border of plaque.[186]

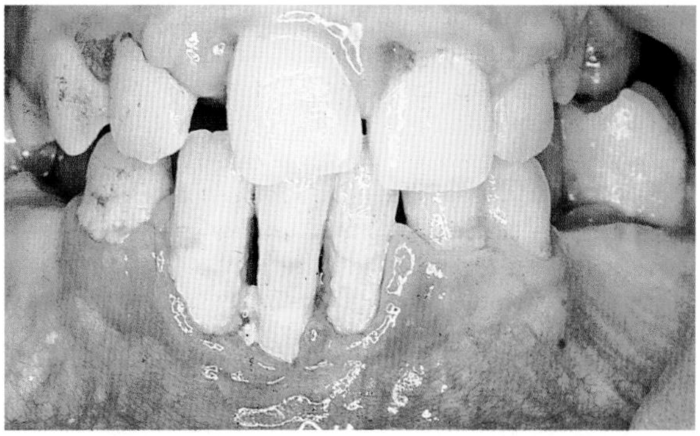

Figure 17-25 Severe periodontal destruction in 14-year-old patient with Down syndrome.

No significant alterations have been found in peripheral blood lymphocytes and PMNs.[164]

Down Syndrome

Down syndrome (mongolism, trisomy 21) is a congenital disease caused by a chromosomal abnormality and characterized by mental deficiency and growth retardation. The prevalence of periodontal disease in Down syndrome is high (occurring in almost 100% of patients younger than 30 years). Although plaque, calculus, and local irritants (e.g., diastemata, crowding of teeth, high frenum attachments, malocclusion) are present and oral hygiene is poor, the severity of periodontal destruction exceeds that explainable by local factors alone.[36,40,174]

Periodontal disease in Down syndrome is characterized by formation of deep periodontal pockets associated with substantial plaque accumulation and moderate gingivitis (Figure 17-25). These findings are usually generalized, although they tend to be more severe in the lower anterior region; marked recession is also sometimes seen in this region, apparently associated with high frenum attachment. The disease progresses rapidly. Acute necrotizing lesions are a frequent finding.

The high prevalence and increased severity of periodontal destruction associated with Down syndrome is most likely explained by poor PMN chemotaxis and phagocytosis.[44,90] Increased numbers of *P. intermedia* have been reported in the mouths of children with Down syndrome.[111]

Antibody Deficiency Disorders

Agammaglobulinemia

Agammaglobulinemia, or *hypogammaglobulinemia,* is an immune deficiency resulting from inadequate antibody production caused by a deficiency in B cells. It can be congenital (X-linked or Bruton's agammaglobulinemia) or acquired (common variable immunodeficiency).

Congenital agammaglobulinemia is caused by an X-linked, recessive gene (Bruton's tyrosine kinase). It affects approximately 1:100,000 population. Because the defect is recessive and linked to the X chromosome, only males have the disease. The gene is responsible for B-cell development. In the absence of mature B cells, patients lack lymphoid tissue and fail to develop plasma cells.

Thus, production of antibodies is deficient. Germinal centers where B cells proliferate and differentiate are poorly developed in all lymphoid tissues. Tonsils, adenoids, and peripheral lymph nodes are small or absent.

Acquired or *late-onset* agammaglobulinemia is most often known as *common variable immunodeficiency disease* (CVID). The disorder is characterized by the onset of recurrent bacterial infections in the second and third decades of life, resulting from drastic decrease in immunoglobulin and antibody levels. The basic immunologic defect in CVID is failure of B-lymphocyte differentiation into plasma cells. In contrast to patients with the X-linked form of the disease, patients with CVID typically have an enlarged spleen and swollen glands or lymph nodes. Along with other autoimmune problems, some patients develop autoantibodies against their blood cells. Causes of the disease are unknown. Unlike the X-linked early-onset form of the disease, CVID is not genetic, and both males and females are susceptible.

T-cell function remains normal in agammaglobulinemia. The disease (congenital or acquired) is characterized by recurrent bacterial infections, especially ear, sinus, and lung infections. Patients are also susceptible to periodontal infections. Aggressive periodontitis is a common finding in children diagnosed with agammaglobulinimia (see Figure 17-22).

Acquired Immunodeficiency Syndrome

Acquired immunodeficiency syndrome (AIDS) is caused by the human immunodeficiency virus (HIV) and is characterized by destruction of lymphocytes, rendering the patient susceptible to opportunistic infections, including destructive periodontal lesions and malignancies (see Chapter 34).

STRESS AND PSYCHOSOMATIC DISORDERS

Psychologic conditions, particularly psychosocial stress, have been implicated as risk indicators for periodontal disease.[64] The most notable example is the documented relationship between stress (e.g., experienced by soldiers at war or by students during examinations) and acute necrotizing ulcerative gingivitis (NUG) (see Chapters 24 and 32). The presence of NUG in soldiers stressed by wartime conditions in the trenches led to one of the early diagnostic terms used to describe this condition, "trench mouth." Despite the well-known association between stress and NUG, *confirming* the connection between psychologic conditions such as stress and other forms of periodontal disease (e.g., chronic periodontitis) has been elusive. These relationships may be difficult to elucidate because, as with many common diseases, the etiology and pathogenesis of periodontal disease are multifactorial, and the role of individual factors (e.g., stress) is difficult to define.

Some studies have failed to recognize a relationship between psychologic conditions and periodontal disease despite specific efforts to identify them. In a study of 80 patients (40 with aggressive periodontitis and 40 with chronic periodontitis), Monteiro da Silva et al.[130] failed to find psychologic factors that could be associated with periodontal disease.[130] They identified depression and smoking as *marginally* significant in the aggressive periodontitis group. The lack of significant differences in psychologic characteristics between the two groups in this study may be attributed to all individuals having some form of periodontitis. In an earlier study, Monteiro da Silva et al.[131] identified depression and loneliness as significant factors associated with aggressive periodontal disease in 50 patients compared with 50 periodontally healthy individuals and 50 individuals with chronic periodontitis.

Psychosocial Stress, Depression, and Coping

Recently, several clinical studies have documented the relationship between psychosocial stress and chronic forms of periodontal disease. In case-controlled studies, individuals with stable lifestyles (based on family structure and employment status) and minimal negative life events had less periodontal disease destruction than individuals with less stable lifestyles (e.g., unmarried, unemployed) and more negative life events.[43] Interestingly, it is now becoming apparent that the effect is not simply matter of the presence of stress versus a lack of stress but rather the type of stress as well as the ability of the individual to cope with stress that correlate with destructive periodontal disease.

All individuals experience stress, but these events do not invariably result in destructive periodontitis. The types of stress that lead to periodontal destruction appear to be more chronic or long term and less likely to be controllable by the individual. Life events such as the loss of a spouse or family member, a failed relationship, loss of employment, and financial difficulties are examples of stressful life events that are typically not controllable by the individual or not perceived by the individual as being under his or her control, rendering the person with a feeling of "helplessness." The duration of the stressful life event will also have an influence on the total impact of the stress-induced disease destruction.

Financial stress is an example of a long-term, constant pressure that may exacerbate periodontal destruction in susceptible individuals. Genco et al.[66] found that individuals with high levels of financial stress and poor coping skills had twice as much periodontal disease as those with minimal stress and good coping skills. Psychologic tests were used to identify and weigh the causes of stress, such as children, spouse, finances, single life, and work, and to measure individual coping skills. Individuals with problem-focused (practical) coping skills fared better than individuals with emotion-focused (avoidance) coping skills with respect to periodontal disease. As part of their analysis, the researchers also found that chronic stress and inadequate coping could lead to changes in daily habits, such as poorer oral hygiene, clenching and grinding, decreased saliva flow, and suppressed immunity.

Comparing 89 patients with periodontal disease to 63 periodontally healthy individuals, Wimmer et al.[192] found that patients with defensive (emotional) coping skills were more likely to refuse responsibility and downplay their condition. All patients completed a comprehensive stress assessment questionnaire (German language) to evaluate their coping behavior. Patients with periodontal disease were less likely to use "active" coping skills (i.e., situation control) and more likely to cope with stress by averting blame (emotional) than were periodontally healthy individuals.

These studies support the conclusion that one of the most important aspects related to the influence of stress on periodontal disease destruction is the manner in which the individual copes with the stress. Emotional coping methods appear to render the host more susceptible to the destructive effects of periodontal disease than do practical coping methods. Furthermore, emotional coping is more common in situations that must be accepted, and by individuals who feel helpless in the situation.

Stress-Induced Immunosuppression

Stress and psychosomatic disorders most likely impact the periodontal health through changes in the individual's behavior and through complex interactions among the nervous, endocrine, and immune systems. Individuals under stress may have poorer oral hygiene, may start or increase clenching and grinding of their teeth, and may smoke more frequently. All these behavioral changes increase their susceptibility to periodontal disease destruction. Likewise, individuals under stress may be less likely to seek professional care.

In addition to the many behavioral changes that may influence periodontal disease destruction, psychosocial stress may also impact the disease through alterations in the immune system. The influence of stress on the immune system and systemic health conditions such as cardiovascular disease is well known. Stress-related immune system changes clearly have the potential to affect the pathogenesis of periodontal disease as well. One possible mechanism involves the production of cortisol. Stress increases cortisol production from the adrenal cortex by stimulating an increase in the release of ACTH from the pituitary gland. Increased cortisol suppresses the immune response directly through suppression of neutrophil activity, IgG production, and salivary IgA secretion. All these immune responses are critical for the normal immunoinflammatory response to periodontal pathogens (see Chapter 12). The resulting "stress-induced" immunosuppression increases the potential for destruction by periodontal pathogens. Stress may also affect the cellular immune response directly through an increased release of neurotransmitters, including epinephrine, norepinephrine, neurokinin, and substance P, which interact directly with lymphocytes, neutrophils, and monocytes/macrophages via receptors causing an increase in their tissue-destructive function. Thus, in a manner similar to cortisol production, the "stress-induced" release of these neurotransmitters results in an immunosuppression that increases the potential for destruction by periodontal pathogens.

It is important to remember that although stress may predispose an individual to more destruction from periodontitis, the presence of periodontal pathogens remains as the essential etiologic factor (i.e., stress alone does not cause or lead to periodontitis in the absence of periodontal pathogens).

Influence of Stress on Periodontal Therapy Outcomes

Psychologic conditions such as stress and depression may also influence the outcome of periodontal therapy. In a large-scale retrospective study, Elter et al.[51] evaluated 1299 dental records from a health maintenance organization (HMO) database. More than half (697) of the patient records were complete enough for a comprehensive evaluation, including both periodontal diagnosis and psychologic profiles. The 85 individuals with depression had posttherapy outcomes that were less favorable (below median) compared to those without depression. The authors concluded that depression might have a negative effect on periodontal treatment outcomes.

In another study, Axtelius et al.[7] compared the psy chiatric characteristics of individuals with different outcomes to periodontal therapy. Two groups were compared to evaluate the psychologic characteristics of 11 individuals who were responsive to periodontal treatment compared with 11 individuals who were not responsive to periodontal treatment. The responsive group had a more rigid personality, whereas the nonresponsive group had a more passive, dependent personality. Furthermore, the nonresponsive group reported more stressful life events in their past.

Therefore, both stressful life events and the individual's personality and coping skills are factors to consider in assessing the risk of periodontal disease destruction and the potential for successful periodontal therapy. If these patients are identified (i.e., patients with emotional or defensive coping skills), care should be taken to ensure that they receive information in a manner that does not elicit a "defensive" reaction.

Psychiatric Influence of Self-Inflicted Injury

Psychosomatic disorders may result in harmful effects to the health of tissues in the oral cavity through the development of habits that are injurious to the periodontium. Neurotic habits, such as grinding or clenching the teeth, nibbling on foreign objects (e.g., pencils, pipes), nail biting, and excessive use of tobacco, are all potentially injurious to the teeth and the periodontium. Self-inflicted gingival injuries such as gingival recession have been described in both children and adults (Figure 17-26). However, Sandhu et al.[159] recently reported that these types of self-inflicted, factitious injuries are not common in psychiatric patients.

NUTRITIONAL INFLUENCES

Some clinicians enthusiastically adhere to the theory in periodontal disease that assigns a key role to nutritional deficiencies and imbalances. Research conducted up to the present in general does not support this view, but numerous problems in experimental design and data

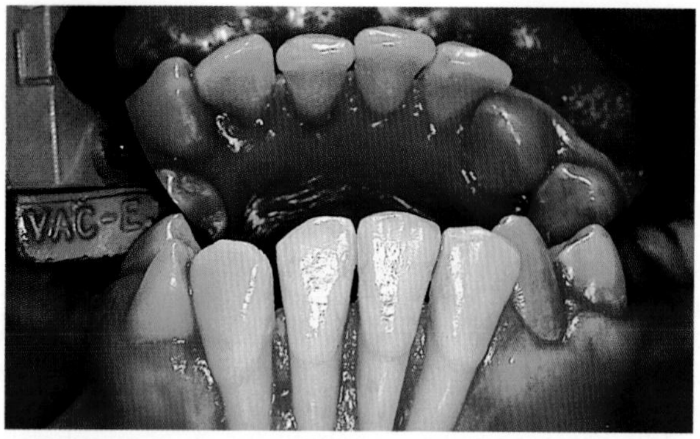

Figure 17-26 Severe gingival recession of all lower incisors, which was discovered under general anesthesia in an uncooperative, institutionalized adult with mental disorders. The patient was known to pace around the home with all four fingers inside his lower lip.

interpretation may render these research findings inadequate.[4,158] The majority of opinions and research findings on the effects of nutrition on oral and periodontal tissues point to the following:

1. *There are no nutritional deficiencies that by themselves can cause gingivitis or periodontitis.* However, nutritional deficiencies can affect the condition of the periodontium and thereby may accentuate the deleterious effects of plaque-induced inflammation in susceptible individuals. Theoretically, one might presume that an individual with a nutritional deficiency is less able to defend against a bacterial challenge compared with a nutritionally competent individual.
2. *There are nutritional deficiencies that produce changes in the oral cavity.* These changes include alterations of tissues of the lips, oral mucosa, gingiva, and bone. These alterations are considered to be periodontal and oral manifestations of nutritional disease.

This section reviews the existing knowledge in the field of nutrition as it relates to oral and periodontal changes as well as gingival and periodontal disease.

Fat-Soluble Vitamin Deficiency

Vitamins A, D, and E are fat-soluble vitamins required in the human diet.

Vitamin A Deficiency

A major function of vitamin A is to maintain the health of epithelial cells of the skin and mucous membranes. Deficiency of vitamin A results in dermatologic, mucosal, and ocular manifestations. In the absence of vitamin A, degenerative changes occur in epithelial tissues, resulting in a keratinizing metaplasia. Because epithelial tissues provide a primary barrier function to protect against invading microorganisms, vitamin A may play an important role in protecting against microbial invasion by maintaining epithelial integrity.

Little information is available regarding the effects of vitamin A deficiency on the oral structures in humans. Several epidemiologic studies have failed to demonstrate any relation between this vitamin and periodontal disease in humans.[188]

In experimental animals, vitamin A deficiency results in hyperkeratosis and hyperplasia of the gingiva with a tendency for increased periodontal pocket formation. The following periodontal changes have been reported in vitamin A–deficient rats: hyperplasia and hyperkeratinization of the gingival epithelium, with proliferation of the junctional epithelium, and retardation of gingival wound healing.[61] In the presence of local factors, vitamin A–deficient rats develop periodontal pockets that are deeper than those in animals not deficient in vitamin A and exhibit associated epithelial hyperkeratosis.[20,71]

Vitamin D Deficiency

Vitamin D, or calciferol, is essential for the absorption of calcium from the gastrointestinal tract and the maintenance of the calcium-phosphorus balance. Deficiency in vitamin D and imbalance in calcium-phosphorus intake result in rickets in young children and osteomalacia in adults. No studies demonstrate a relationship between vitamin D deficiency and periodontal disease.

The effect of vitamin D deficiency or imbalance on the periodontal tissues of young dogs results in osteoporosis of alveolar bone; osteoid that forms at a normal rate but remains uncalcified; failure of osteoid to resorb, which leads to its excessive accumulation; reduction in the width of the periodontal ligament space; a normal rate of cementum formation, but defective calcification and some cementum resorption; and distortion of the growth pattern of alveolar bone.[12,191]

In osteomalacic animals, there is rapid, generalized, severe osteoclastic resorption of alveolar bone; proliferation of fibroblasts that replace bone and marrow; and new bone formation around the remnants of unresorbed bony trabeculae.[48] Radiographically, there is generalized partial to complete disappearance of the lamina dura and reduced density of the supporting bone, loss of trabeculae, increased radiolucency of the trabecular interstices, and increased prominence of the remaining trabeculae. Microscopic and radiographic changes in the periodontium are almost identical with those seen in experimentally induced hyperparathyroidism.

Vitamin E Deficiency

Vitamin E serves as an antioxidant to limit free-radical reactions and to protect cells from lipid peroxidation. Cell membranes, which are high in polyunsaturated lipids, are the major site of damage in vitamin E deficiency. No relationship has been demonstrated between deficiencies in vitamin E and oral disease, but systemic vitamin E appears to accelerate gingival wound healing in the rat.[97,143]

Water-Soluble Vitamin Deficiency

Vitamins B and C are water-soluble vitamins required in the human diet.

B-Complex Deficiency

The vitamin B complex includes thiamin, riboflavin, niacin, pyridoxine (B_6), biotin, folic acid, and cobalamin

(B_{12}). Oral disease is rarely caused by a deficiency in just one component of the B-complex group; the deficiency is generally multiple.

Oral changes common to B-complex deficiencies are gingivitis, glossitis, glossodynia, angular cheilitis, and inflammation of the entire oral mucosa. The gingivitis in vitamin B deficiencies is nonspecific because it is caused by bacterial plaque rather than by the deficiency, but gingivitis is subject to the deficiency's modifying effect.

The human manifestations of **thiamin deficiency,** called *beriberi,* are characterized by paralysis; cardiovascular symptoms, including edema; and loss of appetite. Frank beriberi is rare in the United States. Oral disturbances that have been attributed to thiamin deficiency include hypersensitivity of the oral mucosa; minute vesicles (simulating herpes) on the buccal mucosa, under the tongue, or on the palate; and erosion of the oral mucosa.[77,117]

The symptoms of **riboflavin deficiency** *(ariboflavinosis)* include glossitis, angular cheilitis, seborrheic dermatitis, and a superficial vascularizing keratitis. The glossitis is characterized by a magenta discoloration and atrophy of the papillae. In mild to moderate cases the dorsum exhibits a patchy atrophy of the lingual papillae and engorged fungiform papillae, which project as pebblelike elevations.[197] In severe deficiency the entire dorsum is flat, with a dry and often fissured surface. Changes observed in riboflavin-deficient monkeys include severe lesions of the gingiva, periodontal tissues, and oral mucosa, including noma.[31,180]

Angular cheilitis begins as an inflammation of the commissure of the lips, followed by erosion, ulceration, and fissuring. Riboflavin deficiency is not the only cause of angular cheilitis. Loss of vertical dimension, together with drooling of saliva into the angles of the lips, may produce a condition similar to angular cheilitis. Candidiasis may develop in the commissures of debilitated persons; this lesion has been termed *perlèche.*[75] Supplemental riboflavin is ineffective to resolve cases of glossitis and angular cheilitis that are not caused by vitamin deficiency.[197]

Niacin deficiency results in *pellagra,* which is characterized by dermatitis, gastrointestinal disturbances, neurologic and mental disturbances (dermatitis, diarrhea, dementia), glossitis, gingivitis, and generalized stomatitis. This condition is rare but may occasionally result from malabsorption or alcoholism. Glossitis and stomatitis may be the earliest clinical signs of niacin deficiency.[118] The gingiva may be involved in *aniacinosis* with or without tongue changes.[98] The most common finding is NUG, usually in areas of local irritation.

Oral manifestations of vitamin B–complex and niacin deficiency in experimental animals include black tongue and gingival inflammation, with destruction of the gingiva, periodontal ligament, and alveolar bone.[13,45] Necrosis of the gingiva and other oral tissues and leukopenia are terminal features of niacin deficiency in experimental animals.

Folic acid deficiency results in macrocytic anemia with megaloblastic erythropoiesis, accompanied by oral changes, gastrointestinal lesions, diarrhea, and intestinal malabsorption.[47] Folic acid–deficient animals demonstrate necrosis of the gingiva, periodontal ligament, and alveolar bone without inflammation.[166] The absence of inflammation is the result of deficiency-induced granulocytopenia. In humans with sprue and other folic acid deficiency states, generalized stomatitis occurs, which may be accompanied by ulcerated glossitis and cheilitis. Ulcerative stomatitis is an early indication of the toxic effect of folic acid antagonists (e.g., methotrexate) used in the treatment of leukemia.

In a series of human studies, Vogel et al.[184,185] reported a significant reduction of gingival inflammation after systemic or local use of folic acid compared with placebo. This reduction occurred with no change in plaque accumulation. The authors also postulated that the gingival changes associated with pregnancy and oral contraceptives may be partly related to suboptimal levels of folic acid in the gingiva.[183] In a clinical study of pregnant women, a reduction in gingival inflammation occurred with the use of topical folate mouth rinses; no change was found with systemic folic acid.[139] A relationship has also been suggested between phenytoin-induced gingival overgrowth and folic acid, based on the interference of folic acid absorption and utilization of phenytoin.[182] However, a more recent double-blind, randomized, placebo-controlled study of 20 institutionalized epileptic adults taking phenytoin found no difference in gingival conditions (gingival overgrowth, health or plaque index) between the group taking 3 mg folic acid daily versus the placebo group at 4-week intervals over a 16-week period.[22]

Vitamin C (Ascorbic Acid) Deficiency

Severe vitamin C deficiency in humans results in *scurvy,* a disease characterized by hemorrhagic diathesis and delayed wound healing. Vitamin C is required in the human diet as well as in other primates, guinea pigs, and some rare flying mammals.[41] Because vitamin C is abundant in fruits and vegetables, scurvy is uncommon in developed countries. It may occur in infants in their first year of life if formulas are not fortified with vitamins and in older persons, especially those living alone and with restricted diets.[41] Malnutrition associated with alcoholism may predispose an individual to scurvy.

Scurvy results in defective formation and maintenance of collagen, impairment or cessation of osteoid formation, and impaired osteoblastic function.[58,194] Vitamin C deficiency is also characterized by increased capillary permeability, susceptibility to traumatic hemorrhages, hyporeactivity of the contractile elements of the peripheral blood vessels, and sluggishness of blood flow.[104] Clinical manifestations of scurvy include hemorrhagic lesions into the muscles of the extremities, the joints, and sometimes the nail beds; petechial hemorrhages, often around hair follicles; increased susceptibility to infections; and impaired wound healing.[41] Bleeding, swollen gingiva and loosened teeth are common features of scurvy.

Possible Etiologic Factors. Ascorbic acid may play a role in periodontal disease through one or more of the following suggested mechanisms[195]:

1. *Low levels of ascorbic acid influence the metabolism of collagen within the periodontium, affecting the ability of the tissue to regenerate and repair itself.* No experimental evidence supports this view of the role of ascorbic acid. Furthermore, it has been shown that collagen

fibers in the periodontal ligament of scorbutic monkeys are the last affected before death of the animals.[187]

2. *Ascorbic acid deficiency interferes with bone formation, leading to loss of periodontal bone.* Changes that do occur in alveolar bone and other bones as a result of failure of the osteoblasts to form osteoid take place very late in the deficiency state.[69] Osteoporosis of alveolar bone in scorbutic monkeys results from increased osteoclastic resorption and is not associated with periodontal pocket formation.[187]
3. *Ascorbic acid deficiency increases the permeability of the oral mucosa to tritiated endotoxin and tritiated inulin and of normal human crevicular epithelium to tritiated dextran.*[5,6] Optimal levels of vitamin C therefore would maintain the epithelium's barrier function to bacterial products.
4. *Increasing levels of ascorbic acid enhance both the chemotactic and the migratory action of leukocytes without influencing their phagocytic activity.*[73] Megadoses of vitamin C seem to impair the bactericidal activity of leukocytes.[167] The significance of these findings for the pathogenesis and treatment of periodontal diseases is not understood.
5. An optimal level of ascorbic acid is apparently required to maintain the integrity of the periodontal microvasculature, as well as the vascular response to bacterial plaque and wound healing.[26]
6. *Depletion of vitamin C may interfere with the ecologic equilibrium of bacteria in plaque and thus increase its pathogenicity.* However, no evidence demonstrates this effect.

Epidemiologic Studies. Several studies in large populations have analyzed the relationship between gingival or periodontal status and ascorbic acid levels.[188] These studies used different methods for the biochemical analysis of ascorbic acid and various indices for the assessment of periodontal changes; they were made in persons of different socioeconomic status, different races, and various ages. All the epidemiologic surveys failed to establish a causal relationship between the levels of vitamin C and the prevalence or severity of periodontal disease.[25,53,156] Megadoses of ascorbic acid have also been found to be unrelated to better periodontal health.[89,196]

Gingivitis. The legendary association of severe gingival disease with scurvy led to the presumption that vitamin C deficiency is an etiologic factor in gingivitis, which is common at all ages. Gingivitis with enlarged, hemorrhagic, bluish red gingiva is described as one of the classic signs of vitamin C deficiency, but *gingivitis is not caused by vitamin C deficiency.* Vitamin C–deficient patients do not necessarily have gingivitis. Acute vitamin C deficiency does not cause or increase the incidence of gingival inflammation, but it does increase its severity.[32,69,70] Gingivitis in vitamin C–deficient patients is caused by bacterial plaque. Vitamin C deficiency may aggravate the gingival response to plaque and worsen the edema, enlargement, and bleeding. In addition, although correcting the deficiency may reduce the severity of the disorder, gingivitis will remain as long as bacterial factors are present.

Periodontitis. Changes in the supporting periodontal tissues and gingiva in vitamin C deficiency have been documented extensively in experimental animals.[69,187] Acute vitamin C deficiency results in edema and hemorrhage in the periodontal ligament, osteoporosis of the alveolar bone, and tooth mobility; hemorrhage, edema, and degeneration of collagen fibers occur in the gingiva. Vitamin C deficiency also impairs gingival healing. The periodontal fibers that are least affected by vitamin C deficiency are those just below the junctional epithelium and above the alveolar crest, which explains the infrequent apical downgrowth of the epithelium.[187]

Vitamin C deficiency alone does not cause periodontal destruction; local bacterial factors are required for increased probing depth and attachment loss to occur. How-ever, acute vitamin C deficiency accentuates the destructive effect of gingival inflammation on the underlying periodontal ligament and alveolar bone.[70]

Experimental studies conducted in humans failed to show the dramatic clinical changes that have traditionally been described in scurvy.[42,85,151] A case report by Charbeneau and Hurt[32] showed worsening of a preexisting moderate periodontitis with the development of scurvy. In a retrospective analysis of 12,419 adults studied in the third National Health and Nutrition Examination Survey (NHANES III), Nishida et al.[134] found that there was a weak but statistically significant dose-response relationship between the levels of dietary vitamin C intake and periodontal disease in current and former smokers as measured by clinical attachment. This suggests that vitamin C deficiency has its greatest impact on periodontal disease when preexisting disease and other co-destructive factors are present.

Summary. Analysis of the literature indicates that the microscopic signs of vitamin C deficiency are quite different from those that occur in plaque-induced periodontal disease in humans. Patients with acute or chronic vitamin C–deficient states and no plaque accumulation show minimal, if any, changes in their gingival health status.

Protein Deficiency

Protein depletion results in hypoproteinemia with many pathologic changes, including muscular atrophy, weakness, weight loss, anemia, leukopenia, edema, impaired lactation, decreased resistance to infection, slow wound healing, lymphoid depletion, and reduced ability to form certain hormones and enzyme systems. Protein deprivation has been shown to cause changes in the periodontium of experimental animals.[33] The following observations have been made in protein-deprived animals: degeneration of the connective tissue of the gingiva and periodontal ligament, osteoporosis of alveolar bone, impaired deposition of cementum, delayed wound healing, and atrophy of the tongue epithelium.[28,169,170] Similar changes occur in the periosteum and bone in other nonoral areas. Osteoporosis results from reduced deposition of osteoid, reduction in the number of osteoblasts, and impairment in the morphodifferentiation of connective tissue cells to form osteoblasts, rather than from increased osteoclastic activity.

These observations are of interest in that they reveal a loss of alveolar bone resulting from the inhibition of normal bone-forming activity rather than from the introduction of destructive factors. Protein deficiency also accentuates the destructive effects of bacterial plaque and occlusal trauma on the periodontal tissues, but the initiation of gingival inflammation and its severity depend on the bacterial plaque.[170] In other words, protein deprivation results in periodontal tissues that lack integrity and, as a result, are more vulnerable to breakdown when challenged by bacteria.

OTHER SYSTEMIC CONDITIONS

Hypophosphatasia

Hypophosphatasia is a rare familial skeletal disease characterized by rickets, poor cranial bone formation, craneostenosis, and premature loss of primary teeth, particularly the incisors. Patients have a low level of serum alkaline phosphatase, and phosphoethanolamine is present in serum and urine.

Teeth are lost with no clinical evidence of gingival inflammation and show reduced cementum formation.[17] In patients with minimal bone abnormalities, premature loss of deciduous teeth may be the only symptom of hypophosphatasia. In adolescents, this disease resembles localized "juvenile" (aggressive) periodontitis.[198]

Congenital Heart Disease

Congenital heart disease occurs in about 1% of live births. Approximately 40% of individuals born with heart defects would die without treatment. However, the prognosis has been dramatically improved with advances in cardiac surgery. Cardiac defects can involve the heart, the adjacent vessels, or a combination of both. The most striking feature of congenital heart disease is cyanosis caused by shunting of deoxygenated blood from the right to left, resulting in a return of poorly oxygenated blood to systemic circulation. In severe cases, cyanosis is obvious at birth, particularly in Tetralogy of Fallot. Chronic hypoxia causes impaired development, compensatory poly-cythemia (increase in RBCs/hemoglobin) and clubbing edema of toes and fingers (Figure 17-27). Polycythemia is significant because it can result in hemorrhagic or thrombotic tendencies. Patients with congenital heart defects are often at risk of infective endocarditis because of turbulent blood flow in the heart and associated cardiovascular defects. The need for prophylactic antibiotics should be evaluated before dental therapy.

In addition to the obvious cyanosis of lips and oral mucosa, oral abnormalities associated with cyanotic congenital heart disease include delayed eruption of both deciduous and permanent dentitions, increased positional abnormalities, and enamel hypoplasia. The teeth often have a bluish white appearance with an increased pulp vascular volume. Gingival disease and other oral symptoms have been reported in children with congenital heart disease.[19,94] Reports seem to indicate more severe caries and periodontal disease in patients with cyanotic congenital heart defects. However, the apparent increase in dental disease may be attributed to poor oral hygiene and a general lack of dental care rather than a disease-related etiology.

Tetralogy of Fallot

As its name implies, tetralogy of Fallot is characterized by four cardiac defects: (1) ventricular septal defect, (2) pulmonary stenosis, (3) malposition of the aorta to the right, and (4) compensatory right ventricular enlargement. Clinical features include severe cyanosis, audible heart murmurs, and breathlessness. Cyanosis and breathlessness cause cerebral anoxia and syncope. Oral changes include a purplish red discoloration of the lips and gingiva. Severe marginal gingivitis and periodontal destruction have been reported (Figure 17-28). The discoloration of the lips and gingiva corresponds to the general degree of cyanosis and returns to normal after corrective heart surgery. The tongue appears coated, fissured, and edematous, and there is extreme reddening of the fungiform and filiform papillae. The number of subepithelial capillaries is increased but also returns to normal after heart surgery.[60]

Eisenmenger's Syndrome

Among patients with ventricular septal defects, about half with large defects (>1.5 cm in diameter) develop Eisenmenger's syndrome. This syndrome is distinguished by a greater blood flow from the stronger left ventricle

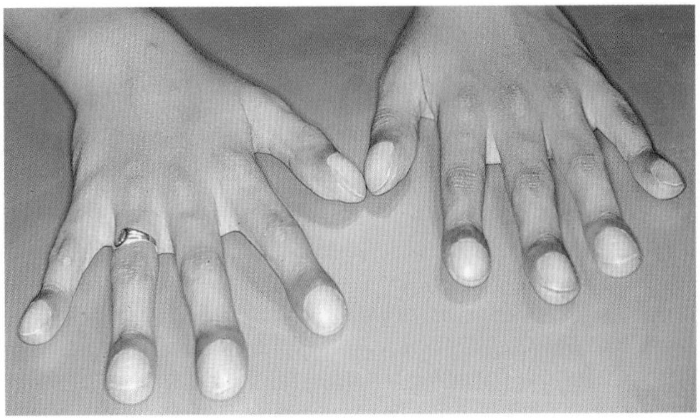

Figure 17-27 Characteristic clubbing of the fingers in adolescent patient with tetralogy of Fallot, consistent with untreated congenital cyanotic heart disease.

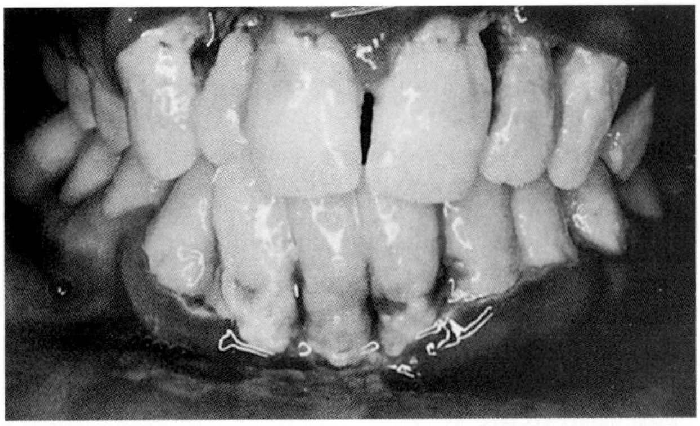

Figure 17-28 Extensive marginal inflammation with ulceronecrotic lesions and periodontal destruction in patient shown in Figure 17-27.

to the right ventricle (backward flow) through the septal defect causing increased pulmonary blood flow, which in turn leads to progressive pulmonary fibrosis, small-vessel occlusion, and high pulmonary vascular resistance. With increasing pulmonary resistance, the right ventricle hypertrophies, the shunt becomes bidirectional, and ultimately blood flow is reversed (right to left). The increased vascular resistance builds pressure in the right ventricle, causing right ventricular hypertrophy, and a reverse in the direction of the blood flow, resulting in a right-to-left shunt.

The natural history of a patient with untreated Eisenmenger's syndrome is a gradual increase in cyanosis over many years, eventually leading to cardiac failure. Cyanosis of the lips, cheeks, and buccal mucous membranes is observed in these patients but is much less severe than in those with tetralogy of Fallot. Severe, generalized periodontitis has been reported in patients with Eisenmenger's syndrome.[34] However, similar to patients with other types of congenital heart disease, the incidence of periodontal disease reported in those with Eisenmenger's syndrome may be related more to poor oral hygiene and a general lack of dental care than to any specific, syndrome-related etiology.

Metal Intoxication

The ingestion of metals such as mercury, lead, and bismuth in medicinal compounds and through industrial contact may result in oral manifestations caused by either intoxication or absorption without evidence of toxicity.

Bismuth Intoxication

Chronic bismuth intoxication is characterized by gastrointestinal disturbances, nausea, vomiting, and jaundice, as well as by an ulcerative gingivostomatitis, generally with pigmentation and accompanied by a metallic taste and burning sensation of the oral mucosa. The tongue may be sore and inflamed. Urticaria, different types of exanthematous eruptions, bullous and purpuric lesions, and herpes zoster–like eruptions and pigmentation of the skin and mucous membranes are among the dermatologic lesions attributed to bismuth intoxication. *Acute* bismuth intoxication, which is seen less frequently, is accompanied by methemoglobin formation, cyanosis, and dyspnea.[83]

Bismuth pigmentation in the oral cavity usually appears as a narrow, bluish black discoloration of the gingival margin in areas of preexisting gingival inflammation (Figure 17-29) (see Chapter 22). Such pigmentation results from the precipitation of particles of bismuth sulfide associated with vascular changes in inflammation; it is not evidence of intoxication but simply indicates the presence of bismuth in the bloodstream. Bismuth pigmentation in the oral cavity also occurs in cases of intoxication; it assumes a linear form if the marginal gingiva is inflamed.

Lead Intoxication

Lead is slowly absorbed, and toxic symptoms are not particularly definitive when they do occur.[91] There is pallor of the face and lips and gastrointestinal symptoms

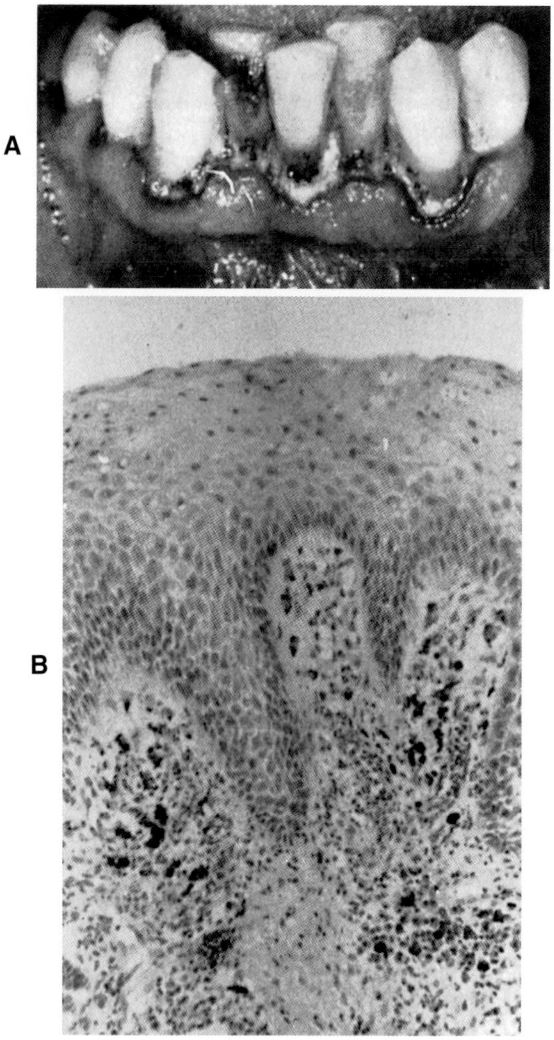

Figure 17-29 Bismuth line. **A,** Linear discoloration of the gingival in relation to local irritation in a patient receiving bismuth therapy. **B,** Biopsy specimen showing bismuth particles engulfed by monocytes/macrophages.

consisting of nausea, vomiting, loss of appetite, and abdominal colic. Peripheral neuritis, psychologic disorders, and encephalitis have been reported. Oral signs include salivation, coated tongue, a peculiar sweetish taste, gingival pigmentation, and ulceration. *Gingival pigmentation is linear (burtonian line), steel gray, and associated with local inflammation. Oral signs may occur without toxic symptoms.*

Mercury Intoxication

Mercury intoxication is characterized by headache, insomnia, cardiovascular symptoms, pronounced salivation (ptyalism), and a metallic taste.[3] *Gingival pigmentation in linear form results from the deposition of mercuric sulfide. The chemical also acts as an irritant, which accentuates the preexisting inflammation and often leads to notable ulceration of the gingiva and adjacent mucosa and destruction of the underlying bone.* Mercurial pigmentation of the gingiva also occurs in areas of local irritation in patients without symptoms of intoxication.

SCIENCE TRANSFER

A wide variety of systemic abnormalities affect the host response to bacterial plaque that is central to periodontal disease. The systemic diseases that play a role in loss of periodontal health need to be considered in the initial diagnosis, and in some cases, periodontal changes may be the initial presenting sign of disease, such as the gingival bleeding and ecchymosis seen in leukemia.

Of particular note is diabetes, which affects 5% to 9% of the U.S. population. Diabetic patients have increased bone destruction, increased incidence of periodontal abscesses, and often an exaggerated, acute inflammatory reaction to plaque. *Because half of diabetic individuals are undiagnosed, clinicians may detect suspect patients based on their periodontal status and refer the patient for appropriate blood tests for definitive diagnosis of diabetes.* Treatment outcomes are generally poorer in diabetic patients; therefore, treatment plans need to be instituted at times of optimum control of circulating glucose, and antimicrobial protocols are needed to control posttreatment infections.

In the past, systemic diseases were known to influence periodontal disease, but more recently, periodontal disease has been shown to influence systemic health. Thus it is important to understand possible relationships between multiple factors that may alter the periodontal tissues, and vice versa. One well-described relationship is the interaction between the bacterial plaque and the host's first line of defense, the polymorphonuclear leukocyte (PMN). Several conditions demonstrate that interference with the host's ability to neutralize the bacteria in plaque results in periodontal tissue destruction. In a severe example, when leukocytes lack a certain cell receptor that allows the cell to adhere to the blood vessel wall near an infection (e.g., in leukocyte adhesion deficiency), the condition can be lethal. In addition, stressful life events can influence periodontal disease, and this appears to be related to the individual's personality and coping skills. *Thus, assessing the risk of periodontal disease must be comprehensive, and similarly, informing the patient of potential risk to systemic health must be broad in scope.*

Other Chemicals

Other chemicals, such as phosphorus, arsenic, and chromium, may cause necrosis of the alveolar bone with loosening and exfoliation of the teeth.[105,163] Inflammation and ulceration of the gingiva are usually associated with destruction of the underlying tissues. Benzene intoxication is accompanied by gingival bleeding and ulceration with destruction of the underlying bone.[163]

REFERENCES

1. Adler P, Wegner H, Bohatka A: Influence of age and duration of diabetes on dental development in diabetic children, *J Dent Res* 52:535, 1973.
2. Ainamo J, Lahtinen A, Vitto VJ: Rapid periodontal destruction in adult humans with poorly controlled diabetes: a report of two cases, *J Clin Periodontol* 17:22, 1990.
3. Akers LH: Ulcerative stomatitis following therapeutic use of mercury and bismuth, *J Am Dent Assoc* 23:781, 1936.
4. Alfano MC: Controversies, perspectives and clinical implications of nutrition in periodontal disease, *Dent Clin North Am* 20:519, 1976.
5. Alfano MC, Miller SA, Drummond JF: Effect of ascorbic acid deficiency on the permeability and collagen biosynthesis of oral mucosal epithelium, *Ann NY Acad Sci* 258:253, 1975.
6. Alvares O, Siegel I: Permeability of gingival sulcular epithelium in the development of scorbutic gingivitis, *J Oral Pathol* 10:40, 1981.
7. Axtelius B, Soderfeldt B, Nilsson A, et al: Therapy-resistant periodontitis: psychosocial characteristics, *J Clin Periodontol* 25:482, 1998.
8. Babior BM: Disorders of neutrophil function. In Wyngaarden JB, Smith LHJ, editors: *Cecil textbook of medicine,* ed 18, Philadelphia, 1988, Saunders.
9. Barnett ML, Baker RL, Yancey JM, et al: Absence of periodontitis in a population of insulin-dependent diabetes mellitus (IDDM) patients, *J Periodontol* 55:402, 1984.
10. Barrett P: Gingival lesions in leukemia: a classification, *J Periodontol* 55:585, 1984.
11. Bartolucci EG, Parkes RB: Accelerated periodontal breakdown in uncontrolled diabetes: pathogenesis and treatment, *Oral Surg Oral Med Oral Pathol* 52:387, 1981.
12. Becks H, Collins DA, Freytog RM: Changes in oral structures of the dog persisting after chronic overdoses of vitamin D, *Am J Orthod* 32:463, 1946.
13. Becks H, Wainwright WW, Morgan AF: Comparative study of oral changes in dogs due to deficiencies of pantothenic acid, nicotinic acid and unknowns of B vitamin complex, *Am J Orthod* 29:183, 1943.
14. Been V, Engel D: The effects of immunosuppressive drugs on periodontal inflammation in human renal allograft patients, *J Periodontol* 53:245, 1982.
15. Bergmann OJ, Ellegaard B, Dahl M, et al: Gingival status during chemical plaque control with or without prior mechanical plaque removal in patients with acute myeloid leukemia, *J Clin Periodontol* 19:169, 1992.
16. Bernick SM, Cohen DW, Baker L, et al: Dental disease in children with diabetes mellitus, *J Periodontol* 46:241, 1975.
17. Beumer J III, Trowbridge HO, Silverman S Jr, et al: Childhood hypophosphatasia and the premature loss of teeth, *Oral Surg Oral Med Oral Pathol* 35:631, 1973.
18. Biro S: Studies regarding the influence of pregnancy upon caries, *Vierteljahrschr Zahnheilk* 14:371, 1898.
19. Blitzer B, Sznajder N, Carranza FA Jr: Hallazgos clinicos periodontales en ninos con cardiopatias congenitas [Periodontal disease risks in children with congenital cardiopathies], *Rev Assoc Odont Argent* 63:169, 1975.
20. Boyle PE: Effect of vitamin A deficiency on the periodontal tissues, *Am J Orthod* 33:744, 1947.

21. Brown LR, Roth GD, Hoover D, et al: Alveolar bone loss in leukemic and nonleukemic mice, *J Periodontol* 40:725, 1969.
22. Brown RS, Di Stanislao PT, Beaver WT, Bottomley WK: The administration of folic acid to institutionalized epileptic adults with phenytoin-induced gingival hyperplasia: a double-blind, randomized, placebo-controlled, parallel study, *Oral Surg Oral Med Oral Pathol* 71:565, 1991.
23. Brownlee M: Glycation and diabetic complications, *Diabetes* 43:836, 1994.
24. Bullon P, Pascual A, Fernandez-Novoa MC, et al: Late onset Papillon-Lefèvre syndrome? *J Clin Periodontol* 20:662, 1993.
25. Buzina R, Brodarec A, Jusic M, et al: Epidemiology of angular stomatitis and bleeding gums, *Int J Vitam Nutr Res* 43:401, 1973.
26. Cabrini RL, Carranza FA Jr: Adenosine triphosphatase in normal and scorbutic wounds, *Nature* 200:1113, 1963.
27. Campbell MJ: Epidemiology of periodontal disease in the diabetic and the nondiabetic, *Aust Dent J* 17:274, 1972.
28. Carranza FA Jr, Gravina O, Cabrini RL: Periodontal and pulpal pathosis in leukemic mice, *Oral Surg* 20:374, 1965.
29. Carranza FA Jr, Cabrini RL, Lopez Otero R, et al: Histometric analysis of interradicular bone in protein deficient animals, *J Periodontal Res* 4:292, 1969.
30. Carvel RI: Palmar-plantar hyperkeratosis and premature periodontal destruction, *J Oral Med* 24:73, 1969.
31. Chapman OD, Harris AE: Oral lesions associated with dietary deficiencies in monkeys, *J Infect Dis* 69:7, 1941.
32. Charbeneau TD, Hurt WC: Gingival findings in spontaneous scurvy: a case report, *J Periodontol* 54:694, 1983.
33. Chawla TN, Glickman I: Protein deprivation and the periodontal structures of the albino rat, *Oral Surg* 4:578, 1951.
34. Chung EM, Sung EC, Sakurai KL: Dental management of the Down and Eisenmenger syndrome patient, *J Contemp Dent Pract* 5:70, 2004.
35. Cianciola LJ, Park BH, Bruck E, et al: Prevalence of periodontal disease in insulin-dependent diabetes mellitus (juvenile diabetes), *J Am Dent Assoc* 104:653, 1982.
36. Cichon P, Crawford L, Grimm WD: Early-onset periodontitis associated with Down's syndrome—clinical interventional study, *Ann Periodontol* 3:370, 1998.
37. Cohen DW, Friedman LA, Shapiro J, et al: Diabetes mellitus and periodontal disease: two year longitudinal observations. Part I, *J Periodontol* 41:709, 1970.
38. Cohen DW, Morris AL: Periodontal manifestations of cyclic neutropenia, *J Periodontol* 32:159, 1961.
39. Cohen DW, Shapiro J, Friedman L, et al: A longitudinal investigation of the periodontal changes during pregnancy and fifteen months postpartum, *J Periodontol* 42:653, 1971.
40. Cohen MM, Winer RA, Schwartz S, et al: Oral aspects of mongolism. Part I. Periodontal disease in mongolism, *Oral Surg Oral Med Oral Pathol* 14:92, 1961.
41. Cotran RS, Kumar V, Robbins SR: *Robbins' pathologic basis of disease,* ed 4, Philadelphia, 1989, Saunders.
42. Crandon JH, Lund CC, Dill DB: Experimental human scurvy, *N Engl J Med* 223:353, 1940.
43. Croucher R, Marcenes WS, Torres MC, et al: The relationship between life-events and periodontitis: a case-control study, *J Clin Periodontol* 24(1):39, 1997.
44. Cutler CW, Wasfy MO, Ghaffar K, et al: Impaired bactericidal activity of PMN from two brothers with necrotizing ulcerative gingivo-periodontitis, *J Periodontol* 65:357, 1994.
45. Denton J: A study of tissue changes in experimental black tongue of dogs compared with similar changes in pellagra, *Am J Pathol* 4:341, 1928.
46. Diabetes and oral health, *J Am Dent Assoc* 115:741, 1987.
47. Dreizen S: Oral manifestations of human nutritional anemias, *Arch Environ Health* 5:66, 1962.
48. Dreizen S, Levy BM, Bernick S, et al: Studies of the biology of the periodontium of marmosets. III. Periodontal bone changes in marmosets with osteomalacia and hyperparathyroidism, *Isr J Med Sci* 3:731, 1967.
49. Dreizen S, McCredie KB, Keating MJ, et al: Malignant gingival and skin infiltrates in adult leukemia, *Oral Surg* 55:572, 1983.
50. El-Ashiry GM, El-Kafrawy AH, Nasr MF, et al: Comparative study of the influence of pregnancy and oral contraceptives on the gingivae, *Oral Surg* 30:472, 1970.
51. Elter JR, White BA, Gaynes BN, Bader JD: Relationship of clinical depression to periodontal treatment outcome, *J Periodontol* 73(4):441, 2002.
52. Emrich LJ, Shlossman M, Genco RJ: Periodontal disease in non–insulin-dependent diabetes mellitus, *J Periodontol* 62:123, 1991.
53. Enwonwu CO, Edozien JC: Epidemiology of periodontal disease in western Nigerians in relation to socioeconomic status, *Arch Oral Biol* 15:1231, 1970.
54. Falk H, Hugoson A, Thorstensson H: Number of teeth, prevalence of caries and periapical lesions in insulin-dependent diabetics, *Scand J Dent Res* 97:198, 1989.
55. Fardal O, Drangsholt E, Olsen I: Palmar plantar keratosis and unusual periodontal findings: observations from a family of 4 members, *J Clin Periodontol* 25:181, 1998.
56. Farzim I, Edalat M: Periodontitis with hyperkeratosis palmaris et plantaris (Papillon-Lefèvre syndrome), *J Periodontol* 45:316, 1974.
57. Ficara AI, Levin MP, Grover MF, et al: A comparison of the glucose and protein content of gingival fluid from diabetics and nondiabetics, *J Periodontal Res* 10:171, 1975.
58. Follis RH: *The pathology of nutritional disease,* Springfield, Ill, 1948, Charles C Thomas.
59. Formicola AJ, Weatherford T, Grupe H Jr: The uptake of H3-estradiol by the oral tissues in rats, *J Periodont Res* 5:269, 1970.
60. Forsslund G: Occurrence of subepithelial gingival blood vessels in patients with morbus caeruleus (tetralogy of Fallot), *Acta Odontol Scand* 20:301, 1962.
61. Frandsen AM: Periodontal tissue changes in vitamin A deficient young rats, *Acta Odontol Scand* 21:19, 1963.
62. Friedman LA: Horizontal tooth mobility and the menstrual cycle, *J Periodontal Res* 7:125, 1972.
63. Galea H, Aganovic I, Anganovic M: The dental caries and periodontal disease experience of patients with early-onset insulin-dependent diabetes, *Int Dent J* 36:219, 1986.
64. Genco RJ: Current view of risk factors for periodontal diseases, *J Periodontol* 67(suppl):1041, 1996.
65. Genco RJ, Shlossman M, Zambon JJ: Immunologic studies of periodontitis patients with type II diabetes, *J Dent Res* 66:257, 1987 (abstract).
66. Genco RJ, Ho AW, Grossi SG, et al: Relationship of stress, distress and inadequate coping behaviors to periodontal disease, *J Periodontol* 70:711, 1999.
67. Glavind L, Lund B, Löe H: The relationship between periodontal state and diabetes duration, insulin dosage and retinal changes, *J Periodontol* 39:341, 1968.
68. Glickman I: The periodontal structures in experimental diabetes, *NY J Dent* 16:226, 1946.
69. Glickman I: Acute vitamin C deficiency and periodontal disease. I. The periodontal tissues of the guinea pig in acute vitamin C deficiency, *J Dent Res* 27:9, 1948.
70. Glickman I: Acute vitamin C deficiency and the periodontal tissues. II. The effect of acute vitamin C deficiency upon the response of the periodontal tissues of the

guinea pig to artificially induced inflammation, *J Dent Res* 27:201, 1948.
71. Glickman I, Stoller M: The periodontal tissues of the albino rat in vitamin A deficiency, *J Dent Res* 27:758, 1948.
72. Glickman I, Stone IC, Chawla TN: The effect of cortisone acetate upon the periodontium of white mice, *J Periodontol* 24:161, 1953.
73. Goetzl EJ: Enhancement of random migration and chemotactic response of human leukocytes by ascorbic acid, *J Clin Invest* 53:813, 1974.
74. Goldman HM: Acute aleukemic leukemia, *Am J Orthod* 26:89, 1940.
75. Goodman MH: Perlèche: a consideration of its etiology and pathology, *Bull Johns Hopkins Hosp* 51:263, 1943.
76. Gottsegen R: Dental and oral considerations in diabetes mellitus, *NY J Med* 62:389, 1962.
77. Govier WM, Grieg ME: Prevention of oral lesions in B1 avitaminotic dogs, *Science* 98:216, 1943.
78. Greenberg MS, Cohen SB, Boosz B, et al: Oral herpes infections in patients with leukemia, *J Am Dent Assoc* 114:483, 1987.
79. Grossi SG, Zambon JJ, Ho AW, et al: Assessment of risk for periodontal disease. I. Risk indicators for attachment loss, *J Periodontol* 65:260, 1994.
80. Gusberti F, Grossman N, Loesche W: Puberty gingivitis in insulin-dependent diabetes, *J Dent Res* 61:201, 1982 (abstract).
81. Hayden P, Buckley LA: Diabetes mellitus and periodontal disease in an Irish population, *J Periodontal Res* 24:298, 1989.
82. Henrikson PA: Periodontal disease and calcium deficiency in the dog, *Acta Odontol Scand* 26(suppl 50):1, 1968.
83. Higgins WH: Systemic poisoning with bismuth, *JAMA* 66:648, 1916.
84. Hirschfeld I: Periodontal symptoms associated with diabetes, *J Periodontol* 5:37, 1934.
85. Hodges RE, Baker EM, Hood J, et al: Experimental scurvy in man, *Am J Clin Nutr* 22:535, 1969.
86. Holm-Pederson P, Löe H: Flow of gingival exudate as related to menstruation and pregnancy, *J Periodontal Res* 2:13, 1967.
87. Hugoson A: Gingival inflammation and female sex hormones, *J Periodontal Res* 5(suppl), 1970.
88. Iacopino AM: Periodontitis and diabetes interrelationships: role of inflammation, *Ann Periodontol* 6:125, 2001.
89. Ismail AI, Burt BA, Eklund SA: Relation between ascorbic acid intake and periodontal disease in the United States, *J Am Dent Assoc* 107:927, 1983.
90. Izumi Y, Sugiyama S, Shinozuka O, et al: Defective neutrophil chemotaxis in Down's syndrome patients and its relationship to periodontal disease, *J Periodontol* 60:238, 1989.
91. Jones RR: Symptoms in early stages of industrial plumbism, *JAMA* 104:195, 1935.
92. Jung JR, Carranza FA Jr, Newman MG: Scanning electron microscopy of plaque in Papillon-Lefèvre syndrome, *J Periodontol* 52:442, 1981.
93. Kalkwarf KL: Effect of oral contraceptive therapy on gingival inflammation in humans, *J Periodontol* 49:560, 1978.
94. Kaner A, Losch P, Green M: Oral manifestations of congenital heart disease, *J Pediatr* 29:269, 1946.
95. Kardachi BJR, Newcomb GM: A clinical study of gingival inflammation in renal transplant patients taking immunosuppressive drugs, *J Periodontol* 49:307, 1978.
96. Kastlin G: Agranulocytic angina, *Am J Med Sci* 173:799, 1927.
97. Kim JE, Shklar G: The effect of vitamin E on the healing of gingival wounds in rats, *J Periodontol* 54:305, 1983.
98. King JD: Vincent's disease treated with nicotinic acid, *Lancet* 2:32, 1940.
99. Knight GM, Wade AB: The effects of hormonal contraceptives on the human periodontium, *J Periodontal Res* 9:18, 1974.
100. Kolodzinski E, Munoa N, Malatesta E: Clinical study of gingival tissue in pregnant women, *J Dent Res* 53:693, 1974 (abstract).
101. Kornman KS, Loesche WJ: The subgingival microbial flora during pregnancy, *J Periodontal Res* 1980; 15:111.
102. Kracke RR: Granulopenia as associated with amidopyrine administration. Presented at Annual Session of American Medical Association, 1934.
103. Krohn S: The effect of the administration of steroid hormones on the gingival tissues, *J Periodontol* 29:300, 1958.
104. Lee RE, Lee NZ: The peripheral vascular system and its reactions in scurvy: an experimental study, *Am J Physiol* 149:465, 1947.
105. Liberman H: Chrome ulcerations of the nose and throat, *N Engl J Med* 225:132, 1941.
106. Lindhe J, Attstrom R: Gingival exudation during the menstrual cycle, *J Periodontal Res* 2:194, 1967.
107. Lindhe J, Bjorn AL: Influence of hormonal contraceptives on the gingiva of women, *J Periodontal Res* 2:64, 1967.
108. Lindhe J, Branemark PI: Changes in microcirculation after local application of sex hormones, *J Periodontal Res* 2:185, 1967.
109. Löe H: Periodontal changes in pregnancy, *J Periodontol* 36:209, 1965.
110. Löe H: Periodontal disease: the sixth complication of diabetes mellitus, *Diabetes Care* 16:329, 1993.
111. Loesche WJ, Hockett RN, Syed SA: The predominant cultivable flora of tooth surface plaque removed from institutionalized subjects, *Arch Oral Biol* 17:1311, 1972.
112. Loushine RJ, Weller RN, Kimbrough WF, Liewehr FR: Secondary hyperparathyroidism: a case report, *J Endod* 29:272, 2003.
113. Lundgren T, Renvert S, Papapanou PN, et al: Subgingival microbial profile of Papillon-Lefèvre patients assessed by DNA probes, *J Clin Periodontol* 25:624, 1998.
114. Lynch MA, Ship I: Initial oral manifestations of leukemia, *J Am Dent Assoc* 75:932, 1967.
115. Madison FW, Squier TL: Primary granulocytopenia after administration of benzene chain derivatives, *JAMA* 102:755, 1934.
116. Maier AW, Orban B: Gingivitis in pregnancy, *Oral Surg* 2:234, 1949.
117. Mann AW, Spies TD, Springer M: Oral manifestations of vitamin B complex deficiencies, *J Dent Res* 20:269, 1941.
118. Manson-Bahr P, Ransford ON: Stomatitis of vitamin B2 deficiency treated with nicotinic acid, *Lancet* 2:426, 1938.
119. Mark HA: Agranulocytic angina: its oral manifestations, *J Am Dent Assoc* 21:119, 1934.
120. Martinez Lalis RR, Lopez Otero R, Carranza FA Jr: A case of Papillon-Lefèvre syndrome, *Periodontics* 3:292, 1965.
121. Mascola B: The oral manifestations of diabetes mellitus: a review, *NY Dent J* 36:139, 1970.
122. Mashimo P, Yamamoto Y, Slots J, et al: The periodontal microflora of juvenile diabetes: culture, immunofluorescence and serum antibody studies, *J Periodontol* 54:420, 1983.
123. Massler M, Henry J: Oral manifestations during the female climacteric, *Alpha Omegan,* September 1950, p 105.
124. McCarthy P, Shklar G: Diseases of the oral mucosa, ed 2, Philadelphia, 1980, Lea & Febiger.
125. McMullen JA, van Dyke TE, Horozewicz HU, et al: Neutrophil chemotaxis in individuals with advanced periodontal

disease and a genetic predisposition to diabetes mellitus, *J Periodontol* 52:167, 1981.
126. Mealey BL: Influence of periodontal infections on systemic health, *Periodontology 2000* 21:197, 1999.
127. Mealey BL, Moritz AJ: Hormonal influences: effects of diabetes mellitus and endogenous female sex steroid hormones on the periodontium, *Periodontol 2000* 32:59, 2003.
128. Meyer A: Agranulocytosis: report of a case caused by sulfadiazine, *Calif West Med J* 61:54, 1944.
129. Mohammed AH, Waterhouse JP, Friederici HH: The microvasculature of the rat gingiva as affected by progesterone: an ultrastructural study, *J Periodontol* 45:50, 1974.
130. Monteiro da Silva AM, Newman HN, Oakley DA, O'Leary R: Psychosocial factors, dental plaque levels and smoking in periodontitis patients, *J Clin Periodontol* 25:517, 1998.
131. Monteiro da Silva AM, Oakley DA, Newman HN, et al: Psychosocial factors and adult onset rapidly progressive periodontitis, *J Clin Periodontol* 23:789, 1996.
132. National Diabetes Data Group: *Diabetes in America,* ed 2, NIH No 95-1468, Bethesda, Md, 1995, National Institutes of Health.
133. Nichols C, Laster AA, Bodak Gyovai LZ: Diabetes mellitus and periodontal disease, *J Periodontol* 49:85, 1978.
134. Nishida M, Grossi SG, Dunford RG, et al: Dietary vitamin C and the risk for periodontal disease, *J Periodontol* 71:1215, 2000.
135. Novaes AB Jr, Pereira ALA, Moraes N, et al: Manifestations of insulin-dependent diabetes mellitus in the periodontium of young Brazilian patients, *J Periodontol* 62:116, 1991.
136. O'Leary TM, Shannon I, Prigmore JR: Clinical and systemic findings in periodontal disease, *J Periodontol* 32:243, 1962.
137. O'Neil TCA: Maternal T-lymphocyte response and gingivitis in pregnancy, *J Periodontol* 50:178, 1979.
138. Oshrain HI, Mender S, Mandel ID: Periodontal status of patients with reduced immunocapacity, *J Periodontol* 50:185, 1979.
139. Pack A, Thomson M: Effects of topical and systemic folic acid supplementation on gingivitis in pregnancy, *J Clin Periodontol* 7:402, 1980.
140. Page RC: The pathobiology of periodontal diseases may affect systemic diseases: inversion of a paradigm, *Ann Periodontol* 3:108, 1998.
141. Page RC, Bowen T, Altman L, et al: Prepubertal periodontitis. I. Definition of a clinical disease entity, *J Periodontol* 54:257, 1983.
142. Page RC, Schroeder HE: *Periodontitis in man and other animals a comparative review,* Basel, 1982, Karger.
143. Parrish JH Jr, DeMarco TJ, Bissada NF: Vitamin E and periodontitis in the rat, 44:210, 1977.
144. Patrone F, Dallegri F, Rebora A, Sacchetti C: Lazy leukocyte syndrome, *Blut* 39:265, 1979.
145. Perry DA: Oral contraceptives and periodontal health, *J West Soc Periodontol* 29:72, 1981.
146. Phair J: Neutrophil dysfunction in diabetes mellitus, *J Lab Clin Med* 85:26, 1975.
147. Prout RES, Hopps RM: A relationship between human oral bacteria and the menstrual cycle, *J Periodontol* 41:98, 1970.
148. Rada RE, Bronny AT, Hasiakos PS: Sickle cell crisis precipitated by periodontal infection, *J Am Dent Assoc* 11:799, 1987.
149. Randall CL: Granulocytopenia following barbiturates and amidopyrine, *JAMA* 102:1137, 1934.
150. Rateitschak KH: Tooth mobility changes in pregnancy, *J Periodontal Res* 2:199, 1967.
151. Restarski JS, Pijoan M: Gingivitis and vitamin C, *J Am Dent Assoc* 31:1323, 1944.
152. Richman JJ, Abarbanel AR: Effects of estradiol, testosterone, diethylstilbestrol and several of their derivatives upon the human mucous membrane, *J Am Dent Assoc* 30:913, 1943.
153. Robbins SL, Cotran RS, Kumar V: *Pathologic basis of disease,* ed 4, Philadelphia, 1989, Saunders.
154. Robertson HD, Polk HC Jr: The mechanism of infection in patients with diabetes mellitus: a review of leukocyte malfunction, *Surgery* 75:123, 1974.
155. Rosenberg EH, Guralnick WC: Hyperparathyroidism, *Oral Surg* 15(suppl 2):84, 1962.
156. Russell AL: International nutrition surveys: a summary of preliminary dental findings, *J Dent Res* 42:233, 1963.
157. Safkan-Seppala B, Ainamo J: Periodontal conditions in insulin-dependent diabetes mellitus, *J Clin Periodontol* 19:24, 1992.
158. Salvi GE, Lawrence HP, Offenbacher S, Beck JD: Influence of risk factors on the pathogenesis of periodontitis, *Periodontol 2000* 14:173, 1997.
159. Sandhu HS, Sharma V, Sidhu GS: Role of psychiatric disorders in self-inflicted periodontal injury: a case report, *J Periodontol* 68:1136, 1997.
160. Sastrowijoto SH, Hillemans P, van Steenbergen TJM, et al: Periodontal condition and microbiology of healthy and diseased periodontal pockets in type I diabetes mellitus patients, *J Clin Periodontol* 16:316, 1989.
161. Schmidt AM, Weidman E, Lalla E: Advanced glycation endproducts (AGEs) induce oxidant stress in the gingiva: a potential mechanism underlying accelerated periodontal disease associated with diabetes, *J Periodontal Res* 31:508, 1996.
162. Schneir M, Imberman M, Ramamurthy N, et al: Streptozotocin-induced diabetes and the rat periodontium: decreased relative collagen production, *Coll Relat Res* 8:221, 1988.
163. Schour I, Sarnat BG: Oral manifestations of occupational origin, *JAMA* 120:1197, 1942.
164. Schroeder HE, Seger RA, Keller HU, et al: Behavior of neutrophilic granulocytes in a case of Papillon-Lefèvre syndrome, *J Clin Periodontol* 10:618, 1983.
165. Scully CE, MacFayden A, Campbell A: Oral manifestations in cyclic neutropenia, *Br J Oral Surg* 20:96, 1982.
166. Shaw JH: The relation of nutrition to periodontal disease, *J Dent Res* 41(suppl 1):264, 1962.
167. Shilotri PG, Bhat KS: Effect of megadoses of vitamin C on bacterial activity of leukocytes, *Am J Clin Nutr* 30:1077, 1977.
168. Silverman S, Gordon G, Grant T, et al: The dental structures in primary hyperparathyroidism, *Oral Surg* 15:426, 1962.
169. Stahl SS: The effect of a protein-free diet on the healing of gingival wounds in rats, *Arch Oral Biol* 7:551, 1962.
170. Stahl SS, Sandler HC, Cahn L: The effects of protein deprivation upon the oral tissues of the rat and particularly upon the periodontal structures under irritation, Oral Surg 8:760, 1955.
171. Strock MS: The mouth in hyperparathyroidism, *N Engl J Med* 224:1019, 1945.
172. Sutcliffe P: A longitudinal study of gingivitis and puberty, *J Periodont Res* 7:52, 1972.
173. Svanberg G, Lindhe J, Hugoson A, et al: Effect of nutritional hyperparathyroidism on experimental periodontitis in the dog, *Scand J Dent Res* 81:155, 1973.
174. Sznajder N, Carraro JJ, Otero E, Carranza FA Jr: Clinical periodontal finding in trisomy 21 (mongolism), *J Periodontal Res* 3:1, 1968.
175. Sznajder N, Carraro JJ, Rugna S, et al: Periodontal findings in diabetic and nondiabetic patients, *J Periodontol* 49:445, 1978.

176. Tan JS, Anderson JL, Watanakunakorn C, Phair J: Neutrophil dysfunction in diabetes mellitus, *J Lab Clin Med* 85:26, 1975.
177. Telsey B, Beube FE, Zegarelli EV, et al: Oral manifestations of cyclical neutropenia associated with hypergammaglobulinemia, *Oral Surg* 15:540, 1962.
178. Tervonen T, Knuuttila M, Pohjamo L, et al: Immediate response to non-surgical periodontal treatment in subjects with diabetes mellitus, *J Clin Periodontol* 18:65, 1991.
179. Tollefsen T, Saltvedt E, Koppang HS: The effect of immunosuppressive agents on periodontal disease in man, *J Periodontal Res* 13:240, 1978.
180. Topping NH, Fraser HF: Mouth lesions associated with dietary deficiencies in monkeys, *Public Health Rep* 54:416, 1939.
181. Turesky S, Fisher B, Glickman I: A histochemical study of the attached gingiva in pregnancy, *J Dent Res* 37:1115, 1958.
182. Vogel, R: Relationship of folic acid to phenytoin-induced gingival overgrowth. In Hassell TM, Johnson M, Dudley K, editors: *Phenytoin-induced teratology and gingival pathology,* New York, 1980, Raven Press.
183. Vogel R, Deasy M, Alfano M, et al: The effect of folic acid on gingival health of women taking oral contraceptives, *J Prev Dent* 6:221, 1980.
184. Vogel R, Fink R, Frank O, et al: The effect of topical application of folic acid on gingival health, *J Oral Med* 33:20, 1978.
185. Vogel R, Fink R, Schneider L, et al: The effect of folic acid on gingival health, *J Periodontol* 47:667, 1976.
186. Vrahopoulos TP, Barber P, Liakoni H, et al: Ultrastructure of the periodontal lesion in a case of Papillon-Lefèvre syndrome (PLS), *J Clin Periodontol* 15:17, 1988.
187. Waerhaug J: Effect of C-avitaminosis on the supporting structures of the teeth, *J Periodontol* 29:87, 1958.
188. Waerhaug J: Epidemiology of periodontal disease: review of the literature. In *World Workshop in Periodontics,* Ann Arbor, 1966, American Academy of Periodontology, University of Michigan Press.
189. Waldrop TC, Anderson DC, Hallmon WW, et al: Periodontal manifestations of the heritable Mac-1, LFA-1, deficiency syndrome: clinical, histopathologic and molecular characteristics, *J Periodontol* 58:400, 1987.
190. Weinmann JP, Schour I: The effect of parathyroid hormone on the alveolar bone and teeth of the normal and rachitic rat, *Am J Pathol* 21:857, 1945.
191. Weinmann JP, Schour I: Experimental studies in calcification, *Am J Pathol* 21:821, 1945.
192. Wimmer G, Janda M, Wieselmann-Penkner K, et al: Coping with stress: its influence on periodontal disease, *J Periodontol* 73:1343, 2002.
193. Wingrove FA, Rubright WC, Kerber PE: Influence of ovarian hormone situation on atrophy, hypertrophy, and/or desquamation of human gingiva in premenopausal and postmenopausal women, *J Periodontol* 50:445, 1979.
194. Wolbach SB, Bessey OA: Tissue changes in vitamin deficiencies, *Physiol Rev* 22:233, 1942.
195. Woolfe SN, Hume WR, Kenney EB: Ascorbic acid and periodontal disease: a review of the literature, *J West Soc Periodontol* 28:44, 1980.
196. Woolfe SN, Kenney EB, Hume WR, et al: Relationship of ascorbic acid levels of blood and gingival tissue with response to periodontal therapy, *J Clin Periodontol* 11:159, 1984.
197. Wray D, Lowe, GDO, Dagg JH, et al: Systemic disease: oral manifestations and effects on oral health. In *Textbook of general and oral medicine,* Edinburgh, 1999, Churchill Livingstone.
198. Yendt ER: The parathyroids and calcium metabolism. In Volpe R, editor: *Clinical medicine,* Vol 8. Endocrinology, Philadelphia, 1986, Harper & Row.
199. Zambon JJ, Reynolds H, Fisher JB, et al: Microbiological and immunological studies of adult periodontitis in patients with non–insulin-dependent diabetes mellitus, *J Periodontol* 59:23, 1988.
200. Ziskin DE, Blackberg SN: A study of the gingivae during pregnancy, *J Dent Res* 13:253, 1933.
201. Ziskin DE, Blackberg SN, Stout A: The gingivae during pregnancy: an experimental study and a histopathological interpretation, *Surg Gynecol Obstet* 57:719, 1933.

Periodontal Medicine: Impact of Periodontal Infection on Systemic Health

18 CHAPTER

Brian L. Mealey and Perry R. Klokkevold

CHAPTER OUTLINE

Advances in science and technology over the last century have greatly expanded our knowledge of the pathogenesis of periodontal diseases. Periodontal disease is an infectious disease, but environmental, physical, social, and host stresses may affect and modify disease expression. Certain systemic conditions clearly may affect the initiation and progression of gingivitis and periodontitis (see Chapters 11 and 17). Systemic disorders affecting neutrophil, monocyte/macrophage, and lymphocyte function result in altered production or activity of host inflammatory mediators.[74] These alterations may manifest clinically as early onset of periodontal destruction or a more rapid rate of destruction than would occur in the absence of such disorders.

Evidence has also shed light on the converse side of the relationship between systemic health and oral health, that is, the potential effects of periodontal disease on a wide range of organ systems. This field of periodontal medicine addresses the following important questions:

- Can bacterial infection of the periodontium, commonly known as *periodontitis,* have an effect remote from the oral cavity?
- Is periodontal infection a risk factor for systemic diseases or conditions that affect human health?

PATHOBIOLOGY OF PERIODONTITIS

Our understanding of the pathogenesis of periodontitis has changed remarkably over the last 30 years.[78] Nonspecific accumulation of bacterial plaque was once thought to be the cause of periodontal destruction, but it is now recognized that periodontitis is an infectious disease associated with a small number of predominantly gram-negative microorganisms that exist in a subgingival biofilm.[31] Furthermore, the importance of the host in disease initiation and progression is clearly recognized. Although pathogenic bacteria are necessary for periodontal disease, they are not sufficient alone to cause the disease. A susceptible host is also imperative. In a host who is not susceptible to disease, pathogenic bacteria may have no clinical effect. Conversely, the susceptible host experiences clinical signs of periodontitis in the presence of pathogenic bacteria.

Recognition of the importance of host susceptibility opens a door to understanding the differences in the onset, natural history, and progression of periodontitis seen throughout the scientific literature. Because of differences in host susceptibility, not all individuals are equally vulnerable to the destructive effects of periodontal pathogens. Thus patients may not necessarily have similar disease expression despite the presence of similar bacteria. Likewise, the response to periodontal treatment may vary depending on the wound-healing capacity and susceptibility of the host to further disease progression. The importance of host susceptibility is clearly evident in the medical literature. For example, respiratory tract pathogens may have minimal effect on many individuals, but in a susceptible host such as an elderly patient, these same pathogens may cause life-threatening respiratory tract illnesses.

Many of the systemic conditions discussed in Chapters 11 and 17 serve to modify the host's susceptibility to periodontitis. For example, patients with immune suppression may not be able to mount an effective host response to subgingival microorganisms, resulting in more rapid and severe periodontal destruction. Although the potential impact of many systemic disorders on the periodontium is well documented, recent evidence suggests that periodontal infection may significantly enhance the risk for certain systemic diseases or alter the natural course of systemic conditions.[66] Conditions in which the influences of periodontal infection are documented include coronary heart disease (CHD) and CHD-related events such as angina and infarction, atherosclerosis, stroke, diabetes mellitus, preterm labor, low-birth-weight delivery, and respiratory conditions such as chronic obstructive pulmonary disease[66,79] (Box 18-1).

BOX 18-1

Organ Systems and Conditions Possibly Influenced by Periodontal Infection

Cardiovascular/Cerebrovascular System
Atherosclerosis
Coronary heart disease (CHD)
Angina
Myocardial infarction (MI)
Cerebrovascular accident (stroke)

Endocrine System
Diabetes mellitus

Reproductive System
Preterm low-birth-weight (LBW) infants
Preeclampsia

Respiratory System
Chronic obstructive pulmonary disease (COPD)
Acute bacterial pneumonia

FOCAL INFECTION THEORY REVISITED

Research in the area of periodontal medicine marks a resurgence in the concept of focal infection. In 1900, William Hunter, a British physician, first developed the idea that oral microorganisms were responsible for a wide range of systemic conditions that were not easily recognized as being infectious in nature.[22,71] He claimed that restoration of carious teeth instead of extraction resulted in the trapping of infectious agents under restorations. In addition to caries, pulpal necrosis, and periapical abscesses, Hunter also identified gingivitis and periodontitis as foci of infection. He advocated extraction of teeth with these conditions to eliminate the source of sepsis. Hunter believed that teeth were liable to septic infection primarily because of their structure and their relationship to alveolar bone. He stated that the degree of systemic effect produced by oral sepsis depended on the virulence of the oral infection and the individual's degree of resistance. He also believed that oral organisms had specific actions on different tissues and that these organisms acted by producing toxins, resulting in low-grade "subinfection," which produced systemic effects over prolonged periods. Finally, Hunter believed that the connection between oral sepsis and resulting systemic conditions could be shown by removal of the causative sepsis through tooth extraction and observation of the improvement in systemic health. Because it explained a wide range of disorders for which there was no known explanation at the time, Hunter's theory became widely accepted in Britain and eventually the United States, leading to wholesale extraction of teeth.

The focal infection theory fell into disrepute in the 1940s and 1950s when widespread extraction, often of the entire dentition, failed to reduce or eliminate the systemic conditions to which the supposedly infected dentition had been linked. The theory, while offering a possible explanation for perplexing systemic disorders, had been based on very little, if any, scientific evidence. Hunter and other advocates of the theory were unable to explain how focal oral sepsis produced these systemic maladies. They were also unable to elucidate possible interactive mechanisms between oral and systemic health. Furthermore, the suggested intervention of tooth extraction often had no effect on the systemic conditions for which patients sought relief. However, Hunter's ideas did encourage extensive research in microbiology and immunology.

EVIDENCE-BASED CLINICAL PRACTICE

Many of the precepts of the focal infection theory are being revived today in light of recent research demonstrating links between oral and systemic health. However,

TABLE 18-1

Evaluation of Evidence

Type of Study	Strength of Evidence	Comments
Case report	+/−	Provides relatively weak, retrospective anecdotal evidence. May suggest further study is needed.
Cross-sectional study	+	Compares groups of subjects at a single point in time. Stronger than case report. Fairly easy to conduct. Relatively inexpensive to conduct.
Longitudinal study	++	Follows groups of subjects over time. Stronger than cross-sectional study. Studies with control group are much stronger than studies without controls. More difficult and expensive to conduct.
Intervention trial	+++	Examines effects of some interventions. Studies with control group (i.e., placebo) much stronger than studies without controls. Strongest form of evidence is randomized controlled intervention trial. Difficult and expensive to conduct.

in order for the "hypothesis not to fall into disrepute for a second time, there must be no unsubstantiated attributions, no theories without evidence."[71] Today's era of evidence-based medicine and dentistry provides an excellent environment in which to examine the possible relationships between oral infection and systemic disorders.[24]

To establish a relationship between conditions A and B, different levels of evidence must be examined. All scientific evidence is not given the same weight.[72,73] The stronger the evidence, the more likely it is that a true relationship exists between the conditions. Table 18-1 describes these various levels of evidence.

For example, in examining the relationship between elevated cholesterol levels and CHD-related events, the literature might initially consist entirely of *case reports* or similar anecdotal information in which individual patients with recent myocardial infarction (MI) are found to have elevated cholesterol levels. These anecdotal reports suggest a possible relationship between elevated cholesterol and MI, but the evidence is weak. The case reports may lead to *cross-sectional studies* in which a large subject population is examined to determine whether those individuals who had an MI have higher cholesterol levels than other individuals (control subjects) who did not have an MI. Ideally, these cross-sectional studies are controlled for other potential causes or factors associated with MI, such as age, gender, and smoking history. In other words, the subjects with a previous MI would be retrospectively "matched" with subjects of similar age, gender, and smoking history. Then their cholesterol levels would be examined for similarities or differences. Significantly higher cholesterol level in subjects with a previous MI compared with those without MI offers stronger evidence than case reports, and it further substantiates a possible link between elevated cholesterol and MI.

Even stronger evidence is provided by *longitudinal studies,* in which subject populations are examined over time. For example, a group of subjects might periodically have cholesterol levels evaluated over several years. If individuals with elevated cholesterol levels have a significantly higher rate of MI over time compared with subjects with normal cholesterol levels, even stronger evidence is available to substantiate the link between cholesterol and MI. Finally, *intervention trials* may be designed to alter the potentially causative condition and to determine the effect of this change on the resultant condition. For example, patients with elevated cholesterol may be divided into two groups: a group who uses a cholesterol-lowering drug or diet and a control group who has no intervention. These two groups might also be compared with a third group with normal cholesterol levels. Over time, the rate of MI in each group would be determined. If the group receiving the cholesterol-lowering regimen has a significantly lower rate of MI than the group with continued elevations in cholesterol level, strong evidence of a link between cholesterol and MI would be established.

At each level of evidence, it is important to determine whether a biologically plausible link exists between conditions A and B. For example, if case reports, cross-sectional studies, longitudinal studies, and intervention trials all support the link between cholesterol levels and MI, the following questions remain:

- How is cholesterol related to myocardial infarction?
- What are the mechanisms by which cholesterol affects the cardiovascular system and thus increases the risk for infarction?

These studies provide explanatory data that further substantiate the link between the two conditions.

The focal infection theory, as proposed and defended in the early part of the twentieth century, was based on almost no evidence. Only the occasional case report and other anecdotes were available to substantiate the theory. Although explanatory mechanisms were proposed, none was validated with scientific research. Unfortunately, this theory predated current concepts of evidence-based clinical practice, leading to unnecessary extraction of millions of teeth. Currently, in reexamining the potential associations between oral infections and systemic conditions, it is important to determine what evidence (1) is available, (2) is still needed to substantiate the associations, and (3) validates the possible mechanisms of association. This chapter reviews current knowledge relating periodontal infection to overall systemic health.

SUBGINGIVAL ENVIRONMENT AS RESERVOIR OF BACTERIA

The subgingival microbiota in patients with periodontitis provides a significant and persistent gram-negative bacterial challenge to the host (see Chapters 9 and 13). These organisms and their products, such as *lipopolysaccharide* (LPS), have ready access to the periodontal tissues and to the circulation via the sulcular epithelium, which is frequently ulcerated and discontinuous. Even with treatment, complete eradication of these organisms is difficult, and their reemergence is often rapid. The total surface area of pocket epithelium in contact with subgingival bacteria and their products in a patient with generalized moderate periodontitis has been estimated to be approximately the size of the palm of an adult hand, with even larger areas of exposure in cases of more advanced periodontal destruction.[78] Bacteremias are common after mechanical periodontal therapy and also occur frequently during normal daily function and oral hygiene procedures.[26,33,65] Just as the periodontal tissues mount an immunoinflammatory response to bacteria and their products, systemic challenge with these agents also induces a major vascular response. This host response may offer explanatory mechanisms for the interactions between periodontal infection and a variety of systemic disorders.

PERIODONTAL DISEASE AND MORTALITY

The ultimate medical outcome measure is mortality. The Normative Aging Study examined 2280 healthy men every 3 years for more than 30 years after baseline clinical, radiographic, laboratory, and electrocardiographic examinations. A subset of this population was examined in the Veterans Affairs (VA) Dental Longitudinal Study to determine age-related changes in the oral cavity and to identify risk factors for oral disease. Clinical examinations were performed and alveolar bone level measurements determined from full-mouth radiographs. The mean percentage of alveolar bone loss and the mean probing depth were determined for each subject.

A recent study of data from this subject population sought to determine whether periodontal disease status was a significant predictor of mortality independent of other baseline characteristics within the population.[25] From the original sample of 804 dentate, medically healthy subjects, a total of 166 died during the study. Periodontal status at the baseline examination was a significant predictor of mortality independent of other factors, such as smoking, alcohol use, cholesterol levels, blood pressure, family history of heart disease, education level, and body mass. For those subjects with the most alveolar bone loss, averaging more than 21% alveolar bone loss at baseline, the risk of dying during the follow-up period was 70% higher than for all other subjects. Interestingly, alveolar bone loss increased the risk of mortality more than smoking (52% increased risk), a well-known risk factor for mortality.

In the previous study, periodontitis preceded and increased the risk of mortality. However, this only establishes an association, not causation. It is possible that periodontal disease reflects other health behaviors not evaluated in this study, rather than acting as a specific cause of mortality. In other words, patients with poor periodontal health may also have other risk factors that increase mortality rate (e.g., smoking).

In examining research that suggests oral health status as a possible risk factor for systemic conditions, it is important to recognize when other known risk factors for those systemic conditions have been accounted for in the analysis. Host susceptibility factors that place individuals at risk for periodontitis may also place them at risk for systemic diseases such as cardiovascular disease. In these patients the association may actually be between the risk factors rather than between the diseases. For example, periodontitis and cardiovascular disease share such risk factors as smoking, age, race, male gender, and stress. Genetic risk factors may also be shared.[76] In the VA Dental Longitudinal Study, smoking was an independent risk factor for mortality. When examining the data to determine if periodontal status was a risk factor, smoking status and other known risk factors for mortality were removed from the equation to allow independent evaluation of periodontal status. Other studies support the association between poor oral health and an increased risk for mortality.[46]

PERIODONTAL DISEASE AND CORONARY HEART DISEASE/ATHEROSCLEROSIS

To further explore the periodontal disease and CHD/atherosclerosis association, investigators have studied specific systemic disorders and medical outcomes to determine their relationship to periodontal status. CHD-related events are a major cause of death. Myocardial infarction has been associated with acute systemic bacterial and viral infections, and MI is sometimes preceded by influenza-like symptoms.[58,94] Is it possible that oral infection is similarly related to MI? Traditional risk factors such as smoking, dyslipidemia, hypertension, and diabetes mellitus do not explain the presence of coronary atherosclerosis in a large number of patients. Localized infection resulting in a chronic inflammatory reaction has been suggested as a mechanism underlying CHD in these individuals.[68]

In cross-sectional studies of patients with acute MI or confirmed CHD compared with age- and gender-matched control patients, MI patients had significantly worse dental health (periodontitis, periapical lesions, caries, pericoronitis) than did controls.[45,59,60] This association between poor dental health and MI was independent of known risk factors for heart disease, such as age, cholesterol levels, hypertension, diabetes, and smoking. Because atherosclerosis is a major determinant of CHD-related events, dental health has also been related to coronary atheromatosis. Mattila et al.[61] performed oral radiographic examinations and diagnostic coronary angiography on men with known CHD and found significant correlation between the severity of dental disease and the degree of coronary atheromatosis. This relationship remained significant after accounting for other known risk factors for coronary artery disease (CAD). Similarly, Malthaner et al.[57] found an increased risk of angiographically defined CAD in subjects with greater bone loss and attachment loss; however, after adjusting for other known cardiovascular risk factors, the relationship between periodontal status and CAD was no longer statistically significant. There is evidence that the extent of periodontal disease may be associated with CHD. For example, there may be a greater risk for CHD-related events such as MI when periodontitis affects a greater number of teeth in the mouth, compared with subjects having periodontitis at fewer teeth.[5]

Cross-sectional studies thus suggest a possible link between oral health and CHD; however, such studies cannot determine causality in this relationship. Rather, dental diseases may be indicators of general health practices. For example, periodontal disease and CHD are both related to lifestyle and share numerous risk factors, including smoking, diabetes, and low socioeconomic status. Bacterial infections have significant effects on endothelial cells, blood coagulation, lipid metabolism, and monocytes/macrophages. The research of Mattila et al.[59] showed that dental infections were the only factors, other than the classic and well-recognized coronary risk factors, that were associated independently with the severity of coronary atherosclerosis.

Longitudinal studies provide compelling data on this relationship. In a 7-year follow-up study of the patients from the study of Mattila and colleagues, dental disease was significantly related to the incidence of new fatal and nonfatal coronary events, as well as to overall mortality.[62] In a prospective study of a national sample of adults, subjects with periodontitis had a 25% increase in the risk for CHD compared with those with no or minimal periodontal disease, after adjusting for other known risk factors.[20] Among younger males (age 25-49), periodontitis increased the risk of CHD by 70%. The level of oral hygiene was also associated with heart disease. Patients with poor oral hygiene, as indicated by higher debris and calculus scores, had a twofold increased risk for CHD.

In another large prospective study, 1147 men were followed for 18 years.[8] During that time, 207 men (18%) developed CHD. When periodontal status at baseline was related to the presence or absence of CHD-related events during follow-up, a significant relationship was found. Subjects with greater than 20% mean bone loss had a 50% increased risk of CHD compared with those with up to 20% bone loss. The extent of sites with probing depth greater than 3 mm was strongly related to the incidence of CHD. Subjects with probing depths greater than 3 mm on at least half their teeth had a twofold increased risk, whereas those with probing depths greater than 3 mm on all teeth had more than a threefold increased risk of CHD. This study and others in which the periodontal condition is known to have preceded the CHD-related events support the concept that periodontal disease is a risk factor for CHD, independent of other classic risk factors. Not all studies, however, support this concept; some show little independent effect of periodontal status on the risk for CHD, after adjusting for commonly accepted cardiovascular risk factors.[41,42] It is particularly difficult to control for smoking as a confounding variable in these studies because it is such an important risk factor for both periodontal disease and cardiovascular disease. This confounding influence of smoking makes it difficult to clarify the significance of the relationship between the diseases.

Perhaps the best evidence available comes from *systematic reviews* of studies examining the relationship between periodontal infection and cardiovascular diseases. Janket et al.[44] performed a meta-analysis of periodontal disease as a risk factor for future cardiovascular events and found an overall 19% increased risk of such events in individuals with periodontitis. The increase in risk was greater (44%) in people under age 65. Although this increased risk is fairly modest, the extensive prevalence of periodontal disease in the population may increase the significance of the risk from a public health perspective. An extensive systematic review by Scannapieco et al.[87] concluded that a moderate degree of evidence exists to support an association between periodontal disease and atherosclerosis, MI, and cardiovascular disease, but that causality is unclear. Importantly, insufficient evidence exists to show that treatment of periodontal disease has any impact on the risk of heart disease. Intervention trials are needed to make this determination.

Effect of Periodontal Infection

Periodontal infection may affect the onset or progression of atherosclerosis and CHD through certain mechanisms. Periodontitis and atherosclerosis both have complex etiologic factors, combining genetic and environmental influences. In addition to smoking, the diseases share many risk factors and have distinct similarities in basic pathogenic mechanisms.

Ischemic Heart Disease. Ischemic heart disease is associated with the processes of atherogenesis and thrombogenesis (Figure 18-1). Increased viscosity of blood may promote major ischemic heart disease and cerebrovascular accident (stroke) by increasing the risk of thrombus formation.[56] *Fibrinogen* is probably the most important factor in promoting this hypercoagulable state. Fibrinogen is the precursor to fibrin, and increased fibrinogen levels increase blood viscosity. Increased plasma fibrinogen is a recognized risk factor for cardiovascular events and peripheral vascular disease[55] (Figure 18-2). Elevated white blood cell (WBC) count is also a predictor of heart disease and stroke, and circulating leukocytes may promote occlusion of blood vessels. Coagulation factor VIII/von Willebrand factor (vWF) has

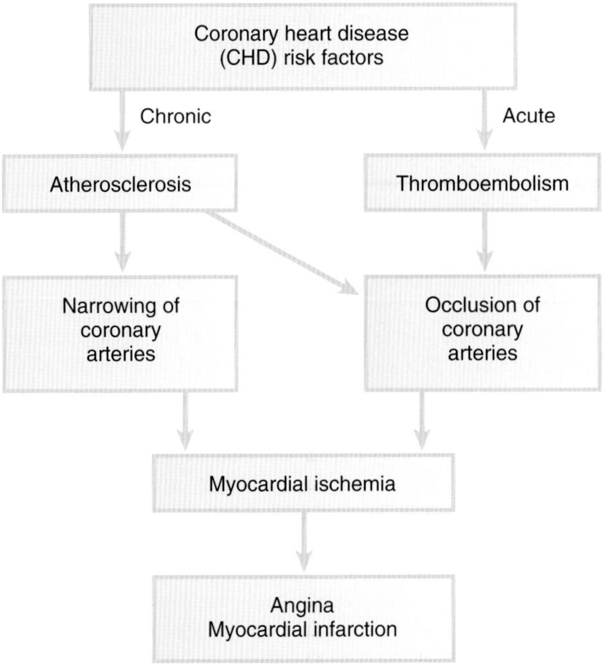

Figure 18-1 Acute and chronic pathways to ischemic heart disease. CHD-related events such as angina or myocardial infarction may be precipitated by either pathway or both pathways.

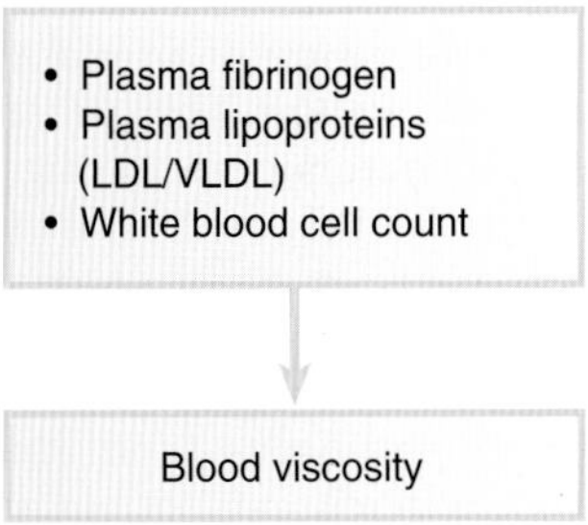

Figure 18-2 Factors affecting blood viscosity in health.

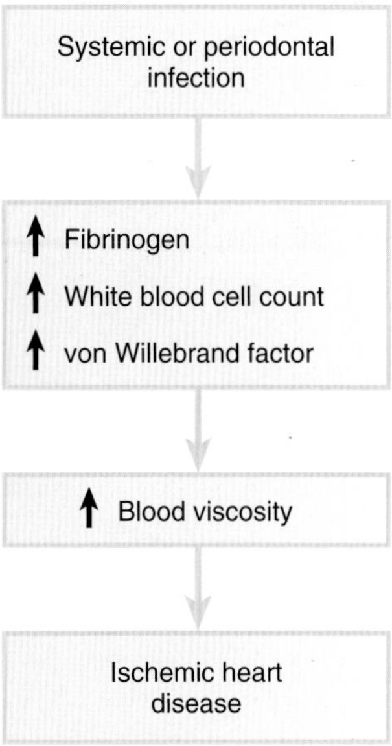

Figure 18-3 Effect of infection on blood viscosity. Increased plasma fibrinogen and von Willebrand factor cause hypercoagulability. When combined with increased white blood cell count, blood viscosity increases, increasing the risk of coronary ischemia.

likewise been associated with the risk of ischemic heart disease.[82]

Systemic Infections. Systemic infections are known to induce a hypercoagulable state and to increase blood viscosity (Figure 18-3). Fibrinogen levels and WBC counts are often increased in patients with periodontal disease.[12,50] Individuals with poor oral health may also have significant elevations in coagulation factor VIII/vWF antigen, increasing the risk of thrombus formation. Thus, periodontal infection may also promote increased blood viscosity and thrombogenesis, leading to an increased risk for central and peripheral vascular disease.

Daily Activity. Routine daily activities such as mastication and oral hygiene procedures result in frequent bacteremia with oral organisms. The exposure time to bacteremia from routine daily chewing and toothbrushing is much greater than from dental procedures.[33] Periodontal disease may predispose the patient to an increased incidence of bacteremia, including the presence of virulent gram-negative organisms associated with periodontitis. An estimated 8% of all cases of infective endocarditis are associated with periodontal or dental disease, without a preceding dental procedure.[21] Recognition of this fact is implicit in the American Heart Association recommendations on prevention of bacterial endocarditis, which stress the importance of establishing and maintaining "the best possible oral health to reduce potential sources of bacterial seeding."[18]

The periodontium, when affected by periodontitis, also acts as a reservoir of *endotoxin* (LPS) from gram-negative organisms. Endotoxin can pass readily into the systemic circulation during normal daily function, precipitating many negative cardiovascular effects. In a study of the incidence of endotoxemia after simple chewing, subjects with periodontitis were four times more likely to have endotoxin present in the bloodstream than subjects without periodontitis. Furthermore, the concentration of endotoxin present was more than fourfold greater in those with periodontitis than in healthy subjects.[26]

Thrombogenesis. Platelet aggregation plays a major role in thrombogenesis, and most cases of acute MI are precipitated by thromboembolism. Oral organisms may be involved in coronary thrombogenesis. Platelets selectively bind some strains of *Streptococcus sanguis,* a common component of supragingival plaque, and *Porphyromonas gingivalis,* a pathogen closely associated with periodontitis.[37] Aggregation of platelets is induced by the *platelet aggregation–associated protein* (PAAP) expressed on some strains of these bacteria.[36] In animal models,

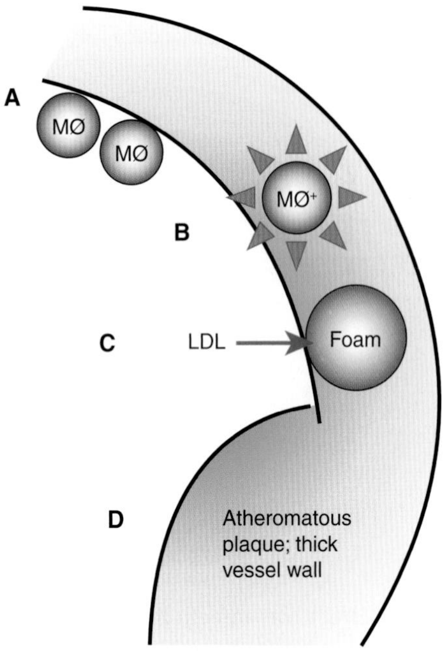

Figure 18-4 Pathogenesis of atherosclerosis. **A,** Monocytes/macrophages adhere to vascular endothelium. **B,** Monocytes/macrophages penetrate into arterial media, producing proinflammatory cytokines and growth factors. **C,** Ingestion of oxidized low-density lipoprotein *(LDL)* enlarges monocytes to form foam cells. **D,** Smooth muscle proliferation and plaque formation thicken vessel wall and narrow lumen. *MØ⁺,* Hyperinflammatory monocyte/macrophage phenotype.

intravenous infusion of PAAP-positive bacterial strains resulted in alterations of heart rate, blood pressure, cardiac contractility, and electrocardiogram (ECG) readings consistent with MI. Platelet accumulation also occurred in the lungs, leading to tachypnea. No such changes were seen with infusion of PAAP-negative strains. PAAP-positive bacteria caused aggregation of circulating platelets, resulting in formation of thromboemboli and the resultant cardiac and pulmonary changes. Thus, periodontitis-associated bacteremia with certain strains of *S. sanguis* and *P. gingivalis* may promote acute thromboembolic events through interaction with circulating platelets.

Atherosclerosis. Atherosclerosis is a focal thickening of the arterial *intima,* the innermost layer lining the vessel lumen, and the *media,* the thick layer under the intima consisting of smooth muscle, collagen, and elastic fibers[84] (Figure 18-4). Early in the formation of atherosclerotic plaques, circulating monocytes adhere to the vascular endothelium. This adherence is mediated through several adhesion molecules on the endothelial cell surface, including intercellular adhesion molecule-1 (ICAM-1), endothelial leukocyte adhesion molecule-1 (ELAM-1), and vascular cell adhesion molecule-1 (VCAM-1).[6,49] These adhesion molecules are upregulated by a number of factors, including bacterial LPS, prostaglandins, and proinflammatory cytokines. After binding to the endothelial cell lining, monocytes penetrate the endothelium and migrate under the arterial intima. The monocytes ingest circulating low-density lipoprotein (LDL) in its oxidized state and become engorged, forming foam cells characteristic of atheromatous plaques.

Once within the arterial media, monocytes may also transform to macrophages. A host of proinflammatory cytokines, such as interleukin-1 (IL-1), tumor necrosis factor alpha (TNF-α), and prostaglandin E_2 (PGE_2) are then produced, which propagate the atheromatous lesion. Mitogenic factors, such as fibroblast growth factor and platelet-derived growth factor, stimulate smooth muscle and collagen proliferation within the media, thickening the arterial wall.[55] Atheromatous plaque formation and thickening of the vessel wall narrow the lumen and dramatically decrease blood flow through the vessel.[84] Arterial thrombosis often occurs after an atheromatous plaque ruptures. Plaque rupture exposes circulating blood to arterial collagen and tissue factor from monocytes/macrophages that activate platelets and the coagulation pathway. Platelet and fibrin accumulation forms a thrombus that may occlude the vessel, resulting in ischemic events such as angina or MI. The thrombus may separate from the vessel wall and form an *embolus,* which may also occlude vessels, again leading to acute events such as MI or cerebral infarction (stroke).

Role of Periodontal Disease in Myocardial or Cerebral Infarction

In animal models, gram-negative bacteria and the associated LPS cause infiltration of inflammatory cells into the arterial wall, proliferation of arterial smooth muscle, and intravascular coagulation. These changes are identical to those seen in naturally occurring atheromatosis. Patients with periodontitis are at increased risk for thickening of the walls of major coronary arteries.[7] In several studies of atheromas obtained from humans during endarterectomy, more than half the lesions contained periodontal pathogens, and many atheromas contained multiple different periodontal species.[11,34] Periodontal diseases result in chronic systemic exposure to products of these organisms. Low-level bacteremia may initiate host responses that alter coagulability, endothelial and vessel wall integrity, and platelet function, resulting in atherogenic changes and possible thromboembolic events (Figure 18-5).

Research has clearly shown a wide variation in host response to bacterial challenge. Some individuals with heavy plaque accumulation and high proportions of pathogenic organisms appear relatively resistant to bone and attachment loss. Others develop extensive periodontal destruction in the presence of small amounts of plaque and low proportions of putative pathogens. Patients with abnormally exuberant inflammatory responses often have a hyperinflammatory monocyte/macrophage phenotype (MØ⁺). Monocytes/macrophages from these individuals secrete significantly increased levels of proinflammatory mediators (e.g., IL-1, TNF-α, PGE_2) in response to bacterial LPS compared with patients with a normal monocyte/macrophage phenotype. Patients with aggressive periodontitis, refractory periodontitis, and type 1 diabetes mellitus often possess the MØ⁺ phenotype.[9]

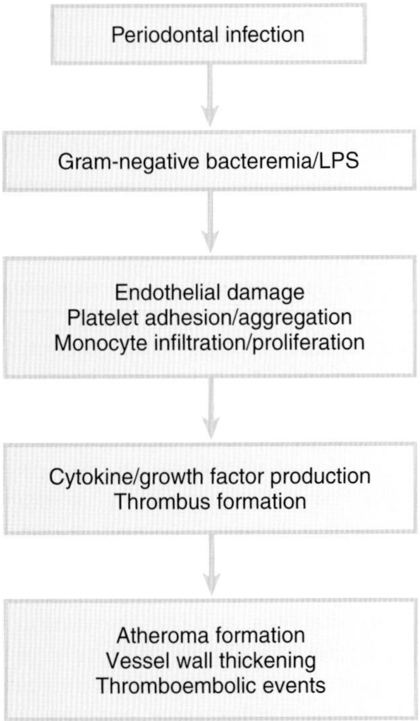

Figure 18-5 Influence of periodontal infection on atherosclerosis. Periodontal pathogens and their products result in damage to vascular endothelium. Monocytes/macrophages enter vessel wall, producing cytokines that further increase inflammatory response and propagate the atheromatous lesion. Growth factor production leads to smooth muscle proliferation in the vessel wall. Damaged endothelium also activates platelets, resulting in platelet aggregation and potentiating thromboembolic events. *LPS,* Lipopolysaccharide.

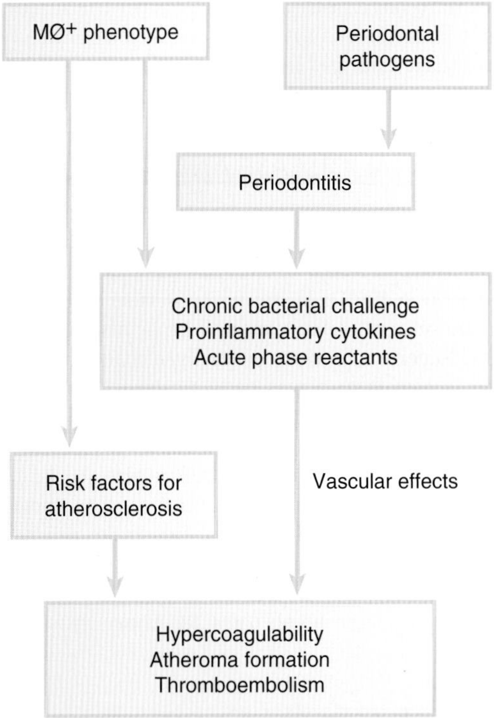

Figure 18-6 Cardiovascular and periodontal consequences of hyperresponsive monocyte/macrophage phenotype. In combination with other risk factors, the MØ$^+$ phenotype predisposes to both atherosclerosis and periodontitis. Bacterial products and inflammatory mediators associated with periodontitis affect vascular endothelium, monocytes/macrophages, platelets, and smooth muscle and may increase blood coagulability. This may further increase atherosclerosis and result in thromboembolism and ischemic events.

This monocyte/macrophage phenotype appears to be under both genetic and environmental control.[9] The monocyte/macrophage cell line is intimately involved in the pathogenesis of both periodontal disease and atherosclerosis. Diet-induced elevations in serum LDL levels upregulate monocyte/macrophage responsiveness to bacterial LPS. Thus, elevated LDL levels, a known risk factor for atherosclerosis and CHD, may increase secretion of destructive and inflammatory cytokines by monocytes/macrophages. This may result not only in propagation of atheromatous lesions, but also in enhanced periodontal destruction in the presence of pathogenic organisms. This is one example of a potential shared mechanism in the pathogenesis of cardiovascular and periodontal diseases. The presence of an MØ$^+$ phenotype may place patients at risk for both CHD and periodontitis (Figure 18-6). Periodontal infections may contribute to atherosclerosis and thromboembolic events by repeatedly challenging the vascular endothelium and arterial wall with bacterial LPS and proinflammatory cytokines. Vascular monocytes/macrophages in patients with an MØ$^+$ phenotype meet this challenge with an abnormally elevated inflammatory response that may directly contribute to atherosclerosis and may precipitate thromboembolic events.[66]

Cardiovascular diseases are increasingly recognized as having a major systemic inflammatory component, further emphasizing possible similarities with periodontal inflammatory diseases.[84] As such, detection of systemic inflammatory markers plays an increasingly important role in risk assessment for vascular events such as MI and cerebral infarction. Acute-phase proteins such as *C-reactive protein* (CRP) and fibrinogen are produced in the liver in response to inflammatory or infectious stimuli and act as inflammatory markers. CRP induces monocytes/macrophages to produce tissue factor, which stimulates the coagulation pathway and increases blood coagulability. Increased fibrinogen levels may contribute to this process. CRP also stimulates the complement cascade, further exacerbating inflammation.

Elevations in serum CRP and fibrinogen levels are well-accepted risk factors for cardiovascular disease.[83] The question often asked is, "When clinically evident infection is absent, what is the source of inflammation that triggers elevated acute-phase protein production?" Recent efforts have focused on periodontitis as a potential trigger for systemic inflammation. Serum CRP and fibrinogen levels are often elevated in subjects with periodontitis compared with nonperiodontitis subjects.[16,52,103] These acute-phase proteins may act as intermediary steps in the pathway from periodontal infection to cardiovascular disease (see Figures 18-5 and 18-6). Thus, periodontal diseases may have both direct effects on the major blood vessels (e.g., atheroma formation) as well as indirect effects that stimulate changes in the cardiovascular system (e.g., elevation of systemic inflammatory responses).

PERIODONTAL DISEASE AND STROKE

Ischemic cerebral infarction, or stroke, is often preceded by systemic bacterial or viral infection.[96] In one study, patients with cerebral ischemia were five times more likely to have had a systemic infection within 1 week before the ischemic event than were nonischemic control subjects. Recent infection was a significant risk factor for cerebral ischemia and was independent of other known risk factors, such as hypertension, history of a previous stroke, diabetes, smoking, and CHD.[27] Interestingly, the presence of systemic infection before the stroke resulted in significantly greater ischemia and a more severe post-ischemic neurologic defect than did stroke not preceded by infection.[28] Stroke patients with a preceding infection had slightly higher levels of plasma fibrinogen and significantly higher levels of CRP than those without infection.

Periodontal Infection Associated with Stroke

In case-control studies, poor dental health was a significant risk factor for cerebrovascular ischemia. In one study, bleeding on probing, suppuration, subgingival calculus, and the number of periodontal or periapical lesions were significantly greater in male stroke patients than in controls.[97] Overall, 25% of all stroke patients had significant dental infections versus only 2.5% of controls. This study supports an association between poor oral health and stroke in men under age 50. In another study, men and women age 50 and older who had a stroke had significantly more severe periodontitis and more periapical lesions than nonstroke controls.[29] Poor dental health was an independent risk factor for stroke. In a longitudinal study over 18 years, subjects with greater than 20% mean radiographic bone loss at baseline were almost three times as likely to have a stroke than subjects with less than 20% bone loss.[5] Periodontitis was a greater risk factor for stroke than was smoking and was independent of other known risk factors. Both large epidemiologic studies and systematic reviews of the evidence suggest an approximate threefold increased risk of stroke in subjects with periodontitis.[44,104]

Most cases of stroke are caused by thromboembolic events, whereas others are related to cerebrovascular atherosclerosis. As previously discussed, periodontal infection may contribute directly to the pathogenesis of atherosclerosis by providing a persistent bacterial challenge to arterial endothelium, contributing to the monocyte/macrophage-driven inflammatory process that results in atheromatosis and narrowing of the vessel lumen. Furthermore, periodontal infection may stimulate a series of indirect systemic effects, such as elevated production of fibrinogen and CRP, which serve to increase the risk of stroke (see Figures 18-5 and 18-6). Finally, bacteremia with PAAP-positive bacterial strains from the supragingival and subgingival plaque can increase platelet aggregation, contributing to thrombus formation and subsequent thromboembolism, the leading cause of stroke.[66]

PERIODONTAL DISEASE AND DIABETES MELLITUS

The relationship between diabetes mellitus and periodontal disease has been extensively examined. It is clear from epidemiologic research that diabetes increases the risk for and severity of periodontal diseases.[80] The biologic mechanisms through which diabetes influences the periodontium are discussed in Chapter 17. The increased prevalence and severity of periodontitis typically seen in patients with diabetes, especially those with poor metabolic control, led to the designation of periodontal disease as the "sixth complication of diabetes."[51] In addition to the five "classic" complications of diabetes (Box 18-2), the American Diabetes Association has officially recognized that periodontal disease is common in patients with diabetes, and the Association's Standards of Care include taking a history of current or past dental infections as part of the physician's examination.[3,4]

Although many studies have examined the effects of diabetes on the periodontium, few have attempted to examine the effect of periodontal infection on control of diabetes. The following questions remain:

- Does the presence or severity of periodontal disease affect the metabolic state in diabetic patients?
- Does periodontal treatment aimed at reducing the bacterial challenge and minimizing inflammation have a measurable effect on glycemic (blood glucose) control?

In a longitudinal study of patients with type 2 (non–insulin-dependent) diabetes, severe periodontitis was associated with significant worsening of glycemic control over time.[98] Individuals with severe periodontitis at the baseline examination had a greater incidence of worsening glycemic control over a 2- to 4-year period than did those without periodontitis at baseline. In this study, periodontitis is known to have preceded the worsening of glycemic control. Periodontitis has also been associated with the classic complications of diabetes. Diabetic adults with severe periodontitis at baseline had a significantly greater incidence of kidney and macrovascular complications over the subsequent 1 to 11 years than did diabetic adults with only gingivitis or mild

BOX 18-2

Complications of Diabetes Mellitus

1. Retinopathy
2. Nephropathy
3. Neuropathy
4. Macrovascular disease
5. Altered wound healing
6. Periodontal disease

From: Löe H: *Diabetes Care* 16(suppl 1):329, 1993.

periodontitis.[99] This was true despite that both groups had similar glycemic control. One or more cardiovascular complications occurred in 82% of patients with severe periodontitis versus 21% of patients without severe periodontitis. Again, severe periodontitis preceded the onset of clinical diabetic complications in these subjects.

In diabetic patients with periodontitis, periodontal therapy may have beneficial effects on glycemic control.[66,67] This may be especially true for patients with relatively poor glycemic control and more advanced periodontal destruction before treatment.[30] More than 40 years ago, the potential benefits of periodontal therapy were first described in young adults with diabetes and severe periodontitis.[102] Treatment with scaling and root planing, surgery, selected tooth extraction, and systemic antibiotics resulted in decreased insulin demand. In a more recent evaluation of scaling and root planing combined with systemic doxycycline therapy for 2 weeks, type 1 (insulin-dependent) diabetic patients with improved periodontal health also had significant improvement in glycemic control (Figure 18-7).[69] Conversely, those individuals who demonstrated little beneficial clinical effect from periodontal treatment had no change in glycemic control.

In a placebo-controlled study of poorly controlled individuals with type 2 diabetes and severe periodontitis, scaling and root planing combined with systemic doxycycline for 14 days was compared with similar treatment combined with systemic placebo.[32] All patient groups had significant improvements in periodontal status, with reduced probing depths and bleeding on probing. Those treated with doxycycline had a greater reduction in the prevalence of *P. gingivalis,* which was more sustained over time. The doxycycline-treated patients also demonstrated significant improvement in glycemic control 3 months after treatment, which gradually reverted to baseline levels at 6 months. Placebo-treated subjects had no significant improvement in glycemic control. These studies suggest that the combination of subgingival mechanical debridement and systemic doxycycline may result in short-term improvement in glycemia in diabetic patients with severe periodontitis and poor metabolic control.

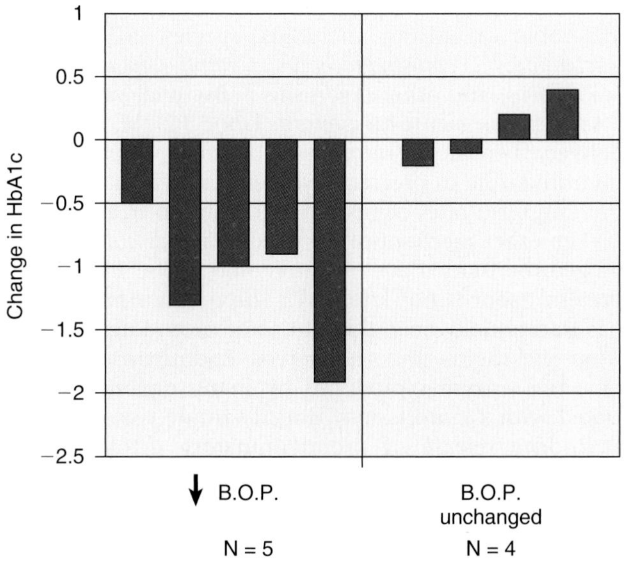

Figure 18-7 Periodontal treatment: effects on glycemic control. In five patients, reductions in periodontal inflammation after mechanical therapy combined with systemic doxycycline were accompanied by improved glycemic control (decreased glycated hemoglobin values, HbA1c). In four patients with no improvement in periodontal health, no improvement in glycemic control occurred. *B.O.P.,* Bleeding on probing (a measure of periodontal inflammation). (From Miller LS, Manwell MA, Newbold D, et al: *J Periodontol* 63:843, 1992.)

Conversely, individuals with moderately well-controlled or well-controlled diabetes and periodontitis who are treated by mechanical therapy alone may demonstrate no significant changes in glycemic control, despite improvement in their periodontal condition. In studies of subjects treated by mechanical therapy without adjunctive use of antibiotics, significant changes in glycemic control are less common.[1,13,32,93] Many patients in these studies had relatively good glycemic control before treatment, so less benefit on metabolic control might be expected. Although routine use of systemic antibiotics in treatment of chronic periodontitis is not justified, patients with poorly controlled diabetes and severe periodontitis may constitute one patient group for whom such therapy is appropriate. Antibiotics remain an adjunct to the necessary mechanical removal of plaque and calculus.

The mechanisms by which adjunctive antibiotics may induce positive changes in glycemic control when combined with mechanical debridement are unknown at this time. Systemic antibiotics may eliminate residual bacteria after scaling and root planing, further decreasing the bacterial challenge to the host. Tetracyclines are also known to suppress glycation of proteins and to decrease activity of tissue-degrading enzymes such as matrix metalloproteinases (MMPs). These changes may contribute to improvement in metabolic control of diabetes. A low-dose form of doxycycline (20 mg) has been introduced with the specific purpose of reducing the production of collagen-degrading MMPs (see Chapter 52). This dose has no antibiotic effects and does not induce antimicrobial resistance with long-term use. Because diabetes is associated with greatly elevated production of collagenase, low-dose doxycycline has been used in treatment of periodontitis in diabetic subjects. Preliminary evidence suggests that low-dose doxycycline, in conjunction with scaling and root planing, may improve clinical periodontal parameters compared with scaling and root planing alone in diabetic patients. Furthermore, short-term improvements in glycemic control have been demonstrated with combination therapy, whereas no change in glycemic control was seen when mechanical therapy alone was used.[2,23] Further research is indicated to determine the adjunctive benefit of such host modulation therapies in the diabetic population.

Periodontal Infection Associated with Glycemic Control in Diabetes

An understanding of the effects of other infections is useful in delineating the mechanisms by which periodontal

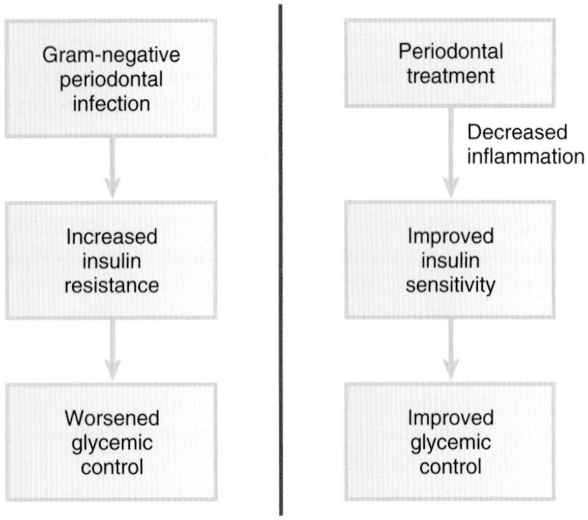

Figure 18-8 Potential effects of periodontal infection and periodontal therapy on glycemia in patients with diabetes.

infection influences glycemia. Acute bacterial and viral infections have been shown to increase insulin resistance and aggravate glycemic control.[85,105] This occurs in individuals with and without diabetes. Systemic infections increase tissue resistance to insulin, preventing glucose from entering target cells, causing elevated blood glucose levels, and requiring increased pancreatic insulin production to maintain normoglycemia. Insulin resistance may persist for weeks or even months after the patient has recovered clinically from their illness. In the individual with type 2 diabetes, who already has significant insulin resistance, further tissue resistance to insulin induced by infection may considerably exacerbate poor glycemic control. In type 1 patients, normal insulin doses may be inadequate to maintain good glycemic control in the presence of infection-induced tissue resistance. It is possible that chronic gram-negative periodontal infections may also result in increased insulin resistance and poor glycemic control.[31] In patients with periodontitis, persistent systemic challenge with periodontopathic bacteria and their products may act similar to well-recognized systemic infections (Figure 18-8). This mechanism would explain the worsening of glycemic control associated with severe periodontitis. Periodontal treatment designed to decrease the bacterial insult and reduce inflammation might restore insulin sensitivity over time, resulting in improved metabolic control. The improved glycemic control seen in several studies of periodontal therapy would support such a hypothesis.

PERIODONTAL DISEASE AND PREGNANCY OUTCOME

Low-birth-weight (LBW) infants (<2500 g at birth) are 40 times more likely to die in the neonatal period than normal-birth-weight (NBW) infants.[63] Although about 7% of all infants weigh less than 2500 g at birth, they account for two thirds of neonatal deaths. LBW infants who survive the neonatal period are at increased risk for congenital anomalies, respiratory disorders, and neurodevelopmental disabilities. The social and financial costs of LBW infants are enormous, and an emphasis on prevention of low birth weight is preferred to the high-cost intensive care often required to allow survival of LBW infants.

The primary cause of LBW deliveries is *preterm labor* or *premature rupture of membranes* (PROM). Factors such as smoking, alcohol, or drug use during pregnancy, inadequate prenatal care, race, low socioeconomic status, hypertension, high or low maternal age, diabetes, and genitourinary tract infections increase the risk of preterm LBW delivery. However, these risk factors are not present in approximately one fourth of preterm LBW cases, leading to a continued search for other causes.[76]

Research has examined the relationship between maternal infection and preterm labor, PROM, and LBW delivery. The true extent of this relationship is difficult to determine because the majority of maternal infections may be subclinical. Genitourinary tract infections have been associated with adverse pregnancy outcomes. Women with bacteriuria have increased rates of preterm delivery, and antibiotic treatment of bacteriuria has resulted in a significant decrease in preterm delivery rates compared with placebo treatment.[40,76] Vaginal colonization with group B streptococci or *Bacteroides* species increases the risk of PROM, preterm delivery, and LBW infants.[64]

Bacterial Vaginosis

Bacterial vaginosis is the most common vaginal disorder in women of reproductive age. It is caused by changes in the vaginal microflora in which normally predominant facultative lactobacilli are replaced by *Gardnerella vaginalis;* anaerobic organisms, including species of *Prevotella, Bacteroides, Peptostreptococcus, Porphyromonas,* and *Mobiluncus;* and other organisms.[38] Bacterial vaginosis is a known risk factor for preterm labor, PROM, and LBW delivery.[31] In fact, treatment of bacterial vaginosis with metronidazole in pregnant women resulted in decreased preterm birth rates compared with placebo treatment.[70]

The exact mechanism by which vaginal colonization or genitourinary tract infection may cause PROM and preterm labor is not known.[101] The primary mechanism has traditionally been thought to be ascending infection from the vagina and endocervix. Endotoxin (LPS) and bioactive enzymes produced by many organisms associated with vaginosis may directly injure tissue, as well as induce release of proinflammatory cytokines and prostaglandins. Throughout normal gestation, amniotic prostaglandin levels rise steadily until a sufficient threshold is reached that induces labor and delivery. Maternal infection may cause increased prostaglandin production and may result in labor-inducing levels being achieved before full gestation. In addition to prostaglandins, various proinflammatory cytokines (e.g., IL-1, IL-6, TNF) have been found in the amniotic fluid of women with preterm labor.

Women with preterm labor often have culture-positive amniotic fluid, even in the absence of clinical infection. Of culture-positive patients, the species most often isolated is *Fusobacterium nucleatum.*[40] Although *F. nucleatum* is occasionally isolated from the vaginal flora in bacterial vaginosis, its prevalence in women with preterm labor is much greater than in vaginosis. *F. nucleatum* is even less frequently isolated from the vaginal flora of women without bacterial vaginosis. Many of the other species isolated from amniotic fluid in women with preterm labor are those often found in bacterial vaginosis, which supports an ascending route of infection. However, the frequency of *F. nucleatum* detection suggests other possible routes of infection. Some investigators have suggested infection by a hematogenous route from a location in which the organism is often detected.[40] *F. nucleatum* is a common oral species highly prevalent in patients with periodontitis and could reach the amniotic fluid by hematogenous spread from the oral cavity. This route is also suggested by the occasional isolation of *Capnocytophaga* species in the amniotic fluid of women with preterm labor, an organism rarely isolated from the vagina but common in the oral cavity. Hill[39] found that the species and subspecies of *F. nucleatum* isolated from amniotic fluid cultures in women with preterm labor more closely matched those found in subgingival plaque than strains identified from the lower genital tract. In addition to hematogenous spread, another possible route of infection is by oral-genital contact, with transfer of oral organisms to the vagina.[40]

Although direct effects of microorganisms may play an important role in many cases of preterm labor, PROM, and LBW delivery, indirect mechanisms may also be operative.[66,76] Bacterial infection of the chorioamnion, or extraplacental membrane, may lead to *chorioamnionitis,* a condition strongly associated with PROM and preterm delivery. However, many cases of histologic chorioamnionitis demonstrate negative bacterial cultures, indicating that infection is not the sole cause of this condition. It is likely that an indirect mechanism may be active in which the cascade of host products produced in response to infection is often responsible for preterm labor. Maternal infection may lead to the presence of amniotic bacterial products, such as LPS from gram-negative organisms, which stimulate production of host-derived cytokines in the amnion and decidua (Figure 18-9). These cytokines, including IL-1, TNF-α, and IL-6, stimulate increased prostaglandin production from the amnion and decidua, leading to onset of preterm labor. A premature rise in PGE_2 and $PGF_{2\alpha}$ is characteristic of preterm labor, regardless of whether clinical or subclinical maternal genitourinary tract infection is detected.

The question then arises as to what stimulates the increased cytokine levels and resultant increased prostaglandin levels seen in preterm delivery in patients with no evidence of genitourinary infection. Many cases of preterm LBW could result from infections of unknown origin, that is, infections originating in areas other than the genitourinary tract.

Role of Periodontitis

Periodontitis is a remote gram-negative infection that may play a role in LBW infants. As discussed previously, periodontopathic organisms and their products may have wide-ranging effects, most likely mediated through

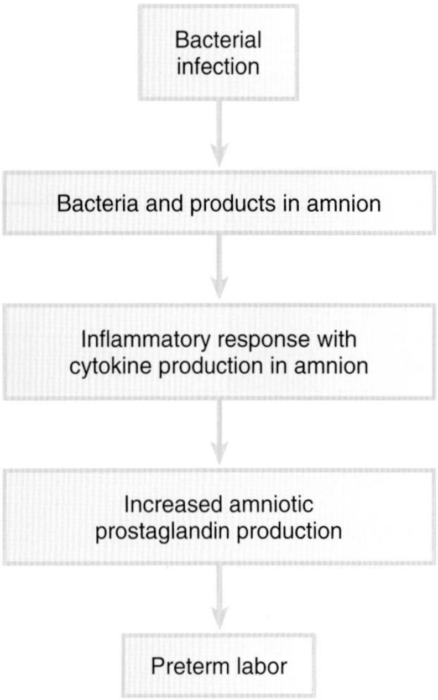

Figure 18-9 Mechanisms by which infection may induce preterm labor.

stimulation of host cytokine production in target tissues. Animal studies suggest that remote reservoirs of gram-negative organisms and their products may have a negative impact on pregnancy outcome. *P. gingivalis* implanted in subcutaneous chambers during gestation caused significant increases in TNF-α and PGE_2 levels.[14] This localized subcutaneous infection resulted in a significant increase in fetal death and a decrease in fetal birth weight for those that remained viable, compared with control animals that were not inoculated. There was a significant correlation between both TNF-α and PGE_2 levels, as well as fetal death and growth retardation. These data suggest that a remote, nondisseminated infection with *P. gingivalis* may result in abnormal pregnancy outcomes in this model.

Decreased fetal birth weight and increased fetal death were also seen after intravenous injections with LPS derived from *P. gingivalis.*[15] This effect was greatly increased when *P. gingivalis* LPS was administered before mating and during gestation, indicating that repeated immunization with *P. gingivalis* LPS does not provide protection during pregnancy, but potentiates the negative effects of LPS exposure during gestation. *P. gingivalis*–induced experimental periodontitis in animal models resulted in decreased fetal birth weight and increased amniotic fluid levels of TNF-α and PGE_2 (Figure 18-10).[76] This provides direct evidence that periodontal infection can affect the fetal environment and pregnancy outcome.

These animal studies have led to examination of the potential effects of periodontitis on pregnancy outcome in humans. In an initial case-control study of 124 women (93 cases with at least one LBW delivery and 31 controls with at least one NBW delivery), Offenbacher et al.[75] found that women having LBW infants had greater clinical attachment loss than women having NBW infants.

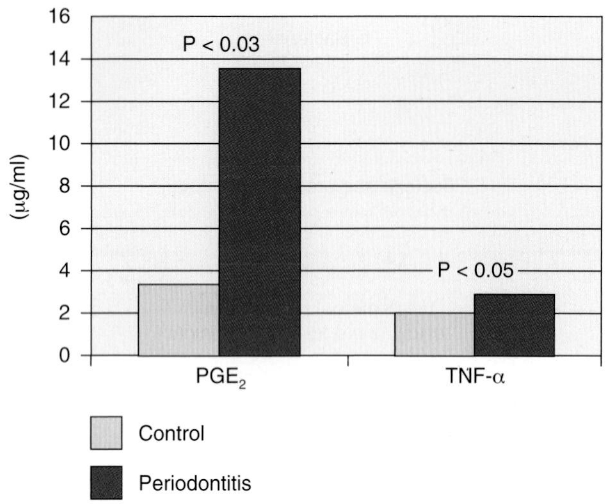

Figure 18-10 Amniotic fluid levels in experimental periodontitis. Experimental periodontitis resulted in increased amniotic fluid levels of tumor necrosis factor alpha (*TNF-α*) and prostaglandin E_2 (*PGE_2*) in the pregnant hamster model, providing evidence that periodontal infection can affect the fetal environment. (From Offenbacher S, Jarad HL, O'Reilly PG, et al: *Ann Periodontol* 3:233, 1998.)

After adjusting for known risk factors for LBW delivery, women with periodontitis resulting in greater than 3 mm of attachment loss in at least 60% of sites had a 7.5-fold increased risk of having a LBW infant. In fact, periodontitis contributed to more preterm LBW cases than did smoking or alcohol use during pregnancy. In a large prospective study of more than 1300 pregnant women, subjects with generalized periodontitis had a fivefold increased risk of preterm birth before 35 weeks of gestation and a sevenfold increased risk of delivery before 32 weeks compared with women without periodontitis.[47] These studies and others[19,53] indicate a strong association between periodontal infection and adverse pregnancy outcomes.

In a cross-sectional study, women having LBW infants had significantly higher levels of *Actinobacillus actinomycetemcomitans, Tannerella forsythia, P. gingivalis,* and *Treponema denticola* in their subgingival plaque than did the control women having NBW infants.[76] Women having LBW infants also had higher levels of gingival crevicular fluid (GCF) PGE_2 and IL-1. In primiparous women (those experiencing a first birth), GCF levels of PGE_2 were inversely related to their infants' birth weight. Women with higher PGE_2 levels in GCF had smaller and more premature infants. GCF levels of IL-1 and PGE_2 have been shown to correlate highly with intraamniotic IL-1 and PGE_2 levels. In fact, measuring GCF levels of these inflammatory mediators has been suggested as a less invasive means of screening expectant mothers for elevated amniotic IL-1 and PGE_2 levels than amniocentesis.[76] Thus, women having LBW infants have a higher prevalence and severity of periodontitis, more gingival inflammation, higher levels of putative periodontal pathogens, and an elevated subgingival inflammatory response compared with women having NBW infants.

Periodontal disease may also increase the risk for *preeclampsia.* This hypertensive disorder affects about 5% to 10% of pregnancies and is a major cause of perinatal and maternal morbidity and mortality. Preeclampsia has multiple potential etiologies, several of which involve vascular changes in the placenta that are similar to those seen in atherosclerosis. The presence of periodontitis during pregnancy or a worsening of periodontal disease during pregnancy may increase the risk for preeclampsia 2- to 2.5-fold.[10]

Several intervention trials have examined the effects of treating periodontal disease during gestation, rather than waiting until after parturition to provide needed care. In a study of 351 pregnant women with periodontitis, Lopez et al.[54] found that women who received scaling and root planing before 28 weeks' gestation, followed by prophylaxis every 2 weeks until parturition, had a LBW rate of 1.8%. Conversely, women who did not receive periodontal therapy during gestation but instead were treated after parturition had a LBW rate of 10.1%. Similarly, Jeffcoat et al.[48] found a reduced preterm birth rate in women who received mechanical periodontal therapy during gestation.

When combined with animal studies showing adverse effects of experimental periodontitis on the fetus and data supporting biologically plausible interactive mechanisms, the evidence strongly suggests that periodontal infection may have significant negative impact on pregnancy outcome in some women. A recent systematic review of the human evidence concluded that a moderate level of evidence suggested that periodontal disease is associated with adverse pregnancy outcome; however, it was unclear whether periodontal disease played a causal role in those adverse outcomes.[88]

PERIODONTAL DISEASE AND CHRONIC OBSTRUCTIVE PULMONARY DISEASE

Chronic obstructive pulmonary disease (COPD) is characterized by airflow obstruction resulting from chronic bronchitis or emphysema. Bronchial mucous glands enlarge, and an inflammatory process occurs in which neutrophils and mononuclear inflammatory cells accumulate within the lung tissue.[35,100] About 14 million Americans have COPD, and tobacco smoking is the primary risk factor.

COPD shares similar pathogenic mechanisms with periodontal disease. In both diseases, a host inflammatory response is mounted in response to chronic challenge: by bacteria in periodontal disease and by factors such as cigarette smoke in COPD. The resulting neutrophil influx leads to release of oxidative and hydrolytic enzymes that cause tissue destruction directly. Recruitment of monocytes and macrophages leads to further release of proinflammatory mediators.

Less is known about the clinical relationship between periodontal disease and COPD compared with CHD and other systemic conditions. In analyzing data from a longitudinal study of more than 1100 men, alveolar bone loss was associated with the risk for COPD.[35] Over a 25-year period, 23% of subjects were diagnosed with COPD. Subjects with more severe bone loss at the baseline dental examination had a significantly increased risk of subsequently developing COPD compared with subjects with less bone loss. The increase in risk was independent of age, smoking status, and other known risk factors for COPD. Individuals with poor oral hygiene have also been found to be at increased risk for chronic respiratory diseases such as bronchitis and emphysema.[90] Conversely, a large epidemiologic study revealed no significant overall association between periodontal disease and COPD.[43] In nonsmokers and former smokers, even severe periodontitis did not increase the risk for COPD. In current smokers, however, the presence of severe periodontitis was associated with an increased risk of COPD. These results suggest that smoking may act as a major "effect modifier" in the relationship between COPD and periodontal disease, and that this modifier's presence may be required to generate an effect. A recent systematic review of available evidence stated that insufficient evidence exists on the potential association between COPD and periodontal disease.[89] Therefore, more research is needed in this area.

SCIENCE TRANSFER

Periodontal disease has a proven relationship with several systemic diseases, including coronary artery disease, diabetes, and stroke, as well as delivery of low-birth-weight infants. Therefore, clinicians have a responsibility to reduce the degree of exposure for all patients, not only to enhance dental health, but also to reduce the risk of these systemic diseases and LBW delivery. This relationship is not likely to affect all individuals, but it certainly affects some. In these patients, periodontal infection is suggested to be a risk factor for systemic disease just as high cholesterol is a risk factor for coronary heart disease. Periodontitis may initiate systemic inflammation. Individuals with significant systemic inflammation can be monitored with inflammatory markers such as C-reactive protein or fibrinogen levels; these are accepted risk factors for cardiovascular disease. This initiation could be a direct consequence of the oral microbiotic flora or an indirect effect through other proteins or molecules stimulated by the periodontal infection. In the case of LBW infants, significant reduction in risk has been reported after periodontal treatment. Also, some diabetic patients have improved their diabetic status and reduced their need for insulin after periodontal therapy combined with systemic doxycycline.

PERIODONTAL DISEASE AND ACUTE RESPIRATORY INFECTIONS

The upper respiratory passages are often contaminated with organisms derived from the oral, nasal, and pharyngeal regions. Conversely, the lower airways, where gas exchange occurs, are generally maintained free of microorganisms by a combination of host immune factors and mechanical clearance through the cough reflex, ciliary transport of aspirated contaminants, and movement of secretions from the lower airways into the trachea.[66]

Pneumonia is an infection of the lungs caused by bacteria, viruses, fungi, or mycoplasma and is broadly categorized as either community-acquired or hospital-acquired pneumonia. A wide variety of bacteria may cause pneumonia, and the spectrum of offending organisms differs greatly between community-acquired and hospital-acquired infections.

Community-acquired bacterial pneumonia is caused primarily by inhalation of infectious aerosols or by aspiration of oropharyngeal organisms. *Streptococcus pneumoniae* and *Haemophilus influenzae* are most common, although numerous other species may be found, including anaerobic bacteria.[77] Antibiotic therapy is highly successful in resolution of most cases of community-acquired bacterial pneumonia. To date, no associations have been found between oral hygiene or periodontal disease and the risk for acute respiratory conditions such as pneumonia in community-dwelling individuals.[90]

The same cannot be said for individuals in the hospital setting. *Hospital-acquired (nosocomial) bacterial pneumonia* has a very high morbidity and mortality rate. Approximately 20% to 50% of patients with nosocomial pneumonia die.[17] The incidence of nosocomial pneumonia is highest in severely ill patients such as those in intensive care units or on ventilatory support. More than half of patients on mechanical ventilation for several days or more acquire pneumonia. Although nosocomial pneumonia is most often caused by gram-negative aerobic organisms, many cases are the result of infection by anaerobic bacteria, including those typically found in the subgingival environment.

Hospital-acquired pneumonia is usually caused by aspiration of oropharyngeal contents. Oropharyngeal colonization with *potential respiratory pathogens* (PRPs) increases during hospitalization; the longer the hospital stay, the greater the prevalence of PRPs.[66] PRPs are found predominantly in the gastrointestinal tract and may be passed through esophageal reflux into the oropharynx, where they colonize. Subsequent aspiration may lead to pneumonia. Patients whose posterior oropharynx becomes colonized with PRPs have a significantly increased risk of developing nosocomial pneumonia compared with those without oropharyngeal colonization by PRPs.[91]

Selective decontamination is a technique that combines systemic antibiotics with orally administered nonabsorbable antibiotics in an attempt to eradicate PRPs from the digestive tract and oropharynx and thereby minimize the risk of nosocomial respiratory infections. The technique is used primarily in patients who are intubated and on mechanical ventilators. Selective decontamination significantly decreases the incidence of nosocomial pneumonia.[92] Decontamination of only the digestive tract does not reduce the incidence of pneumonia, but decontamination of the oropharynx alone does.[81,95] This provides further evidence that the oropharynx is the primary site of PRP colonization, with subsequent aspiration of causative organisms leading to pneumonia.

PRPs may also originate in the oral cavity, with dental plaque serving as a reservoir of these organisms. Poor oral hygiene is common in the hospital and nursing home settings, especially in severely ill patients.[91] PRPs are more often isolated from supragingival plaque and buccal mucosa of patients in intensive care units than in outpatient settings.[86] Thus, organisms that are not routinely found in dental plaque become plaque colonizers after prolonged hospitalization. Subgingival plaque may also harbor PRPs, and putative periodontal pathogens have been associated with nosocomial pneumonia. Furthermore, anaerobic organisms from periodontal pockets may serve as the primary inoculum for suppurative respiratory diseases (e.g., pulmonary abscesses) that have significant morbidity and mortality.

In a systematic review of the evidence, Scannapieco et al.[89] concluded that interventions used to improve oral hygiene, such as mechanical toothbrushing and chemical antimicrobial rinses, have the potential to decrease the risk of nosocomial pneumonia in high-risk patients, such as those in intensive care units or those on ventilators. This conclusion was based on at least five randomized controlled intervention trials that showed consistent positive effects of antiinfective oral therapy on the rate of nosocomial pneumonia.

PERIODONTAL MEDICINE IN CLINICAL PRACTICE

The concept of periodontal diseases as localized entities affecting only the teeth and supporting apparatus is oversimplified and in need of revision. Rather than being confined to the periodontium, periodontal diseases may have wide-ranging systemic effects. In most persons, these effects may be relatively inconsequential or at least not clinically evident. In susceptible individuals, however, periodontal infection may act as an independent risk factor for systemic disease and may be involved in the basic pathogenic mechanisms of these conditions. Furthermore, periodontal infection may exacerbate existing systemic disorders.

Periodontal Disease and Systemic Health

Proper use of the knowledge of potential relationships between periodontal disease and systemic health requires the dental professional to expand his or her horizons, to step back from the technically demanding aspects of the dental art, and to recognize the oral cavity as one of many interrelated organ systems. An infection the size of one's palm on the leg of a pregnant woman would be a major concern to the patient and her health care provider, given the potential negative consequences of this localized infection on fetal and maternal health. A similar suppurating infection on the foot of a person with diabetes would be cause for immediate evaluation and aggressive treatment, knowing the effects of such infections on metabolic control of diabetes.

Periodontal infection must be viewed in a similar manner. Periodontitis is a gram-negative infection resulting in severe inflammation, with potential intravascular dissemination of microorganisms and their products throughout the body. However, periodontitis tends to be a "silent" disease, until destruction results in acute symptoms. Most patients, as well as many medical professionals, do not recognize the potential infection that may exist within the oral cavity.

Patient Education

Patient education is a priority. Only 30 years ago, the factors involved in CHD were unclear. At present, however, it would be difficult to find an individual who was unfamiliar with the link between cholesterol and heart disease. This change was precipitated by research clearly demonstrating the increased risk for heart disease in individuals with high cholesterol levels, followed by intensive education efforts to spread the message from the scientific community to the public at large. It is important to recognize that high cholesterol levels have not been shown to cause heart disease in all individuals, but rather significantly increase the risk of disease. Cholesterol has also been demonstrated to have a biologically plausible role in the pathogenesis of CHD.

Similarly, patient education efforts in the realm of periodontal medicine must emphasize the nature of periodontal infections, the increased risk for systemic disease associated with the infection, and the biologically plausible role periodontal infection may play in systemic disease. Few individuals had their cholesterol levels evaluated until the knowledge of the link between cholesterol and heart disease became widespread. Likewise, increased appreciation of the potential effects of periodontal infection on systemic health may result in increased patient demand for periodontal evaluation.

Enhanced community awareness may be derived from newspapers, magazines, and other lay sources. However, the most reliable origin of information should be the dental and medical professions through daily contact with patients. The pregnant woman usually knows that infections may adversely affect her pregnancy. Persons with diabetes generally know that infections impair glycemic control. However, many of these patients do not know that occult periodontal infections can have the same effect as more clinically evident infections. The dentist is responsible for diagnosing periodontal infections, providing appropriate treatment, and preventing disease recurrence or progression. Because many medical professionals are unfamiliar with the oral cavity and oral health research, dentists must reach out to the medical community to improve patient care through education and communication. Likewise, patients must be educated in disease prevention. Just as patients know that lowering cholesterol levels may decrease their risk for heart disease, prevention of periodontal infection should be emphasized. A physician would be remiss if he or she did not provide education on decreasing cholesterol, losing weight, and ceasing a smoking habit to a patient at risk for CHD. Likewise, controlling the risk factor of periodontal infection requires the dentist to emphasize personal and professional preventive measures focused on thorough oral hygiene and regular recall.

SUMMARY

Does periodontal disease cause CHD, COPD, or adverse pregnancy outcomes? This question may only be answered based on the evidence currently available, with the full knowledge that conclusions may change as future evidence dictates. Periodontal disease may increase the risk for many systemic disorders. Biologically plausible mechanisms support the role of periodontal infection in these conditions, but periodontal infection should not be presented as the cause of such systemic diseases any more than cholesterol is said to cause heart disease. Periodontal infection is one of many potential risk factors for a number of systemic conditions. Fortunately, it is a readily modifiable risk factor, unlike age, gender, and genetic influences.

The focal infection theory of the early twentieth century was widely and appropriately discredited when treatment based on the theory, tooth extraction, had no effect on the underlying diseases that oral sepsis supposedly caused. Similarly, the clinical utility of our current knowledge base is only now evolving. Future research will further delineate the role of periodontal infection in systemic health. The associations between periodontal infection and conditions such as LBW delivery, diabetes, cardiovascular and cerebrovascular diseases, and respiratory diseases may be further substantiated. Longitudinal studies and intervention trials are needed before any causative role can be assigned.

The emerging field of periodontal medicine offers new insights into the concept of the oral cavity as one system interconnected with the whole human body. For many years the dental profession has recognized the effects of systemic conditions on the oral cavity. Only now, however, are dental professionals beginning to understand more fully the impact of the periodontium on systemic health.

REFERENCES

1. Aldridge JP, Lester V, Watts TLP, et al: Single-blind studies of the effects of improved periodontal health on metabolic control in type 1 diabetes mellitus, *J Clin Periodontol* 22:271, 1995.
2. Al-Ghazi MN, Ciancio SG, Aljada A, et al: Evaluation of efficacy of administration of sub-antimicrobial-dose doxycycline in the treatment of generalized adult periodontitis in diabetics, *J Dent Res* 82(A):1752, 2003.
3. American Diabetes Association: Standards of medical care for patients with diabetes mellitus, *Diabetes Care* 21(suppl 1):523, 1998.
4. American Diabetes Association: Report of the Expert Committee on the Diagnosis and Classification of Diabetes Mellitus, *Diabetes Care* 26(suppl 1):5, 2003.
5. Arbes SJ Jr, Slade GD, Beck JD: Association between extent of periodontal attachment loss and self-reported history of heart attack: an analysis of NHANES III data, *J Dent Res* 78:1777, 1999.
6. Beck JD, Offenbacher S: The association between periodontal diseases and cardiovascular diseases: a state-of-the-art review, *Ann Periodontol* 6:9, 2001.
7. Beck JD, Elter JR, Heiss G: Relationship of periodontal disease to carotid artery intima-media wall thickness: the Atherosclerosis Risk in Communities (ARIC) study, *Arterioscler Thromb Vasc Biol* 21:1816, 2001.
8. Beck JD, Garcia RG, Heiss G, et al: Periodontal disease and cardiovascular disease, *J Periodontol* 67:1123, 1996.
9. Beck JD, Offenbacher S, Williams R, et al: Periodontitis: a risk factor for coronary heart disease? *Ann Periodontol* 3:127, 1998.
10. Bogess KA, Lieff S, Murtha AP, et al. Maternal periodontal disease is associated with an increased risk for preeclampsia, *Obstet Gynecol* 101:227, 2003.
11. Chiu B: Multiple infections in carotid atherosclerotic plaques, *Am Heart J* 138(suppl):534, 1999.
12. Christan C, Dietrich T, Hagewald S, et al: White blood cell count in generalized aggressive periodontitis after non-surgical therapy, *J Clin Periodontol* 29:201, 2002.
13. Christgau M, Pallitzsch KD, Schmalz G, et al: Healing response to non-surgical periodontal therapy in patients with diabetes mellitus: clinical, microbiological and immunological results, *J Clin Periodontol* 25:112, 1998.
14. Collins JG, Windley III HW, Arnold RR, et al: Effects of a *Porphyromonas gingivalis* infection on inflammatory mediator response and pregnancy outcome in hamsters, *Infect Immun* 62:4356, 1994.
15. Collins JG, Smith MA, Arnold RR, et al: Effects of a *Escherichia coli* and *Porphyromonas gingivalis* lipopolysaccharide on pregnancy outcome in the golden hamster, *Infect Immun* 62:4652, 1994.
16. Craig RG, Yip JK, So MK, et al: Relationship of destructive periodontal disease to the acute-phase response, *J Periodontol* 74:1007, 2003.
17. Craven DE, Steger KE, Barber TW: Preventing nosocomial pneumonia: state of the art and perspectives for the 1990s, *Am J Med* 91(suppl 3B):44, 1991.
18. Dajani AS, Taubert KA, Wilson W, et al: Prevention of bacterial endocarditis: recommendations by the American Heart Association, *JAMA* 277:1794, 1997.
19. Dasanayake AP: Poor periodontal health of the pregnant woman as a risk factor for low birth weight, *Ann Periodontol* 3:202, 1998.
20. DeStefano F, Andra RF, Kahn HS, et al: Dental disease and risk of coronary heart disease and mortality, *Br Med J* 306:688, 1993.
21. Drangsholt MT: A new causal model of dental diseases associated with endocarditis, *Ann Periodontol* 3:184, 1998.
22. Dussault G, Shieham A: Medical theories and professional development: the theory of focal sepsis and dentistry in early twentieth century Britain, *Soc Sci Med* 16:1405, 1982.
23. Engerbretson SP, Hey-Hadavi J, Celenti R, Lamster IB: Low-dose doxycycline treatment reduces glycosylated hemoglobin in patients with type 2 diabetes: a randomized controlled trial, *J Dent Res* 82(A):1445, 2003.
24. Evidence-Based Medicine Working Group: Evidence-based medicine: a new approach to teaching the practice of medicine, *JAMA* 268:2420, 1992.
25. Garcia RI, Krall EA, Vokonas PS: Periodontal disease and mortality from all causes in the VA Dental Longitudinal Study, *Ann Periodontol* 3:339, 1998.
26. Geerts SO, Nys M, De MP, et al: Systemic release of endotoxins induced by gentle mastication: association with periodontitis severity, *J Periodontol* 73:73, 2002.
27. Grau AJ, Buggle F, Heindl S, et al: Recent infection as a risk factor for cerebrovascular ischemia, *Stroke* 26:373, 1995.
28. Grau AJ, Buggle F, Steichen-Wiehn C, et al: Clinical and biochemical analysis in infection-associated stroke, *Stroke* 26:1520, 1995.
29. Grau AJ, Buggle F, Ziegler C, et al: Association between acute cerebrovascular ischemia and chronic and recurrent infection, *Stroke* 28:1724, 1997.

30. Grossi SG, Genco RJ: Periodontal disease and diabetes mellitus: a two-way relationship, *Ann Periodontol* 3:51, 1998.
31. Grossi SG, Mealey BL, Rose LF: Effect of periodontal infection on systemic health and well-being. In Rose LF, Mealey BL, Genco RJ, Cohen DW, editors: *Periodontics: medicine, surgery and implants,* St Louis, 2004, Elsevier.
32. Grossi SG, Skrepcinski FB, DeCaro T, et al: Treatment of periodontal disease in diabetics reduces glycated hemoglobin, *J Periodontol* 68:713, 1997.
33. Guntheroth WG: How important are dental procedures as a cause of infective endocarditis? *Am J Cardiol* 54:797, 1984.
34. Haraszthy VI, Zambon JJ, Trevisan M, et al: Identification of periodontal pathogens in atheromatous plaques, *J Periodontol* 71:1554, 2000.
35. Hayes C, Sparrow D, Cohen M, et al: The association between alveolar bone loss and pulmonary function: the VA Dental Longitudinal Study, *Ann Periodontol* 3:257, 1998.
36. Herzberg MC, Meyer MW: Effects of oral flora on platelets: possible consequences in cardiovascular disease, *J Periodontol* 67:1138, 1996.
37. Herzberg MC, Meyer MW: Dental plaque, platelets and cardiovascular diseases, *Ann Periodontol* 3:151, 1998.
38. Hill GB: The microbiology of bacterial vaginosis, *Am J Obstet Gynecol* 169:450, 1993.
39. Hill GB: Investigating the source of amniotic fluid isolates of fusobacteria, *Clin Infect Dis* 16(suppl 4):423, 1993.
40. Hill GB: Preterm birth: associations with genital and possibly oral microflora, *Ann Periodontol* 3:222, 1998.
41. Hujoel PP, Drangsholt M, Spiekerman C, DeRouen TA: Periodontal disease and coronary heart disease risk, *JAMA* 284:1406, 2000.
42. Hujoel PP, Drangsholt M, Spiekerman C, Derouen TA: Examining the link between coronary heart disease and the elimination of chronic dental infections, *J Am Dent Assoc* 132:883, 2001.
43. Hyman JJ, Reid BC: Cigarette smoking, periodontal disease, and chronic obstructive pulmonary disease, *J Periodontol* 75:9, 2004.
44. Janket S, Baird AE, Chuang S, Jones JA: Meta-analysis of periodontal disease and risk of coronary heart disease and stroke, *Oral Surg Oral Med Oral Pathol Oral Radiol Endod* 95:559, 2003.
45. Janket S, Qvarnstrom M, Muerman JH, et al: Asymptomatic dental score and prevalent coronary heart disease, *Circulation* 109:1095, 2004.
46. Jansson L, Lavstedt S, Frithiof L: Relationship between oral health and mortality rate, *J Clin Periodontol* 29:1029, 2002.
47. Jeffcoat MK, Guers NC, Reddy MS, et al: Periodontal infection and preterm birth: results of a prospective study, *J Am Dent Assoc* 132:875, 2001.
48. Jeffcoat MJ, Hauth JC, Guers N, et al: Periodontal disease and preterm birth: results of a pilot intervention study, *J Periodontol* 74:1214, 2003.
49. Kinane DF: Periodontal disease's contributions to cardiovascular disease: an overview of potential mechanisms, *Ann Periodontol* 3:142, 1998.
50. Kweider M, Lowe GD, Murray GD, et al: Dental disease, fibrinogen and white cell counts: links with myocardial infarction? *Scott Med J* 38:73, 1993.
51. Löe H: Periodontal disease: the sixth complication of diabetes mellitus, *Diabetes Care* 16(suppl 1):329, 1993.
52. Loos BG, Craandijk J, Hoek FJ, et al: Elevation of systemic markers related to cardiovascular diseases in the peripheral blood of periodontitis patients, *J Periodontol* 71:1528, 2000.
53. Lopez NJ, Smith PC, Gutierrez J: Higher risk of preterm birth and low birth weight in women with periodontal disease, *J Dent Res* 81:58, 2002.
54. Lopez NJ, Smith PC, Gutierrez J: Periodontal therapy may reduce the risk of preterm low birth weight in women with periodontal disease: a randomized controlled trial, *J Periodontol* 73:911, 2002.
55. Lowe GD: Etiopathogenesis of cardiovascular disease: hemostasis, thrombosis, and vascular medicine, *Ann Periodontol* 3:121, 1998.
56. Lowe GD, Lee AJ, Rumley A, et al: Blood viscosity and risk of cardiovascular events: the Edinburg Artery Study, *Br J Haematol* 96:168, 1997.
57. Malthaner SC, Moore S, Mills M, et al: Investigation of the association between angiographically defined coronary artery disease and periodontal disease, *J Periodontol* 73:1169, 2002.
58. Mattila KJ: Viral and bacterial infections in patients with acute myocardial infarction, *J Intern Med* 225:293, 1989.
59. Mattila KJ, Nieminen MS, Valtonen VV, et al: Association between dental health and acute myocardial infarction, *Br Med J* 298:779, 1989.
60. Mattila KJ: Dental infections as a risk factor for acute myocardial infarction, *Eur Heart J* 14:51, 1993.
61. Mattila KJ, Valle MS, Nieminen MS, et al: Dental infections and coronary atherosclerosis, *Atherosclerosis* 103:205, 1993.
62. Mattila KJ, Valtonen VV, Nieminen M, et al: Dental infection and the risk of new coronary events: prospective study of patients with documented coronary artery disease, *Clin Infect Dis* 20:588, 1995.
63. McCormick MC: The contribution of low birth weight to infant mortality and childhood morbidity, *N Engl J Med* 312:82, 1985.
64. McDonald HM, O'Loughlin JA, Jolley P, et al: Vaginal infections and preterm labour, *Br J Obstet Gynecol* 98:427, 1991.
65. Mealey BL: Periodontal implications: medically compromised patients, *Ann Periodontol* 1:256, 1996.
66. Mealey BL: Influence of periodontal infections on systemic health, *Periodontol 2000* 21:197, 1999.
67. Mealey BL: Diabetes mellitus. In Rose LF, Genco RJ, Mealey BL, et al, editors: *Periodontal medicine,* Toronto, 2000, BC Decker.
68. Mehta JL, Saldeen TG, Rand K: Interactive role of infection, inflammation and traditional risk factors in atherosclerosis and coronary artery disease, *J Am Coll Cardiol* 31:1217, 1998.
69. Miller LS, Manwell MA, Newbold D, et al: The relationship between reduction in periodontal inflammation and diabetes control: a report of 9 cases, *J Periodontol* 63:843, 1992.
70. Morales WJ, Schorr S, Albritton J: Effect of metronidazole in patients with preterm birth in preceding pregnancy and bacterial vaginosis: a placebo-controlled double-blind study, *Am J Obstet Gynecol* 171:345, 1994.
71. Newman HN: Focal infection, *J Dent Res* 75:1912, 1996.
72. Newman MG: Improved clinical decision making using the evidence-based approach, *Ann Periodontol* 1:i, 1996.
73. Newman MG, Caton JG, Gunsolley JC: The use of the evidence-based approach in a periodontal therapy contemporary science workshop, *Ann Periodontol* 8:1, 2003.
74. Offenbacher S: Periodontal diseases: pathogenesis, *Ann Periodontol* 1:821, 1996.
75. Offenbacher S, Katz V, Fertik G, et al: Periodontal disease as a possible risk factor for preterm low birth weight, *J Periodontol* 67:1103, 1996.
76. Offenbacher S, Jarad HL, O'Reilly PG, et al: Potential pathogenic mechanisms of periodontitis-associated pregnancy complications, *Ann Periodontol* 3:233, 1998.
77. Ostergaard L, Anderson PL: Etiology of community-acquired pneumonia: evaluation by transtracheal aspiration, blood culture, or serology, *Chest* 104:1400, 1993.

78. Page RC: The pathobiology of periodontal diseases may affect systemic diseases: inversion of a paradigm, *Ann Periodontol* 3:108, 1998.
79. Page RC, Beck JD: Risk assessment for periodontal diseases, *Int Dent J* 47:61, 1997.
80. Papapanou PN: Periodontal diseases: epidemiology, *Ann Periodontol* 1:1, 1996.
81. Pugin J, Auckenthaler R, Lew DP, et al: Oropharyngeal decontamination decreases incidence of ventilator-associated pneumonia: a randomized, placebo-controlled, double-blind clinical trial, *JAMA* 265:2704, 1991.
82. Ridker PM: Fibrinolytic and inflammatory markers for arterial occlusion: the evolving epidemiology of thrombosis and hemostasis, *Thromb Haemost* 78:53, 1997.
83. Ridker PM, Rifai N, Rose L, et al: Comparison of C-reactive protein and low-density lipoprotein cholesterol levels in the prediction of first cardiovascular events, *N Engl J Med* 347:1557, 2002.
84. Ross RL: Atherosclerosis—an inflammatory disease, *N Engl J Med* 342:115, 1999.
85. Sammalkorpi K: Glucose intolerance in acute infections, *J Intern Med* 225:15, 1989.
86. Scannapieco FA, Mylotte JM: Relationships between periodontal disease and bacterial pneumonia, *J Periodontol* 67:1114, 1996.
87. Scannapieco FA, Bush RB, Paju S: Associations between periodontal disease and risk for atherosclerosis, cardiovascular disease, and stroke: a systematic review, *Ann Periodontol* 8:38, 2003.
88. Scannapieco FA, Bush RB, Paju S: Periodontal disease as a risk factor for adverse pregnancy outcomes: a systematic review, *Ann Periodontol* 8:70, 2003.
89. Scannapieco FA, Bush RB, Paju S: Associations between periodontal disease and risk for nosocomial bacterial pneumonia and chronic obstructive pulmonary disease: a systematic review, *Ann Periodontol* 8:54, 2003.
90. Scannapieco FA, Papandonatos GD, Dunford RG: Associations between oral conditions and respiratory disease in a national sample survey population, *Ann Periodontol* 3:251, 1998.
91. Scannapieco FA, Stewart EM, Mylotte JM: Colonization of dental plaque by respiratory pathogens in medical intensive care patients, *Crit Care Med* 20:740, 1992.
92. Selective Decontamination of the Digestive Tract Trialist's Collaborative Group: Meta-analysis of randomised controlled trials of selective decontamination of the digestive tract, *Br Med J* 307:525, 1993.
93. Smith GT, Greenbaum CJ, Johnson BD, et al: Short-term responses to periodontal therapy in insulin-dependent diabetic patients, *J Periodontol* 67:794, 1996.
94. Spodick DH, Flessas AP, Johnson MM: Association of acute respiratory symptoms with onset of acute myocardial infarction: prospective investigation of 150 consecutive patients and matched control patients, *Am J Cardiol* 53:481, 1984.
95. Stoutenbeek CP, van Saene HK, Miranda DR, et al: The effect of oropharyngeal decontamination using topical nonabsorbable antibiotics on the incidence of nosocomial respiratory tract infections in multiple trauma patients, *J Trauma* 27:357, 1987.
96. Syrjanen J, Valtonen VV, Iivanainen M, et al: Preceding infection as an important risk factor for ischemic brain infarction in young and middle aged patients, *Br Med J* 296:1156, 1988.
97. Syrjanen J, Peltola J, Valtonen V, et al: Dental infections in association with cerebral infarction in young and middle-aged men, *J Intern Med* 225:179, 1989.
98. Taylor GW, Burt BA, Becker MP, et al: Severe periodontitis and risk for poor glycemic control in patients with non–insulin-dependent diabetes mellitus, *J Periodontol* 67:1085, 1996.
99. Thorstensson H, Kuylensteirna J, Hugoson A: Medical status and complications in relation to periodontal disease experience in insulin-dependent diabetics, *J Clin Periodontol* 23:194, 1996.
100. Travis J, Pike R, Imamura T, et al: The role of proteolytic enzymes in the development of pulmonary emphysema and periodontal disease, *Am J Respir Crit Care Med* 150:143, 1994.
101. Williams C, Davenport E, Sterne J, et al: Mechanisms of risk in preterm low-birthweight infants, *Periodontology 2000* 23:142, 2000.
102. Williams RC, Mahan CJ: Periodontal disease and diabetes in young adults, *JAMA* 172:776, 1960.
103. Wu T, Trevisan M, Genco RJ, et al: Examination of the relation between periodontal health status and cardiovascular risk factors: serum total and high density lipoprotein cholesterol, C-reactive protein, and plasma fibrinogen, *Am J Epidemiol* 151:273, 2000.
104. Wu T, Trevisan M, Genco RJ, et al: Periodontal disease and risk of cerebrovascular disease: the first National Health and Nutrition Examination Survey and its follow-up study, *Arch Intern Med* 160:2749, 2000.
105. Yki-Jarvinen H, Sammalkorpi K, Koivisto VA, et al: Severity, duration and mechanism of insulin resistance during acute infections, *J Clin Endocrinol Metab* 69:317, 1989.

19 CHAPTER

Oral Malodor

Marc Quirynen and Daniel van Steenberghe

CHAPTER OUTLINE

Breath odor can be defined as the subjective perception after smelling someone's breath. It can be pleasant, unpleasant, or even disturbing, if not repulsive. If unpleasant, the terms *breath malodor, halitosis,* or *bad breath* can be applied. These terms, however, are not synonymous with *oral malodor,* which has its origin in the oral cavity. This is not always the case for all breath malodors. The term "oral malodor" is thus too restrictive.

Breath malodor should not be confused with the momentarily disturbing odor caused by food intake (e.g., garlic) or smoking because these odors do not reveal a health problem. The same is true for "morning" bad breath, as habitually experienced on awakening. This malodor is caused by decreased salivary flow and increased putrefaction during the night and spontaneously disappears after breakfast or oral hygiene. A persistent breath malodor, by definition, does reflect some pathology.

EPIDEMIOLOGY

Breath malodor is a considerable social problem, and its incidence remains poorly documented in most countries. Several studies in industrialized countries report an incidence as high as 50%, with a various degree of intensity.[5,48,50,73] Almost $1 billion a year is spent in the United States on deodorant-type mouth (oral) rinses, mints, and related over-the-counter products to manage bad breath.[44] It would be preferable to spend this money on a proper diagnosis and etiologic care instead of short-term and even inefficient masking attempts. A large-scale Japanese study of more than 2500 subjects age 18 to 64 years reported that the volatile sulfur components (a measure for bad breath) increased with age, tongue coating, and periodontal inflammation. About one in four subjects exhibited values higher than 75 parts per billion (ppb), which is considered the limit for social acceptance.[100]

From large-scale inventories in two multidisciplinary outpatient clinics for breath odor, no gender predominance seems to exist for bad breath, and age can range from 5 to over 80 years.[18,96] Most of the patients had been complaining about breath malodor for several years before seeking proper advice. In the vast majority (85%) the cause originated from the oral cavity. Gingivitis, periodontitis, and tongue coating were the predominant causative factors.[58,59,99,100] Because more than 90% of the population has gingivitis or periodontitis, there is a risk that a plaque-related inflammatory condition is too easily considered the cause while more important pathologies are overlooked. Indeed, for a minority of patients, extraoral causes can be identified, including ear-nose-throat (ENT) pathology, systemic diseases (e.g., diabetes), metabolic or hormonal problems, hepatic or renal insufficiency, bronchial carcinoma, or gastroenterologic pathology.[18,52,63,92,96]

In a special patient category, subjects imagine they have breath malodor; this is called *imaginary breath odor* or *halitophobia*.[56] The latter has been associated with obsessive-compulsive disorders and hypochondria. Well-established personality disorder questionnaires (e.g., SCL-90) allow the clinician to assess the patient's tendency for illusional breath malodor.[19,21,22] The presence of a psychologist or psychiatrist at the malodor consultation can be especially helpful for such patients. Because of the complexity of this pathology, a malodor consultation preferably is multidisciplinary, combining the knowledge of a periodontist or dentist, an ENT specialist, eventually a gastroenterologist, and a psychologist or psychiatrist. If this approach is not feasible, an intense trial therapy focusing on possible intraoral causes should allow a differential diagnosis.

ETIOLOGY

The unpleasant smell of breath mainly originates from *volatile sulfide compounds* (VSCs), especially hydrogen sulfide (H_2S), methylmercaptan (CH_3SH), and dimethylsulfide [$(CH_3)_2S$], as first discovered by Tonzetich.[89] However, other compounds in mouth air may also be offensive, such as diamines (e.g., putrescine, cadaverine), indole, skatole, and butyric or propionic acid.[29] Most of these compounds result from the proteolytic degradation by oral microorganisms of peptides present in saliva (sulfide-containing or non–sulfide-containing amino acids, Figure 19-1), shed epithelium, food debris, gingival crevicular fluid (GCF), interdental plaque, postnasal drip, and blood. In particular, gram-negative, anaerobic bacteria possess such proteolytic activity. Thus, wherever the cause is located, a common pathophysiology is tissue destruction and putrefaction of amino acids by bacteria.

Volatile fatty acids such as valerate, butyrate, and propionate are also malodorous. When hormonal, gastrointestinal, renal, or metabolic pathologies are the cause, additional malodorous molecules can be produced; these circulate in the blood and are expressed through the expired air or the GCF. It is important to consider not only the unpleasantness of the odor of the molecule itself, but also its substantivity and dilution capacity. Most malodorous compounds express themselves only when they become volatile, a phenomenon similar to the perception of perfumes.

Intraoral Causes

Dentition. Possible causes within the dentition are deep carious lesions with food impaction and putrefaction, extraction wounds filled with a blood clot, and purulent discharge leading to important putrefaction. Interdental food impaction in large interdental areas and crowding of teeth favor food entrapment and accumulation of debris. Acrylic dentures, especially when kept in the mouth at night or not regularly cleaned, can also produce a typical smell associated with candidiasis. The denture surface facing the gingiva is porous and retentive for bacteria, yeasts, debris, and all factors that cause putrefaction.

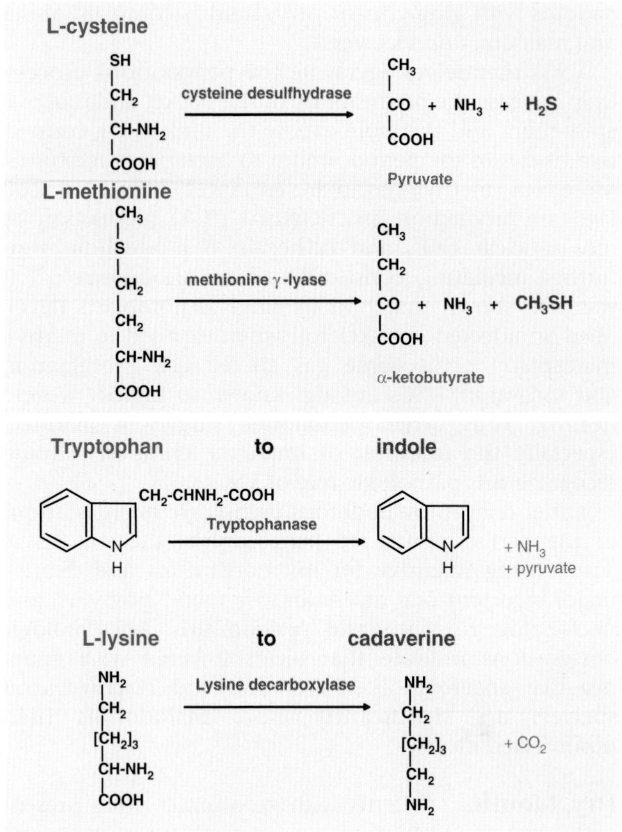

Figure 19-1 Proteolytic degradation by oral microorganisms of four amino acids (two sulfur containing and two non–sulfur containing) to malodorous compounds.

Periodontal Infections. Bacteria associated with gingivitis and periodontitis are almost all gram negative (*Porphyromonas gingivalis, Prevotella intermedia/nigrescens, Actinobacillus actinomycetemcomitans, Campylobacter rectus, Fusobacterium nucleatum, Peptostreptococcus micros, Tannerella forsythia, Eubacterium* species, spirochetes) and are known to produce VSCs.* It is thus understandable that the VSC levels in the mouth correlate positively with the depth of periodontal pockets (the deeper the pocket, the more bacteria, particularly anaerobic species) and that the amount of VSCs in breath increases with the number, depth, and bleeding tendency of the periodontal pockets.[14,57,100] The low oxygen tension in deep periodontal pockets also results in a low pH and an activation of the decarboxylation of the amino acids (e.g., lysine, ornithine) to cadaverine and putrescine, two malodorous diamines. Thus, in the presence of gingivitis or periodontitis, besides the prominent role of VSCs, other molecules might play a significant role. However, not all

*References 36, 51, 53, 58, 59, 89.

patients with gingivitis or periodontitis complain about oral malodor, and vice versa.[5]

VSCs themselves aggravate the periodontitis process; they increase the permeability of the pocket and mucosal epithelium and therefore expose the underlying connective tissues of the periodontium to bacterial metabolites. Moreover, methylmercaptan enhances interstitial collagenase production, interleukin-1 (IL-1) production by mononuclear cells, and cathepsin B production, thus further mediating connective tissue breakdown.[43,70] It was also shown that human gingival fibroblasts developed an affected cytoskeleton when exposed to methylmercaptan[8,70]; the same gas altered cell proliferation and migration. VSCs are also known to impede wound healing. Thus, when periodontal surgery is planned, especially the insertion of implants, clinicians should recognize this pathologic role of VSCs.

Other relevant malodorous pathologic manifestations of the periodontium are pericoronitis (the soft tissue "cap" being retentive for microorganisms and debris), major recurrent oral ulcerations, herpetic gingivitis, and necrotizing gingivitis and periodontitis. Microbiologic observations indicate that ulcers infected with gram-negative anaerobes (i.e., *Prevotella* and *Porphyromonas* species) are significantly more malodorous than noninfected ulcers.[6]

Dry Mouth. Patients with xerostomia often present with large amounts of plaque on teeth, prostheses, and tongue dorsum. The increased microbial load and the escape of VSCs as gases when saliva is drying up explain the strong breath malodor.[36]

Tongue and Tongue Coating. The dorsal tongue mucosa, with an area of 25 cm^2, shows a very irregular surface topography.[15,84] The posterior part exhibits a number of oval cryptolymphatic units, which roughen the surface of this area. The anterior part is even rougher because of the high number of papillae: the filiform papillae with a core of 0.5 mm in length, a central crater, and uplifted borders; the fungiform papillae, 0.5 to 0.8 mm in length; the foliate papillae, located at the edge of the tongue, separated by deep folds; and the vallate papillae, 1 mm in height and 2 to 3 mm in diameter. These innumerable depressions in the tongue surface are ideal niches for bacterial adhesion and growth, sheltered from cleaning actions.[17,99] Also, however, desquamated cells and food remnants remain trapped in these retention sites and consequently can be putrefied by the bacteria.[5] A *fissurated tongue* (deep fissures on dorsum, also called scrotal tongue or lingua plicata) and a *hairy tongue* (lingua villosa) have an even rougher surface (Figure 19-2).

The accumulation of food remnants intermingled with exfoliated cells and bacteria causes a coating on the tongue dorsum. The latter cannot be easily removed because of the retention offered by the irregular surface of the tongue dorsum (Figure 19-2). As such, the two factors essential for putrefaction are united. The dorsum of the tongue has therefore long been considered as a primary source of oral malodor.[5,14,17,76] Indeed, high correlations have been reported between tongue coating and odor formation.[5,17,50,99] The prevalence of tongue coating is six times higher in patients with periodontitis.[99]

Extraoral Causes

Ear-Nose-Throat. The ENT causes include acute pharyngitis (viral or bacterial), purulent sinusitis (when clearance of bacteria into the nose is impaired), and postnasal drip. Postnasal drip is often associated with chronic sinusitis or regurgitation esophagitis, in which the acidic content of the stomach reaches the nasopharynx and causes mucositis. This rather common condition is perceived by patients as a liquid flow in the throat, originating from the nasal cavity.[76] Ozena (caused by *Klebsiella ozenae*) is a rare atrophic condition of the nasal mucosa with the appearance of crusts and causing a very strong breath malodor. During chronic or purulent tonsillitis, the deep crypts of the tonsils accumulate debris and bacteria, especially periopathogens, resulting in putrefaction. In the crypts of the tonsils, even calculus (e.g., subgingivally) can be formed (tonsilloliths). Finally, a foreign body in a nasal or sinus cavity can cause local

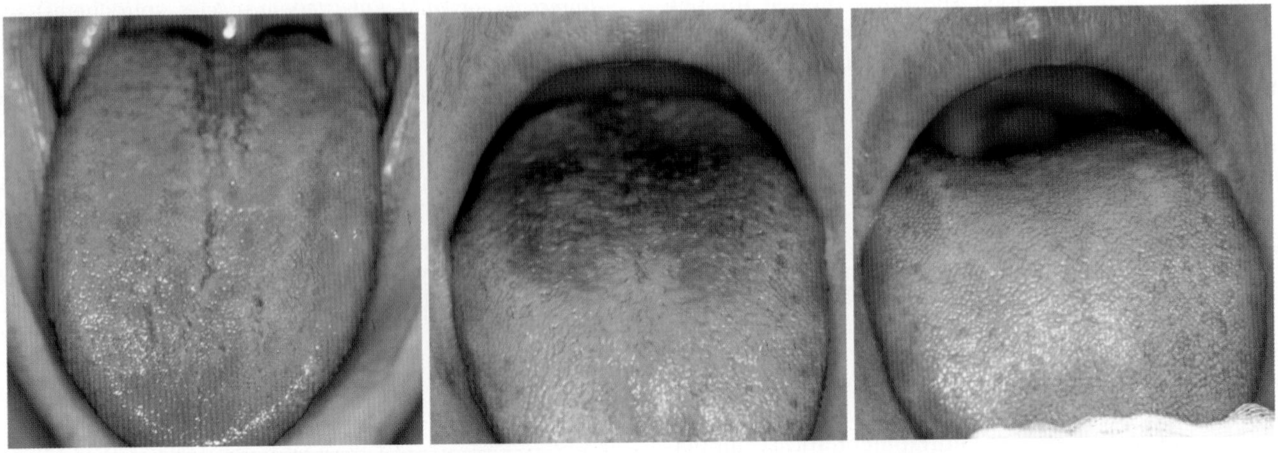

Figure 19-2 Different clinical pictures of heavily coated tongues.

irritation, ulceration, and subsequent putrefaction (e.g., children and mentally handicapped persons tend to put objects such as peas or wet paper in the nose).

Bronchi and Lungs. Pulmonary causes include chronic bronchitis, bronchiectasis (infection of standing mucus secretion in cystic dilations through walls of bronchioles), and bronchial carcinoma.[45,46]

Gastrointestinal Tract. In contrast to common public opinion, even among medical physicians, gastrointestinal pathologies are rarely responsible for bad breath.[55] The following pathologies might be responsible for less than 1% of malodor cases:

- Zenker's diverticulum (hernia in esophagal wall, allowing accumulation of food and debris and thus putrefaction) can cause a significant breath odor because it is not separated from the oral cavity by any sphincter.[16]
- Gastric hernia (fundus of stomach protrudes through diaphragm with relative sphincter insufficiency, allowing gases to escape or contents to flow back in esophagus) can cause reflux of the gastric contents up to the oropharynx. This is sometimes combined with ructus, where air from the stomach suddenly regurgitates.
- Regurgitation esophagitis (ulceration of mucosal lining of esophagus by acidic stomach contents flowing back because of improper function of sphincter).
- Intestinal gas production, because some gases (e.g., dimethylsulfide) are absorbed but not metabolized by the intestinal endothelium and thus transported by the blood. These gases are exhaled through the lungs.[86]

There is no convincing evidence that breath malodor can be linked to *Helicobacter pylori* infection and gastritis.

Liver. In patients with liver insufficiency, such as cirrhosis, ammonium will accumulate in the blood and will be exhaled.[9]

Kidney. Kidney insufficiency, primarily caused by chronic glomerulonephritis, will lead to an increased uric acid level in the blood, which is expressed in the expired air with a typical ammonium-like breath.[85]

Systemic Metabolic Disorders. Type 1 (insulin-dependent) diabetes in particular can result in the accumulation of ketones. The lack of glucose leads to breakdown of fat and proteins, resulting in ketone bodies such as acetoacetate and hydroxybutyrate. Type 2 (non–insulin-dependent) diabetes often remains undiagnosed for years; perception of breath malodor may provide a clue to its diagnosis.

Trimethylaminuria. This hereditary metabolic disorder leads to a typical fishy odor of breath, urine, sweat, expired air, and other bodily secretions.[49] Trimethylaminura is an enzymatic defect that prevents the transformation of trimethylamine to trimethylaminoxide, resulting in abnormal amounts of this molecule. The prevalence is unknown but approaches 1% in the United Kingdom.

Hormonal Causes. With increased progesterone levels during the menstrual cycle, a typical breath odor can develop; partners are often well aware of this odor. Evidence also indicates that VSC levels in the expired air are increased twofold to fourfold about the day of ovulation and in the perimenstrual period. Increases in VSC are smaller in midfollicular phases.

Medications. Some drugs, such as metronidazole, can cause breath malodor. Metronidazole, an antimicrobial, also leads to the patient's perception of a metallic taste, which is often confused with breath odor. Eucalyptus-containing medications impart a melonlike odor. Arsenic smells of rotten onions.

PHYSIOLOGY OF MALODOR DETECTION

The expired air of nonhalitosis patients contains up to 150 different molecules.[61] The perception of these molecule depends on the following factors[30]:

1. The odor itself *(olfactory response)* can be pleasant, unpleasant, or even repulsive.
2. Each particular molecule has its specific concentration before it can be detected *(threshold concentration).*
3. The *odor power* is the extent of concentration that must be increased before a malodor judge will give it a higher odor score.
4. The *volatility* of the compound is the concentration at which it escapes from the liquid phase into the air.

Table 19-1 provides an overview of these essential characteristics for the key malodorous compounds, clearly highlighting large interproduct variations. The odor power is strongest for H_2S, CH_3SH, and CH_3SCH_3; that is, if the concentration of these products increases fivefold to tenfold, the odor will receive a higher *organoleptic rating.* For the other compounds, increases of 25 to 100 times are needed to reach a similar effect. Skatole and methylmercaptan are detected at the lowest concentrations. The three sulfide products have the lowest volatility (i.e., will escape the liquid phase first).

The olfactory response, rated by an organoleptic scale, follows an exponential curve when correlated with the concentration of different gases. In other words, when concentrations of molecules were compared to their organoleptic outcome, an optimal fit was only obtained when the concentrations of the gas were transformed to log values. The latter implies that all types of breath "measurements" (GC, GC-MS, Halimeter, sulfide sensors, HPLC) require log transformation to be comparable with organoleptic scores.[30]

DIAGNOSIS OF MALODOR

Medical History

The proper diagnostic approach to a malodor patient starts with a thorough questioning about the medical history. Asking about all the relevant pathologies for

TABLE 19-1

Odor Threshold and Odor Power of Key Malodorous Compounds

	ODOR THRESHOLDS		ODOR POWER	VOLATILITY (HENRY'S CONSTANTS)
Compound	Greenman* ($mol.dm^{-3}$)	Devos† ($mol.dm^{-3}$)	Greenman* (x increase to "up" score 1 unit)	Volatility (Kcc)‡ in H_2O at 20° C
Butyrate	2.3×10^{-10}	2.4×10^{-10}	10-fold	3.9×10^{4}
Isovalerate	1.8×10^{-11}	2.5×10^{-11}	42-fold	2.5×10^{4}
Skatole	7.2×10^{-13}	1.0×10^{-12}	8-fold	4.1×10^{5}
Trimethylamine	1.8×10^{-11}	1.5×10^{-11}	96-fold (low affinity)	2.0×10^{2}
Putrescine	9.1×10^{-10}	1.0×10^{-9}	27-fold	4.1×10^{1}
CH_3SCH_3	5.9×10^{-8}	5.0×10^{-8}	10-fold	1.7×10^{1}
H_2S	6.4×10^{-10}	5.0×10^{-10}	4.8-fold	$\approx 1.7 \times 10^{1}$
CH_3SH	1.0×10^{-11}	1.0×10^{-11}	7.2-fold	$\approx 1.7 \times 10^{1}$

*Greenman J, Duffield J, Spencer P, et al: *J Dent Res* 83:81, 2004.
†Devos M, Patte F, Roualt J, et al: *Standardized human olfactory thresholds,* Oxford, 1990, IRL Press at Oxford University Press.
‡*Kcc,* Unit for Henry's Law constant.

breath malodor just discussed is not time-consuming; it may save time and expenses to achieve a proper differential diagnosis. As often repeated, "Listen to the patient, and the patient will tell you the diagnosis." This should take place at the clinician's desk in private and before any clinical examination (*not* in a dental chair). This will encourage the proper confidence needed by these patients. The patient's history should be discretely and intermittently noted. The clinician should ask about the frequency (e.g., every month), time of appearance within the day (e.g., after meals can indicate a stomach hernia), whether others (nonconfidants) have identified the problem (excludes imaginary breath odor), what medications are taken, and whether the patient has dryness of the mouth or other symptoms.

Clinical and Laboratory Examination

Self-Examination. It can be worthwhile to involve the patient in monitoring the results of therapy by self-examination, especially when an intraoral cause has been identified. For example, this can motivate the patient to continue the oral hygiene instructions. The following self-testing can be used:

- Smelling a metallic or nonodorous plastic spoon after scraping the back of the tongue.
- Smelling a toothpick after introducing it in an interdental area.
- Smelling saliva spit in a small cup or spoon (especially when allowed to dry for a few seconds so that putrefaction odors can escape from the liquid).
- Licking the wrist and allowing it to dry (reflects the saliva contribution to malodor).

Removing the odorous substances from the body allows a less emotional and thus more objective assessment. Smelling one's own breath by expiring in the hands kept in front of the mouth is not relevant because the smell of the skin and soaps used for handwashing may interfere. Analyzing the tongue coating and interdental debris, two major causes of putrefaction, will immediately provide good insight on the possible intraoral causes.

Organoleptic Rating. Even though instruments are available, organoleptic assessment by a judge is still the "gold standard" in the examination of breath malodor. In organoleptic evaluation, a trained "judge" sniffs the expired air and assesses whether or not this is unpleasant using an intensity rating, normally from 0 to 5, as proposed by Rosenberg and McCulloch.[78] It is solely based on the olfactory organs of the clinician: 0 = no odor present, 1 = barely noticeable odor, 2 = slight but clearly noticeable odor, 3 = moderate odor, 4 = strong offensive odor, and 5 = extremely foul odor.

Before acting as a judge, persons must ensure they do not have *anosmia* (lost or impaired smelling capacity). A significant fraction of the adult population has partial loss of smelling acuity. After age 60, a decline of smelling acuity is common. Candidate odor judges should test their capacity to smell and recognize different odors (qualitative assessment) as well as their capacity to detect odors at low concentrations (quantitative assessment).[20] The first aspect can be checked by using a commercially available test (Smell Identification test, Sensonic) that establishes a response curve based on the capacity to recognize and discriminate among smells. After scratching an odorous surface in a booklet, several options of smells are proposed. If a subject lacks the capacity to recognize certain odors, it will reveal a partial anosmia. The second aspect is tested by sniffing a series of dilutions of substances, such as isovaleric acid, phenethyl alcohol, thiophene, and pyridine, which are inexpensive organic components. These are presented to the candidate judge as dilutions, in one-log dilution steps, from 1 to 10^{-19}. Concentrations of the odorous substance are presented in ascending order until the subject detects the substance, then in descending order until the person no longer detects it. This is the "psychophysical staircase method" for determination of threshold level. The threshold corresponds to the average between ascending and descending levels. Clinicians can thus find out if their smelling threshold level is normal. Abnormalities in the capacity to judge or perceive odors can be caused by a viral infection of the nasal cavities, a concussion, and smoking. Whereas infection can have transient effects on olfactory performance, concussion and smoking have permanent effects.

The use of any fragrance, shampoo, or body lotion; smoking; and consumption of alcohol or garlic are prohibited 12 hours before the organoleptic assessment is made; this applies to both the patient and the judge. The judge also should not wear rubber gloves. Assessments should be repeated because breath odor can fluctuate from day to day. The patient should be encouraged to bring a confidant to the consultations who can identify whether the perceived odor is the one previously noticed. The judge smells a series of different air samples (Figure 19-3), as follows:

1. *Oral cavity odor.* The subject opens the mouth and refrains from breathing while the judge places his or her nose close to the mouth opening. (Smelling the air while the patient counts from 1 to 20 reveals the same but favors oral malodor because drying of the palatal and tongue mucosa will occur, which promotes the expression of VSCs thus far soluble in the salivary coating.)
2. *Breath odor.* The subject expires through the mouth while the judge smells both at the beginning (determined by the oral cavity and systemic factors) and at the end (originating from the bronchi and lungs) of the expiration.
3. *Tongue coating.* The judge smells a tongue scraping. This is also presented to the patient or the confidant to evaluate whether this smell is similar to the experienced malodor.
4. *Nasal breath odor.* The subject expires through the nose, keeping the mouth closed. When the nasal expiration is malodorous, whereas the air expired through the mouth is not, a nasal/paranasal cause can be suspected.

Specific Character of Breath Odor

- A "rotten eggs" smell is indicative of VSCs.
- A sweet odor, which some describe as that of "dead mice," has been associated with liver insufficiency; besides VSCs, aliphatic acids (butyric, isobutyric, propionic) accumulate.
- The smell of "rotten apples" has been associated with unbalanced insulin-dependant diabetes, which leads to the accumulation of ketones.
- A "fish odor" can suggest kidney insufficiency characterized by uremia and accumulation of dimethylamine and trimethylamine (trimethylaminuria, a rare metabolic disease).

Portable Volatile Sulfide Monitor. This electronic device (Halimeter, Interscan, Chatsworth, Calif) analyzes the concentration of hydrogen sulfide and methylmercaptan, but without discriminating them (Figure 19-4). The examination should preferably be done after at least 4 hours of fasting and after keeping the mouth closed for 3 minutes. The mouth air is aspirated by inserting a drinking straw fixed on the flexible tube of the instrument. The straw is kept about 2 cm behind the lips, without touching any surface and while the subject keeps the mouth slightly open and breathes normally. The sulfide meter uses a voltametric sensor that generates a signal when exposed to sulfur-containing gases, especially hydrogen sulfide. Absence of breath malodor leads to readings of 100 ppb or lower. Patients with elevated concentrations of VSCs easily reach 300 to 400 ppb. This device can only reveal sulfur-containing gases, which explains the poor correlation with organoleptic measurements. Even if a large extent of the breath malodor originating from the oral cavity is dominated by VSCs, gases such as putrescine and cadaverine, which can also have an intraoral origin, will remain unnoticed by this device.[40] The monitor needs regular calibration and replacement of the sensors biannually.

Gas Chromatography. This device can analyze air, (incubated) saliva, or crevicular fluid for any volatile component[29] (Figure 19-5). About 100 compounds have been isolated from saliva and tongue coating, with most identified, from ketones to alkanes and sulfur-containing compounds to phenyl compounds.[13,61] Elaborate gas chromatography is only available in specialized centers but is especially useful for identifying nonoral causes.[34,60,86] Recently a small, portable gas chromatograph (OralChroma, Abilit, Henderson, Nevada) has been introduced, which makes this technique available for periodontal clinics (Figure 19-6). It has the capacity to measure the concentration of the three key sulfides separately.

Dark-Field or Phase-Contrast Microscopy. Gingivitis and periodontitis are typically associated with a higher incidence of motile organisms and spirochetes, so shifts in these proportions allow monitoring of therapeutic progress. Another advantage of direct microscopy is that the patient becomes aware of bacteria being present in plaque, tongue coating, and saliva. Too often, patients confuse plaque with food remnants. High proportions of spirochetes in plaque have been associated with a specific acidic malodor.

Saliva Incubation Test. The analysis of the headspace above incubated saliva by gas chromatography reveals *hydrogen sulfide, methylmercaptan, dimethylsulfide, indole, skatole,* lactic acid, *methylamine, diphenylamine, cadaverine,* putrescine, urea, ammonia, *dodecanol, tetradecanol,* and others. The components in italics are elevated in the presence of periodontitis, although this does not necessarily prove they play a role in odor production. By adding some proteins, such as lysine or cysteine, the production of cadaverine or hydrogen sulfide is dramatically increased. Organoleptic evaluation of the saliva headspace offers promising perspectives for monitoring treatment results.[64] It is a less invasive test, especially for the patient, than smelling breath in front of the oral cavity.

For clinical practice, 0.5 ml of unstimulated saliva is collected in a glass tube (diameter 1.5 cm), and the tube

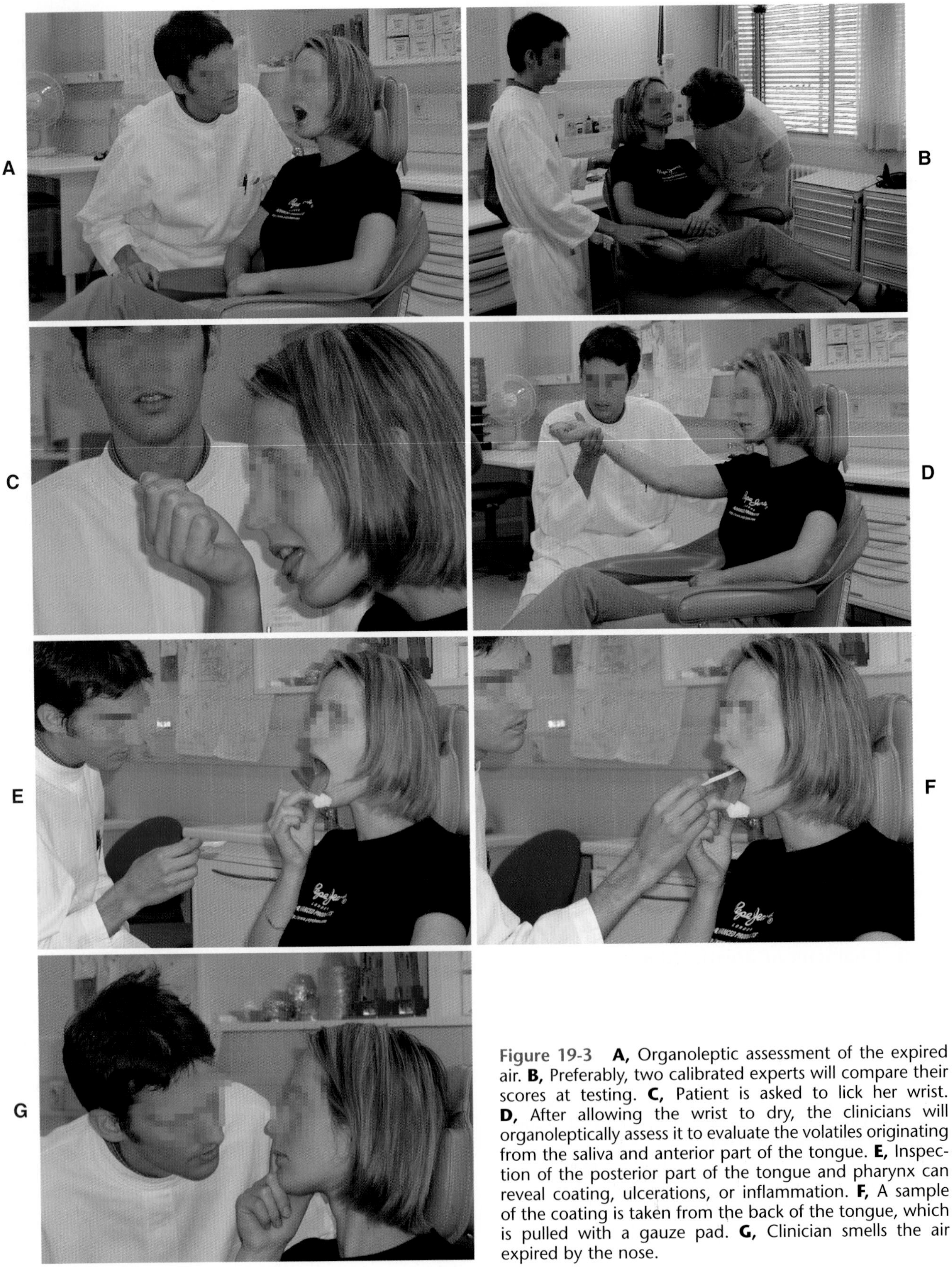

Figure 19-3 **A,** Organoleptic assessment of the expired air. **B,** Preferably, two calibrated experts will compare their scores at testing. **C,** Patient is asked to lick her wrist. **D,** After allowing the wrist to dry, the clinicians will organoleptically assess it to evaluate the volatiles originating from the saliva and anterior part of the tongue. **E,** Inspection of the posterior part of the tongue and pharynx can reveal coating, ulcerations, or inflammation. **F,** A sample of the coating is taken from the back of the tongue, which is pulled with a gauze pad. **G,** Clinician smells the air expired by the nose.

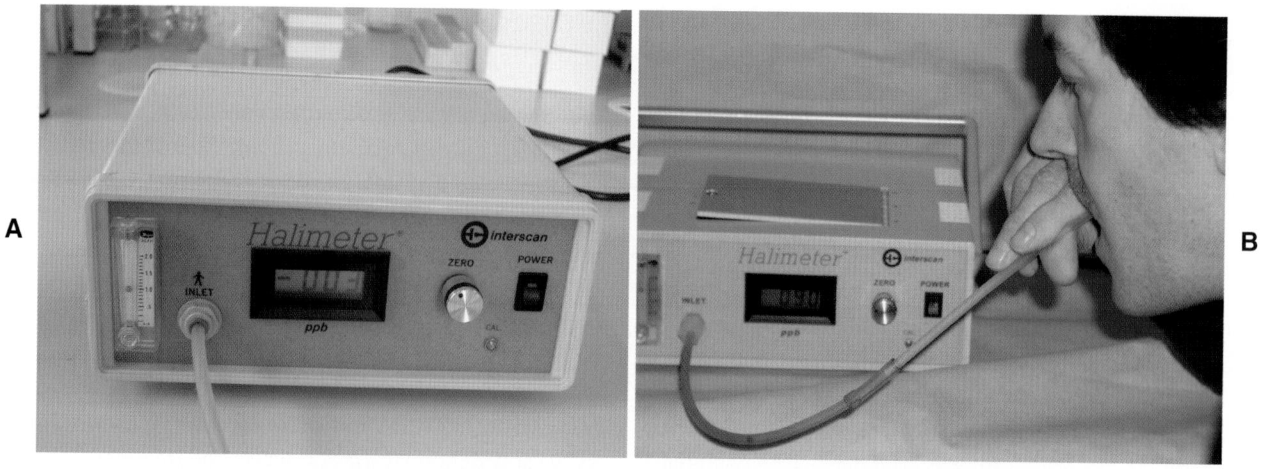

Figure 19-4 **A,** Portable sulfide monitor. **B,** Patient holds the aspirating tube in his mouth. Digital reading reveals the total amount of volatile sulfide compounds (VSCs) in parts per billion (ppb).

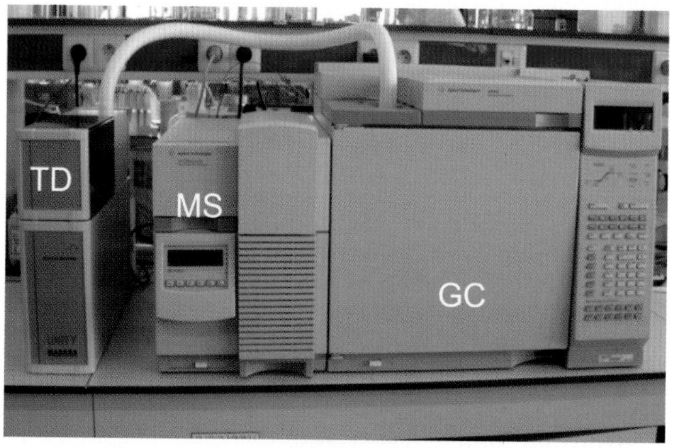

Figure 19-5 Gas chromatography machinery, including thermodisorber (*TD,* to release molecules trapped in special collectors), gas chromatograph (*GC,* for separation of molecules), and mass spectrometer (*MS,* for identification of molecules).

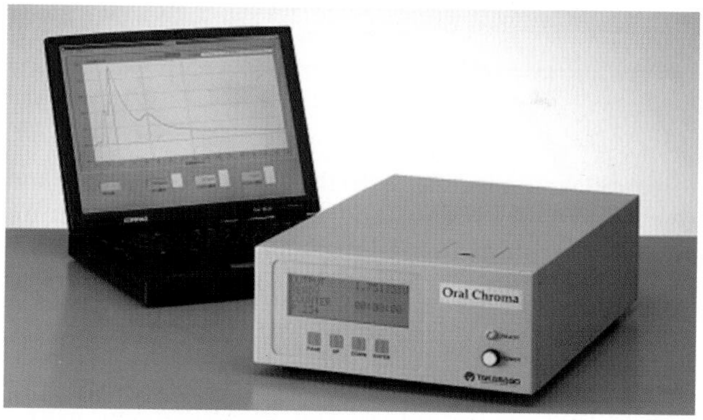

Figure 19-6 Portable gas chromatograph (GC). Small amount of the breath sample, aspirated with a plastic syringe, is injected into the input port of the GC. The computer displays the detection and amount of the three important VSCs (in ppb) within 8 minutes. (Courtesy OralChroma, Henders, Nevada.)

is flushed with carbon dioxide (CO_2) and sealed. The sealing prevents inflow from outside air, and the glass prevents the smell of the hardware. It is incubated at 37° C in an anaerobic chamber under an atmosphere of 80% nitrogen, 10% carbon dioxide, and 10% hydrogen over 3 hours. The organoleptic ratings highly correlate with VSC and organoleptic rating of the patient's breath.[64] The discrimination power for the effect of oral rinses even appears superior to intraoral registrations. It was calculated that for discriminating between different oral therapies, applying the saliva incubation test instead of organoleptic ratings can reduce the number of patients needed to reach statistical significance of 50%.

Electronic Nose. An artificial nose that has the same capacities as the human nose would be ideal. Currently, although significant improvements still need to be made, the first trials thus far with an electronic nose have been promising.[88]

TREATMENT OF ORAL MALODOR

The treatment of oral malodor (thus of intraoral origin) should preferably be cause related. Because oral malodor is caused by the metabolic degradation of available proteins to malodorous gases by certain oral microorganisms, the following general treatment strategies can be applied:

- Mechanical reduction of intraoral nutrients and microorganisms
- Chemical reduction of oral microbial load
- Rendering malodorous gases nonvolatile
- Masking the malodor

Mechanical Reduction of Intraoral Nutrients and Microorganisms

Because of the extensive accumulation of bacteria on the dorsum of the tongue, tongue cleaning has been emphasized.[11,99] Previous investigations demonstrated that

SCIENCE TRANSFER

Dental clinicians have the responsibility to diagnose and treat oral malodor. At least 85% of breath malodors have an oral source. The gram-negative anaerobic bacteria associated with gingivitis and periodontitis cause oral malodor by their proteolysis, which produces foul-smelling volatile sulfide compounds (VSCs). *Similar processes in the bacterial coating of the tongue are also significant.* Although diagnostic machines can detect VSCs, clinicians can be trained to be even more accurate, using their olfactory sense to categorize halitosis on a scale of 0 to 5.

Treatment should be centered on reducing the bacterial load by effective mechanical oral hygiene procedures, including tongue scraping. Periodontal disease should be treated and controlled, and as an auxiliary aid, oral rinses containing chlorhexidine and other ingredients may further reduce the oral malodor. If breath malodor persists after these approaches, other sources of the malodor, such as tonsils, lung disease, gastrointestinal disease, and metabolic abnormalities (e.g., diabetes) should be investigated.

Issues related to oral malodor emphasize the clinician's need for good diagnostic skills and stipulate an appreciation of chemistry. First, the etiology of breath malodor can be from a large variety of intraoral and extraoral causes, and much can be gained from a careful patient history before any oral or extraoral examination. Second, knowledge of the potential volatile substances and gases (e.g., VSCs) and their formation, sources, power, substantivity, and dilution capacity allows for treatment options and rational therapeutic interventions. Furthermore, this knowledge allows the dental clinician to help predict the outcome of therapeutic interventions, such as the short-term effectiveness of masking oral malodor and the longer-term effect of mechanically and chemically reducing the oral microbial load.

tongue cleaning reduces both the amount of coating (and thus bacterial nutrients) and the number of organisms and thereby improves oral malodor effectively.[17,27,28,32,69] Other reports indicated that the reduction in microbial load on the tongue after cleaning is negligible, and that the malodor reduction probably results from the reduction of the bacterial nutrients.[47,68]

Cleansing of the tongue can be carried out with a normal toothbrush, but preferably with a tongue scraper if a coating is established. This should be gentle cleaning to prevent soft tissue damage. It is best to clean as far backward as possible; the posterior portion of the tongue has the most coating.[77] Tongue cleaning should be repeated until almost no coating material can be removed.[12] Gagging reflexes often are elicited, especially when using brushes[68,81]; practice helps to prevent this.[10] It can also be helpful to pull the tongue out with a gauze pad. Tongue cleaning has the additional benefit of improving taste sensation.[68,98]

Interdental cleaning and toothbrushing are essential mechanical means of dental plaque control. Both remove residual food particles and organisms that cause putrefaction. A combination of tooth and tongue brushing or toothbrushing alone has a beneficial effect on bad breath for up to 1 hour (73% and 30% reduction in VSCs, respectively).[90]

Because periodontitis causes chronic oral malodor, professional periodontal therapy is needed.[5,14,57,100] A one-stage full-mouth disinfection, combining scaling and root planing with the application of chlorhexidine, reduced the organoleptic malodor levels up to 90%.[65]

Chewing gum may control bad breath temporarily because it can stimulate salivary flow.[72] The salivary flow itself also has a mechanical cleaning capability. Not surprisingly, therefore, subjects with extremely low salivary flow rate have higher VSC ratings and tongue-coating scores than those with normal saliva production.[39]

On the other hand, clinicians can use bacterial nutrients to provoke malodor, to prove an intraoral origin of the bad breath, for example, or to test the efficacy of different oral rinses. Rinsing with amino acids (e.g., cysteine challenge test) can result in a dramatic increase in hydrogen sulfide[37] (see Figure 19-1).

Chemical Reduction of Oral Microbial Load

Mouth rinsing has become a common practice in patients with oral malodor.[25] The active ingredients in oral rinses are usually antimicrobial agents such as chlorhexidine, cetylpyridinium chloride (CPC), essential oils, chlorine dioxide, hydrogen peroxide, and triclosan. All these agents have only a temporary reducing effect on the total number of microorganisms in the oral cavity.

Chlorhexidine. Chlorhexidine is considered the most effective antiplaque and antigingivitis agent.[1-4,35] Its antibacterial action can be explained by disruption of bacterial cell membrane by the chlorhexidine molecules, increasing its permeability and resulting in cell lysis and death.[35,42] Because of its strong antibacterial effects and superior substantivity in the oral cavity, chlorhexidine rinsing provides significant reduction in VSC levels and organoleptic ratings.[17,66,78-80,95,102] Rosenberg et al.[80] showed that a 0.2% chlorhexidine regimen produced a 43% reduction in VSC values and a greater than 50% reduction in organoleptic mouth odor ratings. De Boever and Loesche[17] reported that a 1-week rinsing with 0.12% chlorhexidine gluconate, in combination with tooth and tongue brushing, significantly reduced VSC levels, mouth odor, and tongue odor, by 73%, 69%, and 78%, respectively. Morning halitosis was reduced up to 90%.[66,95] Halita, a new solution (0.05% chlorhexidine, 0.05% CPC, 0.14% zinc lactate, no alcohol) has been even more efficient than chlorhexidine alone, suggesting that the other compounds are also important.[66,74,95] This is explained by a synergistic effect between chlorhexidine and CPC on one hand and by the Zn^{++} on the other hand (see following discussion).

Essential Oils. Previous studies evaluated the short-term effect (3 hours) of a Listerine rinse (which contains essential oils) compared with a placebo rinse.[62] Listerine was found to be only relatively effective against oral malodor (±25% reduction vs. 10% for placebo) and caused a sustained reduction in the levels of odorigenic bacteria.

Chlorine Dioxide. Chlorine dioxide (ClO_2) is a powerful oxidizing agent that can eliminate bad breath by oxidation of hydrogen sulfide, methylmercaptan, and the amino acids methionine and cysteine. A recent study demonstrated that single use of a chlorine dioxide–containing oral rinse slightly reduces mouth odor.[23,24]

Two-Phase Oil-Water Rinse. Rosenberg et al.[79] designed a two-phase oil-water rinse containing CPC that was shown to result in daylong reduction in oral malodor. The efficacy of oil-water-CPC formulation is thought to result from the adhesion of a high proportion of oral microorganisms to the oil droplets, which is further enhanced by the CPC. A twice-daily rinse with this product (before bedtime and in the morning) showed reductions in both VSC levels and organoleptic ratings. These reductions were almost comparable to chlorhexidine, superior to Listerine, and significantly superior to a placebo.[41,79]

Triclosan. Triclosan, a broad-spectrum antibacterial agent, has been found to be effective against most oral bacteria and has a good compatibility with other compounds used for oral home care. A pilot study demonstrated that an experimental mouth rinse containing 0.15% triclosan and 0.84% zinc produced a more prolonged reduction in mouth odor than a Listerine rinse.[71] The anti-VSC effect of triclosan, however, seems strongly dependent on the solubilizing agents.[101]

Aminefluoride/Stannous Fluoride. The association of aminefluoride with stannous fluoride (AmF/SnF_2) resulted in encouraging reductions of morning breath odor, even when oral hygiene is insufficient.[67]

Hydrogen Peroxide. Suarez et al.[87] reported that rinsing with 3% hydrogen peroxide (H_2O_2) produced impressive reductions (±90%) in sulfur gas that persisted for 8 hours.

Oxidizing Lozenges. Greenstein et al.[31] reported that sucking a lozenge with oxidizing properties reduces tongue dorsum malodor for 3 hours. This antimalodor effect may be caused by the activity of dehydroascorbic acid, which is generated by peroxide-mediated oxidation of ascorbate present in the lozenges.

Conversion of Volatile Sulfide Compounds

Metal Salt Solutions. Metal ions with affinity for sulfur are rather efficient in capturing the sulfur-containing gases. Zinc is an ion with two positive charges (Zn^{++}), which will bind to the twice–negatively loaded sulfur radicals, and thus can reduce the expression of the VSCs. The same applies for other metal ions, such as mercury and copper. Clinically, the VSC inhibitory effect was $CuCl_2 > SnF_2 > ZnCl_2$. In vitro, the inhibitory effect was $HgCl_2 = CuCl_2 = CdCl_2 > ZnCl_2 > SnF_2 > SnCl_2 > PbCl_2$.[103]

Compared with other metal ions, Zn^{++} is relatively nontoxic and noncumulative and gives no visible discoloration. Thus, Zn^{++} has been one of the most-studied ingredients for the control of oral malodor.[103] Schmidt and Tarbet[83] already reported that a rinse containing zinc chloride was remarkably more effective than a saline rinse (or no –treatment) in reducing the levels of both VSCs (±80% reduction) and organoleptic scores (±40% reduction) for 3 hours.

As mentioned, Halita, a rinse containing 0.05% chlorhexidine, 0.05% CPC, and 0.14% zinc lactate, has been even more efficient than a 0.2% chlorhexidine formulation in reducing the VSC levels and organoleptic ratings.[64,95] The special effect of Halita may result from the VSC conversion ability of zinc, besides its antimicrobial action. The combination Zn^{++} and chlorhexidine seems to act synergistically.[102]

Toothpastes. Baking soda dentifrices have been shown to be effective, with a 44% reduction of VSC levels 3 hours after toothbrushing versus a 31% reduction for a fluoride dentifrice.[7,53] The mechanisms by which baking soda produces its inhibition of oral malodor might be related to its bactericidal effects and its transformation of VSCs to a nonvolatile state.

Gerlach et al.[26] compared the antimalodor efficacy of three different toothpastes, 3 and 8 hours after use, and reported a slightly better outcome, especially for an SnF_2-containing paste (50% reduction), when compared to water (35% reduction). In a study of Hoshi and van Steenberghe,[33] a zinc citrate/triclosan toothpaste applied to the tongue dorsum appeared to control morning breath malodor for 4 hours. If the flavor oil was removed, however, the antimalodor efficacy of the active ingredients decreased. Another clinical study reported up to a 41% reduction in VSC levels after 7 days' use of a dentifrice containing triclosan and a copolymer, but the benefit compared with a placebo was relatively small (17% reduction).[54]

Chewing Gum. Chewing gum can be formulated with antibacterial agents, such as fluoride or chlorhexidine, thus helping in reducing oral malodor through both mechanical and chemical approaches. Tsunoda et al.[91] investigated the beneficial effect of chewing gum containing tea extracts for its deodorizing mechanism. *Epigallocatchin* (EGCg) is the main deodorizing agent among the tea catechins. The chemical reaction between EGCg and CH_3SH results in nonvolatile product. Waler[97] compared different concentrations of zinc in a chewing gum and found that a 2-mg Zn^{++} acetate–containing chewing gum that remained in the mouth for 5 minutes resulted in an immediate reduction in the VSC levels of up to 45%, but the long-term effect was not mentioned.

Masking the Malodor

Treatments with rinses, mouth sprays, and lozenges containing volatiles with a pleasant odor have only a short-term effect.[72,73] A typical example is mint-containing lozenges. Another pathway is to increase the solubility of malodorous compounds in the saliva by lowering the pH of the saliva (low pH increases the solubility of VSCs) or simply increase the secretion of saliva; a larger volume allows the retention of larger volumes of soluble VSCs.[38] The latter can also be achieved by ensuring a proper liquid intake or by using a chewing gum; chewing triggers the periodontal-parotid reflex, at least when the lower (pre)molars are still present. To lower the pH, an orange juice may be sufficient, but the effect is short term.

SUMMARY

Breath malodor has important socioeconomic consequences and can reveal important diseases. A proper diagnosis and determination of the etiology allow initiation of the proper etiologic treatment. Although gingivitis, periodontitis, and tongue coating are by far the most common causes of malodor, a clinician cannot take the risk of overlooking other, more challenging diseases. This can be done by either a trial therapy to deal quickly with intraoral causes (the full-mouth one-stage disinfection, including the use of proper mouth rinses and toothpastes) or by a multidisciplinary consultation. For more detailed information, the reader is encouraged to consult van Steenberghe[93] and recent review papers.[75,82,94]

REFERENCES

1. Addy M, Moran JM: Clinical indications for the use of chemical adjuncts to plaque control: chlorhexidine formulations, *Periodontol 2000* 15:52, 1997.
2. Addy M, Renton-Harper P: The role of antiseptics in secondary prevention. In Lang NP, Karring T, editors: *Proceedings of the Second European Workshop in Periodontology,* London, 1997, Quintessence.
3. Addy M, Moran J, Wade W: Chemical plaque control in the prevention of gingivitis and periodontitis. In Lang NP, Karring T, editors: *Proceedings of the 1st European Workshop in Periodontology,* London, 1994, Quintessence.
4. Bollen CM, Quirynen M: Microbiological response to mechanical treatment in combination with adjunctive therapy: a review of the literature, *J Periodontol* 67:1143, 1996.
5. Bosy A, Kulkarni GV, Rosenberg M, et al: Relationship of oral malodor to periodontitis: evidence of independence in discrete subpopulations, *J Periodontol* 65:37, 1994.
6. Bowler PG, Davies BJ, Jones SA: Microbial involvement in chronic wound malodour, *J Wound Care* 8:216, 1999.
7. Brunette DM, Proskin HM, Nelson BJ: The effects of dentifrice systems on oral malodor, *J Clin Dent* 9:76, 1998.
8. Brunette DM, Ouyang Y, Glass-Brudzinski J, et al: Effects of methyl mercaptan on human gingival fibroblast shape, cytoskeleton and protein synthesis and the inhibition of its effect by Zn^{++}. In van Steenberghe D, Rosenberg M, editors: *Bad breath: a multidisciplinary approach,* Leuven, Belgium, 1996, Leuven University Press.
9. Chen S, Zieve L, Mahadevan V: Mercaptans and dimethyl sulfide in the breath of patients with cirrhosis of the liver: effect of feeding methionine, *J Lab Clin Med* 75:628, 1970.
10. Christensen GJ: Why clean your tongue? *J Am Dent Assoc* 129:1605, 1998.
11. Cicek Y, Orbak R, Tezel A, et al: Effect of tongue brushing on oral malodor in adolescents, *Pediatr Int* 45:719, 2003.
12. Clark GT, Nachnani S, Messadi DV: Detecting and treating oral and nonoral malodors, *J Calif Dent Assoc* 25:133, 1997.
13. Claus D, Geypens B, Rutgeers P, et al: Where gastroenterology and periodontology meet: determination of oral volatile organic compounds using closed-loop trapping and high-resolution gas chromatography-ion trap detection. In van Steenberghe D, Rosenberg M, editors: *Bad breath: a multidisciplinary approach,* Leuven, Belgium, 1996 Leuven University Press.
14. Coil J, Tonzetich J: Characterization of volatile sulfure compounds production at individual gingival cervicular sites in humans, *J Clin Dent* 3:97, 1992.
15. Collins LM, Dawes C: The surface area of the adult human mouth and thickness of the salivary film covering the teeth and oral mucosa, *J Dent Res* 66:1300, 1987;
16. Crescenzo DG, Trastek VF, Allen MS, et al: Zenker's diverticulum in the elderly: is operation justified? *Ann Thorac Surg* 66:347, 1998.
17. De Boever EH, Loesche WJ: Assessing the contribution of anaerobic microflora of the tongue to oral malodor, *J Am Dent Assoc* 126:1384, 1995.
18. Delanghe G, Ghyselen J, van Steenberghe D, et al: Multidisciplinary breath-odour clinic, *Lancet* 350:187, 1997.
19. Derogatis LR, Lipman RS, Covi L: SCL-90: an outpatient psychiatric rating scale—preliminary report, *Psychopharmacol Bull* 9:13, 1973.
20. Doty RL, Shaman P, Dann M: Development of the University of Pennsylvania Smell Identification Test: a standardized microencapsulated test of olfactory function, *Physiol Behav* 32:489, 1984.
21. Eli I, Baht R, Koriat H, et al: Self-perception of breath odor, *J Am Dent Assoc* 132:621, 2001.
22. Eli I, Baht R, Kozlovsky A, et al: The complaint of oral malodor: possible psychopathological aspects, *Psychosom Med* 58:156, 1996.
23. Frascella J, Gilbert R, Fernandez P: Odor reduction potential of a chlorine dioxide mouthrinse, *J Clin Dent* 9:39, 1998.
24. Frascella J, Gilbert RD, Fernandez P, et al: Efficacy of a chlorine dioxide–containing mouthrinse in oral malodor, *Compend Contin Educ Dent* 21:241, 2000.
25. Gagari E, Kabani S: Adverse effects of mouthwash use: a review, *Oral Surg Oral Med Oral Pathol Oral Radiol Endod* 80:432, 1995.
26. Gerlach RW, Hyde JD, Poore CL, et al: Breath effects of three marketed dentifrices: a comparative study evaluating single and cumulative use, *J Clin Dent* 9:83, 1998.
27. Gilmore EL, Bhaskar SN: Effect of tongue brushing on bacteria and plaque formed in vitro, *J Periodontol* 43:418, 1972.
28. Gilmore EL, Gross A, Whitley R: Effect of tongue brushing on plaque bacteria, *Oral Surg Oral Med Oral Pathol* 36:201, 1973.
29. Goldberg S, Kozlovsky A, Gordon D, et al: Cadaverine as a putative component of oral malodor, *J Dent Res* 73:1168, 1994.
30. Greenman J, Duffield J, Spencer P, et al: Study on the organoleptic intensity scale for measuring oral malodor, *J Dent Res* 83:81, 2004.

31. Greenstein RB, Goldberg S, Marku-Cohen S, et al: Reduction of oral malodor by oxidizing lozenges, *J Periodontol* 68:1176, 1997.
32. Gross A, Barnes GP, Lyon TC: Effects of tongue brushing on tongue coating and dental plaque scores, *J Dent Res* 54:1236, 1975.
33. Hoshi K, van Steenberghe D: The effect of tongue brushing or toothpaste application on oral malodour reduction. In van Steenberghe D, Rosenberg M, editors: *Bad breath: a multidisciplinary approach,* Leuven, Belgium, 1996, Leuven University Press.
34. Hunter CM, Niles HP, Lenton PA, et al: Breath-odor evaluation by detection of volatile sulfur compounds: correlation with organoleptic odor ratings, *Compend Contin Educ Dent* 24:25, 2003.
35. Jones CG: Chlorhexidine: is it still the gold standard? *Periodontol 2000* 15:55, 1997.
36. Kleinberg I, Codipilly M: The biological basis of oral malodor formation. In Rosenberg M, editor: *Bad breath: research perspectives,* Tel Aviv, 1995, Ramot Publishing.
37. Kleinberg I, Codipilly M: Cysteine challenge testing: a powerful tool for examining oral malodour processes and treatments in vivo, *Int Dent J* 52:221, 2002.
38. Kleinberg I, Wolff MS, Codipilly DM: Role of saliva in oral dryness, oral feel and oral malodour, *Int Dent J* 52(suppl 3): 236, 2002.
39. Koshimune S, Awano S, Gohara K, et al: Low salivary flow and volatile sulfur compounds in mouth air, *Oral Surg Oral Med Oral Pathol Oral Radiol Endod* 96:38, 2003.
40. Kostelc JG, Preti G, Zelson PR, et al: Volatiles of exogenous origin from the human oral cavity, *J Chromatogr* 226:315, 1981.
41. Kozlovsky A, Goldberg S, Natour I, et al: Efficacy of a 2-phase oil: water mouthrinse in controlling oral malodor, gingivitis, and plaque, *J Periodontol* 67:577, 1996.
42. Kuyyakanond T, Quesnel LB: The mechanism of action of chlorhexidine, *FEMS Microbiol Lett* 79:211, 1992.
43. Lancero H, Niu J, Johnson PW: Exposure of periodontal ligament cells to methyl mercaptan reduces intracellular pH and inhibits cell migration, *J Dent Res* 75:1994, 1996.
44. Loesche WJ: The effects of antimicrobial mouthrinses on oral malodor and their status relative to US Food and Drug Administration regulations, *Quintessence Int* 30:311, 1999.
45. Lorber B: "Bad breath": presenting manifestation of anaerobic pulmonary infection, *Am Rev Respir Dis* 112:875, 1975.
46. McGregor IA, Watson JD, Sweeney G, et al: Tinidazole in smelly oropharyngeal tumours, *Lancet* 1:110, 1982.
47. Menon MV, Coykendall AL: Effect of tongue scraping, *J Dent Res* 73:1492, 1994.
48. Meskin LH: A breath of fresh air, *J Am Dent Assoc* 127:1282, 1996.
49. Mitchell SC, Smith RL: Trimethylaminuria: the fish malodor syndrome, *Drug Metab Dispos* 29:517, 2001.
50. Miyazaki H, Sakao S, Katoh Y, et al: Correlation between volatile sulphur compounds and certain oral health measurements in the general population, *J Periodontol* 66:679, 1995.
51. Nakano Y, Yoshimura M, Koga T: Correlation between oral malodor and periodontal bacteria, *Microbes Infect* 4:679, 2002.
52. Newman MG: The role of periodontitis in oral malodor: clinical perspectives. In van Steenberghe D, Rosenberg M, editors: *Bad breath: a multidisciplinary approach,* Leuven, Belgium, 1996, Leuven University Press.
53. Niles HP, Gaffar A: Advances in mouth odor research. In Rosenberg M, editor: *Bad breath: research perspectives,* Tel Aviv, 1995, Ramot Publishing.
54. Niles HP, Vazquez J, Rustogi KN, et al: The clinical effectiveness of a dentifrice containing triclosan and a copolymer for providing long-term control of breath odor measured chromatographically, *J Clin Dent* 10:135, 1999.
55. Norfleet RG: *Helicobacter* halitosis, *J Clin Gastroenterol* 16:274, 1993.
56. Oxtoby A, Field EA: Delusional symptoms in dental patients: a report of four cases, *Br Dent J* 176:140, 1994.
57. Persson S, Hydrogen sulfide and methyl mercaptan in periodontal pockets, *Oral Microbiol Immunol* 7:378, 1992.
58. Persson S, Claesson R, Carlsson J: The capacity of subgingival microbiotas to produce volatile sulfur compounds in human serum, *Oral Microbiol Immunol* 4:169, 1989.
59. Persson S, Edlund MB, Claesson R, et al: The formation of hydrogen sulfide and methyl mercaptan by oral bacteria, *Oral Microbiol Immunol* 5:195, 1990.
60. Phillips M, Cataneo RN, Cheema T, et al: Increased breath biomarkers of oxidative stress in diabetes mellitus, *Clin Chim Acta* 344:189, 2004.
61. Phillips M, Herrera J, Krishnan S, et al: Variation in volatile organic compounds in the breath of normal humans, *J Chromatogr B Biomed Sci Appl* 729:75, 1999.
62. Pitts G, Brogdon C, Hu L, et al: Mechanism of action of an antiseptic, anti-odor mouthwash, *J Dent Res* 62:738, 1983.
63. Preti G, Lawley HJ, Hormann CA: Non-oral and oral aspects of oral malodor. In Rosenberg M, editor: *Bad breath: research perspectives,* Tel Aviv, 1995, Ramot Publishing.
64. Quirynen M, Zhao H, van Steenberghe D: Review of the treatment strategies for oral malodour, *Clin Oral Invest* 6:1, 2002.
65. Quirynen M, Mongardini C, van Steenberghe D: The effect of a 1-stage full-mouth disinfection on oral malodor and microbial colonization of the tongue in periodontitis: a pilot study, *J Periodontol* 69:374, 1998.
67. Quirynen M, Avontroodt P, Soers C, et al: The efficacy of amine fluoride/stannous fluoride in the suppression of morning breath odour, *J Clin Periodontol* 29:944, 2002.
68. Quirynen M, Avontroodt P, Soers C, et al: Impact of tongue cleansers on microbial load and taste, *J Clin Periodontol* 31:506, 2004.
69. Ralph WJ: Oral hygiene—why neglect the tongue? *Aust Dent J* 33:224, 1988.
70. Ratkay LG, Tonzetich J, Waterfield JD: The effect of methyl mercaptan on the enzymatic and immunological activity leading to periodontal tissue destruction. In van Steenberghe D, Rosenberg M, editors: *Bad breath: a multidisciplinary approach,* Leuven, Belgium, 1996, Leuven University Press.
71. Raven S, Matheson JR, Huntington E, et al: The efficacy of combined zinc and triclosan system in the prevention of oral malodour. In van Steenberghe D, Rosenberg M, editors: *Bad breath: a multidisciplinary approach,* Leuven, Belgium, 1996, Leuven University Press.
72. Reingewirtz Y, Girault O, Reingewirtz N, et al: Mechanical effects and volatile sulfur compound–reducing effects of chewing gums: comparison between test and base gums and a control group, *Quintessence Int* 30:319, 1999.
73. Replogle WH, Beebe DK: Halitosis, *Am Fam Physician* 53:1215, 1996.
74. Roldan S, Herrera D, Sanz M: Clinical and microbiological efficiency efficacy of an antimicrobial mouthrinse on oral halitosis, *J Clin Periodontol* 27:24, 2000.
75. Roldan S, Herrera D, Sanz M: Biofilms and the tongue: therapeutical approaches for the control of halitosis, *Clin Oral Invest* 7:189, 2003.
76. Rosenberg M: Clinical assessment of bad breath: current concepts, *J Am Dent Assoc* 127:475, 1996.
77. Rosenberg M, Leib E: Experiences of an Israeli malodor clinic. In Rosenberg M, editor: *Bad breath: research perspectives,* Tel Aviv, 1995, Ramot Publishing.

78. Rosenberg M, McCulloch CA: Measurement of oral malodor: current methods and future prospects, *J Periodontol* 63:776, 1992.
79. Rosenberg M, Gelernter I, Barki M, et al: Day-long reduction of oral malodor by a two-phase oil:water mouthrinse as compared to chlorhexidine and placebo rinses, *J Periodontol* 63:39, 1992.
80. Rosenberg M, Kulkarni GV, Bosy A, et al: Reproducibility and sensitivity of oral malodor measurements with a portable sulphide monitor, *J Dent Res* 70:1436, 1991.
81. Rowley EJ, Schuchman LC, Tishk MN, et al: Tongue brushing versus tongue scraping, *Clin Prev Dent* 9:13, 1987.
82. Sanz M, Roldan S, Herrera D: Fundamentals of breath malodour, *J Contemp Dent Pract* 2:1, 2001.
83. Schmidt NF, Tarbet WJ: The effect of oral rinses on organoleptic mouth odor ratings and levels of volatile sulfur compounds, *Oral Surg Oral Med Oral Pathol* 45(6): 876-83, 1978.
84. Schroeder HE: Oral mucosa. In Schroeder HE, editor: *Oral structural biology,* New York, 1991, Thieme Medical Publishers.
85. Simenhoff ML, Burke JF, Saukkonen JJ, et al: Biochemical profile or uremic breath, *N Engl J Med* 297:132, 1977.
86. Suarez F, Springfield J, Furne J, et al: Differentiation of mouth versus gut as site of origin of odoriferous breath gases after garlic ingestion, *Am J Physiol* 276:G425, 1999.
87. Suarez FL, Furne JK, Springfield J, et al: Morning breath odor: influence of treatments on sulfur gases, *J Dent Res* 79:1773, 2000.
88. Tanaka M, Anguri H, Nonaka A, et al: Clinical assessment of oral malodor by the electronic nose system, *J Dent Res* 83:317, 2004.
89. Tonzetich J: Production and origin of oral malodor: a review of mechanisms and methods of analysis, *J Periodontol* 48:13, 1977.
90. Tonzetich J, Ng SK: Reduction of malodor by oral cleansing procedures, *Oral Surg Oral Med Oral Pathol* 42:172, 1976.
91. Tsunoda M, Yamada S, Yasuda H: Deodorizing mechanism of epigallocatechin and chewing gum containing tea extracts. In van Steenberghe D, Rosenberg M, editors: *Bad breath: a multidisciplinary approach,* Leuven, Belgium, 1996, Leuven University Press.
92. van Steenberghe D: Breath malodor, *Curr Opin Periodontol* 4:137, 1997.
93. van Steenberghe D, editor. *Breath malodor: a step-by-step approach,* Copenhagen, 2004, Quintessence.
94. van Steenberghe D, Quirynen M: Breath malodor. In Lindhe J, Karring T, Lang NP, editors: *Clinical periodontology and implant dentistry,* Oxford, 2003, Blackwell.
95. van Steenberghe D, Avontroodt P, Peeters W, et al: Effect of different mouthrinses on morning breath, *J Periodontol* 72:1183, 2001.
96. Vandekerckhove B, Quirynen M, Warren PR, et al: The safety and efficacy of a powered toothbrush on soft tissues in patients with implant-supported fixed prostheses, *Clin Oral Invest,* 8(4):206-210 2004.
97. Waler SM: The effect of zinc-containing chewing gum on volatile sulfur-containing compounds in the oral cavity, *Acta Odontol Scand* 55:198, 1997.
98. Winkler S, Garg AK, Mekayarajjananonth T, et al: Depressed taste and smell in geriatric patients, *J Am Dent Assoc* 130:1759, 1999.
99. Yaegaki K, Sanada K: Biochemical and clinical factors influencing oral malodor in periodontal patients, *J Periodontol* 63:783, 1992.
100. Yaegaki K, Sanada K: Volatile sulfur compounds in mouth air from clinically healthy subjects and patients with periodontal disease, *J Periodontal Res* 27:233, 1992.
101. Young A, Jonski G, Rolla G: A study of triclosan and its solubilizers as inhibitors of oral malodour, *J Clin Periodontol* 12:1078, 2002.
102. Young A, Jonski G, Rolla G: Inhibition of orally produced volatile sulfur compounds by zinc, chlorhexidine or cetylpyridinium chloride: effect of concentration, *Eur J Oral Sci* 5:400, 2003.
103. Young A, Jonski G, Rolla G, et al: Effects of metal salts on the oral production of volatile sulfur-containing compounds (VSC), *J Clin Periodontol* 28:776, 2001.

PART 6

Periodontal Pathology

Fermin A. Carranza

Thorough knowledge of the microscopic tissue changes in disease is essential to comprehend the biologic nature of the periodontal responses to injury and healing. This knowledge also provides an indispensable basis for the understanding and interpretation of the clinical and radiographic findings encountered in dental patients.

This part of the text provides information of the gingival diseases (Section I) and periodontal diseases (Section II). The latter section also includes chapters with detailed descriptions of the different diseases that can affect the periodontium.

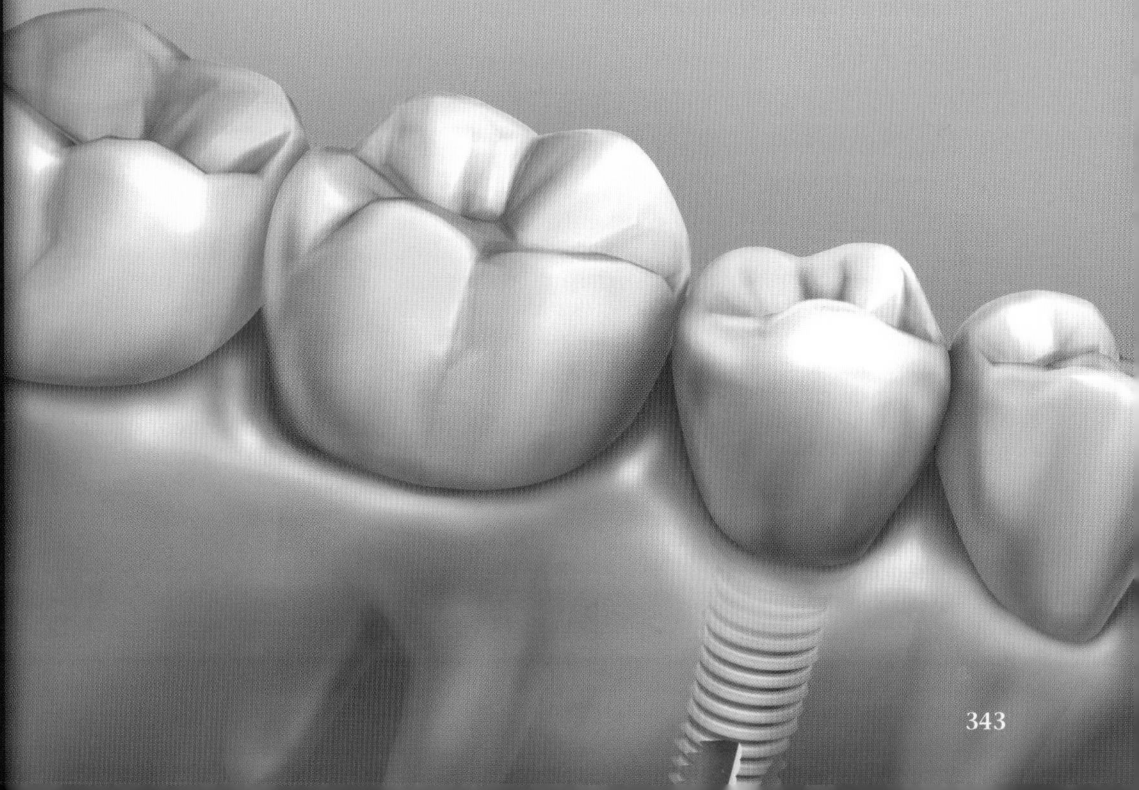

SECTION ▪ I ▪ *Gingival Disease*

20 CHAPTER

Defense Mechanisms of the Gingiva

Jaime Bulkacz and Fermin A. Carranza

CHAPTER OUTLINE

The gingival tissue is constantly subjected to mechanical and bacterial aggressions. The saliva, the epithelial surface, and the initial stages of the inflammatory response provide resistance to these actions. Chapter 4 reviews the role of the epithelium, through its degree of keratinization and turnover rate. This chapter describes the permeability of the junctional and sulcular epithelia and the role of sulcular fluid, leukocytes, and saliva.

SULCULAR FLUID

The presence of sulcular fluid, or *gingival crevicular fluid* (GCF), has been known since the nineteenth century, but its composition and possible role in oral defense mechanisms were elucidated by the pioneering work of Waerhaug[121] and Brill and Krasse[14] in the 1950s. The latter investigators introduced filter paper into the gingival sulci of dogs previously injected intramuscularly with fluorescein; within 3 minutes the fluorescent material was recovered on the paper strips. This indicated the passage of fluid from the bloodstream through the tissues and exiting via the gingival sulcus.

In subsequent studies, Brill[11,12] confirmed the presence of GCF in humans and considered it a "transudate." However, others[73,122] demonstrated that GCF is an inflammatory *exudate,* not a continuous transudate. In strictly normal gingiva, little or no fluid can be collected.

More recently, interest in the development of tests for the detection or prediction of periodontal disease has resulted in numerous research papers on the components, origin, and function of GCF.

Methods of Collection

The most difficult hurdle to overcome when collecting GCF is the scarcity of material that can be obtained from the sulcus. Many collection methods have been tried.* These methods include the use of absorbing paper strips, twisted threads placed around and into the sulcus, micropipettes, and intracrevicular washings.

The absorbing paper strips are placed within the sulcus (intrasulcular method) or at its entrance (extrasulcular method) (Figure 20-1). The placement of the filter paper strip in relation to the sulcus or pocket is important. The Brill technique inserts it into the pocket until resistance is encountered (Figure 20-1, *A*). This method introduces a degree of irritation of the sulcular epithelium that can, by itself, trigger the flow of fluid.

To minimize this irritation, Löe and Holm-Pedersen[73] placed the filter paper strip just at the entrance of the pocket or over the pocket entrance (Figure 20-1, *B* and *C*). In this way, fluid seeping out is picked up by the strip, but the sulcular epithelium is not in contact with the paper.

Preweighed twisted threads were used by Weinstein et al.[122] The threads were placed in the gingival crevice around the tooth, and the amount of fluid collected was estimated by weighing the sample thread.

The use of micropipettes permits the collection of fluid by capillarity. Capillary tubes of standardized length and diameter are placed in the pocket, and their content is later centrifuged and analyzed.[10,12,13]

Crevicular washings can be used to study GCF from clinically normal gingiva. One method uses an appliance consisting of a hard acrylic plate covering the maxilla with soft borders and a groove following the gingival margins; it is connected to four collection tubes. The washings are obtained by rinsing the crevicular areas from one side to the other, using a peristaltic pump.[21]

A modification of the previous method uses two injection needles fitted one within the other such that during sampling, the inside (ejection) needle is at the bottom of the pocket, and the outside (collecting) needle is at the gingival margin. The collection needle is drained into a sample tube by continuous suction.[101]

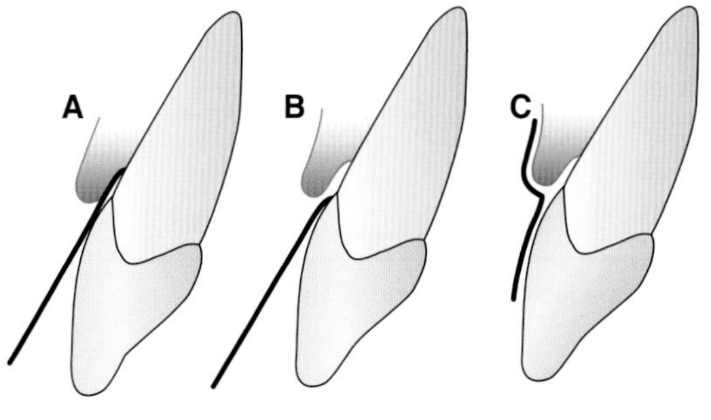

Figure 20-1 Placement of filter strip in gingival sulcus for collection of fluid. **A,** Intrasulcular method. **B** and **C,** Extrasulcular methods.

*References 10, 13, 59, 63, 75, 76, 101.

Permeability of Junctional and Sulcular Epithelia

The initial studies by Brill and Krasse[14] with fluorescein were later confirmed with substances such as India ink[95] and saccharated iron oxide.[21] Substances shown to penetrate the sulcular epithelium include albumin,[94] endotoxin,[93,98] thymidine,[49] histamine,[28] phenytoin,[114] and horseradish peroxidase.[79] These findings indicate permeability to substances with a molecular weight of up to 1000 kD.

Squier and Johnson[113] reviewed the mechanisms of penetration through an intact epithelium. Intercellular movement of molecules and ions along intercellular spaces appears to be a possible mechanism. Substances taking this route do not traverse the cell membranes.

Amount

The amount of GCF collected on a paper strip can be evaluated in a variety of ways. The wetted area can be made more visible by staining with ninhydrin; it is then measured planimetrically on an enlarged photograph or with a magnifying glass or a microscope.

An electronic method has been devised for measuring the fluid collected on a "blotter" (Periopaper), employing an electronic transducer (Periotron, Harco Electronics, Winnipeg, Manitoba, Canada) (Figure 20-2). The wetness of the paper strip affects the flow of an electronic current and gives a digital readout. A comparison of the ninhydrin-staining method and the electronic method performed in vitro revealed no significant differences between the two techniques.[116]

The amount of GCF collected is extremely small. Measurements performed by Cimasoni[21] showed that a strip of paper 1.5 mm wide and inserted 1 mm within the gingival sulcus of a slightly inflamed gingiva absorbs about 0.1 mg of GCF in 3 minutes. Challacombe[19] used an isotope dilution method to measure the amount of GCF present in a particular space at any given time. His calculations in human volunteers with a mean gingival index of less than 1 showed that the mean GCF volume

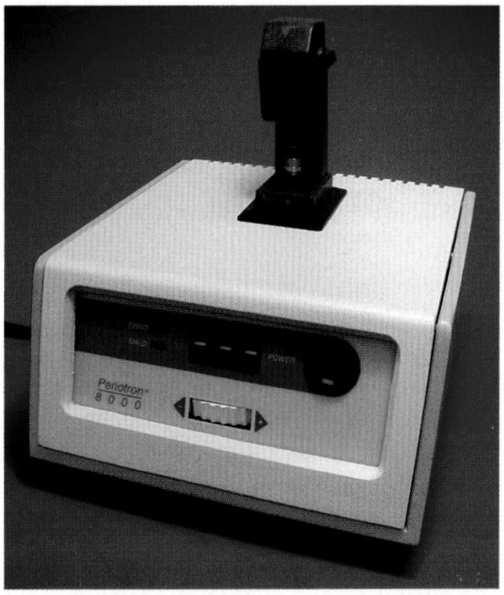

Figure 20-2 Electronic device for measuring the amount of fluid collected on filter paper.

in proximal spaces from molar teeth ranged from 0.43 to 1.56 μl.

Composition

The components of GCF can be characterized according to individual proteins,[73,85,103] specific antibodies, antigens,[35,92] and enzymes of several specificities.[15] The GCF also contains cellular elements.[28,31,124]

Many research efforts have attempted to use GCF components to detect or diagnose active disease or to predict patients at risk for periodontal disease.[2] So far, more than 40 compounds found in GCF have been analyzed,[89] but their origin is not known with certainty. These compounds can be host derived or produced by the bacteria in the gingival crevice, but their source can be difficult to elucidate; examples include β-glucuronidase, a lysosomal enzyme, and lactic acid dehydrogenase, a cytoplasmic enzyme. The source for collagenases may be fibroblasts or polymorphonuclear leukocytes (PMNs, neutrophils),[87] or collagenases may be secreted by bacteria.[35] Phospholipases are lysosomal and cytoplasmic enzymes but are also produced by microorganisms.[15] The majority of GCF elements detected thus far have been enzymes, but there are nonenzymatic substances as well (Box 20-1).

Cellular Elements. Cellular elements found in GCF include bacteria, desquamated epithelial cells, and leukocytes (PMNs, lymphocytes, monocytes/macrophages), which migrate through the sulcular epithelium.[28,31]

Electrolytes. Potassium, sodium, and calcium have been studied in GCF. Most studies have shown a positive correlation of calcium and sodium concentrations and the sodium/potassium ratio with inflammation.[56-58] (For further information, see references 12 and 13 and Box 20-2.)

Organic Compounds. Both carbohydrates and proteins have been investigated. Glucose hexosamine and hexuronic acid are two of the compounds found in GCF.[47] Blood glucose levels do not correlate with GCF glucose levels; glucose concentration in GCF is three to four times greater than that in serum.[47] This is interpreted not only as a result of metabolic activity of adjacent tissues, but also as a function of the local microbial flora.

The total protein content of GCF is much less than that of serum.[13,14] No significant correlations have been found between the concentration of proteins in GCF and the severity of gingivitis, pocket depth, or extent of bone loss.[7]

Metabolic and bacterial products identified in GCF include lactic acid,[48] urea,[42] hydroxyproline,[91] endotoxins,[109] cytotoxic substances, hydrogen sulfide,[112] and antibacterial factors.[27] Many enzymes have also been identified (see Boxes 20-1 and 20-2).

The methodology used for the analysis of GCF components is as varied as the diversity of those components. Examples include fluorometry for the detection of metalloproteinases[28]; enzyme-linked immunoabsorbent assay (ELISA) to detect enzyme levels and interleukin-1 beta (IL-1β)[71]; radioimmunoassays for detecting cyclooxygenase derivatives[86] and procollagen III[117]; high-pressure liquid chromatography (HPLC) to detect timidazole[67]; and direct and indirect immunodot tests for detection of acute-phase proteins.[108]

BOX 20-1

Enzymes and Other Compounds Reported in Gingival Crevicular Fluid*

- Acid phosphatase[42]
- Alkaline phosphatase[37]
- α1-Antitrypsin[2]
- Arylsulfatase[29]
- Aspartate aminotransferase[25]
- Chondroitin sulfatase[44]
- Citric acid[33]
- Cystatins[20]
- Cytokines (interleukins)[12,24,34]
  - IL-1α
  - IL-1β
  - IL-6 and IL-8
- Endopeptidases:
  - Cathepsin D[21]
  - Cathepsin B/L[14]
  - Cathepsin G[13,14]
  - Elastase[13,14]
  - Plasminogen activator[5]
  - Collagenase[15,32]
  - Tryptaselike enzyme[14]
  - Trypsinlike enzyme[14]
  - Dipeptydilpeptidase IV–like enzyme[14]
  - Elastase–α1-proteinase inhibitor[19]
- Exopeptidases[40]
- Fibrin[43]
- Fibronectin[43]
- β-Glucuronidase[29,30]
- Glycosidases[3,44]
  - α1-Fucosidase
  - Sialidase
  - β-*N*-acetylglucosaminidase
  - β-Galactosidase
  - β-Mannosidase
- Hyaluronidase[45]
- Immunoglobulins (IgG, IgA, IgG4, IgM)[17]
- Lactate dehydrogenase[29]
- Lactoferrin[22]
- Lactic acid[31]
- Lysozyme[31]
- α2-Macroglobulins[2]
- Medullasin[28]
- Myeloperoxidase[26]
- Prostaglandin E_2 (PGE_2)[28,36]
- Transferrin[2]
- Thromboxane[28,36]

*References are listed at the end of the chapter.

BOX 20-2

Compounds and Enzymes (Products) of Possible Bacterial Origin Detected in Gingival Crevicular Fluid*

Acid phosphatase[38,39]
Alkaline phosphatase[37]
Aminopeptidases[37]
Chondroitin sulfatase[46]
Chymotrypsin-like product[47]
Collagenase[16]
Deoxyribonuclease (DNase)[38]
Dipeptidylaminopeptidase IV–like enzyme[1]
Fibrinolysin[14,35]
Glucosidases[38]
Hemolysin[11]
Hyaluronidase[45]
Iminopeptidases[4]
Immunoglobulinases[18,27]
β-Lactamase[38,39]
Lysophospholipase[6,9]
Phospholipase A[6]
Phospholipase C[7,10]
Prostaglandin-like product[8]
Trypsinlike enzyme[38,40]

*References are listed at the end of the chapter.

Cellular and Humoral Activity in Gingival Crevicular Fluid

Monitoring periodontal disease is a complicated task because very few noninvasive procedures can follow the initiation and progress of the disease. Analysis of GCF constituents in health and disease may be extremely useful because of GCF's simplicity and because GCF can be obtained with noninvasive methods.

Analysis of GCF has identified cell and humoral responses in both healthy individuals and those with periodontal disease.[64] The cellular immune response includes the appearance of cytokines in GCF (see Box 20-1), but there is no clear evidence of a relationship between cytokines and disease. However, interleukin-1 alpha (IL-1α) and IL-1β are known to increase the binding of PMNs and monocytes/macrophages to endothelial cells, stimulate the production of prostaglandin E_2 (PGE_2) and release of lysosomal enzymes, and stimulate bone resorption.[68] Preliminary evidence also indicates the presence of interferon-α in GCF,[64] which may have a protective role in periodontal disease because of its ability to inhibit the bone resorption activity of IL-1β.[44]

Because the amount of fluid recoverable from gingival crevices is small, only the use of very sensitive immunoassays permits the analysis of the specificity of antibodies.[27] A study comparing antibodies in different crevices with serum antibodies directed at specific microorganisms did not provide any conclusive evidence about the significance of the antibody presence in GCF in periodontal disease.[64]

Even though the role of antibodies in the gingival defense mechanisms is difficult to ascertain, the consensus is that in a patient with periodontal disease, (1) a reduction in antibody response is detrimental, and (2) an antibody response plays a protective role.[65]

Clinical Significance

As mentioned previously, GCF is an inflammatory exudate.[73] Its presence in clinically normal sulci can be explained because gingiva that appears clinically normal invariably exhibits inflammation when examined microscopically.

The amount of GCF is greater when inflammation is present[34,106] and is sometimes proportional to the severity of inflammation.[88] GCF production is not increased by trauma from occlusion[78] but is increased by mastication of coarse foods, toothbrushing and gingival massage, ovulation,[71] hormonal contraceptives,[70] and smoking.[80] Other factors that influence the amount of GCF are circadian periodicity and periodontal therapy.

Circadian Periodicity. There is a gradual increase in GCF amount from 6 AM to 10 PM and a decrease afterward.[9]

Sex Hormones. Female sex hormones increase GCF flow, probably because they enhance vascular permeability.[68] Pregnancy, ovulation,[67] and hormonal contraceptives[69] all increase gingival fluid production.

Mechanical Stimulation. Chewing[12] and vigorous gingival brushing stimulate the flow of GCF. Even the minor stimuli represented by intrasulcular placement of paper strips increases the production of fluid.

Smoking. Smoking produces an immediate transient but marked increase in GCF flow.[80]

Periodontal Therapy. There is an increase in GCF production during the healing period after periodontal surgery.[3]

Drugs in Gingival Crevicular Fluid

Drugs that are excreted through the GCF may be used advantageously in periodontal therapy. Bader and Goldhaber[6] demonstrated in dogs that tetracyclines are excreted through the GCF; this finding triggered extensive research that showed a concentration of tetracyclines in GCF compared with serum.[43] Metronidazole is another antibiotic that has been detected in human GCF[32] (see Chapter 52).

LEUKOCYTES IN THE DENTOGINGIVAL AREA

Leukocytes have been found in clinically healthy gingival sulci in humans and experimental animals. The leukocytes found are predominantly PMNs. They appear in small numbers extravascularly in the connective tissue adjacent to the bottom of the sulcus; from there, they travel across the epithelium[18,45] to the gingival sulcus, where they are expelled (Figures 20-3 and 20-4).

SCIENCE TRANSFER

Teeth penetrate the integument as a structure that emerges from inside the body to outside the body. The gingival sulcular tissue is an area that provides a biologic seal, but it is also the area where the plaque bacteria challenge the host. This microbial challenge can result in a homeostasis with the host response, or it can overwhelm the host and cause tissue destruction, resulting eventually in periodontal disease. The host, however, has exquisite defense mechanisms that involve saliva and gingival crevicular fluid (GCF), both of which have multiple capacities to interact with the bacterial challenge. These capacities range from enzymes to antibodies to polymorphonuclear leukocytes. The contribution of each of these components is unknown, although each appears to be important in the host defense to bacterial plaque. For example, decreased salivary secretion (xerostomia) results in increased gingival disease and caries. Future therapeutic approaches may be directed at stimulating components of saliva or GCF.

The defense mechanisms of GCF, leukocytes, saliva, and the epithelial barrier of the gingival sulcus are generally effective in controlling the deleterious effects of the heavy concentration of bacteria found in dental plaque. If this balance between host and parasite is slightly changed, the result can be progressive periodontal breakdown. *Small clinical alterations, such as an overcontoured restoration or an open subgingival restorative margin, can allow the bacteria to gain a small advantage over the host defenses, resulting in increased gingival inflammation and eventual loss of attachment.* The bacteria can lodge in an open margin and thus may be less vulnerable to leukocytes and the flushing action of GCF, and bulbous contours of restorations can make regular oral hygiene procedures less able to contact the biofilm of plaque.

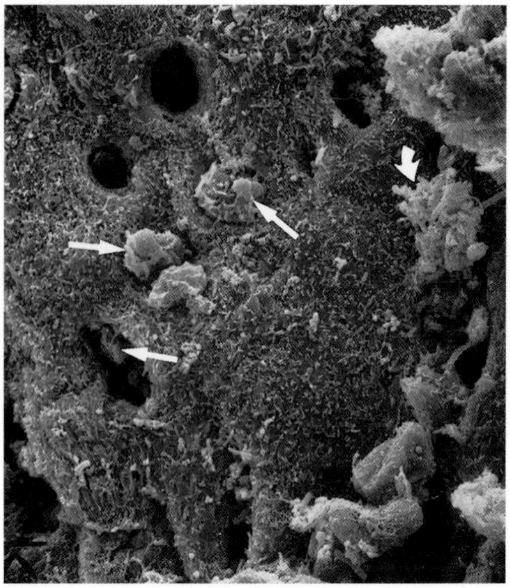

Figure 20-3 Scanning electron microscope view of periodontal pocket wall. Several leukocytes are emerging *(straight arrows),* some partially covered by bacteria *(curved arrow).* Empty holes correspond to tunnels through which leukocytes have emerged.

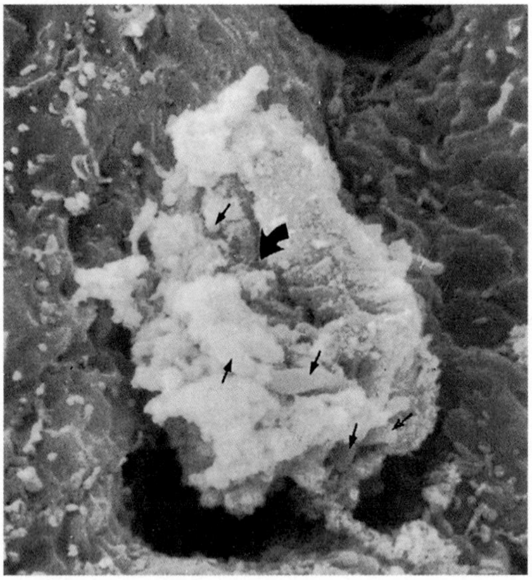

Figure 20-4 Scanning electron microscope view at higher magnification than Figure 20-3. A leukocyte emerging from the pocket wall is covered with bacteria *(small arrows).* The large curved arrow points to a phagosomal vacuole through which bacteria are being engulfed.

Leukocytes are present in sulci even when histologic sections of adjacent tissue are free of inflammatory infiltrate. Differential counts of leukocytes from clinically healthy human gingival sulci have shown 91.2% to 91.5% PMNs and 8.5% to 8.8% mononuclear cells.[111,124]

Mononuclear cells were identified as 58% B lymphocytes, 24% T lymphocytes, and 18% mononuclear phagocytes. The ratio of T lymphocytes to B lymphocytes was found to be reversed from the normal ratio of about 3:1 found in peripheral blood to about 1:3 in GCF.[124]

Leukocytes are attracted by different plaque bacteria[54,123] but can also be found in the dentogingival region of germ-free adult animals.[74,100] Leukocytes were reported in the gingival sulcus in nonmechanically irritated (resting) healthy gingiva, indicating that their migration may be independent of an increase in vascular permeability.[5] The majority of these cells are viable and have phagocytic and killing capacity.[62,90,96] Therefore, leukocytes constitute a major protective mechanism against the extension of plaque into the gingival sulcus.

Leukocytes are also found in saliva (see following discussion). The main port of entry of leukocytes into the oral cavity is the gingival sulcus.[104]

TABLE 20-1

Role of Saliva in Oral Health

Function	Salivary Components	Probable Mechanism
Lubrication	Glycoproteins, mucoids	Coating similar to gastric mucin
Physical protection	Glycoproteins, mucoids	Coating similar to gastric mucin
Cleansing	Physical flow	Clearance of debris and bacteria
Buffering	Bicarbonate and phosphate	Antacids
Tooth integrity maintenance	Minerals	Maturation, remineralization
	Glycoprotein pellicle	Mechanical protection
Antibacterial action	Immunoglobulin A	Control of bacterial colonization
	Lysozyme	Breaks bacterial cell walls
	Lactoperoxidase	Oxidation of susceptible bacteria

SALIVA

Salivary secretions are protective in nature because they maintain the oral tissues in a physiologic state (Table 20-1). Saliva exerts a major influence on plaque by mechanically cleansing the exposed oral surfaces, by buffering acids produced by bacteria, and by controlling bacterial activity.

Antibacterial Factors

Saliva contains numerous inorganic and organic factors that influence bacteria and their products in the oral environment. Inorganic factors include ions and gases, bicarbonate, sodium, potassium, phosphates, calcium, fluorides, ammonium, and carbon dioxide. Organic factors include lysozyme, lactoferrin, myeloperoxidase, lactoperoxidase, and agglutinins such as glycoproteins, mucins, β2-macroglobulins, fibronectins,[117] and antibodies.

Lysozyme is a hydrolytic enzyme that cleaves the linkage between structural components of the glycopeptide muramic acid–containing region of the cell wall of certain bacteria in vitro. Lysozyme works on both gram-negative and gram-positive organisms[50]; its targets include *Veillonella* species and *Actinobacillus actinomycetemcomitans*. It probably repels certain transient bacterial invaders of the mouth.[53]

The lactoperoxidase-thiocyanate system in saliva has been shown to be bactericidal to some strains of *Lactobacillus* and *Streptococcus*[82,99] by preventing the accumulation of lysine and glutamic acid, both of which are essential for bacterial growth. Another antibacterial finding is lactoferrin, which is effective against *Actinobacillus* species.[55]

Myeloperoxidase, an enzyme similar to salivary peroxidase, is released by leukocytes and is bactericidal for *Actinobacillus*[81] but has the added effect of inhibiting the attachment of *Actinomyces* strains to hydroxyapatite.[16]

Salivary Antibodies

As with GCF, saliva contains antibodies that are reactive with indigenous oral bacterial species. Although immunoglobulins G (IgG) and M (IgM) are present, the preponderant immunoglobulin found in saliva is *immunoglobulin A* (IgA). However, IgG is more prevalent in GCF.[115] Major and minor salivary glands contribute all the secretory IgA (sIgA) and lesser amounts of IgG and IgM. GCF contributes most of the IgG, complement, and PMNs that, in conjunction with IgG or IgM, inactivate or opsonize bacteria.

Salivary antibodies appear to be synthesized locally, because they react with strains of bacteria indigenous to the mouth but not with organisms characteristic of the intestinal tract.[36,38] Many bacteria found in saliva have been shown to be coated with IgA, and the bacterial deposits on teeth contain both IgA and IgG in quantities greater than 1% of their dry weight.[37] It has been shown that IgA antibodies present in parotid saliva can inhibit the attachment of oral *Streptococcus* species to epithelial cells.[33,121] Gibbons et al.[36-38] suggested that antibodies in secretions may impair the ability of bacteria to attach to mucosal or dental surfaces.

The *enzymes* normally found in the saliva are derived from the salivary glands, bacteria, leukocytes, oral tissues, and ingested substances; the major enzyme is *parotid amylase*. Certain salivary enzymes have been reported in increased concentrations in periodontal disease: hyaluronidase and lipase,[17] β-glucuronidase and chondroitin sulfatase,[41] amino acid decarboxylases,[41] catalase, peroxidase, and collagenase.[60]

Proteolytic enzymes in the saliva are generated by both the host and oral bacteria. These enzymes have been recognized as contributors to the initiation and progression of periodontal disease.[49,77] To combat these enzymes, saliva contains antiproteases that inhibit cysteine proteases such as cathepsins[51] and antileukoproteases that inhibit elastase.[87] Another antiprotease, identified as a tissue inhibitor of matrix metalloproteinase (TIMP), has been shown to inhibit the activity of collagen-degrading enzymes.[26]

High-molecular-weight mucinous *glycoproteins* in saliva bind specifically to many plaque-forming bacteria. The glycoprotein-bacteria interactions facilitate bacterial accumulation on the exposed tooth surface.[33,36-38,123] The specificity of these interactions has been demonstrated. The interbacterial matrix of human plaque appears to contain polymers similar to salivary glycoproteins that may aid in maintaining the integrity of plaque. In addition, these glycoproteins selectively adsorb to the hydroxyapatite to make up part of the acquired pellicle. Other salivary glycoproteins inhibit the sorption of some bacteria to the tooth surface and to epithelial cells of the oral mucosa. This activity appears to be associated with the glycoproteins that possess blood group reactivity.[1,33,36,38,121] Another effect of mucin is the deletion of bacterial cells from the oral cavity by aggregation with mucin-rich films.

Glycoproteins and a glycolipid present on mammalian cell surfaces appear to serve as receptors for the attachment of some viruses and bacteria. Thus the close similarity between glycoproteins of salivary secretions and components of the epithelial cell surface suggests that the secretions can competitively inhibit antigen sorption and therefore may limit pathologic alterations.

Salivary Buffers and Coagulation Factors

The maintenance of physiologic hydrogen ion concentration (pH) at the mucosal epithelial cell surface and the tooth surface is an important function of salivary buffers. Their primary effect has been studied in relationship to dental caries. In saliva the most important salivary buffer is the bicarbonate–carbonic acid system.[76]

Saliva also contains coagulation factors (factors VIII, IX, and X; plasma thromboplastin antecedent [PTA]; Hageman factor) that hasten blood coagulation and protect wounds from bacterial invasion.[66] An active fibrinolytic enzyme may also be present.

Leukocytes

In addition to desquamated epithelial cells, the saliva contains all forms of leukocytes, of which the principal cells are PMNs. The number of PMNs varies from person to person at different times of the day and is increased in gingivitis. PMNs reach the oral cavity by migrating through the lining of the gingival sulcus. Living PMNs in saliva are sometimes referred to as *orogranulocytes,* and their rate of migration into the oral cavity is termed the *orogranulocytic migratory rate.* Some investigators believe the rate of migration correlates with the severity of gingival inflammation and is therefore a reliable index for assessing gingivitis.[111]

Role in Periodontal Pathology

Saliva exerts a major influence on plaque initiation, maturation, and metabolism. Salivary flow and composition also influence calculus formation, periodontal disease, and caries. The removal of the salivary glands in experimental animals significantly increases the incidence of dental caries[39] and periodontal disease[46] and delays wound healing.[107]

In humans, an increase in inflammatory gingival diseases, dental caries, and rapid tooth destruction associated with cervical or cemental caries is partially a consequence of decreased salivary gland secretion *(xerostomia).* Xerostomia may result from sialolithiasis, sarcoidosis, Sjögren's syndrome, Mikulicz's disease, irradiation, surgical removal of the salivary glands, and other factors (see Chapters 44 and 45).

REFERENCES

1. Adinolri M, Mollison PL, Polley MJ, et al: A blood group antibodies, *J Exp Med* 123:951, 1966.
2. Armitage G: Diagnostic tests for periodontal diseases, *Curr Opin Dent* 2:53, 1992.
3. Arnold R, Lunstad, G, Bissada, N, et al: Alterations in crevicular fluid flow during healing following gingival surgery, *J Periodontal Res* 1:303, 1966.
4. Attstrom R: Presence of leukocytes in the crevices of healthy and clinically inflamed gingiva, *J Periodontol* 5:42, 1970.
5. Attstrom R, Egelberg J: Emigration of blood neutrophils and monocytes into the gingival crevices, *J Periodontal Res* 5:48, 1970.
6. Bader HJ, Goldhaber P: The passage of intravenously administered tetracycline in the gingival sulcus of dogs, *J Oral Ther* 2:324, 1966.
7. Bang J, Cimasoni G: Total protein in human crevicular fluid, *J Dent Res* 50:1683, 1971.
8. Birkedal-Hansen H, Taylor RE, Zambon JJ, et al: Characterization of collagenolytic activity from strains of *Bacteroides gingivalis, J Periodontal Res* 23:258, 1988.
9. Bissada NF, Schaffer EM, Haus E: Circadian periodicity of human crevicular fluid, *J Periodontol* 38:36, 1967.
10. Bjorn HL, Koch G, Lindhe J: Evaluation of gingival fluid measurements, *Odont Rev* 16:300, 1965.
11. Brill N: The gingival pocket fluid: studies of its occurrence, composition and effect, *Acta Odontol Scand* 20(suppl 32):159, 1969.
12. Brill N: Effect of chewing on flow of tissue fluid into gingival pockets, *Acta Odontol Scand* 17:277, 1959.
13. Brill N, Bronnestam R: Immunoelectrophoretic study of tissue fluid from gingival pockets, *Acta Odontol Scand* 18:95, 1960.
14. Brill N, Krasse B: The passage of tissue fluid into the clinically healthy gingival pocket, *Acta Odontol Scand* 16:223, 1958.
15. Bulkacz J: Enzymatic activities in gingival fluid with special emphasis on phospholipases, *J West Soc Periodontol* 36:145, 1986.
16. Camargo PM de, Miyasaki KT, Wolinsky LE: Host modulation of adherence: the effect of human neutrophil myeloperoxidase on the attachment of *Actinomyces viscosus* and *naeslundii* to saliva coated hydroxyapatite, *J Periodontal Res* 23:334, 1988.
17. Carlsson J, Egelberg J: Local effect of diet on plaque formation and development of gingivitis in dogs. II. Effect of high carbohydrate versus high protein/fat diets, *Odont Rev* 16:42, 1965.
18. Cattoni M: Lymphocytes in the epithelium of healthy gingiva, *J Dent Res* 30:627, 1951.
19. Challacombe SJ: Passage of serum immunoglobulin into the oral cavity. In Lehner T, Cimasoni G, editors: *Borderland between caries and periodontal disease,* vol 2, London, 1980, Academic Press.
20. Cimasoni G: The crevicular fluid. In Myers H, editor: *Monographs in oral science,* vol 3, Basel, 1974, S Karger.
21. Cimasoni G: Crevicular fluid updated. In Myers H, editor: *Monographs in oral science,* vol 12, Basel, 1983, S Karger.
22. Cobb CM, Brown LR: The effects of exudate from the periodontal pocket on cell culture, *Periodontics* 5:5, 1967.
23. Dawes C: The chemistry and physiology of saliva. In Shaw JH, Sweeney EA, Cappuccino CC, et al, editors: *Textbook of oral biology,* Philadelphia, 1978, Saunders.

24. Dawes C, Jenkins GM, Tonge CH: The nomenclature of the integuments of the enamel surface of teeth, *Br Dent J* 115:65, 1963.
25. Dinarello CA: Interleukin-1 and its biologically related cytokines. In Cohen S, editor: *Lymphokines and the immune response,* Boca Raton, Fla, 1990, CRC Press.
26. Drouin L, Overall CM, Sodek J: Identification of matrix metallo-endoproteinase inhibitor (TIMP) in human parotid and submandibular saliva: partial purification and characterization, *J Periodontal Res* 23:370, 1988.
27. Ebersole JL, Taubman MA, Smith DJ: Gingival crevicular fluid antibody to oral microorganisms. II. Distribution and specificity of local antibody responses, *J Periodontal Res* 20:349, 1985.
28. Egelberg J: Cellular elements in gingival pocket fluid, *Acta Odontol Scand* 21:283, 1963.
29. Egelberg J: Gingival exudate measurements for evaluation of inflammatory changes of the gingiva, *Odont Rev* 15:381, 1964.
30. Egelberg J: Permeability of the dentogingival vessels. II. Clinically healthy gingiva, *J Periodontal Res* 1:276, 1966.
31. Egelberg J, Attstrom R: Presence of leukocytes within crevices of healthy and inflamed gingiva and their immigration from the blood, *J Periodontal Res* 4(suppl):23, 1969.
32. Eisenberg L, Suchow R, Coles RS, et al: The effects of metronidazole administration on clinical and microbiologic parameters of periodontal disease, *Clin Prev Dent* 13:28, 1991.
33. Ellen RP, Gibbons RJ: Protein associated adherence of *Streptococcus pyogenes* to epithelial surfaces: prerequisite for virulence, *Infect Immun* 5:826, 1972.
34. Garnick JJ, Pearson R, Harrell D: The evaluation of the Periotron, *J Periodontol* 50:424, 1979.
35. Genco RJ, Zambon JJ, Murray PA: Serum and gingival fluid antibodies as an adjunct in the diagnosis of *Actinobacillus actinomycetemcomitans*–associated periodontal disease, *J Periodontol* 56:41, 1985.
36. Gibbons RJ, van Houte J: Selective bacterial adherence to oral epithelial surfaces and its role as an ecological determinant, *Infect Immun* 3:567, 1971.
37. Gibbons RJ, van Houte J: On the formation of dental plaques, *J Periodontol* 44:347, 1973.
38. Gibbons RJ, van Houte J, Liljemark WF: Some parameters that affect the adherence of *S. salivarius* to oral epithelial surfaces, *J Dent Res* 51:424, 1972.
39. Gilda JE, Keyes PH: Increased dental caries activity in the Syrian hamster following desalivation, *Proc Soc Exp Biol Med* 66:28, 1947.
40. Glas JE, Krasse B: Biophysical studies on dental calculus from germ-free and conventional rats, *Acta Odontol Scand* 20:127, 1962.
41. Gochman N, Meyer RK, Blackwell RQ, et al: The amino acid decarboxylase of salivary sediment, *J Dent Res* 38:998, 1959.
42. Golub LM, Borden SM, Kleinberg K: Urea content of gingival crevicular fluid and its relation to periodontal disease in humans, *J Periodontal Res* 6:243, 1971.
43. Gordon JM, Walker CB, Goodson JM, et al: Sensitive assay for measuring tetracycline levels in gingival crevice fluid, *Antimicrob Agents Chemother* 17:193, 1980.
44. Gowan M, Mundy GR: Actions of recombinant interleukin 1, interleukin 2 and interferon-gamma on bone resorption in vitro, *J Immunol* 136:2478, 1986.
45. Grant DA, Orban BJ: Leukocytes in the epithelial attachment, *J Periodontol* 31:87, 1960.
46. Gupta OH, Blechman H, Stahl SS: The effects of desalivation on periodontal tissues of the Syrian hamster, *Oral Surg* 13:470, 1960.
47. Hara K, Löe H: Carbohydrate components of the gingival exudate, *J Periodontal Res* 4:202, 1969.
48. Hasegawa K: Biochemical study of gingival fluid: lactic acid in gingival fluid, *Bull Tokyo Med Dent Univ* 14:359, 1967.
49. Holt SC, Bramanti TE: Factors in virulence expression and their role on periodontal disease pathogenesis, *Crit Rev Oral Biol Med* 2:177, 1991.
50. Iacono VC, Bolot PR, Mackay JB, et al: Lytic sensitivity of *Actinobacillus actinomycetemcomitans* to lysozyme, *Infect Immun* 40:773, 1983.
51. Isemura S, Ando K, Nakashizoka T, et al: Cystatin S: a cystein-proteinase inhibitor of human saliva, *J Biochem* 96:1311, 1984.
52. Jensen RL, Folke LEA: The passage of exogenous tritiated thymidine into gingival tissues, *J Periodontol* 45:786, 1974.
53. Jolles P, Petit JF: Purification and analysis of human saliva lysozyme, *Nature* 200:168, 1963.
54. Kahnberg KE, Lindhe J, Helden J: Initial gingivitis induced by topical application of plaque extract: a histometric study in dogs with normal gingiva, *J Periodontal Res* 11:218, 1976.
55. Kalmar JP, Arnold RP: Killing of *Actinobacillus actinomycetemcomitans* by human lactoferrin, *Infect Immun* 56:2552, 1988.
56. Kaslick RS, Mandel ID, Chasens AJ, et al: Concentration of inorganic ions in gingival fluid, *J Dent Res* 49:887, 1970.
57. Kaslick RS, Chasens AI, Mandel ID, et al: Quantitative analysis of sodium, potassium and calcium in gingival fluid from gingiva in varying degrees of inflammation, *J Periodontol* 41:93, 1970.
58. Kaslick RS, Chasens AI, Mandel ID, et al: Sodium, potassium and calcium in gingival fluid: a study of the relationship of the ions to one another, to circadian rhythms, gingival bleeding, purulence, and to conservative periodontal therapy, *J Periodontol* 41:442, 1970.
59. Kaslik RS, Chasens AI, Weinstein O, et al: Ultramicromethods for the collection of gingival fluid and quantitative analysis of its sodium content, *J Dent Res* 47:1192, 1986.
60. King JD: Experimental investigation of periodontal disease in the ferret and in man, with special reference to calculus formation, *Dent Pract* 4:157, 1954.
61. Kiroshita JJ, Muhlemann HR: Effect of sodium ortho and pyrophosphate on supragingival calculus, *Helv Odontol Acta* 10:46, 1966.
62. Kowolik MJ, Raeburn JA: Functional integrity of gingival crevicular neutrophil polymorphonuclear leukocytes as demonstrated by nitroblue tetrazolium reduction, *J Periodontal Res* 15:483, 1980.
63. Krekeler G: Quantitative determination of the gingival sulcus fluid by means of microcapillaries, *Dtsch Zahnaertzl Z* 30:544, 1975.
64. Lamster IB, Novak MJ: Host mediators in gingival crevicular fluid: implications for the pathogenesis of periodontal disease, *Crit Rev Oral Biol Med* 3:31, 1992.
65. Lamster IB, Celenti R, Ebersole J: The relationship of serum IgG antibody titers to periodontal pathogens to indicators of the host response in gingival crevicular fluid, *J Clin Periodontol* 17:419, 1990.
66. Leung SW, Jensen AT: Factors controlling the deposition of calculus, *Int Dent J* 8:613, 1958.
67. Liew V, Mack G, Tseng P, et al: Single-dose concentrations of timidazole in gingival crevicular fluid, serum and gingival tissue in adults with periodontitis, *J Dent Res* 70:910, 1991.
68. Life JS, Johnson NW, Powell JR, et al: Interleukin-1 beta (IL-1β) levels in gingival crevicular fluid from adults without previous evidence of destructive periodontitis: a cross sectional study, *J Clin Periodontol* 19:53, 1992.

69. Lindhe J, Attstrom R: Gingival exudation during the menstrual cycle, *J Periodontal Res* 2:194, 1967.
70. Lindhe J, Bjorn AL: Influence of hormonal contraceptives on the gingiva of women, *J Periodontal Res* 2:1, 1967.
71. Lindhe J, Attstrom R, Bjorn AL: Influence of sex hormones on gingival exudate of gingivitis-free female dogs, *J Periodontal Res* 3:273, 1968.
72. Lisanti VF: Hydrolytic enzymes in periodontal tissues, *Ann NY Acad Sci* 85:461, 1960.
73. Löe H, Holm-Pedersen P: Absence and presence of fluid from normal and inflamed gingiva, *Periodontics* 3:171, 1965.
74. Magnusson B: Mucosal changes at erupting molars in germ-free rats, *J Periodontal Res* 4:181, 1969.
75. Marcus ER, Jooste CP, Driver HS, Hatting J: The quantification of individual proteins in crevicular gingival fluid, *J Periodontal Res* 20:444, 1985.
76. Mandel I: Relation of saliva and plaque to caries, *J Dent Res* 53(suppl):246, 1974.
77. Mandel ID: Markers of periodontal disease susceptibility and activity derived from saliva. In Johnson NW, editor: *Risk markers of oral diseases,* vol 3, New York, 1991, Cambridge University Press.
78. Martin LP, Noble WH: Gingival fluid in relation to tooth mobility and occlusal interferences, *J Periodontol* 45:444, 1974.
79. McDougall WA: Pathways of penetration and effects of horseradish peroxidase in rat molar gingiva, *Arch Oral Biol* 15:621, 1970.
80. McLaughlin WS, Lovat FM, Macgregor IDM, et al: The immediate effects of smoking on gingival fluid flow, *J Clin Periodontol* 20:448, 1993.
81. Miyasaki KT, Wilson ME, Genco RJ: Killing of *Actinobacillus actinomycetemcomitans* by the human peroxide chloride system, *Infect Immun* 53:161, 1986.
82. Muhlemann HR, Schroeder H: Dynamics of supragingival calculus formation, *Adv Oral Biol* 1:175, 1964.
83. Nagao M: Influence of prosthetic appliances upon the flow of crevicular tissue fluid. I. Relation between crevicular tissue fluid and prosthetic appliances, *Bull Tokyo Med Dent Univ* 14:241, 1967.
84. Nakamura M, Slots J: Salivary enzymes: origin and relationship to periodontal disease, *J Periodontal Res* 18:559, 1983.
85. Novaes AB Jr, Ruben MP, Kramer GM: Proteins of the gingival exudate: a review and discussion of the literature, *J West Soc Periodontol* 27:12, 1979.
86. Offenbacher S, Williams RC, Jeffcoat MK, et al: Effects of NSAIDs on beagle crevicular cyclo-oxygenase metabolites and periodontal bone loss, *J Periodontal Res* 27:207, 1992.
87. Ohlsson M, Rosengreen M, Tegner H, et al: Quantification of granulocyte elastase inhibitor in human mixed saliva and in pure parotid secretion, *Phys Chem* 364:1323, 1983.
88. Orban JE, Stallard RE: Gingival crevicular fluid: a reliable predictor of gingival health? *J Periodontol* 40:231, 1969.
89. Page RC: Host response tests designed for diagnosing periodontal disease, *J Periodontol* 63:356, 1992.
90. Passo SA, Tsai CC, McArthur WP, et al: Interaction of inflammatory cells and oral microorganisms. IX. The bacterial effect of human PMN leukocytes on isolated plaque microorganisms, *J Periodontal Res* 15:470, 1980.
91. Paunio K: On the hydroxyproline-containing components in the gingival exudate, *J Periodontal Res* 6:115, 1971.
92. Pollock JJ, Andors L, Gulumoglu A: Direct measurement of hepatitis B virus antibody and antigen markers in gingival crevicular fluid, *Oral Surg Oral Med Oral Pathol* 57:499, 1984.
93. Ranney RR, Montgomery EH: Vascular leakage resulting from topical application of endotoxin to the gingiva of the beagle dog, *Arch Oral Biol* 18:963, 1973.
94. Ranney RR, Zander HA: Allergic periodontal disease in sensitized squirrel monkeys, *J Periodontol* 41:12, 1970.
95. Ratcliff P: Permeability of healthy gingival epithelium by microscopically observable particles, *J Periodontol* 37:291, 1966.
96. Renggli HH: Phagocytosis and killing by crevicular neutrophils. In Lehner T, editor: *The borderland between caries and periodontal disease,* New York, 1977, Grune & Stratton.
97. Renggli HH, Regolatti B: Intracrevicular sampling of leukocytes using plastic strips, *Helv Odont Acta* 16:93, 1972.
98. Rizzo AA: Histologic and immunologic evaluation of antigen penetration with oral tissues after topical application, *Periodontics* 41:210, 1970.
99. Rosebury R, Karshan M: *Salivary calculus: dental science and dental art,* Philadelphia, 1938, Lea & Febiger.
100. Rovin S, Costich ER, Gordon HA: The influence of bacteria and irritation in the initiation of periodontal disease in germfree and conventional rats, *J Periodontal Res* 1:193, 1966.
101. Salonen JI, Paunio KU: An intracrevicular washing method for collection of intracrevicular contents, *Scand J Dent Res* 99:406, 1961.
102. Sandalli P, Wade AB: Alterations in crevicular fluid flow during healing following gingivectomy and flap procedures, *J Periodontal Res* 4:314, 1969.
103. Sano K, Nakao M, Shiba A, et al: An ultra-micro assay for proteins in biological fluids other than blood using a combination of agarose gel isoelectric focusing and silver staining, *Clin Chim Acta* 137:115, 1984.
104. Schiott CR, Löe H: The origin and variation in the number of leukocytes in the human saliva, *J Periodontal Res* 4(suppl):24, 1969.
105. Schultz-Haudt S, Bibby BG, Bruce MA: Tissue destructive products of gingival bacteria from nonspecific gingivitis, *J Dent Res* 33:624, 1954.
106. Shapiro L, Goldman H, Bloom A: Sulcular exudate flow in gingival inflammation, *J Periodontol* 50:301, 1979.
107. Shen LS, Ghavamzadeh G, Shklar G: Gingival healing in sialadenectomized rats, *J Periodontol* 50:533, 1979.
108. Sibraa PD, Reinhardt AA, Dyer JK, et al: Acute-phase protein detection and quantification in gingival crevicular fluid by direct and indirect immuno-dot, *J Clin Periodontol* 18:101, 1991.
109. Simon B, Goldman HM, Ruben MP, et al: The role of endotoxin in periodontal disease. III. Correlation of the amount of endotoxin with the histologic degree of inflammation, *J Periodontol* 42:210, 1971.
110. Skapski H, Lehner T: A crevicular washing method for investigating immune components of crevicular fluid in man, *J Periodontal Res* 11:19, 1976.
111. Skougaard MR, Bay I, Kilnkhammer JM: Correlation between gingivitis and orogranulocytic migratory rate, *J Dent Res* 48:716, 1994.
112. Solis Gaffar MC, Rustogi KN, Gaffar A: Hydrogen sulfide production from gingival crevicular fluid, *J Periodontol* 51:603, 1980.
113. Squier CA, Johnson NW: Permeability of oral mucosa, *Br Med Bull* 31:169, 1975.
114. Steinberg AD, Steinberg J, Allen P, et al: The effect of alteration in the sulcular environment upon the movement of 14C-diphenylhydantoin through rabbit sulcular tissues, *J Periodontal Res* 11:47, 1976.
115. Sueda T, Bang J, Cimasoni G: Collection of gingival fluid for quantitative analysis, *J Dent Res* 48:159, 1969.
116. Suppipat W, Suppipat N: Evaluation of an electronic device for gingival fluid quantitation, *J Periodontol* 48:388, 1977.
117. Talonopoika JT, Hamalainen MM: Collagen III aminoterminal propeptide in gingival crevicular fluid before and after periodontal disease, *Scand J Dent Res* 100:107, 1992.

118. Tomasi TB, Bienenstock J: Secretory immunoglobulins, *Adv Immunol* 9:1, 1968.
119. Van Winkelhoff AJ, van Steenberger TJM, de Graaff J: The role of black-pigmented *Bacteroides* in human oral infections, *J Clin Periodontol* 15:145, 1988.
120. Vogel JJ, Amdur BH: Inorganic pyrophosphate in parotid saliva, *Arch Oral Biol* 12:159, 1967.
121. Waerhaug J: The gingival pocket: anatomy, pathology deepening and elimination, *Odont Tidskaift* 60(suppl 1):1, 1952.
122. Weinstein E, Mandel ID, Salkind A, et al: Studies of gingival fluid, *Periodontics* 5:161, 1967.
123. Williams RW, Gibbons RG: Inhibition of bacterial adherence by secretory immunoglobulin A: a mechanism of antigen disposal, *Science* 177:697, 1972.
124. Wilton JMA, Renggli HH, Lehner T: The isolation and identification of mononuclear cells from the gingival crevice in man, *J Periodontal Res* 11:243, 1976.

REFERENCES FOR BOXES 20-1 AND 20-2

1. Abiko Y, Hayakawa M, Murai S, et al: Glycylpropyl dipeptidyl amino-peptidase from *Bacteroides gingivalis, J Clin Periodontol* 64:106, 1985.
2. Adonogianaki E, Mooney J, Kinane DF: The ability of acute gingival crevicular fluid phase proteins to distinguish gingivitis and periodontitis sites, *J Clin Periodontol* 19:98, 1992.
3. Beighton D, Radford JR, Naylor MN: Glycosidase activity in gingival crevicular fluid in subjects with adult periodontitis or gingivitis, *Arch Oral Biol* 37:43, 1992.
4. Brandtzaeg P, Mann WA: A comparative study of the lysozyme activity of human gingival pocket fluid, serum and saliva, *Acta Odont Scand* 29:441, 1964.
5. Buduneli N, Buduneli E, Ciotanar S et al: Plasminogen activators and plasminogen activator inhibitors in gingival crevicular fluid of cyclosporine A–treated patients, *J Clin Periodontol* 31:556, 2004.
6. Bulkacz J: Enzymatic activities in gingival fluid with special emphasis on phospholipases, *J West Soc Periodontol* 36:145, 1986.
7. Bulkacz J, Erbland JF: Exocellular phospholipase activity from a strain of *Propionibacterium acnes* isolated from a periodontal pocket, *J Periodontol* 68:369, 1997.
8. Bulkacz J, Grenett H: Synthesis of prostaglandin-like substances by oral gram negative rods, *J Dent Res* 60(abstract 421), 1981.
9. Bulkacz J, Erbland JF, MacGregor: Phospholipase activity in supernatants from cultures of *Bacteroides melaninogenicus, Biochem Biophys Acta* 664:148, 1981.
10. Bulkacz J, Garnick J, Barclay JE: Detection of phospholipase activity in crevicular fluid, *J Dent Res* 60(abstract 1187), 1981.
11. Chu L, Bramanti TE, Holt SC, et al: Hemolytic activity in the periodontopathogen *Porphyromonas gingivalis:* kinetics of enzyme formation and localization, *Infect Immun* 59:1932, 1991.
12. Chung RM, Grbic JT, Lamster IB: Interleukin-8 and beta-glucuronidase in gingival crevicular fluid, *J Clin Periodontol* 24:146, 1997.
13. Cimasoni G: Crevicular fluid updated. In Myers H, editor: *Monographs in oral science,* vol 12, Basel, 1983, S Karger.
14. Eley BM, Cox SW: Cathepsin B/L–, elastase-, tryptase-, trypsin- and dipeptidyl peptidase IV–like activities in gingival crevicular fluid: a comparison of levels before and after periodontal surgery in chronic periodontitis patients, *J Periodontol* 63:412, 1992.
15. Fullmer, HM, Gibson WA: Collagenolytic activity in gingiva in man, *Nature* 209:728, 1966.
16. Gibbons RJ, MacDonald JB: Degradation of collagenous substrates by *Bacteroides melaninogenicus, J Bacteriol* 81:614, 1964.
17. Grbic JT, Singer RE, Jans HH, et al: Immunoglobulin isotypes in gingival crevicular fluid: possible protective of IgA, *J Periodontol* 66:55, 1995.
18. Gregory RL, Kim DE, Kindel JC, et al: Immunoglobulin-degrading enzymes in localized juvenile periodontitis, *J Periodontal Res* 27:176, 1992.
19. Huynk C, Roch-Arveiller M, Meyer J, et al: Gingival crevicular fluid of patients with gingivitis or periodontal disease: evaluation of elastase–alpha 1 proteinase inhibitor complexes, *J Clin Periodontol* 19:187, 1992.
20. Ichimaru E, Imura K, Hara Y, et al: Cystatin activity in gingival crevicular fluid from periodontal disease patients, measured by a new quantitative analysis method, *J Periodontal Res* 27:119, 1992.
21. Ishikawa I, Cimasoni G, Ahmad-Zadeh C: Possible roles of lysosomal enzymes in the pathogenesis of periodontitis: a study in cathepsin D in human gingival fluid, *Arch Oral Biol* 17:111, 1972.
22. Jentsch H, Sievert Y, Gocke R: Lactoferrin and other markers from gingival crevicular fluid and saliva before and after periodontal treatment, *J Clin Periodontol* 31:511, 2004.
23. Jin L, Yu C, Corbet EF: Granulocyte elastase activity in static and flow gingival crevicular fluid, *J Periodontal Res* 38:303, 2003.
24. Jin L, Yu C, Corbet EF: Interleukin-8 and granulocyte elastase in gingival crevicular fluid in relation to periodonyto-pathogens in untreated adult periodontitis, *J Periodontol* 71:929, 2000.
25. Kamma JJ, Nakou M, Persson RG: Association of early onset periodontitis microbiota with aspartate aminotransferase activity in gingival crevicular fluid, *J Clin Periodontol* 28:1096, 2001.
26. Karhuvaara L, Tenovuo J, Sievers G: Crevicular fluid myeloperoxidase: an indicator of acute gingival inflammation, *Proc Finish Dent Soc* 86:3, 1990.
27. Killian M: Degradation of immunoglobulins A1, A2, and G by suspected principal periodontal pathogens, *Infect Immun* 34:757, 1981.
28. Kunamitsu K, Ichimaru E, Kato I, et al: Granulocyte medullasin levels in gingival crevicular fluid from chronic adult periodontitis patients and experimental gingivitis subjects, *J Periodontal Res* 25:352, 1990.
29. Lamster IB, Vogel RI, Hartley LJ, et al: Lactate dehydrogenase, beta-glucuronidase, and arylsulfatase activity in gingival crevicular fluid associated with experimental gingivitis in man, *J Periodontol* 56:139, 1985.
30. Lamster IB, Kaufman E, Grbic JT, et al: Beta-glucuronidase activity in saliva, *J Periodontol* 74: 353, 2003.
31. Life JS, Johnson NW, Powell JR, et al: Interleukin-1 beta (IL-1β) levels in gingival crevicular fluid from adults without previous evidence of destructive periodontitis: a cross sectional study, *J Clin Periodontol* 19:53, 1992.
32. Mancini S, Romanelli R, Laschinger CA, et al: Assessment of a novel screening test for neutrophil collagenase activity in the diagnosis of periodontal disease, *J Periodontol* 70:1292, 1999.
33. Miyajima K, Ohmo Y, Iwata T, et al: The lactic acid and citric acid content in the gingival fluid of orthodontic patients, *Aichi Gakuin Dent Sci* 4:75, 1991.
34. Mogi M, Otogoto J, Ota N, et al: Interleukin 1 beta, interleukin 6, beta 2-microglobulin, and transforming growth factor-alpha in gingival crevicular fluid from human periodontal disease, *Arch Oral Biol* 44:535, 1999.
35. Nitzan D, Sperry JF, Wilkins TD: Fibrinolytic activity of oral anaerobic bacteria, *Arch Oral Biol* 23:465, 1978.

36. Page RC: Host response tests designed for diagnosing periodontal diseases, *J Periodontol* 63:356, 1992.
37. Perinetti G, Paolantonio M, Serra E, et al: Longitudinal monitoring of subgingival colonization by *Actinobacillus actinomycetemcomitans,* and crevicular alkaline phosphatase and aspartate aminotransferase activities around orthodontically treated teeth, *J Clin Periodontol* 31:60, 2004.
38. Slots J: Enzymatic characterization of some oral and non-oral gram-negative bacteria with the API ZYM system, *J Clin Microbiol* 14:288, 1981.
39. Slots J, Dahlen G: Subgingival microorganisms and bacterial virulence factors in periodontitis, *Scand J Dent Res* 93:119, 1985.
40. Smalley J, Birss AJ, Kay HM, et al: The distribution of trypsin-like enzyme activity in cultures of a virulent and an avirulent strain of *Bacteroides gingivalis* W50, *Oral Microbiol Immunol* 4:178, 1989.
41. Soell M, Elkaim R, Tenembaum H: Cathepsin C, matrix metalloproteinases, and their tissue inhibitors in gingival and gingival crevicular fluid from periodontitis-affected patients, *J Dent Res* 81:174, 2002.
42. Sueda T, Cimasoni G, Held AJ: High levels of acid phosphatase in human crevicular fluid, *Arch Oral Biol* 12:1205, 1967.
43. Talonopoika J: Characterization of fibrin(ogen) fragments in gingival crevicular fluid, *Scand J Periodontal Res* 99:40, 1991.
44. Tipler LS, Emberg G: Glycosaminoglycan depolimerizing enzymes form oral microorganisms, *Arch Oral Biol* 30:391, 1985.
45. Tynelius-Brathall G: Hyaluronidase activity in gingival crevicular fluid and in peritoneal exudate leukocytes in dogs, *J Periodontal Res* 7:307, 1972.
46. Uito VJ: Degradation of basement membrane collagen by proteinases from human gingiva, leukocytes and bacterial plaque, *J Periodontol* 54:740, 1983.
47. Uito VJ, Grenier D, Chan ECS, et al: Isolation of a chymotrypsin-like enzyme from *Treponema denticola, Infect Immun* 56:2717, 1988.

21 CHAPTER

Gingival Inflammation

Joseph P. Fiorellini, Satoshi O. Ishikawa, and David M. Kim

Chapter Outline

Pathologic changes in gingivitis are associated with the presence of oral microorganisms attached to the tooth and perhaps in or near the gingival sulcus. These organisms are capable of synthesizing products (e.g., collagenase, hyaluronidase, protease, chondroitin sulfatase, endotoxin) that cause damage to epithelial and connective tissue cells, as well as to intercellular constituents, such as collagen, ground substance, and glycocalyx (cell coat). The resultant widening of the spaces between the junctional epithelial cells during early gingivitis may permit injurious agents derived from bacteria, or bacteria themselves, to gain access to the connective tissue.[10,45,49]

Microbial products activate monocytes/macrophages to produce vasoactive substances such as prostaglandin E_2 (PGE_2), interferon (IFN), tumor necrosis factor (TNF), and interleukin-1 (IL-1).[23,35]

Morphologic and functional changes in the gingiva during plaque accumulation have been thoroughly investigated, especially in beagle dogs and in humans.[36] A useful framework for organization and consideration of these data has been devised based on histopathologic, radiographic, and ultrastructural features and biochemical measurements.[37,39] The sequence of events cumulating in clinically apparent gingivitis is categorized into *initial, early,* and *established stages*, with periodontitis designated as the *advanced stage*[38] (Table 21-1). One stage evolves into the next, with no clear-cut dividing lines.

Despite extensive research, we still cannot distinguish definitively between normal gingival tissue and the

TABLE 21-1

Stages of Gingivitis

Stage	Time (Days)	Blood Vessels	Junctional and Sulcular Epithelia	Predominant Immune Cells	Collagen	Clinical Findings
I. Initial lesion	2-4	Vascular dilation Vasculitis	Infiltration by PMNs	PMNs	Perivascular loss	Gingival fluid flow
II. Early lesion	4-7	Vascular proliferation	Same as stage I Rete pegs Atrophic areas	Lymphocytes	Increased loss around infiltrate	Erythema Bleeding on probing
III. Established lesion	14-21	Same as stage II, plus blood stasis	Same as stage II but more advanced	Plasma cells	Continued loss	Changes in color, size, texture, etc.

PMNs, Polymorphonuclear leukocytes (neutrophils).

SCIENCE TRANSFER

The body responds to an infection by developing an inflammatory response. The gingiva is no exception, and inflammation in the gingiva is termed *gingivitis.* Early work investigating gingival inflammation described the progression from a state of health to a state of inflammation and tissue loss and divided the progression into four stages. This often-quoted process undoubtedly simplifies a complex process in which a host of cells and inflammatory molecules play important roles. An example is the critical role of monocytes/macrophages, which release interleukin-1 (IL-1) and tumor necrosis factor alpha (TNF-α). Inhibition of these two molecules significantly inhibits the inflammatory response and the subsequent tissue changes, emphasizing their role in gingivitis.

Gingival inflammation has two components: the *acute* inflammatory component, with vasodilation, edema, and polymorphonuclear infiltration, and the *chronic* inflammatory component, with B and T lymphocytes and capillary proliferation forming a granulomatous response. Each gingival region can have varying amounts of the acute or chronic component. For patients in whom acute inflammatory changes predominate, clinicians can expect a more dramatic response to initial therapy, whereas for patients with the established or advanced lesion in whom chronic inflammation and tissue damage dominate, such a significant tissue response will not occur. *The more inflamed a gingival unit appears clinically, the better the chances of therapeutic measures resulting in a return to normal gingival health.*

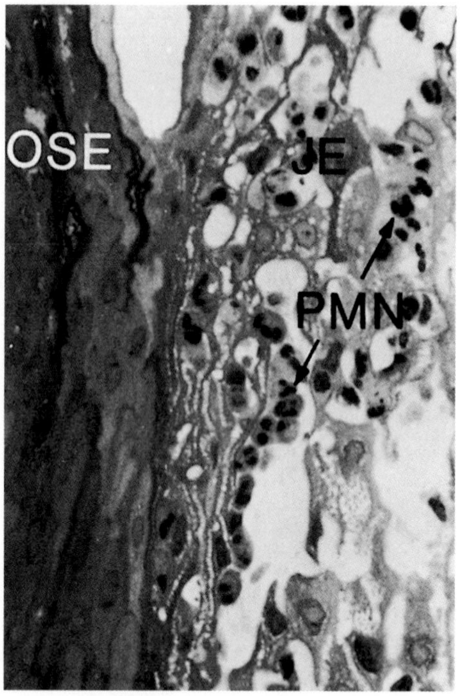

Figure 21-1 Human biopsy sample, experimental gingivitis. After 4 days of plaque accumulation, the blood vessels immediately adjacent to the junctional epithelium are distended and contain polymorphonuclear leukocytes (PMNs, neutrophils). Neutrophils have also migrated between the cells of the junctional epithelium. *OSE,* Oral sulcular epithelium. (Magnification ×500.) (From Payne WA, Page RC, Ogilvie AL, et al: *J Periodontal Res* 10:51, 1975.)

initial stage of gingivitis.[36] Most biopsies of clinically normal human gingiva contain inflammatory cells consisting predominantly of T cells, with very few B cells or plasma cells.[36,50,51] These cells do not create tissue damage, but they appear to be important in the day-to-day host response to bacteria and other substances to which the gingiva is exposed.[36] Under normal conditions, therefore, a constant stream of neutrophils is migrating from the vessels of the gingival plexus through the junctional epithelium, to the gingival margin, and into the gingival sulcus and oral cavity.[43]

STAGE I GINGIVITIS: THE INITIAL LESION

The first manifestations of gingival inflammation are vascular changes consisting of dilated capillaries and increased blood flow. These initial inflammatory changes occur in response to microbial activation of resident leukocytes and the subsequent stimulation of endothelial cells. Clinically, this initial response of the gingiva to bacterial plaque (*subclinical gingivitis*[26]) is not apparent.

Microscopically, some classic features of acute inflammation can be seen in the connective tissue beneath the junctional epithelium. Changes in blood vessel morphologic features (e.g., widening of small capillaries or venules) and adherence of neutrophils to vessel walls (margination) occur within 1 week and sometimes as early as 2 days after plaque has been allowed to accumulate[18,41] (Figure 21-1). Leukocytes, mainly polymorphonuclear neutrophils (PMNs), leave the capillaries by migrating through the walls (diapedesis, emigration)[25,51,52] (Figure 21-2). They can be seen in increased quantities in the connective tissue, the junctional epithelium, and the gingival sulcus* (Figures 21-3 and 21-4). Exudation of fluid from the gingival sulcus[18] and extravascular proteins are present.[20,21]

However, these findings are not accompanied by manifestations of tissue damage perceptible at the light microscopic or ultrastructural level; they do not form an infiltrate, and their presence is not considered to indicate pathologic change.[36]

*References 2, 3, 24, 34, 41, 46, 47.

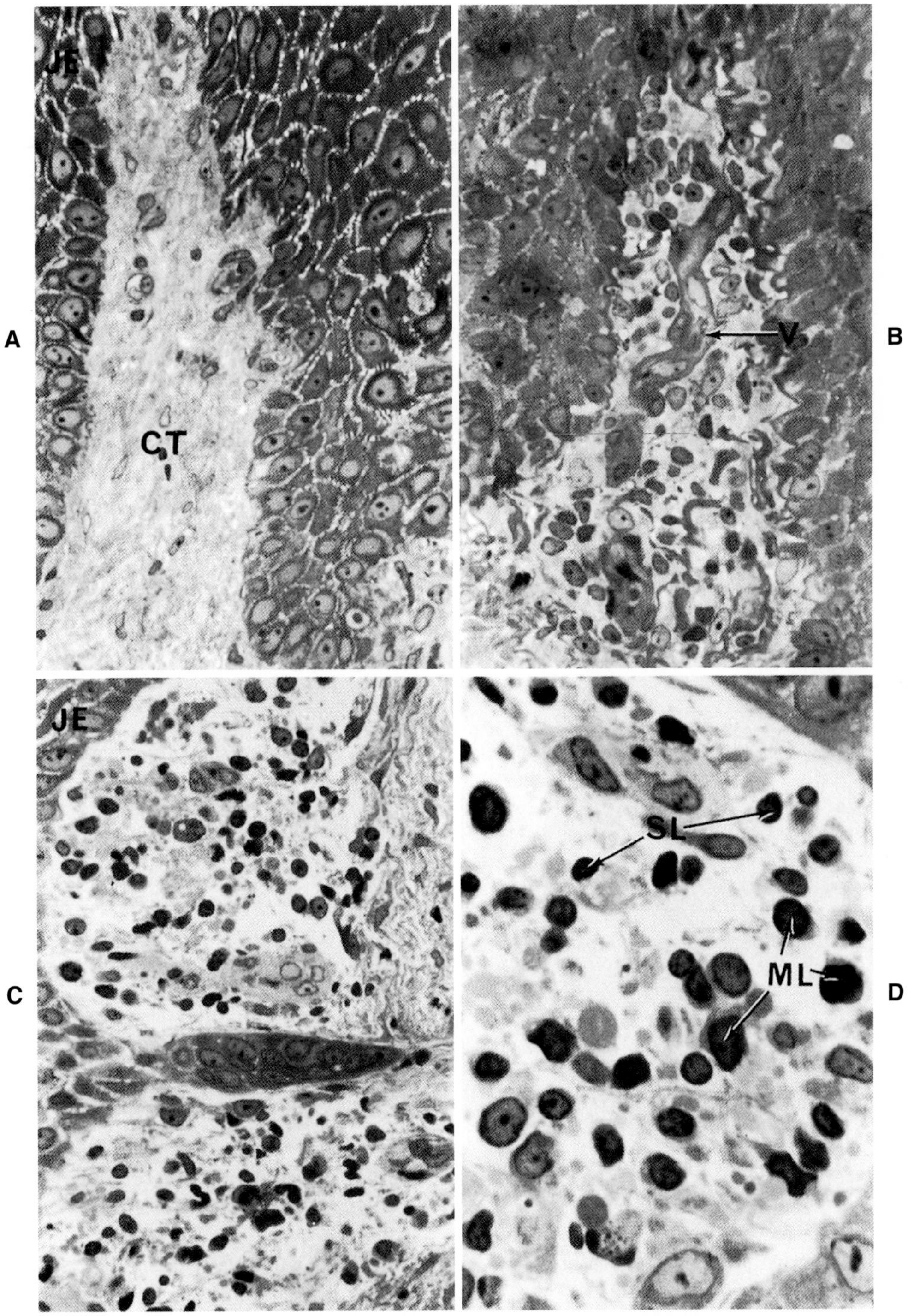

Figure 21-2 Human biopsy, experimental gingivitis. **A,** Control biopsy specimen from a patient with good oral hygiene and no detectable plaque accumulation. The junctional epithelium is at the left. The connective tissue *(CT)* shows few cells other than fibroblasts, blood vessels, and a dense background of collagen fibers. (×500.) **B,** Biopsy specimen taken after 8 days of plaque accumulation. The connective tissue is infiltrated with inflammatory cells, which displace the collagen fibers. A distended blood vessel *(V)* is seen in the center. (×500.) **C,** After 8 days of plaque accumulation, the connective tissue next to the junctional epithelium at the base of the sulcus shows a mononuclear cell infiltrate and evidence of collagen degeneration (clear spaces around cellular infiltrate) (×500). **D,** The inflammatory cell infiltrate at higher magnification. After 8 days of plaque accumulation, numerous small *(SL)* and medium-sized *(ML)* lymphocytes are seen within the connective tissue. Most of the collagen fibers around these cells have disappeared, presumably as a result of enzymatic digestion. (×1250.) (From Payne WA, Page RC, Ogilvie AL, et al: *J Periodontal Res* 10:51, 1975.)

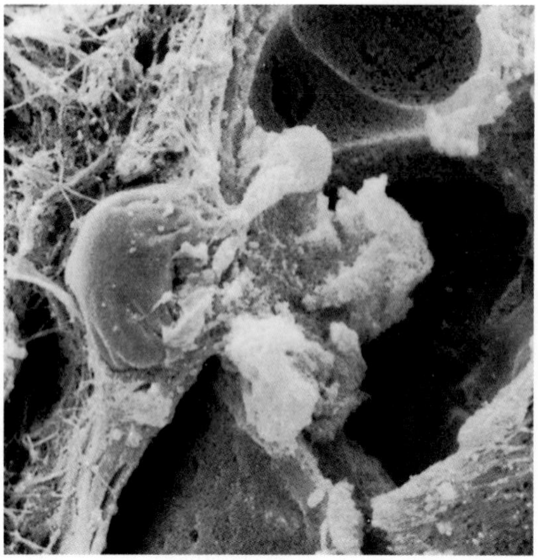

Figure 21-3 Scanning electron micrograph showing a leukocyte traversing the vessel wall to enter into the gingival connective tissue.

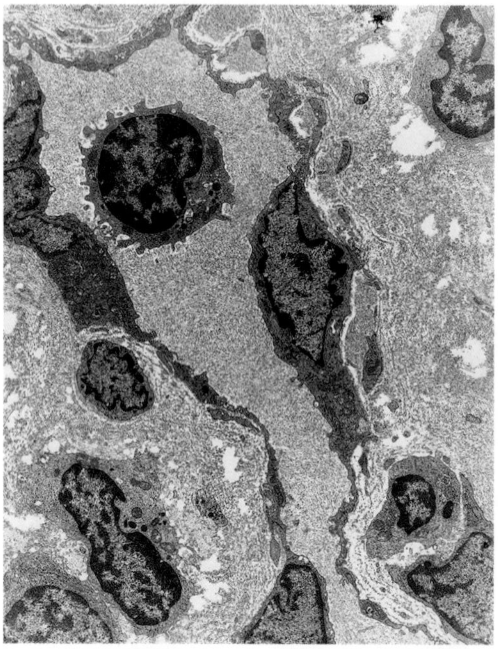

Figure 21-4 Early human gingivitis lesion. Area of lamina propria subjacent to the crevicular epithelium showing a capillary with several extravascular lymphocytes and one lymphocyte within the lumen. The specimen also exhibits considerable loss of perivascular collagen density. (×2500.) (Courtesy Dr. Charles Cobb, Kansas City, Mo.)

Subtle changes can also be detected in the junctional epithelium and perivascular connective tissue at this early stage. For example, the perivascular connective tissue matrix becomes altered, and there is exudation and deposition of fibrin in the affected area.[36] Also, lymphocytes soon begin to accumulate (see Figure 21-2, *D*). The increase in the migration of leukocytes and their accumulation within the gingival sulcus may be correlated

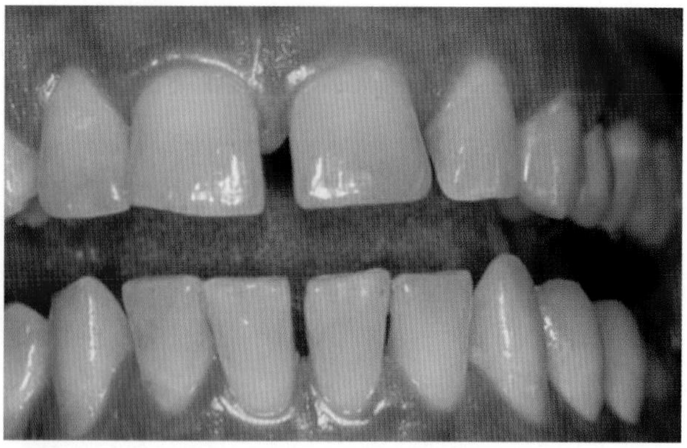

Figure 21-5 Marginal gingivitis and irregular gingival contour.

with an increase in the flow of gingival fluid into the sulcus.[4]

The character and intensity of the host response determine whether this *initial lesion* resolves rapidly, with the restoration of the tissue to a normal state, or evolves into a chronic inflammatory lesion. If the latter occurs, an infiltrate of macrophages and lymphoid cells appears within a few days.

STAGE II GINGIVITIS: THE EARLY LESION

The *early lesion* evolves from the *initial lesion* within about 1 week after the beginning of plaque accumulation.[35,41] Clinically, the early lesion may appear as early gingivitis, and it overlaps with and evolves from the initial lesion with no clear-cut dividing line. As time goes on, clinical signs of erythema may appear, mainly because of the proliferation of capillaries and increased formation of capillary loops between rete pegs or ridges (Figure 21-5). Bleeding on probing may also be evident.[1] Gingival fluid flow and the numbers of transmigrating leukocytes reach their maximum between 6 and 12 days after the onset of clinical gingivitis.[26]

Microscopic examination of the gingiva reveals a leukocyte infiltration in the connective tissue beneath the junctional epithelium, consisting mainly of lymphocytes (75%, with the majority T cells),[41,48] but also composed of some migrating neutrophils, as well as macrophages, plasma cells, and mast cells. All the changes seen in the *initial lesion* continue to intensify with the *early lesion*.[15,28,30,35,48] The junctional epithelium becomes densely infiltrated with neutrophils, as does the gingival sulcus, and the junctional epithelium may begin to show development of rete pegs or ridges.

The amount of collagen destruction increases[11,28,48]; 70% of the collagen is destroyed around the cellular infiltrate. The main fiber groups affected appear to be the circular and dentogingival fiber assemblies. Alterations in blood vessel morphologic features and vascular bed patterns have also been described.[18,19]

Polymorphonuclear leukocytes (PMNs) that have left the blood vessels in response to chemotactic stimuli

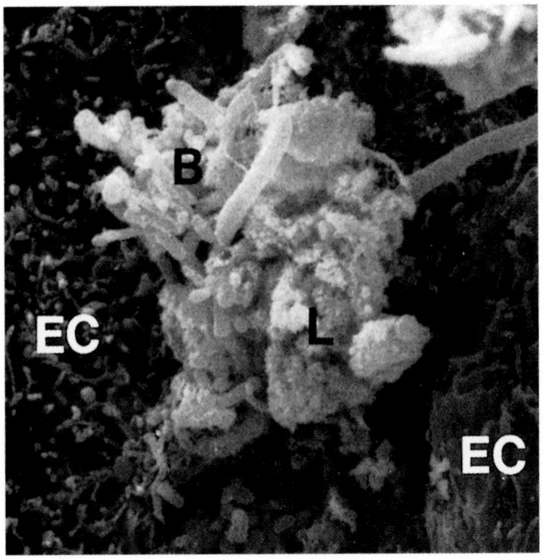

Figure 21-6 Scanning electron micrograph of leukocyte emerging to pocket wall and covered with bacteria and extracellular lysosomes. *EC,* Epithelial cells; *B,* bacteria; *L,* lysosomes.

from plaque components travel to the epithelium, cross the basement lamina, and are found in the epithelium, emerging in the pocket area (see Figure 21-3). PMNs are attracted to bacteria and engulf them in the process of phagocytosis (Figure 21-6). PMNs release their lysosomes in association with the ingestion of bacteria.[22] Fibroblasts show cytotoxic alterations,[40] with a decreased capacity for collagen production.

STAGE III GINGIVITIS: THE ESTABLISHED LESION

Over time, the *established lesion* evolves, characterized by a predominance of plasma cells and B lymphocytes and probably in conjunction with the creation of a small gingival pocket lined with a pocket epithelium.[47] The B cells found in the established lesion are predominantly of the immunoglobulin G1 (IgG1) and G3 (IgG3) subclasses.[36]

In chronic gingivitis, which occurs 2 to 3 weeks after the beginning of plaque accumulation, the blood vessels become engorged and congested, venous return is impaired, and the blood flow becomes sluggish (Figure 21-7). The result is localized gingival *anoxemia,* which superimposes a somewhat bluish hue on the reddened gingiva.[17] Extravasation of erythrocytes into the connective tissue and breakdown of hemoglobin into its component pigments can also deepen the color of the chronically inflamed gingiva. The established lesion can be described as moderately to severely inflamed gingiva.

In histologic sections, an intense, chronic inflammatory reaction is observed. Several detailed cytologic studies have been performed on chronically inflamed gingiva.* A key feature that differentiates the *established lesion* is the increased number of plasma cells, which become the preponderant inflammatory cell type. Plasma cells invade the connective tissue not only immediately below the junctional epithelium, but also deep into the connective tissue, around blood vessels, and between bundles of collagen fibers.[6] The junctional epithelium reveals widened intercellular spaces filled with granular cellular debris, including lysosomes derived from disrupted neutrophils, lymphocytes, and monocytes (Figure 21-8). The lysosomes contain acid hydrolases that can destroy tissue components. The junctional epithelium develops rete pegs or ridges that protrude into the connective tissue, and the basal lamina is destroyed in some areas. In the connective tissue, collagen fibers are destroyed around the infiltrate of

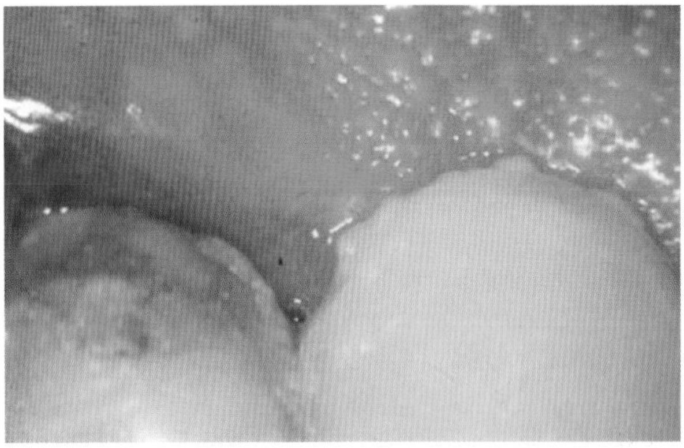

Figure 21-7 Marginal supragingival plaque and gingivitis.

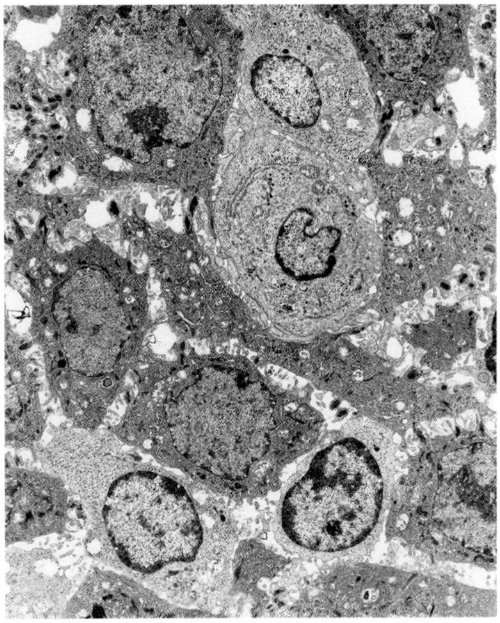

Figure 21-8 Established gingivitis in a human subject. Area of crevicular epithelium exhibiting enlarged intercellular spaces with numerous microvilli and desmosomal junctions. Several lymphocytes, both small and large, are seen migrating through the epithelial layer. (×3000.)

*References 12, 14, 15, 40, 47, 50, 54.

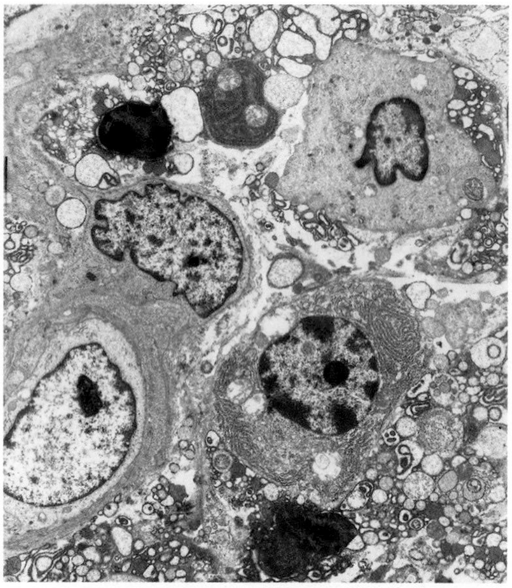

Figure 21-9 Advanced gingivitis in a human subject. Specimen from the lamina propria exhibiting plasma cell degeneration, with abundant cellular debris visible. (×3000.) (Courtesy Dr. Charles Cobb, Kansas City, Mo.)

intact and disrupted plasma cells, neutrophils, lymphocytes, monocytes, and mast cells (Figure 21-9).

The predominance of plasma cells is thought to be a primary characteristic of the established lesion. However, several studies of human experimental gingivitis have failed to demonstrate plasma cell predominance in the affected connective tissues,[7,8,50] including one study of 6 months' duration.[1] Increases in the proportions of plasma cells were evident with long-standing gingivitis, but the time for the development of the classic "established lesion" may exceed 6 months.

An inverse relationship appears to exist between the number of intact collagen bundles and the number of inflammatory cells.[52] Collagenolytic activity is increased in inflamed gingival tissue[16] by the enzyme *collagenase.* Collagenase is normally present in gingival tissues[5] and is produced by some oral bacteria and by PMNs.

Enzyme histochemistry studies have shown that chronically inflamed gingivae have elevated levels of acid and alkaline phosphatase,[56] β-glucuronidase, β-glucosidase, β-galactosidase, esterases,[29] aminopeptidase[33,42] and cytochrome oxidase.[9] Neutral mucopolysaccharide levels are decreased,[54] presumably as a result of degradation of the ground substance.

Established lesions of two types appear to exist; some remain stable and do not progress for months or years,[32,33,53] and others seem to become more active and to convert to progressively destructive lesions. Also, the established lesions appear to be reversible in that the sequence of events occurring in the tissues as a result of successful periodontal therapy seems to be essentially the reverse of the sequence of events observed as gingivitis develops. As the flora reverts from that characteristically associated with destructive lesions to that associated with periodontal health, the percentage of plasma cells decreases greatly, and the lymphocyte population increases proportionately.[27,31]

STAGE IV GINGIVITIS: THE ADVANCED LESION

Extension of the lesion into alveolar bone characterizes a fourth stage known as the *advanced lesion*[40] or *phase of periodontal breakdown.*[28] This is described in detail in Chapters 27 and 28.

Microscopically, there is fibrosis of the gingiva and widespread manifestations of inflammatory and immunopathologic tissue damage.[36] In general at this advanced stage, plasma cells continue to dominate the connective tissues, and neutrophils continue to dominate the junctional epithelium and gingival crevice.

Gingivitis will progress to periodontitis only in individuals who are susceptible. However, whether periodontitis can occur without a precursor of gingivitis is not known at this time.

REFERENCES

1. Amato R, Caton J, Polson A, et al: Interproximal gingival inflammation related to the conversion of a bleeding to a nonbleeding state, *J Periodontol* 57:63, 1986.
2. Attström R: Studies on neutrophil polymorphonuclear leukocytes at the dento-gingival junction in gingival health and disease, *J Periodontal Res* 8(suppl):1, 1971.
3. Attström R: The roles of gingival epithelium and phagocytosing leukocytes in gingival defense, *J Clin Periodontol* 2:25, 1975.
4. Attström R, Egelberg J: Emigration of blood neutrophils and monocytes into the gingival crevices, *J Periodontal Res* 5:48, 1970.
5. Beutner EH, Triftshauser C, Hazen SP: Collagenase activity of gingival tissue from patients with periodontal disease, *Proc Soc Exp Biol Med* 121:1082, 1966.
6. Brecx MC: Histophysiology and histopathology of the gingiva, *J West Soc Periodontol* 39:33, 1991.
7. Brecx MC, Frohlicher I, Gehr P, et al: Stereological observations on long-term experimental gingivitis in man, *J Clin Periodontol* 15:621, 1988.
8. Brecx MC, Lehmann B, Siegwart CM, et al: Observations on the initial stages of healing following human experimental gingivitis: a clinical and morphometric study, *J Clin Periodontol* 15:123, 1988.
9. Burstone MS: Histochemical study of cytochrome oxidase in normal and inflamed gingiva, *Oral Surg Oral Med Oral Pathol* 13:1501, 1960.
10. Caffesse RG, Nasjleti CE: Enzymatic penetration through intact sulcular epithelium, *J Periodontol* 47:391, 1976.
11. Flieder DE, Sun CN, Schneider BC: Chemistry of normal and inflamed human gingival tissues, *Periodontics* 4:302, 1966.
12. Freedman HL, Listgarten MA, Taichman NS: Electron microscopic features of chronically inflamed human gingiva, *J Periodontal Res* 3:313, 1968.
13. Fullmer HM, Gibson W: Collagenolytic activity in gingivae of man, *Nature* 209:728, 1966.
14. Garant PR, Mulvihill JE: The fine structure of gingivitis in the beagle. III. Plasma cell infiltration of the subepithelial connective tissue. J Periodontal Res 1971; 7:161.

15. Gavin JB: Ultrastructural features of chronic marginal gingivitis, *J Periodontal Res* 5:19, 1970.
16. Hancock EB, Cray RJ, O'Leary TJ: The relationship between gingival crevicular fluid and gingival inflammation: a clinical and histologic study, *J Periodontol* 50:13, 1979.
17. Hanioka T, Shizukuishi S, Tsunemitsu A: Changes in hemoglobin concentration and oxygen saturation in human gingiva with decreasing inflammation, *J Periodontol* 62:366, 1991.
18. Hock J, Nuki K: A vital microscopy study of the morphology of normal and inflamed gingiva, *J Periodontal Res* 6:81, 1971.
19. Kindlova M: Changes in the vascular bed of the marginal periodontium in periodontitis, *J Dent Res* 44:456, 1965.
20. Lamster IB, Hartley LJ, Vogel RI: Development of a biochemical profile for gingival crevicular fluid: methodological considerations and evaluation of collagen-degrading and ground substance–degrading enzyme activity during experimental gingivitis, *J Periodontol* 56:13, 1985.
21. Lamster IB, Vogel RI, Hartley LJ, et al: Lactate dehydrogenase, beta-glucuronidase and arylsulfatase activity in gingival crevicular fluid associated with experimental gingivitis in man, *J Periodontol* 56:139, 1985.
22. Lange D, Schroeder HE: Cytochemistry and ultrastructure of gingival sulcus cells, *Helv Odontol Acta* 15:65, 1971.
23. Lindemann RA, Economou JS: *Actinobacillus actinomycetemcomitans* and *Bacteroides gingivalis* activate human peripheral monocytes to produce interleukin-1 and tumor necrosis factor, *J Periodontol* 59:728, 1988.
24. Levy BM, Taylor AC, Bernick S: Relationship between epithelium and connective tissue in gingival inflammation, *J Dent Res* 48:625, 1969.
25. Lindhe J, Socransky SS: Chemotaxis and vascular permeability produced by human periodontopathic bacteria, *J Periodontal Res* 14:138, 1979.
26. Lindhe J, Hamp SE, Löe H: Experimental periodontitis in the beagle dog, *Int Dent J* 23:432, 1973.
27. Lindhe J, Parodi R, Liljenberg B, et al: Clinical and structural alterations characterizing healing gingiva, *J Periodontal Res* 13:410, 1978.
28. Lindhe J, Schroeder HE, Page RC, et al: Clinical and stereologic analysis of the course of early gingivitis in dogs, *J Periodontal Res* 9:314, 1974.
29. Lisanti VF: Hydrolytic enzymes in periodontal tissues, *Ann NY Acad Sci* 85:461, 1960.
30. Listgarten MA, Ellegaard B: Experimental gingivitis in the monkeys: relationship of leukocyte counts in junctional epithelium, sulcus depth, and connective tissue inflammation scores, *J Periodontal Res* 8:199, 1973.
31. Listgarten MA, Hellden L: Relative distribution of bacteria at clinically healthy and periodontal diseased sites in humans, *J Clin Periodontol* 5:115, 1978.
32. Lovdal A, Arno A, Waerhaug J: Incidence of clinical manifestations of periodontal disease in light of oral hygiene and calculus formation, *J Am Dent Assoc* 56:21, 1958.
33. Mori M, Kishiro A: Histochemical observation of aminopeptidase activity in the normal and inflamed oral epithelium, *J Osaka Univ Dent School* 1:39, 1961.
34. Oliver RC, Holm-Pederen P, Löe H: The correlation between clinical scoring, exudate measurements and microscopic evaluation of inflammation in the gingiva, *J Periodontol* 40:201, 1969.
35. Page RC: The role of inflammatory mediators in the pathogenesis of periodontal disease, *J Periodontal Res* 26:230, 1991.
36. Page RC: Gingivitis, *J Clin Periodontol* 13:345, 1986.
37. Page RC, Schroeder HE: Pathogenesis of inflammatory periodontal disease: a summary of current work, *Lab Invest* 34:235, 1976.
38. Page RC, Schroeder, HE: Pathogenic mechanisms. In Schluger S, Youdelis R, Page RC, editors: *Periodontal disease: basic phenomena, clinical management and restorative interrelationships,* Philadelphia, 1977, Lea & Febiger.
39. Page RC, Schroeder HE: *Periodontitis in man and other animals: a comparative review,* Basel, 1982, S Karger.
40. Page RC, Simpson DM, Ammons WF: Host tissue response in chronic inflammatory periodontal disease. IV. The periodontal and dental status of a group of aged great apes, *J Periodontol* 46:144, 1975.
41. Payne WA, Page RC, Ogilvie AL, et al: Histopathologic features of the initial and early stages of experimental gingivitis in man, *J Periodontal Res* 10:51, 1975.
42. Quintarelli G: Histochemistry of the gingiva. III. The distribution of amino-peptidase in normal and inflammatory conditions, *Arch Oral Biol* 2:271, 1960.
43. Ryder MI: Histological ultrastructural characteristics of the periodontal syndrome in the rice rat. I. General light microscopic observations and ultrastructural observations of initial inflammatory changes, *J Periodontal Res* 15:502, 1980.
44. Saglie R, Newman MG, Carranza FA Jr: Scanning electron microscopy study of leukocytes and their interaction with bacteria in human periodontitis, *J Periodontol* 53:752, 1982.
45. Saglie R, Newman MG, Carranza FA Jr, et al: Bacterial invasion of gingiva in advanced periodontitis in humans, *J Periodontol* 53:217, 1982.
46. Schroeder HE: Transmigration and infiltration of leucocytes in human junctional epithelium, *Helv Odontol Acta* 17:6, 1973.
47. Schroeder HE, Graf-de Beer M, Attström R: Initial gingivitis in dogs, *J Periodontal Res* 10:128, 1975.
48. Schroeder HE, Munzel-Pedrazzoli S, Page RC: Correlated morphometric and biochemical analysis of gingival tissue in early chronic gingivitis in man, *Arch Oral Biol* 18:899, 1973.
49. Schwartz J, Stinson FL, Parker RB: The passage of tritiated bacterial endotoxin across intact gingival crevicular epithelium, *J Periodontol* 43:270, 1972.
50. Seymour GJ, Powell RN, Aitken JF: Experimental gingivitis in humans: a clinical and histological investigation, *J Periodontol* 54:522, 1983.
51. Seymour GJ, Powell RN, Cole KL, et al: Experimental gingivitis in humans: a histochemical and immunological characterization of the lymphoid cell subpopulations, *J Periodontal Res* 18:375, 1983.
52. Simpson DM, Avery BE: Histopathologic and ultrastructural features of inflamed gingiva in the baboon, *J Periodontol* 45:500, 1974.
53. Suomi JD, Smith LW, McClendon BJ: Marginal gingivitis during a sixteen-week period, *J Periodontol* 42:268, 1971.
54. Thilander H: Epithelial changes in gingivitis. an electron microscopic study, *J Periodontal Res* 3:303, 1968.
55. Wennstrom J, Heijl L, Lindhe J, et al: Migration of gingival leukocytes mediated by plaque bacteria, *J Periodontal Res* 15:363, 1980.
56. Winer RA, O'Donnell LJ, Chauncey HH, et al: Enzyme activity in periodontal disease, *J Periodontol* 41:449, 1970.

Clinical Features of Gingivitis

Joseph P. Fiorellini, David M. Kim, and Satoshi O. Ishikawa

22

CHAPTER

■ ■ ■

CHAPTER OUTLINE

COURSE AND DURATION
DESCRIPTION
CLINICAL FINDINGS
 Gingival Bleeding on Probing
 Gingival Bleeding Caused by Local Factors
 Gingival Bleeding Associated with Systemic Factors

Color Changes in the Gingiva
Color Changes Associated with Systemic Factors
Changes in Consistency of the Gingiva
Changes in Surface Texture of the Gingiva
Changes in Position of the Gingiva
Changes in Gingival Contour

Experimental gingivitis studies provided the first empiric evidence that accumulation of microbial biofilm on clean tooth surfaces results in the development of an inflammatory process around gingival tissue.[38,64] Research has also shown that the local inflammation will persist as long as the microbial biofilm is present adjacent to the gingival tissues, and that the inflammation may resolve subsequent to a meticulous removal of the biofilm.[64]

The prevalence of gingivitis is evident worldwide. For example, epidemiologic studies indicate that more than 82% of U.S. adolescents have overt gingivitis and signs of gingival bleeding. A similar or higher prevalence of gingivitis is reported for children and adolescents in other parts of the world.[7] A significant percentage of adults also show signs of gingivitis; more than half the U.S. adult population estimated to exhibit gingival bleeding, and other populations show even higher levels of gingival inflammation.[3,5,6,8,61]

In general, clinical features of gingivitis may be characterized by the presence of any of the following clinical signs: redness and sponginess of the gingival tissue, bleeding on provocation, changes in contour, and presence of calculus or plaque with no radiographic evidence of crestal bone loss.[10] Histologic examination of inflamed gingival tissue reveals ulcerated epithelium. The presence of inflammatory mediators negatively affects epithelial

function as a protective barrier. Repair of this ulcerated epithelium depends on the proliferative or regenerative activity of the epithelial cells. Removal of the etiologic agents triggering the gingival breakdown is essential.

COURSE AND DURATION

Gingivitis can occur with sudden onset and short duration and can be painful. A less severe phase of this condition can also occur.

Recurrent gingivitis reappears after having been eliminated by treatment or disappearing spontaneously.

Chronic gingivitis is slow in onset and of long duration. It is painless, unless complicated by acute or subacute exacerbations, and is the type most often encountered (Figure 22-1). Chronic gingivitis is a fluctuating disease in which inflammation persists or resolves and normal areas become inflamed.[30,34]

DESCRIPTION

Localized gingivitis is confined to the gingiva of a single tooth or group of teeth, whereas *generalized gingivitis* involves the entire mouth. *Marginal gingivitis* involves the gingival margin and may include a portion of the contiguous attached gingiva. *Papillary gingivitis* involves the interdental papillae and often extends into the adjacent

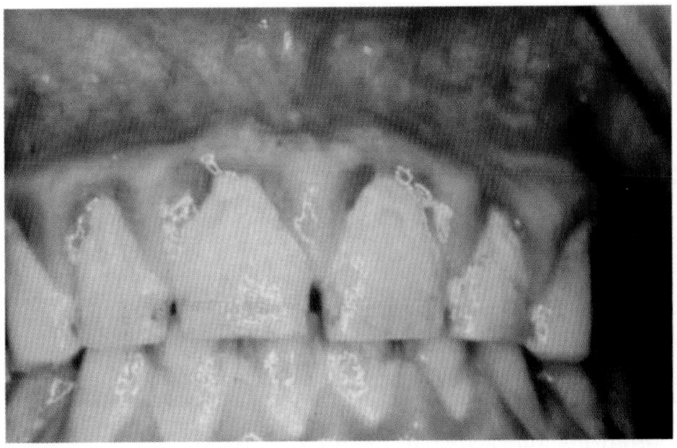

Figure 22-1 Chronic gingivitis. The marginal and interdental gingivae are smooth, edematous, and discolored. Isolated areas of acute response are seen.

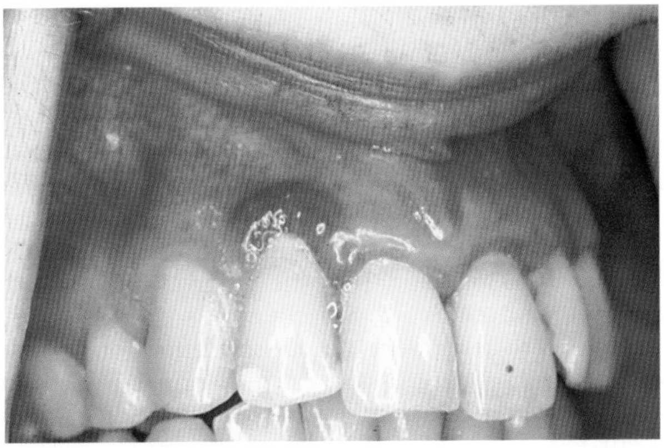

Figure 22-2 Localized, diffuse, intensely red area facial of tooth #7 and dark-pink marginal changes in remaining anterior teeth.

portion of the gingival margin. Papillae are involved more frequently than the gingival margin, and the earliest signs of gingivitis often occur in the papillae. *Diffuse gingivitis* affects the gingival margin, the attached gingiva, and the interdental papillae. Gingival disease in individual cases is described by combining the preceding terms as follows:

- *Localized marginal gingivitis* is confined to one or more areas of the marginal gingiva (Figure 22-2).
- *Localized diffuse gingivitis* extends from the margin to the mucobuccal fold in a limited area (Figure 22-3).
- *Localized papillary gingivitis* is confined to one or more interdental spaces in a limited area (Figure 22-4).
- *Generalized marginal gingivitis* involves the gingival margins in relation to all the teeth. The interdental papillae are usually affected (Figure 22-5).
- *Generalized diffuse gingivitis* involves the entire gingiva. The alveolar mucosa and attached gingiva are affected, so the mucogingival junction is sometimes obliterated (Figure 22-6). Systemic conditions can be involved in the cause of generalized diffuse gingivitis and should be evaluated if suspected as an etiologic cofactor.

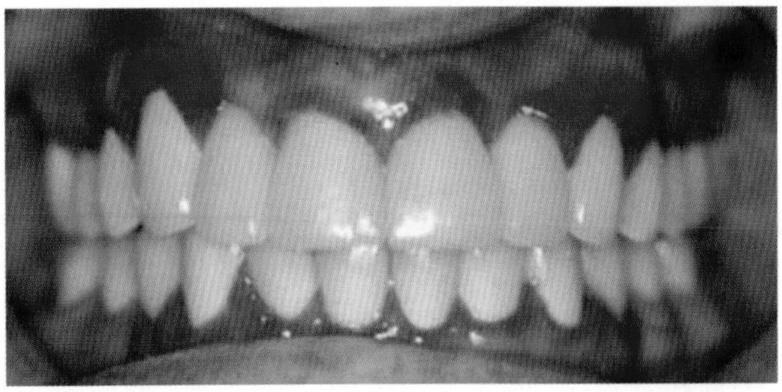

Figure 22-3 Generalized marginal gingivitis in the upper jaw with areas of diffuse gingivitis.

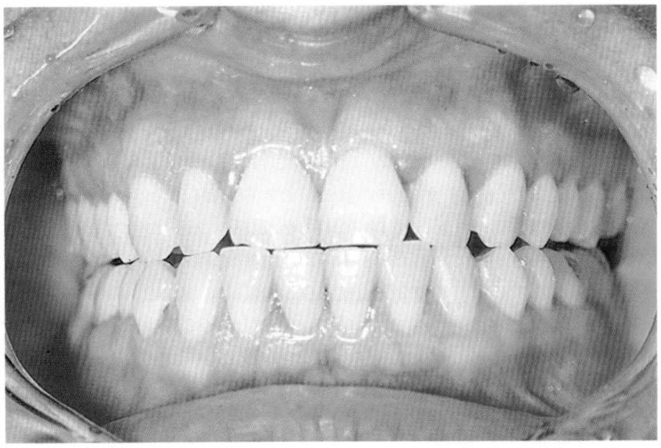

Figure 22-4 Generalized papillary gingivitis.

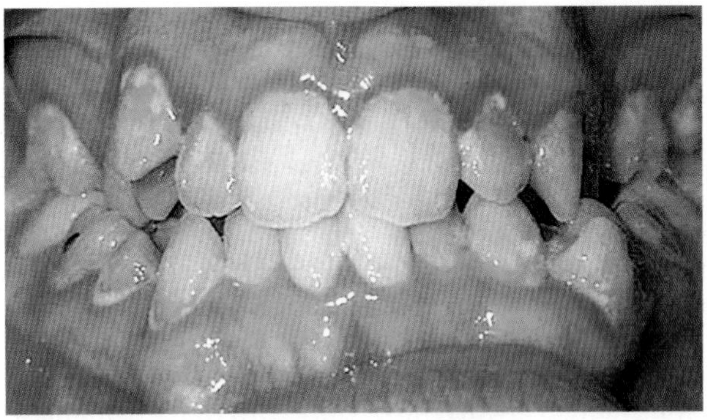

Figure 22-5 Generalized marginal and papillary gingivitis.

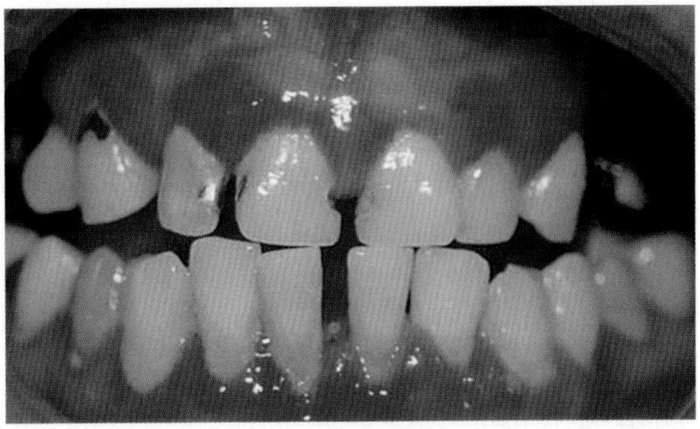

Figure 22-6 Generalized diffuse gingivitis involves the marginal, papillary, and attached gingivae.

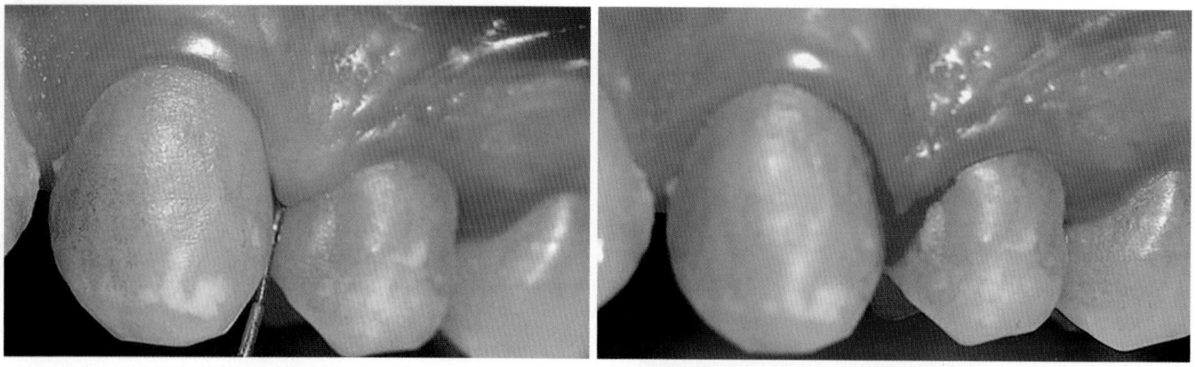

Figure 22-7 Bleeding on probing. **A,** Mild edematous gingivitis; a probe has been introduced to the bottom of the gingival sulcus. **B,** Bleeding appears after a few seconds.

CLINICAL FINDINGS

A *systematic* approach is required in evaluation for the clinical features of gingivitis. The clinician should focus on subtle tissue alterations because these may be of diagnostic significance. A systematic clinical approach requires an orderly examination of the gingiva for color, contour, consistency, position, and ease and severity of bleeding and pain. This section discusses these clinical characteristics and the microscopic changes responsible for each.

Gingival Bleeding on Probing

The two earliest signs of gingival inflammation preceding established gingivitis are (1) increased gingival crevicular fluid production rate and (2) bleeding from the gingival sulcus on gentle probing (Figure 22-7). Chapter 20 discusses gingival crevicular fluid in detail.

Gingival bleeding varies in severity, duration, and ease of provocation. Bleeding on probing is easily detected clinically and therefore is of value for the early diagnosis and prevention of more advanced gingivitis. It has been shown that bleeding on probing appears earlier than a change in color or other visual signs of inflammation[34,35,42]; in addition, the use of bleeding rather than color changes to diagnose early gingival inflammation is advantageous in that bleeding is a more objective sign that requires less subjective estimation by the examiner. For example, it is estimated that 53.2 million (50.3%) of U.S. adults 30 years and older exhibit gingival bleeding.[6] Probing pocket depth measurements by themselves are of limited value for the assessment of the extent and severity of gingivitis. For example, gingival recession may result in reduction of the probing depth and thus cause an inaccurate assessment of the periodontal status.[4] Therefore, bleeding on probing is widely used by clinicians and epidemiologists to measure disease prevalence and progression, to measure outcomes of treatment, and to motivate patients with their home care.[24] Several gingival indices based on bleeding have been developed,[2,16,49] as described in Chapter 8. (For further considerations on probing, see Chapter 35.)

In general, gingival bleeding on probing indicates an inflammatory lesion both in the epithelium and in the connective tissue that exhibits specific histologic differences compared with healthy gingiva.[25] Even though gingival bleeding on probing may not be a good diagnostic indicator for clinical attachment loss, its absence is an excellent negative predictor of future attachment loss.[33] Therefore the absence of gingival bleeding on probing is desirable and implies a low risk of future clinical attachment loss.

Interestingly, numerous studies show that current cigarette smoking suppresses the gingival inflammatory response, and smoking was found to exert a strong, chronic, dose-dependent suppressive effect on gingival bleeding on probing in the third National Health and Nutrition Examination Survey (NHANES III).[19] In addition, recent research reveals an increase in gingival bleeding on probing in patients who quit smoking.[50] Thus, people who are committed to a smoking cessation program should be informed about the possibility of an increase in gingival bleeding associated with smoking cessation.

Gingival Bleeding Caused by Local Factors

Contributing factors to plaque retention that may lead to gingivitis include anatomic and developmental tooth variations, caries, frenum pull, iatrogenic factors, malpositioned teeth, mouth breathing, overhangs, partial dentures, lack of attached gingiva, and recession.[72]

Chronic and Recurrent Bleeding. The most common cause of abnormal gingival bleeding on probing is chronic inflammation.[46] The bleeding is chronic or recurrent and is provoked by mechanical trauma (e.g., from toothbrushing, toothpicks, or food impaction) or by biting into solid foods such as apples.

In gingival inflammation, histopathologic alterations that result in abnormal gingival bleeding include dilation and engorgement of the capillaries and thinning or ulceration of the sulcular epithelium (Figure 22-8). Because the capillaries are engorged and closer to the surface, and the thinned, degenerated epithelium is less protective, stimuli that are normally innocuous cause rupture of the capillaries and gingival bleeding.

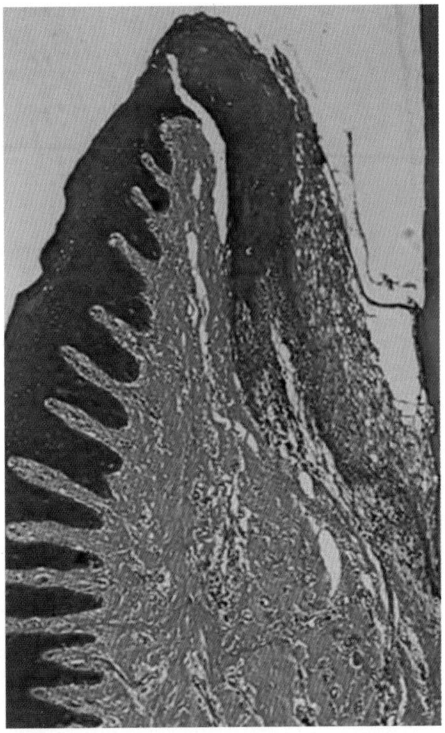

Figure 22-8 Microscopic view of interdental space in a human autopsy specimen. Note inflammatory infiltrate and thinned epithelium in area adjacent to the tooth, as well as collagenous tissue in outer half of the section.

Sites that bleed on probing have a greater area of inflamed connective tissue (i.e., cell-rich, collagen-poor tissue) than sites that do not bleed. In most cases the cellular infiltrate of sites that bleed on probing is predominantly lymphocytic (a characteristic of stage II, or early, gingivitis).[9,17,25]

The severity of the bleeding and the ease of its provocation depend on the intensity of the inflammation. After the vessels are damaged and ruptured, interrelated mechanisms induce hemostasis.[67] The vessel walls contract, and blood flow is diminished; blood platelets adhere to the edges of the tissue; and a fibrous clot is formed, which contracts and results in approximation of the edges of the injured area. Bleeding recurs when the area is irritated.

In cases of moderate or advanced periodontitis, the presence of bleeding on probing is considered a sign of active tissue destruction (see Chapter 27).

Acute episodes of gingival bleeding are caused by injury and can occur spontaneously in gingival disease. Laceration of the gingiva by toothbrush bristles during aggressive toothbrushing or by sharp pieces of hard food can cause gingival bleeding even in the absence of gingival disease. Gingival burns from hot foods or chemicals increase the ease of gingival bleeding.

Spontaneous bleeding or bleeding on slight provocation can occur in acute necrotizing ulcerative gingivitis. In this condition, engorged blood vessels in the inflamed connective tissue are exposed by ulceration of the necrotic surface epithelium.

SCIENCE TRANSFER

Gingival bleeding on probing is an important diagnostic factor for clinicians to use in planning periodontal therapy. It is associated with inflammation and ulceration of the epithelium lining the gingival sulcus. The presence of plaque for only 2 days can initiate gingival bleeding on probing, whereas once established, it may take 7 days or more after continued plaque control and treatment to eliminate gingival bleeding. Thus the absence of plaque and the presence of gingival bleeding may indicate improvement in plaque control that may have occurred immediately before the examination. *The presence of bleeding is an indication of active gingival inflammation, and until it is controlled, the patient is at a risk of continuing periodontal disease and tissue destruction.*

Gingival Bleeding Associated with Systemic Changes

In some systemic disorders, gingival hemorrhage occurs spontaneously or after irritation and is excessive and difficult to control. These hemorrhagic diseases represent a wide variety of conditions that vary in etiologic factors and clinical manifestations. Such conditions have the common feature of a hemostatic mechanism failure and result in abnormal bleeding in the skin, internal organs, and other tissues, including the oral mucosa.[65]

Hemorrhagic disorders in which abnormal gingival bleeding is encountered include vascular abnormalities (vitamin C deficiency or allergy, e.g., Schönlein-Henoch purpura), platelet disorders[27] (thrombocytopenic purpura), hypoprothrombinemia (vitamin K deficiency), other coagulation defects (hemophilia, leukemia, Christmas disease), deficient platelet thromboplastic factor (PF3) resulting from uremia,[43] multiple myeloma[12] and postrubella purpura.[30]

The effects of hormonal replacement therapy, oral contraceptives, pregnancy, and the menstrual cycle are also reported to affect gingival bleeding.[39,60,73,74] In addition, changes in androgenic hormones have long been established as significant modifying factors in gingivitis, especially among adolescents. Several reports have shown notable effects of fluctuating estrogen/progesterone levels on the periodontium, starting as early as puberty.[1,51] Among pathologic endocrine changes, diabetes is an endocrine condition with a well-characterized effect on gingivitis.[72]

Several medications have also been found to have adverse effects on the gingiva. For example, anticonvulsants, antihypertensive calcium channel blockers, and the immunosuppressant drugs are known to cause gingival enlargement, which secondarily can cause gingival bleeding. The American Heart Association has recommended over-the-counter aspirin as a therapeutic agent for cardiovascular disease, and aspirin is often prescribed for rheumatoid arthritis, osteoarthritis, rheumatic fever, and other inflammatory joint diseases.[28] Thus it is important to consider aspirin's effect on bleeding during a routine dental examination to avoid false-positive readings, which could result in an inaccurate patient diagnosis.[62] (Chapter 17 discusses periodontal involvement in hematologic disorders.)

Color Changes in the Gingiva

The color of the gingiva is determined by several factors, including the number and size of blood vessels, epithelial thickness, quantity of keratinization, and pigments within the epithelium.[70]

Color Changes in Gingivitis. *Change in color is an important clinical sign of gingival disease.* The normal gingival color is "coral pink" and is produced by the tissue's vascularity and modified by the overlying epithelial layers. For this reason, the gingiva becomes red when vascularization increases or the degree of epithelial keratinization is reduced or disappears. The color becomes pale when vascularization is reduced (in association with fibrosis of the corium) or epithelial keratinization increases.

Thus, chronic inflammation intensifies the red or bluish red color because of vascular proliferation and reduction of keratinization. Additionally, venous stasis will contribute a bluish hue. The gingival color changes with increasing chronicity of the inflammatory process. The changes start in the interdental papillae and gingival margin and spread to the attached gingiva (see Figure 22-1). Proper diagnosis and treatment require an understanding of the tissue changes that alter the color of the gingiva at the clinical level.

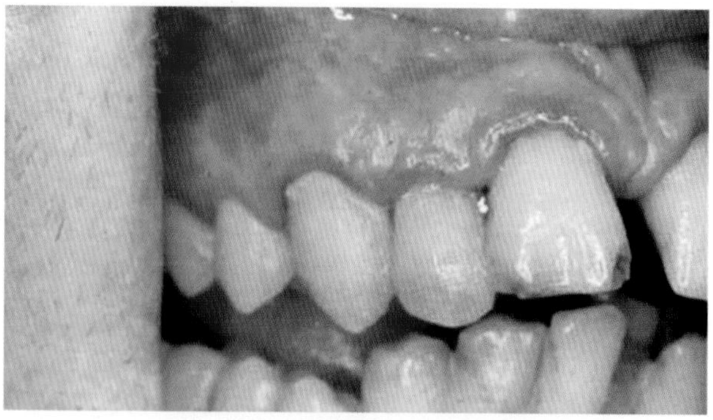

Figure 22-9 Bismuth gingivitis. Note linear black discoloration of the gingiva in a patient receiving bismuth therapy.

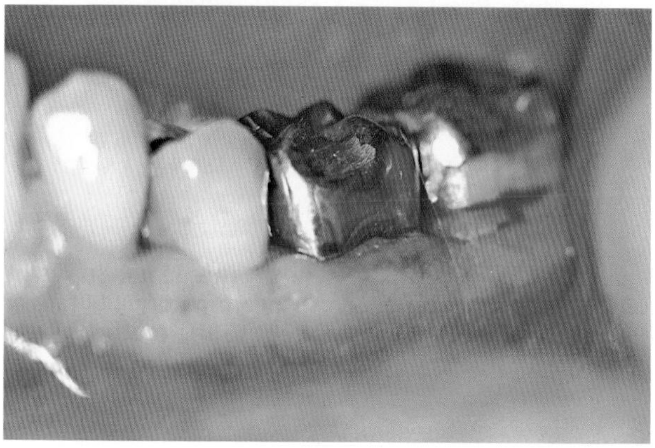

Figure 22-10 Discoloration of the gingiva caused by embedded metal particles (amalgam).

Color changes in acute gingival inflammation differ in both nature and distribution from those in chronic gingivitis. The color changes may be marginal, diffuse, or patchlike, depending on the underlying acute condition. In acute necrotizing ulcerative gingivitis, the involvement is marginal; in herpetic gingivostomatitis, it is diffuse; and in acute reactions to chemical irritation, it is patchlike or diffuse.

Color changes vary with the intensity of the inflammation. Initially, there is an increase in erythema. If the condition does not worsen, this is the only color change until the gingiva reverts to normal. In severe acute inflammation, the red color gradually becomes a dull, whitish gray. The gray discoloration produced by tissue necrosis is demarcated from the adjacent gingiva by a thin, sharply defined erythematous zone. Chapter 24 provides detailed descriptions of the clinical and pathologic features of the various forms of acute gingivitis.

Metallic Pigmentation. Heavy metals (bismuth, arsenic, mercury, lead and silver) absorbed systemically from therapeutic use or occupational or household environments may discolor the gingiva and other areas of the oral mucosa.[41] These changes are rare but still should be ruled out in suspected cases.

Typically, metals produce a black or bluish line in the gingiva that follows the contour of the margin (Figure 22-9). The pigmentation may also appear as isolated black blotches involving the interdental marginal and attached gingiva. This differs from the tattooing produced by the accidental embedding of amalgam or other metal fragments[15] (Figure 22-10).

Gingival pigmentation from systemically absorbed metals results from perivascular precipitation of metallic sulfides in the subepithelial connective tissue. Gingival pigmentation is not a result of systemic toxicity. It occurs only in areas of inflammation, where the increased permeability of irritated blood vessels permits seepage of the metal into the surrounding tissue. In addition to inflamed gingiva, mucosal areas irritated by biting or abnormal chewing habits (e.g., inner surface of lips, cheek at level of occlusal line, lateral border of tongue) are common sites of pigmentation. Pigmentation can be eliminated by treating the inflammatory changes without necessarily discontinuing the metal-containing medication.

Color Changes Associated with Systemic Factors

Many systemic diseases may cause color changes in the oral mucosa, including the gingiva.[22] In general, these abnormal pigmentations are nonspecific and should stimulate further diagnostic efforts or referral to the appropriate specialist.[63]

Endogenous oral pigmentations can be caused by melanin, bilirubin, or iron.[41] *Melanin* oral pigmentations can be normal physiologic pigmentations and are often found in highly pigmented ethnic groups (see Chapter 4). Diseases that increase melanin pigmentation include the following:

- *Addison's disease* is caused by adrenal dysfunction and produces isolated patches of discoloration varying from bluish black to brown.
- *Peutz-Jeghers syndrome* produces intestinal polyposis and melanin pigmentation in the oral mucosa and lips.
- *Albright's syndrome (polyostotic fibrous dysplasia)* and *von Recklinghausen's disease* (neurofibromatosis) produce areas of oral melanin pigmentation.

Skin and mucous membranes can also be stained by *bile pigments*. Jaundice is best detected by examination of the sclera, but the oral mucosa may also acquire a yellowish color. The deposition of *iron* in hemochromatosis may produce a blue-gray pigmentation of the oral mucosa. Several endocrine and metabolic disturbances, including diabetes and pregnancy, may result in color changes. Blood dyscrasias such as anemia, polycythemia, and leukemia may also induce color changes.

Exogenous factors capable of producing color changes in the gingiva include atmospheric irritants, such as coal and metal dust, and coloring agents in food or lozenges. Tobacco causes hyperkeratosis of the gingiva and also may induce a significant increase in melanin pigmentation of the oral mucosa.[52] Localized bluish black areas of pigment are often caused by amalgam implanted in the mucosa (see Figure 22-10).

In recent years the need for esthetics in dentistry has increased, with a growing demand for a pleasing smile. This has made many individuals more aware of their gingival pigmentation that may be apparent during smiling and speech.[20,21] Traditionally, gingival depigmentation has been carried out using nonsurgical and surgical procedures, such as chemical, cryosurgical, and electrosurgical techniques. However, those techniques were met with skepticism because of varying degrees of success. More recently, lasers have been used to ablate cells producing the melanin pigment; a nonspecific laser beam destroys the epithelial cells, including those at the basal layer. In addition, selective ablation using a laser beam with a wavelength that is specifically absorbed in melanin effectively destroys the pigmented cells without damaging the nonpigmented cells. In both cases, radiation energy is transformed into ablation energy, resulting in cellular rupture and vaporization with minimal heating of the surrounding tissue.[70]

Changes in Consistency of the Gingiva

Both chronic and acute inflammations produce changes in the normal firm and resilient consistency of the gingiva. As previously noted, in chronic gingivitis, both destructive (edematous) and reparative (fibrotic) changes

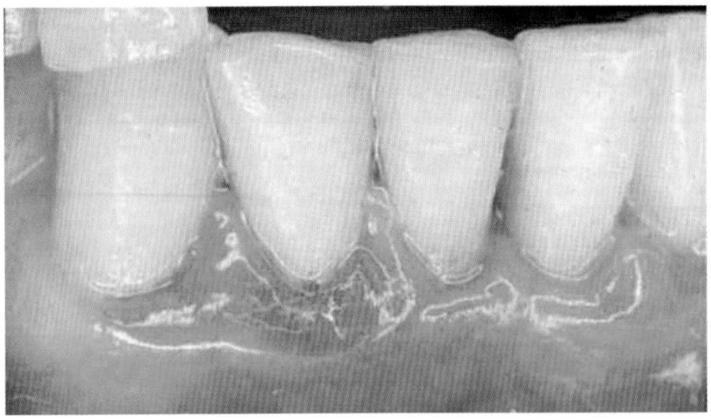

Figure 22-11 Chronic gingivitis. Swelling, loss of stippling, and discoloration occur when inflammatory exudate and edema are the predominant microscopic changes. The gingiva is soft and friable and bleeds easily.

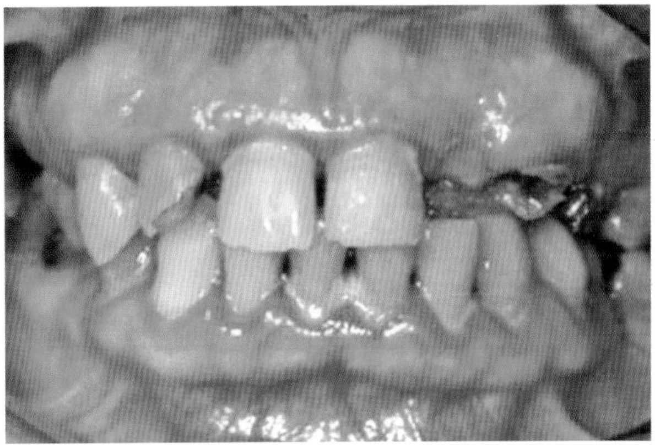

Figure 22-12 Chronic gingivitis. Firm gingiva is produced when fibrosis predominates in the inflammatory process.

coexist, and the consistency of the gingiva is determined by their relative predominance (Figures 22-11 and 22-12). Table 22-1 summarizes the clinical alterations in the consistency of the gingiva and the microscopic changes that produce them.

Calcified Masses in the Gingiva. Calcified microscopic masses may be found in the gingiva.[14,48] They can occur alone or in groups and vary in size, location, shape, and structure. Such masses may be calcified material removed from the tooth and traumatically displaced into the gingiva during scaling,[48] root remnants, cementum fragments, or cementicles (Figure 22-13). Chronic inflammation and fibrosis, and occasionally foreign body, giant cell activity, occur in relation to these masses. They are sometimes enclosed in an osteoid-like matrix. Crystalline foreign bodies have also been described in the gingiva, but their origin has not been determined.[55]

Toothbrushing. Toothbrushing has various effects on the consistency of the gingiva, such as promoting keratinization of the oral epithelium, enhancing capillary gingival circulation, and thickening alveolar bone.[40,45,71] In animal studies, mechanical stimulation by toothbrushing was found to increase the proliferative activity

TABLE 22-1

Clinical and Histopathologic Changes in Gingival Consistency

Clinical Changes	Underlying Microscopic Features
Chronic Gingivitis	
1. Soggy puffiness that pits on pressure.	1. Infiltration by fluid and cells of inflammatory exudate.
2. Marked softness and friability, with ready fragmentation on exploration with probe and pinpoint surface areas of redness and desquamation.	2. Degeneration of connective tissue and epithelium associated with injurious substances that provoke the inflammation and inflammatory exudate; change in connective tissue–epithelium relationship, with inflamed, engorged connective tissue expanding to within a few epithelial cells of surface, thinning of epithelium and degeneration associated with edema and leukocyte invasion, separated by areas in which rete pegs are elongated to connective tissue.
3. Firm, leathery consistency.	3. Fibrosis and epithelial proliferation associated with long-standing chronic inflammation.
Acute Forms of Gingivitis	
1. Diffuse puffiness and softening.	1. Diffuse edema of acute inflammatory origin, fatty infiltration in xanthomatosis.
2. Sloughing with grayish, flakelike particles of debris adhering to eroded surface.	2. Necrosis with formation of pseudomembrane composed of bacteria, polymorphonuclear leukocytes, and degenerated epithelial cells in fibrinous meshwork.
3. Vesicle formation.	3. Intercellular and intracellular edema with degeneration of nucleus and cytoplasm and rupture of cell wall.

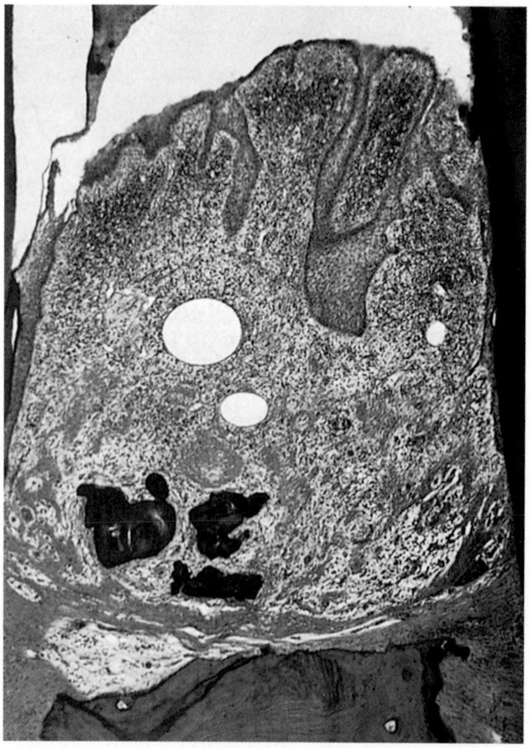

Figure 22-13 Cementicles found in a gingival human specimen; these are asymptomatic.

of the junctional basal cells in dog gingiva by 2.5 times compared with using a scaler.[31] These findings may indicate that toothbrushing causes an increased turnover rate and desquamation of the junctional epithelial surfaces. This process may repair small breaks in the junctional epithelium and prevent direct access to the underlying tissue by periodontal pathogen.[75]

Changes in Surface Texture of the Gingiva

The surface of normal gingiva usually exhibits numerous small depressions and elevations, giving the tissue an orange-peel appearance referred as *stippling*.[13] Stippling is restricted to the attached gingiva and is predominantly localized to the subpapillary area, but it extends to a variable degree into the interdental papilla.[56] Although the biologic significance of gingival stippling is not known, some investigators conclude that loss of stippling is an early sign of gingivitis.[32,56] However, clinicians must take into consideration that its pattern and extent vary in different mouth areas, among patients, and with age.

In chronic inflammation the gingival surface is either smooth and shiny or firm and nodular, depending on whether the dominant changes are exudative or fibrotic. Smooth surface texture is also produced by epithelial atrophy in atrophic gingivitis, and peeling of the surface occurs in chronic desquamative gingivitis. Hyperkeratosis results in a leathery texture, and drug-induced gingival overgrowth produces a nodular surface.

Changes in Position of the Gingiva

Traumatic Lesions. One of the unique features of the most recent gingival disease classification is the recognition of non–plaque-induced traumatic gingival lesions as distinct gingival conditions.[11] Traumatic lesions, whether chemical, physical, or thermal, are among the most common lesions in the mouth. Sources of chemical injuries include aspirin, hydrogen peroxide, silver nitrate, phenol, and endodontic materials. Physical injuries can include lip, oral, and tongue piercing, which can result in gingival recession. Thermal injuries can result from hot drinks and foods. In acute cases, the appearance of slough (necrotizing epithelium), erosion, or ulceration and the accompanying erythema are common features. In chronic cases, permanent gingival defects are usually present in the form of gingival recession. Typically, the localized nature of the lesions and the lack of symptoms readily eliminate them from the differential diagnosis of systemic conditions that may be present with erosive or ulcerative oral lesions.[59]

Gingival Recession. Gingival recession is a common finding. The prevalence, extent, and severity of gingival recession increase with age and are more prevalent in males.[6]

Positions of the Gingiva. By clinical definition, *recession* is exposure of the root surface by an apical shift in the position of the gingiva. To understand recession, it helps to distinguish between the actual and apparent positions of the gingiva. The *actual position* is the level of the epithelial attachment on the tooth, whereas the *apparent position* is the level of the crest of the gingival margin (Figure 22-14). *The severity of recession is determined by the* actual position *of the gingiva, not its apparent position.* For example, in periodontal disease, the inflamed pocket wall covers part of the denuded root; thus some of the recession is hidden, and some may be visible. The total amount of recession is the sum of the two.

Recession refers to the location of the gingiva, not its condition. Receded gingiva can be inflamed but may be normal except for its position (Figure 22-15). Recession may be localized to one tooth or a group of teeth, or it may be generalized throughout the mouth.

Etiologic Factors. Gingival recession increases with age; the incidence varies from 8% in children to 100% after age 50 years.[77] This has led some investigators to assume that recession may be a physiologic process related to aging. However, no convincing evidence has been presented for a physiologic shift of the gingival attachment.[36] The gradual apical shift is most likely the result of the cumulative effect of minor pathologic involvement and repeated minor direct trauma to the gingiva. In some populations without access to dental care, however, recession may be the result of increasing periodontal disease.[29,37]

The following etiologic factors have been implicated in gingival recession: faulty toothbrushing technique (gingival abrasion), tooth malposition, friction from soft tissues (gingival ablation),[66] gingival inflammation, abnormal frenum attachment, and iatrogenic dentistry. Trauma from occlusion has been suggested in the past, but its mechanism of action has never been demonstrated. For example, a deep overbite has been associated with gingival inflammation and recession. Excessive incisal overlap may result in a traumatic injury to the gingiva. Orthodontic movement in a labial direction in monkeys has been shown to result in loss of marginal bone and connective tissue attachment, as well as in gingival recession.[68]

Standard oral hygiene procedures, whether toothbrushing or flossing, may lead to a frequent transient and minimal gingival injury.[18,57] Although toothbrushing is important for gingival health, faulty toothbrushing technique or brushing with hard bristles may cause significant injury. This type of injury may present as lacerations, abrasions, keratosis and recession, with the facial marginal gingiva most affected.[59] Thus, in these cases, recession tends to be more frequent and severe in patients with clinically healthy gingiva, little bacterial plaque, and good oral hygiene.[23,53,54]

Susceptibility to recession is also influenced by the position of teeth in the arch,[76] the root-bone angle, and

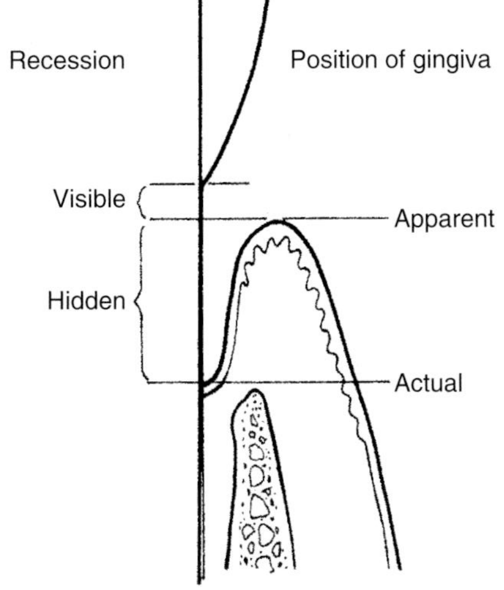

Figure 22-14 Diagram of apparent and actual positions of the gingiva and visible and hidden recession.

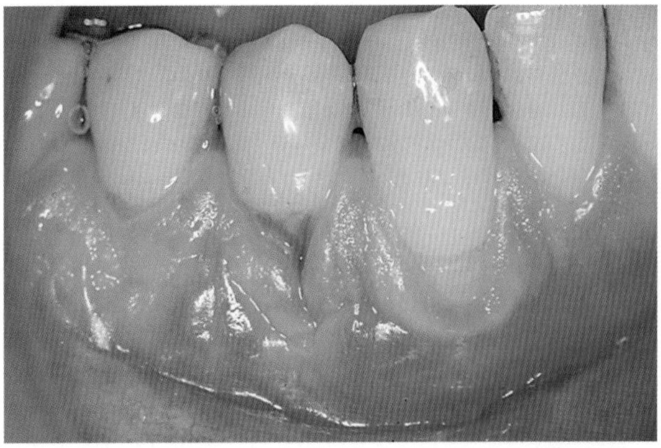

Figure 22-15 Different degrees of recession. Recession is slight in teeth #26 and #29 and marked in #27 and #28. The change in gingival contour and the recession, as seen in tooth #28, are referred to as Stillman's clefts.

the mesiodistal curvature of the tooth surface.[47] On rotated, tilted, or facially displaced teeth, the bony plate is thinned or reduced in height. Pressure from mastication or moderate toothbrushing damages the unsupported gingiva and produces recession. The effect of the angle of the root in the bone on recession is often observed in the maxillary molar area. If the lingual inclination of the palatal root is prominent or the buccal roots flare outward, the bone in the cervical area is thinned or shortened, and recession results from repeated trauma of the thin, marginal gingiva.

The health of the gingival tissue also depends on properly designed and placed restorative materials. Pressure from a poorly designed partial denture, such as ill-fitting denture clasp, can cause gingival trauma and recession.[78] Overhanging dental restorations have long been viewed as a contributing factor to gingivitis because of plaque retention. In addition, there is general agreement that placing restorative margins within the biologic width frequently leads to gingival inflammation, clinical attachment loss, and eventually, bone loss. Clinically, the violation of biologic width typically manifests as gingival inflammation, deepened periodontal pockets, or gingival recession.

A relationship may exist between smoking and gingival recession (see Chapter 14). The multifactorial mechanisms may include reduced gingival blood flow and altered immune response but are not, as yet, conclusive.[26,58]

Clinical Significance. Several aspects of gingival recession make it clinically significant. Exposed root surfaces are susceptible to caries. Abrasion or erosion of the cementum exposed by recession leaves an underlying dentinal surface that can be sensitive. Hyperemia of the pulp and associated symptoms may also result from excessive exposure of the root surface.[44] Interproximal recession creates oral hygiene problems and resulting plaque accumulation.

Changes in Gingival Contour

Changes in gingival contour are primarily associated with gingival enlargement (see Chapter 23), but such changes may also occur in other conditions.

Of historical interest are the descriptions of indentations of the gingival margin referred to as *Stillman's clefts* (see Figure 22-15)[69] and the *McCall festoons.* The term "Stillman's clefts" has been used to describe a specific type of gingival recession consisting of a narrow, triangular-shaped gingival recession. As the recession progresses apically, the cleft becomes broader, exposing the cementum of the root surface. When the lesion reaches the mucogingival junction, the apical border of oral mucosa is usually inflamed because of the difficulty in maintaining adequate plaque control at this site. The term "McCall festoons" has been used to describe a rolled, thickened band of gingiva usually seen adjacent to the cuspids when recession approaches the mucogingival junction. Initially, Stillman's clefts and McCall festoons were attributed to traumatic occlusion, and the recommended treatment was occlusal adjustment. However, this association was never proved, and these indentations merely represent peculiar inflammatory changes of the marginal gingiva.[14]

REFERENCES

1. Addy M, Hunter ML, Kingdon A, et al: An 8-year study of changes in oral hygiene and periodontal health during adolescence, *Int J Paediatr Dent* 4:75, 1994.
2. Ainamo J, Bay I: Problems and proposals for recording gingivitis and plaque, *Int Dent J* 25:229, 1975.
3. Albandar JM: Periodontal diseases in North America, *Periodontol 2000* 29:31, 2002.
4. Albandar JM, Rams TE: Global epidemiology of periodontal diseases: an overview, *Periodontol 2000* 29:7, 2002.
5. Albandar JM, Tinoco EM: Global epidemiology of periodontal diseases in children and young persons, *Periodontol 2000* 29:153, 2002.
6. Albandar JM, Brunelle JA, Kingman A: Destructive periodontal disease in adults 30 years of age and older in the United States, 1988-1994, *J Periodontol* 70:13, 1999.
7. Albandar JM, Brown LJ, Brunelle JA, et al: Gingival state and dental calculus in early-onset periodontitis, *J Periodontol* 67:953, 1996.
8. Albandar JM, Kingman A, Brown LJ, et al: Gingival inflammation and subgingival calculus as determinants of disease progression in early-onset periodontitis, *J Clin Periodontol* 25:231, 1998.
9. Amato R, Caton J, Polson A, et al: Interproximal gingival inflammation related to the conversion of a bleeding to a nonbleeding state, *J Periodontol* 57:63, 1986.
10. American Academy of Periodontology: Parameter on plaque-induced gingivitis, *J Periodontol* 71:851, 2000.
11. Armitage GC: Development of a classification system for periodontal diseases and conditions, *Ann Periodontol* 4:1, 1999.
12. Bennett JH, Shankar S: Gingival bleeding as the presenting feature of multiple myeloma, *Br Dent J* 157:101, 1984.
13. Bergström J: The topography of papillary gingiva in health and early gingivitis, *J Clin Periodontol* 11:423, 1984.
14. Box HK: Gingival clefts and associated tracts, *NY State Dent J* 16:3, 1950.
15. Buchner A, Hansen LS: Amalgam pigmentation (amalgam tattoo) of the oral mucosa: a clinicopathologic study of 268 cases, *Oral Surg Oral Med Oral Pathol* 49:139, 1980.
16. Carter HG, Barnes GP: The gingival bleeding index, *J Periodontol* 45:801, 1974.
17. Cooper PG, Caton JG, Polson AM: Cell populations associated with gingival bleeding, *J Periodontol* 54:497, 1983.
18. Danser MM, Timmerman MF, IJzerman Y, et al: Evaluation of the incidence of gingival abrasion as a result of toothbrushing, *J Clin Periodontol* 25:701, 1998.
19. Dietrich T, Bernimoulin JP, Glynn RJ: The effect of cigarette smoking on gingival bleeding, *J Periodontol* 75:16, 2004.
20. Dummett CO: Oral pigmentation: first symposium on oral pigmentation, *J Periodontol* 31:356, 1960.
21. Dummett CO: Overview of normal oral pigmentations, *Ala J Med Sci* 16:262, 1979.
22. Dummett CO: Oral tissue color changes, *Ala J Med Sci* 16:274, 1979.
23. Gorman WJ: Prevalence and etiology of gingival recession, *J Periodontol* 38:316, 1967.
24. Greenstein G: The role of bleeding upon probing in the diagnosis of periodontal disease: a literature review, *J Periodontol* 55:684, 1984.
25. Greenstein G, Caton J, Polson AM: Histologic characteristics associated with bleeding after probing and visual signs of inflammation, *J Periodontol* 52:420, 1981.

26. Gunsolley JC, Quinn SM, Tew J, et al: The effect of smoking on individuals with minimal periodontal destruction, *J Periodontol* 69:165, 1998.
27. Haeb HP: Postrubella thrombocytopenic purpura: a report of eight cases with discussion of hemorrhagic manifestations of rubella, *Clin Pediatr* 7:350, 1968.
28. Hennekens CH, Dyken ML, Fuster V: Aspirin as a therapeutic agent in cardiovascular disease: a statement for healthcare professionals from the American Heart Association, *Circulation* 96:2751, 1997.
29. Hirschfeld I: A study of skulls in the American Museum of Natural History in relation to periodontal disease, *J Dent Res* 5:241, 1923.
30. Hoover DR, Lefkowitz W: Fluctuation in marginal gingivitis, *J Periodontol* 36:310, 1965.
31. Horiuchi M, Yamamoto T, Tomofuji T, et al: Toothbrushing promotes gingival fibroblast proliferation more effectively than removal of dental plaque, *J Clin Periodontol* 29:791, 2002.
32. King JD: Gingival disease in Dundee, *Dent Rec* 56:9, 1945.
33. Lang NP, Adler R, Joss A, et al: Absence of bleeding upon probing: an indicator of periodontal stability, *J Clin Periodontol* 17:714, 1990.
34. Larato DC, Stahl SS, Brown R Jr, et al: The effect of a prescribed method of toothbrushing on the fluctuation of marginal gingivitis, *J Periodontol* 40:142, 1969.
35. Lenox JA, Kopczyk RA: A clinical system for scoring a patient's oral hygiene performance, *J Am Dent Assoc* 86:849, 1973.
36. Löe H: The structure and physiology of the dentogingival junction. In Miles AE, editor: *Structural and chemical organization of teeth,* vol 2, New York, 1967, Academic Press.
37. Löe H, Anerud A, Boysen H: The natural history of periodontal disease in man: prevalence, severity and extent of gingival recession, *J Periodontol* 63:489, 1992.
38. Löe H, Theilade E, Jensen SB: Experimental gingivitis in man, *J Periodontol* 36:177, 1965.
39. Machtei EE, Mahler D, Sanduri H, et al: The effect of menstrual cycle on periodontal health, *J Periodontol* 75:408, 2004.
40. Mackenzie IC: Does toothbrushing affect gingival keratinization? *Proc R Soc Med* 65:1127, 1972.
41. McCarthy FP, Shklar G: *Diseases of the oral mucosa,* New York, 1964, McGraw-Hill.
42. Meitner SW, Zander H, Iker HP, et al: Identification of inflamed gingival surfaces, *J Clin Periodontol* 6:93, 1979.
43. Merril A, Peterson LJ: Gingival hemorrhage secondary to uremia: review and report of a case, *Oral Surg Oral Med Oral Pathol* 29:530, 1970.
44. Merritt AA: Hyperemia of the dental pulp caused by gingival recession, *J Periodontol* 4:30, 1933.
45. Miake K, Agematsu H, Fukayama M, et al: An experimental study on histological changes occurring in rat-incisor alveolar bone during toothbrushing. In Ishikawa J, Kawasaki H, Ikeda K, et al, editors: *Recent advances in clinical periodontology,* Amsterdam, 1988, Elsevier.
46. Milne AM: Gingival bleeding in 848 army recruits: an assessment, *Br Dent J* 122:111, 1967.
47. Morris ML: The position of the margin of the gingiva, *J Oral Surg* 11:969, 1958.
48. Moskow BS: Calcified material in human gingival tissue, *J Dent Res* 40:644, 1961.
49. Muhlemann HR, Son S: Gingival sulcus bleeding: a leading symptom in initial gingivitis, *Helv Odontol Acta* 15:107, 1971.
50. Nair P, Sutherland G, Palmer RM, et al: Gingival bleeding on probing increases after quitting smoking, *J Clin Periodontol* 30:435, 2003.
51. Nakagawa S, Fujii H, Machida Y, et al: A longitudinal study from prepuberty to puberty of gingivitis: correlation between the occurrence of *Prevotella intermedia* and sex hormones, *J Clin Periodontol* 21:658, 1994.
52. Neville BW, Damm DD, Allen CM, et al: *Oral and maxillofacial pathology,* Philadelphia, 1995, Saunders.
53. O'Leary TJ, Drake RB, Crump PP, et al: The incidence of recession in young males: further study, *J Periodontol* 42:264, 1971.
54. O'Leary TJ, Drake RV, Jividen GJ, et al: The incidence of recession in young males: relationship to gingival and plaque scores, SAM-TR-67-97, *Tech Rep* SAM-TR, 1967, p 1.
55. Orban B: Gingival inclusions, *J Periodontol* 16:16, 1945.
56. Orban B: Clinical and histological study of the surface characteristics of the gingiva, *Oral Surg Oral Med Oral Pathol Oral Radiol Endod* 1:827, 1948.
57. Pearlman BA: A mistaken health belief resulting in gingival injury: a case report, *J Periodontol* 65:284, 1994.
58. Preber H, Bergstrom J: Occurrence of gingival bleeding in smokers and non-smoker patients, *Acta Odontol Scand* 43:315, 1985.
59. Rawal SY, Claman LJ, Kalmar JR, et al: Traumatic lesions of the gingiva: a case series, *J Periodontol* 75:762, 2004.
60. Reinhardt RA, Payne JB, Maze CA, et al: Influence of estrogen and osteopenia/osteoporosis on clinical periodontitis in postmenopausal women, *J Periodontol* 70:823, 1999.
61. Rose G: *The strategy of preventive medicine,* Oxford, 1992, Oxford University Press.
62. Royzman D, Recio L, Badovinac RL, et al: The effect of aspirin intake on bleeding on probing in patients with gingivitis, *J Periodontol* 75:679, 2004.
63. Shklar G, McCarthy PL: *The oral manifestations of systemic disease,* Boston, 1976, Butterworth.
64. Silness J, Löe H: Periodontal disease in pregnancy. II. Correlation between oral hygiene and periodontal condition, *Acta Odontol Scand* 22:121, 1964.
65. Sodeman WA Jr, Sodeman WA: *Pathologic physiology: mechanisms of disease,* ed 7, Philadelphia, 1985, Saunders.
66. Sognnaes RF: Periodontal significance of intraoral frictional ablation. *J West Soc Periodontol Periodontal Abstr* 25:112, 1977.
67. Stefanini M, Dameshek W: *The hemorrhagic disorders,* ed 2, New York, 1962, Grune & Stratton.
68. Steiner GG, Pearson JK, Ainamo J: Changes of the marginal periodontium as a result of labial tooth movement in monkeys, *J Periodontol* 52:314, 1981.
69. Stillman PR: Early clinical evidences of disease in the gingiva and pericementum, *J Dent Res* 3:25, 1921.
70. Tal H, Oegiesser D, Tal M: Gingival depigmentation by erbium:YAG laser: clinical observations and patient responses, *J Periodontol* 74:1660, 2003.
71. Tanaka M, Hanioka T, Kishimoto M, et al: Effect of mechanical toothbrush stimulation on microcirculatory functions in inflamed gingiva of dogs, *J Clin Periodontol* 25:561, 1998.
72. Tatakis DN, Trombelli L: Modulation of clinical expression of plaque-induced gingivitis. I. Background review and rationale, *J Clin Periodontol* 31:229, 2004.
73. Tilakaratne A, Soory M, Ranasinghe AW, et al: Effects of hormonal contraceptives on the periodontium, in a population of rural Sri-Lankan women, *J Clin Periodontol* 27:753, 2000.
74. Tilakaratne A, Soory M, Ranasinghe AW, et al: Periodontal disease status during pregnancy and 3 months post-partum, in a rural population of Sri-Lankan women, *J Clin Periodontol* 27:787, 2000.
75. Tomofuji T, Morita M, Horiuchi M, et al: The effect of duration and force of mechanical toothbrushing stimulation on proliferative activity of the junctional epithelium, *J Periodontol* 73:1149, 2002.

76. Trott JR, Love B: An analysis of localized gingival recession in 766 Winnipeg High School students, *Dent Pract Dent Rec* 16:209, 1966.
77. Woofter C: The prevalence and etiology of gingival recession, *Periodontal Abstr* 17:45, 1969.
78. Zlataric DK, Celebic A, Valentic-Peruzovic M: The effect of removable partial dentures on periodontal health of abutment and non-abutment teeth, *J Periodontol* 73:137, 2002.

Gingival Enlargement

Fermin A. Carranza and Eva L. Hogan

23

CHAPTER

CHAPTER OUTLINE

Increase in size of the gingiva is a common feature of gingival disease. Accepted current terminology for this condition is *gingival enlargement* or *gingival overgrowth*. These are strictly clinical descriptive terms and avoid the erroneous pathologic connotations of terms used in the past, such as "hypertrophic gingivitis" or "gingival hyperplasia."

The many types of gingival enlargement can be classified according to etiologic factors and pathologic changes as follows:

I. Inflammatory enlargement
  A. Chronic
  B. Acute
II. Drug-induced enlargement
III. Enlargements associated with systemic diseases or conditions
  A. Conditioned enlargement
    1. Pregnancy
    2. Puberty
    3. Vitamin C deficiency
    4. Plasma cell gingivitis
    5. Nonspecific conditioned enlargement (pyogenic granuloma)
  B. Systemic diseases causing gingival enlargement
    1. Leukemia
    2. Granulomatous diseases (e.g., Wegener's granulomatosis, sarcoidosis)
IV. Neoplastic enlargement (gingival tumors)
  A. Benign tumors
  B. Malignant tumors
V. False enlargement

Using the criteria of location and distribution, gingival enlargement is designated as follows:

- *Localized:* Limited to the gingiva adjacent to a single tooth or group of teeth.
- *Generalized:* Involving the gingiva throughout the mouth.
- *Marginal:* Confined to the marginal gingiva.
- *Papillary:* Confined to the interdental papilla.
- *Diffuse:* Involving the marginal and attached gingivae and papillae.
- *Discrete:* An isolated sessile or pedunculated, tumorlike enlargement.

The degree of gingival enlargement can be scored as follows[16]:

- *Grade 0:* No signs of gingival enlargement.
- *Grade I:* Enlargement confined to interdental papilla.
- *Grade II:* Enlargement involves papilla and marginal gingiva.
- *Grade III:* Enlargement covers three quarters or more of the crown.

INFLAMMATORY ENLARGEMENT

Gingival enlargement may result from chronic or acute inflammatory changes; chronic changes are much more common. In addition, inflammatory enlargements usually are a secondary complication to any of the other types of enlargement, creating a combined gingival enlargement. In these cases it is important to understand the double etiology and treat them adequately.

Chronic Inflammatory Enlargement

Clinical Features. Chronic inflammatory gingival enlargement originates as a slight ballooning of the interdental papilla and marginal gingiva. In the early stages it produces a life preserver–shaped bulge around the involved teeth. This bulge can increase in size until it covers part of the crowns. The enlargement may be localized or generalized and progresses slowly and painlessly, unless it is complicated by acute infection or trauma (Figures 23-1 and 23-2).

Occasionally, chronic inflammatory gingival enlargement occurs as a discrete sessile or pedunculated mass resembling a tumor. It may be interproximal or on the marginal or attached gingiva. The lesions are slow-growing masses and usually painless. They may undergo spontaneous reduction in size, followed by exacerbation and continued enlargement. Painful ulceration sometimes occurs in the fold between the mass and the adjacent gingiva.

Histopathology. Chronic inflammatory gingival enlargements show the exudative and proliferative features of chronic inflammation (Figure 23-3). Lesions that are clinically deep red or bluish red are soft and friable with a smooth, shiny surface, and they bleed easily. They also have a preponderance of inflammatory cells and fluid, with vascular engorgement, new capillary formation, and associated degenerative changes. Lesions that are relatively firm, resilient, and pink have a greater fibrotic component with an abundance of fibroblasts and collagen fibers.

Etiology. Chronic inflammatory gingival enlargement is caused by prolonged exposure to dental plaque. Factors that favor plaque accumulation and retention[54] include poor oral hygiene, as well as irritation by anatomic abnormalities and improper restorative and orthodontic appliances.

Gingival Changes Associated with Mouth Breathing. Gingivitis and gingival enlargement are often seen in mouth breathers.[74] The gingiva appears red and edematous, with a diffuse surface shininess of the exposed area. The maxillary anterior region is the common site of such involvement. In many cases the altered gingiva is clearly demarcated from the adjacent

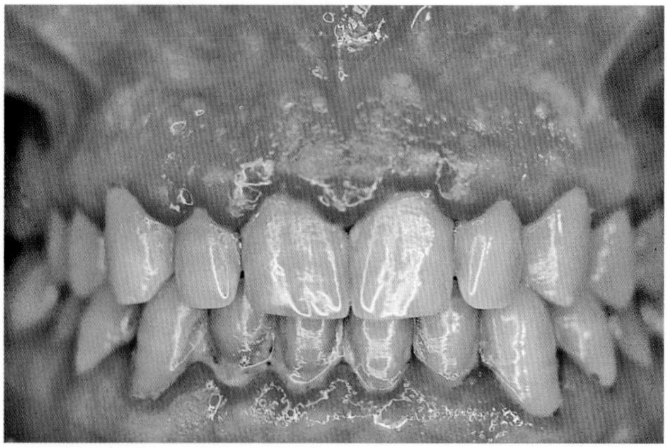

Figure 23-1 Chronic inflammatory gingival enlargement localized to the anterior region.

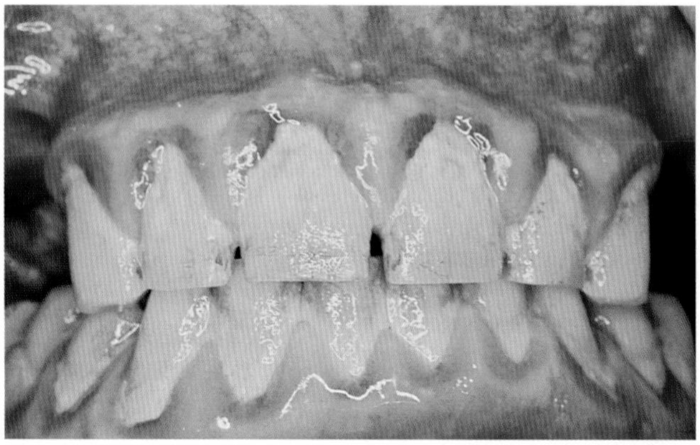

Figure 23-2 Chronic inflammatory gingival enlargement.

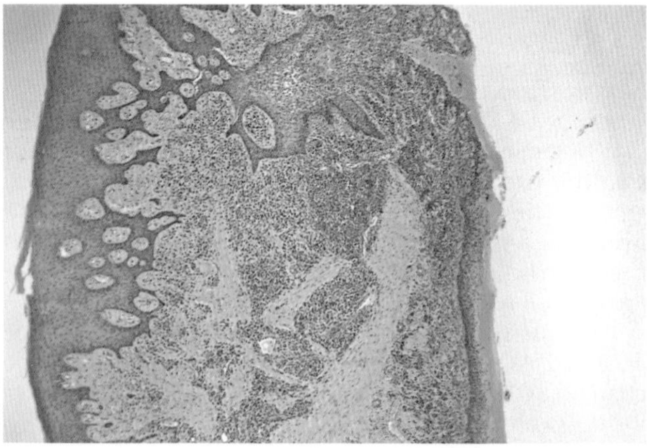

Figure 23-3 Survey section of chronic inflammatory gingival enlargement showing the inflamed connective tissue core and strands of proliferating epithelium.

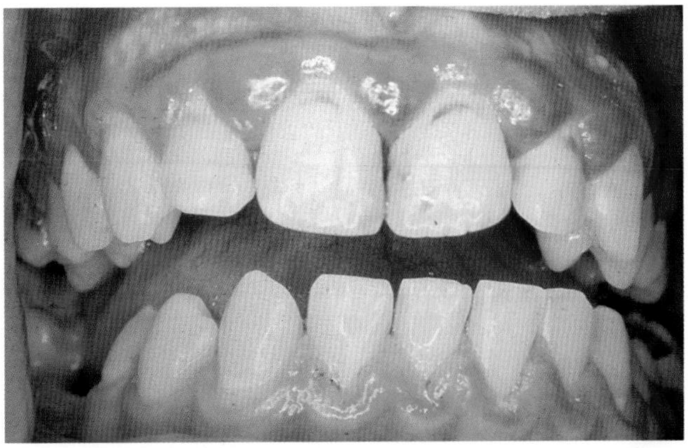

Figure 23-4 Gingival enlargement in a mouth breather. Note the lesion sharply circumscribed to anterior marginal and papillary areas.

SCIENCE TRANSFER

Gingival enlargement can be caused by a wide variety of etiologies. The clinician can often diagnose the cause by a careful history (e.g., drug-induced or pregnancy-induced enlargement), by location (e.g., mouth-breathing enlargement, around anterior teeth), or by the clinical presentation (e.g., generalized enlargement with gingival hematoma formation seen in leukemia). Plaque-induced inflammation can be the sole cause of gingival enlargement or can be a secondary cause, so in all patients, therapy to control gingival inflammation is essential. If there is a localized lesion, biopsy may be needed to correctly diagnose and treat the gingival enlargement.

unexposed normal gingiva (Figure 23-4). The exact manner in which mouth breathing affects gingival changes has not been demonstrated. Its harmful effect is generally attributed to irritation from surface dehydration. However, comparable changes could not be produced by air-drying the gingiva of experimental animals.[67]

Acute Inflammatory Enlargement

Gingival Abscess. A gingival abscess is a localized, painful, rapidly expanding lesion that is usually of sudden onset (Figure 23-5). It is generally limited to the marginal gingiva or interdental papilla. In its early stages it appears as a red swelling with a smooth, shiny surface. Within 24 to 48 hours, the lesion usually becomes fluctuant and pointed with a surface orifice from which a purulent exudate may be expressed. The adjacent teeth are often sensitive to percussion. If permitted to progress, the lesion generally ruptures spontaneously.

Histopathology. The gingival abscess consists of a purulent focus in the connective tissue, surrounded by a diffuse infiltration of polymorphonuclear leukocytes (PMNs), edematous tissue, and vascular engorgement. The surface epithelium has varying degrees of intracellular and extracellular edema, invasion by leukocytes, and sometimes ulceration.

Etiology. Acute inflammatory gingival enlargement results from bacteria carried deep into the tissues when a foreign substance (e.g., toothbrush bristle, piece of apple core, lobster shell fragment) is forcefully embedded into the gingiva. The lesion is confined to the gingiva and should not be confused with periodontal or lateral abscesses.

Periodontal (Lateral) Abscess. Periodontal abscesses generally produce enlargement of the gingiva, but they also involve the supporting periodontal tissues. (For a detailed description of periodontal abscesses, see Chapter 27.)

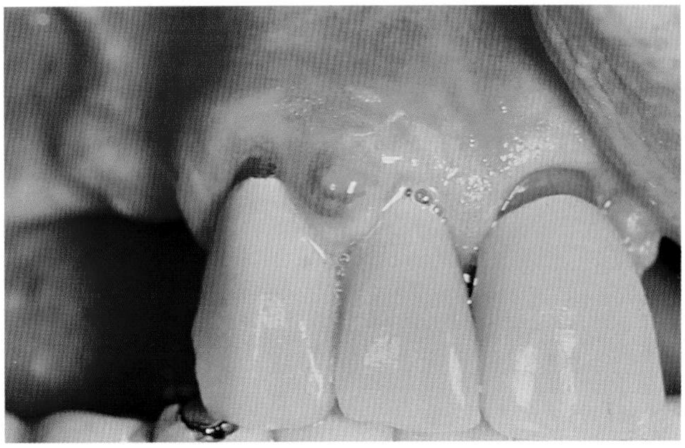

Figure 23-5 Gingival abscess on facial gingival surface, in space between cuspid and lateral incisor, unrelated to the gingival sulcus area.

DRUG-INDUCED GINGIVAL ENLARGEMENT

Gingival enlargement is a well-known consequence of the administration of some anticonvulsants, immunosuppressants, and calcium channel blockers and may create speech, mastication, tooth eruption, and aesthetic problems.

Clinical and microscopic features of the enlargements caused by the different drugs are similar.[23,110] These are presented first, followed by a description of the particular features of each drug.

General Information

Clinical Features. The growth starts as a painless, beadlike enlargement of the interdental papilla and extends to the facial and lingual gingival margins (Figure 23-6). As the condition progresses, the marginal and papillary enlargements unite; they may develop into a massive tissue fold covering a considerable portion of the crowns, and they may interfere with occlusion (Figure 23-7).

A

B

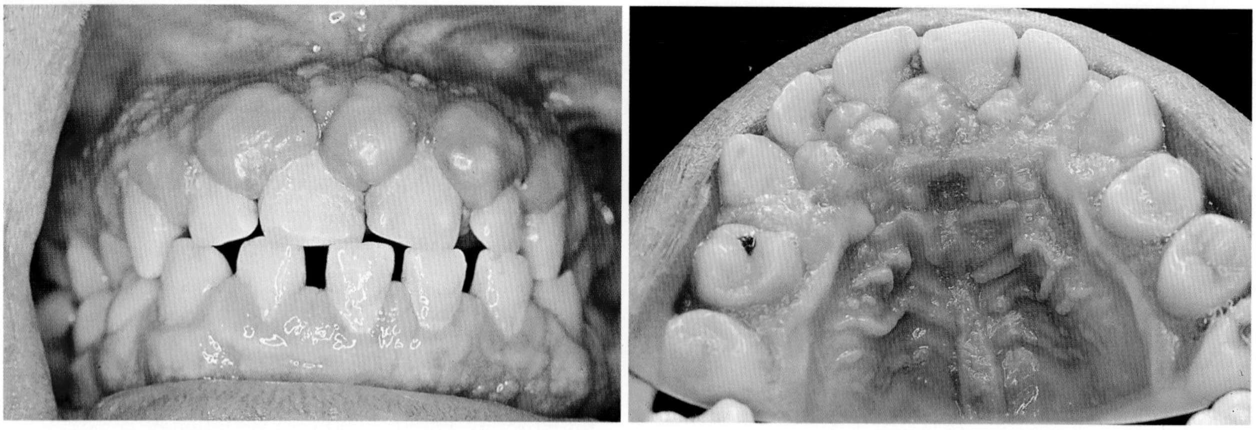

Figure 23-6 Gingival enlargement associated with phenytoin therapy. **A,** Facial view; note the prominent papillary lesions and the firm, nodular surface. **B,** Occlusal view of upper jaw.

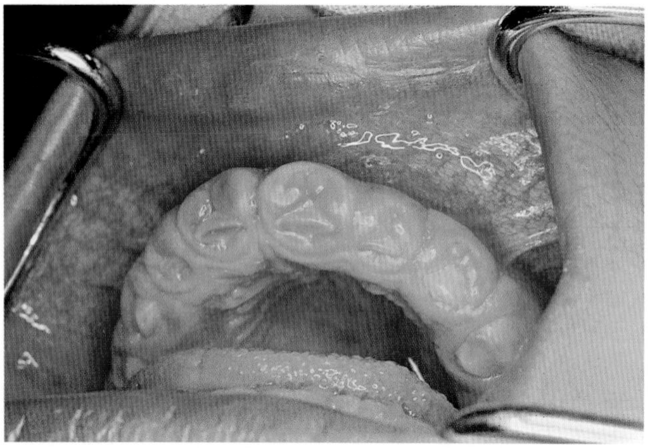

Figure 23-7 Gingival enlargement in a 5-year-old child covering most of the clinical crowns of teeth.

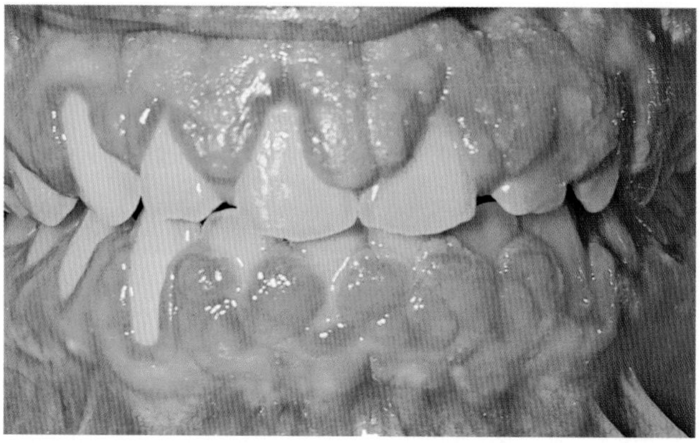

Figure 23-8 Combined gingival enlargement resulting from the inflammatory involvement of a phenytoin-induced overgrowth.

When uncomplicated by inflammation, the lesion is mulberry shaped, firm, pale pink, and resilient, with a minutely lobulated surface and no tendency to bleed. The enlargement characteristically appears to project from beneath the gingival margin, from which it is separated by a linear groove. However, the presence of the enlargement makes plaque control difficult, often resulting in a secondary inflammatory process that complicates the gingival overgrowth caused by the drug.

The resultant enlargement then becomes a combination of the increase in size caused by the drug and the complicating inflammation caused by bacteria. Secondary inflammatory changes not only add to the size of the lesion caused by the drug, but also produce a red or bluish red discoloration, obliterate the lobulated surface demarcations, and increase bleeding tendency (Figure 23-8).

The enlargement is usually generalized throughout the mouth but is more severe in the maxillary and mandibular anterior regions. It occurs in areas in which teeth are present, not in edentulous spaces, and the enlargement disappears in areas from which teeth are extracted. Hyperplasia of the mucosa in edentulous mouths has been reported but is rare.[31,32]

Drug-induced enlargement may occur in mouths with little or no plaque and may be absent in mouths with abundant deposits. Some investigators, however, believe that inflammation is a prerequisite for development of the enlargement, which therefore could be prevented by plaque removal and fastidious oral hygiene.[26,43,66,91,116] Oral hygiene by means of toothbrushing[34] or use of a chlorhexidine toothpaste[103] reduces the inflammation but does not lessen or prevent the overgrowth. Hassell et al.[50] have hypothesized that in noninflamed gingiva, fibroblasts are less active or even quiescent and do not respond to circulating phenytoin, whereas fibroblasts within inflamed tissue are in an active state as a result of the inflammatory mediators and the endogenous growth factors present.

A genetic predisposition is a suspected factor[51,96] in determining whether a person treated with phenytoin will develop gingival enlargement or not.

The enlargement is chronic and slowly increases in size. When surgically removed, it recurs. Spontaneous

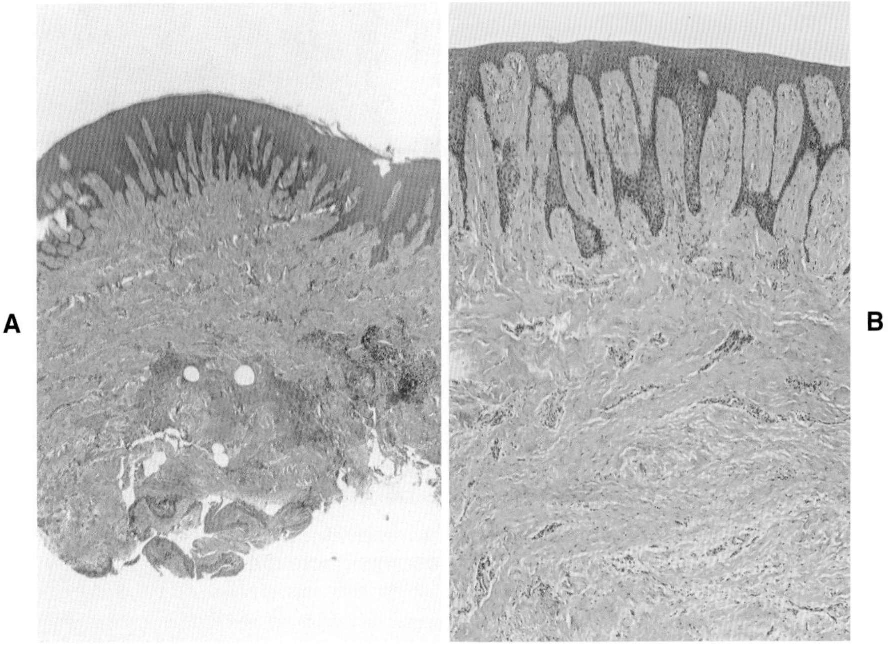

Figure 23-9 Microscopic view of gingival enlargement associated with phenytoin therapy. **A,** Hyperplasia and acanthosis of the epithelium and densely collagenous connective tissue, with evidence of inflammation in the area adjacent to the gingival sulcus (pocket). **B,** Higher-power view showing extension of deep rete pegs into the connective tissue.

disappearance occurs within a few months after discontinuation of the drug (see Chapter 63).

Histopathology. Drug-induced gingival enlargement consists of a pronounced hyperplasia of the connective tissue and epithelium (Figure 23-9). There is acanthosis of the epithelium, and elongated rete pegs extend deep into the connective tissue, which exhibits densely arranged collagen bundles with an increase in the number of fibroblasts and new blood vessels. An abundance of amorphous ground substance has also been reported.[78] Structural changes in the outer epithelial cell surface have been reported in cyclosporine-induced enlargements.[4]

The enlargement begins as a hyperplasia of the connective tissue core of the marginal gingiva and increases by its proliferation and expansion beyond the crest of the gingival margin. An inflammatory infiltrate may be found at the bottom of the sulcus, or pocket. Cyclosporine enlargements usually have a more highly vascularized connective tissue with foci of chronic inflammatory cells,[87] particularly plasma cells.[75]

The "mature" phenytoin enlargement has a fibroblast/collagen ratio equal to that of normal gingiva from normal individuals, suggesting that at some point in the development of the lesion, fibroblastic proliferation must have been abnormally high.[49] Oxytalan fibers are numerous beneath the epithelium and in areas of inflammation.[9]

Recurring phenytoin enlargements appear as granulation tissue composed of numerous young capillaries and fibroblasts and irregularly arranged collagen fibrils with occasional lymphocytes (Figure 23-10).

Anticonvulsants

The first drug-induced gingival enlargements reported were those produced by phenytoin (Dilantin). Dilantin is a hydantoin, introduced by Merritt and Putnam[80] in 1938 for the treatment of all forms of epilepsy, except petit mal. Shortly thereafter, its relationship with gingival enlargement was reported.[40,65]

Other hydantoins known to induce gingival enlargement are ethotoin (Paganone) and mephenytoin (Mesantoin). Other anticonvulsants that have the same side effect are the succinimides (ethosuximide [Zerontin], methsuxinimide [Celontin]), and valproic acid ([Depakene]).[44]

Gingival enlargement occurs in about 50% of patients receiving the drug,[110] although different authors have reported incidences from 3% to 84.5%.[3,40,92] It occurs more often in younger patients.[6] Its occurrence and severity are not necessarily related to the dosage after a threshold level has been exceeded.[110] Phenytoin appears in the saliva. There is no consensus, however, on whether the severity of the overgrowth is related to the levels of phenytoin in plasma or saliva.[3,6,7,133] Some reports indicate a relation between the drug dosage and the degree of gingival overgrowth.[60,66]

Tissue culture experiments indicate that phenytoin stimulates proliferation of fibroblast-like cells[111] and epithelium.[112] Two analogs of phenytoin (1-allyl-5-phenylhydantoinate and 5-methyl-5-phenylhydantoinate) have a similar effect on fibroblast-like cells.[112] Fibroblasts from a phenytoin-induced gingival overgrowth show increased synthesis of sulfated glycosaminoglycans in vitro.[59] Phenytoin may induce a decrease in collagen

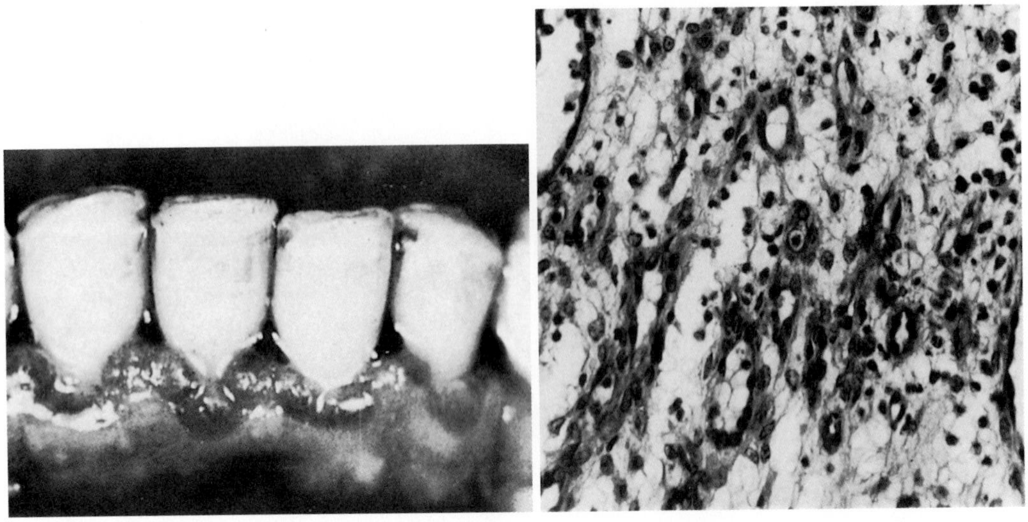

Figure 23-10 Enlarged gingiva in patient receiving phenytoin therapy. **A,** Early recurrence after surgical removal. **B,** Biopsy specimen; note the abundance of new blood vessels.

degradation as a result of the production of an inactive fibroblastic collagenase.[48]

Experimental attempts to induce gingival enlargement with phenytoin administration in laboratory animals have been successful only in the cat,[56] the ferret, and the *Macaca speciosa monkey.*[118] In experimental animals, phenytoin causes gingival enlargement that is independent of local inflammation.

In cats, one of the metabolic products of phenytoin is 5-(parahydroxyphenyl)-5-phenylhydantoin; administration of this metabolite to cats also induces gingival enlargement in some cases. This led Hassell and Page[49] to hypothesize that gingival enlargement may result from the genetically determined ability or inability of the host to deal effectively with prolonged administration of phenytoin.

Systemic administration of phenytoin accelerates the healing of gingival wounds in nonepileptic humans[114] and increases the tensile strength of healing abdominal wounds in rats.[31,113] The administration of phenytoin may precipitate a megaloblastic anemia[76] and folic acid deficiency.[119]

In conclusion, the pathogenesis of gingival enlargement induced by phenytoin is not known, but some evidence links it to a direct effect on specific, genetically predetermined subpopulations of fibroblasts, inactivation of collagenase, and plaque-induced inflammation.

Immunosuppressants

Cyclosporine is a potent immunosuppressive agent used to prevent organ transplant rejection and to treat several diseases of autoimmune origin.[24] Its exact mechanism of action is not well known, but it appears to selectively and reversibly inhibit helper T cells, which play a role in cellular and humoral immune responses. Cyclosporin A (Sandimmune, Neoral) is administered intravenously or by mouth, and dosages greater than 500 mg/day have been reported to induce gingival overgrowth.[29]

Cyclosporine-induced gingival enlargement is more vascularized than phenytoin enlargement (Figure 23-11 and 23-12). Its occurrence varies according to different studies from 25% to 70%,[100] it affects children more frequently, and its magnitude appears to be related more to the plasma concentration than to the patient's periodontal status.[109] Gingival enlargement is greater in patients who are medicated with both cyclosporine and calcium channel blockers.[116,127,128]

The microscopic finding of many plasma cells plus the presence of an abundant amorphous extracellular substance has suggested that the enlargement is a hypersensitivity response to the cyclosporine.[78]

In experimental animals (rats), oral administration of cyclosporine was reported also to induce abundant formation of new cementum.[5]

In addition to gingival enlargement, cyclosporine induces other major side effects, such as nephrotoxicity, hypertension, and hypertrichosis. Another immunosuppressive drug, *tacrolimus,* has been used effectively and is also nephrotoxic, but it results in much less severe hypertension, hypertrichosis, and gingival overgrowth.[8,82,117]

Calcium Channel Blockers

Calcium channel blockers are drugs developed for the treatment of cardiovascular conditions such as hypertension, angina pectoris, coronary artery spasms, and cardiac arrhythmias. They inhibit calcium ion influx across the cell membrane of heart and smooth muscle cells, blocking intracellular mobilization of calcium. This induces direct dilation of the coronary arteries and arterioles, improving oxygen supply to the heart muscle; it also reduces hypertension by dilating the peripheral vasculature.

These drugs are the *dihydropyridine derivatives* (amlodipine [Lotrel, Norvasc], felodipine [Plendil], nicardipine [Cardene], nifedipine [Adalat, Procardia]); the

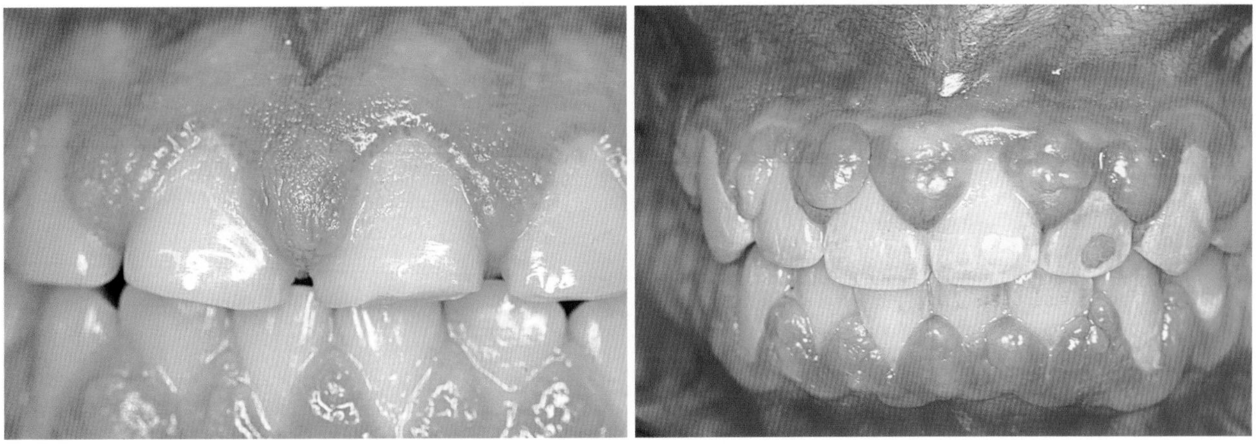

Figure 23-11 Cyclosporine-associated gingival enlargement. **A,** Mild involvement located particularly on papillae between teeth #9 and #10 and #10 and #11. **B,** Advanced generalized enlargement.

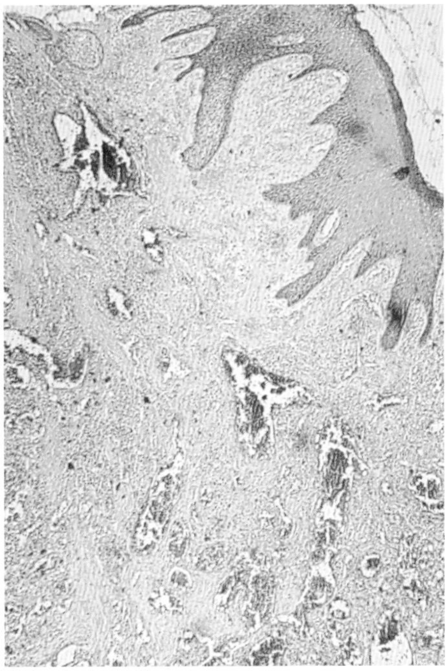

Figure 23-12 Microscopic view of cyclosporine-associated gingival enlargement. Note the epithelial hyperplasia and fibrous stroma with abundant vascularization.

benzothiazine derivatives (diltiazem [Cardizem, Dilacor XR, Tlazac]); and the *phenylalkylamine derivatives* (verapamil [Calan, Isoptin, Verelan, Covera HS]).[44]

Some of these drugs can induce gingival enlargement. Nifedipine, one of the most often used,[73,75,89] induces gingival enlargement in 20% of patients.[10] Diltiazem, felodipine, nitrendipine, and verapamil also induce gingival enlargement.[17,52] The dihydropyridine derivative isradipidine can replace nifedipine in some cases and does not induce gingival overgrowth.[132]

Nifedipine is also used with cyclosporine in kidney transplant recipients, and the combined use of both drugs induces larger overgrowths.[16] Nifedipine gingival enlargement has been induced experimentally in rats, where it appears to be dose dependent;[37] in humans, however, this dose dependency is not clear.

IDIOPATHIC GINGIVAL ENLARGEMENT

Idiopathic gingival enlargement is a rare condition of undetermined cause. It has been designated by such terms as gingivomatosis, elephantiasis, idiopathic fibromatosis, hereditary gingival hyperplasia, and congenital familial fibromatosis.

Clinical Features. The enlargement affects the attached gingiva, as well as the gingival margin and interdental papillae, in contrast to phenytoin-induced overgrowth, which is often limited to the gingival margin and interdental papillae. The facial and lingual surfaces of the mandible and maxilla are generally affected, but the involvement may be limited to either jaw. The enlarged gingiva is pink, firm, and almost leathery in consistency and has a characteristic minutely pebbled surface (Figure 23-13). In severe cases the teeth are almost completely covered, and the enlargement projects into the oral vestibule. The jaws appear distorted because of the bulbous enlargement of the gingiva. Secondary inflammatory changes are common at the gingival margin.

Histopathology. Idiopathic gingival enlargement shows a bulbous increase in the amount of connective tissue that is relatively avascular and consists of densely arranged collagen bundles and numerous fibroblasts. The surface epithelium is thickened and acanthotic with elongated rete pegs.

Etiology. The cause is unknown, and thus the condition is designated as "idiopathic." Some cases have a hereditary basis,[35,136,137] but the genetic mechanisms involved are not well understood. A study of several families found the mode of inheritance to be autosomal recessive in some cases and autosomal dominant in others.[58,96] In some families the gingival enlargement may be linked to impairment of physical development.[64]

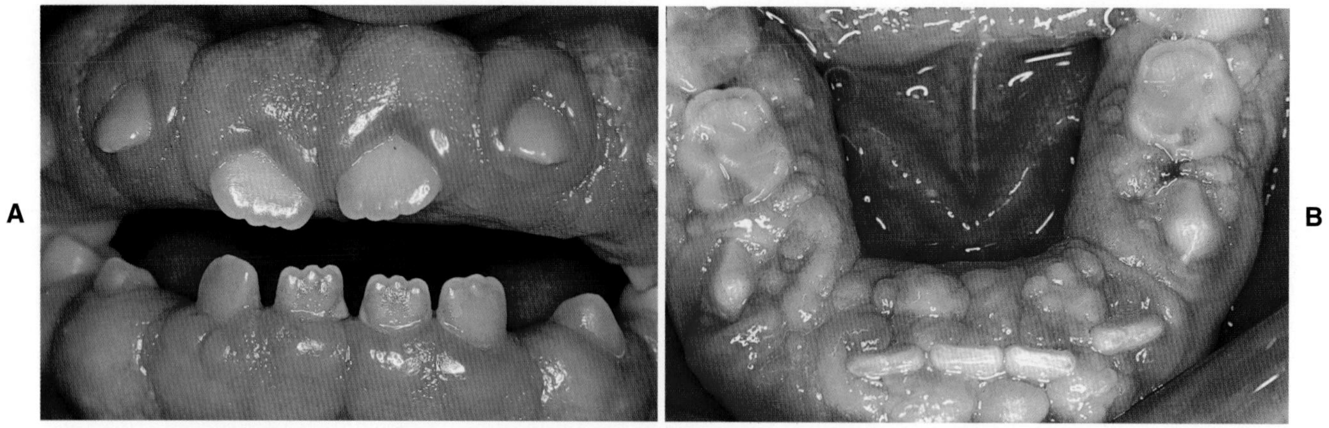

Figure 23-13 Idiopathic gingival enlargement in 14-year-old white male patient. **A,** Facial view; gingiva is firm, with nodular, pebbled surface and partially covers the crowns of the teeth. **B,** Occlusal view of lower jaw.

The enlargement usually begins with the eruption of the primary or secondary dentition and may regress after extraction, suggesting that the teeth (or the plaque attached to them) may be initiating factors. The presence of bacterial plaque is a complicating factor. Gingival enlargement has been described in *tuberous sclerosis,* which is an inherited condition characterized by a triad of epilepsy, mental deficiency, and cutaneous angiofibromas.[121,126]

ENLARGEMENTS ASSOCIATED WITH SYSTEMIC DISEASES

Many systemic diseases can develop oral manifestations that may include gingival enlargement. These diseases and conditions can affect the periodontium by two different mechanisms, as follows:

1. *Magnification of an existing inflammation initiated by dental plaque.* This group of diseases, discussed below under "Conditioned Enlargements," includes some hormonal conditions (e.g., pregnancy and puberty), nutritional diseases such as vitamin C deficiency, and some cases in which the systemic influence is not identified (nonspecific conditioned enlargement).
2. *Manifestation of the systemic disease independently of the inflammatory status of the gingiva.* This group is described under Systemic Diseases Causing Gingival Enlargement and Neoplastic Enlargement (Gingival Tumors).

Conditioned Enlargement

Conditioned enlargement occurs when the systemic condition of the patient exaggerates or distorts the usual gingival response to dental plaque. The specific manner in which the clinical picture of conditioned gingival enlargement differs from that of chronic gingivitis depends on the nature of the modifying systemic influence. *Bacterial plaque is necessary for the initiation of this type of enlargement.* However, plaque is not the sole determinant of the nature of the clinical features.

The three types of conditioned gingival enlargement are *hormonal* (pregnancy, puberty), *nutritional* (associated with vitamin C deficiency), and *allergic.* Nonspecific conditioned enlargement is also seen.

Enlargement in Pregnancy. Pregnancy gingival enlargement may be marginal and generalized or may occur as single or multiple tumor-like masses (see Chapters 17 and 43).

During pregnancy there is an increase in levels of both progesterone and estrogen, which, by the end of the third trimester, reach levels 10 and 30 times the levels during the menstrual cycle, respectively.[2] These hormonal changes induce changes in vascular permeability, leading to gingival edema and an increased inflammatory response to dental plaque. The subgingival microbiota may also undergo changes, including an increase in *Prevotella intermedia.*[69,95]

Marginal Enlargement. Marginal gingival enlargement during pregnancy results from the aggravation of previous inflammation, and its incidence has been reported as 10%[23] and 70%.[138] The gingival enlargement does not occur without the presence of bacterial plaque.

The clinical picture varies considerably. The enlargement is usually generalized and tends to be more prominent interproximally than on the facial and lingual surfaces. The enlarged gingiva is bright red or magenta, soft, and friable and has a smooth, shiny surface. Bleeding occurs spontaneously or on slight provocation.

Tumorlike Gingival Enlargement. The so-called pregnancy tumor is not a neoplasm; it is an inflammatory response to bacterial plaque and is modified by the patient's condition. It usually appears after the third month of pregnancy but may occur earlier. The reported incidence is 1.8% to 5%.[77]

The lesion appears as a discrete, mushroomlike, flattened spherical mass that protrudes from the gingival margin or more often from the interproximal space and is attached by a sessile or pedunculated base (Figure 23-14). It tends to expand laterally, and pressure from the tongue and the cheek perpetuates its flattened appearance. Generally dusky red or magenta, it has a

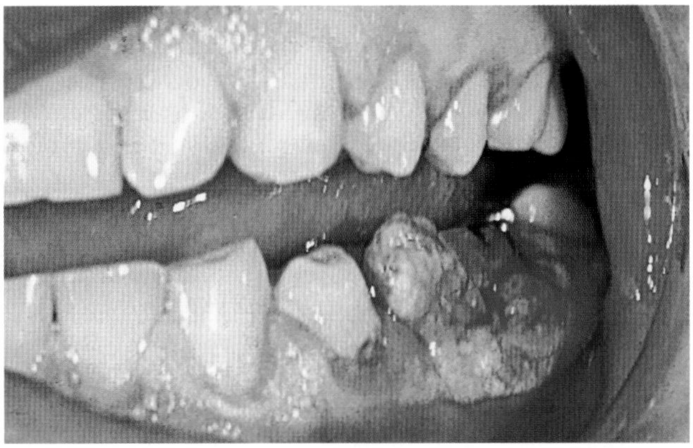

Figure 23-14 Localized gingival enlargement in a 27-year-old pregnant patient.

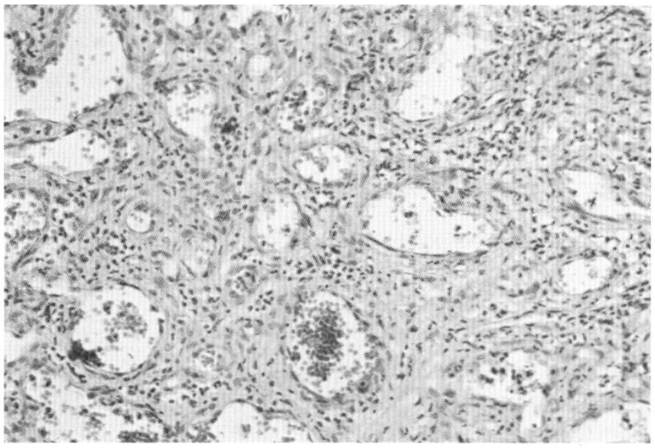

Figure 23-15 Microscopic view of gingival enlargement in pregnant patient showing abundance of blood vessels and interspersed inflammatory cells.

smooth, glistening surface that often exhibits numerous deep-red, pinpoint markings. It is a superficial lesion and usually does not invade the underlying bone. The consistency varies; the mass is usually semifirm, but it may have various degrees of softness and friability. It is usually painless unless its size and shape foster accumulation of debris under its margin or interfere with occlusion, in which case, painful ulceration may occur.

Histopathology. Gingival enlargement in pregnancy is called *angiogranuloma*. Both marginal and tumorlike enlargements consist of a central mass of connective tissue, with numerous diffusely arranged, newly formed, and engorged capillaries lined by cuboid endothelial cells (Figure 23-15), as well as a moderately fibrous stroma with varying degrees of edema and chronic inflammatory infiltrate. The stratified squamous epithelium is thickened, with prominent rete pegs and some degree of intracellular and extracellular edema, prominent intercellular bridges, and leukocytic infiltration.

Although the microscopic findings are characteristic of gingival enlargement in pregnancy, they are not pathognomonic because they cannot be used to differentiate pregnant and nonpregnant patients.[77]

Most gingival disease during pregnancy can be prevented by the removal of plaque and calculus, as well as the institution of fastidious oral hygiene at the outset. In pregnancy, treatment of the gingiva that is limited to the removal of tissue without complete elimination of local irritants is followed by recurrence of gingival enlargement. Although spontaneous reduction in the size of gingival enlargement typically follows the termination of pregnancy, complete elimination of the residual inflammatory lesion requires the removal of all plaque deposits and factors that favor its accumulation.

Enlargement in Puberty. Enlargement of the gingiva is sometimes seen during puberty (see Chapters 17 and 43). It occurs in both male and female adolescents and appears in areas of plaque accumulation.

The size of the gingival enlargement greatly exceeds that usually seen in association with comparable local factors. It is marginal and interdental and is characterized by prominent bulbous interproximal papillae (Figure 23-16). Often, only the facial gingivae are enlarged, and the lingual surfaces are relatively unaltered; the mechanical action of the tongue and the excursion of food prevent a heavy accumulation of local irritants on the lingual surface.

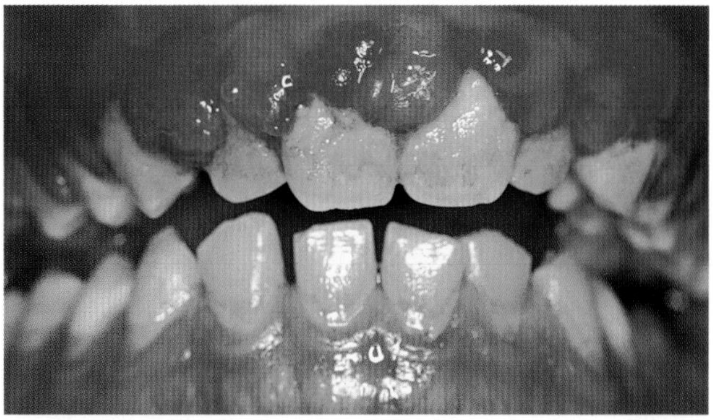

Figure 23-16 Conditioned gingival enlargement in puberty in a 13-year-old boy.

Gingival enlargement during puberty has all the clinical features generally associated with chronic inflammatory gingival disease. It is the *degree* of enlargement and the tendency to develop *massive recurrence* in the presence of relatively scant plaque deposits that distinguish pubertal gingival enlargement from uncomplicated chronic inflammatory gingival enlargement. After puberty the enlargement undergoes spontaneous reduction but does not disappear until plaque and calculus are removed.

A longitudinal study of 127 children 11 to 17 years of age showed a high initial prevalence of gingival enlargement that tended to decline with age.[122] When the mean number of inflamed gingival sites per child was determined and correlated with the time at which the maximum number of inflamed sites was observed and with the oral hygiene index at that time, a pubertal peak in gingival inflammation unrelated to oral hygiene factors clearly occurred. A longitudinal study of subgingival microbiota of children between ages 11 and 14 and their association with clinical parameters has implicated *Capnocytophaga* species in the initiation of pubertal gingivitis.[83] Other studies have reported that hormonal changes coincide with an increase in the proportion of *Prevotella intermedia* and *Prevotella nigrescens*.[85,134]

Histopathology. The microscopic appearance of gingival enlargement in puberty is chronic inflammation with prominent edema and associated degenerative changes.

Enlargement in Vitamin C Deficiency. Enlargement of the gingiva is generally included in classic descriptions of *scurvy*. Acute vitamin C deficiency itself does not cause gingival inflammation, but it does cause hemorrhage, collagen degeneration, and edema of the gingival connective tissue. These changes modify the response of the gingiva to plaque to the extent that the normal defensive delimiting reaction is inhibited, and the extent of the inflammation is exaggerated,[38,39] resulting in the massive gingival enlargement seen in scurvy (Figure 23-17) (see Chapter 17).

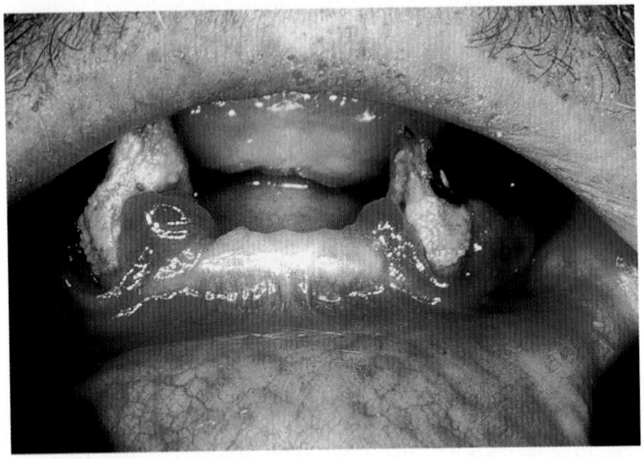

Figure 23-17 Gingival enlargement in patient with vitamin C deficiency. Note the prominent hemorrhagic areas. (Courtesy Dr. Gerald Shklar, Boston.)

Gingival enlargement in vitamin C deficiency is marginal; the gingiva is bluish red, soft, and friable and has a smooth, shiny surface. Hemorrhage, occurring either spontaneously or on slight provocation, and surface necrosis with pseudomembrane formation are common features.

Histopathology. In vitamin C deficiency the gingiva has a chronic inflammatory cellular infiltration with a superficial acute response. There are scattered areas of hemorrhage, with engorged capillaries. Marked diffuse edema, collagen degeneration, and scarcity of collagen fibrils or fibroblasts are striking findings.

Plasma Cell Gingivitis. Plasma cell gingivitis, also referred to as *atypical gingivitis* and *plasma cell gingivostomatitis,* often consists of a mild marginal gingival enlargement that extends to the attached gingiva. A localized lesion, referred to as *plasma cell granuloma,* has also been described.[15]

The gingiva appears red, friable, and sometimes granular and bleeds easily; usually it does not induce a loss of attachment (Figure 23-18). This lesion is located in the oral aspect of the attached gingiva and therefore differs from plaque-induced gingivitis.

Histopathology. In plasma cell gingivitis the oral epithelium shows spongiosis and infiltration with inflammatory cells; ultrastructurally, there are signs of damage in the lower spinous layers and the basal layers. The underlying connective tissue contains a dense infiltrate of plasma cells that also extends to the oral epithelium, inducing a dissecting type of injury.[88]

An associated cheilitis and glossitis have been reported.[63,106] Plasma cell gingivitis is thought to be allergic in origin, possibly related to components of chewing gum, dentifrices, or various diet components. Cessation of exposure to the allergen brings resolution of the lesion.

In rare instances, marked inflammatory gingival enlargements with a predominance of plasma cells can appear, associated with rapidly progressive periodontitis.[90]

A

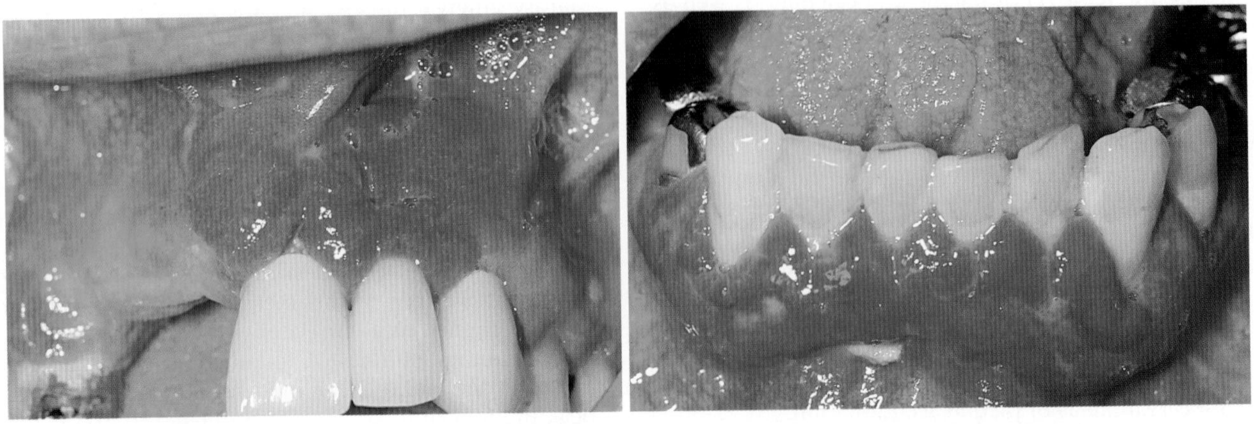

B

Figure 23-18 Plasma cell gingivitis. **A,** Diffuse lesions on facial surface of the anterior maxilla. **B,** Mandibular lesions. (Courtesy Dr. Kim D. Zussman, Thousand Oaks, Calif.)

Nonspecific Conditioned Enlargement (Pyogenic Granuloma). Pyogenic granuloma is a tumorlike gingival enlargement that is considered an exaggerated conditioned response to minor trauma (Figure 23-19). The exact nature of the systemic conditioning factor has not been identified.[62]

The lesion varies from a discrete spherical, tumorlike mass with a pedunculated attachment to a flattened, keloidlike enlargement with a broad base. It is bright red or purple and either friable or firm, depending on its duration; in the majority of cases it presents with surface ulceration and purulent exudation. The lesion tends to involute spontaneously to become a fibroepithelial papilloma, or it may persist relatively unchanged for years.

Histopathology. Pyogenic granuloma appears as a mass of granulation tissue with chronic inflammatory cellular infiltration. Endothelial proliferation and the formation of numerous vascular spaces are the prominent features. The surface epithelium is atrophic in some areas and hyperplastic in others. Surface ulceration and exudation are common features.

Treatment consists of removal of the lesions plus the elimination of irritating local factors. The recurrence rate is about 15%.[14] Pyogenic granuloma is similar in clinical and microscopic appearance to the conditioned gingival enlargement seen in pregnancy. Differential diagnosis is based on the patient's history.

Systemic Diseases That Cause Gingival Enlargement

Several systemic diseases may result in gingival enlargement through different mechanisms. These are uncommon cases and are only briefly discussed.

Leukemia

Leukemic enlargement may be diffuse or marginal and localized or generalized (see Chapter 17). It may appear as a diffuse enlargement of the gingival mucosa, an oversized extension of the marginal gingival (Figure 23-20; see also Figure 17-11), or a discrete tumorlike interproximal mass. In leukemic enlargement the gingiva is generally bluish red and has a shiny surface. The consistency is moderately firm, but there is a tendency toward friability and hemorrhage, occurring either spontaneously or on slight irritation. Acute painful necrotizing ulcerative inflammatory involvement sometimes occurs in the crevice formed at the junction of the enlarged gingiva and the contiguous tooth surfaces.

Patients with leukemia may also have a simple chronic inflammation without the involvement of leukemic cells and may present with the same clinical and microscopic features seen in patients without the disease. Most cases reveal features of both simple chronic inflammation and leukemic infiltrate.

True leukemic enlargement often occurs in acute leukemia but may also be seen in subacute leukemia. It seldom occurs in chronic leukemia.

Histopathology. Gingival enlargements in leukemic patients show various degrees of chronic inflammation. Mature leukocytes and areas of connective tissue are infiltrated with a dense mass of immature and proliferating leukocytes, the specific nature of which varies with the type of leukemia. Engorged capillaries, edematous and degenerated connective tissue, and epithelium with various degrees of leukocytic infiltration and edema are found. Isolated surface areas of acute necrotizing inflammation with a pseudomembranous meshwork of fibrin, necrotic epithelial cells, PMNs, and bacteria are often seen.

Granulomatous Diseases

Wegener's Granulomatosis. Wegener's granulomatosis is a rare disease characterized by acute granulomatous necrotizing lesions of the respiratory tract, including nasal and oral defects. Renal lesions develop, and acute necrotizing vasculitis affects the blood vessels. The initial manifestations of Wegener's granulomatosis may involve the orofacial region and include oral mucosal ulceration, gingival enlargement, abnormal tooth mobility, exfoliation of teeth, and delayed healing response.[20]

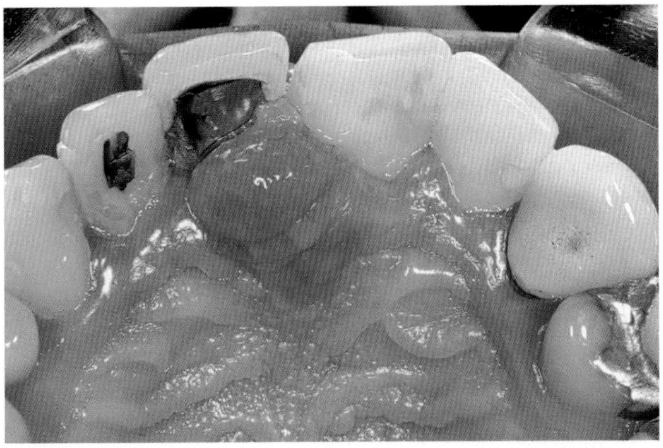

Figure 23-19 Pyogenic granuloma in a young woman. (Courtesy Dr. Silvia Oreamuno, San José, Costa Rica.)

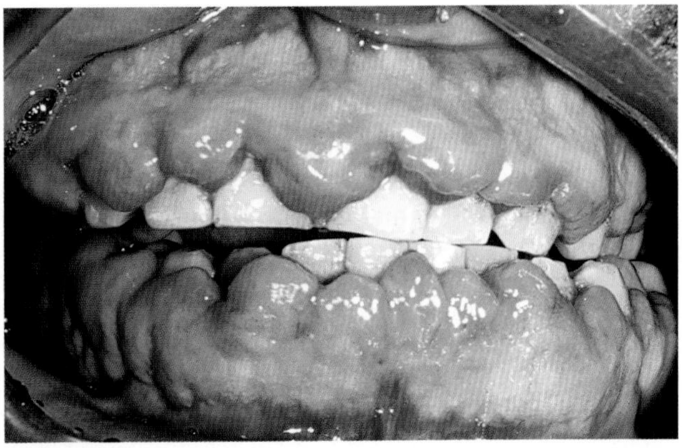

Figure 23-20 Leukemic gingival enlargement (acute myelocytic leukemia). (Courtesy Dr. Spencer Wolfe, Dublin, Ireland.)

The granulomatous papillary enlargement is reddish purple and bleeds easily on stimulation (see Figure 26-31).

Histopathology. Chronic inflammation occurs, with scattered giant cells and foci of acute inflammation and microabscesses covered by a thin, acanthotic epithelium. Vascular changes have not been described with gingival enlargement in Wegener's granulomatosis, probably because of the small size of the gingival blood vessels.[57]

The cause of Wegener's granulomatosis is unknown, but the condition is considered an immunologically mediated tissue injury.[27] At one time the usual outcome was death from kidney failure within a few months, but more recently the use of immunosuppressive drugs has produced prolonged remissions in more than 90% of patients.[68]

Sarcoidosis. Sarcoidosis is a granulomatous disease of unknown etiology. It starts in individuals in their 20s or 30s, predominantly affects blacks, and can involve almost any organ, including the gingiva, where a red, smooth, painless enlargement may appear.

Histopathology. Sarcoid granulomas consist of discrete, noncaseating whorls of epithelioid cells and multinucleated, foreign body–type giant cells with peripheral mononuclear cells.[99]

NEOPLASTIC ENLARGEMENT (GINGIVAL TUMORS)

This section provides only a brief description of some of the more common neoplastic and pseudoneoplastic lesions of the gingiva. The reader is referred to texts on oral pathology for more comprehensive coverage.[87,99,104]

Benign Tumors of the Gingiva

Epulis is a generic term used clinically to designate all discrete tumors and tumorlike masses of the gingiva. It serves to locate the tumor but not to describe it. Most lesions referred to as "epulis" are inflammatory rather than neoplastic.

Neoplasms account for a comparatively small proportion of gingival enlargements and make up a small percentage of the total number of oral neoplasms. In a survey of 257 oral tumors, approximately 8% occurred on the gingiva.[81] In another study of 868 growths of the gingiva and palate, of which 57% were neoplastic and the remainder inflammatory, the following incidence of tumors was noted: carcinoma, 11.0%; fibroma, 9.3%; giant cell tumor, 8.4%; papilloma, 7.3%; leukoplakia, 4.9%; mixed tumor (salivary gland type), 2.5%; angioma, 1.5%; osteofibroma, 1.3%; sarcoma, 0.5%; melanoma, 0.5%; myxoma, 0.45%; fibropapilloma, 0.4%; adenoma, 0.4%; and lipoma, 0.3%.[12]

Fibroma. Fibromas of the gingiva arise from the gingival connective tissue or from the periodontal ligament. They are slow-growing, spherical tumors that tend to be firm and nodular but may be soft and vascular. Fibromas are usually pedunculated. Hard fibromas of the gingiva are rare; most of the lesions diagnosed clinically as "fibromas" are inflammatory enlargements.[105]

Histopathology. Fibromas are composed of bundles of well-formed collagen fibers with a scattering of fibrocytes and a variable vascularity.

The so-called giant cell fibroma contains multinucleated fibroblasts. In another variant, mineralized tissue (bone, cementum-like material, dystrophic calcifications) may be found; this type of fibroma is called *peripheral ossifying fibroma*.

Papilloma. Papillomas are benign proliferations of surface epithelium associated with the human papillomavirus (HPV). Viral subtypes HPV-6 and HPV-11 have been found in most cases of oral papillomas. Gingival papillomas appear as solitary, wartlike or cauliflower-like protuberances (Figure 23-21). They may be small and discrete or broad, hard elevations with minutely irregular surfaces.

Histopathology. The papilloma lesion consists of fingerlike projections of stratified squamous epithelium, often hyperkeratotic, with a central core of fibrovascular connective tissue.

Peripheral Giant Cell Granuloma. Giant cell lesions of the gingiva arise interdentally or from the gingival margin, occur most frequently on the labial surface, and may be sessile or pedunculated. They vary in appearance from smooth, regularly outlined masses to irregularly shaped, multilobulated protuberances with surface indentations (Figure 23-22). Ulceration of the margin is occasionally seen. The lesions are painless, vary in size, and may cover several teeth. They may be firm or spongy, and the color varies from pink to deep red or purplish blue. There are no pathognomonic clinical features whereby these lesions can be differentiated from other forms of gingival enlargement. Microscopic examination is required for definitive diagnosis.

In the past, giant cell lesions of the gingiva have been referred to as "peripheral reparative giant cell tumors." These lesions, however, are essentially responses to local injury and are not neoplasms; and their reparative nature has not been proved. Therefore, they are now referred to as *peripheral giant cell granulomas*. The prefix peripheral is needed to differentiate them from comparable lesions that originate within the jawbone (*central* giant cell granulomas).

In some cases the giant cell granuloma of the gingiva is locally invasive and causes destruction of the underlying bone (Figure 23-23). Complete removal leads to uneventful recovery.

Histopathology. The giant cell granuloma has numerous foci of multinuclear giant cells and hemosiderin particles in a connective tissue stroma.

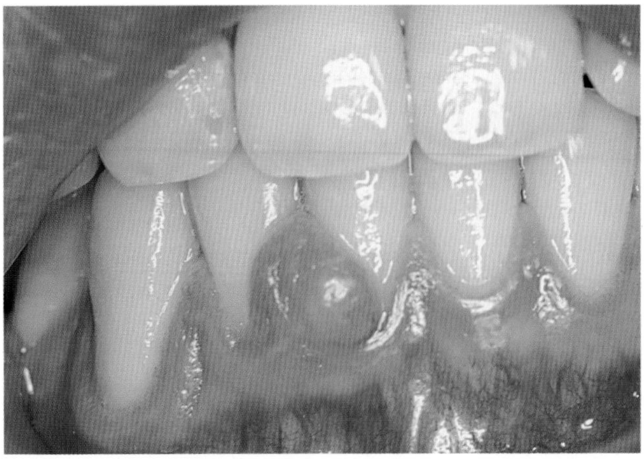

Figure 23-21 Papilloma of the gingiva in 26-year-old man.

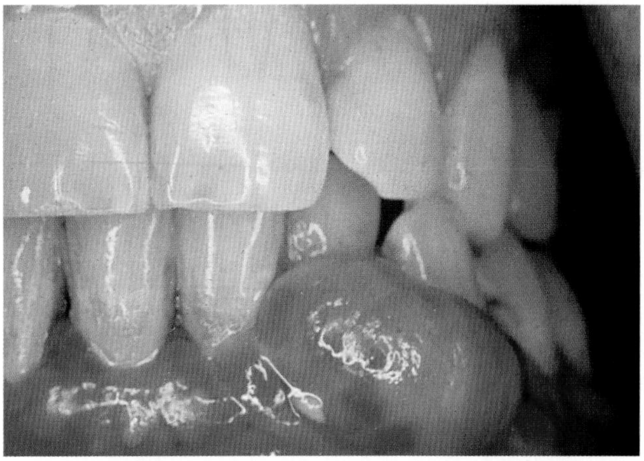

Figure 23-22 Gingival giant cell granuloma.

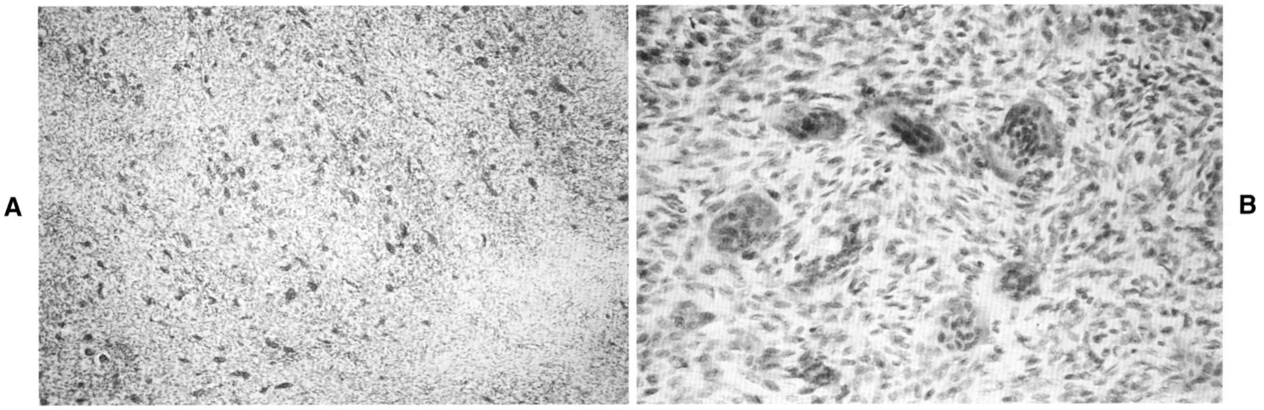

Figure 23-23 **A,** Microscopic survey of peripheral giant cell granuloma. **B,** High-power study of the lesion demonstrating the giant cells and intervening stroma that make up the major portion of the mass.

Areas of chronic inflammation are scattered throughout the lesion, with acute involvement occurring at the surface. The overlying epithelium is usually hyperplastic, with ulceration at the base. Bone formation occasionally occurs within the lesion (Figure 23-24).

Central Giant Cell Granuloma. These lesions arise within the jaws and produce central cavitation. They occasionally create a deformity of the jaw that makes the gingiva appear enlarged.

Mixed tumors, salivary gland type of tumors, and plasmacytomas of the gingiva have also been described but are not often seen.

Leukoplakia. *Leukoplakia* is a strictly clinical term defined by the World Health Organization as a white patch or plaque that does not rub off and cannot be diagnosed as any other disease. The cause of leukoplakia remains obscure, although it is associated to the use of tobacco (smoke or smokeless). Other probable factors are *Candida albicans,* HPV-16 and HPV-18, and trauma. Leukoplakia of the gingiva varies in appearance from

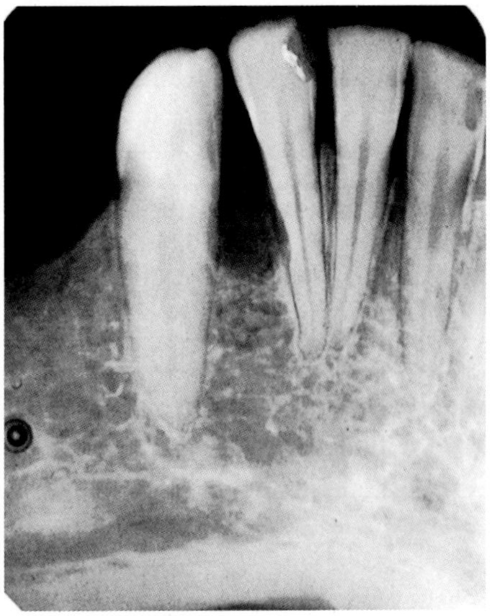

Figure 23-24 Bone destruction in the interproximal space between the canine and lateral incisor caused by the extension of a peripheral giant cell reparative granuloma of the gingiva. (Courtesy Dr. Sam Toll.)

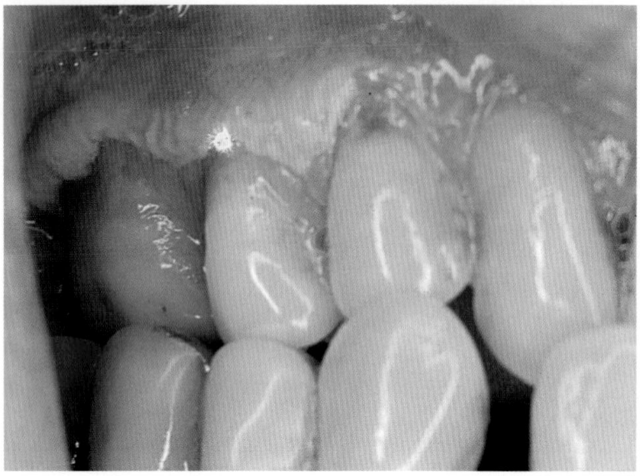

Figure 23-25 Leukoplakia of the gingiva.

a grayish white, flattened, scaly lesion (Figure 23-25) to a thick, irregularly shaped, keratinous plaque.

Most leukoplakias (80%) are benign; the remaining 20% are malignant or premalignant, and only 3% of these are invasive carcinomas.[36] Biopsy of all leukoplakias is necessary, selecting the most suspicious area, to arrive at a correct diagnosis and institute proper therapy.[36,87]

> Histopathology. Leukoplakia exhibits hyperkeratosis and acanthosis. Premalignant and malignant cases have a variable degree of atypical epithelial changes that may be mild, moderate, or severe, depending on the extent of involvement of the epithelial layers. When dysplastic changes involve all layers, it is diagnosed as a *carcinoma in situ,* and this may become invasive carcinoma when the basement membrane is breached.[36] Inflammatory involvement of the underlying connective tissue is a common associated finding.

Gingival Cyst. Gingival cysts of microscopic proportions are common, but they seldom reach a clinically significant size.[84] When they do, they appear as localized enlargements that may involve the marginal and attached gingiva. The cysts occur in the mandibular canine and premolar areas, most often on the lingual surface. They are painless, but with expansion, they may cause erosion of the surface of the alveolar bone. However, gingival cyst should be differentiated from the lateral periodontal cyst (see Chapter 27), which arises within the alveolar bone, adjacent to the root, and is developmental in origin. Gingival cysts develop from odontogenic epithelium or from surface or sulcular epithelium traumatically implanted in the area. Removal is followed by uneventful recovery.

> Histopathology. A gingival cyst cavity is lined by a thin, flattened epithelium with or without localized areas of thickening. Less frequently, the following types of epithelium can be found: unkeratinized stratified squamous epithelium, keratinized stratified squamous epithelium, and parakeratinized epithelium with palisading basal cells.[19]

Other Benign Masses. Other benign tumors have also been described as rare or infrequent findings in the gingiva. They include nevus,[13] myoblastoma,[42,61] hemangioma,[12,123] neurilemoma,[36] neurofibroma,[94] mucus-secreting cysts (mucoceles),[129] and ameloblastoma.[120]

Malignant Tumors of the Gingiva

Carcinoma. Oral cancer accounts for less than 3% of all malignant tumors in the body but is the sixth most common cancer in males and the twelfth in females.[87] The gingiva is not a frequent site of oral malignancy (6% of oral cancers[70]).

Squamous cell carcinoma is the most common malignant tumor of the gingiva. It may be *exophytic,* presenting as an irregular outgrowth, or *ulcerative,* appearing as flat, erosive lesions. It is often symptom free, going unnoticed until complicated by inflammatory changes that may mask the neoplasm but cause pain; sometimes it becomes evident after tooth extraction. These masses are locally invasive, involving the underlying bone and periodontal ligament of adjoining teeth and the adjacent mucosa (Figure 23-26). Metastasis is usually confined to the region above the clavicle; however, more extensive involvement may include the lung, liver, or bone.

Malignant Melanoma. Malignant melanoma is a rare oral tumor that tends to occur in the hard palate and maxillary gingiva of older persons.[87] It is usually darkly pigmented and is often preceded by localized pigmentation.[25] It may be flat or nodular and is characterized by rapid growth and early metastasis. It arises from melanoblasts in the gingiva, cheek, or palate. Infiltration into the underlying bone and metastasis to cervical and axillary lymph nodes are common.

Sarcoma. Fibrosarcoma, lymphosarcoma, and reticulum cell sarcoma of the gingiva are rare; only isolated cases have been described in the literature.[41,46,123] Kaposi's sarcoma often occurs in the oral cavity of patients with acquired immunodeficiency syndrome (AIDS), particularly in the palate and the gingiva (see Chapter 34).

Metastasis. Tumor metastasis to the gingiva occurs infrequently. Such metastasis has been reported with various tumors, including adenocarcinoma of the colon,[55] lung carcinoma, primary hepatocellular carcinoma,[125] renal cell carcinoma,[18] hypernephroma,[93] chondrosarcoma,[124] and testicular tumor.[35]

The low incidence of oral malignancy should not mislead the clinician. Ulcerations that do not respond to therapy in the usual manner, as well as all gingival tumors and tumorlike lesions, must be biopsied and submitted for microscopic diagnosis (see Chapter 35).

The reader is referred to oral pathology textbooks for more complete information on benign and malignant tumors of the gingiva.[87,104]

FALSE ENLARGEMENT

False enlargements are not true enlargements of the gingival tissues but may appear as such as a result of increases in size of the underlying osseous or dental tissues. The gingiva usually presents with no abnormal

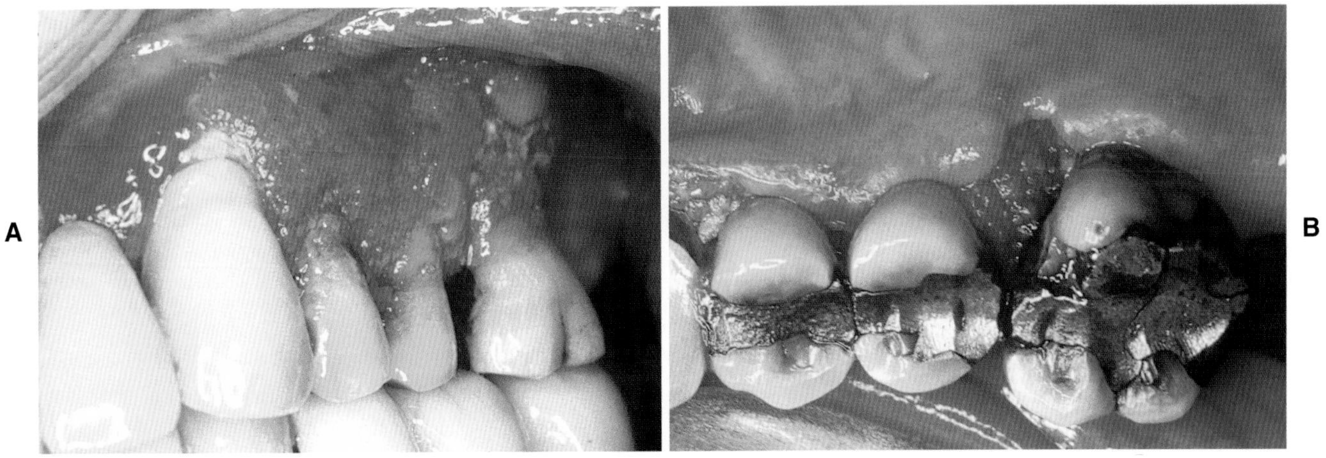

Figure 23-26 Squamous cell carcinoma of the gingiva. **A,** Facial view. Note the extensive verrucous involvement. **B,** Palatal view. Note the mulberry-like tissue emerging between the second premolar and the first molar.

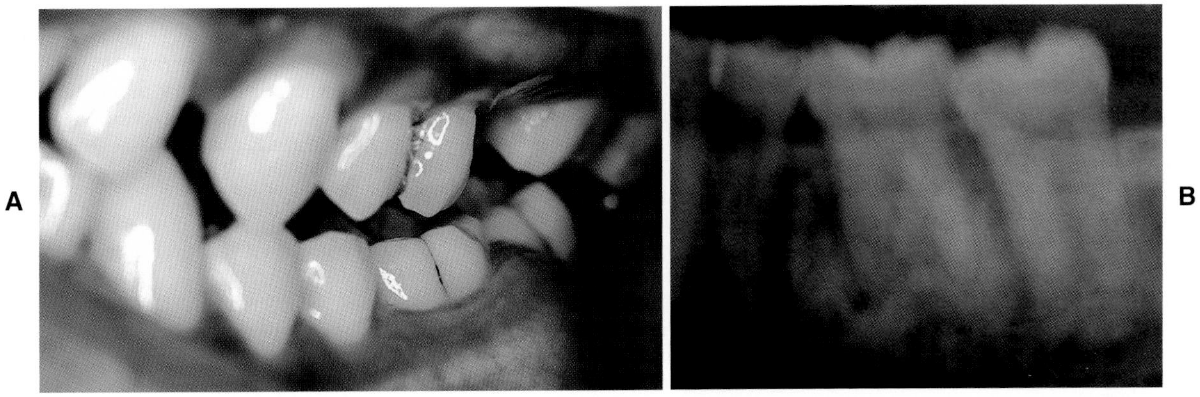

Figure 23-27 **A,** Apparent gingival enlargement associated with bone augmentation in patient with fibrous dysplasia. **B,** Radiograph of case shown in *A,* depicting a ground-glass, mottled pattern.

clinical features except the massive increase in size of the area.

Underlying Osseous Lesions

Enlargement of the bone subjacent to the gingival area occurs most often in *tori* and *exostoses,* but it can also occur in Paget's disease, fibrous dysplasia, cherubism, central giant cell granuloma, ameloblastoma, osteoma, and osteosarcoma. Figure 23-27 shows fibrous dysplasia (florid type) in a 38-year-old black female that induced an osseous enlargement in the mandibular molar area appearing as a gingival enlargement. The gingival tissue can appear normal or may have unrelated inflammatory changes.

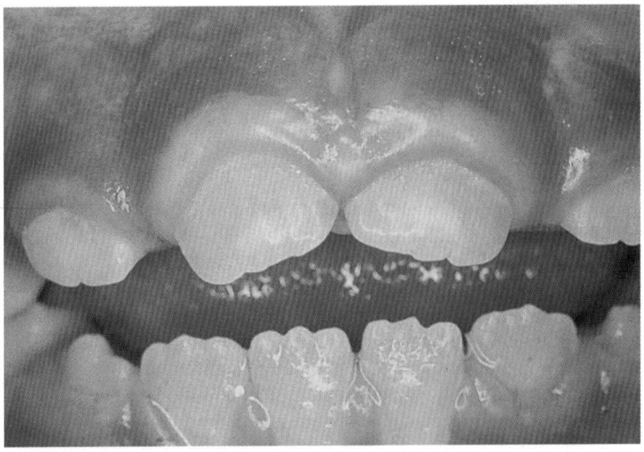

Figure 23-28 Developmental gingival enlargement. The normal bulbous contour of the gingiva around the incompletely erupted anterior teeth is accentuated by chronic inflammation.

Underlying Dental Tissues

During the various stages of eruption, particularly of the primary dentition, the labial gingiva may show a bulbous marginal distortion caused by superimposition of the bulk of the gingiva on the normal prominence of the enamel in the gingival half of the crown. This enlargement has been termed *developmental enlargement* and often persists until the junctional epithelium has migrated from the enamel to the cementoenamel junction.

In a strict sense, developmental gingival enlargements are physiologic and usually present no problems. However, when such enlargement is complicated by marginal inflammation, the composite picture gives the impression of extensive gingival enlargement (Figure 23-28). Treatment to alleviate the marginal inflammation, rather than resection of the enlargement, is sufficient in these patients.

REFERENCES

1. Aas E: *Hyperplasia gingivae diphenylhydantoinea,* Oslo, 1963, Universitetsforlaget.
2. Amar S, Chung KM: Influence of hormonal variation on the periodontium in women, *Periodontol 2000* 6:79, 1994.
3. Angelopoulos AP, Goaz PW: Incidence of diphenylhydantoin gingival hyperplasia, *Oral Surg* 34:898, 1972.
4. Ashrafi SH, Slaski K, Thu K, et al: Scanning electron microscopy of cyclosporine-induced gingival overgrowth, *Scan Microsc* 10:219, 1996.
5. Ayanoglou, CM, Lesty C: New cementum formation induced by cyclosporin A: a histological, ultrastructural and histomorphometric study in the rat, *J Periodontol* 32:543, 1997.
6. Babcock JR: Incidence of gingival hyperplasia associated with dilantin therapy in a hospital population, *J Am Dent Assoc* 71:1447, 1965.
7. Babcock JR, Nelson GH: Gingival hyperplasia and dilantin content of saliva, *J Am Dent Assoc* 68:195, 1964.
8. Bader G, Lejeune S, Messner M: Reduction of cyclosporine-induced gingival overgrowth following a change to tacrolimus: a case history involving a liver transplant patient, *J Periodontol* 69:729, 1988.
9. Baratieri A: The oxytalan connective tissue fibers in gingival hyperplasia in patients treated with sodium diphenylhydantoin, *J Periodontal Res* 2:106, 1967.
10. Barclay S, Thomason JM, Idle JR, et al: The incidence and severity of nifedipine-induced gingival overgrowth, *J Clin Periodontol* 19:311, 1992.
11. Bellinger DH: Blood and lymph vessel tumors involving the mouth, *J Oral Surg* 2:141, 1944.
12. Bernick S: Growth of the gingiva and palate. II. Connective tissue tumors, *Oral Surg* 1:1098, 1948.
13. Bernier JL, Tiecke RW: Nevus of the gingiva, *J Oral Surg* 8:165, 1950.
14. Bhaskar SN, Jacoway JR: Pyogenic granuloma: clinical features, incidence, histology and result of treatment, *J Oral Surg* 24:391, 1966.
15. Bhaskar SN, Levin MP, Frisch J: Plasma cell granuloma of periodontal tissues: report of 45 cases, *Periodontics* 6:272, 1988.
16. Bökenkamp A, Bohnhorst B, Beier C, et al: Nifedipine aggravates cyclosporine A–induced hyperplasia, *Pediatr Nephrol* 8:181, 1994.
17. Brown RS, Sein P, Corio R, et al: Nitrendipine-induced gingival hyperplasia, *Oral Surg* 70:593, 1990.
18. Buchner A, Begleiter A: Metastatic renal cell carcinoma in the gingiva mimicking a hyperplastic lesion, *J Periodontol* 51:413, 1980.
19. Buchner A, Hansen AS: The histomorphologic spectrum of the gingival cyst in the adult, *Oral Surg* 48:532, 1979.
20. Buckley DJ, Barrett AP, Bilous AM, et al: Wegener's granulomatosis—are gingival lesions pathognomonic? *J Oral Med* 42:169, 1987.
21. Buckner HJ: Diffuse fibroma of the gums, *J Am Dent Assoc* 24:2003, 1937.
22. Burket LW: *Oral medicine,* Philadelphia, 1946, Lippincott.
23. Butler RT, Kalkwarf KL, Kaldhal WB: Drug-induced gingival hyperplasia: phenytoin, cyclosporine and nifedipine, *J Am Dent Assoc* 114:56, 1987.
24. Calne R, Rolles K, White DJ, et al: Cyclosporin-A initially as the only immunosuppressant in 34 recipients of cadaveric organs: 32 kidneys, 2 pancreas and 2 livers, *Lancet* 2:1033, 1979.
25. Chaudry AP, Hampel A, Gorlin RJ: Primary malignant melanoma of the oral cavity: a review of 105 cases, *Cancer* 11:923, 1958.
26. Ciancio SG, Yaffe SJ, Catz CC: Gingival hyperplasia and diphenylhydantoin, *J Periodontol* 43:411, 1972.
27. Cotran RS, Kumar V, Robbins SL: *Robbins' pathologic basis of disease,* ed 4, Philadelphia, 1989, Saunders.
28. Daley TD, Nartey NO, Wysocki GP: Pregnancy tumor: an analysis, *Oral Surg* 72:196, 1991.
29. Daley TD, Wysocki GP, Day C: Clinical and pharmacologic correlations in cyclosporine-induced gingival hyperplasia, *Oral Surg* 62:417, 1986.
30. DaCosta ML, Regan MC, al Sader M, et al: Diphenyl hydantoin sodium promotes early and marked angiogenesis and results in increased collagen deposition and tensile strength in healing wounds, *Surgery* 123:287, 1988.
31. Dallas BM: Hyperplasia of the oral mucosa in an edentulous epileptic, *NZ Dent J* 59:54, 1963.
32. Dreyer WP, Thomas CJ: DPH-induced hyperplasia of the masticatory mucosa in an edentulous epileptic patient, *Oral Surg* 45:701, 1978.
33. Elzay RP, Swenson HM: Effect of an electric toothbrush on Dilantin sodium induced gingival hyperplasia, *NY J Dent* 34:13, 1964.
34. Emerson TG: Hereditary gingival hyperplasia: a family pedigree of four generations, *Oral Surg* 19:1, 1965.
35. Fantasia JE, Chen A: A testicular tumor with gingival metastasis, *Oral Surg* 48:64, 1979.
36. Fowler CB: Benign and malignant neoplasms of the periodontium, *Periodontol 2000* 21:33, 1999.
37. Fu E, Nieh S, Hiao CT, et al: Nifedipine-induced gingival overgrowth in rats: brief review and experimental study, *J Periodontol* 69:765, 1988.
38. Glickman I: The periodontal tissues of the guinea pig in vitamin C deficiency, *J Dent Res* 27:9, 1948.
39. Glickman I: The effect of acute vitamin C deficiency upon the response of the periodontal tissues of the guinea pig to artificially induced inflammation, *J Dent Res* 27:201, 1948.
40. Glickman I, Lewitus M: Hyperplasia of the gingiva associated with Dilantin (sodium diphenyl hydantoinate) therapy, *J Am Dent Assoc* 28:1991, 1941.
41. Goldman HM: Sarcoma, *Am J Orthod* 30:311, 1944.
42. Hagen JD, Soule EH, Gores RJ: Granular cell myoblastoma of the oral cavity, *Oral Surg* 14:454, 1961.
43. Hall WB: Dilantin hyperplasia: a preventable lesion, *J Periodontal Res* 4(suppl):36, 1969.
44. Hallmon WW, Rossmann JA: The role of drugs in the pathogenesis of gingival overgrowth, *Periodontol 2000* 21:176, 1999.
45. Hancock RH, Swan RH: Nifedipine-induced gingival overgrowth, *J Clin Periodontol* 19:12, 1992.
46. Hardman FG: Secondary sarcoma presenting clinical appearance of fibrous epulis, *Br Dent J* 86:109, 1949.

47. Hassell TM: Epilepsy and the oral manifestations of phenytoin therapy. In *Monographs in oral science,* vol 9, New York, 1981, S Karger.
48. Hassell TM: Evidence for production of an inactive collagenase by fibroblasts from phenytoin-enlarged human gingiva, *J Oral Pathol* 11:310, 1982.
49. Hassell TM, Burtner AP, McNeal D, et al: Oral problems and genetic aspects of individuals with epilepsy, *Periodontol 2000* 6:68, 1994.
50. Hassell TM, Page RC: The major metabolite of phenytoin (Dilantin) induces gingival overgrowth in cats, *J Periodontal Res* 13:280, 1978.
51. Hassell TM, Page RC, Lindhe J: Histologic evidence of impaired growth control in diphenylhydantoin gingival overgrowth in man, *Arch Oral Biol* 23:381, 1978.
52. Heijl L, Sundin Y: Nitrendipine-induced gingival overgrowth in dogs, *J Periodontol* 60:104, 1989.
53. Henefer EP, Kay LA: Congenital idiopathic gingival fibromatosis in the deciduous dentition, *Oral Surg* 24:65, 1967.
54. Hirschfeld I: Hypertrophic gingivitis: its clinical aspect, *J Am Dent Assoc* 19:799, 1932.
55. Humphrey AA, Amos NH: Metastatic gingival adenocarcinoma from primary lesion of colon, *Am J Cancer* 28:128, 1936.
56. Ishikawa J, Glickman I: Gingival response to the systemic administration of sodium diphenyl hydantoinate (Dilantin) in cats, *J Periodontol* 32:149, 1961.
57. Israelson H, Binnie WH, Hurt WC: The hyperplastic gingivitis of Wegener's granulomatosis, *J Periodontol* 52:81, 1981.
58. Jorgenson RJ, Cocker ME: Variation in the inheritance and expression of gingival fibromatosis, *J Periodontol* 45:472, 1974.
59. Kantor ML, Hassell TM: Increased accumulation of sulfated glycosaminoglycans in cultures of human fibroblasts from phenytoin-induced gingival overgrowth, *J Dent Res* 62:383, 1983.
60. Kapur RN, Grigis S, Little TM, et al: Diphenylhydantoin-induced gingival hyperplasia: its relation to dose and serum level, *Dev Med Child Neurol* 15:483, 1973.
61. Kerr DA: Myoblastic myoma, *Oral Surg* 2:41, 1949.
62. Kerr DA: Granuloma pyogenicum, *Oral Surg* 4:155, 1951.
63. Kerr DA, McClatchey KD, Regezi JA: Allergic gingivostomatitis (due to gum chewing), *J Periodontol* 42:709, 1971.
64. Kilpinen E, Raeste AM, Collan Y: Hereditary gingival hyperplasia and physical maturation, *Scand J Dent Res* 86:118, 1978.
65. Kimball O: The treatment of epilepsy with sodium diphenylhydantoinate, *JAMA* 112:1244, 1939.
66. Klar LA: Gingival hyperplasia during Dilantin therapy: a survey of 312 patients, *J Public Health Dent* 33:180, 1973.
67. Klingsberg J, Cancellaro LA, Butcher EO: Effects of air drying in rodent oral mucous membrane: a histologic study of simulated mouth breathing, *J Periodontol* 32:38, 1961.
68. Kornblut AD, Wolff SM, de Fries HE, et al: Wegener's granulomatosis, *Laryngoscope* 90:1453, 1980.
69. Kornman KS, Loesche WJ: The subgingival microbial flora during pregnancy, *J Periodontal Res* 15:111, 1980.
70. Krolls SO, Hoffman S: Squamous cell carcinomas of the oral soft tissues: a statistical analysis of 14,253 cases by age, sex and race of patients, *J Am Dent Assoc* 92:571, 1976.
71. Lamborghini Deliliers G, Santoro F, Polli N, et al: Light and electron microscopic study of cyclosporin-A induced gingival hyperplasia, *J Periodontol* 57:771, 1986.
72. Larmas LA, Mackinen KK, Paunio KU: A histochemical study of amylaminopeptidase in hydantoin-induced hyperplastic, healthy and inflamed human gingiva. *J Periodontal Res* 8:21, 1973.
73. Lederman D, Lummerman H, Reuben S, et al: Gingival hyperplasia associated with nifedipine therapy, *Oral Surg* 57:620, 1984.
74. Lite T, Dimaio DJ, Burman LR: Gingival patterns in mouth breathers: a clinical and histopathologic study and a method of treatment, *Oral Surg* 8:382, 1955.
75. Lucas RM, Howell LP, Wall RA: Nifedipine-induced gingival hyperplasia: a histochemical and ultrastructural study, *J Periodontol* 56:211, 1985.
76. Lustberg A, Goldman D, Dreskin OH: Megaloblastic anemia due to Dilantin therapy, *Ann Intern Med* 54:153, 1961.
77. Maier AW, Orban B: Gingivitis in pregnancy, *Oral Surg* 2:334, 1949.
78. Mariani G, Calastrini C, Carinci F, et al: Ultrastructural features of cyclosporine A–induced gingival hyperplasia, *J Periodontol* 64:1092, 1993.
79. Mealy BL: Periodontal implications: medically compromised patients, *Ann Periodontol* 1:256, 1996.
80. Merritt H, Putnam T: Sodium diphenylhydantoinate in the treatment of convulsive disorders, *JAMA* 111:1068, 1938.
81. McCarthy FP: A clinical and pathological study of oral disease, *JAMA* 116:16, 1941.
82. Mihatsch MJ, Kyo M, Morozumi K, et al: The side-effects of cyclosporine-A and tacrolimus, *Clin Nephrol* 49:356, 1988.
83. Mombelli A, Lang NP, Burgin WB, et al: Microbial changes associated with the development of puberty gingivitis, *J Periodontal Res* 25:331, 1990.
84. Moskow BS: The pathogenesis of the gingival cyst, *Periodontics* 4:23, 1966.
85. Nakagawa S, Fujii H, Machida Y, et al: A longitudinal study from prepuberty to puberty of gingivitis: correlation between the occurrence of *Prevotella intermedia* and sex hormones, *J Periodontol* 21:658, 1994.
86. Nease WJ: Effect of sodium diphenylhydantoinate on tissue cultures of human gingiva, *J Periodontol* 36:22, 1965.
87. Neville BW, Damm DD, Allen CM, et al: *Oral and maxillofacial pathology,* Philadelphia, 1995, Saunders.
88. Newcomb GM, Seymour GJ, Adkins KF: An unusual form of chronic gingivitis: an ultrastructural, histochemical and immunologic investigation, *Oral Surg* 53:488, 1982.
89. Nishikawa S, Tada H, Hamasaki A, et al: Nifedipine-induced gingival hyperplasia: a clinical and in vitro study, *J Periodontol* 62:30, 1991.
90. Nitta H, Kameyama Y, Ishikawa I: Unusual gingival enlargement with rapidly progressive periodontitis: report of a case, *J Periodontol* 64:1008, 1993.
91. Nuki K, Cooper SH: The role of inflammation in the pathogenesis of gingival enlargement during the administration of diphenylhydantoin sodium in cats, *J Periodontal Res* 7:91, 1972.
92. Panuska HJ, Gorlin RJ, Bearman JE, et al: The effect of anticonvulsant drugs upon the gingiva: a series of 1048 patients, *J Periodontol* 32:15, 1961.
93. Persson PA, Wallenino K: Metastatic renal carcinoma (hypernephroma) in the gingiva of the lower jaw, *Acta Odontol Scand* 19:289, 1961.
94. Pollack RP: Neurofibroma of the palatal mucosa: a case report, *J Periodontol* 61:456, 1990.
95. Raber-Durlacher JE, van Steenbergen TJM, van der Velde U, et al: Experimental gingivitis during pregnancy and postpartum: clinical, endocrinological and microbiological aspects, *J Clin Periodontol* 21:549, 1994.
96. Raeste AM, Collan Y, Kilpinen E: Hereditary fibrous hyperplasia of the gingiva with varying penetrance and expressivity, *Scand J Dent Res* 86:357, 1978.

97. Rateitschak-Pluss EM, Hefti A, Lortscher R, et al: Initial observation that cyclosporin A induces gingival enlargement in man, *J Clin Periodontol* 10:237, 1983.
98. Rees TD: Drugs and oral disorders, *Periodontology 2000* 18:21, 1998.
99. Rees TD, editor: Disorders affecting the periodontium, *Periodontol 2000* 21:145, 1999.
100. Romito GA, Pustiglioni FE, Saraiva L, et al: Relationship of subgingival and salivary microbiota to gingival overgrowth in heart transplant patients following cyclosporine A therapy, *J Periodontol* 75:918, 2004.
101. Rostock MH, Fry HR, Turner JE: Severe gingival overgrowth associated with cyclosporine therapy, *J Periodontol* 57:294, 1986.
102. Rushton MA: Hereditary or idiopathic hyperplasia of the gums, *Dent Pract* 7:136, 1957.
103. Russell BJ, Bay LM: Oral use of chlorhexidine gluconate toothpaste in epileptic children, *Scand J Dent Res* 86:52, 1978.
104. Sapp JP, Eversole LR, Wysocki GP: *Contemporary oral and maxillofacial pathology,* St Louis, 2004, Elsevier.
105. Schneider LC, Weisinger E: The true gingival fibroma: an analysis of 129 fibrous gingival lesions, *J Periodontol* 49:423, 1978.
106. Serio FG, Siegel MA, Slade BE: Plasma cell gingivitis of unusual origin: a case report, *J Periodontol* 49:423, 1978.
107. Setia AP: Severe bleeding from a pregnancy tumor, *Oral Surg* 36:192, 1973.
108. Seymour RA, Jacobs DJ: Cyclosporine and the gingival tissues, *J Clin Periodontol* 19:1, 1992.
109. Seymour RA, Smith DG, Rogers SR: The comparative effects of azathioprine and cyclosporine on some gingival health parameters of renal transplant patients, *J Clin Periodontol* 14:610, 1987.
110. Seymour RA, Thomason JM, Ellis JS: The pathogenesis of drug-induced gingival overgrowth, *J Clin Periodontol* 23:165, 1996.
111. Shafer WG: Effect of Dilantin sodium analogues on cell proliferation in tissue culture, *Proc Soc Exp Biol Med* 106:205, 1960.
112. Shafer WG: Effect of Dilantin sodium on various cell lines in tissue culture, *Proc Soc Exp Biol Med* 108:694, 1961.
113. Shafer WG, Beatty RE, Davis WB: Effect of Dilantin sodium on tensile strength of healing wounds, *Proc Soc Exp Biol Med* 98:348, 1958.
114. Shapiro M: Acceleration of gingival wound healing in nonepileptic patients receiving diphenylhydantoin sodium, *Exp Med Surg* 16:41, 1958.
115. Silverman S Jr, Lozada F: An epilogue to plasma cell gingivostomatitis (allergic gingivostomatitis), *Oral Surg* 43:211, 1977.
116. Slavin J, Taylor J: Cyclosporine, nifedipine and gingival hyperplasia, *Lancet* ii:739, 1987.
117. Spencer CM, Goa KL, Gillis JC: Tacrolimus: an update of its pharmacology and drug efficacy in the management of organ transplantation, *Drugs* 54:925, 1997.
118. Staple PH, Reed MJ, Mashimo PA: Diphenylhydantoin gingival hyperplasia in *Macaca arctoides:* a new human model, *J Periodontol* 48:325, 1977.
119. Stein GM, Lewis H: Oral changes in a folic acid deficient patient precipitated by anticonvulsant drug therapy, *J Periodontol* 44:645, 1973.
120. Stevenson ARL, Austin BW: A case of ameloblastoma presenting as an exophytic gingival lesion, *J Periodontol* 61:378, 1990.
121. Stirrups D, Inglis J: Tuberous sclerosis with nonhydantoin gingival hyperplasia: report of a case, *Oral Surg* 49:211, 1980.
122. Sutcliffe P: A longitudinal study of gingivitis and puberty, *J Periodontal Res* 7:52, 1972.
123. Sznajder N, Dominguez FV, Carraro JJ, Lis G: Hemorrhagic hemangioma of the gingiva: report of a case, *J Periodontol* 44:579, 1973.
124. Taicher S, Mazar A, Hirschberg A, et al: Metastatic chondrosarcoma of the gingiva mimicking a reactive exophytic lesion: a case report, *J Periodontol* 623:223, 1991.
125. Thoma KH, Holland DJ, Woodbury HW, et al: Malignant lymphoma of the gingiva, *Oral Surg* 1:57, 1948.
126. Thomas D, Rapley J, Strathman R, et al: Tuberous sclerosis with gingival overgrowth, *J Periodontol* 63:713, 1992.
127. Thomason JM, Seymour RA, Rice N: The prevalence and severity of cyclosporine and nifedipine-induced gingival overgrowth, *J Clin Periodontol* 20:37, 1993.
128. Thomason JM, Seymour RA, Ellis JS, et al: Determinants of gingival overgrowth severity in organ transplant patients, *J Clin Periodontol* 23:628, 1996.
129. Traeger KA: Cyst of the gingiva (mucocele): report of a case, *Oral Surg* 14:243, 1961.
130. Varga E, Lennon MA, Mair LH: Pre-transplant gingival hyperplasia predicts severe cyclosporin-induced gingival overgrowth in renal transplant patients, *J Clin Periodontol* 25:225, 1988.
131. Wedgwood D, Rusen D, Balk S: Gingival metastases from primary hepatocellular carcinoma, *Oral Surg* 47:263, 1979.
132. Westbrook P, Bednarczyk EM, Carlson M, et al: Regression of nifedipine-induced gingival hyperplasia following switch to a same class calcium channel blocker, isradipine, *J Periodontol* 68:645, 1997.
133. Westphal P: Salivary secretion and gingival hyperplasia in diphenylhydantoin-treated guinea pigs, *Sven Tandlak Tidskr* 62:505, 1969.
134. Wojcicki CJ, Harper DS, Robinson PJ: Differences in periodontal-disease associated microorganisms in prepubertal, pubertal and postpubertal children, *J Periodontol* 58:219, 1987.
135. Wysocki G, Gretsinger HA, Laupacis A, et al: Fibrous hyperplasia of the gingiva: a side effect of cyclosporin A therapy, *Oral Surg* 55:274, 1983.
136. Zackin SJ, Weisberger D: Hereditary gingival fibromatosis, *Oral Surg* 14:828, 1961.
137. Ziskin DE, Zegarelli E: Idiopathic fibromatosis of the gingivae, *Ann Dent* 2:50, 1943.
138. Ziskin DE, Blackberg SM, Stout AP: The gingivae during pregnancy, *Surg Gynecol Obstet* 57:719, 1933.

Acute Gingival Infections

Phillip T. Marucha

24

CHAPTER

CHAPTER OUTLINE

NECROTIZING ULCERATIVE GINGIVITIS

Necrotizing ulcerative gingivitis (NUG) is a microbial disease of the gingiva in the context of an impaired host response. It is characterized by the death and sloughing of gingival tissue and presents with characteristic signs and symptoms.

Clinical Features

Classification. NUG is usually identified as an *acute* disease. NUG often undergoes a diminution in severity without treatment, leading to a *subacute* stage with milder clinical symptoms. Thus, patients may have a history of repeated remissions and exacerbations. Recurrence of the condition in previously treated patients can also occur. Involvement may be limited to a single tooth or group of teeth (Figure 24-1, *A, B,* and *C*) or may be widespread throughout the mouth (Figure 24-1, *D*).

NUG can cause tissue destruction involving the periodontal attachment apparatus, especially in patients with long standing disease or severe immunosuppression. When bone loss occurs, the condition is called *necrotizing ulcerative periodontitis* (NUP) (see Chapter 32).

History. NUG is characterized by sudden onset of symptoms, sometimes following an episode of debilitating disease or acute respiratory tract infection. A change in living habits, protracted work without adequate rest, poor nutrition, tobacco use, and psychologic stress are frequent features of the patient's history.

Oral Signs. Characteristic lesions are *punched-out, craterlike depressions at the crest of the interdental papillae,* subsequently extending to the marginal gingiva and rarely to the attached gingiva and oral mucosa. The surface of the gingival craters is covered by a *gray, pseudomembranous slough,* demarcated from the remainder of the gingival mucosa by a pronounced *linear erythema* (see Figure 24-1, *A*). In some cases the lesions are denuded of the surface pseudomembrane, exposing the gingival margin, which is red, shiny, and hemorrhagic. The characteristic lesions may progressively destroy the gingiva and underlying periodontal tissues (see Figure 24-1, *B*).

Spontaneous gingival hemorrhage or pronounced bleeding after the slightest stimulation are additional characteristic clinical signs (see Figure 24-1, *B* and *C*). Other signs often found are fetid odor and increased salivation.

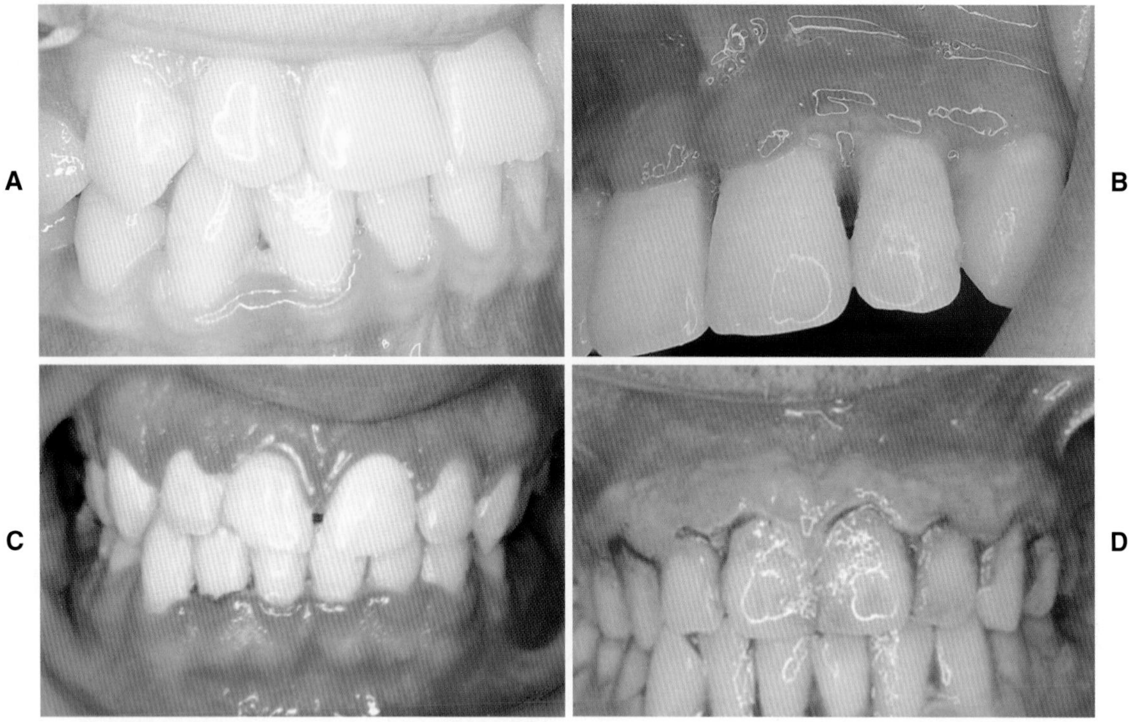

Figure 24-1 Necrotizing ulcerative gingivitis. **A,** Typical punched-out papilla between mandibular canine and lateral incisor, covered by grayish white pseudomembrane. **B,** More advanced case showing destruction of papillae resulting in irregular marginal contour. **C,** Typical lesions with spontaneous hemorrhage. **D,** Generalized involvement of papillae and marginal gingiva, with whitish necrotic lesions.

NUG can be superimposed on chronic gingivitis or periodontal pockets. However, NUG or NUP does not usually lead to periodontal pocket formation because the necrotic changes involve the marginal gingiva, causing recession rather than pocket formation.

Oral Symptoms. The lesions are extremely sensitive to touch, and the patient often complains of a constant radiating, gnawing pain that is intensified by eating spicy or hot foods and chewing. There is a "metallic" foul taste, and the patient is conscious of an excessive amount of "pasty" saliva.

Extraoral and Systemic Signs and Symptoms. Patients are usually ambulatory and have a minimum of systemic symptoms. Local lymphadenopathy and a slight elevation in temperature are common features of the mild and moderate stages of the disease. In severe cases, there may be high fever, increased pulse rate, leukocytosis, loss of appetite, and general lassitude. Systemic reactions are more severe in children. Insomnia, constipation, gastro-intestinal disorders, headache, and mental depression sometimes accompany the condition.

In very rare cases, severe sequelae such as gangrenous stomatitis and noma have been described[2,3,19,35] (Figure 24-2).

Clinical Course. The clinical course can vary. If untreated, NUG may lead to NUP with a progressive destruction of the periodontium and gingival recession, accompanied by an increase in the severity of systemic complications (see Chapter 32).

Pindborg et al.[53] have described these stages in the progress of NUG: (1) erosion of only the tip of the interdental papilla; (2) the lesion extending to marginal gingiva and causing a further erosion of the papilla and potentially a complete loss of the papilla; (3) the attached gingiva also being affected; and (4) exposure of bone.

Horning and Cohen[33] extended the staging of these oral necrotizing diseases as follows (% incidence among cases of NUG in the authors' series):

Stage 1: Necrosis of the tip of the interdental papilla (93%) (Figure 24-1, *A*)
Stage 2: Necrosis of the entire papilla (19%) (Figure 24-1, *B*)
Stage 3: Necrosis extending to the gingival margin (21%) (Figure 24-1, *B* and *C*)
Stage 4: Necrosis extending also to the attached gingiva (1%)
Stage 5: Necrosis extending into buccal or labial mucosa (6%)
Stage 6: Necrosis exposing alveolar bone (1%) (Figure 24-2, *A*)
Stage 7: Necrosis perforating skin of cheek (0%) (Figure 24-2, *B*)

According to Horning and Cohen,[33] stage 1 is NUG, stage 2 may be either NUG or NUP because attachment loss may have occurred, stages 3 and 4 would correspond to NUP, stages 5 and 6 would correspond to necrotizing stomatitis, and stage 7 would be noma (see Chapter 32).

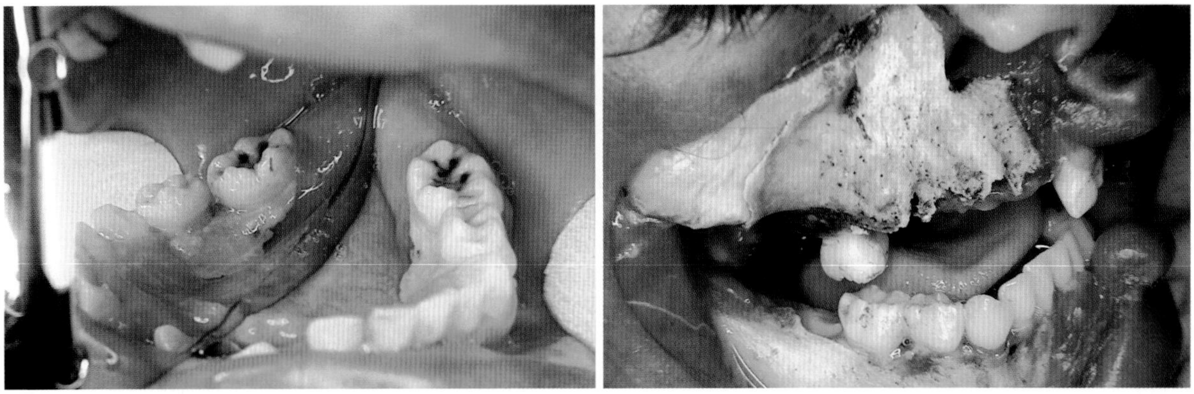

Figure 24-2 Severe sequelae of necrotizing gingivitis in children with severe malnutrition. **A,** Gangrenous stomatitis with exposure of marginal bone in 5-year-old child. **B,** Noma with advanced destruction of facial tissues in 4$^1/_2$-year-old child. (From Jimenez M, Baer PN: *J Periodontol* 46:715, 1975.)

Histopathology. Microscopically, the NUG lesion is acute necrotizing inflammation of the gingival margin, involving both the stratified squamous epithelium and the underlying connective tissue. The surface epithelium is destroyed and replaced by a meshwork of fibrin, necrotic epithelial cells, polymorphonuclear leukocytes (PMNs, neutrophils), and various types of microorganisms (Figure 24-3). This is the zone that appears clinically as the surface pseudomembrane. At the immediate border of the necrotic pseudomembrane, the epithelium is edematous, and the individual cells exhibit varying degrees of hydropic degeneration. In addition, there is an infiltration of PMNs in the intercellular spaces.

The underlying connective tissue is extremely hyperemic, with numerous engorged capillaries and a dense infiltration of PMNs. This acutely inflamed zone appears clinically as the linear erythema beneath the surface pseudomembrane. Numerous plasma cells may appear in the periphery of the infiltrate; this is interpreted as an area of established chronic gingivitis on which the acute lesion became superimposed.[32]

The epithelium and connective tissue alterations decrease as the distance from the necrotic gingival margin increases, blending gradually with the uninvolved gingiva.

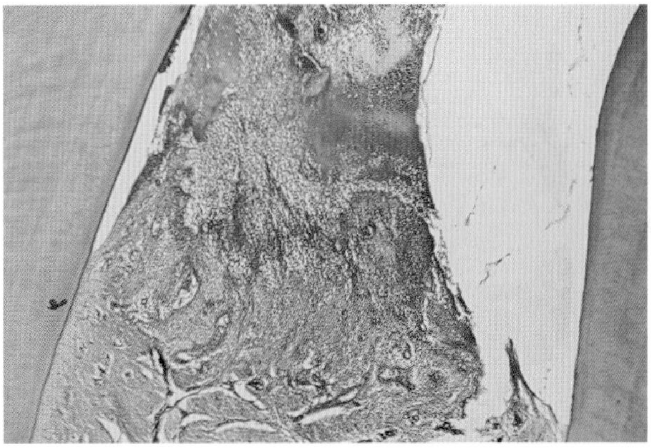

Figure 24-3 Survey section of interdental papilla in necrotizing ulcerative gingivitis. Top portion of the section shows the necrotic tissue that forms the gray marginal pseudomembrane. In lower portion, note the ulceration and accumulation of leukocytes and fibrin.

Relation of Bacteria to Characteristic Lesion

Light and electron microscopy have been used to study the relationship of bacteria to the characteristic lesion of NUG. Light microscopy shows that the exudate on the surface of the necrotic lesion contains microorganisms that morphologically resemble cocci, fusiform bacilli, and spirochetes.[77] The layer between the necrotic and the living tissue contains enormous numbers of fusiform bacilli and spirochetes, in addition to leukocytes and fibrin. Spirochetes and other bacteria[5,12,17,38] invade the underlying living tissue.

Spirochetes have been found as deep as 300 µm from the surface. The majority of spirochetes in the deeper zones are morphologically different from cultivated strains of *Treponema microdentium*. They occur in nonnecrotic tissue before other types of bacteria and may be present in high concentrations intercellularly in the epithelium adjacent to the ulcerated lesion and in the connective tissue[37] (Figure 24-4).

Diagnosis

Diagnosis is based on clinical findings of gingival pain, ulceration, and bleeding. A bacterial smear is not necessary or definitive because the bacterial picture is not appreciably different from that in marginal gingivitis, periodontal pockets, pericoronitis, or primary herpetic gingivostomatitis.[59] Bacterial studies are useful, however, in the differential diagnosis of NUG and specific infections of the oral cavity, such as diphtheria, thrush, actinomycosis, and streptococcal stomatitis.

Microscopic examination of a biopsy specimen is not sufficiently specific to be diagnostic. It can be used to differentiate NUG from specific infections such as tuberculosis or from neoplastic disease, but it does not

TABLE 24-1

Differentiation between Necrotizing Ulcerative Gingivitis and Primary Herpetic Gingivostomatitis

Necrotizing Ulcerative Gingivitis	Primary Herpetic Gingivostomatitis
Etiology: interaction between host and bacteria, most probably fusospirochetes	Specific viral etiology
Necrotizing condition	Diffuse erythema and vesicular eruption
Punched-out gingival margin; pseudomembrane that peels off, leaving raw areas	Vesicles rupture and leave slightly depressed oval or spherical ulcer.
Marginal gingiva affected; other oral tissues rarely affected	Diffuse involvement of gingiva; may include buccal mucosa and lips
Uncommon in children	Occurs more frequently in children
No definite duration	Duration of 7 to 10 days
No demonstrated immunity	Acute episode results in some degree of immunity.
Contagion not demonstrated	Contagion

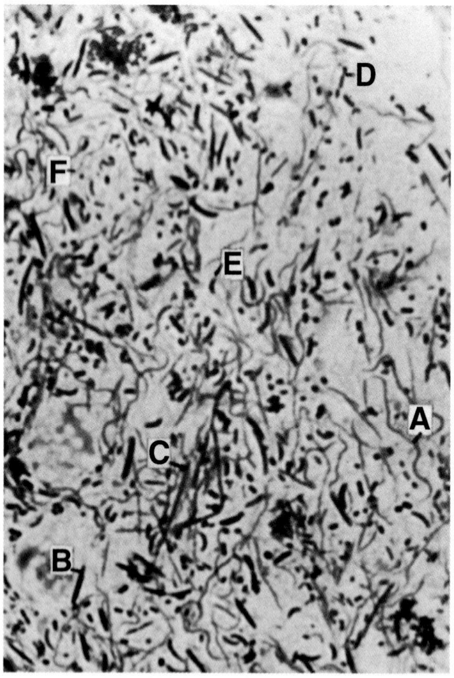

Figure 24-4 Bacterial smear from lesion in necrotizing ulcerative gingivitis. *A,* Spirochete; *B, Bacillus fusiformis; C,* filamentous organism *(Actinomyces* or *Leptotrichia); D, Streptococcus; E, Vibrio; F, Treponema microdentium.*

SCIENCE TRANSFER

The diagnosis of acute gingival infections can often be made on the basis of the clinical presentation. Thus, necrotizing ulcerative lesions of interdental papillae and marginal gingiva together with halitosis indicate acute necrotizing gingivitis, or *necrotizing ulcerative gingivitis* (NUG), and vesicular lesions of keratinized mucosa, including gingiva, together with elevated temperature indicate *primary herpetic gingivostomatitis.*

When necrotizing lesions fail to respond to local and antibiotic therapy, there may be an underlying etiology of depressed immune response. *In all cases of acute gingival infections, the clinician should investigate the patient's history to determine if immunosuppressive diseases are present* (e.g., AIDS, leukemia, cyclic neutropenia).

differentiate between NUG and other necrotizing conditions of nonspecific origin, such as those produced by trauma or caustic medications.

NUG should be differentiated from other conditions that resemble it in some respects, such as herpetic gingivostomatitis (Table 24-1); chronic periodontitis; desquamative gingivitis (Table 24-2); streptococcal gingivostomatitis; aphthous stomatitis; gonococcal gingivostomatitis; diphtheritic and syphilitic lesions (Table 24-3); tuberculous gingival lesion; candidiasis, agranulocytosis, dermatoses (pemphigus, erythema multiforme, lichen planus); and stomatitis venenata. Treatment options for these diseases vary dramatically, and improper treatment may exacerbate the condition. In the case of primary herpetic gingivostomatitis, early diagnosis may result in treatment with antiviral drugs that would be ineffective for NUG, whereas treatment of a case of herpes with the debridement required for NUG could exacerbate herpes. (See Chapter 26 for a description of most of these conditions.)

Streptococcal gingivostomatitis is a rare condition characterized by a diffuse erythema of the gingiva and other areas of the oral mucosa.[43] In some cases it is confined as a marginal erythema with marginal hemorrhage. Necrosis of the gingival margin is not a feature of this disease, and there is no notably fetid odor. Bacterial smears show a preponderance of streptococcal forms, which were identified as *Streptococcus viridans,* but more recent studies report it to be group A β-hemolytic streptococcus.[39]

TABLE 24-2

Differentiation among Necrotizing Ulcerative Gingivitis, Chronic Desquamative Gingivitis, and Chronic Periodontal Disease

Necrotizing Ulcerative Gingivitis	Desquamative Gingivitis	Chronic Destructive Periodontal Disease
Bacterial smears show fusospirochetal complex.	Bacterial smears reveal numerous epithelial cells, few bacterial forms.	Bacterial smears are variable.
Marginal gingiva affected	Diffuse involvement of marginal and attached gingivae and other areas of oral mucosa	Marginal gingiva affected
Acute history	Chronic history	Chronic history
Painful	May or may not be painful	Painless if uncomplicated
Pseudomembrane	Patchy desquamation of gingival epithelium	Generally no desquamation, but purulent material may appear from pockets.
Pupillary and marginal necrotic lesions	Papillae do not undergo necrosis.	Papillae do not undergo noticeable necrosis.
Affects adults of both genders, occasionally children	Affects adults, most often women	Generally in adults, occasionally in children
Characteristic fetid odor	None	Some odor present but not strikingly fetid

TABLE 24-3

Differentiation among Necrotizing Ulcerative Gingivitis, Diphtheria, and Secondary Stage of Syphilis

Necrotizing Ulcerative Gingivitis	Diphtheria	Secondary Stage of Syphilis (Mucous Patch)
Etiology: interaction between host and bacteria, most probably fusospirochetes	Specific bacterial etiology: *Corynebacterium diphtheriae*	Specific bacterial etiology: *Treponema pallidum*
Affects marginal gingiva	Rarely affects marginal gingiva	Rarely affects marginal gingiva
Membrane removal easy	Membrane removal difficult	Membrane not detachable
Painful condition	Less painful	Minimal pain
Marginal gingivae affected	Throat, fauces, and tonsils affected	Any part of mouth affected
Serologic findings normal	Serologic findings normal	Serologic findings abnormal*
Immunity not conferred	Immunity conferred by an attack	Immunity not conferred
Doubtful contagiousness	Contagion	Only direct contact will communicate disease.
Antibiotic therapy relieves symptoms.	Antibiotic treatment has minimal effect.	Antibiotic therapy has excellent results.

*Wassermann, Kahn, Venereal Disease Research Laboratories (VDRL).

Agranulocytosis is characterized by a marked decrease in the number of circulating PMNs, lesions of the throat and other mucous membranes, and ulceration and necrosis of the gingiva, which may resemble that of NUG. The oral condition in agranulocytosis is primarily necrotizing. Because of the diminished innate defense mechanisms in agranulocytosis, the clinical picture is not marked by the severe inflammatory reaction seen in NUG. Blood studies serve to differentiate between NUG and the gingival necrosis in agranulocytosis.

Vincent's angina is a fusospirochetal infection of the oropharynx and throat, as distinguished from NUG, which affects the marginal gingiva. Patients with Vincent's angina have a painful membranous ulceration of the throat, with edema and hyperemic patches breaking down to form ulcers covered with pseudomembranous material. The process may extend to the larynx and middle ear.

NUG in the patient with *leukemia* is not produced by leukemia itself but may result from the reduced host defense mechanisms seen with leukemia. Also, NUG may be superimposed on gingival tissue alterations caused by leukemia. The differential diagnosis consists not in distinguishing between NUG and leukemic gingival changes, but rather in determining whether leukemia is a predisposing factor in a mouth with NUG. For example, if a patient with necrotizing involvement of the gingival margin also has generalized diffuse discoloration and edema of the attached gingiva, the possibility of an underlying, systemically induced gingival change should be considered. Leukemia is one of the conditions that would need to be ruled out (see Chapter 17).

NUG in the patient with *HIV infection* has the same clinical features, although it follows an extremely destructive course leading to NUP, with loss of soft tissue and bone and formation of bony sequestra[29] (see Chapter 34). Importantly, NUG can be a presenting symptom of HIV infection.

Etiology

Role of Bacteria. Plaut[54] (1894) and Vincent[79] (1896) introduced the concept that NUG is caused by specific bacteria: fusiform bacillus and a spirochetal organism.

Opinions still differ regarding whether bacteria are the primary causative factors in NUG. Several observations support this concept, including that spirochetal organisms and fusiform bacilli are always found in the disease, with other organisms also involved. Rosebury et al.[59] described a fusospirochetal complex consisting of *T. microdentium,* intermediate spirochetes, vibrios, fusiform bacilli, and filamentous organisms, in addition to several *Borrelia* species.

Loesche et al.[40] described a predominant constant flora and a variable flora associated with NUG. The constant flora is composed of *Prevotella intermedia,* in addition to *Fusobacterium, Treponema,* and *Selenomonas* species. The variable flora consists of a heterogeneous array of bacterial types.

Treatment with metronidazole results in a significant reduction of *Treponema* species, *P. intermedia,* and *Fusobacterium,* with resolution of the clinical symptoms.[16,40] The antibacterial spectrum of this drug provides evidence for the anaerobic members of the flora as etiologic agents.

These bacteriologic findings have been supported by immunologic data from Chung et al.[9] These investigators reported increased immunoglobulin (IgG and IgM) antibody titers for medium-sized spirochetes and *P. intermedia* in NUG patients compared with titers in those with chronic gingivitis and healthy controls.

Role of the Host Response. Regardless of whether specific bacteria are implicated in the etiology of NUG, the presence of these organisms is insufficient to cause the disease. Exudates from NUG lesions produce fusospirochetal abscesses, rather than typical NUG, when inoculated subcutaneously in experimental animals.[58] Local intracutaneous injection of a hyaluronidase- and chondroitinase-containing cell-free filtrate of oral microaerophilic diphtheroid bacilli aggravated spirochetal lesions that were produced by oral treponemes.[31] Only in one animal experiment has the transmission of lesions comparable with those seen in humans been reported.[2]

The role of an impaired host response in NUG has long been recognized. Even during its early descriptions over the last 2000 years, NUG has been associated with physical and emotional stress[60] and decreased resistance to infection. NUG has not been produced experimentally in humans or animals by just inoculation of bacterial exudates from the lesions. In the animal model, local or systemic immunosuppression with glucocorticoids (e.g., ketaconazole) results in more characteristic lesions of NUG in infected animals. Furthermore, NUG is not found in well-nourished individuals with a fully functional immune system. All the predisposing factors for NUG are associated with immunosuppression. Cogen et al.[10] described a depression in host defense mechanisms, particularly in polymorphonuclear leukocyte (PMN) chemotaxis and phagocytosis, in NUG patients. (For further details on the host-bacteria interactions in NUG, see Chapters 9, 13, and 15.)

It is essential for the clinician to determine the predisposing factors leading to immunodeficiency in NUG in order to address the continued susceptibility of the patient and to determine whether an underlying systemic disease is present. Immunodeficiency may be related to varying levels of nutritional deficiency, fatigue caused by chronic sleep deprivation, other health habits (e.g., alcohol or drug abuse), psychosocial factors, or systemic disease. Importantly, NUG may be the presenting symptom for patients with immunosuppression related to human immunodeficiency (HIV) infection.

Local Predisposing Factors. Preexisting gingivitis, injury to the gingiva, and smoking are important predisposing factors. Although NUG may appear in an otherwise disease-free mouth, it most often occurs superimposed on preexisting chronic gingival disease and periodontal pockets. Deep periodontal pockets and pericoronal flaps are particularly vulnerable areas because they offer a favorable environment for the proliferation of anaerobic fusiform bacilli and spirochetes. Areas of the gingiva traumatized by opposing teeth in malocclusion, such as the palatal surface behind the maxillary incisors and the labial gingival surface of the mandibular incisors, may predispose to NUG.

The relationship between NUG and *smoking* has often been mentioned in the literature. Pindborg[52] reported that 98% of his patients with NUG were smokers and that the frequency of this disease increases with an increasing exposure to tobacco smoke. The effect of smoking on periodontal disease in general has been the subject of numerous studies in the past two decades, and smoking has been established as a high risk factor for disease (see Chapter 14).

Systemic Predisposing Factors. NUG is not found in a well-nourished individual with a fully functional immune system. Therefore, it is important for the clinician to determine the predisposing factors leading to immunodeficiency. Again, immunodeficiency may be related to varying levels of nutritional deficiency; fatigue caused by chronic sleep deficiency; other health habits (e.g., alcohol or drug abuse), and systemic disease (e.g., diabetes, debilitating infection).

Nutritional Deficiency. Necrotizing gingivitis has been produced by giving animals nutritionally deficient diets.[7,36,46,75,78] Several researchers found an increase in the fusospirochetal flora in the mouths of the experimental animals, but the bacteria were regarded as opportunists, proliferating only when the tissues were altered by the deficiency. A poor diet has been cited as a predisposing factor in NUG and its sequelae in developing African countries, although the effects appear primarily to diminish the effectiveness of the immune response.[19,20,33]

Nutritional deficiencies (e.g., vitamin C, vitamin B_2) accentuate the severity of the pathologic changes induced when the fusospirochetal bacterial complex is injected into animals.[70]

Debilitating Disease. Debilitating systemic disease may predispose patients to the development of NUG. Such systemic disturbances include chronic diseases (e.g., syphilis, cancer), severe gastrointestinal disorders (e.g., ulcerative colitis), blood dyscrasias (e.g., leukemia, anemia), and acquired immunodeficiency syndrome (AIDS). Nutritional deficiency resulting from debilitating disease may be an additional predisposing factor. Experimentally induced leukopenia in animals may produce ulcerative gangrenous stomatitis.[46,73,74,76] Ulceronecrotic lesions appear in the gingival margins of hamsters exposed to total-body irradiation;[41] these lesions can be prevented with systemic antibiotics.[42]

Psychosomatic Factors. Psychologic factors appear to be important in the etiology of NUG. The disease often occurs in association with stressful situations (e.g., induction into the armed forces, school examinations).[26] Psychologic disturbances,[27] as well as increased adrenocortical secretion,[65] are common in patients with the disease.

Significant correlation between disease incidence and two personality traits, dominance and abasement, suggests the presence of an NUG-prone personality.[23] The mechanisms whereby psychologic factors create or predispose to gingival damage have not been established, but alterations in digital and gingival capillary responses suggesting increased autonomic nervous activity have been demonstrated in patients with NUG.[25]

Cohen-Cole et al.[11] suggested that a psychiatric disturbance (e.g., trait anxiety, depression, psychopathic deviance) and the impact of negative life events (stress) may lead to activation of the hypothalamic-pituitary-adrenal axis. This results in elevation of serum and urine cortisol levels, which is associated with a depression of lymphocyte and PMN function that may predispose to NUG.

It can be concluded that opportunistic bacteria are the primary etiologic agents of NUG in patients who demonstrate immunosuppression. Stress, smoking, and preexisting gingivitis are common predisposing factors.

Epidemiology and Prevalence

NUG often occurs in groups in an epidemic pattern. At one time, it was considered contagious, but this has not been substantiated.[62]

The prevalence of NUG appears to have been rather low in the United States and Europe before 1914. During World Wars I and II, numerous "epidemics" broke out among the Allied troops, but German soldiers did not seem to have been similarly affected. Epidemic-like outbreaks have also occurred among civilian populations. A study at a dental clinic in Prague, Czech Republic, reported the incidence of NUG as 0.08% in patients age 15 to 19 years, 0.05% in those age 20 to 24, and 0.02% in those age 25 to 29.[68]

NUG occurs at all ages,[13] with the highest incidence reported between ages 20 and 30 years[14,71] and ages 15 and 20 years.[68] It is not common in children in the United States, Canada, and Europe, but it has been reported in children from low socioeconomic groups in underdeveloped countries.[35] In India, 54%[52] and 58%[53] of the patients in two studies were under age 10 years. In a random school population in Nigeria, NUG occurred in 11.3% of children between ages 2 and 6 years,[66] and in a Nigerian hospital population, it was present in 23% of children under age 10 years.[18] It has been reported in several members of the same family in low socioeconomic groups. NUG is more common in children with Down syndrome than in other children with mental deficiencies.[4]

Opinions differ as to whether NUG is more common during the winter,[50] summer, or fall[68] and whether there is a peak seasonal incidence.[15]

Communicability

A distinction must be made between "communicability" and "transmissibility" when referring to the characteristics of disease. The term *transmissible* denotes a capacity for the maintenance of an infectious agent in successive passages through a susceptible animal host.[57] The term *communicable* signifies a capacity for the maintenance of infection by natural modes of spread, such as direct contact through drinking water, food, and eating utensils; via the airborne route; or by means of arthropod vectors. A disease that is communicable is described as *contagious.* It has been demonstrated that disease associated with the fusospirochetal bacterial complex is transmissible; *however, it has not been shown to be communicable or contagious.*

Attempts have been made to spread NUG from human to human, without success.[63] King[36] traumatized an area in his gingiva and introduced debris from a patient with a severe case of NUG. There was no response until he happened to fall ill shortly thereafter; subsequent to his illness, he observed the characteristic lesion in the experimental area. It may be inferred with reservation from this experiment that systemic debility is a prerequisite for the contagion of NUG.

It is a common impression that, because NUG often occurs in groups using the same kitchen facilities, the disease is spread by bacteria on eating utensils. Growth of fusospirochetal organisms requires carefully controlled conditions and an anaerobic environment; they do not ordinarily survive on eating utensils.[31]

The occurrence of NUG in epidemic-like outbreaks does not necessarily mean that it is contagious. The affected groups may be afflicted by the disease because of common predisposing factors rather than because of its spread from person to person. In all likelihood, both a predisposed immunocompromised host and the presence of appropriate bacteria are necessary for the production of this disease.

PRIMARY HERPETIC GINGIVOSTOMATITIS

Primary herpetic gingivostomatitis is an infection of the oral cavity caused by the herpes simplex virus type 1 (HSV-1).[15,44] It occurs most often in infants and children younger than 6 years of age,[6,64] but it is also seen in adolescents and adults. It occurs with equal frequency in male and female patients. In most persons, however, the primary infection is asymptomatic.

As part of the primary infection, the virus ascends through sensory and autonomic nerves, where it persists as latent HSV in neuronal ganglia that innervate the site. In approximately one third of the world's population, secondary manifestations result from various stimuli, such as sunlight, trauma, fever, and stress. These secondary manifestations include herpes labialis (Figure 24-5), herpetic stomatitis, herpes genitalis, ocular herpes, and herpetic encephalitis. Secondary herpetic stomatitis can occur as a result of dental treatment and may present as pain away from the site of treatment 2 to 4 days later. Careful inspection for characteristic vesicles may be diagnostic (Figure 24-6).

Clinical Features

Oral Signs. Primary herpetic gingivostomatitis appears as a diffuse, erythematous, shiny involvement of the gingiva and the adjacent oral mucosa, with varying degrees of edema and gingival bleeding. In its initial stage, it is characterized by the presence of discrete, spherical gray vesicles, which may occur on the gingiva, labial and buccal mucosae, soft palate, pharynx, sublingual mucosa, and tongue (Figure 24-7). After approximately 24 hours, the vesicles rupture and form painful, small ulcers with a red, elevated, halo-like margin and a depressed, yellowish or grayish white central portion. These occur either in widely separated areas or in clusters, where confluence occurs (Figure 24-8).

Occasionally, primary herpetic gingivitis may occur without overt vesiculation. The clinical picture consists of diffuse, erythematous, shiny discoloration and edematous enlargement of the gingivae with a tendency toward bleeding.

The course of the disease is limited to 7 to 10 days. The diffuse gingival erythema and edema that appear early

A

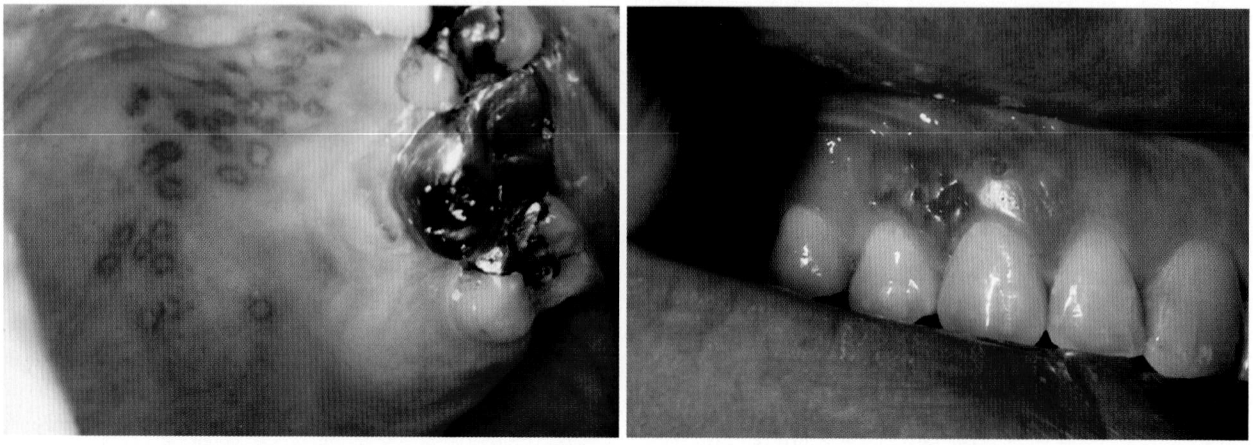

B

Figure 24-5 Recurrent intraoral herpetic vesicles in the palate **(A)** and in the gingiva **(B)**. The latter location is rare. (From Sapp JP, Eversole, LR, Wysocki GP: *Contemporary oral and maxillofacial pathology,* ed 2, St Louis, 2002, Mosby.)

A

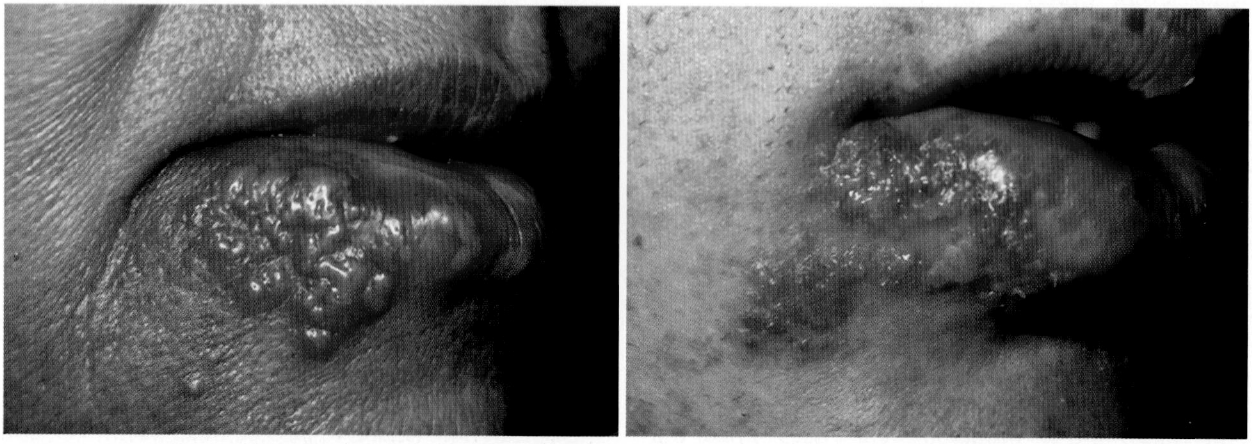

B

Figure 24-6 Recurrent herpetic vesicles in the lip. **A,** Early stage. **B,** Late stage showing brownish crusted lesions. (From Sapp JP, Eversole, LR, Wysocki GP: *Contemporary oral and maxillofacial pathology,* ed 2, St Louis, 2002, Mosby.)

in the disease persist for several days after the ulcerative lesions have healed. Scarring does not occur in the areas of healed ulcerations.

Oral Symptoms. The disease is accompanied by generalized "soreness" of the oral cavity, which interferes with eating and drinking. The ruptured vesicles are the focal sites of pain and are particularly sensitive to touch, thermal changes, foods such as condiments and fruit juices, and the action of coarse foods. In infants the disease is marked by irritability and refusal to take food.

Extraoral and Systemic Signs and Symptoms. Cervical adenitis, fever as high as 101° F to 105° F (38.3° C to 40.6° C), and generalized malaise are common.

History. Primary herpetic gingivostomatitis is the result of an acute infection by HSV and has an acute onset.

Histopathology. The virus targets the epithelial cells, which show "ballooning degeneration" consisting of acantholysis, nuclear clearing, and nuclear enlargement. These cells are called *Tzanck cells.* Infected cells fuse, forming multinucleated cells, and intercellular edema leads to formation of an intraepithelial vesicles that rupture and develop a secondary inflammatory response with a fibropurulent exudate[48] (Figure 24-9). Discrete ulcerations resulting from rupture of the vesicles have a central portion of acute inflammation, with varying degrees of purulent exudate, surrounded by a zone rich in engorged blood vessels.

Diagnosis

It is critical to arrive at a diagnosis as early as possible in primary herpetic infections. Treatment with antiviral medications can dramatically alter the course of the disease, reducing symptoms and potentially reducing recurrences (see Chapter 47). The diagnosis is usually established from the patient's history and the clinical findings. Material may be obtained from the lesions and submitted to the laboratory for confirmatory tests, including virus culture and immunologic tests using monoclonal antibodies or DNA hybridization techniques.[6,24,55] This should not delay treatment if strong clinical evidence exists for primary gingivostomatitis.

Differential Diagnosis

Primary herpetic gingivostomatitis should be differentiated from several conditions.

NUG can be differentiated in different ways (see Table 24-1).

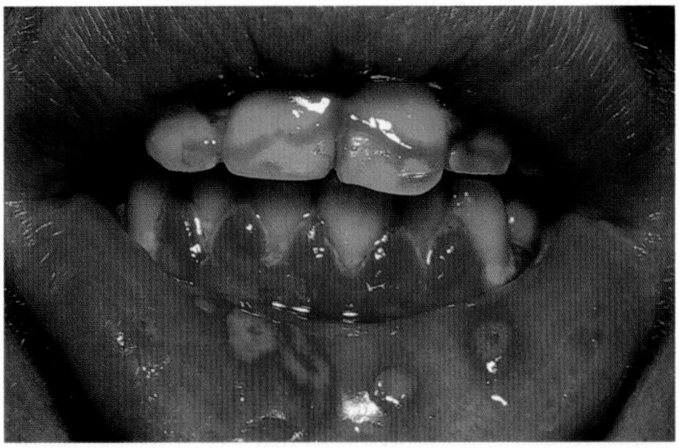

Figure 24-7 Primary herpetic gingivostomatitis in 12-year-old boy, with diffuse erythematous involvement of the gingiva and spherical gray vesicle in the lip. (Courtesy Dr. Heddie Sedano, University of California, Los Angeles, and University of Minnesota.)

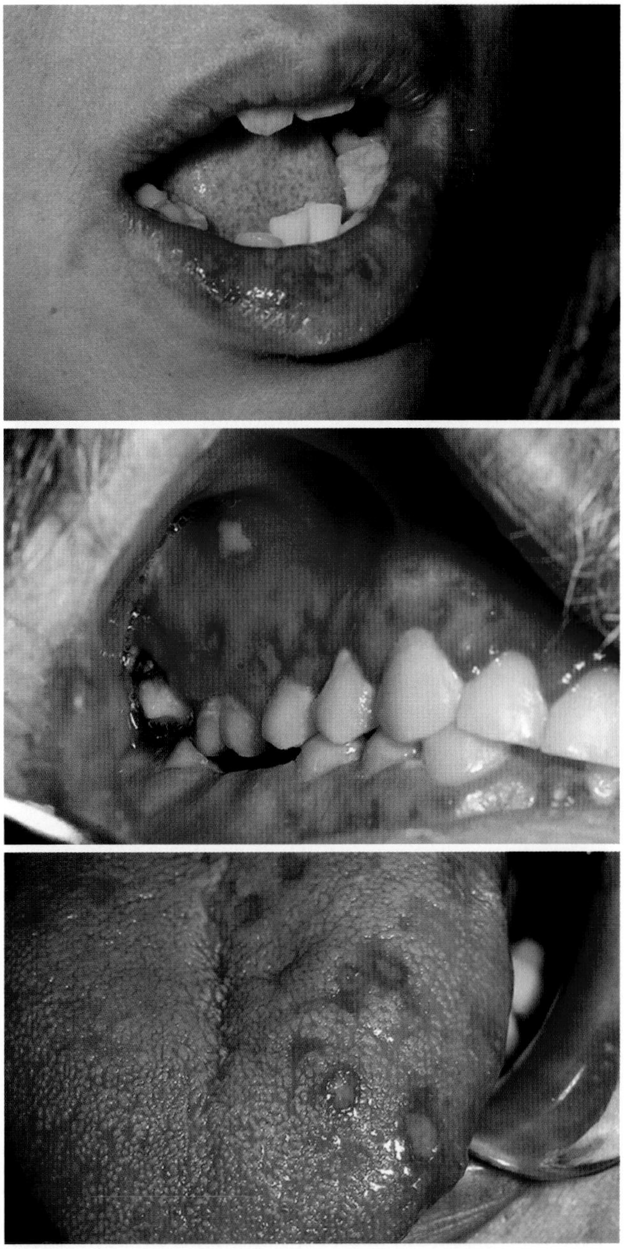

Figure 24-8 Involvement of the lip, gingiva, and tongue in primary herpetic gingivostomatitis. (From Sapp JP, Eversole, LR, Wysocki GP: *Contemporary oral and maxillofacial pathology,* ed 2, St Louis, 2002, Mosby.)

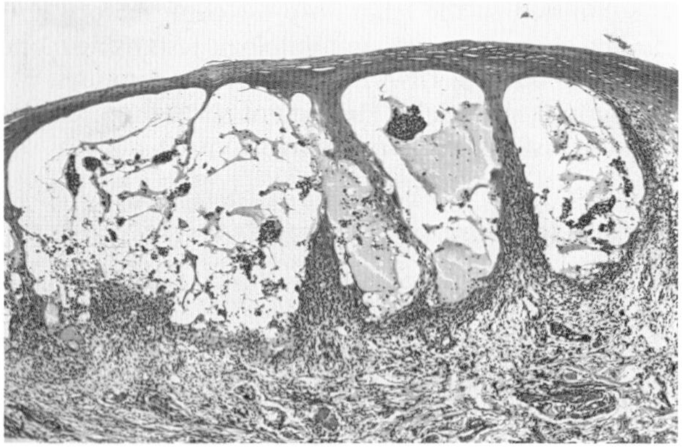

Figure 24-9 Biopsy showing intraepithelial viral vesicles, containing fluid and debris, with large number of viruses and virally altered epithelial cells. (Courtesy Dr. Heddie Sedano, University of California, Los Angeles, and University of Minnesota.)

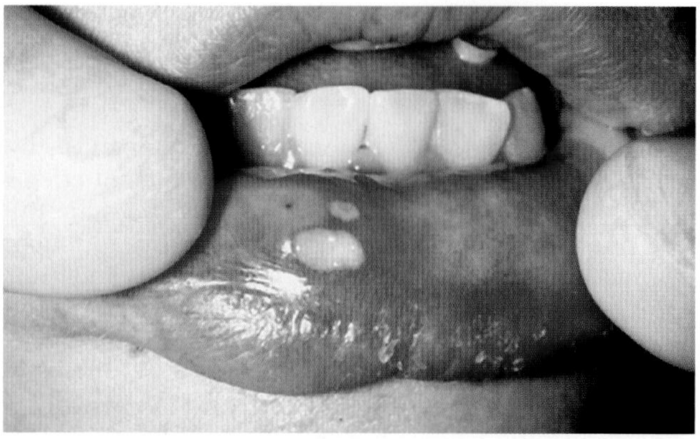

Figure 24-10 Aphthous lesion in the lip. The depressed gray center is surrounded by an elevated red border. (From Sapp JP, Eversole, LR, Wysocki GP: *Contemporary oral and maxillofacial pathology,* ed 2, St Louis, 2002, Mosby.)

Erythema multiforme can be differentiated because its vesicles are generally more extensive than those in primary herpetic gingivostomatitis and on rupture demonstrate a tendency toward pseudomembrane formation. In addition, the tongue is usually very involved in erythema multiforme, with infection of the ruptured vesicles resulting in varying degrees of ulceration. Oral involvement in erythema multiforme may be accompanied by skin lesions. The duration of erythema multiforme may be comparable with that of primary herpetic gingivostomatitis, but prolonged involvement may occur for weeks.

Stevens-Johnson syndrome is a comparatively rare form of erythema multiforme, characterized by vesicular hemorrhagic lesions in the oral cavity, hemorrhagic ocular lesions, and bullous skin lesions.

Bullous lichen planus is a very rare and painful condition. It is characterized by large blisters on the tongue and cheek that rupture and undergo ulceration; it runs a prolonged, indefinite course. Patches of linear, gray, lacelike lesions of lichen planus are often interspersed among the bullous eruptions. Lichen planus involvement of the skin may coexist with the oral lesions and facilitate differential diagnosis.

Desquamative gingivitis is characterized by diffuse involvement of the gingiva, with varying degrees of "peeling" of the epithelial surface and exposure of the underlying tissue. It is a chronic condition (see Chapter 26).

Lesions of *recurrent aphthous stomatitis* (RAS)[21] range from occasional small (0.5-1 cm in diameter), well-defined, round or ovoid, shallow ulcers with a yellowish gray central area surrounded by an erythematous halo, which heal in 7 to 10 days without scarring, to larger (1-3 cm in diameter) oval or irregular ulcers, which persist for weeks and heal with scarring (Figure 24-10). The cause is unknown, although immunopathologic mechanisms appear to play a role. RAS is a different clinical entity from primary herpetic gingivostomatitis. The ulcerations may look the same in the two conditions, but diffuse erythematous involvement of the gingiva and acute toxic systemic symptoms do not occur in RAS. A history of previous episodes of painful mucosal ulcerations suggests RAS rather than primary HSV.

Communicability

Primary herpetic gingivostomatitis is contagious.[8,39] Most adults have developed immunity to HSV as the result of infection during childhood, which in most cases is subclinical. For this reason, acute herpetic gingivostomatitis usually occurs in infants and children. Recurrent herpetic gingivostomatitis has been reported,[30] although it is not often of clinical significance unless immunity is destroyed by debilitating systemic disease. Recent studies demonstrating HSV in periodontal pockets suggest more recurrence of viral replication than previously recognized.[69] Secondary herpetic infection of the skin, such as herpes labialis, does recur.[67]

PERICORONITIS

The term *pericoronitis* refers to inflammation of the gingiva in relation to the crown of an incompletely erupted tooth (Figure 24-11). It occurs most often in the mandibular third molar area. Pericoronitis may be acute, subacute, or chronic.

Clinical Features

The partially erupted or impacted mandibular third molar is the most common site of pericoronitis. The space between the crown of the tooth and the overlying gingival flap (operculum) is an ideal area for the accumulation of food debris and bacterial growth. Even in patients with no clinical signs or symptoms, the gingival flap is often chronically inflamed and infected and has varying degrees of ulceration along its inner surface. Acute inflammatory involvement is a constant possibility and may be exacerbated by trauma, occlusion, or a foreign body trapped underneath the tissue flap (e.g., popcorn husk, nut fragment).

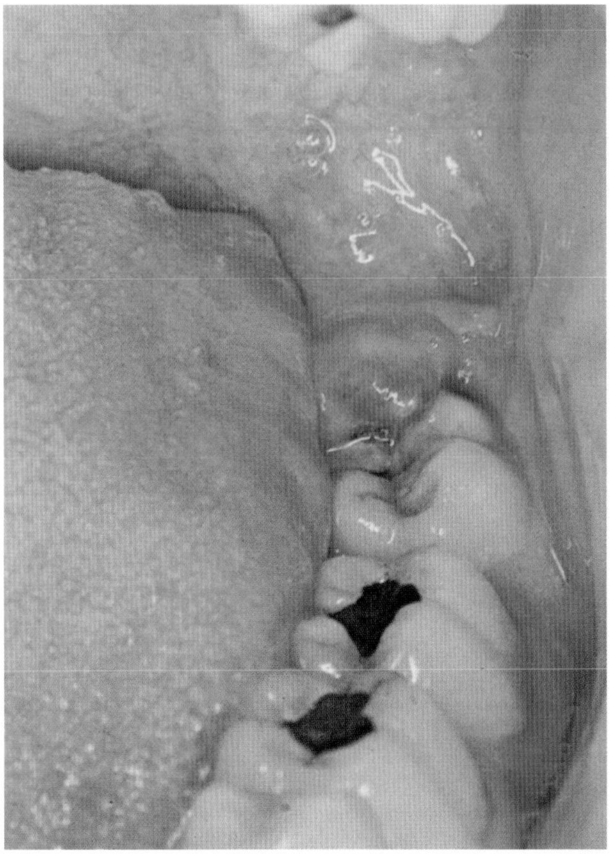

Figure 24-11 Pericoronitis. Inflamed coronal flap covering disto-occlusal surface of impacted mandibular third molar. Note swelling and redness. (From Glickman I, Smulow J: *Periodontal disease: clinical, radiographic and histopathologic features,* Philadelphia, 1974, Saunders.)

Acute pericoronitis is identified by varying degrees of inflammatory involvement of the pericoronal flap and adjacent structures, as well as by systemic complications. The inflammatory fluid and cellular exudate increase the bulk of the flap, which then may interfere with complete closure of the jaws and can be traumatized by contact with the opposing jaw, aggravating the inflammatory involvement.

The resultant clinical picture is that of a red, swollen, suppurating lesion that is exquisitely tender, with radiating pains to the ear, throat, and floor of the mouth. The patient is extremely uncomfortable because of a foul taste and an inability to close the jaws, in addition to the pain. Swelling of the cheek in the region of the angle of the jaw and lymphadenitis are common findings. Trismus may also be a presenting complaint. The patient may also have systemic complications, such as fever, leukocytosis, and malaise.

Complications

The involvement may be localized in the form of a pericoronal abscess. It may spread posteriorly into the oropharyngeal area and medially to the base of the tongue, making it difficult for the patient to swallow. Depending on the severity and extent of the infection, there is involvement of the submaxillary, posterior cervical, deep cervical, and retropharyngeal lymph nodes.[34,51] Peritonsillar abscess formation, cellulitis, and Ludwig's angina are infrequent but potential sequelae of acute pericoronitis.

REFERENCES

1. Barnes GP, Bowles WF III, Carter HG: Acute necrotizing ulcerative gingivitis: a survey of 218 cases, *J Periodontol* 44:35, 1973.
2. Berke JD: Experimental study of acute ulcerative stomatitis, *J Am Dent Assoc* 63:86, 1961.
3. Box HK: *Necrotic gingivitis,* Toronto, 1930, University of Toronto Press.
4. Brown RH: Necrotizing ulcerative gingivitis in mongoloid and nonmongoloid retarded individuals, *J Periodontal Res* 8:290, 1973.
5. Cahn LR: The penetration of the tissue by Vincent's organisms: a report of a case, *J Dent Res* 9:695, 1929.
6. Cawson RA: Infections of the oral mucous membrane. In Cohen B, Kramer IRH, editors: *Scientific foundations of dentistry,* Chicago, 1976, YearBook Medical Publishers.
7. Chapman OD, Harris AE: Oral lesions associated with dietary deficiencies in monkeys, *J Infect Dis* 69:7, 1941.
8. Chilton NW: Herpetic stomatitis, *Am J Orthod Oral Surg* 30:335, 1944.
9. Chung CP, Nisengard RJ, Slots J, et al: Bacterial IgG and IgM antibody titers in acute necrotizing ulcerative gingivitis, *J Periodontol* 54:557, 1983.
10. Cogen RB, Stevens AW Jr, Cohen-Cole SA, et al: Leukocyte function in the etiology of acute necrotizing ulcerative gingivitis, *J Periodontol* 54:402, 1983.
11. Cohen-Cole SA, et al: Psychiatric, psychosocial and endocrine correlates of acute necrotizing ulcerative gingivitis (trench mouth): a preliminary report, *Psychiatr Med* 1:215, 1983.
12. Curtois GJ III, Cobb CM, Killoy WJ: Acute necrotizing ulcerative gingivitis: a transmission electron microscope study, *J Periodontol* 54:671, 1983.
13. Daley FH: Studies of Vincent's infection at the clinic of Tufts College Dental School from October 1926 to February 1928, *J Dent Res* 8:408, 1928.
14. Dean HT, Singleton JE Jr: Vincent's infection—a wartime disease, *Am J Public Health* 35:433, 1945.
15. Dodd, K, Johnston LM, Budding GJ: Herpetic stomatitis, *J Pediatr* 12:95, 1938.
16. Duckworth R, Waterhouse JP, Britton DG, et al: Acute ulcerative gingivitis: a double blind controlled clinical trial with metronidazole, *Br Dent J* 120:599, 1966;
17. Ellerman V: Vincent's organisms in tissue, *Z Hyg Infekt Pr* 56:453, 1907.
18. Emslie RD: Cancrum oris, Dent Pract 13:481, 1963.
19. Enwonwu CO: Epidemiological and biochemical studies of necrotizing ulcerative gingivitis and noma (cancrum oris) in Nigerian children, *Arch Oral Biol* 17:1357, 1972.
20. Enwonwu CO: Cellular and molecular effects of malnutrition and their relevance to periodontal diseases, *J Clin Periodontol* 21:643, 1994.
21. Eversole LR: Diseases of the oral mucous membranes. Review of the literature. In Millard HD, Mason DK, editors: *World workshop on oral medicine,* Chicago, 1989, YearBook Medical Publishers.
22. Falkler WA Jr, Martin SA, Vincent JW, et al: A clinical, demographic and microbiologic study of NUG patients in an urban dental school, *J Clin Periodontol* 14:307, 1987.

23. Formicola AJ, Witte ET, Curran PM: A study of personality traits and acute necrotizing ulcerative gingivitis, *J Periodontol* 41:36, 1970.
24. Gardner PS, McQuillin J, Black MM, et al: Rapid diagnosis of herpesvirus hominis infections in superficial lesions by immunofluorescent antibody techniques, *Br Med J* 4:89, 1968.
25. Giddon DB: Psychophysiology of the oral cavity, *J Dent Res* 45 (Suppl 6):1627, 1966.
26. Giddon DB, Zackin SJ, Goldhaber P: Acute necrotizing gingivitis in college students, *J Am Dent Assoc* 68:381, 1964.
27. Goldhaber P, Giddon DB: Present concepts concerning the etiology and treatment of acute necrotizing ulcerative gingivitis, *Int Dent J* 14:468, 1964.
28. Greenberg MS, Brightman VJ, Ship II: Clinical and laboratory differentiation of recurrent intraoral herpes simplex virus infections following fever, *J Dent Res* 48:385, 1969.
29. Greenspan D, Pindborg JJ, Greenspan JS, et al: *AIDS and the dental team,* Copenhagen, 1986, Munksgaard.
30. Griffin JW: Recurrent intraoral herpes simplex virus infection, *Oral Surg* 19:209, 1965.
31. Hampp EG, Mergenhagen SE: Experimental infection with oral spirochetes, *J Infect Dis* 109:43, 1961.
32. Hooper PA, Seymour GJ: The histopathogenesis of acute ulcerative gingivitis, *J Periodontol* 50:419, 1979.
33. Horning GM, Cohen ME: Necrotizing ulcerative gingivitis, periodontitis and stomatitis: clinical staging and predisposing factors, *J Periodontol* 66:990, 1995.
34. Jacobs MH: Pericoronal and Vincent's infections: bacteriology and treatment, *J Am Dent Assoc* 30:392, 1953.
35. Jimenez M, Baer PN: Necrotizing ulcerative gingivitis in children: a 9-year clinical study, *J Periodontol* 46:715, 1975.
36. King JD: Nutritional and other factors in trench mouth with special reference to the nicotinic acid component of vitamin B complex, *Br Dent J* 74:113, 1943.
37. Listgarten MA: Electron microscopic observations on the bacterial flora of acute necrotizing ulcerative gingivitis, *J Periodontol* 36:328, 1965.
38. Listgarten MA, Lewis DW: The distribution of spirochetes in the lesion of acute necrotizing ulcerative gingivitis: an electron microscopic and statistical survey, *J Periodontol* 38:379, 1967.
39. Littner MM, Dayan D, Kaffe I, et al: Acute streptococcal gingivostomatitis: report of five cases, *Oral Surg Oral Med Oral Pathol Oral Radiol Endod* 53:144, 1982.
40. Loesche WJ, Syed SA, Langhorn BE, Stoll J: The bacteriology of acute necrotizing ulcerative gingivitis, *J Periodontol* 53:223, 1982.
41. Mayo J, Carranza FA Jr, Cabrini RL: Comparative study of the effect of antibiotics, bone marrow and cysteamine on oral lesions produced in hamsters by total body irradiation, *Experientia* 20:403, 1964.
42. Mayo J, Carranza FA Jr, Epper CE, et al: The effect of total-body irradiation on the oral tissues of the Syrian hamster, *Oral Surg* 15:739, 1962.
43. McCarthy PL, Shklar G: Diseases of the oral mucosa, ed 2, Philadelphia, 1980, Lea & Febiger.
44. McNair ST: Herpetic stomatitis, *J Dent Res* 29:647, 1950.
45. Miglani DC, Sharma OP: Incidence of acute necrotizing gingivitis and periodontosis among cases seen at the government hospital, Madras, *J All India Dent Assoc* 37:183, 1965.
46. Miller DK, Rhoads CP: The experimental production in dogs of acute stomatitis associated with leukopenia and a maturation defect of the myeloid elements of the bone marrow, *J Exp Med* 61:173, 1935.
47. Nathanson I, Morin GE: Herpetic stomatitis: an aid in the early diagnosis of infectious mononucleosis, *Oral Surg* 6:1284, 1953.
48. Neville BW, Damm DD, Allen CM, et al: *Oral and maxillofacial pathology,* Philadelphia, 1995, Saunders.
49. Park NH: Virology. In: Newman MG, Nisengard R, editors: *Oral microbiology and immunology,* Philadelphia, 1988, Saunders.
50. Pedler JA, Radden BG: Seasonal influence of acute ulcerative gingivitis, *Dent Pract* 8:23, 1957.
51. Perkins AE: Acute infections around erupting mandibular third molar, *Br Dent J* 76:199, 1944.
52. Pindborg JJ: Gingivitis in military personnel with special reference to ulceromembranous gingivitis, *Odontol Tidskr* 59:407, 1951.
53. Pindborg JJ, Bhat M, Devanath KR, et al: Occurrence of acute necrotizing gingivitis in South Indian children, *J Periodontol* 37:14, 1966.
54. Plaut HC: Studienzur bakterielle diagnostik der diphtheriae un der aginen, *Dtsch Med Wochenschr* 20:920, 1894.
55. Regezi JA, Sciubba JJ: *Oral pathology: clinico-pathologic correlations,* Philadelphia, 1989, Saunders.
56. Rivera-Hidalgo F, Stanford TW: Oral mucosal lesions caused by infective microorganisms. I. Virus and bacteria, *Periodontol 2000* 21:106, 1999.
57. Rosebury T: Is Vincent's infection a communicable disease? *J Am Dent Assoc* 29:823, 1942.
58. Rosebury T, Foley G: Experimental Vincent's infection, *J Am Dent Assoc* 26:1978, 1939.
59. Rosebury T, MacDonald JB, Clark A: A bacteriologic survey of gingival scrapings from periodontal infections by direct examination, guinea pig inoculation and anaerobic cultivation, *J Dent Res* 29:718, 1950.
60. Rowland R: Necrotizing ulcerative gingivitis, *Ann Periodontol* 4:65, 1999;.
61. Roy S, Wolman L: Electron microscopic observations on the virus particles in herpes simplex encephalitis, *J Clin Pathol* 22:51, 1969.
62. Schluger S: Necrotizing ulcerative gingivitis in the army: incidence, communicability, and treatment, *J Am Dent Assoc* 38:174, 1949.
63. Schwartzman J, Grossman L: Vincent's ulceromembranous gingivostomatitis, *Arch Pediatr* 58:515, 1941.
64. Scott TFM, Steigman AS, Convey JH: Acute infectious gingivostomatitis: etiology, epidemiology, and clinical picture of common disorders caused by virus of herpes simplex, *JAMA* 117:999, 1941.
65. Shannon IL, Kilgore WG, Leary TJ: Stress as a predisposing factor in necrotizing ulcerative gingivitis, *J Periodontol* 40:240, 1969.
66. Sheiham A: An epidemiological study of oral disease in Nigerians, *J Dent Res* 44:1184, 1965.
67. Ship II, Brightman VJ, Laster LL: The patient with recurrent aphthous ulcers and the patient with recurrent herpes labialis: a study of two population samples, *J Am Dent Assoc* 75:645, 1967.
68. Skach M, Zabrodsky S, Mrklas L: A study of the effect of age and season on the incidence of ulcerative gingivitis, *J Periodontal Res* 5:187, 1970.
69. Slots J, Contreras A: Herpesviruses: a unifying causative factor in periodontitis? *Oral Microbiol Immunol* 5:277, 2000.
70. Smith DT: *Spirochetes and related organisms in fusospirochetal disease,* Baltimore, 1932, Williams & Wilkins.
71. Stammers AF: Vincent's infection, *Br Dent J* 76:171, 1944.
72. Stevens AWJ, Cogen RB, Cohen-Cole SA, et al: Demographic and clinical data associated with acute necrotizing ulcerative gingivitis in a dental school population, *J Clin Periodontol* 11:487, 1984.

73. Swenson HM: Induced Vincent's infection in dogs, *J Dent Res* 23:190, 1944.
74. Swenson HM, Muhler, JC: Induced fusospirochetal infection in dogs, *J Dent Res* 26:161, 1947.
75. Topping NH, Fraser HF: Mouth lesions associated with dietary deficiencies in monkeys, *US Public Health Rep* 54:431, 1939.
76. Tunnicliff R, Hammond C: Abscess production by fusiform bacilli in rabbits and mice by the use of scillaren-B or mucin, *J Dent Res* 16:479, 1937.
77. Tunnicliff R, Fink EB, Hammond C: Significance of fusiform bacilli and spirilla in gingival tissue, *J Am Dent Assoc* 23:1959, 1936.
78. Underhill FP, Mendel LB: Further experiments on the pellagra-like syndrome in dogs, *Am J Physiol* 83:589, 1928.
79. Vincent H: Sur l'etiologie et sur les lesions anatomopathologiques de la pourritute d'hopital, *Ann l'Inst Pasteur* 10:448, 1896.
80. Wilton JM, Ivanyi A, Lehner T: Cell-mediated immunity and humoral antibodies in acute ulcerative gingivitis, *J Periodontal Res* 6:9, 1971.

Gingival Diseases in Childhood

Donald Duperon and Henry H. Takei

25

CHAPTER

■ ■ ■

CHAPTER OUTLINE

PERIODONTIUM OF THE DECIDUOUS DENTITION
PHYSIOLOGIC GINGIVAL CHANGES ASSOCIATED
 WITH TOOTH ERUPTION
 Preeruption Bulge
 Gingival Margin

TYPES OF GINGIVAL DISEASE
 Chronic Marginal Gingivitis
 Acute Gingival Infections
TRAUMATIC CHANGES IN THE PERIODONTIUM
ORAL MUCOUS MEMBRANE IN CHILDHOOD DISEASES

*I*t is postulated that periodontal disease in adults is, at least in part, precipitated by gingival inflammation in the formative years of childhood and early adolescence. The nondestructive gingival inflammations of childhood, without appropriate intervention, may progress to the more significant periodontal diseases seen in the adult population.

The exchange of dentition from primary to permanent and the hormonal changes associated with puberty offer unique conditions in the periodontal structures and the ability of the structures to resist destructive changes. Therefore, after reviewing anatomic and physiologic changes in the periodontium and dentition, this chapter presents the periodontal problems associated with childhood and adolescence.

PERIODONTIUM OF THE DECIDUOUS DENTITION

The normal gingiva of the deciduous dentition is pale pink, but not as pale as that of the adult attached gingiva, because the thinness of the keratinized layer causes the underlying vessels to be more visible.[21] Stippling appears at about 3 years of age and occurs in 35% of children between ages 5 and 15 years.[31] Studying children ages 1 to 10 years, Bimstein et al.[4] found 56.4% with stippling (Figure 25-1).

The interdental gingiva is broad buccolingually and narrow mesiodistally to conform to the morphology of the deciduous dentition. Its structure and composition are similar to the adult gingiva.

The gingival sulcular depth is shallower in the deciduous dentition than in the permanent dentition. The mean sulcus depth for the primary dentition is 2.1 mm

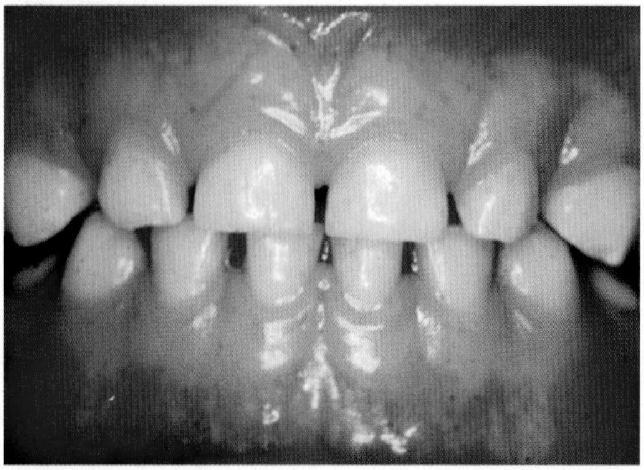

Figure 25-1 Normal gingiva of 5-year-old child showing light stippling and flattened interproximal gingiva in areas of physiologic spacing.

(±0.2 mm).[29] The attached gingiva varies in width anteroposteriorly, being the widest in the incisor area, narrowing over the cuspids, and widening again over the posterior molars[32] (Figure 25-2). The attached gingiva normally increases with age.[1,33] The free gingival collar has fewer collagen bundles and is more easily retracted away from the deciduous tooth surface.

Radiographically, the lamina dura is prominent in the deciduous dentition, with a wider periodontal space than in the permanent dentition. The marrow spaces of the bone are larger, and the crests of the interdental bony septa are flat, with the bony crests within 1 to 2 mm of the cementoenamel junction[8] (Figure 25-3).

Oral flora and dental plaque in childhood are discussed in Chapter 9.

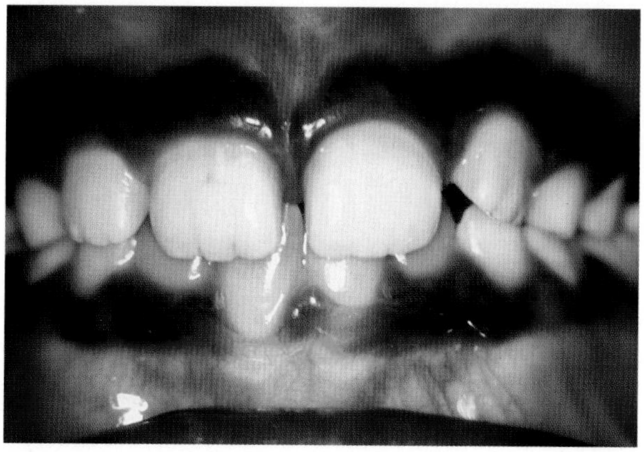

Figure 25-2 Normal gingiva demonstrating width of the attached gingiva, as illustrated by the pigmentation that occurs only in the attached gingival area. This 6-year-old African-American youngster has erupting lower central incisors. As the incisors erupt, the attached gingiva will widen as the alveolus grows.

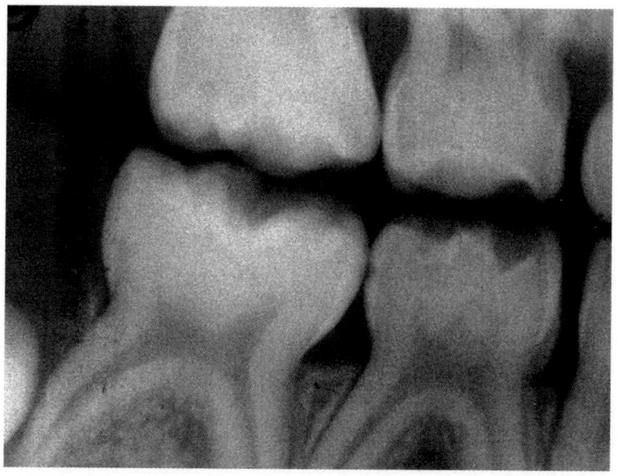

Figure 25-3 Bite-wing radiograph of 5-year-old child illustrating the flattened interseptal bone, which is normal in the deciduous dentition.

PHYSIOLOGIC GINGIVAL CHANGES ASSOCIATED WITH TOOTH ERUPTION

Significant changes occur in the periodontium as the dentition changes from the deciduous to the permanent teeth. Most of the changes are associated with eruption and are physiologic in nature. These changes should be distinguished from gingival disease, which may occur simultaneously.

Preeruption Bulge

Before eruption of the permanent tooth, the gingiva reveals a bulge that is firm and pink or blanched secondary to the underlying permanent crown (Figure 25-4). If the primary tooth has been prematurely lost, or if a first molar is erupting behind the deciduous second molar, an eruption cyst may form. These cysts present as a bluish enlargement of the gingiva over the erupting tooth. Occasionally, the cyst may be filled with blood and present a dark-blue or deep-red appearance. The most common sites are the permanent lower incisors and the first molars. Many resolve without treatment but may be marsupialized if they are painful or interfere with occlusion.[6]

Gingival Margin

Formation. As the tooth erupts, the gingival margin and sulcus develop. At this point the margin is rounded, edematous, and reddened.

Normal Prominence. During the period of active tooth eruption, it is normal for the marginal gingiva surrounding partially erupted teeth to appear prominent; this is most evident in the maxillary anterior region. The prominence is caused by the height from the contour of the erupting tooth and the mild inflammation from mastication. With poor oral hygiene, significant gingivitis may develop in the unprotected gingival areas.

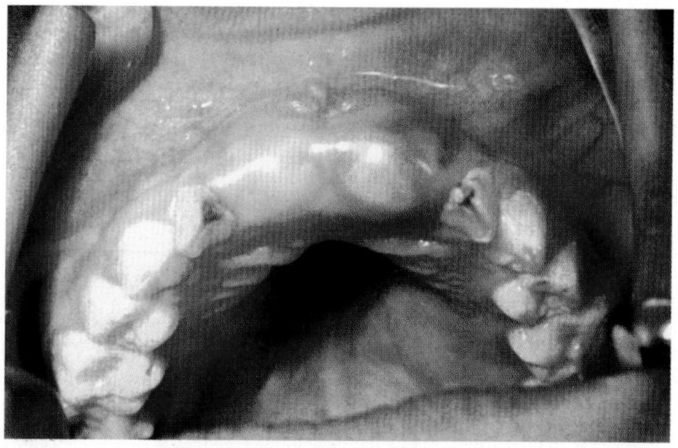

Figure 25-4 On the right side, the central incisor bulge is evident and is normal at this stage of eruption. On the left side, an eruption cyst is evident. These cysts may show the blue color illustrated here or may be hemorrhagic in nature.

SCIENCE TRANSFER

Observations of the gingiva during childhood reveal that the body responds physiologically and pathologically in similar ways as the adult gingiva. For example, not only does inflammation occur as a reaction to plaque, as in the adult (although perhaps not as directly), but trauma, in this case as a result of tooth eruption, causes redness and swelling as well. In another similarity between the child and adult, the reaction of the gingiva is amplified when specific hormonal levels are increased. This occurs in the child during puberty and in the adult during pregnancy. Thus the reactions of the gingiva, both in the child and in the adult, can be interpreted in physiologic and pathologic (e.g., inflammation) terms.

Periodontal evaluation of children's teeth should be an integral part of the dental examination, beginning with eruption of the deciduous dentition. Recordings of pocket depth, gingival recession, and measurements of gingival inflammation (e.g., bleeding on probing) should be made at least annually.

Gingival diseases that begin in childhood require early detection and nonsurgical treatment to maintain gingival health and to prevent initiating periodontal problems that may be difficult to treat later. Occasionally, mucogingival surgery may be needed in the incisor regions to correct problems of inadequate keratinized gingiva and aberrant frenum so that future gingival recession can be prevented.

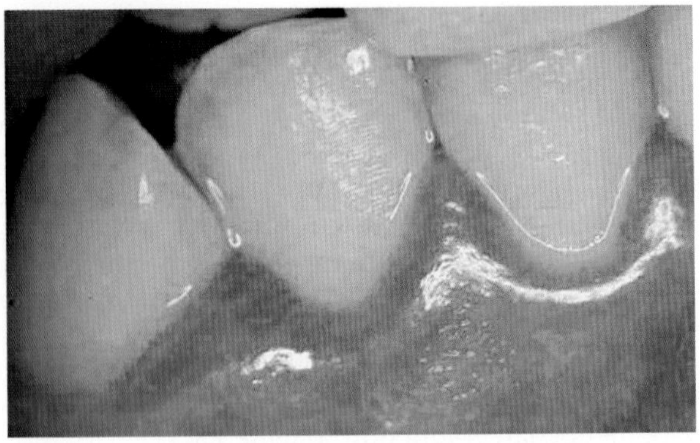

Figure 25-5 Chronic marginal gingivitis secondary to poor oral hygiene and crowding of the erupting teeth.

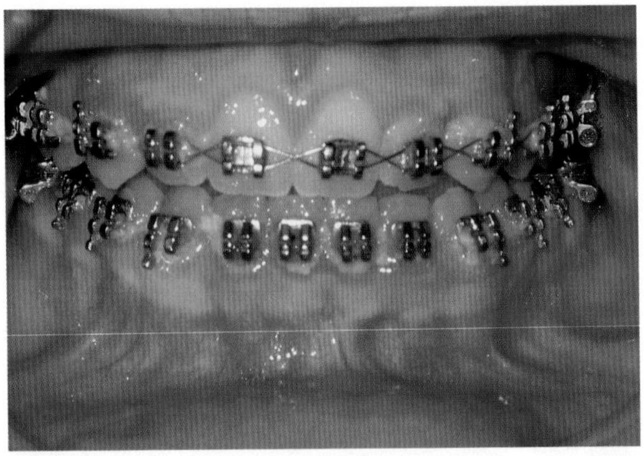

Figure 25-6 Chronic marginal gingivitis secondary to orthodontic therapy and inadequate oral hygiene. Improved hygiene coupled with chlorhexidine mouthwash may help to reduce the inflammation in this patient.

TYPES OF GINGIVAL DISEASE

Chronic Marginal Gingivitis

The most prevalent type of gingival disease in childhood is chronic marginal gingivitis. The gingiva exhibits changes in color, size, consistency, and surface texture similar to chronic inflammation in the adult. The red, linear inflammation is accompanied by underlying chronic changes, including swelling, increased vascularization, and hyperplasia. Bleeding and increased pocket depth are not found as often in children as in adults[4] (Figure 25-5).

Histopathology. Chronic gingivitis in children is characterized by the loss of collagen in the area around the junctional epithelium, an important vascular component, and an infiltrate consisting mostly of lymphocytes and small numbers of polymorphonuclear leukocytes, plasma cells, monocytes, and mast cells. Plasma cells do not appear in large amounts, and therefore the lesion resembles the early lesion seen in adults, which is nondestructive and nonprogressive.

The inflammatory response in children is different from that of adults in that few B lymphocytes and plasma cells are present in children. The response in dominated by T lymphocytes. This difference could explain why gingivitis in children rarely progresses to periodontitis.[14,16,17,20,31]

Puberty Gingivitis. The incidence of marginal gingivitis peaks at 11 to 13 years of age, then decreases slightly after puberty. The most frequent manifestations in adolescents is bleeding and inflammation in the interproximal areas. This is usually the result of hormonal changes that magnify the tissue inflammatory response to dental plaque. It occurs in both males and females and reduces in severity after puberty[22] (see Chapters 23 and 43). This inflammatory response is also seen during orthodontic therapy, when oral hygiene becomes more problematic (Figure 25-6).

During puberty, gingivitis and gingival enlargement may be more prevalent: this is often referred to as *pubertal* (or puberty) *gingivitis*. The most common findings include interproximal bleeding and inflammatory gingival enlargement. This may be a result of the hormonal changes in puberty and affects both males and females. It usually resolves as the person matures (Figure 25-7).

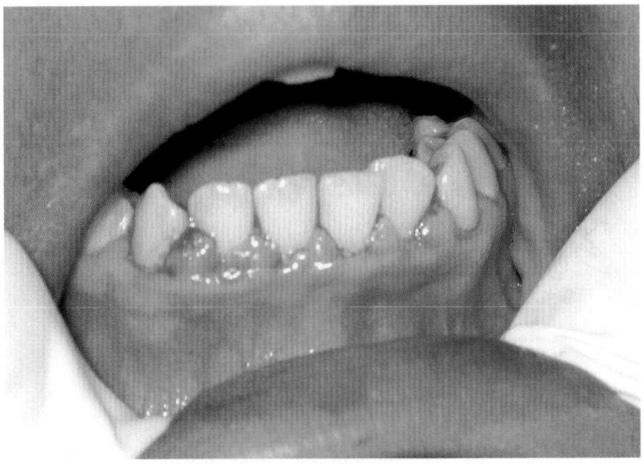

Figure 25-7 Gingival enlargement around erupting incisors. The enlargement will subside as the teeth erupt further.

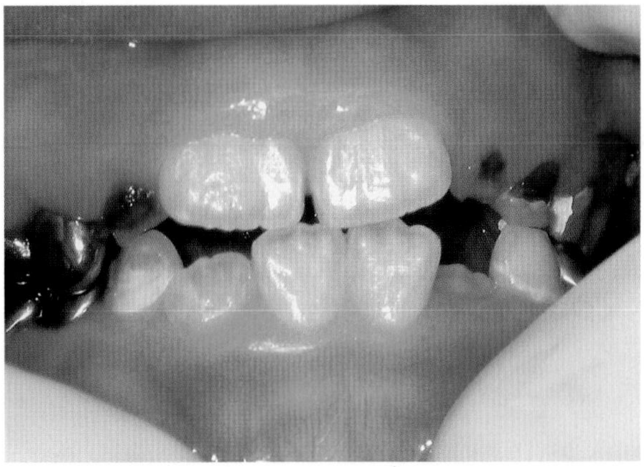

Figure 25-8 Eruption gingivitis complicated with severe marginal gingivitis secondary to the illustrated poor oral hygiene.

Etiology. In children, as in adults, the primary cause of gingivitis is *dental plaque,* which is favored by poor oral higiene. The relationship between plaque and the gingival index, however, is not clear, and only a weak relationship exists between plaque indexes and gingivitis in children.[19,20]

Samples of dental plaque in children indicated that 71% of 18- to 48-month-old children were infected with at least one periodontal pathogen; 68% were infected with *Porphyromonas gingivalis* and 20% with *Bacteroides forsythus (Tannerella forsythia).*[36] A moderate correlation can be found between *B. forsythus* in the child and periodontal disease in the mother. Also, gingival bleeding in children was associated with *B. forsythus.* In a similar study, 60% of children between 2 and 18 years of age had detectable levels of *P. gingivalis* in their plaque; 75% of children also showed similar levels of *Actinobacillus actinomycetemcomitans.* The presence of *P. gingivalis* was most strongly associated with the progression of gingivtis and the onset of periodontitis in healthy children.[24]

Calculus deposits are uncommon in infants and toddlers but increase with age. About 9% of 4- to 6-year-old children show calculus deposits. By age 7 to 9 years, 18% of children present with calculus deposits, and by age 10 to 15 years, 33% to 43% have some calculus formation. In children with cystic fibrosis the incidence of calculus in much higher and the deposits are greater; this may be caused by increased calcium and phosphate concentrations in the saliva.[25] Children fed exclusively with a gastric or nasogastric tube show significant calculus buildup secondary to lack of function and increased oral pH.

Gingivitis associated with tooth eruption is so common that the term "eruption gingivitis" has come into common use. Tooth eruption in itself does not cause gingivitis. Inflammation results from plaque accumulation around the erupting teeth,[10] perhaps secondary to discomfort caused by brushing these friable areas. The gingiva around erupting teeth may appear reddened because the gingival margins have not yet keratinized fully and the sulcus has not developed (Figure 25-8). Figure 25-9 shows erupting incisors with overlying gingivitis caused by poor oral hygiene.

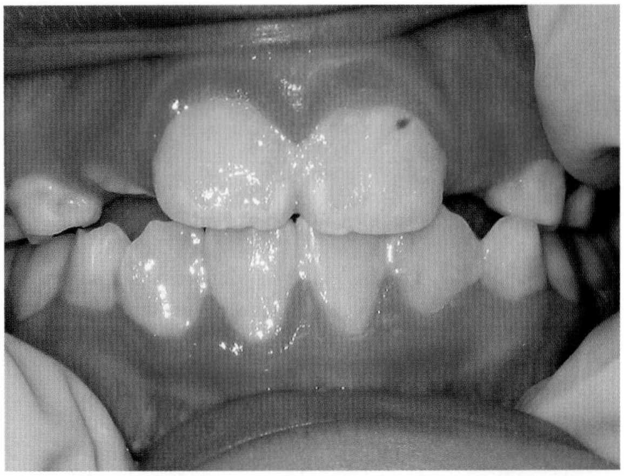

Figure 25-9 Gingivitis secondary to crowding and poor oral hygiene.

Exfoliating and severely carious deciduous teeth often will cause an associated gingivitis. The gingivitis is caused by plaque accumulation from pain during brushing or by food impaction in areas of tooth breakdown. The discomfort of chewing on severely infected teeth forces unilateral chewing and increased food and plaque accumulation on the affected side.

Dental crowding in the mixed dentition can often lead to an increased incidence of gingivitis because of the difficulty of adequately cleansing the area of plaque and food debris (Figure 25-10). Severe changes may include gingival enlargement, discoloration, and occasionally, ulceration and the formation of deep pockets or pseudopockets. Generally, gingival health is restored by orthodontic correction, with surgical removal of the enlarged tissue when necessary.

Gingival inflammation is also increased in children exhibiting *increased overbite* and *overjet, nasal obstruction,* and subsequent *mouth-breathing habit* (Figure 25-11).

According to Maynard and Wilson,[21] *mucogingival problems* start in the primary dentition as a consequence of developmental aberrations in eruption and deficiencies in the thickness of the periodontium. If there is also inadequate plaque control or excessive toothbrushing

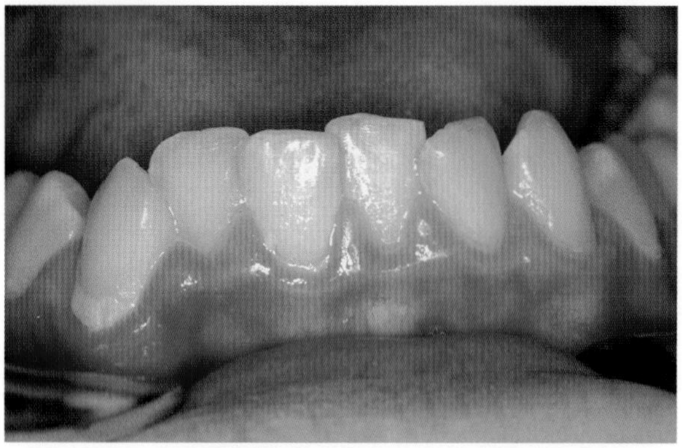

Figure 25-10 Patient with gingivitis secondary to compulsive mouth-breathing secondary to allergic rhinitis. This is a typical gingival response to chronic desiccation in adolescent patients. This was originally diagnosed as "allergic gingivitis" by the patient's pediatrician because it subsided when he gave the patient antihistamines. Of course, the antihistamines simply allowed him to breathe through his nose so he could keep his mouth closed.

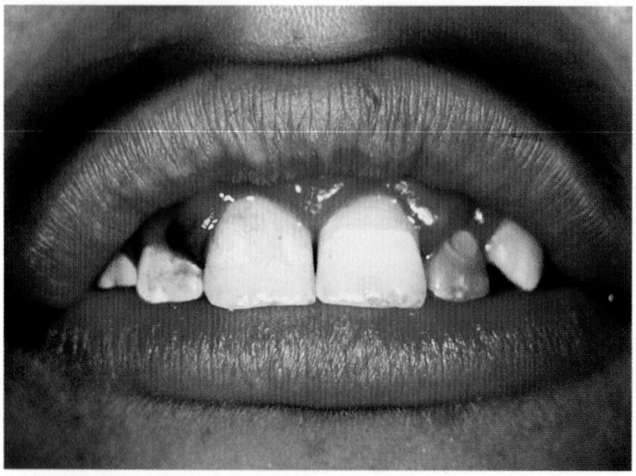

Figure 25-11 Mucosal injury secondary to excessive toothbrushing by the parent. Both the mucosa and the bone have receded more than two thirds of the root length. When the practice was discontinued, some healing occurred.

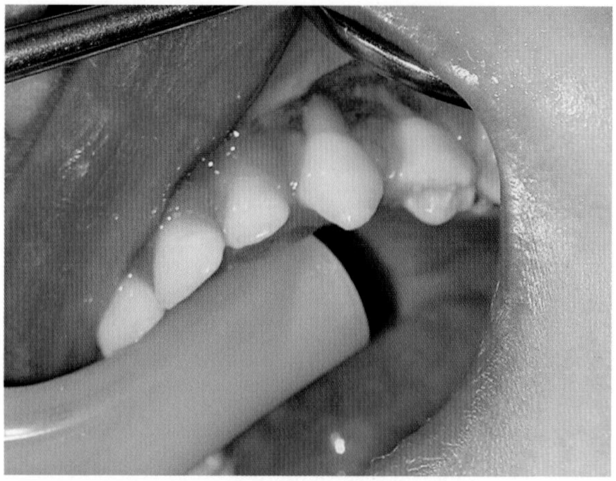

Figure 25-12 Labial stripping secondary to a class II growth pattern and lower incisor crowding. The labially erupting lower incisor demonstrates an associated gingivitis from poor oral hygiene. Immediate orthodontic treatment should be undertaken followed by appropriate grafting, if necessary.

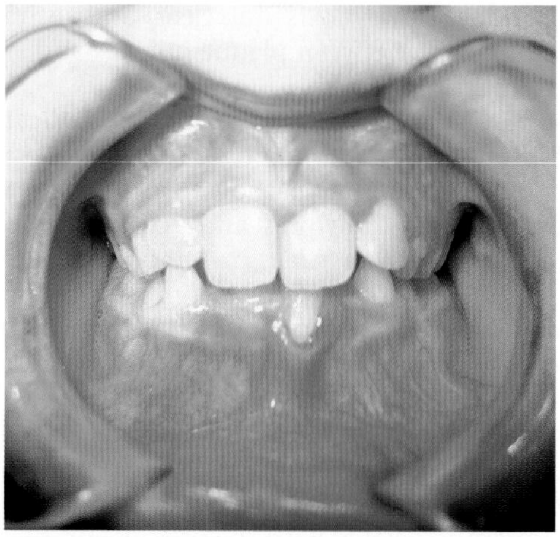

Figure 25-13 Pubertal gingival inflammation and enlargement secondary to poor oral hygiene and hormonal influences. Little or no calculus was found when the child was scaled. This most often clears with improved oral hygiene and natural stabilization of estrogen and testosterone levels.

trauma, a mucogingival problem develops. However, the width of the attached gingiva increases with age, and these problems may resolve.

The prevalence of mucogingival problems and recession in children ranges from 1% to 19%, depending on the criteria used to assess the condition.[15] In the mixed dentition, recession is most often found on the facial aspect of the mandibular permanent incisors. This may be secondary to rotations or to labial positioning secondary to insufficient arch length. Although erupting permanent lower incisors often show minimal attached gingiva, this often increases as the tooth erupts and stimulates the development of bone.

Mucogingival problems can also result from factitious habits or excessive toothbrushing either by the parent or the child (Figure 25-12).

Localized gingival recession may be caused by eruption problems in the lower incisor and upper cuspid regions and can be a source of concern. In children this is most often caused by teeth erupting in labioversion and teeth tilted or rotated secondary to space problems. An anterior open bite may increase the incidence of recession secondary to labial inclination of the teeth.[18] Orthodontic treatment and realignment may be necessary to protect the integrity of the attached gingiva (Figure 25-13).

Acute Gingival Infections

Primary Herpetic Gingivostomatitis. This acute-onset viral infection occurs early in childhood, with a heightened incidence from 1 to 3 years of age. Of children with primary infections, 99% are symptom free,

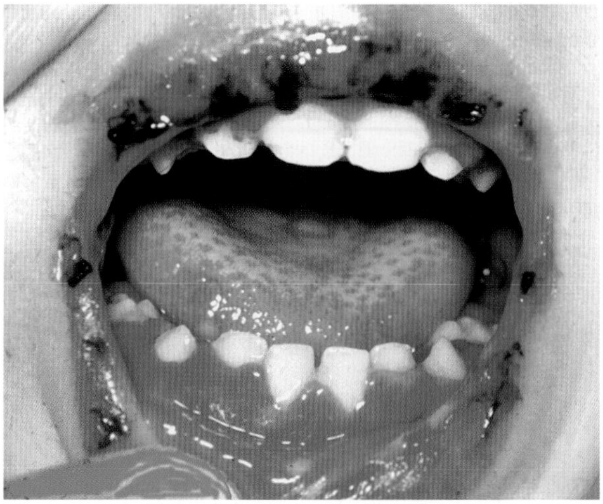

Figure 25-14 Acute herpetic gingivo-stomatitis in an 18-month-old child. Several active lesions still exist on the tongue. The gingiva demonstrates the typical red, swollen appearance associated with the herpes virus. The infection is mostly limited to the attached gingiva, tongue, palate and lips. It is most important to control hydration with bland, non-acetic fluids. Hospitalization may be necessary for re-hydration in severe cases.

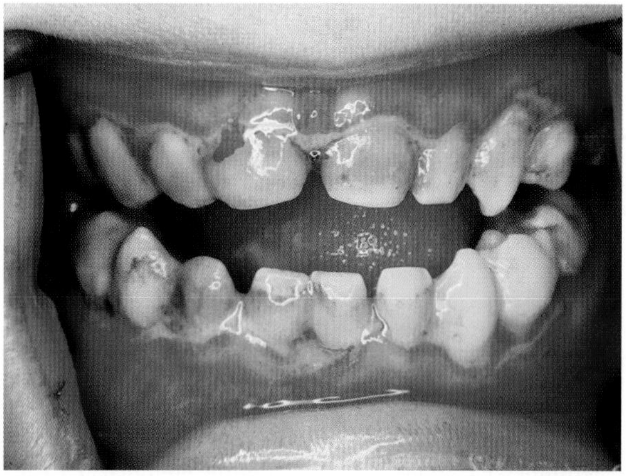

Figure 25-15 Acute necrotizing ulcerative gingivitis in a preschool child. This condition is very rarely seen except in cases of primary or secondary immune suppression, Down syndrome, or severe malnutrition. The breath is fetid, and the child complains of pain and discomfort when eating.

or the symptoms are attributed to teething. The remaining 1% can develop significant gingival inflammation and ulceration of the lips and mucous membranes[12,26] (Figure 25-14) (see Chapter 24).

Candidiasis. This infection occurs as a result of an overgrowth of *Candida albicans*, usually after a course of antibiotics or as a result of congenital or acquired immunodeficiencies (see Chapter 26).

Necrotizing Ulcerative Gingivitis. The incidence of acute necrotizing ulcerative gingivitis (NUG) is low in children, except in those with severe illness or chronic malnutrition.[11,29] Children with Down syndrome often demonstrate an increased tendency to develop NUG[34] (Figure 25-15) (see Chapters 24 and 47).

TRAUMATIC CHANGES IN THE PERIODONTIUM

The changes resulting from the exfoliation of deciduous teeth and the eruption of their successors can lead to trauma to the underlying tissues. Normal functional forces may be injurious to the remaining supporting tissues.[3] Shifting exfoliating teeth may lead to changes in occlusion, which will place significant additional trauma to the periodontium of existing and erupting teeth. As eruption proceeds, malalignments caused by spacing and skeletal relationships may also lead to significant trauma secondary to the malocclusion involved.

Microscopically, minor traumatic changes may demonstrate compression, ischemia, and hyalinization of the periodontal ligament.[13,27] With more severe injury, crushing and necrosis of the periodontal ligament may occur.

In most patients, these injuries are spontaneously resolved as teeth exfoliate, erupt, and align in the normal process of growth. In the mixed-dentition period, the periodontal ligament of and erupting permanent tooth may be injured by masticatory forces on the exfoliating deciduous tooth it is replacing.[9] External trauma, as well as occlusal trauma, may result in ankylosis of deciduous teeth and occasionally of permanent teeth. These teeth appear to be intruded or sunken. Ankylosed deciduous teeth may interfere with alveolar bone growth around erupting permanent teeth and may prevent their timely emergence into the oral cavity. Ankylosed deciduous first molars often clear spontaneously as the bicuspid erupts; however, a significant number of ankylosed second deciduous molars will prevent the eruption of the underlying bicuspid and should be managed appropriately before the completion of root development of the bicuspid.

ORAL MUCOUS MEMBRANE IN CHILDHOOD DISEASES

Some childhood diseases may demonstrate alterations or lesions on the oral mucosa and underlying tissues, such as rubeola (rubella, measles), varicella (chickenpox), diphtheria, and scarlatina (scarlet fever). For a more thorough discussion of this topic, the reader is referred to texts on oral and pediatric pathology.

REFERENCES

1. Ainamo J, Talari A: The increase with age of the width of the attached gingiva, *J Periodontal Res* 11:82, 1976.
2. Albandar JM, Buischi AP, Mayer MP, Axelsson P: Long-term effect of two preventive programs on the incidence of plaque and gingivitis in adolescents, *J Periodontol* 65:605, 1994.
3. Bernick S, Freedman N: Microscopic studies of the periodontium of the primary dentitions of monkeys. II. Posterior teeth during the mixed dentitional period, *Oral Surg Oral Med Oral Pathol* 70:322, 1954.

4. Bimstein E, Lustmann J, Soskolne WA: A clinical and histometric study of gingivitis associated with the human deciduous dentition, *J Periodontol* 56:293, 1985.
5. Bimstein E, Petetz B, Holan G: Prevalence of gingival stippling in children, *J Clin Pediatr Dent* 27:163, 2003.
6. Bodner L, Goldstein J, Sarnat H: Eruption cysts: a clinical report of 24 new cases, *J Clin Pediatr Dent* 28:183, 2004.
7. Gillett R, Cruckley A, Johnson NW: The nature of the inflammatory infiltrates in childhood gingivitis, juvenile periodontitis and adult periodontitis: immunocytochemical studies using monoclonal antibody to HLA, *J Clin Periodontol* 13:281, 1986.
8. Griffen AL: Preventive oral health. In Pinkham JR, Cassamassimo PS, Field HW, et al: *Pediatric dentistry in infancy through adolescence,* ed 3, Philadelphia, 1999, Saunders.
9. Grimmer EA: Trauma in an erupting premolar, *J Dent Res* 18:267, 1939.
10. Hock J: A clinical study of gingivitis of deciduous and succedaneous teeth in dogs, *J Periodontal Res* 13:68, 1978.
11. Jimenez M, Ramos J, Garrington G et al: The familial occurrence of acute necrotizing gingivitis in Colombia, *J Periodontol* 40:414, 1969.
12. King DL, Steinhauer W, Garcia-Godoy F, et al: Herpetic gingivostomatitis and teething difficulty in infants, *Pediatr Dent* 14:82, 1992.
13. Kronfeld R, Weinmann J: Traumatic changes in the periodontal tissues of deciduous teeth, *J Dent Res* 19:441, 1940.
14. Lindhe J, Liljenberg B, Listgarten M: Some microbiological and histopathological features of periodontal disease in man, *J Periodontol* 51:264, 1980.
15. Löe H, Anerud A, Bousen H: The natural history of periodontal disease in man: prevalence, severity and extent of gingival recession, *J Periodontol* 63:489, 1992.
16. Longhurst P, Johnson NW, Hopps RM: Differences in lymphocyte and plasma cell densities in inflamed gingiva from adults and young children, *J Periodontol* 48:705, 1977.
17. Longhurst P, Gillett R, Johnson NW: Electron microscope quantification of inflammatory infiltrates in childhood gingivitis, *J Periodontal Res* 15:255, 1980.
18. Machtei EE, Zubery Y, Bimstein E, et al: Anterior open bite and gingival recession in children and adolescents, *Int Dent J* 40:369, 1990.
19. Mackler SB, Crawford JJ: Plaque development in the primary dentition, *J Periodontol* 44:18, 1973.
20. Mattson L: Development of gingivitis in preschool children and young adults: a comparative experimental study, *J Clin Periodontol* 5:24, 1978.
21. Maynard JG, Wilson RD: Diagnosis and management of mucogingival problems in children, *Dent Clin North Am* 24:683, 1980.
22. Modeer T, Wondimu B: Periodontal diseases in children and adolescents, *Dent Clin North Am* 44: 633, 2000.
23. Mombelli R, Gusberti FR, van Oosten MA, et al: Gingival health and gingivitis development during puberty: a 4-year longitudinal study, *J Clin Periodontol* 16:44, 1989.
24. Morinushi T, Lopatin DE, Van Poperin N, Ueda Y: The relationship between gingivitis and colonization by *Porphyromonas gingivalis* and *Actinobacillus actinomycetemcomitans* in children, *J Periodontol* 71:403, 2000.
25. Notman S, Mandel ID, Mercadante J: Calculus in normal children and children with cystic fibrosis. Presented at International Association of Dental Research Program and Abstracts 48th General Meeting, 1970.
26. Oh TJ, Eber R, Wang HL: Periodontal diseases in the child and adolescent, *J Clin Periodontol* 29:400, 2002.
27. Orban B, Weinmann J: Signs of traumatic occlusion in average human jaws, *J Dent Res* 13:216, 1933.
28. Peretz B, Machtei EM, Bimstein E: Periodontal status in childhood and early adolescence: three-year follow-up, *J Clin Pediatr Dent* 20:229, 1996.
29. Pinborg JJ, Bhat M, Devanath KR et al: Occurrence of acute necrotizing gingivitis in South India children, *J Periodontol* 37:14, 1966.
30. Rosenblum FN: Clinical study of the depth of the gingival sulcus in the primary dentition, *J Dent Child* 5:289, 1966.
31. Seymour GJ, Crouch MS, Powell RN: The identification of lymphoid cell subpopulations in sections of human lymphoid tissue and gingivitis in children using monoclonal antibodies, *J Periodontal Res* 17:247, 1982.
32. Soni NN, Silberkweit M, Hayes RL: Histological characteristics of stippling in children, *J Periodontol* 34:31, 1963.
33. Srivastava B, Chandra S, Jhaiswal JS, et al: Cross-sectional study to evaluate variations in attached gingiva and gingival sulcus in the three periods of dentition, *J Clin Pediatr Dent* 15:17, 1990.
34. Sznajder N, Carraro JJ, Otero E, Carranza FA Jr: Clinical periodontal findings in trisomy 21 (mongolism), *J Periodontal Res* 3:1, 1968.
35. Taiwo JO: Severity of necrotizing ulcerative gingivitis in Nigerian children, *Periodontal Clin Invest* 17:24, 1995.
36. Yang EY, Tanner AC, Milgrom P, et al: Periodontal pathogen detection in gingiva/tooth and tongue flora samples from 18-48-month-old children and periodontal status of their mothers, *Oral Microbiol Immunol* 17:55, 2002.

Desquamative Gingivitis

Alfredo Aguirre, Jose Luis Tapia Vazquez, and Russell J. Nisengard

26

CHAPTER

CHAPTER OUTLINE

CHRONIC DESQUAMATIVE GINGIVITIS

Although first recognized and reported in 1894,[138] the term *chronic desquamative gingivitis* was coined in 1932 by Prinz[106] to describe a peculiar condition characterized by intense erythema, desquamation, and ulceration of the free and attached gingiva (Figure 26-1). Patients may be asymptomatic; when symptomatic, however, their complaints range from a mild burning sensation to an intense pain. Approximately 50% of desquamative gingivitis cases are localized to the gingiva, although patients can have involvement of the gingiva plus other intraoral and even extraoral sites.[97] Initially, the cause of this condition was unclear, with a variety of possibilities suggested. Because most cases were diagnosed in women in the fourth to fifth decades of life (although desquamative gingivitis may occur as early as puberty or as late as the seventh or eighth decade), a hormonal derangement was suspected. In 1960, however, McCarthy et al.[81] suggested that *desquamative gingivitis was not a specific disease entity, but a gingival response associated with a variety of conditions.* This concept has been further supported by numerous immunopathologic studies.[65,98,113,132]

Use of clinical and laboratory parameters have revealed that approximately 75% of desquamative gingivitis cases have a dermatologic genesis. Cicatricial pemphigoid and lichen planus account for more than 95% of the dermatologic cases.[95] However, many other mucocutaneous autoimmune conditions such as bullous pemphigoid, pemphigus vulgaris, linear immunoglobulin A (IgA) disease, dermatitis herpetiformis, lupus erythematosus, and chronic ulcerative stomatitis can clinically manifest as desquamative gingivitis.[118]

Other conditions that must be considered in the differential diagnosis of desquamative gingivitis include chronic bacterial, fungal, and viral infections, as well as reactions to medications, mouthwashes, and chewing gum. Although less common, Crohn's disease, sarcoidosis, some leukemias, and even factitious lesions have also been reported to present clinically as desquamative gingivitis.[118,142]

Therefore it is of paramount importance to ascertain the identity of the disease responsible for desquamative gingivitis to establish the appropriate therapeutic approach and management. To achieve this goal, the clinical examination must be coupled with a thorough history and routine histologic and immunofluorescence studies.[142] Despite this diagnostic approach, however, the cause of desquamative gingivitis cannot be elucidated in up to one third of the cases.[108]

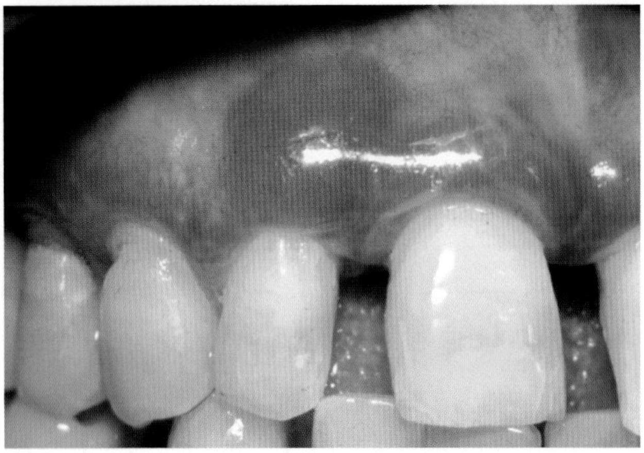

Figure 26-1 Chronic desquamative gingivitis. Irregular, conspicuous erythema involves the free and attached gingival tissues.

DIAGNOSIS OF DESQUAMATIVE GINGIVITIS: A SYSTEMATIC APPROACH

As stated, *desquamative gingivitis* is only a clinical term that describes a peculiar clinical picture. This term is not a diagnosis per se, and once it is rendered, a series of laboratory procedures should be used to arrive to a final diagnosis. Thus the success of any given therapeutic approach depends on the establishment of an accurate final diagnosis. The following discussion represents a systematic approach to elucidate the disease triggering desquamative gingivitis (Figure 26-2).

Clinical History. A thorough clinical history is mandatory to begin the assessment of desquamative gingivitis. Data regarding the symptomatology associated with this condition, as well as its historical aspects (i.e., when did the lesion start, has it worsened, is there a habit that exacerbates the condition), provide the foundation for a thorough examination. Information regarding previous therapy to alleviate the condition should also be documented.

Clinical Examination. Recognition of the pattern of distribution of the lesions (i.e., focal or multifocal, with or without confinement to the gingival tissues) provides leading information to begin the formulation of a differential diagnosis. In addition, a simple clinical maneuver such as Nikolsky's sign offers insight into the plausibility of the presence of a vesiculobullous disorder.

Biopsy. Given the extent and number of lesions that may be present in a given individual, an incisional biopsy is the best alternative to begin the microscopic and immunologic evaluation. An important consideration is selection of the biopsy site. A perilesional incisional biopsy should avoid areas of ulceration because necrosis and epithelial denudation severely hamper the diagnostic process. Once the tissue is excised from the oral cavity, the specimen can be bisected and then submitted for microscopic examination. Buffered formalin (10%) should be used to fix the tissue for conventional hematoxylin and eosin (H&E) evaluation. Michell's buffer (ammonium sulfate buffer, pH 7.0) is used as transport solution for immunofluorescence assessment. In general, an incisional biopsy of uninvolved (normal) mucosa will show the same immunofluorescent findings as the biopsy of the perilesional tissue. However, there are notable exceptions, such as in lichen planus and subacute lupus erythematosus, where only the lesional tissue will exhibit the corresponding immunologic markers. (See Table 26-1.)

Microscopic Examination. Approximately 5-μm sections of formalin-fixed, paraffin-embedded tissue stained with conventional H&E are obtained for light microscopy examination.

Immunofluorescence. For *direct* immunofluorescence, unfixed frozen sections are incubated with a variety of fluorescein-labeled, antihuman serum (anti-IgG, anti-IgA, anti-IgM, antifibrin and anti-C3). With *indirect* immunofluorescence, unfixed frozen sections of oral or esophageal mucosa from an animal such as a

SCIENCE TRANSFER

The multiplicity of causes of desquamative gingival lesions with a focus on dermatologic disease makes it imperative that clinicians develop diagnostic skills and good communication with physicians such as internists and dermatologists. *Because microscopic evaluation is the foundation for diagnosis of desquamative gingival lesions, clinicians must take the responsibility to biopsy all desquamative lesions.*

Recent findings show that in patients with erosive lichen planus, the use of chlorhexidine mouthwashes are helpful in resolving the lesions. In all desquamative lesions, however, mechanical oral hygiene procedures can add to the tissue damage and pain. Thus the clinician must customize a nontraumatic plaque removal program to augment the other treatment modalities used to treat desquamative gingivitis.

A variety of conditions affect the gingiva, either in part or totally. The gingiva consists of the epithelium, the connective tissue, and the basement membrane, which separates the two. Consequently, various conditions can involve each component specifically, totally, or in some cases, specific aspects of each component, such as certain layers of the epithelium. In many of these conditions, some type of inflammatory process is involved, either acute or chronic. Autoimmune mechanisms appear to be a prominent aspect of etiology in many patients. Thus, similar to periodontal disease, inflammation and the immune response are involved in the pathogenesis of the mucocutaneous lesions of the gingiva.

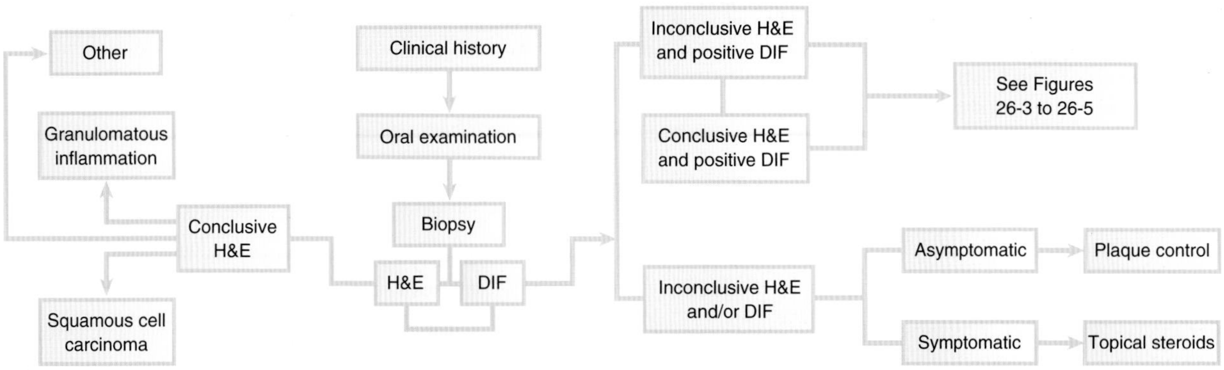

Figure 26-2 Diagnostic approach for desquamative gingivitis. *H&E,* Hematoxylin and eosin; *DIF,* direct immunofluorescence.

TABLE 26-1

Histopathologic, Direct, and Indirect Immunofluorescence Findings in Select Conditions That May Present Clinically as Desquamative Gingivitis

		DIRECT IMMUNOFLUORESCENCE		INDIRECT IMMUNOFLUORESCENCE
Disease	**Histopathology**	**Biopsy Perilesional Mucosa**	**Biopsy Uninvolved Mucosa**	**Serum**
Pemphigus	Intraepithelial clefting above basal cell layer; basal cells have characteristic "tombstone" appearance; acantholysis present.	Intercellular deposits in epithelium; IgG in all cases, C3 in most cases.	Same as for perilesional mucosa.	Intercellular (IgG) antibodies in ≥90% of cases.
Cicatricial pemphigoid	Subepithelial clefting with epithelial separation from underlying lamina propria, leaving intact basal layer.	Linear deposits of C3, with or without IgG at basement membrane zone in almost all cases.	Same as for perilesional mucosa.	Basement membrane zone (IgG) antibodies in 10% of cases.
Bullous pemphigoid	Subepithelial clefting with epithelial separation from underlying lamina propria, leaving intact basal layer.	Linear deposits of C3, with or without IgG at basement membrane zone in almost all cases.	Same as for perilesional mucosa.	Basement membrane zone in 40%-70% of cases.
Epidermolysis bullosa acquisita	Similar to bullous and cicatricial pemphigoid.	Linear deposits of IgG and C3 at basement membrane zone in almost cases.	Same as for perilesional mucosa.	Basement membrane zone (IgG) antibodies in 25% of cases.
Lichen planus	Hyperkeratosis, hydropic degeneration of basal layer, sawtooth rete pegs; lamina propria exhibits dense, bandlike infiltrate primarily of T lymphocytes; colloid bodies present.	Fibrillar deposits of fibrin at dermal-epidermal junction.	Negative.	Negative.
Chronic ulcerative stomatitis	Similar to erosive lichen planus; hyperkeratosis, acanthosis, basal cell layer liquefaction, subepithelial clefting, lymphohistiocytic chronic infiltrate in bandlike configuration.	IgG deposits in nuclei of basal layer of epithelial cells.	Same as for perilesional mucosa.	ANA specific for basal cells of stratified squamous epithelium.

Continued

TABLE 26-1

Histopathologic, Direct, and Indirect Immunofluorescence Findings in Select Conditions That May Present Clinically as Desquamative Gingivitis—cont'd

		DIRECT IMMUNOFLUORESCENCE		INDIRECT IMMUNOFLUORESCENCE
Disease	**Histopathology**	**Biopsy Perilesional Mucosa**	**Biopsy Uninvolved Mucosa**	**Serum**
Linear IgA disease	Similar to erosive lichen planus.	Linear deposits of IgA at basement membrane zone.	Same as for perilesional mucosa.	IgA basement membrane zone (IgA) antibodies in 30% of cases.
Dermatitis herpetiformis	Collection of neutrophils, eosinophils, and fibrin in connective tissue papillae.	IgA deposits in dermal papillae in 85% of cases.	IgA deposits in dermal papillae in 100% of cases.	IgA endomysial antibodies in 70% of cases; gliadin antibodies in 30% of cases.
Systemic lupus erythematosus	Hyperkeratosis, basal cell degeneration, epithelial atrophy, perivascular inflammation.	IgG or IgM, with or without C3 deposits at dermal-epidermal junction.	Same as for perilesional mucosa.	ANA in >95% of cases; DNA and ENA antibodies in >50% of cases.
Chronic cutaneous erythematosus	Hyperkeratosis, basal cell degeneration, epithelial atrophy, perivascular inflammation.	IgG or IgM, with or without C3 deposits at dermal-epidermal junction.	Negative.	Usually negative.
Subacute lupus erythematosus	Less inflammatory cell infiltrate than systemic and chronic cutaneous forms, but with similar microscopic features.	IgG or IgM, with or without C3 deposits at dermal-epidermal junction in 60% of cases; granular IgG deposits in basal cell cytoplasm in 30% of cases.	Same as for perilesional mucosa.	ANA in 60%-90%, Ro (SSA) in 80%, RF in 30%, and anti-RNP in 10% of cases

Modified from Rinaggio J, Neiders ME, Aguirre A, et al: *Compendium* 20:943, 1999.
IgA, Immunoglobulin A; *ANA,* antinuclear antibodies; *DNA,* deoxyribonucleic acid; *ENA,* extractable nuclear antigens; *RF,* rheumatoid factor; *RNP,* ribonucleoprotein.

monkey are first incubated with the patient's serum to allow attachment of any serum antibodies to the mucosal tissue. The tissue is then incubated with fluorescein-labeled antihuman serum. Immunofluorescence tests are positive if a fluorescent signal is observed in the epithelium, its associated basement membrane, or the underlying connective tissue. (See Table 26-1.)

Management. Once the diagnosis is established, the dentist must choose the optimum management for the patient. This is accomplished according to three factors: (1) practitioner's experience, (2) systemic impact of the disease, and (3) systemic complications of the medications.

A detailed consideration of these three factors dictates three different scenarios. In the first scenario the dental practitioner takes direct and exclusive responsibility for the treatment of the patient, as with erosive lichen planus that is responsive to topical steroids (Figure 26-3). In the second scenario the dentist collaborates with another health care provider to evaluate and/or treat a patient concurrently. The classic example is seen in cicatricial pemphigoid, where dentists and ophthalmologists work together (Figure 26-4). Although the dentist addresses the oral lesions, the ophthalmologist monitors the integrity of the ocular conjunctiva. In the third scenario the patient is immediately referred to a dermatologist for further evaluation and treatment. This occurs in conditions where the systemic impact of the disease transcends the boundaries of the oral cavity and results in significant morbidity and even mortality. Pemphigus vulgaris is a clear example of a condition that, once diagnosed by the dentist, requires immediate referral to a dermatologist (Figure 26-5). In addition, the complications of chronically administered systemic medications that are indicated for the management of diseases such as pemphigus vulgaris or nonresponsive mucous membrane pemphigoid (e.g., diabetes mellitus, osteoporosis, methemoglobinemia) warrant the referral to a dermatologist or a specialist in internal medicine.

When oral treatment is provided, periodic evaluation is needed to monitor the response of the patient to the selected therapy. Initially, the patient should be evaluated

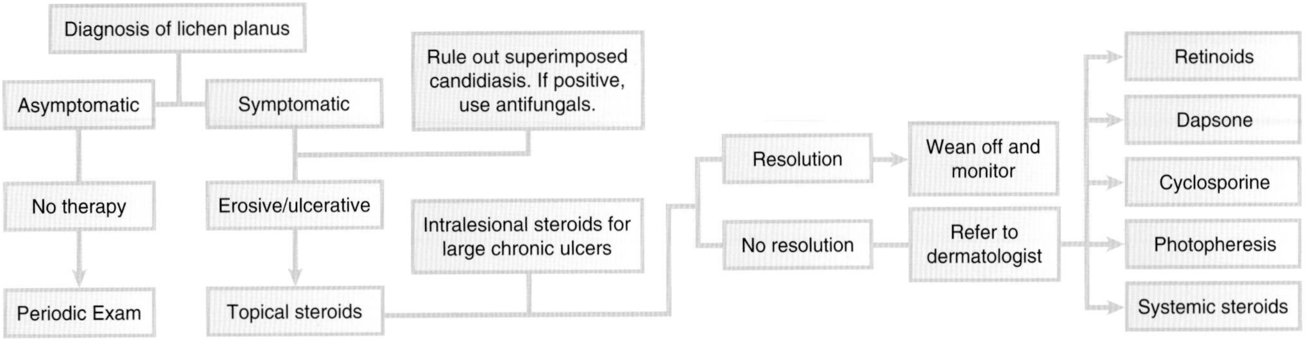

Figure 26-3 Treatment of lichen planus.

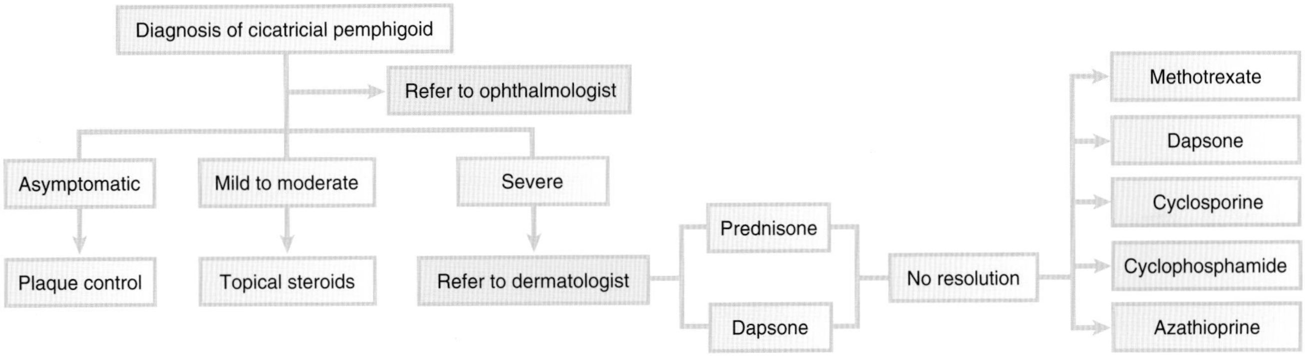

Figure 26-4 Treatment of cicatricial pemphigoid.

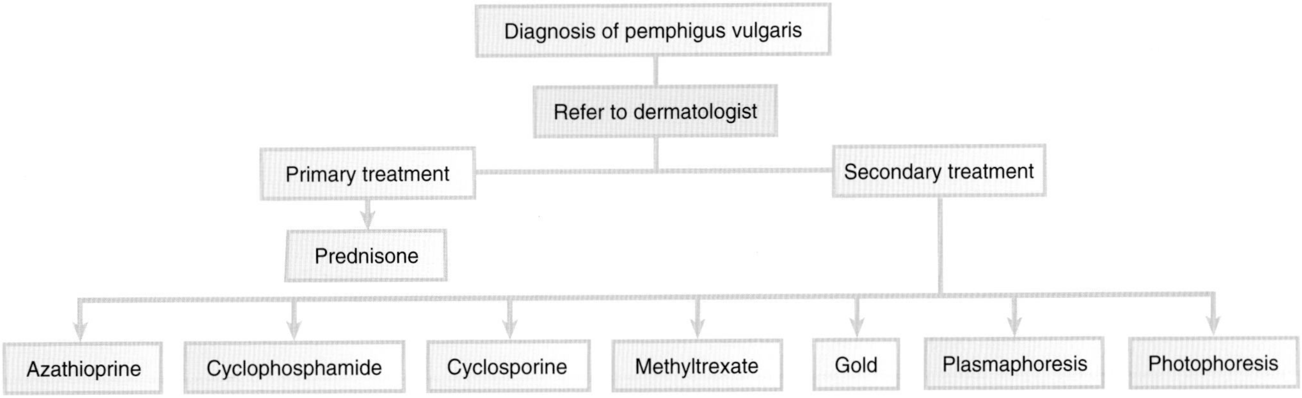

Figure 26-5 Treatment of pemphigus vulgaris.

at 2 to 4 weeks after beginning treatment to ensure that the condition is under control. This observation should continue until the patient is free of discomfort. Appointments every 3 to 6 months would then be appropriate. Doses of medication(s) are usually adjusted during this interval.

Table 26-2 summarizes suggested contemporary therapeutic approaches used to treat select conditions that clinically present as desquamative gingivitis. Dentists clearly play an important role in the diagnosis and management of desquamative gingivitis. The importance of being able to recognize and properly diagnose this condition is accentuated by the fact that a serious and life-threatening disease may initially manifest as desquamative gingivitis.

DISEASES CLINICALLY PRESENTING AS DESQUAMATIVE GINGIVITIS

Lichen Planus

Lichen planus is an inflammatory mucocutaneous disorder that may involve mucosal surfaces, (e.g., oral cavity, genital tract, other mucosae), and the skin (including the scalp and the nails).[114] The current evidence suggests that lichen planus is an immunologically mediated

TABLE 26-2

Accepted Contemporary Therapeutic Approaches Used to Treat Select Conditions That Clinically Present as Desquamative Gingivitis

Disease	Therapy
Erosive lichen planus	*Mild cases:* Delivery of therapeutic agent can be enhanced with use of vacuum-formed custom trays. **Rx:** Lidex (0.05% fluocinonide) gel **Disp:** One tube 1.5 g **Sig:** Apply to affected area pc and hs. Monitoring patient's oral cavity is warranted because candidiasis may develop after a few weeks of topical steroid use; concomitant use of antifungal may be necessary. **Rx:** Nystatin oral pastilles (100,000 IU) **Disp:** 60 pastilles **Sig:** Dissolve in mouth bid, then expectorate for 30 consecutive days. *Recalcitrant cases:* **Rx**: Protopic (0.1% tacrolimus) ointment **Disp:** One tube 15 gm **Sig:** Apply to affected area bid. *Severe or refractory cases:* Refer to dermatologist for management with systemic corticosteroids.
Cicatricial pemphigoid	*Mild cases:* **Rx:** Lidex (0.05% fluocinonide) gel **Disp:** One tube 1.5 g **Sig:** Apply to affected area pc and hs. **Rx:** Temovate (0.05% clobetasol propionate) **Disp:** One tube 1.5 g **Sig:** Apply to affected area qid. *Severe or refractory cases:* Refer to a dermatologist for management with prednisone (20-30 mg/day); concomitant use of azathioprine may be needed; dapsone, sulfonamide, and tetracycline are other alternatives.
Pemphigus	Refer to dermatologist for management with prednisone (20-30 mg/day); concomitant use of azathioprine may be needed.
Chronic ulcerative stomatitis	*Mild cases:* **Rx:** Lidex (0.05% fluocinonide) gel **Disp:** One tube 1.5 g **Sig:** Apply to affected area qid. **Rx:** Temovate (0.05% clobetasol propionate) **Disp:** One tube 1.5 g **Sig:** Apply to affected area qid.

Abbreviations: *g*, grams; *pc*, after meals; *hs*, at bedtime; *IU*, international units; *bid*, twice daily; *qid*, four times daily.

mucocutaneous disorder in which host T lymphocytes play a central role.[9,56,79] Although the oral cavity may present lichen planus lesions with a distinct clinical configuration and distribution, the clinical presentation sometimes may simulate other mucocutaneous disorders. Therefore a clinical diagnosis of oral lichen planus should be accompanied by a broad differential diagnosis. Numerous epidemiologic studies have shown that oral lichen planus presents in 0.1% to 4% of the population.[119,121] The majority of patients with oral lichen planus are middle-aged and older females, with a 2:1 ratio of females to males. Children are rarely affected. In a dental setting, cutaneous lichen planus is observed in about one third of the patients diagnosed with oral lichen planus.[76] In contrast, two thirds of patients seen in dermatologic clinics exhibit oral lichen planus.[117]

Oral Lesions. Although there are several clinical forms of oral lichen planus (reticular, patch, atrophic, erosive, and bullous), the most common are the reticular and erosive subtypes. The typical *reticular* lesions are asymptomatic and bilateral and consist of interlacing white lines on the posterior region of the buccal mucosa. The lateral border and dorsum of the tongue, hard palate, alveolar ridge, and gingiva may also be affected. In addition, the reticular lesions may have an erythematous background, a feature associated with coexisting candidiasis. Oral lichen planus lesions follow a chronic course

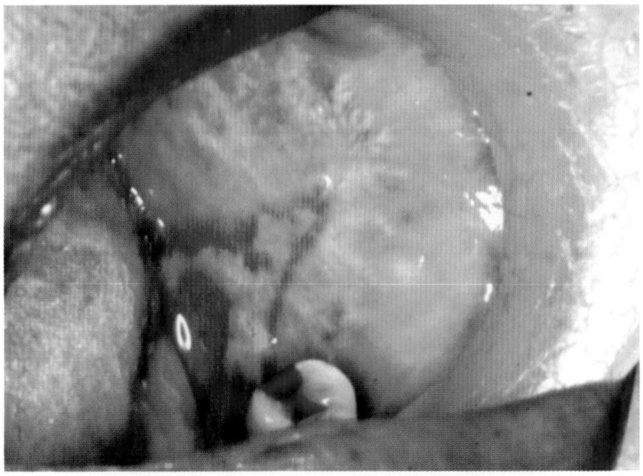

Figure 26-6 Erosive lichen planus. Large ulcerative lesion on the left buccal mucosa exhibits bordering erythema. The typical white striations of lichen planus are evident in the periphery of the ulcer.

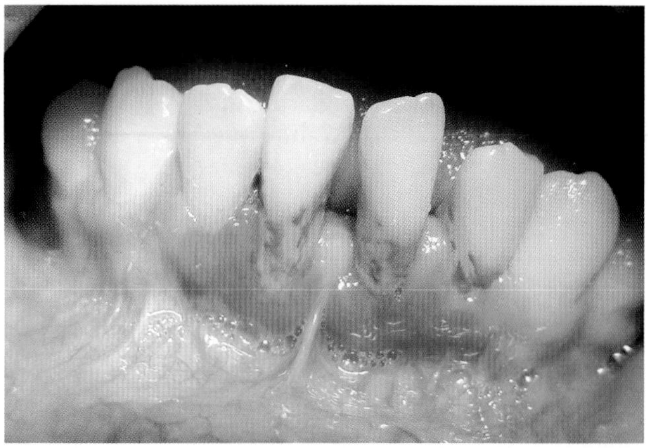

Figure 26-7 Erosive lichen planus presenting as desquamative gingivitis. The gingival tissues are erythematous, ulcerated, and painful. (Courtesy Dr. Luis Gaitan, Oral Pathology Laboratory, Faculty of Odontology, National Autonomous University of Mexico (UNAM), Mexico City.)

and have alternating, unpredictable periods of quiescence and flare-ups.

The *erosive* subtype of lichen planus is often associated with pain and clinically manifests as atrophic, erythematous, and often, ulcerated areas. Fine, white radiating striations are observed bordering the atrophic and ulcerated zones. These areas may be sensitive to heat, acid, and spicy foods (Figure 26-6).

Gingival Lesions. Up to 10% of patients with oral lichen planus have lesions restricted to the gingival tissue[117] that may occur as one or more types of four distinctive patterns, as follows:

1. *Keratotic lesions.* These raised white lesions may present as groups of individual papules, linear or reticular lesions, or plaquelike configurations.
2. *Erosive or ulcerative lesions.* These extensive erythematous areas with a patchy distribution may present as focal or diffuse hemorrhagic areas. These lesions are exacerbated by slight trauma (e.g., toothbrushing) (Figure 26-7).
3. *Vesicular or bullous lesions.* These raised, fluid-filled lesions are uncommon and short lived on the gingiva, quickly rupturing and leaving an ulceration.
4. *Atrophic lesions.* Atrophy of the gingival tissues with ensuing epithelial thinning results in erythema confined to the gingiva.

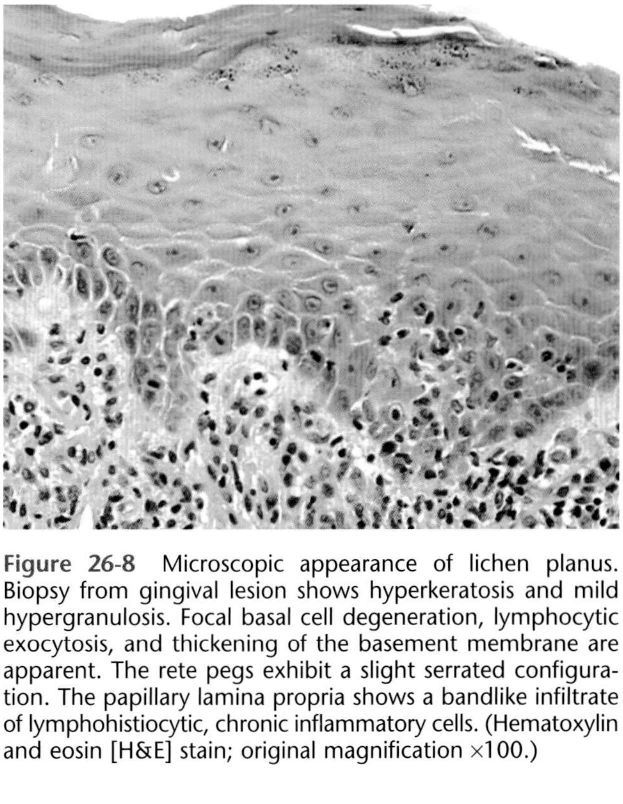

Figure 26-8 Microscopic appearance of lichen planus. Biopsy from gingival lesion shows hyperkeratosis and mild hypergranulosis. Focal basal cell degeneration, lymphocytic exocytosis, and thickening of the basement membrane are apparent. The rete pegs exhibit a slight serrated configuration. The papillary lamina propria shows a bandlike infiltrate of lymphohistiocytic, chronic inflammatory cells. (Hematoxylin and eosin [H&E] stain; original magnification ×100.)

Histopathology. Microscopically, three main features characterize oral lichen planus: (1) hyperkeratosis or parakeratosis, (2) hydropic degeneration of the basal layer, and (3) a dense, bandlike infiltrate primarily of T lymphocytes in the lamina propria (Figure 26-8). Classically, the epithelial rete ridges have a "sawtooth" configuration. Hydropic degeneration of the basal layer of the epithelium may be sufficiently extensive that the epithelium becomes thin and atrophic or detaches off the underlying connective tissue and produces either a subepithelial vesicle or an ulcer. Colloid bodies (Civatte bodies) are often seen at the epithelium–connective tissue interface. A microscopic diagnosis of oral lichen planus is straightforward in the keratotic lesions, and biopsy specimens should be obtained from these areas if possible. However, these classic histologic features may be obscured in the areas of ulceration, making a conclusive diagnosis of oral lichen planus difficult based solely on conventional microscopy.

Electron microscopic studies indicate that lichen planus can be divided into three stages: (1) degeneration of the cytoplasm of the epithelial cells, (2) loss of collagen fibers in the superficial lamina propria, and (3) degeneration and necrosis of the basal and parabasal layers of the epithelium. The superficial lamina propria is also degenerated and necrotic, and the basement lamina is no longer visible. Separation of the basal lamina from the basal cell layer is an early manifestation of lichen planus.[106]

It is noteworthy that oral lesions of lichen planus may change in pattern, and in certain unusual cases, a second or even a third biopsy may be necessary to arrive at a definitive diagnosis. More importantly, controversy exists about the malignant potential of oral lichen planus. In some studies, it has been estimated that oral cancer emerges in 0.4% to 5.6% of patients with oral lichen planus.[55,37,131] In contrast, other researchers reject or question the connection between oral lichen planus and oral cancer.[38,74,107] Despite this controversy, biopsy and close follow-up are warranted in these patients.

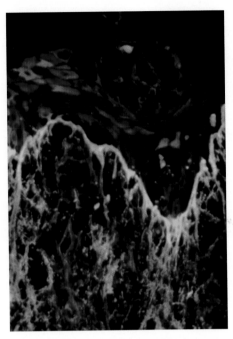

Figure 26-9 Direct immunofluorescence of lichen planus. Fibrin deposits along the basement membrane of the epithelium exhibit a "shaggy" configuration.

Immunopathology. Direct immunofluorescence of both lesional and perilesional oral lichen planus biopsy specimens reveal linear fibrillar deposits of fibrin in the basement membrane zone (Figure 26-9), along with scattered, immunoglobulin-staining cytoid bodies in the upper areas of the lamina propria (Figure 26-10). Serum tests using indirect immunofluorescence are negative in lichen planus (see Table 26-1).

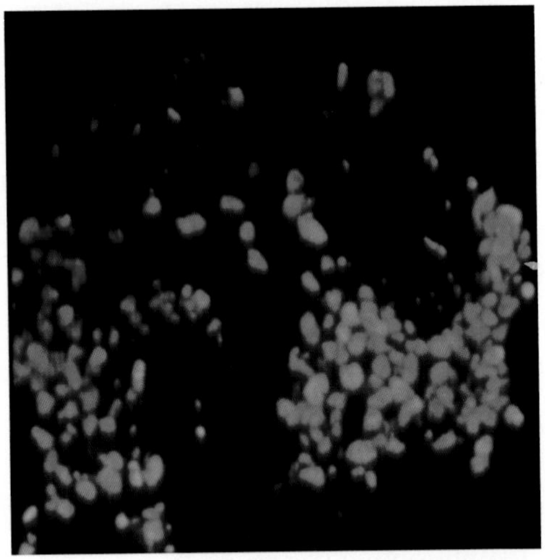

Figure 26-10 Direct immunofluorescence of lichen planus. Clusters of cytoid bodies exhibit immunoglobulin M (IgM) deposits in the lamina propria.

Differential Diagnosis. The classic clinical presentation of oral lichen planus can be simulated by other conditions, mainly by lichenoid mucositis. When an erosive component is present, lupus erythematosus and chronic ulcerative stomatitis should be included in the differential diagnosis. If oral lichen planus is confined to the gingival tissues (erosive oral lichen planus), the identification of fine, white radiating striations bordering the erosive areas support a clinical diagnosis of oral lichen planus. If the white striations are absent, the differential diagnosis should primarily include cicatricial pemphigoid and pemphigus vulgaris. Other, less common possibilities include linear IgA disease and chronic ulcerative stomatitis.

Therapy. The keratotic lesions of oral lichen planus are asymptomatic and do not require treatment once the microscopic diagnosis is established. However, follow-up of the patient every 6 to 12 months is warranted to monitor suspicious clinical changes and the emergence of an erosive component.

In contrast, the erosive, bullous, or ulcerative lesions of oral lichen planus are treated with high-potency topical steroids, such as 0.05% fluocinonide ointment (Lidex, three times daily). Lidex can also be mixed 1:1 with carboxymethyl cellulose (Orabase) paste or other adhesive ointment. A gingival tray can also be used to deliver 0.05% clobetasol proprionate with 100,000 IU/ml of nystatin in Orabase. Three 5-minute applications of this mixture daily appear to be effective in controlling erosive lichen planus.[50] Intralesional injections of triamcinolone acetonide (10-20 mg) or short-term regimens of 40 mg of prednisone daily for 5 days, followed by 10 to 20 mg daily for an additional 2 weeks, have also been used in more severe cases.[97] Because of the potential side effects, administration of systemic steroids should be prescribed and monitored by a dermatologist. Other treatment modalities (e.g., retinoids, hydroxychloroquine, cyclosporine, azathioprine, cyclophosphamide, free gingival grafts) have also been used.[97,103] A promising therapeutic agent, tacrolimus (0.1% Protopic ointment, twice daily), is an immunosuppressant that is effective in controlling lesions of erosive lichen planus.[89,122]

Because candidiasis is often associated with symptomatic oral lichen planus, therapy should also include a topical antifungal agent.[15,46]

Pemphigoid

The term *pemphigoid* applies to a number of cutaneous, immune-mediated, subepithelial bullous diseases characterized by a separation of the basement membrane zone, including bullous pemphigoid, mucous membrane pemphigoid, and pemphigoid (herpes) gestationis.[102,120] Among these conditions, bullous pemphigoid and mucous membrane pemphigoid, also known as *benign mucous membrane pemphigoid* and *cicatricial pemphigoid,* have received considerable attention. Current molecular findings on these two diseases clearly indicate that they are separate entities.[120] However, considerable histologic and immunopathologic overlap exists between the two diseases such that their differentiation may be impossible based on these two criteria.[102] In many cases the clinical findings are probably the best cognitive element to discriminate them. Accordingly, the term *bullous pemphigoid* is preferred when the disease is nonscarring and mainly affects the skin. The term *cicatricial pemphigoid* is favored when scarring occurs and the disease is mainly confined to mucous membranes (although scarring may be absent in some subtypes of mucous membrane pemphigoid).[139] Until more research allows better understanding of this family of diseases, bullous pemphigoid and mucous membrane pemphigoid are discussed separately.

Bullous Pemphigoid. Bullous pemphigoid is a chronic, autoimmune, subepidermal bullous disease with tense bullae that rupture and become flaccid in the skin (Figure 26-11). Oral involvement occurs in about a third of the patients.[129] Although the skin lesions clinically resemble those of pemphigus, the microscopic picture is quite distinct. There is no evidence of acantholysis, and the developing vesicles are subepithelial rather than intraepithelial. The epithelium separates from the underlying connective tissue at the basement membrane zone. Electron microscopic studies show an actual horizontal splitting or replication of the basal lamina. The separating epithelium remains relatively intact, and the basal layer is present and appears to be regular. The two major antigenic determinants for bullous pemphigoid are the 230-kD protein plaque known as *BP1* and the 180-kD collagen-like transmembrane protein *BP2*.[90,112]

Immunofluorescence. Immunologically, bullous pemphigoid is characterized by immunoglobulin G (IgG) and complement 3 (C3) immune deposits along epithelial basement membranes and circulating IgG antibodies to the epithelial basement membrane.[60,94] Direct immunofluoresence is positive in 90% to 100% of these patients, whereas indirect immunofluorescence is positive in 40% to 70% of affected patients[95] (see Table 26-1).

Oral Lesions. Oral lesions have been reported to occur secondarily in up to 40% of cases. There is an erosive or desquamative gingivitis presentation and occasional vesicular or bullous lesions.[129]

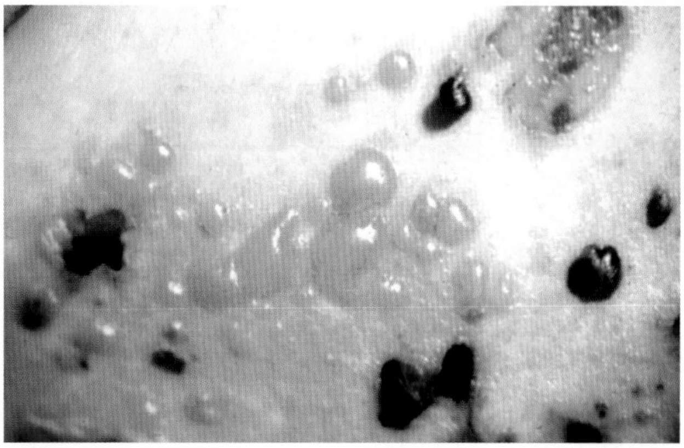

Figure 26-11 Bullous pemphigoid. Coalescing cutaneous bullae are seen, with some hemorrhagic. Rupture of bullae leads to formation of serpiginous ulcers.

Therapy. Because its etiologic factors are unknown, treatment of bullous pemphigoid is designed to control its signs and symptoms.[60,94] The primary treatment is a moderate dose of systemic prednisone. Steroid-sparing strategies (prednisone plus other immunomodulator drugs) are used when high doses of steroids are needed or the steroid alone fails to control the disease.[34] For localized lesions of bullous pemphigoid, high-potency topical steroids or tetracycline with or without nicotinamide can be effective.[96]

Mucous Membrane Pemphigoid (Cicatricial Pemphigoid). Mucous membrane pemphigoid, also known as cicatricial pemphigoid, is a chronic, vesiculobullous autoimmune disorder of unknown cause that predominantly affects women in the fifth decade of life. Although rare, it has been reported in young children.[20,91,120]

Cicatricial pemphigoid involves the oral cavity, conjunctiva, and the mucosa of the nose, vagina, rectum, esophagus, and urethra. In about 20% of patients, however, the skin may also be involved. Recent investigations suggest that cicatricial pemphigoid encompasses a group of heterogeneous conditions with distinct clinical and molecular features.[30,86,115] An elaborate cascade of events is involved in the pathogenesis of cicatricial pemphigoid. Initially, antigen-antibody complexing occurs at the basement membrane zone, followed by complement activation and subsequent leukocyte recruitment. Next, proteolytic enzymes are released and dissolve or cleave the basement membrane zone, usually at the level of the lamina lucida.[40] The two major antigenic determinants for cicatricial pemphigoid are bullous pemphigoid 1 and 2 (BP1 and BP2). Most cases of cicatricial pemphigoid are the result of an immune response directed against BP2 and less often against BP1, epiligrin (laminin-5, a lamina lucida protein in basement membrane of stratified epithelium) and β-4 integrins.[6,18,30] Current research strongly suggests that there are at least five subtypes of cicatricial pemphigoid: oral pemphigoid, antiepiligrin pemphigoid,

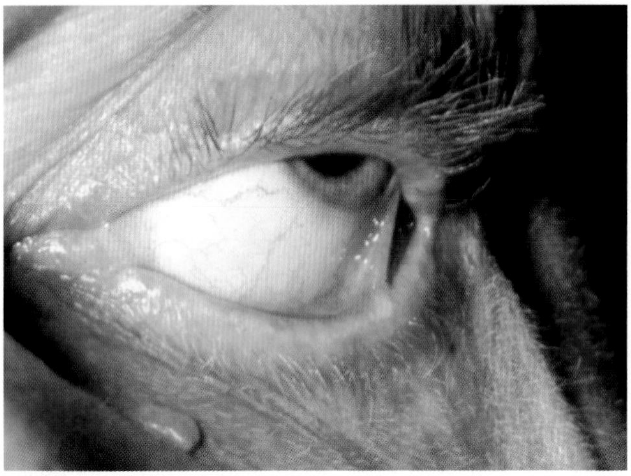

Figure 26-12 Mucous membrane pemphigoid. Characteristic ocular lesion (symblepharon) in a patient presenting with cicatricial pemphigoid. (Courtesy Dr. Carl Allen, Ohio State University, Columbus.)

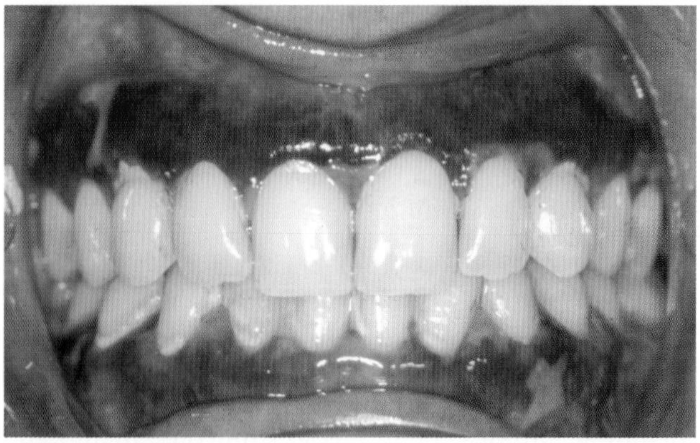

Figure 26-13 Gingival mucous membrane pemphigoid. Lesions are confined to the gingival tissues, producing a typical desquamative gingivitis appearance. (Courtesy Dr. Stuart L. Fischman, State University of New York at Buffalo.)

anti–BP antigen mucosal pemphigoid, ocular pemphigoid, and multiple-antigens pemphigoid.[120]

Ocular Lesions. In cases presenting first to the dentist (mainly desquamative gingivitis), the eyes are affected in approximately 25% of patients.[95] In contrast, in cases presenting first to the dermatologist, 66% of patients present with conjunctival lesions, whereas in ophthalmic studies, 100% of the patients have ocular involvement.[45,69,87,88] The initial lesion is characterized by unilateral conjunctivitis that becomes bilateral within 2 years. Subsequently, there may be adhesions of eyelid to eyeball *(symblepharon)* (Figure 26-12). Adhesions at the edges of the eyelids *(ankyloblepharon)* may lead to a narrowing of the palpebral fissure. Small vesicular lesions may develop on the conjunctiva, which may eventually produce scarring, corneal damage, and blindness.

Oral Lesions. The most characteristic feature of oral involvement is the presence of desquamative gingivitis, typically with areas of erythema, desquamation, ulceration, and vesiculation, of the attached gingiva[47,125] (Figure 26-13). Vesiculobullous lesions may occur elsewhere in the mouth.[47] The bullae tend to have a relatively thick roof and rupture in 2 to 3 days, leaving irregularly shaped areas of ulceration. Healing of the lesions may take up to 3 weeks or longer.

Histopathology. The microscopic appearance of the oral lesions, although not completely diagnostic for mucous membrane pemphigoid, is sufficiently distinctive that a tentative diagnosis can be considered. A striking subepithelial vesiculation, with the epithelium separated from the underlying lamina propria, leaves an intact basal layer (Figure 26-14). The separation of the epithelium and the connective tissue occurs at the basement membrane zone. Electron microscopic studies demonstrate a split in the basal lamina.[136] A mixed inflammatory infiltrate (lymphocytes, plasma cells, neutrophils, and scarce eosinophils) is observed in the underlying fibrous connective tissue.

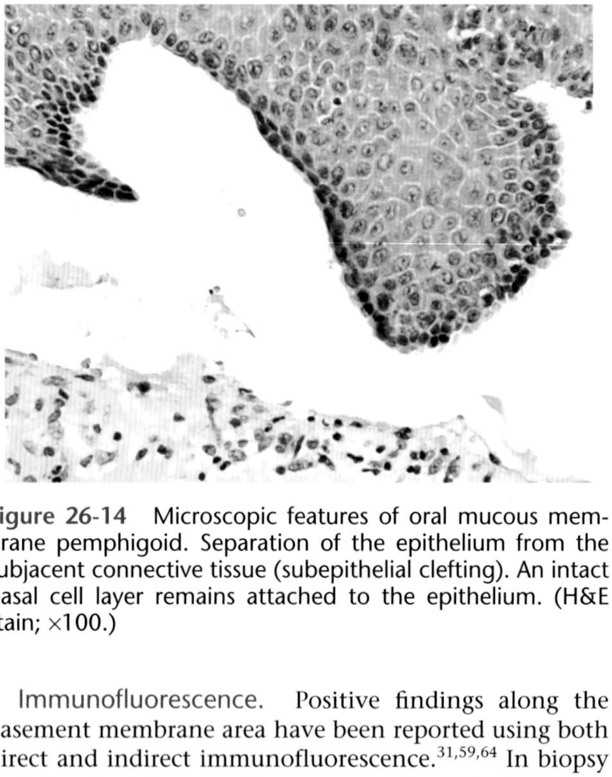

Figure 26-14 Microscopic features of oral mucous membrane pemphigoid. Separation of the epithelium from the subjacent connective tissue (subepithelial clefting). An intact basal cell layer remains attached to the epithelium. (H&E stain; ×100.)

Immunofluorescence. Positive findings along the basement membrane area have been reported using both direct and indirect immunofluorescence.[31,59,64] In biopsy tests by direct immunofluorescence, the main immunoreactants are IgG and C3, which are confined to the basement membrane (Figure 26-15). Some studies indicate that positive indirect immunofluorescence is rare in these patients (<25%).[96] The lack of indirect immunofluorescence findings may be caused by an earlier diagnosis of mucous membrane pemphigoid, resulting in the identification of patients with less extensive disease.[1,67] In any event, circulating autoantibodies do not appear to play a role in the pathogenesis of the disease.

Differential Diagnosis. Several disease entities present with similar clinical and histologic (subepithelial bulla) features.[36] These include bullous pemphigoid, bullous lichen planus, dermatitis herpetiformis, linear IgA disease, erythema multiforme, herpes gestationis, and epidermolysis bullosa acquisita.

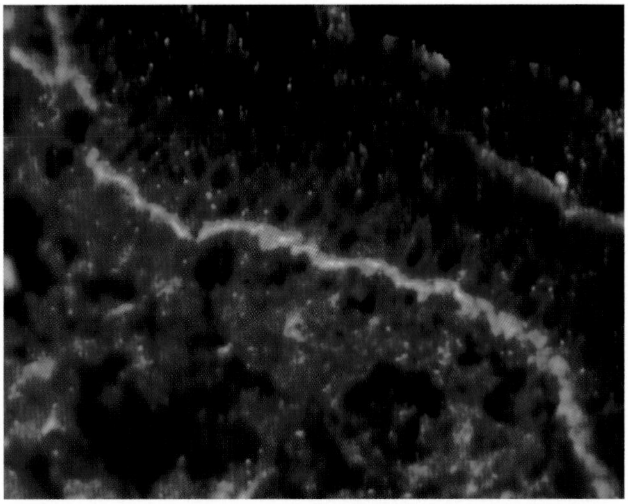

Figure 26-15 Direct immunofluorescence of mucous membrane pemphigoid. C3 deposits confined along the basement membrane.

Pemphigus may be confined to the oral cavity in its early stage, and the vesicular and ulcerative lesions may resemble those of mucous membrane pemphigoid. An erosive or desquamative gingivitis may also be seen in pemphigus as a rare manifestation. Biopsy studies can quickly rule out pemphigus by revealing the absence or presence of acantholytic changes. In erythema multiforme, there are obvious vesiculobullous lesions, but the onset is usually acute rather than chronic, labial involvement is severe, and the gingivae are usually not affected. Desquamative gingivitis is an unusual finding in erythema multiforme, although occasional vesicular lesions may develop. A biopsy study of an oral lesion reveals an unusual degeneration of the upper stratum spinosum, characteristically seen in oral erythema multiforme lesions.

Cicatricial pemphigoid must be differentiated from epidermolysis bullosa acquisita, which can present with similar histopathology and immunopathology. When the biopsy is treated with salt to separate the dermis from the epidermis, basement membrane immunodeposits occur on the epidermal side in pemphigoid and the dermal side in epidermolysis bullosa acquisita.[39]

Therapy. Topical steroids are the mainstay of treatment for mucous membrane pemphigoid, particularly when localized lesions are present. Fluocinonide (0.05%) and clobetasol propionate (0.05%) in an adhesive vehicle can be used three times a day for up to 6 months. When the oral lesions of mucous membrane pemphigoid are confined to the gingival tissues, topical corticosteroids are effectively delivered with vacuum-formed custom trays or veneers.[120] Optimal oral hygiene is essential because local irritants on the tooth surface result in an exaggerated gingival inflammatory response. Gingival irritation from any dental prosthesis should also be minimized.

If the disease is not severe and symptoms are mild, systemic corticosteroids may be omitted. If ocular involvement exists, systemic corticosteroids are indicated.

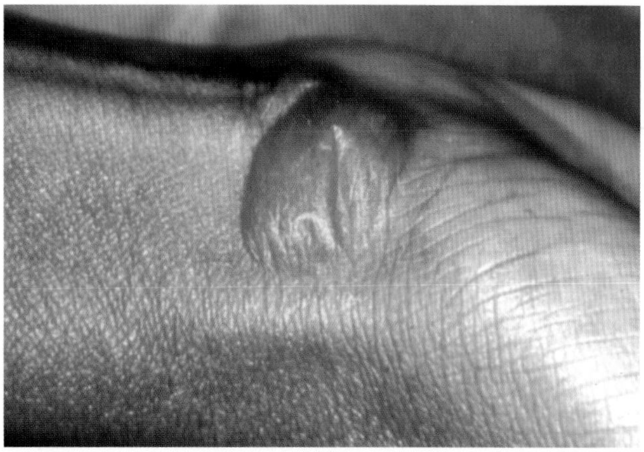

Figure 26-16 Cutaneous lesion of patient with pemphigus vulgaris. A large bulla is present in the flexor surface of the wrist.

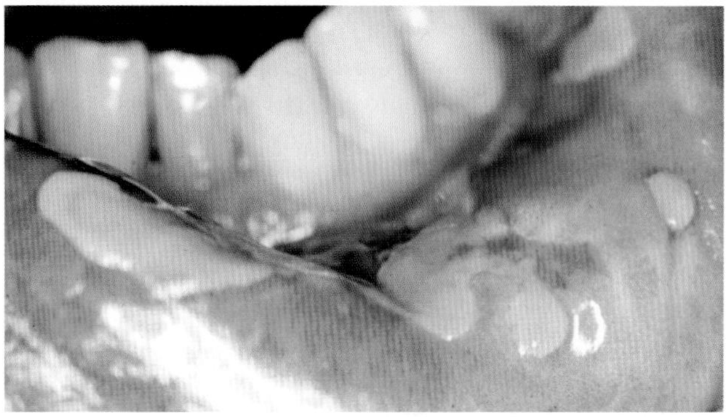

Figure 26-17 Pemphigus vulgaris of the oral cavity. Multiple and coalescent areas of ulceration are covered by pseudomembranes of necrotic epithelium. This patient presented with large ulcers in the labial mucosa, tongue, and soft palate.

When lesions do not respond to steroids, systemic dapsone (4-4′-diaminodiphenylsulfone) has proved to be effective.[25,43,86,93] Because of the systemic side effects to dapsone, including hemolysis and methemoglobulinemia, particularly in patients with glucose-6-phosphate dehydrogenase deficiency, referral to a dermatologist is often indicated.[99] Some authors also advocate sulfonamides and tetracycline; surgery, although not a treatment for mucous membrane pemphigoid, is used in some patients to prevent blindness as well as esophageal and upper airways stenosis.[120] Connective tissue grafting to alleviate root surface sensitivity and improve esthetics has been used with success to manage gingival recession in a cicatricial pemphigoid patient.[72]

Pemphigus Vulgaris

The pemphigus diseases are a group of autoimmune bullous disorders that produce cutaneous and mucous membranes blisters (Figures 26-16 and 26-17). Pemphigus vulgaris is the most common of the pemphigus diseases, which also include pemphigus foliaceous, pemphigus vegetants, and pemphigus erythematosus.[111] Pemphigus vulgaris is a potentially lethal, chronic condition (10% mortality rate) with a worldwide incidence of 0.1 to 0.5 cases per year per 100,000 individuals.[10,111,116] A predilection in women, usually after the fourth decade of life, has been observed.[96] However, pemphigus vulgaris has also been reported in unusually young children and even in newborns.[23,111,140]

The epidermal and mucous membrane blisters occur when the cell-to-cell adhesion structures are damaged by the action of circulating and in vivo binding of autoantibodies to the pemphigus vulgaris antigens, which are cell surface glycoproteins present in keratinocytes. These pemphigus vulgaris glycoproteins are members of the *desmoglein* (DSG) subfamily of the cadherin superfamily of cell-cell adhesion molecules, which are present in desmosomes.[66] Whereas high levels of desmoglein 3 (DSG3) autoantibodies correlate with severity of oral disease in patients with pemphigus vulgaris, elevated levels of desmoglein 1 (DSG1) autoantibodies are associated with severity of cutaneous disease.[53] Recent evidence suggests that DSG3, the gene coding for pemphigus vulgaris, is located in chromosome 18.

Most cases of pemphigus vulgaris are idiopathic. However, medications such as penicillamine and captopril can produce drug-induced pemphigus, which is usually reversible on withdrawal of the causative drug. Paraneoplastic pemphigus is antigenically distinct from pemphigus vulgaris and is associated with underlying malignancies.[92]

In approximately 60% of patients with pemphigus vulgaris, the oral lesions are the first sign of the disease and may herald the dermatologic involvement by a year or more.[84,130]

Oral Lesions. ange from small vesicles to large bullae. When the bullae rupture, they leave extensive areas of ulceration (Figure 26-18). Virtually any region of the oral cavity can be involved, but multiple lesions often develop at sites of irritation or trauma. The soft palate is more often involved (80%), followed by the buccal mucosa (46%), ventral aspect or dorsum of tongue (20%), and lower labial mucosa (10%). Oral lesions of pemphigus vulgaris are confined less often to the gingival tissues.[63] In these patients a clinical diagnosis of erosive gingivitis or desquamative gingivitis is seen as the sole manifestation of oral pemphigus.

Histopathology. Lesions of pemphigus demonstrate a characteristic intraepithelial separation, which occurs above the basal cell layer. The intraepithelial vesiculation begins as a microscopic alteration (Figure 26-19) and gradually results in a grossly visible, fluid-filled bulla. Occasionally the entire superficial layers of epithelium are lost, leaving only the basal cells attached to the underlying lamina propria, conferring a characteristic "tombstone" appearance to the epithelial cells. *Acantholysis,* a separation of the epithelial cells of the lower stratum spinosum, takes place and is characterized by the presence of round rather than polyhedral epithelial cells. The intercellular bridges are lost, and the nuclei are large and hyperchromatic.[29,68,143] The underlying connective tissue usually presents as a mild to moderate, chronic inflammatory cell infiltrate. As the vesicle or bulla ruptures, the ulcerated lesion becomes infiltrated with polymorphonuclear leukocytes (PMNs), and the surface may show suppuration.

Cytology. Cytologic smears of oral pemphigus lesions represent a preliminary test and should not replace the histologic and immunopathologic examinations. Cytologic examination may be used as corroborating evidence for a definitive diagnosis. A positive smear reveals large numbers of rounded acantholytic cells with serrated borders and large, hyperchromatic nuclei.[13,124]

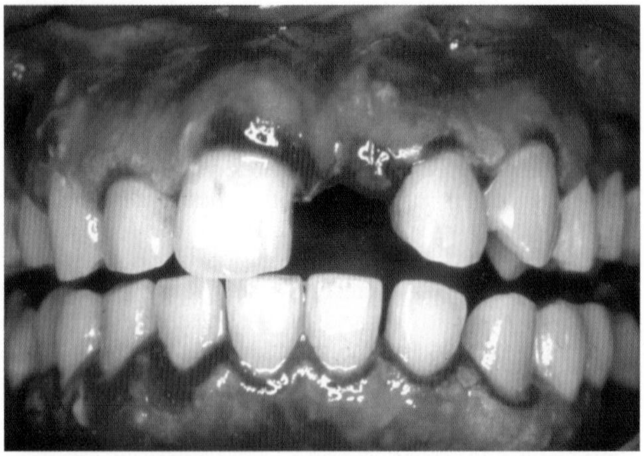

Figure 26-18 Pemphigus vulgaris of the gingiva. Clinical appearance of patient with oral lesions confined to the gingivae that were clinically diagnosed as "consistent with desquamative gingivitis." (Courtesy Dr. Luis Gaitan, Oral Pathology Laboratory, Faculty of Odontology, National Autonomous University of Mexico (UNAM), Mexico City.)

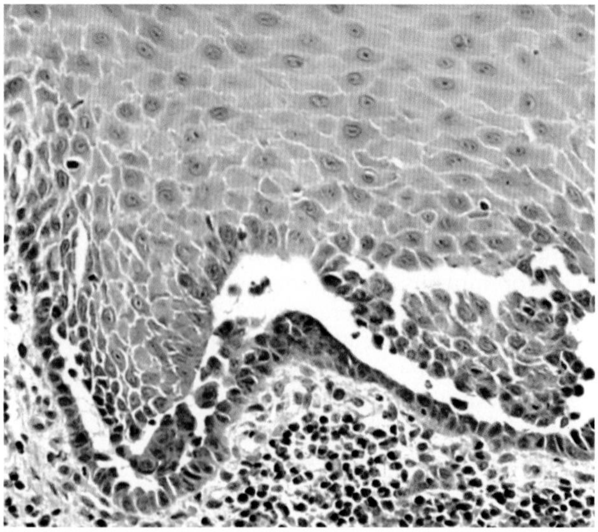

Figure 26-19 Microscopic features of pemphigus vulgaris. Typical intraepithelial clefting with "tombstone" appearance of basal cells, which remain attached to subjacent basement membrane and fibrous connective tissue. Acantholysis of epithelial cells with formation of "Tzanck" cells is seen in the intraepithelial cleft. (H&E stain; ×100.)

Electron Microscopy. Electron microscopic studies indicate that breakdown of the epithelial intercellular cement substance is the first stage in the development of acantholysis. Other investigations suggest that the destruction starts in the tonofilaments[45] or in the desmosomes[128] (Figure 26-20).

Immunofluorescence. The presence of autoantibodies can be demonstrated in the oral mucosa of patients with oral pemphigus by the use of immunofluorescence techniques. For direct immunofluorescence, perilesional unfixed frozen sections are incubated with fluorescein-labeled human anti-IgG. In indirect immunofluorescence, unfixed frozen sections of oral or esophageal mucosa from an animal such as a monkey is first incubated with the patient's serum to allow attachment of any serum antibodies to the mucosal tissue. The tissue is then incubated with fluorescein-labeled, antihuman IgG serum. The test is positive if immunofluorescence is observed in the intercellular spaces of the stratified squamous epithelium of the mucosa (Figure. 26-21). The indirect technique is less sensitive than the direct technique and may be negative in early stages of the disease, particularly in localized forms (see Table 26-1). In most cases, however, the indirect immunofluorescence titers are helpful to monitor disease activity and have prognostic value.

Differential Diagnosis. The oral lesions of pemphigus vulgaris may be similar to those seen in erythema multiforme. In erythema multiforme, however, recurrent active episodes of comparatively short duration are followed by long intervals free of skin or oral lesions. Erythema multiforme affects the lips with considerable severity. Microscopic examination with conventional H&E and direct immunofluorescence can discriminate oral lesions of pemphigus from those of erythema multiforme. Pemphigus vulgaris will show characteristic intraepithelial clefting at the basal-spinous cell layers interface with acantholysis, whereas erythema multiforme shows microvesiculation of the superficial epithelial layers and numerous necrotic keratinocytes. Pemphigus vulgaris shows an intercellular and intraepithelial signal with direct immunofluorescence. In contrast, erythema multiforme exhibits negative immunofluorescence.

Pemphigoid may clinically resemble pemphigus when it is confined to the mouth. Microscopic examination and direct immunofluorescence studies are needed to establish a correct diagnosis. Bullous pemphigoid and mucous membrane pemphigoid exhibit detachment of the epithelium from the underlying connective tissue ("lifting off"), instead of the acantholytic lesion characteristic of pemphigus.

Bullous lichen planus must also be considered in the differential diagnosis. The primary lesion of pemphigus may be of a bullous character, followed by erosion with associated pain and discomfort. In lichen planus, however, the characteristic reticular lesions are invariably found associated with the bullae. Microscopic examination and direct immunofluorescence studies are necessary to differentiate this condition from pemphigus. Bullous lichen planus shows separation of the epithelium from the underlying fibrous connective tissue, "sawtooth" rete pegs, and a bandlike, chronic inflammatory infiltrate

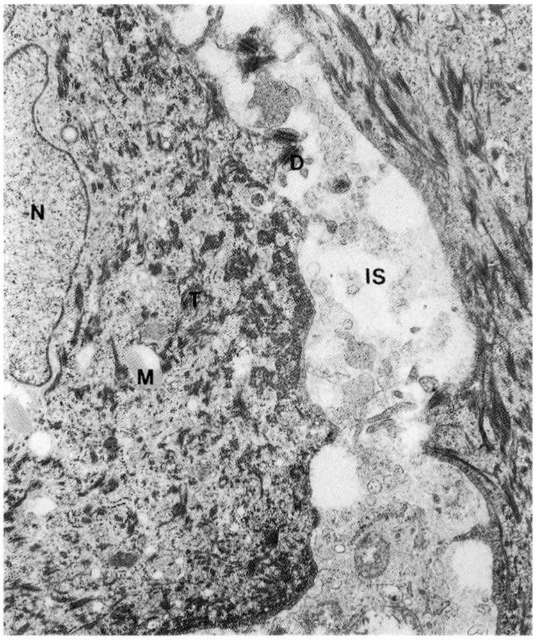

Figure 26-20 Oral pemphigus. Electron micrograph of acantholytic cells showing the disappearance of desmosomes *(D)* and the separation of cells by widening of the intracellular space *(IS)*. Tonofibrils *(T)* show clumping, and mitochondria *(M)* are degenerating. The nucleus *(N)* is intact.

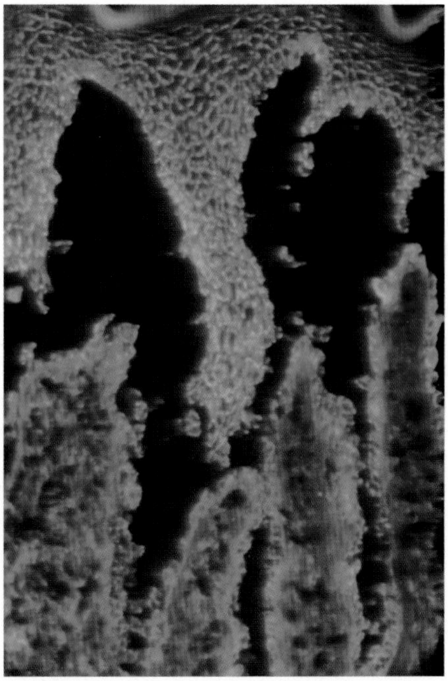

Figure 26-21 Direct immunofluorescence of oral pemphigus. Positive intercellular signal for immunoglobulin G (IgG) deposits is seen in keratinocytes of the stratified squamous epithelium.

in the lamina propria. Direct immunofluorescence reveals linear fibrillar deposits of fibrin in the basement membrane of bullous lichen planus, whereas pemphigus vulgaris has intercellular immunoglobulin deposition within the epithelium.

If the oral lesions of pemphigus vulgaris are restricted to the gingival tissues, erosive lichen planus, pemphigoid, linear IgA disease, and chronic ulcerative stomatitis should be ruled out.

Therapy. The main therapy for pemphigus vulgaris is systemic corticosteroids with or without the addition of other immunosuppressive agents.[130] Initially, when only steroids were employed, high initial and maintenance doses of steroids were necessary to control the disease.[70] Currently, if the patient responds well to corticosteroids, the dosage can be gradually reduced, but a low maintenance dosage is usually necessary to prevent or minimize the recurrence of lesions. Many dermatologists monitor the dose of steroids by periodic indirect immunofluorescence for changes in titer. Increasing titers are often associated with an impending exacerbation and warrant an increase of the steroid dose. A decrease in the indirect immunofluorescence titer justifies a reduction of the steroid dose.[95] In patients not responsive to corticosteroids or who gradually adapt to them, "steroid-sparing" therapies are used; these consist of combinations of steroids plus other medications, such as azathioprine, cyclophosphamide, cyclosporine, dapsone, gold, and methotrexate, as well as photoplasmapheresis and plasmapheresis.[96]

The maintenance phase aims to control the disease with the lowest dose of medication. To minimize the risk of morbidity associated with the long-term use of steroids, alternate-day steroid therapy, steroid-sparing drugs, and topical steroids can be combined. Because topical steroids may promote the development of candidiasis, topical antifungal medication may also be needed.[78]

Minimizing oral irritation is important in patients with oral pemphigus vulgaris. Optimal oral hygiene is essential because there is usually widespread involvement of the marginal and attached gingivae in pemphigus vulgaris, as well as other areas of the mouth, which can be exacerbated by plaque-associated gingivitis and periodontitis. Periodontal care is an important issue of the overall management of patients with pemphigus vulgaris. To prevent flare-ups, patients in the maintenance phase should receive prednisone before professional oral prophylaxis and periodontal surgery.[111] In addition, the fit and design of removable prosthetic appliances should receive special attention, because even slight irritation from these prostheses can cause severe inflammation with vesiculation and ulceration.

Chronic Ulcerative Stomatitis

First reported in 1990,[57] chronic ulcerative stomatitis clinically presents with chronic oral ulcerations and has a predilection for women in their fourth decade of life. The erosions and ulcerations present predominantly in the oral cavity, with only a few cases exhibiting cutaneous lesions.[22,71,141]

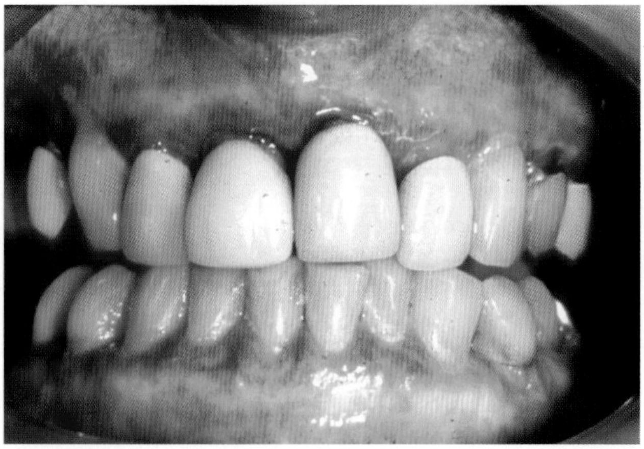

Figure 26-22 Chronic ulcerative stomatitis. Erythema and ulceration of the gingiva consistent with a clinical diagnosis of desquamative gingivitis. Direct and indirect immunofluorescence studies demonstrated the presence of stratified epithelium–specific antinuclear antibodies (SES-ANA). (Courtesy Dr. Douglas Damm, University of Kentucky, Lexington.)

Oral Lesions. Painful, solitary small blisters and erosions with surrounding erythema are present mainly on the gingiva and the lateral border of the tongue. Because of the magnitude and clinical features of the gingival lesions, a diagnosis of desquamative gingivitis is considered (Figure 26-22). The hard palate may also present similar lesions.

Histopathology. The microscopic features of chronic ulcerative stomatitis are similar to those observed in erosive lichen planus. Hyperkeratosis, acanthosis, and liquefaction of the basal cell layer with areas of subepithelial clefting are prominent features of the epithelium. The underlying lamina propria exhibits a lymphohistiocytic, chronic infiltrate in a bandlike configuration.

Immunofluorescence. Direct immunofluorescence of normal and perilesional tissues reveal typical stratified epithelium–specific antinuclear antibodies (SES-ANA). These are nuclear deposits of IgG with a speckled pattern, mainly in the basal cell layer of the normal epithelium (Figure 26-23). In addition, fibrin deposits are visualized at the epithelial tissue–connective tissue interface. Indirect immunofluorescence studies using an esophageal substrate also reveal the presence of SES-ANA.[133]

Diagnosis. Chronic ulcerative stomatitis is clinically similar to erosive lichen planus. In addition, pemphigus vulgaris, mucous membrane pemphigoid, linear IgA disease, bullous pemphigoid, and lupus erythematosus have to be included in the clinical differential diagnosis. Microscopic examination usually reduces the number of possibilities to chronic ulcerative stomatitis, linear IgA disease, and erosive lichen planus. Direct and indirect immunofluorescence are needed to arrive at the correct diagnosis.

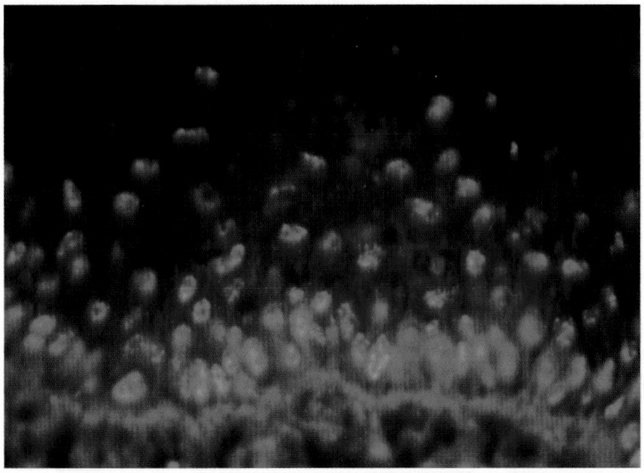

Figure 26-23 Direct immunofluorescence of chronic ulcerative stomatitis. Nuclear deposits of IgG are prominent in the basal cell layer and fade toward the superficial layers. (Courtesy Dr. Douglas Damm, University of Kentucky, Lexington.)

Treatment. For mild cases, topical steroids (fluocinonide, clobetasol propionate) and topical tetracycline may produce clinical improvement; however, recurrences are common.[73] For severe cases, a high dose of systemic corticosteroids is needed to achieve remission. Unfortunately, reduction of the corticosteroid dose results in relapse of the lesions. Hydroxychloroquine sulfate at a dosage of 200 to 400 mg per day seems to be the treatment of choice to produce complete, long-lasting remission.[11,24,57] However, a long-term follow-up study demonstrated that combined therapy (small doses of corticosteroids and chloroquine) may be required, because the initial good response to chloroquine ceases after several months or even years of treatment.[22]

Linear IgA Disease (Linear IgA Dermatosis)

Linear immunoglobulin A (IgA) disease (LAD), also known as linear IgA dermatosis, is an uncommon mucocutaneous disorder with a predilection for women. The etiopathogenic aspects of LAD are not fully understood, although drug-induced LAD triggered by angiotensin-converting enzyme (ACE) inhibitors has been reported.[42] LAD clinically presents as a pruritic vesiculobullous rash, usually during middle to late age, although younger individuals may be affected. Characteristic plaques or crops with an annular presentation surrounded by a peripheral rim of blisters affect the skin of the upper and lower trunk, shoulders, groin, and lower limbs. The face and perineum may also be affected. Mucosal involvement, including the oral mucosa, ranges from 50% to 100% of the cases published.[26,58]

LAD may mimic lichen planus both clinically and histologically. Immunofluorescence studies are needed to establish the correct diagnosis.

Oral Lesions. Oral manifestations of LAD consist of vesicles, painful ulcerations or erosions, and erosive gingivitis/cheilitis. The hard and soft palates are affected more often; tonsillar pillars, buccal mucosa, tongue, and gingiva follow in frequency. Rarely, oral lesions may be the only manifestation of LAD for several years before the presentation of cutaneous lesions.[19] In addition, oral lesions of LAD have been clinically reported as desquamative gingivitis[33,104,105] (Figure 26-24).

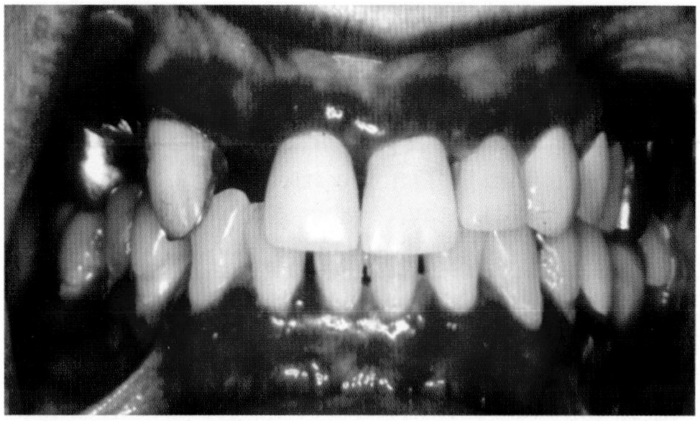

Figure 26-24 Linear IgA disease. Intense erythema and ulceration of the gingiva consistent with desquamative gingivitis.

Histopathology. The microscopic features of linear immunoglobulin A (IgA) disease are similar to those observed in erosive lichen planus.

Immunofluorescence. Linear deposits of IgA are observed at the epithelial tissue–connective tissue interface. They differ from the granular pattern observed in dermatitis herpetiformis.

Differential Diagnosis. The differential diagnosis of LAD includes erosive lichen planus, chronic ulcerative stomatitis, pemphigus vulgaris, bullous pemphigoid, and lupus erythematosus. Microscopic examination and immunofluorescence studies are necessary to establish the correct diagnosis.

Treatment. The primary treatment for LAD is a combination of sulfones and dapsone. Small amounts of prednisone (10-30 mg/day) can be added if the initial response is inadequate.[21] Alternatively, tetracycline (2 g/day) combined with nicotinamide (1.5 g/day) have shown promising results.[101]

Dermatitis Herpetiformis

Dermatitis herpetiformis is a chronic condition that usually develops in young adults (ages 20-30 years) and has a slight predilection for men.[35] Currently, evidence indicates that dermatitis herpetiformis is a cutaneous manifestation of *celiac disease*. Approximately 25% of patients with celiac disease have dermatitis herpetiformis. The etiology of celiac disease is obscure; however, tissue transglutaminase seems to be the predominant autoantigen in the intestine, skin, and sometimes mucosae.[28] Gluten enteropathy can be severe in about two thirds of patients and mild or subclinical in the remaining third.

In severe cases, patients may complain of dysphagia, weakness, diarrhea, and weight loss.[80]

Clinically, dermatitis herpetiformis presents with bilateral and symmetric pruritic papules or vesicles primarily restricted to the extensor surfaces of the extremities. The sacrum, buttocks, and occasionally the face, as well as the oral cavity, may be also affected.[14,35] The name "herpetic" derives from the initial presentation of this disease, in which clusters of vesicles or papules arise on the skin. These vesicles or papules eventually resolve and are followed by hyperpigmentation of the skin, which ultimately wanes. The oral lesions of dermatitis herpetiformis are characterized by the presence of painful ulcerations preceded by the collapse of ephemeral vesicles or bullae.

Histopathology. Microscopic examination of the initial lesions of dermatitis herpetiformis reveals focal aggregates of neutrophils and eosinophils among deposits of fibrin at the apices of the dermal pegs.[146]

Immunofluorescence. Direct immunofluorescence show that IgA and C3 are present at the dermal papillary apices. These findings are present in perilesional and normal, uninvolved tissue. In contrast, biopsies taken from lesional sites may fail to exhibit IgA or C3, resulting in false-negative results.[146] Although no circulating autoantibodies to epithelial basement membrane are present in dermatitis herpetiformis, almost 80% of patients have antiendomysial and gliadin antibodies.[11]

Treatment. A gluten-free diet is essential in the treatment of celiac disease and dermatitis herpetiformis. Oral dapsone is usually needed in newly detected dermatitis herpetiformis to alleviate symptoms promptly.[28]

Lupus Erythematosus

Lupus erythematosus is an autoimmune disease with three different clinical presentations: systemic, chronic cutaneous, and subacute cutaneous.

Systemic Lupus Erythematosus. Systemic lupus erythematosus (SLE) is a severe disease with a predilection for women over men (10:1) that affects vital organs such as kidneys and heart, as well as the skin and mucosa. Its diagnosis is usually hampered by an insidious presentation during the early stages of the disease. However, fever, weight loss, and arthritis are common. The classic cutaneous lesions are characterized by the presence of a rash on the malar area with a butterfly distribution (Figure 26-25). The oral lesions of SLE are usually ulcerative or similar to lichen planus. Oral ulcerations present in 36% of SLE patients. In about 4% of patients, hyperkeratotic plaques reminiscent of lichen planus appear on the buccal mucosa and palate.[16] In extremely rare cases, lupus erythematosus may occur on the oral mucous membrane without skin lesions. Direct immunofluorescence of the perilesional and normal tissue reveals immunoglobulins and C3 deposits at the dermal-epidermal interface. Antinuclear antibodies (ANA) are present in more than 95% of cases, whereas deoxyribonucleic acid (DNA) and extractable nuclear antigen (ENA) antibodies are present in more than 50% of patients (see Table 26-1).

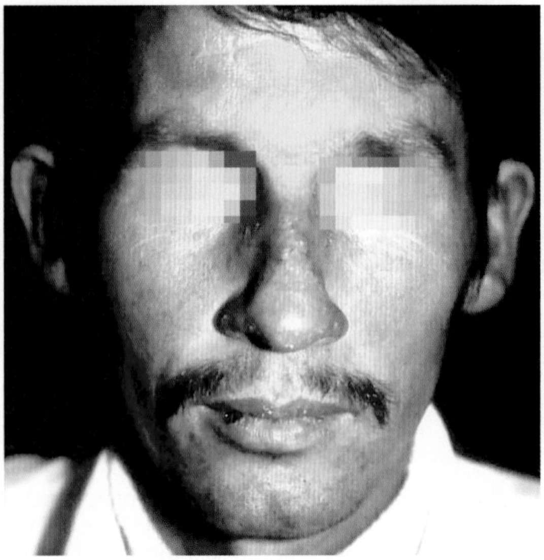

Figure 26-25 Systemic lupus erythematosus producing erythema on bridge of the nose with a "butterfly" pattern. (Courtesy Dr. Luis Gaitan, Oral Pathology Laboratory, Faculty of Odontology, National Autonomous University of Mexico (UNAM), Mexico City.)

Chronic Cutaneous Lupus Erythematosus. Chronic cutaneous lupus erythematosus (CCLE) usually has no systemic signs or symptoms, with lesions being limited to skin or mucosal surfaces. The skin lesions are referred to as *discoid lupus erythematosus* (DLE). It is important to recognize that the term *DLE* refers to a specific skin lesion, not a subset of SLE. DLE merely describes the chronic scarring, atrophy-producing lesion that may develop into hyperpigmentation or hypopigmentation of the healing area (Figure 26-26). In contrast, the subacute cutaneous lupus erythematosus skin lesions do not produce scarring or atrophy.[17]

In the oral cavity, about 9% of patients with CCLE present lichen planus–like plaques on the palate and buccal mucosa.[4,16] The lesions are usually localized and at their borders; numerous dilated blood vessels in a radial arrangement may extend into the surrounding tissue, coupled with whitish, pinhead papules. In the early stages the center of the lesion is slightly depressed and eroded and is covered with a bluish red epithelial surface showing scarring. In older lesions the erythematous border becomes less elevated and is transformed into a whitish or bluish white peripheral zone of thickened epithelium. White lines with the same diverging radial arrangement replace the dilated vessels. On the tongue the disease occurs as circumscribed, smooth, reddened areas in which the papillae are lost or as patches with a whitish sheen resembling leukoplakia.

On the lip the lesions are somewhat similar to those in the mouth, and in most cases the lip is involved by direct extension from perioral skin lesions. Localized patches may be present, or the entire lip may be involved.

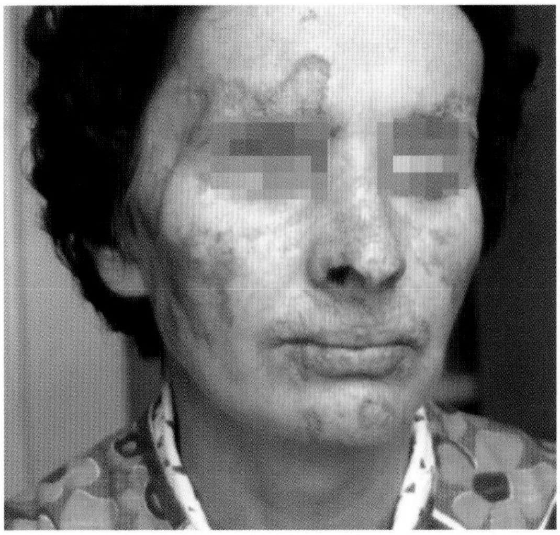

Figure 26-26 Chronic cutaneous lupus erythematosus. Multiple facial lesions with irregular hyperpigmented borders, some of which exhibit central scarring with cutaneous atrophy. Other lesions consist of hyperpigmented cutaneous patches.

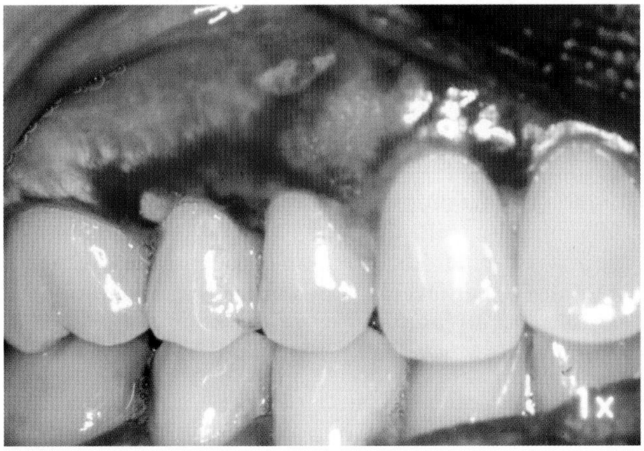

Figure 26-27 Lupus erythematosus of the oral cavity presenting as desquamative gingivitis. Intense erythema with ulceration is bordered by white radial lines. (Courtesy Dr. Stuart L. Fischman, State University of New York at Buffalo.)

Early in the disease the lip is swollen, bluish red, and often everted. The lip lesions may be covered with adherent scales and crusts, which remain localized and are rarely diffuse. At the margins of the patches, dilated capillaries or fine, branching radial lines may be seen. The lip is tender and sensitive, and on removal of the adherent scales, bleeding from the raw surface is noted. Depressed scars may follow healing of the deeper lesions. The gingiva may be affected and clinically present as desquamative gingivitis (Figure 26-27).

Periods of activity and quiescence occur. The lesions enlarge by peripheral extension and are accompanied by fresh erosions and superficial ulcerations, followed by atrophic changes. Some burning sensation occurs in the erosions and deeper ulcerations.

Histopathology. The histopathology of the oral lesions of chronic cutaneous lupus erythematosus consists of hyperkeratosis or parakeratosis, alternated acanthosis and atrophy, and hydropic degeneration of the basal layer of the epithelium. In addition, the lamina propria exhibits a chronic inflammatory cell infiltrate similar to that observed in lichen planus. However, a more diffuse and deeper inflammatory infiltrate with a perivascular pattern is typically observed.[126]

Direct immunofluorescence of lesional tissue reveals immunoglobulins and C3 deposits at the dermal-epidermal junction of the lesional or perilesional tissue but not in normal tissue. This seems to differentiate SLE from DLE. Indirect immunofluorescence reveals the presence of ANAs in more than 95% of patients, whereas DNA- and ENA-circulating antibodies are present in more than 50%.

Subacute Cutaneous Lupus Erythematosus. Subacute cutaneous lupus erythematosus (SCLE) has been used to describe a group of patients who have a characteristic cutaneous lesion that has similarities to DLE but lacks the development of scarring and atrophy.[17] In addition, arthritis/arthralgia, low-grade fever, malaise, and myalgia may present in up to 50% of SCLE patients.[17,137] Direct immunofluorescence reveals immunoglobulins and C3 deposits at the dermal-epidermal junction in 60% of cases, and granular IgG deposits in the cytoplasm of basal cells in 30%. About 80% of patients with SCLE have Ro (SSA) antibodies to nuclear antigens, whereas 25% to 30% have La (SSB) antibodies to nuclear antigens. Rheumatoid factor (RF) is positive in about 30% of these patients, ANA is positive in 60% to 90%, and 10% of cases have antiribonucleoprotein (anti-RNP) antibodies to nuclear antigens (see Table 26-1).

Differential Diagnosis. Diagnosis usually depends on the identification of the accompanying skin lesions. The diagnosis of DLE confined to the oral cavity is difficult to make, but microscopic studies may suggest the characteristic histopathology.[3] Erosive lichen planus, erythema multiforme, and pemphigus vulgaris may sometimes simulate the lesions observed in lupus erythematosus. Biopsy studies (H&E and direct immunofluorescence) aid in differentiating between lupus erythematosus and other erosive diseases.

Treatment. The therapy for SLE depends on the severity and extent of the disease. Cutaneous rashes are treated with topical steroids, sunscreens, and hydroxychloroquine. For arthritis and mild pleuritis, a nonsteroidal antiinflammatory drug (NSAID) or hydroxychloroquine is used. For severe systemic organ involvement, moderate to high doses of prednisone are effective. For severe cases of SLE or when side effects to prednisone develop, immunosuppressive drugs such as cytotoxic agents (cyclophosphamide and azathioprine) and plasmapheresis alone or with steroids are useful.[96] For CCLE, topical steroids are effective to manage the cutaneous and oral lesions. For patients resistant to topical therapy, systemic antimalarial drugs may be used with good results.[95]

Erythema Multiforme

Erythema multiforme is an acute bullous and macular inflammatory mucocutaneous disease in which a series of immunopathologic mechanisms occur. The genesis of ulcerative lesions affecting the skin and mucosa is believed to reside in the development of immune complex vasculitis. This is followed by complement fixation, leading to leukocytoclastic destruction of vascular walls and small vessel occlusion. The culmination of these events produces ischemic necrosis of the epithelium and underlying connective tissue.[40] Target or "iris" lesions with central clearing are the "hallmark" of erythema multiforme. It may be a mild condition *(erythema multiforme minor)* or a severe, possibly life-threatening condition (*erythema multiforme major,* or *Stevens-Johnson syndrome*). An underdiagnosed type of erythema multiforme is the oral form, where most patients have chronic or recurrent oral lesions only.[5]

Erythema multiforme minor lasts approximately 4 weeks and exhibits a moderate cutaneous and mucosal involvement. Stevens-Johnson syndrome may last a month or longer and involves the skin, conjunctiva, oral mucosa, and genitalia, requiring more aggressive therapy. Some researchers consider toxic epidermal necrolysis as the most severe form of erythema multiforme; however, other investigators believe that these are unrelated entities.[8] The three most common etiologic factors for the development of erythema multiforme are (1) herpes simplex infection, (2) mycoplasma infection, and (3) drug reactions. The most common causative drugs are sulfonamides, penicillins, phenylbutazone, and phenytoin.[135]

Oral lesions in erythema multiforme are common and present in more than 70% of patients with skin involvement.[41,77,82] In rare instances, however, erythema multiforme may be confined to the mouth.[5,74,118]

Oral Lesions. The oral lesions consist of multiple, large, shallow, painful ulcers with an erythematous border. They may affect the entire oral mucosa in approximately 20% of erythema multiforme patients. The lesions are so painful that chewing and swallowing are impaired (Figure 26-28). The buccal mucosa and tongue are the most frequently affected sites, followed by the labial mucosa. Less often affected are the floor of the mouth, hard and soft palate, and the gingiva.[41] There are rare instances in which erythema multiforme may be confined exclusively to the gingival tissues, resulting in a clinical diagnosis of desquamative gingivitis.[7] Hemorrhagic crusting of the vermilion border of the lips may occur and is helpful in arriving at a clinical diagnosis of erythema multiforme.

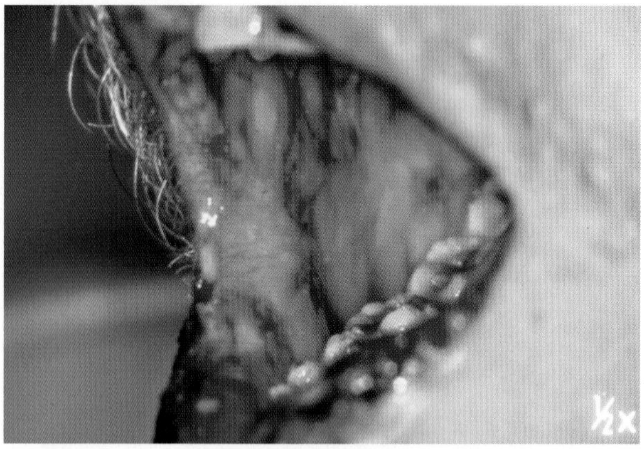

Figure 26-28 Erythema multiforme. Large, shallow, and painful ulcers involving the labial and buccal mucosae. Hemorrhagic crusting of the mandibular vermilion border of the lips is observed. (Courtesy Dr. Stuart L. Fischman, State University of New York at Buffalo.)

Histopathology. A wide spectrum of tissue changes occurs in erythema multiforme. In some cases the value of the microscopic examination is to rule out other conditions. Common microscopic findings of erythema multiforme include liquefaction degeneration of the upper epithelium and development of intraepithelial microvesicles, but without the acantholysis that occurs in pemphigus.[123] In addition, acanthosis, pseudoepitheliomatous hyperplasia, and necrotic keratinocytes are observed in the epithelium. Degenerative changes also occur in the basement membrane. In some cases the junction between the epithelium and the lamina propria is indistinct because of a dense, inflammatory cell infiltrate. Edema of the lamina propria, vascular dilation, and congestion are also present. Deeper layers of the connective tissue stroma exhibit a perivascular, chronic inflammatory cell infiltrate. However, neutrophils and eosinophils may also be present.

Immunofluorescence. Immunofluorescence examination is negative in erythema multiforme. Its value resides in ruling out other vesiculobullous and ulcerative disorders.

Treatment. There is no specific treatment for erythema multiforme. Some cases may even resolve spontaneously, and erythematous lesions may require no treatment. In contrast, patients exhibiting bullous or ulcerative lesions require intervention. For mild symptoms, systemic and local antihistamines together with topical anesthetics and debridement of lesions with an oxygenating agent are adequate. In patients with severe symptoms, corticosteroids are considered the drug of choice, although its use is controversial and not completely accepted.[97]

DRUG ERUPTIONS

An increase in the incidence of skin and oral manifestations of hypersensitivity to drugs has been noted since the advent of the sulfonamides, barbiturates, and various antibiotics. The eruptive skin and oral lesions are

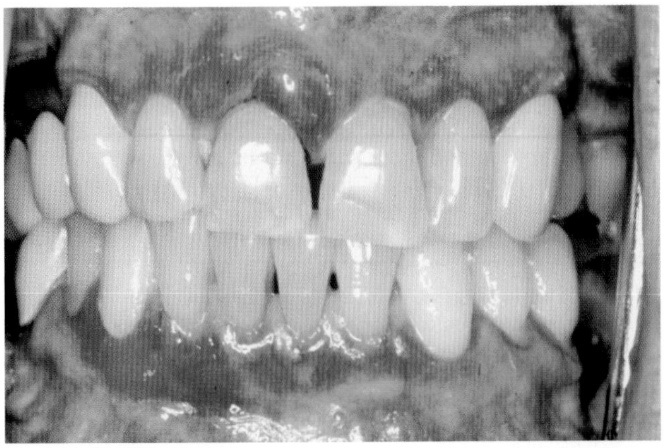

Figure 26-29 Plasma cell gingivitis. The gingiva presents a band of moderate to severe inflammation reminiscent of desquamative gingivitis.

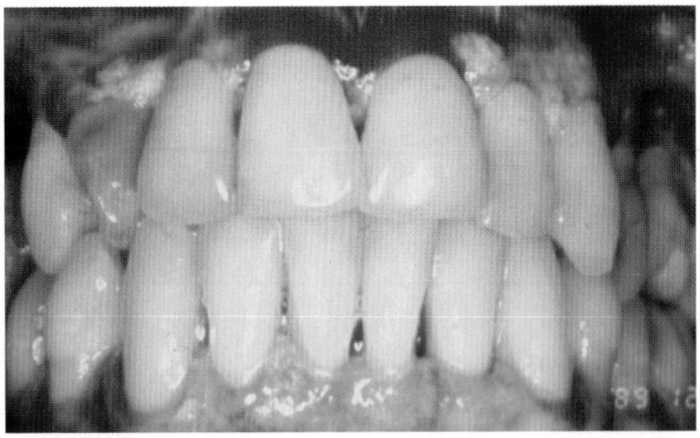

Figure 26-30 Graft-versus-host disease in recipient of allogeneic bone marrow transplant. The maxillary gingiva exhibits features consistent with desquamative gingivitis. (Courtesy Dr. Linda Lee, University of Toronto.)

attributed to the drug acting as an allergen, either alone or in combination, sensitizing the tissues and then causing the allergic reaction.

Eruptions in the oral cavity resulting from sensitivity to drugs that have been taken by mouth or parenterally are termed *stomatitis medicamentosa.* The local reaction from the use of a medicament in the oral cavity (e.g., aspirin burn, stomatitis resulting from topical penicillin) is referred to as *stomatitis venenata* or *contact stomatitis.* Such changes may result either from the irritating local action of the drug or from drug sensitivity. In many cases, skin eruptions may accompany the oral lesions.

In general, drug eruptions in the oral cavity are multiform. Vesicular and bullous lesions occur most often, but pigmented or nonpigmented macular lesions are also frequently observed. Erosions, often followed by deep ulceration with purpuric lesions, may also occur. The lesions are seen in different areas of the oral cavity, with the gingiva often affected.[48]

The development of gingival lesions caused by contact allergy to mercurial compounds present in dental amalgam has been clearly documented.[61] Because of financial considerations, biopsy and patch testing may be indicated before the indiscriminate replacement of dental amalgam restorations. Similarly, desquamative gingivitis has been reported with the use of tartar control toothpaste. Pyrophosphates and flavoring agents have been identified as the main causative agents of this unusual condition.[32] Oral reactions to cinnamon compounds (cinnamon oil, cinnamic acid, cinnamic aldehyde) used to mask the taste of pyrophosphates in tartar control toothpaste include an intense erythema of the attached gingival tissues characteristic of plasma cell gingivitis[2,62] (Figure 26-29). A thorough clinical history usually discloses the source of the gingival disturbance. Elimination of the offending agent (e.g., tartar control toothpaste) leads to resolution of the gingival lesions within a week. Challenge with the offending agent leads to recurrence of the oral lesions.

MISCELLANEOUS CONDITIONS MIMICKING DESQUAMATIVE GINGIVITIS

Another group of heterogeneous conditions may masquerade as desquamative gingivitis. Factitious lesions, candidiasis, graft-versus-host disease, Wegener's granulomatosis, foreign body gingivitis, Kindler syndrome, and even squamous cell carcinoma can divert the attention of the clinician and result in a diagnostic challenge.

Factitious lesions are consciously and intentionally produced injuries without a clear motive, although, guilt, seeking sympathy, or monetary compensation may be the driving force behind this abnormal behavior. Factitious desquamative gingivitis has been reported in the literature and may be difficult to diagnose and may become apparent only after extensive and costly laboratory tests fail to reveal the genesis of the lesions.[83]

Rarely, *candidiasis* may be limited to the gingival tissues and may simulate desquamative gingivitis.

Graft-versus-host disease may occur in recipients of allogenic bone marrow transplants, whose oral lesions may occasionally resemble desquamative gingivitis (Figure 26-30).

Wegener's granulomatosis is a systemic disease that may initially present with striking alterations that are confined to the gingival tissues (see Chapter 23). Classically, the gingival tissues exhibit erythema and enlargement and are typically described as "strawberry gums"[27] (Figure 26-31).

Foreign body gingivitis is clinically characterized by red or red and white chronic lesions that may be painful and are reminiscent of desquamative gingivitis. This condition does not have a gingival site predilection and is more common in women approaching the fifth decade of life. Microscopic analysis reveals small (<5 μm in diameter) foreign bodies associated with a chronic inflammatory cell response that may exhibit granulomatous and lichenoid characteristics. Energy-dispersive x-ray microanalysis has revealed that in this condition, most foreign bodies are of dental material origin (more specifically, abrasives and restorative material).[51,52]

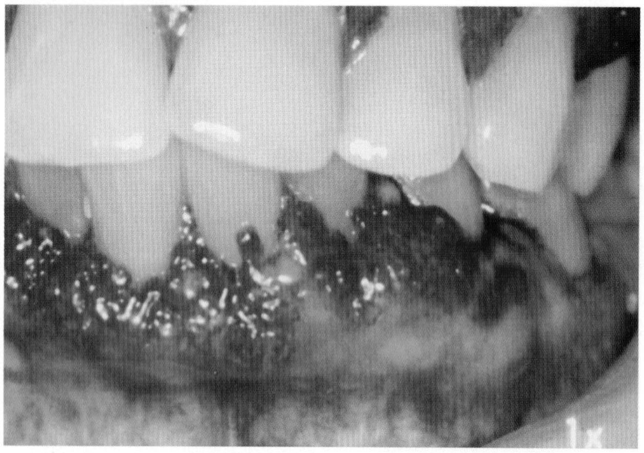

Figure 26-31 Wegener's granulomatosis affecting gingival tissues. The classic "strawberry gums" appearance of the mandibular gingiva is seen in this patient. A slight resemblance with desquamative gingivitis is evident.

Kindler syndrome (cutaneous neonatal bullae, poikiloderma, photosensitivity, and acral atrophy) may also present with oral lesions that are clinically consistent with desquamative gingivitis.[109]

Failure to evaluate properly and systematically a patient with a clinical condition that is consistent with desquamative gingivitis can lead to unpleasant outcomes. This is particularly true when therapy for a putative desquamative gingivitis is established before a biopsy of the lesional tissue is obtained. Every year we see in our laboratory at least two examples of clinically diagnosed desquamative gingivitis for which microscopic and immuno fluorescence studies were not performed to rule out the genesis of the gingival lesions. In these cases the patients have been either "carefully" followed up or prescribed topical steroids for several months. The lack of response of the gingival tissues impels the clinician to obtain a biopsy, which reveals that the gingival lesions are *squamous cell carcinomas*. Thus the clinician should be alert to the possibility of squamous cell carcinoma of the gingival tissues presenting initially as desquamative gingivitis.

REFERENCES

1. Ahmed AR, Kurgis BS, Rogers RS: Cicatricial pemphigoid, *J Am Acad Dermatol* 24:987, 1991.
2. Allen CM, Blozis GG: Oral mucosal reactions to cinnamon-flavored chewing gum, *J Am Dent Assoc* 116:664, 1988.
3. Andreasen JO, Poulsen HE: Oral manifestations in discoid and systemic lupus erythematosus: histologic investigation, *Acta Odontol Scand* 22:389, 1964.
4. Archard HO, Roebuck NF, Stanley HR: Oral manifestations of chronic discoid lupus erythematosus, *Oral Surg* 16:696, 1963.
5. Ayangco L, Rogers RS 3rd: Oral manifestations of erythema multiforme, *Dermatol Clin* 21:195, 2003.
6. Balding SD, Prost C, Diaz LA: Cicatricial pemphigoid autoantibodies react with multiple sites on the BP 180 extracellular domain, *J Invest Dermatol* 106:141, 1996.
7. Barrett AW, Scully C, Eveson JW: Erythema multiforme involving gingiva, *J Periodontol* 64:910, 1993.
8. Bastuji-Garin S, Rzany B, Stern RS, et al: Clinical classification of cases of toxic epidermal necrolysis, Stevens-Johnson syndrome, and erythema multiforme, *Arch Dermatol* 129:92, 1993.
9. Baudet-Pommel M, Janin-Mercier A, Souteyrand P: Sequential immunopathologic study of oral lichen planus treated with tretinoin and etretinate, Oral Surg 71:197, 1991.
10. Becker BA, Gaspari AA: Pemphigus vulgaris and vegetants, *Dermatol Clin* 11:453, 1993.
11. Beutner EH, Chorzelski TP, Parodi A, et al: Ten cases of chronic ulcerative stomatitis with stratified epithelium-specific antinuclear antibody, *J Am Acad Dermatol* 24:781, 1991.
12. Beutner EH, Chorzelski TP, Reunala TL, et al: Immunopathology of dermatitis herpetiformis, *Clin Dermatol* 9:295, 1992.
13. Blank H, Burgoon CF: Abnormal cytology of epithelial cells in pemphigus vulgaris: a diagnostic aid, *J Invest Dermatol* 18:213, 1952.
14. Boh EE, Milikan LE: Vesiculobullous diseases with prominent immunologic features, *JAMA* 268:2893, 1992.
15. Brown RS, Bottomley WK, Puente E, et al: A retrospective evaluation of 193 patients with oral lichen planus, *J Oral Pathol Med* 22:69, 1993.
16. Burge SM, Frith PA, Juniper RP, et al: Mucosal involvement in systemic and chronic cutaneous lupus erythematosus, *Br J Dermatol* 121:727, 1989.
17. Callen JP, Kulick KB, Stelzer G, et al: Subacute cutaneous lupus erythematosus: clinical, serologic, and immunogenetic studies on 49 patients seen in a non-referral setting, *J Am Acad Dermatol* 15:1227, 1986.
18. Challacombe SJ, Setterfield J, Shirlaw P, et al: Immunodiagnosis of pemphigus and mucous membrane pemphigoid, *Acta Odontol Scand* 59:226, 2001.
19. Chan LS, Regezi JA, Cooper KD: Oral manifestations of linear IgA disease, *J Am Acad Dermatol* 22:362, 1990.
20. Chan LS, Ahmed AR, Anhalt GJ, et al: The first international consensus on mucous membrane pemphigoid: definition, diagnostic criteria, pathogenic factors, medical treatment, and prognostic indicators, *Arch Dermatol* 138:370, 2002.
21. Chorzelski T, Jablonska S, Maciejowska E: Linear IgA bullous dermatosis of adults, *Clin Dermatol* 9:383, 1992.
22. Chorzelski T, Olszewska M, Jarzabek-Chorzelska M, et al: Is chronic ulcerative stomatitis an entity? Clinical and immunological findings in 18 cases, *Eur J Dermatol* 8:261, 1998.
23. Chowdhury MM, Natarajan S: Neonatal pemphigus vulgaris associated with mild oral pemphigus vulgaris in the mother during pregnancy, *Br J Dermatol* 139:500, 1998.
24. Church LF Jr, Schosser RH: Chronic ulcerative stomatitis associated with stratified epithelial specific antinuclear antibodies: a case report of a newly described disease entity, *Oral Surg Oral Med Oral Pathol* 73:579, 1992.
25. Ciarrocca KN, Greenberg MS: A retrospective study of the management of oral mucous membrane pemphigoid with dapsone, *Oral Surg Oral Med Oral Pathol Oral Radiol Endod* 88:159, 1999.
26. Cohen DM, Bhattacharyya I, Zunt SL, et al: Linear IgA disease histopathologically and clinically masquerading as lichen planus, *Oral Surg Oral Med Oral Pathol Oral Radiol Endod* 88:196, 1999.
27. Cohen RE, Cardoza TT, Drinnan AJ, et al: Gingival manifestations of Wegener's granulomatosis, *J Periodontol* 61:705, 1990.
28. Collin P, Reunala T: Recognition and management of the cutaneous manifestations of celiac disease: a guide for dermatologists, *Am J Clin Dermatol* 4:13, 2003.

29. Combes FL, Canizares O: Pemphigus vulgaris, a clinicopathological study of one hundred cases, *Arch Dermatol Syph* 62:786, 1950.
30. Dabelsteen E: Molecular biological aspects of acquired bullous diseases, *Crit Rev Oral Biol Med* 9:162, 1998.
31. Dabelsteen E, Ullman S, Thomson K, et al: Demonstration of basement membrane autoantibodies in patients with benign mucous membrane pemphigoid, *Acta Dermatol Venereol Stockh* 54:189, 1974.
32. DeLattre V: Factors contributing to adverse soft tissue reactions due to the use of tartar control toothpastes: report of a case and literature review, *J Periodontol* 70:803, 1999.
33. Del Valle AE, Martinez-Sahuquillo A, Padron JR, et al: Two cases of linear IgA disease with clinical manifestations limited to the gingiva, *J Periodontol* 74:879, 2003.
34. De Vita S, Neri R, Bombardieri S: Cyclophosphamide pulses in the treatment of rheumatic diseases: an update, *Clin Exp Rheumatol* 9:179, 1991.
35. Economopoulou P, Laskaris G: Dermatitis herpetiformis: oral lesions as an early manifestation, *Oral Surg Oral Med Oral Pathol* 62:77, 1986.
36. Eisen D, Ellis CN, Duell GA, et al: Effect of topical cyclosporin rinse on oral lichen planus, *N Engl J Med* 323:290, 1990.
37. Eisenberg E: Lichen planus and oral cancer: is there a connection between the two? *J Am Dent Assoc* 123:104, 1992.
38. Eisenberg E, Krutchkoff DJ: Lichenoid lesions of oral mucosa: diagnostic criteria and their importance in the alleged relationship to oral cancer, *Oral Surg Oral Med Oral Pathol* 73:699, 1992.
39. Engel M, Ray HG, Orban B: The pathogenesis of desquamative gingivitis, *J Dent Res* 29:410, 1950.
40. Eversole LR: Immunopathology of oral mucosal ulcerative, desquamative and bullous diseases, *Oral Surg Oral Med Oral Pathol* 77:55, 1994.
41. Farthing PM, Margou P, Coates M, et al: Characteristics of the oral lesions in patients with cutaneous recurrent erythema multiforme, *J Oral Pathol Med* 24:9, 1995.
42. Femiano F, Scully C, Gombos F: Linear IgA dermatosis induced by a new angiotensin-converting enzyme inhibitor, *Oral Surg Oral Med Oral Pathol Oral Radiol Endod* 95:169, 2003.
43. Fine JD: Management of acquired bullous diseases, *N Engl J Med* 5:33, 1995.
44. Foss CL, Grupe HE, Orban B: Gingivosis, *J Periodontol* 24:207, 1953.
45. Foster CS: Cicatricial pemphigoid, *Trans Am Ophthalmol Soc* 84:527, 1986.
46. Fotos PG, Vincent SD, Hellstein JW: Oral candidosis: clinical, historical and therapeutic features of 100 cases, *Oral Surg* 74:41, 1992.
47. Gallagher G, Shklar G: Oral involvement in mucous membrane pemphigoid, *Clin Dermatol* 5:19, 1987.
48. Gallagher GT: Oral mucous membrane reactions to drugs and chemicals, *Curr Opin Dent* 1:777, 1991.
49. Goadby K: *Diseases of the gums and oral mucous membrane,* London, 1923, Henry Froude and Hodder & Staughton.
50. Gonzalez-Moles MA, Ruiz-Avila I, Rodriguez-Archilla A, et al: Treatment of severe erosive gingival lesions by topical application of clobetasol propionate in custom trays, *Oral Surg Oral Med Oral Pathol Oral Radiol Endod* 95:688, 2003.
51. Gordon SC, Daley TD: Foreign body gingivitis: clinical and microscopic features of 61 cases, *Oral Surg Oral Med Oral Pathol Oral Radiol Endod* 83:562, 1997.
52. Gordon SC, Daley TD: Foreign body gingivitis: identification of the foreign material by energy-dispersive x-ray microanalysis, *Oral Surg Oral Med Oral Pathol Oral Radiol Endod* 83:571, 1997.
53. Harman KE, Seed PT, Gratian MJ, et al: The severity of cutaneous and oral pemphigus is related to desmoglein 1 and 3 antibody levels, *Br J Dermatol* 144:775, 2001.
54. Hashimoto K, Dibella R, Shklar G, et al: Electron microscopic studies of oral lichen planus, *G Ital Dermatol* 107:765, 1966.
55. Holmstrup P: The controversy of a premalignant potential of lichen planus is over, *Oral Surg Oral Med Oral Pathol* 73:704, 1992.
56. Ishii T: Immunohistochemical demonstration of T cell subsets and accessory cells in oral lichen planus, *J Oral Pathol* 15:268, 1987.
57. Jaremko WM, Beutner EH, Kumar V, et al: Chronic ulcerative stomatitis associated with a specific immunologic marker, *J Am Acad Dermatol* 22:215, 1990.
58. Kelly SE, Frith PA, Millard PR, et al: A clinicopathological study of mucosal involvement in linear IgA disease, *Br J Dermatol* 119:161, 1988.
59. Komori A, Welton NA, Kelln EE: The behavior of the basement membrane of skin and oral lesions in patients with lichen planus, erythema multiforme, lupus erythematosus, pemphigus vulgaris, pemphigoid and epidermolysis bullosa, *Oral Surg* 22:752, 1966.
60. Korman NJ: Bullous pemphigoid, *Dermatol Clin* 11:483, 1993.
61. Laine J, Kalimo K, Happonen R: Contact allergy to dental restorative materials in patients with oral lichenoid lesions, *Contact Dermatitis* 36:141, 1997.
62. Lamey PJ, Lewis MAO, Ress TD, et al: Sensitivity reaction to the cinnamonaldehyde component of toothpaste, *Br Dent J* 168:115, 1990.
63. Lamey PJ, Rees TD, Binnie WH, et al: Oral presentation of pemphigus vulgaris and its response to systemic steroid therapy, *Oral Surg Oral Med Oral Pathol* 74:54, 1992.
64. Laskaris G, Angelopoulos A: Cicatricial pemphigoid: direct and indirect immunofluorescent studies, *Oral Surg* 51:48, 1981.
65. Laskaris G, Demetrou N, Angelopoulos A: Immunofluorescent studies in desquamative gingivitis, *J Oral Pathol* 10:398, 1981.
66. Lenz P, Amagai M, Volc-Platzer B, et al: Desmoglein 3-ELISA: a pemphigus vulgaris specific diagnostic tool, *Arch Dermatol* 135:142, 1999.
67. Leonard J: Immunofluorescent studies in ocular cicatricial pemphigoid, *Br J Dermatol* 118:209, 1988.
68. Lever WF: Pemphigus, *Medicine* 32:1, 1953.
69. Lever WF: Pemphigus and pemphigoid: a review of the advances made since 1964, *J Am Acad Dermatol* 1979; 1:2.
70. Lever WF, Schaumburg-Lever G: Immunosuppressants and prednisone in pemphigus vulgaris, *Arch Dermatol* 113:1236, 1977.
71. Lewis JE, Beutner EH, Rostami R, et al: Chronic ulcerative stomatitis with stratified epithelium-specific antinuclear antibodies, *Int J Dermatol* 35:272, 1996.
72. Lorenzana ER, Rees TD, Hallmon WW: Esthetic management of multiple recession defects in a patient with cicatricial pemphigoid, *J Periodontol* 72:230, 2001.
73. Lorenzana ER, Rees TD, Glass M, et al: Chronic ulcerative stomatitis: a case report, *J Periodontol* 71:104, 2000.
74. Lozada F, Silverman S: Erythema multiforme: clinical characteristics and natural history in fifty patients, *Oral Surg* 46:628, 1978.
75. Lozada-Nur F: Oral lichen planus and oral cancer: is there enough epidemiologic evidence? *Oral Surg Oral Med Oral Pathol Oral Radiol Endod* 89:265, 2000.

76. Lozada-Nur F, Miranda C: Oral lichen planus: epidemiology, clinical characteristics, and associated diseases, *Semin Cutan Med Surg* 16:273, 1997.
77. Lozada-Nur F, Gorsky M, Silverman S Jr: Oral erythema multiforme: clinical observations and treatment of 95 patients, Oral Surg Oral Med Oral Pathol 67:36, 1989.
78. Lozada-Nur F, Miranda C, Maliski R: Double-blind clinical trial of 0.05% clobetasole propionate ointment in orabase and 0.05% fluocinonide ointment in orabase in the treatment of patients with vesiculoerosive diseases, *Oral Surg Oral Med Oral Pathol* 77:598, 1994.
79. Malmstrom M, Kontinnen YT, Jungell P, et al: Lymphocyte activation in oral lichen planus in situ, *Am J Clin Pathol* 89:329, 1988.
80. Marsh MN: The natural history of gluten sensitivity: defining, refining and re-defining, *Q J Med* 85:9, 1995.
81. McCarthy FP, McCarthy PL, Shklar G: Chronic desquamative gingivitis: a reconsideration, *Oral Surg* 13:1300, 1960.
82. McCarthy PL, Shklar G: *Diseases of the oral mucosa,* ed 2, Philadelphia, 1980, Lea & Febiger.
83. McGrath KG, Pick R, Leboff-Ries E, Patterson R: Factitious desquamative gingivitis simulating a possible immunologic disease, *J Allergy Clin Immunol* 75:44, 1985.
84. Mignogna MD, Lo Muzio L, Bucci E: Clinical features of gingival pemphigus vulgaris, *J Clin Periodontol* 28:489, 2001.
85. Merritt AH: Chronic desquamative gingivitis, *J Periodontol* 4:30, 1933.
86. Mobini N, Nagarwalla N, Ahmed AR: Oral pemphigoid: subset of cicatricial pemphigoid? *Oral Surg Oral Med Oral Pathol Oral Radiol Endod* 85:37, 1998.
87. Mondino BJ, Brown SI: Ocular cicatricial pemphigoid. Ophthalmology 1981; 99:95.
88. Mondino BJ, Linstone FA: Ocular pemphigoid, *Clin Dermatol* 5:28, 1987.
89. Morrison L, Kratochvil FJ 3rd, Gorman A: An open trial of topical tacrolimus for erosive oral lichen planus, *J Am Acad Dermatol* 47: 617, 2002.
90. Muller S, Klaus-Kovtun V, Stanley JR: A 230-kD basic protein is the major bullous pemphigoid antigen, *J Invest Dermatol* 92:33, 1989.
91. Musa NJ, Kumar V, Humphreys L, et al: Oral pemphigoid masquerading as necrotizing ulcerative gingivitis in a child, *J Periodontol* 73:657, 2002.
92. Mutasim DF, Pelc DJ, Anhalt GJ: Paraneoplastic pemphigus, *Dermatol Clin* 11:473, 1993.
93. Mutasim DF, Pelc NJ, Anhalt GJ: Cicatricial pemphigoid, *Dermatol Clin* 11:499, 1993.
94. Nemeth AJ, Klein AD, Gould EW, et al: Childhood bullous pemphigoid: Clinical and immunologic features, treatment, and prognosis, *Arch Dermatol* 127:378, 1991.
95. Neville BW, Damm DD, Allen C, et al: Dermatologic disease. In Neville BW, Damm DD, Allen C, Bouquot JE, editors: *Oral and maxillofacial pathology,* Philadelphia, 1995 Saunders.
96. Nisengard R: Periodontal implications: mucocutaneous disorders, *Ann Periodontol* 1:401, 1996.
97. Nisengard R, Levine R: Diagnosis and management of desquamative gingivitis, *Periodontal Insights* 2:4, 1995.
98. Nisengard RJ, Neiders M: Desquamative lesions of the gingiva, *J Periodontol* 52:500, 1981.
99. Nisengard RJ, Rogers RS III: The treatment of desquamative gingival lesions, *J Periodontol* 58:167, 1987.
100. O'Regan E, Bane A, Flint S, et al. Linear IgA disease presenting as desquamative gingivitis: a pattern poorly recognized in medicine, *Arch Otolaryngol Head Neck Surg* 130:469, 2004.
101. Peoples D, Fivenson DP: Linear IgA bullous dermatosis: successful treatment with tetracycline and nicotinamide, *J Am Acad Dermatol* 26:498, 1992.
102. Pleyer U, Bruckner-Tuderman L, Friedmann A, et al: The immunology of bullous oculo-muco-cutaneous disorders, *Immunol Today* 17:111, 1996.
103. Popovsky JL, Camisa C. New and emerging therapies for diseases of the oral cavity, *Dermatol Clin* 18:113, 2000.
104. Porter SR, Bain SE, Scully CM: Linear IgA disease manifesting as recalcitrant desquamative gingivitis, *Oral Surg Oral Med Oral Pathol* 74:179, 1992.
105. Porter SR, Scully C, Midda M, et al: Adult linear immunoglobulin A: a disease manifesting as desquamative gingivitis, *Oral Surg Oral Med Oral Pathol* 70:450, 1990.
106. Prinz H: Chronic diffuse desquamative gingivitis, *Dent Cosmos* 74:331, 1932.
107. Ramer MA, Altchek A, Deligdisch L, et al: Lichen planus and the vulvovaginal-gingival syndrome, *J Periodontol* 74:1385, 2003.
108. Rees TD: Adjunctive therapy. In *Proceedings of the World Workshop in Clinical Periodontics,* Chicago, 1989, American Academy of Periodontology.
109. Ricketts DN, Morgan CL, McGregor JM, et al: Kindler syndrome: a rare cause of desquamative lesions of the gingiva, *Oral Surg Oral Med Oral Pathol Oral Radiol Endod* 84:488, 1997.
110. Rinaggio J, Neiders ME, Aguirre A, et al: Using immunofluorescence in the diagnosis of chronic ulcerative lesions of the oral mucosa, *Compendium* 20:943, 1999.
111. Robinson JC, Lozada-Nur F, Frieden I: Oral pemphigus vulgaris: a review of the literature and a report on the management of 12 cases, *Oral Surg Oral Med Oral Pathol Oral Radiol Endod* 84:349, 1997.
113. Robledo MA, Soo-Chan K, Korman NJ, et al: Studies of the relationship of the 230-kD and 180-kD bullous pemphigoid antigens, *J Invest Dermatol* 94:793, 1990.
113. Rogers RS, Sheridan PJ, Jordon RC: Desquamative gingivitis: clinical, histopathologic and immunopathologic investigations, *Oral Surg* 42:316, 1976.
114. Rogers RS 3rd, Eisen D: Erosive oral lichen planus with genital lesions: the vulvovaginal-gingival syndrome and the peno-gingival syndrome, *Dermatol Clin* 21:91, 2003.
115. Sciubba JJ: Autoimmune aspects of pemphigus vulgaris and mucosal pemphigoid, *Adv Dent Res* 10:52, 1996.
116. Scully C, Challacombe SJ: Pemphigus vulgaris: update on etiopathogenesis, oral manifestations, and management, *Crit Rev Oral Biol Med* 13:397, 2002.
117. Scully C, El-Kom M: Lichen planus: review and update on pathogenesis, *J Oral Pathol* 14:431, 1985.
118. Scully C, Porter SR: The clinical spectrum of desquamative gingivitis, *Semin Cutan Med Surg* 16:308, 1997.
119. Scully C, Beyli M, Ferreiro MC, et al: Update on oral lichen planus: etiopathogenesis and management, *Crit Rev Oral Biol Med* 9:86, 1998.
120. Scully C, Carrozzo M, Gandolfo S, et al: Update on mucous membrane pemphigoid: a heterogeneous immune-mediated subepithelial blistering entity, *Oral Surg Oral Med Oral Pathol Oral Radiol Endod* 88:56, 1999.
121. Setterfield JF, Black MM, Challacombe SJ: The management of oral lichen planus, *Clin Exp Dermatol* 25:176, 2000.
122. Shen JT, Pedvis-Leftick A: Mucosal staining after using topical tacrolimus to treat erosive oral lichen planus, *J Am Acad Dermatol* 50:326, 2004.
123. Shklar G: Oral lesions of erythema multiforme: histologic and histochemical observations, *Arch Dermatol* 92:495, 1965.
124. Shklar G, Cataldo E: Histopathology and cytology of oral pemphigus vulgaris, *Arch Dermatol* 101:36, 1970.
125. Shklar G, McCarthy PL: The oral lesions of mucous membrane pemphigoid: a study of 85 cases, *Arch Otolaryngol* 93:354, 1971.

126. Shklar G, McCarthy PL: Histopathology of oral lesions of chronic discoid lupus erythematosus, *Arch Dermatol* 114:1031, 1978.
127. Shklar G, Flynn E, Szabo G: Basement membrane changes in oral lichen planus, *J Invest Dermatol* 70:45, 1978.
128. Shklar G, Frim S, Flynn E: Gingival lesions of pemphigus, *J Periodontol* 49:428, 1978.
129. Shklar G, Meyer I, Zacarian S: Oral lesions in bullous pemphigoid, *Arch Dermatol* 99:663, 1969.
130. Siegel MA, Balciunas BA: Oral presentation and management of vesiculobullous disorders, *Semin Dermatol* 13:78, 1994.
131. Silverman S, Shachi B: Oral lichen planus update: clinical characteristics, treatment responses, and malignant transformation, *Am J Dent* 10:259, 1997.
132. Sklavounou A, Laskaris G: Frequency of desquamative gingivitis in skin disease, *Oral Surg Oral Med Oral Pathol* 56:141, 1983.
133. Solomon LW, Aguirre A, Neiders M, et al: Chronic ulcerative stomatitis: clinical, histopathologic, and immunopathologic findings, *Oral Surg Oral Med Oral Pathol Oral Radiol Endod* 96:718, 2003.
134. Sorrin S: Chronic desquamative gingivitis, *J Am Dent Assoc* 27:250, 1940.
135. Stampien TM, Schwartz RA: Erythema multiforme, *Am Fam Physician* 46:1171, 1992.
136. Susi FR, Shklar G: Histochemistry and fine structure of oral lesions of mucous membrane pemphigoid, *Arch Dermatol* 104:244, 1971.
137. Tan EM, Cohen AS, Fries JR, et al: The 1982 revised criteria for the classification of systemic lupus erythematosus, *Arthritis Rheum* 25:1271, 1982.
138. Tomes J, Tomes G: *Dental surgery,* ed 4, London, 1894, Churchill.
139. Venning VA, Frith PA, Bron AJ, et al: Mucosal involvement in bullous and cicatricial pemphigoid: a clinical and immunopathological study, *Br J Dermatol* 118:7, 1988.
140. Weston WL, Morelli JG, Huff JC: Misdiagnosis, treatments and outcomes in the immunobullous diseases in children, *Pediatr Dermatol* 14:164, 1997.
141. Worle B, Wollenberg A, Schaller M, et al: Chronic ulcerative stomatitis, *Br J Dermatol* 137:262, 1997.
142. Yih WY, Maier T, Kratochvil FJ, et al: Analysis of desquamative gingivitis using direct immunofluorescence in conjunction with histology, *J Periodontol* 69:678, 1998.
143. Zegarelli DJ, Zegarelli EV: Intraoral pemphigus vulgaris, *Oral Surg* 44:384, 1977.
144. Ziskin D, Silvers HF: Report of a case of desquamative gingivitis and lichen planus, *J Periodontol* 16:7, 1945.
145. Ziskin D, Zegarelli EV: Chronic desquamative gingivitis, *Am J Orthod* 33:756, 1947.
146. Zone JJ, Meyer LJ, Petersen MJ: Deposition of granular IgA relative to clinical lesions in dermatitis herpetiformis, *Arch Dermatol* 132:912, 1996.

CHAPTER 27

The Periodontal Pocket

Fermin A. Carranza and Paulo M. Camargo

CHAPTER OUTLINE

The periodontal pocket, defined as a pathologically deepened gingival sulcus, is one of the most important clinical features of periodontal disease. All different types of periodontitis, as outlined in Chapter 7, share histopathologic features, such as tissue changes in the periodontal pocket, mechanisms of tissue destruction, and healing mechanisms. They differ, however, in their etiology, natural history, progression, and response to therapy.[36]

CLASSIFICATION

Deepening of the gingival sulcus may occur by coronal movement of the gingival margin, apical displacement of the gingival attachment, or a combination of the two processes (Figure 27-1). Pockets can be classified as follows:

Gingival pocket *(pseudopocket)*. This type of pocket is formed by gingival enlargement without destruction of the underlying periodontal tissues. The sulcus is deepened because of the increased bulk of the gingiva (Figure 27-2, *A*).

Periodontal pocket. This type of pocket occurs with destruction of the supporting periodontal tissues. Progressive pocket deepening leads to destruction of the supporting periodontal tissues and loosening and exfoliation of the teeth. The remainder of this chapter refers to this type of pocket.

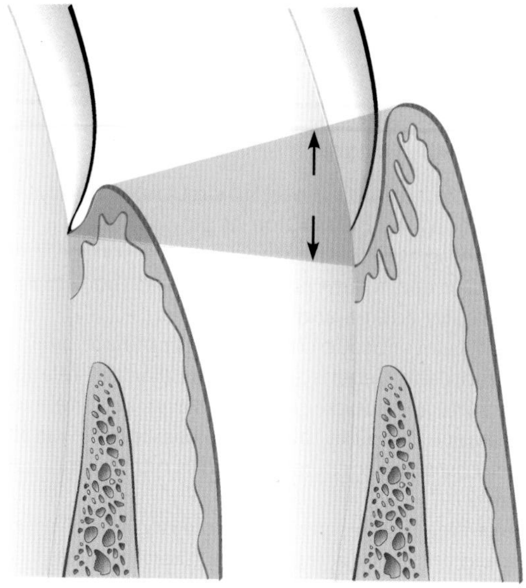

Figure 27-1 Illustration of pocket formation indicating expansion in two directions *(arrows)* from the normal gingival sulcus *(left)* to the periodontal pocket *(right)*.

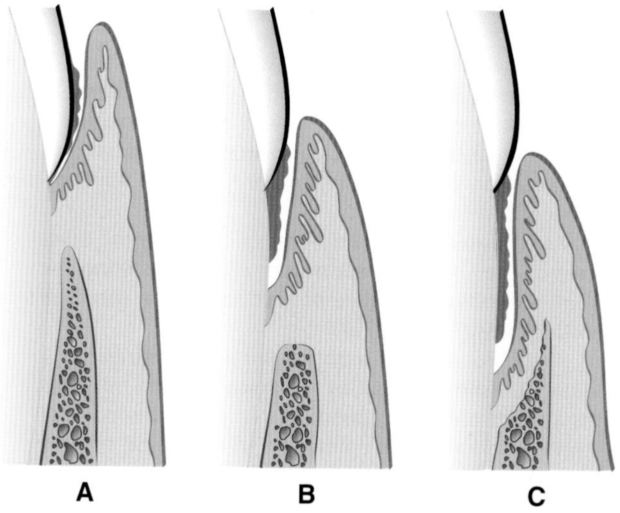

Figure 27-2 Different types of periodontal pockets. **A,** Gingival pocket. There is no destruction of the supporting periodontal tissues. **B,** Suprabony pocket. The base of the pocket is coronal to the level of the underlying bone. Bone loss is horizontal. **C,** Intrabony pocket. The base of the pocket is apical to the level of the adjacent bone. Bone loss is vertical.

Two types of periodontal pockets exist, as follows:

Suprabony (*supracrestal* or *supraalveolar*), in which the bottom of the pocket is coronal to the underlying alveolar bone (Figure 27-2, *B*).

Intrabony (*infrabony, subcrestal,* or *intraalveolar*), in which the bottom of the pocket is apical to the level of the adjacent alveolar bone. In this second type, the lateral pocket wall lies between the tooth surface and the alveolar bone (Figure 27-2, *C*).

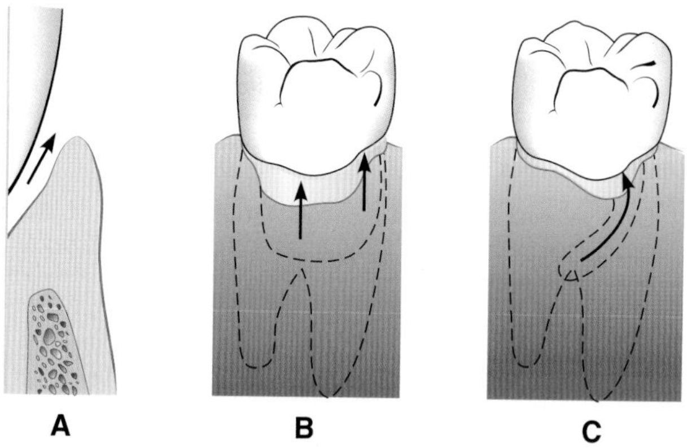

Figure 27-3 Classification of pockets according to involved tooth surfaces. **A,** Simple pocket. **B,** Compound pocket. **C,** Complex pocket.

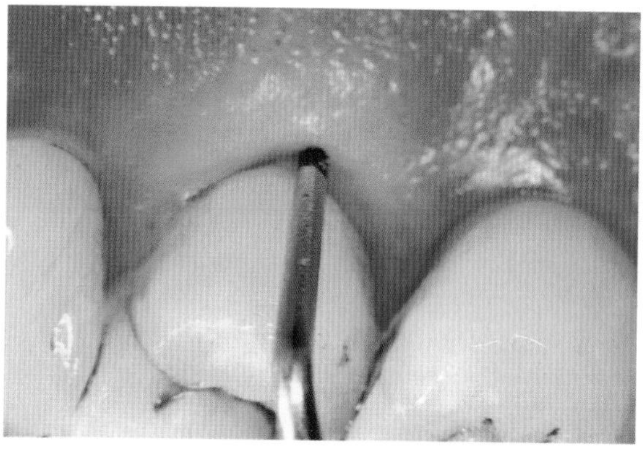

Figure 27-4 Probing of a deep periodontal pocket. Entire length of the periodontal probe has been inserted to the base of the pocket in palatal surface of first premolar.

Pockets can involve one, two, or more tooth surfaces and can be of different depths and types on different surfaces of the same tooth and on approximating surfaces of the same interdental space.[32,42] Pockets can also be spiral (i.e., originating on one tooth surface and twisting around the tooth to involve one or more additional surfaces) (Figure 27-3). These types of pockets are most common in furcation areas.

CLINICAL FEATURES

Clinical signs that suggest the presence of periodontal pockets include a bluish red, thickened marginal gingiva; a bluish red, vertical zone from the gingival margin to the alveolar mucosa; gingival bleeding and suppuration; tooth mobility; diastema formation; and symptoms such as localized pain or pain "deep in the bone." The only reliable method of locating periodontal pockets and determining their extent is careful probing of the gingival margin along each tooth surface (Figure 27-4 and Table 27-1). On the basis of depth alone, however, it is sometimes difficult to differentiate between a deep normal sulcus and a shallow periodontal pocket. In such borderline cases, pathologic changes in the gingiva distinguish the two conditions.

TABLE 27-1

Correlation of Clinical and Histopathologic Features of the Periodontal Pocket

Clinical Features	Histopathologic Features
1. Gingival wall of pocket presents various degrees of bluish red discoloration; flaccidity; a smooth, shiny surface; and pitting on pressure.	1. The discoloration is caused by circulatory stagnation; the flaccidity, by destruction of gingival fibers and surrounding tissues; the smooth, shiny surface, by atrophy of epithelium and edema; and the pitting on pressure, by edema and degeneration.
2. Less frequently, gingival wall may be pink and firm.	2. In such cases, fibrotic changes predominate over exudation and degeneration, particularly in relation to outer surface of pocket wall. However, despite external appearance of health, inner wall of pocket invariably presents some degeneration and is often ulcerated (see Figure 27-15).
3. Bleeding is elicited by gently probing soft tissue wall of pocket.	3. Ease of bleeding results from increased vascularity, thinning and degeneration of epithelium, and proximity of engorged vessels to inner surface.
4. When explored with a probe, inner aspect of pocket is generally painful.	4. Pain on tactile stimulation is caused by ulceration of inner aspect of pocket wall.
5. In many cases, pus may be expressed by applying digital pressure.	5. Pus occurs in pockets with suppurative inflammation of inner wall.

For a more detailed discussion of the clinical aspects of periodontal pockets, see Chapter 35.

PATHOGENESIS

The initial lesion in the development of periodontitis is the inflammation of the gingiva in response to a bacterial challenge. Changes involved in the transition from the normal gingival sulcus to the pathologic periodontal pocket are associated with different proportions of bacterial cells in dental plaque. Healthy gingiva is associated with few microorganisms, mostly coccoid cells and straight rods. Diseased gingiva is associated with increased numbers of spirochetes and motile rods.[44,45,47] However, the microbiota of diseased sites cannot be used as a predictor of future attachment or bone loss because their presence alone is not sufficient for disease to start or progress.[39]

Pocket formation starts as an inflammatory change in the connective tissue wall of the gingival sulcus. The cellular and fluid inflammatory exudate causes degeneration of the surrounding connective tissue, including the gingival fibers. Just apical to the junctional epithelium, collagen fibers are destroyed,[21,65] and the area becomes occupied by inflammatory cells and edema (Figure 27-5).

Two mechanisms are considered to be associated with collagen loss: (1) collagenases and other enzymes secreted by various cells in healthy and inflamed tissue, such as fibroblasts,[78] polymorphonuclear leukocytes (PMNs),[77] and macrophages,[57] become extracellular and destroy collagen; these enzymes that degrade collagen and other matrix macromolecules into small peptides are called *matrix metalloproteinases*[79]; and (2) fibroblasts phagocytize collagen fibers by extending cytoplasmic processes to the ligament-cementum interface and degrade the inserted collagen fibrils and the fibrils of the cementum matrix.[21,22]

As a consequence of the loss of collagen, the apical cells of the junctional epithelium proliferate along the root, extending fingerlike projections two or three cells in thickness (Figure 27-6).

The coronal portion of the junctional epithelium detaches from the root as the apical portion migrates. As a result of inflammation, PMNs invade the coronal end of the junctional epithelium in increasing numbers (Figure 27-7). The PMNs are not joined to one another or to the remaining epithelial cells by desmosomes. When the relative volume of PMNs reaches approximately 60% or more of the junctional epithelium, the tissue loses cohesiveness and detaches from the tooth surface. Thus the sulcus bottom shifts apically, and the oral sulcular epithelium occupies a gradually increasing portion of the sulcular (pocket) lining.[66]

The initial deepening of the pocket has been described as occurring between the junctional epithelium and the tooth[33,34,65] or by an intraepithelial cleavage within the junctional epithelium.[10,24,46,78]

Extension of the junctional epithelium along the root requires the presence of healthy epithelial cells. Marked degeneration or necrosis of the junctional epithelium impairs rather than accelerates pocket formation. Degenerative changes seen in the junctional epithelium at the base of periodontal pockets are usually less severe than those in the epithelium of the lateral pocket wall (see Figure 27-7). Because migration of the junctional

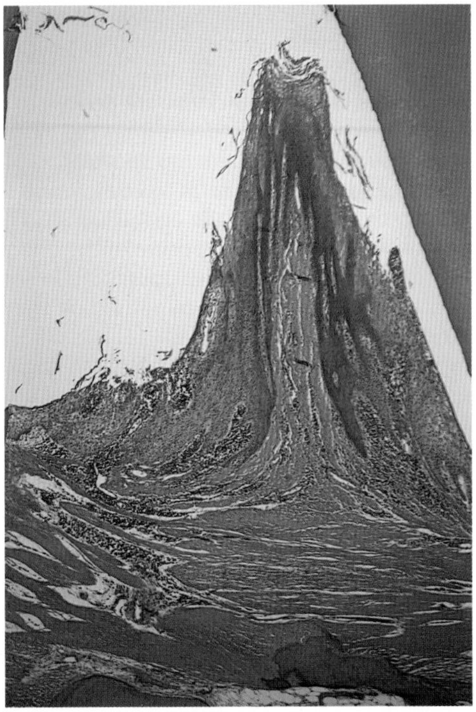

Figure 27-5 Interdental papilla with suprabony pockets on proximal tooth surfaces. Note the densely inflamed connective tissue, with the infiltrate extending between the collagen fibers, and the proliferating and ulcerated pocket epithelium.

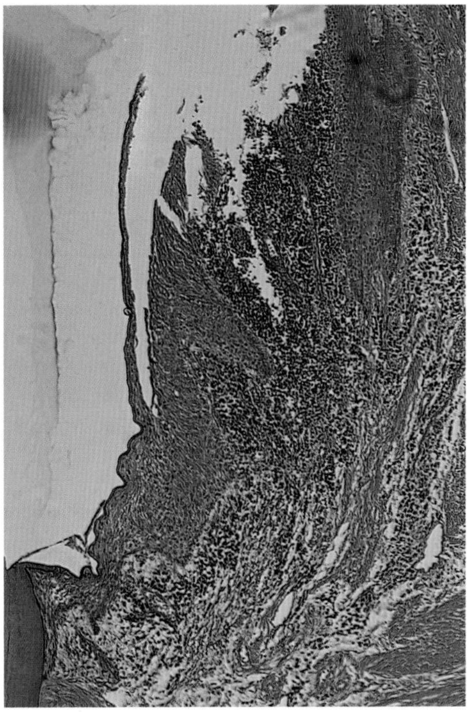

Figure 27-7 High-power view of base of periodontal pocket. The lateral epithelial wall is ulcerated. Note the extension of epithelial cells and the dense accumulation of leukocytes within the epithelium and in the connective tissue.

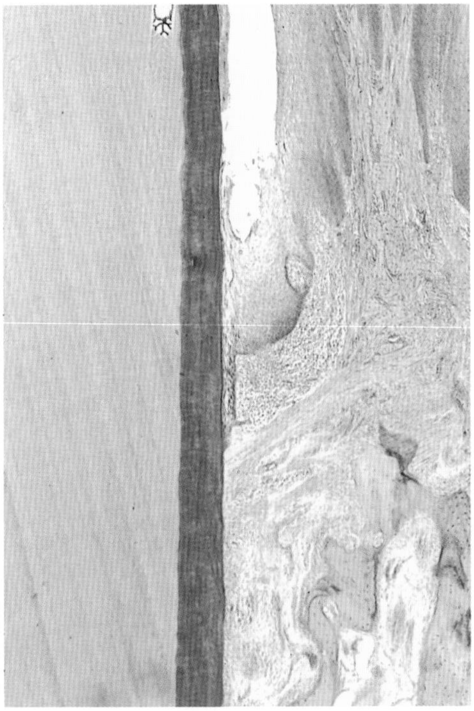

Figure 27-6 Low-power view of base of periodontal pocket and apical area. Note the dense inflammatory infiltrate on area of destroyed collagen fibers and the thin, fingerlike extension of epithelium covering the cementum denuded of fibers.

epithelium requires healthy, viable cells, it is reasonable to assume that the degenerative changes seen in this area occur after the junctional epithelium reaches its position on the cementum.

The degree of leukocyte infiltration of the junctional epithelium is independent of the volume of inflamed connective tissue, and thus this process may occur in gingiva with only slight signs of clinical inflammation.[65]

With continued inflammation, the gingiva increases in bulk, and the crest of the gingival margin extends coronally. The junctional epithelium continues to migrate along the root and separate from it. The epithelium of the lateral wall of the pocket proliferates to form bulbous, cordlike extensions into the inflamed connective tissue. Leukocytes and edema from the inflamed connective tissue infiltrate the epithelium lining the pocket, resulting in various degrees of degeneration and necrosis.

The transformation of a gingival sulcus into a periodontal pocket creates an area where plaque removal becomes impossible, and a feedback mechanism is established. The rationale for pocket reduction is based on the need to eliminate areas of plaque accumulation.

HISTOPATHOLOGY

Changes occurring in the initial stages of gingival inflammation are presented in Chapter 21. Once the pocket is formed, several microscopic features are present, as discussed in this section.

Soft Tissue Wall

The connective tissue is edematous and densely infiltrated with plasma cells (approximately 80%),[86] lymphocytes, and a scattering of PMNs. The blood vessels are increased in number, dilated, and engorged, particularly in the subepithelial connective tissue layer.[11] The connective tissue exhibits varying degrees of degeneration. Single or multiple necrotic foci are occasionally present.[56] In addition to exudative and degenerative changes, the connective tissue shows proliferation of the endothelial cells, with newly formed capillaries, fibroblasts, and collagen fibers (see Figure 27-5).

The junctional epithelium at the base of the pocket is usually much shorter than that of a normal sulcus. Although marked variations are found as to length, width, and condition of the epithelial cells, usually the coronoapical length of the junctional epithelium is reduced to only 50 to 100 μm.[15] The cells may be well formed and in good condition or may exhibit slight to marked degeneration (see Figures 27-6 and 27-8, *B*).

The most severe degenerative changes in the periodontal pocket occur along the lateral wall (see Figure 27-7). The epithelium of the lateral wall of the pocket presents striking proliferative and degenerative changes. Epithelial buds or interlacing cords of epithelial cells project from the lateral wall into the adjacent inflamed connective tissue and may extend farther apically than the junctional epithelium (Figures 27-8, *A*, and 27-9). These epithelial projections, as well as the remainder of the lateral epithelium, are densely infiltrated by leukocytes and edema from the inflamed connective tissue. The cells undergo vacuolar degeneration and rupture to form vesicles. Progressive degeneration and necrosis of the epithelium lead to ulceration of the lateral wall, exposure of the underlying inflamed connective tissue, and suppuration. In some cases, acute inflammation is superimposed on the underlying chronic changes.

A comparative study of gingival histopathologic changes in rapidly progressive (aggressive) and adult periodontitis (chronic) revealed more pronounced degenerative changes in the epithelium of aggressive cases with more open intercellular spaces, with microclefts and necrotic areas.[39]

The severity of the degenerative changes is not necessarily related to pocket depth. Ulceration of the lateral wall may occur in shallow pockets, and deep pockets are occasionally observed in which the lateral epithelium is relatively intact or shows only slight degeneration.

The epithelium at the gingival crest of a periodontal pocket is generally intact and thickened, with prominent rete pegs.

For a detailed electron microscopic study of the pocket epithelium in experimentally induced pockets in dogs, see Müller-Glauser and Schröder.[53]

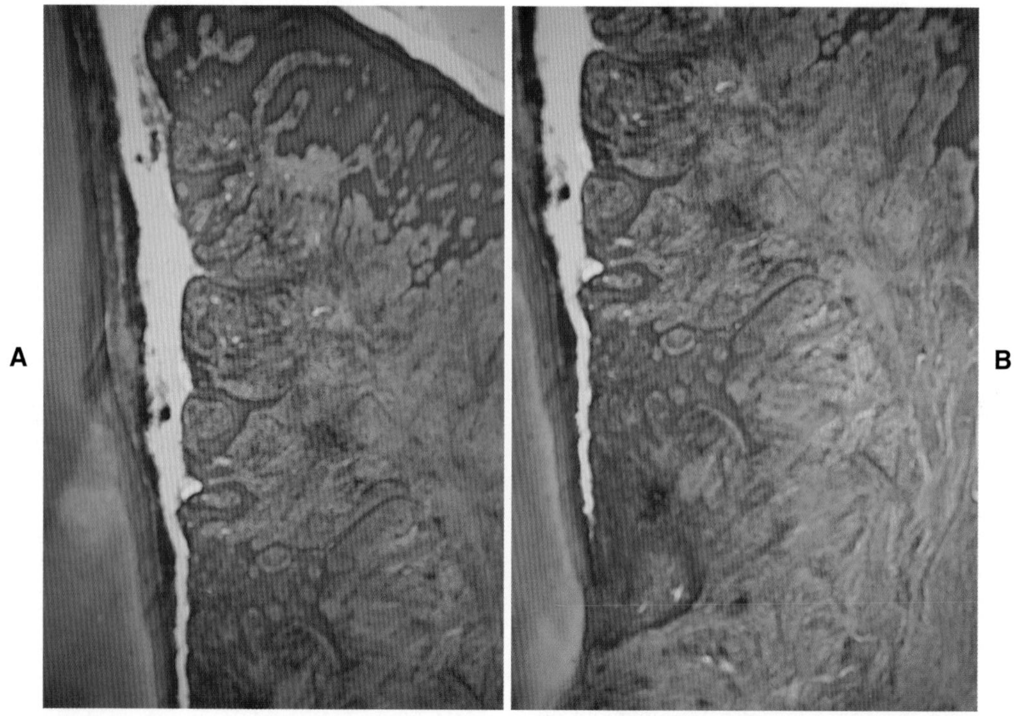

Figure 27-8 **A,** Lateral wall of periodontal pocket showing epithelial proliferative and atrophic changes and marked inflammatory infiltrate and destruction of collagen fibers. **B,** Slightly apical view of the same case showing the shortened junctional epithelium.

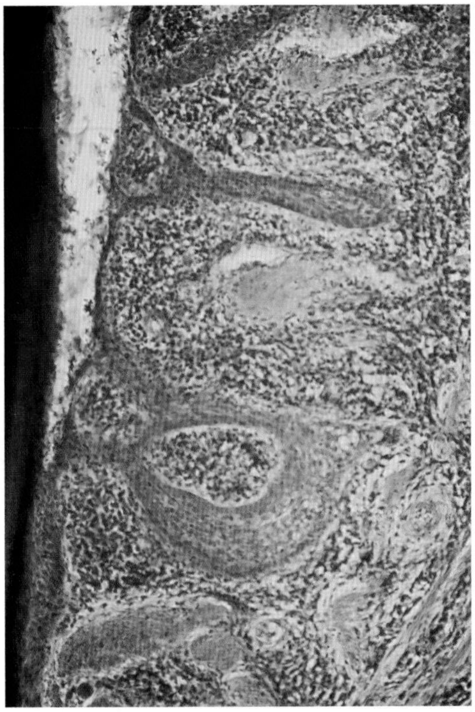

Figure 27-9 Base of periodontal pocket showing extensive proliferation of lateral epithelium next to atrophic areas, dense inflammatory infiltrate, remnants of destroyed collagen fibers, and the junctional epithelium, apparently in a less altered state than lateral pocket epithelium.

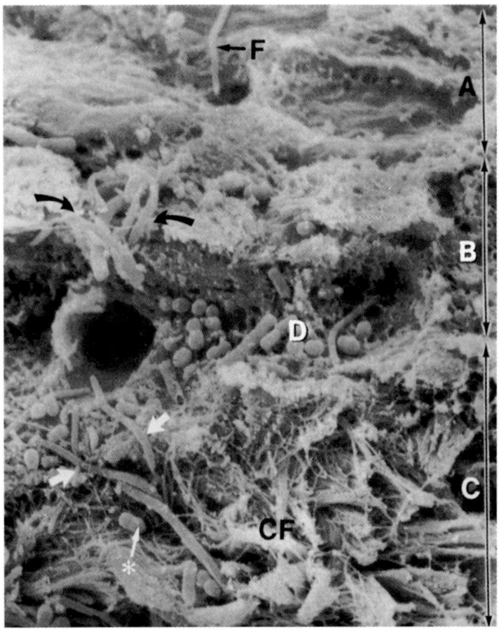

Figure 27-10 Electron micrograph of section of pocket wall in advanced periodontitis in human specimen, showing bacterial penetration into the epithelium and connective tissue. Scanning electron microscope view of surface of pocket wall *(A)*, sectioned epithelium *(B)*, and sectioned connective tissue *(C)*. Curved arrows point to areas of bacterial penetration into the epithelium. Thick white arrows point to bacterial penetration into the connective tissue through a break in the continuity of the basal lamina. *CF*, Connective tissue fibers; *D*, accumulation of bacteria (rods, cocci, filaments) on basal lamina; *F*, filamentous organism on surface of epithelium. Asterisk points to coccobacillus in connective tissue.

Bacterial Invasion

Bacterial invasion of the apical and lateral areas of the pocket wall has been described in human chronic periodontitis. Filaments, rods, and coccoid organisms with predominant gram-negative cell walls have been found in intercellular spaces of the epithelium.[27,28] Hillmann et al.[39] have reported the presence of *Porphyromonas gingivalis* and *Prevotella intermedia* in the gingiva of aggressive periodontitis cases. *Actinobacillus actinomycetemcomitans* has also been found in the tissues.[17,51,62]

Bacteria may invade the intercellular space under exfoliating epithelial cells, but they are also found between deeper epithelial cells and accumulating on the basement lamina. Some bacteria traverse the basement lamina and invade the subepithelial connective tissue[64] (Figures 27-10 and 27-11).

The presence of bacteria in the gingival tissues has been interpreted by different investigators as bacterial invasion or as "passive translocation" of plaque bacteria. This important point has significant clinicopathologic implications and has not yet been clarified.[18,43,47]

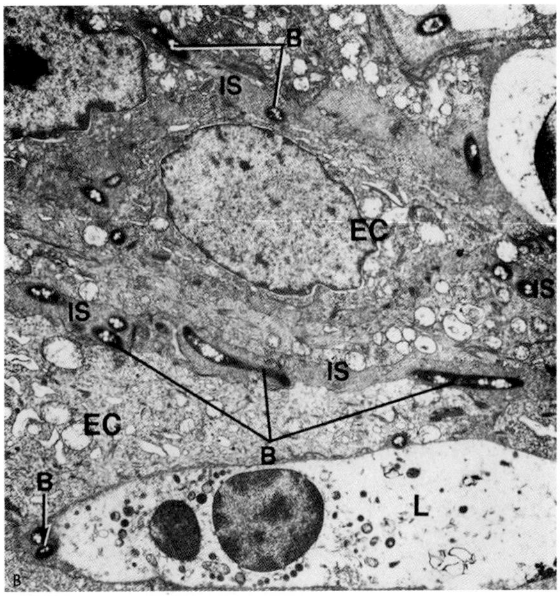

Figure 27-11 Transmission electron micrograph of the epithelium in the periodontal pocket wall showing bacteria in the intercellular spaces. *B*, Bacteria; *EC*, epithelial cell; *IS*, intercellular space; *L*, leukocyte about to engulf bacteria. (×8000.)

Microtopography of Gingival Wall

Scanning electron microscopy has permitted the description of several areas in the soft tissue (gingival) wall of the periodontal pocket where different types of activity take place.[60] These areas are irregularly oval or elongated and adjacent to one another and measure about 50 to 200 μm. These findings suggest that the pocket wall is constantly changing as a result of the interaction between the host and the bacteria. The following areas have been noted:

1. *Areas of relative quiescence,* showing a relatively flat surface with minor depressions and mounds and occasional shedding of cells (Figure 27-12, area *A*).
2. *Areas of bacterial accumulation,* which appear as depressions on the epithelial surface, with abundant debris and bacterial clumps penetrating into the enlarged intercellular spaces. These bacteria are mainly cocci, rods, and filaments, with a few spirochetes (Figure 27-12, area *B*).
3. *Areas of emergence of leukocytes,* where leukocytes appear in the pocket wall through holes located in the intercellular spaces (Figure 27-13).
4. *Areas of leukocyte-bacteria interaction,* where numerous leukocytes are present and covered with bacteria in an apparent process of phagocytosis. Bacterial plaque associated with the epithelium is seen either as an organized matrix covered by a fibrinlike material in contact with the surface of cells or as bacteria penetrating into the intercellular spaces (Figure 27-12, area *C*).
5. *Areas of intense epithelial desquamation,* which consist of semiattached and folded epithelial squames, sometimes partially covered with bacteria (Figure 27-12, area *D*).
6. *Areas of ulceration,* with exposed connective tissue (Figure 27-14).
7. *Areas of hemorrhage,* with numerous erythrocytes.

SCIENCE TRANSFER

The histopathologic aspects of pocket formation provide a basis for clinical therapy. The presence of bleeding on probing indicates that bacterial subgingival plaque is causing inflammation and ulceration of the epithelial lining of the pocket and that periodontal breakdown is active. The evidence of a purulent exudate is another indicator of disease activity. If these signs are present, antiplaque mechanical and/or antimicrobial therapy should be implemented immediately, regardless of pocket depth. Although bleeding on probing is an early sign of gingivitis, occurring within 2 days of plaque-initiating disease, it is also often present throughout disease progression. Elimination of gingivitis-induced gingival bleeding on probing can be accomplished within 7 to 10 days of initial therapy and with the patient's control of plaque. *In deep pockets associated with bone loss and periodontitis, initial therapy will need to be followed by surgical therapy so that pockets are reduced to a level where the patient's oral hygiene can systematically remove subgingival plaque, and epithelial ulceration and gingival bleeding are resolved.*

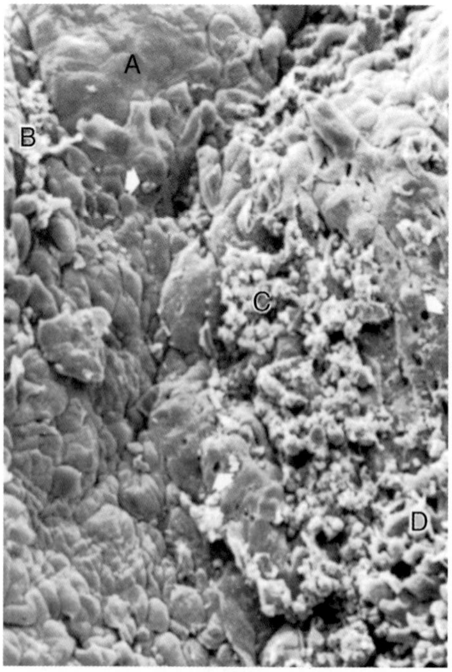

Figure 27-12 Scanning electron frontal micrograph of the periodontal pocket wall. Different areas can be seen in the pocket wall surface. *A,* Area of quiescence; *B,* bacterial accumulation; *C,* bacterial-leukocyte interaction; *D,* intense cellular desquamation. Arrows point to emerging leukocytes and holes left by leukocytes in the pocket wall. (×800.)

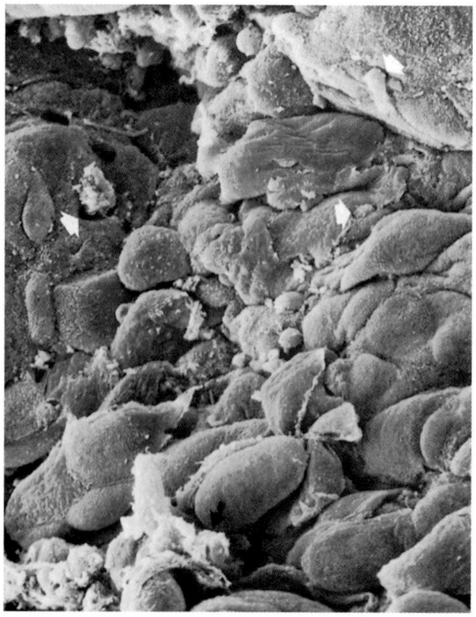

Figure 27-13 Scanning electron micrograph of the periodontal pocket wall, frontal view, in a patient with advanced periodontitis. Note the desquamating epithelial cells and leukocytes *(white arrows)* emerging onto the pocket space. Scattered bacteria can also be seen *(black arrow).* (×1500.)

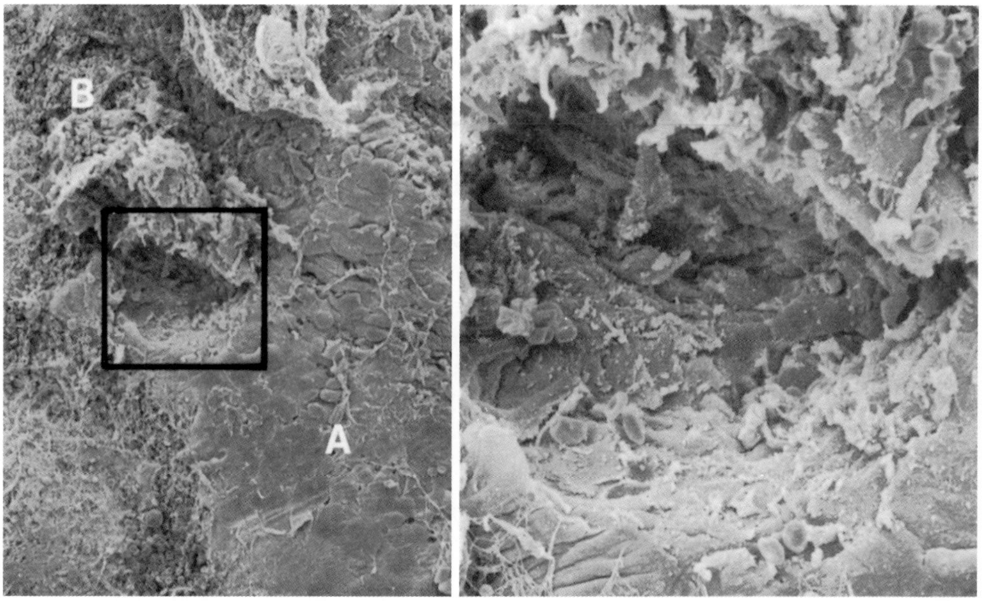

Figure 27-14 *Left,* Area of ulceration in the lateral wall of a deep periodontal pocket in a human specimen. *A,* Surface of pocket epithelium in a quiescent state; *B,* area of hemorrhage. (×800.) *Right,* Magnification of the square on left. Connective tissue fibers and cells can be seen in the bottom of the ulcer. (Scanning electron microscopy, ×3000.)

The transition from one area to another could result from bacteria accumulating in previously quiescent areas and triggering the emergence of leukocytes and the leukocyte-bacteria interaction. This would lead to intense epithelial desquamation and finally to ulceration and hemorrhage.

Periodontal Pockets as Healing Lesions

Periodontal pockets are chronic inflammatory lesions and thus are constantly undergoing repair. Complete healing does not occur because of the persistence of the bacterial attack, which continues to stimulate an inflammatory response, causing degeneration of the new tissue elements formed in the continuous effort at repair.

The condition of the soft tissue wall of the periodontal pocket results from the interplay of the destructive and constructive tissue changes. Their balance determines clinical features such as color, consistency, and surface texture of the pocket wall. If the inflammatory fluid and cellular exudate predominate, the pocket wall is bluish red, soft, spongy, and friable, with a smooth, shiny surface; at the clinical level, this is generally referred to as an *edematous pocket wall.* If there is a relative predominance of newly formed connective tissue cells and fibers, the pocket wall is more firm and pink, clinically referred to as a *fibrotic pocket wall* (see Table 27-1 and Chapter 35).

Edematous and fibrotic pockets represent opposite extremes of the same pathologic process, not different disease entities. They are subject to constant modification, depending on the relative predominance of exudative and constructive changes.

Fibrotic pocket walls may be misleading because they do not necessarily reflect what is taking place throughout the pocket wall. The most severe degenerative changes in periodontal tissues occur adjacent to the tooth surface and subgingival plaque. In some cases, inflammation and ulceration on the inside of the pocket are walled off by fibrous tissue on the outer aspect (Figure 27-15). Externally the pocket appears pink and fibrotic, despite the inflammatory changes occurring internally.

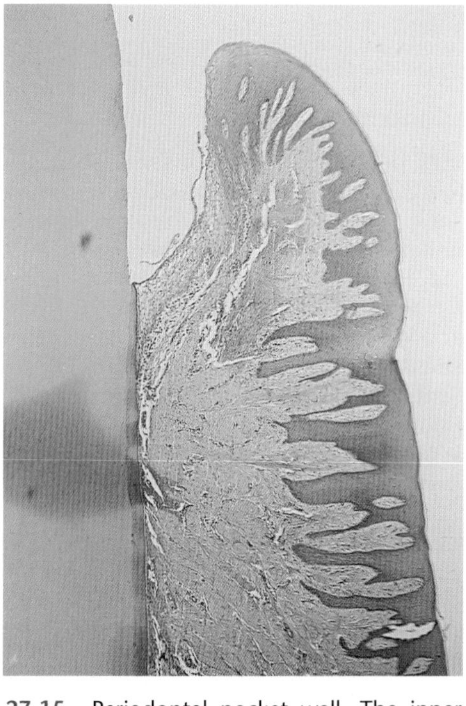

Figure 27-15 Periodontal pocket wall. The inner half is inflamed and ulcerated; the outer half is densely collagenous.

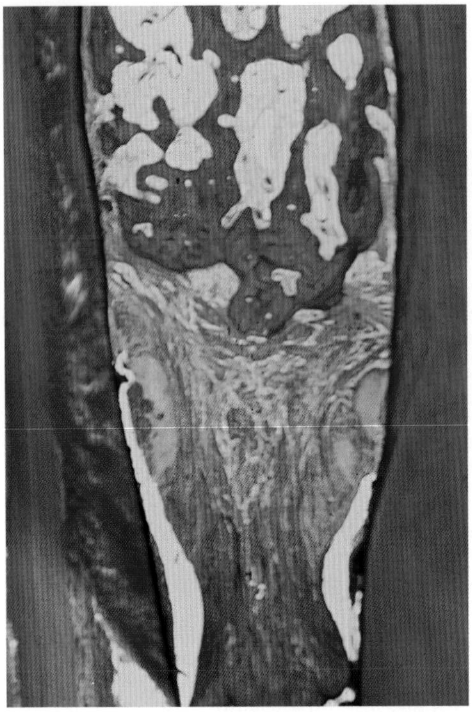

Figure 27-16 Interdental papilla with ulcerated suprabony periodontal pockets on its mesial and distal aspects. Calculus is present on the approximal tooth surfaces and within the gingiva.

Pocket Contents

Periodontal pockets contain debris consisting principally of microorganisms and their products (enzymes, endotoxins, and other metabolic products), gingival fluid, food remnants, salivary mucin, desquamated epithelial cells, and leukocytes. Plaque-covered calculus usually projects from the tooth surface (Figure 27-16). Purulent exudate, if present, consists of living, degenerated, and necrotic leukocytes; living and dead bacteria; serum; and a scant amount of fibrin.[50] The contents of periodontal pockets filtered free of organisms and debris have been demonstrated to be toxic when injected subcutaneously into experimental animals.[35]

Significance of Pus Formation. There is a tendency to overemphasize the importance of the purulent exudate and to equate it with severity of periodontal disease. Because it is a dramatic clinical finding, early observers assumed that it was responsible for the loosening and exfoliation of the teeth. *Pus is a common feature of periodontal disease, but it is only a secondary sign.* The presence of pus or the ease with which it can be expressed from the pocket merely reflects the nature of the inflammatory changes in the pocket wall. It is not an indication of the depth of the pocket or the severity of the destruction of the supporting tissues. Extensive pus formation may occur in shallow pockets, whereas deep pockets may exhibit little or no pus.

Localized accumulation of pus constitutes an abscess, discussed later in this chapter.

Root Surface Wall

The root surface wall of periodontal pockets often undergoes changes that are significant because they may perpetuate the periodontal infection, cause pain, and complicate periodontal treatment.

As the pocket deepens, collagen fibers embedded in the cementum are destroyed and cementum becomes exposed to the oral environment. Collagenous remnants of Sharpey's fibers in the cementum undergo degeneration, creating an environment favorable to the penetration of bacteria. Viable bacteria have been found in the roots of 87% of periodontally diseased noncarious teeth.[2] Bacterial penetration into the cementum can be found as deep as the cementodentinal junction[1,19] and may also enter the dentinal tubules[31] (Figure 27-17).

Pathologic granules[9] have been observed with light and electron microscopy[6,7] and may represent areas of collagen degeneration or areas where collagen fibrils have not been fully mineralized initially.

Penetration and growth of bacteria leads to fragmentation and breakdown of the cementum surface and result in areas of necrotic cementum, separated from the tooth by masses of bacteria (Figure 27-18).

In addition, bacterial products such as endotoxins[3,5] have also been detected in the cementum wall of periodontal pockets. When root fragments from teeth with periodontal disease are placed in tissue culture, they induce irreversible morphologic changes in the cells of the culture. Such changes are not produced by normal roots.[37] Diseased root fragments also prevent the in vitro attachment of human gingival fibroblasts, whereas normal root surfaces allow the cells to attach freely.[4] When reimplanted in the oral mucosa of the patient, diseased root fragments induce an inflammatory response even if they are autoclaved.[48]

These changes manifest clinically as softening of the cementum surface, which is usually asymptomatic, but painful when a probe or explorer penetrates the area. They also constitute a possible reservoir for reinfection of the area after treatment. In the course of treatment, these necrotic areas are removed by root planing until a hard, smooth surface is reached. Cementum is very thin in the cervical areas, and scaling and root planing often remove it entirely, exposing the underlying dentin. Sensitivity to cold may result until secondary dentin is formed by the pulp tissue.

Decalcification and Remineralization of Cementum. Areas of *increased mineralization*[69] are probably a result of an exchange, on exposure to the oral cavity, of minerals and organic components at the cementum-saliva interface. The mineral content of exposed cementum increases.[68] Minerals that are increased in diseased root surfaces include calcium,[71] magnesium,[54,71] phosphorus,[54] and fluoride.[54] Microhardness, however, remains unchanged.[59,85] The development of a highly mineralized superficial layer may increase the tooth resistance to decay.[4]

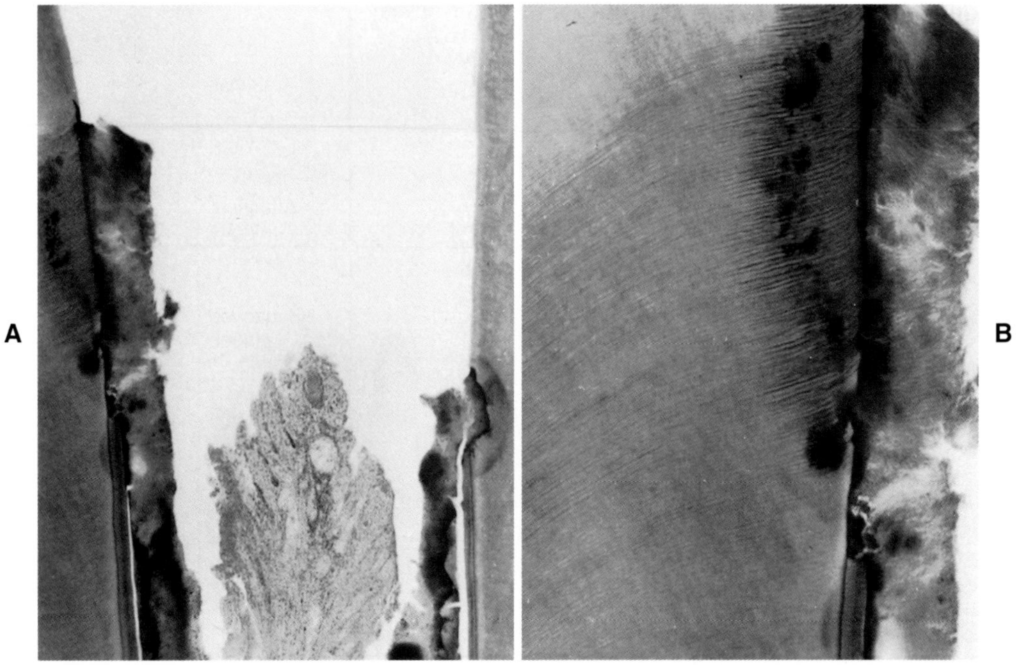

Figure 27-17 Caries on root surfaces exposed by periodontal disease. **A,** Interdental space, showing inflamed gingiva and caries on proximal tooth surfaces. **B,** Caries of cementum and dentin, showing bacterial invasion of dentinal tubules. Note the filamentous structure of the dental plaque and darker staining of calculus adherent to the root.

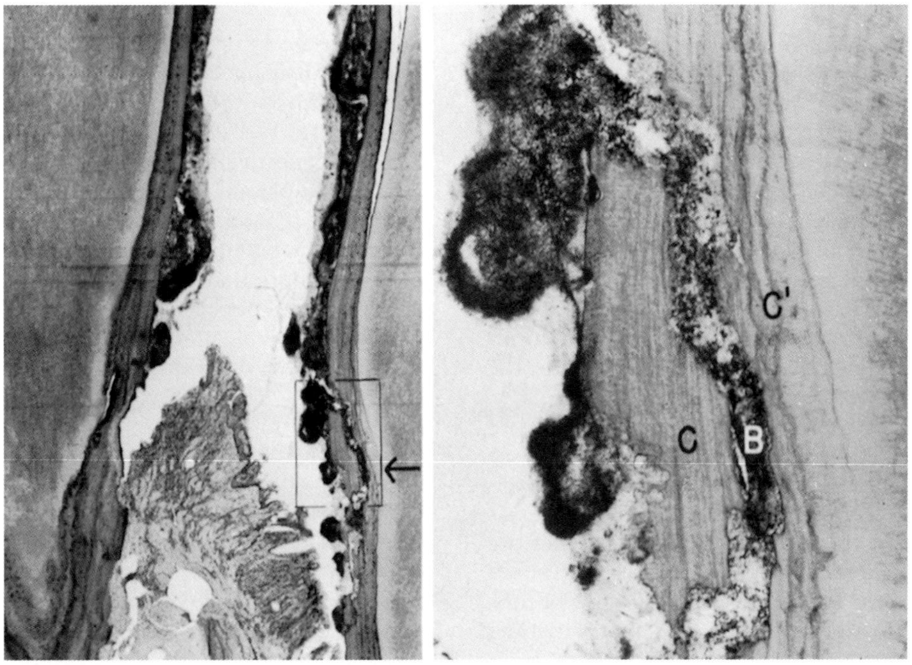

Figure 27-18 *Left,* Mesiodistal section through an interdental space in a patient with extensive periodontal destruction. An area of cementum necrosis is enclosed within the rectangle designated by the arrow. *Right,* Detailed section of the rectangular area showing a necrotic fragment of cementum *(C)* separated from lamellated cementum *(C′)* by clumps of bacteria *(B).*

The hypermineralized zones are detectable by electron microscopy and are associated with increased perfection of the crystal structure and organic changes suggestive of a subsurface cuticle.[68,69] These zones have also been seen in microradiographic studies[70] as a layer 10 to 20 μm thick, with areas as thick as 50 μm. No decrease in mineralization was found in deeper areas, thereby indicating that increased mineralization does not come from adjacent areas. A loss of, or reduction in, the cross-banding of collagen near the cementum surface[29,30] and a subsurface condensation of organic material of exogenous origin[68] have also been reported.

Areas of demineralization are often related to **root caries.** Exposure to oral fluid and bacterial plaque results in proteolysis of the embedded remnants of Sharpey's fibers; the cementum may be softened and may undergo fragmentation and cavitation.[38] Unlike enamel caries, root surface caries tend to progress around rather than into the tooth.[52] Active root caries lesions appear as well-defined yellowish or light-brown areas, are frequently covered by plaque, and have a softened or leathery consistency on probing. Inactive lesions are well-defined darker lesions with a smooth surface and a harder consistency on probing.[26]

The dominant microorganism in root surface caries is *Actinomyces viscosus,*[76] although its specific role in the development of the lesion has not been established.[26] Other bacteria, such as *Actinomyces naeslundii, Streptococcus mutans, Streptococcus salivarius, Streptococcus sanguis,* and *Bacillus cereus,* have been found to produce root caries in animal models. Quirynen et al.[58] reported that when plaque levels and pocket depths decrease after periodontal therapy (both conservative and surgical), a shift in oral bacteria occurs, leading to a reduction in periodontal pathogens and an increase in *S. mutans* and the development of root caries.

A prevalence rate study of root caries in 20- to 64-year-old individuals revealed that 42% had one or more root caries lesions and that these lesions tended to increase with age.[41]

The tooth may not be painful, but exploration of the root surface reveals the presence of a defect, and penetration of the involved area with a probe causes pain. Caries of the root, however, may lead to pulpitis, sensitivity to sweets and thermal changes, or severe pain. Pathologic exposure of the pulp occurs in severe cases. Root caries may be the cause of toothache in patients with periodontal disease and no evidence of coronal decay.

Caries of the cementum requires special attention when the pocket is treated. The necrotic cementum must be removed by scaling and root planing until firm tooth surface is reached, even if this entails extension into the dentin.

Areas of cellular resorption of cementum and dentin are common in roots unexposed by periodontal disease[72] (see Figure 27-18). These areas are of no particular significance because they are symptom free, and as long as the root is covered by the periodontal ligament, they are likely to undergo repair. However, if the root is exposed by progressive pocket formation before repair occurs, these areas appear as isolated cavitations that penetrate into the dentin. These areas can be differentiated from caries of the cementum by their clear-cut outline and hard surface. They may be sources of considerable pain, requiring placement of a restoration.

Surface Morphology of Tooth Wall.* The following zones can be found in the bottom of a periodontal pocket (Figure 27-19):

1. *Cementum covered by calculus,* where all the changes described in the preceding paragraphs can be found.

*References 8, 13, 40, 60, 61, 82.

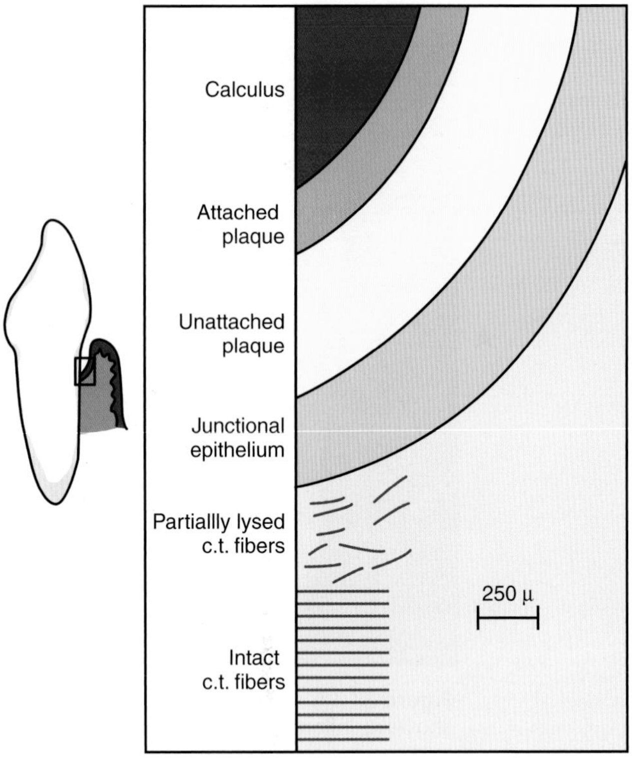

Figure 27-19 Diagram of the area at the bottom of a pocket; *c.t.,* connective tissue.

2. *Attached plaque,* which covers calculus and extends apically from it to a variable degree, probably 100 to 500 μm.
3. The zone of *unattached plaque* that surrounds attached plaque and extends apically to it.
4. The zone of *attachment of junctional epithelium to the tooth.* The extension of this zone, which in normal sulci is more than 500 μm, is usually reduced in periodontal pockets to less than 100 μm.
5. A zone of *semidestroyed connective tissue fibers* may be apical to the junctional epithelium (see Pathogenesis).

Zones 3, 4, and 5 make up the "plaque-free zone" seen in extracted teeth. The total width of the plaque-free zone varies according to the type of tooth (wider in molars than in incisors) and the depth of the pocket (narrower in deeper pockets).[60] It is important to remember that the term *plaque-free zone* refers only to attached plaque because unattached plaque contains a variety of gram-positive cocci and various gram-negative morphotypes, including cocci, rods, filaments, fusiforms, and spirochetes. The most apical zone contains predominantly gram-negative rods and cocci.[80]

PERIODONTAL DISEASE ACTIVITY

For many years the loss of attachment produced by periodontal disease was thought to be a slow but continuously progressive phenomenon. More recently, as a result of studies on the specificity of plaque bacteria, the concept of periodontal disease activity has evolved.

According to this concept, periodontal pockets go through periods of exacerbation and quiescence, resulting from episodic bursts of activity followed by periods of remission. *Periods of quiescence* are characterized by a reduced inflammatory response and little or no loss of bone and connective tissue attachment. A buildup of unattached plaque, with its gram-negative, motile, and anaerobic bacteria (see Chapter 9), starts a *period of exacerbation* in which bone and connective tissue attachment are lost and the pocket deepens. This period may last for days, weeks, or months and is eventually followed by a period of remission or quiescence in which gram-positive bacteria proliferate and a more stable condition is established. Based on a study of radioiodine ^{125}I absorptiometry, McHenry et al.[49] confirmed that bone loss in untreated periodontal disease occurs in an episodic manner.

These periods of quiescence and exacerbation are also known as *periods of inactivity* and *periods of activity.* Clinically, active periods show bleeding, either spontaneously or with probing, and greater amounts of gingival exudate. Histologically, the pocket epithelium appears thin and ulcerated, and an infiltrate composed predominantly of plasma cells,[20] polymorphonuclear leukocytes (PMNs),[57] or both are seen. Bacterial samples from the pocket lumen analyzed with dark-field microscopy show high proportions of motile organisms and spirochetes.[47] Over time, loss of bone should be detected radiographically.

Methods to detect periods of activity or inactivity are currently being investigated (see Chapter 37).

SITE SPECIFICITY

Periodontal destruction does not occur in all parts of the mouth at the same time but rather on a few teeth at a time or even only some aspects of some teeth at any given time. This is referred to as the *site specificity* of periodontal disease. Sites of periodontal destruction are often found next to sites with little or no destruction. Therefore the severity of periodontitis increases with the development of new disease sites and the increased breakdown of existing sites.

PULP CHANGES ASSOCIATED WITH PERIODONTAL POCKETS

The spread of infection from periodontal pockets may cause pathologic changes in the pulp. Such changes may give rise to painful symptoms or may adversely affect the response of the pulp to restorative procedures. Involvement of the pulp in periodontal disease occurs through either the apical foramen or the lateral canals in the root after infection spreads from the pocket through the periodontal ligament. Atrophic and inflammatory pulpal changes occur in such cases (see Chapters 58 and 68).

RELATIONSHIP OF ATTACHMENT LOSS AND BONE LOSS TO POCKET DEPTH

Pocket formation causes loss of attachment of the gingiva and denudation of the root surface. The severity of the attachment loss is generally, but not always, correlated with the depth of the pocket. This is because the degree of attachment loss depends on the location of the base of the pocket on the root surface, whereas the pocket depth is the distance between the base of the pocket and the crest of the gingival margin. Pockets of the same depth may be associated with different degrees of attachment loss (Figure 27-20), and pockets of different depths may be associated with the same amount of attachment loss (Figure 27-21).

Severity of bone loss is generally, but not always, correlated with pocket depth. Extensive attachment and bone loss may be associated with shallow pockets if the attachment loss is accompanied by recession of the gingival margin, and slight bone loss can occur with deep pockets.

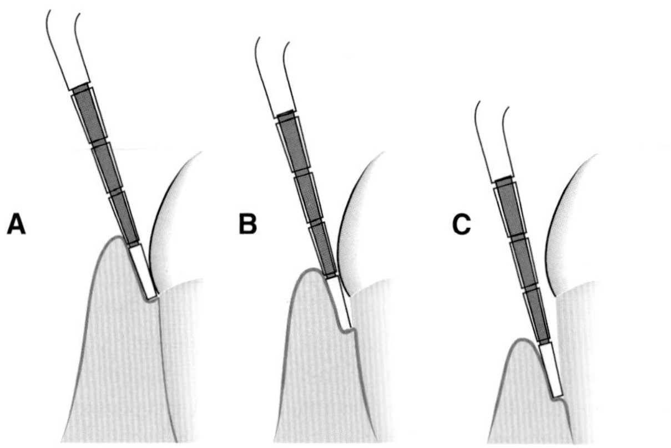

Figure 27-20 Same pocket depth with different amounts of recession. **A,** Gingival pocket with no recession. **B,** Periodontal pocket of similar depth as in *A,* but with some degree of recession. **C,** Pocket depth same as in *A* and *B,* but with still more recession.

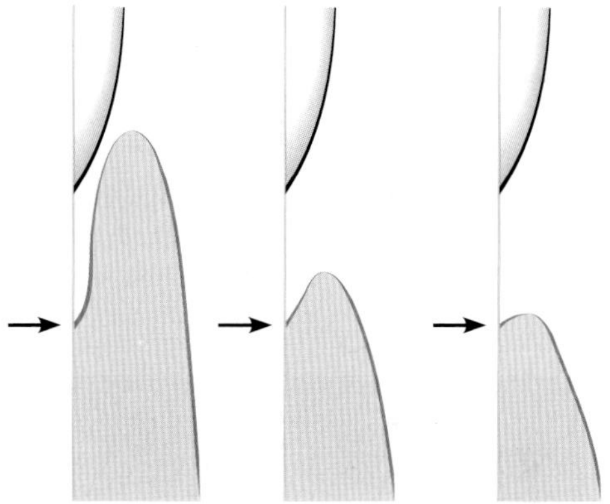

Figure 27-21 Different pocket depths with the same amount of attachment loss. Arrows point to bottom of the pocket. The distance between the arrow and the cementoenamel junctions remains the same despite different pocket depths.

AREA BETWEEN BASE OF POCKET AND ALVEOLAR BONE

Normally, the distance between the apical end of the junctional epithelium and the alveolar bone is relatively constant. The distance between the apical extent of calculus and the alveolar crest in human periodontal pockets is most constant, having a mean length of 1.97 mm (±33.16%).[75,81]

The distance from attached plaque to bone is never less than 0.5 mm and never more than 2.7 mm.[81,82] These findings suggest that the bone-resorbing activity induced by the bacteria is exerted within these distances. However, the finding of isolated bacteria or clumps of bacteria in the connective tissue[64] and on the bone surface[28] may modify these considerations.

RELATIONSHIP OF POCKET TO BONE

In intrabony pockets, the base of the pocket is apical to the crest of the alveolar bone, and the pocket wall lies between the tooth and the bone. Intrabony pockets most often occur interproximally but may be located on the facial and lingual tooth surfaces. Most often the pocket spreads from the surface on which it originated to one or more contiguous surfaces. The base of the suprabony pocket is coronal to the crest of the alveolar bone.

The inflammatory, proliferative, and degenerative changes in intrabony and suprabony pockets are the same, and both types lead to destruction of the supporting periodontal tissues.

Differences between Intrabony and Suprabony Pockets

The principal differences between intrabony and suprabony pockets are the relationship of the soft tissue wall of the pocket to the alveolar bone, the pattern of bone destruction, and the direction of the transseptal fibers of the periodontal ligament[16] (Figures 27-22, 27-23, and 27-24).

When loss of attachment and bone occur as a result of suprabony pockets, the alveolar crest and the periodontal ligament gradually attain a more apical position in relation to the tooth but retain their general morphology and architecture. This is usually associated with a horizontal pattern of bone loss. In intrabony pockets the morphology of the alveolar crest changes completely, with the formation of angular bony defects as a result of vertical bone loss. This may affect the function of the area.[14]

Table 27-2 summarizes The distinguishing features of suprabony and intrabony pockets. The morphologic features of the intrabony pocket are important because they necessitate modification in treatment techniques (see Chapters 65 through 67). The classification of intrabony pockets is discussed in Chapter 28.

PERIODONTAL ABSCESS

A periodontal abscess is a localized purulent inflammation in the periodontal tissues (Figure 27-25). It is also known as a *lateral abscess* or *parietal abscess.* Abscesses localized in the gingiva, caused by injury to the outer surface of the gingiva, and not involving the supporting structures are called *gingival abscesses.* Gingival abscesses may occur in the presence or absence of a periodontal pocket (see Chapter 23).

A

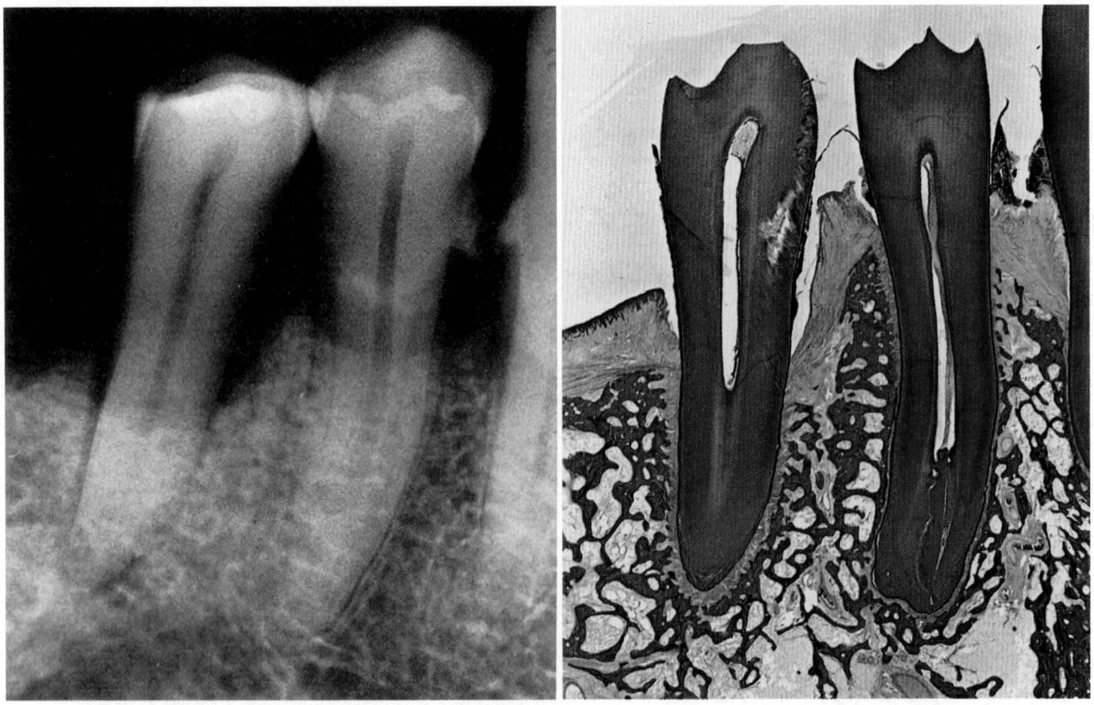

B

Figure 27-22 Radiographic and microscopic features of intrabony pockets. **A,** Radiograph of mandibular canine and premolar area, showing angular bone loss mesial to second premolar. Type of bone loss between first premolar and canine is not radiographically apparent. **B,** Mesiodistal histologic section of teeth seen in *A,* showing intrabony pocket mesial to second premolar, as well as suprabony pockets distal to second premolar and mesial and distal to first premolar. The mesial suprabony pocket of first premolar appears coronal to a vertical bone loss.

C D E F

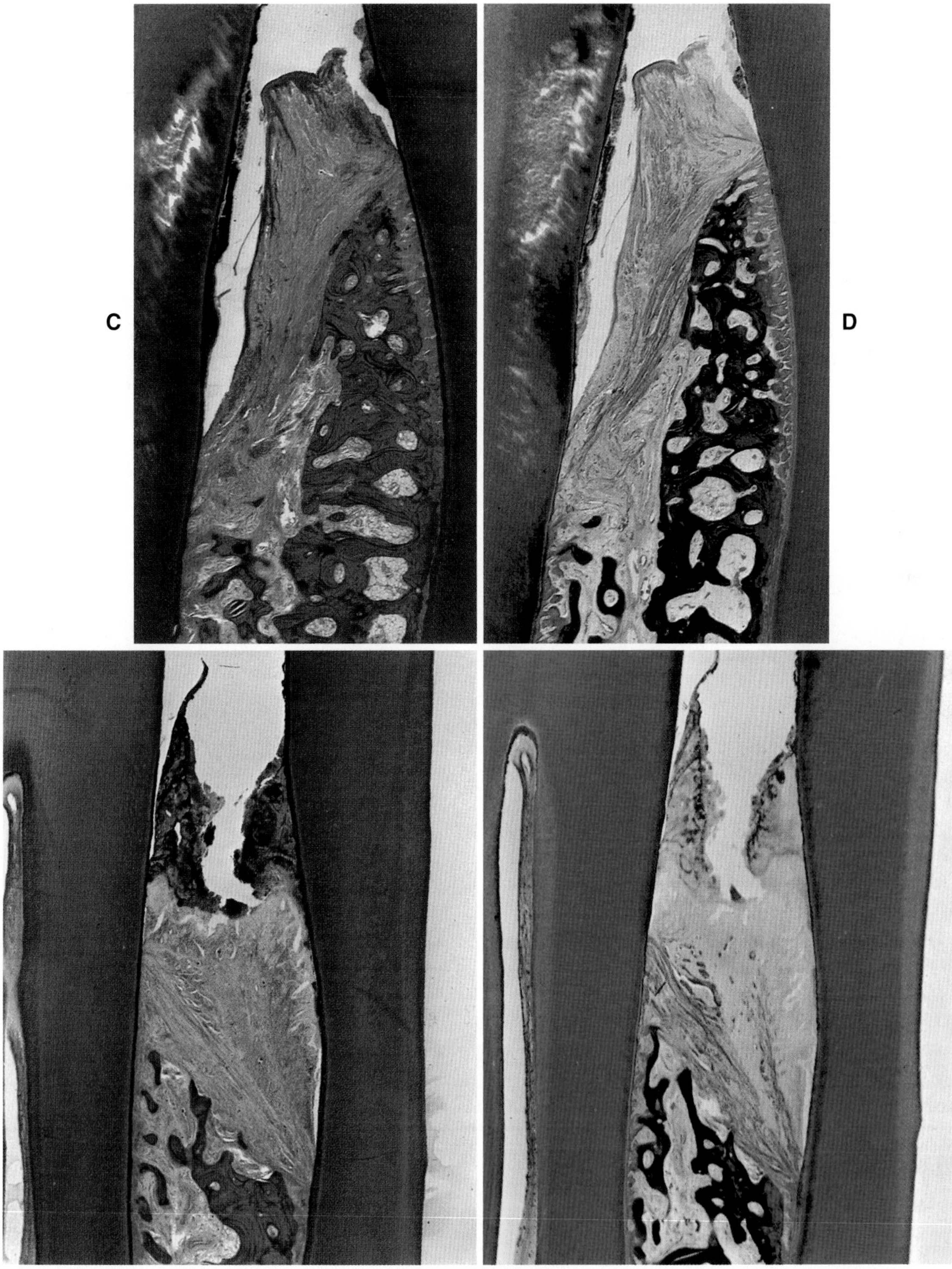

Figure 27-22, cont'd **C,** Higher-power view of area between the premolars. Note the angular bone loss and transseptal fibers covering the bone. **D,** Higher-power view of area between the premolars, stained with Mallory connective tissue stain, clearly showing the direction of transseptal fibers. **E,** Higher-power view of area between first premolar and canine. Note the abundant calculus, dense leukocytic infiltration of the gingiva, and angulation of transseptal fibers and bone. The pocket is still suprabony. **F,** Mallory stain of similar area as in *E.* Note destruction of the gingival fibers caused by inflammation and the angular fibers formed over angular bone loss and less affected by the inflammation. Transseptal fibers extend from distal surface of premolar over crest of alveolar bone into the intrabony pocket. Note the leukocytic infiltration of the transseptal fibers. (From Glickman I, Smulow J: *Periodontal disease: clinical, radiographic and histopathologic features,* Philadelphia, 1974, Saunders.)

Periodontal abscess formation may occur in the following ways:

1. Extension of infection from a periodontal pocket deeply into the supporting periodontal tissues, and localization of the suppurative inflammatory process along the lateral aspect of the root.
2. Lateral extension of inflammation from the inner surface of a periodontal pocket into the connective tissue of the pocket wall. Localization of the abscess results when drainage into the pocket space is impaired (Figure 27-26).
3. Formation in a pocket with a tortuous course around the root. A periodontal abscess may form in the cul-de-sac, the deep end of which is shut off from the surface.
4. Incomplete removal of calculus during treatment of a periodontal pocket. The gingival wall shrinks, occluding the pocket orifice, and a periodontal abscess occurs in the sealed-off portion of the pocket.
5. After trauma to the tooth, or with perforation of the lateral wall of the root in endodontic therapy. In these situations, a periodontal abscess may occur in the absence of periodontal disease.

Periodontal abscesses are classified according to location as follows:

1. Abscess in the *supporting periodontal tissues* along the lateral aspect of the root. In this condition, a sinus

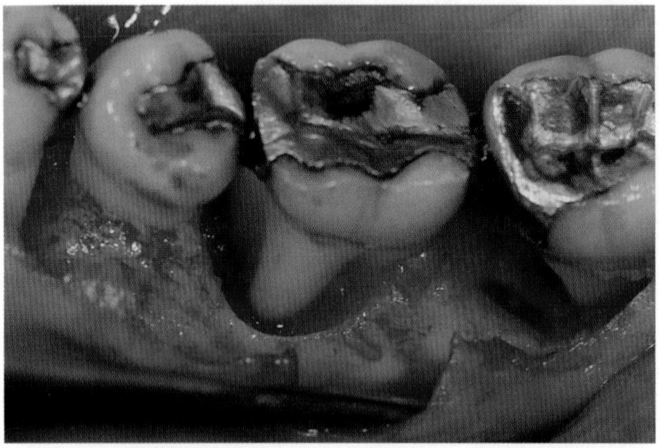

Figure 27-23 After raising a flap for the treatment of the infrabony pockets, the vertical bone loss around the mesial roots of the mandibular first and second molars can be seen.

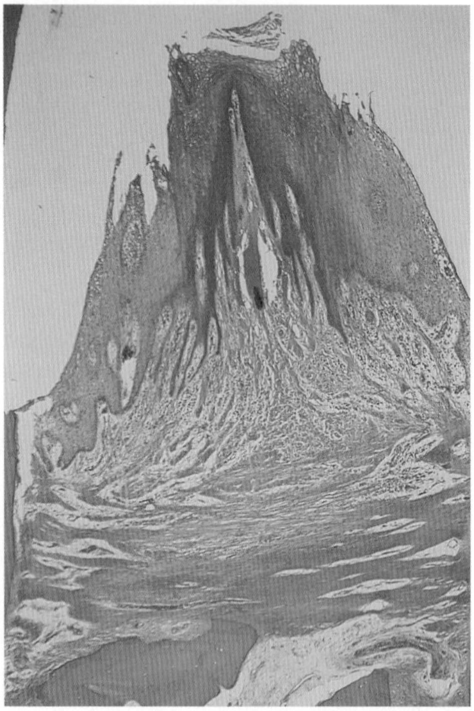

Figure 27-24 Two suprabony pockets in an interdental space. Note the normal horizontal arrangement of the transseptal fibers.

TABLE 27-2

Distinguishing Features of Suprabony and Intrabony Periodontal Pockets

Suprabony Pocket	Intrabony Pocket
1. Base of pocket is coronal to level of alveolar bone.	1. Base of pocket is apical to crest of alveolar bone so that the bone is adjacent to soft tissue wall (see Figure 27-2).
2. Pattern of destruction of underlying bone is horizontal.	2. Pattern of bone destruction is vertical (angular) (see Figures 27-22 and 27-23).
3. Interproximally, transseptal fibers that are restored during progressive periodontal disease are arranged horizontally in the space between base of pocket and alveolar bone (see Figure 27-24).	3. Interproximally, transseptal fibers are oblique rather than horizontal. They extend from cementum beneath base of pocket along alveolar bone and over crest to cementum of adjacent tooth (see Figure 27-22).
4. On facial and lingual surfaces, periodontal ligament fibers beneath pocket follow their normal horizontal-oblique course between the tooth and bone.	4. On facial and lingual surfaces, periodontal ligament fibers follow angular pattern of adjacent bone. They extend from cementum beneath base of pocket along alveolar bone and over crest to join with outer periosteum.

generally occurs in the bone that extends laterally from the abscess to the external surface.
2. Abscess in the *soft tissue wall* of a deep periodontal pocket.

Microscopically, an abscess is a localized accumulation of viable and nonviable PMNs within the periodontal pocket wall. The PMNs liberate enzymes that digest the cells and other tissue structures, forming the liquid product known as *pus,* which constitutes the center of the abscess. An acute inflammatory reaction surrounds the purulent area, and the overlying epithelium exhibits intracellular and extracellular edema and invasion of leukocytes (Figure 27-27).

The localized acute abscess becomes a chronic abscess when its purulent content drains through a fistula into the outer gingival surface or into the periodontal pocket and the infection causing the abscess is not resolved.

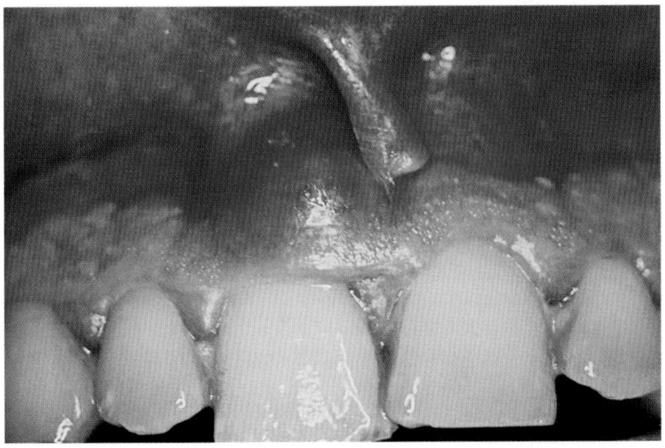

Figure 27-25 Periodontal abscess on an upper right central incisor.

Bacterial invasion of tissues has been reported in abscesses; the invading organisms were identified as gram-negative cocci, diplococci, fusiforms, and spirochetes. Invasive fungi were also found and were interpreted as being "opportunistic invaders."[23] Microorganisms that colonize the periodontal abscess have been reported to be primarily gram-negative anaerobic rods.[55]

PERIODONTAL CYST

The periodontal cyst is an uncommon lesion that produces localized destruction of the periodontal tissues along a lateral root surface, most often in the mandibular canine–premolar area.[25,73]

The following possible etiologies have been suggested:

1. Odontogenic cyst caused by proliferation of the epithelial rests of Malassez; the stimulus initiating the cellular activity is not known.
2. Lateral dentigerous cyst retained in the jaw after tooth eruption.
3. Primordial cyst of supernumerary tooth germ.
4. Stimulation of epithelial rests of the periodontal ligament by infection from a periodontal abscess or the pulp through an accessory root canal.

A periodontal cyst is usually asymptomatic, without grossly detectable changes, but it may present as a localized, tender swelling. Radiographically, an interproximal periodontal cyst appears on the side of the root as a radiolucent area bordered by a radiopaque line. Its radiographic appearance cannot be differentiated from that of a periodontal abscess.

A

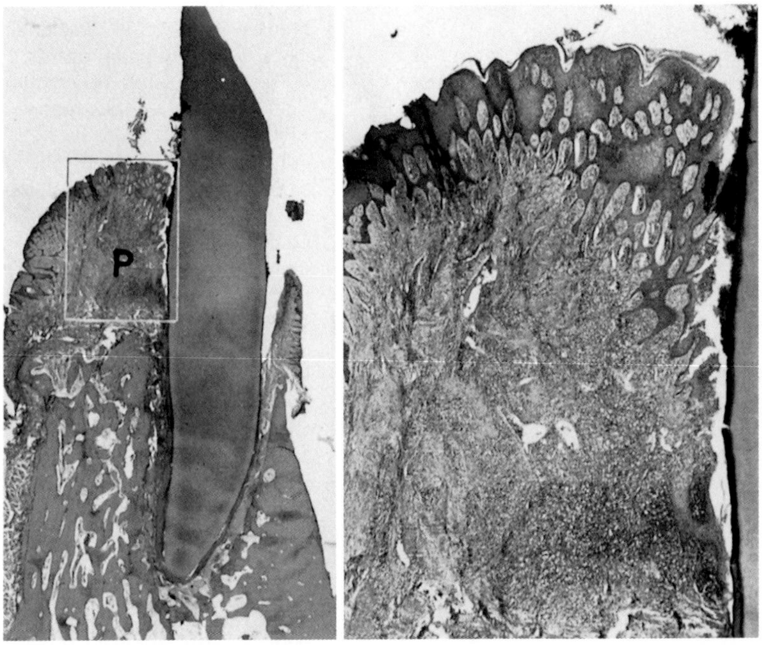

B

Figure 27-26 **A,** Periodontal abscess (*P,* enclosed in rectangle) on lingual surface of mandibular incisor. **B,** Detailed view of periodontal abscess showing dense leukocytic infiltration and suppuration.

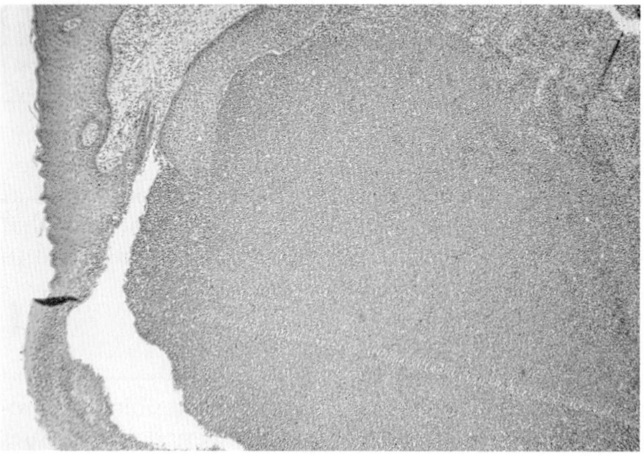

Figure 27-27 Microscopic view of a periodontal abscess showing dense accumulation of polymorphonuclear leukocytes (PMNs) covered by squamous epithelium.

Microscopically, the cystic lining may be (1) a loosely arranged, nonkeratinized, thickened, proliferating epithelium; (2) a thin, nonkeratinized epithelium; or (3) an odontogenic keratocyst.[25]

REFERENCES

1. Adriaens, PA, DeBoever JA: Ultrastructural study of bacterial invasion in roots of periodontally diseased, caries-free human teeth, *J Dent Res* 65:770, 1986.
2. Adriaens PA, DeBoever JA, Loesche WJ: Bacterial invasion in root cementum and radicular dentin of periodontally diseased teeth in humans: a reservoir of periodontopathic bacteria, *J Periodontol* 59:222, 1988.
3. Aleo JJ, Vandersall DC: Cementum: recent concepts related to periodontal disease therapy, *Dent Clin North Am* 24:627, 1980.
4. Aleo JJ, DeRenzis FA, Farber PA: In vitro attachment of human gingival fibroblasts to root surfaces, *J Periodontol* 46:639, 1975.
5. Aleo JJ, DeRenzis FA, Farber PA, et al: The presence and biologic activity of cementum-bound endotoxin, *J Periodontol* 45:672, 1974.
6. Armitage GC, Christie TM: Structural changes in exposed cementum. I. Light microscopic observations, *J Periodontal Res* 8:343, 1973.
7. Armitage GC, Christie TM: Structural changes in exposed cementum. II. Electronmicroscopic observations, *J Periodontal Res* 8:356, 1973.
8. Bass CC: A demonstrable line on extracted teeth indicating the location of the outer border of the epithelial attachment, *J Dent Res* 25:401, 1946.
9. Bass CC: A previously undescribed demonstrable pathologic condition in exposed cementum and the underlying dentine, *Oral Surg* 4:641, 1951.
10. Becks H: Normal and pathologic pocket formation, *J Am Dent Assoc* 16:2167, 1929.
11. Bonakdar MPS, Barber PM, Newman HN: The vasculature in chronic adult periodontitis: a qualitative and quantitative study, *J Periodontol* 68:50, 1997.
12. Bosshardt DD, Selvig KA: Dental cementum: the dynamic tissue covering the root, *Periodontol 2000* 13:41, 1997.
13. Brady JM: A plaque-free zone on human teeth: Scanning and transmission electron microscopy, *J Periodontol* 44:416, 1973.
14. Carranza FA, Carranza FA Jr: The management of alveolar bone in the treatment of the periodontal pocket, *J Periodontol* 27:29, 1956.
15. Carranza FA Jr: Histometric evaluation of periodontal pathology: a review of recent studies, *J Periodontol* 38:741, 1967.
16. Carranza FA Jr, Glickman I: Some observations on the microscopic features of the infrabony pockets, *J Periodontol* 28:33, 1957.
17. Christersson LA, Albini B, Zambon JJ, et al: Tissue localization of *Actinobacillus actinomycetemcomitans* in human periodontitis. I. Light, immunofluorescence and electron-microscopic studies, *J Periodontol* 58:529, 1987.
18. Coons DB, Charbeneau TD, Rivera-Hidalgo F: Quantification of bacterial penetration in spontaneous periodontal disease in beagle dogs, *J Periodontol* 60:23, 1989.
19. Daly CG, Seymour GJ, Kieser JB, et al: Histological assessment of periodontally involved cementum, *J Clin Periodontol* 9:266, 1982.
20. Davenport RH Jr, Simpson DM, Hassell TM: Histometric comparison of active and inactive lesions of advanced periodontitis, *J Periodontol* 53:285, 1982.
21. Deporter DA, Brown DJ: Fine structural observations on the mechanisms of loss of attachment during experimental periodontal disease in the rat, *J Periodontal Res* 15:304, 1980.
22. Deporter DA, Ten Cate AR: Collagen resorption by periodontal ligament fibroblasts at the hard tissue–ligament interfaces of the mouse molar periodontium, *J Periodontol* 51:429, 1980.
23. DeWitt GV, Cobb CM, Killoy WJ: The acute periodontal abscess: microbial penetration of the soft tissue wall, *Int J Periodont Restor Dent* 5:39, 1985.
24. Euler H: Der Epithelansatz in neuere Beleuchtung, *Vjschr Zahnheilk* 29:103, 1923.
25. Fantasia JE: Lateral periodontal cyst: an analysis of 46 cases, *Oral Surg Oral Med Oral Pathol* 48:237, 1979.
26. Fejerskov O, Nyvad B: Pathology and treatment of dental caries in the aging individual. In Holm-Pedersen P, Löe H, editors: *Geriatric dentistry,* Copenhagen, 1986, Munksgaard.
27. Frank RM: Bacterial penetration in the apical wall of advanced human periodontitis, *J Periodontal Res* 15:563, 1980.
28. Frank RM, Voegel RC: Bacterial bone resorption in advanced cases of human periodontitis, *J Periodontal Res* 13:251, 1978.
29. Furseth R: Further observations on the fine structure of orally exposed carious human dental cementum, *Arch Oral Biol* 16:71, 1971.
30. Furseth R, Johanson E: The mineral phase of sound and carious human dental cementum studies by electron microscopy, *Acta Odontol Scand* 28:305, 1970.
31. Giuliana G, Ammatuna P, Pizzo G, et al: Occurrence of invading bacteria in radicular dentin of periodontally diseased teeth: microbiological findings, *J Clin Periodontol* 24:478, 1997.
32. Glickman I, Smulow JB: *Periodontal disease: clinical, radiographic, and histopathologic features,* Philadelphia, 1974, Saunders.
33. Gottlieb B: Der Epithelansatz am Zahne, *Dtsch Monatsschr Zahnheilk* 39:142, 1921.
34. Gottlieb B: Biology of the cementum, *J Periodontol* 13:13, 1942.
35. Graham JW: Toxicity of sterile filtrate from parodontal pockets, *Proc R Soc Med* 30:1165, 1937.
36. Greenstein G, Lamster I: Changing periodontal paradigms: therapeutic implications, *Int J Periodont Restor Dent* 20:337, 2000.
37. Hatfield CG, Baumhammers A: Cytotoxic effects of periodontally involved surfaces of human teeth, *Arch Oral Biol* 16:465, 1971.
38. Herting HC: Electron microscope studies of the cementum surface structures of periodontally healthy and diseased teeth, *J Dent Res* 46(suppl):127, 1967.

39. Hillmann G, Dogan S, Gewrtsen W: Histopathological investigation of gingival tissue from patients with rapidly progressive periodontitis, *J Periodontol* 69:195, 1998.
40. Hoffman ID, Gold W: Distances between plaque and remnants of attached periodontal tissues on extracted teeth, *J Periodontol* 42:29, 1971.
41. Katz RV, Hazen SP, Chilton NW, et al: Prevalence and intraoral distribution of root caries in an adult population, *Caries Res* 16:265, 1982.
42. Krayer JW, Rees TD: Histologic observations on the topography of a human periodontal pocket viewed in transverse step-serial sections, *J Periodontol* 64:585, 1993.
43. Liakoni H, Barber P, Newman HN: Bacterial penetration of pocket soft tissues in chronic adult and juvenile periodontitis cases: an ultrastructural study, *J Clin Periodontol* 14:22, 1987.
44. Lindhe J, Liljenberg B, Listgarten MA: Some microbiological and histopathological features of periodontal disease in man, *J Periodontol* 52:264, 1980.
45. Listgarten MA: Structure of the microbial flora associated with periodontal health and disease in man, *J Periodontol* 47:1, 1976.
46. Listgarten MA: Pathogenesis of periodontitis, *J Clin Periodontol* 13:418, 1986.
47. Listgarten MA, Hellden L: Relative distributions of bacteria at clinically healthy and periodontally diseased sites in humans, *J Clin Periodontol* 5:665, 1978.
48. Lopez NJ, Belvederessi M, de la Sotta R: Inflammatory effects of periodontally diseased cementum studied by autogenous dental root implants in humans, *J Periodontol* 51:582, 1980.
49. McHenry KR, Hausman E, Genco RJ, et al: ^{125}I absorptiometry: alveolar bone mass measurements in untreated periodontal disease, *J Dent Res* 60(suppl A):387, 1981 (abstract).
50. McMillan L, Burrill DY, Fosdick LS: An electron microscope study of particulates in periodontal exudate, J Dent Res 37:51, 1958 (abstract).
51. Meyer DH, Screenivasan PK, Fives-Taylor PM: Evidence for the invasion of a human oral cell line by *Actinobacillus actinomycetemcomitans, Infect Immun* 59:2719, 1991.
52. Mount GJ: Root surface caries: a recurrent dilemma, *Aust Dent J* 31:288, 1986.
53. Müller-Glauser W, Schröder HE: The pocket epithelium: a light and electron microscopic study, *J Periodontol* 53:133, 1982.
54. Nakata T, Stepnick R, Zipkin I: Chemistry of human dental cementum: the effect of age and exposure on the concentration of F, Ca, P and Mg, *J Periodontol* 43:115, 1972.
55. Newman MG, Sims TN: The predominant cultivable microbiota of the periodontal abscess, *J Periodontol* 50:350, 1979.
56. Orban B, Ray AG: Deep necrotic foci in the gingiva, *J Periodontol* 19:91, 1948.
57. Page RC, Schroeder HH: Structure and pathogenesis. In Schluger S, Youdelis R, Page R, editors: *Periodontal disease,* Philadelphia, 1977, Lea & Febiger.
58. Quirynen M, Gizani S, Mongardini C, et al: The effect of periodontal therapy on the number of cariogenic bacteria in different intraoral niches, *J Clin Periodontol* 26:322, 1999.
59. Rautiola CA, Craig RG: The micro hardness of cementum and underlying dentin of normal teeth and teeth exposed to periodontal disease, *J Periodontol* 32:113, 1961.
60. Saglie FR, Johansen JR, Flotra L: The zone of completely and partially destroyed periodontal fibers in pathologic pockets, *J Clin Periodontol* 2:198, 1975.
61. Saglie FR, Johansen JR, Tollefsen T: Plaque-free zones on human teeth in periodontitis, *J Clin Periodontol* 2:190, 1975.
62. Saglie FR, Marfany A, Camargo P: Intragingival occurrence of *Actinobacillus actinomycetemcomitans* and *Bacteroides gingivalis* in active destructive periodontal lesions, *J Periodontol* 59:259, 1988.
63. Saglie FR, Carranza FA Jr, Newman MG, et al: Scanning electron microscopy of the gingival wall of deep periodontal pockets in humans, *J Periodontal Res* 17:284, 1982.
64. Saglie FR, Newman MG, Carranza FA Jr, et al: Bacterial invasion of gingiva in advanced periodontitis in humans, *J Periodontol* 53:217, 1982.
65. Schroeder HE: Quantitative parameters of early human gingival inflammation, *Arch Oral Biol* 15:383, 1970.
66. Schroeder HE, Attstrom R: *The borderland between caries and periodontal disease,* vol 2, London, 1980, Grune & Stratton.
67. Schroeder HE, Listgarten MA: Fine structure of the developing epithelial attachment of human teeth. In *Monographs in developmental biology,* vol 2, Basel, 1977, S Karger.
68. Selvig KA: Ultrastructural changes in cementum and adjacent connective tissue in periodontal disease, *Acta Odontol Scand* 24:459, 1966.
69. Selvig KA: Biological changes at the tooth-saliva interface in periodontal disease, *J Dent Res* 48(suppl):846, 1969.
70. Selvig KA, Hals E: Periodontally diseased cementum studied by correlated microradiography, electron probe analysis and electron microscopy, *J Periodontal Res* 12:419, 1977.
71. Selvig KA, Zander HA: Chemical analysis and microradiography of cementum and dentin from periodontally diseased human teeth, *J Periodontol* 33:303, 1962.
72. Sottosanti JS: A possible relationship between occlusion, root resorption, and the progression of periodontal disease, *J West Soc Periodontol* 25:69, 1977.
73. Spouge JD: A new look at the rests of Malassez: a review of their embryological origin, anatomy, and possible role in periodontal health and disease, *J Periodontol* 51:437, 1980.
74. Standish SN, Shafer WG: The lateral periodontal cyst, *J Periodontol* 29:27, 1958.
75. Stanley HR: The cyclic phenomenon of periodontitis, *Oral Surg Oral Med Oral Pathol* 8:598, 1955.
76. Syed SA, Loesche WJ, Pape HL, et al: Predominant cultivable flora isolated from human root surface caries plaque, *Infect Immun* 11:727, 1975.
77. Taichman N: Potential mechanisms of tissue destruction in periodontal disease, *J Dent Res* 47:928, 1968.
78. Takada T, Donath K: The mechanism of pocket formation: a light microscopic study of undecalcified human material, *J Periodontol* 59:215, 1988.
79. Ten Cate AR: Fibroblasts and their products. In Ten Cate JR, editor: *Oral histology: development, structure, and function,* ed 4, St Louis, 1994, Mosby.
80. Vrahopoulos TP, Barber PM, Newman HN: The apical border plaque in severe periodontitis: an ultrastructural study, *J Periodontol* 66:113, 1995.
81. Wade AB: The relation between the pocket base, the epithelial attachment and the alveolar process. In *Les Parodontopathies,* 16th ARPA Congress, Vienna, 1960.
82. Waerhaug J: The gingival pocket, *Odont Tidsk* 60(suppl 1), 1952.
83. Waerhaug J: The angular bone defect and its relationship to trauma from occlusion and downgrowth of subgingival plaque, *J Clin Periodontol* 6:61, 1979.
84. Waerhaug J: The infrabony pocket and its relationship to trauma from occlusion and subgingival plaque, *J Periodontol* 50:355, 1979.
85. Warren EB, Hanse NM, Swartz ML, et al: Effects of periodontal disease and of calculus solvents on microhardness of cementum, *J Periodontol* 35:505, 1964.
86. Wittwer JW, Dickler EH, Toto PD: Comparative frequencies of plasma cells and lymphocytes in gingivitis, *J Periodontol* 40:274, 1969.
87. Zander HA: The attachment of calculus to root surfaces, *J Periodontol* 24:16, 1953.

Bone Loss and Patterns of Bone Destruction

Fermin A. Carranza and Henry H. Takei

28

CHAPTER

CHAPTER OUTLINE

Although periodontitis is an infectious disease of the gingival tissue, changes that occur in bone are crucial because the destruction of bone is responsible for tooth loss.

The height and density of the alveolar bone are normally maintained by an equilibrium, regulated by local and systemic influences[12,15] between bone formation and bone resorption. When resorption exceeds formation, both bone height and bone density may be reduced.

The level of bone is the consequence of past pathologic experiences, whereas changes in the soft tissue of the pocket wall reflect the present inflammatory condition. Therefore the degree of bone loss is not necessarily correlated with the depth of periodontal pockets, severity of ulceration of the pocket wall, or presence or absence of pus.

BONE DESTRUCTION CAUSED BY EXTENSION OF GINGIVAL INFLAMMATION

The most common cause of bone destruction in periodontal disease is the extension of inflammation from the marginal gingiva into the supporting periodontal tissues. The inflammatory invasion of the bone surface and the initial bone loss that follows mark the transition from gingivitis to periodontitis.

Periodontitis is always preceded by gingivitis, but not all gingivitis progresses to periodontitis. Some cases of gingivitis apparently never become periodontitis, and other cases go through a brief gingivitis phase and rapidly develop into periodontitis. The factors that are responsible for the extension of inflammation to the supporting structures and that initiate the conversion of gingivitis to periodontitis are not known at this time.

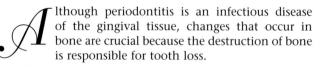

The transition from gingivitis to periodontitis is associated with changes in the composition of bacterial plaque. In advanced stages of disease, the number of motile organisms and spirochetes increases, whereas the number of coccoid rods and straight rods decreases.[36]

The cellular composition of the infiltrated connective tissue also changes with increasing severity of the lesion (see Chapter 21). Fibroblasts and lymphocytes predominate in stage I gingivitis, whereas the number of plasma cells and blast cells increases gradually as the disease progresses. Seymour et al.[66,67] have postulated a stage of "contained" gingivitis in which T lymphocytes are preponderant; they believe that as the lesion becomes a B-lymphocyte lesion, it becomes progressively destructive.

Heijl et al.[24] were able to convert a confined, naturally occurring chronic gingivitis into a progressive periodontitis in experimental animals by placing a silk ligature into the sulcus and tying it around the neck of the tooth. This induced ulceration of the sulcular epithelium, a shift in the connective tissue population from predominantly plasma cells to predominantly polymorphonuclear leukocytes (PMNs), and osteoclastic resorption of the alveolar crest. The recurrence of episodes of acute destruction over time may be one mechanism leading to progressive bone loss in marginal periodontitis.

The extension of inflammation to the supporting structures of a tooth may be modified by the pathogenic potential of plaque or the resistance of the host. The latter includes immunologic activity and other tissue-related mechanisms, such as the degree of fibrosis of the gingiva, probably the width of the attached gingiva, and the reactive fibrogenesis and osteogenesis that occur peripheral to the inflammatory lesion. A fibrin-fibrinolytic system has been mentioned as "walling off" the advancing lesion.[59] The pathway of the spread of inflammation is critical because it affects the pattern of bone destruction in periodontal disease. Considerable controversy exists about the possible changes in the pathway of gingival inflammation caused by trauma from occlusion. The suggested change in the pathway of inflammation, going toward the periodontal ligament rather than to the bone,[13,39] has not been confirmed.[8,68]

Histopathology. Gingival inflammation extends along the collagen fiber bundles and follows the course of the blood vessels through the loosely arranged tissues around them into the alveolar bone[77] (Figure 28-1). Although the inflammatory infiltrate is concentrated in the marginal periodontium, the reaction is a much more diffuse one, often reaching the bone and eliciting a response before evidence of crestal resorption or loss of attachment exists.[45] In the upper molar region, inflammation can extend to the maxillary sinus, resulting in thickening of the sinus mucosa.[44]

Interproximally, inflammation spreads to the loose connective tissue around the blood vessels, through the fibers, and then into the bone through vessel channels that perforate the crest of the interdental septum at the center of the crest (Figure 28-2), toward the side of the crest (Figure 28-3), or at the angle of the septum. Also, inflammation may enter the bone through more than one channel. Less frequently, the inflammation spreads from the gingiva directly into the periodontal ligament and from there into the interdental septum[1] (Figure 28-4).

Facially and lingually, inflammation from the gingiva spreads along the outer periosteal surface of the bone (see Figure 28-4) and penetrates into the marrow spaces through vessel channels in the outer cortex.

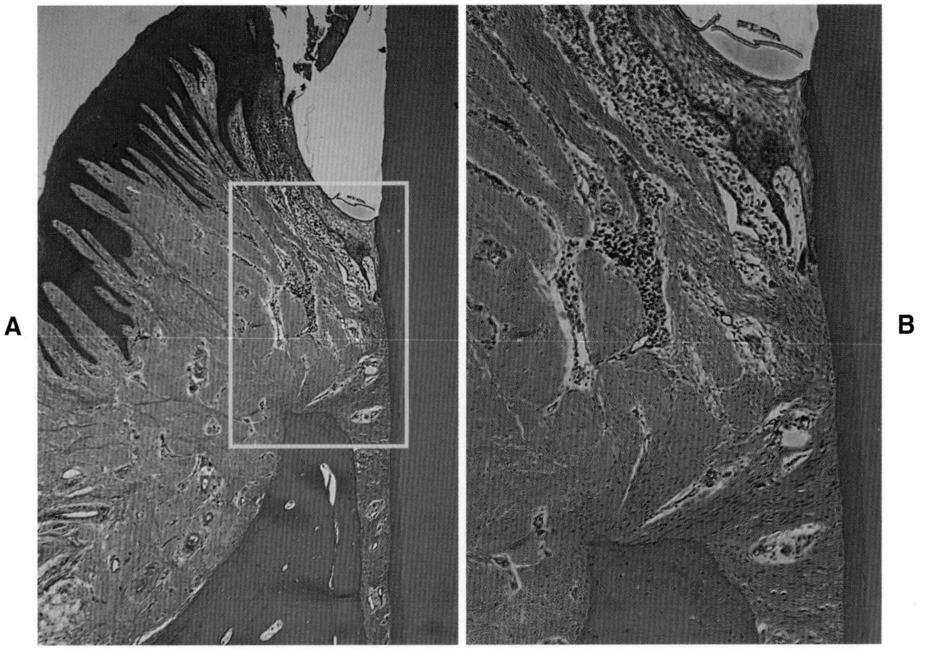

Figure 28-1 **A,** Area of inflammation extending from the gingiva into the suprabony area. **B,** Extension of inflammation along blood vessels and between collagen bundles.

Along its course from the gingiva to the bone, the inflammation destroys the gingival and transseptal fibers, reducing them to disorganized granular fragments interspersed among the inflammatory cells and edema.[49] However, there is a continuous tendency to recreate transseptal fibers across the crest of the interdental septum farther along the root as the bone destruction progresses (Figure 28-5). As a result, transseptal fibers are present, even in cases of extreme periodontal bone loss.

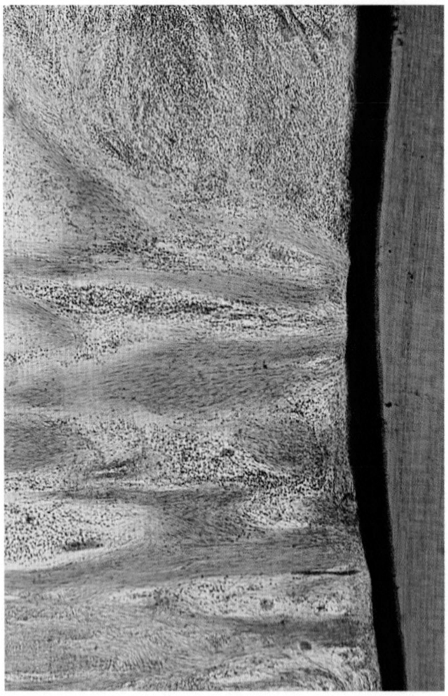

Figure 28-2 Inflammation extending from the pocket area *(top)* between the collagen fibers, which are partially destroyed.

The dense transseptal fibers are of clinical importance when surgical procedures are used to eradicate periodontal pockets. They form a firm covering over the bone, which is encountered after the superficial granulation tissue is removed.[54]

After inflammation reaches the bone by extension from the gingiva (Figure 28-6), it spreads into the marrow spaces and replaces the marrow with a leukocytic and fluid exudate, new blood vessels, and proliferating fibroblasts (Figure 28-7). Multinuclear osteoclasts and mononuclear phagocytes increase in number, and the bone surfaces appear, lined with Howship lacunae (Figure 28-8).

In the marrow spaces, resorption proceeds from within, causing a thinning of the surrounding bony trabeculae and enlargement of the marrow spaces, followed by destruction of the bone and a reduction in bone height. Normally fatty bone marrow is partially or totally replaced by a fibrous type of marrow in the vicinity of the resorption (see Figure 28-8).

Bone destruction in periodontal disease is not a process of bone necrosis.[29] It involves the activity of living cells along viable bone. When tissue necrosis and pus are present in periodontal disease, they occur in the soft tissue walls of periodontal pockets, not along the resorbing margin of the underlying bone.

A 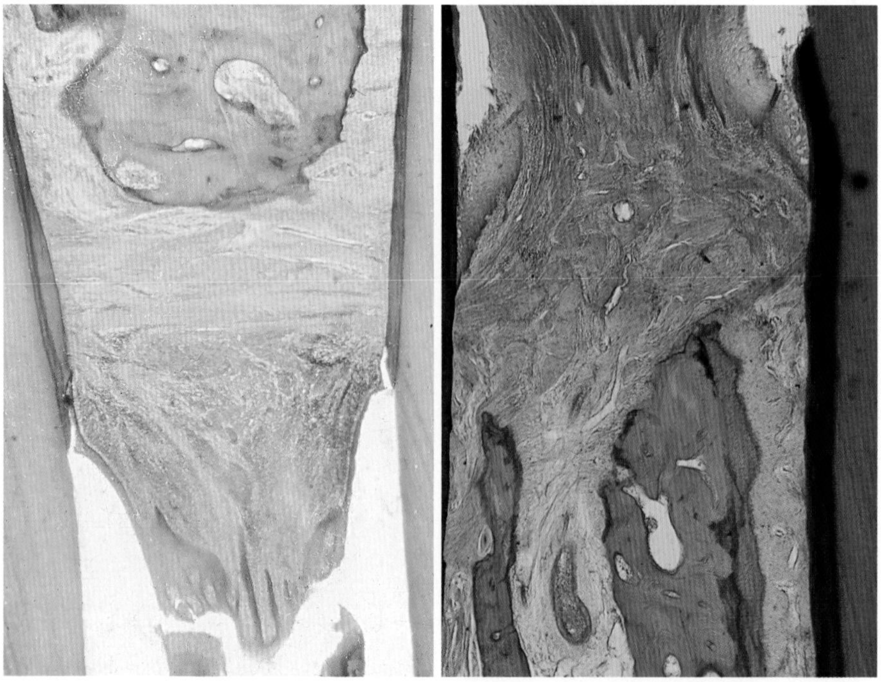 B

Figure 28-3 **A,** Extension of inflammation into the center of the interdental septum. Inflammation from the gingiva penetrates the transseptal fibers and enters the bone around blood vessel in the center of the septum. **B,** Cortical layer at the top of the septum has been destroyed, and the inflammation penetrates into the marrow spaces.

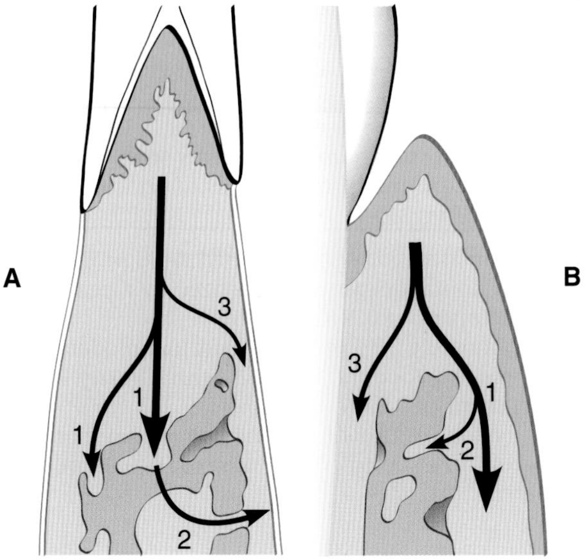

Figure 28-4 Pathways of inflammation from the gingiva into the supporting periodontal tissues in periodontitis. **A,** Interproximally, from the gingiva into the bone *(1)*, from the bone into the periodontal ligament *(2)*, and from the gingiva into the periodontal ligament *(3)*. **B,** Facially and lingually, from the gingiva along the outer periosteum *(1)*, from the periosteum into the bone *(2)*, and from the gingiva into the periodontal ligament *(3)*.

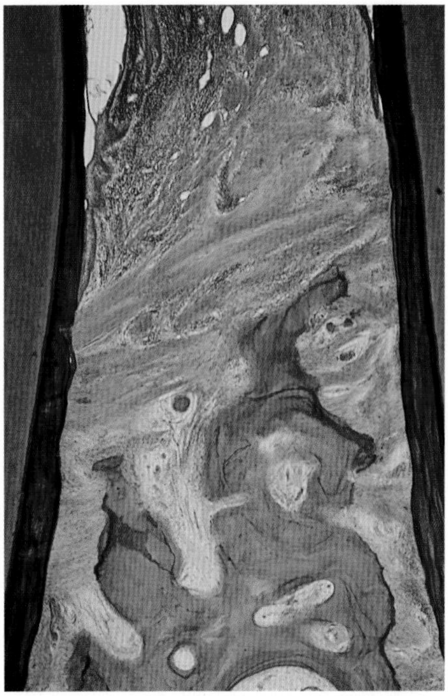

Figure 28-5 Re-formation of transseptal fibers. Mesiodistal section through interdental septum showing gingival inflammation and bone loss. Recreated transseptal fibers can be seen above the bone margin, partially infiltrated by the inflammatory process.

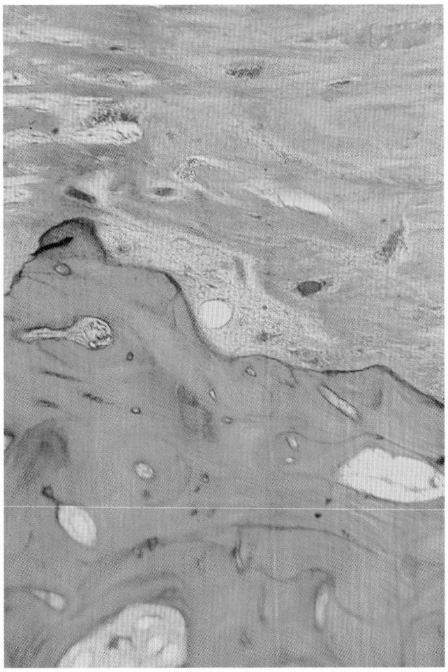

Figure 28-6 Extension of inflammation has reached the crestal bone surface.

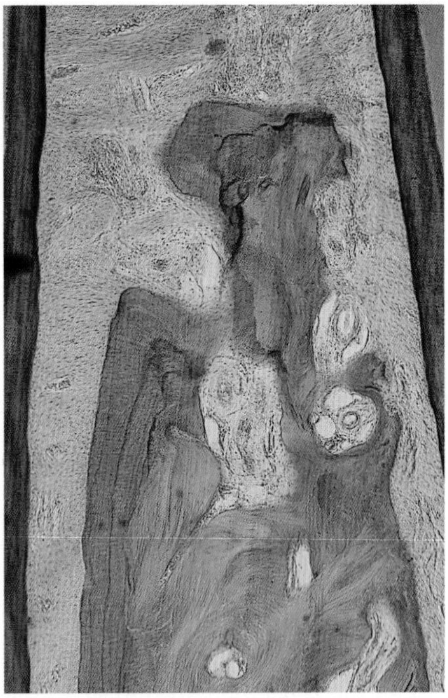

Figure 28-7 Interdental septum in human autopsy section. Extensive inflammatory infiltrate has invaded the marrow spaces, entering from both the mesial and the distal aspect. Fatty bone marrow has been replaced by inflammatory cells and fibrous marrow.

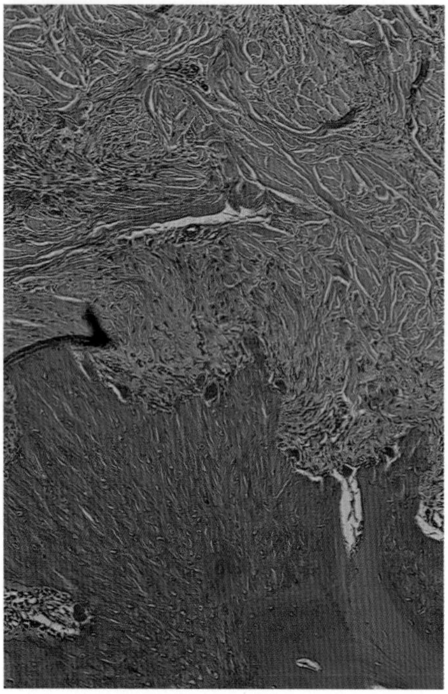

Figure 28-8 Osteoclasts and Howship lacunae in the resorption of crestal bone.

> The amount of inflammatory infiltrate correlates with the degree of bone loss but not with the number of osteoclasts. However, the distance from the apical border of the inflammatory infiltrate to the alveolar bone crest correlates with both the number of osteoclasts on the alveolar crest and the total number of osteoclasts.[58] Similar findings have been reported in experimentally induced periodontitis in animals.[34]

Radius of Action

Garant and Cho[11] suggested that locally produced bone resorption factors may need to be present in the proximity of the bone surface to exert their action. Page and Schroeder,[53] on the basis of Waerhaug's measurements made on human autopsy specimens,[74,75] postulated a range of effectiveness of about 1.5 to 2.5 mm within which bacterial plaque can induce loss of bone. Beyond 2.5 mm there is no effect; interproximal angular defects can appear only in spaces that are wider than 2.5 mm because narrower spaces would be destroyed entirely. Tal[70] corroborated this with measurements in human patients.

Large defects greatly exceeding a distance of 2.5 mm from the tooth surface (as described in aggressive types of periodontitis) may be caused by the presence of bacteria in the tissues.[6,10,62]

Rate of Bone Loss

In a study of Sri Lankan tea laborers with no oral hygiene and no dental care, Löe et al.[37] found the rate of bone loss to average about 0.2 mm a year for facial surfaces and about 0.3 mm a year for proximal surfaces when periodontal disease was allowed to progress untreated.[37] However, the rate of bone loss may vary, depending on the type of disease present. Löe et al.[38] identified the following three subgroups of patients with periodontal disease based on interproximal loss of attachment* and tooth mortality:

1. Approximately 8% of persons had rapid progression of periodontal disease, characterized by a yearly loss of attachment of 0.1 to 1.0 mm.
2. Approximately 81% of individuals had moderately progressive periodontal disease, with a yearly loss of attachment of 0.05 to 0.5 mm.
3. The remaining 11% of persons had minimal or no progression of destructive disease (0.05-0.09 mm yearly).

Periods of Destruction

Periodontal destruction occurs in an episodic, intermittent manner, with periods of inactivity or quiescence. The destructive periods result in loss of collagen and alveolar bone with deepening of the periodontal pocket. The reasons for the onset of destructive periods have not been totally elucidated, although the following theories have been offered:

1. Bursts of destructive activity are associated with subgingival ulceration and an acute inflammatory reaction, resulting in rapid loss of alveolar bone.[53,64]
2. Bursts of destructive activity coincide with the conversion of a predominantly T-lymphocyte lesion to one with a predominantly B-lymphocyte–plasma cell infiltrate.[67]
3. Periods of exacerbation are associated with an increase of the loose, unattached, motile, gram-negative, anaerobic pocket flora, and periods of remission coincide with the formation of a dense, unattached, nonmotile, gram-positive flora with a tendency to mineralize.[47]
4. Tissue invasion by one or several bacterial species is followed by an advanced local host defense that controls the attack.[61]

Mechanisms of Bone Destruction

The factors involved in bone destruction in periodontal disease are bacterial and host mediated. Bacterial plaque products induce the differentiation of bone progenitor cells into osteoclasts and stimulate gingival cells to release mediators that have the same effect.[23,65] Plaque products and inflammatory mediators can also act directly on osteoblasts or their progenitors, inhibiting their action and reducing their numbers.

In addition, in rapidly progressing diseases such as aggressive periodontitis, bacterial microcolonies or single bacterial cells may be present between collagen fibers and over the bone surface, suggesting a direct effect.[6,65]

*Loss of attachment can be equated with loss of bone, although attachment loss precedes bone loss by about 6 to 8 months.[21]

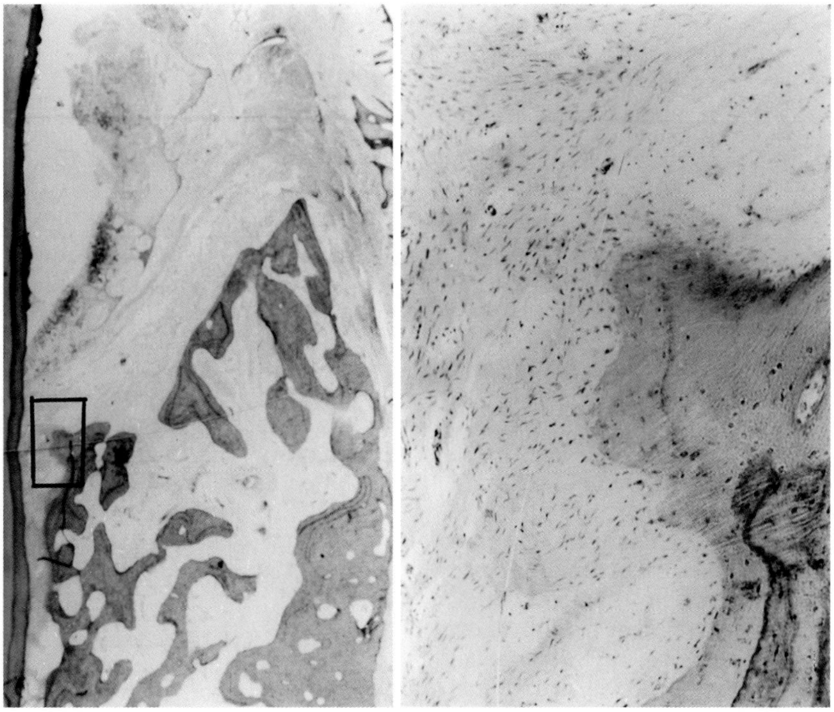

Figure 28-9 Bone formation in untreated periodontal disease. **A,** Section showing an intrabony pocket with deep angular bone loss. **B,** Magnification of the rectangular area in *A,* showing newly formed bone at bottom of defect.

Several host factors released by inflammatory cells are capable of inducing bone resorption in vitro and can play a role in periodontal disease. These include host-produced prostaglandins and their precursors, interleukin-1α (IL-1α) and IL-β, and tumor necrosis factor alpha (TNF-α).

When injected intradermally, prostaglandin E_2 (PGE_2) induces the vascular changes seen in inflammation; when injected over a bone surface, PGE_2 induces bone resorption in the absence of inflammatory cells and with few multinucleated osteoclasts.[18,28] In addition, nonsteroidal antiinflammatory drugs (NSAIDs), such as flurbiprofen and ibuprofen, inhibit PGE_2 production, slowing bone loss in naturally occurring periodontal disease in beagle dogs and humans. This effect occurs without changes in gingival inflammation and rebounds 6 months after cessation of drug administration.[27,78] (See also Chapters 9, 12, 13 and 15.)

Bone Formation in Periodontal Disease

Areas of bone formation are also found immediately adjacent to sites of active bone resorption (Figure 28-9) and along trabecular surfaces at a distance from the inflammation, in an apparent effort to reinforce the remaining bone (buttressing bone formation). This osteogenic response is clearly found in experimentally produced periodontal bone loss in animals.[7] In humans, it is less obvious but has been confirmed by histometric[4,5] and histologic studies.[14]

The response of alveolar bone to inflammation includes bone formation and resorption; thus, bone loss in periodontal disease is not simply a destructive process but results from the predominance of resorption over formation. New bone formation impairs the rate of bone loss, compensating in some degree for the bone destroyed by inflammation.

Autopsy specimens from individuals with untreated disease occasionally show areas where bone resorption has ceased and new bone is being formed on previously eroded bone margins. This confirms the intermittent character of bone resorption in periodontal disease and is consistent with the varied rates of progression observed clinically in untreated periodontal disease.

These periods of remission and exacerbation (or inactivity and activity, respectively) appear to coincide with the quiescence or exacerbation of gingival inflammation, manifested by changes in the extent of bleeding, amount of exudate, and composition of bacterial plaque (see Chapter 26).

The presence of bone formation in response to inflammation, even in active periodontal disease, has an effect on the outcome of treatment. The basic aim of periodontal therapy is the elimination of inflammation to remove the stimulus for bone resorption and therefore allow the inherent constructive tendencies to predominate.

BONE DESTRUCTION CAUSED BY TRAUMA FROM OCCLUSION

Another cause of periodontal destruction is trauma from occlusion, which can produce bone destruction in the absence or presence of inflammation (see Chapter 29).

In the absence of inflammation, the changes caused by trauma from occlusion vary from increased compression

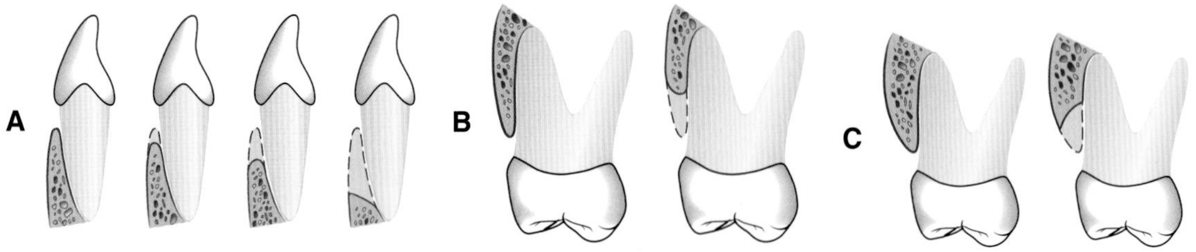

Figure 28-10 **A,** Lower incisor with thin labial bone. Bone loss can become vertical only when it reaches thicker bone in apical areas. **B,** Upper molars with thin facial bone, where only horizontal bone loss can occur. **C,** Upper molar with a thick facial bone, allowing for vertical bone loss.

and tension of the periodontal ligament and increased osteoclasis of alveolar bone to necrosis of the periodontal ligament and bone and the resorption of bone and tooth structure. These changes are reversible in that they can be repaired if the offending forces are removed. However, persistent trauma from occlusion results in funnel-shaped widening of the crestal portion of the periodontal ligament, with resorption of the adjacent bone.[35] These changes, which may cause the bony crest to have an angular shape, represent adaptation of the periodontal tissues aimed at "cushioning" increased occlusal forces, but the modified bone shape may weaken tooth support and cause tooth mobility.

When combined with inflammation, trauma from occlusion aggravates the bone destruction caused by the inflammation[35] and results in bizarre bone patterns.

BONE DESTRUCTION CAUSED BY SYSTEMIC DISORDERS

Local and systemic factors regulate the physiologic equilibrium of bone. When a generalized tendency toward bone resorption exists, bone loss initiated by local inflammatory processes may be magnified.

This systemic influence on the response of alveolar bone, as envisioned by Glickman[12] in the early 1950s, considers a systemic component in all cases of periodontal disease. In addition to the amount and virulence of plaque bacteria, the nature of the systemic component, not its presence or absence, influences the severity of periodontal destruction. This concept of a role played by systemic defense mechanisms has been validated, particularly by studies of immune deficiencies in severely destructive types of periodontitis.

In recent years, interest has increased in the possible relationship between periodontal bone loss and osteoporosis. *Osteoporosis* is a physiologic condition of postmenopausal women, resulting in loss of bone mineral content and structural bone changes. Periodontitis and osteoporosis share a number of risk factors (e.g., aging, smoking, diseases, medications that interfere with healing). Few studies on the relationship between periodontitis and osteoporosis are available, and some show relationships between skeletal density and oral bone density and between crestal height and residual ridge resorption. In 1968, Groen et al.[20] reported relationships between osteopenia and periodontal disease, tooth mobility, and tooth loss. Several more recent studies have indicated that such an association may exist, but final proof is lacking[25,26,62,73] (see Chapter 43).

Periodontal bone loss may also occur in generalized skeletal disturbances (e.g., hyperparathyroidism, leukemia, Langerhans cell histiocytosis) by mechanisms that may be totally unrelated to the usual periodontal problem.

FACTORS DETERMINING BONE MORPHOLOGY IN PERIODONTAL DISEASE

Normal Variation in Alveolar Bone

Considerable normal variation exists in the morphologic features of alveolar bone (see Chapter 5), which affects the osseous contours produced by periodontal disease. The anatomic features that substantially affect the bone-destructive pattern in periodontal disease include the following:

- The thickness, width, and crestal angulation of the interdental septa
- The thickness of the facial and lingual alveolar plates
- The presence of fenestrations and dehiscences
- The alignment of the teeth
- Root and root trunk anatomy
- Root position within the alveolar process
- Proximity with another tooth surface

For example, angular osseous defects cannot form in thin facial or lingual alveolar plates, which have little or no cancellous bone between the outer and inner cortical layers. In such cases the entire crest of the plate is destroyed, and the height of the bone is reduced (Figure 28-10).

Exostoses

Exostoses are outgrowths of bone of varied size and shape. Palatal exostoses have been found in 40% of human skulls.[46] They can occur as small nodules, large nodules, sharp ridges, spike-like projections, or any combination of these (Figure 28-11). Exostoses have been described in rare cases as developing after the placement of free gingival grafts.[50]

Trauma from Occlusion

Trauma from occlusion may be a factor in determining the dimension and shape of bone deformities. It may

A 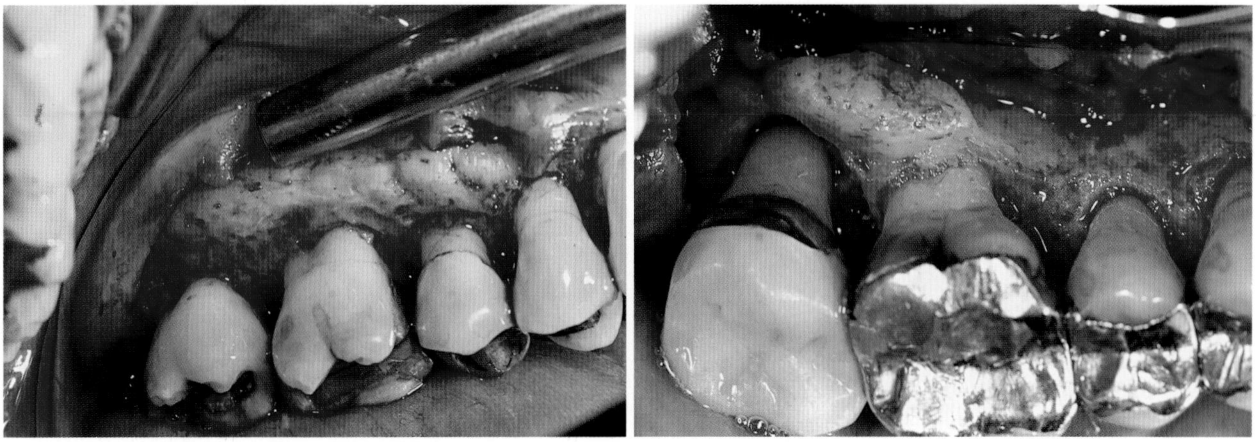 B

Figure 28-11 **A,** Exostosis in the facial aspect of upper second premolar and molars. **B,** Exostosis in the palatal aspect of first and second molars. Note also the circumferential defect in the second molar (left).

cause a thickening of the cervical margin of alveolar bone or a change in the morphology of the bone (e.g., angular defects, buttressing bone) on which inflammatory changes will later be superimposed.

Buttressing Bone Formation (Lipping)

Bone formation sometimes occurs in an attempt to buttress bony trabeculae weakened by resorption. When it occurs within the jaw, it is termed *central buttressing bone formation.* When it occurs on the external surface, it is referred to as *peripheral buttressing bone formation.*[14] The latter may cause bulging of the bone contour, termed *lipping,* which sometimes accompanies the production of osseous craters and angular defects (Figure 28-12).

Food Impaction

Interdental bone defects often occur where proximal contact is abnormal or absent. Pressure and irritation from food impaction contribute to the inverted bone architecture. In some cases the poor proximal relationship may result from a shift in tooth position because of extensive bone destruction preceding food impaction. In such patients, food impaction is a complicating factor rather than the cause of the bone defect.

Aggressive Periodontitis

A vertical or angular pattern of alveolar bone destruction is found around the first molars in aggressive periodontitis. The cause of the localized bone destruction in this type of periodontal disease is unknown (see Chapter 33).

BONE DESTRUCTION PATTERNS IN PERIODONTAL DISEASE

Periodontal disease alters the morphologic features of the bone in addition to reducing bone height. An understanding of the nature and pathogenesis of these alterations is essential for effective diagnosis and treatment.

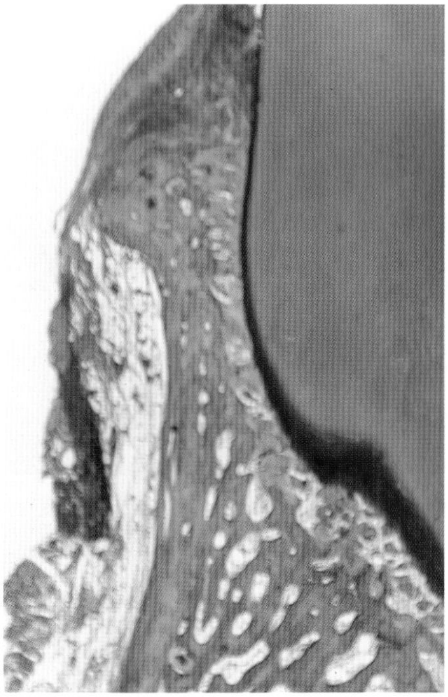

Figure 28-12 Lipping of facial bone. Peripheral buttressing bone formation along external surface of the facial bony plate and at the crest. Note the deformity in the bone produced by the buttressing bone formation and the bulging of the mucosa.

Horizontal Bone Loss

Horizontal bone loss is the most common pattern of bone loss in periodontal disease. The bone is reduced in height, but the bone margin remains approximately perpendicular to the tooth surface. The interdental septa and facial and lingual plates are affected, but not necessarily to an equal degree around the same tooth (Figure 28-13, *A*).

A B

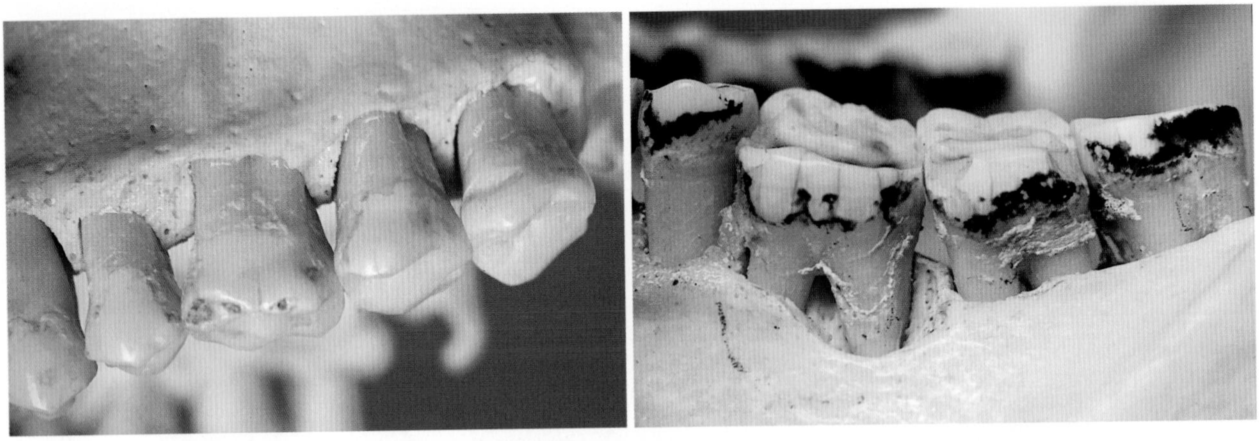

Figure 28-13 **A,** Horizontal bone loss. Note the reduction in height of the marginal bone, exposing cancellous bone and reaching the furcation of the second molar. **B,** Vertical (angular) bone loss on the distal root of the first molar.

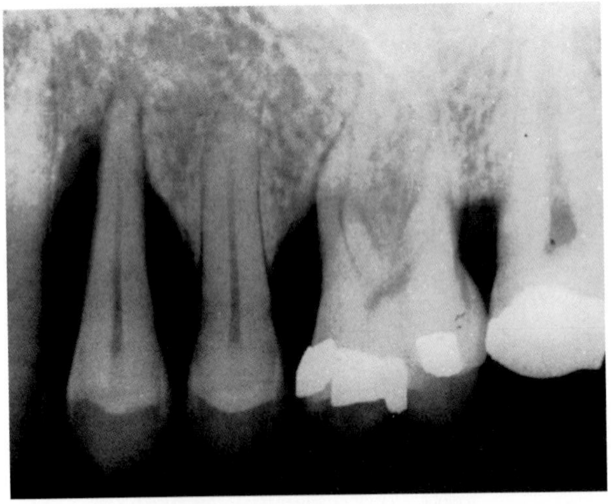

Figure 28-14 Angular (vertical) defects of different depths.

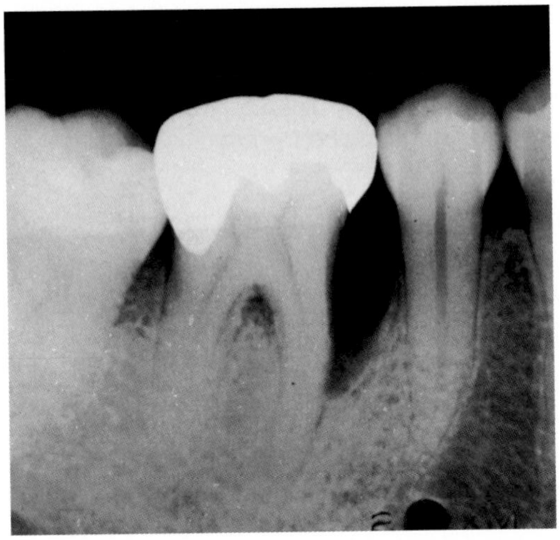

Figure 28-15 Angular defect on mesial surface of the first molar. Note also the furcation involvement.

Bone Deformities (Osseous Defects)

Different types of bone deformities can result from periodontal disease. These usually occur in adults and have been reported in human skulls with deciduous dentitions.[30] Their presence may be suggested on radiographs, but careful probing and surgical exposure of the areas are required to determine their exact conformation and dimensions.

Vertical or Angular Defects

Vertical or angular defects are those that occur in an oblique direction, leaving a hollowed-out trough in the bone alongside the root; the base of the defect is located apical to the surrounding bone (Figures 28-13, *B*; 28-14; and 28-15). In most instances, angular defects have accompanying intrabony periodontal pockets; intrabony pockets, however, always have an underlying angular defect.

Angular defects are classified on the basis of the number of osseous walls.[17] Angular defects may have one, two, or three walls (Figures 28-16 to 28-19). The number of walls in the apical portion of the defect may be greater than that in its occlusal portion, in which case the term *combined osseous defect* is used (Figure 23-20).

Vertical defects occurring interdentally can generally be seen on the radiograph, although thick, bony plates sometimes may obscure them. Angular defects can also appear on facial and lingual or palatal surfaces, but these defects are not seen on radiographs. Surgical exposure is the only sure way to determine the presence and configuration of vertical osseous defects.

Vertical defects increase with age.[48,52,79] Approximately 60% of persons with interdental angular defects have only a single defect.[48] Vertical defects detected radiographically have been reported to appear most often on the distal surfaces[48] and mesial surfaces.[52,79] However, three-wall defects are more frequently found on the mesial surfaces of upper and lower molars.[31]

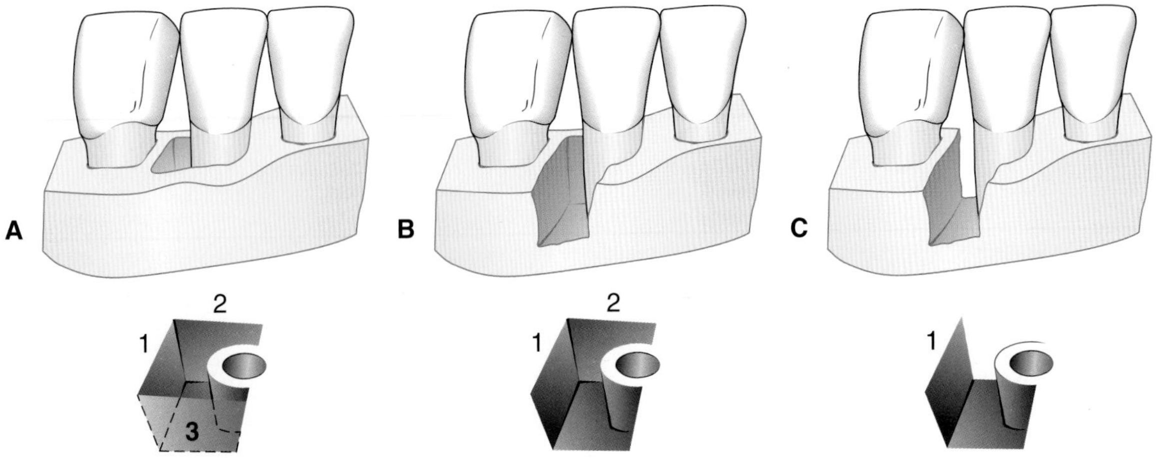

Figure 28-16 One-, two-, and three-walled vertical defects on right lateral incisor. **A,** Three bony walls: distal *(1)*, lingual *(2)*, and facial *(3)*. **B,** Two-wall defect: distal *(1)* and lingual *(2)*. **C,** One-wall defect: distal wall only *(1)*.

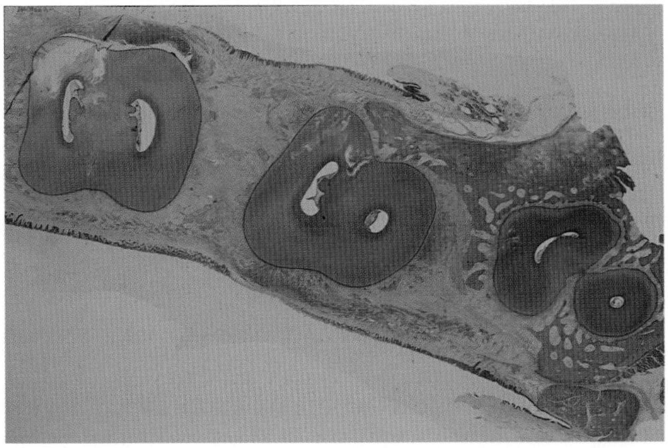

Figure 28-17 Horizontal section of lower molars at midroot level, showing a two-wall osseous defect distal to second molar.

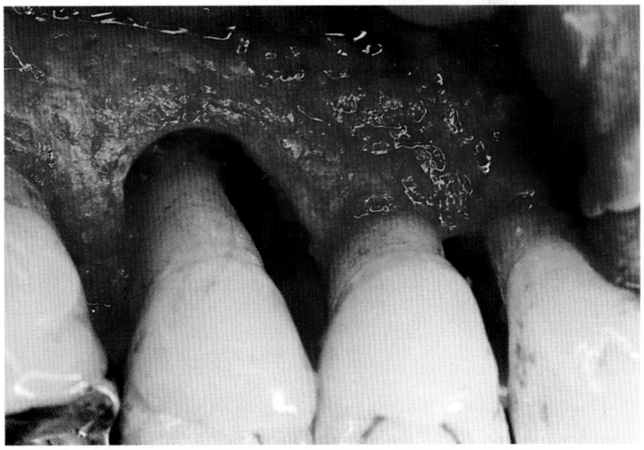

Figure 28-19 Circumferential vertical defect in relation to the upper premolar and canine.

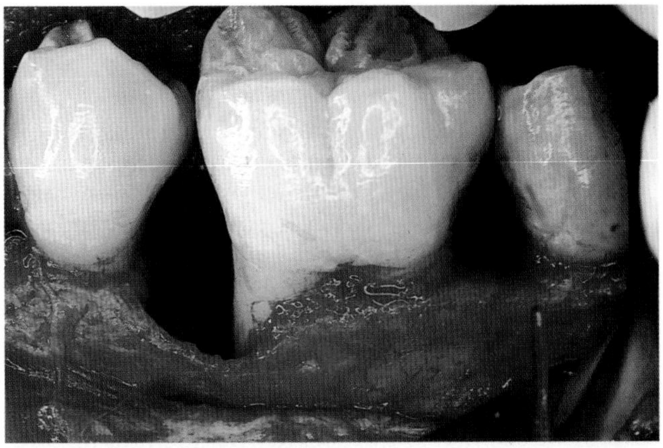

Figure 28-18 One-wall vertical defect on mesial surface of the left lateral incisor and one-wall defect (distal wall and half of labial wall) on distal surface of the right lateral incisor.

SCIENCE TRANSFER

A variety of bone loss patterns occur in periodontitis. Although the amount of bone loss in patients with untreated periodontal disease averages 0.2 to 0.3 mm per year, approximately 8% of the population has aggressive, rapid bone loss, and 11% has minimal bone destruction. *Clinicians need to treat patients who have aggressive bone loss with a prompt and extensive plan of therapy focusing on periodontal surgery, whereas those who have minimal bone-destructive activity can be treated with therapies focusing on periodontal maintenance.*

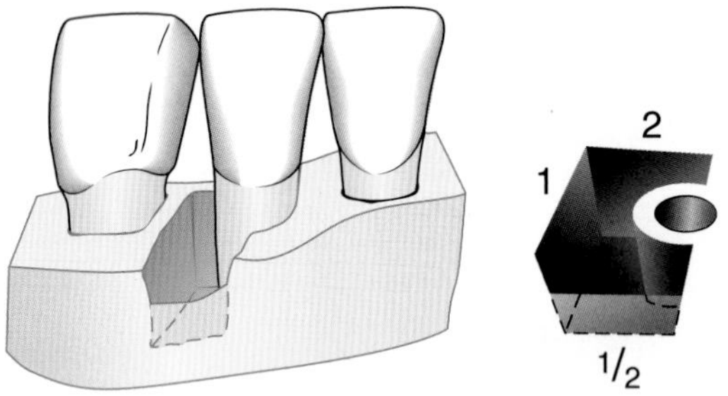

Figure 28-20 Combined type of osseous defect. Because the facial wall is half the height of the distal *(1)* and lingual *(2)* walls, this is an osseous defect with three walls in its apical half and two walls in the occlusal half.

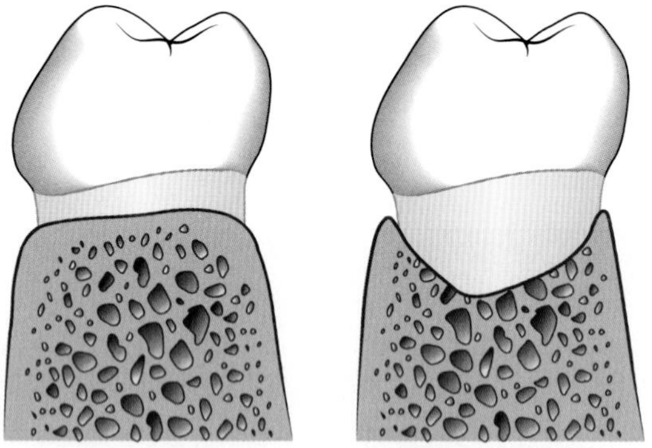

Figure 28-21 Diagrammatic representation of an osseous crater in a faciolingual section between two lower molars. *Left,* Normal bone contour. *Right,* Osseous crater.

The three-wall vertical defect was originally called an *intrabony defect.** This defect appears most frequently on the mesial aspects of second and third maxillary and mandibular molars. The one-wall vertical defect is also called a *hemiseptum.*

Osseous Craters

Osseous craters are concavities in the crest of the interdental bone confined within the facial and lingual walls (Figure 28-21). Craters have been found to make up about one third (35.2%) of all defects and about two thirds (62%) of all mandibular defects and occur twice as often in posterior segments as in anterior segments.[42,43]

The heights of the facial and lingual crests of a crater have been found to be identical in 85% of cases, with the remaining 15% being almost equally divided between higher facial crests and higher lingual crests.[60] The following reasons for the high frequency of interdental craters have been suggested[40,41,60]:

- The interdental area collects plaque and is difficult to clean.
- The normal flat or even concave faciolingual shape of the interdental septum in lower molars may favor crater formation.
- Vascular patterns from the gingiva to the center of the crest may provide a pathway for inflammation.

*The term *intrabony* was later expanded to designate all vertical defects.

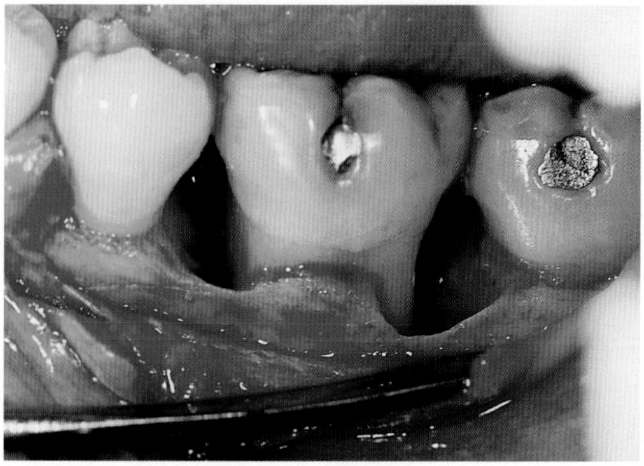

Figure 28-22 Reversed architecture. Elevated flap shows irregular bone margin.

Bulbous Bone Contours

Bulbous bone contours are bony enlargements caused by exostoses (see Figure 28-11), adaptation to function, or buttressing bone formation. They are found more frequently in the maxilla than in the mandible.

Reversed Architecture

Reversed architecture defects are produced by loss of interdental bone, including the facial plates and lingual plates, without concomitant loss of radicular bone, thereby reversing the normal architecture (Figure 28-22). Such defects are more common in the maxilla.[48]

Ledges

Ledges are plateaulike bone margins caused by resorption of thickened bony plates (Figure 28-23).

Furcation Involvement

The term *furcation involvement* refers to the invasion of the bifurcation and trifurcation of multirooted teeth by periodontal disease. The prevalence of furcation-involved molars is not clear.[9,51] Whereas some reports indicate that the mandibular first molars are the most common sites and the maxillary premolars are the least common,[32] other studies have found higher prevalence in upper molars.[70] The number of furcation involvements increases with age.[32,33]

The denuded furcation may be visible clinically or covered by the wall of the pocket. The extent of involvement is determined by exploration with a blunt probe, along with a simultaneous blast of warm air to facilitate visualization (Figure 28-24).

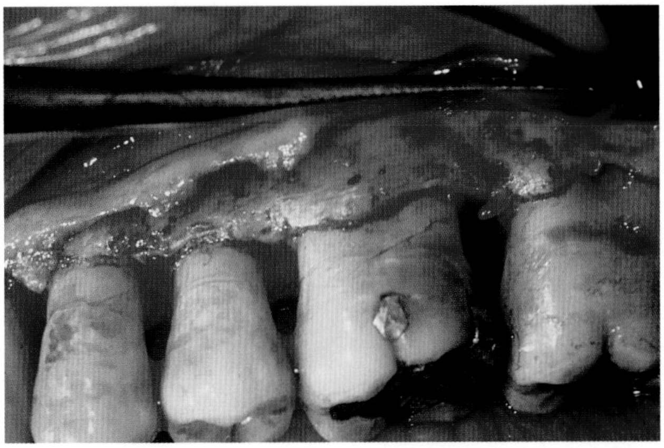

Figure 28-23 Ledge produced by interproximal resorption.

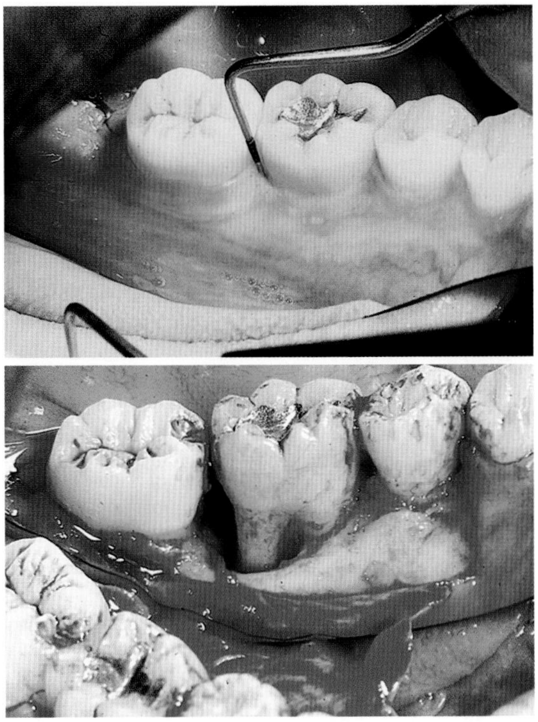

Figure 28-24 **A,** Molar with slightly inflamed gingiva clinically; however, it has a deep distal pocket. **B,** Flap elevation reveals extensive bone loss and furcation involvement. (Courtesy Dr. Terry Fiori, Palo Alto, Calif.)

Furcation involvements have been classified as grades I, II, III, and IV according to the amount of tissue destruction. Grade I is incipient bone loss, grade II is partial bone loss (cul-de-sac), and grade III is total bone loss with through-and-through opening of the furcation. Grade IV is similar to grade III, but with gingival recession exposing the furcation to view.

Microscopically, furcation involvement presents no unique pathologic features. It is simply a phase in the rootward extension of the periodontal pocket. In its early stages, a widening of the periodontal space occurs, with cellular and fluid inflammatory exudation, followed by epithelial proliferation into the furcation area from an adjoining periodontal pocket. Extension of the inflammation into the bone leads to resorption and reduction in bone height. The bone-destructive pattern may produce horizontal loss, or angular osseous defects associated with intrabony pockets may exist (Figure 28-25). Plaque, calculus, and bacterial debris occupy the denuded furcation space.

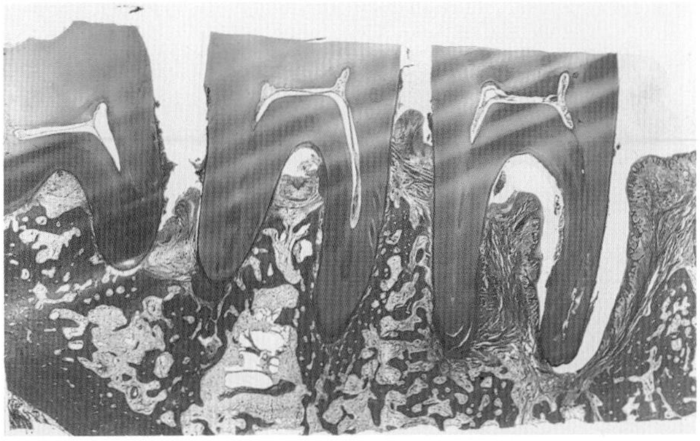

Figure 28-25 Different degrees of furcation involvement in human autopsy specimen. Moderate involvement is found in the third molar, a more advanced lesion in the second molar, and an extremely severe lesion in the first molar, exposing almost the entire mesial root.

The destructive pattern in a furcation involvement varies in different cases and with the degree of involvement. Bone loss around each individual root may be horizontal or angular, and frequently a crater develops in the interradicular area (Figure 28-26). Probing to determine the presence of these destructive patterns must be done horizontally and vertically around each involved root and in the crater area to establish the depth of the vertical component.

Furcation involvement is a stage of progressive periodontal disease and has its same etiology. The difficulty and sometimes the impossibility[2,3] of controlling plaque in furcations are responsible for the presence of extensive lesions in this area.[76]

The role of trauma from occlusion in the etiology of furcation lesions is controversial. Some assign a key role to trauma, believing that furcation areas are most sensitive to injury from excessive occlusal forces.[16] Others deny the initiating effect of trauma and consider that inflammation and edema caused by plaque in the furcation area tend to extrude the tooth, which then becomes traumatized and sensitive.[76]

Trauma from occlusion has been suspected as a contributing etiologic factor in cases of furcation involvement with craterlike or angular deformities in the bone and especially when bone destruction is localized to one of the roots.

Other factors that may play a role are the presence of enamel projections into the furcation,[42] which occurs in about 13% of multirooted teeth, and the proximity

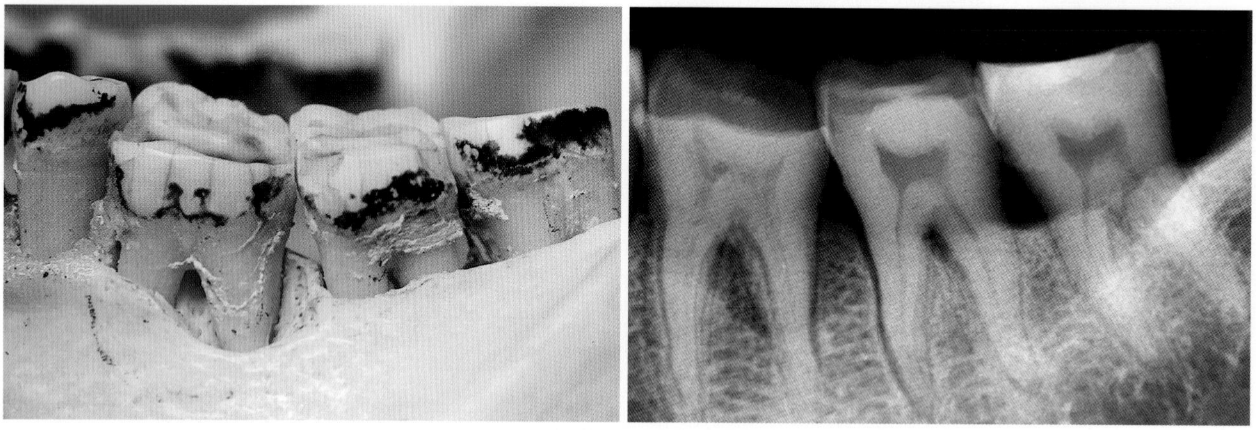

Figure 28-26 Photograph **(A)** and radiograph **(B)** of different degrees of bone loss in a skull. Furcation involvements in the first and second molar; deep angular bone loss in the distal root of the first molar; and interradicular and interdental craters in the second molar and between the second and third molars, respectively.

of the furcation to the cementoenamel junction, which occurs in about 75% of cases of furcation involvement.[33]

The presence of accessory pulpal canals in the furcation area may extend pulpal inflammation to the furcation.[21] This possibility should be carefully explored, particularly when mesial and distal bone retain their normal height. Accessory canals connecting the pulp chamber floor to the furcation have been found in 36% of maxillary first molars, 12% of maxillary second molars, 32% of mandibular first molars, and 24% of mandibular second molars.[72]

The diagnosis of furcation involvement is made by clinical examination and careful probing with a specially designed probe (see Chapter 35). Radiographic examination of the area is helpful, but lesions can be obscured by angulation of the beam and the radiopacity of neighboring structures (see Chapter 36).

For more detailed clinical considerations in the diagnosis and treatment of furcation involvement, see Chapters 35 and 68.

REFERENCES

1. Akiyoshi M, Mori K: Marginal periodontitis: a histological study of the incipient stage, *J Periodontol* 38:45, 1967.
2. Bower RC: Furcation morphology relative to periodontal treatment: furcation entrance architecture, *J Periodontol* 50:23, 1979.
3. Bower RC: Furcation morphology relative to periodontal treatment: furcation root surface anatomy, *J Periodontol* 50:366, 1979.
4. Carranza FA Jr: Histometric evaluation of periodontal pathology: a review of recent studies, *J Periodontol* 38:741, 1967.
5. Carranza FA Jr, Cabrini RL: Histometric studies of periodontal tissues, *Periodontics* 5:308, 1967.
6. Carranza FA Jr, Saglie R, Newman MG: Scanning and transmission electron microscopy study of tissue invading microorganisms in juvenile periodontitis, *J Periodontol* 54:598, 1983.
7. Carranza FA Jr, Simes RJ, Mayo J, et al: Histometric evaluation of periodontal bone loss in rats, *J Periodontal Res* 6:65, 1971.
8. Comar MD, Kollar JD, Gargiulo AW: Local irritation and occlusal trauma as cofactors in the periodontal disease process, *J Periodontol* 40:193, 1969.
9. Easley JR, Drennan GA: Morphological classification of the furca, *J Can Dent Assoc* 35:104, 1969.
10. Frank RM, Voegel JC: Bacterial bone resorption in advanced cases of human periodontitis, *J Periodontal Res* 13:251, 1978.
11. Garant PR, Cho MJ: Histopathogenesis of spontaneous periodontal disease in conventional rats. I. Histometric and histologic study, *J Periodontal Res* 14:297, 1979.
12. Glickman I: The experimental basis for the "bone factor" concept in periodontal disease, *J Periodontol* 20:7, 1951.
13. Glickman I, Smulow JB: Alterations in the pathway of gingival inflammation into the underlying tissues induced by excessive occlusal forces, *J Periodontol* 33:7, 1962.
14. Glickman I, Smulow J: Buttressing bone formation in the periodontium, *J Periodontol* 36:365, 1965.
15. Glickman I, Wood H: Bone histology in periodontal disease, *J Dent Res* 21:35, 1942.
16. Glickman I, Stein RS, Smulow JB: The effects of increased functional forces upon the periodontium of splinted and nonsplinted teeth, *J Periodontol* 32:290, 1961.
17. Goldman HM, Cohen DW: The intrabony pocket: classification and treatment, *J Periodontol* 29:272, 1958.
18. Goodson JM, Haffajee AD, Socransky SS: The relationship between attachment level loss and alveolar bone loss, *J Clin Periodontol* 11:348, 1984.
19. Goodson JM, McClatchy K, Revell C: Prostaglandin-induced resorption of the adult calvarium, *J Dent Res* 53:670, 1974.
20. Groen JJ, Menczel J, Shapiro S: Chronic destructive periodontal disease in patients with presenile osteoporosis, *J Periodontol* 39:19, 1968.
21. Gutman JL: Prevalence, location and patency of accessory canals in the furcation region of permanent molars, *J Periodontol* 49:21, 1978.
22. Hausmann E: Potential pathways for bone resorption in human periodontal disease, *J Periodontol* 45:338, 1974.
23. Hausmann E, Raisz LG, Miller WA: Endotoxin: stimulation of bone resorption in tissue culture, *Science* 168:793, 1970.
24. Heijl L, Rifkin BR, Zander HA: Conversion of chronic gingivitis to periodontitis in squirrel monkeys, *J Periodontol* 47:710, 1976.
25. Jeffcoat MK: Osteoporosis: a possible modifying factor in oral bone loss, *Ann Periodontol* 3:312, 1998.

26. Jeffcoat MK, Lewis CE, Reddy MS, et al: Post-menopausal bone loss and its relationship to oral bone loss, *Periodontol 2000* 23:94, 2000.
27. Jeffcoat MK, Williams RC, Wachter WJ, et al: Flurbiprofen treatment of periodontal disease in beagles, *J Periodontal Res* 21:624, 1986.
28. Klein DC, Raisz LG: Prostaglandins: stimulation of bone resorption in tissue culture, *Endocrinology* 86:1436, 1970.
29. Kronfeld R: Condition of alveolar bone underlying periodontal pockets, *J Periodontol* 6:22, 1935.
30. Larato DC: Periodontal bone defects in the juvenile skull, *J Periodontol* 41:473, 1970.
31. Larato DC: Intrabony defects in the dry human skull, *J Periodontol* 41:496, 1970.
32. Larato DC: Furcation involvements: incidence of distribution, *J Periodontol* 41:499, 1970.
33. Larato DC: Some anatomical factors related to furcation involvements, *J Periodontol* 46:608, 1975.
34. Lindhe J, Ericsson I: Effect of ligature placement and dental plaque on periodontal tissue breakdown in the dog, *J Periodontol* 49:343, 1978.
35. Lindhe J, Svanberg G: Influence of trauma from occlusion on progression of experimental periodontitis in beagle dogs, *J Clin Periodontol* 1:3, 1974.
36. Lindhe J, Liljenberg B, Listgarten MA: Some microbiological and histopathological features of periodontal disease in man, *J Periodontol* 51:264, 1980.
37. Löe H, Anerud A, Boysen H, et al: Natural history of periodontal disease in man: rapid, moderate and no loss of attachment in Sri Lankan laborers 14 to 46 years of age, *J Clin Periodontol* 13:431, 1986.
38. Löe H, Anerud A, Boysen H, et al: The natural history of periodontal disease in man: the rate of periodontal destruction before 40 years of age, *J Periodontol* 49:607, 1978.
39. Macapanpan LC, Weinmann JP: The influence of injury to the periodontal membrane on the spread of gingival inflammation, *J Dent Res* 33:263, 1954.
40. Manson JD: Bone morphology and bone loss in periodontal disease, *J Clin Periodontol* 3:14, 1976.
41. Manson JD, Nicholson K: The distribution of bone defects in chronic periodontitis, *J Periodontol* 45:88, 1974.
42. Masters DH, Hoskins SW: Projection of cervical enamel into molar furcations, *J Periodontol* 35:49, 1963.
43. Melcher AH, Eastoe JE: *Biology of the periodontium,* New York, 1969, Academic Press.
44. Moskow BS: A histomorphologic study of the effects of periodontal inflammation on the maxillary sinus mucosa, *J Periodontol* 63:674, 1992.
45. Moskow BS, Polson AM: Histologic studies on the extension of the inflammatory infiltrate in human periodontitis, *J Clin Periodontol* 18:534, 1991.
46. Nery EB, Corn H, Eisenstein IL: Palatal exostoses in the molar region, *J Periodontol* 48:663, 1977.
47. Newman MG: The role of *Bacteroides melaninogenicus* and other anaerobes in periodontal infections, *Rev Infect Dis* 1:313, 1979.
48. Nielsen JI, Glavind L, Karring T: Interproximal periodontal intrabony defects: prevalence, localization and etiological factors, *J Clin Periodontol* 7:187, 1980.
49. Ooya K, Yamamoto H: A scanning electron microscopic study of the destruction of human alveolar crest in periodontal disease, *J Periodont Res* 13:498, 1978.
50. Pack ARC, Gaudie WM, Jennings AM: Bony exostosis as a sequela to free gingival grafting: two case reports, *J Periodontol* 62:269, 1991.
51. Papapanou PN, Tonetti MS: Diagnosis and epidemiology of periodontal osseous lesions, *Periodontol 2000* 22:8, 2000.
52. Papapanou PN, Wennström JL, Grondahl K: Periodontal status in relation to age and tooth type: a cross-sectional radiographic study, *J Clin Periodontol* 15:469, 1988.
53. Page RC, Schroeder HE: *Periodontitis in man and other animals: a comparative review,* Basel, 1982, S Karger.
54. Prichard JF: *Periodontal surgery: practical dental monographs,* Chicago, 1961, Year Book Medical.
55. Raisz LG, Sandberg AL, Goodson JM, et al: Complement-dependent stimulation of prostaglandin synthesis and bone resorption, *Science* 185:789, 1974.
56. Rifkin BR, Heijl L: The occurrence of mononuclear cells at sites of osteoclastic bone resorption in experimental periodontitis, *J Periodontol* 50:636, 1979.
57. Rizzo AA, Mergenhagen SE: Histopathologic effects of endotoxin injected into rabbit oral mucosa, *Arch Oral Biol* 9:659, 1964.
58. Rowe DJ, Bradley LS: Quantitative analyses of osteoclasts, bone loss and inflammation in human periodontal disease, *J Periodontal Res* 16:13, 1981.
59. Ruben M, Cooper SJ: Tissue factors modifying the spread of periodontal inflammation: a perspective, *Contin Educ Dent* 2:387, 1981.
60. Saari JT, Hurt WC, Briggs NL: Periodontal bony defects on the dry skull, *J Periodontol* 39:278, 1968.
61. Saglie RF, Rezende M, Pertuiset J, et al: Bacterial invasion during disease activity as determined by significant loss of attachment, *J Periodontol* 58:336, 1987 (abstract).
62. Salvi GE, Lawrence HP, Offenbacher S, et al: Sequence of risk factors on the pathogenesis of periodontitis, *Periodontol 2000* 14:173, 1997.
63. Schroeder HE: Discussion: pathogenesis of periodontitis, *J Clin Periodontol* 13:426, 1986.
64. Schroeder HE, Lindhe J: Conditions and pathological features of rapidly destructive experimental periodontitis in dogs, *J Periodontol* 51:6, 1980.
65. Schwartz Z, Goultschin J, Dean DD, et al: Mechanisms of alveolar bone destruction in periodontitis, *Periodontol 2000* 14:158, 1997.
66. Seymour GJ, Dockrell HM, Greenspan JS: Enzyme differentiation of lymphocyte subpopulations in sections of human lymph nodes, tonsils, and periodontal disease, *Clin Exp Immunol* 32:169, 1978.
67. Seymour GJ, Powell RN, Davies WJR: Conversion of a stable T cell lesion to a progressive B cell lesion in the pathogenesis of chronic inflammatory periodontal disease: a hypothesis, *J Clin Periodontol* 6:267, 1979.
68. Stahl SS: The response of the periodontium to combined gingival inflammation and occlusofunctional stresses in four surgical specimens, *Periodontics* 6:14, 1968.
69. Svärdström G, Wennström JL: Prevalence of furcation involvements in patients referred for periodontal treatment, *J Clin Periodontol* 23:1093, 1996.
70. Tal H: Relationship between interproximal distance of roots and the prevalence of intrabony pockets, *J Periodontol* 55:604, 1984.
71. Ubios AM, Costa OR, Cabrini RL: Early steps in bone resorption in experimental periodontitis: a histomorphometric study, *Acta Odont Lat Am* 7:45, 1993.
72. Vertucci FJ, Anthony RL: An SEM investigation of accessory foramina in the furcation and pulp chamber floor of molar teeth, *Oral Surg* 62:319, 1986.
73. Wactawski-Wende J, Grossi SG, Trevisan M, et al: The role of osteopenia in oral bone loss and periodontal disease, *J Periodontol* 67:1076, 1996.
74. Waerhaug J: The angular bone defect and its relationship to trauma from occlusion and downgrowth of subgingival plaque, *J Clin Periodontol* 6:61, 1979.

75. Waerhaug J: The infrabony pocket and its relationship to trauma from occlusion and subgingival plaque, *J Periodontol* 50:355, 1979.
76. Waerhaug J: The furcation problem: etiology, pathogenesis, diagnosis, therapy and prognosis, *J Clin Periodontol* 7:73, 1980.
77. Weinmann JP: Progress of gingival inflammation into the supporting structures of the teeth, *J Periodontol* 12:71, 1941.
78. Williams RC, Jeffcoat MK, Kaplan ML, et al: Flurbiprofen: a potent inhibitor of alveolar bone resorption in beagles, *Science* 227:640, 1985.
79. Wouters FR, Salonen LE, Helldén LB, et al: Prevalence of interproximal periodontal infrabony defects in an adult population in Sweden: a radiographic study, *J Clin Periodontol* 16:144, 1989.

Periodontal Response to External Forces

Fermin A. Carranza

29

CHAPTER

CHAPTER OUTLINE

ADAPTIVE CAPACITY OF THE PERIODONTIUM TO OCCLUSAL FORCES

The periodontium attempts to accommodate to the forces exerted on the crown. This adaptive capacity varies in different persons and in the same person at different times. The effect of occlusal forces on the periodontium is influenced by the magnitude, direction, duration, and frequency of the forces.

When the **magnitude** of occlusal forces is increased, the periodontium responds with a widening of the periodontal ligament space, an increase in the number and width of periodontal ligament fibers, and an increase in the density of alveolar bone.

Changing the **direction** of occlusal forces causes a reorientation of the stresses and strains within the periodontium (Figure 29-1).[32] The principal fibers of the periodontal ligament are arranged so that they best accommodate occlusal forces along the long axis of the tooth. *Lateral* (horizontal) forces and *torque* (rotational) forces are more likely to injure the periodontium.

The response of alveolar bone is also affected by the **duration** and **frequency** of occlusal forces. Constant pressure on the bone is more injurious than intermittent forces. The more frequent the application of an intermittent force, the more injurious is the force to the periodontium.

TRAUMA FROM OCCLUSION

An inherent "margin of safety" common to all tissues permits some variation in occlusion without adversely affecting the periodontium. However, *when occlusal forces exceed the adaptive capacity of the tissues, tissue injury results.*[13,35,53,54] The resultant injury is termed *trauma from occlusion.**

Thus, *trauma from occlusion refers to the tissue injury, not the occlusal force.* An occlusion that produces such injury is called a *traumatic occlusion.*[2] Excessive occlusal forces may also disrupt the function of the masticatory musculature and cause painful spasms, injure the temporomandibular joints, or produce excessive tooth wear. However, the term *trauma from occlusion* is generally used in connection with injury in the periodontium.

*This term is used to designate periodontal tissue injury produced by occlusal forces. It is also known as *traumatism* and *occlusal trauma.*

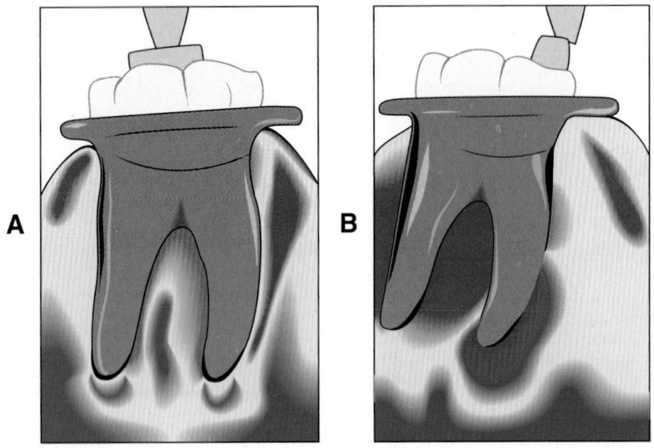

Figure 29-1 Stress patterns around the roots changed by shifting the direction of occlusal forces (experimental model using photoelastic analysis). **A,** Buccal view of an ivorine molar subjected to an axial force. The shaded fringes indicate that the internal stresses are at the root apices. **B,** Buccal view of ivorine molar subjected to a mesial tilting force. The shaded fringes indicate that the internal stresses are along the mesial surface and at the apex of the mesial root. (From Glickman I, Roeber F, Brion M, et al: *J Periodontol* 41:30, 1970.)

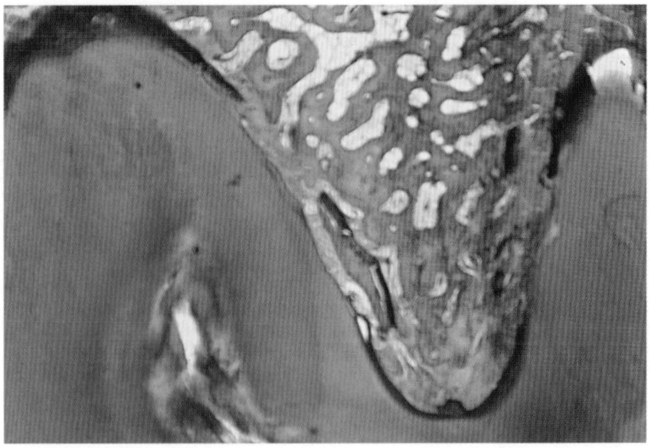

Figure 29-2 Cemental tear presumably caused by acute trauma from occlusion in human autopsy specimen. Note the repair process depositing bone on the displaced, torn cementum and recreating a periodontal ligament.

Acute and Chronic Trauma

Trauma from occlusion may be acute or chronic. *Acute trauma from occlusion* results from an abrupt occlusal impact, such as that produced by biting on a hard object (e.g., olive pit). Restorations or prosthetic appliances that interfere with or alter the direction of occlusal forces on the teeth may also induce acute trauma.

Acute trauma results in tooth pain, sensitivity to percussion, and increased tooth mobility. If the force is dissipated by a shift in the position of the tooth or by wearing away or correction of the restoration, the injury heals and the symptoms subside. Otherwise, periodontal injury may worsen and develop into necrosis, accompanied by periodontal abscess formation, or may persist as a symptom-free, chronic condition. Acute trauma can also produce cementum tears (Figure 29-2) (see Chapter 5).

Chronic trauma from occlusion is more common than the acute form and is of greater clinical significance. It most often develops from gradual changes in occlusion produced by tooth wear, drifting movement, and extrusion of teeth, combined with parafunctional habits such as bruxism and clenching, rather than as a sequela of acute periodontal trauma (see Chapter 30). The features of chronic trauma from occlusion and their significance are discussed next.

The criterion that determines if an occlusion is traumatic is whether it produces periodontal injury, not how the teeth occlude. Any occlusion that produces periodontal injury is traumatic. Malocclusion is not necessary to produce trauma; periodontal injury may occur when the occlusion appears normal. The dentition may be anatomically and aesthetically acceptable but functionally injurious. Similarly, not all malocclusions are necessarily injurious to the periodontium. Traumatic occlusal relationships are referred to by such terms as *occlusal disharmony, functional imbalance,* and *occlusal dystrophy.* These terms refer to the effect of the occlusion on the periodontium, not to the position of the teeth. Because trauma from occlusion refers to the tissue injury rather than the occlusion, an increased occlusal force is not traumatic if the periodontium can accommodate it.

Primary and Secondary Trauma from Occlusion

Trauma from occlusion may be caused by alterations in occlusal forces, reduced capacity of the periodontium to withstand occlusal forces, or both. When trauma from occlusion is the result of alterations in occlusal forces, it is called "primary trauma from occlusion." When it results from reduced ability of the tissues to resist the occlusal forces, it is known as "secondary trauma from occlusion."

Primary trauma from occlusion occurs if trauma from occlusion is considered the primary etiologic factor in periodontal destruction and if the only local alteration to which a tooth is subjected is from occlusion. Examples include periodontal injury produced around teeth with a previously healthy periodontium after the (1) insertion of a "high filling," (2) insertion of a prosthetic replacement that creates excessive forces on abutment and antagonistic teeth, (3) drifting movement or extrusion of teeth into spaces created by unreplaced missing teeth, and (4) orthodontic movement of teeth into functionally unacceptable positions. Most studies on experimental animals of the effect of trauma from occlusion have examined the primary type of trauma. Changes produced by primary trauma do not alter the level of connective tissue attachment and do not initiate pocket formation. This is probably because the supracrestal gingival fibers are not affected and therefore prevent apical migration of the junctional epithelium.[58]

Secondary trauma from occlusion occurs when the adaptive capacity of the tissues to withstand occlusal forces is impaired by bone loss resulting from marginal

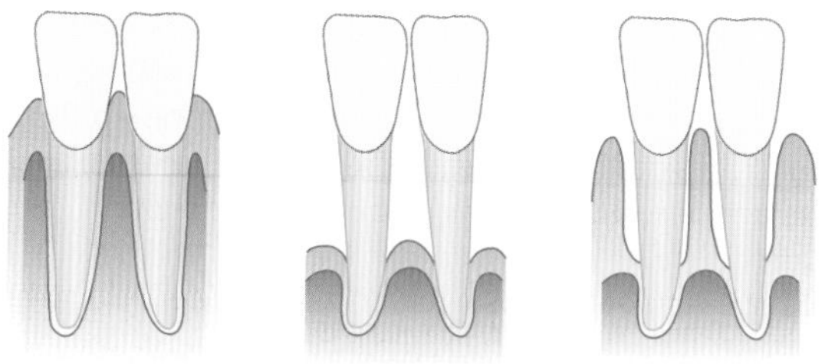

Figure 29-3 Traumatic forces can occur on **A,** normal periodontium with normal height of bone; **B,** normal periodontium with reduced height of bone; or **C,** marginal periodontitis with reduced height of bone.

inflammation. This reduces the periodontal attachment area and alters the leverage on the remaining tissues. The periodontium becomes more vulnerable to injury, and previously well-tolerated occlusal forces become traumatic.

Figure 29-3 depicts three different situations on which excessive occlusal forces can be superimposed, as follows:

1. Normal periodontium with normal height of bone
2. Normal periodontium with reduced height of bone
3. Marginal periodontitis with reduced height of bone

The first case is an example of primary trauma from occlusion, whereas the last two represent secondary trauma from occlusion. The effects of trauma from occlusion in these different situations are analyzed in the following discussion.

It has been found in experimental animals that systemic disorders can reduce tissue resistance and that previously tolerable forces may become excessive.[30,61,72] This could theoretically represent another mechanism by which tissue resistance to increased forces is lowered, resulting in secondary trauma from occlusion.

STAGES OF TISSUE RESPONSE TO INCREASED OCCLUSAL FORCES

Tissue response occurs in three stages[9,15]: injury, repair, and adaptive remodeling of the periodontium.

Stage I: Injury

Tissue injury is produced by excessive occlusal forces. The body then attempts to repair the injury and restore the periodontium. This can occur if the forces are diminished or if the tooth drifts away from them. If the offending force is chronic, however, the periodontium is remodeled to cushion its impact. The ligament is widened at the expense of the bone, resulting in angular bone defects without periodontal pockets, and the tooth becomes loose.

Under the forces of occlusion, a tooth rotates around a fulcrum or axis of rotation, which in single-rooted teeth is located in the junction between the middle third and the apical third of the clinical root (Figure 29-4). This creates areas of pressure and tension on opposite sides of the fulcrum. Different lesions are produced by different degrees of pressure and tension. If jiggling forces are exerted, these different lesions may coexist in the same area.

SCIENCE TRANSFER

The periodontium has a remarkable adaptive response to external forces. In the absence of inflammation or past periodontal disease, the tissue response appears to be mediated through forces exerted on the periodontal ligament fibers. When tension is exerted through the fibers to the bone, bone formation is initiated. However, in areas where tension is decreased, bone resorption occurs. These responses are observed in orthodontic movement and in cases where the occlusal forces exceed the adaptive ability of the periodontium. Inflammation and a history of periodontal disease with bone loss modify the adaptive ability of the periodontium. The mechanisms for tissue change in response to forces on the ligament are likely mediated through the extracellular matrix and the attachment apparatus between the matrix and the resident cells in the tissue.

Trauma from occlusion causes vascular changes in the periodontium within 30 minutes. The stasis and vasodilation are accompanied by pain, and in some cases, these changes even cause pulpal pain and hypersensitivity. Later changes result in loss of bone lining the socket, with a resultant widened periodontal ligament and increased tooth mobility. *It is unlikely that trauma from occlusion can initiate pocket formation, but when there is plaque-induced progressive periodontal bone loss and pocketing, the widened periodontal ligament space and the hyalinization of periodontal ligament fibers caused by traumatic occlusion can accentuate the loss of bone support.* Clinicians should evaluate and treat trauma from occlusion as part of the overall approach to periodontal therapy.

Slightly excessive pressure stimulates resorption of the alveolar bone, with a resultant widening of the periodontal ligament space. Slightly excessive tension causes elongation of the periodontal ligament fibers and apposition of alveolar bone. In areas of increased pressure, the blood vessels are numerous and reduced in size; in areas of increased tension, they are enlarged.[79]

Greater pressure produces a gradation of changes in the periodontal ligament, starting with compression of the fibers, which produces areas of hyalinization.[64-66] Subsequent injury to the fibroblasts and other connective tissue cells leads to necrosis of areas of the ligament.[62,66] Vascular changes are also produced: within 30 minutes, impairment and stasis of blood flow occur; at 2 to 3 hours, blood vessels appear to be packed with

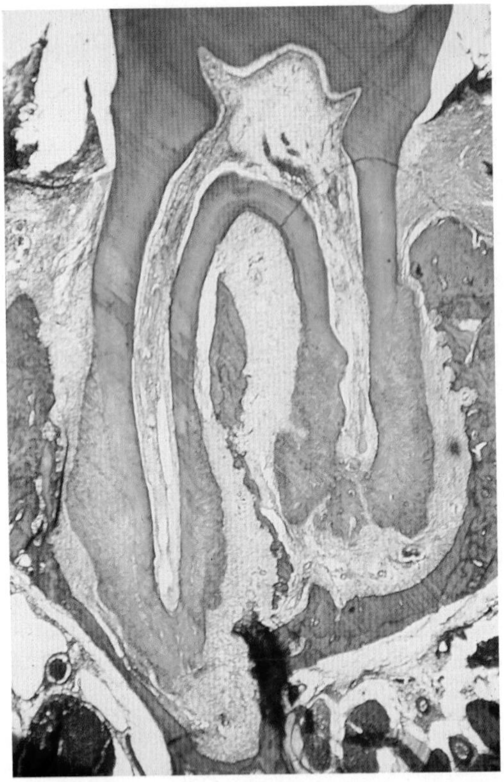

Figure 29-4 Areas of tension and pressure in opposite sites of the periodontal ligament caused by experimentally induced orthodontic movement in a rat molar.

erythrocytes, which start to fragment; and between 1 and 7 days, disintegration of the blood vessel walls and release of the contents into the surrounding tissue occur.[63] In addition, increased resorption of alveolar bone and resorption of the tooth surface occur[39,44] (Figure 29-5).

Severe tension causes widening of the periodontal ligament, thrombosis, hemorrhage, tearing of the periodontal ligament, and resorption of alveolar bone.

Pressure severe enough to force the root against bone causes necrosis of the periodontal ligament and bone. The bone is resorbed from viable periodontal ligament adjacent to necrotic areas and from marrow spaces, a process called *undermining resorption.*[34,53]

The areas of the periodontium most susceptible to injury from excessive occlusal forces are the furcations.[31]

Injury to the periodontium produces a temporary depression in mitotic activity and the rate of proliferation and differentiation of fibroblasts,[73] in collagen formation, and in bone formation.[39,71,73] These return to normal levels after dissipation of the forces.

Stage II: Repair

Repair is constantly occurring in the normal periodontium, and trauma from occlusion stimulates increased reparative activity.

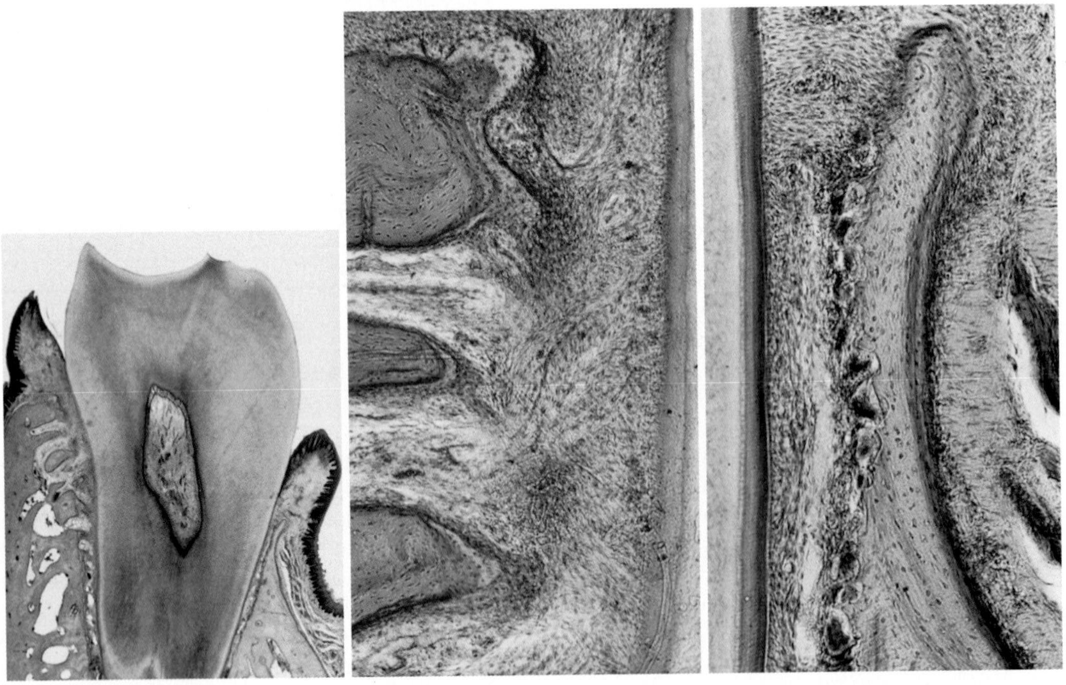

A B C

Figure 29-5 Periodontal accommodation to lateral forces. **A,** Mandibular premolar. **B,** Lingual surface, showing new bone formation in response to tension on the periodontal ligament. Note the pale-staining osteoid bordered by osteoblasts and the incremental lines indicative of previous additions to the bone. **C,** Facial surface shows compression of the periodontal ligament and osteoclastic resorption of the bony plate. Note the new bone formed on the external surface. This is peripheral buttressing bone, which reinforces the resorbing facial plate. Note also that the buttressing bone has produced a bulge in the bony contour.

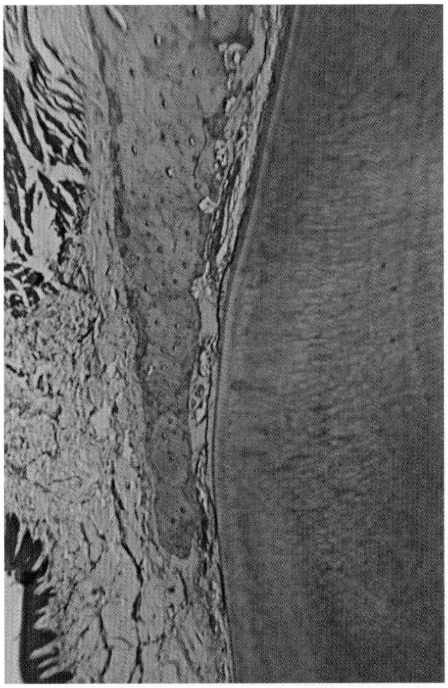

Figure 29-6 Experimental occlusal trauma in rats. Area of necrosis of the marginal periodontal ligament and resorption and remodeling in more apical periodontal sites.

The damaged tissues are removed, and new connective tissue cells and fibers, bone, and cementum are formed in an attempt to restore the injured periodontium (Figure 29-6). Forces remain traumatic only as long as the damage produced exceeds the reparative capacity of the tissues.

When bone is resorbed by excessive occlusal forces, the body attempts to reinforce the thinned bony trabeculae with new bone (Figure 29-7). This attempt to compensate for lost bone is called *buttressing bone formation* and is an important feature of the reparative process associated with trauma from occlusion.[27] It also occurs when bone is destroyed by inflammation or osteolytic tumors.

Buttressing bone formation occurs within the jaw (central buttressing) and on the bone surface (peripheral buttressing). In *central buttressing* the endosteal cells deposit new bone, which restores the bony trabeculae and reduces the size of the marrow spaces. *Peripheral buttressing* occurs on the facial and lingual surfaces of the alveolar plate. Depending on its severity, peripheral buttressing may produce a shelflike thickening of the alveolar margin, referred to as "lipping" (Figure 29-8; see also Figure 29-5), or a pronounced bulge in the contour of the facial and lingual bone[15,25] (see Chapter 28).

Cartilage-like material sometimes develops in the periodontal ligament space as an aftermath of the trauma.[21] Formation of crystals from erythrocytes has also been shown.[67]

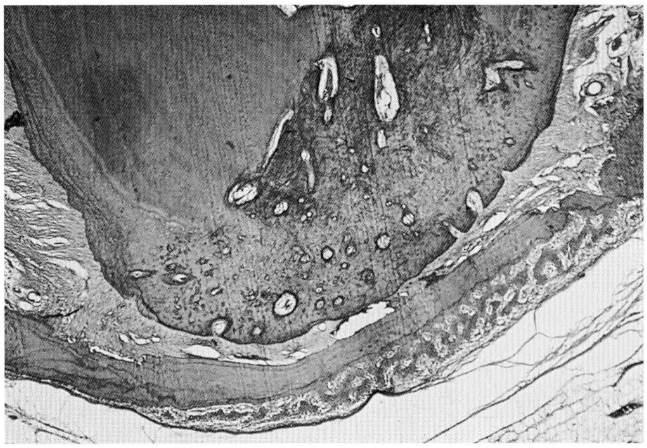

Figure 29-7 Experimental occlusal trauma in a dog, causing intrusion of a premolar and areas of necrosis in the apical periodontal ligament. Note the active bone formation on the outer aspect of the bone and the resorptive activity in the periphery of the necrotic site.

Stage III: Adaptive Remodeling of the Periodontium

If the repair process cannot keep pace with the destruction caused by the occlusion, the periodontium is remodeled in an effort to create a structural relationship in which the forces are no longer injurious to the tissues. *This results in a thickened periodontal ligament, which is funnel shaped at the crest, and angular defects in the bone, with no pocket formation. The involved teeth become loose.*[78] Increased vascularization has also been reported.[16]

The three stages in the evolution of traumatic lesions have been differentiated histometrically by the relative amounts of periodontal bone surface undergoing resorption or formation[10,15] (Figure 29-9). The injury phase shows an increase in areas of resorption and a decrease in bone formation, whereas the repair phase demonstrates decreased resorption and increased bone formation. After adaptive remodeling of the periodontium, resorption and formation return to normal.

EFFECTS OF INSUFFICIENT OCCLUSAL FORCE

Insufficient occlusal force may also be injurious to the supporting periodontal tissues.[11,46] Insufficient stimulation causes thinning of the periodontal ligament, atrophy of the fibers, osteoporosis of the alveolar bone, and reduction in bone height. Hypofunction can result from an open-bite relationship, an absence of functional antagonists, or unilateral chewing habits that neglect one side of the mouth.

REVERSIBILITY OF TRAUMATIC LESIONS

Trauma from occlusion is reversible. When trauma is artificially induced in experimental animals, the teeth move away or intrude into the jaw. When the impact of the artificially created force is relieved, the tissues undergo repair. Although trauma from occlusion is reversible under such conditions, it does not always

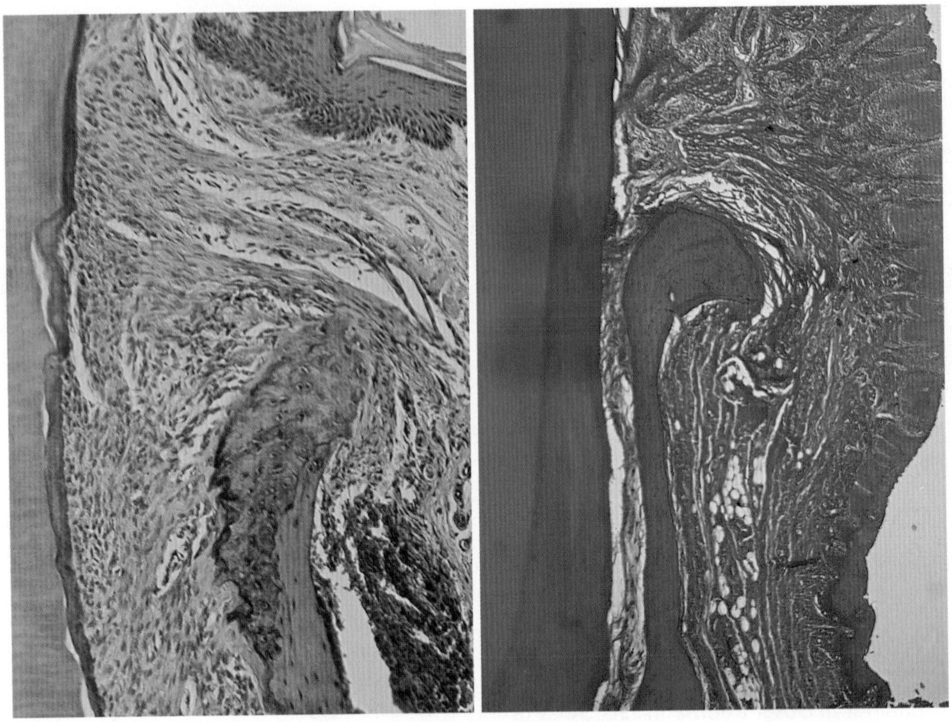

Figure 29-8 **A,** Widening of the periodontal ligament space in cervical area and a change in the shape of marginal alveolar bone as a result of chronic prolonged trauma from occlusion in rats. **B,** Comparable change in shape of marginal bone found in a human autopsy case.

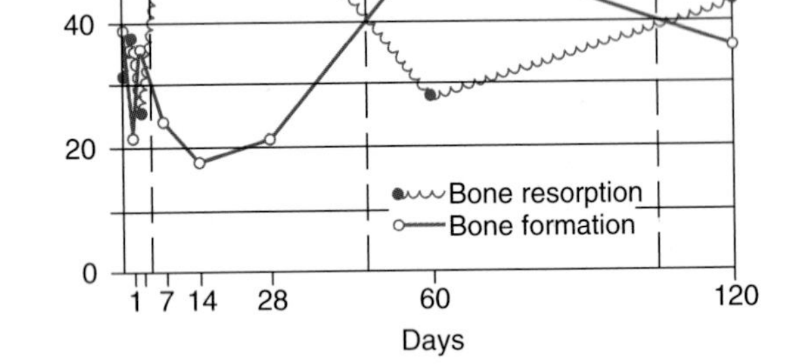

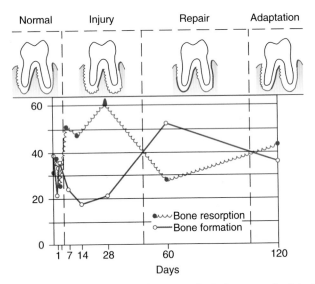

Figure 24-9 Evolution of traumatic lesions as depicted experimentally in rats by variations in relative amounts of areas of bone formation and bone resorption in periodontal bone surfaces. *Horizontal axis,* Days after initiation of traumatic interference. *Vertical axis,* Percentage of bone surface undergoing resorption or formation. The stages in the evolution of the lesions are represented in the top drawings, which show the average amount of bone activity for each group. (See references 9, 16, and 39.)

correct itself, and therefore it is not always temporary or of limited clinical significance. The injurious force must be relieved for repair to occur.[31,59] If conditions in humans do not permit the teeth to escape from or adapt to excessive occlusal force, periodontal damage persists and worsens.

The presence of inflammation in the periodontium as a result of plaque accumulation may impair the reversibility of traumatic lesions.[40,59]

EFFECTS OF EXCESSIVE OCCLUSAL FORCES ON DENTAL PULP

The effects of excessive occlusal forces on the dental pulp have not been established. Some clinicians report the disappearance of pulpal symptoms after correction of excessive occlusal forces. Pulpal reactions have been noted in animals subjected to increased occlusal forces[14,45] but did not occur when the forces were minimal and occurred over short periods.[45]

INFLUENCE OF TRAUMA FROM OCCLUSION ON PROGRESSION OF MARGINAL PERIODONTITIS

The clinical impressions of early investigators and clinicians assigned an important role to trauma from occlusion in the etiology of periodontal lesions. Since then, numerous studies have been performed attempting to determine the mechanisms by which trauma from occlusion may affect periodontal disease.

Initial studies involved the placement of high crowns or restorations on the teeth of dogs or monkeys, resulting in a continuous or intermittent force in one direction.[2,29] These investigations provided an orthodontic type of force and gave clear descriptions of changes occurring in pressure zones and tension zones. These procedures usually resulted in tooth displacement and consolidation in a new, nontraumatized position.

Trauma from occlusion in humans, however, is the result of forces that act alternatively in opposing directions. These were analyzed in experimental animals with "jiggling forces," usually produced by a high crown combined with an orthodontic appliance that would bring the traumatized tooth back to its original position when the force was dissipated by separating the teeth. In another method the teeth were separated by wooden or elastic material wedged interproximally to displace a tooth toward the opposite proximal side. After 48 hours the wedge was removed, and the procedure was repeated on the opposite side.

These studies resulted in a combination of changes produced by pressure and tension on both sides of the tooth, with an increase in the width of the ligament and increased tooth mobility. None of these methods caused gingival inflammation or pocket formation, and the results essentially represented different degrees of functional adaptation to increased forces.[58,79]

To mimic the problem in humans more closely, studies were then conducted on the effect produced by jiggling trauma and simultaneous plaque-induced gingival inflammation.

The accumulation of bacterial plaque that initiates gingivitis and results in periodontal pocket formation affects the marginal gingiva, but trauma from occlusion occurs in the supporting tissues and does not affect the gingiva (Figure 29-10). The marginal gingiva is unaffected by trauma from occlusion because its blood supply is not affected, even when the vessels of the periodontal ligament are obliterated by excessive occlusal forces.[33] It has been repeatedly proved that *trauma from occlusion does not cause pockets or gingivitis,** nor does it increase gingival fluid flow.[37,43,51] Furthermore, experimental trauma in dogs does not influence bacterial repopulation of pockets after scaling and root planing.[41] However, mobile teeth in humans harbor significantly higher proportions of *Campylobacter rectus* and *Peptostreptococcus micros* than nonmobile teeth.[36]

As long as inflammation is confined to the gingiva, the inflammatory process is not affected by occlusal forces.[42] When inflammation extends from the gingiva into the supporting periodontal tissues (i.e., when gingivitis becomes periodontitis), plaque-induced inflammation enters the zone influenced by occlusion, which Glickman has called the *zone of co-destruction.*[23,24,26]

*References 2, 29, 39, 60, 77, 78, 80.

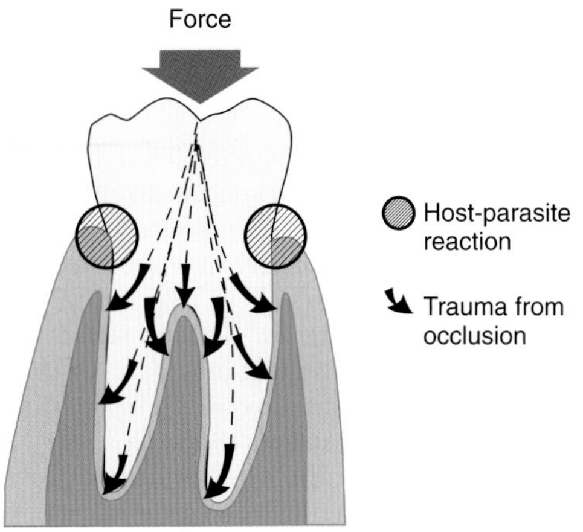

Figure 29-10 The reaction between dental plaque and the host takes place in the gingival sulcus region. Trauma from occlusion appears in the tissues supporting the tooth.

Two groups have studied this topic experimentally with conflicting results, probably because of the different methods used. The Eastman Dental Center group in Rochester, NY, used squirrel monkeys, produced trauma by repetitive interdental wedging, and added mild to moderate gingival inflammation; experimental times were up to 10 weeks. They reported that the presence of trauma did not increase the loss of attachment induced by periodontitis.[52,55-57] The University of Gothenburg group in Sweden used beagle dogs, produced trauma by placing cap splints and orthodontic appliances, and induced severe gingival inflammation; experimental times were up to 1 year. This group found that occlusal stresses increase the periodontal destruction induced by periodontitis.[18,19,49]

When trauma from occlusion is eliminated, a substantial reversal of bone loss occurs, except in the presence of periodontitis. This indicates that inflammation inhibits the potential for bone regeneration.[40,48,58,59] *Thus it is important to eliminate the marginal inflammatory component in cases of trauma from occlusion because the presence of inflammation affects bone regeneration after the removal of the traumatizing contacts.*[40] It also has been shown in experimental animals that trauma from occlusion does not induce progressive destruction of the periodontal tissues in regions kept healthy after the elimination of preexisting periodontitis.[18]

Trauma from occlusion also tends to change the shape of the alveolar crest. The change in shape consists of a widening of the marginal periodontal ligament space, a narrowing of the interproximal alveolar bone, and a shelflike thickening of the alveolar margin.[16,49,52] Therefore, although trauma from occlusion does not alter the inflammatory process, it changes the architecture of the area around the inflamed site.[15,49] *Thus, in the absence of inflammation, the response to trauma from occlusion is limited to adaptation to the increased forces. In the presence of inflammation, however, the changes in the shape of the alveolar crest may be conducive to angular bone loss, and existing pockets may become intrabony.*

Other theories that have been proposed to explain the interaction of trauma and inflammation include the following:

- Trauma from occlusion may alter the pathway of extension of gingival inflammation to the underlying tissues. This may be favored by the reduced collagen density and increased number of leukocytes, osteoclasts, and blood vessels in the coronal portion of increasingly mobile teeth.[3] Inflammation then may proceed to the periodontal ligament rather than to the bone. Resulting bone loss would be angular, and pockets could become intrabony.*
- Trauma-induced areas of root resorption uncovered by apical migration of the inflamed gingival attachment may offer a favorable environment for the formation and attachment of plaque and calculus and therefore may be responsible for the development of deeper lesions.[69]
- Supragingival plaque can become subgingival if the tooth is tilted orthodontically or migrates into an edentulous area, resulting in the transformation of a suprabony pocket into an intrabony pocket.[17,20]
- Increased mobility of traumatically loosened teeth may have a pumping effect on plaque metabolites, increasing their diffusion.[76]

Clinical and Radiographic Signs of Trauma from Occlusion Alone

The most common clinical sign of trauma to the periodontium is *increased tooth mobility*. In the injury stage of trauma from occlusion, destruction of periodontal fibers occurs, which increases tooth mobility. In the final stage the accommodation of the periodontium to increased forces entails a widening of the periodontal ligament, which also leads to increased tooth mobility. Although this tooth mobility is greater than the so-called normal mobility, it cannot be considered pathologic because it is an adaptation and not a disease process. When it becomes progressively worse, it can be considered pathologic.

Other causes of increased tooth mobility include advanced bone loss, inflammation of the periodontal ligament of periodontal or periapical origin, and some systemic causes (e.g., pregnancy). The destruction of surrounding alveolar bone, such as occurs in osteomyelitis or jaw tumors, may also increase tooth mobility (see Chapter 35).

Radiographic signs of trauma from occlusion may include the following:

1. Increased width of the periodontal space, often with thickening of the lamina dura along the lateral aspect of the root, in the apical region, and in bifurcation areas. These changes do not *necessarily* indicate destructive changes because they may result from thickening and strengthening of the periodontal ligament and alveolar bone, constituting a favorable response to increased occlusal forces (Figure 29-11).
2. A "vertical" rather than "horizontal" destruction of the interdental septum.
3. Radiolucency and condensation of the alveolar bone.
4. Root resorption (see Chapter 27).

In summary, *trauma from occlusion does not initiate gingivitis or periodontal pockets, but it may constitute an additional risk factor for the progression and severity of the disease.* An understanding of the effect of trauma from occlusion on the periodontium is useful in the clinical management of periodontal problems.

PATHOLOGIC TOOTH MIGRATION

Pathologic migration refers to tooth displacement that results when the balance among the factors that maintain physiologic tooth position is disturbed by periodontal disease. Pathologic migration is relatively common and may be an early sign of disease, or it may occur in association with gingival inflammation and pocket formation as the disease progresses.

Pathologic migration occurs most frequently in the anterior region, but posterior teeth may also be affected. The teeth may move in any direction, and the migration is usually accompanied by mobility and rotation. Pathologic migration in the occlusal or incisal direction is termed *extrusion*. All degrees of pathologic migration are encountered, and one or more teeth may be affected (Figure 29-12). It is important to detect migration in its early stages and prevent more serious involvement by eliminating the causative factors. Even in the early stage, some degree of bone loss occurs.

Pathogenesis

Two major factors play a role in maintaining the normal position of the teeth: the health and normal height of the periodontium and the forces exerted on the teeth. The latter includes the forces of occlusion and pressure from the lips, cheeks, and tongue. Factors that are important in relation to the forces of occlusion include (1) tooth morphologic features and cuspal inclination; (2) the presence of a full complement of teeth; (3) a physiologic tendency toward mesial migration; (4) the nature and location of contact point relationships; (5) proximal, incisal, and occlusal attrition; and (6) the axial inclination of the teeth. Alterations in any of these factors start an interrelated sequence of changes in the environment of a single tooth or group of teeth that results in pathologic migration. Thus, pathologic migration occurs under conditions that weaken the periodontal support, increase or modify the forces exerted on the teeth, or both.

Weakened Periodontal Support

The inflammatory destruction of the periodontium in periodontitis creates an imbalance between the forces maintaining the tooth in position and the occlusal and muscular forces the tooth ordinarily needs to bear. The tooth with weakened support is unable to maintain its normal position in the arch and moves away from the opposing force unless it is restrained by proximal contact. The force that moves the weakly supported tooth may be

*References 1, 23, 25, 26, 28, 50.

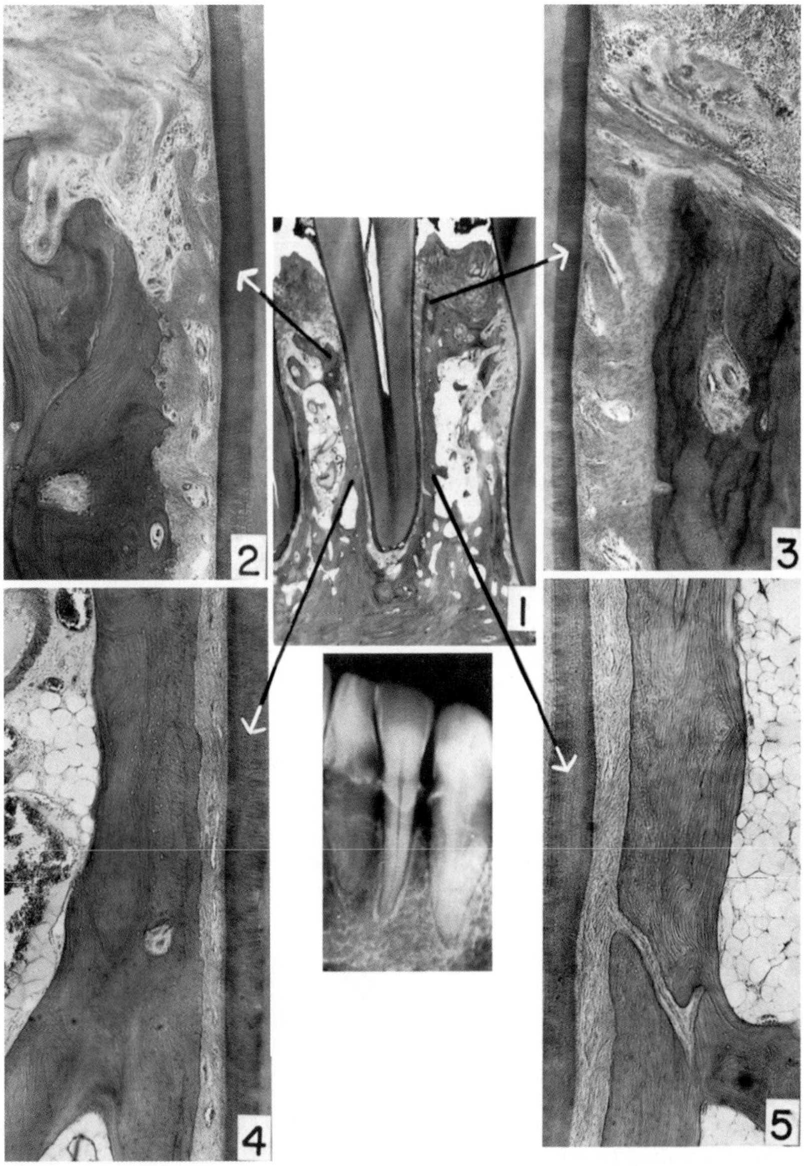

Figure 29-11 Widened periodontal space produced by two types of tissue response to increased occlusal forces. Radiograph shows thickening of periodontal space and lamina dura around the lateral incisor. *1,* Survey microscopic section of the lateral incisor. *2,* Mesial surface widening of the periodontal space has resulted from resorption of alveolar bone associated with pressure. *3,* Distal surface widening of the periodontal space has resulted from thickening of the periodontal ligament, which is a favorable response to increased tension. *4* and *5,* Thinned periodontal ligament at axis of rotation, one-third the distance from the apex.

A 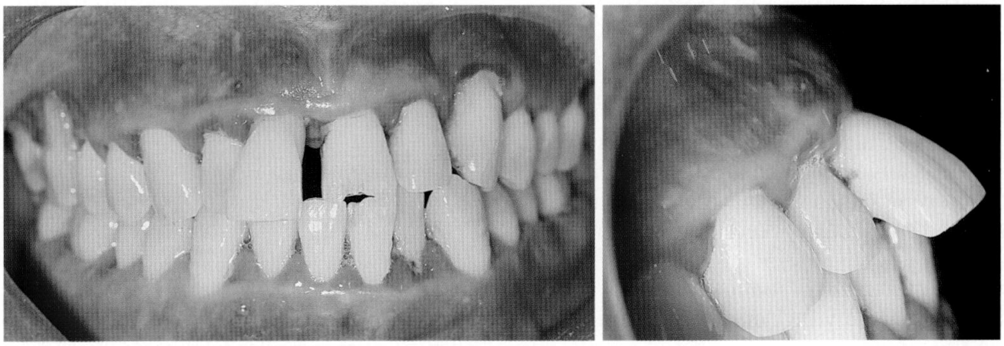 B

Figure 29-12 Labial migration of maxillary central incisors, especially the right incisor. **A,** Frontal view. **B,** Lateral view.

created by factors such as occlusal contacts or pressure from the tongue.

It is important to understand that the abnormality in pathologic migration rests with the weakened periodontium; the force itself is not necessarily abnormal. Forces that are acceptable to an intact periodontium become injurious when periodontal support is reduced, as in the tooth with abnormal proximal contacts. Abnormally located proximal contacts convert the normal anterior component of force to a wedging force that moves the tooth occlusally or incisally. The wedging force, which can be withstood by the intact periodontium, causes the tooth to extrude when the periodontal support is weakened by disease. *As its position changes, the tooth is subjected to abnormal occlusal forces, which aggravate the periodontal destruction and the tooth migration.*

Pathologic migration may continue after a tooth no longer contacts its antagonist. Pressures from the tongue, the food bolus during mastication, and proliferating granulation tissue provide the force.

Pathologic migration is also an early sign of localized aggressive periodontitis. Weakened by loss of periodontal support, the maxillary and mandibular anterior incisors drift labially and extrude, creating diastemata between the teeth (see Chapter 33).

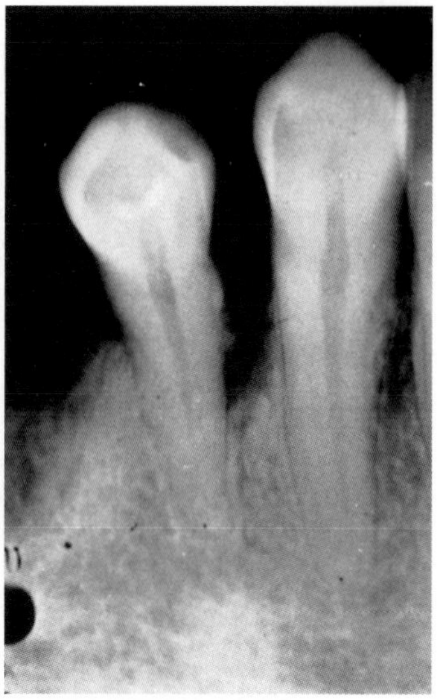

Figure 29-13 Calculus and bone loss on the mesial surface of a canine that has drifted distally.

Changes in the Forces Exerted on the Teeth

Changes in the magnitude, direction, or frequency of the forces exerted on the teeth can induce pathologic migration of a tooth or group of teeth. These forces do not have to be abnormal to cause migration if the periodontium is sufficiently weakened. Changes in the forces may result from unreplaced missing teeth, failure to replace first molars, or other causes.

Unreplaced Missing Teeth. Drifting of teeth into the spaces created by unreplaced missing teeth often occurs. Drifting differs from pathologic migration in that it does not result from destruction of the periodontal tissues. However, it usually creates conditions that lead to periodontal disease, and thus the initial tooth movement is aggravated by loss of periodontal support (Figure 29-13).

Drifting generally occurs in a mesial direction, combined with tilting or extrusion beyond the occlusal plane. The premolars frequently drift distally (Figure 29-14). Although drifting is a common sequela when missing teeth are not replaced, it does not always occur (Figure 29-15).

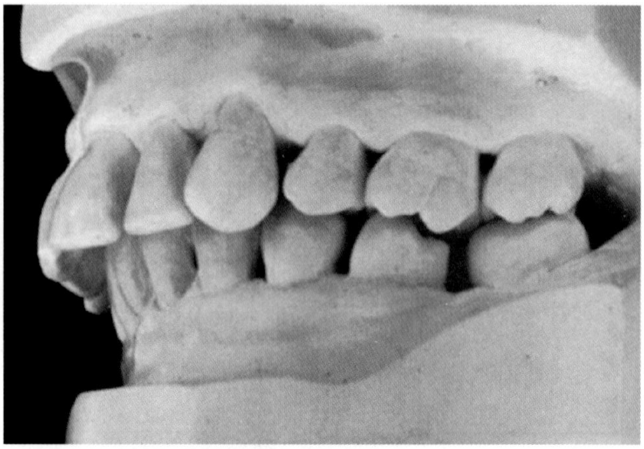

Figure 29-14 Maxillary first molar tilted and extruded into the space created by a missing mandibular tooth.

Failure to Replace First Molars. The pattern of changes that may follow failure to replace missing first molars is characteristic. In extreme cases it consists of the following:

1. The second and third molars tilt, resulting in a decrease in vertical dimension (Figure 29-16).
2. The premolars move distally, and the mandibular incisors tilt or drift lingually. While drifting distally, the mandibular premolars lose their intercuspating relationship with the maxillary teeth and may tilt distally.
3. Anterior overbite is increased. The mandibular incisors strike the maxillary incisors near the gingiva or traumatize the gingiva.

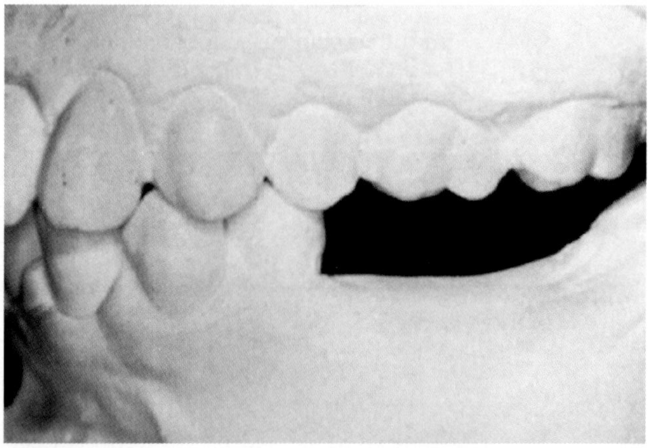

Figure 29-15 No drifting or extrusion despite 4 years' absence of mandibular teeth.

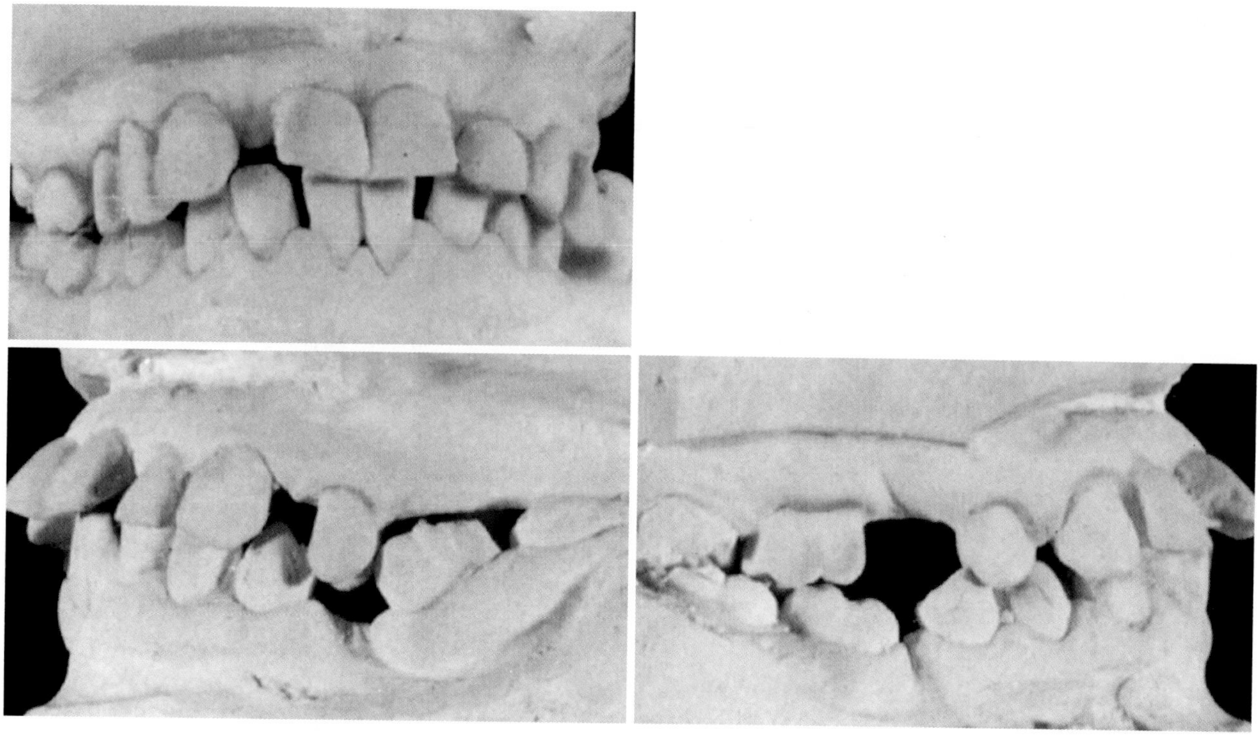

Figure 29-16 Examples of mutilation of occlusion associated with unreplaced missing teeth. Note pronounced pathologic migration, disturbed proximal contacts, and functional relationships with closing of the bite.

4. The maxillary incisors are pushed labially and laterally (Figure 29-17).
5. The anterior teeth extrude because the incisal apposition has largely disappeared.
6. Diastemata are created by the separation of the anterior teeth (see Figure 29-16).

The disturbed proximal contact relationships lead to food impaction, gingival inflammation, and pocket formation, followed by bone loss and tooth mobility. Occlusal disharmonies created by the altered tooth positions traumatize the supporting tissues of the periodontium and aggravate the destruction caused by the inflammation. Reduction in periodontal support leads to further migration of the teeth and mutilation of the occlusion.

Other Causes. *Trauma from occlusion* may cause a shift in tooth position either by itself or in combination with inflammatory periodontal disease. The direction of movement depends on the occlusal force.

Pressure from the tongue may cause drifting of the teeth in the absence of periodontal disease or may contribute to pathologic migration of teeth with reduced periodontal support (Figure 29-18).

In tooth support weakened by periodontal destruction, *pressure from the granulation tissue of periodontal pockets* has been mentioned as contributing to pathologic migration.[38] The teeth may return to their original positions after the pockets are eliminated, but if more destruction has occurred on one side of a tooth than the other, the healing tissues tend to pull in the direction of the lesser destruction.

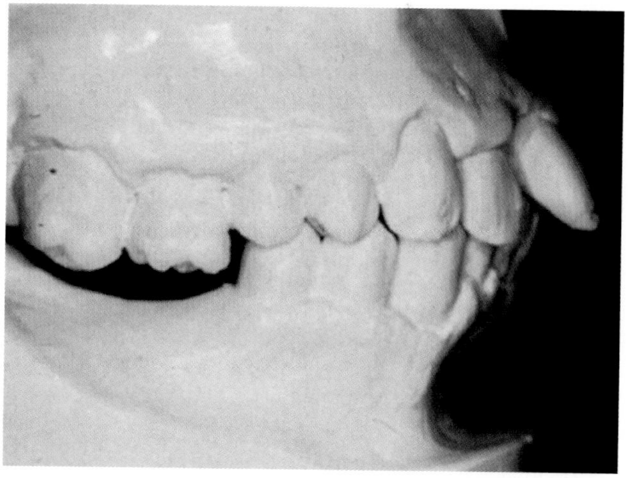

Figure 29-17 Maxillary incisors pushed labially in patient with bilateral unreplaced mandibular molars. Note extrusion of the maxillary molars.

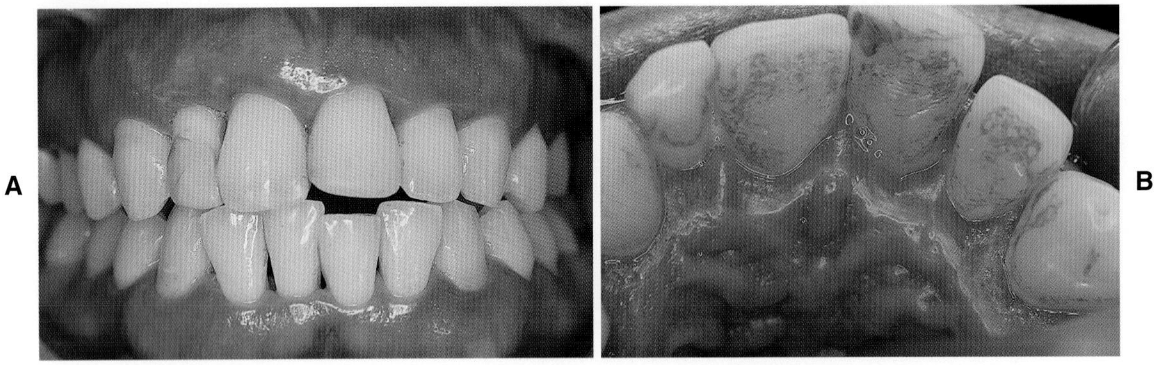

Figure 29-18 Pathologic migration associated with tongue pressure. **A**, Facial view. **B**, Palatal view.

REFERENCES

1. Ballbe R, Carranza FA, Erausquin R: Los paradencios del caso ocho, *Rev Odont (Buenos Aires)* 26:606, 1938.
2. Bhaskar SN, Orban B: Experimental occlusal trauma, *J Periodontol* 26:270, 1955.
3. Biancu S, Ericsson I, Lindhe J: Periodontal ligament tissue reactions to trauma and gingival inflammation: an experimental study in the beagle dog, *J Clin Periodontol* 22:772, 1995.
4. Box HK: Traumatic occlusion and traumatogenic occlusion, *Oral Health* 20:642, 1930.
5. Box HK: Experimental traumatogenic occlusion in sheep, *Oral Health* 25:9, 1935.
6. Box HK: *Twelve periodontal studies,* Toronto, 1940, University of Toronto Press.
7. Budtz-Jorgensen E: Bruxism and trauma from occlusion, *J Clin Periodontol* 7:149, 1980.
8. Burgett FG: Trauma from occlusion: periodontal concerns, *Dent Clin North Am* 39:301, 1995.
9. Carranza FA Jr: Histometric evaluation of periodontal pathology, *J Periodontol* 38:741, 1970.
10. Carranza FA Jr, Cabrini RL: Histometric studies of periodontal tissues, *Periodontics* 5:308, 1967.
11. Cohn SA: Disuse atrophy of the periodontium in molar teeth of mice, *J Dent Res* 40:707, 1961.
12. Comar MD, Kollar JA, Gargiulo AW: Local irritation and occlusal trauma as cofactors in the periodontal disease process, *J Periodontol* 40:193, 1969.
13. Coolidge ED: Traumatic and functional injuries occurring in the supporting tissues on human teeth, *J Am Dent Assoc* 25:343, 1938.
14. Cooper MB, Landay MA, Seltzer S: The effects of excessive occlusal forces on the pulp. II. Heavier and longer term forces, *J Periodontol* 42:353, 1971.
15. Dotto CA, Carranza FA Jr, Itoiz ME: Efectos mediatos del trauma experimental en ratas, *Rev Asoc Odontol Argent* 54:48, 1966.
16. Dotto CA, Carranza FA Jr, Cabrini RL, et al: Vascular changes in experimental trauma from occlusion, *J Periodontol* 38:183, 1967.
17. Ericsson I: The combined effects of plaque and physical stress on periodontal tissues, *J Clin Periodontol* 13:918, 1986.
18. Ericsson I, Lindhe J: Lack of effect of trauma from occlusion on the recurrence of experimental periodontitis, *J Clin Periodontol* 4:115, 1977.
19. Ericsson I, Lindhe J: Effect of longstanding jiggling on experimental marginal periodontitis in the beagle dog, *J Clin Periodontol* 9:497, 1982.
20. Ericsson I, Thilander B, Lindhe J, et al: The effect of orthodontic tilting movements on the periodontal tissues of infected and noninfected dentitions in dogs, *J Clin Periodontol* 4:278, 1977.
21. Everett FG, Bruckner RJ: Cartilage in the periodontal ligament space, *J Periodontol* 41:165, 1970.
22. Gher ME: Changing concepts: the effects of occlusion on periodontitis, *Dent Clin North Am* 42:285, 1998.
23. Glickman I: Occlusion and the periodontium, *J Dent Res* 46(suppl):53, 1967.
24. Glickman I, Smulow JB: Alterations in the pathway of gingival inflammation into the underlying tissues induced by excessive occlusal forces, *J Periodontol* 33:7, 1962.
25. Glickman I, Smulow JB: Buttressing bone formation in the periodontium, *J Periodontol* 36:365, 1965.
26. Glickman I, Smulow JB: Effect of excessive occlusal forces upon the pathway of gingival inflammation in humans, *J Periodontol* 36:141, 1965.
27. Glickman I, Smulow JB: Adaptive alterations in the periodontium of the rhesus monkey in chronic trauma from occlusion, *J Periodontol* 39:101, 1968.
28. Glickman I, Smulow JB: The combined effects of inflammation and trauma from occlusion to periodontitis, *Int Dent J* 19:393, 1969.
29. Glickman I, Weiss L: Role of trauma from occlusion in initiation of periodontal pocket formation in experimental animals, *J Periodontol* 26:14, 1955.
30. Glickman I, Smulow JB, Moreau J: Effect of alloxan diabetes upon the periodontal response to excessive occlusal forces, *J Periodontol* 37:146, 1966.
31. Glickman I, Stein RS, Smulow JB: The effects of increased functional forces upon the periodontium of splinted and nonsplinted teeth, *J Periodontol* 32:290, 1961.
32. Glickman I, Roeber F, Brion M, et al: Photoelastic analysis of internal stresses in the periodontium created by occlusal forces, *J Periodontol* 41:30, 1970.
33. Goldman H: Gingival vascular supply in induced occlusal traumatism, *Oral Surg Oral Med Oral Pathol* 9:939, 1956.
34. Gottlieb B, Orban B: *Changes in the tissue due to excessive force upon the teeth,* Leipzig, 1931, G Thieme.
35. Gottlieb B, Orban B: Tissue changes in experimental traumatic occlusion with special reference to age and constitution, *J Dent Res* 11:505, 1931.
36. Grant DA, Grant DA, Flynn MJ, et al: Periodontal microbiota of mobile and nonmobile teeth, *J Periodontol* 66:386, 1985.
37. Hakkarainen K: Relative influence of scaling and root influence and occlusal adjustment on sulcular fluid flow, *J Periodontol* 57:681, 1986.

38. Hirschfeld I: The dynamic relationship between pathologically migrating teeth and inflammatory tissue in periodontal pockets: a clinical study, *J Periodontol* 4:35, 1933.
39. Itoiz ME, Carranza FA Jr, Cabrini RL: Histologic and histometric study of experimental occlusal trauma in rats, *J Periodontol* 34:305, 1963.
40. Kantor M, Polson AN, Zander HA: Alveolar bone regeneration after removal of inflammatory and traumatic factors, *J Periodontol* 46:687, 1976.
41. Kaufman H, Carranza FA Jr, Enders B, et al: The influence of trauma from occlusion on the bacterial repopulation of periodontal pockets in dogs, *J Periodontol* 55:86, 1984.
42. Kenney EB: A histopathologic study of incisal dysfunction and gingival inflammation in the rhesus monkey, *J Periodontol* 42:3, 1971.
43. Kobayashi K, Kobayashi K, Soeda W, et al: Gingival crevicular pH in experimental gingivitis and occlusal trauma in man, *J Periodontol* 69:1036, 1998.
44. Kvam E: Scanning electron microscopy of tissue changes on the pressure surface of human premolars following tooth movement, *Scand J Dent Res* 80:357, 1972.
45. Landay MA, Nazimov H, Seltzer S: The effects of excessive occlusal forces on the pulp, *J Periodontol* 41:3, 1970.
46. Levy G, Mailland ML: Etude quantitative des effets de l'hypofonction occlusale sur la largeur desmodontale et la resorption osteoclastique alveolaire chez le rat, *J Biol Buccale* 8:17, 1980.
47. Lindhe J, Ericsson I: The influence of trauma from occlusion on reduced but healthy periodontal tissues in dogs, *J Clin Periodontol* 3:110, 1976.
48. Lindhe J, Ericsson I: The effect of elimination of jiggling forces on periodontally exposed teeth in the dog, *J Periodontol* 53:562, 1982.
49. Lindhe J, Svanberg G: Influence of trauma from occlusion on progression of experimental periodontitis in the beagle dog, *J Clin Periodontol* 1:3, 1974.
50. Macapanpan LC, Weinmann JP: The influence of injury to the periodontal membrane on the spread of gingival inflammation, *J Dent Res* 33:263, 1954.
51. Martin LP, Noble WH: Gingival fluid in relation to tooth mobility and occlusal interferences, *J Periodontol* 45:444, 1974.
52. Meitner S: Co-destructive factors of marginal periodontitis and repetitive mechanical injury, *J Dent Res* 54:C78, 1975.
53. Orban B: Tissue changes in traumatic occlusion, *J Am Dent Assoc* 15:2090, 1928.
54. Orban B, Weinmann JP: Signs of traumatic occlusion in average human jaws, *J Dent Res* 13:216, 1933.
55. Polson AM: Trauma and progression of marginal periodontitis in squirrel monkeys. II. Codestructive factors of periodontitis and mechanically produced injury, *J Periodontal Res* 9:108, 1974.
56. Polson AM: The relative importance of plaque and occlusion in periodontal disease, *J Clin Periodontol* 13:923, 1986.
57. Polson AM, Zander HA: Effect of periodontal trauma upon intrabony pockets, *J Periodontol* 54:586, 1983.
58. Polson AM, Meitner SW, Zander HA: Trauma and progression of marginal periodontitis in squirrel monkeys. III. Adaption of interproximal alveolar bone to repetitive injury, *J Periodontal Res* 11:279, 1976.
59. Polson AM, Meitner SW, Zander HA: Trauma and progression of marginal periodontitis in squirrel monkeys. IV. Reversibility of bone loss due to trauma alone and trauma superimposed upon periodontitis, *J Periodontal Res* 11:290, 1976.
60. Ramfjord SP, Kohler CA: Periodontal reaction to functional occlusal stress, *J Periodontol* 30:95, 1959.
61. Rothblatt JM, Waldo CM: Tissue response to tooth movement in normal and abnormal metabolic states, *J Dent Res* 32:678, 1953.
62. Rygh P: Ultrastructural cellular reactions in pressure zones of rat molar periodontium incident to orthodontic movement, *Acta Odontol Scand* 30:575, 1972.
63. Rygh P: Ultrastructural vascular changes in pressure zones of rat molar periodontium incident to orthodontic movement, *Scand J Dent Res* 80:307, 1972.
64. Rygh P: Ultrastructural changes in pressure zones of human periodontium incident to orthodontic tooth movement, *Acta Odontol Scand* 31:109, 1973.
65. Rygh P: Ultrastructural changes of the periodontal fibers and their attachment in rat molar periodontium incident to orthodontic tooth movement, *Scand J Dent Res* 81:467, 1973.
66. Rygh P: Elimination of hyalinized periodontal tissues associated with orthodontic tooth movement, *Scand J Dent Res* 82:57, 1974.
67. Rygh P, Selvig KA: Erythrocytic crystallization in rat molar periodontium incident to tooth movement, *Scand J Dent Res* 81:62, 1973.
68. Solt CW, Glickman I: A histologic and radioautographic study of healing following wedging interdental injury in mice, *J Periodontol* 39:249, 1968.
69. Sottosanti JS: A possible relationship between occlusion, root resorption and the progression of periodontal disease, *J West Soc Periodontol* 25:69, 1977.
70. Stahl SS: The responses of the periodontium to combined gingival inflammation and occlusofunctional stresses in four human surgical specimens, *Periodontics* 6:14, 1968.
71. Stahl SS: Accommodation of the periodontium to occlusal trauma and inflammatory periodontal disease, *Dent Clin North Am* 19:531, 1975.
72. Stahl SS, Miller SC, Goldsmith ED: The effects of vertical occlusal trauma on the periodontium of protein deprived young adult rats, *J Periodontol* 28:87, 1957.
73. Stallard RE: The effect of occlusal alterations on collagen formation within the periodontium, *Periodontics* 2:49, 1964.
74. Stones HH: An experimental investigation into the association of traumatic occlusion with paradontal disease, *Proc Soc Med* 31:479, 1938.
75. Svanberg G, Lindhe J: Vascular reactions to the periodontal ligament incident to trauma from occlusion, *J Clin Periodontol* 1:58, 1974.
76. Vollmer WH, Rateitschak KH: Influence of occlusal adjustment by grinding on gingivitis and mobility of traumatized teeth, *J Clin Periodontol* 2:113, 1975.
77. Waerhaug J, Hansen ER: Periodontal changes incidental to prolonged occlusal overload in monkeys, *Acta Odontol Scand* 24:91, 1966.
78. Wentz FM, Jarabak J, Orban B: Experimental occlusal trauma imitating cuspal interferences, *J Periodontol* 29:117, 1958.
79. Zaki AE, Van Huysen G: Histology of the periodontium following tooth movement, *J Dent Res* 42:1373, 1963.
80. Zander HA, Muhlemann HR: The effect of stresses on the periodontal structures, *Oral Surg Oral Med Oral Pathol* 9:380, 1956.

Masticatory System Disorders

Michael J. McDevitt

30

CHAPTER

CHAPTER OUTLINE

The masticatory system consists of the temporomandibular joints (TMJs), masticatory muscles, teeth in occlusion, and neurologic and vascular supplies supporting all these structures.

Research suggests that masticatory system disorders include many varied conditions with multiple possible contributing factors, rather than different manifestations of a single disease or syndrome.[2,72,111] The ability to understand the anatomy and function of the masticatory system and correctly interpret relevant diagnostic information is a prerequisite to fulfilling comprehensive standards of care. Our diagnostic process must be broad based and inclusive enough to determine the most appropriate cause of masticatory dysfunction.[118]

TEMPOROMANDIBULAR JOINT

Harmonious function of the TMJs is a product of the coordination of the muscles of mastication by intricate mechanisms of neurologic control. Understanding the dynamics and the relationship of the TMJ to the associated muscles and nerves provides the working knowledge required for effective assessment and diagnosis.

The TMJ is one of the most complex joints in the human body. It is capable of providing both hinging *(rotation)* and gliding *(translation)* movements and sustaining incredible forces of mastication. The TMJ is formed by the head of the condyle of the mandible as it fits into the articular fossa of the temporal bone (Figure 30-1). The body of the mandible effectively connects both condyles so that neither condyle functions independently of the other. Interposed between the head of the condyle and the articular surface of the temporal bone is the *articular disc,* consisting of dense connective tissue, resulting in a compound joint with two joint cavities (Figure 30-2). The articulating surfaces of the osseous structures are essentially convex in a healthy situation, so the biconcave configuration of the articular disc compensates for the opposing convexities. The articular surfaces of the condyles and temporal bones consist of fibrous connective tissue, rendering them resistant to breakdown and capable of repair. Deep to the superficial connective tissue layer, articular cartilage provides the cellular and structural basis for the response to the functional loading and movement of the TMJs.[72,118,163] The discal ligaments and attachments to the capsule, along with the disc itself, become the means of separating the joint into superior and inferior joint spaces (Figures 30-1 and 30-2). Synovial lubrication of the articular surfaces is a function of synovial fluid production by endothelial cells along the borders of each joint cavity and at the anterior extent of the retrodiscal tissues.*

*References 38, 72, 118, 158, 160, 163.

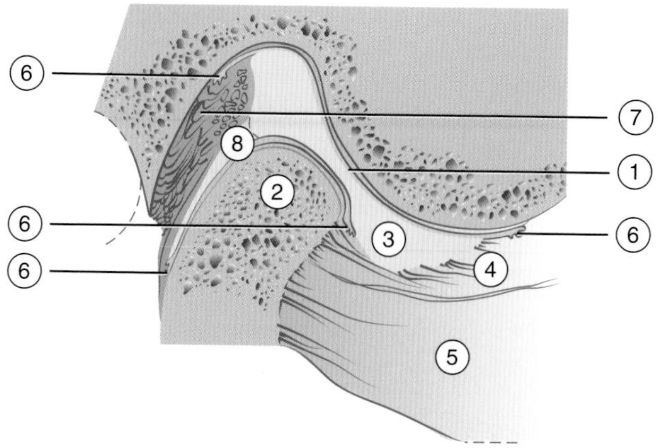

Figure 30-1 Lateral view of cross section through temporomandibular joint. *1,* Posterior slope of articular eminence of temporal bone; *2,* head of condyle; *3,* articular disc (note biconcave shape); *4,* superior lateral pterygoid muscle (note attachment to both head of condyle and articular disc); *5,* inferior lateral pterygoid muscle; *6,* synovial tissue; *7,* retrodiscal tissue; *8,* discal ligament attachment to the posterior surface of head of condyle. (Modified from Dawson PE: *Evaluation, diagnosis, and treatment of occlusal problems,* ed 2, St Louis, 1989, Mosby.)

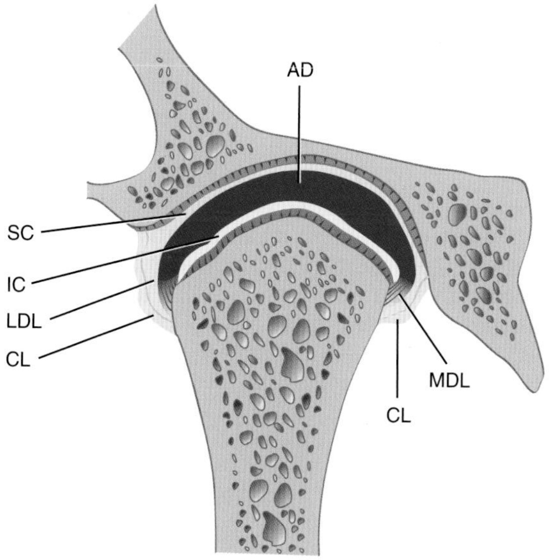

Figure 30-2 Temporomandibular joint (anterior view), showing collateral ligaments. *AD,* Articular disc; *CL,* capsular ligament; *IC,* inferior joint cavity; *LDL,* lateral discal ligament; *MDL,* medial discal ligament; *SC,* superior joint cavity. (From Okeson JP: *Management of temporomandibular joint disorders and occlusion,* ed 4, St Louis, 1998, Mosby.)

MUSCLES AND NERVES OF THE MASTICATORY SYSTEM

The muscles and nerves of the masticatory system are extensively reviewed elsewhere and are only briefly discussed here for the purpose of understanding the mechanisms involved. Appropriate references are provided for further reading.

The muscles of mastication consist principally of two groups: the *elevator* muscles and *depressor* muscles. The muscles responsible for elevating the mandible are the masseter, internal pterygoid, and much of the temporal muscle. The posteriorly oriented fibers of the temporal muscle also retrude the mandible. The superficial muscle bundle of the masseter muscle may also assist in protruding the mandible while the deeper bundle serves to stabilize the condylar head against the articular eminence. Juxtaposed with the masseter muscle, the medial pterygoid forms a muscular support for the mandible at its angle. Although the primary function of this muscle is elevation of the mandible, it is also active during protrusion.[72,118] The *lateral pterygoid muscle* is now known to function as two distinct muscles, the inferior and superior lateral pterygoid muscles, having independent and almost opposite functions.[6,14] The inferior lateral pterygoid muscle depresses and protrudes the mandible. The superior lateral pterygoid muscle does not contract during depression of the mandible but rather contracts along with the elevator muscles, bracing the condyle anteromedially.[98,106,116,118,138]

Physiologic mandibular posture and movement are products of harmonious muscular contraction among masticatory and supportive muscles. The neurologic input to produce synergy of complementary and antagonistic muscles is extremely complex. Motor and sensory innervation of the TMJs and the rest of the masticatory system are provided by structures of the trigeminal nerve. Mechanoreceptors in the skin, muscle, and ligamentous structures, especially the periodontal ligament, discern pressure differences at sensitive degrees of discrimination. Painful stimuli are perceived by nociceptors and result in both pain perception and reflex responses. The innervation of both the capsular ligaments and the discal ligaments provide essential proprioceptive input with regard to joint position. Efferent or motor neurons cause muscle contraction in response to central cortical stimulation and in response to afferent stimuli in reflex activity.[38,118,163]

Sensory input from the *periodontal ligament* (PDL) offers the potential to be an important component of the complex neurologic management of the masticatory system. Currently, little evidence of the existence of proprioceptive sensory organs within the neuroanatomy of the PDL is available, although it was once considered likely. Pain perception causes the nociceptive reflex to open the mouth rapidly through contraction of depressor muscles and suppression of elevator muscles, consistent with other protective reflexes within the musculoskeletal system.[118] Protective reflexes may be suppressed in individuals experiencing *chronic occlusal parafunction* (clenching or grinding of teeth).[24,46] Pressure perception is a function of the numerous mechanoreceptors within the PDL of teeth in contact. Discrimination within the dentition based on specific teeth in contact, direction of force, and intensity of force and their influence on muscle activity have been demonstrated in human study populations and animal studies.[22,35,89,97,141] Both research and clinical observations suggest that elevator muscle contraction is suppressed when anterior teeth promote *disclusion* or separation of posterior teeth during excursive mandibular movements.[159] Loss of attachment resulting from periodontitis involves the loss of some

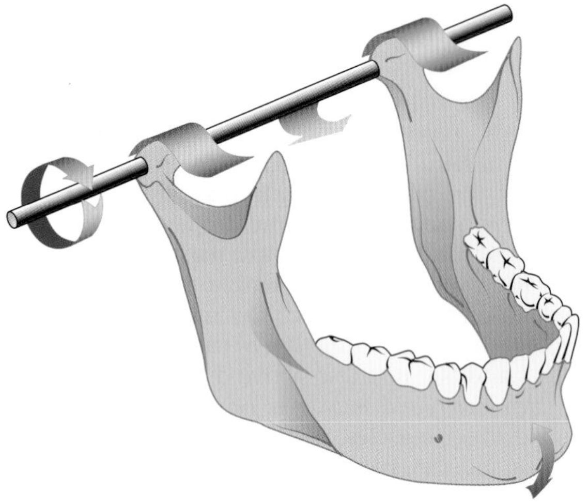

Figure 30-3 In centric relation, condyles can rotate on a fixed axis. As long as the rotational axis stays fixed at the most superior position against the eminentiae, the mandible can open or close and still be in centric relation. If the condyle axis moves forward, it is no longer in centric relation. (From Dawson PE: *Evaluation, diagnosis, and treatment of occlusal problems,* ed 2, St Louis, 1989, Mosby.)

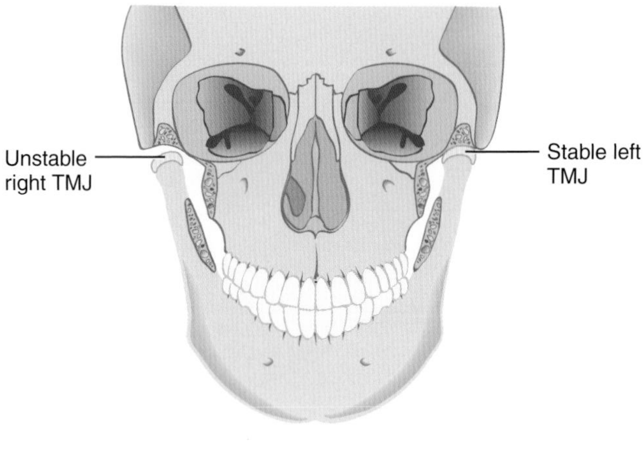

Figure 30-4 Example of orthopedic instability. Note that with the teeth in their stable position (maximum intercuspation), the left temporomandibular joint *(TMJ)* is in a stable relationship with the fossa. The right TMJ, however, is not in a stable position in the fossa. When the elevator muscles contract, the right condyle moves superiorly, seeking a more stable relationship with the articular disc and fossa (the musculoskeletally stable position). This type of loading can lead to an intracapsular disorder. (From Okeson JP: *Management of temporomandibular joint disorders and occlusion,* ed 4, St Louis, 1998, Mosby.)

mechanoreceptors. Patients with significant bone loss, significant inflammatory disruption of the integrity of the PDL, or chronic occlusal parafunction may experience compromised regulation of muscle activity.*

CENTRIC RELATION

The mandible is suspended from the cranial base by ligaments and muscles. Understanding mandibular movement begins from an initial reference point for each condyle, usually referred to as *centric relation.* This clinically determined relationship of the mandible to the maxilla occurs when both condyle-disc assemblies are positioned in their most superior position in the maxillary (or glenoid) fossa and against the slope of the articular eminence of the temporal bone. Verification of centric relation is obtained by loading the TMJs bilaterally with the teeth apart, using the bimanual mandibular manipulation technique advocated by Dawson and others.[38,39,151] When both condyles are in this relationship, rotation or hinging action occurs around an axis defined by the medial poles of each condyle (Figure 30-3). The term *centric relation* is limited to the rotation axis through both condyles while they are seated in their respective glenoid fossae. The only occlusal consideration relative to centric relation occurs when rotation of the mandible initiates the first contact of opposing occlusal surfaces. The term *initial contact in centric relation* can be used to define this relationship (see Chapter 56). If the contraction of elevator muscles occurs at the point of initial occlusal contact, resulting in the distraction of one or both condyle-disc assemblies from their seated relationship, centric relation is no longer occurring.[38,39]

*References 2, 23, 46, 69, 72, 111, 118, 136.

For TMJs to maintain orthopedic stability, the condyles must remain fully seated in their respective fossae when the teeth occlude in maximal intercuspation. Orthopedic instability occurs when the occlusal relationships are such that contraction of elevator muscles is required to achieve stable occlusion in maximal intercuspal position, resulting in the unseating of one or both condyles from their respective fossae (Figure 30-4). The strain on the discal ligaments caused by a loaded joint being displaced from the fossa can lead to internal derangement of that joint, as described later. Postural and parafunctional stress can also be a source of orthopedic instability of a TMJ. An individual's susceptibility to masticatory system disorders determines whether that person adapts with minimal consequence or develops dysfunction or degeneration.[23,38,118,151]

BIOMECHANICS OF THE MASTICATORY SYSTEM

Biomechanics of mandibular movement are a function of neurologic input from cortical and stomatognathic sources acting to initiate or restrict muscular contraction. Muscular action either stabilizes the condyle against the articular eminence or directs its rotational and translational movements relative to each respective temporal bone. The position and functional movement of one condyle always depend on the status or activity of the other. Because the maxillary teeth have a fixed relationship to the cranial base, just as mandibular teeth have a fixed relationship to the condyle, contact of their respective occlusal surfaces may directly influence condylar position or movement.[38,118]

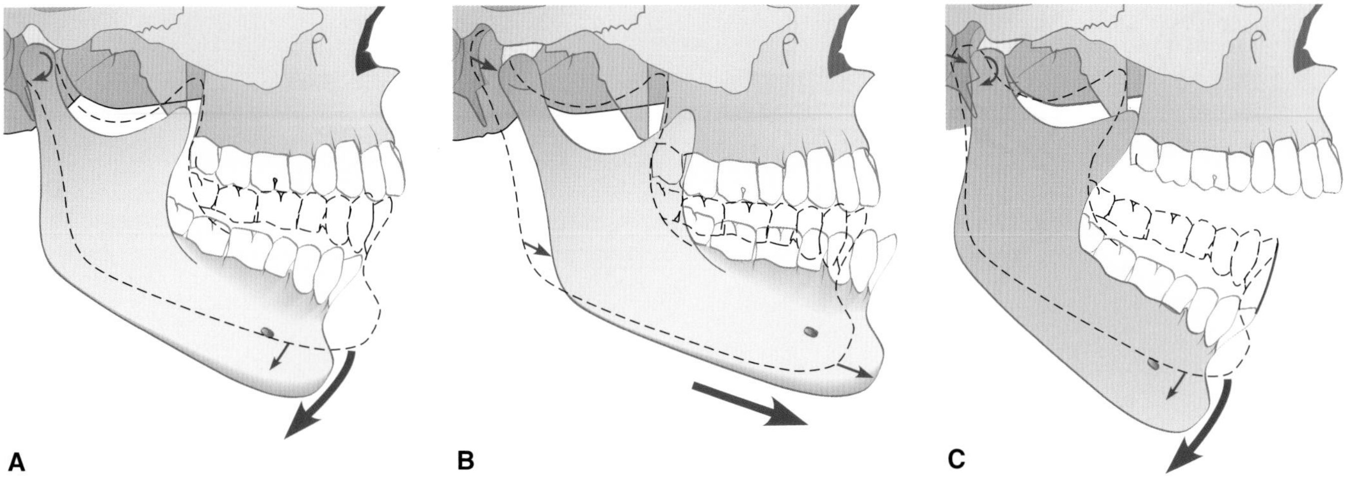

Figure 30-5 **A,** Rotational movement of mandible with condyles in centric relation. This pure rotational opening can occur until the anterior teeth are about 20 to 25 mm apart. **B,** Translational movement of the condyle-disc assembly during protrusion of the mandible. **C,** Second stage of rotational movement during opening. Note the dual activity relative to the articular disc. *1,* Rotation of the condylar head, relative to the disc, occurs in the inferior space. *2,* Movement of the disc anteriorly and inferiorly along the articular surface of the temporal bone. The articular disc moves anteriorly and inferiorly with the head of the condyle, which continues to rotate against the disc. Translation occurs in the superior joint space, and rotation occurs in the inferior joint space. (From Okeson JP: *Management of temporomandibular joint disorders and occlusion,* ed 4, St Louis, 1998, Mosby.)

The mandible can move within a range of motion that is limited by skeletal, muscular, and ligamentous structures. Pure rotation of up to approximately 25 mm can occur before translation of the condyle is required to continue toward maximal opening of the jaw. Movement of the condyle is relative to the disc, so rotation effectively occurs within the inferior joint space (Figure 30-5, *A*). Strict translation protrudes the mandible while the condyle-disc assembly moves anterior and inferior toward the articular eminence of the temporal bone. The disc moves relative to the temporal bone, and movement occurs within the upper joint space (Figure 30-5, *B*). In combination translation/rotation movement of the condyle, the axis of rotation for each condyle changes as the condyle translates down the articular eminence to a position inferior to its fossa (Figure 30-5, *C*). Harmonious muscle function and ligament attachments keep the condyle-disc assembly properly related so that the articular disc remains loaded in its concave, avascular central portion between the condyle and the articular surface of the temporal bone. The elasticity and vascularity of the retrodiscal tissues permit anterior movement of the disc during translation of each respective condyle. Rotation and translation of the condyle can occur in the absence of any tooth-to-tooth contact because the condyle-disc assembly can be supported by the muscles of mastication against the articular eminence during rotation, translation, and combination movements. When the teeth are in contact, their ability to influence both the position and the direction of movement of condyle-disc assemblies is defined by the intensity of muscle activity and the steepness of the inclines of those teeth.[38,66,76,92,118]

DYSFUNCTION AND DETERIORATION

Ideally, function never exceeds the integrity or adaptive limits of the structural elements of the masticatory system. Clinical experience shows that the tolerance of the components of the masticatory system can be exceeded by both acute trauma and chronic trauma.

Acute trauma to the head and neck region can range from a distinct event, such as an accident or a blow to the face, to a sustained overuse experience, such as a long dental appointment. Acute trauma can serve as an initiating event leading toward a chronic condition, so accurate documentation and careful monitoring may prove extremely valuable should symptoms or dysfunction persist.[12,19,41]

Chronic trauma is defined as any experience that repeatedly exceeds the tolerances of the affected masticatory system structure. Postural stresses and parafunctional occlusal habits, with or without occlusal discrepancies, may produce musculoskeletal disharmony and orthopedic instability of the TMJ. Occlusal relationships that disrupt the condyle during physiologic movement of rotation or translation require muscular and TMJ compensation. The extent to which the repeated loading of the teeth and the condyles during function and parafunction exceeds the tolerance of an individual will determine whether structural or muscular compromise occurs.[118]

In the absence of prospective research, it is somewhat difficult to associate defined occlusal patterns with specific muscle or joint disorders; however, retrospective studies and clinical experience still offer valuable perspectives. When TMJ dysfunction could be correlated with specific occlusal relationships, the trend was to recognize

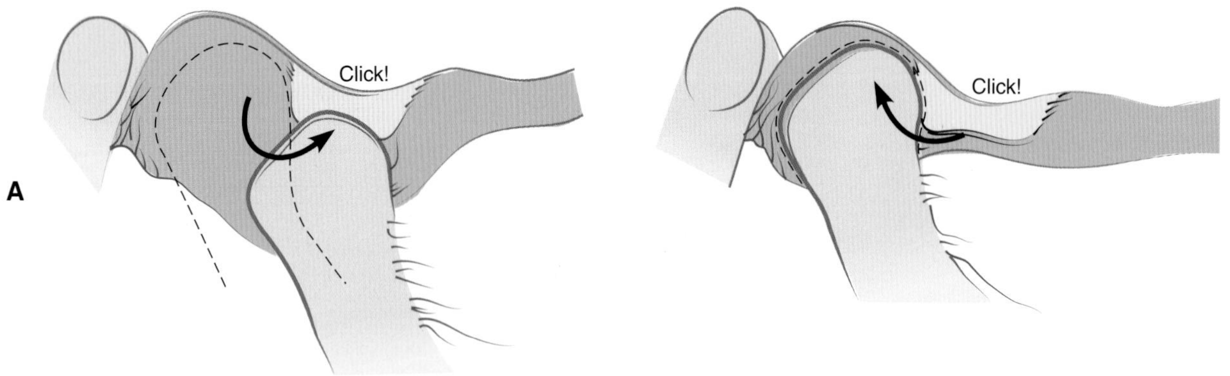

Figure 30-6 Reciprocal click. **A,** Reciprocal click occurs when the condyle moves onto the articular disc from a position behind the posterior band of the disc and then, **B,** clicks off the disc when the condyle moves back. This occurs as the condyle translates forward and back in the opening and closing movements. (From Dawson PE: *Evaluation, diagnosis, and treatment of occlusal problems,* ed 2, St Louis, 1989, Mosby.)

that when inclines of posterior teeth dominated occlusal function, masticatory system harmony was disrupted.* Other researchers have found that various occlusal interferences and relationships are common among individuals with and without masticatory system disorders. They could not distinguish a particular occlusal feature as a specific etiologic or predisposing factor to the development of masticatory system disorders, although some found that several factors occurring together encouraged dysfunction.[33,65,127,128,150] There seems to be less correlation between static references, such as class of malocclusion, and masticatory system disorders than when functional or extrafunctional occlusal forces exceed the tolerance of the TMJ and masticatory musculature.[118,140]

The general terms for occlusal parafunction used in this text include *bruxism,* or grinding of the teeth, and *clenching,* where a person holds the teeth firmly together with significant force. Bruxism is usually confirmed by observing excessive tooth wear. Clenching type of parafunction can be distinguished from grinding the teeth and seems to be more often associated with masticatory system disorders than does bruxism.† Discrimination between occlusal function–related or parafunction-related masticatory system disorders and those with other etiology requires exacting standards of occlusal evaluation. If sufficient evidence exists to suspect that the occlusal relationships in function or parafunction may have exceeded the tolerances of that individual's masticatory system, responsible intervention or monitoring can be initiated.[39,56,121,128]

Disruption of the relationship or alignment of the condyle, disc, and articular surface of the temporal bone is typically called an *intracapsular disorder* or *internal derangement* of the TMJ. The articular disc can be displaced as a result of an acute blow to the jaw, chronic trauma, or uncoordinated contraction of the lateral pterygoid muscle. When the disc cannot return to its normal relationship to the condyle on full closure of the mouth, it is considered to be *displaced* or *dislocated.* Progressive disc displacement most often occurs in an anterior and medial direction because of the insertion of muscle fibers into the anteromedial aspect of the disc and the reported variability in resistance of the attachment of the lateral aspect of the disc.[11,142] Stretching of the retrodiscal tissues and collateral ligaments permits the disc to be displaced and function to be limited because of pain resulting from compressive forces on retrodiscal tissues. At some stage of opening, the remaining elasticity of the retrodiscal tissues and tension of the capsular ligaments can pull the disc onto the head of the condyle, often with a discernible sound. Closing then results in the disc again becoming dislocated anteriorly, with a common joint sound often referred to as a *reciprocal click** (Figure 30-6).

When the disc remains anterior to the head of the condyle during rotation and the limited range of translation possible, the condition is called *closed lock* or *disc displacement (dislocation) without reduction* (Figure 30-7). The entire disc need not be locked anterior to the head of the condyle for this condition to limit function and cause pain. The lateral aspect of the disc would be more likely than the medial aspect to be displaced anteriorly if a *partial anterior disc displacement without reduction* were to occur. A history of joint sounds is usually reported, although this state of the condyle-disc assembly may not result in currently discernible sounds.[38,118]

The vascular portion of the retrodiscal tissues being loaded (between the condyle and the articular surface of the eminentia) accounts for most current pain or a history of pain originating within the TMJ. Adaptation of the retrodiscal tissues to completely nonvascular fibrous tissue or perforation of the disc may account for cessation of the painful symptoms.[122]

The presence of abnormal anatomic features of the condyle and fossa results in deviation in the shape of the affected articular surface, to which the disc then must adapt its normal anatomy, resulting in a deviation in form and function. If this type of functional limitation

*References 1, 27, 39, 61, 65, 70, 109, 118, 157, 159.
†References 28, 52, 54, 71, 121, 126.

*References 9, 38, 39, 118, 129, 153.

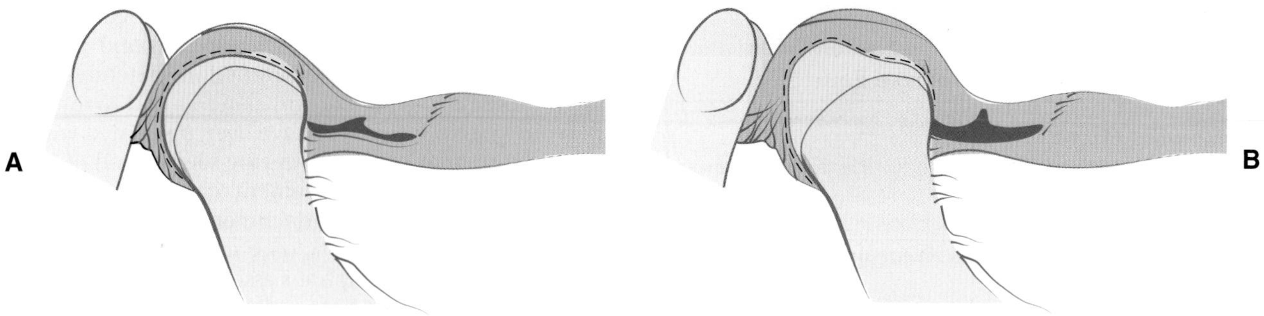

Figure 30-7 Anterior disc displacement without reduction. **A,** Condyle positioned in the fossa on retrodiscal tissues with the disc remaining anterior to head of condyle. **B,** During translation, the disc is further misshapen, restricting full opening of the mandible.

or irregularity is observed at a consistently occurring point in jaw opening and closing, it is often within the compensatory mechanisms of the patient and should be distinguished from the disc derangements described previously.[118]

When the intensity and duration of the functional and dysfunctional loading of the TMJs result in injury, molecular agents appear to be active in the degeneration of joints. Free radicals, various catabolic enzymes, neuropeptides, estrogen, cytokines, and prostaglandins are implicated in inflammatory reactions that have an impact on the articular surfaces and synovial fluid.* Loss of the ability of the synovial fluid to lubricate articular surfaces can result in adherence of the disc. Limitation of rotation occurs with adherence between the disc and the condyle, whereas fixation of the disc against the fossa permits rotation but does not allow the disc to move forward during translation.[118]

Hypermobility *(subluxation)* of the TMJ can permit the condyle to translate beyond the eminentia with both the disc and the condyle beyond its prominence. The combination of anatomic features that predisposes individuals to subluxation, often allows for self-reduction of the condyles. When condyles translate beyond the eminentia but the discs are trapped posteriorly, the combined steepness of the disc and the eminentia prevents reduction of each condyle, and the mandible is locked open.[118]

OROFACIAL PAIN

Discomfort associated with masticatory system disorders falls under the larger umbrella of orofacial pain. Pain associated with TMJ dysfunction is most frequently muscular in origin.[38] Working knowledge of even the uncommon sources of pain perceived in the region of the masticatory system is essential to providing comprehensive diagnosis and treatment. Sources of dental or periodontal pain should be identified by clinical, radiographic, and historical information. Nondental sources of pain include TMJ structures, muscles, cervical structures, neuropathies, vascular inflammation, all types of headache, sleep disorders, systemic disorders, and psychoimmune neurologic sources.[117] A survey of 45,700 American households revealed that 22% of respondents had experienced some type of orofacial pain in the previous 6 months, establishing a meaningful probability that the periodontal patient's list of symptoms includes pain.[94] Box 30-1 provides the current list of possible sources of orofacial pain, prepared by the American Academy of Orofacial Pain.[117]

Headache pain is perceived primarily within the trigeminal nerve pathways, although other cranial and cervical nerves may offer painful sensory input.[72,117] Pain originating in masticatory system structures, which are also innervated by the trigeminal nerve, requires diagnostic differentiation from headache pain.[140] Headache can present in a myriad of forms and can influence perception of pain and diagnosis of origin of pain.[72,117] Pain of dental and periodontal origin must be clearly defined and differentiated from heart attack, sinus pain, and myofascial pain.[117,118] Pain originating in pulpal or periodontal nocioceptors would be differentiated with a comprehensive clinical and radiographic evaluation. Orofacial pain originating in the TMJs or the muscles of mastication can result from neoplasm, macrotrauma, repeated microtrauma, systemic disease, and anatomic predisposition. Within the joint structures, inflammation and compression of vascularized components are the direct sources of pain. Synovitis or capsulitis, with or without osteoarthritis, and the polyarthritides are characterized by local pain, which increases with function while limiting range of motion of the affected TMJ. In addition to the potential for pain, symptoms of arthritis can include limited mandibular opening, disruption of other jaw mechanics, and joint sounds characteristic of degenerative change to and direct contact between articular surfaces.*

Orofacial pain originating in the muscles of mastication may be perceived in that region or may be referred to other structures, such as individual teeth. Similarly, pain referral to the region of certain muscles requires definition of origin. Because local provocation at the origin of pain should produce symptoms at the site of pain perception, movement of the jaw would be expected to elicit pain in painful muscles of mastication. Cranial

*References 50, 59, 80, 83, 85, 107, 108, 114, 132, 144.

*References 42, 45, 55, 57, 67, 81, 82, 96, 99, 101, 117, 164.

BOX 30-1

Differential Diagnosis of Orofacial Pain

Intracranial Pain Disorders[64,72,117,123]
Neoplasm, aneurysm, abscess, hemorrhage, hematoma, edema

Primary Headache Disorders (Neurovascular Disorders)[86,118]
Migraine, migraine variants, cluster headache, paroxysmal hemicrania, cranial arteritis, carotidynia, tension-type headache[79,117,118,139]

Neurogenic Pain Disorders
Paroxysmal neuralgias: Trigeminal, glossopharyngeal, nervus intermedius, and superior laryngeal neuralgias[155]
Continuous pain disorders: Deafferentation pain syndromes (peripheral neuritis, postherpetic neuritis, posttraumatic and postsurgical neuralgia, neuralgia-inducing cavitation osteonecrosis[16,17])
Sympathetically maintained pain

Intraoral Pain Disorders
Dental pulp, periodontium, mucogingival tissues, tongue[13,104]

Temporomandibular Disorders
Masticatory muscle, temporomandibular joint, associated structures

Associated Structures[117,118]
Ears, eyes, nose, paranasal sinuses, throat, lymph nodes, salivary glands, neck

Axis II Mental Disorders
Somatoform disorders
Pain syndromes of psychogenic origin
Compiled by American Academy of Orofacial Pain.

nerves experience referral on the same side, whereas skeletal nerve referral can occur to the opposite side; both sources generally refer pain centrally or superiorly.[72,118,145]

The muscles of mastication are subject to a variety of disorders and dysfunction, many of which can be painful. The American Academy of Orofacial Pain designates myofascial pain, myositis, muscle spasm (myospasm), local myalgia, and myofibrotic contracture as major categories of these conditions. Muscle palpation that reveals a taut band of muscle or fascia and that results in pain, which is also frequently referred, is virtually diagnostic for *myofascial pain. Myostitis* of masticatory muscles arises from direct trauma or infection close to muscle. Associated pain increases with mandibular movement, thereby limiting range of motion. *Muscle spasm* is the sustained involuntary contraction resulting in pain and dramatic shortening of the affected muscle. Myospasm of masticatory muscles greatly limits mandibular movement and can change occlusion suddenly because of its rapid onset. *Local myalgia,* or pain specific to individual muscles, may result from ischemia or fatigue and may present as delayed-onset muscle soreness and protective co-contraction. Occlusal parafunction, extended dental appointments, metabolic imbalances, and sympathetic nervous system influences have been associated with this painful muscular reaction. An extended period of limited range of mandibular movement can result in fibrosis of the muscle and related attachments, creating a painless condition called *myofibrotic contracture.*[117]

Otolaryngologic symptoms associated with masticatory system disorders have been reported and include degrees of deafness, tinnitus, and vertigo.* Trauma and postural stress in the cervical spine can be responsible for both the perception and the origin of pain within the masticatory system.[12,19,72,118]

Determination of a specific origin or source of pain can become more difficult with pain referral and modulation of painful experiences by the central nervous system. Sensitization of peripheral nocioceptors by higher neural centers and inflammation at the site of origin of pain can alter pain perception. Persistent inflammation therefore may be a contributing factor to chronic pain.[73,100,143] Systemic conditions that may contribute to or predispose an individual to compromised pain regulation include sleep disorders, fibromyalgia, chronic depression, chronic fatigue syndrome, hypothyroidism, insufficient thyroid receptor activity, prolactin feedback disorder, epinephrine sensitivity related to mitral valve prolapse, premenstrual syndrome, androgen excess in women, and posttraumatic stress disorder. Although some of these situations exhibit gender bias because of hormonal factors, the influence of stress on pain experiences and the effect of variable coping skills are reported for both genders.†

COMPREHENSIVE EVALUATION

Patient History and Interview

The written history and personal interview should be designed to invite open-ended responses and reflection by the patient on past experiences and the current condition. Standard dental or medical history forms may require modification to include questions regarding any history of limited or painful jaw movement, noise in either joint, and masticatory muscle symptoms (Box 30-2). These issues should be documented with regard to timing, duration, frequency, and relationship to any history of trauma.[117]

Clinical Examination

The clinical examination continues the interview process through co-discovery of the patient's masticatory system status. The dentist leads the patient to understand the meaning of signs and symptoms of dysfunction or deterioration, seeking opportunities to expand the patient's responses to questions. The physical examination actually

*References 15, 21, 25, 26, 34, 36, 51, 75, 112, 118, 120, 134, 135, 162.
†References 5, 20, 91, 115, 117, 137, 148.

SCIENCE TRANSFER

Stability in centric relation is an important determinant of orthopedic stability of the masticatory system because it allows for the condyles to be fully seated in their glenoid fossae. After identifying centric relation, as described in this chapter, the dentist employs procedures for establishing tooth contact by using interocclusal, hard occlusal splints and occlusal adjustment. In addition to stable centric relation, the masticatory system requires an intercuspal position that is tolerated by the joints, ligaments, and muscles and ideally, anterior disclusion to limit the contact of posterior teeth during functional and parafunctional mandibular movements. When any of these requirements is compromised, dysfunction of the masticatory system becomes more likely.

The masticatory system consists of the temporomandibular joints, masticatory muscles, oral structures, and all their corresponding vascular and neurologic components. As such, many conditions exist where various aspects of these structures change because of wear or inflammation. As changes occur, various components are affected, and in many cases, pain results. Unfortunately, however, the pain is often diffuse and not well localized. This makes definitive diagnosis extremely difficult, and although improved, imaging of masticatory structures is still problematic. *Thus, masticatory system disorders remain a difficult area for diagnosis and treatment.*

BOX 30-2

Examples of Questions Involving Masticatory System to Include in Patient History

Are you now experiencing or have you ever experienced:

1. Pain in either jaw joint or pain when opening or closing your mouth?[8]
2. Acute or direct trauma to the face, jaw, head, or neck, such as during an accident?
3. Any locking or restricted movement of either jaw joint?[44,146]
4. Inability to bite or close teeth together completely without discomfort in one or both jaw joints?
5. Earache without infection, especially if it is recurring?
6. Ringing or rushing sounds in either ear?
7. Any type of neuralgia (nerve pain), especially with trigger points?[8] Tooth pain without diagnosed dental problem or after tooth removal?[102,103,161]
9. Fibromyalgia (muscle pain)?[37,125,130]
10. Sleep apnea or any sleep disturbance?
11. Any sounds, such as clicks or pops, in either jaw joint, especially when opening or while eating?
12. Chronic or frequently recurring headaches, especially migraine or cluster type of headache?[4]
13. Shingles or any painful infection of face or neck?
14. Having to "adjust" the jaw or manipulate jaw joint with your hand to be able to open or close your mouth?
15. An occupation or activity that requires regular stressful posture, such as cradling a telephone between head and shoulder, working at a computer, playing a musical instrument, or scuba diving?[149,165]
16. Awareness of frequently keeping your teeth together, maintaining a clenched jaw, or holding your jaw in an assumed position, such as holding a pipe?
17. Lyme disease?[60]
18. Neck muscles that are often tired or sore?
19. Sleep position or posture that maintains pressure on your lower jaw?

begins during the interview, when asymmetries in facial form, head posture, and mandibular movement patterns can be observed. Clinical evaluation of the various structures of the masticatory system, although individual to each practitioner, should include the following[9,38,118]:

1. Observation and measurement of full range of motion (ROM) of the mandible.
2. Auscultation and light palpation of each TMJ in its full ROM.
3. Load testing of each TMJ.
4. Palpitation of each muscle of mastication and related head and neck muscles.
5. Evaluation of all the soft tissues of the face, oral cavity, and oropharynx.
6. Periodontal and dental examinations.
7. Complete occlusal analysis, including accurately mounted diagnostic models.

Evaluation of the TMJ begins with *ROM analysis*. Observation of departure from a straight path of opening and closing the mandible suggests an intracapsular disorder or masticatory muscle incoordination.[38,118] An average maximal opening of 50 mm is common; findings of less than 40 mm of opening suggest limited opening caused by a masticatory system disorder. The range of right and left lateral excursions is usually about 9 mm, and protrusion of mandible is typically 7 mm. Limitation in ROM may be normal for some patients, but for most, these observations are of diagnostic value.[9,44,63,118,146] *Auscultation* of the joint by listening with a stethoscope or Doppler instrument, which amplifies joint sound for both the patient and the dentist, can reveal noises diagnostic for numerous conditions. The intensity and nature of any sounds, clicks, pops, or crepitus (grinding, grating, or rubbing sounds) should be recorded accurately. Any sound detected as part of the initial evaluation should be tracked consistently to detect any change. Diagnostic interpretation and management based on specific sounds correlated with status of the TMJ can be found in other references.[7,9,38,118,156]

Firm palpation of the TMJ with the mouth closed can be uncomfortable to the patient with inflammation in joint structures or superficial muscles. Palpation while opening may become more uncomfortable if retrodiscal tissues are also inflamed. Load testing of the TMJ is essentially a means to palpate the head of the condyle, surface of the glenoid fossa, and tissue interposed between them, except in the case of bone-to-bone contact. With bimanual mandibular manipulation, the dentist loads the joints equally and may detect resistance or tension on either side. The patient is in a supine position in the dental chair to minimize postural influence on muscle activity. The patient's head is braced by the support of the chair and by being cradled against the dentist's arm or abdomen. The dentist's middle fingers locate the notch in the mandible just anterior to the angle, and the thumbs are placed near the midline in the mental region of the mandible (Figure 30-8). Initially, the dentist provides very gentle guidance to the hinging action of the mandible, with a slight lifting force applied by the fingers and slight depressing force applied with the thumbs. If the patient remains comfortable, increasing force can be applied at both points, ultimately with enough pressure to load-test the joints. With the avascular fibrous discs interposed, the condyles are in centric relation, and the loading of both joints is comfortable. Discomfort may occur with muscle incoordination or bracing or with an anterior displaced disc and attempted loading of vascular retrodiscal tissues of either TMJ. When performed properly, the patient can bite firmly as part of guided loading of the TMJs and report the nature or absence of pain or tension.[9,38,58,118]

Muscle palpation is also a learned technique that requires both experience and expertise to derive the most reliable information. Too little pressure is not diagnostic of modest muscle pain or spasm, whereas too much pressure can hurt even when normal musculature is palpated.[53] Externally, the muscles palpated include the anterior, middle, and posterior temporalis; superficial masseter; anterior and posterior digastric; sternocleidomastoid; trapezeius; posterior cervical muscles; and insertion of the medial pterygoid muscle. Intraorally, the deep masseter is tested with moderate squeezing pressure, and the medial pterygoid muscle is palpated directly in the general region of the insertion point for local anesthesia with mandibular block. The lateral pterygoid is difficult to palpate because of the dominance of the medial pterygoid in the same region. Its palpation superior and distal to the palpation point for the medial pterygoid can be attempted distal to the maxillary tuberosity. Offering manual resistance to the patient's efforts to protrude the mandible is also a test of the lateral pterygoid muscle. Neither method of evaluation of the possible soreness of the lateral pterygoid muscle is completely reliable, although both provide some insight into muscle status.*

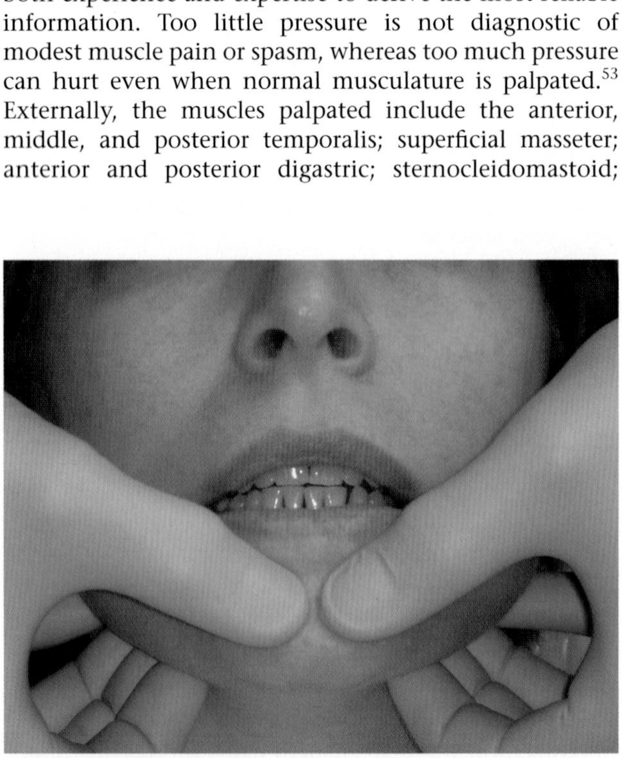

Figure 30-8 Bimanual manipulation load testing in centric relation with the teeth apart.

During muscle palpation, the dentist may be able to detect a particularly taut and uncomfortable band of muscle fibers. This condition represents *regional myofascial pain* or *trigger point myalgia,* which can be responsible for referral of pain to the teeth and other orofacial regions. Diagnostic injection of local anesthesia can be effective in identifying trigger point pain and pain referral patterns.[118,145]

The *occlusal analysis* is a logical extension of the evaluation of the teeth and periodontium. Tooth mobility is assessed in both static and dynamic modes. Pressure applied to a tooth with a firm object allows detection of movement through both visual and tactile evaluation (see Chapter 35). Asking the patient to move in excursions of the mandible while maintaining firm contact of opposing teeth also permits visual and tactile assessment. Sources of tooth mobility include inadequate periodontal support, inflammation of the periodontium, and excessive occlusal loading of the teeth with adequate periodontium, resulting in adaptive mobility. The physical evaluation of the teeth and any restorations can reflect history of trauma or wear. Visual observation, registration with marking paper or wax, and electronic assessment of tooth contacts as the patient moves in all excursions may reveal disharmonies sufficient to cause orthopedic instability of either TMJ. If the teeth are found to be relatively firm, the relationship between the maxillary and mandibular teeth may influence the direction of condylar movement as soon as tooth-to-tooth contact is made.

While maintaining centric relation, the dentist continues the physical examination by positioning the condyles in a fully seated relationship without tooth-to-tooth contact, using bimanual manipulation or a leaf gauge technique. The mandible is manually guided to close until the first tooth-to-tooth contact is made. If that position is also maximum intercuspation, optimum seating of the condyles is maintained. If the initial contact in centric relation is *not* maximum intercuspation, the condyles will be directed from a fully seated position to an inferior position relative to their respective fossae, resulting in an orthopedic instability. The direction and extent of the accommodation of the mandible should be carefully measured and recorded at the initial evaluation

*References 3, 9, 38, 47, 49, 72, 118, 147.

and consistently evaluated at subsequent appointments to discover any trend.*

To increase the reliability of this evaluation, a muscle-deprogramming effort may be employed. The simplest approach is to use cotton rolls placed between the anterior teeth for 5 to 15 minutes to allow possible muscle relaxation through avoidance of proprioceptive or pressure neurologic input. A prefabricated or directly fabricated acrylic or composite bite stop for anterior teeth offers the same advantage.[9,10,118] A more complex means of confirming the seating of the condyles in centric relation is achieved with a maxillary or mandibular muscle relaxation occlusal appliance. These appliances provide full coverage for the respective arch and occlusal contact for at least one cusp or incisal edge of the opposing teeth so that teeth are protected from spontaneous shifting. The occlusal design provides immediate disclusion of all the posterior teeth in every protrusive or lateral excursion. This allows for the progressive deprogramming of muscles through the advantage of reduced muscle contractions and limited noxious neurologic input.[39,87,159]

Models of the dentition must be accurately mounted to be diagnostic. The *facebow transfer* relates the maxillary cast to the axis of rotation of the articulator as the maxillary teeth relate to the cranial case. With careful bimanual manipulation or the use of an anterior bite stop, a transfer wafer is generated with the condyles fully seated in their glenoid fossa. The maxillary and mandibular teeth of each diagnostic model then relate to one another in centric relation, as determined by condylar position. They may reveal an occlusal discrepancy in centric relation, which would require compensation by the patient.[9,38]

Imaging

When the clinical evaluation and patient history indicate the possibility of structural masticatory system disorders or the possible presence of pathology, especially neoplasm, appropriate imaging of the TMJ is warranted. The state-of-the-art technique for imaging of soft tissue, especially the articular disc, is magnetic resonance imaging (MRI). The current highest standard for imaging of hard tissue, such as the condyle or the temporal bone, is computed tomography (CT). Both techniques are usually reserved for more difficult or strategic diagnoses, such as when joint surgery is being considered. Their interpretation usually requires specialized training for the clinician or access to a radiologist. Although arthrography is still being used for certain diagnostic situations, such as suspected perforation of the articular disc, CT and MRI are being increasingly utilized.[9,18,74,88,124]

Although plain-film tomography is occasionally a feature of some of the newer radiographic equipment, the technique most readily available to a majority of practitioners is *panoramic radiography.* The image produced depicts only general relationships and gross anatomy, so the information provided should be used only for screening purposes. When pathology or marked deformation is suggested by a panoramic radiograph, further diagnostic imaging and procedures may be warranted.[18,72]

DIAGNOSTIC DECISION MAKING

Complete evaluation of every patient's periodontal status must include the diagnostic components required to reveal any form of masticatory system disorder. The existence of factors responsible for historical, current, or potential impairment of masticatory system function can be integrated into a comprehensive treatment plan. Patients who require substantial periodontal therapy or have advanced periodontal disease may be at increased risk for masticatory system disorders, so diagnostic processes must remain consistently thorough and inclusive for all patients.[23,136] For the patient presenting with a symptomatic masticatory system disorder, the diagnostic strategy would logically begin with the inclusion of all potential sources of pain or dysfunction, followed by the systematic exclusion of possible causative or contributing factors, beginning with the least likely. When no symptoms are reported, the history and clinical examination still need to be thorough because some patients tend to tolerate modest dysfunction or mild transient discomfort. The diagnostic strategy for the patient presenting minimal or no signs and symptoms of masticatory system disorders is to attempt to confirm a stable condition while identifying risk factors. Careful documentation of past or current trauma and disharmony provide the basis for trend analysis and anticipation of possible future problems.*

Consistent professional maintenance care has been clearly demonstrated to be a key ingredient in successful management of a patient's periodontal condition.[62,105] Complementing any treatment sequence, these appointments afford dentists the opportunity at every stage of comprehensive care to provide continuing evaluation of the status of the entire masticatory systemand to provide timely and appropriate intervention when needed (see Chapter 56).

ACKNOWLEDGMENTS

I would like to acknowledge the incredible efforts of Dr. David K. Warfield in helping me compile the numerous references reviewed during the development of this chapter. His encouragement, along with that of Drs. Peter Dawson and Henry Gremillion, was very meaningful and often timely. Drs. Dawson, Gremillion, Parker Mahan, and Okeson provided invaluable foundations through their publications, texts, and lectures. Although there are many others from whom I have learned much, these four exceptional dentists certainly deserve my public appreciation. I would especially like to acknowledge my precious wife, Martha-Anne, whose patience and support were priceless, as always.

*References 9, 29, 30, 38-40, 68, 70, 77, 78, 84, 94, 95, 118, 119, 131, 133, 140, 154.

*References 31, 32, 43, 53, 90, 110, 111, 113, 152.

REFERENCES

1. Al-Hadi LA: Prevalence of temporomandibular disorders in relation to some occlusal parameters, *J Prosthet Dent* 70:345, 1993.
2. Allen EP, Bayne SC, Becker IM, et al: Annual review of selected dental literature: Report of the Committee of Scientific Investigation of the American Academy of Restorative Dentistry, *J Prosthet Dent* 82:39, 1999.
3. Atwood MJ, Dixon DC, Talcott GW, et al: Comparison of two scales in the assessment of muscle and joint palpation tenderness in chronic temporomandibular disorders, *J Orofac Pain* 7:403, 1993.
4. Austin DG: Special considerations in orofacial pain and headache, *Dent Clin North Am* 41:325, 1997.
5. Auvenshine RC: Psychoneuroimmunology and its relationship to the differential diagnosis of temporomandibular disorders, *Dent Clin North Am* 41:279, 1997.
6. Aziz MA, Cowie RJ, Skinner CE, et al: Are the two heads of the human lateral pterygoid separate muscles? A perspective based on their nerve supply, *J Orofac Pain* 12:226, 1998.
7. Bade DM, Lovasko JH, Dimitroff M, et al: Clinical comparison of temporomandibular joint sound auscultation and emission imaging studies, *J Orofac Pain* 8:55, 1994.
8. Bates RE, Gremillion HA, Stewart CM: Degenerative joint disease. Part II. Symptoms and examination findings, *J Craniomandib Pract* 12:88, 1994.
9. Becker IM, Tarantola GJ: *Parameters of care: temporomandibular disorders,* Key Biscayne, Fla, 1994, Pankey Institute of Advanced Dental Education.
10. Becker I, Tarantola G, Zambrano J, et al: Effect of a prefabricated anterior bite stop on electromyographic activity of masticatory muscles, *J Prosthet Dent* 82:22, 1999.
11. Ben Amor F, Carpentier P, Foucart JM, et al: Anatomic and mechanical properties of the lateral disc attachment of the temporomandibular joint, *J Oral Maxillofac Surg* 56:1164, 1998.
12. Benoliel R, Eliav E, Elishoov H, et al: Diagnosis and treatment of persistent pain after trauma to the head and neck. *J Oral Maxillofac Surg* 1994; 52:1138.
13. Bergdahl J, Anneroth G, Anneroth I: Clinical study of patients with burning mouth. Scand J Dent Res 1994; 102:229.
14. Bertilsson O, Ström D: A literature survey of a hundred years of anatomic and functional lateral pterygoid muscle research, *J Orofac Pain* 9:17, 1995.
15. Bjorne A, Agerberg G: Craniomandibular disorders in patients with Ménière's disease: a controlled study, *J Orofac Pain* 10:28, 1996.
16. Bouquot J, Roberts A: NICO (neuralgia-inducing cavitational osteonecrosis): radiographic appearance of the "invisible" osteomyelitis, *Oral Surg* 74:600, 1992.
17. Bouquot JE, Roberts AM, Person P, et al: NICO (neuralgia-inducing cavitational osteonecrosis): osteomyelitis in 224 jawbone samples from patients with facial neuralgias, *Oral Surg* 73:307, 1992.
18. Brooks SL, Brand JW, Gibbs SJ, et al: Imaging of the temporomandibular joint: a position paper of the American Academy of Oral and Maxillofacial Radiology, *Oral Surg Oral Med Oral Pathol Oral Radiol Endod* 83:609, 1997.
19. Burgess JA, Kolbinson DA, Lee PT, et al: Motor vehicle accidents and TMDs: assessing the relationship, *J Am Dent Assoc* 127:1767, 1996.
20. Bush FM, Harkins SW: Pain-related limitation in activities of daily living in patients with chronic orofacial pain: psychometric properties of a disability index, *J Orofac Pain* 9:57, 1995.
21. Bush FM, Harkins SW, Harrington WG: Otalgis and aversive symptoms in temporomandibular disorders, *Ann Otol Rhino Laryngol* 108:884, 1999.
22. Byers MR, Dong WK: Comparison of trigeminal receptor location and structure in the periodontal ligament of different types of teeth from the rat, cat, and monkey, *J Comp Neurol* 279:117, 1989.
23. Carranza FA, Newman MG: *Clinical periodontology,* ed 8, Philadelphia, 1996, Saunders.
24. Cathelineau G, Yardin M: The relationship between tooth vibratory sensation and periodontal disease, *J Periodontol* 53:704, 1982.
25. Chan SWY, Reade PC: Tinnitus and temporomandibular pain-dysfunction disorder, *Clin Otolaryngol* 19:370, 1994.
26. Chole RA, Parker WS: Tinnitus and vertigo in patients with temporomandibular disorder, *Arch Otolaryngol Head Neck Surg* 118:817, 1992.
27. Christensen GJ: Abnormal occlusal conditions: a forgotten part of dentistry, *J Am Dent Assoc* 126:1667, 1995.
28. Christensen GJ: Treating bruxism and clenching, *J Am Dent Assoc* 131:233, 2000.
29. Christensen LV, Rassouli NM: Experimental occlusal interferences. Part I. A review, *J Oral Rehabil* 22:515, 1995.
30. Christensen LV, Rassouli NM: Experimental occlusal interferences. Part V. Mandibular rotations versus hemimandibular translations, *J Oral Rehabil* 22:865, 1995.
31. Christensen LV, McKay DC: TMD diagnostic decision-making and probability theory. Part I, *J Craniomandib Pract* 14:240, 1996.
32. Christensen LV, McKay DC: TMD diagnostic decision-making and probability theory. Part II, *J Craniomandib Pract* 14:312, 1996.
33. Clark GT, Tsukiyama Y, Baba K, et al: Sixty-eight years of experimental occlusal interference studies: what have we learned? *J Prosthet Dent* 82:704, 1999.
34. Ciancaglini R, Loreti P, Radaelli G: Ear, nose, and throat symptoms in patients with TMD: the association of symptoms according to severity of arthropathy, *J Orofac Pain* 8:293, 1994.
35. Coffey JP, Williams WN, Turner GE, et al: Human bite force discrimination using specific maxillary and mandibular teeth, *J Oral Rehabil* 16:529, 1989.
36. Cooper BC, Cooper DL: Recognizing otolaryngologic symptoms in patients with temporomandibular disorders, *J Craniomandib Pract* 11:260, 1993.
37. Dao TTT, Reynolds WJ, Tenenbaum HC: Comorbidity between myofascial pain of the masticatory muscle and fibromyalgia, *J Orofac Pain* 11:232, 1997.
38. Dawson PE: *Evaluation, diagnosis, and treatment of occlusal problems,* ed 2, St Louis, 1989, Mosby.
39. Dawson PE: New definition for relating occlusion to varying conditions of the temporomandibular joint, *J Prosthet Dent* 74:619, 1995.
40. Dawson PE: A classification system that relates maximal intercuspation to the position and condition of the temporomandibular joint, *J Prosthet Dent* 75:60, 1996.
41. De Boever JA, Keersmaeker K: Trauma in patients with temporomandibular disorders: frequency and treatment outcomes, *J Oral Rehabil* 23:91, 1996.
42. De Bont LGM, Stengenga B: Pathology of temporomandibular joint internal derangement and osteoarthrosis, *Int J Oral Maxillofac Surg* 22:71, 1993.
43. De Wijer A, Lobbezoo-Scholte AM, Steenks MH, et al: Reliability of clinical findings in temporomandibular disorders, *J Orofac Pain* 9:181, 1995.
44. Dimitroulis G, Dolwick MF, Gremillion HA: Temporomandibular disorders. 1. Clinical evaluation, *Aust Dent J* 40:301, 1995.

45. Donaldson KW: Rheumatoid diseases and the temporomandibular joint: a review, *J Craniomandib Pract* 13:264, 1995.
46. Dong WK, Shiwaku T, Kawakami Y, et al: Static and dynamic responses of periodontal ligament mechanoreceptors and intradental mechanoreceptors, *J Neurophysiol* 69:1567, 1993.
47. Ehrlich R, Garlick D, Ninio M: The effect of jaw clenching on the electromyographic activities of 2 neck and 2 trunk muscles, *J Orofac Pain* 13:115, 1999.
48. Ferrario VF, Sforza C, Sigurta D, et al: Temporomandibular joint dysfunction and flat lateral guidances: a clinical association, *J Prosthet Dent* 75:534, 1996.
49. Ferrario VF, Sforza C, Colombo A, et al: An electromyographic investigation of masticatory muscle symmetry in normo-occlusion subjects, *J Oral Rehabil* 27:33, 2000.
50. Fu K, Ma X, Zhang Z, et al: Interleukin-6 in synovial fluid and HLA-DR expression in synovium from patients with temporomandibular disorders, *J Orofac Pain* 9:131, 1995.
51. Gelb H, Gelb ML, Wagner ML: The relationship of tinnitus to craniocervical mandibular disorders, *J Craniomandib Pract* 15:136, 1997.
52. Glaros AG, Baharloo L, Glass EG: Effect of parafunctional clenching and estrogen on temporomandibular disorder pain, *J Craniomandib Pract* 16:78, 1998.
53. Glaros AG, Glass EG, Williams KB: Clinical examination findings of temporomandibular disorder patients: a factor analytic study, *J Orofac Pain* 12:193, 1998.
54. Glaros AG, Tabacchi KN, Glass EG: Effect of parafunctional clenching on TMD pain, *J Orofac Pain* 12:145, 1998.
55. Goupille P, FouQuet B, Goga D, et al: The temporomandibular joint in rheumatoid arthritis: correlations between clinical and tomographic features, *J Dent* 21:141, 1993.
56. Gremillion HA: TMD and maladaptive occlusion: does a link exist? *J Craniomandib Pract* 13:205, 1995.
57. Gynther GW, Holmlund AB, Reinholt FP, et al: Temporomandibular joint involvement in generalized osteoarthritis and rheumatoid arthritis: a clinical, arthroscopic, histologic, and immunohistochemical study, *Int J Oral Maxillofac Surg* 26:10, 1997.
58. Harper RP, Schneiderman E: Condylar movement and centric relation in patients with internal derangement of the temporomandibular joint, *J Prosthet Dent* 75:67, 1996.
59. Haskin CL, Milam SB, Cameron IL: Pathogenesis of degenerative joint disease in the human temporomandibular joint, *Crit Rev Oral Biol Med* 6:248, 1995.
60. Heir GM: Differentiation of orofacial pain related to Lyme disease from other dental and facial pain disorders, *Dent Clin North Am* 41:243, 1997.
61. Hickman DM, Cramer R: The effect of different condylar positions on masticatory muscle electromyography activity in humans, *Oral Surg Oral Med Oral Pathol Radiol Endod* 85:18, 1998.
62. Hirschfield L, Wasserman B: A long-term survey of tooth loss in 600 treated periodontal patients, *J Periodontol* 49:225, 1978.
63. Hochstedler JL, Allen JD, Follmar MA: Temporomandibular joint range of motion: a ratio of interincisal opening to excursive movement in a healthy population, *J Craniomandib Pract* 14:296, 1996.
64. Huntley TA, Wiesenfeld D: Delayed diagnosis of the cause of facial pain in patients with neoplastic disease: a report of eight cases, *J Oral Maxillofac Surg* 52:81, 1994.
65. Ingervall B, Hähner R, Kessi S: Pattern of tooth contacts in eccentric mandibular positions in young adults, *J Prosthet Dent* 66:169, 1991.
66. Isberg A, Westesson PL: Steepness of articular eminence and movement of the condyle and disk in asymptomatic temporomandibular joints, *Oral Surg Oral Med Oral Pathol Oral Radiol Endod* 86:152, 1998.
67. Israel HA, Diamond B, Saed-Nejad F, et al: Osteoarthritis and synovitis as major pathoses of the temporomandibular joint: comparison of clinical diagnosis with arthroscopic morphology, *J Oral Maxillofac Surg* 56:1023, 1998.
68. Ito T, Gibbs CH, Marguelles-Bonnet R, et al: Loading on the temporomandibular joints with five occlusal conditions, *J Prosthet Dent* 56:478, 1986.
69. Jacobs R, van Steenberghe D: Role of periodontal ligament receptors in the tactile function of teeth: a review, *J Periodont Res* 29:153, 1994.
70. Kahn J, Tallents RH, Katzberg RW, et al: Association between dental occlusal variables and intraarticular temporomandibular joint disorders: horizontal and vertical overlap, *J Prosthet Dent* 79:658, 1998.
71. Kampe T, Tagdae T, Bader G, et al: Reported symptoms and clinical findings in a group of subjects with longstanding bruxing behavior, *J Oral Rehabil* 24:581, 1997.
72. Kaplan AS, Assaed LA: *Temporomandibular disorders: diagnosis and treatment,* Philadelphia, 1991, Saunders.
73. Katz MA: Approach to the management of nonmalignant pain, *Am J Med* 101(suppl 1A):54S, 1996.
74. Katzberg RW, Westesson P: *Diagnosis of the temporomandibular joint,* Philadelphia, 1993, Saunders.
75. Keersmaeker K, De Boever JA, van Den Berghe L: Otalgia in patients with temporomandibular joint disorders, *J Prosthet Dent* 75:72, 1996.
76. Kenworthy CR, Morrish RB, Mohn C, et al: Bilateral condylar movement patterns in adult subjects, *J Orofac Pain* 11:328, 1997.
77. Kerstein RB: Disclusion time measurement studies: a comparison of disclusion time between chronic myofascial pain dysfunction patients and nonpatients: a population analysis, *J Prosthet Dent* 72:473, 1994.
78. Kerstein R: Disclusion time measurement studies: stability of disclusion time—a 1-year follow-up, *J Prosthet Dent* 72:164, 1994.
79. Kleinegger CL, Lilly GE: Cranial arteritis: a medical emergency with orofacial manifestations, *J Am Dent Assoc* 130:1203, 1999.
80. Kelmetti E, Vainio P, Kroger H: Craniomandibular disorders and skeletal mineral status, *J Craniomandib Pract* 13:89, 1995.
81. Koh ET, Yap AU, Koh CK, et al: Temporomandibular disorders in rheumatoid arthritis, *J Rheumatol* 26:1918, 1999.
82. Könönen M, Wenneberg B, Kallenberg A: Craniomandibular disorders in rheumatoid arthritis, psoriatic arthritis, and ankylosing spondylitis: a clinical study, *Acta Odontol Scand* 50:281, 1992.
83. Kopp S: The influence of neuropeptides, serotonin, and interleukin 1B on temporomandibular joint pain and inflammation, *J Oral Maxillofac Surg* 56:189, 1998.
84. Kuboki T, Azuma Y, Orsini MG, et al: Effects of sustained unilateral molar clenching on the temporomandibular joint space, *Oral Surg Oral Med Oral Pathol Oral Radiol Endod* 82:616, 1996.
85. Kubota E, Kubota T, Matsumoto J, et al: Synovial fluid cytokines and proteinases as markers of temporomandibular joint disease, *J Oral Maxillofac Surg* 56:192, 1998.
86. Kumar KL, Cooney TG: Headaches, *Med Clin North Am* 79:261, 1995.
87. Kurita H, Ikeda K, Kurashina K: Evaluation of the effect of a stabilization splint on occlusal force in patient occlusions with masticatory muscle disorders, *J Oral Rehabil* 27:79, 2000.
88. Larheim TA: Current trends in temporomandibular joint imaging, *Oral Surg Oral Med Oral Pathol Oral Radiol Endod* 80:555, 1995.

89. Lavigne G, Kim JS, Valiquette C, et al: Evidence that periodontal pressoreceptors provide positive feedback to jaw closing muscles during mastication, *J Neurophysiol* 58:342, 1987.
90. Levitt SR, McKinney MW: Appropriate use of predictive values in clinical decision making and evaluating diagnostic tests for TMD, *J Orofac Pain* 8:298, 1994.
91. Levitt SR, McKinney MW: Validating the TMJ scale in the national sample of 10,000 patients: demographic and epidemiologic characteristics, *J Orofac Pain* 8:25, 1994.
92. Lindauer SJ, Sabol G, Isaccson RJ, et al: Condylar movement and mandibular rotation during jaw opening, *Am J Orthod Dentofac Orthop* 107:573, 1995.
93. Lipton JA, Ship JA, Larach-Robinson D: Estimated prevalence and distribution of reported orofacial pain in the United States, *J Am Dent Assoc* 124:115, 1993.
94. Liu ZJ, Yamagata K, Kashara Y, et al: Electromyographic examination of jaw muscles in relation to symptoms and occlusion of patients with temporomandibular joint disorders, *J Oral Rehabil* 26:33, 1999.
95. Lobbezoo F, Lavigne GJ: Do bruxism and temporomandibular disorders have a cause-and-effect relationship? *J Orofac Pain* 11:15, 1997.
96. Locher MC, Felder M, Sailer HF: Involvement of the temporomandibular joints in ankylosing spondylitis (Bechterew's disease), *J Craniomaxillofac Surg* 24:205, 1996.
97. Louca C, Cadden SW, Linden RWA: The roles of periodontal ligament mechanoreceptors in the reflex control of human jaw-closing muscles, *Brain Res* 731:63, 1996.
98. Loughner BA, Gremillion HA, Larkin LH, et al: Muscle attachment to the lateral aspect of the articular disc of the human temporomandibular joint, *Oral Surg Oral Med Oral Pathol Oral Radiol Endod* 82:139, 1996.
99. Lyssy KJ, Escalante A: Perioperative management of rheumatoid arthritis: areas of concern for primary care physicians, *Postgrad Med Rheum Arthritis* 99:191, 1996.
100. Maixner W, Fillingham R, Kincaid S, et al: Relationship between pain sensitivity and resting arterial blood pressure in patients with painful temporomandibular disorders, *Psychosom Med* 59:503, 1997.
101. Major P, Ramos-Remus C, Suarez-Almazor ME, et al: Magnetic resonance imaging and clinical assessment of temporomandibular joint pathology in ankylosing spondylitis, *J Rheumatol* 26:616, 1999.
102. Marbach JL: Is phantom tooth pain a deafferentation (neuropathic) syndrome? *Oral Surg Oral Med Oral Pathol* 75:225, 1993.
103. Marbach JL: Orofacial phantom pain: theory and phenomenology, *J Am Dent Assoc* 127:221, 1996.
104. Marbach JJ: Medically unexplained chronic orofacial pain: temporomandibular pain and dysfunction syndrome, orofacial phantom pain, burning mouth syndrome, and trigeminal neuralgia, *Med Clin North Am* 83:691, 1999.
105. McGuire MK, Nunn ME: Prognosis versus actual outcome: a long-term survey of 100 treated periodontal patients under maintenance care, *J Periodontol* 62:51, 1991.
106. Merida-Velasco JR, Rodriguez-Vazquez JF, Jimenez-Collado J: The relationships between the temporomandibular joint disc and related masticatory muscles in humans, *J Oral Maxillofac Surg* 51:390, 1993.
107. Milam SB, Schmitz JP: Molecular biology of temporomandibular joint disorders: proposed mechanisms of disease, *J Oral Maxillofac Surg* 53:1448, 1995.
108. Milam SB, Zardeneta G, Schmitz JP: Oxidative stress and degenerative temporomandibular joint disease: a proposed hypothesis, *J Oral Maxillofac Surg* 56:214, 1998.
109. Minagi S, Ohtsuki H, Sato T, et al: Effect of balancing-side occlusion on the ipsilateral TMJ dynamics under clenching, *J Oral Rehabil* 24:57, 1997.
110. Mohl ND: Reliability and validity of diagnostic modalities for temporomandibular disorders, *Adv Dent Res* 7:113, 1993.
111. Mohl ND, Ohrbach R: Clinical decision making for temporomandibular disorders, *J Dent Educ* 56:823, 1992.
112. Morgan DH, Goode RL, Christiansen RL, et al: The TMJ-ear connection, *J Craniomandib Pract* 13:42, 1995.
113. Moses AJ: Scientific methodology in temporomandibular disorders. Part I. Epidemiology, *J Craniomandib Pract* 12:114, 1994.
114. Murakami K, Kubota E, Maeda H, et al: Intraarticular levels of prostaglandin E_2, hyaluronic acid, and chrondroitin-4 and -6 sulfates in the temporomandibular joint synovial fluid of patients with internal derangements, *J Oral Maxillofac Surg* 56:199, 1998.
115. Murray H, Locker D, Mock D, et al: Pain and the quality of life in patients referred to a craniofacial pain unit, *J Orofac Pain* 10:316, 1996.
116. Neff PA: *TMJ occlusion and function,* Washington, DC, 1975, Georgetown University School of Dentistry.
117. Okeson JP: *Orofacial pain: guidelines for assessment, diagnosis, and management,* Carol Stream, Ill, 1996, Quintessence.
118. Okeson JP: *Management of temporomandibular joint disorders and occlusion,* ed 4, St Louis, 1998, Mosby.
119. Parker MW: The significance of occlusion in restorative dentistry, *Dent Clin North Am* 37:341, 1993.
120. Parker WS, Chole RA: Tinnitus, vertigo, and temporomandibular disorders, *Am J Orthod Dentofac Orthop* 107:153, 1995.
121. Pavone BW: Bruxism and its effect on the natural teeth, *J Prosthet Dent* 53:692, 1985.
122. Pereira FL, Lundh H, Eriksson L, et al: Microscopic changes in the retrodiscal tissues of painful temporomandibular joints, *J Oral Maxillofac Surg* 54:461, 1996.
123. Pertes RA: Differential diagnosis of orofacial pain, *Mt Sinai J Med* 65:348, 1998.
124. Pharoah MJ: The prescription of diagnostic images for temporomandibular joint disorders, *J Orofac Pain* 13:251, 1999.
125. Pleash O, Wolfe F, Lane N: The relationship between fibromyalgia and temporomandibular disorders: prevalence and symptom severity, *J Rheumatol* 23:1948, 1996.
126. Pullinger AG, Seligman DA: The degree to which attrition characterizes differentiated patient groups of temporomandibular disorders, *J Orofac Pain* 7:196, 1993.
127. Pullinger AG, Seligman DA: Quantification and validation of predictive values of occlusal variables in temporomandibular disorders using multifactorial analysis, *J Prosthet Dent* 83:66, 2000.
128. Pullinger AG, Seligman DA, Gornbein JA: A multiple logistic regression analysis of the risk and relative odds of temporomandibular disorders as a function of common occlusal features, *J Dent Res* 72:968, 1993.
129. Rammelsberg P, Pospiech PR, Jäger L, et al: Variability of disc position in asymptomatic volunteers and patients with internal derangements of the TMJ, *Oral Surg Oral Med Oral Pathol Oral Radiol Endod* 83:393, 1997.
130. Raphael KG, Marbach JJ, Klausner J: Myofascial face pain: clinical characteristics of those with regional versus widespread pain, *J Am Dent Assoc* 131:161, 2000.
131. Rassouli NM, Christensen LV: Experimental occlusal interferences. Part III. Mandibular rotations induced by a rigid interference, *J Oral Rehabil* 22:781, 1995.
132. Ratcliffe A, Israel H, Saed-Nejad F, et al: Proteoglycans in the synovial fluid of the temporomandibular joint as an indicator of changes in cartilage metabolism during primary and secondary osteoarthritis, *J Oral Maxillofac Surg* 56:204, 1998.
133. Raustia AM, Pirttiniemi PM, Pyhtinen J: Correlation of occlusal factors and condyle position asymmetry with

signs and symptoms of temporomandibular disorders in young adults, *J Craniomandib Pract* 13:152, 1995.
134. Ren Y, Isberg A: Tinnitus in patients with temporomandibular joint internal derangement, *J Craniomandib Pract* 13:75, 1995.
135. Rodriguez-Vazquez JF, Merida-Velasco JR, Merida-Velasco JA, et al: Anatomical considerations on the discomalleolar ligament, *J Anat* 192:617, 1998.
136. Rosenbaum RS: The possible effects of periodontal disease on occlusal function, *Curr Opin Periodontol* 163-9, 1993 (review).
137. Ruf S, Cecere F, Kupfer J, et al: Stress-induced changes in the functional electromyographic activity of the masticatory muscles, *Acta Odontol Scand* 55:44, 1997.
138. Sarnat BG, Laskin DM: *The temporomandibular joint: biologic basis for clinical practice,* ed 4, Philadelphia, 1992, Saunders.
139. Schiffman E, Haley D, Baker C, et al: Diagnostic criteria for screening headache patients for temporomandibular disorders, *Headache* 35:121, 1995.
140. Schiffman EL, Fricton JR, Haley D: The relationship of occlusion, parafunctional habits and recent life events to mandibular dysfunction in a nonpatient population, *J Oral Rehabil* 19:201, 1992.
141. Schindler JH, Stengel E, Spiess WE: Feedback control during mastication of solid food textures: a clinical-experimental study, *J Prosthet Dent* 80:330, 1998.
142. Schmolke C: The relationship between the temporomandibular joint capsule, articular disc, and jaw muscles, *J Anat* 184:335, 1994.
143. Sessle BJ: The neural basis of the temporomandibular joint and masticatory muscle pain, *J Orofac Pain* 13:238, 1999.
144. Shibata T, Murakami K, Kubota E, et al: Glycosaminoglycan components in temporomandibular joint synovial fluid as markers of joint pathology, *J Oral Maxillofac Surg* 56:209, 1998.
145. Simons DG, Travell JG, Simons LS: *Myofascial pain and dysfunction: the trigger point manual,* Baltimore, 1999, Williams & Wilkins.
146. Stegenga B, de Bont LGM, de Leeuw R, et al: Assessment of mandibular function impairment associated with temporomandibular joint osteoarthrosis and internal derangement, *J Orofac Pain* 7:183, 1993.
147. Stratmann U, Mokyrs K, Meyer U, et al: Clinical anatomy and palpability of the inferior lateral pterygoid muscle, *J Prosthet Dent* 83:548, 2000.
148. Suvinen TI, Reade PC: Temporomandibular disorders: A critical review of the nature of pain and its assessment, *J Orofacial Pain* 9:317, 1995.
149. Taddey JJ: Musicians and temporomandibular disorders: Prevalence and occupational etiologic considerations, *J Craniomandib Pract* 10:241, 1992.
150. Tanne K, Tanaka E, Sakuda M: Association between malocclusion and temporomandibular disorders in orthodontic patients before treatment, *J Orofacial Pain* 7:156, 1993.
151. Tarantola GJ, Becker IM, Gremillion H: The reproducibility of centric relation: a clinical approach, *J Am Dent Assoc* 128:1245, 1997.
152. Tasaki MM, Westesson P, Isberg AM, et al: Classification and prevalence of temporomandibular joint disc displacement in patients and symptom-free volunteers, *Am J Orthod Dentofac Orthop* 109:249, 1996.
153. Tenenbaum HC, Freeman BV, Psutka DJ, et al: Temporomandibular disorders: disc displacements, *J Orofac Pain* 13:285, 1999.
154. Tsolka P, Walter JD, Wilson RF, et al: Occlusal variables, bruxism and temporomandibular disorders: a clinical and kinesiographic assessment, *J Oral Rehabil* 22:849, 1995.
155. Turp JG, Gobetti JP: Trigeminal neuralgia: an update, *Compendium* 21:279, 2000.
156. Wabeke KB, Spruijt RJ, van der Zaag J: The reliability of clinical methods for recording temporomandibular joint sounds, *J Dent Res* 73:1157, 1994.
157. Watanabe EK, Yatani H, Kuboki T, et al: The relationship between signs and symptoms of temporomandibular disorders and bilateral occlusal contact patterns in lateral excursions, *J Oral Rehabil* 25:409, 1998.
158. Wilkinson TM, Crowley CM: A histologic study of retrodiscal tissues of the human temporomandibular joint in the open and closed position, *J Orofac Pain* 8:7, 1994.
159. Williamson EH, Ludquist DO: Anterior guidance: its effect on electromyographic activity of the temporal and masseter muscles, *J Prosthet Dent* 49:816, 1983.
160. Wish-Baratz S, Ring GD, Hiss J, et al: The microscopic structure and function of the vascular retrodiscal pad of the human temporomandibular joint, *Arch Oral Biol* 38:265, 1993.
161. Wright EF, Bifano SL: Tinnitus improvement through TMD therapy, *J Am Dent Assoc* 128:1424, 1997.
162. Wright EF, Gullickson DC: Identifying acute pulpalgia as a factor in TMD pain, *J Am Dent Assoc* 127:773, 1996.
163. Zarb GA, Carlsson GE, Sessle BJ, et al: *Temporomandibular joint and masticatory muscle disorders,* St Louis, 1994, Mosby.
164. Zarb GA, Carlsson GE: Temporomandibular disorders: osteoarthritis, *J Orofac Pain* 13:295, 1999.
165. Zimers PL, Gobetti JP: Head and neck lesions commonly found in musicians, J Am Dent Assoc 125:1487, 1994.

31 CHAPTER

Chronic Periodontitis

M. John Novak and Karen F. Novak

Chapter Outline

Chronic periodontitis, formerly known as "adult periodontitis" or "chronic adult periodontitis," is the most prevalent form of periodontitis. It is generally considered to be a slowly progressing disease. However, in the presence of systemic or environmental factors that may modify the host response to plaque accumulation, such as diabetes, smoking, or stress, disease progression may become more aggressive. Although chronic periodontitis is most frequently observed in adults, it can occur in children and adolescents in response to chronic plaque and calculus accumulation. This observation underlies the recent name change from "adult" periodontitis, which suggests that chronic, plaque-induced periodontitis is only observed in adults, to a more universal description of "chronic" periodontitis, which can occur at any age (see Chapter 7).

Chronic periodontitis has been defined as "an infectious disease resulting in inflammation within the supporting tissues of the teeth, progressive attachment loss, and bone loss."[2] This definition outlines the major clinical and etiologic characteristics of the disease: (1) microbial plaque formation, (2) periodontal inflammation, and (3) loss of attachment and alveolar bone. Periodontal pocket formation is usually a sequela of the disease process unless gingival recession accompanies attachment loss, in which case pocket depths may remain shallow, even in the presence of ongoing attachment loss and bone loss.

CLINICAL FEATURES

General Characteristics

Characteristic clinical findings in patients with untreated chronic periodontitis may include supragingival and subgingival plaque accumulation (frequently associated with calculus formation), gingival inflammation, pocket formation, loss of periodontal attachment, loss of alveolar bone, and occasional suppuration (Figure 31-1). In patients with poor oral hygiene, the gingiva typically may be slightly to moderately swollen and exhibits alterations in color ranging from pale red to magenta. Loss of gingival stippling and changes in the surface topography may include blunted or rolled gingival margins and flattened or cratered papillae.

In many patients, especially those who perform regular home care measures, the changes in color, contour, and consistency frequently associated with gingival inflammation may not be visible on inspection, and inflammation may be detected only as bleeding of the gingiva in response to examination of the periodontal pocket with a periodontal probe (Figures 31-2, *A*, and 31-3, *A*). Gingival

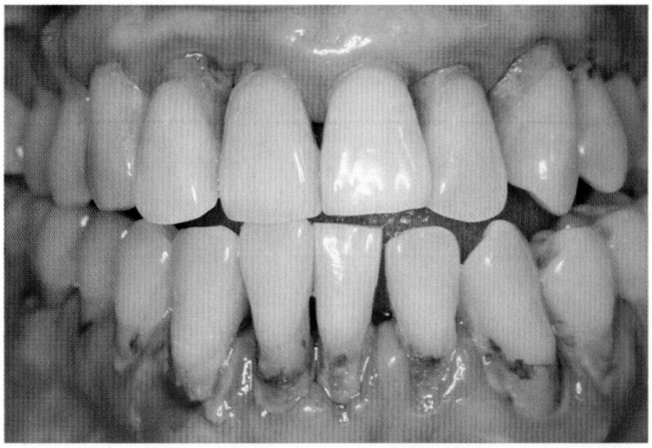

Figure 31-1 Clinical features of chronic periodontitis in 45-year-old patient with poor oral home care and no previous dental treatment. Abundant plaque and calculus are associated with redness, swelling, and edema of the gingival margin. Gingival recession is evident, resulting from loss of attachment and alveolar bone. Spontaneous bleeding is present, and there is visible exudate of gingival crevicular fluid. Gingival stippling has been lost.

bleeding, either spontaneous or in response to probing, is common, and inflammation-related exudates of crevicular fluid and suppuration from the pocket also may be found. In some cases, probably as a result of long-standing, low-grade inflammation, thickened, fibrotic marginal tissues may obscure the underlying inflammatory changes. Pocket depths are variable, and both horizontal and vertical bone loss can be found. Tooth mobility often appears in advanced cases with extensive attachment loss and bone loss.

Chronic periodontitis can be clinically diagnosed by the detection of chronic inflammatory changes in the marginal gingiva, presence of periodontal pockets, and loss of clinical attachment. It is diagnosed radiographically by evidence of bone loss. These findings may be similar to those seen in aggressive disease. A differential diagnosis is based on the age of the patient, rate of disease progression over time, familial nature of aggressive disease, and relative absence of local factors in aggressive disease compared with the presence of abundant plaque and calculus in chronic periodontitis.

A

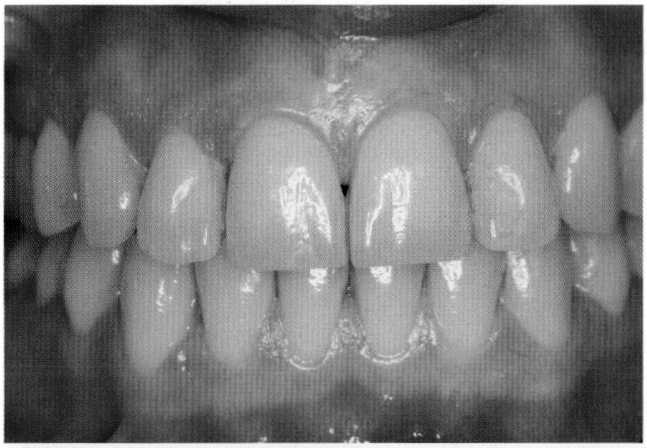

B

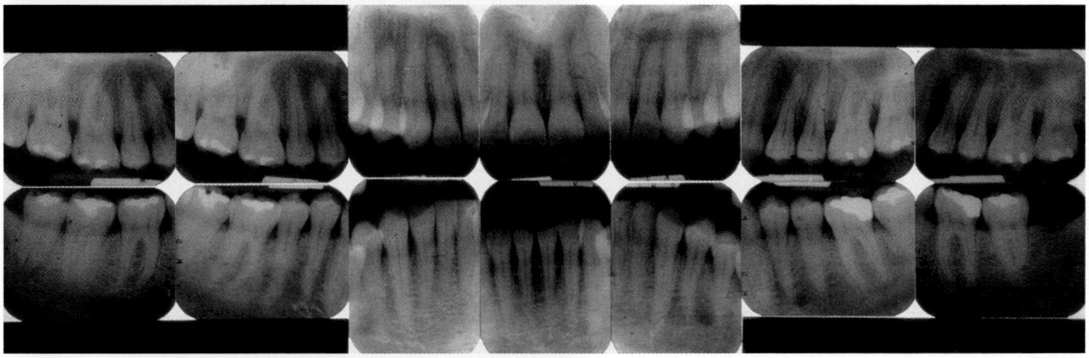

C

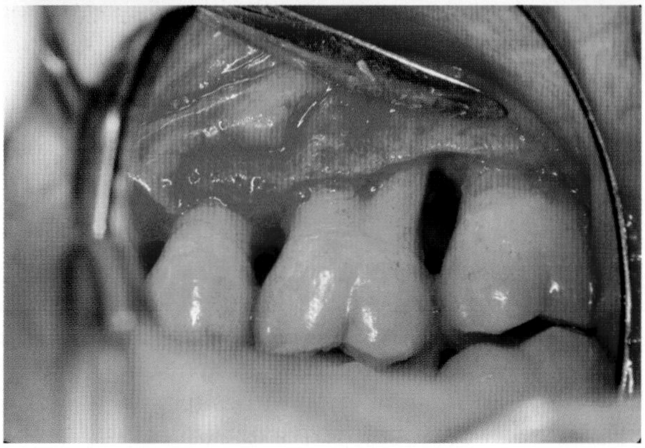

Figure 31-2 Localized chronic periodontitis in 42-year-old woman. **A,** Clinical view of anterior teeth showing minimal plaque and inflammation. **B,** Radiographs showing presence of localized, vertical, angular bone loss on the distal side of the maxillary left first molar. **C,** Surgical exposure of the vertical, angular defect associated with the chronic plaque accumulation and inflammation in the distobuccal furcation.

A

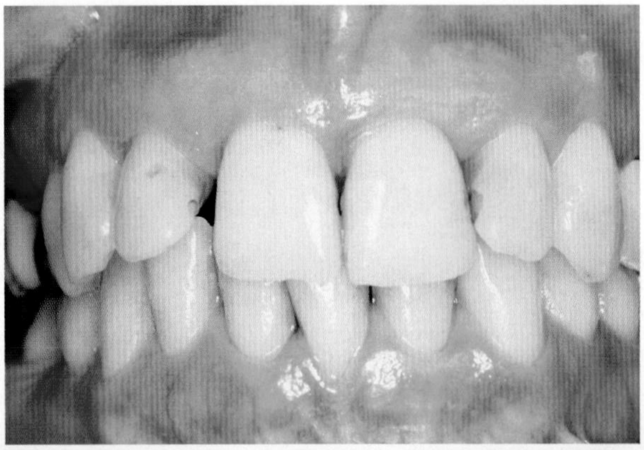

B

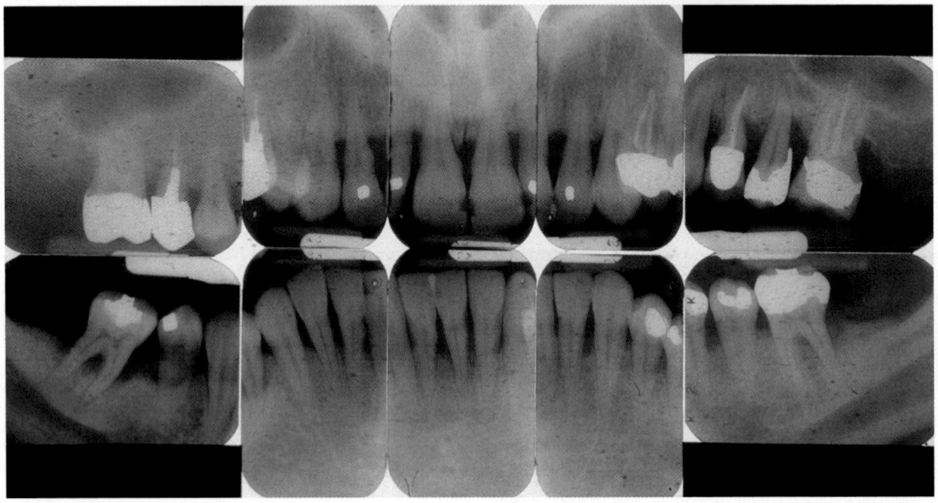

Figure 31-3 Generalized chronic periodontitis in 38-year-old woman with 20-year history of smoking at least one pack of cigarettes per day. **A,** Clinical view showing minimal plaque and inflammation. Probing produced negligible bleeding, which is common with smokers. Patient complained of spacing between the right maxillary incisors, which was associated with advanced attachment and bone loss. **B,** Radiographs showing severe, generalized, horizontal pattern of bone loss. Maxillary and mandibular molars have already been lost through advanced disease and furcation involvement.

Disease Distribution

Chronic periodontitis is considered a *site-specific* disease. The clinical signs of chronic periodontitis—inflammation, pocket formation, attachment loss, and bone loss—are believed to be caused by the direct, site-specific effects of subgingival plaque accumulation. As a result of this local effect, pocketing, attachment, and bone loss may occur on one surface of a tooth while other surfaces maintain normal attachment levels. For example, a proximal surface with chronic plaque accumulation may have loss of attachment, whereas the plaque-free facial surface of the same tooth may be free of disease.

In addition to being site specific, chronic periodontitis may be described as being *localized,* when few sites demonstrate attachment and bone loss, or *generalized,* when many sites around the mouth are affected, as follows:

Localized periodontitis: Periodontitis is considered localized when less than 30% of the sites assessed in the mouth demonstrate attachment loss and bone loss (Figure 31-2).

Generalized periodontitis: Periodontitis is considered generalized when 30% or more of the sites assessed in the mouth demonstrate attachment loss and bone loss (Figure 31-3).

The pattern of bone loss observed in chronic periodontitis may be *vertical,* when attachment and bone loss on one tooth surface is greater than that on an adjacent surface (Figure 31-2, *C*), or *horizontal,* when attachment and bone loss proceeds at a uniform rate on the majority of tooth surfaces (Figure 31-3, *B*). Vertical bone loss is usually associated with angular bony defects and intrabony pocket formation. Horizontal bone loss is usually associated with suprabony pockets (see Chapter 28).

Disease Severity

The severity of destruction of the periodontium that occurs as a result of chronic periodontitis is generally considered a function of time. With increasing age, attachment loss and bone loss become more prevalent and more severe because of an accumulation of destruction (see Chapter 8). Disease severity may be described as being *slight (mild), moderate,* or *severe* (see Chapter 7). These terms may be used to describe the disease severity of the entire mouth or part of the mouth (e.g., quadrant, sextant) or the disease status of an individual tooth, as follows.

Slight (mild) periodontitis: Periodontal destruction is generally considered slight when no more than 1 to 2 mm of clinical attachment loss has occurred.

Moderate periodontitis: Periodontal destruction is generally considered moderate when 3 to 4 mm of clinical attachment loss has occurred.

Severe periodontitis: Periodontal destruction is considered severe when 5 mm or more of clinical attachment loss has occurred.

Symptoms

Patients may first become aware that they have chronic periodontitis when they notice that their gums bleed when brushing or eating; that spaces occur between their teeth as a result of tooth movement; or that teeth have become loose. Because chronic periodontitis is usually painless, however, patients may be totally unaware that they have the disease and may be less likely to seek treatment and accept treatment recommendations. In addition, a negative response to questions such as, "Are you in pain?" is not sufficient to eliminate suspicion of periodontitis. Occasionally, pain may be present in the absence of caries caused by exposed roots that are sensitive to heat, cold, or both. Areas of localized dull pain, sometimes radiating deep into the jaw, have been associated with periodontitis. The presence of areas of food impaction may add to the patient's discomfort. Gingival tenderness or "itchiness" may also be found.

Disease Progression

Patients appear to have the same susceptibility to plaque-induced chronic periodontitis throughout their lives. The rate of disease progression is usually slow but may be modified by systemic or environmental and behavioral factors. Onset of chronic periodontitis can occur at any time, and the first signs may be detected during adolescence in the presence of chronic plaque and calculus accumulation. Because of its slow rate of progression, however, chronic periodontitis usually becomes clinically significant in the mid-30s or later.

Chronic periodontitis does not progress at an equal rate in all affected sites throughout the mouth. Some involved areas may remain static for long periods,[4] whereas others may progress more rapidly. More rapidly progressive lesions occur most frequently in interproximal areas[5] and may also be associated with areas of greater plaque accumulation and inaccessibility to plaque control measures (e.g., furcation areas, overhanging margins, sites of malposed teeth, areas of food impaction).

Several models have been proposed to describe the rate of disease progression.[8] In these models, progression is measured by determining the amount of attachment loss during a given period, as follows:

- The *continuous model* suggests that disease progression is slow and continuous, with affected sites showing a constantly progressive rate of destruction throughout the duration of the disease.
- The *random model,* or *episodic-burst model,* proposes that periodontal disease progresses by short bursts of destruction followed by periods of no destruction. This pattern of disease is random with respect to the tooth sites affected and the chronology of the disease process.
- The *asynchronous, multiple-burst model* of disease progression suggests that periodontal destruction occurs around affected teeth during defined periods of life, and that these bursts of activity are interspersed with periods of inactivity or remission. The chronology of these bursts of disease is asynchronous for individual teeth or groups of teeth.

Prevalence

Chronic periodontitis increases in prevalence and severity with age, generally affecting both genders equally. Periodontitis is an *age-associated,* not an age-related, disease. In other words, it is not the age of the individual that causes the increase in disease prevalence, but rather the length of time that the periodontal tissues are challenged by chronic plaque accumulation. The incidence and prevalence of chronic periodontitis are discussed in detail in Chapter 8.

RISK FACTORS FOR DISEASE

Prior History of Periodontitis

Although not a true risk factor for disease but rather a disease *predictor,* a prior history of periodontitis puts patients at greater risk for developing further loss of attachment and bone, given a challenge from bacterial plaque accumulation.[7] This means that a patient who presents with pocketing, attachment loss, and bone loss will continue to lose periodontal support if not successfully treated. In addition, a chronic periodontitis patient who has been successfully treated will develop continuing disease if plaque is allowed to accumulate. This emphasizes the need for continuous monitoring and maintenance of periodontitis patients to prevent recurrence of disease. The risk factors that contribute to patient susceptibility are discussed in the following sections.

Local Factors

Plaque accumulation on tooth and gingival surfaces at the dentogingival junction is considered the primary initiating agent in the etiology of chronic periodontitis. Attachment and bone loss are associated with an increase in the proportion of gram-negative organisms in the subgingival plaque biofilm, with specific increases in organisms known to be exceptionally pathogenic and virulent. *Porphyromonas gingivalis* (formerly *Bacteroides gingivalis*), *Tannerella forsythia* (formerly *Bacteroides forsythus*), and *Treponema denticola,* otherwise known as the "red complex," are frequently associated with ongoing attachment and bone loss in chronic periodontitis (see Chapters 9 and 13).

SCIENCE TRANSFER

Although chronic periodontitis requires an infection to initiate the host response and subsequent inflammatory reaction, the specific bacteria causing the infection in an individual are unknown. Several different microorganisms apparently are capable of initiating the host response, and a certain combination of species is probably required to overwhelm the host and initiate tissue loss (attachment loss and bone loss). *This provides the basis for periodontal therapy in which periodic monitoring, removal of plaque, and management of risk factors are aimed at keeping the host-bacteria relationship tipped in favor of the host response and control of the disease process.*

Chronic periodontitis is generally slowly progressive, with some patients having increased susceptibility to bone loss and pocketing. Some patients who have a genetic profile that accentuates interleukin-1 production have a 2.9-times increased risk of tooth loss, and if these patients are also smokers, their risk increases to 7.7 times. Diabetes is another factor that often leads to severe and extensive periodontal destruction. Also, a specific group of microorganisms is seen in the subgingival biofilm of patients with ongoing bone loss associated with chronic periodontitis, including *Porphyromonas gingivalis*, *Tannerella forsythia*, and *Treponema denticola*.

The identification and characterization of these and other pathogenic microorganisms and their association with attachment and bone loss have led to the *specific plaque hypothesis* for the development of chronic periodontitis. This hypothesis implies that although a general increase occurs in the proportion of gram-negative microorganisms in the subgingival plaque in periodontitis, it is the presence of increased proportions of members of the red complex, and perhaps other microorganisms, that precipitates attachment and bone loss. The mechanisms by which this occurs have not been clearly delineated, but these bacteria may impart a local effect on the cells of the inflammatory response and the cells and tissues of the host, resulting in a local, site-specific disease process. The interactions between pathogenic bacteria and the host and their potential effects on disease progression are discussed in detail in Chapter 13.

Because plaque accumulation is the primary initiating agent in periodontal destruction, anything that facilitates plaque accumulation or prevents plaque removal by oral hygiene procedures can be detrimental to the patient. *Plaque-retentive factors* are important in the development and progression of chronic periodontitis because they retain plaque microorganisms in proximity to the periodontal tissues, providing an ecologic niche for plaque growth and maturation. *Calculus* is considered the most important plaque-retentive factor because of its ability to retain and harbor plaque bacteria on its rough surface. As a result, calculus removal is essential for the maintenance of a healthy periodontium. Other factors that are known to retain plaque or prevent its removal are subgingival and overhanging margins of restorations; carious lesions that extend subgingivally; furcations exposed by loss of attachment and bone; crowded and malaligned teeth; and root grooves and concavities. These potential risk factors for periodontitis are discussed further in Chapter 38, and their impact on the prognosis of periodontal treatment is discussed in Chapter 40.

Systemic Factors

The rate of progression of plaque-induced chronic periodontitis is generally considered to be slow. However, when chronic periodontitis occurs in a patient who also has a systemic disease that influences the effectiveness of the host response, the rate of periodontal destruction may be significantly increased.

Diabetes is a systemic condition that can increase the severity and extent of periodontal disease in an affected patient. Type 2 diabetes, or non–insulin-dependent diabetes mellitus (NIDDM), is the most prevalent form of diabetes and accounts for 90% of diabetic patients.[1] In addition, type 2 diabetes is most likely to develop in an adult population at the same time as chronic periodontitis. The synergistic effect of plaque accumulation and modulation of an effective host response through the effects of diabetes can lead to severe and extensive periodontal destruction that may be difficult to manage with standard clinical techniques without controlling the systemic condition. An increase in type 2 diabetes in teenagers and young adults has been observed and may be associated with an increase in juvenile obesity. In addition, type 1 diabetes, or insulin-dependent diabetes mellitus (IDDM), is observed in children, teenagers, and young adults and may lead to increased periodontal destruction when it is uncontrolled. It is likely that chronic periodontitis, aggravated by the complications of type 1 and type 2 diabetes, will increase in prevalence in the near future and will provide therapeutic challenges to the clinician.

Environmental and Behavioral Factors

Smoking has been shown to increase the severity and extent of periodontal disease. When combined with plaque-induced chronic periodontitis, an increase in the rate of periodontal destruction may be observed in patients who smoke and have chronic periodontitis. As a result, smokers with chronic periodontitis have more attachment and bone loss, more furcation involvements, and deeper pockets (see Figure 31-3). In addition, they appear to form more supragingival and less subgingival calculus and demonstrate less bleeding on probing than nonsmokers. Initial evidence to explain these effects suggests changes in the subgingival microflora of smokers compared with nonsmokers, in addition to the effects of smoking on the host response. The clinical, microbiologic, and immunologic effects of smoking also appear to influence the response to therapy and the frequency of recurrent disease (see Chapter 14).

Emotional stress has previously been associated with necrotizing ulcerative disease, perhaps because of the effects of stress on immune function. Increasing evidence suggests that emotional stress also may influence the extent and severity of chronic periodontitis, probably through the same mechanisms.

Genetic Factors

Periodontitis is considered to be a multifactorial disease in which the normal balance between microbial plaque and host response is disrupted. This disruption, as described previously, can occur through changes in the plaque composition, changes in the host response, or environmental and behavioral influences on both plaque response and host response. In addition, periodontal destruction is frequently seen among family members and across different generations within a family, suggesting a genetic basis for the susceptibility to periodontal disease. Recent studies have demonstrated a familial aggregation of localized and generalized aggressive periodontitis. In addition, studies of monozygotic twins suggest a genetic component to chronic periodontitis, but the influences of bacterial transmission among family members and environmental effects make it difficult to interpret a complex interaction (see Chapters 11 and 33).

Although no clear genetic determinants have been described for patients with chronic periodontitis, a genetic predisposition to more aggressive periodontal breakdown in response to plaque and calculus accumulation may exist. Recent data indicate that a genetic variation or polymorphism in the genes encoding interleukin-1α (IL-1α) and IL-1β is associated with an increased susceptibility to a more aggressive form of chronic periodontitis in subjects of Northern European origin.[3] In addition, smokers demonstrating the composite IL-1 genotype are at even greater risk for severe disease. One study suggested that patients with the IL-1 genotype increased the risk for tooth loss by 2.7 times; those who were heavy smokers and IL-1 genotype negative increased the risk for tooth loss by 2.9 times. The combined effect of the IL-1 genotype and smoking increased the risk of tooth loss by 7.7 times.[6] With increased characterization of genetic polymorphisms that may exist in other target genes, a complex genotype is likely to be identified for many different clinical forms of periodontitis.

REFERENCES

1. Diagnosis and classification. In Raskin P, editor: *Medical management of non-insulin-dependent (type II) diabetes,* ed 3, Alexandria, Va, 1994, American Diabetes Association.
2. Flemmig TF: Periodontitis, *Ann Periodontol* 4:32, 1999.
3. Kornman KS, di Giovine FS: Genetic variations in cytokine expression: a risk factor for severity of adult periodontitis, *Ann Periodontol* 3:327, 1998.
4. Lindhe J, Okamoto H, Yoneyama T, et al: Longitudinal changes in periodontal disease in untreated subjects, *J Clin Periodontol* 16:662, 1989.
5. Lindhe J, Okamoto H, Yoneyama T, et al: Periodontal loser sites in untreated adult subjects, *J Clin Periodontol* 16:671, 1989.
6. McGuire MK, Nunn ME: Prognosis versus actual outcome. IV. The effectiveness of clinical parameters and IL-1 genotype in accurately predicting prognoses and tooth survival, *J Periodontol* 70:49, 1999.
7. Papapanou PN: Risk assessment in the diagnosis and treatment of periodontal diseases, *J Dent Educ* 62:822, 1998.
8. Socransky SS, Haffajee AD, Goodson JM, et al: New concepts of destructive periodontal disease, *J Clin Periodontol* 11:21, 1984.

Necrotizing Ulcerative Periodontitis

Perry R. Klokkevold

32 CHAPTER

CHAPTER OUTLINE

Necrotizing ulcerative periodontitis (NUP) may be an extension of *necrotizing ulcerative gingivitis* (NUG) into the periodontal structures, leading to periodontal attachment and bone loss. On the other hand, however, NUP and NUG may be different diseases. To date, there is no evidence to support the progression of NUG to NUP or to establish a relationship between the two conditions as a single disease entity. However, numerous clinical descriptions and case reports of NUP clearly demonstrate many clinical similarities between the two conditions. Until a distinction between NUG and NUP can be proved or disproved, it has been suggested that NUG and NUP be classified together under the broader category of *necrotizing periodontal diseases,* although with differing levels of severity.[1,21]

Chapter 24 describes necrotizing ulcerative gingivitis in detail. This chapter describes the clinical features, etiology, and characteristics of necrotizing ulcerative periodontitis, with a prelude on the pertinent clinical and microscopic aspects of NUG.

CLINICAL AND MICROSCOPIC DESCRIPTION OF NECROTIZING ULCERATIVE GINGIVITIS

Necrotizing ulcerative gingivitis (NUG) has been recognized and described in the literature for centuries. Historical descriptions of the disease refer to it by many names, including "Vincent's infection," "trench mouth," and the descriptive term "acute necrotizing ulcerative gingivitis" (ANUG). However, "acute" has been dropped from the latter nomenclature and description because it is understood that the disease has a sudden onset and that there is no chronic form.[1,25]

The features of NUG are distinctly different from those of any other periodontal disease. Areas of ulceration and necrosis of the interdental papilla, covered by a whitish yellow soft layer, or *pseudomembrane,* characterize gingival lesions of NUG. The ulcerated margin is surrounded by an erythematous halo. Lesions are typically painful and bleed easily, often without provocation. The clinical presentation of a patient with ulcerated, "punched out" papilla, pain, and bleeding is pathognomonic for NUG (see Figure 24-1). Patients may also present with oral malodor, localized lymphadenopathy, fever, and malaise.

Microscopically, NUG lesions demonstrate a nonspecific necrotizing inflammation presenting with a predominant polymorphonuclear leukocyte (PMN, neutrophil) infiltrate in the ulcerated areas and an abundant chronic infiltrate of lymphocytes and plasma cells in the peripheral and deeper areas.[32] The classic electron microscopic description of NUG lesions identified four zones[14]: (1) the *bacterial zone,* composed of a large mass of bacteria with various morphotypes, including spirochetes; (2) the *neutrophil-rich zone,* consisting of many leukocytes and a predominance of neutrophils, with many spirochetes and other bacteria interspersed between cells; (3) the *necrotic zone,* composed of dead cells, many spirochetes (large and intermediate size), and other bacteria; and (4) the *spirochetal infiltration zone,* consisting of intact tissue elements infiltrated by spirochetes but no other bacteria. The presence of spirochetes in the deepest zone of the lesion within normal tissue elements is highly suggestive of the primary "invasive" role that spirochetes may play in this disease.

The bacterial flora associated with NUG is well known. The fusiform-spirochete bacterial flora found in NUG lesions was first described by Plaut[23] in 1894 and (independently) by Vincent[31] in 1896. Numerous subsequent studies have described the presence of additional bacteria in NUG lesions, including cocci and rods. Many bacterial species, especially spirochetes, are difficult to isolate and grow in culture; thus the microbes that have been "associated" with the etiology of NUG have been identified either by the frequency of their growth in culture or the regularity of their presence in microscopic evaluations. The constant cultivable flora consists of *Prevotella intermedia* (formerly *Bacteroides melaninogenicus* subsp. *intermedius*) and *Fusobacterium* species, whereas the constant microscopic observations reveal the presence of *Treponema* and *Selenomonas* species. The association of these bacteria with NUG is compelling. However, the bacterial etiology has not been proven because the bacteria have not been able to transfer the disease between healthy animals (i.e., have not been able to fulfill one of Koch's postulates). Interestingly, bacterial isolates have transmitted NUG from animal to animal in the beagle dog with a steroid-induced immunosuppression.[17-19] The ability to transmit NUG with bacteria in an immunosuppressed animal (but not in immunocompetent animals) suggests that the host response or resistance is an important factor in the pathogenesis of NUG.

The lesions of NUG have been described as being confined to the gingiva without loss of periodontal attachment or alveolar bone support, a feature that distinguishes this condition from NUP. In contrast to this view, MacCarthy and Claffey[15] suggested that periodontal attachment loss *is* one of the consequences of NUG lesions. In their evaluation of 13 patients with NUG, the mean probing attachment level for NUG-affected sites (2.2 ± 0.9 mm) was greater than control sites (0.8 ± 0.7 mm). This finding supports the concept that NUG and NUP are similar (or identical) diseases, with differences in host response or resistance rather than differences in bacterial etiology and pathogenesis.

CHARACTERISTIC FEATURES OF NECROTIZING ULCERATIVE PERIODONTITIS

The classification of necrotizing ulcerative "periodontitis" (NUP) was first adopted at the 1989 World Workshop on Clinical Periodontics.[5] It was changed from the 1986 classification of "necrotizing ulcerative gingivo-periodontitis," which represented the condition of recurrent NUG progressing to a chronic form of periodontitis with attachment and bone loss. The 1989 adoption of NUP as a disease classification occurred when there was a heightened awareness and an increase in the number of necrotizing periodontitis cases being diagnosed and described in the literature. Specifically, more cases of NUP were being described in immunocompromised patients, especially those who were human immunodeficiency virus (HIV) positive or had acquired immunodeficiency syndrome (AIDS). In 1999 the subclassifications of NUG and NUP were included as separate diagnoses under the broader classification of "necrotizing ulcerative periodontal diseases."[1] Again, a distinction between the two conditions as separate diseases has not been clarified, but they are distinguished by the presence or absence of attachment and bone loss.

Clinical Presentation

Similar to NUG, clinical cases of NUP are defined by necrosis and ulceration of the coronal portion of the interdental papillae and gingival margin, with a painful, bright-red marginal gingiva that bleeds easily. The distinguishing feature of NUP is the destructive progression of the disease that includes periodontal attachment and bone loss. Deep interdental osseous craters typify periodontal lesions of NUP (Figure 32-1). However, "conventional" periodontal pockets with deep probing depth are not found because the ulcerative and necrotizing nature of the gingival lesion destroys the marginal epithelium and connective tissue, resulting in gingival recession. Advanced lesions of NUP lead to severe bone loss, tooth mobility, and ultimately tooth loss. In addition to these intraoral manifestations, as previously mentioned, NUP patients may present with oral malodor, fever, malaise, or lymphadenopathy.

Microscopic Findings

In an electron microscopy (TEM/SEM) study of the microbial plaque overlying the necrotic gingival papillae, Cobb et al.[3] demonstrated striking histologic similarities between NUP in HIV-positive patients and previous descriptions of NUG lesions in non-HIV patients. Biopsies of involved posterior papillae from 10 male and six female HIV-positive patients with NUP were evaluated. Microscopic examination revealed a surface biofilm composed of a mixed microbial flora with different morphotypes and a subsurface flora with dense aggregations of spirochetes (bacterial zone). Below the bacterial layers were dense aggregations of PMNs (neutrophil-rich zone) and necrotic cells (necrotic zone). The biopsy technique used in this study did not allow observation of the deepest layer and thus was not able to identify the spirochetal infiltration zone, which is classically described in NUG lesions. In addition to the NUG-like microscopic features of NUP described in this study, high levels of yeasts and herpeslike viruses were observed. This latter finding is most likely indicative of the conditions afforded to opportunistic microbes in the immunocompromised host (HIV-positive patients).

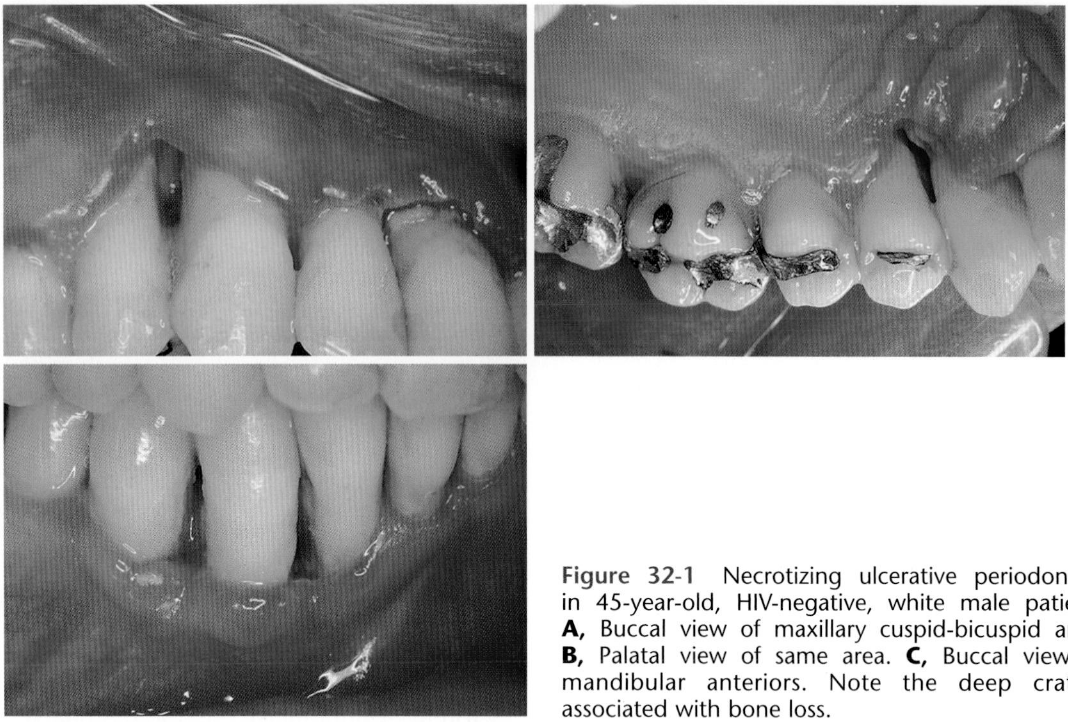

A B C

Figure 32-1 Necrotizing ulcerative periodontitis in 45-year-old, HIV-negative, white male patient. **A,** Buccal view of maxillary cuspid-bicuspid area. **B,** Palatal view of same area. **C,** Buccal view of mandibular anteriors. Note the deep craters associated with bone loss.

HIV/AIDS Patient

Gingival and periodontal lesions with distinctive features are frequently found in patients with HIV infection and AIDS. Many of these lesions are atypical manifestations of inflammatory periodontal diseases that arise in the course of HIV infection and the patient's concomitant immunocompromised state. Linear gingival erythema (LGE), NUG, and NUP are the most common HIV-associated periodontal conditions reported in the literature.[22] Chapter 34 provides detailed descriptions of these and other atypical periodontal diseases that occur in the HIV-infected patient.

NUP lesions found in HIV-positive/AIDS patients can present with similar features to those seen in HIV-negative patients. On the other hand, NUP lesions in HIV-positive/AIDS patients can be much more destructive and frequently result in complications that are extremely rare in non-HIV/AIDS patients. For example, periodontal attachment and bone loss associated with HIV-positive NUP may be extremely rapid. Winkler et al.[33] reported cases of NUP in HIV-positive patients (formerly referred to as "HIV-P") with teeth that lost more than 90% of periodontal attachment and 10 mm of bone over a 3- to 6-month period. Ultimately, many of these lesions resulted in tooth loss. Other complications reported in this population include a progression of the lesions to involve large areas of soft tissue necrosis, with exposure of bone and sequestration of bone fragments. This type of severe, progressive lesion with extension into the vestibular area and the palate is referred to as *necrotizing ulcerative stomatitis* (see Figure 34-31).

The reported prevalence of NUP in HIV-infected patients varies.[7,22,11,24] Riley et al.[24] reported only two cases of NUP in 200 HIV-positive patients (1%), whereas Glick et al.[11] found a prevalence of 6.3% for NUP cases in a prospective study of 700 HIV-positive patients. Variations in reported findings may be related to differences in the populations (e.g., intravenous drug users vs. homosexuals vs. patients with hemophilia) and differences in the immune status of the study subjects.

Necrotizing forms of periodontitis appear to be more prevalent in patients with more severe immunosuppression.[22] Case reports have depicted NUP as a progressive extension of HIV periodontitis (i.e., chronic to necrotic progression).[26] Glick et al.[10,11] found a high correlation between the diagnosis of NUP and immunosuppression in HIV-positive patients. Those patients presenting with NUP were 20.8 times more likely to have CD4+ counts below 200 cells/mm^3 compared with HIV-positive patients without NUP. The authors consider a diagnosis of NUP to be a marker for immune deterioration and a predictor for the diagnosis of AIDS.[11] Others have suggested that NUP may be used as an indicator of HIV infection in undiagnosed patients. Shangase et al.[28] reported that a diagnosis of NUG or NUP in systemically healthy, asymptomatic South Africans was strongly correlated with HIV infection. Of patients presenting with NUG or NUP, 39 of 56 (69.6%) were subsequently found to be HIV positive. (See Chapter 34.)

ETIOLOGY OF NECROTIZING ULCERATIVE PERIODONTITIS

The etiology of NUP has not been determined, although a mixed fusiform-spirochete bacterial flora appears to play a key role. Because bacterial pathogens are not solely responsible for causing the disease, some predisposing "host" factor(s) may be necessary. Numerous predisposing

SCIENCE TRANSFER

Necrotizing forms of periodontitis emphasize the importance of the patient's immune response. In severe immunosuppression, patients can experience extremely rapid and extensive tissue destruction. The tissue destruction usually does not involve significantly deep periodontal pockets because of the necrosis that occurs in the marginal soft tissues. Little is known about the relationship, if any, between necrotizing ulcerative gingivitis (NUG) and necrotizing ulcerative periodontitis (NUP), except for the difference between gingivitis and periodontitis. Further complicating this area of research, many studies on these fairly rare conditions are performed on HIV-positive and AIDS patients with wide variance in disease conditions and treatments. *It is clear, however, that immunosuppression is associated with atypical periodontal diseases.*

NUP is frequently associated with a diagnosis of AIDS or a positive HIV status. Therefore, clinicians should check all patients presenting with NUP to ascertain their HIV status. NUP can progress rapidly and lead to tooth exfoliation, so treatment should include local debridement, local antiplaque agents, and systemic antibiotics. Early diagnosis and treatment of NUP are crucial because the osseous defects that occur in the late stages of the disease are extremely difficult to resolve, even with extensive regenerative surgical procedures. If a child presents with NUP, severe systemic abnormalities, such as advanced malnutrition, are often present.

factors have been attributed to NUG, including poor oral hygiene, preexisting periodontal disease, smoking, viral infections, immunocompromised status, psychosocial stress, and malnutrition.

Microbial Flora

Assessment of the microbial flora of NUP lesions is almost exclusively limited to studies involving HIV-positive and AIDS patients, with some conflicting evidence. Murray et al.[20] reported that cases of NUP in HIV-positive patients demonstrated significantly greater numbers of the opportunistic fungus *Candida albicans* and a higher prevalence of *Actinobacillus actinomycetemcomitans, Prevotella intermedia, Porphyromonas gingivalis, Fusobacterium nucleatum,* and *Campylobacter* species compared with HIV-negative controls. Further, they reported a low or variable level of spirochetes, which is inconsistent with the flora associated with NUG. Citing differences in microbial flora, they refuted the notion that the destructive lesions seen in HIV-positive patients were related to NUG lesions; they suggested that the flora of NUP lesions in HIV-positive patients is comparable to that of "classic" (chronic) periodontitis lesions, thus supporting their concept that necrotizing periodontitis in the HIV-positive patient is an aggressive manifestation of chronic periodontitis in the immunocompromised host.

In contrast to these findings, Cobb et al.[3] reported that the microbial composition of NUP lesions in HIV-positive patients was very similar to that of NUG lesions, as discussed earlier. They described a mixed microbial flora with various morphotypes in 81.3% of specimens. The subsurface microbial flora featured dense aggregations of spirochetes in 87.5% of specimens. They also reported opportunistic yeasts and herpeslike viruses in 65.6% and 56.5% of NUP lesions, respectively.

The differences between these reports may be explained by the limitations in obtaining viable cultures of spirochetes[20] compared with the more definitive electron microscopic observation of spirochetes.[3]

Immunocompromised Status

Clearly, both NUG and NUP lesions are more prevalent in patients with compromised or suppressed immune systems. Numerous studies, particularly those evaluating HIV-positive and AIDS patients, support the concept that a diminished host response is present in those individuals diagnosed with necrotizing ulcerative periodontal diseases. Whereas a compromised immune system ("immune compromise") in the HIV-infected patient is driven by impaired T-cell function and altered T-cell ratios, evidence indicates that other forms of compromised immunity predispose individuals to NUG and NUP as well.

Cutler et al.[7] described impaired bactericidal activity of PMNs in two children with NUP. In a comparative assay of PMNs against periodontal pathogens, two brothers (ages 9 and 14 years) showed significant depression of PMN phagocytosis and killing function compared with gender- and age-matched controls. Further, Batista et al.[2] reported periodontal findings and NUP in an adolescent with a rare genetic disease (multifactorial congenital immunodeficiency, or CVID) that causes impaired secretion of immunoglobulin; the oral lesions resolved with administration of intravenous immunoglobulin (IVIG).

Psychologic Stress

Most clinical and animal studies evaluating the role of stress on necrotizing periodontal disease have evaluated subjects with NUG and thus have not specifically addressed the role of stress on NUP. However, many articles strongly support the suggestion that emotional stress contributes to the development of NUG.[8,12] One of the earliest terms used to name the disease was "trench mouth," which referred to the condition of soldiers in the trenches of war under stress (and unable to change their circumstances).

In a study of 35 patients with NUG and 35 matched controls without signs of NUG, Cohen-Cole et al.[4] found that those with NUG had significantly more anxiety, higher depression scores, a greater magnitude of recent stressful events, more overall distress and adjustments related to these events, and more negative life events. In a study of military personnel, Shields[30] found that a greater number of individuals with NUG reported feeling "run down" and under more emotional stress than healthy controls. Although the role of stress in the development of NUP has not been reported specifically, the many similarities between NUG and NUP would suggest that similar relationships to stress may exist.

The mechanisms that predispose an individual with stress to necrotizing ulcerative periodontal diseases have not been established. However, it is well known that stress increases systemic cortisol levels, and sustained increases in cortisone have a suppressive effect on the immune response. In an investigation of 474 military personnel, Shannon et al.[29] found that urinary levels of 17-hydroxycorticosteroid were higher in subjects with NUG than in all other subjects, diagnosed with periodontal health, gingivitis, or periodontitis. Experimentally, noma-like lesions have been produced in rats by administering cortisone and causing mechanical injury to the gingiva[27] and in hamsters by total body irradiation.[16] Thus, stress-induced immunosuppression may be one mechanism that impairs the host response and leads to necrotizing periodontal disease.

The scientific evidence supporting an etiologic role of stress in chronic periodontitis is not as clear (see Chapter 17).

Malnutrition

Direct evidence of the relationship between malnutrition and necrotizing periodontal disease is limited to descriptions of necrotizing infections in severely malnourished children. Lesions resembling NUG but with progression to become *gangrenous stomatitis,* or *noma,* have been described in children with severe malnutrition in underdeveloped countries. Jimenez and Baer[13] reported cases of NUG in children and adolescents age 2 to 14 years with malnutrition in Colombia. In the advanced stages, NUG lesions extended from the gingiva to other areas of the oral cavity, becoming gangrenous stomatitis (noma) and causing exposure, necrosis, and sequestration of the alveolar bone.

A plausible explanation is that malnutrition, particularly when extreme, contributes to a diminished host resistance to infection and necrotizing disease. It is well documented that many of the host defenses are impaired in malnourished individuals, including phagocytosis, cell-mediated immunity, and complement, antibody, and cytokine production and function.[9] Depletion of nutrients to cells and tissues results in immunosuppression and increases disease susceptibility. Thus, it is reasonable to conclude that malnutrition can predispose an individual to opportunistic infections or intensify the severity of existing oral infections.

SUMMARY

Necrotizing ulcerative periodontitis and NUG share many clinical and microbiologic features, but NUP is distinguished by a more severe condition with periodontal attachment and bone loss. Indeed, some patients with NUP, particularly those with compromised immunity, can have severe and rapidly progressive disease. It appears that an impaired immune response and lowered host resistance to infection are significant factors in the onset and progression of NUP. The best example of an immunocompromised host with a predisposition for NUP is the HIV-positive/AIDS patient. As with the other infection-related complications of HIV/AIDS, the immunocompromised status of these patients renders them vulnerable to opportunistic periodontal infections, including NUP. Several other factors have been identified, specifically in cases of NUG, that may also play a role in NUP, including smoking, viral infections, psychosocial stress, and malnutrition. These additional factors undoubtedly influence host response or resistance to infection as well.

REFERENCES

1. Armitage GC: Development of a classification system for periodontal diseases and conditions, *Ann Periodontol* 4:1, 1999.
2. Batista EL Jr, Novaes AB Jr, Calvano LM, et al: Necrotizing ulcerative periodontitis associated with severe congenital immunodeficiency in a prepubescent subject: clinical findings and response to intravenous immunoglobulin treatment, *J Clin Periodontol* 26:499, 1999.
3. Cobb CM, Ferguson BL, Keselyak NT, et al: A TEM/SEM study of the microbial plaque overlying the necrotic gingival papillae of HIV-seropositive, necrotizing ulcerative periodontitis, *J Periodontal Res* 38:147, 2003.
4. Cohen-Cole SA, Cogen RB, Stevens AW Jr, et al: Psychiatric, psychosocial, and endocrine correlates of acute necrotizing ulcerative gingivitis (trench mouth): a preliminary report, *Psychiatr Med* 1:215, 1983.
5. Consensus report on periodontal diagnosis and diagnostic aids. In *Proceedings of the World Workshop in Clinical Periodontics,* Chicago, 1989, American Academy of Periodontology.
6. Cram S, Rasheed A, Meador H, et al: Objective parameters of refractory periodontitis, *J Dent Res* 68:360, 1989 (special issue, abstract 1428).
7. Cutler CW, Wasfy MO, Ghaffar K, et al: Impaired bactericidal activity of PMN from two brothers with necrotizing ulcerative gingivo-periodontitis, *J Periodontol* 65:357, 1994.
8. Da Silva AM, Newman HN, Oakley DA: Psychosocial factors in inflammatory periodontal diseases: a review, *J Clin Periodontol* 22:516, 1995.
9. Enwonwu CO, Phillips RS, Falkler WA Jr: Nutrition and oral infectious diseases: state of the science, *Compend Contin Educ Dent* 23:431, 2002.
10. Glick M, Muzyka BC, Salkin LM, Lurie D: Necrotizing ulcerative periodontitis: a marker for immune deterioration and a predictor for the diagnosis of AIDS, *J Periodontol* 65:393, 1994.
11. Glick M, Muzyka BC, Lurie D, Salkin LM: Oral manifestations associated with HIV-related disease as markers for immune suppression and AIDS, *Oral Surg Oral Med Oral Pathol* 77:344, 1994.
12. Hildebrand HC, Epstein J, Larjava H: The influence of psychological stress on periodontal disease, *J West Soc Periodontol Periodontal Abstr* 48:69, 2000.
13. Jimenez M, Baer PN: Necrotizing ulcerative gingivitis in children: a 9 year clinical study, *J Periodontol* 46:715, 1975.
14. Listgarten MA: Electron microscopic observations on the bacterial flora of acute necrotizing ulcerative gingivitis, *J Periodontol* 36:328, 1965.
15. MacCarthy D, Claffey N: Acute necrotizing ulcerative gingivitis is associated with attachment loss, *J Clin Periodontol* 18:776, 1991.

16. Mayo J, Carranza FA Jr, Epper CE, et al: The effect of total body irradiation on the oral tissues of the Syrian hamster, *Oral Surg Med Pathol* 15:739, 1962.
17. Mikx F, van Campen GJ: Preliminary evaluation of the microflora in spontaneous and induced necrotizing ulcerative gingivitis in the beagle dog, *J Periodontal Res* 17:460, 1982.
18. Mikx FH, van Campen GJ: Microscopical evaluation of the microflora in relation to necrotizing ulcerative gingivitis in the beagle dog, *J Periodontal Res* 17:576, 1982.
19. Mikx FH, Hug HU, Maltha JC: Necrotizing ulcerative gingivitis in beagle dogs. I. Attempts at unilateral induction and intraoral transmission of NUG: a microbiological and clinical study, *J Periodontal Res* 19:76, 1984.
20. Murray PA, Winkler JR, Sadkowski L, et al: Microbiology of HIV-associated gingivitis and periodontitis. In Robertson PB, Greenspan JS, editors: *Perspectives on oral manifestations of AIDS,* Littleton, Mass, 1988, PSG Publishing.
21. Novak MJ: Necrotizing ulcerative periodontitis, *Ann Periodontol* 4:74, 1999.
22. Pistorius A, Willershausen B: Cases of HIV-associated characteristic periodontal diseases, *Eur J Med Res* 4:121, 1999.
23. Plaut HC: [Bacterial diagnostic studies of diphtheria and oral diseases], *Dtsch Med Wochnschr* 20:920, 1894.
24. Riley C, London JP, Burmeister JA: Periodontal health in 200 HIV-positive patients, *J Oral Pathol Med* 21:124, 1992.
25. Rowland RW: Necrotizing ulcerative gingivitis, *Ann Periodontol* 4:65, 1999.
26. SanGiacomo TR, Tan PM, Loggi DG, Itkin AB: Progressive osseous destruction as a complication of HIV-periodontitis, *Oral Surg Oral Med Oral Pathol* 70:476, 1990.
27. Selye H: Effect of cortisone and somatotrophic hormone upon the development of a noma-like condition in the rat, *Oral Surg Med Pathol* 6:557, 1953.
28. Shangase L, Feller L, Blignaut E: Necrotising ulcerative gingivitis/periodontitis as indicators of HIV infection, *SADJ* 59:105, 2004.
29. Shannon IL, Kilgore WG, O'Leary TJ: Stress as a predisposing factor for necrotizing ulcerative gingivitis, *J Periodontol* 40:240, 1969.
30. Shields WD: Acute necrotizing ulcerative gingivitis: a study of some of the contributing factors and their validity in an Army population, *J Periodontol* 48:346, 1977.
31. Vincent H: [The etiology and the histopathology of hospital rot], *Ann de l'Insti Pastuer* 10:488, 1896.
32. Wade DN, Kerns DG: Acute necrotizing ulcerative gingivitis-periodontitis: a literature review, *Mil Med* 16:337, 1998.
33. Winkler JR, Grassi M, Murray PA: Clinical description and etiology of HIV-associated periodontal diseases. In Robertson PB, Greenspan JS, editors: *Perspectives on oral manifestations of AIDS,* Littleton, Mass, 1988, PSG Publishing.

Aggressive Periodontitis

Karen F. Novak and M. John Novak

33

CHAPTER

CHAPTER OUTLINE

Aggressive periodontitis generally affects systemically healthy individuals less than 30 years old, although patients may be older. Aggressive periodontitis may be universally distinguished from *chronic periodontitis* by the age of onset, the rapid rate of disease progression, the nature and composition of the associated subgingival microflora, alterations in the host's immune response, and a familial aggregation of diseased individuals.[17] In addition, a strong racial influence is observed in the United States; the disease is more prevalent among African Americans.[26]

Aggressive periodontitis describes three of the diseases formerly classified as "early-onset periodontitis." *Localized aggressive periodontitis* was formerly classified as "localized juvenile periodontitis" (LJP). *Generalized aggressive periodontitis* encompasses the diseases previously classified as "generalized juvenile periodontitis" (GJP) and "rapidly progressive periodontitis" (RPP).

LOCALIZED AGGRESSIVE PERIODONTITIS

Historical Background

In 1923, Gottlieb[13] reported a patient with a fatal case of epidemic influenza and a disease that Gottlieb called "diffuse atrophy of the alveolar bone." This disease was characterized by a loss of collagen fibers in the periodontal ligament (PDL) and their replacement by loose connective tissue and extensive bone resorption, resulting in a widened PDL space. The gingiva apparently was not involved. In 1928, Gottlieb[14] attributed this condition to the inhibition of continuous cementum formation, which he considered essential for maintenance of the PDL fibers. He then termed the disease "deep cementopathia" and hypothesized that this was a "disease of eruption" and that cementum initiated a foreign body response. As a result, it was postulated that the host attempted to exfoliate the tooth, resulting in the observed bone resorption and pocket formation.[14]

In 1938, Wannenmacher[49] described incisor–first molar involvement and called the disease "parodontitis marginalis progressiva." Several explanations evolved for the etiology and pathogenesis of this type of disease. Many authors considered this to be a degenerative, noninflammatory disease process[12,34,45] and therefore gave it the name "periodontosis." Other investigators denied the existence of a degenerative type of periodontal disease and attributed the changes observed to trauma from occlusion.[6,33] Finally, in 1966, the World Workshop in Periodontics concluded that the concept of "periodontosis" as a degenerative entity was unsubstantiated and that the term should be eliminated from periodontal nomenclature.[38] The committee did recognize that a clinical entity different from "adult periodontitis" might occur among adolescents and young adults.

The term "juvenile periodontitis" was introduced by Chaput and colleagues in 1967 and by Butler[5] in 1969. In 1971, Baer[2] defined it as "a disease of the periodontium occurring in an otherwise healthy adolescent which is characterized by a rapid loss of alveolar bone about more than one tooth of the permanent dentition. The amount of destruction manifested is not commensurate with the amount of local irritants." In 1989 the World Workshop in Clinical Periodontics categorized this disease as "localized juvenile periodontitis" (LJP), a subset of the broad classification of "early-onset periodontitis" (EOP).[8] Under this classification system, age of onset and distribution of lesions were of primary importance when making a diagnosis of LJP. Most recently, disease with the characteristics of LJP has been renamed *localized aggressive periodontitis*.

Clinical Characteristics

Localized aggressive periodontitis (LAP) usually has an age of onset at about puberty.[22] Clinically, it is characterized as having "localized first molar/incisor presentation with interproximal attachment loss on at least two permanent teeth, one of which is a first molar, and involving no more than two teeth other than first molars and incisors"[22] (Figure 33-1). The localized distribution of lesions in LAP is characteristic but as yet unexplained. The following possible reasons for the limitation of periodontal destruction to certain teeth have been suggested:

1. After initial colonization of the first permanent teeth to erupt (the first molars and incisors), *Actinobacillus actinomycetemcomitans* evades the host defenses by different mechanisms, including production of polymorphonuclear leukocyte (PMN) chemotaxis-inhibiting factors, endotoxin, collagenases, leukotoxin, and other factors that allow the bacteria to colonize the pocket and initiate the destruction of the periodontal tissues. After this initial attack, adequate immune defenses are stimulated to produce opsonic antibodies to enhance the clearance and phagocytosis of invading bacteria and neutralize leukotoxic activity. In this manner, colonization of other sites may be prevented.[51] A strong antibody response to infecting agents is one characteristic of LAP.[22]
2. Bacteria antagonistic to *A. actinomycetemcomitans* may colonize the periodontal tissues and inhibit *A. actinomycetemcomitans* from further colonization of periodontal sites in the mouth. This would localize *A. actinomycetemcomitans* infection and tissue destruction.[19]
3. *A. actinomycetemcomitans* may lose its leukotoxin-producing ability for unknown reasons.[44] If this happens, the progression of the disease may become arrested or impaired, and colonization of new periodontal sites may be averted.
4. A defect in cementum formation may be responsible for the localization of the lesions.[25,35] Root surfaces of teeth extracted from patients with LAP have been found to have hypoplastic or aplastic cementum. This was true not only of root surfaces exposed to periodontal pockets, but also of roots still surrounded by their periodontium.

A striking feature of LAP is the lack of clinical inflammation despite the presence of deep periodontal pockets and advanced bone loss (see Figure 33-1). Furthermore, in many cases the amount of plaque on the affected teeth is minimal, which seems inconsistent with the amount of periodontal destruction present.[22] The plaque that is present forms a thin biofilm on the teeth and rarely mineralizes to form calculus.[48] Although the quantity of plaque may be limited, it often contains elevated levels of *A. actinomycetemcomitans*, and in some patients, *Porphyromonas gingivalis*. The potential significance of the qualitative composition of the microbial flora in LAP is discussed later in the section on risk factors.

As the name suggests, localized aggressive periodontitis progresses rapidly. Evidence suggests that the rate of bone loss is about three to four times faster than in chronic periodontitis.[2] Other clinical features of LAP may include (1) distolabial migration of the maxillary incisors with concomitant diastema formation, (2) increasing mobility of the maxillary and mandibular incisors and first molars, (3) sensitivity of denuded root surfaces to

SCIENCE TRANSFER

Some patients present with either a significant amount of periodontal tissue loss at a young age or a significant amount of tissue loss over a short period. These cases are referred to as "aggressive periodontitis." The tissue loss can occur around selected teeth or in a more generalized manner. These conditions represent a potentially valuable source to study disease etiology and pathogenesis because change occurs rapidly. However, because of their different presentations, the etiology of aggressive cases of periodontitis would appear to be unique. This argument favors a strong genetic influence to the etiology.

Aggressive periodontitis can be either *localized*, with first molars and incisors usually involved at or around puberty, or *generalized*, affecting at least three permanent teeth other than first molars or incisors, generally seen in patients under 30 years of age. The localized form may show decreased destructive activity when the patients are in their 20s. The exact etiology for these aggressive forms of periodontitis is not known, although some patients have decreased function of polymorphonuclear leukocytes (PMNs). Several microorganisms also are suspected as playing a role, particularly *Actinobacillus actinomycetemcomitans*, and an as-yet undetected genetic predisposition may exist as well.

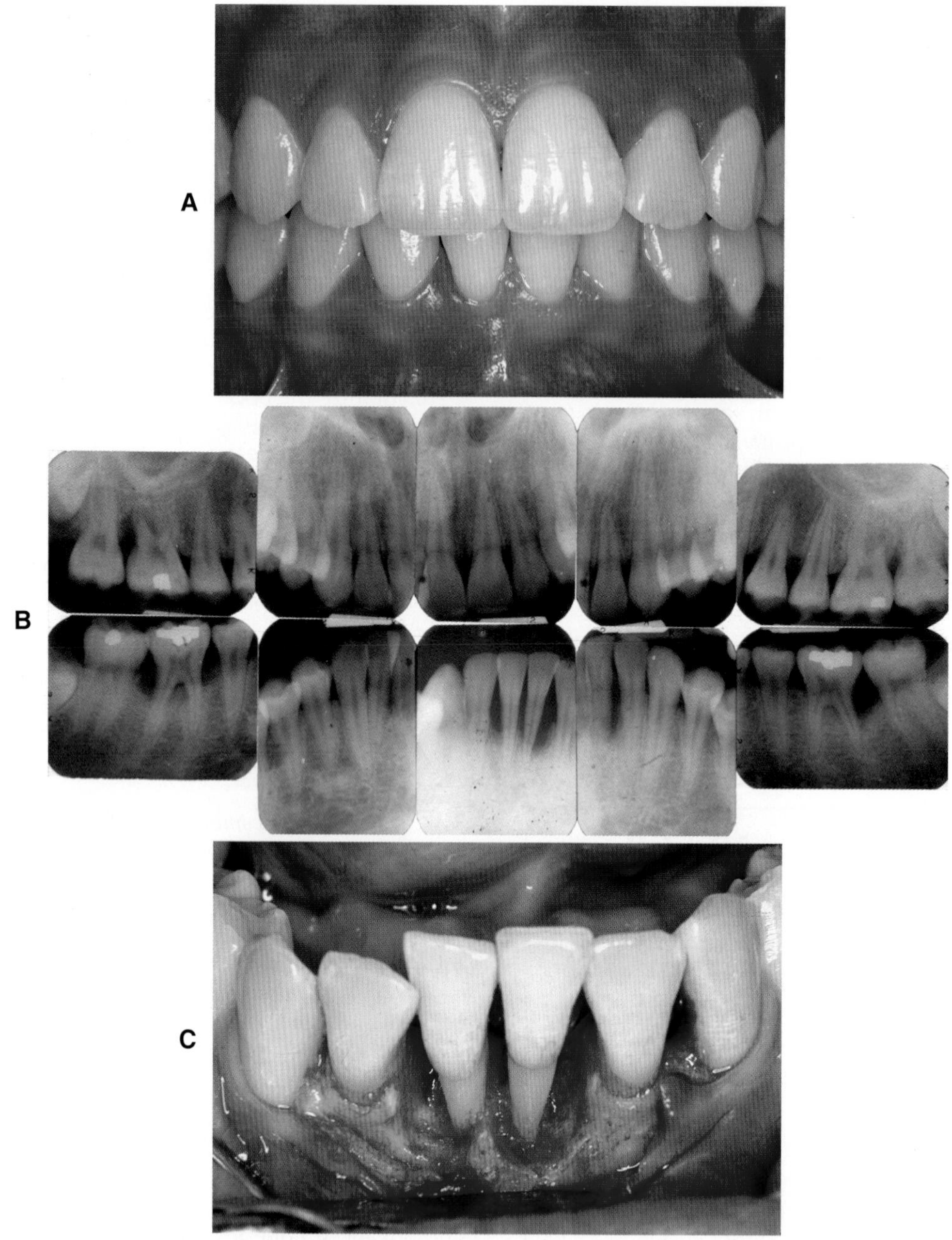

Figure 33-1 Localized aggressive periodontitis in 15-year-old black female patient who had a twin with a similar disease. **A,** Clinical view showing minimal plaque and inflammation except for localized inflammation on the distal side of the maxillary left central incisor and the mandibular right central incisor. **B,** Radiographs showing localized, vertical, angular bone loss associated with the maxillary and mandibular first molars and the mandibular central incisors. The maxillary incisors show no apparent involvement. **C,** Surgical appearance of the localized, vertical, angular bony defects affecting the mandibular incisors. Note the wide circumferential nature of the defects and the lack of calculus on the root surfaces.

thermal and tactile stimuli, and (4) deep, dull, radiating pain during mastication, probably caused by irritation of the supporting structures by mobile teeth and impacted food. Periodontal abscesses may form at this stage, and regional lymph node enlargement may occur.[30]

Not all cases of LAP progress to the degree just described. In some patients the progression of attachment loss and bone loss may be self-arresting.[22]

Radiographic Findings

Vertical loss of alveolar bone around the first molars and incisors, beginning around puberty in otherwise healthy teenagers, is a classic diagnostic sign of LAP. Radiographic findings may include an "arc-shaped loss of alveolar bone extending from the distal surface of the second premolar to the mesial surface of the second molar"[33] (see Figure

33-1, *B*). Bone defects are usually wider than usually seen with chronic periodontitis (see Figure 33-1, *C*).

Prevalence and Distribution by Age and Gender

The prevalence of LAP in geographically diverse adolescent populations is estimated at less than 1%. Most reports suggest a low prevalence, about 0.2%.[26] Two independent radiographic studies of 16-year-old adolescents, one in Finland[41] and the other in Switzerland,[21] followed the strict diagnostic criteria delineated by Baer[2] and reported a prevalence rate of 0.1%. A clinical and radiographic study of 7266 English adolescents 15 to 19 years old also showed a prevalence rate of 0.1%.[40] In the United States a national survey of adolescents age 14 to 17 reported that 0.53% had LAP.[26] Blacks were at much higher risk for LAP, and black male teenagers were 2.9 times more likely to have the disease than black female adolescents. In contrast, white female teenagers were more likely to have LAP than white male adolescents. Several other studies have found the highest prevalence of LAP among black males,[4,32,40] followed in descending order by black females, white females, and white males.[32]

Localized aggressive periodontitis affects both males and females and is seen most frequently in the period between puberty and 20 years of age. Some studies have suggested a predilection for female patients, particularly in the youngest age groups,[20] whereas others report no male-female differences in incidence when studies are designed to correct for ascertainment bias.[18] (For additional epidemiologic data on localized aggressive periodontitis, see Chapter 8.)

GENERALIZED AGGRESSIVE PERIODONTITIS

Clinical Characteristics

Generalized aggressive periodontitis (GAP) usually affects individuals under age 30, but older patients also may be affected.[22] In contrast to LAP, evidence suggests that individuals affected with GAP produce a poor antibody response to the pathogens present. Clinically, GAP is characterized by "generalized interproximal attachment loss affecting at least three permanent teeth other than first molars and incisors."[22] The destruction appears to occur episodically, with periods of advanced destruction followed by stages of quiescence of variable length (weeks to months or years). Radiographs often show bone loss that has progressed since the radiographic examination.

As seen in LAP, patients with GAP often have small amounts of bacterial plaque associated with the affected teeth.[22] Quantitatively, the amount of plaque seems inconsistent with the amount of periodontal destruction. Qualitatively, *P. gingivalis, A. actinomycetemcomitans*, and *Tannerella forsythia* (formerly *Bacteroides forsythus*) frequently are detected in the plaque that is present.[46]

Two gingival tissue responses can be found in cases of GAP. One is a severe, acutely inflamed tissue, often proliferating, ulcerated, and fiery red. Bleeding may occur spontaneously or with slight stimulation. Suppuration may be an important feature. This tissue response is believed to occur in the destructive stage, in which attachment and bone are actively lost. In other cases the gingival tissues may appear pink, free of inflammation, and occasionally with some degree of stippling, although stippling may be absent (Figure 33-2, *A*). However, despite the apparently mild clinical appearance, deep pockets can be demonstrated by probing. Page and Schroeder[36] believe that this tissue response coincides with periods of quiescence in which the bone level remains stationary. Some patients with GAP may have systemic manifestations, such as weight loss, mental depression, and general malaise.[37]

Patients with a presumptive diagnosis of GAP must have their medical histories updated and reviewed. These patients should receive medical evaluations to rule out possible systemic involvement. As seen with LAP, cases of GAP may be arrested spontaneously or after therapy, whereas others may continue to progress inexorably to tooth loss despite intervention with conventional treatment.

Radiographic Findings

The radiographic picture in generalized aggressive periodontitis can range from severe bone loss associated with the minimal number of teeth, as described previously, to advanced bone loss affecting the majority of teeth in the dentition (Figure 33-2, *B*). A comparison of radiographs taken at different times illustrates the aggressive nature of this disease. Page et al.[37] described sites in GAP patients that demonstrated osseous destruction of 25% to 60% during a 9-week period. Despite this extreme loss, other sites in the same patient showed no bone loss.

Prevalence and Distribution by Age and Gender

In a study of untreated periodontal disease conducted in Sri Lanka by Löe et al.,[27] 8% of the population had rapid progression of periodontal disease, characterized by a yearly loss of attachment of 0.1 to 1.0 mm. A U.S. national survey of adolescents age 14 to 17 reported that 0.13% had GAP.[26] In addition, blacks were at much higher risk than whites for all forms of aggressive periodontitis, and male teenagers were more likely to have GAP than female adolescents (see Chapter 8).

RISK FACTORS FOR AGGRESSIVE PERIODONTITIS

Microbiologic Factors

Although several specific microorganisms frequently are detected in patients with localized aggressive periodontitis (*A. actinomycetemcomitans, Capnocytophaga* spp., *Eikenella corrodens, Prevotella intermedia*, and *Campylobacter rectus*), *A. actinomycetemcomitans* has been implicated as the primary pathogen associated with LAP. As summarized by Tonetti and Mombelli,[46] this link is based on the following evidence:

1. *A. actinomycetemcomitans* is found in high frequency (approximately 90%) in lesions characteristic of LAP.

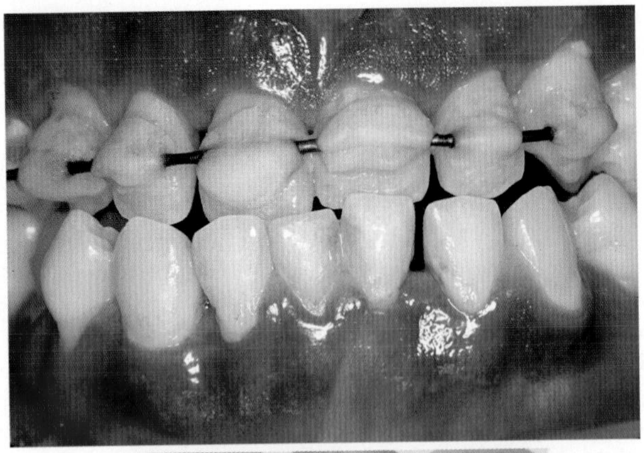

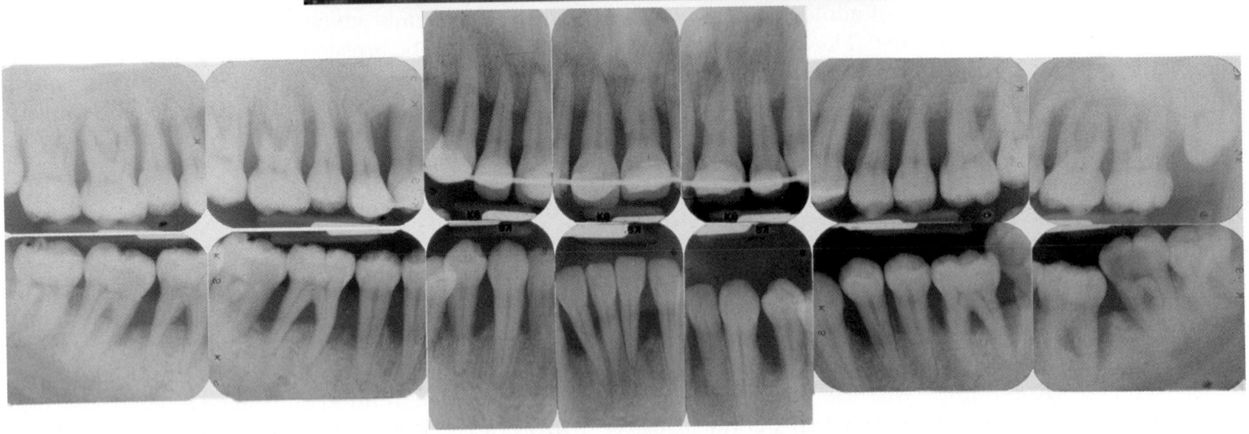

Figure 33-2 Severe generalized aggressive periodontitis in 22-year-old black male patient with a family history of early tooth loss through periodontal disease. **A,** Clinical view showing minimal plaque and inflammation. A provisional wire-and-resin splint had been placed by the general-practice dentist to stabilize the teeth. **B,** Radiographs showing the severe, generalized nature of the disease with all erupted teeth affected.

2. Sites with evidence of disease progression often show elevated levels of *A. actinomycetemcomitans.*
3. Many patients with the clinical manifestations of LAP have significantly elevated serum antibody titers to *A. actinomycetemcomitans.*
4. Clinical studies show a correlation between reduction in the subgingival load of *A. actinomycetemcomitans* during treatment and a successful clinical response.
5. *A. actinomycetemcomitans* produces a number of virulence factors that may contribute to the disease process.

Not all reports support the association of *A. actinomycetemcomitans* and localized aggressive periodontitis. In some studies, *A. actinomycetemcomitans* either could not be detected in patients with this form of disease or could not be detected at the previously reported frequencies. Another study found elevated levels of *P. gingivalis, P. intermedia, Fusobacterium nucleatum, C. rectus,* and *Treponema denticola* in patients with either localized or generalized aggressive disease, but no significant association was found between the presence of aggressive disease and *A. actinomycetemcomitans.* In addition, *A. actinomycetemcomitans* often can be detected in periodontally healthy subjects, suggesting that this microorganism may be part of the normal flora in many individuals (see Chapter 9).

Electron microscopy studies of LAP have revealed bacterial invasion of connective tissue[9,11] that reaches the bone surface.[7] The invading flora has been described as morphologically mixed but composed mainly of gram-negative bacteria, including cocci, rods, filaments, and spirochetes.[11] Using different methods, including immunocytochemistry, several tissue-invading microorganisms have been identified as *A. actinomycetemcomitans, Capnocytophaga sputigena, Mycoplasma* species, and spirochetes.[39]

Immunologic Factors

Some immune defects have been implicated in the pathogenesis of aggressive periodontitis. The human leukocyte antigens (HLAs), which regulate immune responses, have been evaluated as candidate markers for aggressive periodontitis. Although the findings with many HLAs have been inconsistent, HLA A9 and B15 antigens are consistently associated with aggressive periodontitis (see Chapter 11).

Several investigators[10,23,24] have shown that patients with aggressive periodontitis display functional defects of polymorphonuclear leukocytes (PMNs), monocytes, or both. These defects can impair either the chemotactic attraction of PMNs to the site of infection or their ability to phagocytose and kill microorganisms. Current studies have also demonstrated a hyperresponsiveness of monocytes from LAP patients involving their production of prostaglandin E_2 (PGE_2) in response to lipopolysaccharide (LPS).[43] This hyperresponsive phenotype could lead to increased connective tissue or bone loss caused by excessive production of these catabolic factors. Also, poorly functional inherited forms of monocyte FcγRII, the receptor for human immunoglobulin G2 (IgG2) antibodies, have been shown to be disproportionately present in patients with localized aggressive periodontitis.[50] These PMN and monocyte defects may be induced by the bacterial infection or may be genetic in origin. Further studies are needed to characterize the origin of these cellular alterations.

Autoimmunity has a role in generalized aggressive periodontitis, according to Anusaksathien and Dolby,[1] who found host antibodies to collagen, deoxyribonucleic acid (DNA), and IgG. Possible immune mechanisms include an increase in the expression of major histocompatibility complex (MHC) class II molecules, HLA DR4,[3] altered helper or suppressor T-cell function, polyclonal activation of B cells by microbial plaque, and genetic predisposition. (For additional information on the immunology of aggressive periodontitis, see Chapters 7 and 8.)

Genetic Factors

Results from several studies support the concept that all individuals are not equally susceptible to aggressive periodontitis.[46] Specifically, several authors have described a familial pattern of alveolar bone loss and have implicated genetic factors in aggressive periodontitis.[5,28,29,31] Currently, specific genes have not been identified that are responsible for these diseases. However, segregational and linkage analyses of families with a genetic predisposition for localized aggressive periodontitis suggest that a major gene plays a role in LAP, which is transmitted through an autosomal dominant mode of inheritance in U.S. populations.[31] It should be noted that most of the segregational studies were conducted in African American populations, and therefore other modes of inheritance may exist in different populations.

Evidence suggests that some immunologic defects associated with aggressive periodontitis may be inherited. For example, Van Dyke et al.[47] reported a familial clustering of the neutrophil abnormalities seen in localized aggressive periodontitis. This clustering suggests that the defect(s) may be inherited.[46] Studies also have demonstrated that the antibody response to periodontal pathogens, particularly *A. actinomycetemcomitans*, is under genetic control, and that the ability to mount high titers of specific, protective antibody (primarily IgG2) against *A. actinomycetemcomitans* may be race dependent.[15]

In summary, data support the concept that a gene of major effect exists for aggressive periodontitis. Data also support a genetic basis for some of the immunologic defects seen in patients with aggressive periodontitis. However, it is unlikely that all patients affected with aggressive periodontitis have the same genetic defect. As summarized by Tonetti and Mombelli,[46] "It seems that specific genes may be different in various populations and/or ethnic groups and therefore true heterogeneity in disease susceptibility may be present. The role of specific genes remains to be elucidated." (See Chapter 11.)

Environmental Factors

The amount and duration of smoking are important variables that can influence the extent of destruction seen in young adults.[46] Patients with generalized aggressive periodontitis who smoke have more affected teeth and more loss of clinical attachment than nonsmoking patients with GAP.[16] However, smoking may not have the same impact on attachment levels in younger patients with localized aggressive periodontitis.[42] (See Chapter 14.)

REFERENCES

1. Anusaksathien O, Dolby AE: Autoimmunity in periodontal disease, *J Oral Pathol Med* 20:101, 1991.
2. Baer PN: The case for periodontosis as a clinical entity, *J Periodontol* 42:516, 1971.
3. Bonfil JJ, Dillier FL, Mercier P: A "case control" study on the role of HLA DR4 in severe periodontitis and rapidly progressive periodontitis: identification of types and subtypes using molecular biology, *J Clin Periodontol* 26:77, 1999.
4. Burmeister JA, Best AM, Palcanis KG, et al: Localized juvenile periodontitis and generalized severe periodontitis: clinical findings, *J Clin Periodontol* 11:181, 1984.
5. Butler JH: A familial pattern of juvenile periodontitis (periodontosis), *J Periodontol* 40:115, 1969.
6. Carranza FA Sr, Carranza FA Jr: A suggested classification of common periodontal disease, *J Periodontol* 30:140, 1959.
7. Carranza FA Jr, Saglie R, Newman MG: Scanning and transmission electron microscopy study of tissue invading microorganisms in localized juvenile periodontitis, *J Periodontol* 54:598, 1983.
8. Caton J. Consensus report: periodontal diagnosis and diagnostic aids. In *Proceedings of the World Workshop in Clinical Periodontics,* Chicago, 1989, American Academy of Periodontology.
9. Christersson LA, Albini B, Zambon J, et al: Demonstration of *Actinobacillus actinomycetemcomitans* in gingiva in localized juvenile periodontitis in humans, *J Dent Res* 62:255, 1983 (abstract).
10. Clark RA, Page RC, Wilde G: Defective neutrophil chemotaxis in juvenile periodontitis, *Infect Immun* 18:694, 1977.
11. Gillett R, Johnson NW: Bacterial invasion of the periodontium in a case of juvenile periodontitis, *J Clin Periodontol* 9:93, 1982.
12. Goldman HM: Similar condition to periodontosis in two spider monkeys, *Am J Orthod* 33:749, 1947.
13. Gottlieb B: Die diffuse Atrophy des Alveolarknochens, *Z Stomatol* 21:195, 1923.
14. Gottlieb B: The formation of the pocket: diffuse atrophy of alveolar bone, *J Am Dent Assoc* 15:462, 1928.
15. Gunsolley JC, Tew JG, Gooss CM, et al: Effects of race, smoking and immunoglobulin allotypes on IgG subclass concentrations, *J Periodontal Res* 32:381, 1997.
16. Haber J, Wattles J, Crowley M, et al: Evidence for cigarette smoking as a major risk factor for periodontitis, *J Periodontol* 64:16, 1993.
17. Hart TC: Genetic risk factors for early-onset periodontitis, *J Periodontol* 67:355, 1996.

18. Hart TC, Marazita ML, Schenkein HA, et al: No female preponderance in juvenile periodontitis after correction of ascertainment bias, *J Periodontol* 62:745, 1991.
19. Hillman JD, Socransky SS: Bacterial interference in the oral ecology of *Actinobacillus actinomycetemcomitans* and its relationship to human periodontosis, *Arch Oral Biol* 27:75, 1982.
20. Hormand J, Frandsen A: Juvenile periodontitis. localization of bone loss in relation to age, sex, and teeth, *J Clin Periodontol* 6:407, 1979.
21. Kronauer E, Borsa G, Lang NP: Prevalence of incipient juvenile periodontitis at age 16 years in Switzerland, *J Clin Periodontol* 13:103, 1986.
22. Lang N, Bartold PM, Cullinan M, et al: Consensus report: aggressive periodontitis, *Ann Periodontol* 4:53, 1999.
23. Lavine WS, Maderazo EG, Stolman J, et al: Impaired neutrophil chemotaxis in patients with juvenile and rapidly progressing periodontitis, *J Periodontal Res* 14:10, 1979.
24. Leino L, Hurttia H: A potential role of an intracellular signaling defect in neutrophil functional abnormalities and promotion of tissue damage in patients with localized juvenile periodontitis, *Clin Chem Lab Med* 37:215, 1999.
25. Lindskog S, Blomlof L: Cementum hypoplasia in teeth affected by juvenile periodontitis, *J Clin Periodontol* 10:443, 1983.
26. Löe H, Brown LJ: Early-onset periodontitis in the United States of America, *J Periodontol* 62:608, 1991.
27. Löe H, Anerud A, Boysen H, et al: Natural history of periodontal disease in man: rapid, moderate and no loss of attachment in Sri Lankan laborers 14 to 46 years of age, *J Clin Periodontol* 13:431, 1986.
28. Long JC, Nance WE, Waring P, et al: Early onset periodontitis: a comparison and evaluation of two modes of inheritance, *Genet Epidemiol* 4:13, 1987.
29. Lopez NJ: Clinical, laboratory and immunological studies of a family with a high prevalence of generalized prepubertal and juvenile periodontitis, *J Periodontol* 63:457, 1992.
30. Manson JD, Lehner T: Clinical features of juvenile periodontitis (periodontosis), *J Periodontol* 45:636, 1974.
31. Marazita ML, Burmeister JA, Gunsolley JC, et al: Evidence for autosomal dominant inheritance and race-specific heterogeneity in early-onset periodontitis, *J Periodontol* 65:623, 1994.
32. Melvin WL, Sandifer JB, Gray JL: The prevalence and sex ratio of juvenile periodontitis in a young racially mixed population, *J Periodontol* 62:330, 1991.
33. Miller SC: Precocious advanced alveolar atrophy, *J Periodontol* 19:146, 1948.
34. Orban B, Weinmann JP: Diffuse atrophy of alveolar bone, *J Periodontol* 13:31, 1942.
35. Page RC, Baab DA: A new look at the etiology and pathogenesis of early-onset periodontitis: cementopathia revisited, *J Periodontol* 56:748, 1985.
36. Page RC, Schroeder HE: *Periodontitis in man and other animals: a comparative review,* Basel, 1982, S Karger.
37. Page RC, Altman LC, Ebersole JL, et al: Rapidly progressive periodontitis: a distinct clinical condition, *J Periodontol* 54:197, 1983.
38. Ramfjord SP, Ash MM, Kerr DA, editors: *World Workshop in Periodontics,* Ann Arbor, 1966, University of Michigan.
39. Saglie FR, Carranza FA Jr, Newman MG, et al: Identification of tissue invading bacteria in juvenile periodontitis, *J Periodontal Res* 17:452, 1982.
40. Saxby MS: Juvenile periodontitis: an epidemiologic study in the West Midlands of the United Kingdom, *J Clin Periodontol* 14:594, 1987.
41. Saxen L: Prevalence of juvenile periodontitis in Finland, *J Clin Periodontol* 7:177, 1980.
42. Schenkein JA, Gunsolley JC, Koertge TE, et al: Smoking and its effects on early-onset periodontitis, *J Am Dent Assoc* 126:1107, 1995.
43. Shapira L, Soskolone WA, Van Dyke TE, et al: Prostaglandin E_2 secretion, cell maturation, and CD 14 expression by monocyte-derived macrophages from localized juvenile periodontitis patients, *J Periodontol* 67:224, 1996.
44. Slots J, Zambon JJ, Rosling BC, et al: *Actinobacillus actinomycetemcomitans* in human periodontal disease: association, serology, leukotoxicity, and treatment, *J Periodontal Res* 17:447, 1982.
45. Thoma KH, Goldman HM: Wandering and elongation of the teeth and pocket formation in paradontosis, *J Am Dent Assoc* 27:335, 1940.
46. Tonetti MS, Mombelli A: Early-onset periodontitis, *Ann Periodontol* 4:39, 1999.
47. Van Dyke TE, Schweinebraten M, Cinaciola LJ, et al: Neutrophil chemotaxis in families with localized juvenile periodontitis, *J Periodontal Res* 20:503, 1985.
48. Waerhaug J: Subgingival plaque and loss of attachment in periodontosis as well as observed in autopsy material, *J Periodontol* 47:636, 1976.
49. Wannenmacher E: Ursachen auf dem Gebiet der Paradentopathien, *Zbl Gesant Zahn Mund Kieferheilk* 3:81, 1938.
50. Wilson ME, Kalmar JR: FcγRIIa (CD32): a potential marker defining susceptibility to localized juvenile periodontitis, *J Periodontol* 67:323, 1996.
51. Zambon JJ, Christersson LA, Slots J: *Actinobacillus actinomycetemcomitans* in human periodontal disease: prevalence in patient groups and distribution of biotypes and serotypes within families, *J Periodontol* 54:707, 1983.

Pathology and Management of Periodontal Problems in Patients with HIV Infection

Terry D. Rees

34

CHAPTER

CHAPTER OUTLINE

PATHOGENESIS

Acquired immunodeficiency syndrome (AIDS) is characterized by profound impairment of the immune system. The condition was first reported in 1981, and a viral pathogen, the *human immunodeficiency virus* (HIV), was identified in 1984.[184] The condition was originally believed to be restricted to male homosexuals. Subsequently, it was also identified in male and female heterosexuals and bisexuals who participated in unprotected sexual activities or abused injected drugs.[157,179] Currently, sexual activity and drug abuse remain the primary means of transmission.

HIV has a strong affinity for cells of the immune system, most specifically those that carry the CD4 cell surface receptor molecule. Thus, helper T lymphocytes *(T4 cells)* are most profoundly affected, but monocytes, macrophages, Langerhans cells, and some neuronal and glial brain cells may also be involved.[59] Viral replication occurs continuously in the lymphoreticular tissues of lymph nodes, spleen, gut-associated lymphoid cells, and macrophages.[233]

In recent years, combined therapeutic regimens consisting of antiretroviral agents and protease-inhibiting drugs have resulted in marked improvement in the health status of HIV-infected individuals and occasionally a reduction in viral plasma bioloads below detectable levels, although the infection is still transmissible.[63,91,.99,238] Current evidence indicates that the virus is never completely eradicated; rather, it is sequestered at low levels in resting CD4 cells even in individuals with no detectable plasma virus.[37,62] These findings suggest that effective combination drug therapy may be necessary for the lifetime of infected individuals. Long-term control of the infection may be difficult because the antiviral agents currently used have many adverse side effects and readily develop drug-resistant variant strains.[233] In untreated or inadequately treated HIV infection, the overall effect is gradual impairment of the immune system by interference with T4 lymphocytes and other immune cell functions.[234]

B lymphocytes are not infected, but the altered function of infected T4 lymphocytes secondarily results in B-cell dysregulation and altered neutrophil function.[123] This may place the HIV-positive individual at increased risk for malignancy and disseminated infections with microorganisms such as viruses, mycobacterioses, and mycoses.[90,168,176,194] HIV-positive individuals are also at increased risk for adverse drug reactions because of altered antigenic regulation.

> Epithelial cells of the mucosa may become infected and may allow access of the virus into the bloodstream. Most evidence, however, indicates that oral transmucosal viral transmission occurs after mild or severe traumatic injury or punctures of the mucous membranes. This allows for infection of circulating host defense cells, such as lymphocytes, macrophages, and dendritic cells.[9,33,208]

HIV has been detected in most body fluids, although it is found in high quantities only in blood, semen, and cerebrospinal fluid. Transmission occurs almost exclusively by sexual contact, illicit use of injection drugs, or exposure to blood or blood products. Transmission following a human bite has been reported, although the risk is extremely low.[229]

The high-risk population includes homosexual and bisexual men; users of illegal injection drugs; persons with hemophilia or other coagulation disorders; recipients of blood transfusions before April 1985; infants of HIV-infected mothers (in whom transmission occurs by fetal transmission, at delivery, or by breastfeeding); promiscuous heterosexuals; and individuals who engage in unprotected sex with HIV-positive cohorts. Heterosexual transmission is a common cause of AIDS in the world population and is increasing significantly in the United States.[31,161] Transmission is more likely to occur through contact with HIV-infected individuals with a high plasma bioload of the virus.[161,186] HIV transmission has also been reported to occur through organ transplantation and artificial insemination.[36]

EPIDEMIOLOGY AND DEMOGRAPHICS

As of December 31, 2002, 886,575 AIDS cases had been reported in the United States, and 501,669 deaths have been attributed to the syndrome.[31] The increase in numbers of patients with AIDS in the United States and other developed countries has resulted in part from prolonged survival since the advent of multidrug anti-HIV therapy.[18,63,98,163,228] The World Health Organization (WHO) has estimated that as many as 38 million individuals worldwide are infected with one of the 10 known subtypes of HIV.[127] Although the rate of infection has slowed slightly in developed countries, this number has increased to more than 40 million people in the twenty-first century.[101,127] Thus, AIDS represents the most serious medical crisis in world history.[14,100]

AIDS affects individuals of all ages, but more than 98% of cases occur among adults and adolescents over age 12. The majority of adult victims in the United States are men, 54% of whom are homosexuals or bisexuals. Approximately 12% of this group also use illicit injection drugs. An additional 27% contract the infection exclusively through injection drug use, and 15% of all patients with AIDS in the United States contracted the infection through heterosexual contact.[31] More than 19% of AIDS victims are women, the majority of whom are those who have sex with intravenous drug users or bisexual men.[31,161] Other women with AIDS were born in countries such as Haiti or one of several high-incidence African nations where heterosexual contact is the major mode of transmission. Only 1% of individuals contracted AIDS from blood products or blood transfusions in the United States because of stringent blood bank controls. This mode of transmission continues to be a threat, however, in undeveloped countries. A disproportionately high number of black and Hispanic male homosexuals, male and female heterosexuals, and children of affected women have HIV infection. The major risk factor for this disparity appears to be a more frequent history of use of injection drugs and needle sharing and unprotected sexual activity in these groups.[31,128,143]

Transmission from health care workers to patients has been documented on three occasions, with one dentist infecting six patients either accidentally or deliberately.[122,132] Conversely, seroconversion has been documented in 103 health care workers following occupational injury, usually related to management of patients with high plasma viral loads. The majority of these incidents involved nurses, and no *documented* seroconversion has been reported among dental health care workers.[106,132]

CLASSIFICATION AND STAGING

In 1982 the Centers for Disease Control and Prevention (CDC) developed a surveillance case definition for AIDS based on the presence of opportunistic illnesses or malignancies secondary to defective cell-mediated immunity in HIV-positive individuals.[28] This definition was further expanded in 1985, 1987, and 1993.[29] The 1993 revision added invasive cervical cancer in women, bacillary tuberculosis, and recurrent pneumonia into the AIDS designation. Currently, any of 25 specific clinical conditions found in HIV-positive individuals can establish the diagnosis of AIDS (Box 34-1).

The most significant change in the most recent CDC case definition was the inclusion of severe immunodeficiency (T4 lymphocyte count $<200/mm^3$ or T4 lymphocyte percentage <14% of total lymphocytes) as definitive for AIDS. This change was based on recognition that severe immunodeficiency results in increased risk for opportunistic, life-threatening conditions. Many HIV-positive individuals have been designated as patients with AIDS solely because of low T4 cell count or percentage, even in the absence of life-threatening conditions. More recently, HIV plasma bioload has been identified as a significant factor related to the transmissibility and severity of the disease.

The number of individuals living with AIDS in the United States has greatly increased in recent years because of the development of *highly active antiretroviral therapy*

BOX 34-1

CDC AIDS Surveillance Case Definition Conditions

- Candidiasis of bronchi, trachea, or lungs
- Candidiasis, esophageal
- Cervical cancer, invasive
- Coccidioidomycosis, disseminated or extrapulmonary
- Cryptococcosis, extrapulmonary
- Cryptosporidiosis, chronic intestinal (>1 month's duration)
- Cytomegalovirus disease (other than liver, spleen, or nodes)
- Cytomegalovirus retinitis (with loss of vision)
- Encephalopathy, HIV related
- Herpes simplex: chronic ulcer(s) (>1 month's duration) or bronchitis, pneumonitis, or esophagitis
- Histoplasmosis, disseminated or extrapulmonary
- Isosporiasis, chronic intestinal (1 month's duration)
- Kaposi's sarcoma
- Lymphoma, Burkitt's (or equivalent term)
- Lymphoma, immunoblastic (or equivalent term)
- Lymphoma, primary, of brain
- *Mycobacterium avium* complex or *Mycobacterium kansasii,* disseminated or extrapulmonary
- *Mycobacterium tuberculosis,* any site (pulmonary or extrapulmonary)
- *Mycobacterium,* other species or unidentified species, disseminated or extrapulmonary
- *Pneumocystis carinii* pneumonia
- Pneumonia, recurrent
- Progressive multifocal leukoencephalopathy
- *Salmonella* septicemia, recurrent
- Toxoplasmosis of brain
- Wasting syndrome caused by HIV

From Centers for Disease Control: *MMWR* 41:RR-17, 1993.

(HAART), which combines various types of antiretroviral drugs, protease inhibitors, and fusion inhibitors.[93,109] Infected individuals treated with HAART may experience a marked rise in T4 cell levels and a decreased plasma viral load. T4 counts may reach normal levels, and viral bioload may decrease to a point below the level of detection.[63,99] Despite this improvement, these individuals are still considered to have AIDS because the virus is apparently sequestered somewhere in the body. The patient remains potentially infectious to others, and viral activity may resume if medications are discontinued or if the virus becomes drug resistant.[17,91,167,182,238]

A few weeks to a few months after initial exposure, some HIV-infected individuals may experience acute symptoms, such as sudden onset of an acute mononucleosis-like illness characterized by malaise, fatigue, fever, myalgia, erythematous cutaneous eruption, oral candidiasis, oral ulcerations, and thrombocytopenia.[65,224] This acute phase may last for up to 2 weeks, with seroconversion occurring 3 to 8 weeks later.[120,225] However, antigenic viremia may sometimes be present for an extended time before seroconversion occurs.[104,120] Some individuals experience

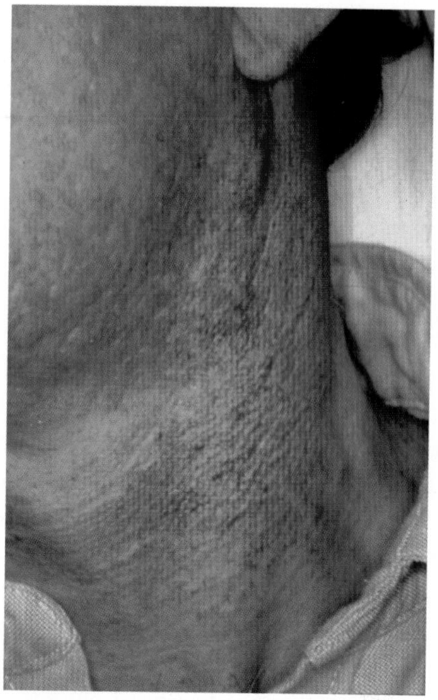

Figure 34-1 Cervical lymphadenopathy in an asymptomatic HIV-positive individual.

asymptomatic HIV infection, whereas others may become asymptomatic after the initial acute infection. In either case, infected individuals eventually become seropositive for HIV antibody, but the mean time from infection until development of AIDS is now estimated to be up to 15 years or more.[120,228]

CDC Surveillance Case Classification

AIDS patients have been grouped as follows, according to the CDC Surveillance Case Classification (1993)[29]:

- **Category A** includes patients with acute symptoms or asymptomatic diseases, along with individuals with persistent generalized lymphadenopathy, with or without malaise, fatigue, or low-grade fever (Figure 34-1).
- **Category B** patients have symptomatic conditions such as oropharyngeal or vulvovaginal candidiasis, herpes zoster, oral hairy leukoplakia, idiopathic thrombocytopenia, or constitutional symptoms of fever, diarrhea, and weight loss.
- **Category C** patients are those with outright AIDS, as manifested by life-threatening conditions or identified through CD4+ T lymphocyte levels of less than 200 cells/mm^3.

The CDC staging categories reflect progressive immunologic dysfunction, but patients do not necessarily progress serially through the three stages, and the predictive value of these categories is not known. However, because HAART drugs may cause severe adverse side effects, many AIDS treatment centers continue to follow these guidelines in determining when to initiate or discontinue multidrug therapy.[13,18,22,25,96,126]

SCIENCE TRANSFER

Patients with human immunodeficiency virus (HIV) can present with a number of oral lesions and conditions that are associated with a compromised immune response. The dentist may be the first professional to make a diagnosis of these common oral lesions. HIV-infected patients can have severe periodontal disease, but this is not always the case. Therefore, although helper T-lymphocyte (T4-cell) alteration and other changes may have a profound effect in some patients, such serious periodontal effects may not be seen in others. Thus, clinicians must be astute in their diagnosis of patients and, in HIV patients, must be cognizant of the therapeutic regimen used for the specific patient and the oral consequences of that treatment (e.g., with opportunistic infections). Furthermore, the exact relationship of HIV infection to severe periodontal conditions (e.g., necrotizing ulcerative periodontitis) is not known at this time.

AIDS patients may require special periodontal therapy, and each patient should be assessed individually and managed carefully using good professional judgment. Infection control measures are mandatory, although no reported cases of seroconversion of dental therapists have been associated with occupational injury while treating an HIV-positive patient.

ORAL AND PERIODONTAL MANIFESTATIONS OF HIV INFECTION

Oral lesions are common in HIV-infected patients, although geographic and environmental variables may exist. Previous reports indicated that most AIDS patients have head and neck lesions,[186] whereas oral lesions are quite common in HIV-positive individuals who do not yet have AIDS.[73,135] Several reports have identified a strong correlation between HIV infection and oral candidiasis, oral hairy leukoplakia, atypical periodontal diseases, oral Kaposi's sarcoma, and oral non-Hodgkin's lymphoma.[50,88,127,200]

Oral lesions less strongly associated with HIV infection include melanotic hyperpigmentation, mycobacterial infections, necrotizing ulcerative stomatitis, miscellaneous oral ulcerations, and viral infections (e.g., herpes simplex virus, herpes zoster, condyloma acuminatum). Lesions seen in HIV-infected individuals but of undetermined frequency include less common viral infections (e.g., cytomegalovirus, molluscum contagiosum); recurrent aphthous stomatitis; and bacillary angiomatosis (epithelioid angiomatosis).[50]

The advent of HAART has resulted in greatly diminished frequency of oral lesions in association with HIV infection and AIDS.[26,95,152,219] However, many current medical protocols delay the use of HAART drugs until immune suppression is relatively severe. These protocols also discontinue HAART if immune stability has been achieved or if the targeted virus becomes drug resistant.[58,139,198,219] Adherence to these protocols suggests that HIV/AIDS patients may experience a greater number of oral manifestations than in the recent past, and the dental practitioner must continue to be prepared to diagnose and manage these conditions in coordination with the patient's physician. Also, an increasing number of HIV-infected individuals are developing viral resistance to drug therapy, and this resistance may even be transmitted to newly infected sexual partners or to newborns of infected mothers.[69]

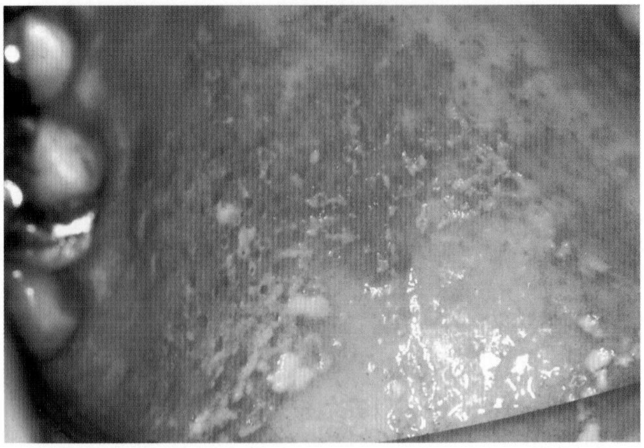

Figure 34-2 Palatal pseudomembraneous candidiasis.

Oral Candidiasis

Candida, a fungus found in normal oral flora, proliferates on the surface of the oral mucosa under certain conditions. A major factor associated with overgrowth of *Candida* is diminished host resistance, as seen in debilitated patients or in patients receiving immunosuppressive therapy. The incidence of candidal infection has been demonstrated to increase progressively in relationship to diminishing immune competency.[1,60,105,130,131] Most oral candidal infections (85%-95%) are associated with *Candida albicans,* but other species of *Candida* may be involved.[97] Currently, at least 11 strains of *Candida* have been identified, and non–*C. albicans* infections are more common among immunocompromised individuals already receiving antifungal therapy for *C. albicans.*[6,129,202]

Candidiasis is the most common oral lesion in HIV diseases and has been found in approximately 90% of AIDS patients.[164] It usually has one of four clinical presentations: pseudomembranous, erythematous, or hyperplastic candidiasis or angular cheilitis.[151]

Pseudomembranous candidiasis ("thrush") presents as painless or slightly sensitive, yellow-white curdlike lesions that can be readily scraped and separated from the surface of the oral mucosa. This type is most common on the hard and soft palate and the buccal or labial mucosa but can occur anywhere in the oral cavity (Figure 34-2).

Erythematous candidiasis may be present as a component of the pseudomembranous type, appearing as red

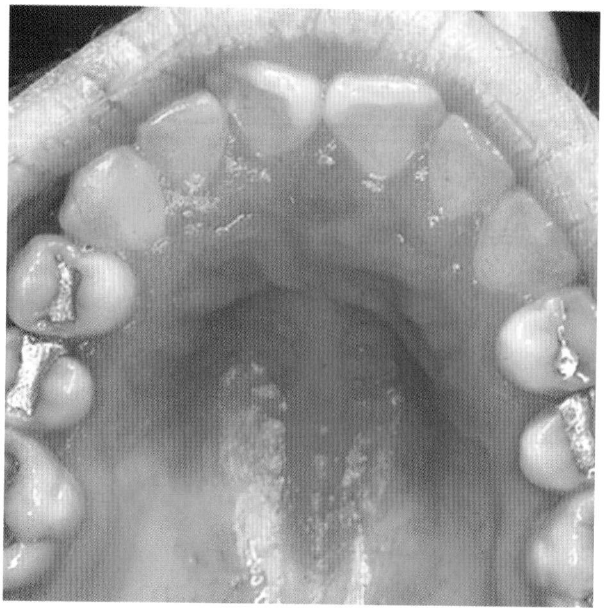

Figure 34-3 Palatal erythematous candidiasis.

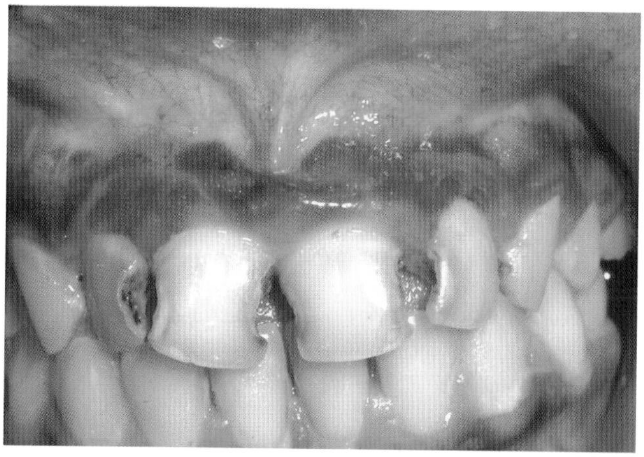

Figure 34-4 Gingival erythematous candidiasis suggestive of desquamative gingivitis.

patches on the buccal or palatal mucosa, or it may be associated with depapillation of the tongue. *If gingiva is affected, it may be misdiagnosed as desquamative gingivitis* (Figures 34-3, 34-4, and 34-5).

Hyperplastic candidiasis is the least common form and may be seen in the buccal mucosa and tongue. It is more resistant to removal than the other types (Figures 34-6 and 34-7).

In *angular cheilitis* the commissures of the lips appear erythematous with surface crusting and fissuring.

Diagnosis of candidiasis is made by clinical evaluation, culture analysis, or microscopic examination of a tissue sample or smear of material scraped from the lesion, which shows hyphae and yeast forms of the organisms (Figure 34-8). When oral candidiasis appears in patients with no apparent predisposing causes, the clinician should be alerted to the possibility of HIV infection.[2] Many patients at risk for HIV infection who present

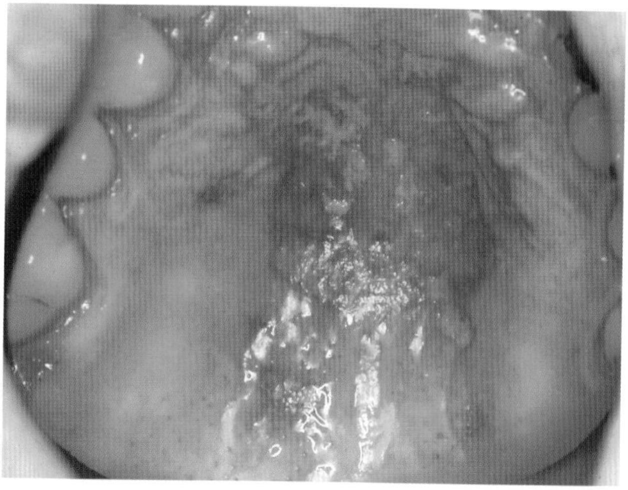

Figure 34-5 Mixed erythematous and pseudomembranous candidiasis of the palate.

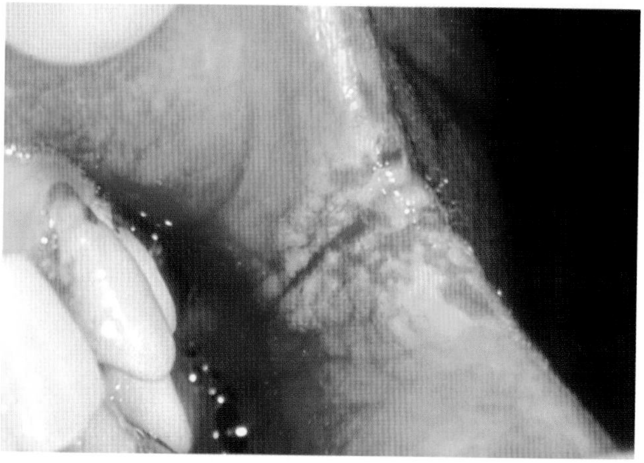

Figure 34-6 Mixed erythematous and hyperplastic candidiasis of corner of mouth.

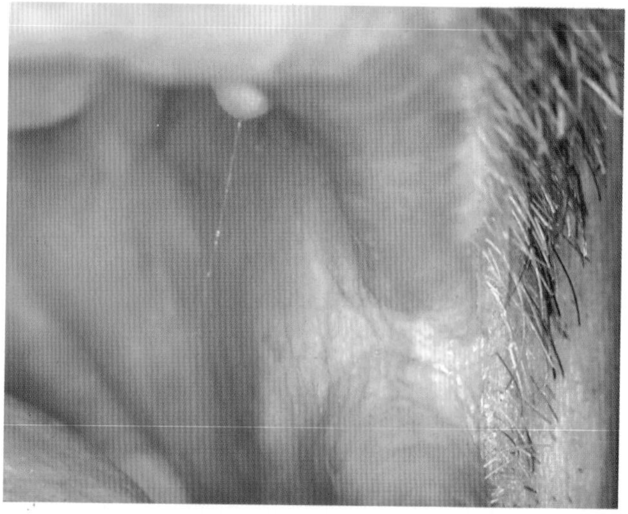

Figure 34-7 Hyperplastic candidiasis in corner of mouth. Lesion has persisted despite use of systemic antifungal drugs.

A

B

C

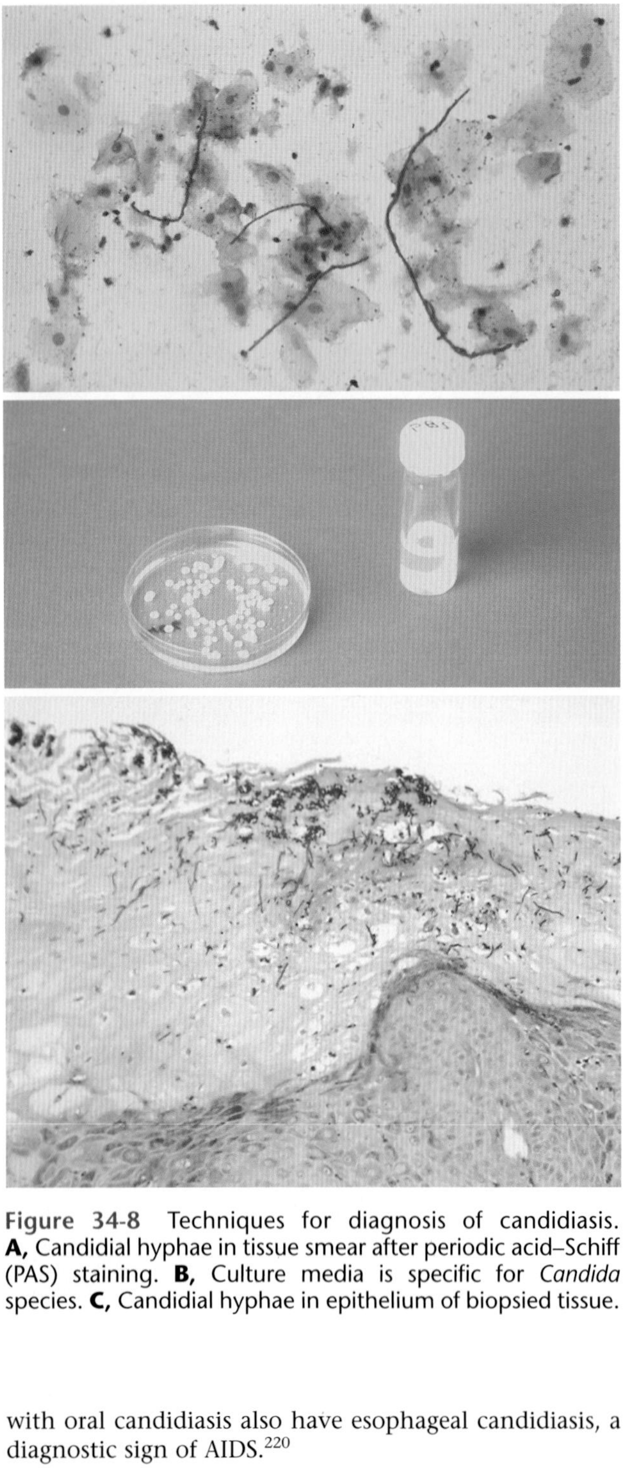

Figure 34-8 Techniques for diagnosis of candidiasis. **A,** Candidial hyphae in tissue smear after periodic acid–Schiff (PAS) staining. **B,** Culture media is specific for *Candida* species. **C,** Candidial hyphae in epithelium of biopsied tissue.

with oral candidiasis also have esophageal candidiasis, a diagnostic sign of AIDS.[220]

Although candidiasis in HIV-infected patients may respond to antifungal therapy, it is often refractory or recurrent. Traditionally, 30% of patients with AIDS-related candidiasis relapse within 4 weeks of treatment and 60% to 80% within 3 months. This relapse may result from decreasing immunocompetency or development of antifungal-resistant candidial strains.[102] As many as 10% of candidial organisms become resistant to long-term fluconazole therapy, and cross-resistance to other antifungal agents may develop to include itraconazole, amphotericin B oral suspension, and intravenous amphotericin B.[111,149,156,165] Resistant candidiasis is more common in individuals who have low CD4 counts at baseline.[106]

Recent reports indicate that the administration of HAART in HIV infections has resulted in a significant decrease in incidence of oropharyngeal candidiasis and oral candidal carriage and has reduced the rate of fluconazole resistance.[27,46,129,152,182] Early oral lesions of HIV-related candidiasis are usually responsive to topical antifungal therapy (Figure 34-9). More advanced lesions, including hyperplastic candidiasis, may require systemic

BOX 34-2

Common Antifungal Therapeutic Agents for Oral Candidiasis

Topical Drugs

1. Clotrimazole (Mycelex), 10-mg tablets: Dissolve in mouth, 3-5 tablets daily for 7-14 days.
2. Nystatin (Mycostatin, Nilstat).
   a. Oral suspension.
      - 100,000 U/ml: Administer 240 ml.
      - Rinse with 1 tsp (5 ml) qid.
   b. Oral suspension (extemporaneous).
      - Administer 2-4 billion U.
      - Mix tsp (500,000 U) in 4 oz water (cup).
      - Rinse qid.
      - *Note*: Extemporaneous nystatin is sucrose free.
   c. Tablets (500,000 U): Dissolve 1 tablet in mouth, 4 or 5 times daily.
   d. Pastilles (200,000 U): Dissolve 1 or 2 pastilles in mouth, 4 or 5 times daily.
   e. Vaginal tablets (100,000 U): Dissolve 1 tablet in mouth tid.
      - *Note*: Vaginal troches are sucrose free.
   f. Ointment (for angular cheilitis), 15-g tube: Apply to affected area tid or qid.
3. Clotrimazole ointment, 15-g tube: Apply to affected area qid.
4. Miconazole 2% ointment, 15-g tube: Apply to affected area qid.
5. Itraconazole oral suspension (Sporanox), 100-200 mg once daily for 7-28 days.
6. Fluconazole oral suspension (Diflucan), 200 mg first day followed by 100 mg once daily for at least 2 weeks.
7. Amphotericin B oral suspension (Fungizone), 100 mg qid for 2 weeks.

Systemic Drugs

1. Ketoconazole (Nizoral), 200-mg tablets: Take 2 tablets immediately, then 1 or 2 tablets daily with food for 5-14 days.
2. Fluconazole (Diflucan), 100-mg tablets: Take 2 tablets immediately, then 1 tablet daily for 7-14 days.
3. Itraconazole (Sporanox), 100-mg capsules: Take 200 mg once daily with meals for 4 weeks (AIDS and neutropenic patients).

U, Units; *qid,* four times daily; *tid,* three times daily; *AIDS, acquired immunodeficiency syndrome.*

A

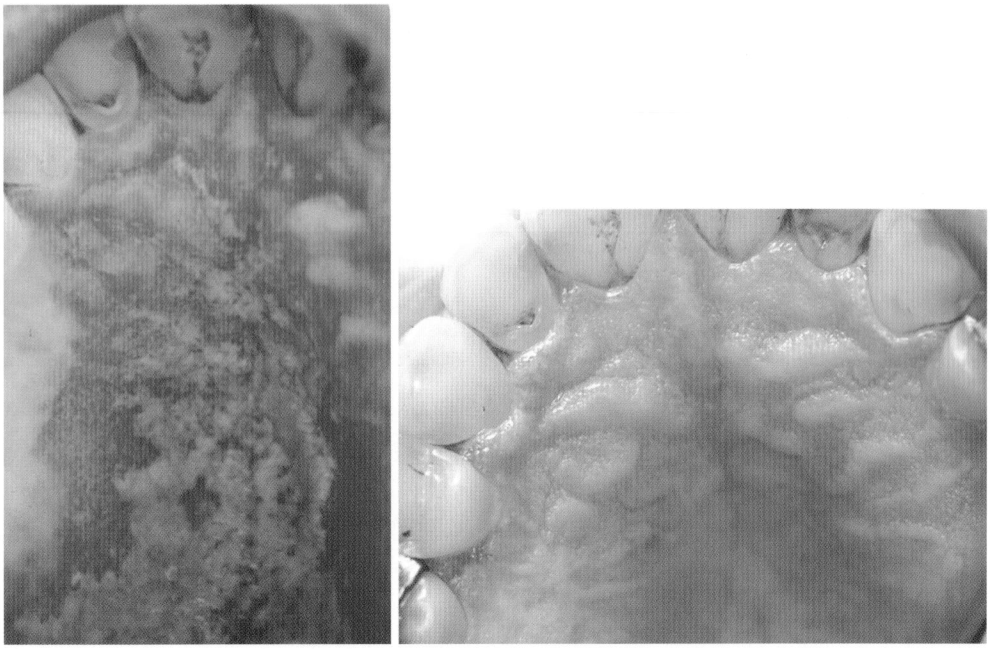

B

Figure 34-9 Palatal pseudomembranous candidiasis. **A,** Before treatment with nystatin oral suspension. **B,** Remission after 2 weeks of treatment.

A

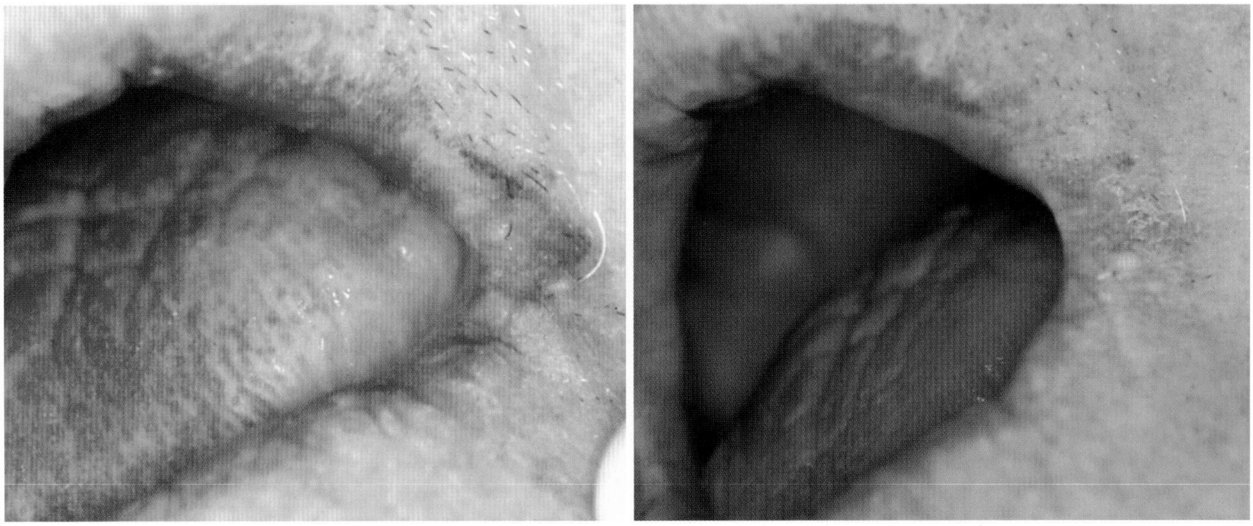

B

Figure 34-10 Severe angular cheilitis. **A,** Before treatment. **B,** After treatment with systemic fluconazole.

antifungal drugs; systemic therapy is mandatory for esophageal candidiasis[201,223] (Figure 34-10).

With any therapy, lesions tend to recur after the drug is discontinued, and resistant strains of candidal organisms have been described, especially with the use of systemic agents.[44,201,220,223] Box 34-2 identifies therapeutic agents often prescribed for treatment of candidal infections. Most oral topical antifungal agents contain large quantities of sucrose, which may be cariogenic after long-term use. For this reason, some authorities recommend oral use of vaginal tablets because they do not contain sucrose. However, such tablets are relatively low in active units (100,000) compared with usual oral dosages of 200,000 to 600,000 units. Sucrose-free nystatin is also available in a powder form, which may be mixed extemporaneously with water at each use (teaspoon powder to glass water). Recently, sucrose-free oral suspensions of itraconazole and amphotericin B oral rinse have become available. To date, no comparative studies have been performed regarding the effectiveness of these products. Amphotericin B oral suspension is more effective against *Candida albicans* than other species. Patients should be instructed to rinse with the oral suspension for several minutes, then swallow.[172] Fluconazole oral suspension has been reported to be more effective as an antifungal than liquid nystatin.[166] Chlorhexidine and cetylpyridinium chloride oral rinses may also be of some prophylactic value against oral candidal infection.[52,70] Long-term prophylactic effectiveness of once-weekly systemic fluconazole also has been described.[52,201]

Systemic antifungal agents such as ketoconazole, fluconazole, itraconazole, and amphotericin B are effective in treatment of oral candidiasis[156] (see Box 34-2). *Ketoconazole* may be the agent of choice when systemic therapy is required.[44,210] As previously mentioned, however, resistant strains of candidal organisms may develop with prolonged use of any systemic agent, potentially rendering the drugs ineffective against life-threatening candidal infections in the later stages of immunosuppression.[24,172] In addition, significant adverse side effects may occur. For example, long-term use of ketoconazole may induce liver damage in individuals with preexisting liver disease. The increased risk of chronic hepatitis B or hepatitis C infection in immunosuppressed individuals may put some patients at risk for ketoconazole-induced liver damage. If ketoconazole is prescribed, patients should receive liver function tests at baseline and at least monthly during therapy. The drug is contraindicated if the patient's aspartate transaminase (AST) level is greater than 2.5 times normal.[223] Ketoconazole absorption also may be impaired by the gastropathy experienced by many HIV-infected individuals.[117]

A

B

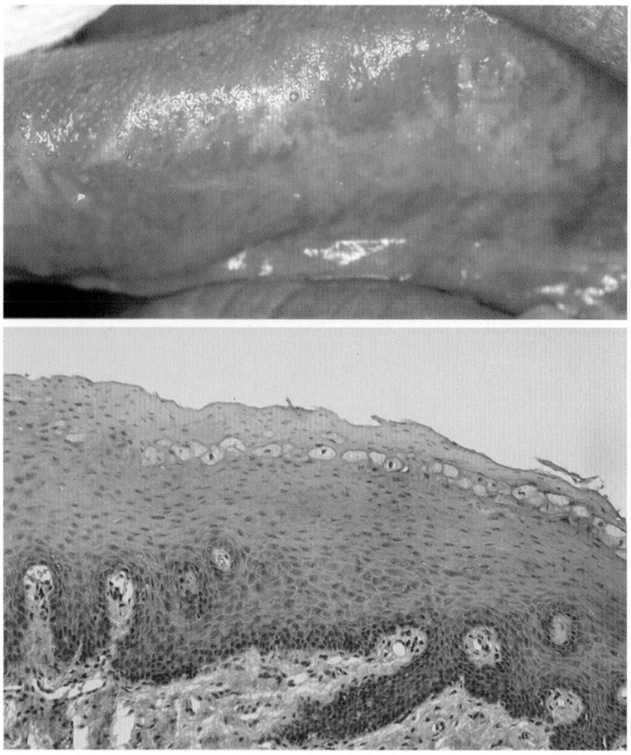

Figure 34-11 Oral hairy leukoplakia on left lateral border of tongue. **A,** Clinical view. **B,** Biopsy confirmation of oral hairy leukoplakia. Note the ballooned epithelial cells near the surface of the epithelium.

Oral Hairy Leukoplakia

Oral hairy leukoplakia (OHL) primarily occurs in persons with HIV infection.[84,86] Found on the lateral borders of the tongue, OHL frequently has a bilateral distribution and may extend to the ventrum. This lesion is characterized by an asymptomatic, poorly demarcated keratotic area ranging in size from a few millimeters to several centimeters (Figure 34-11, *A*). Often, characteristic vertical striations are present, imparting a corrugated appearance, or the surface may be shaggy and appear "hairy" when dried. The lesion does not rub off and may resemble other keratotic oral lesions.

> Microscopically, the OHL lesion shows a hyperparakeratotic surface with projections that often resemble hairs. Beneath the parakeratotic surface, acanthosis and some characteristic "balloon cells" resembling koilocytes are seen (Figure 34-11, *B*). It has been demonstrated that these cells contain viral particles of the human herpesvirus group; these particles have been interpreted as the Epstein-Barr virus (EBV).[84,87]
>
> Epithelial dysplasia is not a feature, and in most OHL lesions, little or no inflammatory infiltrate in the underlying connective tissue is present.[197]

OHL is found almost exclusively on the lateral borders of the tongue, although it has been reported on the dorsum of the tongue, buccal mucosa, floor of the mouth, retromolar area, and soft palate.[57,84,111] In addition, most of these lesions reveal surface colonization by *Candida* organisms, which are secondary invaders and not the cause of the lesion.

OHL was originally believed to be caused by the human papillomavirus, but subsequent evidence indicated an association with Epstein-Barr virus (EBV).[84,86,232] In the late 1980s, so-called pseudo–hairy leukoplakia was described in HIV-negative and EBV-negative individuals with lesions clinically identical to OHL. In addition, several case reports have described OHL in EBV-infected but HIV-negative individuals with a variety of immunosuppressed conditions (e.g., acute myelogenous leukemia) or who develop immunosuppression as a result of organ transplantation or extensive systemic corticosteroid therapy.[85,217] Regardless of cause, biopsy identification of a lesion suggestive of OHL should dictate that HIV testing be performed. It should be emphasized that the severity of the lesion is not correlated with the likelihood of developing AIDS; thus, small lesions are as diagnostically significant as extensive lesions.[197]

The differential diagnosis of OHL includes several white lesions of the mucosa, such as dysplasia, carcinoma, frictional and idiopathic keratosis, lichen planus, tobacco-related leukoplakia, secondary syphilis, psoriasiform lesions (e.g., geographic tongue), and hyperplastic candidiasis.[2,158] The microscopic confirmation of OHL of the tongue in a high-risk patient is considered to be a specific early sign of HIV infection and an indication that the patient will develop AIDS.[86] Before the advent of effective therapy for HIV, survival analysis indicated that 83% of HIV-infected patients with hairy leukoplakia would develop AIDS within 31 months,[85] and the number of patients with hairy leukoplakia who eventually developed AIDS approached 100%.[88] Use of HAART, however, has

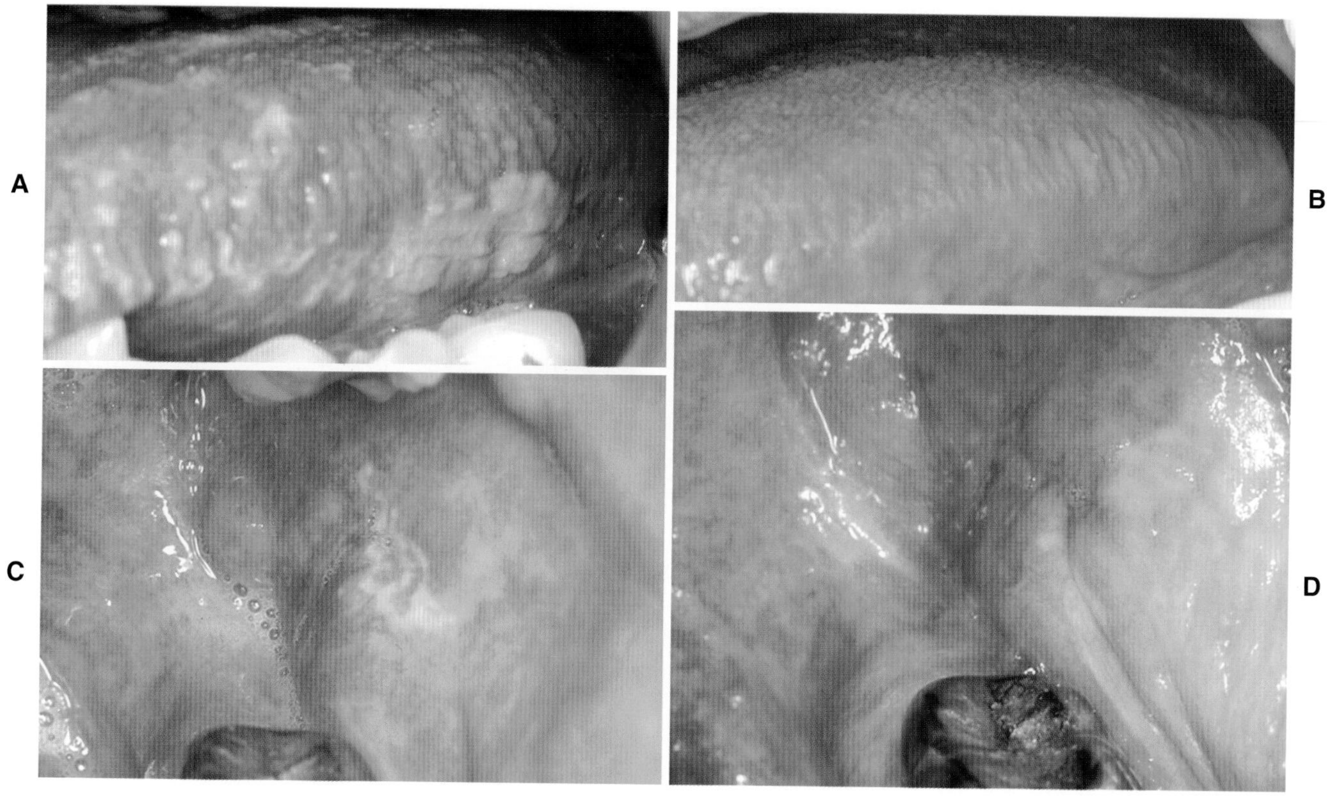

Figure 34-12 **A,** Oral hairy leukoplakia of tongue before initiating highly active antiretroviral therapy (HAART). **B,** Oral hairy leukoplakia of buccal mucosa before initiating HAART. **C,** Tongue lesion in remission after initiation of HAART. **D,** Remission of lesion on buccal mucosa after HAART.

resulted in a greatly diminished incidence of OHL[16,26,58,219] (Figure 34-12).

If OHL occurs despite HAART, it may represent an increasing immunodeficiency resulting from therapeutic failure, failure to take medications as prescribed, or reduced dosage of medications to prevent adverse side effects.[58] Vigorous treatment of OHL is usually not indicated. However, the lesions are often responsive to HIV drug therapy or the use of antiviral agents such as acyclovir or valacyclovir.[231] Lesions can be successfully removed with laser or conventional surgery. Some have advocated the topical application of podophyllin, retinoids, or interferon, but these agents can induce unwanted local or systemic side effects. Regardless of the choice of treatment, OHL lesions tend to recur when therapy is discontinued.[136,231,232]

Kaposi's Sarcoma and Other Malignancies

Oral malignancies occur more frequently in severely immunocompromised individuals than in the general population. An HIV-positive individual with *non-Hodgkin's lymphoma* (NHL) or Kaposi's sarcoma (KS) is categorized as having AIDS (Figure 34-13). Oral lesions are reported in approximately 4% of individuals with NHL, and the gingiva and palate are common sites. The incidence of oral squamous cell carcinoma may also increase in HIV-infected individuals.

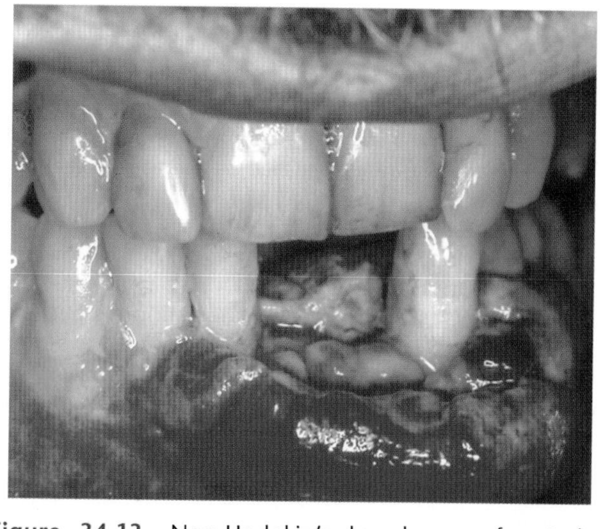

Figure 34-13 Non-Hodgkin's lymphoma of anterior mandibular gingiva.

However, KS is the most common oral malignancy associated with AIDS. This angiomatous tumor is a rare, multifocal, vascular neoplasm; it was originally described in 1872 as occurring in the skin of the lower extremities of older men of Mediterranean origin. Its cause is unknown, although sexually transmitted viral infection has

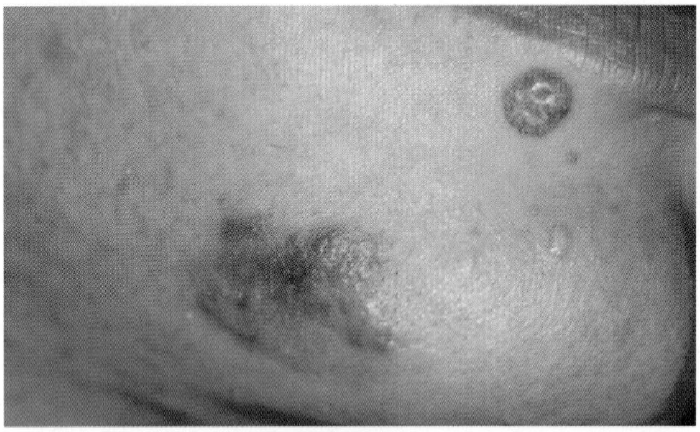

Figure 34-14 Cutaneous Kaposi's sarcoma on right chin.

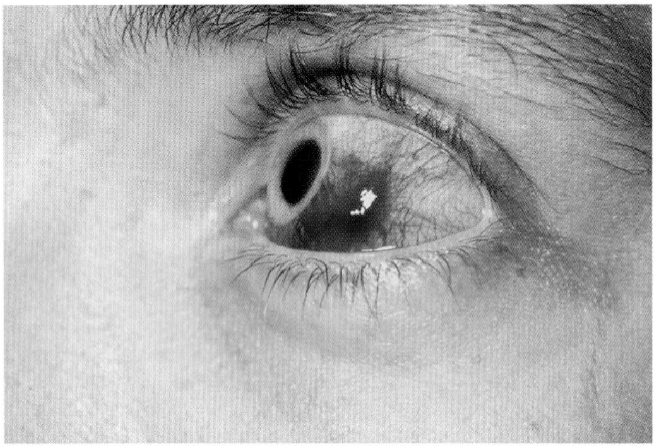

Figure 34-15 Ocular Kaposi's sarcoma causing loss of vision.

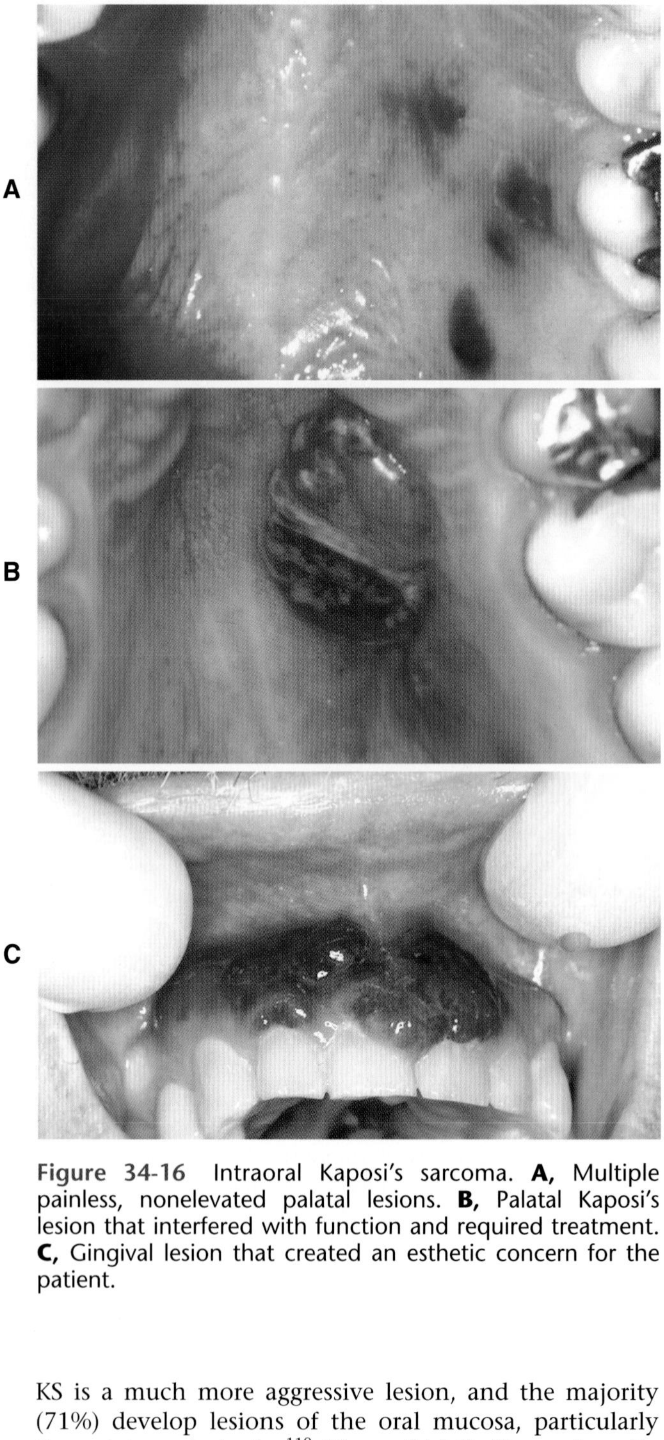

Figure 34-16 Intraoral Kaposi's sarcoma. **A,** Multiple painless, nonelevated palatal lesions. **B,** Palatal Kaposi's lesion that interfered with function and required treatment. **C,** Gingival lesion that created an esthetic concern for the patient.

been suspected. A new strain of herpesvirus identified as closely associated with KS was originally named the *KS-herpesvirus* but is now designated as *human herpesvirus-8* (HHV-8). HHV-8, also called the "Kaposi's sarcoma–associated herpesvirus," has been associated with both AIDS-related and non–AIDS-related KS.[67,188] However, HIV-infected individuals are 7000-fold more likely to develop KS.[63] Despite this strong association, an etiologic association between HHV-8 and KS is not always identified.[67,108,110] The virus has been isolated from 29% of American adults and 8% of children in the non-AIDS general population. It has also been isolated from lesions of NHL, Castleman's disease, other lymphoproliferative disorders, and a variety of additional abnormalities, although these findings may coincide with those of the healthy general population.[78,108,212] In contrast, one study identified HHV-8 in 53 of 54 AIDS-related KS lesions.[114] Thus it appears that decreasing immunocompetence results in activation of latent HHV-8. Although the virus may be sexually transmitted, it may also be transmitted from infected mothers to children.[211]

Although KS is a malignant tumor, in its classic form it is a localized and slowly growing lesion. The KS that occurs in HIV-infected patients presents different clinical features (Figures 34-14 and 34-15). In these individuals, KS is a much more aggressive lesion, and the majority (71%) develop lesions of the oral mucosa, particularly the palate and gingiva[110] (Figure 34-16). The oral cavity may often be the first or only site of the lesion.[11]

In the early stages the oral lesions are painless, reddish purple macules of the mucosa. As they progress, the lesions frequently become nodular and can easily be confused with other oral vascular entities, such as hemangioma, hematoma, varicosity, or pyogenic granuloma (when occurring in the gingiva).[203]

Lesions manifest as nodules, papules, or nonelevated macules that are usually brown, blue, or purple in color, although occasionally the lesions may display normal pigmentation. Diagnosis is based on histologic findings.[116,181]

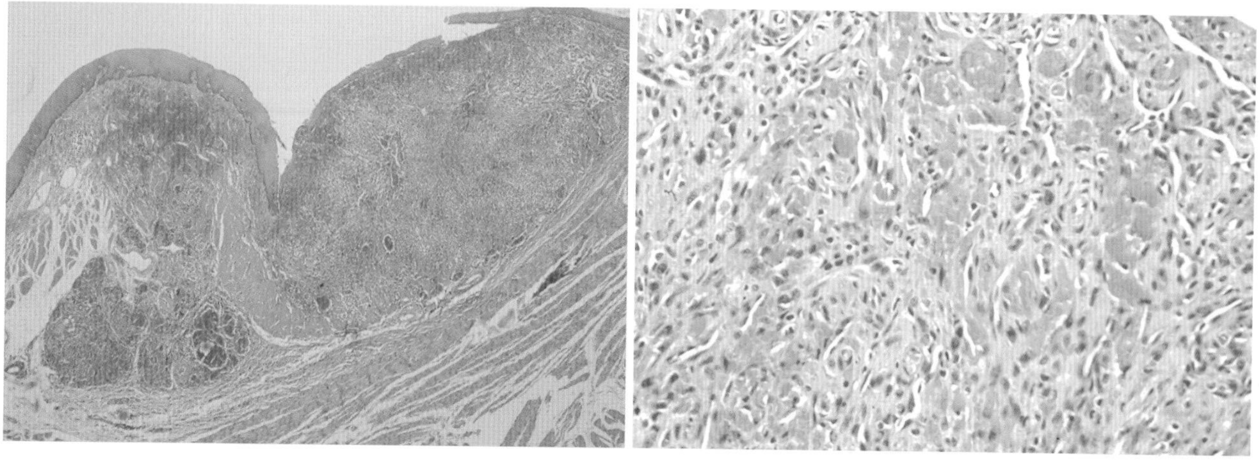

Figure 34-17 **A,** Histologic view of Kaposi's sarcoma. Lesion is exophytic and only minimally inflamed (low magnification). **B,** Note sheets of endothelial cells and numerous small blood vessels (high magnification).

Microscopically, Kaposi's sarcoma consists of four components: (1) endothelial cell proliferation with the formation of atypical vascular channels; (2) extravascular hemorrhage with hemosiderin deposition; (3) spindle cell proliferation in association with atypical vessels; and (4) a mononuclear inflammatory infiltrate consisting mainly of plasma cells[81] (Figure 34-17).

Regional and gender differences are apparent; oral KS is more common in the United States than in Europe, and the male/female ratio is 20:1.[221] The condition has also been reported in patients with lupus erythematosus who are receiving immunosuppressant therapy, as well as in renal transplant patients and other individuals receiving corticosteroid or cyclosporine therapy. Case reports describe gingival KS in HIV-negative patients experiencing cyclosporine-induced gingival enlargement.[175,221] In an HIV-positive individual, the presence of KS signifies transition to outright AIDS. Before the advent of combined drug therapy for AIDS, the median survival time after onset of KS ranged from 7 to 31 months.[37,40]

The differential diagnosis of oral KS includes pyogenic granuloma, hemangioma, atypical hyperpigmentation, sarcoidosis, bacillary angiomatosis, angiosarcoma, pigmented nevi, and cat-scratch disease (skin).[181]

The advent of HAART has resulted in a marked reduction in the incidence of KS. However, the lesions may still be found in severely immunocompromised individuals or those who are unaware of their HIV-positive status.[67] HHV-8 may be found more frequently in saliva of HIV-positive individuals with higher CD4 cell counts, suggesting that viral shedding may occur relatively early in the disease process.[82]

Treatment of oral KS includes antiretroviral agents, laser excision, cryotherapy, radiation therapy, and intralesional injection with vinblastine, interferon-α, sclerosing agents, or other chemotherapeutic drugs.* Nichols et al.[150] described the successful use of intralesional injections of vinblastine at a dose of 0.1 mg/cm^2 using a 0.2 mg/ml solution of vinblastine sulfate in saline (Figure 34-18). In responsive patients, treatment was repeated at 2-week intervals until resolution or stabilization of the lesions. Side effects included some posttreatment pain and occasional ulceration of the lesions, but in general the therapy was well tolerated. Total resolution was achieved in 70% of 82 intraoral KS lesions with one to six treatments. Lesions tended to recur, however, indicating that

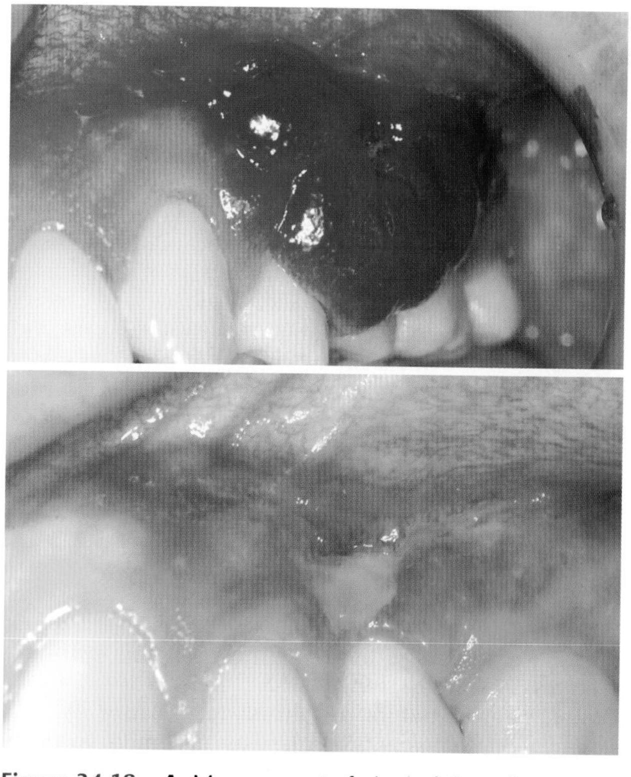

Figure 34-18 **A,** Management of gingival Kaposi's sarcoma interfering with function. **B,** Nearly complete resolution of the lesion after intralesional injection with vinblastine.

*References 13, 53, 55, 61, 195, 207, 221.

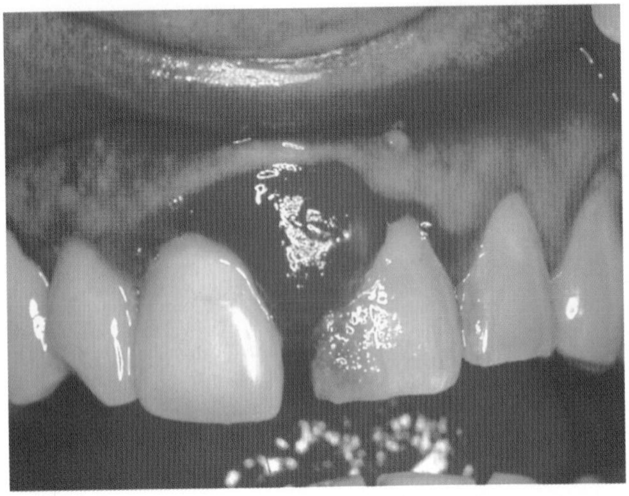

Figure 34-19 Bacillary angiomatosis mimicking Kaposi's sarcoma.

treatment probably should be reserved for oral KS lesions that are easily traumatized or that interfere with chewing or swallowing. Occasionally, treatment may be indicated when KS lesions create an unsightly appearance on the lips or in the anterior oral cavity.

In a double-blind, randomized clinical trial on a small group of patients with oral KS lesions, the authors concluded that vinblastine injections remain the most effective treatment in managing localized lesions.[177] However, comparable results may be obtained using injections of 3% sodium tetradecyl sulfate, a sclerosing agent, previously used in treatment of varicose veins. The sclerosing agent offers the advantage of being relatively inexpensive and easy to use. Destructive periodontitis has also been reported in conjunction with gingival KS. In such patients, scaling and root planing and other periodontal therapy may be indicated in addition to intralesional or systemic chemotherapy.[207,220]

Bacillary (Epithelioid) Angiomatosis

Bacillary (epithelioid) angiomatosis (BA) is an infectious vascular proliferative disease with clinical and histologic features similar to those of KS. BA is believed to be caused by rickettsia-like organisms (e.g., Bartonellaceae, *Rochalimaea quintana*).* Skin lesions are similar to those seen in KS or cat-scratch disease. Gingival BA manifests as red, purple, or blue edematous soft tissue lesions that may cause destruction of periodontal ligament and bone[72] (Figure 34-19). The condition is more prevalent in HIV-positive individuals with low CD4 levels.[138]

Diagnosis of bacillary angiomatosis is based on biopsy, which reveals an "epithelioid" proliferation of angiogenic cells accompanied by an acute inflammatory cell infiltrate. The causative organism in the biopsy specimen may be identified using Warthen-Starry silver staining or electron microscopy.[68]

*References 50, 138, 148, 174, 188, 235.

A

B

C

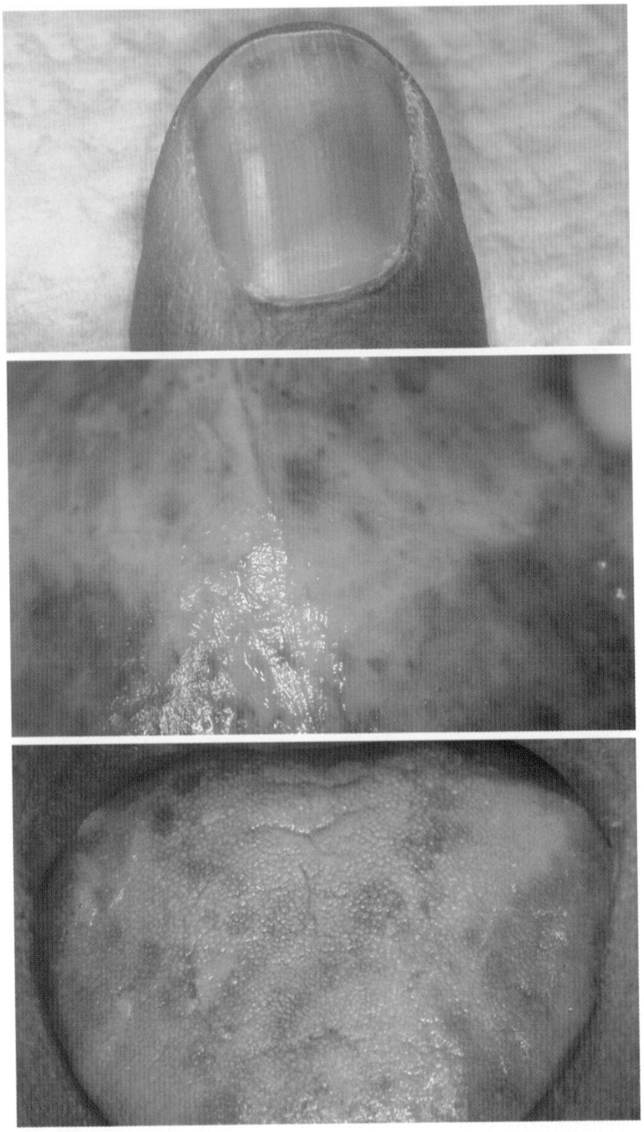

Figure 34-20 Drug-induced hyperpigmentation (zidovudine). **A,** Fingernail bed discoloration. **B,** Same patient, palatal hyperpigmentation. **C,** Same patient, tongue hyperpigmentation. Note similarity between the oral lesions and those caused by adrenal cortex hypofunction (Addison's disease).

Differential diagnosis of BA includes KS, angiosarcoma, hemangioma, pyogenic granuloma, and nonspecific vascular proliferation.[35] Bacillary angiomatosis is usually treated using broad-spectrum antibiotics such as erythromycin or doxycycline. Gingival lesions may be managed using the antibiotic in conjunction with conservative periodontal therapy and possibly excision of the lesion.[72,73,121,178]

Oral Hyperpigmentation

An increased incidence of oral hyperpigmentation has been described in HIV-infected individuals.[115,119] Oral pigmented areas often appear as spots or striations on the buccal mucosa, palate, gingiva, or tongue (Figure 34-20).

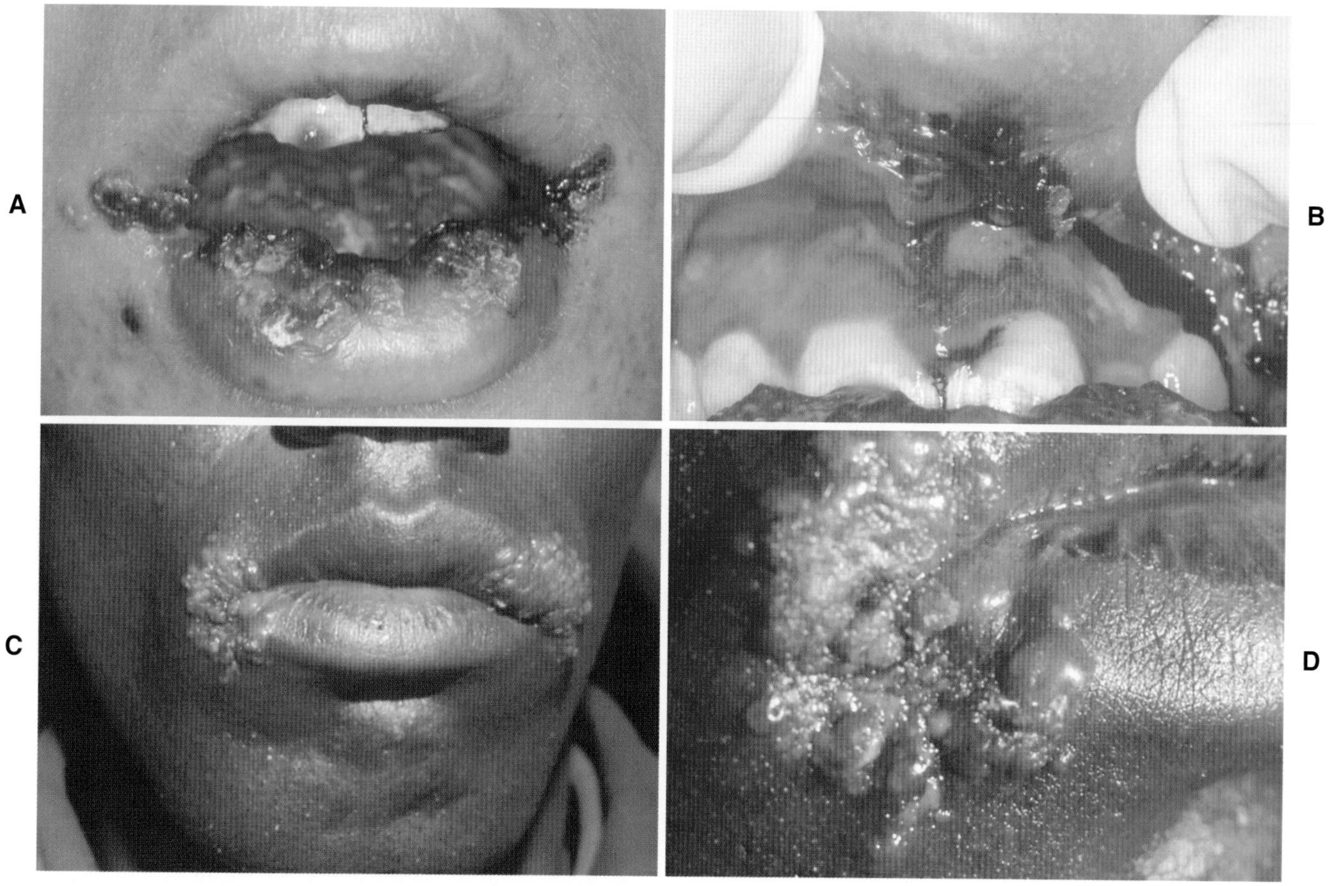

Figure 34-21 Abnormal herpetic lesions in HIV-positive individuals. **A,** Lip crusting of primary herpetic gingivostomatitis. **B,** Same patient, ulcerations of gingiva, alveolar mucosa, and vestibule. **C,** Severe herpes labialis in commissures of lip. **D,** Close-up view of herpes labialis. Note fluid-filled vesicles.

In some cases the pigmentation may relate to prolonged use of drugs such as zidovudine, ketoconazole, or clofazimine.[239] Zidovudine is also associated with excessive pigmentation of the skin and nails, although similar hyperpigmentation has been reported in some individuals who have never taken zidovudine. On occasion, oral pigmentation may be the result of adrenocorticoid insufficiency induced in an HIV-positive individual by prolonged use of ketoconazole or by *Pneumocystis carinii* infection or cytomegalovirus or other viral infections[64] (see Figure 34-11).

Atypical Ulcers

Nonspecific oral ulcerations in HIV-infected individuals may have multiple etiologies that include neoplasms such as lymphoma, KS, and squamous cell carcinoma. Recent case reports suggest that HIV-associated neutropenia may also feature oral ulcerations. Neutropenia has been successfully treated using recombinant human granulocyte colony-stimulating factor (G-CSF) with resultant resolution of oral ulcers.[123] Severe, prolonged oral ulcers have been successfully managed using prednisone or thalidomide, a drug that inhibits tissue necrosis factor alpha (TNF-α). Recurrence is likely, however, if either drug is discontinued.[48,78,79,107,256]

HIV-infected patients have a higher incidence of recurrent herpetic lesions and aphthous stomatitis (see Figures 34-12 and 34-13). Approximately 10% of HIV-infected patients have herpes infection,[164,209] and multiple episodes are common. The CDC HIV classification system indicates that mucocutaneous herpes lasting longer than 1 month is diagnostic of AIDS in HIV infected individuals.[29] Aphthae and aphthalike lesions are common when patients are followed throughout the course of their immunosuppression.[76]

In healthy patients, herpetic and aphthous lesions are self-limiting and relatively easy to diagnose by their characteristic clinical features (i.e., herpes on the keratinizing mucosa, aphthae on the nonkeratinizing surfaces). In HIV-infected patients the clinical presentation and course of these lesions may be altered. Herpes may involve all mucosal surfaces and extend to the skin and may persist for months[56] (Figure 34-21). Atypical large, persistent, nonspecific, painful ulcers are common in immunocompromised individuals. If healing is delayed, these lesions are secondarily infected and may become indistinguishable from persistent herpetic or aphthous lesions.[183]

A wide variety of bacterial and viral infections may produce severe oral ulcerations in HIV-infected individuals. Essentially, immunocompromised individuals are at risk from infectious agents endemic to the patient's geographic location. Atypical or nonhealing ulcers may require biopsy, microbial cultures, or both to determine the etiology. Oral ulcerations have been described in association with enterobacterial organisms such as *Klebsiella pneumoniae, Enterobacter cloacae,* and *Escherichia coli.*[183] Such infections are rare and are usually associated with systemic involvement. Specific antibiotic therapy is indicated, and close coordination of oral therapy with the patient's physician is usually necessary.

Herpes simplex virus (HSV), varicella-zoster virus (VZV), Epstein-Barr virus (EBV), and cytomegalovirus (CMV) are frequently retrieved from nonspecific oral ulcers, indicating a possible etiologic role.[218] Recently, atypical ulcers were found to be co-infected with HSV and CMV or with EBV and CMV.[180,217] These ulcers may be more common in individuals who are neutropenic in conjunction with their HIV infection. Neutropenia may also be induced by drugs such as zidovudine, trimethoprim-sulfamethoxazole, and gancyclovir.[123] Atypical ulcers may be more severe and persistent in individuals with low CD4 cell counts, and the presence of oral CMV-induced ulcers may be indicative of systemic CMV infection.[76]

Herpes labialis in HIV infected individuals may be responsive to topical antiviral therapy (e.g., acyclovir, pencyclovir, doconasol), reducing the healing time of lesions. In other patients, however, oral or labial herpetic lesions may require the use of systemic antiviral agents (e.g., acyclovir, valacyclovir, famciclovir).[51]

Recurrent aphthous stomatitis (RAS) has been described in HIV-infected individuals, but the overall incidence may be no greater than that in the general population.[50] RAS may occur, however, as a component of the initial acute illness of HIV seroconversion.[134] The incidence of major aphthae may be increased, and the oropharynx, esophagus, or other areas of the gastrointestinal tract may be involved[4,5] (Figure 34-22).

Proven methods of treatment for recurrent aphthous stomatitis include topical or intralesional corticosteroids, chlorhexidine or other antimicrobial mouth rinses, oral tetracycline rinses, or topical amlexanox. Systemic corticosteroid therapy may be necessary in some cases. Consequently, in patients with HIV infection and recurrent aphthae, closely coordinated medical and dental therapy may be necessary.[36]

Recent evidence indicates that many nonspecific oral ulcerations may be of viral origin, with HSV, EBV, and CMV being most common[76] (Figure 34-23). For this reason, the practitioner should consider viral culturing of such lesions and the use of antiviral agents in treatment where appropriate.

Oral viral infections in immunocompromised individuals are often treated with acyclovir (200-800 mg administered five times daily for at least 10 days). Subsequent daily maintenance therapy (200 mg two to five times daily) may be required to prevent recurrence. Resistant viral strains are treated with foscarnet, ganciclovir, or valacyclovir.[220,222]

Topical corticosteroid therapy (fluocinonide gel applied three to six times daily) is safe and efficacious for treatment of recurrent aphthous ulcers or other mucosal lesions in immunocompromised individuals.[36] However, topical corticosteroids may predispose immunocompromised individuals to candidiasis. Consequently, prophylactic antifungal medications should be prescribed.

A

B

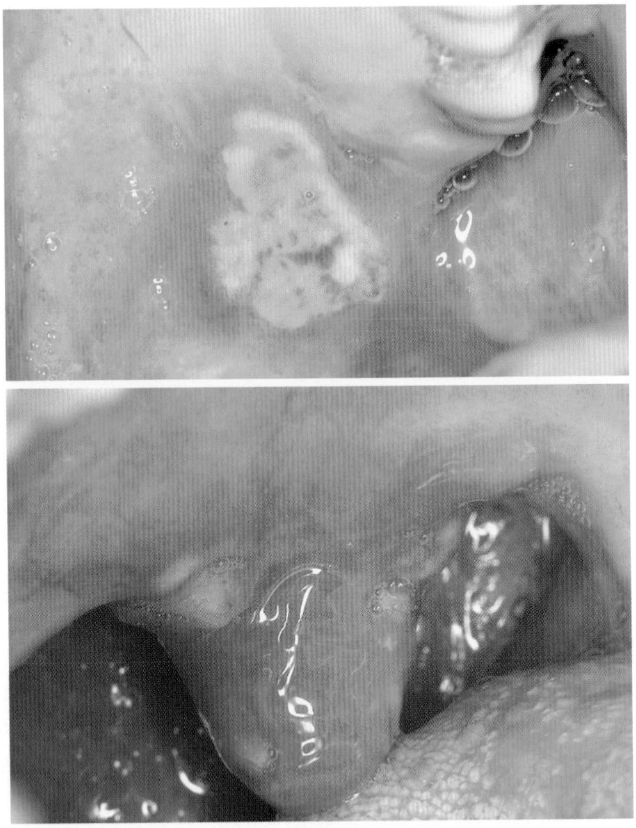

Figure 34-22 Intraoral aphthous stomatitis in AIDS patient. **A,** Major aphthous lesion in left soft palate. **B,** Same patient, ulcerations of uvula.

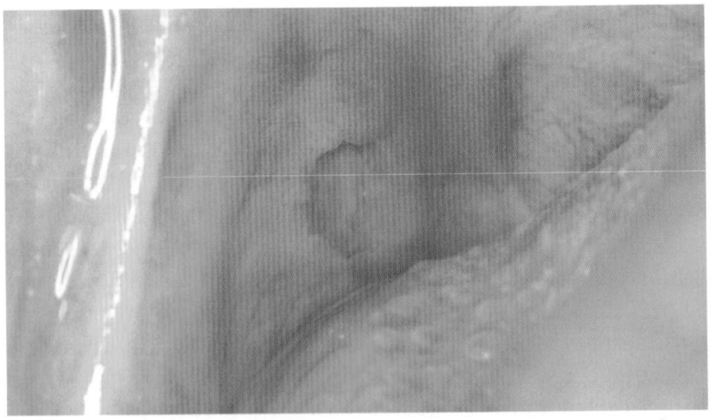

Figure 34-23 Solitary ulcer in soft palate. Culture confirmed presence of cytomegalovirus.

Occasionally, large aphthae in HIV-positive individuals may prove resistant to conventional topical therapy. In these patients, medical consultation is recommended, and administration of systemic corticosteroids (e.g., prednisone, 40-60 mg daily) or alternative therapy (e.g., thalidomide, levamisole, pentoxifylline) should be considered.[34,79,107,209] These agents may have significant side effects, however, and the clinician should remain alert for any evidence suggestive of an adverse drug reaction or interaction with currently prescribed medications.[50] Because virtually all antiviral agents used in treatment of HIV infection have the potential for adverse side effects or drug interactions, the dental clinician should consider topical therapy when appropriate.

DENTAL TREATMENT COMPLICATIONS

Concerns have been expressed regarding the potential for postoperative complications (hemorrhage, infection, delayed wound healing) in individuals with HIV/AIDS. Medically compromised patients must be carefully managed in the dental office to avoid undue treatment complications.[45] However, systematic reviews of the literature indicate that special precautions are not necessary based simply on the HIV status of patients when performing periodontal treatment procedures such as dental prophylaxis, scaling and root planing, periodontal surgery, extractions, and placement of implants. On occasion, however, the poor overall health status of an individual with AIDS may limit periodontal therapy to conservative, minimally invasive procedures, and antibiotic therapy may be required.[8,47,75,160]

Adverse Drug Effects

A number of adverse drug-induced effects have been reported in HIV-positive patients, and the dentist may be the first to recognize an oral drug reaction. Foscarnet, interferon, and 2′-3′-dideoxycytidine (DDC) occasionally induce oral ulcerations, and erythema multiforme has been reported with use of didanosine (DDI).[41] Zidovudine and ganciclovir may induce leukopenia, resulting in oral ulcers.[137] Xerostomia and altered taste sensation have been described in conjunction with diethyldithiocarbamate (Dithiocarb). HIV-positive patients are believed to be generally more susceptible to drug-induced mucositis and lichenoid drug reactions than the general population.[12,41,94,205] In some patients, mouth ulcers and mucositis resolve if drug therapy is continued beyond 2 to 3 weeks, but when drug effects are severe or persistent, alternative therapy with different drugs should be used.

HAART drugs may induce adverse side effects ranging from relatively mild conditions such as nausea to the development of kidney stones. Individuals with hepatitis C and HIV co-infection are susceptible to liver cirrhosis.[182] A newly identified adverse effect is *lipodystrophy*, a condition that features the redistribution of body fat. Affected individuals may develop gaunt facial features yet display excessive abdominal fat or even a fat pad on the rear of the shoulders (buffalo hump). This may be accompanied by severe systemic hyperlipidemia.[13,22,42,124] Other adverse effects of HAART include increased insulin resistance,[96] gynecomastia,[126] toxic epidermal necrolysis, blood dyscrasias,[204] and possibly increased incidence of oral warts.[23,83,173,185,230] Other reported oral or perioral adverse effects include oral lichenoid reactions, xerostomia, altered taste sensation, perioral paresthesia, and exfoliative cheilitis[19,20,25,153,204] (Figures 34-24 and 34-25).

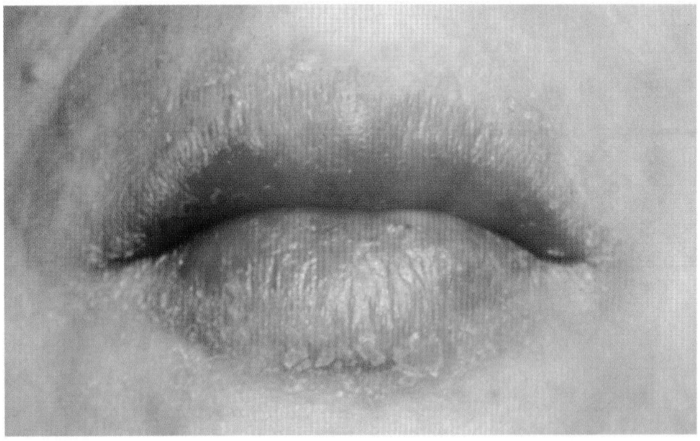

Figure 34-24 Exfoliative cheilitis associated with HAART therapy.

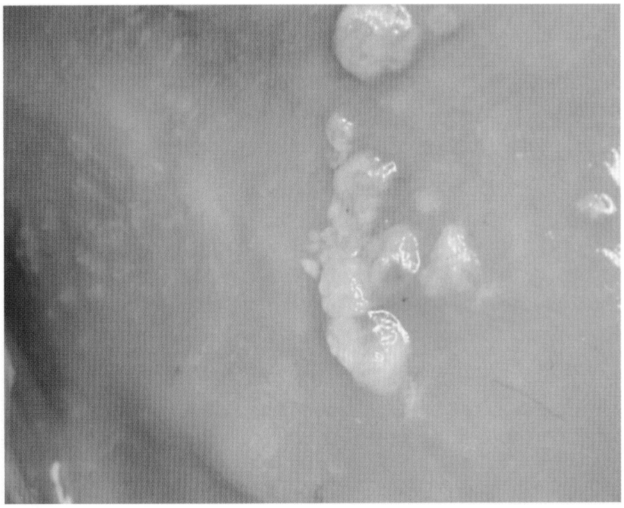

Figure 34-25 Condyloma acuminatum in left buccal mucosa in HIV-positive patient receiving HAART. Available evidence suggests that such human papillomavirus–induced lesions occur with increased frequency after initiation of multidrug therapy for AIDS.

GINGIVAL AND PERIODONTAL DISEASES

Considerable research has focused on the nature and incidence of periodontal diseases in HIV-infected individuals. Some studies suggest that chronic periodontitis is more common in this patient population, but others do not. Periodontal diseases are more common among HIV-infected users of injection drugs, but this may relate to poor oral hygiene and lack of dental care rather than decreased CD4 cell counts.[89,118,164] However, some unusual types of periodontal diseases do seem to occur with greater frequency in HIV-positive individuals.

Linear Gingival Erythema

A persistent, linear, easily bleeding, erythematous gingivitis has been described in some HIV-positive patients. Linear gingival erythema (LGE) may or may not serve as a precursor to rapidly progressive necrotizing ulcerative

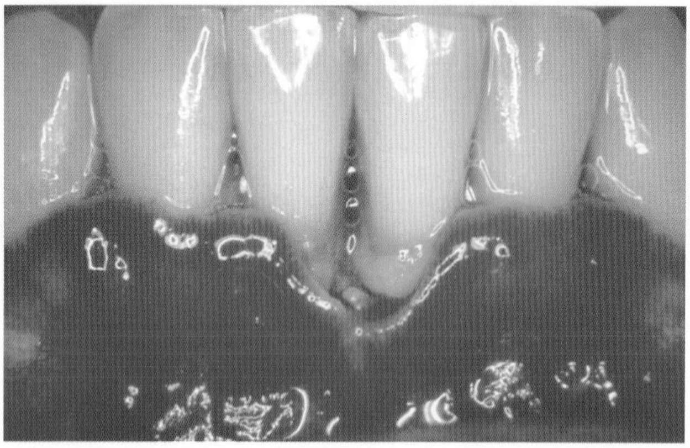

Figure 34-26 Linear gingival erythema (LGE) and necrotizing ulcerative gingivitis (NUG) in AIDS patient.

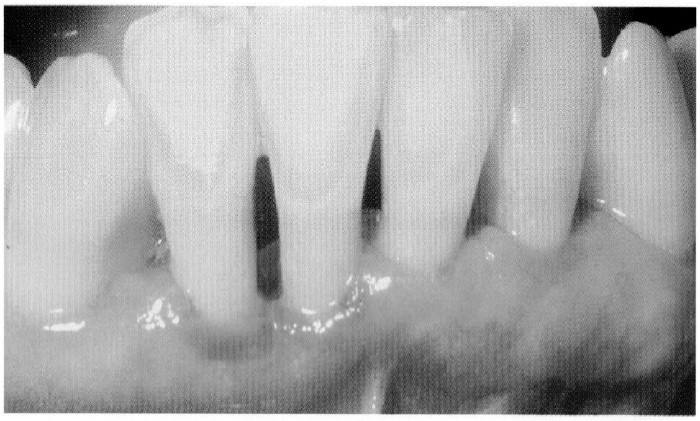

Figure 34-27 Mild LGE. Patient had a T4 count of 9 and a viral load too numerous to count.

periodontitis (NUP)[66,73,135] (Figures 34-26 and 34-27). The microflora of LGE may closely mimic that of periodontitis rather than gingivitis.[41] Linear gingivitis lesions may be localized or generalized in nature. The erythematous gingivitis (1) may be limited to marginal tissue, (2) may extend into attached gingiva in a punctate or a diffuse erythema, or (3) may extend into the alveolar mucosa.

LGE is sometimes unresponsive to corrective therapy, but such lesions may undergo spontaneous remission.[144] Concomitant oral candidiasis and LGE lesions have been identified, suggesting a possible etiologic role for candidial species in LGE.[118] In one study, direct microscopic cultures from LGE lesions implicated *Candida dubliniensis* in four patients, all of whom experienced complete or partial remission after systemic antifungal therapy.[226] It is not yet known whether candidial infections are etiologic in all LGE cases.[52] A recent systematic review indicates that LGE is more common among HIV-infected populations but that most individuals who are HIV positive do not experience LGE.[159]

LGE can often be adequately managed by following the therapeutic principles associated with marginal gingivitis. The affected sites should be scaled and polished. Subgingival irrigation with chlorhexidine or 10% povidone-iodine may be of benefit. The patient should be carefully instructed in performance of meticulous oral hygiene procedures. The condition should be reevaluated 2 to 3 weeks after initial therapy. If the patient is compliant with home care procedures and the lesions persist, the possibility of a candidial infection should be considered. It is doubtful that topical antifungal rinses will reach the base of the gingival crevices. Consequently, the treatment of choice may be the empiric administration of a systemic antifungal agent such as fluconazole for 7 to 10 days.[101]

It is important to remember that LGE may be refractory to treatment. If so, the patient should be carefully monitored for developing signs of more severe periodontal conditions (e.g., NUG, NUP, NUS). The patient should be placed on a 2- to 3-month recall maintenance interval and re-treated as necessary. As mentioned, despite the occasional resistance of LGE to conventional periodontal therapy, spontaneous remission may occur for reasons that are not yet known.

Necrotizing Ulcerative Gingivitis

Some reports have described an increased incidence of necrotizing ulcerative gingivitis (NUG) among HIV-infected individuals, although this has not been substantiated by other studies.[49,77,103,192,216]

There is no consensus on whether the incidence of NUG increases in HIV-positive patients.[159,183] Treatment of NUG condition in these patients does not differ from that in HIV-negative individuals (see Chapter 47). The affected gingiva may be exquisitely painful, and caution must be taken to avoid undue patient discomfort.

Basic treatment may consist of cleaning and debridement of affected areas with a cotton pellet soaked in peroxide after application of a topical anesthetic. Escharotic oral rinses such as hydrogen peroxide should only rarely be used, however, for any patient and are especially contraindicated in immunocompromised individuals. The patient should be seen daily or every other day for the first week; debridement of affected areas is repeated at each visit, and plaque control methods are gradually introduced. A meticulous plaque control program should be taught and started as soon as the sensitivity of the area allows it. After initial healing has occurred, the patient should be able to tolerate scaling and root planing if needed.

The patient should avoid tobacco, alcohol, and condiments. An antimicrobial oral rinse such as chlorhexidine gluconate 0.12% is prescribed.

Systemic antibiotics such as metronidazole or amoxicillin may be prescribed for patients with moderate to severe tissue destruction, localized lymphadenopathy or systemic symptoms, or both. The use of prophylactic antifungal medication should be considered if antibiotics are prescribed.

The periodontium should be reevaluated 1 month after resolution of acute symptoms to assess the results of treatment and determine if further therapy will be necessary.

Necrotizing Ulcerative Periodontitis

A necrotizing, ulcerative, rapidly progressive form of periodontitis occurs more frequently among HIV-positive individuals, although such lesions were described long before the onset of the AIDS epidemic. Necrotizing ulcerative periodontitis (NUP) may represent an extension of NUG in which bone loss and periodontal attachment loss occur.[103,154,206]

NUP is characterized by soft tissue necrosis, rapid periodontal destruction, and interproximal bone loss[73,171] (Figures 34-28, 34-29, and 34-30). Lesions may occur anywhere in the dental arches and are usually localized to a few teeth, although generalized NUP is sometimes present after marked CD4+ cell depletion. Bone is often exposed, resulting in necrosis and subsequent sequestration. NUP is severely painful at onset, and immediate treatment is necessary. Occasionally, however, patients undergo spontaneous resolution of the necrotizing lesions, leaving painless, deep interproximal craters that are difficult to clean and that may lead to conventional periodontitis.[73]

Some evidence suggests slight differences between the microbial flora found in NUP lesions and that found in chronic periodontitis,[142] but most data implicate a similar microbial component in both diseases.[77,145,146,189] An increasing number of studies, however, have identified the presence of candidal organisms and human herpesviruses of various types in individuals with necrotizing ulcerative periodontal diseases. The exact role for these organisms is not yet fully understood.[39,214] As discussed earlier, the reported periodontal health of HIV-infected individuals is subject to wide variations.[187,237] Riley et al.[187] examined 200 HIV-positive patients and found that 85 were periodontally healthy; none had NUG; 59 had gingivitis; 54 were experiencing mild, moderate, or advanced periodontitis; and only two had NUP. Glick et al.[77] reported the prevalence of NUP as 6.3% in an HIV-positive population and described a positive correlation with the presence of NUP and outright AIDS.[76]

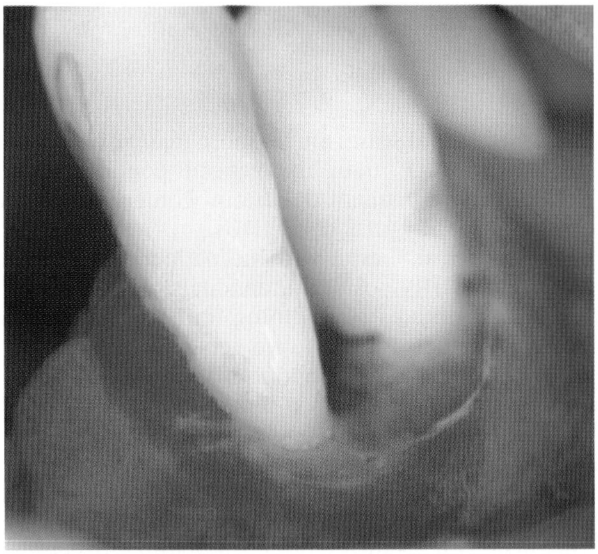

Figure 34-28 Necrotizing ulcerative periodontitis (NUP). Note adjacent LGE.

Therapy for NUP includes local debridement, scaling and root planing, in-office irrigation with an effective antimicrobial agent such as chlorhexidine gluconate or povidone-iodine (Betadine), and establishment of meticulous oral hygiene, including home use of antimicrobial rinses or irrigation.[159,170,193]

This therapeutic approach is based on reports involving only a small number of patients.[78] In severe NUP, antibiotic therapy may be necessary but should be used with caution in HIV-infected patients to avoid an opportunistic and potentially serious, localized candidiasis or even candidal septicemia.[171] If an antibiotic is necessary, metronidazole (250 mg, with two tablets taken immediately and then one tablet four times daily for 5-7 days) is the drug of choice. Prophylactic prescription of a topical or systemic antifungal agent is prudent if an antibiotic is used.

Necrotizing Ulcerative Stomatitis

Necrotizing ulcerative stomatitis (NUS) has occasionally been reported in HIV-positive patients. NUS may be severely destructive and acutely painful and may affect significant areas of oral soft tissue and underlying bone. It may occur separately or as an extension of NUP[103,170] and is often associated with severe suppression of CD4 immune cells. The condition appears to be identical to cancrum oris *(noma)*, a rare destructive process reported in nutritionally deprived individuals, especially in Africa. NUS may be associated with severe immunodeficiency regardless of the cause of onset.[7,15,188]

Treatment for NUS may include an antibiotic such as metronidazole and use of an antimicrobial mouth rinse

A

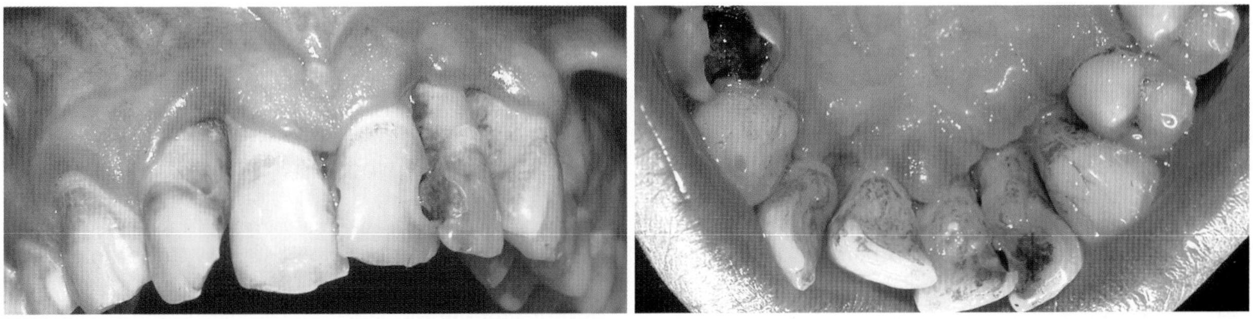

B

Figure 34-29 NUP in otherwise healthy 19-year-old male patient who was HIV negative. **A,** Anterior maxilla. **B,** Palatal view.

A B C D
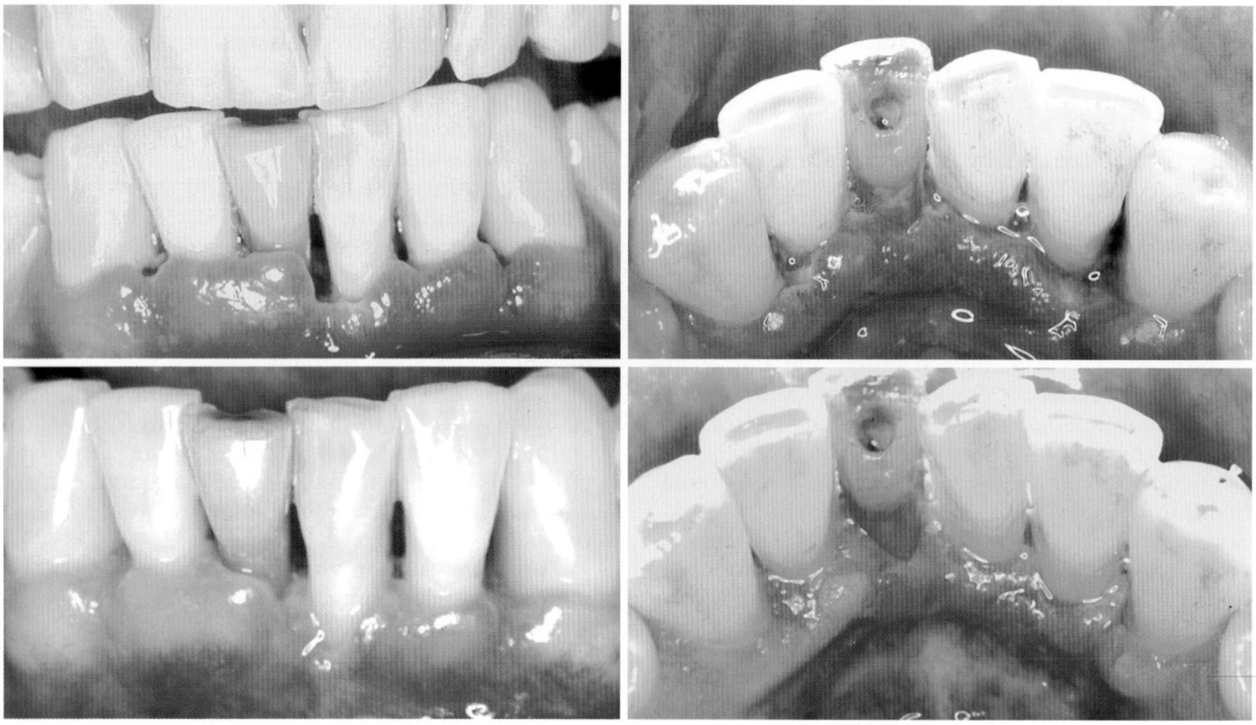

Figure 34-30 Early NUP in patient with AIDS. **A,** Facial view. **B,** Lingual view. **C,** Complete resolution of NUP after treatment, facial view. **D,** Lingual view.

such as chlorhexidine gluconate. If osseous necrosis is present, it is often necessary to remove the affected bone to promote wound healing[223] (Figure 34-31).

Chronic Periodontitis

A number of longitudinal or prevalence studies have suggested that HIV-positive individuals are more likely to experience chronic periodontitis than the general population.* Most studies, however, do not take into account the level of oral hygiene or the degree of immunodeficiency in the population studied or whether the individuals in the study are injection drug users (IDUs); these confounding factors cloud the issue. Lamster et al.[118] compared frequency of oral lesions and periodontal diseases between HIV-positive and HIV-negative individuals, some of whom were IDUs. They concluded that the lifestyle of IDUs may play a larger role in oral disease than the individual's HIV status. They also found that tongue lesions consistent with hairy leukoplakia were most common among seropositive homosexual males, whereas oral candidiasis and LGE were most common among IDUs.

Others have reported that the incidence and severity of chronic periodontitis are similar in HIV-positive and HIV-negative groups.[135,136,191,193] Klein et al.[114] evaluated 181 heterosexuals with AIDS and found a larger percentage of women (91%) than men (73%) with gingivitis or periodontitis. Overall, most heterosexuals with AIDS had only gingivitis (70%), whereas others had moderate (27%) to severe periodontitis (27%). This study suggests that periodontal diseases are no more frequent in heterosexuals with AIDS than the general population. The finding of more frequent disease in women may reflect more women with AIDS being IDUs.

Drinkard et al.[49] evaluated the periodontal status of asymptomatic HIV-positive individuals and those with signs and symptoms of declining immune status. They reported that both groups were generally in good periodontal health, with no significant differences between groups. Others have described similar findings.[185,191,193,196]

A well-controlled study indicated that gingival recession and early attachment loss are more common in HIV groups than matched groups from the general population.[190] This appears to affirm that immunocompromised individuals are slightly more susceptible to chronic periodontitis than those with a robust immune system. The majority of HIV-positive individuals experience gingivitis and chronic periodontitis in a manner similar to the general population. With proper home care and appropriate periodontal treatment and maintenance, HIV-positive individuals can anticipate reasonably good periodontal health throughout the course of their disease. The median period between initial HIV infection and outright AIDS is approximately 15 years, and the life expectancy of persons living with AIDS has been significantly prolonged with current anti-HIV drug therapy.[31] This indicates that HIV-infected patients are potential candidates for conventional periodontal treatment procedures to include periodontal surgery and implant placement. *Treatment decisions should be based on the overall health status of the patient, the degree of periodontal involvement, and the motivation and ability of the patient to perform effective oral hygiene* (Figure 34-32).

*References 10, 54, 80, 133, 136, 147.

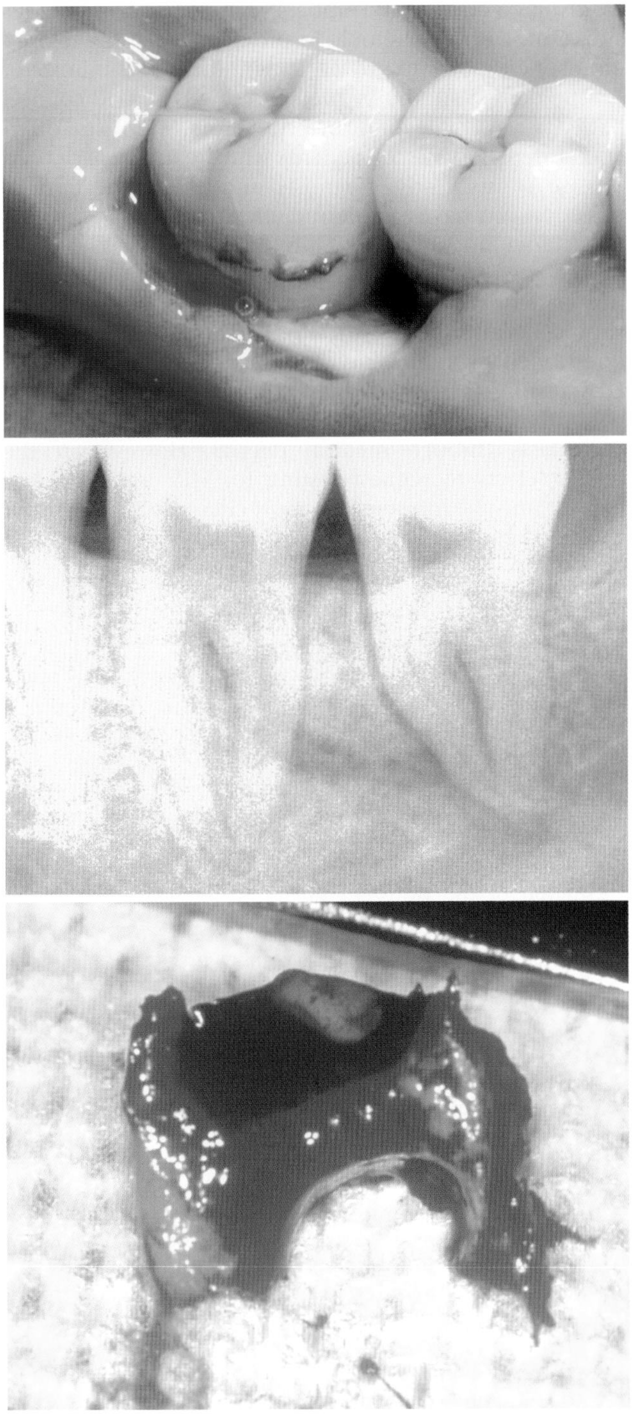

Figure 34-31 **A,** Necrotizing ulcerative stomatitis (NUS) in left mandibular molar area. **B,** Radiographic view. Note large osseous sequestrum. **C,** Osseous sequestrum removed.

Clearly, some less common periodontal diseases do occur more frequently in HIV-positive individuals, but these same conditions are also reported among HIV-negative persons. Consequently, definitions for these conditions and discussion of their management should not be construed as limiting them to individuals with HIV or AIDS.

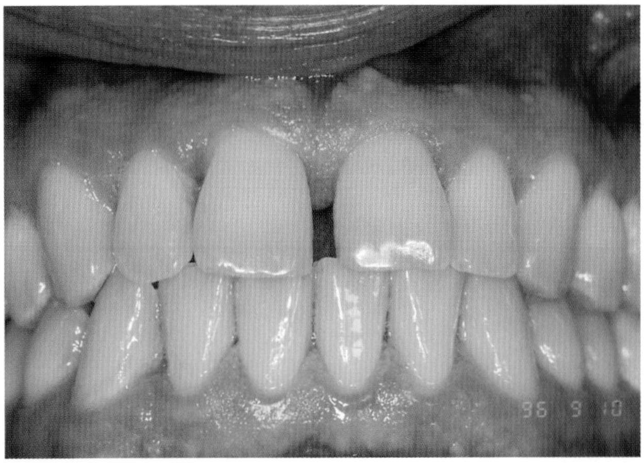

Figure 34-32 Periodontal health in an individual with advanced AIDS.

PERIODONTAL TREATMENT PROTOCOL

It is imperative that medically compromised patients, including those with HIV or AIDS, be safely and effectively managed in dental practice. Several universal treatment considerations are important to ensure that this is achieved.

Health Status

The patient's health status should be determined from the health history, physical evaluation, and consultation with the patient's physician. Treatment decisions will vary depending on the patient's state of health. For example, delayed wound healing and increased risk of postoperative infection are possible complicating factors in AIDS patients, but neither concern should significantly alter treatment planning in an otherwise healthy, asymptomatic, HIV-infected patient with a normal or near-normal CD4 count and a low viral bioload.[92,127,175] It is important to obtain information regarding the patient's immune status with questions such as the following:

- What is the CD4+ T4 lymphocyte level?
- What is the current viral load?
- How do current CD4+ T4 cell and viral load counts differ from previous evaluations? How often are such tests performed?
- How long ago was the HIV infection identified? Is it possible to identify the approximate date of original exposure?
- Is there a history of drug abuse, sexually transmitted diseases, multiple infections, or other factors that might alter immune response? For example, does the patient have a history of chronic hepatitis B, hepatitis C, neutropenia, thrombocytopenia, nutritional deficiency, or adrenocorticoid insufficiency?
- What medications is the patient taking?
- Does the patient describe or present with possible adverse side effects from medications?

Infection Control Measures

Clinical management of HIV-infected periodontal patients requires strict adherence to established methods of infection control, based on guidance from the American Dental Association (ADA) and the CDC.[30] Compliance, especially with universal precautions, will eliminate or minimize risks to patients and the dental staff.[125,155] Immunocompromised patients are potentially at risk for acquiring as well as transmitting infections in the dental office or other health care facility.[122,141,227]

Goals of Therapy

A thorough oral examination will determine the patient's dental treatment needs. The primary goals of dental therapy should be the restoration and maintenance of oral health, comfort, and function. At the very least, periodontal treatment goals should be directed toward control of HIV-associated mucosal diseases, such as chronic candidiasis and recurrent oral ulcerations. Acute periodontal and dental infections should be managed, and the patient should receive detailed instructions in performance of effective oral hygiene procedures.[215] Conservative, nonsurgical periodontal therapy should be a treatment option for virtually all HIV-positive patients, and performance of elective surgical periodontal procedures, including implant placement, has been reported.[71,135,193] NUP or NUS can be severely destructive to periodontal structures, but a history of these conditions does not automatically dictate extraction of involved teeth unless the patient is unable to maintain effective oral hygiene in affected areas. Decisions regarding elective periodontal procedures should be made with the informed consent of the patient and after medical consultation, when possible.

Maintenance Therapy

It is imperative that the patient maintain meticulous personal oral hygiene. In addition, periodontal maintenance recall visits should be conducted at short intervals (2-3 months) and any progressive periodontal disease treated vigorously. As mentioned earlier, however, systemic antibiotic therapy should be administered with caution. Blood and other medical laboratory tests may be required to monitor the patient's overall health status, and close consultation and coordination with the patient's physician are necessary.

Psychologic Factors

HIV infection of neuronal cells may affect brain function and lead to outright dementia. This may profoundly influence the responsiveness of affected patients to dental treatment. However, psychologic factors are numerous in virtually all HIV-infected patients, even in the absence of neuronal lesions. Patients may be greatly concerned with maintenance of medical confidentiality, and such confidentiality must be upheld. Coping with a life-threatening disease may elicit depression, anxiety, and anger in such patients, and this anger may be directed toward the dentist and the staff. It is important to display concern and understanding for the patient's situation. Treatment should be provided in a calm, relaxed atmosphere, and stress to the patient must be minimized.[3]

The dentist should be prepared to advise and counsel patients on their oral health status. Dentists often encounter HIV-infected patients who are unaware of their disease status. Early diagnosis and treatment of HIV infection can have a profound effect on the patient's life expectancy and quality of life, and the dentist should be prepared to assist the patient in obtaining testing.[199] Any patient with oral lesions suggestive of HIV infection should be informed of the findings and, if appropriate, questioned regarding any previous exposure to HIV. If HIV testing is requested, it must be accompanied by patient counseling; therefore, it might be best to obtain such tests through medical referral. However, if the dentist elects to request testing for HIV antibody, the patient must be informed. In most circumstances, written informed consent is desirable before testing.

REFERENCES

1. Aly R, Berger T: Common superficial fungal infections in patients with AIDS, *Clin Infect Dis* 22(suppl 2):S128, 1996.
2. Aquilina C, Viraben R, Denis P: Secondary syphilis simulating oral hairy leukoplakia, *J Am Acad Dermatol* 49:749, 2003.
3. Asher RS, McDowell JD, Winquist H: HIV-related neuropsychiatric changes: concerns for dental professionals, *J Am Dent Assoc* 124:80, 1993.
4. Bach MC, Howell DA, Valenti AJ, et al: Aphthous ulceration of the gastrointestinal tract in patients with the acquired immunodeficiency syndrome (AIDS), *Ann Intern Med* 112:465, 1990.
5. Bach MC, Valenti AJ, Howell DA, et al: Odynophagia from aphthous ulcers of the pharynx and oesophagus in the acquired immunodeficiency syndrome (AIDS), *Ann Intern Med* 108:338, 1988.
6. Baily GG, Moore CB, Essayag SM, et al: *Candida inconspicua,* a fluconazole-resistant pathogen in patients infected with human immunodeficiency virus, *Clin Infect Dis* 25:161, 1997.
7. Barasch A, Gordon S, Geist RY, Geist JR: Necrotizing stomatitis: report of 3 *Pseudomonas aeruginosa*–positive patients, *Oral Surg Oral Med Oral Pathol Oral Radiol Endod* 96:136, 2003.
8. Baron M, Gritsch F, Hansy AM, Haas R: Implants in an HIV-positive patient: a case report, *Int J Oral Maxillofac Implants* 19:425, 2004.
9. Baron P, Bremer J, Wasserman SS, et al: Detection and quantitation of human immunodeficiency virus type 1 in the female genital tract. The Division of AIDS Treatment Research Initiative 009 Study Group, *J Clin Microbiol* 38:3822, 2000.
10. Barr C, Lopez MR, Rua-Dobles A: Periodontal changes by HIV serostatus in a cohort of homosexual and bisexual men, *J Clin Periodontol* 19:794, 1992.
11. Barrett AP, Bilous AM, Buckley DJ, et al: Clinicopathological presentations of oral Kaposi's sarcoma in AIDS, *Aust Dent J* 33:395, 1988.
12. Bayard PJ, Berger TG, Jacobson MA: Drug hypersensitivity reactions and human immunodeficiency virus disease, *J Acquir Immune Defic Syndr* 5:1237, 1992.
13. Behrens GM, Stoll M, Schmidt RE: Lipodystrophy syndrome in HIV infection: what is it, what causes it and how can it be managed? *Drug Saf* 23:57, 2000.

14. Bendick C, Scheifele C, Reichart PA: Oral manifestations in 101 Cambodians with HIV and AIDS, *J Oral Pathol Med* 31:1, 2002.
15. Berthold P: Noma: a forgotten disease, *Dent Clin North Am* 47:559, 2003.
16. Birnbaum W, Hodgson TA, Reichart PA, et al: Prognostic significance of HIV-associated oral lesions and their relation to therapy, *Oral Dis* 8(suppl 2):110, 2002.
17. Blankson JN, Persaud D, Siliciano RF: The challenge of viral reservoirs in HIV-1 infection, *Annu Rev Med* 53:557, 2002.
18. Buve A, Rogers MF: Epidemiology, *AIDS* 12(suppl A):S53, 1998.
19. Calista D, Boschini A: Cutaneous side effects induced by indinavir, *Eur J Dermatol* 10:292, 2000.
20. Calista D, Morri M, Stagno A, Boshini A: Changing morbidity of cutaneous diseases in patients with HIV after introduction of highly active antiretroviral therapy including a protease inhibitor, *Am J Clin Dermatol* 3:59, 2002.
21. Campo-Trapero J, Cano-Sanchez J, del Romero-Guerrero J, et al: Dental management of patients with human immunodeficiency virus, *Quintessence Int* 34:515, 2003.
22. Carr A, Cooper DA: Adverse effects of antiretroviral therapy, *Lancet* 356:1423, 2000.
23. Carr A, Samaras K, Thorisdottir A, et al: Diagnosis, prediction, and natural course of HIV-1 protease-inhibitor–associated lipodystrophy, hyperlipidaemia, and diabetes mellitus: a cohort study, *Lancet* 353:2093, 1999.
24. Casado JL, Quereda C, Oliva J, et al: Candidal meningitis in HIV-infected patients: analysis of 14 cases, *Clin Infect Dis* 25:673, 1997.
25. Casariego Z, Pombo T, Perez H, Patterson P: Eruptive cheilitis: a new adverse effect in reactive HIV-positive patients subjected to high activity antiretroviral therapy (HAART)—presentation of six clinical cases, *Med Oral* 6:19, 2001.
26. Ceballos-Salobrena A, Gaitain-Cepeda LA, Ceballos-Garcia L, Lezama-Del Valle D: Oral lesions in HIV/AIDS patients undergoing highly active antiretroviral treatment including protease inhibitors: a new face of oral AIDS? *AIDS Patient Care STDS* 14:627, 2000.
27. Ceballos-Salobrena A, Gaitain-Cepeda L, Ceballos-Garcia L, Samaranayake LP: The effect of antiretroviral therapy on the prevalence of HIV-associated oral candidiasis in a Spanish cohort, *Oral Surg Oral Med Oral Pathol Oral Radiol Endod* 97:345, 2004.
28. Centers for Disease Control and Prevention: Update on AIDS—United States, *MMWR* 31:507, 1982.
29. Centers for Disease Control and Prevention: 1993 revised classification system for HIV infection and expanded surveillance case definition for AIDS among adolescents and adults, *MMWR* 41:RR-17, 1993.
30. Centers for Disease Control and Prevention: Guidelines for infection control in dental health care settings—2003, *MMWR* 52(RR-17):1, 2003.
31. Centers for Disease Control and Prevention–NCHSTP-DHAP: *HIV/AIDS surveillance report.* Addendum: cases of HIV infection and AIDS in the United States, 2002, Atlanta, 2003, CDC.
32. Chachoua A, Krigel R, Lafleur F, et al: Prognostic factors and staging classification of Kaposi's sarcoma, *J Clin Oncol* 7:774, 1989.
33. Challacombe SJ, Sweet SP: Salivary and mucosal immune responses to HIV and its co-pathogens, *Oral Dis* 3(suppl 1): S79, 1997.
34. Chandrasekhar J, Liem AA, Cox NH, et al: Oxpentifylline in the management of recurrent aphthous oral ulcers, *Oral Surg Oral Med Oral Pathol Oral Radiol Endod* 87:564, 1999.
35. Cheuk W, Wong KO, Wong CS, et al: Immunostaining for human herpesvirus 8 latent nuclear antigen 1 helps distinguish Kaposi sarcoma from its mimickers, *Am J Clin Pathol* 121:335, 2004.
36. Chiasson MA, Stoneburner RL, Joseph SC: Human immunodeficiency virus transmission through artificial insemination, *J Acquir Immune Defic Syndr* 3:69, 1990.
37. Chun T-W, Carruth L, Finzi D, et al: Quantification of latent tissue reservoirs and total body viral load in HIV-1 infection, *Nature* 387:183, 1997.
38. Clerici M, Piconi S, Balotta C, et al: Pentoxifylline improves cell-mediated immunity and reduces human immunodeficiency virus (HIV) plasma viremia in asymptomatic HIV-seropositive persons, *J Infect Dis* 175:1210, 1997.
39. Cobb CM, Ferguson BL, Keselyak NT, et al: A TEM/SEM study of the microbial plaque overlying the necrotic gingival papillae of HIV-seropositive, necrotizing ulcerative periodontitis, *J Periodontal Res* 38:147, 2003.
40. Conant MA, Opp KM, Paretz D, et al: Reduction on Kaposi's sarcoma lesions following treatment of AIDS with ritonavir, *AIDS* 11:1300, 1997.
41. Coopman SA, Stern RS: Cutaneous drug reactions in human immunodeficiency virus infection, *Arch Dermatol* 127:714, 1991.
42. Cossarizza A, Mussini C, Vigano A: Mitochondria in the pathogenesis of lipodystrophy induced by anti-HIV antiretroviral drugs: actors or bystanders? *Bioessays* 23:1070, 2001.
43. Desai N, Mathur M: Selective transmission of multidrug resistant HIV to a newborn related to poor maternal adherence, *Sex Transm Infect* 79:419, 2003.
44. Diz Dios P, Hermida AO, Alvarez CM, et al: Fluconazole-resistant oral candidosis in HIV-infected patients, *AIDS* 9:809, 1995.
45. Diz Dios P, Fernandez Feijoo J, Vazquez Garcia E: Tooth extraction in HIV sero-positive patients, *Int Dent J* 49:317, 1999.
46. Diz Dios P, Ocampo A, Miralles C, et al: Frequency of oropharyngeal candidiasis in HIV-infected patients on protease inhibitor therapy, *Oral Surg Oral Med Oral Pathol Oral Radiol Endod* 87:437, 1999.
47. Dodson TB: HIV status and the risk of post-extraction complications, *J Dent Res* 76:1644, 1997.
48. Domingo P, Ris J, Lopez-Conteras J: Esophageal ulcers in AIDS, *Ann Intern Med* 124:928, 1996.
49. Drinkard CR, Decher L, Little JW, et al: Periodontal status of individuals in early stages of human immunodeficiency virus infection, *Commun Dent Oral Epidemiol* 19:281, 1991.
50. EC-Clearinghouse on Oral Problems Related to HIV Infection, WHO Collaborating Centre on Oral Manifestations of the Immunodeficiency Virus: Classification and diagnostic criteria for oral lesions in HIV infection, *J Oral Pathol Med* 22:289, 1993.
51. Elish D, Singh F, Weinberg JM: Therapeutic options for herpes labialis. I. Oral agents, *Cutis* 74:31, 2004.
52. Epstein JB: Antifungal therapy in oropharyngeal mycotic infections, *Oral Surg Oral Med Oral Pathol* 69:32, 1990.
53. Epstein JB, Scully C: HIV infection: clinical features and treatment of 33 homosexual men with Kaposi's sarcoma, *Oral Med Oral Surg Oral Pathol* 71:38, 1991.
54. Epstein JB, Leziy S, Ransier A: Periodontal pocketing in HIV-associated periodontitis, *Spec Care Dent* 13:236, 1993.
55. Epstein JB, Lozada-Nur F, McLeod A, et al: Oral Kaposi's sarcoma in acquired immunodeficiency syndrome: review of management and report of the efficacy of intralesional vinblastine, *Cancer* 64:2424, 1989.
56. Eversole LR: Viral infections of the head and neck among HIV-seropositive patients, *Oral Surg Oral Med Oral Pathol* 73:155, 1992.

57. Eversole LR, Jacobsen P, Stone CE, et al: Oral condyloma planus (hairy leukoplakia) among homosexual men: a clinico-pathologic study of thirty-six cases, *Oral Surg* 61:249, 1986.
58. Eyeson JD, Tenant-Flowers M, Cooper DJ, et al: Oral manifestations of an HIV-positive cohort in the era of highly active anti-retroviral therapy (HAART) in South London, *J Oral Pathol Med* 31:169, 2002.
59. Fauci AS, Schnittman SM, Poli G, et al: Immunopathogenic mechanisms in human immunodeficiency virus (HIV) infection, *Ann Intern Med* 114:678, 1993.
60. Fetter A, Partisani M, Koenig H, et al: Asymptomatic oral *Candida albicans* carriage in HIV-infection: frequency and predisposing factors, *J Oral Pathol Med* 22:57, 1993.
61. Ficarra G, Berson AM, Silverman S Jr, et al: Kaposi's sarcoma of the oral cavity: a study of 134 patients with a review of the pathogenesis, epidemiology, clinical aspects and treatment, *Oral Surg Oral Med Oral Pathol* 66:543, 1988.
62. Finzi D, Blankson J, Siliciano JD, et al: Latent infection of CD+4 T cells provides a mechanism for lifelong persistence of HIV-1, even in patients on effective combination therapy, *Nature Med* 5:512, 1999.
63. Fleming PL, Ward JW, Karon JM, et al: Declines in AIDS incidence and deaths in the USA: a signal change in the epidemic, *AIDS* 12(suppl A):S55, 1998.
64. Freda PU, Bilezikian JP: The hypothalamus-pituitary-adrenal axis in HIV disease, *AIDS Read* 9:43, 1999.
65. Gaines H, Von Sydow M, Pehrson PO, et al: Clinical picture of primary HIV infection presenting as a glandular-fever-like illness, *Br Med J* 97:1363, 1988.
66. Gandhi M, Koelle DM, Ameli N, et al: Prevalence of human herpesvirus-8 salivary shedding in HIV increases with CD4 count, *J Dent Res* 83:639, 2004.
67. Gazouli M, Papaconstantinou I, Zavos G, et al: Human herpvirus type 8 genotypes in iatrogenic, classic and AIDS-associated Kaposi's sarcoma from Greece, *Anticancer Res* 24:1597, 2004.
68. Ghidoni JJ: Role of *Bartonella henselae* endocarditis in the nucleation of aortic valvular calcification, *Ann Thorac Surg* 77:704, 2004.
69. Girardi E: Epidemiological aspects of transmitted HIV drug resistance, *Scand J Infect Dis Suppl* 35(106):17, 2003.
70. Giuliana G, Pizzo G, Milici ME, et al: In vitro activities of antimicrobial agents against *Candida* species, *Oral Surg Oral Med Oral Pathol Oral Radiol Endod* 87:44, 1999.
71. Glick M: Clinical protocol for treating patients with HIV disease, *Gen Dent* 38:418, 1990.
72. Glick M, Cleveland DB: Oral mucosal bacillary epithelioid angiomatosis in a patient with AIDS associated with rapid alveolar bone loss: a case report, *J Oral Pathol Med* 22:235, 1993.
73. Glick M, Holmstrup P: HIV infection and periodontal diseases. In Genco R, Mealey B, Rose L, editors: *Periodontal medicine,* Hamilton, Canada, 2000, BC Decker.
74. Glick M, Muzyka BC: Alternative therapies for major aphthous ulcers in AIDS patients, *J Am Dent Assoc* 123:61, 1992.
75. Glick M, Abel SN, Muzyka BC, Delorenzo M: Dental complications after treating patients with AIDS, *J Am Dent Assoc* 125:296, 1994.
76. Glick M, Muzyka BC, Lurie D, et al: Oral manifestations associated with HIV disease as markers for immune suppression and AIDS, *Oral Surg Oral Med Oral Pathol* 77:344, 1994.
77. Glick M, Muzyka BC, Salkin LM, et al: Necrotizing ulcerative periodontitis: a marker for immune deterioration and a predictor for the diagnosis of AIDS, *J Periodontol* 65:393, 1994.
78. Gompels UA, Kasolo FC: HHV-8 serology and Kaposi's sarcoma, *Lancet* 348:1587, 1996.
79. Gorin I, Vilette B, Gehanno P, et al: Thalidomide in hyperalgic pharyngeal ulceration of AIDS, *Lancet* 335:1343, 1990.
80. Gornitsky M, Clark DC, Siboo R, et al: Clinical documentation and occurrence of putative periodontopathic bacteria in human immunodeficiency virus–associated periodontal disease, *J Periodontol* 62:576, 1991.
81. Green TS, Beckstead JH, Lozada-Nur F, et al: Histo pathologic spectrum of oral Kaposi's sarcoma, *Oral Surg* 58:306, 1984.
82. Greenblatt RM, Jacobson LP, Levine AM, et al: Human herpesvirus 8 infection and Kaposi's sarcoma among human immunodeficiency virus–infected and –uninfected women, *J Infect Dis* 183:1130, 2001.
83. Greenspan D, Canchola AJ, MacPhail LA, et al: Effect of highly active antiretroviral therapy on frequency of oral warts, *Lancet* 357:1411, 2001.
84. Greenspan D, Conant M, Silverman S Jr, et al: Oral hairy leukoplakia in male homosexuals: evidence of association with both papilloma virus and a herpes-group virus, *Lancet* 2:831, 1984.
85. Greenspan D, Greenspan JS, de Souza Y, et al: Oral hairy leukoplakia in an HIV-negative renal transplant recipient, *J Oral Pathol Med* 18:32, 1989.
86. Greenspan D, Greenspan JS, Hearst NG, et al: Relations of oral hairy leukoplakia with HIV and the risk of developing AIDS, *J Infect Dis* 155:475, 1987.
87. Greenspan JS, Greenspan D, Lennette ET, et al: Replication of Epstein-Barr virus within the epithelial cells of oral hairy leukoplakia, and AIDS associated lesion, *N Engl J Med* 313:1564, 1985.
88. Greenspan D, Pindborg JJ, Greenspan JS, et al: *AIDS and the mouth,* Copenhagen, 1990, Munksgaard.
89. Guarinos J, Bagan JV, Martinez-Canut P: Dental health in patients infected by human immunodeficiency virus (HIV): a study of 94 cases, *Bull Group Int Rech Sci Stomatol Odontol* 39:119, 1996.
90. Gupta G: Viral pathogenesis and opportunistic infections, *CDA J* 21:29, 1993.
91. Haase AT, Schacker TW: Potential for the transmission of HIV-1 despite highly active antiretroviral therapy, *N Engl J Med* 17:339:1846, 1998.
92. Hammer SM: Advances in antiretroviral therapy and viral load monitoring, *AIDS* 10(suppl 3):S1, 1996.
93. Handforth J, Sharland M: Triple nucleoside reverse transcriptase inhibitor therapy in children, *Paediatr Drugs* 6:147, 2004.
94. Harb GE, Alldredge BK, Coleman R, et al: Pharmacoepidemiology of adverse drug reactions in hospitalized patients with human immunodeficiency virus disease, *J Acquir Immune Defic Syndr* 6:919, 1993.
95. Hardy GA, Imami N, Gotch FM: Improving HIV-specific immune responses in HIV-infected patients, *J HIV Ther* 7:40, 2002.
96. Hardy H, Esch LD, Morse GD: Glucose disorders associated with HIV and its drug therapy, *Ann Pharmacother* 35:343, 2001.
97. Hauman CH, Thompson IO, Theunissen F, Wolfaardt P: Oral carriage of *Candida* in healthy and HIV-seropositive persons, *Oral Surg Oral Med Oral Pathol* 76:570, 1993.
98. Hicks JM: Assessing survival in HIV-seropositive individuals with extremely low CD4 counts, *DAAC Forum,* March 1997, p 10.
99. Ho DD, Neumann AU, Perelson AS, et al: Rapid turnover of plasma virions and CD4 lymphocytes in HIV-1 infection, *Nature* 373:123, 1995.

100. Hodgson TA, Rachanis CC: Oral fungal and bacterial infections in HIV-infected individuals: an overview in Africa, *Oral Dis* 8(suppl 2):80, 2002.
101. Hofer D, Hammerle CH, Grassi M, Lang NP: Long-term results of supportive periodontal therapy (SPT) in HIV-seropositive and HIV-seronegative patients, *J Clin Periodontol* 29:630, 2002.
102. Hood SV, Hollis S, Percy M, et al: Assessment of therapeutic response of oropharyngeal and esophageal candidiasis in AIDS with use of a new clinical scoring system: studies with D0870, *Clin Infect Dis* 28:587, 1999.
103. Horning GM, Cohen ME: Necrotizing ulcerative gingivitis, periodontitis and stomatitis: clinical staging and predisposing factors, *J Periodontol* 66:990, 1995.
104. Imagawa DT, Lee MH, Wolinsky SM, et al: Human immunodeficiency virus type 1 infection in homosexual men who remain seronegative for prolonged periods, *N Engl J Med* 320:1458, 1989.
105. Imam N, Carpenter CC, Mayer KH, et al: Hierarchical pattern of mucosal *Candida* infections in HIV-seropositive women, *Am J Med* 89:142, 1990.
106. Ippolito G, Puro V, Heptonstall J, et al: Occupational human immunodeficiency virus infection in health care workers: worldwide cases through September 1997, *Clin Infect Dis* 28:365, 1999.
107. Jacobson JM, Greenspan JS, Spritzler J, et al: Thalidomide for the treatment of oral aphthous ulcers in patients with human immunodeficiency virus infection, *N Engl J Med* 336:1487, 1997.
108. Jaffe HW, Pellett PE: Human herpesvirus 8 and Kaposi's sarcoma—some answers, more questions, *N Engl J Med* 340:1912, 1999.
109. Jamjian MC, McNicholl IR: Enfuvirtide: first fusion inhibitor for treatment of HIV infection, *Am J Health Syst Pharm* 61:1242, 2004.
110. Jin Y-T, Tsai S-T, Yan J-J, et al: Presence of human herpesvirus–like DNA sequence in oral Kaposi's sarcoma, *Oral Surg Oral Med Oral Pathol Oral Radiol Endod* 81:442, 1996.
111. Kabani S, Greenspan D, DeSouza YD, et al: Oral hairy leukoplakia with extensive oral mucosal involvement: report of two cases, *Oral Surg Oral Med Oral Pathol* 67:411, 1989.
112. Kelly SL, Lamb DC, Kelly DE, et al: Resistance to fluconazole and amphotericin in *Candida albicans* from AIDS patients, *Lancet* 348:1523, 1996.
113. King MD, Reznik DA, O'Daniels CM, et al. Human papillomavirus–associated oral warts among human immunodeficiency virus–seropositive patients in the era of highly active antiretroviral therapy: an emerging infection, *Clin Infect Dis* 34:641, 2002.
114. Klein RS, Quart AM, Small CB: Periodontal disease in heterosexuals with acquired immunodeficiency syndrome, *J Periodontol* 62:535, 1991.
115. Kumar SN, Sarswathi TR, Ranganathan K: Intra-oral hypermelanosis in an HIV sero-positive patient: a case report, *Indian J Dent Res* 14:131, 2003.
116. Kuntz AA, Gelderblum HR, Reichart PA: Ultrastructural findings on oral Kaposi's sarcoma (AIDS), *J Oral Pathol* 16:372, 1987.
117. Lake-Bakaar G, Tom W, Lake-Bakaar D, et al: Gastropathy and ketoconazole malabsorption in the acquired immunodeficiency syndrome (AIDS), *Ann Intern Med* 109:471, 1988.
118. Lamster IB, Begg MD, Mitchell-Lewis D, et al: Oral manifestations of HIV infection in homosexual men and intravenous drug users, *Oral Surg Oral Med Oral Pathol* 78:163, 1994.
119. Langford A, Pohle HD, Gelderblum HR, et al: Oral hyperpigmentation in HIV-infected patients, *Oral Surg Oral Med Oral Pathol* 67:301, 1989.
120. Lindhardt BO, Ulrich K, Sindrup JH, et al: Seroconversion to human immunodeficiency virus (HIV) in persons attending an STD clinic in Copenhagen, *Acta Derm Venereol (Stockh)* 68:250, 1998.
121. Lopez de Blanc S, Sambuelli R, Femopase F, et al: Bacillary angiomatosis affecting the oral cavity. report of two cases and review, *J Oral Pathol Med* 29:91, 2000.
122. Lot F, Seguier J-C, Fegueux S, et al: Probable transmission of HIV from an orthopedic surgeon to a patient in France, *Ann Intern Med* 130:1, 1999.
123. Luzzi GA, Jones BJ: Treatment of neutropenic oral ulceration in human immunodeficiency virus infection with G-CSF, *Oral Surg Oral Med Oral Pathol Oral Radiol Endod* 81:53, 1996.
124. Mallon PW, Cooper DA, Carr A: HIV-associated lipodystrophy, *HIV Med* 2:166, 2001.
125. Mandel ID: Occupational risks in dentistry: comforts and concerns, *J Am Dent Assoc* 124:41, 1993.
126. Manfredi R, Calza L, Chiodo F: Gynecomastia associated with highly active antiretroviral therapy, *Ann Pharmacother* 35:438, 2001.
127. Margiotta V, Campisi G, Mancuso S, et al: HIV infection: oral lesions, CD4+ cell count and viral load in an Italian study population, *J Oral Pathol Med* 28:173, 1999.
128. Marmor M, Krasinski K, Sanchez M, et al: Sex, drugs, and HIV infection in a New York City hospital outpatient population, *J Acquir Immune Defic Syndr* 3:307, 1990.
129. Martins MD, Lozano-Chiu M, Rex JH: Declining rates of oropharyngeal candidiasis and carriage of *Candida albicans* associated with trends toward reduced rates of carriage of fluconazole-resistant *C. albicans* in human immunodeficiency virus–infected patients, *Clin Infect Dis* 27:1291, 1998.
130. McCarthy GM: Host factors associated with HIV-related oral candidiasis, *Oral Surg Oral Med Oral Pathol* 73:181, 1992.
131. McCarthy GM, Mackie ID, Koval J, et al: Factors associated with increased frequency of HIV-related oral candidiasis, *J Oral Pathol Med* 20:332, 1991.
132. McCarthy GM, Ssali CS, Bednarsh H, et al: Transmission of HIV in the dental clinic and elsewhere, *Oral Dis* 8(suppl 2):126, 2002.
133. McKaig RG, Patton LL, Thomas JC, et al: Factors associated with periodontitis in an HIV-infected southeast USA study, *Oral Dis* 6:158, 2000.
134. McLeod WA: Dermatologic aspects of HIV in dermatology nursing, *Dermatol Nurs* 4:110, 1992.
135. Mealey BL: Periodontal implications: medically compromised patients, *Ann Periodontol* 1:256, 1996.
136. Mealey BL, Rees TD: Systemic factors impacting the periodontium. In Rose LF, Mealey BL, Genco RJ, Cohen DW, editors: *Periodontics, medicine, surgery, and implants,* St Louis, 2004, Mosby, Elsevier.
137. Medical Letter: Drugs for AIDS and associated infections, *Med Lett* 35:79, 1993.
138. Michael NL, Brown AD, Voigt RF, et al: Rapid disease progression without seroconversion following primary human immunodeficiency virus type 1 infection: evidence for highly susceptible human hosts, *J Infect Dis* 175: 1352, 1997.
139. Modrzejewski KA, Herman RA: Emtricitabine: a once-daily nucleoside reverse transcriptase inhibitor, *Ann Pharmacother* 38:1006, 2004.
140. Mohle-Boetani JC, Koehler JE, Berger TG, et al: Bacillary angiomatosis and bacillary peliosis in patients infected with human immunodeficiency virus: clinical characteristics in a case-control study, *Clin Infect Dis* 22:794, 1996.

141. Molinari JA: HIV, health care workers and patients: how to ensure safety in the dental office, *J Am Dent Assoc* 124:51, 1993.
142. Moore LV, Moore WE, Riley C, et al: Periodontal microflora of HIV-positive subjects with gingivitis or adult periodontitis, *J Periodontol* 64:48, 1993.
143. Mulligan R: The changing profile of the HIV/AIDS epidemic, *CDA J* 21(9):23, 1993.
144. Murray PA: Periodontal diseases in patients infected by human immunodeficiency virus, *Periodontol 2000* 6:50, 1994.
145. Murray PA, Grassi M, Winkler JR: The microbiology of HIV-associated periodontal lesions, *J Clin Periodontol* 16:636, 1989.
146. Murray PA, Winkler JR, Peros WJ, et al: DNA probe detection of periodontal pathogens in HIV-associated periodontal lesions, *Oral Microbiol Immunol* 6:34, 1991.
147. Ndiaye CF, Critchlow CW, Leggot PJ et al: Periodontal status of HIV1 and HIV2 seropositive female commercial sex workers in Senegal, *J Periodontol* 68:827, 1997.
148. Newell AM, Francis N, Nelson MR: Nephrotic syndrome associated with bacillary angiomatosis in a patient with AIDS, *Clin Infect Dis* 25:750, 1997.
149. Nguyen MT, Weiss PJ, LaBarre RC, et al: Orally administered amphotericin B in the treatment of oral candidiasis in HIV-infected patients caused by azole-resistant *Candida albicans, AIDS* 10:1745, 1996.
150. Nichols CM, Flaitz CM, Hicks MJ: Treating Kaposi's lesions in the HIV-infected patient, *J Am Dent Assoc* 124:78, 1993.
151. Nicolatou O, Theodoridou M, Mostrou G, et al: Oral lesions in children with perinatally acquired human immunodeficiency virus infection, *J Oral Pathol Med* 28:49, 1999.
152. Nicolatou-Galitis O, Velegraki A, Paikos S, et al: Effect of PI-HAART on the prevalence or oral lesions in HIV-1 infected patients: a Greek study, *Oral Dis* 10:145, 2004.
153. Nittayananta W, Chanowanna N, Striatanakul S, Winn T: Risk factors associated with oral lesions in HIV-infected heterosexual people and intravenous drug users in Thailand, *J Oral Pathol Med* 30:224, 2001.
154. Novak MJ: Necrotizing ulcerative periodontitis, *Ann Periodontol* 4:74, 1999.
155. Olsen RJ, Lynch P, Coyle MB, et al: Examination gloves as barriers to hand contamination in clinical practice, *JAMA* 270(3):350, 1993.
156. Oude Lashof AM, De Bock R, Herbrecht R, et al: An open multicentre comparative study of the efficacy, safety and tolerance of fluconazole and itraconazole in the treatment of cancer patients with oropharyngeal candidiasis, *Eur J Cancer* 40:1314, 2004.
157. Padian NS, Shiboski SC, Glass SO, et al: Heterosexual transmission of human immunodeficiency virus in northern California: results from a ten-year study, *Am J Epidemiol* 146:350, 1997.
158. Patel AS, Glick M: Oral manifestations associated with HIV infection: evaluation, assessment, and significance, *Gen Dent* 51:153, 2003.
159. Patton LL: HIV disease, *Dent Clin North Am* 47:467, 2003.
160. Patton LL, Shugars DA, Bonito AJ: A systematic review of complication risks for HIV-positive patients undergoing dental treatment, *J Am Dent Assoc* 133:195, 2000.
161. Pedraza MA, del Romero J, Roldan F, et al: Heterosexual transmission of HIV-1 is associated with high plasma viral load levels and a positive viral isolation in the infected partner, *J AIDS* 21:120, 1999.
162. Persaud D, Siberry GK, Ahonkhai A, et al: Continued production of drug-sensitive human immunodeficiency virus type-1 in children on combination antiretroviral therapy who have undetectable viral loads, *J Virol* 78:968, 2004.
163. Pezzotti P, Napoli PA, Acciai S, et al: Increasing survival time after AIDS in Italy: the role of new combination antiretroviral therapies, *AIDS* 13:249, 1999.
164. Phelan JA, Saltzman BR, Friedland GH, et al: Oral findings in patients with acquired immunodeficiency syndrome, *Oral Surg* 64:50, 1987.
165. Phillips P: Refractory mucosal candidiasis in patients with human immunodeficiency virus infection, *Clin Infect Dis* 28:407, 1999.
166. *Physicians' Desk Reference:* Fungisone oral suspension, *Health Care Series* 97:1, 1998.
167. Pierson T, Hoffman T, Blankson J, et al: Characterization of chemokine receptor utilization of viruses in the latent reservoir for human immunodeficiency virus type 1, *J Virol* 74:7824, 2000.
168. Piliero PJ: HIV and hepatitis coinfection, *AIDS Clin Care* 5:93, 102, 1993.
169. Pindborg JJ: Global aspects of the AIDS epidemic, *Oral Surg Oral Med Oral Pathol* 73:138, 1992.
170. Pistorius A, Willershausen B: Cases of HIV-associated characteristic periodontal diseases, *Eur J Med Res* 4:121, 1999.
171. Plemons JM, Benton E, Rankin KV, Steinig TH: Necrotizing ulcerative periodontitis: a case report, *Tex Dent J* 120:508, 2003.
172. Pons V, Greenspan D, Lozada-Nur F, et al: Oropharyngeal candidiasis in patients with AIDS: randomized comparison of fluconazole versus nystatin oral suspensions, *Clin Infect Dis* 24:1204, 1997.
173. Porter SR, Scully C, Luker J: Complications of dental surgery in persons with HIV disease, *Oral Surg Oral Med Oral Pathol* 75:165, 1993.
174. Price DA, Birtles RJ, Levine TS, et al: Bacillary angiomatosis: a role for Phyllobacterium? *AIDS* 11:1186, 1997.
175. Qunibi WY, Akhtar M, Ginn E, et al: Kaposi's sarcoma in cyclosporine-induced gingival hyperplasia, *Am J Kidney Dis* 11:349, 1988.
176. Rahman MA, Kingsley LA, Breinig MK, et al: Enhanced antibody responses to Epstein-Barr virus in HIV-infected homosexual men, *J Infect Dis* 159:472, 1989.
177. Ramirez-Amador V, Esquivel-Pedraza L, Lozada-Nur F, et al: Intralesional vinblastine vs 3% sodium tetradecyl sulfate for the treatment of oral Kaposi's sarcoma: a double blind, randomized clinical trial, *Oral Oncol* 38:460, 2002.
178. Ramirez Ramirez CR, Saavedra S, Ramirez Ronda C: Bacillary angiomatosis: microbiology, histopathology, clinical presentation, diagnosis and management, *Bol Asoc Med P R* 88:46, 1996.
179. Rees TD: Oral effects of drug abuse, *Crit Rev Oral Biol Med* 3:163, 1992.
180. Regezi JA, Eversole LR, Barker BF, et al: Herpes simplex and cytomegalovirus coinfected oral ulcers in HIV-positive patients, *Oral Surg Oral Med Oral Pathol Oral Radiol Endod* 81:55, 1996.
181. Regezi JA, MacPhail LA, Daniels TE, et al: Oral Kaposi's sarcoma: a 10-year retrospective histopathologic study, *J Oral Pathol Med* 22:292, 1993.
182. Reichart PA: Oral manifestations in HIV infection: fungal and bacterial infections, Kaposi's sarcoma, *Med Microbiol Immunol (Berl)* 192:165, 2003.
183. Reichart PA: Oral ulceration and iatrogenic disease in HIV infection, *Oral Surg Oral Med Oral Pathol* 73:212, 1992.
184. Relman AS: Pathogenic human retroviruses, *N Engl J Med* 318:243, 1988.
185. Reznik DA, O'Daniels C: Oral manifestations of HIV/AIDS in the HAART era, 2002, http://www.hivdent.org/oralm/oralmOMHAH052002.htm.

186. Richards JM: Notes on AIDS, *Br Dent J* 158:199, 1985.
187. Riley C, London JP, Burmeister JA: Periodontal health in 200 HIV-positive patients, *J Oral Pathol Med* 21:124, 1992.
188. Rivera-Hidalgo F, Stanford T: Oral mucosal lesions caused by infective microorganisms. 1. Lesions caused by viruses and bacteria, *Periodontal 2000* 21:125, 1999.
189. Robinson P: Periodontal diseases and HIV infection, *J Clin Periodontol* 19:609, 1992.
190. Robinson PG, Boulter A, Birnbaum W, Johnson NW: A controlled study of relative attachment loss in people with HIV infection, *J Clin Periodontol* 25:278, 2000.
191. Robinson PG, Adeghoye A, Rowland RW, et al: Periodontal diseases and HIV infection, *Oral Dis* 8(suppl 2):144, 2002.
192. Rowland RW, Escobar MR, Friedman RB, et al: Painful gingivitis may be an early sign of infection with the human immunodeficiency virus, *Clin Infect Dis* 16:233, 1993.
193. Ryder MI: Periodontal management of HIV-infected patients, *Periodontol 2000* 23:85, 2000.
194. Safai B, Diaz B, Schwartz J: Malignant neoplasms associated with human immunodeficiency virus infection, *AIDS Patient Care,* October 1993, p 262.
195. Saiag P, Pavlovic M, Clerici T, et al: Treatment of early AIDS-related Kaposi's sarcoma with oral all-*trans*-retinoic acid: results of a sequential non-randomized phase II trial, *AIDS* 12:2169, 1998.
196. Scheutz F, Matee Min, Andsager L, et al: Is there an association between periodontal condition and HIV infection? *J Clin Periodontol* 22:580, 1997.
197. Schiodt M, Greenspan D, Daniels TE, et al: Clinical and histologic spectrum of oral hairy leukoplakia, *Oral Surg Oral Med Oral Pathol* 64:716, 1987.
198. Schmidt-Westhausen AM, Priepke F, Bergmann FJ, Reichart PA: Decline in the rate of oral opportunistic infections following introduction of highly active antiretroviral therapy, *J Oral Pathol Med* 29:336, 2000.
199. Schulman DJ: The dentist, HIV and the law, *CDA J* 21(9):45, 1993.
200. Schulten EA, ten Kate RW, van der Waal I: Oral manifestations of HIV infection in 75 Dutch patients, *J Oral Pathol Med* 18:42, 1989.
201. Schuman P, Capps L, Peng G, et al: Weekly fluconazole for the prevention of mucosal candidiasis in women with HIV infection, *Ann Intern Med* 126:689, 1997.
202. Schuman P, Sobel JD, Ohmit SE, et al: Mucosal candidal colonization and candidiasis in women with or without risk for human immunodeficiency virus infection, *Clin Infect Dis* 27:1161, 1998.
203. Sciubba JJ: Recognizing the oral manifestations of AIDS, *Oncology* 6:64, 1992.
204. Scully C, Diz Dios P: Orofacial effects of antiretroviral therapies, *Oral Dis* 7:205, 2001.
205. Scully C, McCarthy G: Management of oral health in persons with HIV infection, *Oral Surg Oral Med Oral Pathol* 73:215, 1992.
206. Shangase L, Feller L, Blignaut E: Necrotising ulcerative gingivitis/periodontitis as indicators of HIV infection, *SADJ* 59:105, 2004.
207. Shibosky CH, Winkler JR: Gingival Kaposi's sarcoma and periodontitis, *Oral Surg Oral Med Oral Pathol* 76:49, 1993.
208. Shugars DC, Wahl SM: The role of the oral environment in HIV-1 transmission, *J Am Dent Assoc* 129:851, 1998.
209. Silverman S: *Color atlas of oral manifestations of AIDS,* Toronto, 1989, BC Decker.
210. Silverman S Jr, Gallo JW, McKnight ML, et al: Clinical characteristics and management responses in 85 HIV-infected patients with oral candidiasis, *Oral Surg Oral Med Oral Pathol Oral Radiol Endod* 82:402, 1996.
211. Sitas F, Newton R, Boshoff C: Increasing probability of mother-to-child transmission of HHV-8 with increasing maternal antibody titer for HHV-8, *N Engl J Med* 340:1923, 1999.
212. Sitas F, Carrara H, Beral V, et al: Antibodies against human herpesvirus 8 in black South African patients with cancer, *N Engl J Med* 340:1863, 1999.
213. Slavkin HC: An update on HIV/AIDS, *J Am Dent Assoc* 127:1401, 1996.
214. Slots J: Update on human cytomegalovirus in destructive periodontal disease, *Oral Microbiol Immunol* 19:217, 2004.
215. Stevenson GC: Removable prosthodontics and the HIV-infected patient: assessment and treatment planning, *Dent Alliance AIDS/HIV Care* 3:8, 1996.
216. Swango PA, Kleinman DV, Konzelman JL: HIV and periodontal health: a study of military personnel with HIV, *J Am Dent Assoc* 122:49, 1991.
217. Syrjanen S, Laine P, Niemela M, et al: Oral hairy leukoplakia is not a specific sign of HIV infection but related to immunosuppression in general, *J Oral Pathol Med* 18:28, 1989.
218. Syrjanen S, Leimola-Virtanen R, Schmidt-Westhausen A, et al: Oral ulcers in AIDS patients frequently associated with cytomegalovirus (CMV) and Epstein-Barr virus (EBV) infection, *J Oral Pathol Med* 28:204, 1999
219. Tappuni AR, Fleming GJ: The effect of antiretroviral therapy on the prevalence of oral manifestations in HIV-infected patients: a UK study, *Oral Surg Oral Med Oral Pathol Oral Radiol Endod* 92:623, 2001.
220. Tavitian A, Raufman JP, Rosenthal LE: Oral candidiasis as a marker for esophageal candidiasis in the acquired immunodeficiency syndrome, *Ann Intern Med* 104:54, 1986.
221. Tomlinson DR, Coker RJ, Fisher M: Management and treatment of Kaposi's sarcoma in AIDS, *Int J STD AIDS* 7:466, 1996.
222. United States Pharmacopeial Convention, Inc: *Drug information for the health care professional,* ed 19, Taunton, Mass, 1999, World Color Book Services.
223. Ustianowski AP, Leake H, Evans S: Outpatient therapy of HIV-associated oral and oesophageal candidosis, *Int J STD AIDS* 8:592, 1997.
224. Vanhems P, Allard R, Toma E, et al: Prognostic value of the CD4-T cell count for HIV-1 infected patients with advanced immunosuppression. *Int J STD AIDS* 1996; 7:495.
225. Vanhems P, Dassa C, Lambert J, et al: Comprehensive classification of symptoms and signs reported among 218 patients with acute HIV-1 infection, *J AIDS* 21:99, 1999.
226. Velegraki A, Nicolatou O, Theodoridou M, et al: Paediatric AIDS-related linear gingival erythema; a form of erythematous candidiasis? *J Oral Pathol Med* 28:178, 1999.
227. Verrusio AC: Risk of transmission of the human immunodeficiency virus to health care workers exposed to HIV-infected patients: a review, *J Am Dent Assoc* 118:339, 1989.
228. Veugelers PJ, Cornelisse PG, Craib KJ, et al: Models of survival in HIV infection and their use in the quantification of treatment benefits, *Am J Epidemiol* 148:487, 1998.
229. Vidmar L, Poljak M, Tomazic J, et al: Transmission of HIV-1 by human bite, *Lancet* 347:1762, 1996.
230. Walli R, Goebel FD: Impaired glucose tolerance and protease inhibitors, *Ann Intern Med* 129:837, 1998.
231. Walling DM, Flaitz CM, Nichols CM: Epstein-Barr virus replication in oral hairy leukoplakia: response, persistence, and resistance to treatment with valacyclovir, *J Infect Dis* 188:883, 2003.
232. Walling DM, Etienne W, Ray AJ, et al: Persistence and transition of Epstein-Barr virus genotypes in the pathogenesis of oral hairy leukoplakia, *J Infect Dis* 190:387, 2004.

233. Wei X, Ghosh SK, Taylor ME, et al: Dynamics in human immunodeficiency virus type 1 infection, *Nature* 12:117, 1995.
234. Weisman Z, Kalinkovich A, Borkow G, et al: Infection by different HIV-1 subtypes (B and C) results in a similar immune activation profile despite distinct immune backgrounds, *J AIDS* 21:157, 1999.
235. Welch DF, Pickett DA, Slater LN, et al: *Rochalimaea henselae* sp. nov., a cause of septicemia, bacillary angiomatosis and parenchymal bacillary peliosis, *J Clin Microbiol* 30:275, 1992.
236. Wilcox CM: Esophageal ulcers in AIDS: in response, *Ann Intern Med* 124:928, 1996.
237. Yeung SC, Stewart GJ, Cooper DA, et al: Progression of periodontal disease in HIV seropositive patients, *J Periodontol* 64:651, 1993.
238. Zhang H, Dornadula G, Beumont M, et al: Human immunodeficiency virus type 1 in the semen of men receiving highly active antiretroviral therapy, *N Engl J Med* 17:339, 1998.
239. Zhang X, Langford A, Gelderblom H, et al: Ultrastructural findings in oral hyperpigmentation of HIV-infected patients, *J Oral Pathol Med* 18:471, 1989.

Treatment of Periodontal Disease

Henry H. Takei

PART 7

Periodontal treatment requires an interrelationship between the care of the periodontium and other phases of dentistry. The concept of total treatment is based on the elimination of gingival inflammation and the factors that lead to it (e.g., plaque accumulation favored by calculus and pocket formation, inadequate restorations, areas of food impaction).

Total treatment requires consideration of systemic aspects, including the possibility of interaction of periodontal disease with other diseases, systemic adjuncts to local treatment, and special precautions in patient management necessitated by systemic conditions. It may also entail consideration of functional aspects for the establishment of optimal occlusal relationships for the entire dentition.

All these aspects are embodied in a master plan, which consists of a rational sequence of dental procedures that includes periodontal and other measures necessary to create a well-functioning dentition in a healthy periodontal environment.

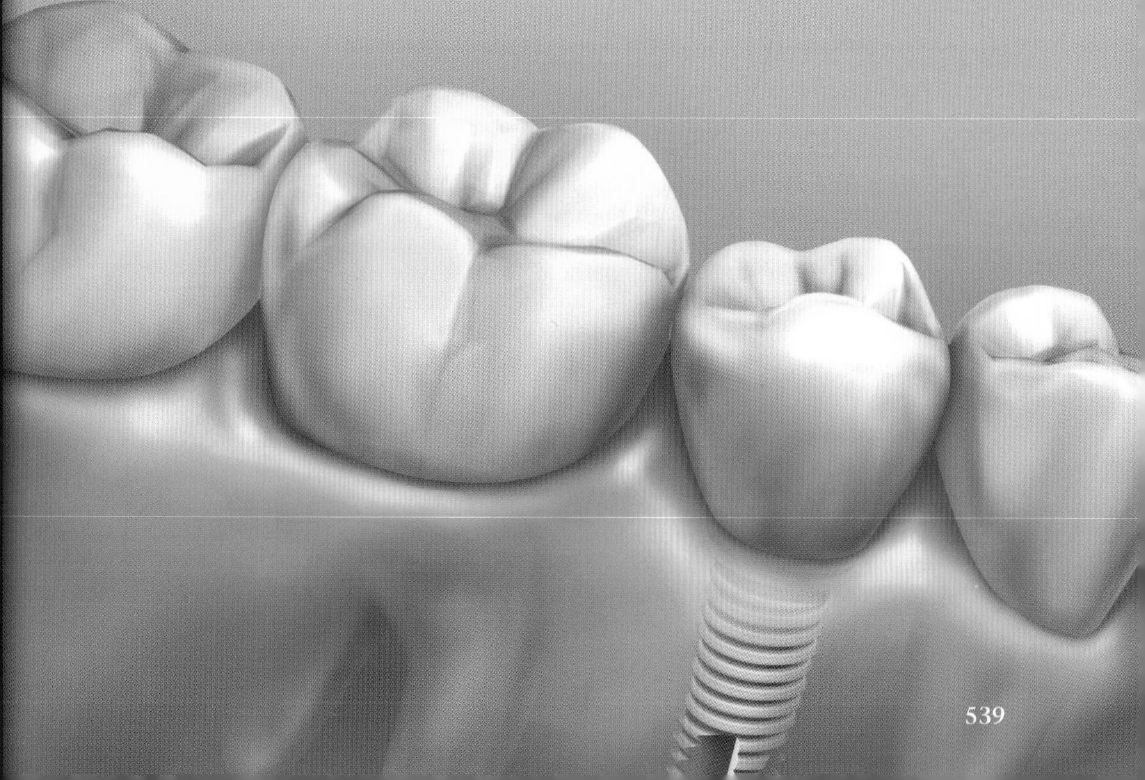

SECTION I

Diagnosis, Prognosis, and Treatment Plan

Henry H. Takei

CHAPTER 35

Clinical Diagnosis

Fermin A. Carranza and Henry H. Takei

CHAPTER OUTLINE

Proper diagnosis is essential to intelligent treatment. Periodontal diagnosis should first determine whether disease is present; then identify its type, extent, distribution, and severity; and finally provide an understanding of the underlying pathologic processes and their cause. Chapters 31 to 34 provide a detailed description of the different diseases that can affect the periodontium. In general, they fall into three broad categories, as follows:

1. Gingival diseases (Box 35-1)
2. Various types of periodontitis (Table 35-1)
3. Periodontal manifestations of systemic diseases

Periodontal diagnosis is determined after careful analysis of the case history and evaluation of the clinical signs and symptoms, as well as the results of various tests (e.g., probing mobility assessment, radiographs, blood tests, and biopsies).

BOX 35-1

Gingival Diseases

- Chronic marginal gingivitis
- Acute necrotizing ulcerative gingivitis
- Acute herpetic gingivostomatitis
- Allergic gingivitis
- Gingivitis associated with skin diseases
- Gingivitis associated with endocrine-metabolic disturbances
- Gingivitis associated with hematologic-immunologic disturbances
- Gingival enlargement associated with medications
- Gingival tumors

TABLE 35-1

Features of Types of Periodontitis

Parameter	Chronic	Aggressive	Prepubertal	LAP	NUP
Age (years)	35+	20-35	<11	11-19	15-35
Calculus	Moderate to abundant	Scanty to moderate	Scanty	Moderate	Scanty
Disease progression	Slow	Rapid	Rapid	Rapid	Rapid
Distribution	Generalized; associated with etiologic factors	Generalized; no consistent pattern	Primary molars and incisors	First molars and incisors, and no more than two other teeth	?
Prevalence	US: >50% Sri Lanka: 81%	US: 4%-5% Sri Lanka: 11%	?	<0.50%	?
Racial predilection	No	No	No	More common in blacks	No
Familial tendency	No	?	Yes	Yes	?
Gender distribution	More severe in men	?	?	?	?
PMN/macrophage defects	No	Yes	Yes	Yes	Yes
Association with systemic problems	No	Some cases	Yes	Yes	Yes
Response to therapy	Very good	Variable	Poor	Good	Variable

Prevalence in adolescents 14 to 17 years of age in the United States.
LAP, Localized aggressive periodontitis (formerly "localized juvenile periodontitis" [LJP]); *NUP,* necrotizing ulcerative periodontitis; *PMN,* polymorphonuclear leukocyte.

The focus of interest should be on the *patient* who has the disease and not simply on the disease itself. Diagnosis must therefore include a general evaluation of the patient and consideration of the oral cavity.

Diagnostic procedures must be systematic and organized for specific purposes; merely assembling facts is insufficient. The findings must be correlated so that they provide a meaningful explanation of the patient's periodontal problem.

The following discussion provides a recommended sequence of procedures for the diagnosis of periodontal diseases.

FIRST VISIT

Overall Appraisal of the Patient

From the first meeting, the clinician should attempt an overall appraisal of the patient. This includes consideration of the patient's mental and emotional status, temperament, attitude, and physiologic age.

Medical History

The medical history is mostly obtained at the first visit and can be supplemented by pertinent questioning at subsequent visits. The health history can be obtained verbally by questioning the patient and recording the responses on paper or by having the patient complete a printed questionnaire.

The importance of the medical history should be explained to the patient because patients often omit information that they cannot relate to their dental problems. The patient should be made aware of the following:

1. The role that some systemic diseases, conditions, or behavioral factors may play in the cause of periodontal disease.
2. The powerful influence that oral infection may have on the occurrence and severity of a variety of systemic diseases and conditions (see Chapters 17 and 18).

The medical history aids the clinician in the diagnosis of oral manifestations of systemic disease. It also assists in the detection of systemic conditions that may be affecting the periodontal tissue response to local factors or that require special precautions or modifications in treatment procedures (see Chapters 43, 44, and 45).

The medical history should address the following areas:

1. Is the patient under the care of a physician? If so, what is the nature and duration of the problem and the therapy? The name, address, and telephone number of the physician should be recorded because direct communication may be necessary.
2. Details on any hospitalization and surgery should be provided, including diagnosis, type of procedure, and untoward events (e.g., anesthetic, hemorrhagic, or infectious complications).
3. A list should be supplied of all the patient's medications and whether they were prescribed or obtained over the counter. All the possible effects of these medications should be carefully analyzed to determine their effect, if any, on the oral tissues and to avoid administering medications that would cause adverse drug interactions. Special inquiry should be

made regarding the dosage and duration of therapy with anticoagulants and corticosteroids.

4. A history should be taken of all the patient's medical problems (e.g., cardiovascular, hematologic, endocrine), including infectious diseases, sexually transmitted diseases, and high-risk behavior for human immunodeficiency virus (HIV) infection.
5. Any possibility of occupational disease should be noted.
6. Abnormal bleeding tendencies should be noted, such as nosebleeds, prolonged bleeding from minor cuts, spontaneous ecchymoses, tendency toward excessive bruising, and excessive menstrual bleeding.
7. Any history of allergy should be recorded, including hay fever, asthma, sensitivity to foods, and sensitivity to drugs (e.g., aspirin, codeine, barbiturates, sulfonamides, antibiotics, procaine, laxatives) or dental materials (e.g., eugenol, acrylic resins).
8. Information should be provided regarding onset of puberty and, for female patients, menopause, menstrual disorders, hysterectomy, pregnancies, and miscarriages.
9. The patient's family medical history should be taken, including bleeding disorders and diabetes.

Dental History

Current Illness. Some patients may be unaware of any problems, but many may report bleeding gums, loose teeth, spreading of the teeth with the appearance of spaces where none previously existed, foul taste in the mouth, and an itchy feeling in the gums relieved by digging with a toothpick. The patient may also have pain of varied types and duration, including constant, dull, gnawing pain; dull pain after eating; deep, radiating pains in the jaws; acute, throbbing pain; sensitivity when chewing; sensitivity to heat and cold; burning sensation in the gums; and extreme sensitivity to inhaled air.

A preliminary oral examination is done to explore the source of the patient's chief complaint and to determine whether immediate emergency care is required. If this is the case, the problem is addressed after consideration of the medical history (see Chapters 47 and 48).

The dental history should address the following areas:

1. A list of dental visits should be supplied, including frequency, date of most recent visit, nature of treatment, and oral prophylaxis or cleaning by a dentist or hygienist, including frequency and date of most recent cleaning.
2. The patient's oral hygiene regimen should be noted, including toothbrushing frequency, time of day, method, type of toothbrush and dentifrice, and duration of use before brush replacement, as well as other methods of mouth care (e.g., mouthwashes, finger massage, interdental stimulation, water irrigation, dental floss).
3. Any orthodontic treatment should be noted, including duration and approximate date of termination.
4. If the patient is experiencing pain in the teeth or gums, its nature and duration and how the pain is provoked, and relieved should be noted.
5. Bleeding gums should be investigated, including when first noted; whether occurring spontaneously, on brushing or eating, at night, or with regular periodicity; whether associated with menstrual period or other specific factors; and duration of the bleeding and how it is stopped.
6. A bad taste in the mouth and areas of food impaction should be recorded.
7. Do the teeth feel "loose" or "unsecured"? Is there difficulty in chewing? Any tooth mobility should be recorded.
8. What are the patient's general dental habits? Any grinding or clenching of the teeth during the day or at night should be noted. Do the teeth or jaw muscles feel "sore" in the morning? Other habits, such as tobacco smoking or chewing, nail biting, or biting on foreign objects, should be recorded.
9. Any history of previous periodontal problems should be noted, including the nature of the condition, any treatment received (surgical or nonsurgical), and approximate termination of previous treatment. If the patient believes the present problem is a recurrence of previous disease, what does the patient think caused it?

Intraoral Radiographic Survey

The radiographic survey should consist of a minimum of 14 intraoral films and four posterior bite-wing films (Figure 35-1).

Panoramic radiographs are a simple and convenient method of obtaining a survey view of the dental arch and surrounding structures (Figure 35-1). These films are helpful for the detection of developmental anomalies, pathologic lesions of the teeth and jaws, and fractures (Figure 35-2), as well as for dental screening of large groups. Panoramic radiographs provide an informative overall picture of the distribution and severity of bone destruction in periodontal disease, but *a complete intraoral series is required for periodontal diagnosis and treatment planning* (see Chapter 36).

Casts

Casts from dental impressions are extremely useful adjuncts in the oral examination. Casts indicate the position of the gingival margins and the position and inclination of the teeth, proximal contact relationships, and food impaction areas. In addition, they provide a view of lingual-cuspal relationships. Casts are important records of the dentition before it is altered by treatment. Finally, casts also serve as visual aids in discussions with the patient and are useful for pretreatment and post-treatment comparisons, as well as for reference at checkup visits.

Clinical Photographs

Color photographs are not essential, but they are useful for recording the appearance of the tissue before and after treatment. Clinicians cannot always rely on photographs for comparing subtle color changes in the gingiva, but

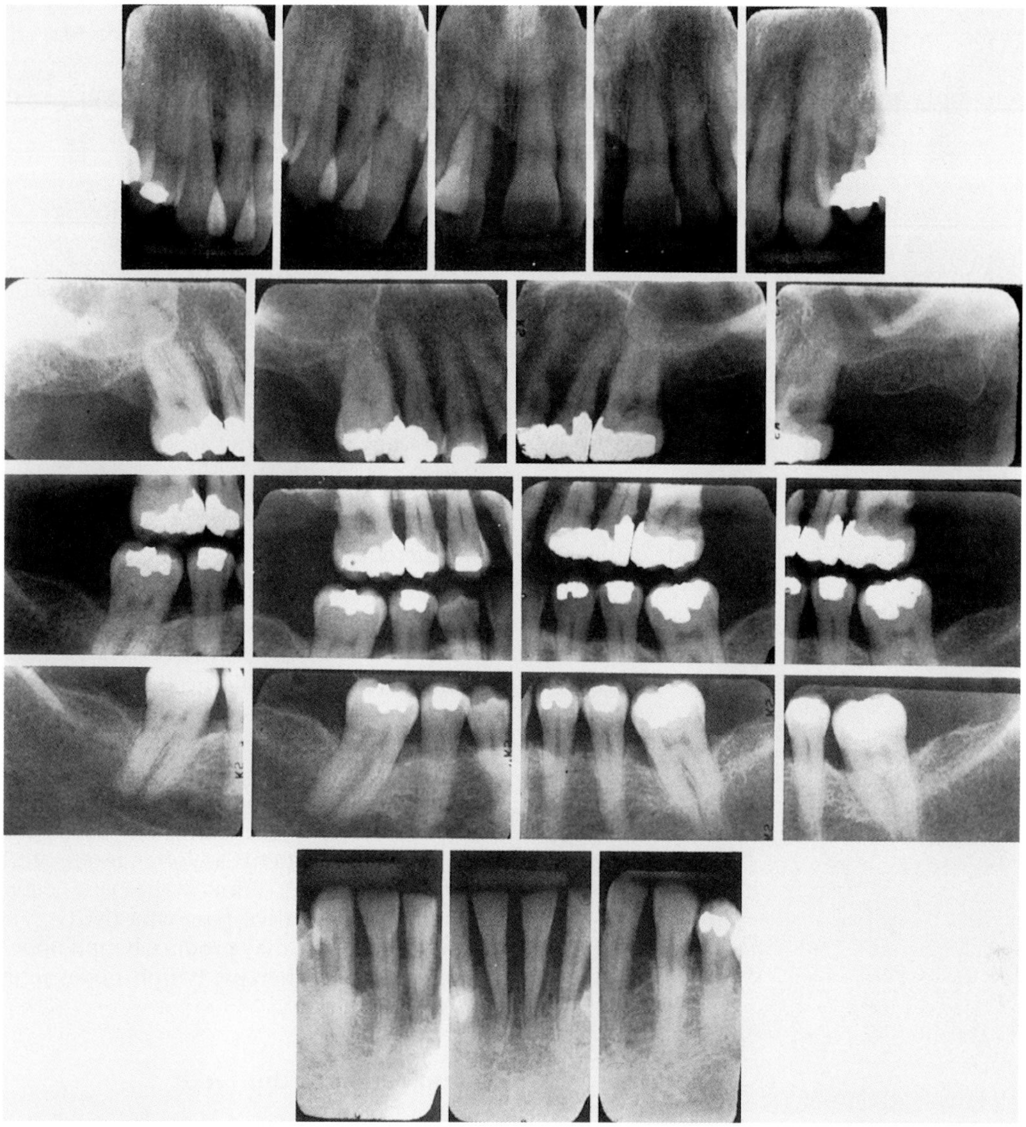

Figure 35-1 Full-mouth intraoral radiographic series (16 periapical films and four bite-wing films) used as an adjunct in periodontal diagnosis.

photos do depict gingival morphologic changes. With the advent of digital clinical photography, record keeping for mucogingival problems has become important (e.g., areas of gingival recession, frenum involvement, papilla loss).

Review of Initial Examination

If no emergency care is required, the patient is dismissed and informed about the second visit. Before then, a correlated examination is made of the radiographs and casts to relate the radiographic changes to unfavorable conditions represented on the casts. The casts are checked for evidence of abnormal wear, plunger cusps, uneven marginal ridges, malposed or extruded teeth, crossbite relationships, or other conditions that could cause occlusal disharmony or food impaction. Such areas are marked on the casts to serve as a reference during the detailed examination of the oral cavity. The radiographs and casts are valuable diagnostic aids; however, *the clinical findings in the oral cavity constitute the basis for diagnosis.*

SECOND VISIT

Oral Examination

Oral Hygiene. The cleanliness of the oral cavity is appraised in terms of the extent of accumulated food debris, plaque, materia alba, and tooth surface stains (Figure 35-3). Disclosing solution may be used to detect plaque that would otherwise be unnoticed. The amount of plaque detected, however, is not necessarily related to the severity of the disease present. For example, aggressive periodontitis is a destructive type of periodontitis in which plaque is scanty. Qualitative assessments of plaque are more meaningful (see Chapter 37).

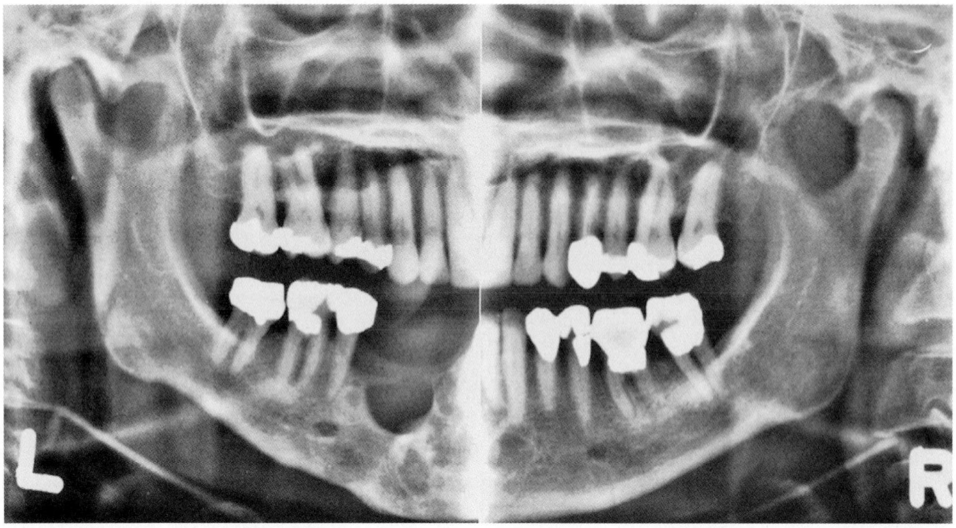

Figure 35-2 Panoramic radiograph showing temporomandibular joints and "cystic" spaces in the jaw. Areas of periodontal bone loss are not seen in detail. (Compare with Figure 35-1.)

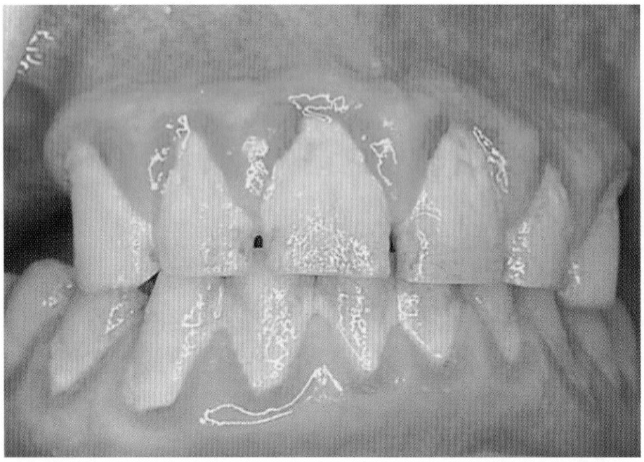

Figure 35-3 Poor oral hygiene. Gingival inflammation associated with plaque, materia alba, and calculus.

Oral Malodor. Oral malodor, also called *fetor ex ore, fetor oris,* and *halitosis,* is foul or offensive odor emanating from the oral cavity. Mouth odors may be of diagnostic significance, and their origin may be oral or extraoral (remote)[51] (see Chapter 19).

Examination of Oral Cavity. The entire oral cavity should be carefully examined. The examination should include the lips, floor of the mouth, tongue, palate, and oropharyngeal region, as well as the quality and quantity of saliva. Although findings may not be related to the periodontal problem, the dentist should detect all pathologic changes present in the mouth. Textbooks on oral medicine and oral diagnosis cover these topics in detail.

Examination of Lymph Nodes. Because periodontal, periapical, and other oral diseases may result in lymph node changes, the diagnostician should routinely examine and evaluate head and neck lymph nodes. Lymph nodes can become enlarged and indurated as a result of an infectious episode, malignant metastases, or residual fibrotic changes.

Inflammatory nodes become enlarged, palpable, tender, and fairly immobile. The overlying skin may be red and warm. Patients are often aware of the presence of "swollen glands." Primary herpetic gingivostomatitis, necrotizing ulcerative gingivitis (NUG), and acute periodontal abscesses may produce lymph node enlargement. After successful therapy, lymph nodes return to normal in days or weeks.

Examination of the Teeth

The teeth are examined for caries, developmental defects, anomalies of tooth form, wasting, hypersensitivity, and proximal contact relationships.

Wasting Disease of the Teeth. *Wasting* is defined as any gradual loss of tooth substance characterized by the formation of smooth, polished surfaces, without regard to the possible mechanism of this loss. The forms of wasting are erosion, abrasion, attrition, and abfraction.

Erosion. Also called *corrosion,* erosion is a sharply defined, wedge-shaped depression in the cervical area of the facial tooth surface.[53] The long axis of the eroded area is perpendicular to the vertical axis of the tooth The surfaces are smooth, hard, and polished. Erosion generally affects a group of teeth. In the early stages, it may be confined to the enamel, but it generally extends to involve the underlying dentin as well as the cementum.

The etiology of erosion is not known. Suggested causes include decalcification by acidic beverages[35] or citrus fruits and the combined effect of acid salivary secretion and friction.[37] Sognnaes[59] refers to these lesions as *dentoalveolar ablations* and attributes them to forceful frictional actions between the oral soft tissues and the adjacent hard tissues. Salivary pH, buffering capacity,

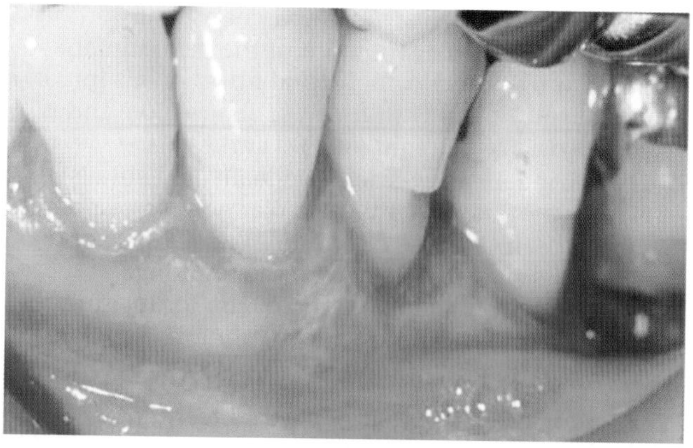

Figure 35-4 Abrasion attributed to aggressive toothbrushing. Involvement of the roots is followed by undermining of the enamel.

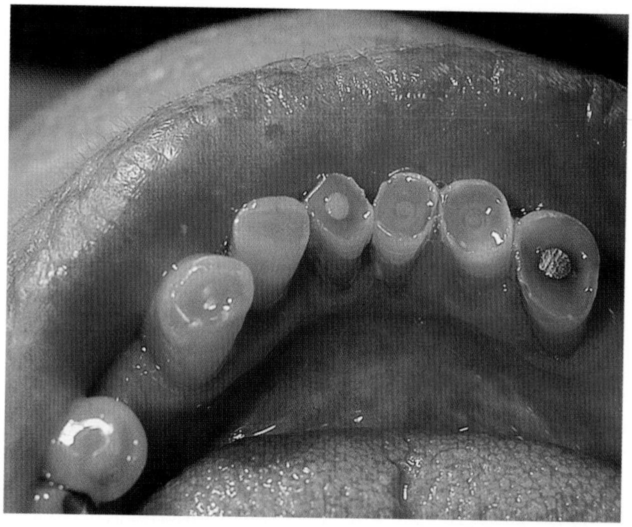

Figure 35-5 Occlusal wear. Flat, shiny, discolored surfaces produced by occlusal wear.

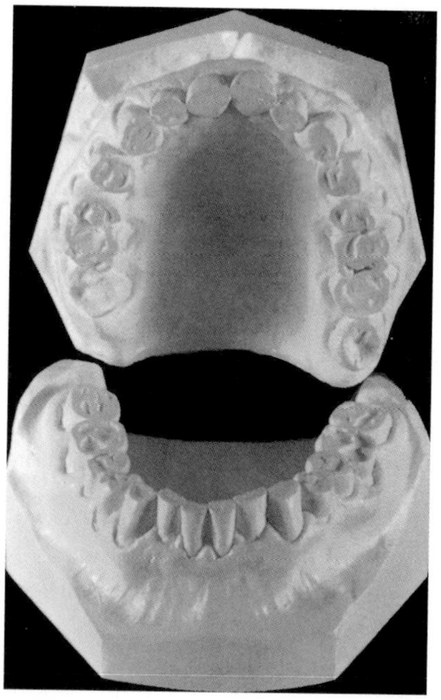

Figure 35-6 Reversed faciolingual occlusal plane. The normal occlusal plane is sometimes reversed by occlusal wear so that in the mandible the occlusal surfaces slope facially instead of lingually and in the maxilla they are inclined lingually. The third molars usually are not affected.

and calcium and phosphorus content have been reported as normal in patients with erosion, and the mucin level is elevated.[34]

Abrasion. Abrasion refers to the loss of tooth substance induced by mechanical wear other than that of mastication. Abrasion results in saucer-shaped or wedge-shaped indentations with a smooth, shiny surface. Abrasion starts on exposed cemental surfaces rather than on the enamel and extends to involve the dentin of the root. A sharp "ditching" around the cementoenamel junction appears because of to the soft cemental surface compared with the hard enamel surface.

Continued exposure to the abrasive agent, combined with decalcification of the enamel by locally formed acids, may result in loss of enamel, followed by loss of the dentin of the crown.

Toothbrushing with an abrasive dentifrice and the action of clasps are common causes of abrasion; brushing is the much more prevalent cause[24] (Figure 35-4). The degree of tooth wear from toothbrushing depends on the abrasive effect of the dentifrice and the angle of brushing.[32,33] Horizontal brushing at right angles to the vertical axis of the teeth results in the severest loss of tooth substance. Occasionally, abrasion of the incisal edges results from habits such as holding objects (e.g., bobby pin, tacks) between the teeth.

Attrition. Attrition is occlusal wear resulting from functional contacts with opposing teeth. Such physical wear patterns may occur on incisal, occlusal, and approximal tooth surfaces. A certain amount of tooth wear is physiologic, but accelerated wear may occur when abnormal anatomic or unusual functional factors are present.

Occlusal or incisal surfaces worn by attrition are called *facets*. When active tooth gnashing occurs, the enamel rods are fractured and become highly reflective to light.[68] Thus, shiny, smooth, and curviplanar facets are usually the best indicator of ongoing frictional activity. If dentin is exposed, a yellowish brown discoloration is frequently present (Figure 35-5). Facets vary in size and location depending on whether they are produced by physiologic or abnormal wear.[10,66] At least one significant wear facet has been reported in 92% of adults,[56] and facet prevalence is almost universal.[10,67] Facets are usually not sensitive to thermal or tactile stimulation.

Facets generally represent functional or parafunctional wear, as well as iatrogenic dental treatment through coronoplasty (occlusal adjustment). Coronoplasty, however, does not appear to contribute to higher ratings of wear.[57] Excessive wear may result in obliteration of the cusps and the formation of either a flat or a cuneiform (cupped-out) occlusal surface. Reversal of the occlusal plane of the premolars and first and second molars occurs in advanced stages of wear (Figure 35-6). Contrary to earlier thought, attrition of young adults from modern societies is not age related.[12,57] This suggests that a significant amount of attrition in young adults is unlikely to occur from functional wear[27] and is probably the result of bruxing activity.[57] Attrition has been correlated with age in older adults.[6,55]

The angle of the facet on the tooth surface may be significant to the periodontium. Horizontal facets tend to direct forces on the vertical axis of the tooth, to which the periodontium can adapt most effectively. Angular facets direct occlusal forces laterally and increase the risk of periodontal damage. However, continuous tooth eruption without alveolar bone growth may compensate for gradual attrition, which is characterized by a lack of inflammatory changes on the alveolar bone surfaces.[63]

Abfraction. A recently studied mechanism of tooth wear, abfraction results from occlusal loading surfaces causing tooth flexure and mechanical microfractures and tooth substance loss in the cervical area.[19]

These four mechanisms of tooth wear—corrosion, abrasion, attrition, and abfraction—can combine with each other, resulting in increased degree of tooth wear.

Dental Stains. These stains are pigmented deposits on the teeth. Dental stains should be carefully examined to determine their origin (see Chapter 10).

Hypersensitivity. Root surfaces exposed by gingival recession may be hypersensitive to thermal changes or tactile stimulation. Patients often direct the operator to the sensitive areas. These may be located by gentle exploration with a probe or cold air.

Proximal Contact Relationships. Slightly open contacts permit food impaction. The dentist should check the tightness of contacts using clinical observation and dental floss. Abnormal contact relationships may also initiate occlusal changes, such as a shift in the median line between the central incisors, labial version of the maxillary canine, buccal or lingual displacement of the posterior teeth, and an uneven relationship of the marginal ridges.

Tooth Mobility. All teeth have a slight degree of physiologic mobility, which varies for different teeth and at different times of the day.[41] Mobility is greatest on arising in the morning and progressively decreases. The increased mobility in the morning is attributed to slight extrusion of the tooth because of limited occlusal contact during sleep. During the waking hours, mobility is reduced by chewing and swallowing forces, which intrude the teeth in the sockets. These 24-hour variations are less marked in persons with a healthy periodontium than in those with occlusal habits such as bruxism and clenching.

Single-rooted teeth have more mobility than multirooted teeth; incisors have the most mobility. Mobility is principally in a horizontal direction, although some axial mobility occurs, but to a much lesser degree.[43]

Tooth mobility occurs in the following two stages:

1. In the initial, or intrasocket, stage the tooth moves within the confines of the periodontal ligament (PDL). This is associated with viscoelastic distortion of the PDL and redistribution of the periodontal fluids, interbundle content, and fibers.[25] This initial movement occurs with forces of about 100 g and is about 0.05 to 0.10 mm (50-100 μm).[38]
2. The secondary stage occurs gradually and entails elastic deformation of the alveolar bone in response to increased horizontal forces.[40] When a force of 500 g is applied to the crown, the resulting displacement is about 100 to 200 μm for incisors, 50 to 90 μm for canines, 8 to 10 μm for premolars, and 40 to 80 μm for molars.[38]

When a force such as that applied to teeth in occlusion is discontinued, the teeth return to their original position in two stages: (1) an immediate, springlike elastic recoil and (2) a slow, asymptomatic recovery movement. The recovery movement is pulsating and is apparently associated with the normal pulsation of the periodontal vessels, which occurs in synchrony with the cardiac cycle.[39]

Many attempts have been made to develop mechanical or electronic devices for the precise measurement of tooth mobility.[39,42,44,56] Even though standardization of the grading of mobility would be helpful in diagnosing periodontal disease and in evaluating the outcome of treatment, these devices are not widely used. As a general rule, mobility is graded clinically with a simple method. The tooth is held firmly between the handles of two metallic instruments or with one metallic instrument and one finger (Figure 35-7), and an effort is made to move it in all directions; abnormal mobility most often occurs faciolingually. Mobility is graded according to the ease and extent of tooth movement, as follows:

- Normal mobility.
- *Grade I:* Slightly more than normal.
- *Grade II:* Moderately more than normal.
- *Grade III:* Severe mobility faciolingually and mesiodistally, combined with vertical displacement.

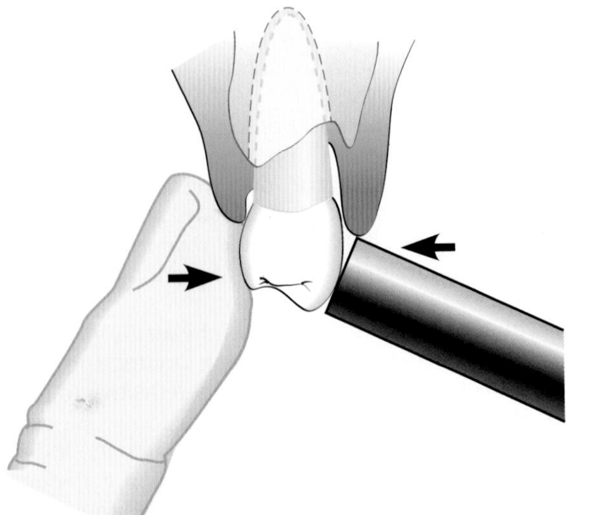

Figure 35-7 Tooth mobility checked with a metal instrument and one finger.

Mobility beyond the physiologic range is termed *abnormal* or *pathologic*. It is pathologic in that it exceeds the limits of normal mobility values; the periodontium is not necessarily diseased at the time of examination.

Increased mobility is caused by one or more of the following factors:

1. *Loss of tooth support* (bone loss) can result in mobility. The amount of mobility depends on the severity and distribution of bone loss at individual root surfaces, the length and shape of the roots, and the root size compared with that of the crown.[45] A tooth with short, tapered roots is more likely to loosen than one with normal-size or bulbous roots with the same amount of bone loss. Because bone loss usually results from a combination of factors and does not occur as an isolated finding, the severity of tooth mobility does not necessarily correspond to the amount of bone loss.
2. *Trauma from occlusion,* or injury produced by excessive occlusal forces or incurred because of abnormal occlusal habits (e.g., bruxism, clenching), is a common cause of tooth mobility. Mobility is also increased by *hypofunction*. Mobility produced by trauma from occlusion occurs initially as a result of resorption of the cortical layer of bone, leading to reduced fiber support, and later as an adaptation phenomenon resulting in a widened periodontal space.
3. *Extension of inflammation* from the gingiva or from the periapex into the PDL results in changes that increase mobility. The spread of inflammation from an acute periapical abscess may increase tooth mobility in the absence of periodontal disease.
4. *Periodontal surgery* temporarily increases tooth mobility for a short period.[47-50]
5. Tooth mobility is increased in *pregnancy* and is sometimes associated with the *menstrual cycle* or the use of *hormonal contraceptives*. Mobility occurs in patients with or without periodontal disease, presumably because of physicochemical changes in the periodontal tissues.
6. *Pathologic processes of the jaws* that destroy the alveolar bone or the roots of the teeth can also result in mobility. Such processes include osteomyelitis and tumors of the jaws.

One study has suggested that pockets around mobile teeth harbor higher proportions of *Campylobacter rectus* and *Peptostreptococcus micros* (and perhaps *Porphyromonas gingivalis*) than nonmobile teeth.[15] This hypothesis needs further verification.

Trauma from Occlusion. Trauma from occlusion refers to *tissue injury* produced by occlusal forces, not to the occlusal forces themselves (see Chapter 29). The criterion that determines if an occlusal force is injurious is whether it causes damage in the periodontal tissues; therefore the diagnosis of trauma from occlusion is made from the condition of the periodontal tissues. The periodontal findings are then used as a guide for locating the responsible occlusal relationships.

Periodontal findings that suggest the presence of trauma from occlusion include excessive tooth mobility, particularly in teeth showing radiographic evidence of a widened periodontal space (see Chapter 36); vertical or angular bone destruction; intrabony pockets; and pathologic migration, especially of the anterior teeth (see following discussion).

Pathologic Migration of the Teeth. Alterations in tooth position should be carefully noted, particularly with a view toward identifying abnormal forces, a tongue-thrusting habit, or other habits that may be contributing factors (see Chapter 29). Premature tooth contacts in the posterior region that deflect the mandible anteriorly contribute to destruction of the periodontium of the maxillary anterior teeth and to pathologic migration (Figure 35-8; see also Figure 29-12). Pathologic migration of anterior teeth in young persons may be a sign of localized aggressive (juvenile) periodontitis.

Sensitivity to Percussion. Sensitivity to percussion is a feature of acute inflammation of the PDL. Gentle percussion of a tooth at different angles to the long axis often aids in localizing the site of inflammatory involvement.

A 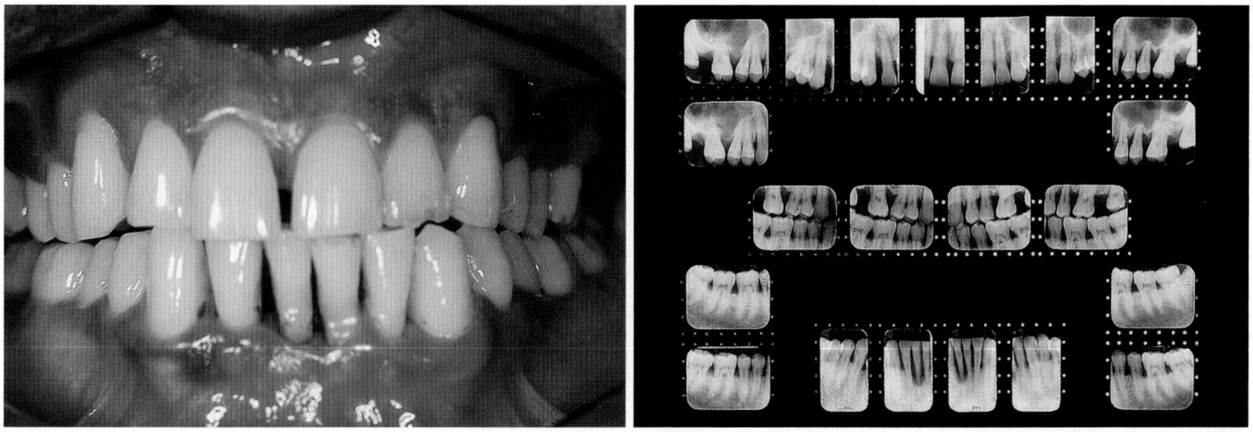 B

Figure 35-8 Periodontal disease with pathologic migration of the anterior teeth. **A,** Clinical photograph. **B,** Radiographic view.

Dentition with the Jaws Closed. Examination of the dentition with the jaws closed can detect conditions such as irregularly aligned teeth, extruded teeth, improper proximal contacts, and areas of food impaction, all of which may favor plaque accumulation.

Excessive *overbite,* seen most often in the anterior region, may cause impingement of the teeth on the gingiva and food impaction, followed by gingival inflammation, gingival enlargement, and pocket formation. The real significance of excessive overbite for gingival health, however, is controversial.[2]

In *open-bite* relationships, abnormal vertical spaces exist between the maxillary and mandibular teeth. The condition occurs most often in the anterior region, although posterior open bite is occasionally seen. Reduced mechanical cleansing by the passage of food may lead to accumulation of debris, calculus formation, and extrusion of teeth.

In *crossbite* the normal relationship of the mandibular teeth to the maxillary teeth is reversed, with the maxillary teeth being lingual to the mandibular teeth. Crossbite may be bilateral or unilateral, or it may affect only a pair of antagonists. Trauma from occlusion, food impaction, spreading of the mandibular teeth, and associated gingival and periodontal disturbances may be caused by crossbite.

Functional Occlusal Relationships. Examination of functional occlusal relationships is an important part of the diagnostic procedure. Dentitions that appear normal when the jaws are closed may present marked functional abnormalities (see Chapter 56).

Examination of the Periodontium

The periodontal examination should be systematic, starting in the molar region in either the maxilla or the mandible and proceeding around the arch. This avoids overemphasis of spectacular findings at the expense of other conditions, which, although less striking, may be equally important. It is important to detect the earliest signs of gingival and periodontal disease.

Charts to record the periodontal and associated findings provide a guide for a thorough examination and record of the patient's condition (Figure 35-9). They are also used for evaluating the response to treatment and for comparison at recall visits. However, excessively complicated mouth charting may lead to identification of a frustrating maze of minutiae rather than clarification of the patient's problem.

In the last decade, electronic clinical records have been developed and are increasingly being used by general dentists and periodontists. Most systems provide rapid and easy access to information and allow the incorporation of digital clinical and radiographic images.[52] Computerized dental examination systems using high-resolution graphics and voice-activated technology permit easy retrieval and comparison of data.[8]

Plaque and Calculus. Many methods are available for assessing plaque and calculus accumulation.[13] The presence of supragingival plaque and calculus can be directly observed and the amount measured with a calibrated probe. For the detection of subgingival calculus, each tooth surface is carefully checked to the level of the gingival attachment with a sharp #17 or #3A explorer (Figure 35-10). Warm air may be used to deflect the gingiva and aid in visualization of the calculus.

Although the radiograph may sometimes reveal heavy calculus deposits interproximally (see Chapter 36) and even on the facial and lingual surfaces, it cannot be used reliably for the thorough detection of calculus.

Gingiva. The gingiva must be dried before accurate observations can be made (Figure 35-11). Light reflection from moist gingiva obscures detail. In addition to visual examination and exploration with instruments, firm but gentle palpation should be used for detecting pathologic alterations in normal resilience, as well as for locating areas of pus formation.

Features of the gingiva to consider are color, size, contour, consistency, surface texture, position, ease of bleeding, and pain (see Chapters 22 and 23). No deviation from the norm should be overlooked. The distribution of gingival disease and its acute or chronic nature should also be noted.

Clinically, gingival inflammation can produce two basic types of tissue response: edematous and fibrotic. *Edematous* tissue response is characterized by a smooth, glossy, soft, red gingiva. In the *fibrotic* tissue response, some of the characteristics of normalcy persist; the gingiva is more firm, stippled, and opaque, although it is usually thicker, and its margin appears rounded.

Use of Clinical Indices in Dental Practice. There has been a tendency to extend the use of indices originally designed for epidemiologic studies into dental practice (see Chapter 8). Of all the indices proposed, the gingival index and the sulcus bleeding index appear to be the most useful and most easily transferred to clinical practice.

The *gingival index* (Löe) provides an assessment of gingival inflammatory status that can be used in practice to compare gingival health before and after Phase I therapy or before and after surgical therapy. It can also be used to compare gingival status at recall visits. Attaining good intraexaminer and interexaminer calibration is imperative in the dental office.

The *sulcus bleeding index* (Mühlemann) provides an objective, easily reproducible assessment of the gingival status. It is extremely useful for detecting early inflammatory changes and the presence of inflammatory lesions located at the base of the periodontal pocket, an area inaccessible to visual examination. Because patients can easily understand it, the sulcus bleeding index can be used to enhance the patient's motivation for plaque control.

Periodontal Pockets. Examination for periodontal pockets must include consideration of the presence and distribution on each tooth surface, pocket depth, level of attachment on the root, and type of pocket (suprabony or intrabony).

Signs and Symptoms. Although probing is the only reliable method of detecting pockets, clinical signs may

A

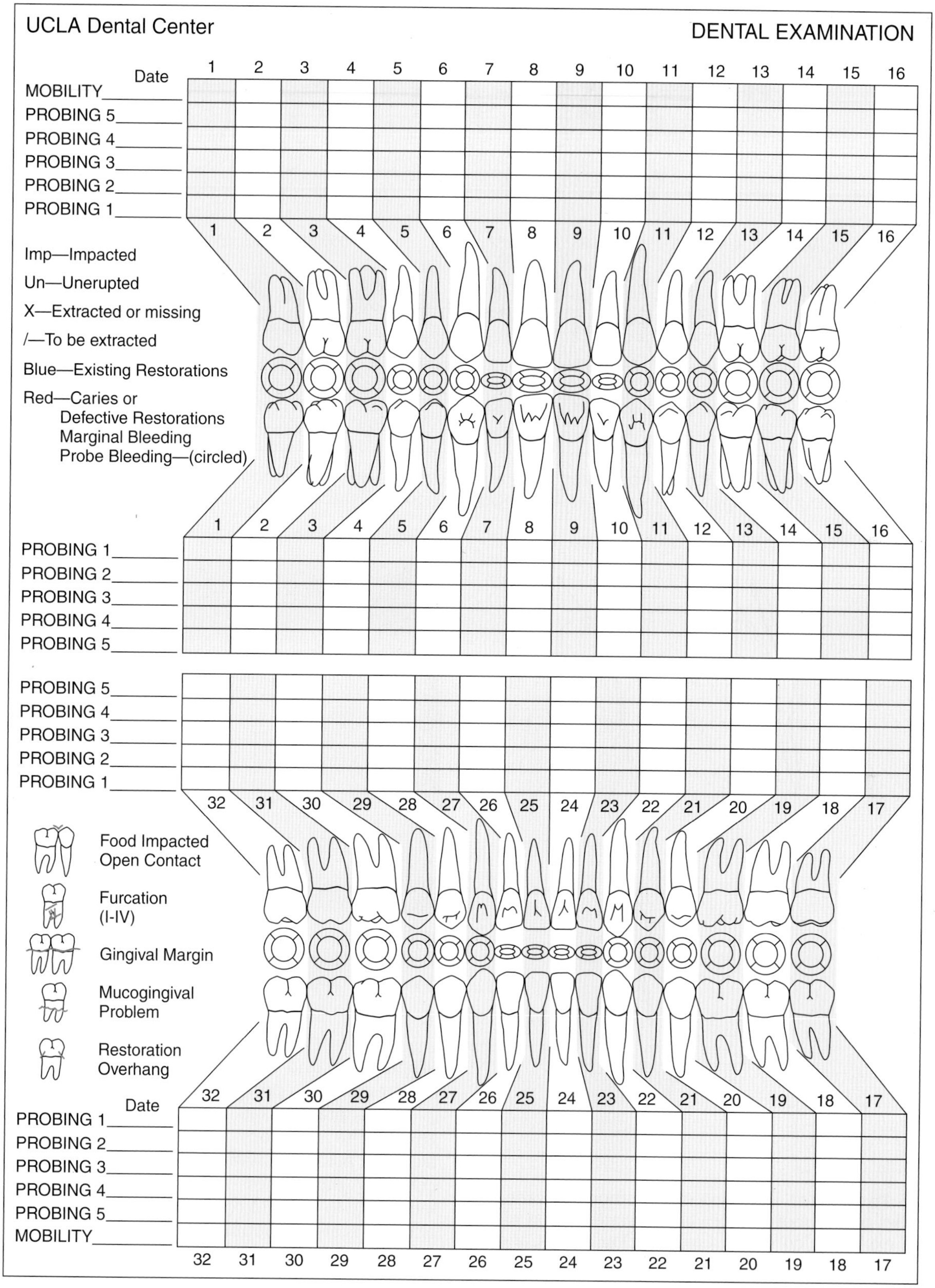

Figure 35-9 **A,** UCLA periodontal chart. (Courtesy University of California, Los Angeles School of Dentistry)

Continued

B

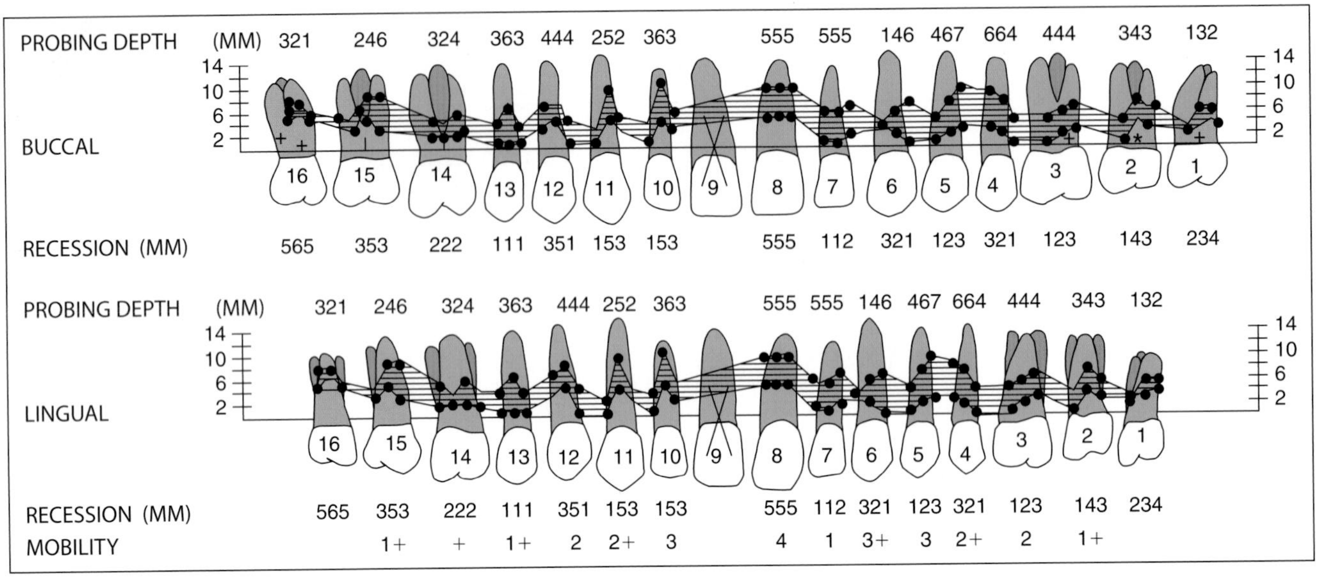

Figure 35-9 **B,** Computerized diagram showing various periodontal parameters. (Courtesy University of California, Los Angeles School of Dentistry)

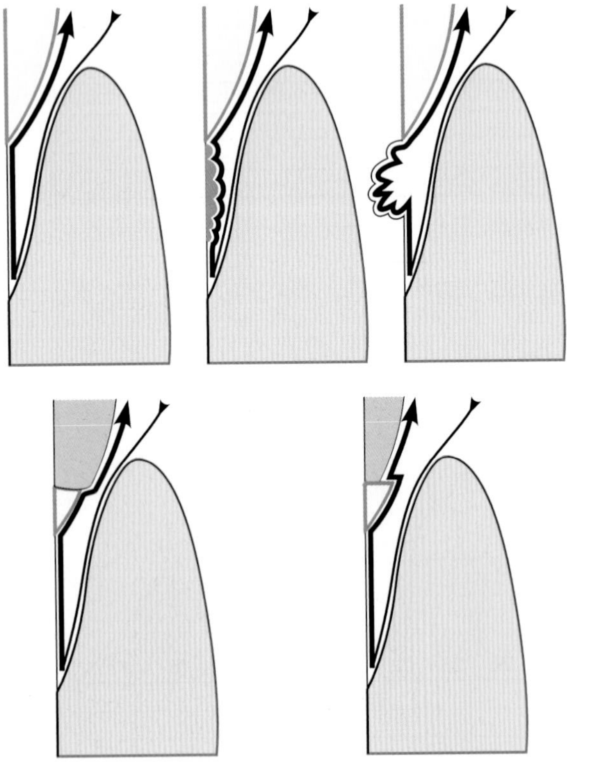

Figure 35-10 *Top left,* Detection of smoothness or various irregularities on the root surface with outward motion of a probe or explorer. *Top center,* Calculus. *Top right,* Caries. *Bottom left and right,* Irregular margins of restorations.

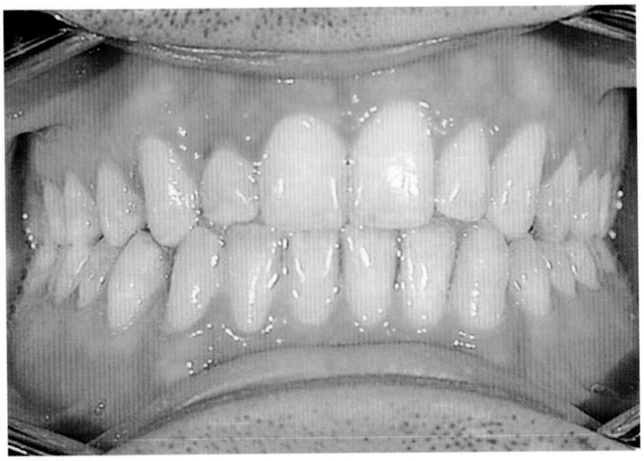

Figure 35-11 Normal gingiva, with incipient gingivitis in tooth #7. Normal surface features are better revealed by drying the gingiva.

suggest their presence, such as color changes (bluish red marginal gingiva or bluish red vertical zone extending from gingival margin to attached gingiva), a "rolled" edge separating the gingival margin from the tooth surface, or an enlarged, edematous gingiva. The presence of bleeding, suppuration, and loose, extruded teeth may also denote the presence of a pocket (Figures 35-12 to 35-15).

Periodontal pockets are generally painless but may give rise to symptoms such as localized or sometimes radiating pain or sensation of pressure after eating, which gradually diminishes. A foul taste in localized areas, sensitivity to hot and cold, and toothache in the absence of caries is also sometimes present.

Detection of Pockets. The only accurate method of detecting and measuring periodontal pockets is careful exploration with a periodontal probe. Pockets are not detected by radiographic examination. The periodontal pocket is a soft tissue change. Radiographs indicate areas of bone loss where pockets may be suspected; they do not show pocket presence or depth, and thus they show no difference before or after pocket elimination unless bone has been modified.

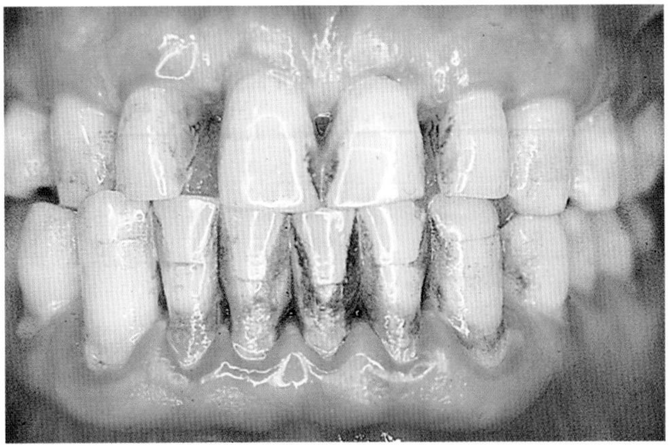

Figure 35-12 Periodontal pockets around lower anterior teeth, showing rolled margins, edematous inflammatory changes, and abundant calculus and materia alba.

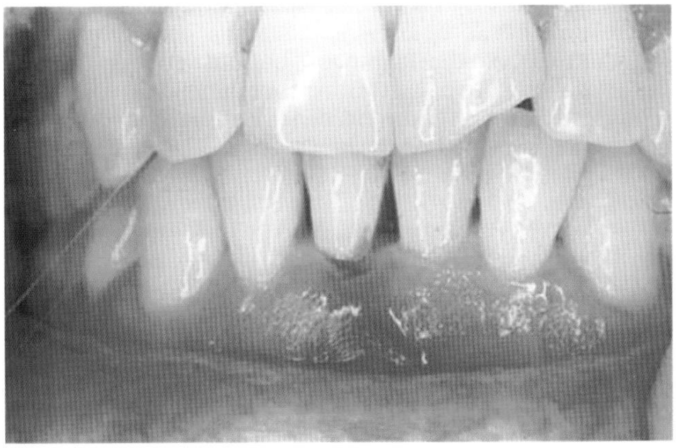

Figure 35-13 Periodontal pocket with vertical discolored zone extending to the alveolar mucosa.

Gutta percha points or calibrated silver points[22] can be used with the radiograph to assist in determining the level of attachment of periodontal pockets (Figure 35-16). They may be used effectively for individual pockets or in clinical research, but their routine use throughout the mouth would be rather cumbersome. Clinical examination and probing are more direct and efficient.

Pocket Probing. There are two different pocket depths: (1) the biologic or histologic depth and (2) the clinical or probing depth[28] (Figure 35-17) (see Chapter 4).

The *biologic depth* is the distance between the gingival margin and the base of the pocket (coronal end of junctional epithelium). This can be measured only in carefully prepared and adequately oriented histologic sections. The *probing depth* is the distance to which an ad hoc instrument (probe) penetrates into the pocket. The depth of penetration of a probe in a pocket depends on such factors as size of the probe, force of its introduction, direction of penetration, resistance of the tissues, and convexity of the crown. Probes presently used are described in Chapter 51.

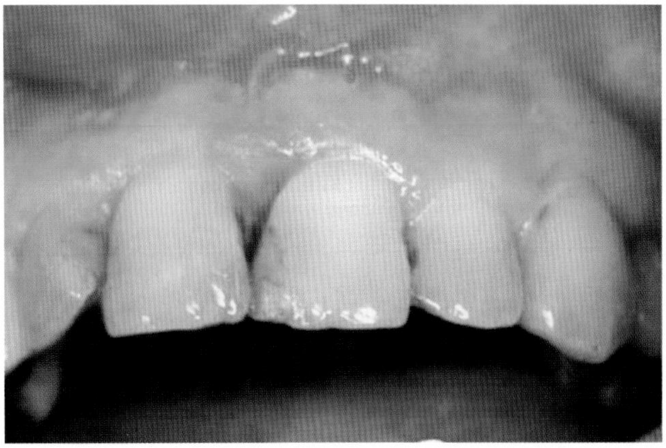

Figure 35-14 Periodontal pocket between upper central incisors produced bluish discoloration extending apically. Probing reveals presence of deep pocket.

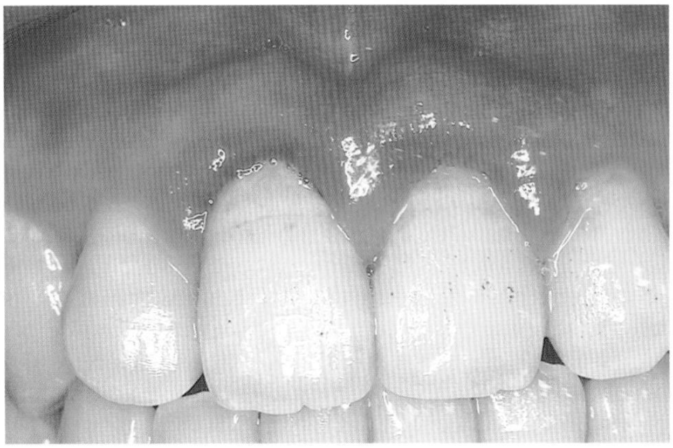

Figure 35-15 Severe generalized gingival inflammation. Note the dark hue in the marginal areas of the central incisors, which is caused in part by dark subgingival calculus and a deep pocket.

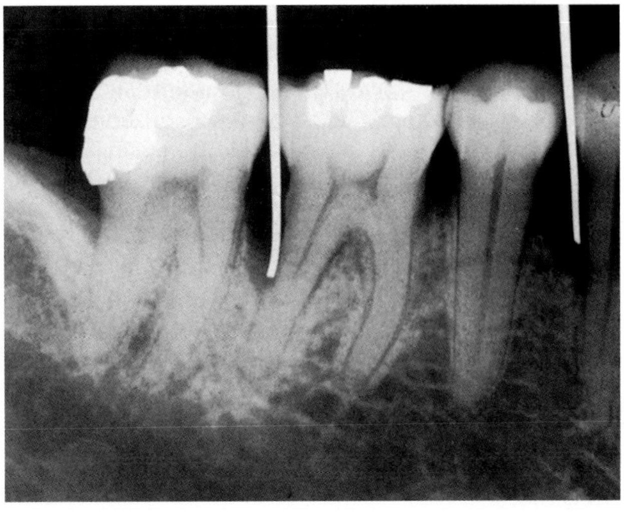

Figure 35-16 Blunted silver points assist in locating the base of pockets.

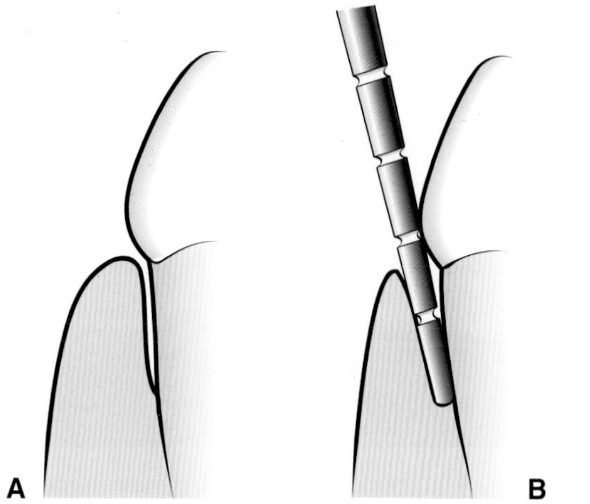

Figure 35-17 **A,** Biologic or histologic pocket depth is the actual distance between the gingival margin and the attached tissues (bottom of pocket). **B,** Probing or clinical pocket depth is the depth of penetration of the probe.

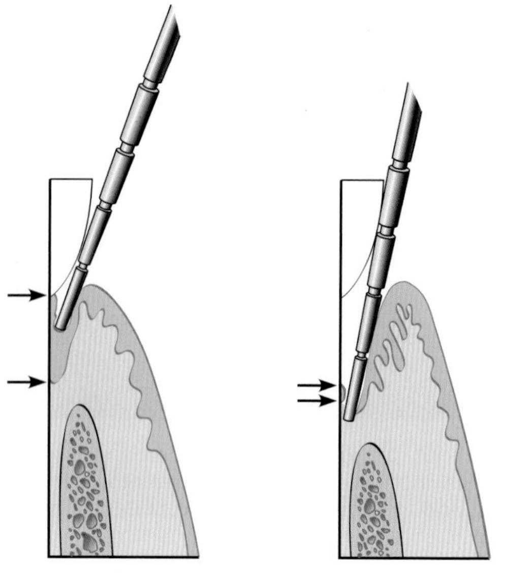

Figure 35-18 **A,** In a normal sulcus with a long junctional epithelium (between *arrows*), the probe penetrates about one-third to half the length of the junctional epithelium. **B,** In a periodontal pocket with a short junctional epithelium (between *arrows*), the probe penetrates beyond the apical end of the junctional epithelium.

Probe penetration can vary depending on the force of introduction, the shape and size of the probe tip, and the degree of tissue inflammation.[4] Several studies have attempted to determine the depth of penetration of a probe in a sulcus or pocket. Armitage et al.[5] used beagle dogs to evaluate the penetration of a probe using a standardized force of 25 grams. In healthy specimens the probe penetrated the epithelium to about two thirds of its length; in gingivitis specimens it stopped 0.1 mm short of its apical end; and in periodontitis specimens the probe tip consistently went past the most apical cells of the junctional epithelium (Figure 35-18).

In humans the probe tip penetrates to the most coronal intact fibers of the connective tissue attachment.[29,60] The depth of penetration of the probe in the connective tissue apical to the junctional epithelium in a periodontal pocket is about 0.3 mm.[29,54,60] This is important in evaluating differences in probing depth before and after treatment, because the reduction in probe penetration may be a result of reduced inflammatory response rather than gain in attachment.[28,30]

The probing forces have been explored by several investigators[14,64,65]; forces of 0.75 N have been found to be well tolerated and accurate.[62] Interexaminer error (depth discrepancies between examiners) was reported to be as much as 2.1 mm (average of 1.5 mm) in the same areas.[21]

Probing Technique. The probe should be inserted parallel to the vertical axis of the tooth and "walked" circumferentially around each surface of each tooth to detect the areas of deepest penetration (Figure 35-19).

In addition, special attention should be directed to detecting the presence of interdental craters and furcation involvements. To detect an *interdental crater,* the probe should be placed obliquely from both the facial and the lingual surface to explore the deepest point of the pocket located beneath the contact point (Figure 35-20). In multirooted teeth the possibility of *furcation involvement* should be carefully explored. The use of specially

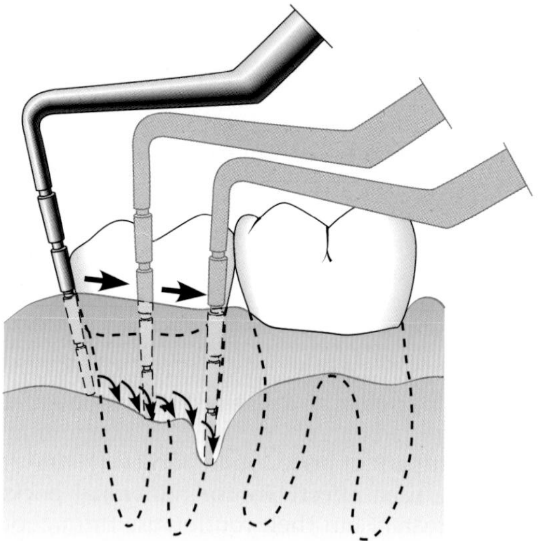

Figure 35-19 "Walking" the probe to explore the entire pocket.

designed probes (e.g., Nabers probe) allows an easier and more accurate exploration of the horizontal component of furcation lesions (Figure 35-21).

Level of Attachment Versus Pocket Depth. *Pocket depth* is the distance between the base of the pocket and the gingival margin. It may change from time to time even in untreated periodontal disease because of changes in the position of the gingival margin, and therefore it may be unrelated to the existing attachment of the tooth.

The *level of attachment,* on the other hand, is the distance between the base of the pocket and a fixed point

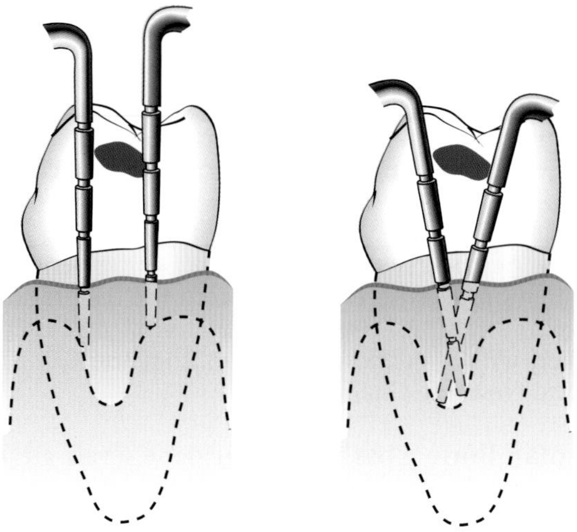

Figure 35-20 Vertical insertion of the probe *(left)* may not detect interdental craters; oblique positioning of the probe *(right)* reaches the depth of the crater.

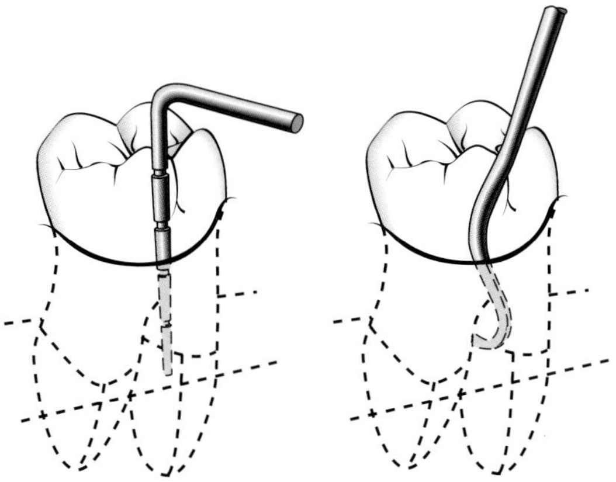

Figure 35-21 Exploring with a periodontal probe *(left)* may not detect furcation involvement; specially designed instruments (Nabers probe) *(right)* can enter the furcation area.

on the crown, such as the cementoenamel junction (CEJ). Changes in the level of attachment can be caused only by gain or loss of attachment and thus provide a better indication of the degree of periodontal destruction. *Shallow pockets attached at the level of the apical third of the root connote more severe destruction than deep pockets attached at the coronal third of the roots* (see Chapter 27 and Figures 27-19 and 27-20).

Determining the level of Attachment. When the *gingival margin is located on the anatomic crown,* the level of attachment is determined by subtracting from the depth of the pocket the distance from the gingival margin to the CEJ. If both are the same, the loss of attachment is zero.

When the *gingival margin coincides with the CEJ,* the loss of attachment equals the pocket depth.

When the *gingival margin is located apical to the CEJ,* the loss of attachment is greater than the pocket depth, and therefore the distance between the CEJ and the gingival margin should be added to the pocket depth. Drawing the gingival margin on the chart where pocket depths are entered helps clarify this important point.

Bleeding on Probing. The insertion of a probe to the bottom of the pocket elicits bleeding if the gingiva is inflamed and the pocket epithelium is atrophic or ulcerated. Noninflamed sites rarely bleed. In most cases, bleeding on probing is an earlier sign of inflammation than gingival color changes[36] (see Chapter 22). In some cases, however, color changes are found with no bleeding on probing.[17] Depending on the severity of inflammation, bleeding can vary from a tenuous red line along the gingival sulcus to profuse bleeding.[1] After successful treatment, bleeding on probing ceases.[3]

To test for bleeding after probing, the probe is carefully introduced to the bottom of the pocket and gently moved laterally along the pocket wall. In some patients, bleeding appears immediately after removal of the probe; in others it may be delayed a few seconds. Therefore the clinician should recheck for bleeding 30 to 60 seconds after probing.

As a single test, bleeding on probing is not a good predictor of progressive attachment loss; however, its absence is an excellent predictor of periodontal stability.[4] When present in multiple sites of advanced disease, bleeding on probing is a good indicator of progressive attachment loss.[4,20] Performing a meta-analysis on this subject to 1996, Armitage[4] concluded that the presence of bleeding on probing in a "treated and maintained patient population" is an important risk predictor for increased loss of attachment.

Insertion of a soft wooden interdental stimulator in the interdental space produces a similar bleeding response.[3] The patient can use this to self-examine the gingiva for inflammation.[11]

When to Probe. Probing of pockets is done at various times for diagnosis and for monitoring the course of treatment and maintenance. The initial probing of moderate or advanced cases is usually hampered by the presence of heavy inflammation and abundant calculus and cannot be done accurately. The purpose of this initial probing, however, together with the clinical and radiographic examination, is to determine whether the tooth can be saved or should be extracted. After the patient has performed adequate plaque control over time and calculus has been removed, the major inflammatory changes disappear, and a more accurate probing of the pockets can be performed. The purpose of this second probing is to establish accurately the level of attachment and degree of involvement of roots and furcations. Data obtained from this probing provide valuable information for treatment decisions.

Later in periodontal treatment, probings are done to determine changes in pocket depth and to ascertain healing progress after different procedures.

Probing Around Implants. Periimplantitis can create pockets around implants, so probing around the implants becomes part of the examination and diagnosis. To prevent scratching of the implant surface, plastic periodontal probes should be used instead of the usual steel probes used for the natural dentition.

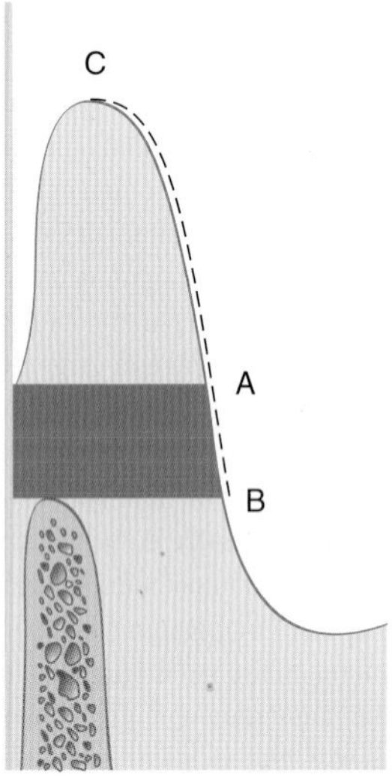

Figure 35-22 Shaded area shows the attached gingiva, which extends between the projection on the external surface of the bottom of the pocket **(A)** and the mucogingival junction **(B)**. The keratinized gingiva may extend from the mucogingival junction **(B)** to the gingival margin **(C)**.

Determination of Disease Activity. The determination of pocket depth or attachment levels does not provide information on whether the lesion is in an active or inactive state. Currently, no sure method exists to determine activity or inactivity of a lesion. Inactive lesions may show little or no bleeding on probing and minimal amounts of gingival fluid; the bacterial flora, as revealed by dark-field microscopy, consists mostly of coccoid cells. Active lesions bleed more readily on probing and have large amounts of fluid and exudate; their bacterial flora shows a greater number of spirochetes and motile bacteria.[18] In patients with aggressive periodontitis, progressing and nonprogressing sites may show no differences in bleeding on probing.[31]

The precise determination of disease activity has a direct influence on diagnosis, prognosis, and therapy. The goals of therapy may change, depending on the state of the periodontal lesion (see Chapter 37).

Amount of Attached Gingiva. It is important to establish the relation between the bottom of the pocket and the mucogingival line. The width of the *attached* gingiva is the distance between the mucogingival junction and the projection on the external surface of the bottom of the gingival sulcus or the periodontal pocket. It should not be confused with the width of the *keratinized* gingiva, which also includes the marginal gingiva (Figure 35-22).

The width of the attached gingiva is determined by subtracting the sulcus or pocket depth from the total width of the gingiva (gingival margin to mucogingival line). This is done by stretching the lip or cheek to demarcate the mucogingival line while the pocket is being probed (Figure 35-23). The amount of attached gingiva is generally considered to be insufficient when stretching of the lip or cheek induces movement of the free gingival margin.

Other methods used to determine the amount of attached gingiva include pushing the adjacent mucosa coronally with a dull instrument or painting the mucosa with Schiller's potassium iodide solution, which stains keratin.

Degree of Gingival Recession. During periodontal examination, it is necessary to record the data regarding the amount of gingival recession. This measurement is taken with a periodontal probe from the CEJ to the gingival crest (see Chapter 22).

Alveolar Bone Loss. Alveolar bone levels are evaluated by clinical and radiographic examination. Probing is helpful for determining (1) the height and contour of the facial and lingual bones obscured on the radiograph by the dense roots and (2) the architecture of the interdental bone. Transgingival probing, performed after the area is anesthetized, is a more accurate method of evaluation and provides additional information on bone architecture[16,25,,62] (see Chapter 66).

Palpation. Palpating the oral mucosa in the lateral and apical areas of the tooth may help locate the origin of radiating pain that the patient cannot localize. Infection deep in the periodontal tissues and the early stages of a periodontal abscess may also be detected by palpation.

Suppuration. The presence of an abundant number of neutrophils in the gingival fluid transforms it into a purulent exudate.[4] Several studies[7,8,11,23] have evaluated the association between suppuration and the progression of periodontitis and reported that this sign is present in a very low percentage of sites with the disease (3%-5%).[4] Therefore, suppuration by itself is not a good indicator.

Clinically, the presence of pus in a periodontal pocket is determined by placing the ball of the index finger along the lateral aspect of the marginal gingiva and applying pressure in a rolling motion toward the crown (Figure 35-24). Visual examination without digital pressure is insufficient; the purulent exudate is formed in the inner pocket wall, and therefore the external appearance may give no indication of its presence. Pus formation does not occur in all periodontal pockets, but digital pressure often reveals it in pockets where its presence is not suspected.

Periodontal Abscess. A periodontal abscess is a localized accumulation of pus within the gingival wall of a periodontal pocket (see Chapter 27). Periodontal abscesses may be acute or chronic.

The *acute periodontal abscess* appears as an ovoid elevation of the gingiva along the lateral aspect of the root (Figures 35-25, 35-26, and 35-27). The gingiva is edematous and red, with a smooth, shiny surface. The shape and consistency of the elevated area vary; the area may be domelike and relatively firm or pointed and soft. In most cases, pus may be expressed from the gingival margin with gentle digital pressure.

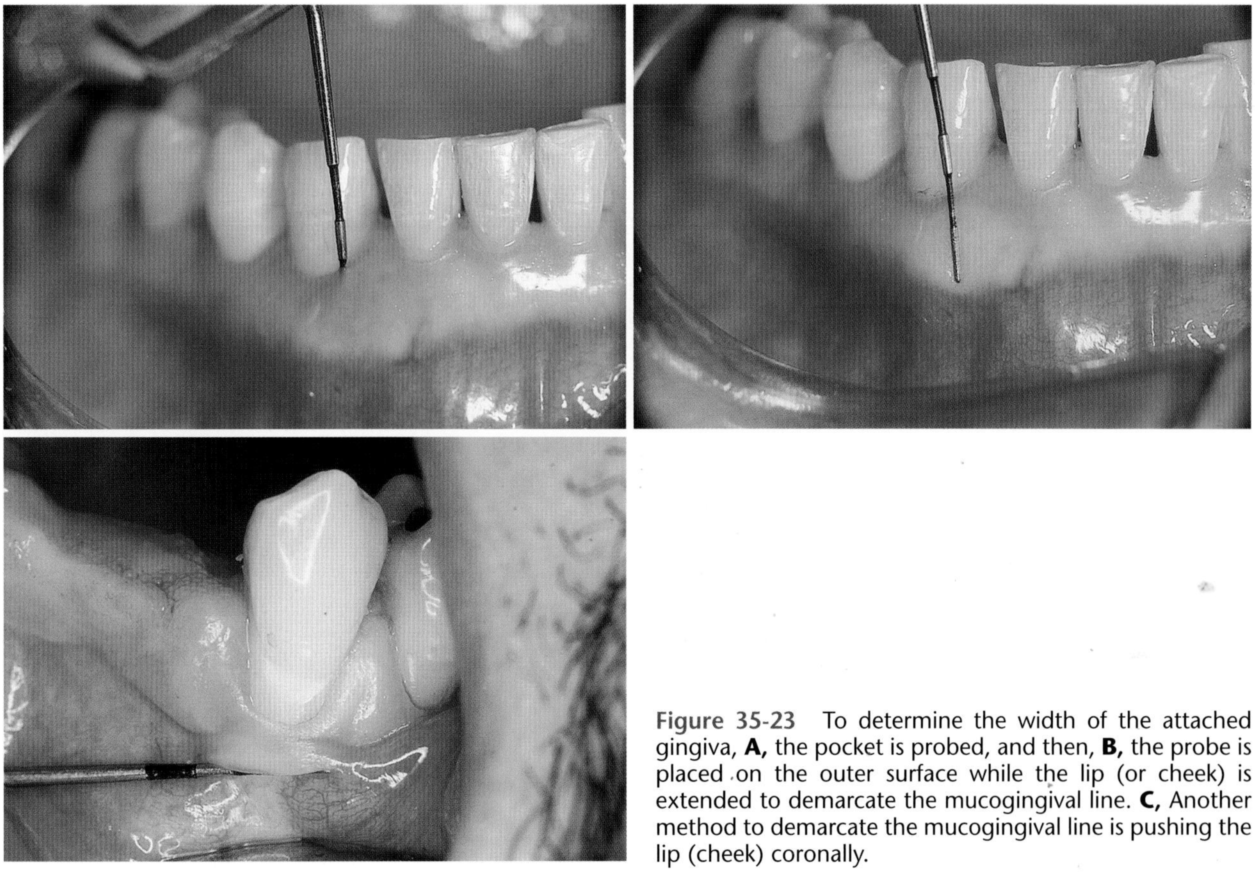
A B C

Figure 35-23 To determine the width of the attached gingiva, **A,** the pocket is probed, and then, **B,** the probe is placed on the outer surface while the lip (or cheek) is extended to demarcate the mucogingival line. **C,** Another method to demarcate the mucogingival line is pushing the lip (cheek) coronally.

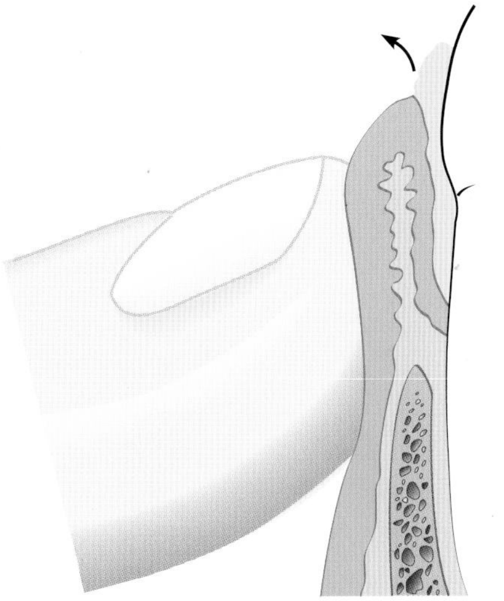

Figure 35-24 Purulent exudate expressed from a periodontal pocket by digital pressure.

The acute periodontal abscess is accompanied by symptoms such as throbbing, radiating pain; exquisite tenderness of the gingiva to palpation; sensitivity of the tooth to palpation; tooth mobility; lymphadenitis; and less frequently, systemic effects such as fever, leukocytosis, and malaise. Occasionally the patient may have symptoms of an acute periodontal abscess without any notable clinical lesion or radiographic changes.

The *chronic periodontal abscess* usually presents a sinus that opens onto the gingival mucosa somewhere along the length of the root. There may be a history of intermittent exudation. The orifice of the sinus may appear as a difficult-to-detect pinpoint opening, which reveals a sinus tract deep in the periodontium when probed (Figure 35-28). The sinus may be covered by a small, pink, beadlike mass of granulation tissue (Figure 35-29).

The chronic periodontal abscess is usually asymptomatic. However, the patient may report episodes of dull, gnawing pain; slight elevation of the tooth; and a desire to bite down on and grind the tooth. The chronic periodontal abscess often undergoes acute exacerbations, with all the associated symptoms.

Diagnosis of the periodontal abscess requires correlation of the history and the clinical and radiographic findings. The suspected area should be probed carefully along the gingival margin in relation to each tooth surface to detect a channel from the marginal area to the deeper periodontal tissues. Continuity of the lesion with the gingival margin is clinical evidence that the abscess is periodontal.

The abscess is not necessarily located on the same surface of the root as the pocket from which it is formed. A pocket at the facial surface may give rise to a periodontal abscess interproximally. A periodontal abscess often is located at a root surface other than the surface along which the pocket originated, because drainage is more likely to be impaired when a pocket follows a tortuous course.

A 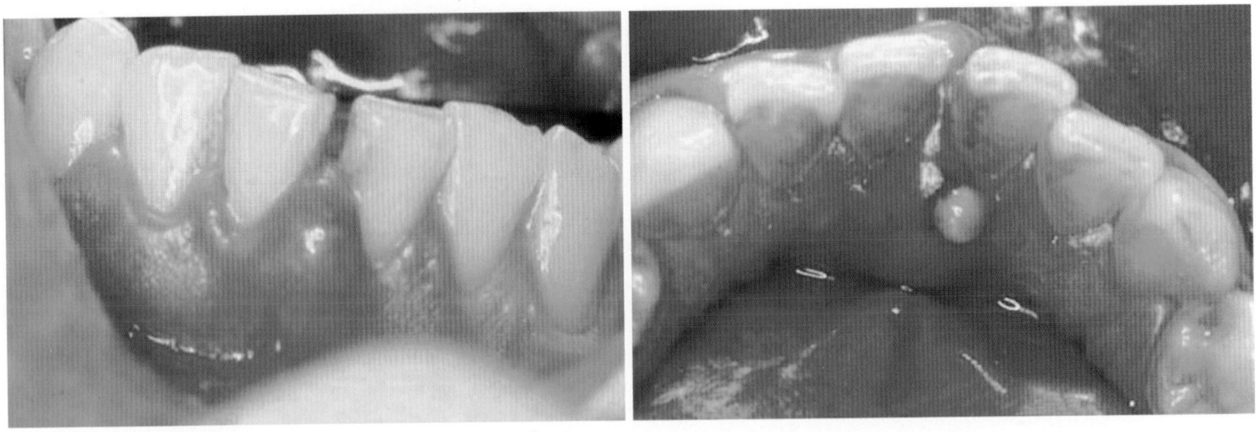 B

Figure 35-25 **A,** Facial view of acute periodontal abscess between the lower central incisors. **B,** Lingual view of the same patient with a suppurating draining sinus.

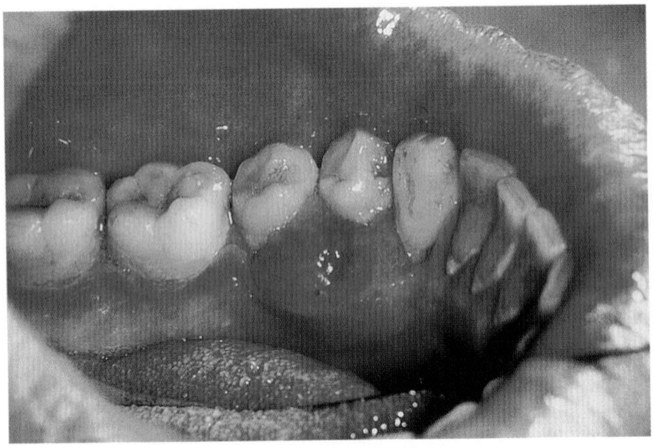

Figure 35-26 Acute periodontal abscess in the wall of a deep pocket in the lingual surface of lower premolars.

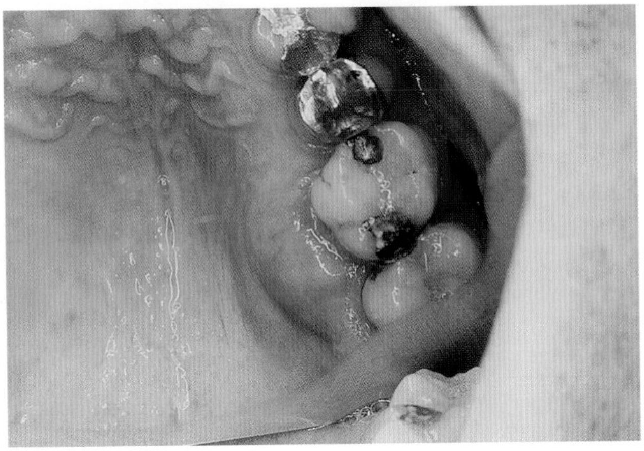

Figure 35-27 Acute periodontal abscess associated with a deep periodontal pocket in palatal area of first and second upper molars. Note how the fibrotic character of the palatal tissue masks the typical changes of the abscess.

A 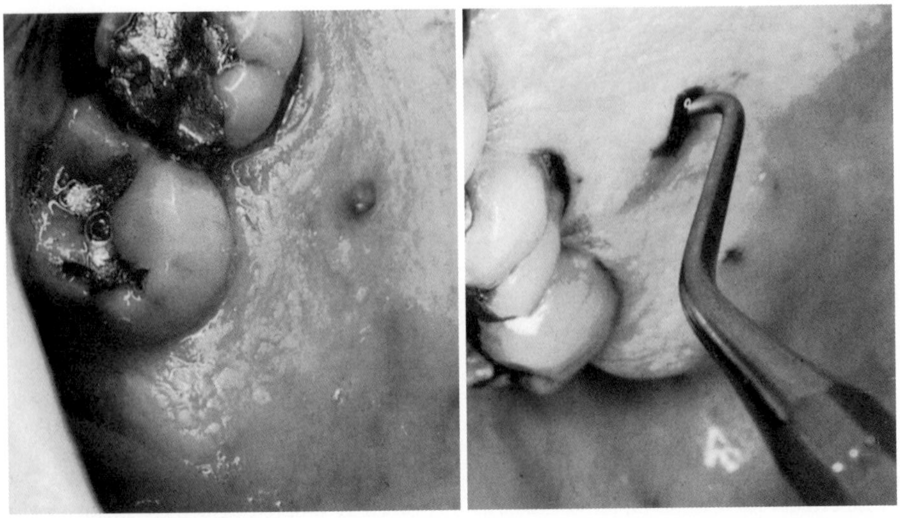 B

Figure 35-28 Sinus orifice from a palatal periodontal abscess. **A,** Pinpoint orifice on the palate indicative of a sinus from a periodontal abscess. **B,** Probe extends into the abscess deep in the periodontium.

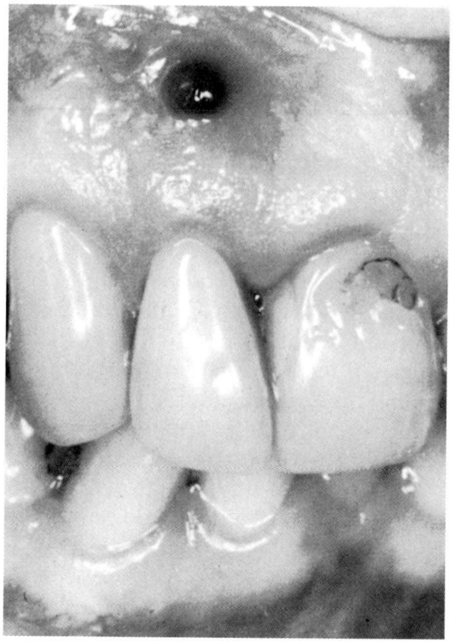

Figure 35-29 Nodular mass at the orifice of a draining sinus.

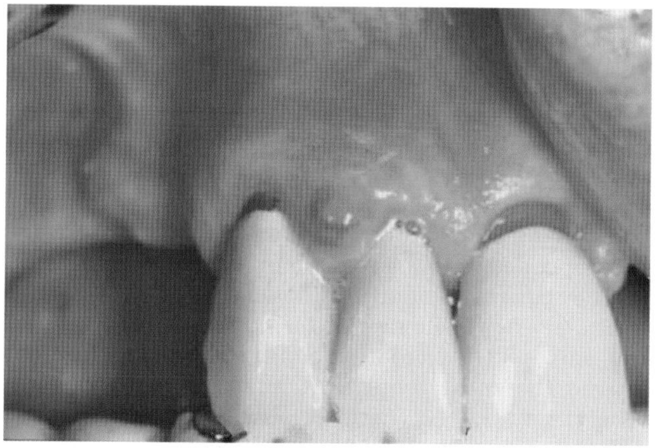

Figure 35-30 Gingival abscess between upper lateral incisor and canine.

In children a sinus orifice along the lateral aspect of a root is usually the result of periapical infection of a deciduous tooth. In the permanent dentition such an orifice may be caused by a periodontal abscess, as well as by apical involvement. The orifice may be patent and draining, or it may be closed and appear as a red, nodular mass (see Figure 35-29). Exploration of such masses with a probe usually reveals a pinpoint orifice that communicates with an underlying sinus.

Periodontal Abscess and Gingival Abscess. The principal differences between the periodontal abscess and the gingival abscess are location and history (see Chapters 23 and 58). The gingival abscess is confined to the marginal gingiva and often occurs in previously disease-free areas (Figure 35-30). Also, the gingival abscess is usually an acute inflammatory response to the forcing of foreign material into the gingiva. The periodontal abscess involves the supporting periodontal structures and generally occurs in the course of chronic destructive periodontitis.

SCIENCE TRANSFER

The evaluation of a patient for periodontal disease must be comprehensive because systemic conditions can influence oral health and periodontal disease can influence systemic health. Thus the evaluation must include medical and dental histories and extraoral and oral examinations. In the oral examination, visual changes, radiographic analyses, and periodontal probing provide valuable information in determining a diagnosis for the patient. Most findings, however, are related to past disease, and it is impossible to determine if the disease is active or inactive on a cross-sectional examination. A major difficulty in diagnosis is the vast area for potential disease; breakdown may occur at any location around any of the teeth. Inflammation is an important aspect of the disease process, however, and thus the general elimination of inflammation is the overriding principle of periodontal treatment.

To detect periodontal disease, each patient must have a thorough periodontal examination. This includes probing data on six surfaces of each tooth, as well as the recording of any gingival recession and bleeding on probing. Other parameters that need to be recorded include mobility, furcation involvement, mucogingival deficiencies, plaque scores, and open contacts. Epidemiologic diagnostic procedures are inadequate for individual patient care and should be restricted to use in population-based surveys.

Periodontal Abscess and Periapical Abscess. Several characteristics can be used as guidelines in differentiating a periodontal abscess from a periapical abscess. If the tooth is nonvital, the lesion is most likely periapical. However, a previously nonvital tooth can have a deep periodontal pocket that can abscess. Moreover, a deep periodontal pocket can extend to the apex and cause pulpal involvement and necrosis.

An apical abscess may spread along the lateral aspect of the root to the gingival margin. However, when the apex and lateral surface of a root are involved by a single lesion that can be probed directly from the gingival margin, the lesion is more likely to have originated in a periodontal abscess.

Radiographic findings are sometimes helpful in differentiating between a periodontal and a periapical lesion (see Chapter 36). Early acute periodontal and periapical abscesses present no radiographic changes. Ordinarily, a radiolucent area along the lateral surface of the root suggests the presence of a periodontal abscess, whereas apical rarefaction suggests a periapical abscess. However, acute periodontal abscesses that show no radiographic changes often cause symptoms in teeth with long-standing, radiographically detectable periapical lesions that are not contributing to the patient's complaint. Clinical findings, such as the presence of extensive caries, pocket formation, lack of tooth vitality, and the existence of continuity between the gingival margin and the abscess area, often prove to be of greater diagnostic value than radiographic appearance.

A draining sinus on the lateral aspect of the root suggests periodontal rather than apical involvement; a sinus from a periapical lesion is more likely to be located farther apically. However, sinus location is not conclusive. In many cases, particularly in children, the sinus from a periapical lesion drains on the side of the root rather than at the apex (see Chapter 58).

LABORATORY AIDS TO CLINICAL DIAGNOSIS

When the dentist detects unusual gingival or periodontal problems that cannot be explained by local causes, the possibility of contributing systemic factors must be explored. The signs and symptoms of oral manifestations of systemic disease must be clearly understood and analyzed and their presence discussed with the patient's physician.

Numerous laboratory tests aid in the diagnosis of systemic diseases. Standard texts on the subject provide descriptions on how these tests are performed and how the findings are interpreted.

Nutritional Status

If the dentist suspects a nutritional deficiency when examining a patient, this suspicion must be corroborated by a medical evaluation of the patient's nutritional status. Nutritional therapy in the treatment of periodontal disturbances must be based on a demonstrated need, which is best determined by a nutritionist.

Certain signs and symptoms have been identified with different nutritional deficiencies. However, many patients with nutritional disease do not exhibit classic signs of deficiency disorders, and different types of deficiency produce comparable clinical findings. Clinical findings are suggestive, but definitive diagnosis of nutritional deficiencies and their nature requires the combined information revealed by the history, clinical and laboratory findings, and therapeutic trial. Clinical findings identified with specific nutritional deficiencies and the oral manifestations of nutritional disorders are described in Chapter 17.

Patients with Special Diets for Medical Reasons

Patients who follow low-residue, nondetergent diets often develop gingivitis because the prescribed foods lack cleansing action, increasing the tendency for plaque and food debris to accumulate on the teeth. Because fibrous foods are contraindicated, special effort is made to compensate for the soft diet by emphasizing the patient's oral hygiene measures. Patients following salt-free diets should not be given saline mouthwashes and should not be treated with saline preparations without consulting their physician. Diabetes, gallbladder disease, and hypertension are examples of conditions in which particular care should be taken to avoid the prescription of contraindicated foodstuffs in the diet.

Blood Tests

Analyses of blood smears, blood cell counts, white blood cell differential counts, and erythrocyte sedimentation rates are used to evaluate the presence of blood dyscrasias and generalized infections. Determination of coagulation time, bleeding time, clot retraction time, prothrombin time, capillary fragility test, and bone marrow studies may be required for some patients. These tests may be useful aids in the differential diagnosis of certain types of periodontal diseases (see hematology texts for further consideration of this subject).

Chapter 44 describes the use of these tests for the evaluation and management of medically compromised patients.

PERIODONTAL SCREENING AND RECORDING SYSTEM*

A method for periodontal screening and recording (PSR) has been developed jointly by the American Academy of Periodontology and the American Dental Association, with the support of the Procter & Gamble Company.[45] This method is designed for easier and faster screening and recording of the periodontal status of a patient by a general practitioner or a dental hygienist. It uses a specially designed probe that has a 0.5-mm ball tip and is color-coded from 3.5 to 5.5 mm (Figure 35-31, *A*).

The patient's mouth is divided into six sextants (maxillary right, anterior, and left; mandibular left, anterior, and right). Each tooth is probed, by walking the probe around the entire tooth to examine at least six points around each tooth: mesiofacial, midfacial, distofacial, and the corresponding lingual/palatal areas. The deepest finding is recorded in each sextant, along with other findings, according to the following codes:

Code 0: In the deepest sulcus of the sextant, the probe's colored band remains completely visible. Gingival tissue is healthy and does not bleed on gentle probing. No calculus or defective margins are found. These patients require only appropriate preventive care.

Code 1: The colored band of the probe remains completely visible in the deepest sulcus of the sextant; no calculus or defective margins are found, but some bleeding after gentle probing is detected. Treatment for these patients consists of subgingival plaque removal and appropriate oral hygiene instructions.

Code 2: The probe's colored band is still completely visible, but there is bleeding on probing, and

*Periodontal Screening & Recording™ and PSR® are service marks and trademarks of the American Dental Association.

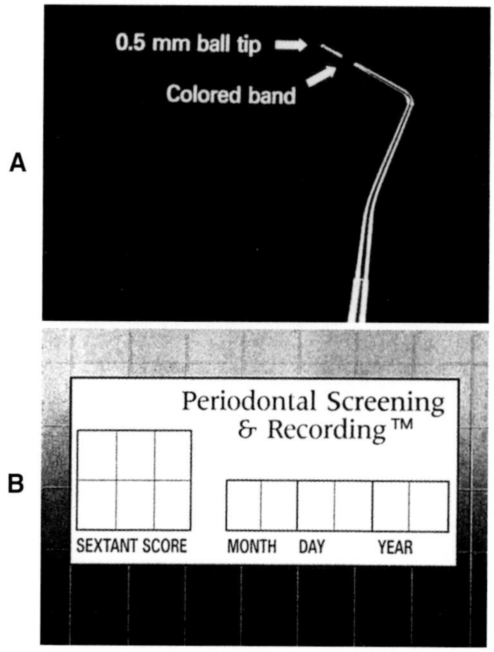

Figure 35-31 **A,** Periodontal probe especially designed for the PSR system. Note the ball tip and the color coding, 3.5 to 5.5 mm from the probe tip. **B,** Special sticker to be placed in the patient's chart with the code for each sextant. (From *Periodontal Screening & Recording training manual,* American Dental Association, American Academy of Periodontology, sponsored by Procter & Gamble, 1992.)

supragingival or subgingival calculus and/or defective margins are found. Treatment should include plaque and calculus removal, correction of plaque-retentive margins of restorations, and oral hygiene instruction.

Code 3: The colored band is partially submerged. This indicates the need for a comprehensive periodontal examination and charting of the affected sextant to determine the necessary treatment plan. If two or more sextants score Code 3, a comprehensive full-mouth examination and charting are indicated.

Code 4: The colored band completely disappears in the pocket, indicating a depth greater than 5.5 mm. A comprehensive full-mouth periodontal examination, charting, and treatment planning are needed.

Code:* When any of the following abnormalities are seen, an asterisk (*) is entered, in addition to the code number: furcation involvement, tooth mobility, mucogingival problem, or gingival recession extending to the colored band of the probe (3.5 mm or greater).

The code finding for each sextant and the date are entered on a sticker (Figure 35-31, *B*), which is placed on the patient's record.

REFERENCES

1. Abrams K, Caton J, Polson AM: Histologic comparisons of interproximal gingival tissues related to the presence or absence of bleeding, *J Periodontol* 55:629, 1984.
2. Alexander AG, Tipnis AK: The effect of irregularity of teeth and the degree of overbite and overjet on the gingival health, *Br Dent J* 128:539, 1970.
3. Amato R, Caton J, Polson A, et al: Interproximal gingival inflammation related to the conversion of a bleeding to a non-bleeding state, *J Periodontol* 57:63, 1986.
4. Armitage GC: Periodontal diseases: diagnosis, *Ann Periodontol* 1:37, 1996.
5. Armitage GC, Svanberg GK, Löe H: Microscopic evaluation of clinical measurements of connective tissue attachment levels, *J Clin Periodontol* 4:173, 1977.
6. Arstad T: *The capsular ligaments of the temporomandibular joint and retrusion facets of the dentition in relationship to mandibular movements,* Oslo, Norway, 1954, Akademisk Forlag.
7. Badersten A, Nilvéus R, Egelberg J: Effect of nonsurgical therapy. VII. Bleeding, suppuration and probing depth in sites with probing attachment loss, *J Clin Periodontol* 12:432, 1985.
8. Badersten A, Nilvéus R, Egelberg J: Scores of plaque, bleeding, suppuration and probing depth to predict probing attachment loss: five years of observation following nonsurgical periodontal therapy, *J Clin Periodontol* 7:102, 1990.
9. Baumgartner HS: A voice-input computerized dental examination system using high resolution graphics, *Compend Contin Educ Dent* 9:446, 1988.
10. Beyron HI: Occlusal changes in the adult dentition, *J Am Dent Assoc* 48:674, 1954.
11. Caton J, Polson A: The interdental bleeding index: a simplified procedure to monitor gingival health, *Compend Contin Educ Dent* 6:89, 1985.
12. Egermark-Erikson I, Carlsson GE, Ingervall B: Prevalence of mandibular dysfunction and orofacial parafunction in 7-, 11-, and 15-year old Swedish children, *Eur J Orthop* 13:163, 1981.
13. Fischman SL, Picozzi A: Review of the literature: the methodology of clinical calculus evaluation, *J Periodontol* 40:607, 1969.
14. Gabathuler H, Hassel TM: A pressure sensitive periodontal probe, *Helv Odontol Acta* 15:114, 1971.
15. Grant DA, Grant DA, Flynn MJ, et al: Periodontal microbiota of mobile and non-mobile teeth, *J Periodontol* 66:386, 1995.
16. Greenberg J, Laster L, Listgarten MA: Transgingival probing as a potential estimator of alveolar bone level, *J Periodontol* 47:514, 1976.
17. Greenstein G: The role of bleeding upon probing in the diagnosis of periodontal disease. A literature review, *J Periodontol* 55:684, 1984.
18. Greenstein G, Caton J, Polson AM: Histologic characteristics associated with bleeding after probing and visual signs of inflammation, *J Periodontol* 52:420, 1981.
19. Grippo JO, Simring M, Schreiner S: Attrition, abrasion, corrosion and adfraction revisited, *J Am Dent Assoc* 135:1109, 2004.
20. Haffajee, AD, Socransky, SS, Lindhe, J et al: Clinical risk indicators for periodontal attachment loss, *J Clin Periodontol* 18:117, 1991.
21. Hassel TM, German MA, Saxer UP: Periodontal probing: interinvestigator discrepancies and correlations between probing force and recorded depth, *Helv Odontol Acta* 17:38, 1973.
22. Hirschfeld L: A calibrated silver point for periodontal diagnosis and recording, *J Periodontol* 24:94, 1953.
23. Kaldahl WB, Kalkwarf KL, Patil KD, et al: Relationship of gingival bleeding, gingival suppuration and supragingival plaque to attachment loss, *J Periodontol* 61:347, 1990.
24. Kitchen PC: The prevalence of tooth root exposure and the relation of the extent of such exposure to the degree of abrasion in differing age classes, *J Dent Res* 20:565, 1941.

25. Kim HY, Yi SW, Choi SH, et al: Bone probing measurement as a reliable evaluation of the bone level in periodontal defects, *J Periodontol* 71:729, 2000.
26. Kurashima K: Viscoelastic properties of periodontal tissue, *Bull Tokyo Med Dent Univ* 12:240, 1965.
27. Lambrechts P, Braem M, Vuylsteke-Wanters M, Vanherle G: Quantitative in vivo wear of human enamel, *J Dent Res* 68:1752, 1989.
28. Listgarten MA: Periodontal probing: what does it mean? *J Clin Periodontol* 7:165, 1980.
29. Listgarten MA, Mao R, Robinson PJ: Periodontal probing: the relationship of the probe tip to periodontal tissues, *J Periodontol* 47:511, 1976.
30. Magnusson I, Listgarten MA: Histological evaluation of probing depth following periodontal treatment, *J Clin Periodontol* 7:26, 1980.
31. Mandell RL, Ebersole JL, Socransky SS: Clinical, immunologic and microbiologic features of active disease sites in juvenile periodontitis, *J Clin Periodontol* 14:534, 1987.
32. Manly RS: Abrasion of cementum and dentin by modern dentifrices, *J Dent Res* 20:583, 1941.
33. Manly RS: Factors influencing tests on the abrasion of dentin by brushing with dentifrices, *J Dent Res* 23:59, 1944.
34. Mannerberg F: Saliva factors in cases of erosion, *Odont Rev* 14:156, 1963.
35. McCay CM, Wills L: Erosion of molar teeth by acid beverages, *J Nutr* 39:313, 1949.
36. Meitner SW, Zander HA, Iker HP, et al: Identification of inflamed gingival surfaces, *J Clin Periodontol* 6:93, 1979.
37. Miller WD: Experiments and observations on the wasting of tooth tissue variously designated as erosion, abrasion, chemical abrasion, denudation, etc., *Dent Cosmos* 49:1, 1907.
38. Mühlemann HR: Ten years of tooth mobility measurements, *J Periodontol* 31:110, 1960.
39. Mühlemann HR: Tooth mobility: a review of clinical aspects and research findings, *J Periodontol* 38:686, 1967.
40. Mühlemann HR, Savdir S, Rateitschak KH: Tooth mobility: its causes and significance, *J Periodontol* 36:148, 1965.
41. O'Leary TJ: Tooth mobility, *Dent Clin North Am* 3:567, 1969.
42. O'Leary TJ, Rudd KD: An instrument for measuring horizontal mobility, *Periodontics* 1:249, 1963.
43. Parfitt GJ: Measurement of the physiologic mobility of individual teeth in an axial direction, *J Dent Res* 39:608, 1960.
44. Parfitt GJ: The dynamics of a tooth in function, *J Periodontol* 32:102, 1961.
45. *Periodontal Screening & Recording training manual,* American Academy of Periodontology, American Dental Association, sponsored by Procter & Gamble, 1992.
46. Perlitsch MJ: A systematic approach to the interpretation of tooth mobility and clinical implications, *Dent Clin North Am* 24:177, 1980.
47. Persson R: Assessment of tooth mobility using small loads. II. Effect of oral hygiene procedures, *J Clin Periodontol* 7:506, 1980.
48. Persson R: Assessment of tooth mobility using small loads. III. Effect of periodontal treatment including a gingivectomy procedure, *J Clin Periodontol* 8:4, 1981.
49. Persson R: Assessment of tooth mobility using small loads. IV. The effect of periodontal treatment including gingivectomy and flap procedures, *J Clin Periodontol* 8:88, 1981.
50. Persson R, Svensson A: Assessment of tooth mobility using small loads. I. Technical devices and calculations of tooth mobility in periodontal health and disease, *J Clin Periodontol* 7:259, 1980.
51. Ratcliff PA, Johnson PW: The relationship between malodor, gingivitis and periodontitis: a review, *J Periodontol* 70:485, 1999.
52. Rhodes PR: The electronic patient record. In Rose LF, Mealey BL, Genco RJ, Cohen DW, editors: *Periodontics: medicine, surgery, and implants,* St Louis, 2004, Mosby, Elsevier.
53. Robinson HB: Abrasion, attrition and erosion of teeth, *Health Center J Ohio State Univ* 3:21, 1949.
54. Saglie R, Johanson JR, Flotra L: The zone of completely and partially destructed periodontal fibers in pathological pockets, *J Clin Periodontol* 2:198, 1975.
55. Salonen L, Hellden L: Prevalence of signs and symptoms of dysfunction in the masticatory system: an epidemiologic study in an adult Swedish population, *J Craniomandib Dis Fac Oral Pain* 4:241, 1990.
56. Schulte W, D'Hoedt B, Scholz F, et al: Periotest-neues Messverfahren der Funktion des Parodontiums, *Zahnarztl Mitt* 73:1229, 1983.
57. Seligman DA, Pullinger AG, Solberg AK: The prevalence of dental attrition and its association with factors of age, gender and TMJ symptomatology, *J Dent Res* 67:1323, 1988.
58. Sivertson JF, Burgett FG: Probing of pockets related to the attachment level, *J Periodontol* 47:281, 1976.
59. Sognnaes RF: Periodontal significance of intraoral frictional ablation, *J West Soc Periodontol* 25:112, 1977.
60. Spray JR, Garnick JJ, Doles LR, et al: Microscopic demonstration of the position of periodontal probes, *J Periodontol* 49:148, 1978.
61. Takenoshita Y, Ikebe T, Yamamoto M, Oka M: Occlusal contacts and temporomandibular symptoms, *Oral Surg Oral Med Oral Pathol Oral Radiol Endod* 72:388, 1991.
62. Tibbetts LS: Use of diagnostic probes for detection of periodontal disease, *J Am Dent Assoc* 78:549, 1969.
63. Van der Bilt A, Olthoff LW, Bosman F, Osterhaven SP: The effect of missing postcanine teeth on chewing performance in man, *Arch Oral Biol* 38:423, 1993.
64. Van der Velden U: Probing force and the relationship of the probe tip to the periodontal tissues, *J Clin Periodontol* 6:106, 1979.
65. Van der Velden U, De Vries JH: Introduction of a new periodontal probe: the pressure probe, *J Clin Periodontol* 5:188, 1978.
66. Weinberg LA: Diagnosis of facets in occlusal equilibration, *J Am Dent Assoc* 52:26, 1956.
67. Woda A, Gourdon AM, Faraj M: Occlusal contact and tooth wear, *J Prosthet Dent* 57:85, 1987.
68. Xhonga FA: Bruxism and its effect on teeth, *J Oral Rehabil* 4:65, 1977.

Radiographic Aids in the Diagnosis of Periodontal Disease

Sotirios Tetradis, Fermin A. Carranza, Robert C. Fazio, and Henry H. Takei

CHAPTER 36

CHAPTER OUTLINE

The radiograph is a valuable aid in the diagnosis of periodontal disease, determination of the prognosis, and evaluation of the outcome of treatment. However, *the radiograph is an adjunct to the clinical examination, not a substitute for it.*

The radiograph reveals alterations in calcified tissue; it does not reveal current cellular activity but shows the effects of past cellular experience on the bone and roots. Special techniques not yet in routine clinical use are required to show changes in the soft tissues of the periodontium.

NORMAL INTERDENTAL SEPTA

Radiographic evaluation of bone changes in periodontal disease is based mainly on the appearance of the interdental septa, because the relatively dense root structure obscures the facial and lingual bony plates. The interdental septum normally presents a thin, radiopaque border that is adjacent to the periodontal ligament (PDL) and at the alveolar crest, referred to as the *lamina dura* (Figure 36-1). This appears radiographically as a continuous white line, but in reality it is perforated by numerous small foramina and traversed by blood vessels, lymphatics, and nerves, which pass between the PDL and the bone. *Because the lamina dura represents the bone surface lining the tooth socket, the shape and position of the root and changes in the angulation of the x-ray beam produce considerable variations in its appearance.*[15]

The width and shape of the interdental septum and the angle of the crest normally vary according to the convexity of the proximal tooth surfaces and the level of the cementoenamel junction (CEJ) of the approximating teeth.[29] The interdental space and therefore the interdental septum between teeth with prominently convex proximal surfaces are wider anteroposteriorly than those between teeth with relatively flat proximal surfaces. The faciolingual diameter of the bone is related to the width of the proximal root surface. The angulation of the crest of the interdental septum is generally parallel to a line between the CEJs of the approximating teeth (Figure 36-1). When there is a difference in the level of the CEJs, the crest of the interdental bone appears angulated rather than horizontal.

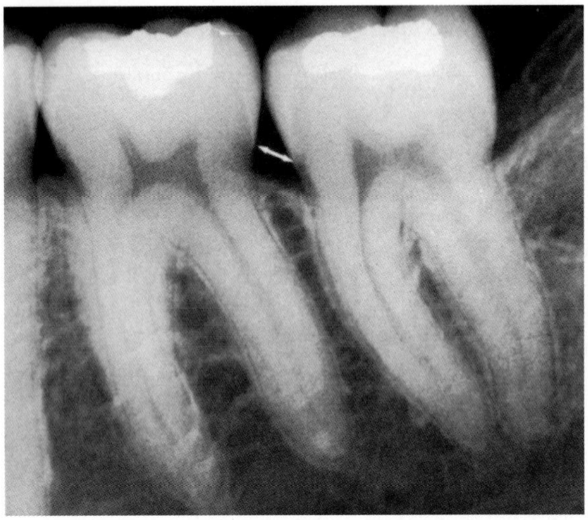

Figure 36-1 Crest of interdental septum normally parallel to a line drawn between the cementoenamel junction of adjacent teeth *(arrow)*. Note also the radiopaque lamina dura around the roots and interdental septum.

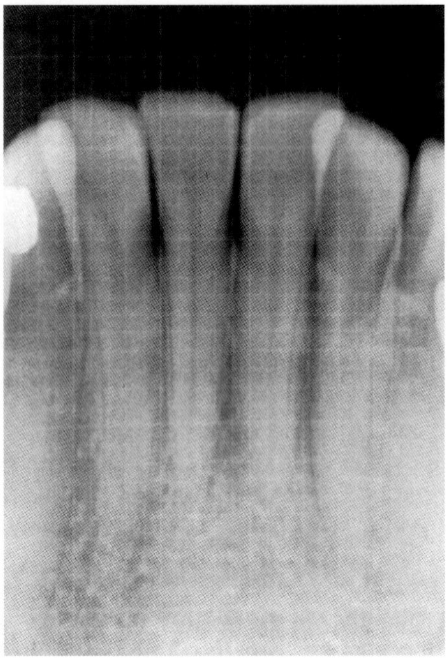

Figure 36-2 Radiograph with superimposed grid calibrated in millimeters.

DISTORTIONS PRODUCED BY VARIATIONS IN RADIOGRAPHIC TECHNIQUE

Variations in technique produce artifacts that limit the diagnostic value of the radiograph. The bone level, pattern of bone destruction, and width of the PDL space,[33] as well as the radiodensity, trabecular pattern, and marginal contour of the interdental septum, are modified by altering the exposure and development time, type of film, and x-ray angulation.[17] Standardized, reproducible techniques are required to obtain reliable radiographs for pretreatment and posttreatment comparisons.[16,24,31] A grid calibrated in millimeters, superimposed on the finished film, is helpful for comparing bone levels in radiographs taken under similar conditions[6] (Figure 36-2).

The effects of *angulation* can be useful in producing diagnostic radiographs. The *long-cone paralleling technique* projects the most realistic image of the level of the alveolar bone[8] (Figure 36-3). The *bisection-of-the-angle technique* increases the projection and makes the bone margin appear closer to the crown; the level of the facial bone margin is distorted more than that of the lingual margin. Shifting the cone mesially or distally without changing the horizontal plane projects the x-rays obliquely and changes the shape of the interdental bone on the radiograph, the radiographic width of the PDL space, and the appearance of the lamina dura. It may also distort the extent of furcation involvement (Figure 36-4).[19]

Prichard[23] established the following four criteria to determine adequate angulation of periapical radiographs:

1. The radiograph should show the tips of molar cusps with little or none of the occlusal surface showing.
2. Enamel caps and pulp chambers should be distinct.
3. Interproximal spaces should be open.
4. Proximal contacts should not overlap unless teeth are out of line anatomically.

Periapical radiographs taken with either the long-cone paralleling or bisection-of-the-angle technique frequently do not reveal the correct relationship between the alveolar bone and the CEJ. This is particularly true in cases of a shallow palate or floor of the mouth that do not allow ideal placement of the periapical film.

An additional intraoral projection that can be used for the evaluation of alveolar crest is the *bite-wing projection.* For bite-wing radiographs, the film is placed behind the crowns of the upper and lower teeth parallel to the long axis of the teeth. The x-ray beam is directed through the contact areas of the teeth and perpendicular to the film.[35] Thus the projection geometry of the bite-wing films allows the evaluation of the relationship between the interproximal alveolar crest and the CEJ without distortion (Figures 36-5 and 36-6). If the periodontal bone loss is severe and the bone level cannot be visualized on regular bite-wing radiographs, films can be placed vertically to cover a larger area of the jaws (Figure 36-7). More than two vertical bite-wing films might be necessary to cover all the interproximal spaces of the area of interest.

BONE DESTRUCTION IN PERIODONTAL DISEASE

The radiograph does not reveal minor destructive changes in bone.[3,4,25] Therefore, slight radiographic changes in the periodontal tissues mean that the disease has progressed beyond its earliest stages. *The earliest signs of periodontal disease must be detected clinically.*

Bone Loss

The radiographic image tends to show less severe bone loss than that actually present.[28] The difference between the alveolar crest height and the radiographic appearance

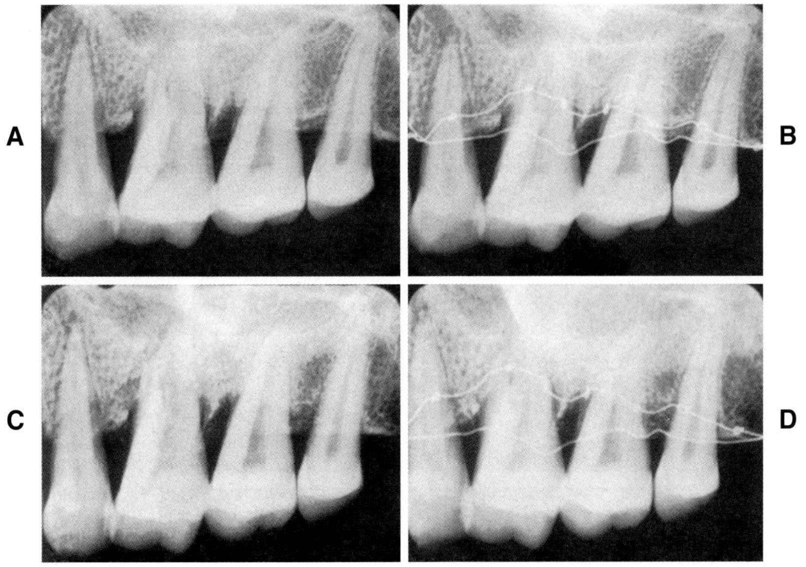

Figure 36-3 Comparison of long-cone paralleling and bisection-of-the-angle techniques. **A,** Long-cone paralleling technique, radiograph of dried specimen. **B,** Long-cone paralleling technique, same specimen as **A.** Smooth wire is on margin of the facial plate and knotted wire is on the lingual plate to show their relative positions. **C,** Bisection-of-the-angle technique, same specimen as **A** and **B. D,** Bisection-of-the-angle technique, same specimen. Both bone margins are shifted toward the crown, the facial margin (smooth wire) more than the lingual margin (knotted wire), creating the illusion that the lingual bone margin has shifted apically. (Courtesy Dr. Benjamin Patur, Hartford, Conn.)

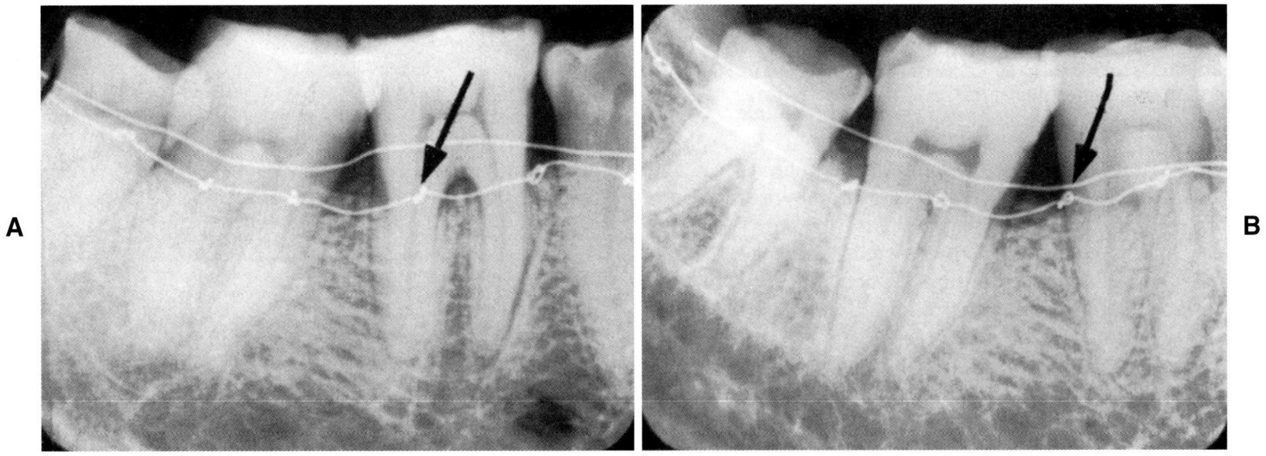

Figure 36-4 Distortion by oblique radiographic projection. **A,** Long-cone paralleling technique. Smooth wire is on the facial bony plate, and knotted wire is on the lingual plate. Note the knot *(arrow)* near the center of the distal root of the first molar, which shows bifurcation involvement. **B,** Long-cone paralleling technique. Cone is placed distally, projecting the x-rays mesially and obliquely. The oblique projection shifts the image of all structures mesially. *The structures closest to the cone shift the most.* This creates the illusion that the knot *(arrow)* has moved distally. Note that the bifurcation involvement shown in **A** is obliterated in **B.** (Courtesy Dr. Benjamin Patur, Hartford, CT.)

ranges from 0 mm to 1.6 mm,[27] mostly accounted for by x-ray angulation.

Amount. The radiograph is an indirect method for determining the amount of bone loss in periodontal disease; it shows the amount of remaining bone rather than the amount lost. The amount of bone lost is estimated to be the difference between the physiologic bone level of the patient and the height of the remaining bone.

The distance from the CEJ to the alveolar crest has been analyzed by several investigators.[12,14,27] Most studies have been conducted in adolescents, and the general consensus seems to be a distance of 2 mm; this distance may be greater in older patients.

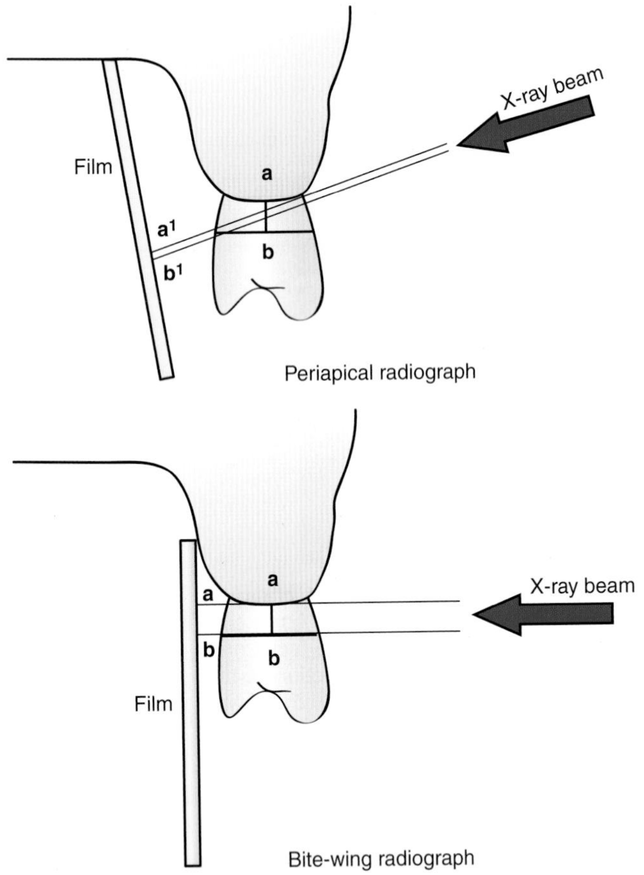

Figure 36-5 Schematic diagram of periapical **(A)** and bite-wing **(B)** radiographs. Angulation of the x-ray beam and the film on the periapical radiograph distort the distance between the alveolar crest and the cementoenamel junction (CEJ) (compare a-b vs. a′-b′). In contrast, the projection geometry of the bite-wing radiograph allows a more accurate depiction (a′-b′) of the distance between the alveolar crest and the CEJ (a-b).

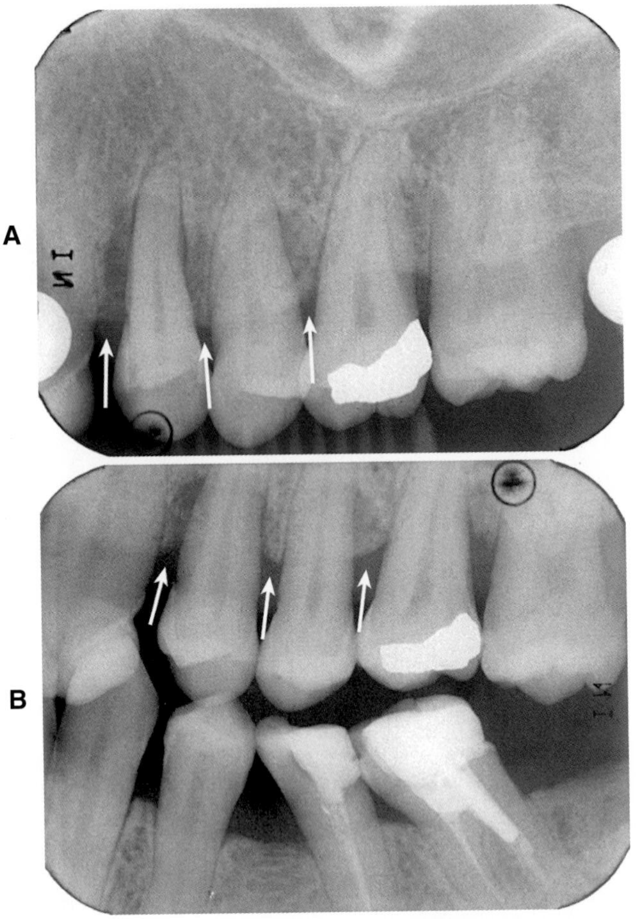

Figure 36-6 Periapical **(A)** and bitewing **(B)** radiographs from full-mouth series of patient with periodontitis. The periapical film clearly underestimates the amount of bone loss *(white arrows)*. Because of appropriate projection geometry, the alveolar crest height is accurately depicted on the bite-wing radiograph *(white arrows)*.

Distribution. The distribution of bone loss is an important diagnostic sign. It points to the location of destructive local factors in different areas of the mouth and in relation to different surfaces of the same tooth.

Pattern of Bone Destruction

In periodontal disease the interdental septa undergo changes that affect the lamina dura, crestal radiodensity, size and shape of the medullary spaces, and height and contour of the bone. The interdental septa may be reduced in height, with the crest horizontal and perpendicular to the long axis of the adjacent teeth (*horizontal* bone loss; Figure 36-8), or the septa may have angular or arcuate defects (*angular,* or *vertical,* bone loss: Figure 36-9) (see Chapter 28).

Radiographs do not indicate the internal morphology or depth of the craterlike interdental defects, which appear as angular or vertical defects. Also, radiographs do not reveal the extent of involvement on the facial and lingual surfaces. Bone destruction of facial and lingual surfaces is obscured by the dense root structure, and bone destruction on the mesial and distal root surfaces may be partially hidden by a dense mylohyoid ridge (Figure 36-10). In most cases it can be assumed that bone losses seen interdentally continue in either the facial or the lingual aspect, creating a troughlike lesion. The true lesion can be detected only by clinically probing the defect.

Dense cortical plates on the facial and lingual surfaces of the interdental septa obscure destruction that occurs in the intervening cancellous bone. Thus it is possible to have a deep crater in the bone between the facial and lingual plates without radiographic indications of its presence. To record destruction of the interproximal cancellous bone radiographically, the cortical bone must be involved. A reduction of only 0.5 to 1.0 mm in the thickness of the cortical plate is sufficient to permit radiographic visualization of destruction of the inner cancellous trabeculae.[20]

Interdental vertical lesions in the posterior area with thick facial or lingual bone may not be isolated in the interdental area but may continue facially and/or

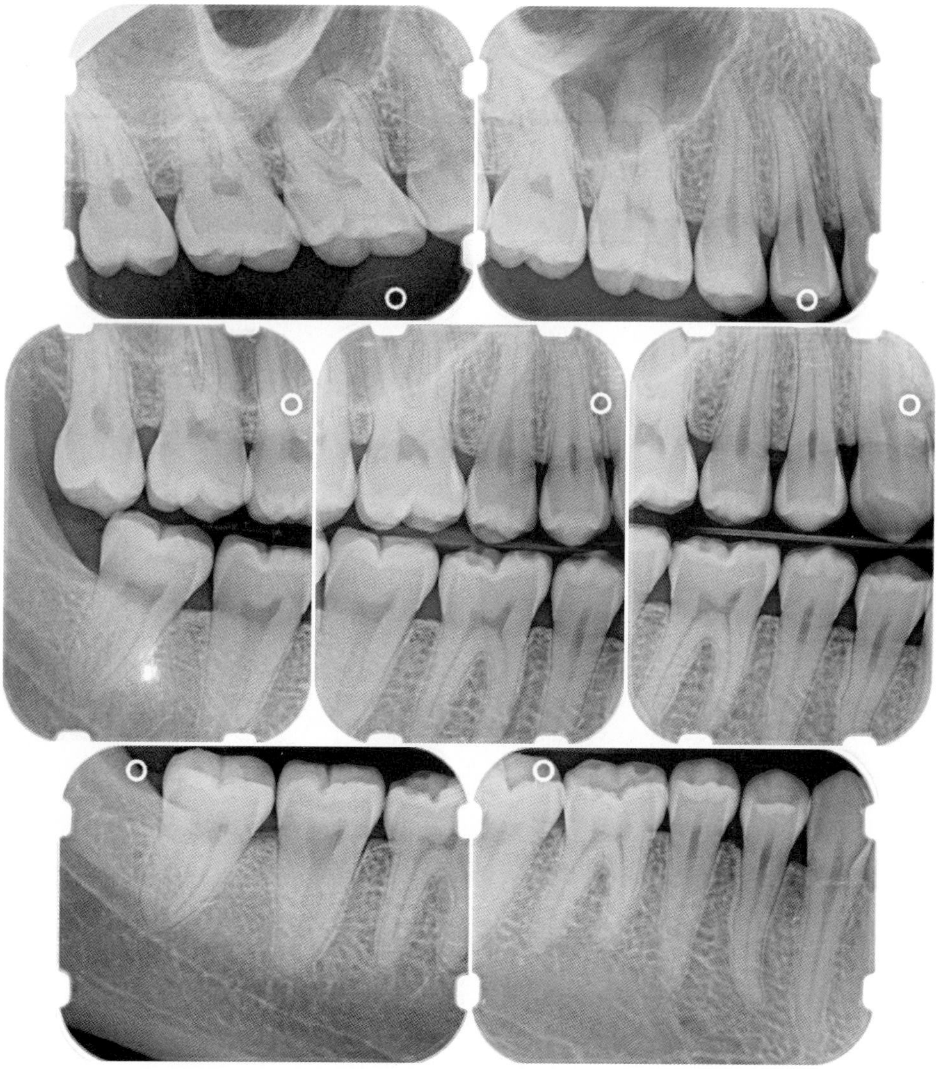

Figure 36-7 Vertical bite-wing films can be used to cover a larger area of the alveolar bone.

lingually to form a troughlike defect that cannot be seen radiographically. These lesions may terminate on the radicular surface or may communicate with the adjacent interdental area to form one continuous lesion (Figure 36-11).

Figure 36-12 shows two adjacent interdental lesions connecting on the radicular surface to form one interconnecting osseous lesion. Along with clinical probing of these lesions, the use of a radiopaque pointer placed in these radicular defects will demonstrate the extent of the bone loss.

Gutta percha packed around the teeth increases the usefulness of the radiograph for detecting the morphologic changes of osseous craters and involvement of the facial and lingual surfaces (Figure 36-13). However, this is a cumbersome technique and is seldom performed. Surgical exposure and visual examination provide the most definitive information regarding the bone architecture produced by periodontal destruction.[22]

RADIOGRAPHIC APPEARANCE OF PERIODONTAL DISEASE

Periodontitis

The sequence of radiographic changes in periodontitis and the causative tissue changes are as follows:

1. *Fuzziness and a break in the continuity of the lamina dura* at the mesial or distal aspect of the crest of the interdental septum have been considered as the earliest radiographic changes in periodontitis (Figure 36-14, *A* and *B*). These result from the extension of gingival inflammation into the bone, causing widening of the vessel channels and a reduction in calcified tissue at the septal margin. These changes, however, depend greatly on the radiographic technique (angulation of tube, placement of film) and on anatomic variations (thickness and density of interdental bone, position

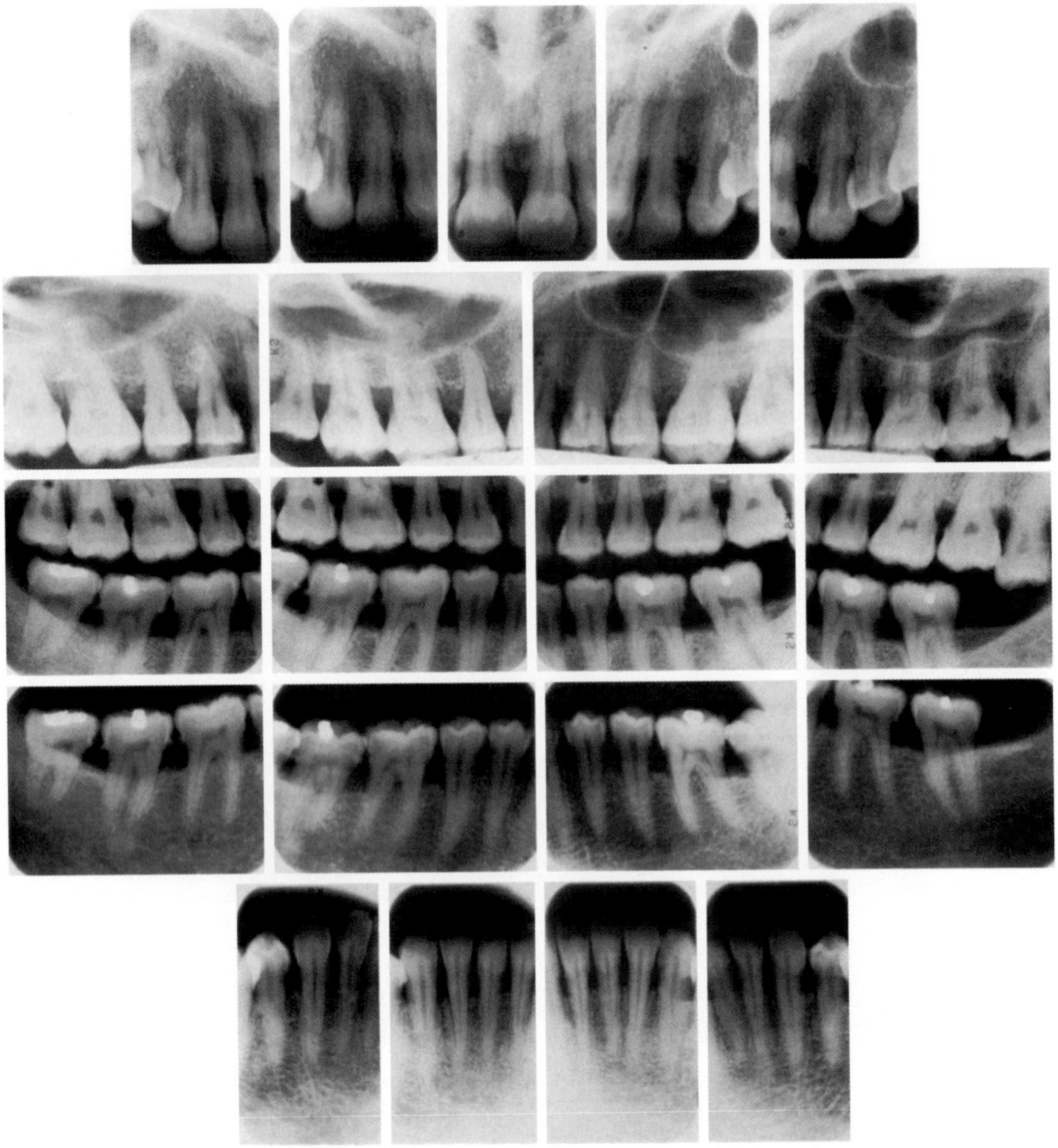

Figure 36-8 Generalized horizontal bone loss.

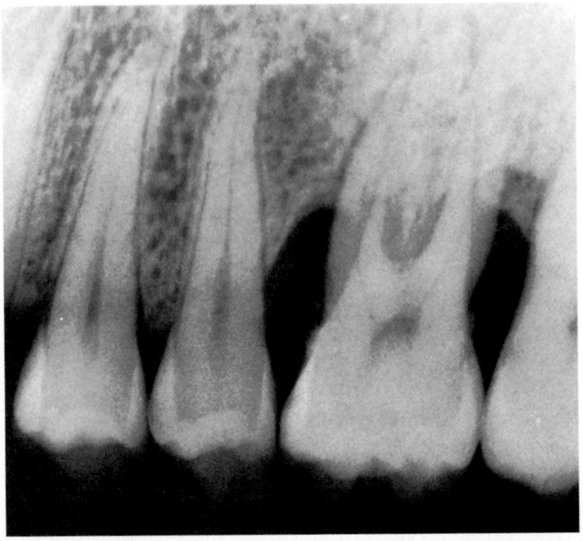

Figure 36-9 Angular bone loss on first molar with involvement of the furcation.

of adjoining teeth). No correlation has been found between crestal lamina dura in radiographs and the presence or absence of clinical inflammation, bleeding on probing, periodontal pockets, or loss of attachment.[11,26] Therefore it can be concluded that the presence of an intact crestal lamina dura may be an indicator of periodontal health, whereas its absence lacks diagnostic relevance.[2]

2. A *wedge-shaped radiolucent area* is formed at the mesial or distal aspect of the crest of the septal bone

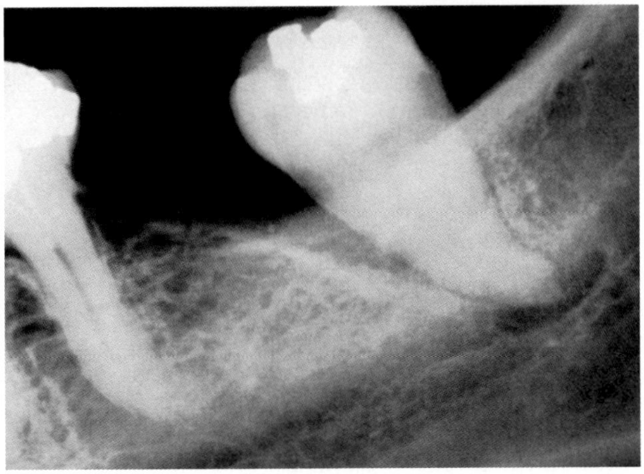

Figure 36-10 Angular bone loss on mandibular molar partially obscured by dense mylohyoid ridge.

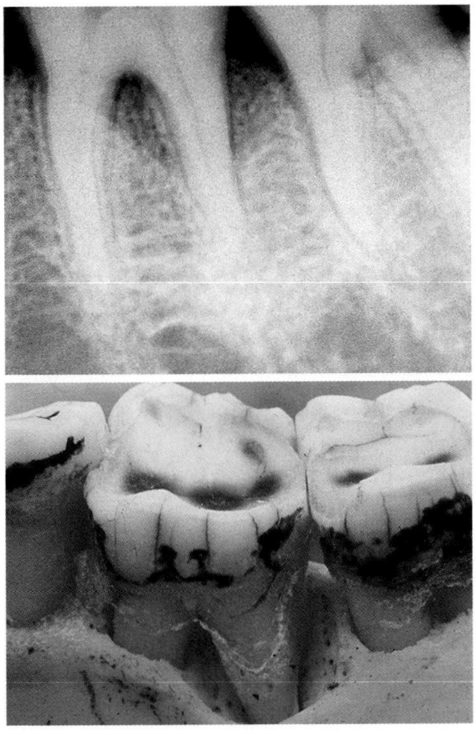

Figure 36-11 Interdental lesion that extends to the facial or lingual surfaces in a troughlike manner.

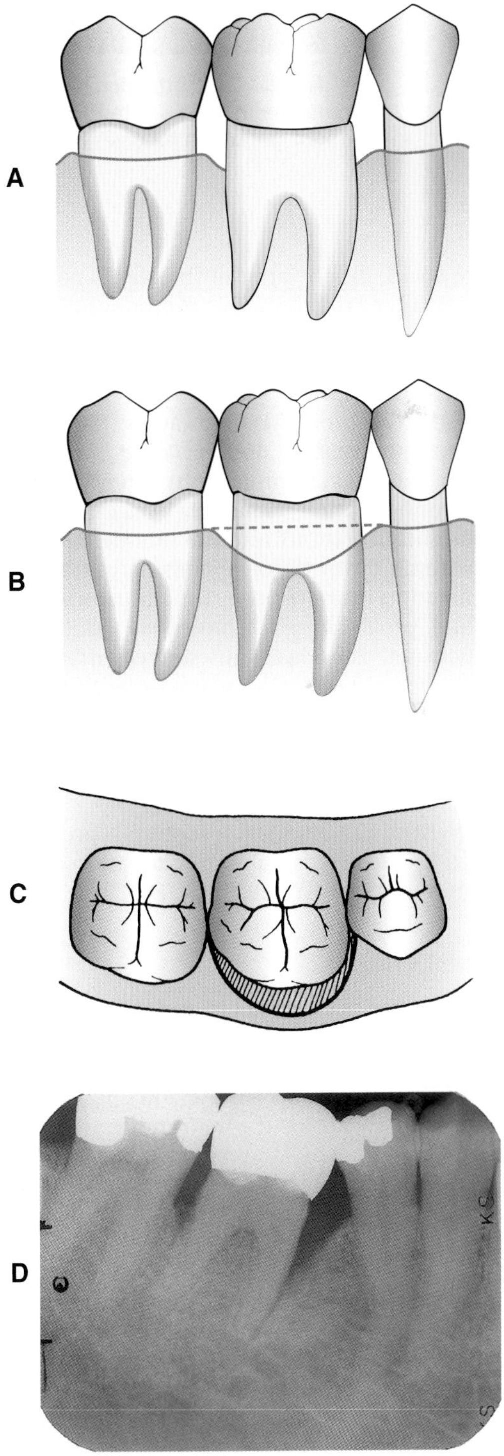

Figure 36-12 **A,** Interdental mesial and distal lesions. **B,** Facial or lingual outlines of actual lesion. **C,** Occlusal view of lesion. **D,** Actual radiograph of mesial and facial lesions.

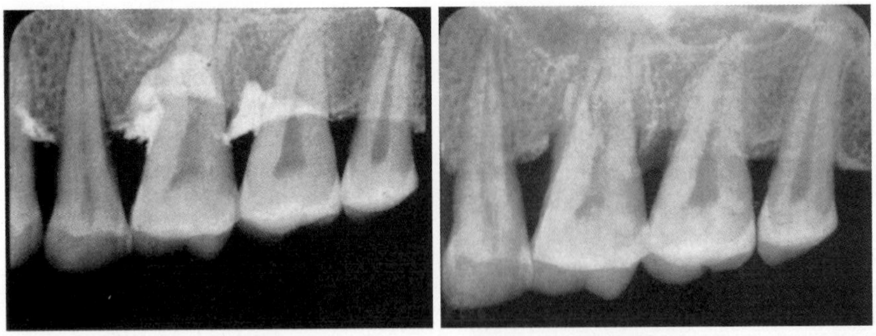

Figure 36-13 Gutta percha aids in detecting bone defects. **A,** Gutta percha packed around teeth shows interproximal and facial and lingual bone loss. **B,** Same area as *A* without gutta percha gives little indication of the extent of bone involvement.

(Figure 36-14, *B*). The apex of the area is pointed in the direction of the root. This is produced by resorption of the bone of the lateral aspect of the interdental septum, with an associated widening of the periodontal space.
3. The destructive process extends across the crest of the interdental septum, and *the height is reduced.* Fingerlike radiolucent projections extend from the crest into the septum (Figure 36-14, *C*). The radiolucent projections into the interdental septum are the result of the deeper extension of the inflammation into the bone. Inflammatory cells and fluid, proliferation of connective tissue cells, and increased osteoclasis cause increased bone resorption along the endosteal margins of the medullary spaces. The radiopaque projections separating the radiolucent spaces are the composite images of the partially eroded bony trabeculae.
4. The height of the interdental septum is progressively reduced by the extension of inflammation and the resorption of bone (Figure 36-14, *D*).

Interdental Craters

Interdental craters are seen as irregular areas of reduced radiopacity on the alveolar bone crests.[28] Craters are generally not sharply demarcated from the rest of the bone, with which they blend gradually. Radiographs do not accurately depict the morphology or depth of interdental craters, which sometimes appear as vertical defects.

Furcation Involvement

Definitive diagnosis of furcation involvement is made by clinical examination, which includes careful probing with a specially designed probe (e.g., Nabers). Radiographs are helpful but show artifacts that allow furcation involvement to be present without detectable radiographic changes.

As a general rule, bone loss is always greater than it appears in the radiograph. Variations in the radiographic technique may obscure the presence and extent of furcation involvement. A tooth may present marked bifurcation involvement in one film (Figure 36-15, *A*) but appear to be uninvolved in another (Figure 36-15, *B*). Radiographs should be taken at different angles to reduce the risk of missing furcation involvement.

The recognition of a large, clearly defined radiolucency in the furcation area presents no problem (Figure 36-15, *A*), but less clearly defined radiographic changes produced by furcation involvement are often overlooked. To assist in the radiographic detection of furcation involvement, the following diagnostic criteria are suggested:

1. The slightest radiographic change in the furcation area should be investigated clinically, especially if there is bone loss on adjacent roots (Figure 36-16).
2. Diminished radiodensity in the furcation area in which outlines of bony trabeculae are visible suggests furcation involvement (Figure 36-17).
3. Whenever there is marked bone loss in relation to a single molar root, it may be assumed that the furcation is also involved (Figures 36-18 and 36-19).

Periodontal Abscess

The typical radiographic appearance of the periodontal abscess is a discrete area of radiolucency along the lateral aspect of the root (Figures 36-20 and 36-21). *However, the radiographic picture is often not typical* (Figure 36-22) because of many variables, such as the following:

1. *The stage of the lesion.* In the early stages the acute periodontal abscess is extremely painful but presents no radiographic changes.
2. *The extent of bone destruction and the morphologic changes of the bone.*
3. *The location of the abscess.* Lesions in the soft tissue wall of a periodontal pocket are less likely to produce radiographic changes than those deep in the supporting tissues. Abscesses on the facial or lingual surface are obscured by the radiopacity of the root; interproximal lesions are more likely to be visualized radiographically.

Therefore the radiograph alone cannot be relied on for the diagnosis of a periodontal abscess.

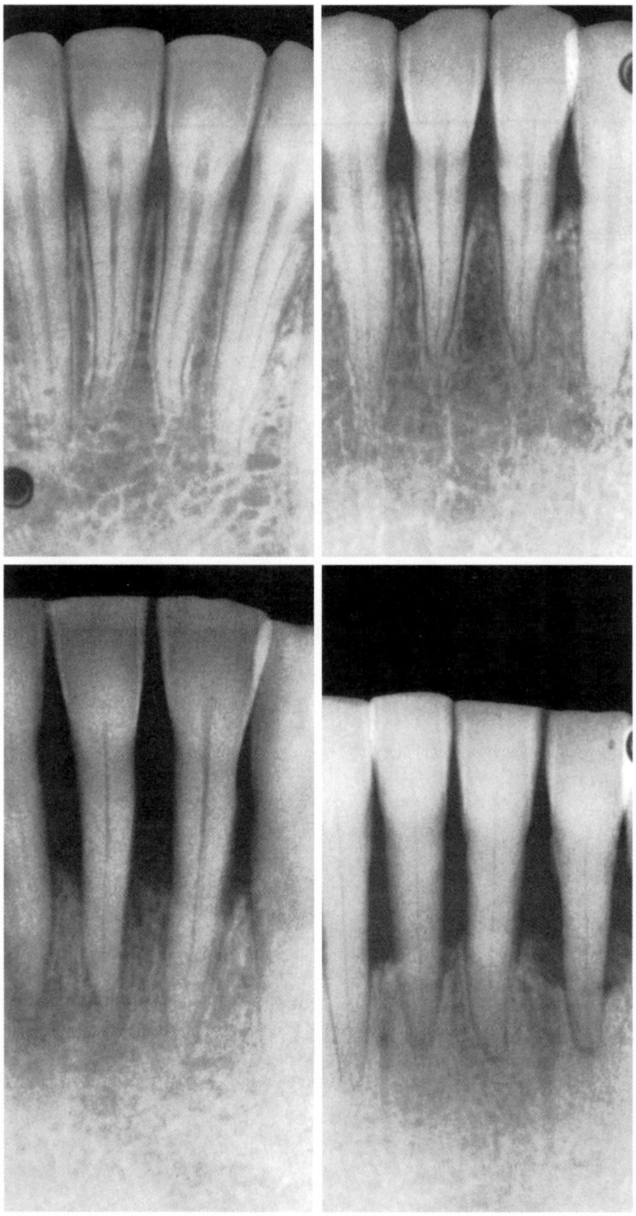

Figure 36-14 Radiographic changes in periodontitis. **A,** Normal appearance of interdental septa. **B,** Fuzziness and a break in the continuity of the lamina dura at the crest of the bone distal to the central incisor *(left).* There are wedge-shaped radiolucent areas at the crests of the other interdental septa. **C,** Radiolucent projections from the crest into the interdental septum indicate extension of destructive processes. **D,** Severe bone loss.

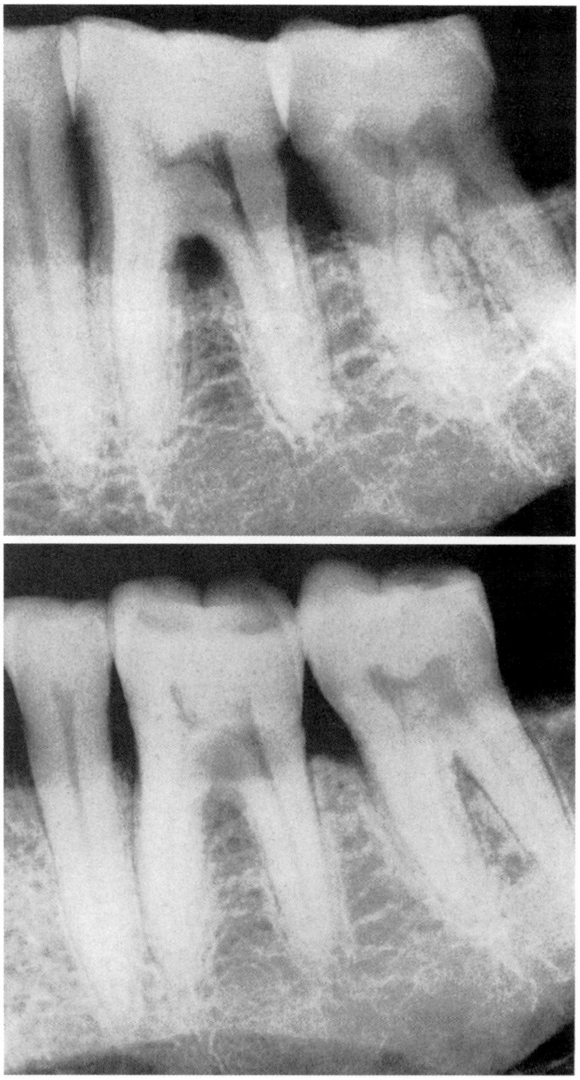

Figure 36-15 **A,** Furcation involvement indicated by triangular radiolucency in bifurcation area of mandibular first molar. The second molar presents only a slight thickening of the periodontal space in the bifurcation area. **B,** Same area as *A,* different angulation. The triangular radiolucency in the bifurcation of the first molar is obliterated, and involvement of the second molar bifurcation is apparent.

Clinical Probing

Regenerative and resective flap designs and incisions require prior knowledge of the underlying osseous topography. Careful probing of these pocket areas after scaling and root planing often require local anesthesia and definitive radiographic evaluation of the osseous lesions. Radiographs taken with periodontal probes or other indicators (e.g., Hirschfeld pointers) placed into the anesthetized pocket show the true extent of the bone lesion. As indicated previously, the attachment level on the radicular surface or interdental lesions with thick facial or lingual bone cannot be visualized in the radiograph. The use of radiopaque indicators is an efficient diagnostic

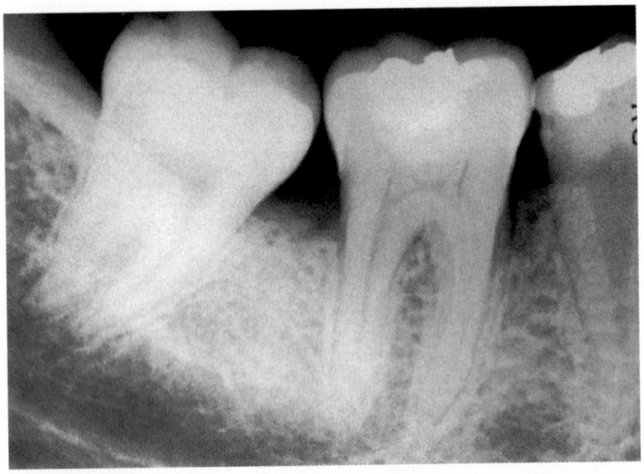

Figure 36-16 Early furcation involvement suggested by fuzziness in the bifurcation of the mandibular first molar, particularly when associated with bone loss on the roots.

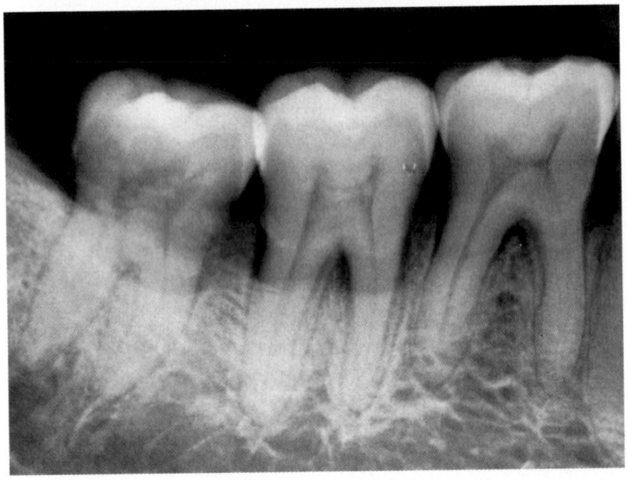

Figure 36-17 Furcation involvement of mandibular first and second molars indicated by thickening of periodontal space in furcation area. The furcation of the third molar is also involved, but the thickening of the periodontal space is partially obscured by the external oblique line.

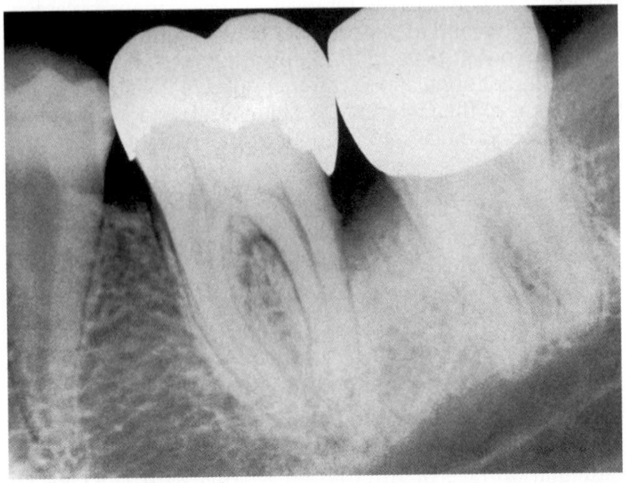

Figure 36-18 Furcation involvement of the first molar, associated with bone loss on the distal root.

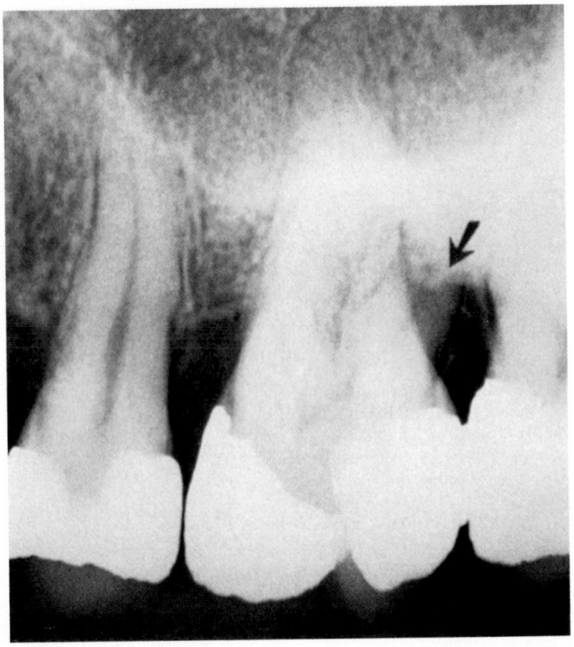

Figure 36-19 Furcation involvement of the first molar partially obscured by the radiopaque lingual root. The horizontal line across the distobuccal root demarcates the apical portion *(arrow),* which is covered by bone, from the remainder of the root, where the bone has been destroyed.

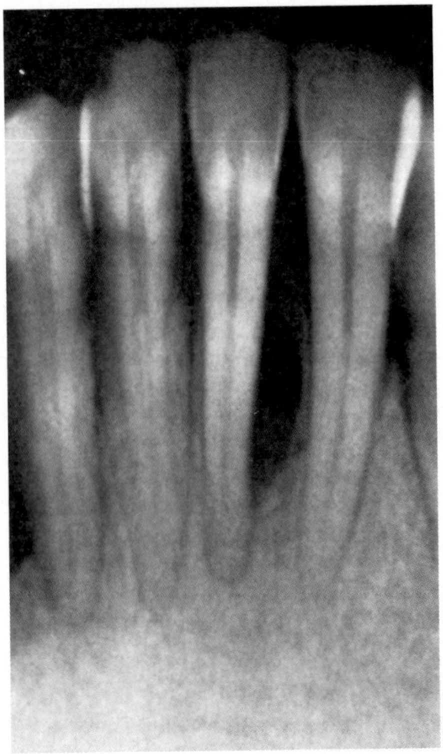

Figure 36-20 Radiolucent area on lateral aspect of root with chronic periodontal abscess.

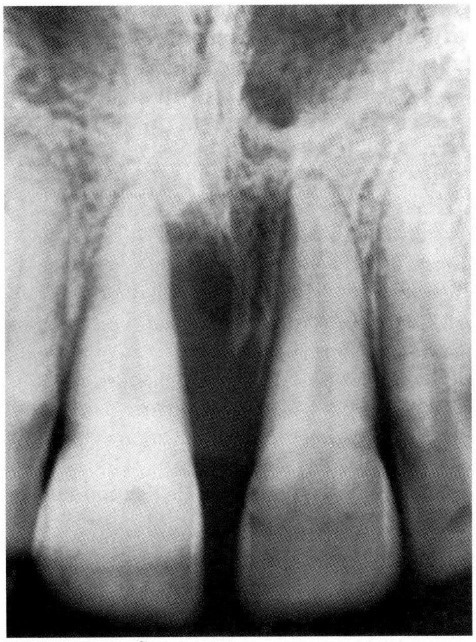

Figure 36-21 Typical radiographic appearance of periodontal abscess on right central incisor.

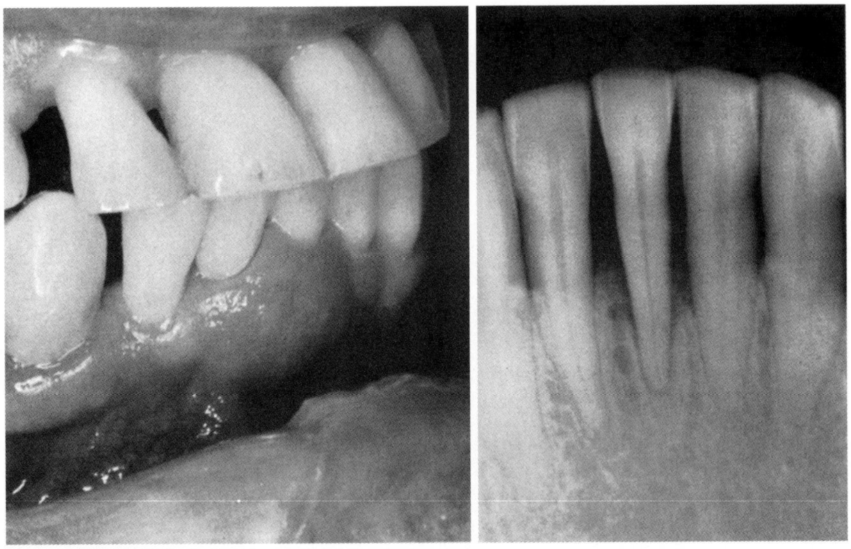

Figure 36-22 Chronic periodontal abscess. **A,** Periodontal abscess in the right central and lateral incisor area. **B,** Extensive bone destruction and thickening of the periodontal ligament space around the right central incisor.

aid for the clinician to better visualize every aspect of the defect. Figure 36-23 provides examples of probes placed in pockets to indicate the bone level.

Localized Aggressive Periodontitis

Localized aggressive (formerly "localized juvenile") periodontitis is characterized by a combination of the following radiographic features:

1. Bone loss may occur initially in the maxillary and mandibular incisor and/or first molar areas, usually bilaterally, and results in vertical, arclike destructive patterns (Figure 36-24).
2. Loss of alveolar bone may become generalized as the disease progresses but remains less pronounced in the premolar areas.

Trauma from Occlusion

Trauma from occlusion can produce radiographically detectable changes in the lamina dura, morphology of the alveolar crest, width of the PDL space, and density of the surrounding cancellous bone.

A

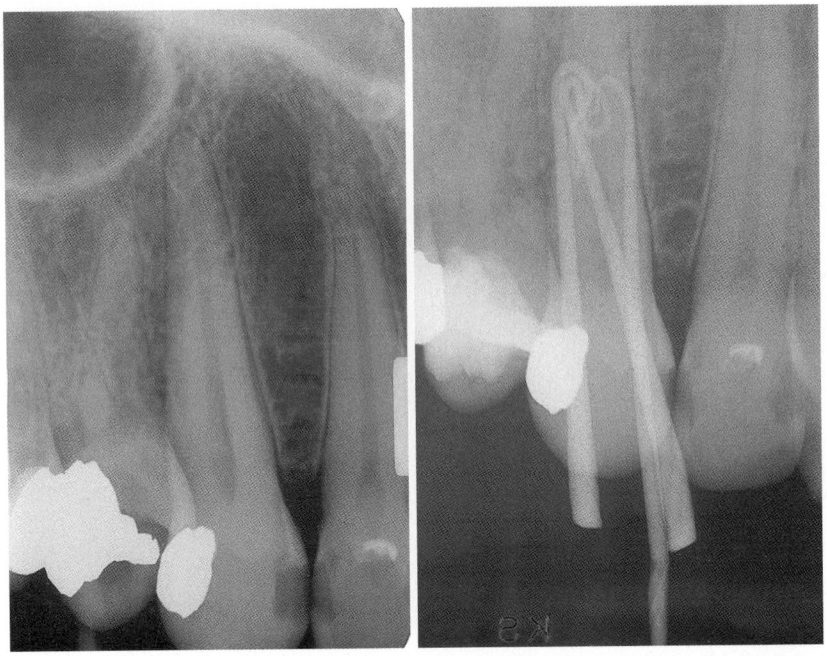

B

Figure 36-23 **A,** Radiograph of maxillary cuspid. This view does not show facial bone loss. **B,** Radiograph of same maxillary cuspid as *A,* with gutta percha points placed in the facial pocket to indicate bone loss.

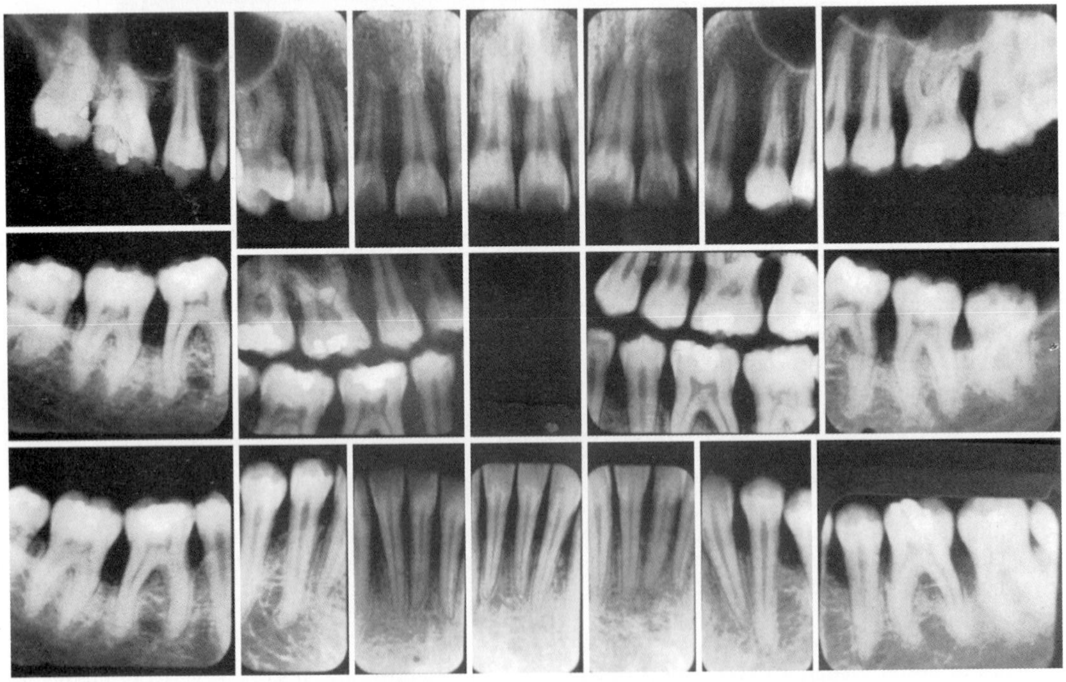

Figure 36-24 Localized aggressive periodontitis. The accentuated bone destruction in the anterior and first molar areas is considered to be characteristic of this disease.

Traumatic lesions manifest more clearly in faciolingual aspects, because mesiodistally the tooth has the added stability provided by the contact areas with adjacent teeth. Therefore, slight variations in the proximal surfaces may indicate greater changes in the facial and lingual aspects. *The radiographic changes listed next are not pathognomonic of trauma from occlusion and must be interpreted in combination with clinical findings,* particularly tooth mobility, presence of wear facets, pocket depth, and analysis of occlusal contacts and habits.

The *injury phase* of trauma from occlusion produces a loss of the lamina dura that may be noted in apices,

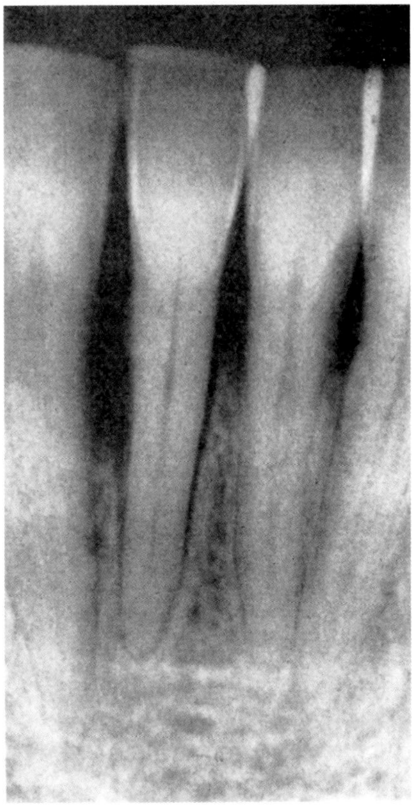

Figure 36-25 Widened periodontal space caused by trauma from occlusion. Note the increased density of the surrounding bone caused by new bone formation in response to increased occlusal forces.

SCIENCE TRANSFER

Diagnosing periodontal disease requires the clinician to use a variety of techniques and skills, and ultimately the combination of these findings allows for a differential diagnosis. Each technique or skill has advantages and disadvantages, and being aware of these can facilitate diagnosis.

Radiographic analysis of periodontal tissues permits accurate evaluation of the results from prior interproximal disease, but it is very limited in regard to evaluating current disease or prior disease on the facial or lingual root surfaces. Another important aspect of radiographic analysis is the ability to detect changes in periodontal structures. Much effort has been expended to increase the sensitivity to detect these changes, and although improvements have been made, limitations persist. The clinician must remember that the metabolic events involved in the loss of periodontal tissues, particularly bone, are the same as those that occur throughout the skeleton; thus, important events occur at the cellular level. Unfortunately, a relatively large amount of demineralization must occur before radiographic changes can be detected.

Interpretation of radiographic images of periodontal disease should be coupled with clinical findings because great variation in the images results from technical factors. Angulation, exposure, and superimposition of buccal and lingual or palatal cortical bone of the alveolar process all add to the complexity of radiographic interpretation. For example, the height of the interdental bone may show a difference of up to 1.6 mm in the radiograph compared with its actual diagnostic height. Also, bony changes in periodontitis are not seen radiographically in the early stages of the disease. Further, bone loss in furcations may be caused by periodontitis or traumatic occlusion, and care must be taken to measure attachment levels clinically to distinguish bone loss caused by periodontitis from that caused by traumatic occlusion. In cases involving only traumatic occlusion, bone loss occurs without any loss of attachment or pocket formation.

furcations, and marginal areas. This loss of lamina dura results in widening of the PDL space (Figure 36-25). This change, particularly when incipient or circumscribed, may easily be confused with technical variations caused by x-ray angulation or malposition of the tooth; it can be diagnosed with certainty only in radiographs of the highest quality.

The *repair phase* of trauma from occlusion results in an attempt to strengthen the periodontal structures to better support the increased loads. Radiographically, this is manifested by a widening of the PDL space, which may be generalized or localized.

Although microscopic measurements have determined that normal variations exist in the width of the PDL space in the different regions of the root, these are generally not detected in radiographs. When variations in width between the marginal area and midroot or between the midroot and apex are detected, it means that the tooth is being subjected to increased forces. Successful attempts to reinforce the periodontal structures by widening of the PDL space is accompanied by increased width of the lamina dura and sometimes by condensation of the perialveolar cancellous bone.

More advanced traumatic lesions may result in deep angular bone loss, which, when combined with marginal inflammation, may lead to intrabony pocket formation. In terminal stages these lesions extend around the root apex, producing a wide, radiolucent periapical image (cavernous lesions).

Root resorption may also result from excessive forces on the periodontium, particularly those caused by orthodontic appliances. Although trauma from occlusion produces many areas of root resorption, these areas are usually of a magnitude insufficient to be detected radiographically.

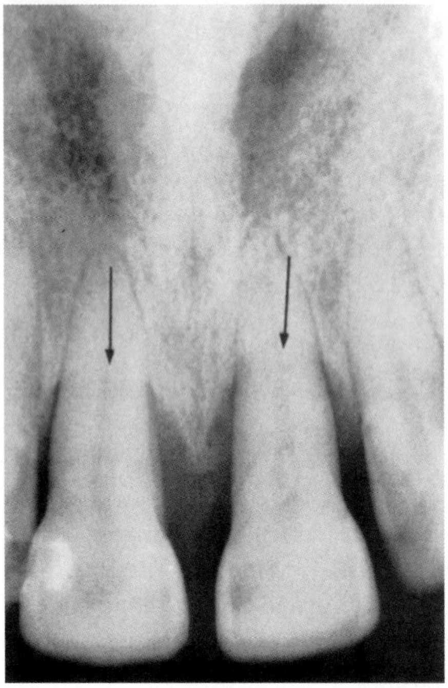

Figure 36-26 Horizontal lines across the roots of the central incisors *(arrows)*. The area of the roots below the horizontal lines is partially or completely denuded of the facial and lingual bony plates.

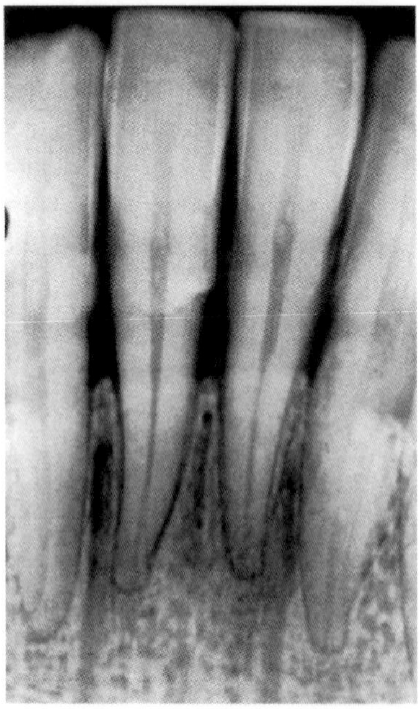

Figure 36-27 Prominent vessel canals in the mandible.

ADDITIONAL RADIOGRAPHIC CRITERIA

The following diagnostic criteria can be used as further aids in the radiographic identification of periodontal disease:

1. *Radiopaque horizontal line across the roots.* This line demarcates the portion of the root where the labial or lingual bony plate has been partially or completely destroyed from the remaining bone-supported portion (Figure 36-26).
2. *Vessel canals in the alveolar bone.* Hirschfeld[13] described linear and circular radiolucent areas produced by interdental canals and their foramina, respectively (Figure 36-27). These canals indicate the course of the vascular supply of the bone and are normal radiographic findings. The radiographic image of the canals is often so prominent, particularly in the anterior region of the mandible, that they might be confused with radiolucency resulting from periodontal disease.
3. *Differentiation between treated and untreated periodontal disease.* It is sometimes necessary to determine whether the reduced bone level is the result of periodontal disease that is no longer destructive (usually after treatment and proper maintenance) or whether destructive periodontal disease is present. Clinical examination is the basic determinant. However, radiographically detectable alterations in the normally clear-cut peripheral outline of the septa are corroborating evidence of destructive periodontal disease.

SKELETAL DISTURBANCES MANIFESTED IN THE JAWS

Skeletal disturbances may produce changes in the jaws that affect the interpretation of radiographs from the periodontal perspective. Destruction of tooth-supporting bone may occur in various diseases.

Osteitis fibrosa cystica (Recklinghausen's disease of bone) develops in advanced primary or secondary hyperparathyroidism and causes osteoclastic resorption of bone with fibrous replacement and hemorrhage with hemosiderin deposition, creating a mass known as *brown tumor*[5] (see Figure 17-6). It often appears as a cystic lesion of the jaw. This disease results in a diffuse granular mottling, scattered cystlike radiolucent areas throughout the jaws, and a generalized disappearance of the lamina dura.[30] Correction of the parathyroid hyperfunction usually results in rapid reversion of the bone to normal.

In *Paget's disease* the normal trabecular pattern is replaced by a hazy, diffuse meshwork of closely knit, fine trabecular markings, with the lamina dura absent (Figure 36-28), or scattered radiolucent areas may contain irregularly shaped radiopaque zones.[10,34]

Fibrous dysplasia may appear as a small radiolucent area at a root apex or as an extensive radiolucent area with irregularly arranged trabecular markings.[9] The cancellous spaces may be enlarged, with distortion of the normal trabecular pattern (ground-glass appearance) and obliteration of the lamina dura (Figure 36-29).

Langerhans cell histiocytosis results from disturbances in immunoregulation, and its different forms comprise the diseases formerly called Hand-Schüller-Christian disease, Letterer-Siwe disease, Gaucher's disease, and eosinophilic granuloma.[5,34] The disease manifestations appear as single or multiple radiolucent areas, which may be unrelated to the teeth or may entail destruction of the tooth-supporting bone (Figure 36-30).

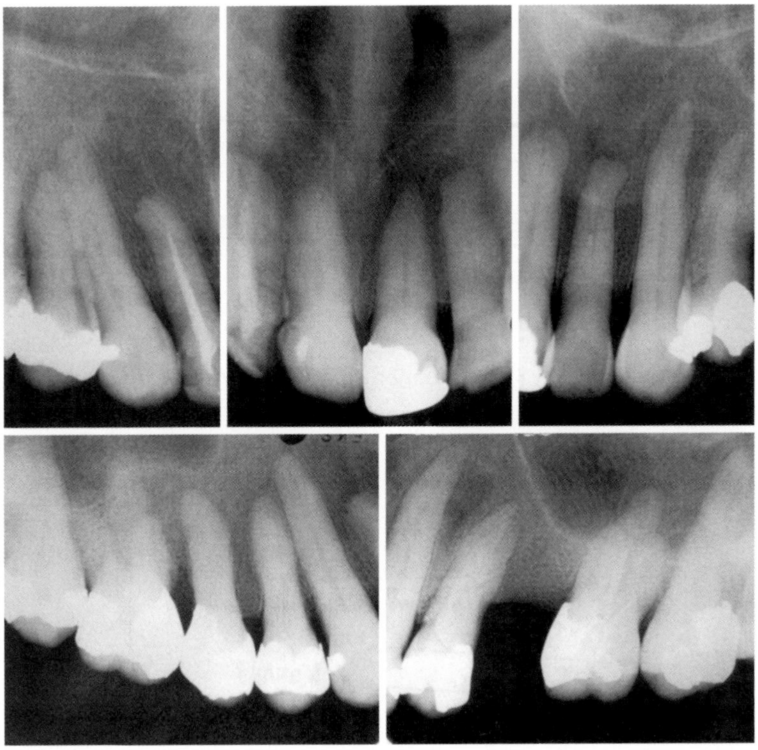

Figure 36-28 Altered trabecular pattern and diminution in the prominence of the lamina dura in Paget's disease.

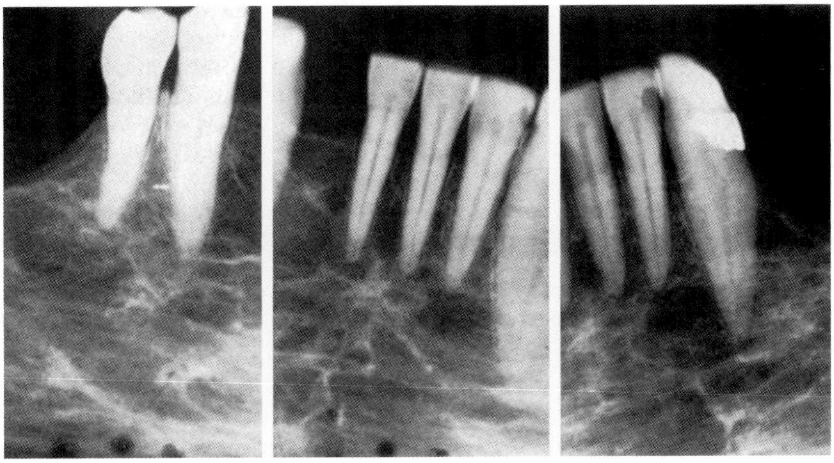

Figure 36-29 Osteoporosis and altered trabecular arrangement in fibrous dysplasia.

Numerous radiolucent areas occur when the jaws are involved by *multiple myeloma.*

In *osteopetrosis* (marble-bone disease, Albers-Schönberg disease)[7,34] the outlines of the roots may be obscured by diffuse radiopacity of the jaws. In less severe cases the increased density is confined to the bone in relation to the nutrient canals and the lamina dura.

In *scleroderma* the PDL is uniformly widened at the expense of the surrounding alveolar bone[1] (Figure 36-31).

Malignancy, both primary and metastatic, can affect the alveolar ridge and often presents as periodontal disease. A uniform widening of the PDL can be an early sign of osteosarcoma. Irregular destruction of the periodontal bone without tooth displacement is frequently the result of squamous cell carcinoma or metastatic carcinoma.[35]

DIGITAL INTRAORAL RADIOGRAPHY

Intraoral digital radiographs offer several advantages over conventional film-based radiographs in clinical dentistry. The number of dentists using intraoral digital radiographs increases steadily, and some practices are now completely digital. Telediagnosis, videoconferencing, rapid

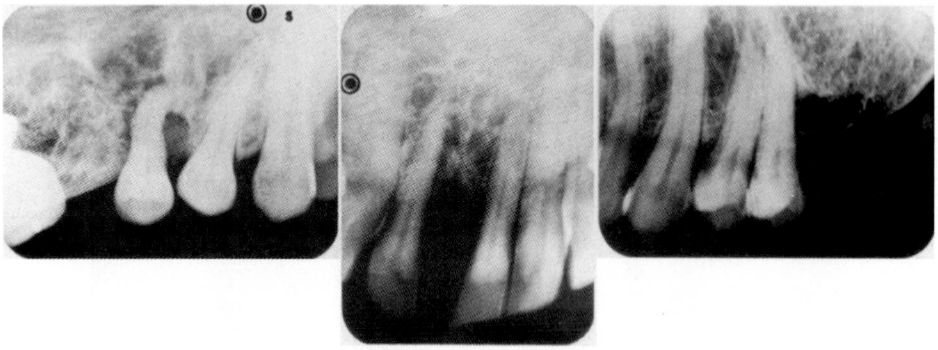

Figure 36-30 Osteoporosis in Gaucher's disease.

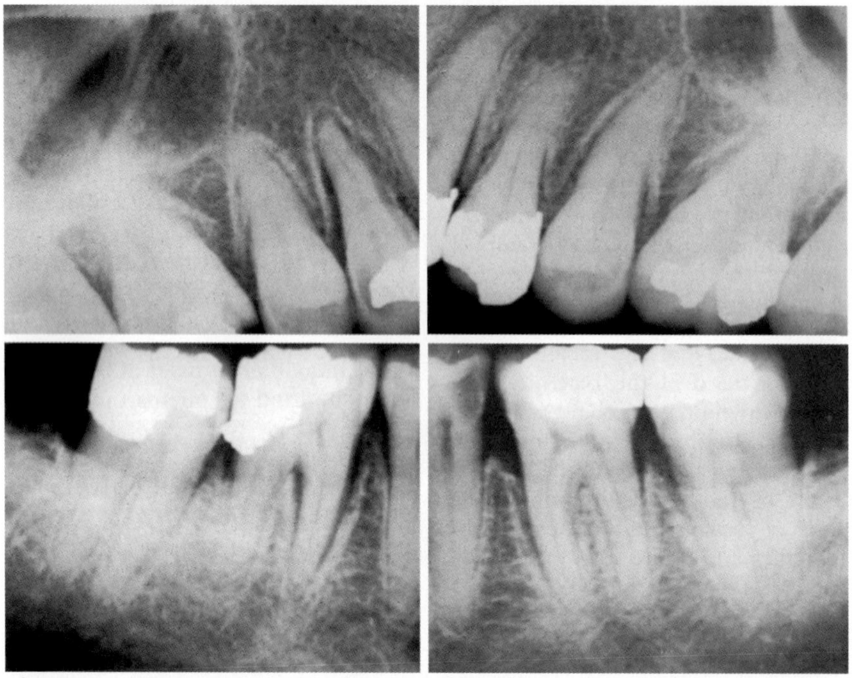

Figure 36-31 Scleroderma, showing typical uniform widening of the periodontal ligament and thickening of the lamina dura. (Courtesy Drs. David F. Mitchell and Anand P. Chaudhry.)

image transmission among dentists and third parties, a seamless electronic patient record, and integration with computer-aided diagnostic software are areas in which digital information is revolutionizing dentistry.[36]

Two major digital intraoral systems are currently available.[18] The first system uses charge-coupled devices (CCDs) or complementary metal oxide semiconductor (CMOS) receptors as detectors. These detectors are placed in the patient's mouth and are linked by a wire to the computer. On radiation exposure, virtually in real time, the radiographic image appears on a computer screen. The detector is then moved to the next position, and so on, until the whole area of interest is imaged. The second system uses photostimulable phosphor (PSP) plates as detectors. PSP plates resemble film with one of the sides lined with a PSP coating. When interacting with x-rays, PSP stores energy, which it then releases on stimulation by light of an appropriate wavelength. PSP plates are placed and exposed similar to regular film. The exposed plates are placed on a plate scanner and scanned by a laser beam, and the radiographic image appears on the computer screen.[18]

Once captured and displayed, computer software can be used to enhance the digital image and increase its diagnostic efficacy.[21] Exposure adjustment provides a balanced image that utilizes the complete scale of gray levels and does not suppress diagnostic information (Figure 36-32, compare A and B). A sharpening (edge enhancement) filter increases the definition and separation of adjacent structures (Figure 36-32, compare B and C). Inversion filters provide a negative of the image that sometimes might reveal disease not seen on the positive image (Figure 36-32, *D*). The ability to magnify the image allows close examination of the area of interest and

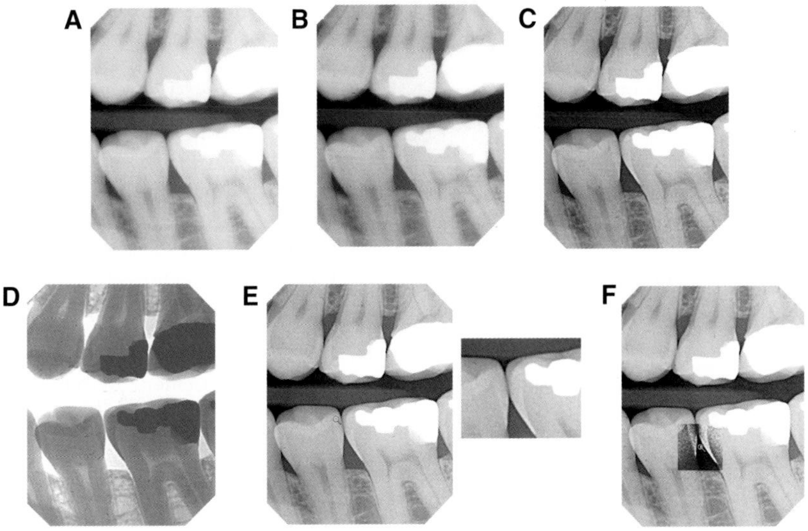

Figure 36-32 Various enhancement features help optimize the appearance of the radiographic image to improve diagnosis. Brightness and contrast of an underexposed image **(A)** is adjusted **(B)** to utilize the full gray scale. **C,** Sharpness of the image is then increased using "clear view" feature. **D,** "Invert" feature provides a negative of the image. **E,** "Zooming" function allows close examination of the interproximal space. **F,** Contrast of the interproximal area is maximized to aid in the diagnosis of possible caries. (Courtesy Dexis Digital Radiography, Alpharetta, Georgia.)

detection of occult disease (Figure 36-32, *E*). Different image qualities allow better detection of dental disease. For example, high-contrast images favor caries detection, whereas low-contrast images permit a more accurate depiction of the alveolar crest. Digital images can be adjusted such that the contrast of the interproximal contacts can be enhanced for caries detection while the remainder of the image is not altered (Figure 36-32, *F*).

Advantages of intraoral digital radiography include the speed of image capture and display; low x-ray exposure; ability to manipulate the image and maximize diagnostic efficacy; use of digital tools, such as linear, angular, and density measurements; improved patient education; ease of storage, transfer, and copying; and seamless integration with electronic patient record management or other software. Most studies conclude that the aid provided by digital radiographs in the diagnosis of common dental diseases such as caries is similar to that of conventional radiographs.

However, the proper use of digital intraoral radiographs requires familiarity with the digital nature of the images and an understanding of the principles of image manipulation by computer software.[35] Although contrast and brightness adjustments can be used to refine the image, they cannot correct a grossly overexposed or underexposed projection. The ease of digital image acquisition should not replace correct detector placement and exposure techniques. Image enhancement should be used with caution and should be task oriented. For example, increased contrast might aid in caries diagnosis but lead to underestimation of the alveolar bone crest height. If properly used, intraoral digital radiography offers great benefits in the diagnosis of dental disease.[35]

REFERENCES

1. Alexandridis C, White SC: Periodontal ligament changes in patients with progressive systemic sclerosis, *Oral Surg* 58:113, 1984.
2. Armitage G: Periodontal diseases: diagnosis, *Ann Periodontol* 1:37, 1996.
3. Bender IB, Seltzer S: Roentgenographic and direct observation of experimental lesions in bone. I, *J Am Dent Assoc* 62:152, 1961.
4. Bender IB, Seltzer S: Roentgenographic and direct observation of experimental lesions in bone. II, *J Am Dent Assoc* 62:708, 1961.
5. Cotran RS, Kumar V, Robbins SL: *Robbins pathologic basis of disease,* ed 5, Philadelphia, 1994, Saunders.
6. Everett FG, Fixott HC: Use of an incorporated grid in the diagnosis of oral roentgenograms, *Oral Surg* 9:1061, 1963.
7. Fairbank HAT: Osteopetrosis, *J Bone Joint Surg* 30:339, 1948.
8. Fitzgerald GM: Dental radiography. IV. The voltage factor (kp), *J Am Dent Assoc* 41:19, 1950.
9. Glickman I: Fibrous dysplasia in alveolar bone, *Oral Surg* 1:895, 1948.
10. Glickman I, Glidden S: Paget's disease of the maxillae and mandible: clinical analysis and case reports, *J Am Dent Assoc* 29:2144, 1942;.
11. Greenstein G, Polson A, Iker H, et al: Associations between crestal lamina dura and periodontal status, *J Periodontol* 52:362, 1981.
12. Hausmann E, Allen K, Clerehugh V: What alveolar crest level on a bite-wing radiograph represents bone loss? *J Periodontol* 62:570, 1991.
13. Hirschfeld I: Interdental canals, *J Am Dent Assoc* 14:617, 1927.
14. Källestål C, Matsson L: Criteria for assessment of interproximal bone loss on bite-wing radiographs in adolescents, *J Clin Periodontol* 16:300, 1989.
15. Manson JD: The lamina dura, *Oral Surg* 16:432, 1963.

16. Nicopoulos-Karayianni K, Mombelli A, Lang NO: Diagnostic problems of periodontitis-like lesions caused by eosinophilic granuloma, *J Clin Periodontol* 16:505, 1989.
17. Parfitt GJ: An investigation of the normal variations in alveolar bone trabeculations, *Oral Surg* 15:1453, 1962.
18. Parks ET, Williamson GF: *Digital radiography: an overview, J Contemp Dent Pract* 3:23, 2002.
19. Patur B, Glickman I: Roentgenographic evaluation of alveolar bone changes in periodontal disease, *J Clin North Am* 4:47, 1960.
20. Pauls V, Trott JR: A radiological study of experimentally produced lesions in bone, *Dent Pract* 16:254, 1966.
21. Preston JD: Digital radiography: not if, but when, *CDA J* 27:935, 1999.
22. Prichard JF: Role of the roentgenogram in the diagnosis and prognosis of periodontal disease, *Oral Med* 14:182, 1961.
23. Prichard JF: *Advanced periodontal disease: surgical and prosthetic management,* ed 2, Philadelphia, 1972, Saunders.
24. Puckett J: A device for comparing roentgenograms of the same mouth, *J Periodontol* 39:38, 1968.
25. Ramadan ABE, Mitchell DF: A roentgenographic study of experimental bone destruction, *Oral Surg* 15:934, 1962.
26. Rams TE, Listgarten MA, Slots J: Utility of radiographic crestal lamina dura for predicting periodontal disease activity, *J Clin Periodontol* 21:571, 1995.
27. Regan JE, Mitchell DF: Roentgenographic and dissection measurements of alveolar crest height, *J Am Dent Assoc* 66:356, 1962.
28. Rees TD, Biggs NL, Collings CK: Radiographic interpretation of periodontal osseous lesions, *Oral Surg Oral Med Oral Pathol* 5:934, 1962.
29. Ritchey B, Orban B: The crests of the interdental septa, *J Periodontol* 24:75, 1953.
30. Rosenberg EH, Guralnick WC: Hyperparathyroidism, *Oral Surg* 15(suppl 2):84, 1962.
31. Rosling B, Hollender L, Nyman S, et al: A radiographic method for assessing changes in alveolar bone height following periodontal therapy, *J Clin Periodontol* 2:211, 1975.
32. Theilade J: An evaluation of the reliability of radiographs in the measurement of bone loss in periodontal disease, *J Periodontol* 31:143, 1960.
33. Van der Linden LWJ, Van Aken J: The periodontal ligament in the roentgenogram, *J Periodontol* 41:243, 1970.
34. Waldron CA: Bone pathology. In Neville BW, Damm DD, Allen CM, et al: *Oral and maxillofacial pathology,* Philadelphia, 1995, Saunders.
35. White SC, Pharoah MJ: *Oral radiology: principles and interpretation,* ed 5, St Louis, 2004, Mosby, Elsevier.
36. White SC, Yoon DC, Tetradis S: Digital radiography in dentistry: what it should do for you? *CDA J* 27:942, 1999.

Advanced Diagnostic Techniques

Mariano Sanz, Michael G. Newman, and Marc Quirynen

37

CHAPTER

■ ■ ■

CHAPTER OUTLINE

LIMITATIONS OF CONVENTIONAL PERIODONTAL
 DIAGNOSIS
 Advances in Clinical Diagnosis
 Gingival Bleeding
 Gingival Temperature
 Periodontal Probing
ADVANCES IN RADIOGRAPHIC ASSESSMENT
 Digital Radiography
 Subtraction Radiography
 Computer-Assisted Densitometric Image Analysis
 System
ADVANCES IN MICROBIOLOGIC ANALYSIS

Bacterial Culturing
Direct Microscopy
Immunodiagnostic Methods
Enzymatic Methods
Diagnostic Assays Based on Molecular Biology
 Techniques
ADVANCES IN CHARACTERIZING THE HOST RESPONSE
 Source of Samples
 Inflammatory Mediators and Products
 Host-Derived Enzymes
 Tissue Breakdown Products
CONCLUSION

LIMITATIONS OF CONVENTIONAL PERIODONTAL DIAGNOSIS

Periodontal diseases are prevalent human diseases defined by the signs and symptoms of gingival inflammation and periodontal tissue destruction. These diseases are conventionally diagnosed by clinical evaluation of the signs of inflammation in the gingiva without periodontal tissue destruction (gingivitis) or by the presence of both inflammation and tissue destruction (periodontitis).

Periodontitis is characterized by a loss of connective tissue attachment that begins at, or just apical to, the cementoenamel junction and extends apically along the root surface. The traditional clinical diagnosis is made by measuring either the loss of connective tissue attachment to the root surface (clinical attachment loss) or the loss of alveolar bone (radiographic bone loss) (Figure 37-1; see Chapters 35 and 36). Disease evaluation, as performed at one point in time, attempts to identify and quantify current clinical signs of inflammation as well as historical evidence of damage, with its extent and severity. However, evaluation cannot reliably identify sites with ongoing periodontal destruction and does not provide any information on the cause of the condition, on the patient's susceptibility to disease, whether the disease is progressing, whether it is in remission, or whether the response to therapy will be positive or negative.

The current view of the natural history of destructive periodontal disease is that disease susceptibility is related to the whole person rather than the local site. This means that a person's susceptibility and host defense mechanisms are generalized. However, the disease process itself is considered to be site specific and has a multifactorial origin in which periodontal pathogens, host response, and genetic, systemic, and behavioral risk factors interplay to develop the disease process. In light of this information, consideration should be given to including microbiologic, immunologic, systemic, genetic, and behavioral factors, in addition to the traditional clinical and radiographic parameters, when assessing patient status. This chapter systematically reviews the advances made in the use of these parameters.[71]

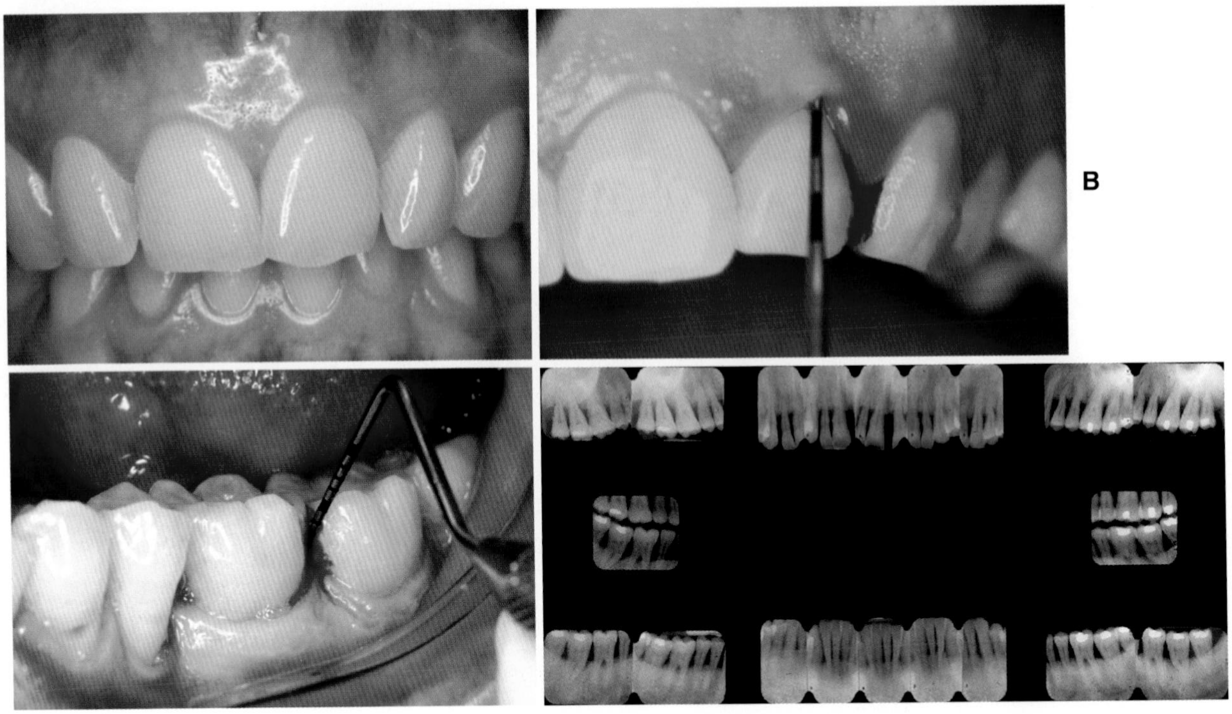

Figure 37-1 Conventional clinical diagnostic tools. **A,** Visual diagnosis. **B,** Periodontal probing. **C,** Bleeding on probing. **D,** Intraoral periapical radiographic series.

SCIENCE TRANSFER

Periodontal disease is considered a site-specific disease characterized by a local inflammatory reaction to bacterial infection. As such, many problems are encountered when attempting to identify a specific site on a tooth undergoing disease. For example:

- The site may occur anywhere around any of the teeth.
- Many bacteria appear to be associated with stimulating infection.
- The host reaction is not unique to a periodontal infection and involves inflammatory molecules and cells observed throughout the body.

Thus, attempts to identify specific bacteria, specific inflammatory cells or molecules, or specific breakdown products unique to periodontal destruction have been unsuccessful despite excellent progress in diagnostic methodology. Conventional efforts evaluating inflammation and past evidence of tissue breakdown remain the standard for disease evaluation. Future efforts will likely identify factors and conditions that place the periodontium at risk for future attachment loss and thus will help focus diagnosis on patients more likely to experience disease progression.

This chapter provides a comprehensive review of current diagnostic techniques, ranging from digital subtraction radiography to polymerase chain reaction (PCR) detection of bacterial DNA and analysis of gingival fluid for markers of periodontal disease activity. Few of these procedures can be applied to individual patient care in a practice setting with any degree of confidence. This is summarized in the conclusion of the chapter: "After all these years of intensive research, we still lack a proven diagnostic test that has demonstrated high predictive value for disease progression, has a proven impact on disease incidence and prevalence, and is simple, safe, and cost-effective." Nevertheless, clinicians are able to use conventional diagnostic methods to identify gingivitis, periodontitis, and other periodontal lesions with a high degree of precision.

Future application of advanced diagnostic techniques will be of value in documenting disease activity and treatment options.

ADVANCES IN CLINICAL DIAGNOSIS

Gingival Bleeding

Clinical evaluation of the degree of gingival inflammation includes assessment of the redness and swelling of the gingiva along with assessment of gingival bleeding. Although the earliest clinical signs of gingivitis consist of color and texture changes, there may be underlying structural alterations without corresponding clinical signs (Figure 37-1, *A*). Gingival bleeding is related to the persistent presence of plaque on the teeth and is regarded as a sign of the associated inflammatory response. Subjects who refrain from normal oral hygiene procedures have a resultant increase in plaque accumulation and demonstrate a concomitant increase in gingival bleeding as gingivitis develops over a 2- to 3-week period.[38] Moreover, the use of gingival bleeding as an indicator of inflammation has the clinical advantage of being more objective, because color changes require a subjective estimation. It has also been shown that gingival bleeding is a good indicator of the presence of an inflammatory lesion in the connective tissue at the base of the sulcus and that the severity of bleeding increases with an increase in size of the inflammatory infiltrate.[38,108] Therefore, clinicians tend to evaluate gingivitis by gingival bleeding alone, with the use of a periodontal probe or a wooden interdental cleaner, instead of using visual signs of both inflammation and bleeding[2] (Figure 37-1, *C*). Besides an indicator of gingival inflammation, some investigators have suggested that gingival bleeding is also an indicator of disease activity[108]; *however, its relationship to disease progression is unclear.*

Lang et al.,[73] in a retrospective study, reported that sites that bled on probing at several visits had a higher probability of losing attachment than those that bled at one visit or did not bleed. However, well-controlled longitudinal studies investigated the predictive values of such clinical signs, trying to correlate them with attachment loss, but failed to demonstrate a significant correlation between bleeding on probing and other clinical signs and subsequent loss of attachment.[8,45] A further limitation of the use of bleeding as an inflammatory parameter is the possibility that healthy sites may bleed on probing. Lang et al.[73] demonstrated that any force greater than 0.25 N may evoke bleeding in healthy sites with an intact periodontium.

In summary, although bleeding on probing may have a limited predictive value for disease progression, its absence indicates periodontal stability with high probability. However, this fact may not be true in heavy smokers. Different studies have reported that tobacco smoking may mask the inflammatory signs of gingivitis and periodontitis, particularly the propensity of the gingivae to bleed on brushing, eating, or after periodontal probing.[10] Similarly, a recent study has shown that despite a significant decrease in plaque scores, subjects had a twofold increase in bleeding on probing after quitting smoking, strongly suggesting that the signs of inflammation were inhibited by the smoking experience.[96] The mechanisms by which smoking may exert a suppressive action on the bleeding responsiveness of the gingivae are not well understood. The clinical effect of reduced bleeding in smokers presumably is caused by the long-standing use of tobacco rather than acute events. It seems likely that the interference of smoking with this property of the periodontal tissues is not caused by a vasoconstrictive action (from nicotine), but a result of a more profound influence on the vasculature and cellular metabolism.[104]

Gingival Temperature

Researchers have attempted to develop other measures of periodontal inflammation that may be useful when the usual clinical signs are unreliable. One such measure is subgingival temperature. Kung et al.[69] claim that thermal probes are sensitive diagnostic devices for measuring early inflammatory changes in the gingival tissues. One commercially available system, the PerioTemp probe (Abiodent), enables the calculation of the temperature differential (*DT*, with a sensitivity of 0.1° C) between the probed pocket and the subgingival temperature (Figure 37-2). This temperature differential is useful because it allows consideration of differences in core temperature between individuals. Individual temperature differences are compared with those expected for each tooth, and higher-temperature pockets are signaled with a red-emitting diode. Studies have demonstrated that the subgingival temperature at diseased sites is increased compared with healthy sites and that a natural anteroposterior temperature gradient exists within the dental arches (posterior sites warmer than anterior sites). In addition, mandibular sites were reported to be warmer than maxillary sites.[69] The reason why temperature increases with probing depth remains unknown. A possible explanation is an increase in cellular and molecular activity caused by increased periodontal inflammation with increasing probing depth.

In subsequent reports, Haffajee et al.[46] also found that elevated subgingival site temperature was particularly related to attachment loss in shallow pockets and that *Prevotella intermedia, Peptostreptococcus micros, Porphyromonas gingivalis, Tannerella forsythia,* and *Actinobacillus*

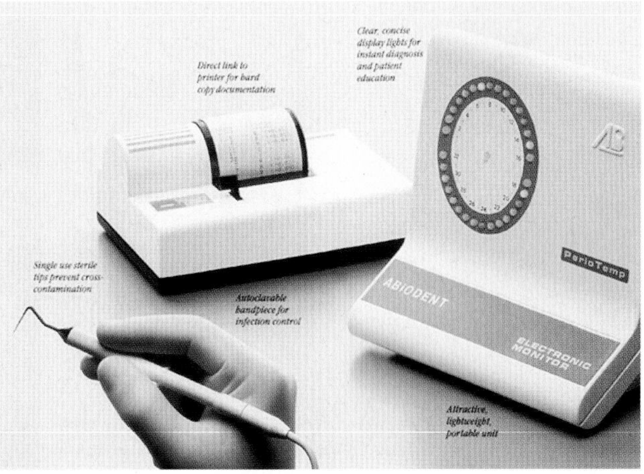

Figure 37-2 Thermal periodontal probe system: PerioTemp electronic monitor. (Courtesy Abiodent, Danvers, Mass.)

actinomycetemcomitans had elevated proportions in the total microbiota in sites with elevated temperatures. Whether the pathogens are responsible for the higher temperature by initiating the inflammatory process, or whether the increased temperature provides an environment susceptible for the pathogens, remains unclear.

Recently, studies have reported differences in the temperature differentials between subgingival temperature and sublingual temperature in smokers compared to nonsmokers.[131] Therefore, smoking and probing depths should be considered when temperature is used as a means of diagnosis or monitoring periodontal health.

Periodontal Probing

The most widely used diagnostic tool for the clinical assessment of connective tissue destruction in periodontitis is the periodontal probe. In fact, increased probing depth and loss of clinical attachment are pathognomonic for periodontitis, and therefore, pocket probing is a crucial and mandatory procedure in diagnosing periodontitis and evaluating periodontal therapy (see Chapter 35). Currently, the "gold standard" for recording changes in periodontal status is longitudinal measurement of clinical attachment levels from the cementoenamel junction or a relative attachment level from a fixed reference point. Reduction of pocket depth and gain of clinical attachment are the major clinical outcome measurements used to determine success of treatment (Figure 37-1, *B*).

However, the use of a periodontal probe presents many problems in terms of sensitivity and reproducibility of the measurements. Readings of clinical pocket depth obtained with the periodontal probe do not normally coincide with the histologic pocket depth because the probe normally penetrates the coronal level of the junctional epithelium,[109] and the precise location of the probe tip depends on the degree of inflammation of the underlying connective tissues. If the tissue is inflamed, it offers less resistance to probe penetration, and the probe tip either coincides with or is apical to the coronal level of connective tissue attachment.[80] Conversely, after use of subgingival instrumentation, healed gingiva demonstrates an increased resistance to periodontal probing.[85] These facts may not be true when making the clinical diagnosis in smokers. The reduced inflammation and bleeding and increased fibrosis reported in smokers might affect clinical probing measurements because of less probe tip penetration. A probing validity study showed that, with a constant-force probe, clinical probing depth at molar sites in smokers was lower than in nonsmokers, which may reflect more closely the true pocket depth and attachment levels with less probe tip penetration of tissue, as shown by the reduced inflammation in smokers compared with non-smokers.[11]

The disparity between measurements also depends on the probing technique, probing force, size of the probe, angle of insertion of the probe, and precision of the probe calibration[80] (Figure 37-3). All these variables contribute to the large standard deviations (0.5-1.3 mm) in clinical probing results, which make detection of small changes difficult.[49]

Since the mid-1980s, different probe prototypes have been developed and tested to overcome these limitations.[134] One of the main problems in reproducibility has been the variation in probing force. Different studies have shown that the penetration of the probe was positively correlated with probing force.[91] This has been solved with the development of *pressure-sensitive probes,* which have a standardized, controlled insertion pressure[133] (Figure 37-3, *B*). These studies have shown that with forces of up to 30 *g*, the tip of the probe seems to remain within the junctional epithelium,[4] and forces of up to 50 *g* are necessary to diagnose periodontal osseous defects.[61] Standardization of probe tips (<1 mm) and the addition of registration stents to maintain reproducible probing angulations have also been used to overcome sources of error.[7] However, fabrication of stents is time-consuming and impractical for clinical diagnosis. In addition, current techniques for data readout and storage are inaccurate and time-consuming as well.

New technology and high-tech computers are becoming the rule rather than the exception during patient treatment. Computer applications and new devices are being developed and marketed to improve diagnosis, enhance

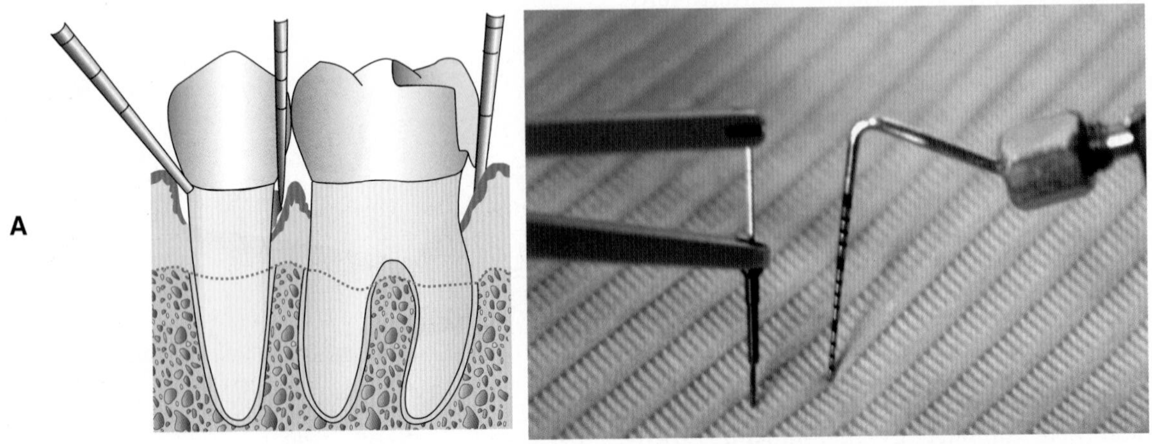

Figure 37-3 **A,** Limitations in periodontal probing. **B,** Probing pressure caused by probe angulation, presence of subgingival calculus, and presence of overhanging restorations. (**A** courtesy Dr. J. Frontan.)

TABLE 37-1

Criteria defined by National Institute of Dental and Craniofacial Research (NIDCR) for overcoming limitations of conventional periodontal probing

LIMITATION	CONVENTIONAL PROBING	NIDCR – CRITERIA
Limitation	**Conventional Probing**	**NIDCR Criteria**
Precision	1 mm	0.1 mm
Range	12 mm	10 mm
Probing force	Nonstandardized	Constant and standardized
Applicability	Noninvasive and easy to use	Noninvasive, lightweight, and easy to use
Reach	Easy to access any location around all teeth	Easy to access any location around all teeth
Angulation	Subjective	A guidance system to ensure proper angulation
Security	Easily sterilized	Complete sterilization of all portions entering the mouth
	Simple stainless steel instrument	No biohazard from material or electric shock
Readout	Depending on voice dictation and recording in writing	Direct electronic reading and digital output

therapy, and monitor treatment outcomes. Additionally, computerization offers the entire dental team the ideal potential to achieve examiner standardization so that future comparison of health and disease becomes simpler and more precise and remains cost-effective. This has resulted in the development of new periodontal probing systems. After a National Institute of Craniofacial Research (NIDCR) workshop on the quantitative evaluation of periodontal diseases by physical measurement techniques,[106] there was a proposal to develop and clinically evaluate an improved periodontal pocket depth–attachment level measurement system that would meet the nine NIDCR criteria shown in Table 37-1.

Following these criteria, the Florida Probe System was developed.[36] This automated probe system consists of a probe handpiece, digital readout, foot switch, computer interface, and computer (Figure 37-4). The end of the probe tip is 0.4 mm in diameter. This probe tip reciprocates through a sleeve, and the edge of the sleeve provides a reference by which measurements are made (Figure 37-5). These measurements are made electronically and transferred automatically to the computer when the foot switch is pressed. Constant probing force is provided by coil springs inside the probe handpiece and digital readout. This probing method combines the advantages of constant probing force with precise electronic measurement and computer storage of data, thus eliminating the potential errors associated with visual reading and the need for an assistant to record the measurements.

These automated probes offer many solutions to the problems of conventional probing but also introduce problems. The probing elements lack tactile sensitivity, mainly because of their independent movement, which forces the operator to predetermine an insertion point and angle. In addition, the use of a fixed-force setting throughout the mouth, regardless of the site or inflammatory status, may generate inaccurate measurements or patient discomfort. One common problem reported in studies comparing the Florida Probe System with conventional probing is the underestimation of deep probing depths by the automated probe.[107] Several studies even suggested that the use of this automated probing system does not offer any advantage over conventional probing, rendering a similar level of reproducibility. However, other studies have clearly shown that with the use of trained operators and performing the "double-pass" method, the measurements taken with the Florida Probe System are significantly less variable (lower standard deviation) than those obtained with a conventional probe.[21,86,113,140] The Florida Probe System obtained mean standard deviations (reproducibility) for clinical attachment level measurements of about 0.3 mm, which is clearly superior to an average of 0.82 mm (range, 0.52-1.30 mm) reported by Haffajee et al.[44] using manual probing.

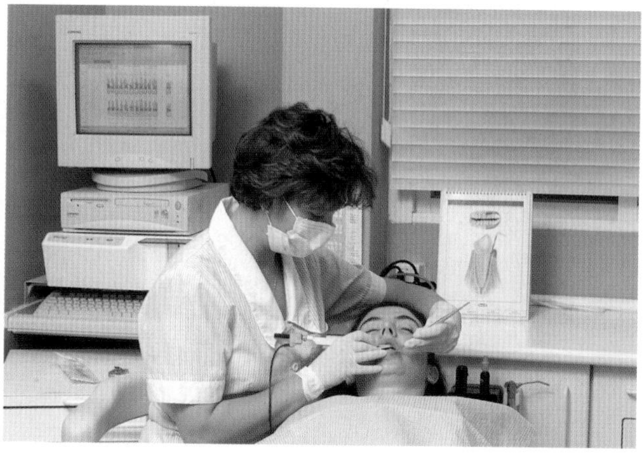

Figure 37-4 Automated periodontal probes: Florida Probe System. Integration of direct electronic measurements with constant probing force with computer storage and online data readout.

Other commercially available electronic probing systems, such as the Interprobe and Periprobe, have also been evaluated (Figure 37-6). They provide constant

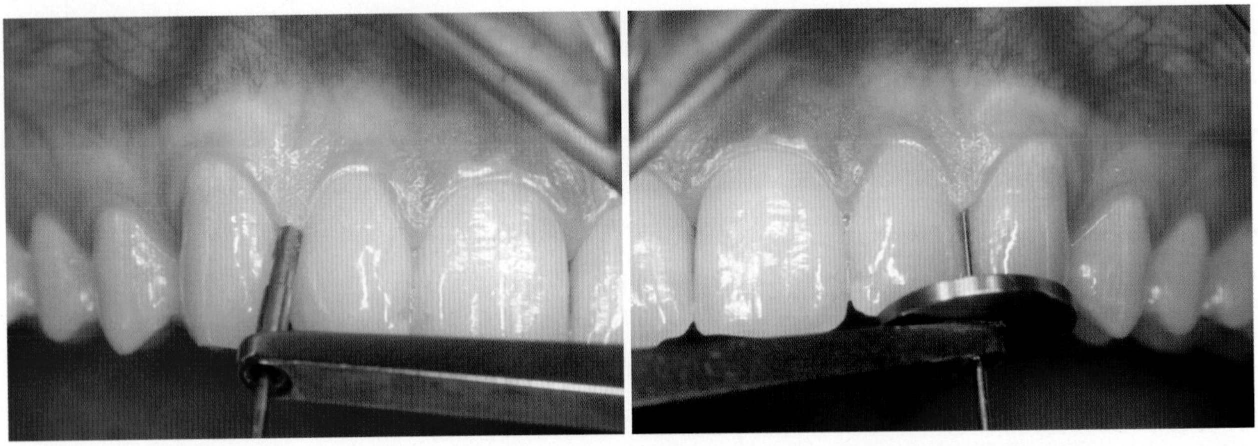

Figure 37-5 Florida Probe System. **A,** Handpiece for assessing probing pocket depths. **B,** Handpiece for assessing relative clinical attachment levels.

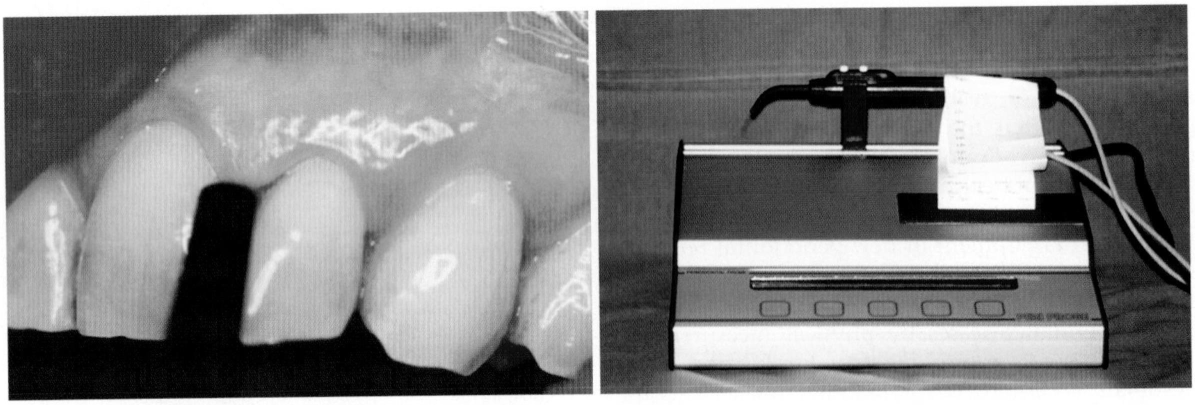

Figure 37-6 Periprobe electronic periodontal probing system. **A,** Measuring device inserted in the sulcus. **B,** Probing unit.

probing force, computer storage of data, and precise electronic management of the resulting inflammation. However, clinical evaluations have reported only slightly improved reproducibility compared with conventional probing, although not clinically significant.[111,133] Other electronic probing systems reported in the literature have never been released for general use. One of these systems is an electronic probe (Foster-Miller) capable of coupling pocket depth measurement with detection of the cementoenamel junction, from which the clinical attachment level is automatically detected.[58,60] Researchers at the University of Toronto have described a probe (Toronto Automated) that, as with the Florida probe, uses the occlusal-incisal surface to measure relative clinical attachment levels.[90] The sulcus is probed with a 0.5-mm nickel-titanium wire that is extended under air pressure. It controls angular discrepancies by means of a mercury-tilt sensor that limits angulation within ±30 degrees, but it requires reproducible positioning of the patient's head and cannot easily measure second or third molars.

The assessment of *clinical attachment level* (CAL) provides information relating to the gain or loss of connective tissue attachment to the root surface, and it is the most practical method of determining that disease is progressing (active) when a significant loss of attachment has occurred over time. The threshold for this change is derived from changes in sequential measurements over time, once the measurement error has been eliminated. Various methods have been used to calculate this threshold, including regression analysis of measurements over time, running medians, the tolerance method, endpoint analysis, and the cumulative sum method.[3,37,58] All these mathematic methods take into account the reproducibility of probing measurements, and therefore the various factors that affect the accuracy of probing, including probing force and position, presence of inflammation, tactile and visual assessment errors, root morphology, and probe design, will affect the calculation of this threshold for change.

Increased precision of periodontal probing is of clinical importance because the reported prevalence of disease activity as identified by CAL change clearly depends on the threshold used for identifying whether loss of attachment (LOA) has occurred.[59] Moreover, although CAL should ideally be measured from the base of the pocket to the cementoenamel junction (CEJ), the detection of this anatomic landmark is usually difficult and not easily reproducible by standard probing methods. Therefore the use of conventional probes to locate the CEJ accurately and reproducibly has been questioned, and currently no commercially available automated probe exists to measure CAL.

The Florida Probe System provides a means of recording relative CAL changes over time. When using the Florida probe, CALs are recorded relative to a fixed reference point, such as the occlusal surfaces of the teeth (disk probe) or a prefabricated stent (stent probe). These measurements are made sequentially over time, and thus differences in relative attachment levels at consecutive examinations must be calculated (see Figure 37-5, *B*). Unfortunately, the use of relative reference points provides no information relating to CALs at a single examination, and further, the reference points may change (a tooth may be restored, or a stent may become distorted). For these reasons, it is desirable to measure CALs using the CEJ as the reference point. A modification of the Florida probe has recently been developed and tested to increase accuracy in detecting the CEJ. This new electronic probe has a modified sleeve, which includes a prominent 0.125-mm edge to facilitate a "catch" of the CEJ. The width of this edge is considered small enough not to interfere with probing-depth measurements, offering clinicians measurement of CAL and probing depth concurrently. This Florida PASHA Probe can reproducibly and reliably identify the CEJ in human skulls[110] and shows promise in measuring CALs in humans.[63] However, longitudinal clinical studies and long-term evaluation of periodontal patients with this new instrument are lacking.

ADVANCES IN RADIOGRAPHIC ASSESSMENT

Dental radiographs are the traditional method used to assess the destruction of alveolar bone associated with periodontitis. Although radiographs cannot accurately reflect the bone morphology buccally and lingually, they provide useful information on interproximal bone levels. Moreover, they provide information on the periodontium that cannot be obtained by other noninvasive methods (e.g., root length, root proximity, presence of periapical lesions, estimates of remaining alveolar bone) (see Figure 37-1, *D*). However, it is well known that substantial volumes of alveolar bone must be destroyed before the loss is detectable in radiographs[37]; specifically, more than 30% of the bone mass at the alveolar crest must be lost for a change in bone height to be recognized on radiographs.[102] *Therefore, conventional radiographs are very specific but lack sensitivity.* (See Chapter 36.)

Numerous cross-sectional and longitudinal epidemiologic studies have used radiographs as the principal method of determining the presence or absence of periodontal destruction. The primary criterion for bone loss in these studies was the distance from the CEJ to the alveolar crest, as measured from bite-wing radiographs. The threshold distance of *bone loss* has varied from 1 to 3 mm, although most of the studies have used greater than 2 mm as the criterion for bone loss.[1] This low degree of sensitivity primarily results from the subjectivity of radiographic assessment and the inherent sources of variability affecting conventional radiographic technique, such as (1) variations in projection geometry; (2) variations in contrast and density caused by differences in film processing, voltage, and exposure time; and (3) masking of osseous changes by other anatomic structures (Figure 37-7). The variations in projection geometry can be reduced by the use of standardized long-cone paralleling radiographic techniques (Figure 37-8). To standardize the radiographic assessment, radiographs should be obtained in a constant and reproducible plane, using film holders with a template containing some type of impression material, which is placed in a constant position on a group of teeth, and an extension arm that can be precisely attached to both the film holder and the x-ray tube[117] (Figure 37-9). The use of a paralleling radiographic technique should be standard to all radiographic assessments for periodontal diagnosis. The use of individualized film holders has been shown to be valid in evaluating bone changes in longitudinal studies and clinical trials.

Digital Radiography

The variations in image quality resulting from the variables inherent to conventional radiography can be reduced with digital intraoral radiography. Digital radiography allows the use of computerized images, which can be stored, manipulated, and corrected for underexposures and overexposures. Digital radiography may yield image properties almost equal to conventional radiographs, but through digital storage and processing, diagnostic information can be enhanced.[52] Moreover, there is a one-third to half reduction in radiation dose obtained with digital radiographs compared with conventional radiographs.

Digital intraoral radiography is in a state of rapid development. Sensors, as well as computer hardware and software, are continually modified and improved. Because of the clear advantage of *real* or *almost-real* images that can be improved and the important educational component of online images presented to the patient, it is expected that digital radiography will soon replace conventional radiography in modern daily practice (Figure 37-10). However, certain improvements should be expected to overcome some of the current limitations (see Chapter 36).

Subtraction Radiography

Subtraction radiography, a well-established technique in medicine, has been introduced as a technique in periodontal diagnosis.[39] This technique relies on the conversion of serial radiographs into digital images. The serially obtained digital images can then be superimposed and the resultant composite viewed on a video screen. Changes in the density and volume of bone can be detected as lighter areas (bone gain) or dark areas (bone loss). Quantitative changes in comparison with the baseline images can be detected using an algorithm for gray-scale levels. This is accomplished by means of computer-assisted subtraction radiography (Figure 37-11). This technique requires a paralleling technique to obtain a standardized geometry and accurate superimposable radiographs.

Studies using this technique have shown (1) a high degree of correlation between changes in alveolar bone

A B C D

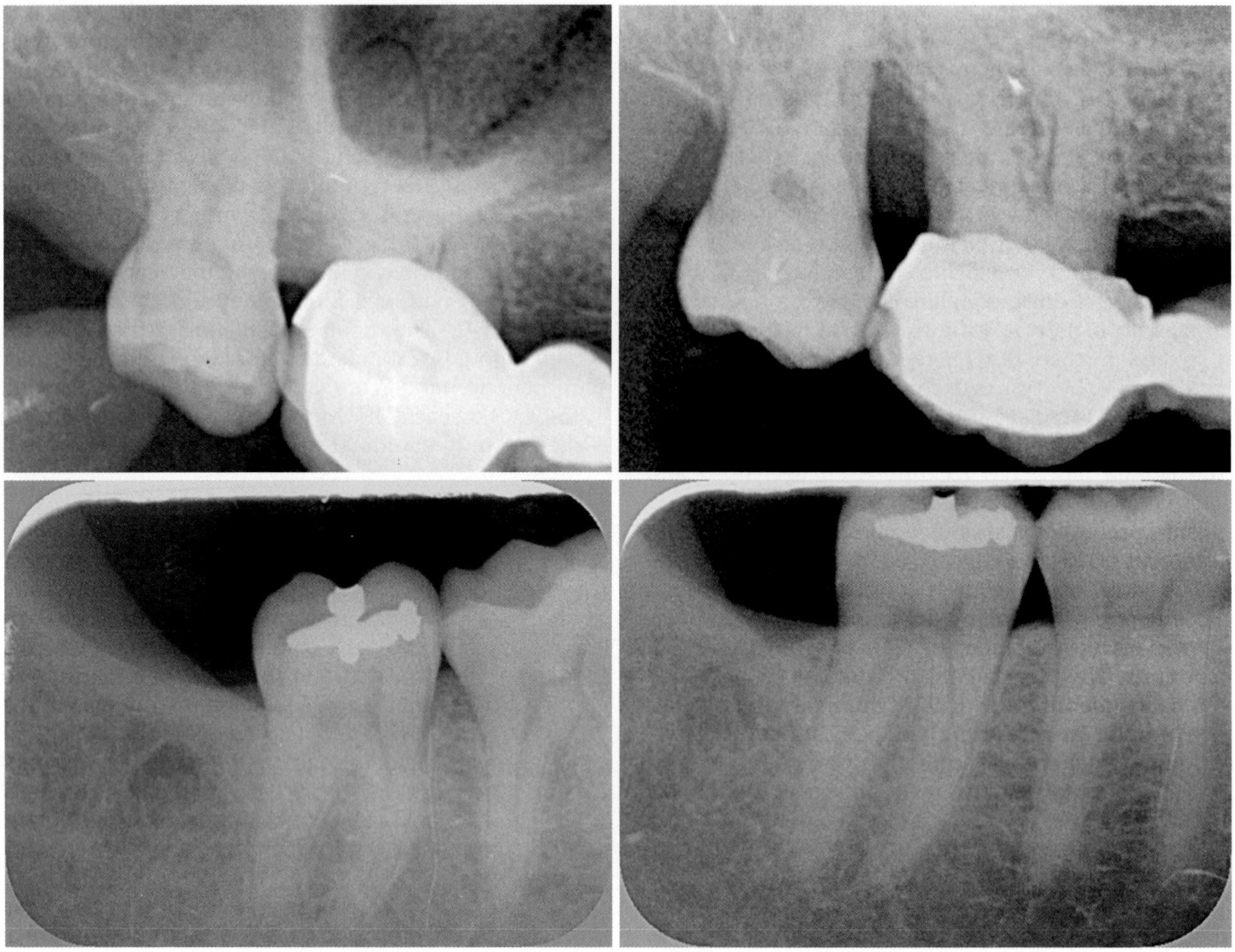

Figure 37-7 Limitations in conventional periapical radiography. Examples of the importance of image projection in the diagnostic utility of oral periapical radiography. **A,** X-ray film taken without a paralleling technique showing a clear distortion of the root length relative to the crown. The alveolar bone height is obscured and fills the interproximal space. **B,** Image of the same tooth in *A* with a proper image projection showing the real alveolar bone height and demonstrating severe bone loss in the distal surface of the upper first molar **C,** X-ray film taken without a paralleling technique showing a clear distortion of the root length relative to the crown, The alveolar bone height is obscured and fills the interproximal space. **D,** Image of the same tooth in *C* with a proper image projection showing the real alveolar bone height and the open interproximal space. (Courtesy Dr. Federico Herrero.)

determined by subtraction radiography and CAL changes in periodontal patients after therapy[54] and (2) increased detectability of small osseous lesions compared with the conventional radiographs from which the subtraction images are produced.[115] Grondahl et al.,[40] using subtraction analysis, showed nearly perfect accuracy at a lesion depth corresponding to 0.49 mm of compact bone, whereas a lesion must be at least three times larger to be detectable with a conventional radiology technique. Subtraction radiography has also been applied to longitudinal clinical studies. Hausmann et al.[53] detected significant differences in crestal bone height of 0.87 mm, and Jeffcoat et al.[59] showed a strong relationship between probing attachment loss detected using sequential measurements made with an automated periodontal probe and bone loss detected with digital subtraction radiography.

Subtraction radiography is a technique that facilitates both qualitative and quantitative visualization of even minor density changes in bone by removing the unchanged anatomic structures from the image. This enhances the detection of bone structures with true density change and significantly improves the sensitivity and accuracy of the evaluation. The main disadvantage of digital subtraction radiography techniques is the need to be almost at identical projection alignment during the exposure of the sequential radiographs, which makes this method impractical in a clinical setting.

Recently, new image subtraction methods, called *diagnostic subtraction radiography* (DSR), have been introduced combining the use of a positioning device during film exposure with specialized software designed for digital image subtraction using conventional personal computers in dental offices (Figure 37-11). This image analysis

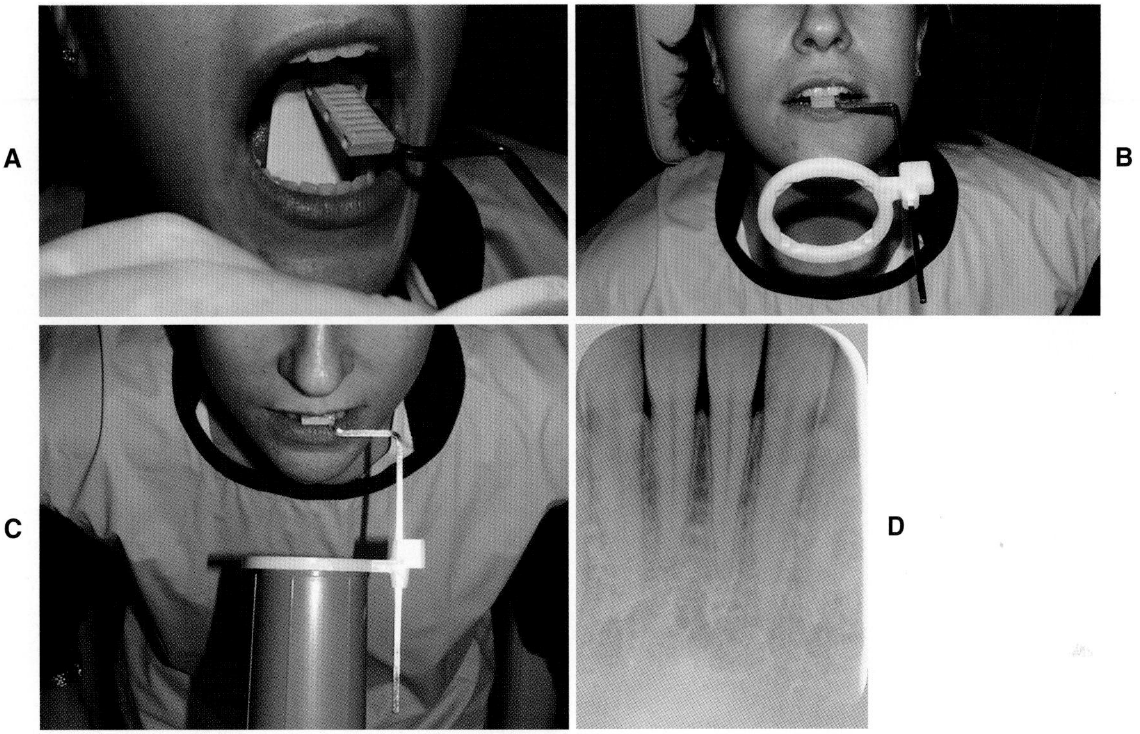

Figure 37-8 Radiographic paralleling technique. **A,** Position of the film holder relative to the teeth. **B,** Position of the film holder relative to the paralleling device. **C,** Position of the paralleling device to the x-ray long-cone tube. **D,** Radiograph obtained with proper image projection. (Courtesy Dr. Federico Herrero.)

software system applies an algorithm that corrects for the effects of angular alignment discrepancies and provides some degree of flexibility in the imaging procedure. Compared with conventional subtraction radiography and conventional intraoral radiography, DSR showed statistically significant gains in diagnostic accuracy over conventional radiographs but no differences with subtraction radiography.[100]

Computer-Assisted Densitometric Image Analysis System

In the computer-assisted densitometric image analysis system (CADIA), a video camera measures the light transmitted through a radiograph, and the signals from the camera are converted into gray-scale images.[15] The camera is interfaced with an image processor and a computer that allow the storage and mathematic manipulation of the images.

CADIA appears to offer an objective method for following alveolar bone density changes quantitatively over time. Also, compared with digital subtraction analysis, CADIA has shown a higher sensitivity and a high degree of reproducibility and accuracy. This technique has also been applied to longitudinal clinical studies. Deas et al.,[26] using replicate measurements of CALs and CADIA, demonstrated that the prevalence of progressing lesions in periodontitis (38% of sites per patient), as detected by this radiographic method, may be much higher than previously thought.

ADVANCES IN MICROBIOLOGIC ANALYSIS

A substantial number of publications have reported that certain microorganisms from the subgingival microbiota, particularly gram-negative anaerobes, are the major etiologic factors of chronic and aggressive periodontitis.[28,98,123] Although the subgingival microenvironment in the periodontal pocket is characterized by a wide diversity of organisms, with more than 300 species isolated from different individuals and as many as 40 from a single site, only a few species have been associated with disease.[94] Despite the difficulty in identifying all the members of the oral microbiota and understanding how they interact with each other and with the host, a limited number of microorganisms have demonstrated a clear etiologic role and have been identified as periodontal pathogens.[33] Evidence for etiology is based on the fulfilment of several criteria, as described by Socransky.[126] Using these criteria, strong evidence has been demonstrated for *Actinobacillus actinomycetemcomitans* (Aa), *Porphyromonas gingivalis* (Pg), and *Tannerella forsythia* (Tf) (formerly *Bacteroides forsythus),* as concluded at a world workshop in 1996.[33] Moderately strong evidence has been demonstrated for other bacteria isolated from the subgingival microbiota, including *Campylobacter rectus* (Cr), *Eubacterium nodatum, Fusobacterium nucleatum* (Fn), *Peptostreptococcus micros* (Pm), *Prevotella intermedia* (Pi) and *Prevotella nigrescens* (Pn), *Streptococcus intermedius,* and various spirochetes, such as *Treponema denticola* (Td), although their etiologic role is less evident.

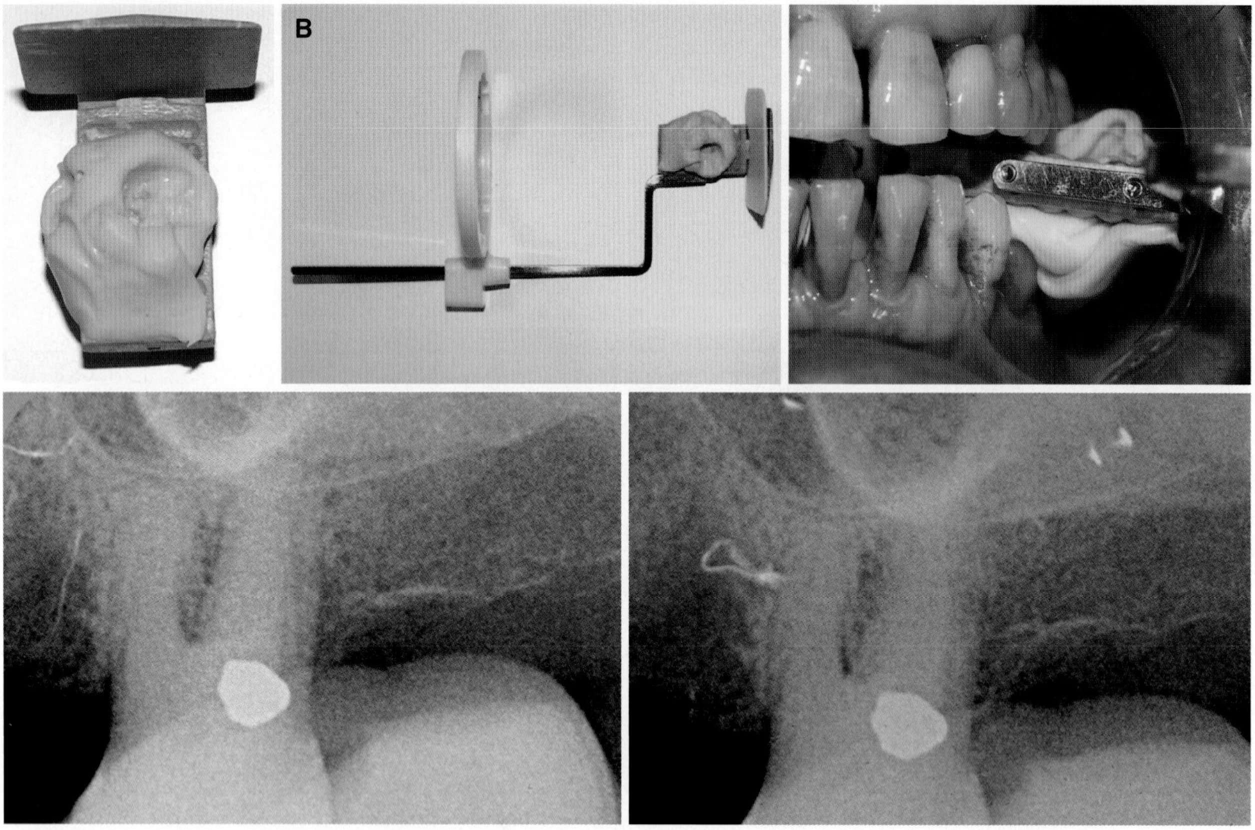

Figure 37-9 Individualized radiographic paralleling technique for the assessment of alveolar bone changes. **A,** Occlusal imprint in film holder. **B,** Individualized film holder in paralleling device. **C,** Individualized paralleling technique in place intraorally. **D** and **E,** Two radiographs obtained 6 months apart demonstrating identical projection geometry. (Courtesy Dr. Federico Herrero.)

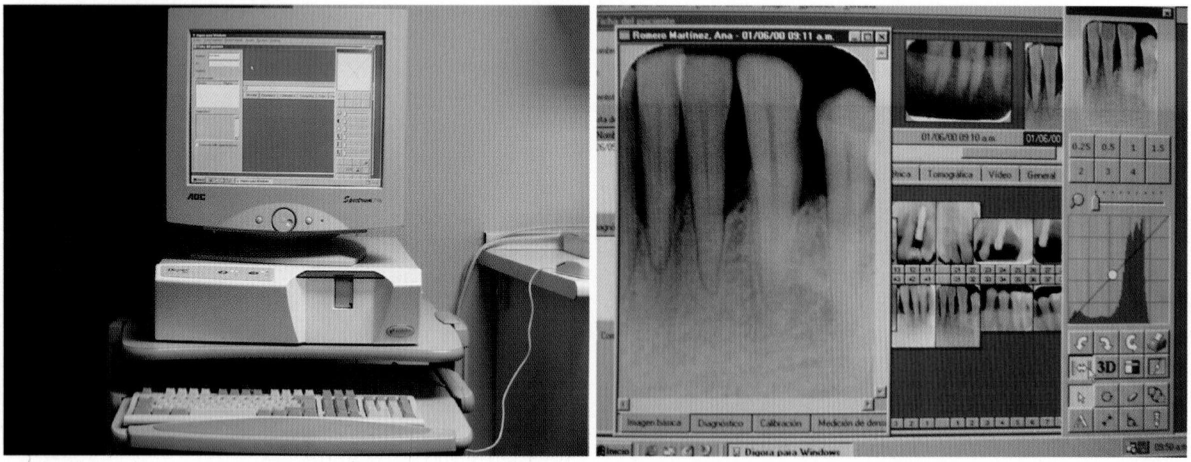

Figure 37-10 Digital radiographic system: Digora.

Even though the etiologic role of *Aa*, *Pg*, and *Tf* in periodontitis seems uncontentious, the use and utility of diagnostic tests aimed to identify and quantify the presence of these bacteria in periodontitits patients remain controversial. Microbiologic tests to identify these putative pathogens have the potential to support the diagnosis of the various forms of periodontal disease, to serve as indicators of disease initiation and progression (i.e., disease activity), and to determine which periodontal sites are at higher risk for active destruction. Microbiologic tests can also be used to monitor periodontal therapy directed at the suppression or eradication of periodontal pathogenic microorganisms.[136]

Microbiologic testing for the presence or absence of *Pg* and *Aa* to distinguish subjects with aggressive periodontitis from those with chronic periodontitis clearly

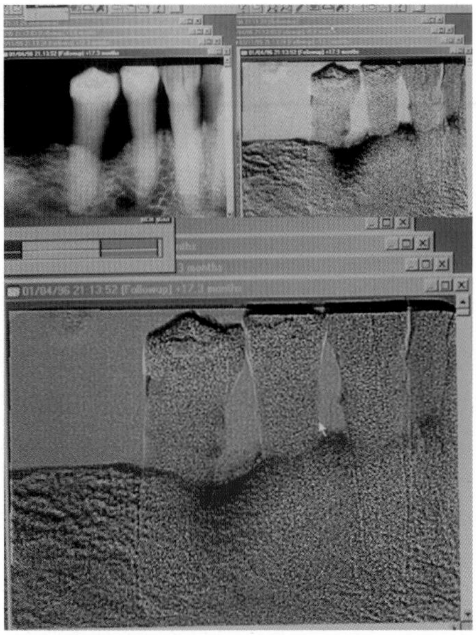

Figure 37-11 Digital subtraction radiography (DSR) analysis can be used to evaluate the effects of therapy on bone density and morphology. The effects of surgical therapy on an angular defect are seen, with the new bone formation represented by the dark area.

showed its limitations in the recent systematic review by Mombelli et al.[92] Although the diagnosis of aggressive periodontitis may be less likely in a subject with no detection of *Aa,* the sensitivity and specificity for a positive clinical diagnosis of aggressive periodontitis in presence of these bacteria is low and heterogeneous. Therefore the mere presence or absence of these putative pathogens cannot be used to discriminate subjects with aggressive periodontitis from those with chronic periodontitis. The utility of microbial identification as an aid in the treatment planning of patients with periodontitis has been tested in a limited number of studies, mostly case reports involving patients with aggressive or nonresponding periodontitis.[30,56,77,114,116] The aim of most of these studies was to guide in the selection of adjunctive antimicrobial therapy based on the microbial data. Only one of these publications reported a controlled study,[77] in which two different groups of periodontists developed their treatment plans based on the results of adjunctive diagnostic microbiology (test) or just on standard clinical diagnosis (controls). The use of microbial diagnosis resulted in using more systemic antibiotics and less periodontal surgery. However, the long-term outcome of these patients was not reported. The other studies involved case reports in which the use of microbial diagnosis guided periodontal therapy. In most of these studies the patients improved after treatment, with some even showing dramatic improvement. The lack of appropriate controls, however, makes the interpretation of these results difficult, and therefore the utility of microbial testing in developing specific treatment plans cannot be ascertained.

The utility of microbiologic testing as an indicator of healing or disease progression has been suggested by several prospective studies, where the detection or lack of detection of putative periodontal pathogens was significantly associated with a different clinical response.* In most of these studies the absence of these pathogens was a better predictor of periodontal health than their presence was a predictor of periodontal disease.[23,137] Some studies showed that the presence of these pathogens above certain critical levels increased the risk for periodontitis recurrence.

Several methods have been employed for the detection of putative periodontal pathogens in subgingival samples. Some of these methods have been strictly used for research purposes, whereas others have been adapted or modified for clinical use. All these methods share the common need for an appropriate subgingival plaque sample. Selecting the proper specimen site and collecting an adequate sample are essential elements in periodontal microbiology. These samples may be difficult to obtain in patients infected by organisms that are unevenly distributed in the dentition. Mombelli et al.[92] have shown that four individual subgingival specimens, each from the deepest periodontal pocket in each quadrant, should be pooled to be able to detect the highest amount of periodontal pathogens. If a microbial culture is contemplated, the sample must be collected and transported in an anaerobic environment, and minimal transport time should be ensured to reach the laboratory and to maintain the growth of the microorganisms sampled. Figure 37-12 shows the standard subgingival sampling technique by means of sterile paper points inserted into the deepest area of the selected periodontal pocket.

Bacterial Culturing

Historically, culture methods have been widely used in studies aimed at characterizing the composition of the subgingival microflora and are still considered the reference method ("gold standard") when determining the performance of new microbial diagnostic methods. Generally, plaque samples are cultivated under anaerobic conditions, and the use of selective and nonselective media, with several biochemical and physical tests, allows the identification of different putative pathogens. The main advantage of this method is that the clinician can obtain relative and absolute counts of the cultured species. Moreover, it is the only in vitro method able to assess for antibiotic susceptibility of the microbes.

However, culture techniques have important shortcomings. Culture methods can only grow live bacteria; therefore, strict sampling and transport conditions are essential. Moreover, some of the putative pathogens, such as *Treponemas* species and *Tf,* are fastidious and difficult to culture. The sensitivity of culture methods is rather low, since the detection limits for selective and nonselective media average 10^3 to 10^4 bacteria, and thus low numbers of a specific pathogen in a pocket are undetected. The most important drawback, however, is that culture requires sophisticated equipment and experienced personnel and is relatively time-consuming and

*References 16, 18, 23, 47-49, 113, 130, 137.

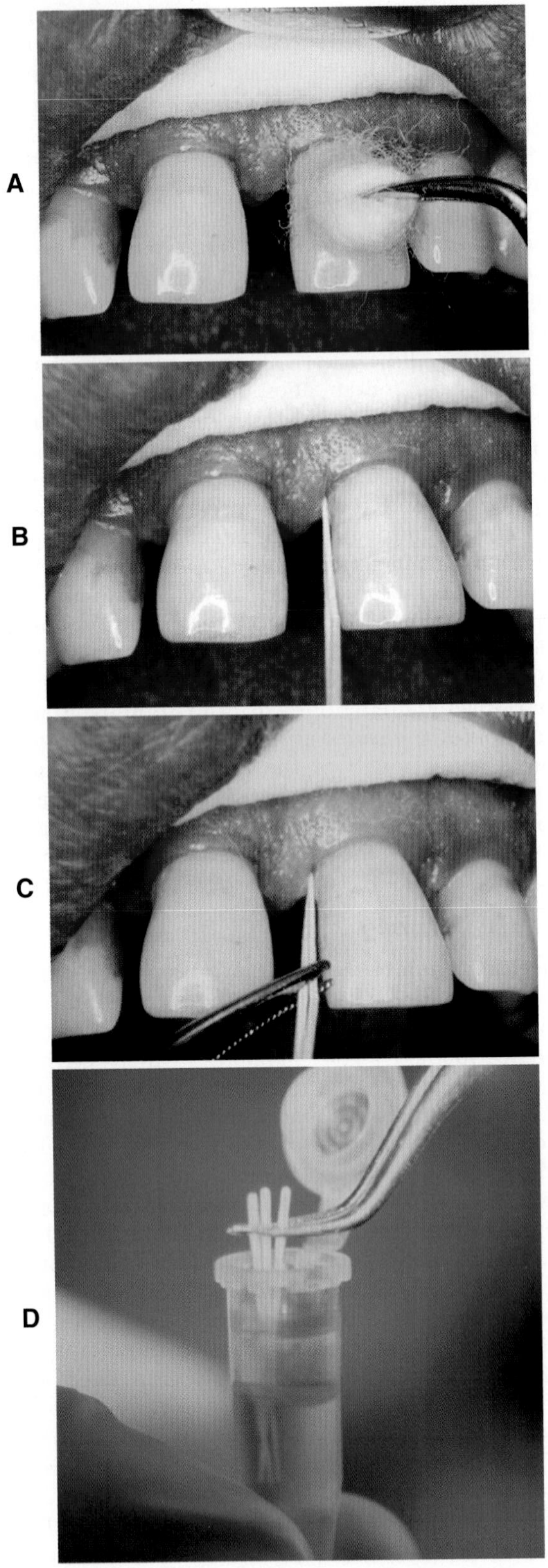

Figure 37-12 Microbial sampling of subgingival microflora. **A** and **B,** Tooth is dried, and supragingival plaque is removed from the sampling site. **C,** Three sterile endodontic paper points are placed subgingivally to the base of the pocket. **D,** The paper points are removed and placed in a vial of anaerobic media for immediate transport to the laboratory for analysis.

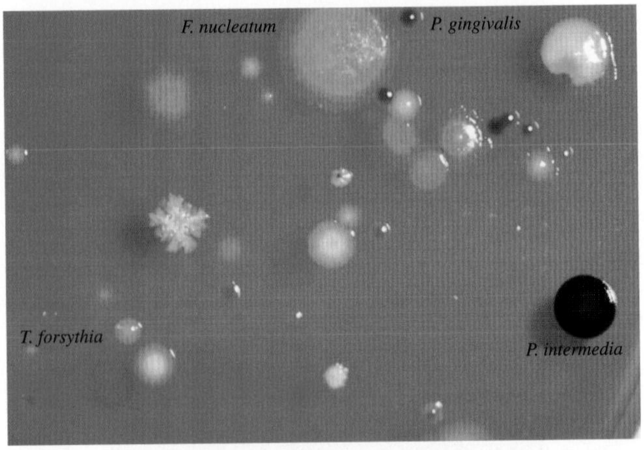

Figure 37-13 Bacteriologic anaerobic culture of the subgingival microflora in a patient with severe periodontitis.

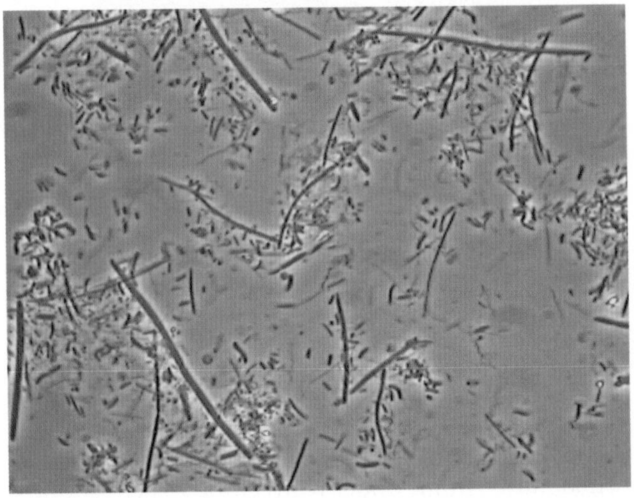

Figure 37-14 Phase-contrast microscopic image showing different bacterial morphotypes.

expensive. When using this method, clinicians must be confident that the laboratory has the appropriate technology and expertise in periodontal microbiology to communicate diagnostically and therapeutically useful information to them (Figure 37-13).

Direct Microscopy

Dark-field or phase-contrast microscopy has been suggested as an alternative to culture methods[80] on the basis of its ability to assess directly and rapidly the morphology and motility of bacteria in a plaque sample (Figure 37-14). However, most of the main putative periodontal pathogens, including *Aa, Pg, Tf, Eikenella corrodens* (Ec), and *Eubacterium* species, are nonmotile, and therefore this technique is unable to identify these species. Microscopy is also unable to differentiate among the various species of *Treponema*. Therefore, dark-field microscopy seems an unlikely candidate as a diagnostic test of destructive periodontal diseases.[81]

Immunodiagnostic Methods

Immunologic assays employ antibodies that recognize specific bacterial antigens to detect target microorganisms. This reaction can be revealed using a variety of procedures, including direct and indirect immunofluorescent (microscopy) assays (IFAs), flow cytometry, enzyme-linked immunosorbent assay, membrane assay, and latex agglutination.

Direct IFA employs both monoclonal and polyclonal antibodies conjugated to a fluorescein marker that binds with the bacterial antigen to form a fluorescent immune complex detectable under a microscope. *Indirect IFA* employs a secondary fluorescein-conjugated antibody that reacts with the primary antigen-antibody complex. Both direct and indirect IFAs are able to identify the pathogen and quantify the percentage of the pathogen directly using a plaque smear. IFA has been used mainly to detect *Aa* and *Pg*. Zambon et al[142] showed that IFA is comparable to bacterial culture in its ability to identify these pathogens in subgingival dental plaque samples. In fact, IFA microscopy may be even more likely to detect them in clinical samples because it does not require viable bacterial cells. Comparative studies indicate that the sensitivity of these assays ranges from 82% to 100% for detection of *Aa* and from 91% to 100% for detection of *Pg*, with specificity values of 88% to 92% and 87% to 89%, respectively.[141]

Cytofluorography or *flow cytometry* for the rapid identification of oral bacteria involves labeling bacterial cells from a patient plaque sample with both species-specific antibody and a second fluorescein-conjugated antibody. The suspension is then introduced into the flow cytometer, which separates the bacterial cells into an almost single-cell suspension by means of a laminar flow through a narrow tube. The sophistication and cost involved in this procedure precludes its wide use.

Enzyme-linked immunosorbent assay (ELISA) is similar in principle to other radioimmunoassays, but instead of the radioisotope, an enzymatically derived color reaction is substituted as the label. The intensity of the color depends on the concentration of the antigen and is usually read photometrically for optimal quantification. ELISA has been used primarily to detect serum antibodies to periodontal pathogens, although it has also been used in research studies to quantify specific pathogens in subgingival samples using specific monoclonal antibodies. A membrane immunoassay has been adapted for chairside clinical diagnostic use (Evalusite). It involves linkage between the antigen and a membrane-bound antibody to form an immunocomplex that is later revealed through a colorimetric reaction. Evalusite has been designed to detect *Aa*, *Pg*, and *Pi*[14,18,125] and found a detection limit of 10^5 for *Aa* and 10^6 for *Pg* (Figure 37-15).

Latex agglutination is a simple immunologic assay based on the binding of protein to latex. Latex beads are coated with the species-specific antibody, and when these beads come in contact with the microbial cell surface antigens or antigen extracts, cross-linking occurs; its agglutination or clumping is then visible, usually in 2 to 5 minutes. Because of their simplicity and rapidity, these assays have great potential for chairside detection of periodontal pathogens. However, these assays have only been tested for research purposes and are not clinically available.

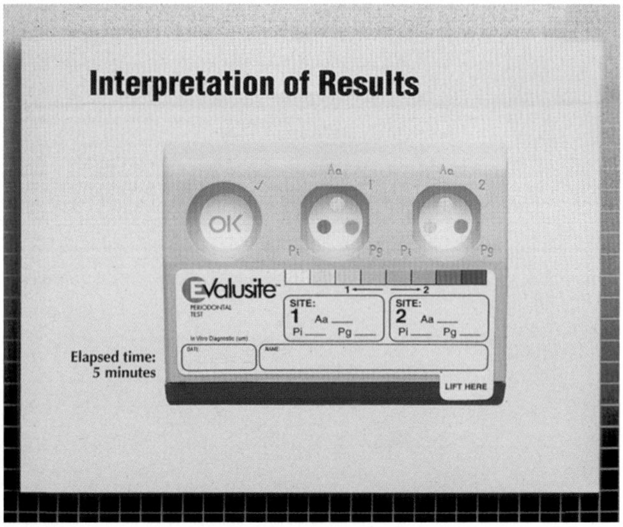

Figure 37-15 Enzyme-linked immunosorbent assay (ELISA, Evalusite) demonstrating positive results for *Actinobacillus actinomycetemcomitans.*

In summary, immunologic assays for oral bacteria provide a quantitative or semiquantitative estimate of target microorganisms. These methods have shown a higher sensitivity and specificity than bacterial culturing for the detection of target microorganisms (*Aa, Pg,* and *Tf*). However, they require the use of monoclonal antibodies to ensure high specificity, and the detection limits are not significantly lower than with bacterial culturing (10^3-10^4). These tests also have the advantage of not requiring stringent sampling and transport methodology to ensure bacterial viability. However, immunologic assays are limited to the number of antibodies tested, are not amenable for studying antibiotic susceptibility, and lack the validity of well-controlled clinical studies.

Enzymatic Methods

Tannerella forsythia (Tf), *Porphyromonas gingivalis* (Pg), the small spirochete *Treponema denticola* (Td), and *Capnocytophaga* species share a common enzymatic profile: all have a trypsinlike enzyme. The activity of this enzyme can be measured with the hydrolysis of the colorless substrate *N*-benzoyl-*d* L-arginine-2-naphthylamide (BANA). When the hydrolysis takes place, it releases the chromophore β-naphthylamide, which turns orange red when a drop of fast garnet is added to the solution. Diagnostic kits have been developed using this reaction for the identification of this bacteria profile in plaque isolates (Perioscan). Loesche[82] proposed the use of this BANA reaction in subgingival plaque samples to detect the presence of any of these periodontal pathogens and thus serve as a marker of disease activity (Figure 37-16). Using probing depths as a measure of periodontal morbidity, Loesche showed that shallow pockets exhibited only 10% positive BANA reactions, whereas deep pockets (7 mm) exhibited 80% to 90% positive BANA reactions. Beck[9] used the BANA test as a risk indicator for periodontal attachment loss.

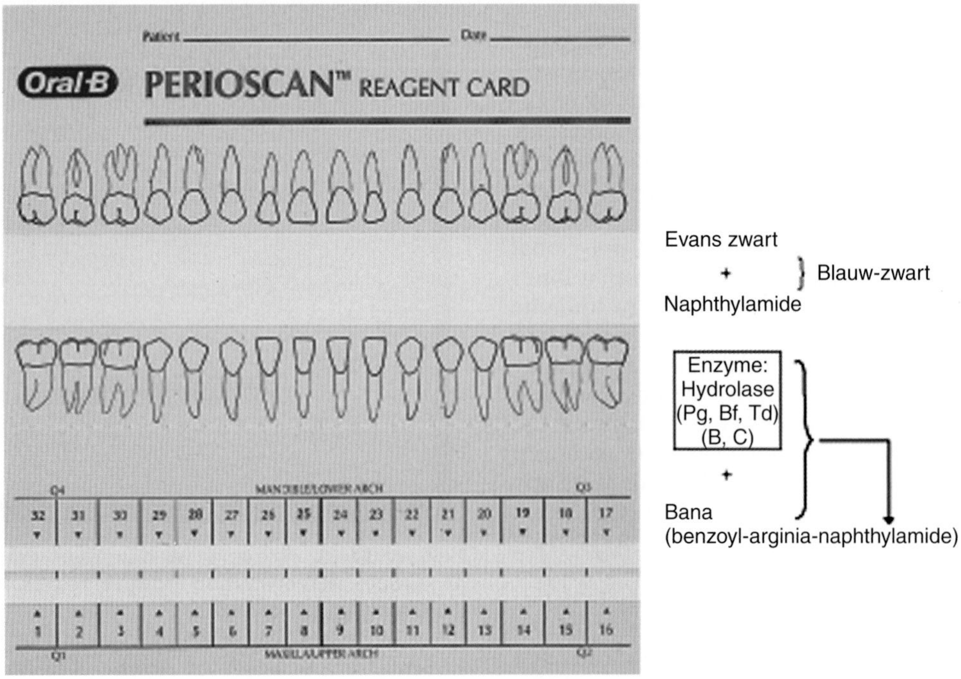

Figure 37-16 Diagnostic kit (Perioscan) developed for the identification of specific bacteria profiles using an enzymatic reaction from plaque isolates. (Courtesy Oral-B, South Boston, Mass.)

Collectively, results using this diagnostic method suggest that positive BANA findings are a good indication that *Td, Pg,* or both are present at sampled sites. One of the potential difficulties of this test is that it may be positive at clinically healthy sites, and whether this test can detect sites undergoing periodontal destruction has yet to be proved. Further, because it only detects a very limited number of pathogens, its negative result does not rule out the presence of other important periodontal pathogens.[83]

Diagnostic Assays Based on Molecular Biology Techniques

The development of techniques in molecular biology aimed at the detection of bacterial pathogens not only has allowed the acquisition of knowledge in microbial genetics, but also has set the bases for the development of improved diagnostic techniques.[36,55,119] The principles of molecular biology techniques reside in the analysis of deoxyribonucleic acid (DNA), ribonucleic acid (RNA), and the structure or function of protein.[25,78] The genetic material of a bacterium is composed of a chromosomal DNA and transferring RNA (tRNA), ribosomal RNA (rRNA), and messenger RNA (mRNA). Chromosomal DNA is dispersed in the bacterial cell without a membrane envelope.[55] Diagnostic assays employing molecular biology techniques require specific DNA fragments that recognize complementary-specific bacterial DNA sequences from target microorganisms. Development of a microbiologic diagnostic test using this technology therefore requires the ability to extract the bacterial DNA from the plaque sample and amplify the specific DNA sequence of the target periodontal pathogens.

Nucleic Acid Probes. A *probe* is a known nucleic acid molecule (DNA or RNA) from a specific microorganism artificially synthesized and labeled for its detection when placed with a plaque sample. DNA probes use segments of a single-stranded nucleic acid, labeled with an enzyme or radioisotope that is able to "hybridize" to the complementary nucleic acid sequence and thus detect the presence of target microorganism. *Hybridization* refers to the pairing of complementary DNA strands to produce a double-stranded nucleic acid. The nucleotide base-pair relationship is so specific that strands cannot anneal unless the respective nucleotide strand sequences are complementary (Figure 37-17). All hybridization methods use radiolabeled or fluorescence-labeled DNA probes that bind to the target DNA of interest, thus allowing its visualization.* DNA probes may target whole genomic DNA or individual genes. Whole genomic DNA is more likely to cross-react with nontarget microorganisms because of the presence of homologous sequences between different bacterial species. Currently, most of the probes used are oligonucleotides ranging from 20 to 30 nucleotides.[99]

Whole genomic probes for the detection of *Aa, Pg, Pi,* and *Td* have been developed and tested and are the bases of commercially available diagnostic methods (e.g., DMDx, Omnigene). When compared to culture, van Steenberghe et al.[135] reported a sensitivity of 96% and specificity of 86% for *Aa* and 60% and 82%, respectively, for *Pg* in pure laboratory isolates. However, when tested in clinical specimens, both sensitivity and specificity

*References 22, 25, 75, 83, 99, 129.

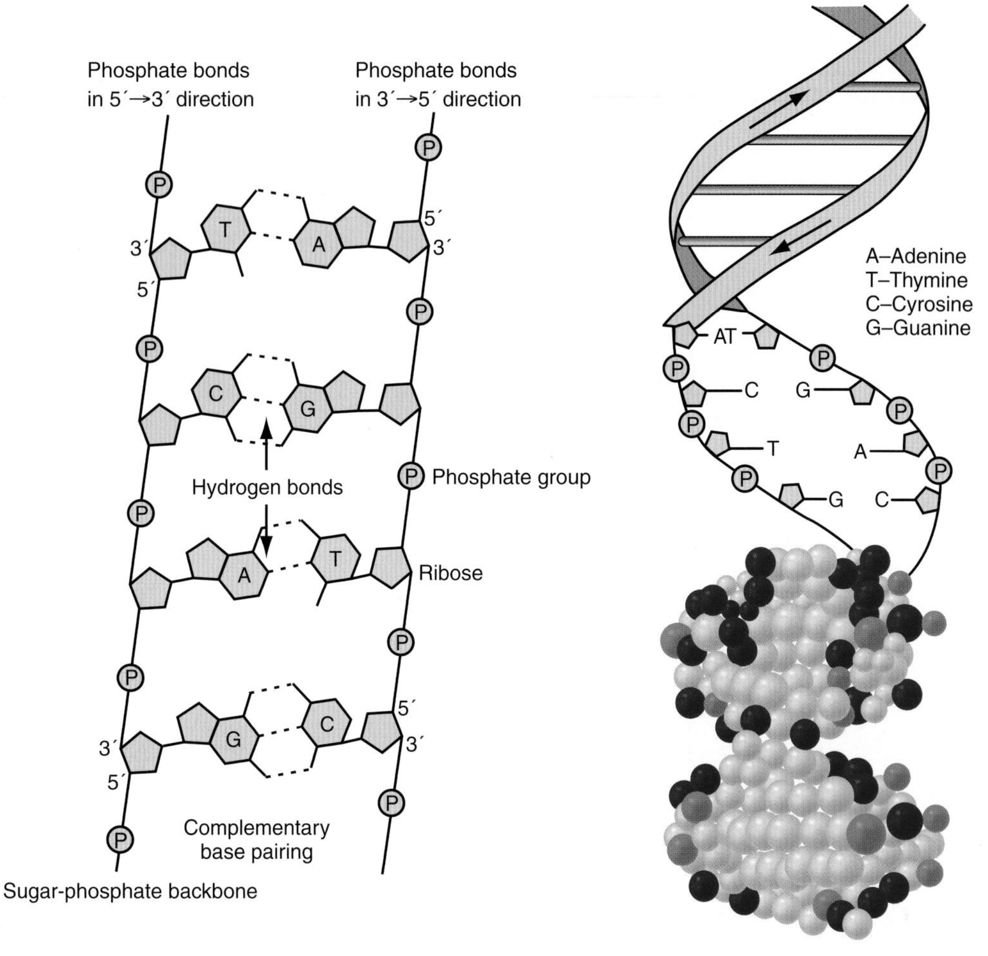

Figure 37-17 The DNA nucleotide base-pair relationship is so specific that strands cannot anneal unless the respective nucleotide strand sequences are complementary.

were reduced significantly, suggesting cross-reactivity with unknown bacteria in subgingival plaque samples. To overcome this drawback, oligonucleotide probes complementary to variable regions of the 16S rRNA bacterial genes have been developed for the detection of various periodontal pathogens. These bacterial 16S rRNA genes contain both regions shared by different bacteria and short stretches of variable regions shared only by specific organisms of the same species or genus.[93] When these oligonuclotide probes where compared with culture in clinical samples for the detection of *Aa, Pg,* and *Pi,* Savitt et al.[120] reported an effectiveness of 100% in detecting *Aa* and *Pi* and of 91% in detecting *Pg,* calculated at culture-positive levels (10^3 cells). However, DNA probes were more sensitive than culture in detecting these pathogens in samples from periodontitis patients; for example, *Aa* was detected by probe analysis in 70% of localized aggressive (juvenile) periodontitis samples, but only detected in 10% by culture analysis. Conversely, when these probes were compared with IFA for the detection of *Pg* and *Tf,* IFA showed significantly higher detection rates and higher sensitivity.

Checkerboard DNA-DNA hybridization Technology. Socransky et al.[127] developed this technique by for the detection and levels of 40 bacterial species often found in the oral cavity. The assay uses whole genomic, digoxigenin-labeled DNA probes and facilitates rapid processing of large numbers of plaque samples with multiple hybridization for up to 40 oral species in a single test (Figure 37-18). The DNA probes used in this technology are usually adjusted to permit detection of 10^4 cells of each species. The method requires sophisticated laboratory equipment and expertise and is highly specific, and thus this assay has not been generalized for diagnostic purposes. It is particularly applicable, however, for epidemiologic research and ecologic studies because it does not require viable bacteria and allows for the assessment of large number of plaque samples and multiple species.* Papapanou et al.[105] made a comparison study between this method and culture for the identification of subgingival bacteria. The checkerboard technology resulted in higher prevalence figures for half the species tested (*Pg, Pi, Pn, Fn,* and *Tf*) and statistically significant higher bacterial counts for the majority of the species. Both techniques showed a reasonable degree of agreement.

*References 31, 49, 50, 51, 77, 138, 139.

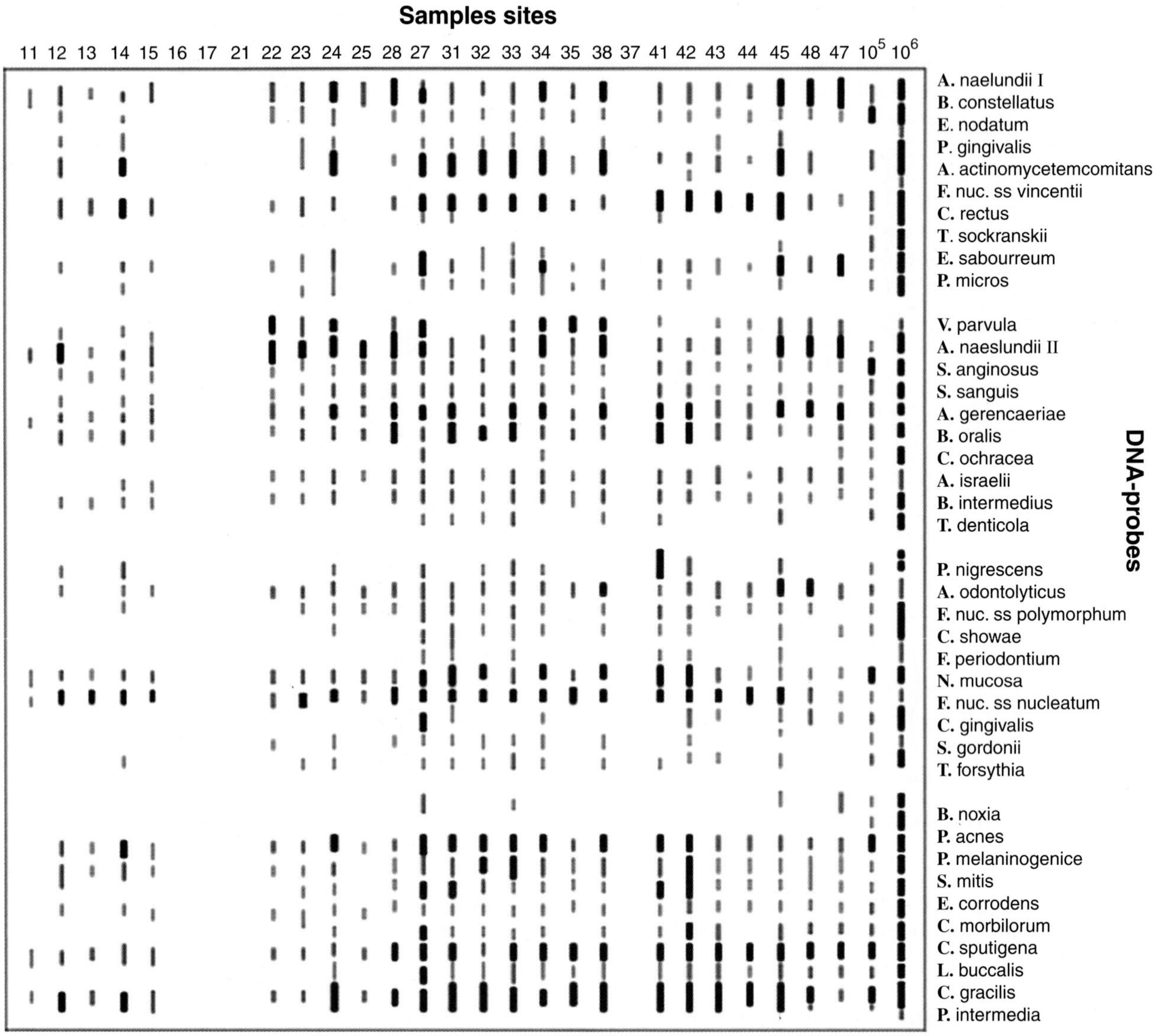

Figure 37-18 Checkerboard DNA-DNA hybridization technology for detecting 40 bacterial species often found in the oral cavity.

Polymerase Chain Reaction. Polymerase chain reaction (PCR) has emerged as the most powerful tool for the amplification of genes and their RNA transcripts. This technique, developed in 1985, is the single technique used almost universally to study DNA and RNA obtained from a variety of tissue sources. PCR allows large quantities of DNA to be obtained in a simplified and automated manner.[25,57,122] PCR typically begins with the isolation of DNA from a fresh tissue specimen. By heating the complementary double strands, DNA splits into single-stranded forms intended to act as the template dictating the nucleotide sequence in vitro. The amplification is followed using a DNA polymerase that requires a *primer,* or known short oligonucleotide sequence corresponding to the border of the region that is amplified. For obtaining amplified fragments of constant length and in large quantities, a second primer, complementary of the opposed chain, must be used to *anneal* (bind) the template and flank the region of interest. This amplification can be performed several times, known as *cycles.* In each cycle the processes of complementary chain denaturation, primer hybridization, and primer extension by means of the polymerase take place. With each cycle there is an exponential increase in the quantity of DNA. Throughout this process the temperature during the cycle is critical to control the double-chain denaturation and the stability of the hybridization between the model fragment and the primer. In 1988 a thermostable DNA polymerase isolated from the organism *Thermus aquaticus,* known as Taq-polymerase, was developed.[119] This Taq-polymerase has allowed automatization of the reaction using specific appliances called *thermocyclers.* This sequenced DNA is then detected and visualized through electrophoresis in agarose gel and ethidium-bromure, obtaining a qualitative signal.[57,97]

Since the advent of PCR technology, different microbiologic tests have been developed for the detection of *Aa, Pg,* and *Tf* using a variety of DNA extraction methods

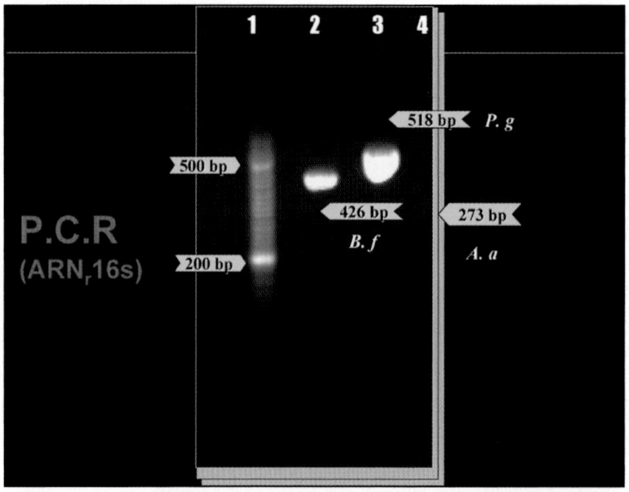

Figure 37-19 Standard PCR technology using 16s rRNA primers for *Actinobacillus actinomycetemcomitans, Porphyromonas gingivalis,* and *Tannerella forsythia.*

and primers. Ashimoto et al.[6] developed a 16S rRNA-based PCR detection method to determine the prevalence of *Aa, Tf, Cr, Ec, Pg, Pi, Pn,* and *Td.* Matched results between PCR and culture occurred in 28% (*Tf*) and 71% (*Aa*) of the samples; the major discrepancy occurred in the PCR-positive/culture-negative category. This probably resulted from the PCR lower detection limit (25-100 cells) compared with culture (10^4-10^5 cells). Eick and Pfister[29] recently compared a commercial multiplex PCR of 16s rRNA for *Aa, Pg, Pi, Tf,* and *Td* with standard culturing. The PCR test was able to detect *Pg* and *Tf* more often than cultivation. *Aa* was detected in similar numbers with both techniques. Although these microbial tests using standard PCR are extremely specific and sensitive, they have a number of important limitations. These PCR tests provide only qualitative information (prevalence of the tested bacteria), and therefore their use for diagnostic and prognostic purposes in clinical use is limited (Figure 37-19).

The importance of a quantitative assessment of the target bacteria has led to the recent development of quantitative PCR methods. The first assays used *endpoint PCR.*[27,32] However, this technique obtains PCR product in the saturated phase, disregarding the early exponential phase; therefore the amount of PCR product obtained shows a weak correlation with the initial DNA quantity. To overcome this limitation, *real-time PCR* assays have been developed. With this technology and by using a single copy of these genes per cell, a good correlation between the fluorescent signal measured and the number of cells has been obtained.[84,121] Morillo et al.[95] tested a real-time PCR assay, based on single-copy gene sequence and on the SYBR Green I chemistry, aimed at the quantification of *Aa* and *Pg* in subgingival plaque samples. This assay demonstrated a high degree of specificity and was a reproducible and consistent method to quantify these pathogenic species. Although demonstrating a high degree of sensitivity, specificity, and reproducible quantification, real-time PCR requires expensive laboratory equipment, which makes this method very expensive for routine diagnostic clinical microbiology.

In summary, standard PCR technology, although demonstrating high sensitivity and specificity for the identification of target periodontal pathogens, is unable to quantify them accurately in clinical samples, and therefore its role as a routine clinical diagnostic tool is limited. However, the advent of quantitative PCR technology may circumvent this limitation and improve some of the shortcomings of standard cultural techniques. These quantitative PCR assays must be validated in clinical studies to demonstrate their diagnostic utility, and cost-benefit evaluation of their use in routine clinical diagnosis must also be done because they require expensive and sophisticated technology.

ADVANCES IN CHARACTERIZING THE HOST RESPONSE

Our understanding of the initiation and progression of periodontal disease and the pathogenic processes involved has expanded enormously in light of advances in clinical and basic science research. Diagnostic tests have been developed that add measures of the inflammatory process to conventional clinical measures. These tests may provide information on the destructive process itself, current activity of the disease, rate of disease progression, patterns of destruction, extent and severity of future breakdown, and likely response to therapy. With this information, clinicians would be able to better individualize their therapeutic approach, thus customizing the recommended treatment.

Assessment of the *host response* refers to the study of mediators, by immunologic or biochemical methods, that are recognized as part of the individual's response to the periodontal infection. These mediators are either specifically identified with the infection, such as antibody to a putative pathogen, or represent a less specific reaction, such as the local release of inflammatory mediators, host-derived enzymes, or tissue breakdown products. The host response in periodontal disease involves aspects of acute and chronic inflammation as well as humoral and cellular immune responses. Mediators representing each of these systems have been evaluated using diagnostic tests in clinical periodontics from samples that usually involve noninvasive or minimally invasive techniques.[103]

Source of Samples

Potential sample sources include saliva, gingival crevicular fluid (GCF), gingival crevicular cells, blood serum, blood cells, and urine. However, analysis of urine shows little promise except for its use in the differential diagnosis of tooth loss related to hypophosphatasia in young children, in whom the presence of phosphoethanolamine in urine is diagnostic of the disease. Most efforts to date have been based on the use of components of GCF and, to a lesser extent, saliva and blood.[103] Different studies have demonstrated a high correlation between clinical and histologic signs of gingivitis and increased amounts of GCF flow.[24] In addition, more than 40 components

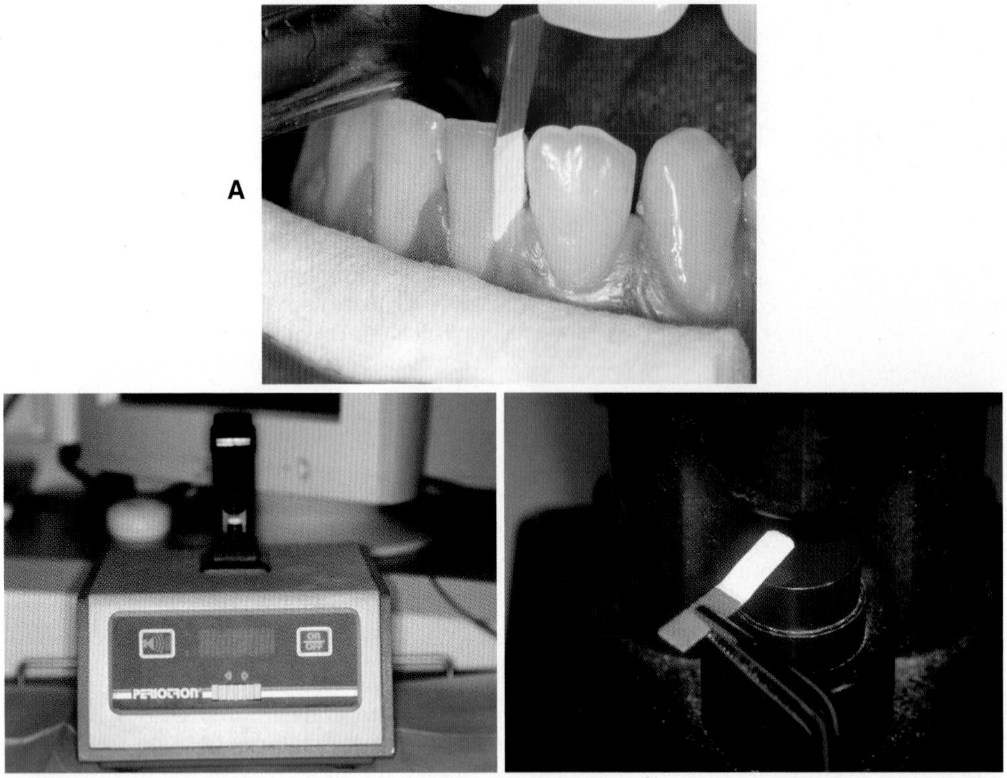

Figure 37-20 Sampling method for gingival crevicular fluid (GCF) analysis (Periotron). **A,** Saliva is removed from the tooth surface with cotton wool before placement of a periopaper strip into the pocket to collect GCF. **B,** The moist paper strip is removed and placed between the jaws of the Periotron for assessment of fluid content. **C,** Periotron device.

of GCF have been studied and can be divided into three main groups: host-derived enzymes, tissue breakdown products, and inflammatory mediators.

For the collection of GCF, a number of approaches have been used, ranging from paper strips, to microcapillary tubes and micropipettes, to microsyringes and plastic strips. The most common method is the use of paper strips. These strips are placed in the gingival sulcus for a standard time until the filter paper is saturated (Figure 37-20, *A*). The fluid volume collected on the strips can be then quantified in a number of ways. At present, the most common way is using the Periotron. This electronic device measures the change in capacitance across the wetted strip, and this change is converted to a digital readout, which can be correlated to the volume of GCF (Figure 37-20, *B* and *C*). Researchers have established that the Periotron 6000 achieves the easiest and quickest measurement and shows high correlation with other clinical gingival indices.[132] Research on GCF has focused on the search for biochemical markers of the progression of periodontitis, as discussed later.

Saliva is another fluid that can be easily collected and may contain both locally and systemically derived markers of periodontal disease, which can be evaluated for diagnostic purposes. Saliva can be collected from the parotid, submandibular, and sublingual glands or as "whole saliva" consisting of a mixture of oral fluids, including secretions from the major and minor salivary glands, in addition to constituents of nonsalivary origin (e.g., GCF, bacteria and bacterial products, desquamated cells, expectorated bronchial secretions). In addition, saliva samples can be collected with or without stimulation. The use of saliva for periodontal diagnosis has been the subject of considerable research activity, although no saliva-based diagnostic tests are available to be used in clinical practice. Proposed diagnostic markers in saliva include proteins and enzymes of host origin, phenotypic markers, host cells, hormones (cortisol), bacteria and bacterial products, volatile compounds, and ions.[64]

Inflammatory Mediators and Products

Cytokines are potent local mediators of inflammation that are produced by a variety of cells. Cytokines that are present in GCF and have been investigated as potential diagnostic markers include tumor necrosis factor alpha (TNF-α),[118] interleukin-1α (IL-1α), interleukin-1β (IL-1β),[128] interleukin-6 (IL-6), and interleukin-8 (IL-8). IL-1, IL-6, and TNF-α are cytokines produced by a variety of cells at inflamed sites. They are potent immunoregulatory molecules with a variety of biologic effects, including metalloproteinase stimulation and bone resorption; therefore they seem good candidates for markers of disease progression (see Chapter 12). Cross-sectional studies have shown good correlation with disease status and severity,[128] but not disease progression. Prostaglandin E_2 (PGE_2) is a product of the cyclooxygenase pathway of the metabolism of arachidonic acid. It is a potent mediator of inflammation and induces bone resorption. In cases of untreated periodontitis, the concentration of PGE_2 found in GCF is increased during active phases of periodontal destruction.[101]

Host-Derived Enzymes

Various enzymes are released from host cells during the initiation and progression of periodontal disease.[13,66]

Matrix components may be dissolved either by extracellular matrix metalloproteinase–dependent or plasmin-dependent cleavage reactions, and the subsequent larger fragments may be disposed of through a phagocytic pathway by way of cleavage by lysosomal proteinases. The proteases and enzymes involved in these processes may have use as diagnostic aids, and thus their role should be considered further.

The breakdown of collagen occurs during inflammation, tissue breakdown, remodeling, and tissue repair or wound healing. This process can occur by two different pathways: an intracellular and an extracellular route. Under nonpathologic conditions, phagocytosis and intracellular digestion of collagen fibrils is a process observed at a high level in dynamic, soft connective tissues such as gingiva and periodontal ligament. In the pathologic conditions of periodontal disease, the balance between synthesis and degradation is disrupted, and the collagen fibrils of the periodontal ligament are broken down, together with the supporting alveolar bone. Different enzymes involved in both the intracellular and the extracellular pathway of tissue destruction have been investigated as potential diagnostic markers of periodontitis.

Among the intracellular destruction enzymes that have received the most attention as possible markers of active periodontal destruction are aspartate aminotransferase, akaline phosphatase, β-glucuronidase, and elastase. These enzymes are released from dead and dying cells of the periodontium, mostly from polymorphonuclear leukocytes (PMNs, neutrophils). Extracellular digestion has been associated with the activity of matrix metalloproteinases. This family of enzymes is produced by inflammatory, epithelial, and connective tissue cells at affected sites.

Aspartate aminotransferase (AST) is an enzyme released from dead cells from a variety of tissues throughout the body, including the heart (after myocardial infarction) and the liver (during hepatitis). Several studies evaluating the association between elevated AST levels in GCF and periodontal disease have demonstrated a marked elevation in AST levels in GCF samples from sites with severe gingival inflammation[17] and sites with a recent history of progressive attachment loss. A rapid chairside test kit for AST has been developed (Periogard). The test involves collection of GCF with a filter paper strip, which is then placed in tromethamine hydrochloride buffer. A substrate reaction mixture containing L-aspartic and α-ketoglutaric acids are added and allowed to react for 10 minutes. In the presence of AST, the aspartate and glutarate are catalyzed to oxalacetate and glutamate. The addition of a dye, such as fast red, results in a color product, the intensity of which is proportional to the AST activity in the GCF sample. A potential problem with the AST test is its inability to discriminate between sites with severe inflammation but with no attachment loss from sites that are losing attachment. It remains to be demonstrated whether this test offers some advantage over existing clinical measures of disease.[17] Using this chairside test, Kamma et al.[62] showed a high degree of correlation between the presence of putative periodontal pathogens and positive AST scores at periodontal sites that clinically were considered to be potentially disease active in patients with aggressive periodontitis.

Alkaline phosphatase (ALP) is an enzyme found in many cells of the periodontium, including osteoblasts, fibroblasts, and neutrophils. Cross-sectional studies show that concentrations of this enzyme in GCF from diseased sites are significantly higher than from healthy sites. Only one longitudinal study has associated whole-mouth ALP levels with the progression of periodontitis,[12] and this study has not been reproduced.

β-Glucuronidase (βG) is a lysosomal enzyme found in the primary (azurophilic) granules of neutrophils. Cross-sectional data clearly show elevated βG activity in sites with more severe periodontal disease. Two longitudinal studies from the same research group have shown that the concentration of βG may have predictive value in identifying patients at higher risk for losing attachment.[70] *Elastase* is a serine protease also stored in the primary granules of neutrophils. Cross-sectional studies clearly indicate that GCF samples taken from sites with periodontitis have significantly higher elastase activity than GCF from healthy or gingivitis sites.[41] A rapid chairside test kit (Periocheck) has been developed to detect neutral proteases in GCF. A limited number of longitudinal studies have evaluated their value as markers of periodontal disease progression.[5] They have shown some predictive value for disease progression in a short-term evaluation of an untreated population, but it remains unclear if its validity can be applied to a treated population in a maintenance program. Similar results have been obtained studying *cathepsins*. These enzymes are a group of acidic lysosomal enzymes that play an important role in intracellular protein degradation. Although they have shown correlation with disease severity and significant decrease after periodontal therapy, they have not been evaluated longitudinally as markers of disease progression.[20]

Matrix metalloproteinases (MMPs) are members of a large subfamily of zinc-dependent and calcium-dependent proteolytic enzymes (proteinases) responsible for remodeling and degradation of extracellular matrix components. The homeostasis of extracellular matrices is regulated by the release of MMPs by different cells, such as fibroblasts and macrophages, and the presence of tissue inhibitors of MMPs (TIMPs) that are widely distributed in tissues and fluids. Different cross-sectional studies have shown that high MMP levels are associated with periodontitis, as are low TIMP levels.

In chronic periodontitis the collagen fibrils of the periodontal ligament are degraded, together with the supporting alveolar bone. In this pathologic condition, collagen degradation is likely to occur through an MMP-mediated pathway. The concerted action of MMP-2 (gelatinase A), MMP-9 (gelatinase B), MMP-8 (collagenase-2), MMP-13 (collagenase-3), and MMP-3 (stromelysin-1) eventually has a significant role in the initial destruction of periodontal extracellular matrix macromolecules. Evidently, MMP activity is associated with inflammation related to gingivitis and especially to periodontitis. The impact on the ability of MMPs to differentiate gingivitis and periodontitis diagnostically will depend on identifying the enzyme that clearly differentiates between gingivitis and peridontitis, as well as between stable and progressive periodontal tissue-destructive conditions.

A substantial body of evidence now indicates that MMPs and TIMPs are produced locally in the periodontium and that MMP-8 plays an important role in periodontal tissue destruction.[67] GCF from periodontitis patients contains pathologically elevated levels of collagenase-2 (MMP-8) in catalytically active form. Association between increased GCF collagenase MMP-8 activity and progressive loss of connective tissue attachment has been demonstrated, and longitudinal studies have shown a significant decrease in GCF MMP-8 activity after successful treatment.[20,67,76,88] The reduction in GCF MMP-8 levels after therapy indicates that MMP-8 is one molecule with potential diagnostic use an indicator of current disease status and possibly as a predictor of future disease. To test this hypothesis, a chairside test stick for detection of MMP-8 in GCF has recently been developed.[89] Studies of periodontitis patients have shown that this diagnostic test is able to differentiate between gingivitis and periodontitis, and significant reductions of this indicator have been demonstrated in response to treatment (scaling and root planing) of periodontitis.[68]

Tissue Breakdown Products

One of the major features of periodontitis is the destruction of collagen and extracellular matrices. The connective tissues of the periodontium are composed of fibrous elements, including proteins such as collagen and elastin, and nonfibrous components, including a variety of glycoproteins (laminin, fibronectin, proteoglycans) as well as minerals, lipids, water, and tissue-bound growth factors. The extracellular matrix of the periodontium is composed of a diverse number of macromolecules; the predominant one is collagen, and the other components include proteoglycan (versican, decorin, biglycan, syndecan) and noncollagen proteins (elastin, fibronectin, laminin, osteocalcin, osteopontin, bone sialoprotein, osteonectin, tenascin). All these matrix components are theoretically detectable and potentially informative in terms of their clinical diagnostic utility.

Analysis of GCF obtained from sites with periodontitis clearly shows elevated levels of hydroxyproline from collagen breakdown and glycosaminoglycans from matrix degradation.[74] Other bone and connective tissue proteins, including osteocalcin and type I collagen peptides, have been correlated with the progression of alveolar bone loss induced in beagle dogs.[34] Both markers gave high positive predictive values and now need to be extended to longitudinal studies in humans.

CONCLUSION

Although there are many potential markers for periodontal disease activity and progression, numerous features still hamper the ability to use them as diagnostic tests of proven utility. There is still a lack of a proven "gold standard" of disease progression, and thus the correlation of these potential markers with proven clinical attachment loss may be a potential confounder in any proposed test. After all these years of intensive research, we still lack a proven diagnostic test that has demonstrated high predictive value for disease progression, has a proven impact on disease incidence and prevalence, and is simple, safe, and cost-effective.

REFERENCES

1. Aas AM, Albandar J, Aasenden R, et al: Variation in prevalence of radiographic alveolar bone loss in subgroups of 14-year old schoolchildren in Oslo, *J Clin Periodontol* 16:300, 1989.
2. Abrams K, Caton J, Polson A: Histologic comparisons of interproximal gingival tissues related to the presence or absence of bleeding, *J Periodontol* 55:629, 1984.
3. Aeppli DM, Pihlstrom BL: Detection of longitudinal changes in periodontitis, *J Periodontal Res* 24:329, 1989.
4. Armitage GC, Svanberg GK, Löe H: Microscopic evaluation of clinical measurements of connective tissue attachment levels, *J Clin Periodontol* 4:173, 1977.
5. Armitage GC, Jeffcoat MK, Chadwick DE, et al: Longitudinal evaluation of elastase as a marker for the progression of periodontitis, *J Periodontol* 65; 120, 1994.
6. Ashimoto A, Chen C, Bakker I, Slots J: Polymerase chain reaction detection of 8 putative periodontal pathogens in subgingival plaque of gingivitis and advanced periodontitis lesions, *Oral Microbiol Immunol* 11:266, 1996.
7. Badersten A, Nilveus R, Egelberg J: Reproducibility of probing attachment level measurements, *J Clin Periodontol* 11:475, 1984.
8. Badersten A, Nilveus R, Egelberg J: Effect of non-surgical periodontal therapy. VII. Bleeding, suppuration and probing depth in sites with probing attachment loss, *J Clin Periodontol* 12:432, 1985.
9. Beck JD: Issues in assessment of diagnostic tests and risk for periodontal diseases, *Periodontol 2000* 7:100, 1995.
10. Bergström J, Boström L: Tobacco smoking and periodontal haemorrhagic responsiveness, *J Clin Periodontol* 28:680, 2001.
11. Biddle AJ, Palmer RM, Wilson RF, Watts TL: Comparison of the validity of periodontal probing measurements in smokers and non-smokers, *J Clin Periodontol* 28:806, 2001.
12. Binder TA, Goodson JM, Socransky SS: Gingival fluid levels of acid and alkaline phosphatase, *J Periodontal Res* 22:14, 1987.
13. Bowers JE, Zahradnik M: Evaluation of a chairside gingival protease test for use in periodontal diagnosis, *J Clin Dent* 1:106, 1989.
14. Boyer BP, Ryerson CC, Reynolds HS, et al: Colonization by *Actinobacillus actinomycetemcomitans, Porphyromonas gingivalis* and *Prevotella intermedia* in adult periodontitis patients as detected by the antibody-based Evalusite Test, *J Clin Periodontol* 23:477, 1996.
15. Brägger U, Pasquali L, Rylander H, et al: Computer assisted densitometric image analysis in periodontal radiography: a methodological study, *J Clin Periodontol* 15:27, 1988.

16. Buchmann R, Muller RF, Heinecke A, Lange DE: *Actinobacillus actinomycetemcomitans* in destructive periodontal disease: three-year follow-up results, *J Periodontol* 71:444, 2000.
17. Chambers DA, Imrey PB, Cohen R, et al: A longitudinal study of aspartate aminotransferase in human gingival crevicular fluid, *J Periodontal Res* 26:65, 1991.
18. Chaves ES, Jeffcoat MK, Ryerson CC, Snyder B: Persistent bacterial colonization of *Porphyromonas gingivalis, Prevotella intermedia,* and *Actinobacillus actinomycetemcomitans* in periodontitis and its association with alveolar bone loss after 6 months of therapy, *J Clin Periodontol* 27:897, 2000.
19. Chen HY, Cox SW, Eley BM: Cathepsin B, α-2 macroglobulin and cytastin levels in gingival crevicular fluid from chronic periodontitis patients, *J Clin Periodontol* 25:34, 1998.
20. Chen HY, Cox SW, Eley BM, et al: Matrix metalloproteinase-8 levels and elastase activities in gingival crevicular fluid from chronic adult periodontitis patients, *J Clin Periodontol* 27:366, 2000.
21. Clark WB, Yang MC, Magnusson I: Measuring clinical attachment: reproducibility and relative measurements with an electronic probe, *J Periodontol* 63:831, 1992.
22. Crockett AO, Wittwer CT: Fluorescein-labeled oligonucleotides for real-time PCR: using the inherent quenching of deoxyguanosine nucleotides, *Anal Biochem* 290:89, 2001.
23. Dahlen G, Rosling B: Identification of bacterial markers by culture technique in evaluation of periodontal therapy, *Int Dent J* 48:104, 1998.
24. Daneshmann H, Wade AB: Correlation between gingival fluid measurements and macroscopic and microscopic characteristics of gingival tissue, *J Periodontal Res* 11:35, 1976.
25. Dawson MT, Powell R, Gannon F: *Gene technology,* Oxford, 1996, BIOS Scientific Publishers.
26. Deas D, Pasquali LA, Yuan CH, et al: The relationship between probing attachment loss and computerized radiographic analysis in monitoring the progression of periodontitis, *J Periodontol* 62:135, 1991.
27. Doungudomdacha S, Rawlinson A, Walsh T, Douglas C: Effect of non-surgical periodontal treatment on clinical parameters and the numbers of *Porphyromonas gingivalis, Prevotella intermedia* and *Actinobacillus actinomycetemcomitans* at adult periodontitis sites, *J Clin Periodontol* 28:437, 2001.
28. Dzink JL, Tanner AC, Haffajee AD, Socransky SS: Gram-negative species associated with active destructive periodontal lesions, *J Clin Periodontol* 12:648, 1985.
29. Eick S, Pfister W: Comparison of microbial cultivation and a commercial PCR-based method for detection of periodontopathogenic species in subgingival plaque samples, *J Clin Periodontol* 29:638, 2002.
30. Eickholz P, Kugel B, Pohl S, et al: Combined mechanical and antibiotic periodontal therapy in a case of Papillon-Lefevre syndrome, *J Periodontol* 72:542, 2001.
31. Feres M, Haffajee AD, Allard K, et al: Change in subgingival microbial profiles in adult periodontitis subjects receiving either systemically administered amoxicillin or metronidazole, *J Clin Periodontol* 28:597, 2001.
32. Fujise O, Hamachi T, Inoue K, et al: Microbiological markers for prediction and assessment of treatment outcome following non-surgical periodontal therapy, *J Periodontol* 73:1253, 2002.
33. Genco RJ: Current view of risk factors for periodontal diseases, *J Periodontol* 67:1041, 1996.
34. Giannobile WV, Lynch SE, Denmark RG, et al: Crevicular fluid osteocalcin and piridoline cross-linked carboxyterminal telopeptide of type I collagen (ICTP) as markers of rapid bone turn over in periodontitis, *J Clin Periodontol* 22:903, 1995.
35. Gibbs CH, Hirschfeld JW, Lee JG, et al: Description and clinical evaluation of a new computerized periodontal probe—the Florida probe, *J Clin Periodontol* 15:137, 1988.
36. Gibbs RA: DNA amplification by the polymerase chain reaction, *Anal Chem* 62:1202, 1990.
37. Goodson JM, Haffajee AD, Socransky SS: The relationship between attachment level loss and alveolar bone loss, *J Clin Periodontol* 11:348, 1984.
38. Greenstein G, Caton J, Polson AM: Histologic characteristics associated with bleeding after probing and visual signs of inflammation, *J Periodontol* 52:420, 1981.
39. Grondahl HG, Grondahl K: Subtraction radiography for the diagnosis of periodontal bone lesions, *Oral Surg* 55:208, 1983.
40. Grondahl K, Kullendorff B, Strid HG, et al: Detectability of artificial marginal bone lesions as a function of lesion depth, *J Clin Periodontol* 15:156, 1988.
41. Gustavsson A, Asman B, Bergstrom KG: Granulocyte elastase in gingival crevicular fluid: a possible discriminator between gingivitis and periodontitis, *J Clin Periodontol* 19:535, 1992.
42. Haffajee AD, Socransky SS: Attachment level changes in destructive periodontal diseases, *J Clin Periodontol* 13:461, 1986.
43. Haffajee AD, Socransky SS: Relationship of cigarette smoking to the subgingival microbiota, *J Clin Periodontol* 28:377, 2001.
44. Haffajee AD, Socransky SS, Goodson JM: Comparisons of different data analysis for detecting changes in attachment level, *J Clin Periodontol* 10:298, 1983.
45. Haffajee AD, Socransky SS, Goodson JM: Clinical parameters as predictors of destructive periodontal activity, *J Clin Periodontol* 10:257, 1983.
46. Haffajee AD, Socransky SS, Goodson JM: Subgingival temperature: relation to future periodontal attachment loss, *J Clin Periodontol* 19:409, 1992.
47. Haffajee AD, Dibart S, Kent RL Jr, Socransky SS: Factors associated with different responses to periodontal therapy, *J Clin Periodontol* 22:628, 1995.
48. Haffajee AD, Socransky SS, Dibart S, Kent RL Jr: Response to periodontal therapy in patients with high or low levels of *P. gingivalis, P. intermedia, P. nigrescens* and *B. forsythus, J Clin Periodontol* 23:336, 1996.
49. Haffajee AD, Socransky SS, Smith C, Dibart S: Microbial risk indicators for periodontal attachment loss, *J Periodontal Res* 26:293, 1991.
50. Haffajee AD, Cugini MA, Dibart S, et al: The effect of SRP on the clinical and microbiological parameters of periodontal diseases, *J Clin Periodontol* 24:324, 1997.
51. Haffajee AD, Smith C, Torresyap G, et al: Efficacy of manual and powered toothbrushes. II. Effect on microbiological parameters, *J Clin Periodontol* 28:947, 2001.
52. Hausmann E: Radiographic and digital imaging in periodontal practice, *J Periodontol* 71:497, 2000.
53. Hausmann E, Allen K, Carpio L, et al: Computerized methodology for detection of alveolar crestal bone loss from serial intraoral radiographs, *J Periodontol* 63:657, 1992.
54. Hausmann E, Christersson L, Dunford R, et al: Usefulness of subtraction radiography in the evaluation of periodontal therapy, *J Periodontol* 56:4, 1985.
55. Holt SC, Progulske A: General microbiology, metabolism and genetics. In Newman MG, Nisengard R, editors: *Oral microbiology and immunology,* Philadelphia, 1988, Saunders.
56. Ishikawa I, Kawashima Y, Oda S, et al: Three case reports of aggressive periodontitis associated with *Porphyromonas gingivalis* in younger patients, *J Periodontal Res* 37, 324, 2002.

57. Jankowski JA, Polak JM: *Clinical gene analysis and manipulation,* New York, 1996, Cambridge University Press.
58. Jeffcoat MK: Diagnosing periodontal disease: new tools to solve old problems, *J Am Dent Assoc* 122:54, 1991.
59. Jeffcoat MK: Radiographic methods for the detection of progressive alveolar bone loss, *J Periodontol* 63:367, 1992.
60. Jeffcoat MK, Jeffcoat RL, Jens SC, et al: A new periodontal probe with automated cemento-enamel junction detection, *J Clin Periodontol* 13:276, 1986.
61. Kalkwarf KL, Kahldal WD, Patil KD: Comparison of manual and pressure controlled periodontal probing, *J Periodontol* 57:467, 1986.
62. Kamma JJ, Nakou M, Persson RG: Association of early onset periodontitis microbiota with aspartate aminotransferase activity in gingival crevicular fluid, *J Clin Periodontol* 28:1096, 2001.
63. Karpinia K, Magnusson I, Gibbs C, et al: Accuracy of probing attachment levels using a CEJ probe versus traditional probes, *J Clin Periodontol* 31:173, 2004.
64. Kaufman E, Lamster IB: Analysis of saliva for periodontal diagnosis: a review, *J Clin Periodontol* 27:453, 2000.
65. Kelly GP, Cain RJ, Knowles JW, et al: Radiographs in clinical periodontal trials, *J Periodontol* 46:381, 1975.
66. Kinane D: Host-based chemical agents in diagnosis. In Lang NP, Karring T, Lindhe J, editors: *Proceedings of the Second European Workshop on Periodontology,* Berlin, 1997, Quintessence.
67. Kinane DF: Regulators of tissue destruction and homeostasis as diagnostic aids in periodontology, *Periodontol 2000* 24:215, 2000.
68. Kinane DF, Darby IB, Said S, et al: Changes in gingival crevicular fluid matrix metalloproteinase-8 levels during periodontal treatment and maintenance, *J Periodontal Res* 38:400, 2003.
69. Kung RT, Ochs B, Goodson JM: Temperature as a periodontal diagnostic, *J Clin Periodontol* 17:557, 1990.
70. Lamster IB, Oshrain RL, Harper CS, et al: Enzyme activity in crevicular fluid for the detection and prediction of clinical attachment loss in patients with chronic adult periodontitis, *J Periodontol* 59:516, 1988.
71. Lang NP, Brägger U: Periodontal diagnosis in the 1990s, *J Clin Periodontol* 18:370, 1991.
72. Lang NP, Joss A, Orsanic T, et al: Bleeding on probing: a predictor for the progression of periodontal disease? *J Clin Periodontol* 13:590, 1986.
73. Lang NP, Nyman S, Senn C, et al: Bleeding on probing as it relates to probing pressure and gingival health, *J Clin Periodontol* 18:257, 1991.
74. Last KS, Stanbury JB, Embery G: Glycosaminoglycans in human gingival sulcus fluid as indicators of active periodontal disease, *Arch Oral Biol* 30:275, 1985.
75. Lawer G, Lippke J, Frey G, et al: Isolation of a DNA probe for tetracycline resistance from *B. intermedius, J Dent Res* 69:376, 1990.
76. Lee W, Aitken S, Sodek J,McCulloch CA: Evidence of a direct relationship between neutrophil collagenase activity and periodontal tissue destruction in vivo: role of active enzyme in human periodontitis, *J Periodontal Res* 30:23, 1995.
77. Levy D, Csima A, Birek P, et al: Impact of microbiological consultation on clinical decision making: a case-control study of clinical management of recurrent periodontitis, *J Periodontol* 64, 1029, 1993.
78. Lewin B: *Genes*, New York, 1993, Oxford University Press.
79. Listgarten MA: Direct microscopy of periodontal pathogens, *Oral Microbiol Immunol* 1:31, 1986.
80. Listgarten MA, Mao R, Robinson PJ: Periodontal probing and the relationship of the probe tip to periodontal tissues, *J Periodontol* 47:511, 1976.
81. Listgarten MA, Schifter CC, Sullivan P, et al: Failure of a microbial assay to reliably predict disease recurrence in a treated periodontitis population receiving regularly scheduled prophylaxis, *J Clin Periodontol* 13:768, 1987.
82. Loesche WJ: The identification of bacteria associated with periodontal disease and dental caries by enzymatic methods, *Oral Microbiol Immunol* 1:65, 1986.
83. Loesche WJ: DNA probe and enzyme analysis in periodontal diagnostics, *J Periodontol* 63:1102, 1992.
84. Lyons SR, Griffen AL, Leys EJ: Quantitative real-time PCR for *Porphyromonas gingivalis* and total bacteria, *J Clin Microbiol* 38:2362, 2000.
85. Magnusson I, Listgarten MA: Histological evaluation of probing depth following periodontal treatment, *J Clin Periodontol* 7:26, 1980.
86. Magnusson I, Fuller WW, Heins PJ, et al: Correlation between electronic and visual readings of pocket depths with a newly developed constant force probe, *J Clin Periodontol* 15:180, 1988.
87. Magnusson I, Persson RG, Page RC et al: A multicenter clinical trial of a new chairside test in distinguishing diseased and healthy periodontal sites, *J Periodontol* 67:589, 1995.
88. Mancini S, Romanelli R, Laschinger CA, et al: Assessment of a novel screening test for neutrophil collagenase activity in the diagnosis of periodontal diseases, *J Periodontol* 70:1292, 1999.
89. Manttila P, Stenman M, Kinane DF, et al: Gingival crevicular fluid collagenase-2 (MMP-8) test stick for chair-side monitoring of periodontitis, *J Periodontal Res* 38:436, 2003.
90. McCulloch CA, Birek P: Automated probe: futuristic technology for diagnosis of periodontal disease, *Univ Toronto Dent J* 4:6, 1991.
91. Mombelli A, Graf H: Depth force patterns in periodontal probing, *J Clin Periodontol* 13:126, 1986.
92. Mombelli A, Casagni F, Madianos PN: Can presence or absence of periodontal pathogens distinguish between subjects with chronic and aggressive periodontitis? A systematic review, *J Clin Periodontol* 29:10, 2002.
93. Moncla BJ, Braham P, Dix K, et al: Use of synthetic oligonucleotide DNA probes for the identification of *Bacteroides gingivalis, J Clin Microbiol* 28:324, 1990.
94. Moore WE, Moore LV: The bacteria of periodontal diseases, *Periodontol 2000* 5:66, 1994.
95. Morillo JM, Lau L, Sanz M, et al: Quantitative real-time PCR based on single-copy gene sequence for detection of *Actinobacillus actinomycetemcomitans* and *Porphyromonas gingivalis, J Periodontal Res* 38:518, 2003.
96. Nair P, Sutherland G, Palmer R, et al: Gingival bleeding on probing increases after quitting smoking, *J Clin Periodontol* 30:435, 2003;.
97. Neumaier M, Braun A, Wagener S (International Federation of Clinical Chemistry, Scientific Division, Committee on Molecular and Biology Techniques): Fundamentals of quality assessment of molecular amplification methods in clinical diagnostics, *Clin Chem* 44:12, 1998.
98. Newman HN: Plaque and chronic inflammatory periodontal disease: a question of ecology, *J Clin Periodontol* 17, 533, 1990.
99. Nicholl DS: *An introduction to genetic engineering,* New York, 1994, Cambridge University Press.
100. Nummikoski PV, Steffensen B, Hamilton K, et al: Clinical validation of a new substraction radiographic technique for periodontal bone loss detection, *J Periodontol* 71:598, 2000.
101. Offenbacher S, Odle BM, Van Dyke TE: The use of crevicular fluid prostaglandin E_2 levels as predictor of periodontal attachment loss, *J Periodontal Res* 21:101, 1986.

102. Ortman LF, McHenry K, Hausmann E: Relationship between alveolar bone measured by ^{125}I absorptiometry with analysis of standardized radiographs, *J Periodontol* 53:311, 1982.
103. Page RC: Host response tests for diagnosing periodontal diseases, *J Periodontol* 63:356, 1992.
104. Palmer RM, Scott DA, Meekin TN, et al: Potential mechanisms of susceptibility to periodontitis in tobacco smokers, *J Periodontal Res* 34:363, 1999.
105. Papapanou PN, Madianos PN, Dahlen G, Sandros J: "Checkerboard" versus culture: a comparison between two methods for identification of subgingival microbiota, *Eur J Oral Sci* 105:389, 1997.
106. Parakkal PF: Proceedings of the workshop on quantitative evaluation of periodontal diseases by physical measurement techniques, *J Dent Res* 58:547, 1979.
107. Perry DA, Taggart EJ, Leung A, et al: Comparison of a conventional probe with electronic and manual pressure–regulated probes, *J Periodontol* 65:908, 1994.
108. Polson AM, Caton JG: Current status of bleeding in the diagnosis of periodontal diseases, *J Periodontol* 56(suppl 11):1, 1985.
109. Polson AM, Caton JG, Yeaple RN, et al: Histological determination of probe tip penetration into gingival sulcus of humans using an electronic pressure-sensitive probe, *J Clin Periodontol* 7:479, 1980.
110. Preshaw PM, Kupp L, Hefti AF, et al: Measurement of clinical attachment levels using a constant-force periodontal probe modified to detect the cemento-enamel junction, *J Clin Periodontol* 26:434, 1999.
111. Quirynen M, Callens A, van Steenberghe D, et al: Clinical evaluation of a constant force electronic probe, *J Periodontol* 64:35, 1993.
112. Rams TE, Slots J: Comparison of two pressure-sensitive periodontal probes and a manual periodontal probe in shallow and deep pockets, *Int J Periodont Restor Dent* 13:521, 1993.
113. Rams TE, Listgarten MA, Slots J: Utility of 5 major putative periodontal pathogens and selected clinical parameters to predict periodontal breakdown in patients on maintenance care, *J Clin Periodontol* 23:346, 1996.
114. Renvert S, Dahlen G, Wikstrom M: Treatment of periodontal disease based on microbiological diagnosis: relation between microbiological and clinical parameters during 5 years, *J Periodontol* 67:562, 1996.
115. Rethman M, Ruttimann U, O'Neal R, et al: Diagnosis of bone lesions by subtraction radiography, *J Periodontol* 56:324, 1985.
116. Rosenberg ES, Torosian JP, Hammond BF, Cutler SA: Routine anaerobic bacterial culture and systemic antibiotic usage in the treatment of adult periodontitis: a 6-year longitudinal study, *Int J Periodont Restor Dent* 13, 213, 1993.
117. Rosling B, Hollender L, Nyman S, et al: A radiographic method for assessing changes in alveolar height following periodontal therapy, *J Clin Periodontol* 2:211, 1975.
118. Rossomando EF, Kennedy JE, Hadjimichael J: Tumor necrosis factor alpha in gingival crevicular fluid as a possible indicator of periodontal disease in humans, *Arch Oral Biol* 35:431, 1990.
119. Saiki R, Gelfand DH, Stoffel S, et al: Primer-directed enzymatic amplification of DNA with thermostable DNA polymerase, *Science* 239:487, 1988.
120. Savitt ED, Strzempko MN, Vaccaro KK, et al: Comparison of cultural methods and DNA probe analyses for the detection of *Actinobacillus actinomycetemcomitans, Bacteroides gingivalis,* and *Bacteroides intermedius* in subgingival plaque samples, *J Periodontol* 59:431, 1988.
121. Shelbourne CE, Prabhu A, Gleason RM, et al: Quantitation of *Bacteroides forsythus* in subgingival plaque: comparison of immunoassay and quantitative polymerase chain reaction, *J Microbiol* 39:97, 2000.
122. Shibata DK: The polymerase chain reaction and the molecular genetic analysis of tissue biopsies. In Herrington CS, McGee JO, editors: *Diagnostic,* Oxford,1992, Oxford University Press.
123. Slots J: Bacterial specificity in adult periodontitis: a summary of recent work, *J Clin Periodontol* 13:912, 1986.
124. Smith AJ, Kinane D: Comparison of polymerase chain reaction and culture methods for detection of Actinobacillus actinomycetemcomitans and *Porphyromonas gingivalis* in subgingival plaque samples, *J Periodontal Res* 31:496, 1996.
125. Snyder B, Ryerson CC, Corona H et al: Analytical performance of an immunologic-based periodontal bacterial test for simultaneous detection and differentiation of *Actinobacillus actinomycetemcomitans, Porphyromonas gingivalis,* and *Prevotella intermedia, J Periodontol* 67:497, 1996.
126. Socransky SS: Relationship of bacteria to the etiology of periodontal disease, *J Dent Res* 49:203, 1970.
127. Socransky SS, Smith C, Martin L, et al: Checkerboard DNA-DNA hybridization, *Biotechniques* 17:788, 1994.
128. Stashenko P, Fujiyoshi P, Obernesser MS, et al: Levels of interleukin-1β in tissue from sites of active periodontal disease, *J Clin Periodontol* 18:548, 1991.
129. Tanner AC, Maiden MF, Zambon J, et al: Rapid chair-side DNA probe assay of *Bacteroides forsythus* and *Porphyromonas gingivalis, J Periodontal Res* 33:105, 1998.
130. Tran SD, Rudney JD, Sparks BS, Hodges JS: Persistent presence of *Bacteroides forsythus* as a risk factor for attachment loss in a population with low prevalence and severity of adult periodontitis, *J Periodontol* 72:1, 2001.
131. Trikilis N, Rawlinson A, Walsh TF: Periodontal probing depth and subgingival temperature in smokers and non-smokers, *J Clin Periodontol* 26:38, 1999.
132. Tsuchida K, Hara K: Clinical significance of gingival fluid measurement by Periotron, *J Periodontol* 52:599, 1981.
133. Tupta-Veselicky L, Famili P, Ceravolo FJ, et al: A clinical study of an electronic constant force periodontal probe, *J Periodontol* 65:616, 1994.
134. Van der Velden U, de Vries JH: Introduction of a new periodontal probe: the pressure probe, *J Clin Periodontol* 5:188, 1978.
135. Van Steenberghe D, Rosling B, Soder PO, et al: A 15-month evaluation of the effects of repeated subgingival minocycline in chronic adult periodontitis, *J Periodontol* 70:657, 1999.
136. Van Winkelhoff AJ, Rams TE, Slots J: Systemic antibiotic therapy in periodontics, *Periodontol 2000* 10:45, 1996.
137. Wennström JL, Dahlen G, Svensson J, Nyman S: *Actinobacillus actinomycetemcomitans, Bacteroides gingivalis* and *Bacteroides intermedius:* predictors of attachment loss? *Oral Microbiol Immunol* 2:158, 1987.
138. Ximenez-Fyvie LA, Haffajee AD, Socransky SS: Comparison of the microbiota of supra- and subgingival plaque in health and periodontitis, *J Clin Periodontol* 27:648, 2000.
139. Ximenez-Fyvie LA, Haffajee AD, Socransky SS: Microbial composition of supra- and subgingival plaque in subjects with adult periodontitis, *J Clin Periodontol* 27:722, 2000.
140. Yang MCK, Marks RG, Clark WB, et al: Predictive power of various models for longitudinal attachment level change, *J Clin Periodontol* 19:77, 1992.
141. Zambon JJ, Haraszthy VI: The laboratory diagnosis of periodontal infections, *Periodontol 2000* 7:69, 1995.
142. Zambon JJ, Bochacki V, Genco RJ: Immunological assays for putative periodontal pathogens, *Oral Microbiol Immunol* 1:39, 1986.

38 CHAPTER

Risk Assessment

Karen F. Novak and M. John Novak

CHAPTER OUTLINE

DEFINITIONS

Risk assessment is defined by numerous components.[2,29] *Risk* is the probability that an individual will develop a specific disease in a given period. The risk of developing the disease will vary from individual to individual.

Risk factors may be environmental, behavioral, or biologic factors that, when present, increase the likelihood that an individual will develop the disease. Risk factors are identified through longitudinal studies of patients with the disease of interest. Exposure to a risk factor or factors may occur at a single point in time; over multiple, separate points in time; or continuously. However, to be identified as a risk factor, the exposure must occur *before* disease onset. Interventions often can be identified and, when implemented, can help modify risk factors.

The term *risk determinant/background characteristic,* which is sometimes substituted for the term *risk factor,* should be reserved for those risk factors that cannot be modified.

Risk indicators are *probable* or *putative* risk factors that have been identified in cross-sectional studies but not confirmed through longitudinal studies.

Risk predictors/markers, although associated with increased risk for disease, do not cause the disease. These factors also are identified in cross-sectional and longitudinal studies.

Box 38-1 lists elements of these categories of risk for periodontal disease.

RISK FACTORS FOR PERIODONTAL DISEASE

Tobacco Smoking

Tobacco smoking is a well-established risk factor for periodontitis.[2,31] A direct relationship exists between smoking and the prevalence of periodontal disease (see Chapter 8). This association is independent of other factors, such as oral hygiene or age.[18] Studies comparing the response to periodontal therapy in smokers, previous smokers, and nonsmokers have shown that smoking has a negative

BOX 38-1

Categories of Risk Elements for Periodontal Disease

Risk Factors
Tobacco smoking
Diabetes
Pathogenic bacteria
Microbial tooth deposits

Risk Determinants/Background Characteristics
Genetic factors
Age
Gender
Socioeconomic status
Stress

Risk Indicators
HIV/AIDS
Osteoporosis
Infrequent dental visits

Risk Markers/Predictors
Previous history of periodontal disease
Bleeding on probing

HIV, Human immunodeficiency virus; *AIDS,* acquired immunodeficiency syndrome.

impact on the response to therapy. However, former smokers respond similarly to nonsmokers.[3] These studies demonstrate the therapeutic impact of intervention strategies on patients who smoke (see Chapter 14).

Diabetes

Diabetes is a clear risk factor for periodontitis.[2] Epidemiologic data demonstrate that the prevalence and severity of periodontitis are significantly higher in patients with type 1 or type 2 diabetes mellitus than in those without diabetes, and that the level of diabetic control is an important variable in this relationship (see Chapter 8).

Pathogenic Bacteria and Microbial Tooth Deposits

It is well documented that accumulation of bacterial plaque at the gingival margin results in the development of gingivitis and that the gingivitis can be reversed with the implementation of oral hygiene measures.[25] These studies demonstrate a causal relationship between accumulation of bacterial plaque and gingival inflammation. However, a causal relationship between plaque accumulation and *periodontitis* has been more difficult to establish. Often, patients with severe loss of attachment have minimal levels of bacterial plaque on the affected teeth, indicating that the *quantity* of plaque is not of major importance in the disease process. However, although quantity may not indicate risk, there is evidence that the composition, or *quality,* of the complex plaque biofilm is of importance.

In terms of quality of plaque, three specific bacteria have been identified as etiologic agents for periodontitis: *Actinobacillus actinomycetemcomitans, Porphyromonas gingivalis,* and *Tannerella forsythia* (formerly *Bacteroides forsythus*).[11] *P. gingivalis* and *T. forsythia* are often found in chronic periodontitis, whereas *A. actinomycetemcomitans* is often associated with aggressive periodontitis. Cross-sectional and longitudinal studies support the delineation of these three bacteria as risk factors for periodontal disease. Additional evidence that these organisms are causal agents includes the following[16]:

1. Their elimination or suppression impacts the success of therapy.
2. There is a host response to these pathogens.
3. Virulence factors are associated with these pathogens.
4. Inoculation of these bacteria into animal models induces periodontal disease.

Although not completely supported by these criteria for causation, moderate evidence also suggests that *Campylobacter rectus, Eubacterium nodatum, Fusobacterium nucleatum, Prevotella intermedia/nigrescens, Peptostreptococcus micros, Streptococcus intermedius,* and *Treponema denticola* are etiologic factors in periodontitis.[11]

Therefore the quantity of plaque present may not be as important as the quality of the plaque in determining risk for periodontitis.

Anatomic factors, such as furcations, root concavities, developmental grooves, cervical enamel projections, enamel pearls, and bifurcation ridges, may predispose the periodontium to disease as a result of their potential to harbor bacterial plaque and present a challenge to the clinician during instrumentation. Similarly, the presence of subgingival and overhanging margins can result in increased plaque accumulation, increased inflammation, and increased bone loss. Although not clearly defined as risk factors for periodontitis, anatomic factors and *restorative factors* that influence plaque accumulation may play a role in disease susceptibility for specific teeth.[7]

The presence of *calculus,* which serves as a reservoir for bacterial plaque, has been suggested as a risk factor for periodontitis. Although the presence of some calculus in healthy individuals receiving routine dental care does not result in significant loss of attachment, the presence of calculus in other groups of patients, such as those not receiving regular care and patients with poorly controlled diabetes, can have a negative impact on periodontal health.[29]

RISK DETERMINANTS/BACKGROUND CHARACTERISTICS FOR PERIODONTAL DISEASE

Genetic Factors

Evidence indicates that genetic differences between individuals may explain why some patients develop periodontal disease and others do not. Studies conducted in twins have shown that genetic factors influence clinical measures of gingivitis, probing pocket depth, attachment loss, and interproximal bone height.[26-28] The familial aggregation seen in localized and generalized aggressive periodontitis also is indicative of genetic involvement in these diseases (see Chapter 33).

Kornman et al.[21] demonstrated that alterations in specific genes encoding the inflammatory cytokines interleukin-1α and interleukin-1β (IL-1α, IL-1β) were associated with severe chronic periodontitis in nonsmoking subjects.[21] However, results of other studies have shown limited association between these altered genes and the presence of periodontitis. Overall, it appears that changes in the IL-1 genes may be only one of several genetic changes involved in the risk for chronic periodontitis. Therefore, although the alteration in the IL-1 genes may be a valid marker for periodontitis in defined populations, its usefulness as a genetic marker in the general population may be limited.[20]

Immunologic alterations, such as neutrophil abnormalities,[17] monocytic hyperresponsiveness to lipopolysaccharide stimulation in patients with localized aggressive periodontitis,[35] and alterations in the monocyte/macrophage receptors for the Fc portion of antibody,[20,45] also appear to be under genetic control. In addition, genetics plays a role in regulating the titer of the protective immunoglobulin G2 (IgG2) antibody response to *A. actinomycetemcomitans* in patients with aggressive periodontitis[15] (see Chapter 11).

Age

Both the prevalence and the severity of periodontal disease increase with age.[8,30,31] It is possible that degenerative changes related to aging may increase susceptibility to periodontitis. However, it also is possible that the attachment loss and bone loss seen in older individuals are the result of prolonged exposure to other risk factors over a person's life, creating a cumulative effect over time. In support of this, studies have shown minimal loss of attachment in aging subjects enrolled in preventive programs throughout their lives.[32,33] Therefore it is suggested that periodontal disease is not an inevitable consequence of the aging process and that aging alone does not increase disease susceptibility. However, it remains to be determined whether changes related to the aging process, such as intake of medications, decreased immune function, and altered nutritional status, interact with other well-defined risk factors to increase susceptibility to periodontitis.

Evidence of loss of attachment may be of more consequence in younger patients. The younger the patient, the longer the patient has for exposure to causative factors. In addition, aggressive periodontitis in young individuals often is associated with an unmodifiable risk factor, such as a genetic predisposition to disease.[31] Therefore, young individuals with periodontal disease may be at greater risk for continued disease as they age.

Gender

Gender plays a role in periodontal disease.[2] National U.S. surveys conducted since 1960 demonstrate that men have more loss of attachment than women.[40,42,43] In addition, men have poorer oral hygiene than women, as evidenced by higher levels of plaque and calculus.[1,41,43]

SCIENCE TRANSFER

Risk factors, when present, increase the probability of having disease. In patients with periodontal disease, some factors have a stronger influence than others, and often the strength of the influence of the risk factor is unknown. In addition, these factors can vary considerably. Even more perplexing is the interaction of risk factors, which theoretically may be inhibitory, additive, or synergistic. Thorough and comprehensive examinations and histories are therefore important. Experience as a clinician is also important because evaluation and assessment of examination findings could lead to a better assimilation of risk factors for individual patients.

The presence of bacterial plaque is a prerequisite for periodontal disease. With increasing amounts of plaque and increasing time of contact, periodontal disease is more advanced. In some patients, additional factors increase the amount of periodontal disease for a given exposure to plaque. These risk factors need to be identified so that a coherent approach to treatment is implemented. Some risk factors, such as qualitative plaque makeup, cigarette smoking, diabetes, and frequency of dental care, affect not only the development of periodontitis but also the response to periodontal therapy. Other risk factors (risk determinants/background characteristics), such as genetic makeup, gender, and socioeconomic status, may play a role in etiology and influence the choice of treatment, but these factors have not been shown to affect short-term treatment outcomes.

Therefore, gender differences in prevalence and severity of periodontitis appear to be are related to preventive practices rather than any genetic factor.

Socioeconomic Status

Gingivitis and poor oral hygiene can be related to lower socioeconomic status (SES).[2,40,42] This can most likely be attributed to decreased dental awareness and decreased frequency of dental visits compared with more educated individuals of higher SES. After adjusting for other risk factors, such as smoking and poor oral hygiene, lower SES alone does not result in increased risk for periodontitis (see Chapter 8).

Stress

The incidence of necrotizing ulcerative gingivitis increases during periods of emotional and physiologic stress, suggesting a link between the two.[10,36] Emotional stress may interfere with normal immune function[6,38] and may result in increased levels of circulating hormones, which can affect the periodontium.[34] Stressful life events such as bereavement and divorce appear to lead to a greater prevalence of periodontal disease,[13] and an apparent association exists between psychosocial factors and risk behaviors such as smoking, poor oral hygiene, and chronic periodontitis.[9] Adult patients with periodontitis who are resistant to therapy are more stressed than those who respond to therapy.[5] Individuals with financial strain, distress, depression, or inadequate coping mechanisms have more severe loss of attachment.[12] Although epidemiologic data on the relationship between stress and periodontal disease are limited, stress may be a putative risk factor for periodontitis.[31]

RISK INDICATORS FOR PERIODONTAL DISEASE

Human Immunodeficiency Virus/Acquired Immunodeficiency Syndrome

It has been hypothesized that the immune dysfunction associated with human immunodeficiency virus (HIV) infection and acquired immunodeficiency syndrome (AIDS) increases susceptibility to periodontal disease. Early reports on the periodontal status of patients with AIDS or individuals who are HIV seropositive revealed that these patients often had severe periodontal destruction characteristic of necrotizing ulcerative periodontitis.[46] More recent reports, however, have failed to demonstrate significant differences in the periodontal status of individuals with HIV infection and healthy controls.[24,39] The apparent discrepancy in these reports may have been caused by the inclusion of patients with AIDS (vs. patients who were exclusively HIV seropositive) in some studies.[31]

Conflicting results also exist in studies examining the level of immunosuppression and severity of periodontal destruction. Some studies support that as the degree of immunosuppression increases in adults with AIDS, periodontal pocket formation and loss of clinical attachment also increase. Results of other studies have found no relationship between periodontal diseases and HIV/AIDS status. Evidence also suggests that AIDS-affected individuals who practice good preventive oral health measures, including effective home care and seeking appropriate professional therapy, can maintain periodontal health.[37] Therefore, although it seems reasonable to hypothesize that HIV infection and immunosuppression are risk factors for periodontal disease, the evidence is not conclusive.[2,31]

Osteoporosis

Osteoporosis has been suggested as another risk factor for periodontitis. Although studies in animal models indicate that osteoporosis does not initiate periodontitis, evidence indicates that the reduced bone mass seen in osteoporosis may aggravate periodontal disease progression.[4,23] However, reports in humans are conflicting. In a study of 12 women with osteoporosis and 14 healthy women, von Wowern et al.[44] reported that the women with osteoporosis had greater loss of attachment than the control subjects. In contrast, Kribbs[22] examined pocket depth, bleeding on probing, and gingival recession in women with and without osteoporosis. Although the two groups had significant differences in bone mass, no differences in periodontal status were noted. However, it appears that a link may exist between osteoporosis and periodontitis, and additional studies may need to be conducted to determine if osteoporosis is a true risk factor for periodontal disease.[14,19]

Infrequent Dental Visits

Identifying failure to visit the dentist regularly as a risk factor for periodontitis is controversial.[29] One study demonstrated an increased risk for severe periodontitis in patients who had not visited the dentist for 3 or more years, whereas another demonstrated that there was no more loss of attachment or bone loss in individuals who did not seek dental care compared with those who did over a 6-year period. However, differences in the ages of the subjects in these two studies may explain the different results. Additional longitudinal and intervention studies are necessary to determine if infrequency of dental visits is a risk factor for periodontal disease.

RISK MARKERS/PREDICTORS FOR PERIODONTAL DISEASE

Previous History of Periodontal Disease

A history of previous periodontal disease is a good clinical predictor of risk for future disease.[29] Patients with the most severe existing loss of attachment are at the greatest risk for future loss of attachment. Conversely, patients currently free of periodontitis have a decreased risk for developing loss of attachment compared with those who currently have periodontitis (see Chapter 8).

Bleeding on Probing

Bleeding on probing is the best clinical indicator of gingival inflammation.[29] Although this indicator alone does not serve as a predictor for loss of attachment, bleeding on probing coupled with increasing pocket depth may serve as an excellent predictor for future loss of attachment. Lack of bleeding on probing does appear to serve as an excellent indicator of periodontal health.

CLINICAL RISK ASSESSMENT FOR PERIODONTAL DISEASE

Information concerning individual risk for developing periodontal disease is obtained through careful evaluation of the patient's demographic data, medical history, dental history, and clinical examination (Box 38-2). The elements that contribute to increased risk that can be identified through the collection of demographic data include the patient's age, gender, and SES. The medical history may reveal elements such as a history of diabetes, smoking, HIV/AIDS, or osteoporosis, as well as the perceived level of stress. The dental history can reveal a family history of early tooth loss (suggestive of a genetic predisposition for aggressive periodontitis), a previous

BOX 38-2

Clinical Risk Assessment for Periodontal Disease

Demographic Data
Age
Duration of exposure to risk elements
Postmenopausal women
Evidence of aggressive disease

Male gender
Preventive practices
Frequency of care

Socioeconomic status
Dental awareness
Frequency of care

Medical History
Diabetes
Tobacco smoking
HIV/AIDS
Osteoporosis
Stress

Dental History
Family history of early tooth loss
  Genetic predisposition to aggressive disease
Previous history of periodontal disease
Frequency of dental care

Clinical Examination
Plaque accumulation
  Microbial sampling for putative periodontal pathogens
Calculus
Bleeding on probing
Extent of loss of attachment
  Aggressive forms of disease
Tooth examination
  Plaque retentive areas
  Anatomic factors
  Restorative factors

history of periodontal disease, and information concerning the frequency of oral health care in the past. Important elements identified during the clinical examination can include the location and extent of bacterial plaque accumulation, presence of plaque-retentive factors (e.g., overhanging restorations, subgingival margins), presence of anatomic plaque-retentive areas (e.g., grooves, furcation involvements), presence of calculus, extent of attachment loss, and presence or absence of bleeding on probing.

Once an at-risk patient is identified and a diagnosis is made, the treatment plan may be modified accordingly (Figure 38-1). For example, patients with a history of cigarette smoking should be informed of the relationship between smoking and periodontitis. They also should be informed of the impact of smoking on their prognosis and the likelihood of success of their periodontal therapy if they continue to smoke. Part of their recommended treatment plan for initial therapy may include referral to a smoking cessation program or implementation of self-administered smoking cessation aids. As another example, a patient diagnosed with severe, chronic periodontitis may be encouraged to be tested for the IL-1–positive genotype. If positive, the patient's treatment may involve the administration of systemic antimicrobial agents and host modifiers that would not be used in a patient without this genetic marker. If alterations in the host response are identified, the prognosis and treatment plan may be modified. Previously identified risk elements also may need to be reassessed at the reevaluation stage of treatment. This is especially important in patients who do not respond favorably to periodontal therapy (see Figure 38-1).

CONCLUSION

Risk assessment involves identifying elements that either may predispose a patient to developing periodontal disease or may influence the progression of disease that already exists. In either case, these patients may require modification of their prognosis and treatment plan. In addition to an evaluation of the factors contributing to their risk, these patients should be educated concerning their risk, and when appropriate, suitable intervention strategies should be implemented.

REFERENCES

1. Abdellatif HM, Burt BA: An epidemiological investigation into the relative importance of age and oral hygiene status as determinants of periodontitis, *J Dent Res* 66:13, 1987.
2. American Academy of Periodontology: Position paper: Epidemiology of periodontal diseases, *J Periodontol* 67:935, 1996.
3. American Academy of Periodontology: Position paper: Tobacco use and the periodontal patient, *J Periodontol* 70:1419, 1999.
4. Aufdemorte TB, Boyan BD, Fox WC, et al: Diagnostic tools and biologic markers: animal models in the study of osteoporosis and oral bone loss, *J Bone Miner Res* 8 (suppl 1):S29, 1993.
5. Axtelius B, Söderfeldt B, Nilsson A, et al: Therapy-resistant periodontitis: psychosocial characteristics, *J Clin Periodontol* 25:482, 1998.
6. Ballieux RE: Impact of mental stress on the immune response, *J Clin Periodontol* 18:427, 1991.
7. Blieden TM: Tooth-related issues, *Ann Periodontol* 4:91, 1999.
8. Burt BA: Periodontitis and aging: reviewing recent evidence, *J Am Dent Assoc* 125:273, 1994.
9. Croucher R, Marcenes WS, Torres MC, et al: The relationship between life-events and periodontitis: a case-control study, *J Clin Periodontol* 24:39, 1997.
10. Enwonwu CO: Epidemiological and biochemical studies of necrotizing ulcerative gingivitis and noma (cancrum oris) in Nigerian children, *Arch Oral Biol* 17:1357, 1972.
11. Genco R, Kornman K, Williams R, et al: Consensus report: Periodontal diseases: pathogenesis and microbial factors, *Ann Periodontol* 1:926, 1996.
12. Genco RJ, Ho AW, Grossi SG, et al: Relationship of stress, distress, and inadequate coping behaviors to periodontal disease, *J Periodontol* 70:711, 1999.
13. Green LW, Tryon WW, Marks B, et al: Periodontal disease as a function of life events stress, *J Stress* 12:32, 1986.

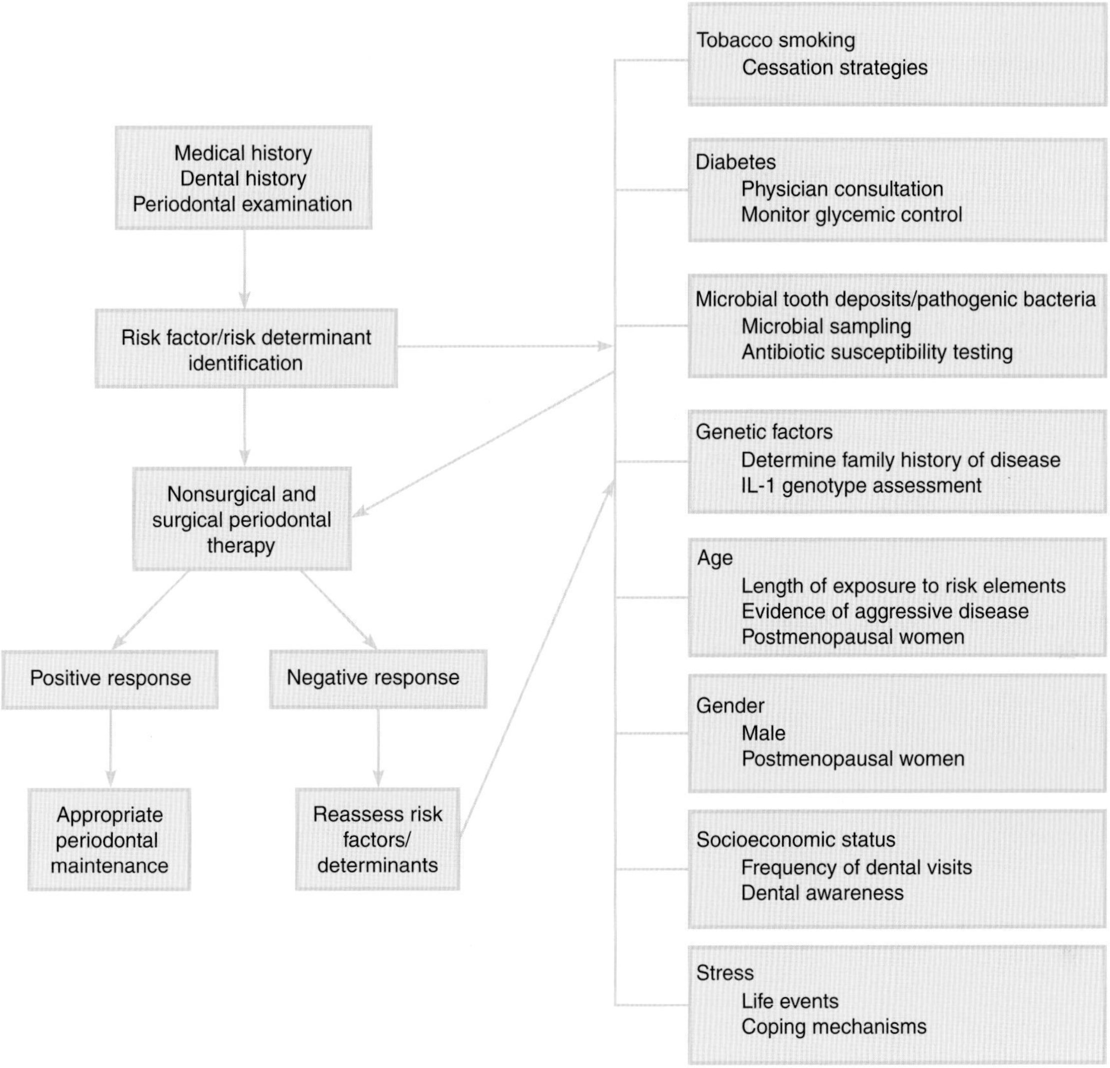

Figure 38-1 Risk assessment in periodontal therapy. The major risk elements to be considered in the diagnosis and treatment of periodontal disease are indicated. The importance of risk assessment before the initiation of therapy is highlighted, as well as the need for reassessment after a negative response to therapy.

14. Guers NC, Lewis CE, Jeffcoat MJ: Osteoporosis and periodontal disease progression, *Periodontol 2000* 32:105, 2003.
15. Gunsolley JC, Tew JG, Gooss CM, et al: Effects of race, smoking and immunoglobulin allotypes on IgG subclass concentrations, *J Periodontal Res* 32:381, 1997.
16. Haffajee AD, Socransky SS: Microbial etiological agents of destructive periodontal diseases, *Periodontol 2000* 5:78, 1994.
17. Hart TC, Shapira L, Van Dyke TE: Neutrophil defects as risk factors for periodontal diseases, *J Periodontol* 65:521, 1994.
18. Ismail AI, Burt BA, Eklund SA: Epidemiologic patterns of smoking and periodontal disease in the United States, *J Am Dent Assoc* 106:617, 1983.
19. Kinane DF: Periodontitis modified by systemic factors, *Ann Periodontol* 4:55, 1999.
20. Kinane DF, Hart TC: Genes and gene polymorphisms associated with periodontal disease, *Crit Rev Oral Biol Med* 14:430, 2003.
21. Kornman KS, Crane S, Wang HY, et al: The interleukin-1 genotype as a severity factor in adult periodontal disease, *J Clin Periodontol* 24:72, 1997.
22. Kribbs PJ: Comparison of mandibular bone in normal and osteoporotic women, *J Prosthet Dent* 63:218, 1990.
23. Krook L, Whalen JP, Lesser GV, et al: Experimental studies on osteoporosis, *Methods Achiev Exp Pathol* 7:72, 1975.
24. Lamster IB, Begg MD, Mitchell L, et al: Oral manifestations of HIV infection in homosexual men and intravenous drug users: study design and relationship of epidemiologic, clinical, and immunologic parameter to oral lesions, *Oral Surg Oral Med Oral Pathol* 78:163, 1994.
25. Löe H, Theilade E, Jensen SB: Experimental gingivitis in man, *J Periodontol* 36:177, 1965.
26. Michalowicz BS, Aeppli DP, Kuba RK, et al: A twin study of genetic variation in proportional radiographic alveolar bone height, *J Dent Res* 70:1431, 1991.
27. Michalowicz BS, Aeppli DP, Virag JG, et al: Risk findings in adult twins, *J Periodontol* 62:293, 1991.
28. Michalowicz BS, Diehl SR, Gunsolley JC, et al: Evidence for a substantial genetic basis for risk of adult periodontitis, *J Periodontol* 71:1699, 2000.
29. Page RC, Beck JD: Risk assessment for periodontal diseases, *Int Dent J* 47:61, 1997.

30. Papapanou PN: Epidemiology and natural history of periodontal disease. In Lang NP, Karring T, editors: *Proceedings of the First European Workshop on Periodontology,* London, 1994, Quintessence.
31. Papapanou PN: Risk assessments in the diagnosis and treatment of periodontal diseases, *J Den Educ* 62:822, 1998.
32. Papapanou PN, Lindhe J: Preservation of probing attachment and alveolar bone levels in two random population samples, *J Clin Periodontol* 19:583, 1992.
33. Papapanou PN, Lindhe J, Sterrett JD, et al: Considerations on the contribution of aging to loss of periodontal tissue support, *J Clin Periodontol* 18:611, 1991.
34. Rose RM: Endocrine responses to stressful psychological events, *Psychiatr Clin North Am* 3:251, 1980.
35. Shapira L, Soskolone WA, Van Dyke TE, et al: Prostaglandin E_2 secretion, cell maturation, and CD14 expression by monocyte-derived macrophages from localized juvenile periodontitis patients, *J Periodontol* 67:224, 1996.
36. Shields WD: Acute necrotizing ulcerative gingivitis: a study of some of the contributing factors and their validity in an Army population, *J Periodontol* 48:346, 1977.
37. Stanford TW, Rees TD: Acquired immune suppression and other risk factors/indicators for periodontal disease progression, *Periodontol 2000* 32:118, 2003.
38. Sternberg EM, Chrousos GP, Wilder RL, et al: The stress response and the regulation of inflammatory disease, *Ann Intern Med* 117:854, 1992.
39. Swango PA, Kleinman DV, Konzelman JL: HIV and periodontal health: a study of military personnel with HIV, *J Am Dent Assoc* 122:49, 1991.
40. US Public Health Service, National Center for Health Statistics: *Periodontal disease in adults, United States, 1960–1962,* PHS Pub No 1000, Series 11, No 12, Washington, DC, 1965, US Government Printing Office.
41. US Public Health Service, National Center for Health Statistics: *Oral hygiene in adults, United States, 1960–1962,* PHS Pub No 1000, Series 11, No 16, Washington, DC, 1966, US Government Printing Office.
42. US Public Health Service, National Center for Health Statistics: *Basic data on dental examination findings of persons 1–74 years, United States, 1971–1974,* DHEW PHS Pub No 79-1662, Series 11, No 214, Washington, DC, 1979, US Government Printing Office.
43. US Public Health Service, National Institute of Dental Research (NIDR): *Oral health of United States adults: national findings,* NIH Pub No 87-2868, Bethesda, Md, 1987, NIDR.
44. von Wowern J, Klausen B, Kollerup G: Osteoporosis: a risk factor in periodontal disease, *J Periodontol* 65:134, 1994.
45. Wilson ME, Kalmar JR: FcγIIa (CD32): a potential marker defining susceptibility to localized juvenile periodontitis, *J Periodontol* 76:323, 1996.
46. Winkler JR, Herrera C, Westenhouse J, et al: Periodontal disease in HIV-infected and uninfected homosexual and bisexual men, *AIDS* 6:1041, 1992 (letter).

Levels of Clinical Significance

Philippe P. Hujoel

39 CHAPTER

Chapter Outline

In a study of periodontal tissue regeneration, investigators reported that a treatment that resulted in a gain of 1.2 mm in clinical attachment level and a reduction of 1 mm in probing pocket depth "may not have a great clinical impact."[4] Another group reported that a treatment that resulted in 0.0 mm gain in clinical attachment level and a reduction of 0.2 mm in probing depth had such clinical significance that it should "be used universally."[26] Different individuals will reach different decisions regarding what is meant by the term 'clinical significance'. As a result, the term "clinical significant" has largely become a useless term, more useful to marketers than to clinicians.

The term *clinically significant* could be made more relevant by recognizing (1) the nature of the benefits (tangible/intangible) and (2) the size of the treatment effect (large/small).These two criteria for classifying clinical significance are now defined.

TANGIBLE VERSUS INTANGIBLE BENEFITS

The clinical significance of a treatment depends on whether the benefits identified are tangible or intangible.

Tangible benefits are those treatment outcomes that reflect how a patient feels, functions, or survives. The word "tangible" is defined as "capable of being precisely identified or realized by the mind." Examples of tangible benefits could include improved oral health–related quality of life,[13,14] a decrease in self-reported symptoms (e.g., bleeding) after brushing, prevention of tooth loss, or elimination of a painful periodontal abscess. These examples of treatment benefits can precisely be identified or realized by the *patient's mind;* that is, they are tangible. Tangible benefits can also be referred to as "clinically relevant" benefits or "clinically meaningful" benefits.

Intangible benefits cannot be realized by the patient's mind. Changes in probing attachment level as a result of scaling, changes in enamel mineralization level as a result of fluorides, and changes in the size of a periapical radiolucency as a result of a root canal treatment are examples of changes the mind cannot identify or realize; thus they are intangible treatment benefits. Intangible treatment benefits can often be measured objectively by the clinician or by laboratory methods.

A first step in assessing the clinical significance of a treatment is to determine whether the documented treatment benefits are tangible or intangible. This distinction is important because intangible benefits do not necessarily translate into tangible benefits. A medication that lowers elevated blood lipid levels (an intangible benefit) may shorten life span (a tangible patient harm).[19] A treatment that increases bone density (an intangible benefit) can increase fracture risk (a tangible patient harm).[10] A treatment that provides extensive periodontal bone regeneration (an intangible benefit) can lead to tooth loss (a tangible harm).[12]

SCIENCE TRANSFER

"Clinical significance" in periodontology has often been debated when evaluating therapeutic options. Factors not often considered in the debate is whether the benefit is tangible and whether the likelihood of obtaining the benefit is large. According to this chapter, if the patient's mind is aware of the benefit from treatment, this is a "tangible" result, whereas if the benefit cannot be realized by the patient's mind, it is "intangible." Clinicians can further judge if a treatment effect is significant based on the likelihood the treatment indeed the delivers the promised benefit. Results may be statistically significant, yet be of little or no clinical value when small intangible changes such as improvement in pocket depths do not translate into tangible benefits such as tooth retention.

TABLE 39-1

Definition of levels of Significance Based on Size and Nature of the benefit

		SIZE OF THE BENEFIT	
Clinical Significance		**Large‡**	**Small§**
Nature of the benefit	*Tangible**	Level 1	Level 2
	Intangible†	Level 3	Level 4

*Tangible benefits are outcomes that directly measure how a patient feels, functions, or survives.
†Intangible benefits are outcomes that are not perceivable by the patient's mind.
‡A large benefit is defined as one that can reliably be identified using epidemiologic methodology.
§A small benefit is defined as one that requires the conduct of randomized controlled trials for reliable identification.

A treatment that has been shown to provide tangible benefits has a higher level of clinical significance than a treatment for which only evidence of intangible benefits exists. The finding that implant-supported dentures improve quality of life[1] has a higher level of clinical significance than the finding that scaling improves probing attachment levels. The finding that an endodontic treatment reliably eliminates tooth pain has a higher level of clinical significance than the finding that chlorhexidine reduces *Streptococcus mutans* levels.

SIZE OF THE TREATMENT EFFECT

A second important criterion for assessing clinical significance is the size of the treatment effect. The size of the treatment effect is a comparison of the success rates of the experimental treatment and the control treatment. This comparison of treatments can be a subtraction of the success rates, a division of the success rates, or some other mathematic operation. The size of the treatment effect, regardless of how it is calculated, has long been been recognized as an important part of assessing clinical significance. The larger the likelihood of obtaining an expected benefit of a treatment (relative to a control treatment), the more clinically significant is the treatment. We suggest that if the odds ratio associated with the treatment comparison is 0.25 or smaller (when compared to the control), the size of the treatment effect may be considered large.

The likelihood of obtaining a treatment benefit (relative to the control) determines to a large extent the methodologic and analytic rigor required to establish treatment effectiveness. At one extreme, in all-or-none situations, reliable evidence may result from observations on a small number of patients. For example, no concurrent controlled trials were conducted to assess the effectiveness of general anesthesia. Determining effectiveness for treatments that achieve a dramatic and immediate effect is straightforward, and only essential scientific principles (e.g., consistency of observations across different operators) are considered sufficient evidence of treatment effectiveness. Reportedly, the words, "Gentleman, this is no humbug," were sufficient to convince an audience that general anesthesia was effective.

At another extreme, if the likelihood of obtaining an expected treatment benefit is small, extreme rigor in both design and analysis of controlled clinical trials is required. The benefit of mammography screening for early detection of breast cancer, the benefit of one "clot-buster" drug over another after a myocardial event, and the benefit of local antibiotics in the treatment of periodontitis are all so small that large, randomized controlled trials are required to provide reliable evidence of whether small benefits indeed are associated with treatment.

The likelihood of obtaining an treatment benefit is a determinant of clinical significance; the larger the likelihood, the more confident a patient can feel that a treatment will be successful. Although it is possible to have a clear, unequivocal definition of what constitutes a tangible benefit associated with treatment, it is *not* possible to have similar rigorous definition of what can be *considered* a large likelihood. We define a "large treatment effect" as an odds ratio of 0.25 which can reliably be identified using good epidemiologic methodology.[5,24]

DEFINING FOUR LEVELS OF CLINICAL SIGNIFICANCE

Based on the nature of the benefit (tangible/intangible) and the size of the treatment effect (large/small), four levels of clinical significance can be defined (Table 39-1).

Clinical Significance Level 1

Treatments of clinical significance level 1 are the "magical bullets," the "miracle cures" in which the treatment provides a tangible benefit and the size of the treatment effect is large. Examples of such treatments include the use of vitamin C to treat scurvy, bone marrow transplantation to treat leukemia, and dental implants to improve the oral-health-related quality of life of edentulous individuals. In all three examples, the benefits of the treatment are tangible, and the size of the treatment effect is large.

An understanding of biologic mechanisms of treatment actions is not required to establish that a treatment has clinical significance level 1. Lemon juice was identified as an effective method to prevent scurvy in 1601, but it was not until the beginning of the twentieth century that vitamin C was isolated.[21] Digitalis was discovered as a treatment for "dropsy" long before physicians became aware of the drug's cardiac effects.[25] Lithium is an effective drug for bipolar disorder, but its mechanism of action remains largely unknown.[23] In contrast, HRT, for which the biologic mechanisms explaining how the drug provided benefits were supposedly so well understood, resulted in more harm than good.[11]

Treatments of clinical significance level 1 are not always immediately accepted or widely used. It took the British Navy 264 years from the time of the observations of Captain James until a universal preventive policy was established to prevent scurvy.[3] This lack of appreciation for this treatment of clinical significance level 1 was unfortunate: "It is estimated that 5000 lives a year were needlessly lost from scurvy during this period: that is a total of nearly 800,000. In the 200 years from 1600 to 1800 nearly 1,000,000 men died of an easily preventable disease. There are in the whole of human history few more notable examples of official indifference and stupidity producing such disastrous consequence to human life."[20] Although it is easy to determine clinical significance level 1 in retrospect, it may be difficult to recognize at the time of discovery.

Clinical Significance Level 2

The term *clinical significance level 2* is used to describe treatments that have been demonstrated to provide a tangible benefit, but for which the likelihood of obtaining the benefit from treatment is small. Because the size of the benefit of one therapy over another is small, randomized controlled trials (RCTs), often large in size and rigorous in execution and analysis, are required to provide unequivocal evidence that the treatment provides tangible patient benefits. Examples of such treatments include the advantage of tissue plasminogen activator (t-PA) over streptokinase[9] and the benefits of penciclovir in the treatment of herpetic lesions.[18]

Determining the clinical relevance of treatments of clinical significance level 2 is an individual choice in which issues such as cost and side effects often play a more important role. For example, the mortality rate with t-PA is 6.3%, whereas the mortality rate with streptokinase is 7.3%.[9] In other words, there is a 1% increased chance for survival associated with t-PA. In the 1990s, when this treatment was introduced, the increased cost for t-PA was $2000. Is a 1% increased survival probability worth $2000? Different individuals, different governments, and different health insurance companies may decide differently on this important question. Indeed, some individuals may believe that if large RCTs are required to determine treatment effectiveness, the clinical significance of the treatment is questionable.

The use of penciclovir in the treatment of herpetic lesions provides another example of a drug of clinical significance level 2. When applying a 1% penciclovir cream, 70% of the patients report lesion healing by day 6. When applying placebo cream, 59% of the patients report lesion healing by day 6.[18] Is an 11% increased probability of lesion healing by day 6 of sufficient magnitude to refer to the treatment as "clinically relevant"? Once again, the answer to this question is highly individual; the cream may be worth its weight in gold for a young teenager when prom night is approaching, but it may be clinically irrelevant for a more sedate adult. By using the terminology "clinical significance level 2," the concept of small, tangible patient benefit can quickly be communicated without becoming trapped in meaningless discussions regarding the clinical relevance of small benefits.

Clinical Significance Level 3

Treatments of clinical significance level 3 are the magical bullets, the miracle cures in the surrogate world where the beneficial but intangible effects of treatment are so convincing that the need for RCTs may appear remote. Examples of such treatments include the use of highly active antiretroviral therapy (HAART) in patients with acquired immunodeficiency syndrome (AIDS)[15] imatinib (Gleevec) in the treatment of chronic myeloid leukemia,[16] and chlorhexidine varnish in the prevention of caries.[22]

With a treatment that has the label of "clinical significance level 3," there is always the uncertainty of whether the intangible benefits translate into real, tangible patient benefits. It has been a common observation that the larger the effect size observed on the surrogate, the more likely the surrogate benefit translates into a real, tangible patient benefit.[6]

For certain treatments, such as HAART for AIDS or Gleevec for chronic leukemia, the opportunity may exist to avoid RCTs, and treatments of clinical significance level 3 can become treatments of clinical significance level 1 by means of epidemiological studies where the tangible benefits associated with the intangible surrogate changes are identified. For example, drastic changes in the viral load of human immunodeficiency virus (HIV) have been shown to lead to large reductions in the risk of AIDS and death. Using historical controls, it was shown that HAART treatment reduced the AIDS risk by 38% and the mortality risk by 34%.[15] A large surrogate benefit (clinical significance level 3) translated into a large survival benefit (clinical significance level 1).

However, assuming that large, intangible treatment benefits invariably translate into tangible treatment benefits remains a dangerous assumption, no matter how large the effect on the surrogate endpoint. A 40% chlorhexidine varnish used for the prevention of caries was reported to result in a 99.9% mutans streptococci reduction in all the 20 subjects treated, and the streptococci stayed below detectable levels for at least 4 weeks in nine subjects. In contrast, the placebo varnish-sealant led to only a 32% mutans streptococci reduction, and none of the 20 subjects had mutans streptococci below detectable levels for 4 weeks.[22] Based on these data, it was reported that, "Chlorzoin will wipe out dental decay much like smallpox." A subsequent RCT in 1240 children at high risk for caries did not translate into a reduction of large cavities in the teeth. The chlorzoin group had 6.8 D3 lesions (standard deviation, 6.2), and the placebo group had 6.4 D3 lesions (standard deviation, 6.4), in other words, fewer lesions.[7] This example shows that even large, intangible treatment benefits do not always translate into tangible treatment benefits.

Clinical Significance Level 4

Treatments of clinical significance level 4 are those treatments which have reliable evidence from large randomized controlled trials of small, intangible treatment benefits. Because the treatment effects are small, epidemiological studies are almost always incapable of identifying treatment of clinical significance level 4. Examples of treatments of clinical significance level 4 include those that cause a small decrease in lipid level, a small drop in blood pressure, or a small decrease in pocket depth. Large leaps of faith are often required to jump from the observations that small changes in surrogate endpoints translate into real, tangible benefits.

The use of clofibrate to lower lipid levels is an example of a drug of clinical significance level 4. Clofibrate reduced the mean cholesterol levels from 324 to 224 mg and the mean value of triglycerides from 271 to 125 (which can be argued are "not so small" mean changes).[2] Clofibrate was the most widely prescribed lipid-lowering agent in the United States, but the uncertainty remained whether clofibrate actually provided a tangible patient benefit. Advertisements that were widely used in medical journals accurately reflected the clinical uncertainty surrounding use of this drug. A text box within the advertisement stated, "It has not been established whether the drug-induced lowering of serum cholesterol or lipid levels has a detrimental, beneficial, or no effect on the mortality and the morbidity due to atherosclerosis or coronary heart disease. Several years will be required before current investigations will yield an answer to this question." A subsequent World Health Organization (WHO) cooperative trial on clofibrate revealed the wisdom of this disclaimer. The trial results showed that clofibrate resulted in excess mortality of 47%, providing yet another example of a misleading surrogate.[19]

Treatment of clinical significance level 4 may cause more harm than good, and there is debate whether the drug-approval process should be changed.[17] If such a change were to occur, it could have significant consequences for periodontal therapies because most approved periodontal therapies are of clinical significance level 4, and minimal information on their long-term safety is available.

SUMMARY

Two important determinants of clinical significance are the nature of benefit (tangible vs. intangible) and the likelihood for obtaining the benefit (when compared to the control treatment). These two characteristics can be used to define 4 hierarchical of clinical significance. Treatments that provide a tangible patient benefit (level 1 or 2) are of greater value and should correspond to a higher level of clinical significance than treatments with evidence of only intangible benefits (level 3 and 4). Similarly, treatments with a large likelihood for clinical improvement (level 1 and 3) are clinically more significant than treatments with a small likelihood for clinical improvement (level 2 and 4). Providing four hierarchical levels of clinical significance may help clinicians and patients communicate more effectively regarding the clinical significance of a treatment.

REFERENCES

1. Awad MA, Locker D, Korner-Bitensky N, Feine JS: Measuring the effect of intra-oral implant rehabilitation on health-related quality of life in a randomized controlled clinical trial, *J Dent Res* 79:1659, 2000.
2. Berkowitz D: Long-term treatment of hyperlipidemic patients with clofibrate, *JAMA* 218:1002, 1971.
3. Berwick DM: Disseminating innovations in health care, *JAMA* 289:1969, 2003.
4. Esposito M, Coulthard P, Worthington HV: Enamel matrix derivative (Emdogain) for periodontal tissue regeneration in intrabony defects, *Cochrane Database Syst Rev* CD003875, 2003.
5. Feinstein AR: Scientific standards in epidemiologic studies of the menace of daily life, *Science* 242:1257, 1988.
6. Fleming TR, Prentice RL, Pepe MS, Glidden D: Surrogate and auxiliary endpoints in clinical trials, with potential applications in cancer and AIDS research, *Stat Med* 13:955, 1994.
7. Forgie AH, Paterson M, Pine CM, et al: A randomised controlled trial of the caries-preventive efficacy of a chlorhexidine-containing varnish in high-caries-risk adolescents, *Caries Res* 34:432, 2000.
8. Giles J: Study warns of "avoidable" risks of CT scans, *Nature* 431:391, 2004.
9. GUSTO investigators: An international randomized trial comparing four thrombolytic strategies for acute myocardial infarction, *N Engl J Med* 329:673, 1993.
10. Haguenauer D, Welch V, Shea B, et al: Fluoride for treating postmenopausal osteoporosis, *Cochrane Database Syst Rev* CD002825, 2000.
11. Hogervorst E: Estrogen plus progestin use did not improve global cognitive function in older postmenopausal women, *Evid Base Obstet Gynecol* 5:189, 2003.
12. Hujoel PP: Endpoints in periodontal trials: the need for an evidence-based research approach, *Periodontol 2000* 36:196, 2004.
13. Leao A, Sheiham A: The development of a socio-dental measure of dental impacts on daily living, *Community Dent Health* 13:22, 1996.
14. McGrath C, Bedi R: An evaluation of a new measure of oral health related quality of life: OHQoL-UK(W), *Community Dent Health* 18:138, 2001.
15. Mocroft A, Ledergerber B, Katlama C, et al: Decline in the AIDS and death rates in the EuroSIDA study: an observational study, *Lancet* 362:22, 2003.
16. O'Brien SG, Deininger MW: Imatinib in patients with newly diagnosed chronic-phase chronic myeloid leukemia, *Semin Hematol* 40:26, 2003.

17. Psaty BM, Weiss NS, Furberg CD, et al: Surrogate end points, health outcomes, and the drug-approval process for the treatment of risk factors for cardiovascular disease, *JAMA* 282:786, 1999.
18. Raborn GW, Martel AY, Lassonde M, et al: Effective treatment of herpes simplex labialis with penciclovir cream: combined results of two trials, *J Am Dent Assoc* 133:303, 2002.
19. Report of the Committee of Principal Investigators: WHO cooperative trial on primary prevention of ischaemic heart disease with clofibrate to lower serum cholesterol: final mortality follow-up, *Lancet* 2:600, 1984.
20. Roddis LH: *A short history of nautical medicine,* New York, 1941, Hoeber.
21. Rosenfeld L: Vitamine—vitamin: the early years of discovery, *Clin Chem* 43:680, 1997.
22. Sandham HJ, Brown J, Chan KH, et al: Clinical trial in adults of an antimicrobial varnish for reducing mutans streptococci, *J Dent Res* 70:1401, 1991.
23. Shaldubina A, Agam G, Belmaker RH: The mechanism of lithium action: state of the art, ten years later, *Prog Neuropsychopharmacol Biol Psychiatry* 25:855, 2001.
24. Taubes G: Epidemiology faces its limits, *Science* 269:164, 1995.
25. Wade OL: Digoxin 1785-1985. I. Two hundred years of digitalis, *J Clin Hosp Pharm* 11:3, 1986.
26. Williams RC, Paquette DW, Offenbacher S, et al: Treatment of periodontitis by local administration of minocycline microspheres: a controlled trial, *J Periodontol* 72:1535, 2001.

Determination of Prognosis

Karen F. Novak, Stephen F. Goodman, and Henry H. Takei

CHAPTER 40

CHAPTER OUTLINE

DEFINITIONS

The **prognosis** is a prediction of the probable course, duration, and outcome of a disease based on a general knowledge of the pathogenesis of the disease and the presence of risk factors for the disease. It is established after the diagnosis is made and before the treatment plan is established. The prognosis is based on specific information about the disease and the manner in which it can be treated, but it also can be influenced by the clinician's previous experience with treatment outcomes (successes and failures) as they relate to the particular case.

Prognosis is often confused with the term *risk*. Risk generally deals with the likelihood that an individual will develop a disease in a specified period (see Chapter 8). *Risk factors* are those characteristics of an individual that put the person at increased risk for developing a disease (see Chapter 38). In contrast, *prognosis* is the prediction of the course or outcome of a disease. *Prognostic factors* are characteristics that predict the outcome of disease once the disease is present. In some cases, risk factors and prognostic factors are the same. For example, patients with diabetes or patients who smoke are more at risk for acquiring periodontal disease, and once they have it, they generally have a worse prognosis.

TYPES OF PROGNOSIS

Although some factors may be more important than others when assigning a prognosis[29,30] (see Box 40-1), consideration of each factor may be beneficial to the clinician. In most cases, careful analysis of these factors allows the clinician to establish one of the following prognoses[28]:

Excellent prognosis: No bone loss, excellent gingival condition, good patient cooperation, no systemic or environmental factors.

Good prognosis: One or more of the following: adequate remaining bone support, adequate possibilities to control etiologic factors and establish a maintainable dentition, adequate patient cooperation, no systemic or environmental factors, or if systemic factors are present, they are well controlled.

Fair prognosis: One or more of the following: less-than-adequate remaining bone support, some tooth mobility, grade I furcation involvement, adequate maintenance possible, acceptable patient cooperation, presence of limited systemic or environmental factors.

Poor prognosis: One or more of the following: moderate to advanced bone loss, tooth mobility, grade I and II furcation involvements, difficult-to-maintain areas or doubtful patient cooperation, presence of systemic or environmental factors.

Questionable prognosis: One or more of the following: advanced bone loss, grade II and III furcation involvements, tooth mobility, inaccessible areas, presence of systemic or environmental factors.

Hopeless prognosis: One or more of the following: advanced bone loss, nonmaintainable areas, extraction(s) indicated, presence of uncontrolled systemic or environmental factors.

It should be recognized that excellent, good, and hopeless prognoses are the only prognoses that can be established with a reasonable degree of accuracy. Fair, poor, and even questionable prognoses depend on a large number of factors that can interact in an unpredictable number of ways.[6,11,42] In many of these cases, it may be advisable to establish a provisional prognosis until Phase I therapy is completed and evaluated.

The *provisional prognosis* allows the clinician to initiate treatment of teeth that have a doubtful outlook in the hope that a favorable response may tip the balance and allow teeth to be retained. The reevaluation phase in the treatment sequence allows the clinician to examine the tissue response to scaling, oral hygiene, and root planing, as well as to the possible use of chemotherapeutic agents where indicated. The patient's compliance with the proposed treatment plan also can be determined.

Overall versus Individual Tooth Prognosis

Prognosis can be divided into overall prognosis and individual tooth prognosis. The *overall prognosis* is concerned with the dentition as a whole. Factors that may influence the overall prognosis include patient age, current severity of disease, systemic factors, smoking, the presence of plaque, calculus and other local factors, patient compliance, and prosthetic possibilities (see Box 40-1). The overall prognosis answers the following questions:

- Should treatment be undertaken?
- Is treatment likely to succeed?
- When prosthetic replacements are needed, are the remaining teeth able to support the added burden of the prosthesis?

The *individual tooth prognosis* is determined after the overall prognosis and is affected by it.[28] For example, in a patient with a poor overall prognosis, the dentist likely would not attempt to retain a tooth that has a questionable prognosis because of local conditions. Many of the factors listed under *Local Factors* and *Prosthetic and Restorative Factors* in Box 40-1 have a direct effect on the prognosis for individual teeth, in addition to any overall systemic or environmental factors that may be present.

FACTORS IN DETERMINATION OF PROGNOSIS

Box 40-1 lists the factors to consider when determining a prognosis.

BOX 40-1

Factors to Consider when Determining a Prognosis

Overall Clinical Factors
Patient age
Disease severity
Plaque control
Patient compliance

Systemic and Environmental Factors
Smoking
Systemic disease or condition
Genetic factors
Stress

Local Factors
Plaque and calculus
Subgingival restorations

Anatomic factors:
- Short, tapered roots
- Cervical enamel projections
- Enamel pearls
- Bifurcation ridges
- Root concavities
- Developmental grooves
- Root proximity
- Furcation involvement

Tooth mobility

Prosthetic and Restorative Factors
Abutment selection
Caries
Nonvital teeth
Root resorption

Overall Clinical Factors

Patient Age. For two patients with comparable levels of remaining connective tissue attachment and alveolar bone, the prognosis is generally better for the older of the two. For the younger patient, the prognosis is not as good because of the shorter time frame in which the periodontal destruction has occurred; the younger patient may have an aggressive type of periodontitis, or disease progression may have increased because of systemic disease or smoking. In addition, although the younger patient would ordinarily be expected to have a greater reparative capacity, the occurrence of so much destruction in a relatively short period would exceed any naturally occurring periodontal repair.

Disease Severity. Studies have demonstrated that a patient's history of previous periodontal disease may be indicative of their susceptibility for future periodontal breakdown (see Chapter 8). Therefore the following variables should be carefully recorded because they are important for determining the patient's past history of periodontal disease: pocket depth, level of attachment, degree of bone loss, and type of bony defect. These factors are determined by clinical and radiographic evaluation (see Chapters 35 and 36).

The determination of the level of clinical attachment reveals the approximate extent of root surface that is devoid of periodontal ligament; the radiographic examination shows the amount of root surface still invested in bone. Pocket depth is less important than level of attachment, because it is not necessarily related to bone loss. In general, a tooth with deep pockets and little attachment and bone loss has a better prognosis than one with shallow pockets and severe attachment and bone loss. However, deep pockets are a source of infection and may contribute to progressive disease.

Prognosis is adversely affected if the base of the pocket (level of attachment) is close to the root apex. The presence of apical disease as a result of endodontic involvement also worsens the prognosis. However, surprisingly good apical and lateral bone repair can sometimes be obtained by combining endodontic and periodontal therapy (see Chapter 58).

The prognosis also can be related to the height of remaining bone. Assuming bone destruction can be arrested, is there enough bone remaining to support the teeth? The answer is readily apparent in extreme cases, that is, when there is so little bone loss that tooth support is not in jeopardy (Figure 40-1), or when bone loss is so severe that the remaining bone is obviously insufficient for proper tooth support (Figure 40-2). Most patients, however, do not fit into these extreme categories. The height of remaining bone is usually somewhere in between, making bone level assessment alone insufficient for determining the overall prognosis.

The type of defect also must be determined. The prognosis for horizontal bone loss depends on the height of the existing bone, because it is unlikely that clinically significant bone height regeneration will be induced by therapy. In the case of angular, intrabony defects, if the contour of the existing bone and the number of osseous walls are favorable, there is an excellent chance that therapy could regenerate bone to approximately the level of the alveolar crest.[40]

When greater bone loss has occurred on one surface of a tooth, the bone height on the less involved surfaces should be taken into consideration when determining the prognosis. Because of the greater height of bone in relation to other surfaces, the center of rotation of the tooth will be nearer the crown (Figure 40-3). This results in a more favorable distribution of forces to the periodontium and less tooth mobility.[44]

In dealing with a tooth with a questionable prognosis, the chances of successful treatment should be weighed against any benefits that would accrue to the adjacent teeth if the tooth under consideration were extracted. Heroic attempts to retain a hopelessly involved tooth may jeopardize the adjacent teeth. Extraction of the questionable tooth may be followed by partial restoration of the bone support of the adjacent teeth (Figure 40-4).

Plaque Control. Bacterial plaque is the primary etiologic factor associated with periodontal disease (see Chapter 9). Therefore, effective removal of plaque on a daily basis by the patient is critical to the success of periodontal therapy and to the prognosis.

Patient Compliance and Cooperation. The prognosis for patients with gingival and periodontal disease is critically dependent on the patient's attitude, desire to retain the natural teeth, and willingness and ability to maintain good oral hygiene. Without these, treatment cannot succeed. Patients should be clearly informed of the important role they must play for treatment to succeed. If patients are unwilling or unable to perform adequate plaque control and to receive the timely periodic maintenance checkups and treatments that the dentist deems necessary, the dentist can (1) refuse to accept the patient for treatment or (2) extract teeth that have a hopeless or poor prognosis and perform scaling and root planing on the remaining teeth. The dentist should make it clear to the patient and in the patient record that further treatment is needed but will not be performed because of a lack of patient cooperation.

Systemic and Environmental Factors

Smoking. Epidemiologic evidence suggests that smoking may be the most important environmental risk factor impacting the development and progression of periodontal disease (see Chapter 8). Therefore it should be made clear to the patient that a direct relationship exists between smoking and the prevalence and incidence of periodontitis. In addition, patients should be informed that smoking affects not only the severity of periodontal destruction, but also the healing potential of the periodontal tissues. As a result, patients who smoke do not respond as well to conventional periodontal therapy as patients who have never smoked.[38,39] Therefore the prognosis in patients who smoke and have slight to moderate periodontitis is generally fair to poor. In patients with severe periodontitis, the prognosis may be poor to hopeless.

However, it should be emphasized that smoking cessation can affect the treatment outcome and therefore the prognosis.[3,14] Patients with slight to moderate periodontitis who stop smoking can often be upgraded to a good prognosis, whereas those with severe periodontitis who stop smoking may be upgraded to a fair prognosis.

Systemic Disease or Condition. The patient's systemic background affects overall prognosis in several ways. For example, evidence from epidemiologic studies clearly demonstrates that the prevalence and severity of periodontitis are significantly higher in patients with type 1 and type 2 diabetes than in those without diabetes, and that the level of control of the diabetes is an important variable in this relationship (see Chapter 8). Therefore, patients at risk for diabetes should be identified as early as possible and informed of the relationship between periodontitis and diabetes. Similarly, patients diagnosed with diabetes must be informed of the impact of diabetic control on the development and progression of periodontitis. It follows that the prognosis in these cases depends on patient compliance relative to both medical

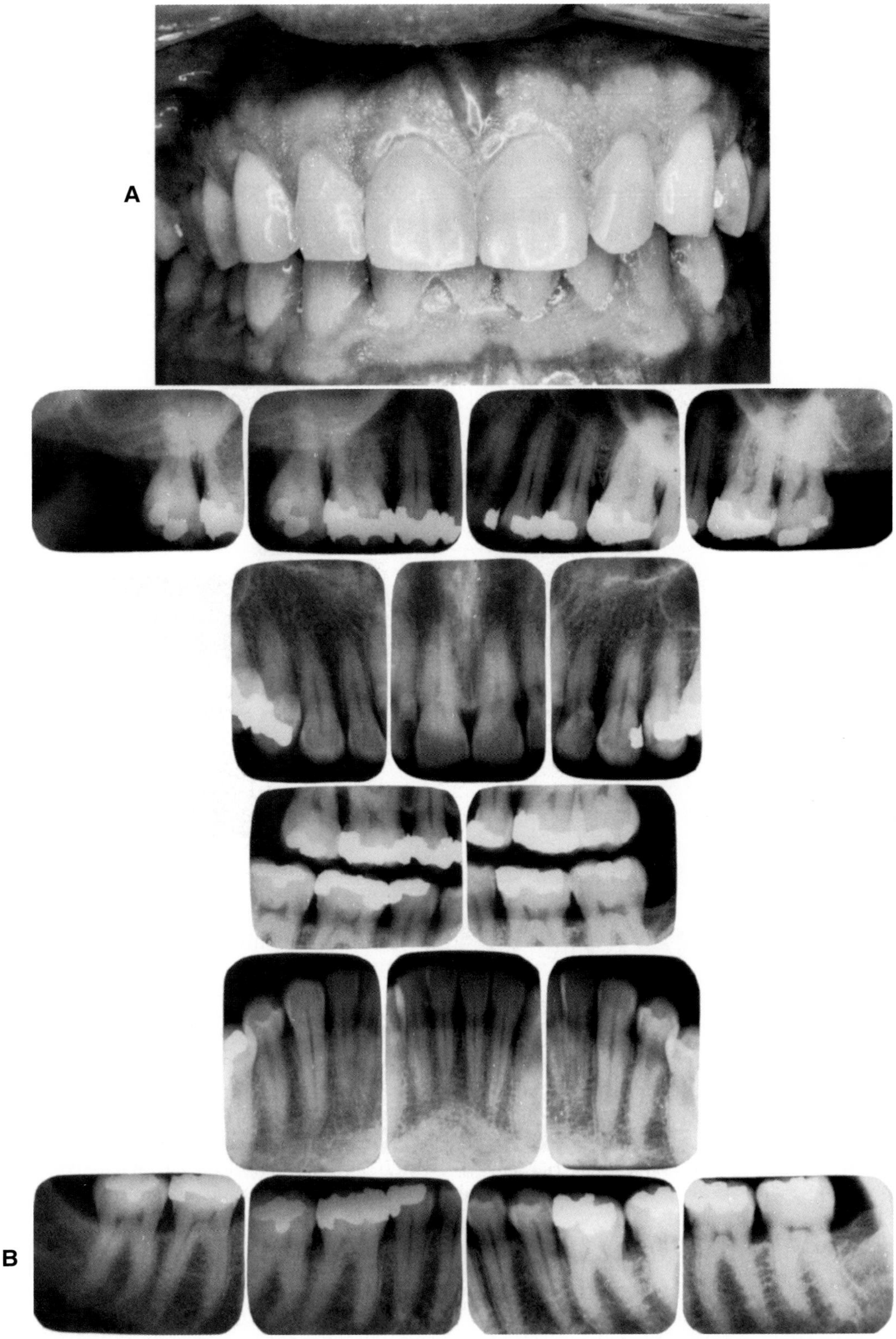

Figure 40-1 Chronic periodontitis in systemically healthy, nonsmoking 42-year-old man; overall prognosis good. **A,** Gingival inflammation, poor oral hygiene, and pronounced anterior overbite. **B,** Although local factors are present, the patient presents with adequate remaining bone support and a good prognosis, provided local factors can be controlled.

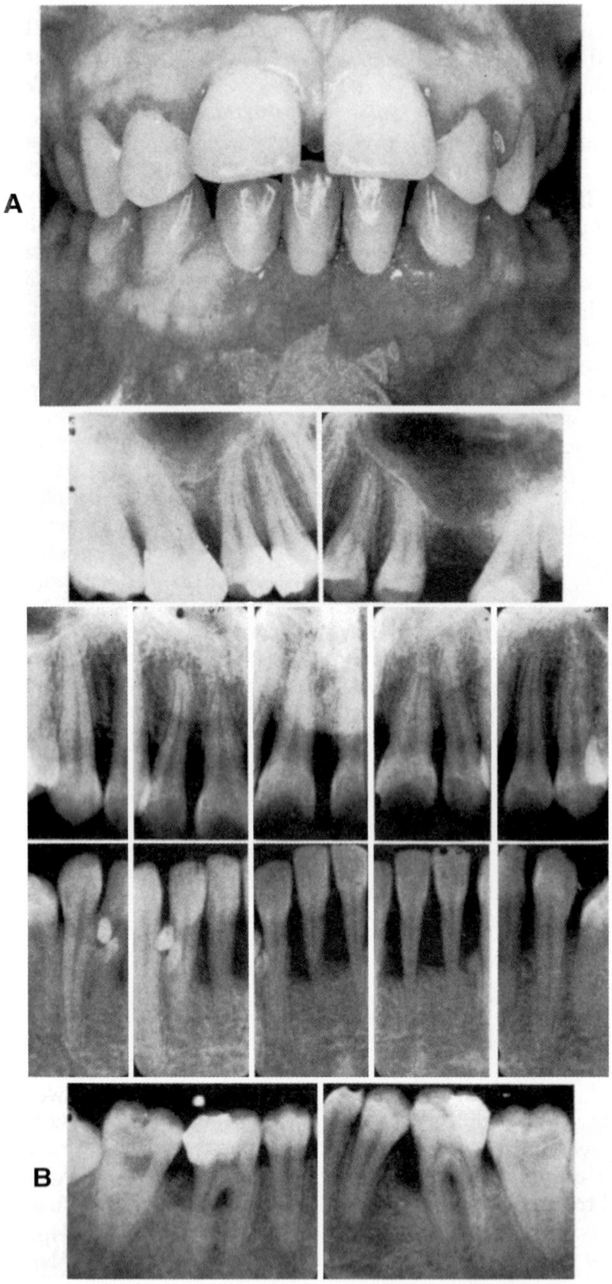

Figure 40-2 Localized aggressive periodontitis in 17-year-old girl; overall prognosis fair. **A,** Gingival inflammation, periodontal pockets, and pathologic migration. **B,** Severe bone destruction.

and dental status. Well-controlled diabetic patients with slight to moderate periodontitis who comply with their recommended periodontal treatment should have a good prognosis. Similarly, in patients with other systemic disorders that could affect disease progression, prognosis improves with correction of the systemic problem.

The prognosis is questionable when surgical periodontal treatment is required but cannot be provided because of the patient's health (see Chapter 44). Incapacitating conditions that limit the patient's performance of oral procedures (e.g., Parkinson's disease) also adversely

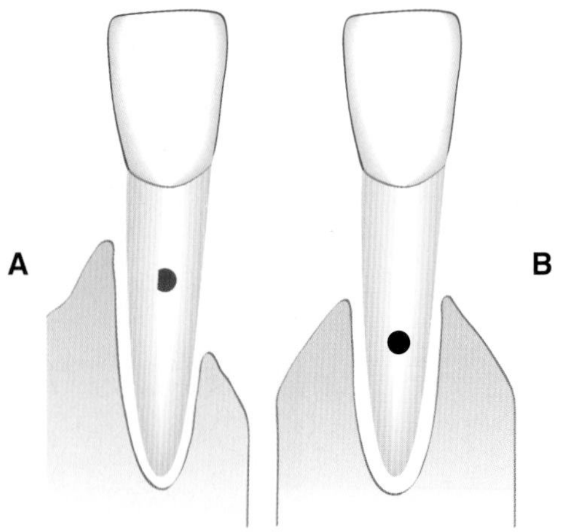

Figure 40-3 Prognosis for tooth **A** is better than for tooth **B,** despite less bone on one of the surfaces of *A.* Because the center of rotation of tooth *A* is closer to the crown, the distribution of occlusal forces to the periodontium is more favorable than in *B.*

affect the prognosis. Newer "automated" oral hygiene devices such as electric toothbrushes may be helpful for these patients and may improve their prognosis (see Chapter 50).

Genetic Factors. Periodontal diseases represent a complex interaction between a microbial challenge and the host's response to that challenge, both of which may be influenced by environmental factors such as smoking. In addition to these external factors, evidence also indicates that genetic factors may play an important role in determining the nature of the host response.[15] Evidence for this type of genetic influence exists for patients with both chronic and aggressive periodontitis. Genetic polymorphisms in the interleukin-1 (IL-1) genes, resulting in increased production of IL-1β, have been associated with a significant increase in risk for severe, generalized, chronic periodontitis.[20,32] It has been demonstrated that knowledge of the patient's IL-1 genotype and smoking status can aid the clinician in assigning a prognosis.[31] Genetic factors also appear to influence serum immunoglobulin G2 (IgG2) antibody titers and the expression of FcγRII receptors on the neutrophil, both of which may be significant in aggressive periodontitis.[15] Other genetic disorders, such as leukocyte adhesion deficiency type 1, can influence neutrophil function, creating an additional risk factor for aggressive periodontitis.[15] Finally, the familial aggregation that is characteristic of aggressive periodontitis indicates that additional, as yet unidentified, genetic factors may be important in susceptibility to this form of disease (see Chapter 33).

The influence of genetic factors on prognosis is not simple. Although microbial and environmental factors can be altered through conventional periodontal therapy and patient education, genetic factors currently cannot be altered. However, detection of genetic variations linked to periodontal disease can potentially influence the prognosis in several ways. First, early detection of patients at risk because of genetic factors can lead to early

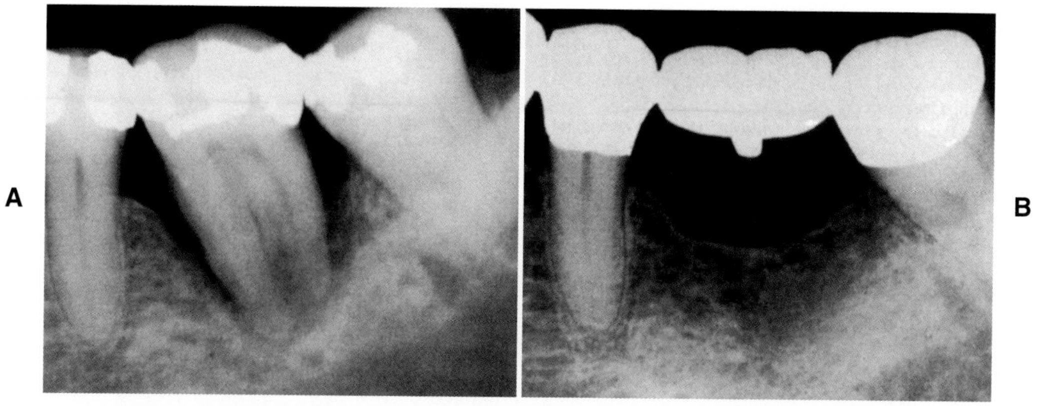

Figure 40-4 Extraction of severely involved tooth to preserve bone on adjacent teeth. **A,** Extensive bone destruction around the mandibular first molar. **B,** Radiograph made 8½ years after extraction of the first molar and replacement by a prosthesis. Note the excellent bone support.

implementation of preventive and treatment measures for these patients. Second, identification of genetic risk factors later in the disease or during the course of treatment can influence treatment recommendations, such as the use of adjunctive antibiotic therapy or increased frequency of maintenance visits. Third, identification of young individuals who have not been evaluated for periodontitis, but who are recognized as being at risk because of the familial aggregation seen in aggressive periodontitis, can lead to the development of early intervention strategies. In each of these cases, early diagnosis, intervention, and alterations in the treatment regimen may lead to an improved prognosis for the patient.

Stress. Physical and emotional stress, as well as substance abuse, may alter the patient's ability to respond to the periodontal treatment performed (see Chapter 8). These factors must be realistically faced in attempting to establish a prognosis.

Local Factors

Plaque and Calculus. The microbial challenge presented by bacterial plaque and calculus is the most important local factor in periodontal diseases. Therefore, in most cases, having a good prognosis depends on the ability of the patient and the clinician to remove these etiologic factors (see Chapters 9 and 10).

Subgingival Restorations. Subgingival margins may contribute to increased plaque accumulation, increased inflammation, and increased bone loss[2,35,43] when compared with supragingival margins. Furthermore, discrepancies in these margins (e.g., overhangs) can negatively impact the periodontium (see Chapter 10). The size of these discrepancies and duration of their presence are important factors in the amount of destruction that occurs. In general, however, a tooth with a discrepancy in its subgingival margins has a poorer prognosis than a tooth with well-contoured supragingival margins.

Anatomic Factors. Anatomic factors that may predispose the periodontium to disease and therefore affect the prognosis include short, tapered roots with large crowns, cervical enamel projections and enamel pearls, intermediate bifurcation ridges, root concavities, and developmental grooves. The clinician must also consider root proximity and the location and anatomy of furcations when developing a prognosis.

Prognosis is poor for teeth with short, tapered roots and relatively large crowns (Figure 40-5). Because of the disproportionate crown-to-root ratio and the reduced root surface available for periodontal support,[17] the periodontium may be more susceptible to injury by occlusal forces.

Cervical enamel projections (CEPs) are flat, ectopic extensions of enamel that extend beyond the normal contours of the cementoenamel junction.[27] CEPs extend into the furcation of 28.6% of mandibular molars and 17% of maxillary molars.[27] CEPs are most likely to be found on buccal surfaces of maxillary second molars.[13,45] *Enamel pearls* are larger, round deposits of enamel that can be located in furcations or other areas on the root surface.[34] Enamel pearls are seen less frequently (1.1%-5.7% of permanent molars; 75% appearing in maxillary third molars[34]) than CEPs. An intermediate bifurcation ridge has been described in 73% of mandibular first molars, crossing from the mesial to the distal root at the midpoint of the furcation.[8] The presence of these enamel projections on the root surface interferes with the attachment apparatus and may prevent regenerative procedures from achieving their maximum potential. Therefore their presence may have a negative effect on the prognosis for an individual tooth.

Scaling with root planing is a fundamental procedure in periodontal therapy. Anatomic factors that decrease the efficiency of this procedure can have a negative impact on the prognosis. Therefore the morphology of the tooth root is an important consideration when discussing prognosis. *Root concavities* exposed through loss of attachment can vary from shallow flutings to deep

A

B

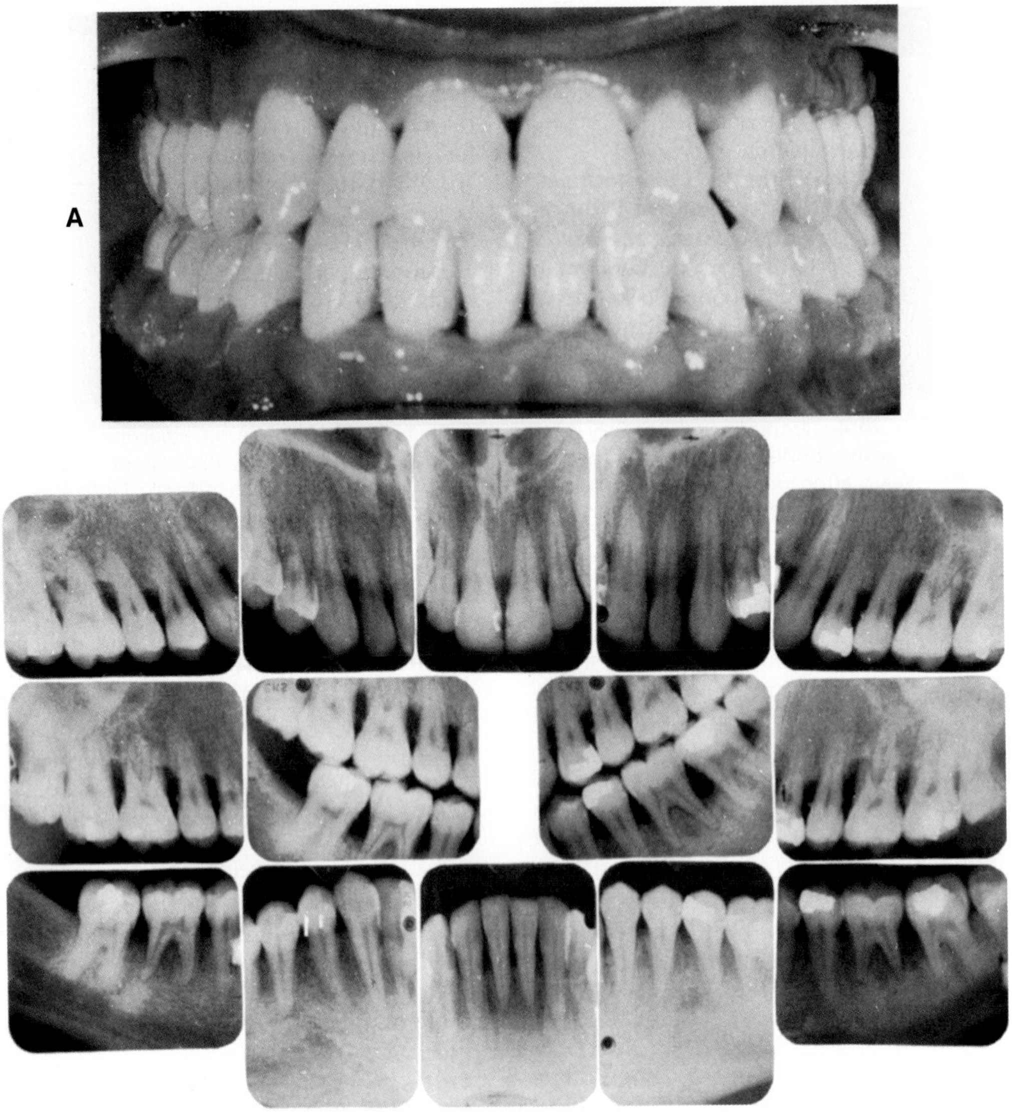

Figure 40-5 Generalized aggressive periodontitis and poor crown-to-root ratio in 24-year-old patient; overall prognosis poor. **A,** Generalized periodontal attachment loss and pocket formation. **B,** Moderate to advanced bone destruction. The contrast between the well-formed crowns and the relatively short, tapered roots worsens the prognosis.

depressions. They appear more marked on maxillary first premolars, the mesiobuccal root of the maxillary first molar, both roots of mandibular first molars, and the mandibular incisors[4,5] (Figures 40-6 and 40-7). Any tooth, however, can have a proximal concavity.[10] Although these concavities increase the attachment area and produce a root shape that may be more resistant to torquing forces, they also create areas that can be difficult for both the dentist and the patient to clean.

Other anatomic considerations that present accessibility problems are developmental grooves, root proximity, and furcation involvements. The presence of any of these can worsen the prognosis. *Developmental grooves,* which sometimes appear in the maxillary lateral incisors (palatogingival groove[46]; Figure 40-8) or in the lower incisors, create an accessibility problem.[7,12] They initiate on enamel and can extend a significant distance on the root surface, providing a plaque-retentive area that is difficult to instrument. These palatogingival grooves are found on 5.6% of maxillary lateral incisors and 3.4% of maxillary central incisors.[19] Similarly, *root proximity* can result in interproximal areas that are difficult for the clinician and patient to access. Finally, *access to the furcation area* is usually difficult to obtain. In 58% of maxillary and mandibular first molars, the furcation entrance diameter is narrower than the width of conventional periodontal curettes[5] (Figure 40-9). Maxillary first premolars present the greatest difficulties, and therefore their prognosis is usually unfavorable when the lesion reaches the mesiodistal furcation. Maxillary molars also present some difficulty; sometimes their prognosis can be improved by resecting one of the buccal roots (see Chapter 68), thereby improving access to the area. When mandibular first molars or buccal furcations of

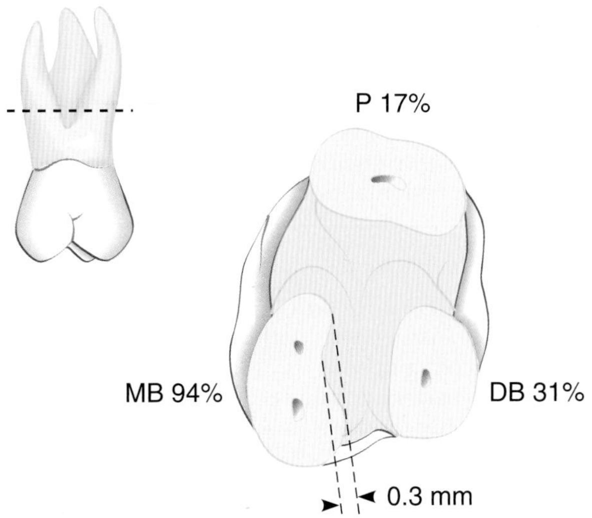

Figure 40-6 Root concavities in maxillary first molars sectioned 2 mm apical to the furca. The furcal aspect of the root is concave in 94% of the mesiobuccal *(MB)* roots, 31% of the distobuccal *(DB)* roots, and 17% of the palatal *(P)* roots. The deepest concavity is found in the furcal aspects of the mesiobuccal root (mean concavity, 0.3 mm). The furcal aspect of the buccal roots diverges toward the palate in 97% of teeth (mean divergence, 22 degrees). (Redrawn from Bower RC: *J Periodontol* 50:366, 1979.)

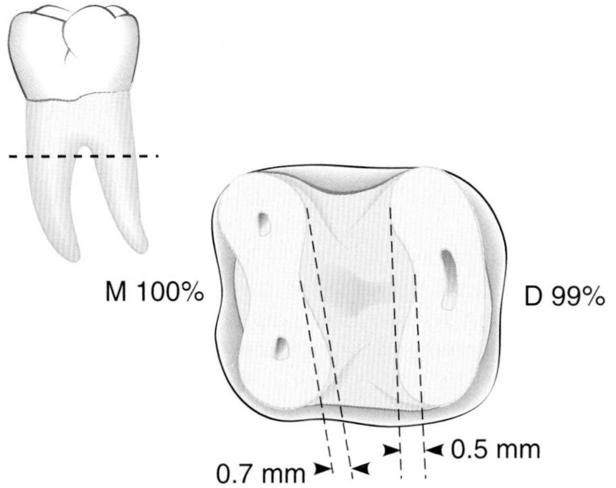

Figure 40-7 Root concavities in mandibular first molars sectioned 2 mm apical to the furca. Concavity of the furcal aspect was found in 100% of mesial *(M)* roots and 99% of distal *(D)* roots. Deeper concavity was found in the mesial roots (mean concavity, 0.7 mm). (Redrawn from Bower RC: *J Periodontol* 50:366, 1979.)

maxillary molars offer good access to the furcation area, their prognosis is usually better.

Tooth Mobility. The principal causes of tooth mobility are loss of alveolar bone, inflammatory changes in the periodontal ligament, and trauma from occlusion. Tooth mobility caused by inflammation and trauma from occlusion may be correctable.[33] However, tooth mobility

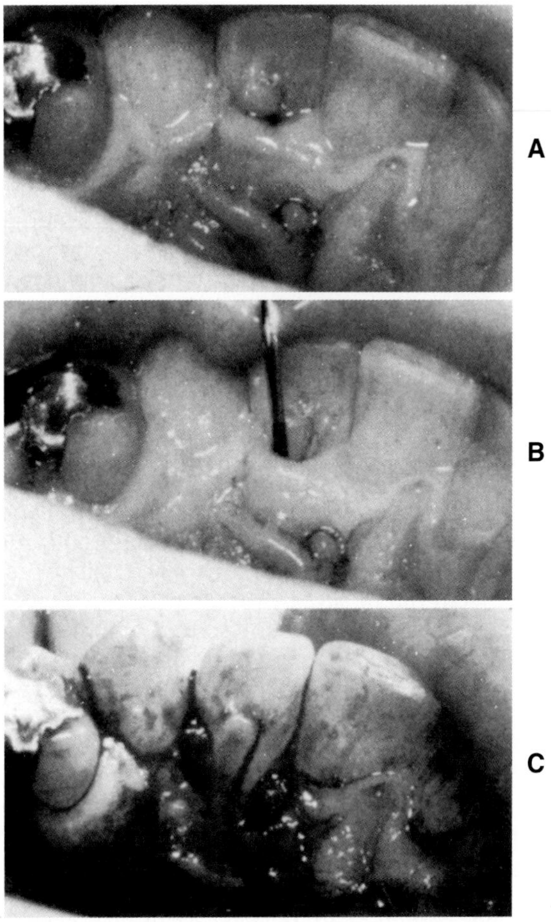

Figure 40-8 Palatogingival groove. **A,** Gingival inflammation and exudate in an area palatal to the upper lateral incisor. **B,** Probing shows deep pocket. **C,** The area is flapped, and the presence of a palatogingival groove is confirmed. (Courtesy Dr. Robert Merin, Woodland Hills, Calif.)

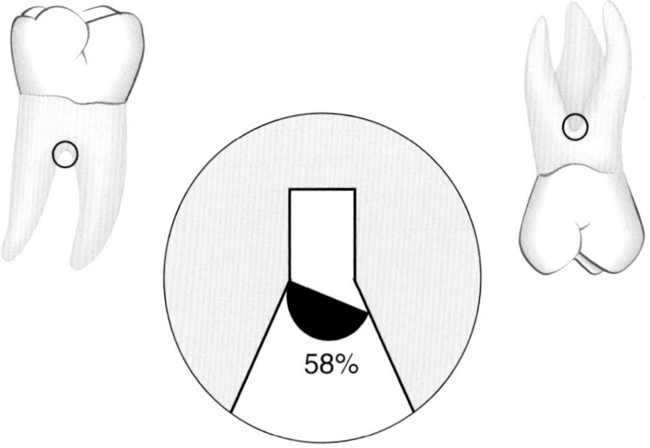

Figure 40-9 The furcation entrance is narrower than a standard curette in 58% of first molars. (Redrawn from Bower RC: *J Periodontol* 50:366, 1979.)

resulting from loss of alveolar bone is not likely to be corrected. The likelihood of restoring tooth stability is inversely proportional to the extent to which mobility is caused by loss of supporting alveolar bone. A longitudinal study of the response to treatment of teeth with different degrees of mobility revealed that pockets on clinically mobile teeth do not respond as well to periodontal therapy as pockets on nonmobile teeth exhibiting the same initial disease severity.[9] Another study, however, in which ideal plaque control was attained, found similar healing in both hypermobile and firm teeth.[40] The stabilization of tooth mobility through the use of splinting may have a beneficial impact on the overall and individual tooth prognosis.

Prosthetic and Restorative Factors

The overall prognosis requires a general consideration of bone levels (evaluated radiographically) and attachment levels (determined clinically) to establish whether enough teeth can be saved either to provide a functional and aesthetic dentition or to serve as abutments for a useful prosthetic replacement of the missing teeth.

At this point, the overall prognosis and the individual tooth prognosis overlap because the prognosis for key individual teeth may affect the overall prognosis for prosthetic rehabilitation. For example, saving or losing a key tooth may determine whether other teeth are saved or extracted or whether the prosthesis used is fixed or removable (see Figure 40-4). When few teeth remain, the prosthodontic needs become more important, and sometimes periodontally treatable teeth may have to be extracted if they are not compatible with the design of the prosthesis.

Teeth that serve as abutments are subjected to increased functional demands. More rigid standards are required when evaluating the prognosis of teeth adjacent to edentulous areas. A tooth with a post that has undergone endodontic treatment is more likely to fracture when serving as a distal abutment supporting a distal removable partial denture. Additionally, special oral hygiene measures must be instituted in these areas.

Caries, Nonvital Teeth, and Root Resorption. For teeth mutilated by extensive caries, the feasibility of adequate restoration and endodontic therapy should be considered before undertaking periodontal treatment. Extensive idiopathic root resorption or root resorption resulting from orthodontic therapy jeopardizes the stability of teeth and adversely affects the response to periodontal treatment. The periodontal prognosis of treated nonvital teeth does not differ from that of vital teeth. New attachment can occur to the cementum of both nonvital and vital teeth.

RELATIONSHIP BETWEEN DIAGNOSIS AND PROGNOSIS

Many of the criteria used in the diagnosis and classification of the different forms of periodontal disease[1] (see Chapter 7) are also used in developing a prognosis (see Box 40-1). Factors such as patient age, severity of disease, genetic susceptibility, and presence of systemic disease are important criteria in the diagnosis of the condition. These are also important in developing a prognosis. These common factors suggest that for any given diagnosis, there should be an expected prognosis under ideal conditions. This section discusses the potential prognoses of the various periodontal diseases outlined in Chapter 7.

Prognosis for Patients with Gingival Disease

Dental Plaque–Induced Gingival Diseases

Gingivitis Associated with Dental Plaque Only. Plaque-induced gingivitis is a reversible disease that occurs when bacterial plaque accumulates at the gingival margin.[24,26] This disease can occur on a periodontium that has experienced no attachment loss or on a periodontium with nonprogressing attachment loss. In either case, the prognosis for patients with gingivitis associated with dental plaque only is good, provided all local irritants are eliminated, other local factors contributing to plaque retention are eliminated, gingival contours conducive to the preservation of health are attained, and the patient cooperates by maintaining good oral hygiene.

Plaque-Induced Gingival Diseases Modified by Systemic Factors. The inflammatory response to bacterial plaque at the gingival margin can be influenced by systemic factors, such as endocrine-related changes associated with puberty, menstruation, pregnancy, and diabetes, and the presence of blood dyscrasias. In many cases the frank signs of gingival inflammation that occur in these patients are seen in the presence of relatively small amounts of bacterial plaque. Therefore the long-term prognosis for these patients depends not only on control of bacterial plaque, but also on control or correction of the systemic factor(s).

Plaque-Induced Gingival Diseases Modified by Medications. Gingival diseases associated with medications include drug-influenced *gingival enlargement,* often seen with phenytoin, cyclosporine, and nifedipine and in oral contraceptive–associated gingivitis. In drug-influenced gingival enlargement, reductions in dental plaque can limit the severity of the lesions. However, plaque control alone does not prevent development of the lesions, and surgical intervention is usually necessary to correct the alterations in gingival contour. Continued use of the drug usually results in recurrence of the enlargement, even after surgical intervention (see Chapter 23). Therefore the long-term prognosis depends on whether the patient's systemic problem can be treated with an alternative medication that does not have gingival enlargement as a side effect.

In oral contraceptive–associated gingivitis, frank signs of gingival inflammation can be seen in the presence of relatively little plaque. Therefore, as seen in plaque-induced gingival diseases modified by systemic factors, the long-term prognosis in these patients depends on not only the control of bacterial plaque, but also on the likelihood of continued use of the oral contraceptive.

Gingival Diseases Modified by Malnutrition. Although malnutrition has been suspected to play a role in the development of gingival diseases, most clinical studies have not shown a relationship between the two.

One possible exception is severe vitamin C deficiency. In early experimental vitamin C deficiency, gingival inflammation and bleeding on probing were independent of plaque levels present. The prognosis in these patients may depend on the severity and duration of the deficiency and on the likelihood of reversing the deficiency through dietary supplementation.

Non–Plaque-Induced Gingival Lesions. Non–plaque-induced gingivitis can be seen in patients with a variety of bacterial, fungal, and viral infections.[16] Since the gingivitis in these patients is not usually attributed to plaque accumulation, prognosis depends on elimination of the source of the infectious agent. Dermatologic disorders such as lichen planus, pemphigoid, pemphigus vulgaris, erythema multiforme, and lupus erythematosus also can manifest in the oral cavity as atypical gingivitis (see Chapter 26). Prognosis for these patients is linked to management of the associated dermatologic disorder. Finally, allergic, toxic, and foreign body reactions, as well as mechanical and thermal trauma, can result in gingival lesions. Prognosis for these patients depends on elimination of the causative agent.

Prognosis for Patients with Periodontitis

Chronic Periodontitis. Chronic periodontitis is a slowly progressive disease associated with well-known local environmental factors.[22] It can present in a localized or generalized form (see Chapter 31). In cases where the clinical attachment loss and bone loss are not very advanced (slight to moderate periodontitis), the prognosis is generally good, provided the inflammation can be controlled through good oral hygiene and the removal of local plaque-retentive factors (see Figure 40-1). In patients with more severe disease, as evidenced by furcation involvement and increasing clinical mobility, or in patients who are noncompliant with oral hygiene practices, the prognosis may be downgraded to fair to poor.

Aggressive Periodontitis. Aggressive periodontitis can present in a localized or a generalized form.[21] Two common features of both forms are (1) rapid attachment loss and bone destruction in an otherwise clinically healthy patient and (2) a familial aggregation. These patients often present with limited microbial deposits that seem inconsistent with the severity of tissue destruction. However, the deposits that are present often have elevated levels of *Actinobacillus actinomycetemcomitans* or *Porphyromonas gingivalis*. These patients also may present with phagocyte abnormalities and a hyperresponsive monocyte/macrophage phenotype. These clinical, microbiologic, and immunologic features would suggest that patients diagnosed with aggressive periodontitis would have a poor prognosis.

However, the clinician should consider additional specific features of the localized form of disease when determining the prognosis (see Figure 40-2). Localized aggressive periodontitis usually occurs around the age of puberty and is localized to first molars and incisors. The patient often exhibits a strong serum antibody response to the infecting agents, which may contribute to localization of the lesions (see Chapter 33). When diagnosed early, these cases can be treated conservatively with oral hygiene instruction and systemic antibiotic therapy,[37] resulting in an excellent prognosis. When more advanced disease occurs, the prognosis can still be good if the lesions are treated with debridement, local and systemic antibiotics, and regenerative therapy.[25,47]

In contrast, although patients with generalized aggressive periodontitis also are young patients (usually under age 30), they present with generalized interproximal attachment loss and a poor antibody response to infecting agents. Secondary contributing factors such as cigarette smoking are often present. These factors, coupled with the alterations in host defense seen in many of these patients, may result in a case that does not respond well to conventional periodontal therapy (scaling with root planing, oral hygiene instruction, and surgical intervention). Therefore these patients often have a fair, poor, or questionable prognosis, and the use of systemic antibiotics should be considered to help control the disease (see Chapter 47).

Periodontitis as a Manifestation of Systemic Diseases. Periodontitis as a manifestation of systemic diseases can be divided into two categories[18,23]:

1. Periodontitis associated with hematologic disorders such as leukemia and acquired neutropenias.
2. Periodontitis associated with genetic disorders such as familial and cyclic neutropenia, Down syndrome, Papillon-Lefèvre syndrome, and hypophosphastasia.

Although the primary etiologic factor in periodontal diseases is bacterial plaque, systemic diseases that alter the ability of the host to respond to the microbial challenge presented may affect the progression of disease and therefore the prognosis for the case. For example, decreased numbers of circulating neutrophils (as in acquired neutropenias) may contribute to widespread destruction of the periodontium. Unless the neutropenia can be corrected, these patients present with a fair to poor prognosis. Similarly, genetic disorders that alter the way the host responds to bacterial plaque (as in leukocyte adhesion deficiency syndrome) also can contribute to the development of periodontitis. Because these disorders generally manifest early in life, the impact on the periodontium may be clinically similar to generalized aggressive periodontitis. The prognosis in these cases will be fair to poor.

Other genetic disorders do not affect the host's ability to combat infections but still affect the development of periodontitis. Examples include hypophosphatasia, in which patients have decreased levels of circulating alkaline phosphatase, severe alveolar bone loss, and premature loss of deciduous and permanent teeth, and the connective tissue disorder Ehlers-Danlos syndrome, in which patients may present with the clinical characteristics of aggressive periodontitis. In both examples the prognosis is fair to poor.

Necrotizing Periodontal Diseases. Necrotizing periodontal disease can be divided into necrotic diseases that affect the gingival tissues exclusively (necrotizing ulcerative gingivitis, NUG) and necrotic diseases that

SCIENCE TRANSFER

Clinicians use a wide variety of variables to establish a prognosis, including anatomic factors, diagnosis of periodontal condition, patient's age, plaque levels, smoking, severity of attachment loss, control of etiologic factors, occlusal loading, and genetic and systemic makeup. *There are no reliable algorithms for prognosis, so clinicians must use their clinical judgment. Constant reviewing of results of treatment coupled with detailed documentation of periodontal status will sharpen the clinician's acumen for accurate assessment of prognosis.*

In advanced cases, prognosis may be better established after reviewing the effectiveness of Phase I therapy.

Determination of the prognosis of a tooth or teeth can be difficult, particularly for teeth with previous disease. Many factors can influence disease progression and the response to therapy, and the specific influence of any one factor is unknown and is likely different from one patient to another. In addition, each patient can respond differently at different times. All these issues make determination of a prognosis difficult.

Therefore the prognosis is often determined after initial treatment is provided, assuming a favorable outcome. The prognosis is delayed until after initial therapy because the etiology depends on the host response. During initial therapy the patient's motivation and commitment also can be determined, acknowledged as critical in all periodontal therapy, as well as the host response and healing capacity of the patient. Clearly, enhancing the host response to plaque's microbial challenge will significantly and positively influence the periodontal prognosis. Likewise, an *inability* to enhance the host response will negatively influence the prognosis. Either outcome, however, will allow the clinician to determine a more accurate prognosis.

affect deeper tissues of the periodontium, resulting in loss of connective tissue attachment and alveolar bone (necrotizing ulcerative periodontitis, NUP).[36,41] In NUG the primary predisposing factor is bacterial plaque. However, this disease is usually complicated by the presence of secondary factors such as acute psychologic stress, tobacco smoking, and poor nutrition, all of which can contribute to immunosuppression. Therefore, superimposition of these secondary factors on a preexisting gingivitis can result in the painful, necrotic lesions characteristic of NUG. With control of both the bacterial plaque and the secondary factors, the prognosis for a patient with NUG is good. However, the tissue destruction in these cases is not reversible, and poor control of the secondary factors may make these patients susceptible to recurrence of the disease. With repeated episodes of NUG, the prognosis may be downgraded to fair.

The clinical presentation of NUP is similar to that of NUG, except the necrosis extends from the gingiva into the periodontal ligament and alveolar bone. In systemically healthy patients, this progression may have resulted from multiple episodes of NUG, or the necrotizing disease may occur at a site previously affected with periodontitis. In these patients the prognosis depends on alleviating the plaque and secondary factors associated with NUG. However, many patients presenting with NUP are immunocompromised through systemic conditions, such as human immunodeficiency virus (HIV) infection. In these patients the prognosis depends on not only reducing local and secondary factors, but also on dealing with the systemic problem (see Chapter 46).

REEVALUATION OF PROGNOSIS AFTER PHASE I THERAPY

A frank reduction in pocket depth and inflammation after Phase I therapy indicates a favorable response to treatment and may suggest a better prognosis than previously assumed. If the inflammatory changes present cannot be controlled or reduced by Phase I therapy, the overall prognosis may be unfavorable. In these patients the prognosis can be directly related to the severity of inflammation. Given two patients with comparable bone destruction, the prognosis may be better for the patient with the greater degree of inflammation, because a larger component of that patient's bone destruction may be attributable to local irritants. In addition, Phase I therapy allows the clinician an opportunity to work with the patient and the patient's physician to control systemic and environmental factors such as diabetes and smoking, which may have a positive effect on prognosis if adequately controlled.

The progression of periodontitis generally occurs in an episodic manner, with alternating periods of quiescence and shorter destructive stages (see Chapter 27). No methods are available at present to determine accurately whether a given lesion is in a stage of remission or exacerbation. Advanced lesions, if active, may progress rapidly to a hopeless stage, whereas similar lesions in a quiescent stage may be maintainable for long periods. Phase I therapy will, at least temporarily, transform the prognosis of the patient with an active advanced lesion, and the lesion should be reanalyzed after completion of Phase I therapy.

REFERENCES

1. Armitage GC: Development of a classification system for periodontal diseases and conditions, *Ann Periodontol* 4:1, 1999.
2. Björn AL, Björn H, Grkovic B: Marginal fit of restorations and its relation to periodontal bone levels. I. Metal fillings, *Odontol Rev* 20:311, 1969.
3. Bolin A, Eklund G, Frithiof L, et al: The effect of changed smoking habits on marginal alveolar bone loss: a longitudinal study, *Swed Dent J* 17:211, 1993.
4. Bower RC: Furcation morphology relative to periodontal treatment: furcation entrance architecture, *J Periodontol* 50:23, 1979.

5. Bower RC: Furcation morphology relative to periodontal treatment–furcation root surface anatomy, *J Periodontol* 50:366, 1979.
6. Chace R Sr, Low SB: Survival characteristics of periodontally involved teeth: a 40-year study, *J Periodontol* 64:701, 1993.
7. Everett FG, Kramer GN: The distolingual groove in the maxillary lateral incisor: a periodontal hazard, *J Periodontol* 43:352, 1972.
8. Everett FG, Jump EB, Holder TD, et al: The intermediate bifurcational ridge: a study of the morphology of the bifurcation of the lower first molar, *J Dent Res* 37:162, 1958.
9. Flezar TJ, Knowles JW, Morrison EC, et al: Tooth mobility and periodontal therapy, *J Clin Periodontol* 7:495, 1980.
10. Fox SC, Bosworth BL: A morphological study of proximal root concavities: a consideration in periodontal therapy, *J Am Dent Assoc* 114:811, 1987.
11. Ghaia S, Bissada NF: Prognosis and actual treatment outcome of periodontally involved teeth, *Periodont Clin Invest* 18:7, 1996.
12. Gher ME, Vernino AR: Root morphology: clinical significance in pathogenesis and treatment of periodontal disease, *J Am Dent Assoc* 101:627, 1980.
13. Grewe JM, Meskin LH, Miller T: Cervical enamel projections: prevalence, location, and extent; with associated periodontal implications, *J Periodontol* 36:460, 1965.
14. Grossi SD, Zambon J, Machtei EE, et al: Effects of smoking and smoking cessation on healing after mechanical therapy, *J Am Dent Assoc* 128:599, 1997.
15. Hart TC, Kornman KS: Genetic factors in the pathogenesis of periodontitis, *Periodontol 2000* 14:202, 1997.
16. Holmstrup P: Non–plaque-induced gingival lesions, *Ann Periodontol* 4:20, 1999.
17. Kay S, Forscher BK, Sackett LM: Tooth root length-volume relationships: an aid to periodontal prognosis. I. Anterior teeth, *Oral Surg* 7:735, 1954.
18. Kinane D: Periodontitis modified by systemic factors, *Ann Periodontol* 4:54, 1999.
19. Kogan SL: The prevalence, location and conformation of palato-radicular grooves in maxillary incisors, *J Periodontol* 57:2312, 1986.
20. Kornman KS, di Giovine FS: Genetic variations in cytokine expression: a risk factor for severity of adult periodontitis, *Ann Periodontol* 3:327, 1998.
21. Lang N, Bartold PM, Cullinan M, et al: Consensus report: aggressive periodontitis, *Ann Periodontol* 4:53, 1999.
22. Lindhe J, Ranney R, Lamster I, et al: Consensus report: chronic periodontitis, *Ann Periodontol* 4:38, 1999.
23. Lindhe J, Ranney R, Lamster I, et al: Consensus report: periodontitis as a manifestation of systemic diseases, *Ann Periodontol* 4:64, 1999.
24. Löe H, Theilade E, Jensen SB: Experimental gingivitis in man, *J Periodontol* 36:177, 1965.
25. Mabry T, Yukna R, Sepe W: Freeze-dried bone allografts with tetracycline in the treatment of juvenile periodontitis, *J Periodontol* 56:74, 1985.
26. Mariotti A: Dental plaque–induced gingival disease, *Ann Periodontol* 4:7, 1999.
27. Masters DH, Hoskins SW: Projection of cervical enamel into molar furcations, *J Periodontol* 35:49, 1964.
28. McGuire MK: Prognosis versus actual outcome: a long-term survey of 100 treated periodontal patients under maintenance care, *J Periodontol* 62:51, 1991.
29. McGuire MK, Nunn ME: Prognosis versus actual outcome. II. The effectiveness of clinical parameters in developing an accurate prognosis, *J Periodontol* 67:658, 1996.
30. McGuire MK, Nunn ME: Prognosis versus actual outcome. III. The effectiveness of clinical parameters in accurately predicting tooth survival, *J Periodontol* 67:666, 1996.
31. McGuire MK, Nunn ME: Prognosis versus actual outcome. IV. The effectiveness of clinical parameters and IL-1 genotype in accurately predicting prognoses and tooth survival, *J Periodontol* 70:49, 1999.
32. Michalowicz BS, Diehl SR, Gunsolley JC, et al: Evidence of a substantial genetic basis for risk of adult periodontitis, *J Periodontol* 71:1699, 2000.
33. Morris ML: The diagnosis, prognosis and treatment of loose tooth, *Oral Surg* 6:1037, 1953.
34. Moskow BS, Canut PM: Studies on root enamel. 2. Enamel pearls: a review of their morphology, localization, nomenclature, occurrence, classification, histogenesis and incidence, *J Clin Periodontol* 17:275, 1990.
35. Newcomb GM: The relationship between the location of subgingival crown margins and gingival inflammation, *J Periodontol* 45:151, 1974.
36. Novak MJ: Necrotizing ulcerative periodontitis, *Ann Periodontol* 4:74, 1999.
37. Novak MJ, Polson AM, Adair SM: Tetracycline therapy in patients with early juvenile periodontitis, *J Periodontol* 59:366, 1988.
38. Preber J, Bergström J: The effect of non-surgical treatment on periodontal pockets in smokers and non-smokers, *J Clin Periodontol* 13:319, 1986.
39. Renvert S, Dahlen G, Wikström M: The clinical and microbiological effects of non-surgical periodontal therapy in smokers and non-smokers, *J Clin Periodontol* 25:153, 1998.
40. Rosling B, Nyman S, Lindhe J: The effect of systematic plaque control on bone regeneration in infrabony pockets, *J Clin Periodontol* 3:38, 1976.
41. Rowland RW: Necrotizing ulcerative gingivitis, *Ann Periodontol* 4:65, 1999.
42. Shapiro N: Retaining periodontally "hopeless" teeth: a case report, *J Am Dent Assoc* 125:596, 1994.
43. Silness J: Periodontal conditions in patients treated with dental bridges. III. The relationship between the location of the crown margin and the periodontal condition, *J Periodontal Res* 5:225, 1970.
44. Sorrin S, Burman LR: A study of cases not amenable to periodontal therapy, *J Am Dent Assoc* 31:204, 1944.
45. Tsatsas B, Mandi F, Kerani S: Cervical enamel projections in the molar teeth, *J Periodontol* 44:312, 1973.
46. Withers JA, Brunsvold MA, Killoy WJ, et al: The relationship of palato-gingival grooves to localized periodontal disease, *J Periodontol* 52:41, 1981.
47. Yukna R, Sepe W: Clinical evaluation of localized periodontosis defects with freeze-dried bone allografts combined with local and systemic tetracyclines, *Int J Periodont Restor Dent* 5:9, 1982.

The Treatment Plan

Fermin A. Carranza and Henry H. Takei

41

CHAPTER

CHAPTER OUTLINE

After the diagnosis and prognosis have been established, the treatment is planned. The treatment plan is the blueprint for case management. It includes all procedures required for the establishment and maintenance of oral health and involves the following decisions:

- Teeth to be retained or extracted.
- Pocket therapy techniques, surgical or nonsurgical, that will be used.
- The need for occlusal correction, before, during, or after pocket therapy.
- The use of implant therapy.
- The need for temporary restorations.
- Final restorations that will be needed after therapy, and which teeth will be abutments if a fixed prosthesis is used.
- The need for orthodontic consultation.
- Endodontic therapy.
- Decisions regarding esthetic considerations in periodontal therapy.
- Sequence of therapy.

Unforeseen developments during treatment may necessitate modification of the initial treatment plan. However, *except for emergencies, no treatment should be started until the treatment plan has been established.*

MASTER PLAN FOR TOTAL TREATMENT

The aim of the treatment plan is *total* treatment, that is, the coordination of all treatment procedures for the purpose of creating a well-functioning dentition in a healthy periodontal environment. The master plan of periodontal treatment encompasses different areas of therapeutic objectives for each patient according to his or her needs. It is based on the diagnosis, disease severity, and other factors outlined in previous chapters and should include a reasoned decision on the possible and desirable therapeutic endpoints and the techniques to be used to reach this objective.

The primary goal is elimination of gingival inflammation and correction of the conditions that cause and perpetuate it. This includes not only elimination of root irritants, but also pocket eradication and reduction, establishment of gingival contours and mucogingival relationships conducive to the preservation of periodontal health, restoration of carious areas, and correction of existing restorations.

Extracting or Preserving a Tooth

Periodontal treatment requires long-range planning. Its value to the patient is measured in years of healthy functioning of the entire dentition, not by the number of teeth retained at the time of treatment. *Treatment is directed to establishing and maintaining the health of the periodontium throughout the mouth rather than to spectacular efforts to "tighten loose teeth."*

The welfare of the dentition should not be jeopardized by a heroic attempt to retain questionable teeth. The periodontal condition of the teeth to be retained is more important than the number of such teeth. Teeth that can be retained with minimal doubt and a maximal margin of safety provide the basis for the total treatment plan. Teeth on the borderline of hopelessness do not contribute to the overall usefulness of the dentition, even if they can be saved in a somewhat precarious state. Such teeth become sources of recurrent annoyance to the patient and detract from the value of the greater service rendered by the establishment of periodontal health in the remainder of the oral cavity.

Removal, retention, or temporary (interim) retention of one or more teeth is a very important part of the overall treatment plan.

A tooth should be extracted when any of the following occurs:

- It is so mobile that function becomes painful.
- It can cause acute abscesses during therapy.
- There is no use for it in the overall treatment plan.

A tooth can be retained temporarily, postponing the decision to extract it until after treatment, when any of the following occurs:

- It maintains posterior stops; the tooth can be removed after treatment when it can be replaced by a prosthesis.
- It maintains posterior stops and may be functional after implant placement in adjacent areas. When the implant is exposed, these teeth can be extracted.
- In anterior esthetic areas, a tooth can be retained during periodontal therapy and removed when treatment is completed, and a permanent restorative procedure can be performed. This approach avoids the need for temporary appliances and can be considered when retention of the tooth will not jeopardize adjacent teeth.
- Removal of hopeless teeth can also be performed during periodontal surgery of neighboring teeth. This approach reduces appointments for surgery in the same area.

In the formulation of the treatment plan, in addition to proper function of the dentition, esthetic considerations play an increasingly important role in many cases. Different patients value esthetics differently according to their age, gender, profession, social status, and other reasons, and the clinician should carefully evaluate and consider a final outcome of treatment that will be acceptable to the patient without jeopardizing the basic consideration of attaining health.

With the predictable use of implants, questionable teeth should be carefully evaluated as to whether their removal and replacement with an implant may be a better and more satisfactory course of therapy.

In complex cases, interdisciplinary consultation with other specialty areas is necessary before a final plan can be made. The opinion of orthodontists and prosthodontists is especially important for the final decision in these patients.

Consideration of occlusal relationships may be in order and may necessitate occlusal adjustment; restorative, prosthetic, and orthodontic procedures; splinting; and correction of bruxism and clamping and clenching habits.

Systemic conditions should be carefully evaluated because they may require special precautions during the course of periodontal treatment and may also affect the tissue response to treatment procedures or threaten the preservation of periodontal health after treatment is completed. Such situations should be taken in conjunction with the patient's physician.

Supportive periodontal care is also of paramount importance for case maintenance. Such care entails all procedures for maintaining periodontal health after it has been attained. It consists of instruction in oral hygiene and checkups at regular intervals, according to the patient's needs, to examine the condition of the periodontium and the status of the restoration as it affects the periodontium.

THERAPEUTIC PROCEDURES

Periodontal therapy is an inseparable part of dental therapy. The list of procedures presented here includes periodontal procedures (in italics) and other procedures not considered to be within the province of the periodontist. They are listed together to emphasize the close relationship of periodontal therapy with other phases of therapy performed by general dentists or other specialists (Box 41-1).

The sequence in which the above phases of therapy are performed may vary to some extent in response to the requirements of the case. However, the preferred sequence, which covers the vast majority of cases, is shown in Figure 41-1.

Although the phases of treatment have been numbered, the recommended sequence does not follow the numbers. Phase I, or the *nonsurgical phase,* is directed to the elimination of the etiologic factors of gingival and periodontal diseases. When successfully performed, this phase stops the progression of dental and periodontal disease.

Immediately after completion of Phase I therapy, the patient should be placed on the *maintenance phase* (Phase IV) to preserve the results obtained and prevent any further deterioration and recurrence of disease. While on the maintenance phase, with its periodic checkups and controls, the patient enters into the *surgical phase* (Phase II) and *restorative* (reparative) *phase* (Phase III) of treatment. These phases include periodontal surgery to repair and improve the condition of the periodontal and surrounding tissues and their esthetics, rebuilding of lost structures, placement of implants, and construction of the necessary restorative work.

EXPLAINING TREATMENT PLAN TO THE PATIENT

The following discussion includes suggestions for explaining the treatment plan to the patient.

Be specific. Tell your patient, "You have gingivitis," or "You have periodontitis," then explain exactly what these conditions are, how they are treated, and prognosis for the patient after treatment. Avoid vague statements such as, "You have trouble with your gums," or "Something should be done about your gums." Patients do not understand the significance of such statements and disregard them.

BOX 41-1

Phases of Periodontal Therapy

Preliminary Phase
Treatment of emergencies:

- Dental or periapical
- *Periodontal*
- Other

Extraction of hopeless teeth and provisional replacement if needed (may be postponed to a more convenient time)

Nonsurgical Phase (Phase I Therapy)
Plaque control and patient education:

- Diet control (in patients with rampant caries)
- *Removal of calculus and root planing*
- *Correction of restorative and prosthetic irritational factors*
- Excavation of caries and restoration (temporary or final, depending on whether a definitive prognosis for the tooth has been determined and on the location of caries)
- *Antimicrobial therapy (local or systemic)*
- *Occlusal therapy*
- *Minor orthodontic movement*
- *Provisional splinting and prosthesis*

Evaluation of response to nonsurgical phase
Rechecking:

- *Pocket depth and gingival inflammation*
- *Plaque and calculus, caries*

Surgical Phase (Phase II Therapy)
Periodontal therapy, including placement of implants
Endodontic therapy

Restorative Phase (Phase III Therapy)
Final restorations
Fixed and removable prosthodontic appliances
Evaluation of response to restorative procedures
Periodontal examination

Maintenance Phase (Phase IV Therapy)
Periodic rechecking:

- *Plaque and calculus*
- *Gingival condition (pockets, inflammation)*
- *Occlusion, tooth mobility*
- Other pathologic changes

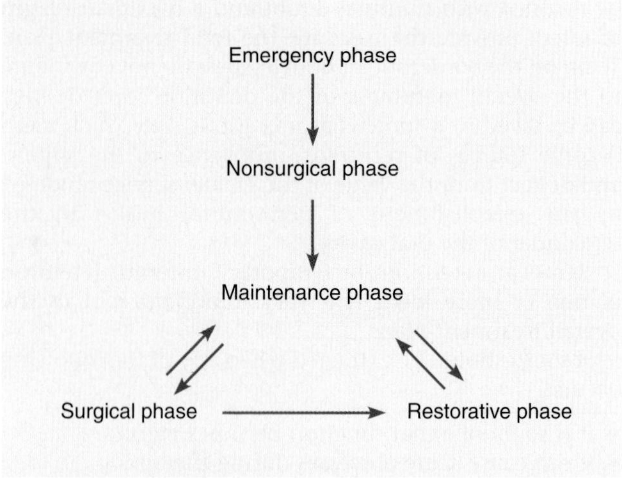

Figure 41-1 Preferred sequence of periodontal therapy.

Begin your discussion on a positive note. Talk about the teeth that can be retained and the long-term service they can be expected to render. Do not begin your discussion with the statement, "The following teeth have to be extracted." This creates a negative impression, which adds to the erroneous attitude of hopelessness the patient already may have regarding his or her mouth. Make it clear that every effort will be made to retain as many teeth as possible, but do not dwell on the patient's loose teeth. Emphasize that the important purpose of the treatment is to prevent the other teeth from becoming as severely diseased as the loose teeth.

Present the entire treatment plan as a unit. Avoid creating the impression that treatment consists of separate procedures, some or all of which may be selected by the patient. Make it clear that dental restorations and prostheses contribute as much to the health of the gums as the elimination of inflammation and periodontal pockets. Do not speak in terms of "having the gums treated and then taking care of the necessary restorations later" as if these were unrelated treatments.

Patients often seek guidance from the dentist with questions such as the following:

- "Are my teeth worth treating?"
- "Would you have them treated if you had my problem?"
- "Why don't I just go along the way I am until the teeth really bother me and then have them all extracted?"

Explain that "doing nothing" or holding onto hopelessly diseased teeth as long as possible is inadvisable for the following reasons:

1. Periodontal disease is a microbial infection, and research has clearly shown it to be an important risk factor for severe life-threatening diseases such as stroke, cardiovascular disease, pulmonary disease, and diabetes, as well as for premature low-birth-weight babies in women of childbearing age. Correcting the periodontal condition eliminates a serious potential risk of systemic disease, which in some cases ranks as high on the danger list as smoking.
2. It is not feasible to place restorations or bridges on teeth with untreated periodontal disease because the usefulness of the restoration would be limited by the uncertain condition of the supporting structures.
3. Failure to eliminate periodontal disease not only results in the loss of teeth already severely involved,

but also shortens the life span of other teeth that, with proper treatment, could serve as the foundation for a healthy, functioning dentition.

Therefore the dentist should make it clear to the patient that if the periodontal condition is treatable, the best results are obtained by prompt treatment. If the condition is not treatable, the teeth should be just as promptly extracted.

It is the dentist's responsibility to advise the patient of the importance of periodontal treatment. However, if treatment is to be successful, the patient must be sufficiently interested in retaining the natural teeth to maintain the necessary oral hygiene. Individuals who are not particularly perturbed by the thought of losing their teeth are generally not good candidates for periodontal treatment.

SCIENCE TRANSFER

An objective of the overall treatment plan is the creation and maintenance of oral health, function, and esthetics. The outcome is thus long term and in most cases requires the coordination of several disciplines of dentistry. *A motivated patient is a prerequisite, and success will depend on this motivation being sustained through maintenance care.* A large part of therapy is eliminating inflammation. This is important not only to preserve periodontal tissues, but also to eliminate an oral source of inflammation contributing to overall systemic health. One way to measure systemic inflammation is to monitor C-reactive protein levels. Future objectives of overall care may include the monitoring of oral and systemic levels of inflammation as the relationship between these two factors becomes better understood.

Treatment planning should focus on the list of diagnoses for the patient. Treatment should be planned in phases. At the completion of each phase, the patient should be reevaluated to assess response to treatment, and the treatment plan may be modified based on this assessment.

Rationale for Periodontal Treatment

Fermin A. Carranza and Henry H. Takei

CHAPTER

42

■ ■ ■

CHAPTER OUTLINE

WHAT DOES PERIODONTAL THERAPY ACCOMPLISH?
 Local Therapy
 Systemic Therapy
FACTORS THAT AFFECT HEALING
 Local Factors
 Systemic Factors

HEALING AFTER PERIODONTAL THERAPY
 Regeneration
 Repair
 New Attachment
PERIODONTAL RECONSTRUCTION

WHAT DOES PERIODONTAL THERAPY ACCOMPLISH?

The effectiveness of periodontal therapy is made possible by the remarkable healing capacity of the periodontal tissues. Periodontal therapy can restore chronically inflamed gingiva so that, from a clinical and structural point of view, it is almost identical with gingiva that has never been exposed to excessive plaque accumulation[20] (see Chapter 83).

Properly performed, periodontal treatment can be relied on to accomplish the following: eliminate pain, eliminate gingival inflammation[27] and gingival bleeding, reduce periodontal pockets and eliminate infection, stop pus formation, arrest the destruction of soft tissue and bone,[28] reduce abnormal tooth mobility,[7] establish optimal occlusal function, restore tissue destroyed by disease in some cases, reestablish the physiologic gingival contour necessary for the preservation of periodontal health, prevent the recurrence of disease, and reduce tooth loss[24] (Figure 42-1).

Local Therapy

The cause of periodontitis and gingivitis is bacterial plaque accumulation on the tooth surface close to the gingival tissue. The accumulation of plaque can be favored by a variety of local factors, such as calculus, overhanging margins of restorations, and food impaction. *The removal of plaque and of all the factors that favor its accumulation is therefore the primary consideration in local therapy.*

Abnormal forces on the tooth increase tooth mobility. The thorough elimination of plaque and the prevention of its new formation, by themselves, maintain periodontal health, even if traumatic forces are allowed to persist.[18,19] However, the elimination of trauma may increase the chances of bone regeneration and gain of attachment.[15] Although this point is not widely accepted,[25] it appears that creating occlusal relationships that are more tolerable to the periodontal tissues increases the margin of safety of the periodontium to minor buildup of plaque, in addition to reducing tooth mobility. It should be remembered that total plaque elimination as obtained in experimental studies may not be possible in all human subjects.

Systemic Therapy

Systemic therapy may be employed as an adjunct to local measures and for specific purposes, such as the control of systemic complications from acute infections, chemotherapy to prevent harmful effects of posttreatment bacteremia, and the control of systemic diseases that

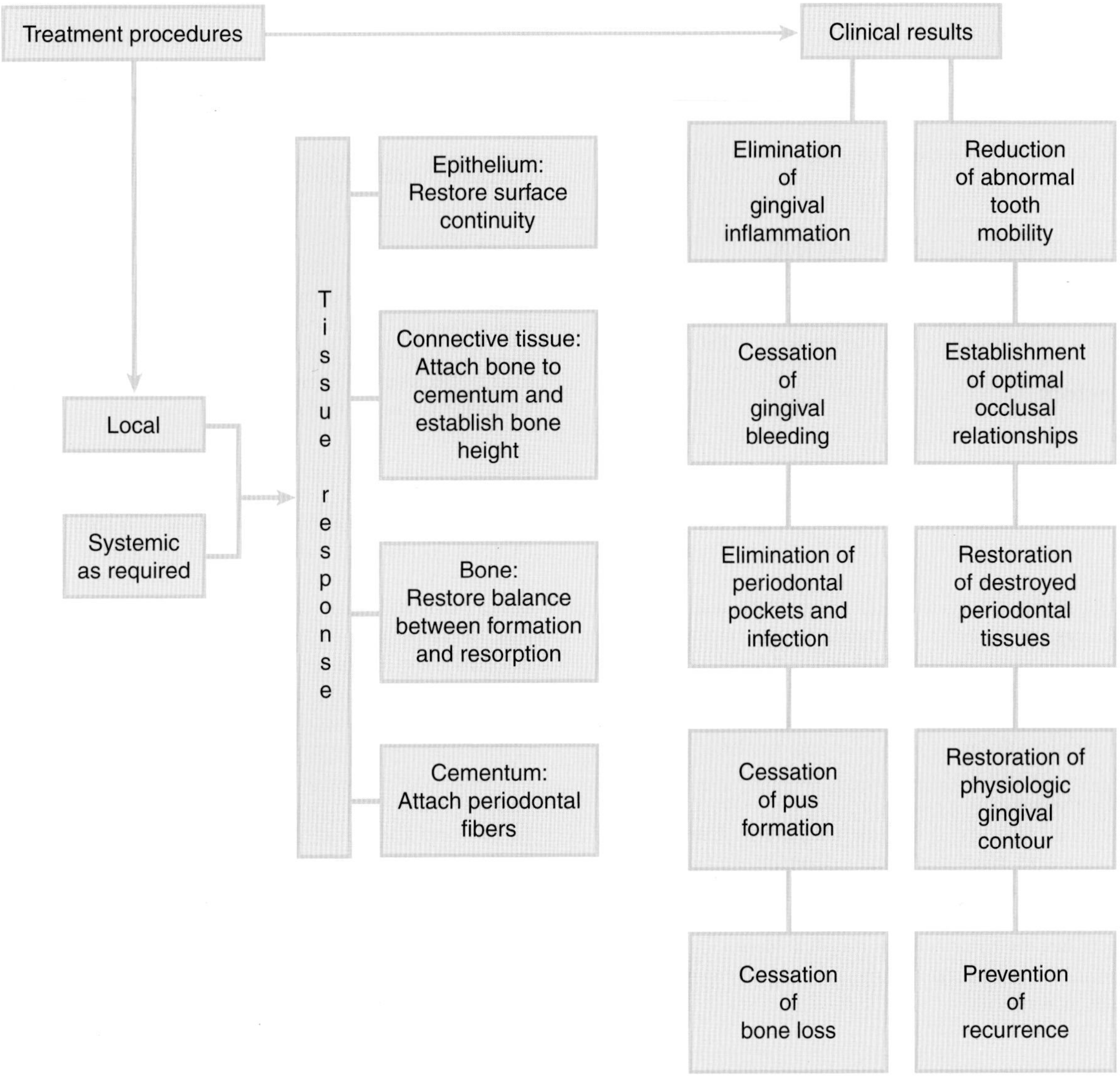

Figure 42-1 Tissue response and clinical results after periodontal treatment.

aggravate the patient's periodontal condition or necessitate special precautions during treatment (see Chapters 43, 44, and 45).

Systemic therapy for treatment of the periodontal condition and in conjunction with local therapy is indicated in patients with aggressive periodontitis. In these diseases, systemic antibiotics are used to eliminate the bacteria that invade the gingival tissues and can repopulate the pocket after scaling and root planing (see Chapters 46 and 52).

In addition, periodontal manifestations of systemic diseases (see Chapter 17) are treated primarily by interventions other than local measures. However, local therapy may still be indicated to reduce or prevent complicating gingival inflammation.

In the late twentieth century the concept of *host modulation* was introduced as a medical approach to periodontal treatment. The classic 1979 paper by Nyman, Schroeder, and Lindhe[23] showed how it was possible to block periodontal bone loss in animals with the aspirin-like drug indomethacin. Evidence was then presented that some *nonsteroidal antiinflammatory drugs* (NSAIDs), such as flurbiprofen and ibuprofen, can slow down the development of experimental gingivitis,[9] as well as the loss of alveolar bone in periodontitis.[11,33-35] These drugs are propionic acid derivatives and act by inhibiting the cyclooxygenase pathway of arachidonic acid metabolism, thereby reducing prostaglandin formation. These NSAIDs can be administered by mouth[13] or applied topically.[33]

Another drug that has a strong inhibitory effect on bone resorption is alendronate, a *bisphosphonate,* which is currently used to treat metabolic diseases in humans, such as Paget's disease or hypercalcemia of malignancy, which result in bone resorption. Experimental studies in monkeys have shown that alendronate reduced the bone loss associated with periodontitis.[3,31]

Host modulation is still in experimental stages, and protocols for its clinical use have not been established. However, it shows that future treatment modalities may attempt not only to control the bacterial cause of the disease, but also to suppress the self-destructive components of the host inflammatory response[11] (see Chapter 16 and 53).

FACTORS THAT AFFECT HEALING

In the periodontium, as elsewhere in the body, healing is affected by local and systemic factors.

Local Factors

Systemic conditions that impair healing may reduce the effectiveness of local periodontal treatment and should be corrected before or during local procedures. However, local factors, particularly plaque microorganisms, are the most common deterrents to healing after periodontal treatment.

Healing is also delayed by (1) excessive tissue manipulation during treatment, (2) trauma to the tissues, (3) the presence of foreign bodies, and (4) repetitive treatment procedures that disrupt the orderly cellular activity in the healing process. An adequate blood supply is needed for the increased cellular activity during healing; if this is impaired or insufficient, areas of necrosis will develop and delay the healing process.

Healing is improved by debridement (removal of degenerated and necrotic tissue), immobilization of the healing area, and pressure on the wound. The cellular activity in healing entails an increase in oxygen consumption, but healing of the gingiva is not accelerated by artificially increasing the oxygen supply beyond the normal requirements.[8]

Systemic Factors

The effects of systemic conditions on healing have been extensively documented in animal experiments but are less clearly defined in humans. Healing capacity diminishes with age,[4,10] probably because of the atherosclerotic vascular changes common in aging and the resulting reduction in blood circulation. Healing is delayed in patients with generalized infections and in those with diabetes and other debilitating diseases.

Healing is impaired by insufficient food intake; bodily conditions that interfere with the use of nutrients; and deficiencies in vitamin C,[1,30] proteins,[29] and other nutrients. However, the nutrient requirements of the healing tissues in minor wounds, such as those created by periodontal surgical procedures, are usually satisfied by a well-balanced diet.

Healing is also affected by hormones. Systemically administered glucocorticoids such as cortisone hinder repair by depressing the inflammatory reaction or by inhibiting the growth of fibroblasts, the production of collagen, and the formation of endothelial cells. Systemic stress,[29] thyroidectomy, testosterone, adrenocorticotropic hormone (ACTH), and large doses of estrogen suppress the formation of granulation tissue and impair healing.[4] Progesterone increases and accelerates the vascularization of immature granulation tissue[17] and appears to increase the susceptibility of the gingiva to mechanical injury by causing dilation of the marginal vessels.[12]

HEALING AFTER PERIODONTAL THERAPY

The basic healing processes are the same after all forms of periodontal therapy. These processes consist of the removal of degenerated tissue debris and the replacement of tissues destroyed by disease. This implies regeneration and repair of the periodontal structures but not necessarily a gain in attachment. Techniques to gain attachment and bone level are discussed under New Attachment and Periodontal Reconstruction.

Regeneration

Regeneration is the *natural renewal of a structure, produced by growth and differentiation of new cells and intercellular substances to form new tissues or parts.* Regeneration occurs through growth from the same type of tissue that has been destroyed or from its precursor. In the periodontium, gingival epithelium is replaced by epithelium, and the underlying connective tissue and periodontal ligament are derived from connective tissue. Bone and cementum are replaced by connective tissue, which is the precursor of both. Undifferentiated connective tissue cells develop into osteoblasts and cementoblasts, which form bone and cementum.

Regeneration of the periodontium is a continuous physiologic process. Under normal conditions, new cells and tissues are constantly being formed to replace those that mature and die; this is termed "wear and tear" repair.[16] It is manifested by (1) mitotic activity in the epithelium of the gingiva and the connective tissue of the periodontal ligament, (2) the formation of new bone, and (3) the continuous deposition of cementum.

Regeneration is occurring even during destructive periodontal disease. Most gingival and periodontal diseases are chronic inflammatory processes and, as such, are *healing* lesions. Regeneration is part of healing. However, bacteria and bacterial products that perpetuate the disease process, along with the resulting inflammatory exudate, are injurious to the regenerating cells and tissues, thus preventing completion of the healing process.

By removing bacterial plaque and creating the conditions to prevent its new formation, periodontal treatment removes the obstacles to regeneration and enables the patient to benefit from the inherent regenerative capacity of the tissues. A brief "spurt" in regenerative activity occurs immediately after periodontal treatment, but no local treatment procedures promote or accelerate regeneration.

Repair

Repair simply restores the continuity of the diseased marginal gingiva and reestablishes a normal gingival sulcus at the same level on the root as the base of the preexisting periodontal pocket (Figure 42-2, *B*). This process, called "healing by scar,"[26] arrests bone destruction but

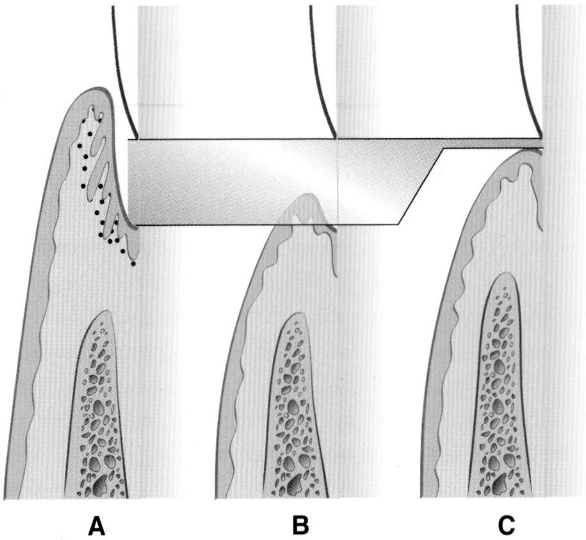

Figure 42-2 Two possible outcomes of pocket elimination. **A,** Periodontal pocket before treatment. **B,** Normal sulcus reestablished at the level of the base of the pocket. **C,** Periodontium restored on the root surface previously denuded by disease; this is called *new attachment.* Shaded areas show denudation caused by periodontal disease.

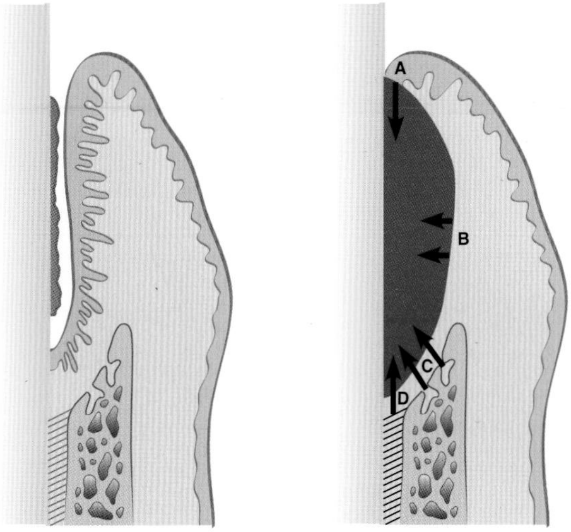

Figure 42-3 Sources of regenerating cells in the healing stages of a periodontal pocket. *Left,* Intrabony pocket. *Right,* After therapy the clot formed is invaded by cells from *A,* the marginal epithelium; *B,* the gingival connective tissue; *C,* the bone marrow; and *D,* the periodontal ligament.

does not result in gain of gingival attachment or bone height. This return of the destroyed periodontium to health involves regeneration and mobilization of epithelial and connective tissue cells into the damaged area and increased local mitotic divisions to provide sufficient numbers of cells (Figure 42-3).

For the diseased gingiva and attachment apparatus to regain (totally or partially) their level on the root (Figure 42-2, *C*), therapy must include special materials and techniques. If these are not used or are not successful, tissues undergo only repair, which involves regeneration of tissue to remodel the attachment apparatus, but does not include regaining attachment level or new bone height. For this reason, we prefer to use the term *reconstruction of the periodontium* to refer to the crucial therapeutic techniques that seek to rebuild the periodontium and result in a significant gain of attachment and bone height (see Chapter 67).

New Attachment

New attachment is the embedding of new periodontal ligament fibers into new cementum and the attachment of the gingival epithelium to a tooth surface previously denuded by disease.

The critical phrase in this definition is "tooth surface previously denuded by disease" (Figure 42-4, area *B*). The attachment of the gingiva or the periodontal ligament to areas of the tooth from which they have been removed in the course of treatment (or during preparation of teeth for restorations) represents simple healing or reattachment of the periodontium, not new attachment.[14] The term *reattachment* refers to repair in areas of the root not previously exposed to the pocket, such as after surgical detachment of the tissues or following traumatic tears

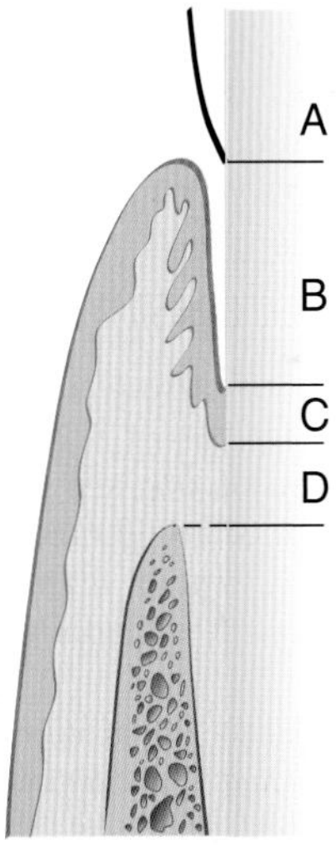

Figure 42-4 *A,* Enamel surface. *B,* Area of cementum denuded by pocket formation. *C,* Area of cementum covered by junctional epithelium. *D,* Area of cementum apical to junctional epithelium. The term *new attachment* refers to a new junctional epithelium and attached connective tissue fibers formed on zone *B.*

in the cementum, tooth fractures, or the treatment of periapical lesions (Figure 42-4, area *D*).

Epithelial adaptation differs from new attachment in that it is the close apposition of the gingival epithelium to the tooth surface, with no gain in height of gingival fiber attachment. The pocket is not completely obliterated, although it may not permit passage of a probe (Figure 42-5). However, studies have shown that these deep sulci lined by long, thin epithelium may be as resistant to disease as true connective tissue attachments.[2,21] The absence of bleeding or secretion on probing, the absence of clinically visible inflammation, and the absence of

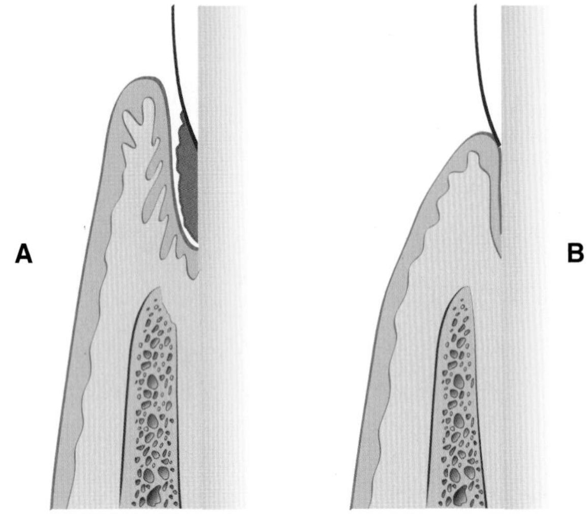

Figure 42-5 Epithelial adaptation after periodontal treatment. **A,** Periodontal pocket. **B,** After treatment. The pocket epithelium is closely adapted to, but not attached to, the root.

stainable plaque on the root surface when the pocket wall is deflected from the tooth may indicate that the "deep sulcus" persists in an inactive state, causing no further loss of attachment.[5,35] A posttherapy depth of 4 or even 5 mm may therefore be acceptable in these cases.

PERIODONTAL RECONSTRUCTION

As just discussed, we use the term *periodontal reconstruction* to refer to the process of regeneration of cells and fibers and remodeling of the lost periodontal structures that results in (1) gain of attachment level, (2) formation of new periodontal ligament fibers, and (3) a level of alveolar bone significantly coronal to that present before treatment.

A technique to attain these ideal results has been a constant but elusive goal of periodontal therapy for centuries.[6] Since the 1970s, renewed laboratory and clinical research efforts have resulted in new concepts and techniques that have moved us much closer to attaining this ideal result of therapy. Melcher[22] pointed out that the regeneration of the periodontal ligament is the key to periodontal reconstruction because it "provides continuity between the alveolar bone and the cementum and also because it contains cells that can synthesize and remodel the three connective tissues of the alveolar part of the periodontium."

During the healing stages of a periodontal pocket, the area is invaded by cells from four different sources (see Figure 42-3): oral epithelium, gingival connective tissue, bone, and periodontal ligament.

The final outcome of periodontal pocket healing depends on the sequence of events during the healing stages.[22] If the epithelium proliferates along the tooth surface before the other tissues reach the area, the result will be a long junctional epithelium. If the cells from the gingival connective tissue are the first to populate the area, the result will be fibers parallel to the tooth surface and remodeling of the alveolar bone with no attachment to the cementum. If bone cells arrive first, root resorption and ankylosis may occur. Finally, only when cells from the periodontal ligament proliferate coronally is there new formation of cementum and periodontal ligament.[22]

Several methods, based on different concepts and resulting in various techniques, have been recommended to improve the likelihood of gaining new attachment and increased bone levels, as discussed in Chapter 67.

SCIENCE TRANSFER

It is well recognized that tissue loss in periodontal disease does not involve only the microbial plaque that initiates inflammation, but also the host's reaction to that inflammation. Thus *the rationale for treatment must focus on two aspects: (1) the removal of plaque that is initiating the inflammation and (2) the ability of the host to respond to inflammation.* In addition to the mechanical removal of plaque and calculus by surgical and nonsurgical therapies, local and systemic therapies can be used to inhibit tissue loss and enhance the host's ability to fight infection and decrease inflammation. Likewise, new therapies to gain tissues lost to disease are being developed using strategies to harness the host's cellular activities that result in new tissue formation.

The main rationale for periodontal therapy is to optimize the dentition so that functional and esthetic needs are stabilized. This means that restoration of periodontal health by repair, regeneration, or reconstruction provides the means for retaining damaged teeth. However, recent information shows that active periodontal disease increases the susceptibility to systemic problems, such as atherosclerosis, lung infections, strokes, and low-birth-weight, premature infants. *Therefore the rationale for periodontal treatment is much wider than optimizing the dentition, and patients need to be informed of the broader benefits of obtaining periodontal health.*

REFERENCES

1. Barr CE: Oral healing in ascorbic acid deficiency, *Periodontics* 3:286, 1965.
2. Beaumont RH, O'Leary TJ, Kafrawy AH: Relative resistance of long junctional epithelial adhesions and connective tissue attachments to plaque-induced inflammation, *J Periodontol* 55:213, 1984.
3. Brunsvold MA, Chaves ES, Kornman KS, et al: Effects of a bisphosphonate on experimental periodontitis in monkeys, *J Periodontol* 63:825, 1992.
4. Butcher EO, Klingsberg J: Age, gonadectomy, and wound healing in the palatal mucosa, *J Dent Res* 40:694, 1961.
5. Caffesse RG, Ramfjord SP, Nasjleti CE: Reverse bevel periodontal flaps in monkeys, *J Periodontol* 39:219, 1968.
6. Carranza F, Shklar G: *History of periodontology,* Chicago, 2003, Quintessence.

7. Ferris RT: Quantitative evaluation of tooth mobility following initial periodontal therapy, *J Periodontol* 37:190, 1966.
8. Glickman I, Turesky SS, Manhold J: The oxygen consumption of healing gingiva, *J Dent Res* 29:429, 1950.
9. Heasman PA, Seymour RA: The effect of a systemically administered non-steroidal anti-inflammatory drug (flurbiprofen) on experimental gingivitis in humans, *J Clin Periodontol* 16:551, 1989.
10. Holm-Pedersen P, Löe H: Wound healing in the gingiva of young and old individuals, *Scand J Dent Res* 79:40, 1971.
11. Howell TH, Williams RC: Nonsteroidal antiinflammatory drugs as inhibitors of periodontal disease progression, *Crit Rev Oral Biol Med* 4:177, 1993.
12. Hugoson A: Gingival inflammation and female sex hormones, *J Periodontal Res* 5(suppl):1, 1970.
13. Jeffcoat MK, Williams RC, Reddy MS, et al: Flurbiprofen treatment of human periodontitis: effect on alveolar bone height and metabolism, *J Periodontal Res* 23:381, 1988.
14. Kalkwarf KL: Periodontal new attachment without the placement of osseous potentiating grafts, *Periodont Abstr* 22:53, 1974.
15. Kantor M, Polson AM, Zander HA: Alveolar bone regeneration after removal of inflammatory and traumatic factors, *J Periodontol* 47:687, 1976.
16. Leblond CP, Walker BE: Renewal of cell populations, *Physiol Rev* 36:255, 1956.
17. Lindhe J, Branemark PI: The effect of sex hormones on vascularization of a granulation tissue, *J Periodontal Res* 3:6, 1968.
18. Lindhe J, Ericsson I: The influence of trauma from occlusion on reduced but healthy periodontal tissues in dogs, *J Clin Periodontol* 3:110, 1976.
19. Lindhe J, Nyman S: The effect of plaque control and surgical pocket elimination on the establishment and maintenance of periodontal health: a longitudinal study of periodontal therapy in cases of advanced periodontal disease, *J Clin Periodontol* 2:67, 1975.
20. Lindhe J, Parodi R, Liljenberg B, et al: Clinical and structural alterations characterizing healing gingiva, *J Periodontal Res* 13:410, 1978.
21. Magnusson I, Runstad L, Nyman S, et al: A long junctional epithelium: a locus minoris resistentiae in plaque infection? *J Clin Periodontol* 10:33, 1983.
22. Melcher AH: On the repair potential of periodontal tissues, *J Periodontol* 47:256, 1976.
23. Nyman S, Schroeder HE, Lindhe J: Suppression of inflammation and bone resorption by indomethacin during experimental periodontitis in dogs, *J Periodontol* 50:450, 1979.
24. Oliver RC: Tooth loss with and without periodontal therapy, *Periodont Abstr* 17:8, 1969.
25. Polson AM: Interrelationship of inflammation and tooth mobility (trauma) in pathogenesis of periodontal disease, *J Clin Periodontol* 7:351, 1980.
26. Ratcliff PA: An analysis of repair systems in periodontal therapy, *Periodont Abstr* 14:57, 1966.
27. Rateitschak K: The therapeutic effect of local treatment on periodontal disease assessed upon evaluation of different diagnostic criteria. 2. Changes in gingival inflammation, *J Periodontol* 35:155, 1964.
28. Rateitschak K, Engelberger A, Marthaler TM: The therapeutic effect of local treatment on periodontal disease assessed upon evaluation of different diagnostic criteria. 3. Radiographic changes in appearance of bone, *J Periodontol* 35:263, 1964.
29. Stahl SS: Healing gingival injury in normal and systemically stressed young adult male rats, *J Periodontol* 32:63, 1961.
30. Stahl SS: The effect of a protein-free diet on the healing of gingival wounds in rats, *Arch Oral Biol* 7:551, 1962.
31. Turesky SS, Glickman I: Histochemical evaluation of gingival healing in experimental animals on adequate and vitamin C deficient diets, *J Dent Res* 33:273, 1954.
32. Weinreb M, Quartuccio H, Seedor JG, et al: Histomorphometrical analysis of the effects of the bisphosphonate alendronate on bone loss caused by experimental periodontitis in monkeys, *J Periodontal Res* 29:35, 1994.
33. Williams RC, Jeffcoat MK, Howell TH, et al: Topical flurbiprofen treatment of periodontitis in beagles, *J Periodontal Res* 23:166, 1988.
34. Williams RC, Jeffcoat MK, Howell H, et al: Altering the progression of human alveolar bone loss with the non-steroidal anti-inflammatory drug flurbiprofen, *J Periodontol* 60:485, 1989.
35. Williams RC, Jeffcoat MK, Kaplan ML, et al: Flurbiprofen: a potent inhibitor of alveolar bone resorption in beagles, *Science* 227:640, 1985.
36. Yukna RA: A clinical and histologic study of healing following the excisional new attachment procedure in rhesus monkeys, *J Periodontol* 47:701, 1976.

Periodontal Therapy in the Female Patient

43

CHAPTER

Joan Otomo-Corgel

CHAPTER OUTLINE

Throughout a woman's life cycle, hormonal influences affect therapeutic decision making in periodontics. Historically, therapies have been gender biased. However, the advent of new research has provided keener appreciation of the unique systemic influences on oral, periodontal, and implant tissues. Oral health care professionals have greater awareness of, and better capabilities for dealing with, hormonal influences associated with the reproductive process. Periodontal and oral tissue responses may be altered, creating diagnostic and therapeutic dilemmas. Therefore it is imperative that the clinician recognize, customize, and appropriately alter periodontal therapy according to the individual woman's needs based on the stage of her life cycle.

This chapter reviews phases of the female life cycle from puberty through menopause. Periodontal manifestations, systemic effects, and clinical management are presented.

PUBERTY

Puberty occurs between the average ages of 11 to 14 in most women. The production of sex hormones (estrogen and progesterone) increases, then remains relatively constant during the remainder of the reproductive phase.

Also, the prevalence of gingivitis increases, without an increase in the amount of plaque. Gram-negative anaerobes, especially *Prevotella intermedia,* have been implicated in association with puberty gingivitis. Kornman and Loesche[42] postulated that this anaerobic organism may use ovarian hormone as a substitute for vitamin K growth factor. Levels of black-pigmented *Bacteroides,* especially *P. intermedia* (formerly known as *Bacteroides intermedius*), are thought to increase with increased levels of gonadotropic hormones in puberty. *Capnocytophaga* species also increase in incidence as well as in proportion. These organisms have been implicated in the increased bleeding tendency observed during puberty.[33] Recent studies associated with puberty gingivitis indicate proportionately elevated motile rods, spirochetes, and *P. intermedia.*[59] Statistically significant increases in gingival inflammation and in the proportions of *P. intermedia* and *Prevotella nigrescens* have been seen in puberty gingivitis.[62]

During puberty, periodontal tissues may have an exaggerated response to local factors. A hyperplastic reaction of the gingiva may occur in areas where food debris, materia alba, plaque, and calculus are deposited. The inflamed tissues become erythematous, lobulated, and retractable. Bleeding may occur easily with mechanical debridement of the gingival tissues. Histologically, the appearance is consistent with inflammatory hyperplasia.

During the reproductive years, women tend to have a more vigorous immune response, including higher immunoglobulin concentrations, stronger primary and secondary responses, increased resistance to the induction of immunologic tolerance, and a greater ability to reject tumors and homografts.[85] Allergy sensitivity and asthma occur more often in young men, but after puberty, women become more susceptible than their male counterparts.

Management

During puberty, education of the parent or caregiver is part of successful periodontal therapy. Preventive care, including a vigorous program of oral hygiene, is also vital. Milder gingivitis cases respond well to scaling and root planing, with frequent oral hygiene reinforcement.[4] Severe cases of gingivitis may require microbial culturing, antimicrobial mouthwashes and local site delivery, or antibiotic therapy. Periodontal maintenance appointments may need to be more frequent when periodontal instability is noted.

The clinician should recognize the intraoral effects of chronic regurgitation of gastric contents on intraoral tissues because this age group also is susceptible to eating disorders, namely, bulimia and anorexia nervosa. *Perimylosis* (smooth erosion of enamel and dentin), typically on the lingual surfaces of maxillary anterior teeth, varies with the duration and frequency of the behavior.[13] Also, enlargement of the parotid glands (occasionally sublingual glands) has been estimated to occur in 10% to 50% of patients who "binge and purge."[55] Therefore a diminished salivary flow rate may also be present, which will increase oral mucous membrane sensitivity, gingival erythema, and caries susceptibility.

MENSES

Periodontal Manifestations

During the reproductive years, the ovarian cycle is controlled by the anterior pituitary gland. The gonadotropins follicle-stimulating hormone (FSH) and luteinizing hormone (LH) are produced from the anterior pituitary gland. The secretion of gonadotropins also depends on the hypothalamus. Ongoing changes in the concentration of the gonadotropins and ovarian hormones occur during the monthly menstrual cycle (Figure 43-1). Under the influence of FSH and LH, estrogen and progesterone are steroid hormones produced by the ovaries during the menstrual cycle. During the reproductive cycle, the purpose of estrogen and progesterone is to prepare the uterus for implantation of the egg.

The monthly reproductive cycle has two phases. The first phase is referred to as the *follicular phase.* Levels of FSH are elevated, and estradiol (E_2), the major form of estrogen, is synthesized by the developing follicle and peaks approximately 2 days before ovulation. The effect of estrogen stimulates the egg to move down the fallopian tubules (ovulation) and stimulates proliferation of the stroma cells, blood vessels, and glands of the endometrium.

The second phase is called the *luteal phase.* The developing corpus luteum synthesizes both estradiol and progesterone. Estrogen peaks at 0.2 ng/ml and progesterone at 10.0 ng/ml to complete the rebuilding of the endometrium for implantation of the fertilized egg. The corpus

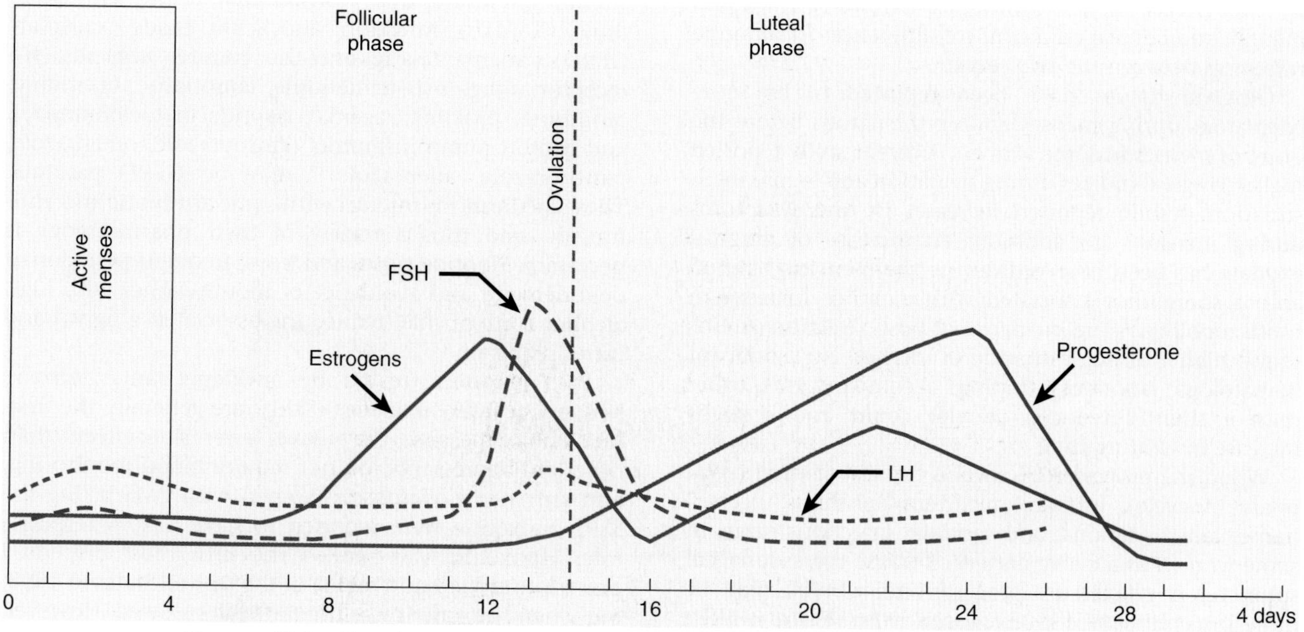

Figure 43-1 Female reproductive cycle. Note the peak levels of progesterone and estrogen compared with follicle-stimulating hormone *(FSH)* and luteinizing hormone *(LH).*

luteum involutes, ovarian hormone levels drops, and menstruation ensues.

It has been postulated that ovarian hormones may increase inflammation in gingival tissues and exaggerate the response to local irritants. Gingival inflammation seems to be aggravated by an imbalance or increase in sex hormones. Numerous studies have demonstrated in vitro and in vivo that sex hormones affect and modify the actions of cells of the immune system. In addition, evidence suggests that the interaction between estrogen and cells of the immune system can have nonimmune regulatory effects.[5,16] Possible mechanisms have been suggested for the increase in hormonal gingival interaction in the menstrual cycle. Tumor necrosis factor alpha (TNF-α), which fluctuates during the menstrual cycle[11]; elevated prostaglandin E_2 (PGE_2) synthesis[56]; and angiogenetic factors, endothelial growth factors, and receptors may be modulated by progesterone and estrogen, contributing to increases in gingival inflammation during certain stages of the menstrual cycle.

Progesterone has been associated with increased permeability of the microvasculature, altering the rate and pattern of collagen production in the gingiva,[52] increasing folate metabolism,[70,90] and altering the immune response. During menses, progesterone increases from the second week, peaks at approximately 10 days, and dramatically drops before menstruation. (Note that this is based on a 28-day cycle; individual cycles are variable.) Progesterone plays a role in stimulating the production of prostaglandins that mediate the body's response to inflammation. PGE_2 is one of the major secretory products of monocytes and is increased in inflamed gingiva. Miyagi et al.[57] found that the chemotaxis of polymorphonuclear leukocytes (PMNs, neutrophils) was enhanced by progesterone but reduced by estradiol. Testosterone did not have a measurable effect on PMN chemotaxis. The researchers suggested that the altered PMN chemotaxis associated with gingival inflammation may be caused by the effects of sex hormones. Physiologic, experimental, and clinical data confirm differences in immune responses between the two sexes.[96]

Gingival tissues have been reported to be more edematous during menses and erythematous before the onset of menses in some women. A recent study reported higher gingival indices during ovulation and before menstruation despite reported increases in oral symptoms during menses.[53] In addition, an increase of gingival exudate has been observed during the menstrual period and is sometimes associated with a minor increase in tooth mobility.[31] The incidence of postextraction osteitis is also higher during initiation of menses. No significant hematologic laboratory findings accompany this, other than a slightly reduced platelet count and a slight increase in clotting time.

When the progesterone level is highest (during luteal phase of cycle), intraoral recurrent aphthous ulcers,[25] herpes labialis lesions, and candidal infections occur in some women as a cyclic pattern. Because the esophageal sphincter is relaxed by progesterone, women may be more susceptible to *gastroesophageal reflux disease* (GERD) during this time of the cycle as well. Symptoms of GERD include heartburn, regurgitation, and chest pain, and when reflux is severe, some patients develop unexplained coughing, hoarseness, sore throat, gingivitis, and asthma.[82]

During the peak level of progesterone (about 7-10 days before menstruation), *premenstrual syndrome* (PMS) may also occur. There appears to be no significant difference in the estrogen and progesterone levels between women with PMS and those without PMS. However, women with PMS seem to have lower levels of certain neurotransmitters, such as enkephalins, endorphins, gamma-aminobutyric acid (GABA), and serotonin. Depression, irritability, mood swings, and difficulty with memory and concentration may be symptoms of neurotransmitter reduction. Patients are more sensitive and less tolerant of procedures, have a heightened gag reflex, and may have an exaggerated response to pain.

Management

Increased gingival bleeding and tenderness associated with the menstrual cycle require closer periodontal monitoring. Periodontal maintenance should be titrated to the individual patient's need and, if problematic, 3- to 4-month intervals should be recommended. An antimicrobial oral rinse before cyclic inflammation may be indicated. Emphasis should be placed on oral hygiene.

For the patient with a history of excessive postoperative hemorrhage or menstrual flow, scheduling surgical visits after cyclic menstruation is prudent. Anemia is common, and appropriate consultation with a physician and recent laboratory tests, when indicated, should be maintained.

During PMS, many women exhibit physical symptoms that include fatigue, sweet and salty food cravings, abdominal bloating, swollen hands or feet, headaches, breast tenderness, nausea, and gastrointestinal upset.[96] GERD may make it more uncomfortable for the patient to lay fully supine, especially after a meal, and the woman may have a more sensitive gag reflex. The clinician should be aware that nonsteroidal antiinflammatory drugs (NSAIDs), infection, and acidic foods exacerbate GERD. Patients taking over-the counter antacids, H_2-receptor antagonists (cimetidine, famotidine, nizatidine, ranitidine), prokinetic agents (cisapride, metoclopramide), and proton pump inhibitors (lansoprazole, omeprazole, pantoprazole, abeprazole)[83] may be GERD patients. These medications interact with some antibiotic and antifungals, and thus a review of their pharmacology is necessary. Fluoride rinses and trays, frequent periodontal debridement, and avoidance of mouthwashes with high alcohol content may reduce the associated gingival and caries sequelae.

PMS is often treated by antidepressants. *Selective serotonin reuptake inhibitors* (SSRIs) are generally the first-line choice because they have fewer side effects than other antidepressants, do not require blood monitoring, and are safe in overdoses. Women with PMS taking the SSRI fluoxetine were reported to have a 70% response rate. Fluoxetine was ranked the fifth most dispensed prescription (new and refills) in the United States in 1998, but when the patent was lifted its sales slowed. However, overall SSRIs ranked second in total dollar sales in the 2000s. (Sertraline was ranked twelfth and is the drug of choice for treatment of PMS).[101] The clinician should be aware that patients taking fluoxetine have increased side effects with highly protein-bound drugs (e.g., aspirin), and the half-life of diazepam and other central nervous system (CNS) depressants is increased. Additional common SSRIs are fluvoxamine, paroxetine, and citalopram. Other antidepressants that may be prescribed are the selective serotonin and norepinephrine reuptake inhibitors (SNRIs), tricyclics, trazodone, mirtazapine, nefazodone, and maprotiline.

The PMS patient may be difficult to treat because of emotional and physiologic sensitivity. The dentist should treat the gingival and oral mucosal tissues gently. Gauze pads or cotton rolls should be moistened with a lubricant, chlorhexidine rinse, or water before placing them in the aphtha-prone patient. Careful retraction of the oral mucosa, cheeks, and lips is necessary in patients prone to aphthous or herpetic lesions. Because the hypoglycemic threshold is elevated, the clinician should advise the patient to have a light snack before her appointment. Of menstruating women, 70% have PMS symptoms, but only 5% meet the strict diagnostic criteria.

PERIODONTAL MANIFESTATIONS OF PREGNANCY

The link between pregnancy and periodontal inflammation has been known for many years. In 1778, Vermeeren discussed "toothpains" in pregnancy. In 1818, Pitcarin[75] described gingival hyperplasia in pregnancy. Despite awareness regarding pregnancy and its effect on periodontal disease, only recently has evidence indicated an inverse relationship to systemic health. Current research implies periodontal disease may alter the systemic health of the patient and adversely affect the well-being of the fetus by elevating the risk for low-birth-weight, preterm infants.

Periodontal Diseases

In 1877, Pinard[74] recorded the first case of "pregnancy gingivitis." Only recently has periodontal research begun to focus on causative mechanisms. The occurrence of pregnancy gingivitis is extremely common, occurring in 30% to 100% of all pregnant women.[34,46,50,84] It is characterized by erythema, edema, hyperplasia, and increased bleeding. Histologically, the description is the same as for gingivitis. However, the etiologic factors are different despite clinical and histologic similarities. Cases range from mild to severe inflammation (Figure 43-2), which can progress to severe hyperplasia, pain, and bleeding (Figures 43-3 and 43-4). Other growths that resemble pregnancy granulomas must be ruled out, such as central giant cell granulomas or underlying systemic diseases. Periodontal status before pregnancy may influence the progression or severity as the circulating hormones fluctuate. The anterior region of the mouth is affected more often, and interproximal sites tend to be most involved.[20] Increased tissue edema may lead to increased pocket depths and may be associated with transient tooth mobility.[76] Anterior site inflammation may be exacerbated by increased mouth breathing, primarily in the third

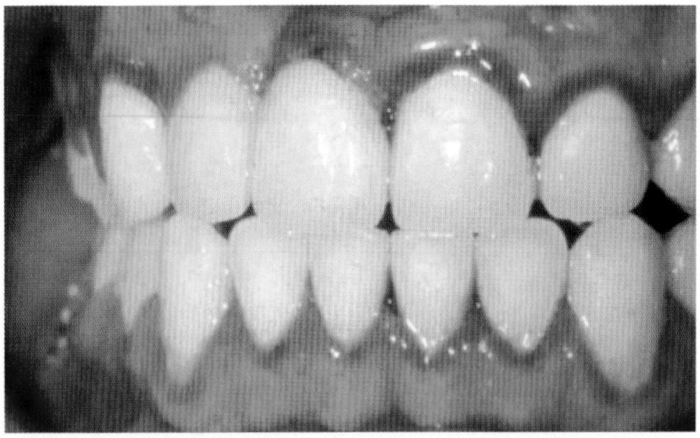

Figure 43-2 Moderate form of pregnancy gingivitis.

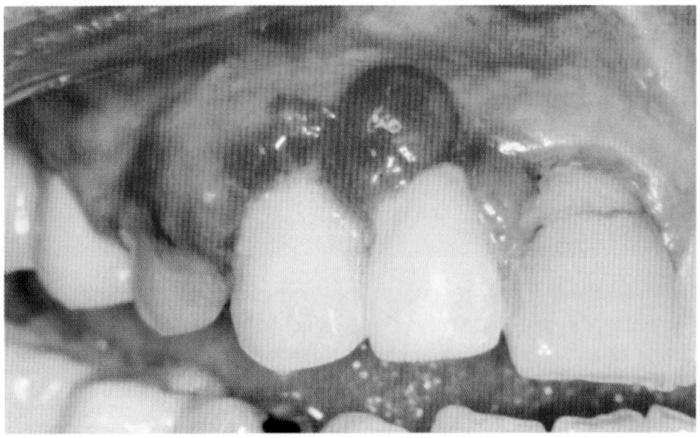

Figure 43-3 Pyogenic granuloma of pregnancy ("pregnancy tumor").

trimester, from pregnancy rhinitis. The gingiva is the most common site involved (approximately 70% of all cases), followed by the tongue and lips, buccal mucosa, and palate.[8]

Pyogenic granulomas ("pregnancy tumors," pregnancy epulides) occur in 0.2% to 9.6% of pregnancies. They are clinically and histologically indistinguishable from pyogenic granulomas occurring in nonpregnant women or in men. Pyogenic granulomas appear most often during the second or third month of pregnancy. Clinically, they bleed easily and become hyperplastic and nodular. When excised, the lesions usually do not leave a large defect. They may be sessile or pedunculated and ulcerated, ranging in color from purplish red to deep blue, depending on the vascularity of the lesion and degree of venous stasis. The lesion classically occurs in an area of gingivitis and is associated with poor oral hygiene and calculus. Alveolar bone loss is usually not associated with pyogenic granulomas of pregnancy.

Role of Pregnancy Hormones

Subgingival Plaque Composition. Epidemiologic studies indicate a relationship between the level of home care and the severity of gingival inflammation. It appears that the association between signs of gingival inflammation and the amount of plaque is greater after parturition

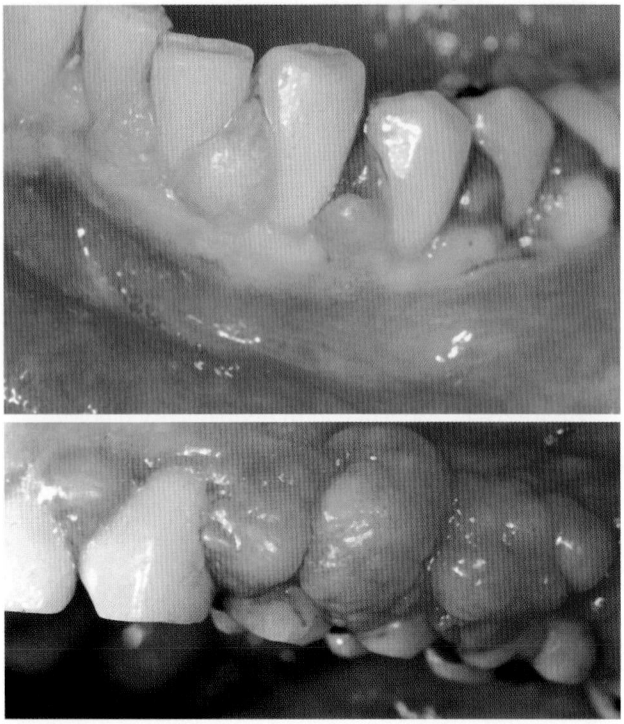
A
B

Figure 43-4 Severe pregnancy gingivitis with hyperplasia in patients with poorly controlled non–insulin-dependent diabetes mellitus. **A,** Moderate gingival enlargement. **B,** Severe gingival enlargement.

than during pregnancy. An alteration in the compositions of subgingival plaque occurs during pregnancy. As mentioned, Kornman and Loesche[43] found that during the second trimester, gingivitis and gingival bleeding increased, without an increase in plaque levels. Bacterial anaerobic/aerobic ratios increased, in addition to proportions of *Bacteroides melaninogenicus* and *Prevotella intermedia* (2.2%-10.1%). The authors suggested that estradiol or progesterone can substitute for menadione (vitamin K) as an essential growth factor for *P. intermedia* but not *Porphyromonas gingivalis* or *Eikenella corrodens*. There was also an increase in *P. gingivalis* during the 21st through 27th weeks of gestation, but this was not statistically significant. The relative increase in the numbers of *P. intermedia* may be a more sensitive indicator of an altered systemic hormonal situation than clinical parameters of gingivitis.[87]

Periodontal Disease and Preterm, Low-Birth-Weight Infants. Offenbacher et al.[66] have provided evidence that untreated periodontal disease in pregnant women may be a significant risk factor for preterm (<37 weeks' gestation), low-birth-weight (<2500 g) infants. The relationship between genitourinary tract infection and preterm, low-birth-weight (PLBW) infants is well documented in human and animal studies. Periodontal researchers, suspecting periodontal disease as another source of infection, found that otherwise low-risk mothers of PLBW infants had significantly more periodontal attachment loss than control mothers having normal-weight infants at birth.

The current opinion is that the correlation of periodontal disease to PLBW births occurs as a result of infection and is mediated indirectly, principally by the translocation of bacterial products such as endotoxin (lipopolysaccharide, LPS) and the action of maternally produced inflammatory mediators.[28] Biologically active molecules such as PGE_2 and TNF-α, which are normally involved in normal parturition, are raised to artificially high levels by the infection process, which may foster premature labor.[2] Gram-negative bacteria in periodontal diseases therefore may permit selective overgrowth or invasion of gram-negative bacteria within the genitourinary tract.

Recently, gingival crevicular fluid (GCF) levels of PGE_2 were positively associated with intraamniotic PGE_2 levels (p = 0.018), suggesting that gram-negative periodontal infection may present a systemic challenge sufficient to initiate the onset of premature labor as a source of LPS, or through stimulation of secondary inflammatory mediators such as PGE_2 and interleukin-1β (IL-1β).[17] Ongoing research supports the association of periodontal disease and PLBW.[18,19] Offenbacher et al.[65] suggested a dose-response relationship for increasing GCF PGE_2 as a marker of current periodontal disease activity and decreasing birth weight. Four organisms associated with mature plaque and progressing periodontitis—*Tannerella forsythia, P. gingivalis, Actinobacillus actinomycetemcomitans*, and *Treponema denticola*—were detected at higher levels in PLBW mothers compared with normal-birth-weight controls (see Chapter 13).

Maternal Immunoresponse

The maternal immune system is thought to be suppressed during pregnancy. This response may allow the fetus to survive as an allograft. Documentation of immunosuppressive factors in the sera of pregnant women can be noted by marked increase of monocytes (which in large numbers inhibit in vitro proliferative responses to mitogens, allogenic cells, and soluble antigen),[92] and pregnancy-specific β_I-glycoproteins contribute to diminished lymphocyte responsiveness to mitogens and antigens.[9] In addition, a decrease in the ratio of peripheral T helper cells to T suppressor cells (CD4/CD8) has been reported to occur throughout pregnancy.[87]

These changes in maternal immunoresponsiveness suggest an increased susceptibility to developing gingival inflammation. In one study, the gingival index was higher, but percentages of T3, T4, and B cells appeared to decrease in peripheral blood and gingival tissues during pregnancy compared with a control group.[1] Other studies report decreased PMN (neutrophil) chemotaxis, depression of cell-mediated immunity, phagocytosis, and a decreased T-cell response with elevated ovarian hormone levels, especially progesterone.[77] Decreased in vitro responses of peripheral blood lymphocytes to several mitogens and to a preparation of *P. intermedia* have been reported.[10,51,64] Also, evidence suggests a decrease in the absolute numbers of CD4+ cells in peripheral blood during pregnancy compared with the number of these cells postpartum.[78,87] Lapp et al.[44] suggest that high levels of progesterone during pregnancy affect the development of localized inflammation by downregulation of interleukin-6 (IL-6) production, rendering the gingiva less efficient at resisting the inflammatory challenges produced by the bacteria.

Also, ovarian hormone stimulates the production of prostaglandins, in particular PGE_1 and PGE_2, which are potent mediators of the inflammatory response. With the prostaglandin acting as an immunosuppressant, gingival inflammation may increase when the mediator level is high.[23,67] Kinnby et al.[40] found that high progesterone levels during pregnancy influenced plasminogen activator inhibitor type 2 (PAI-2) and disturbed the balance of the fibrinolytic system. Because PAI-2 serves as an important inhibitor of tissue proteolysis, this research implies that components of the fibrinolytic system may be involved in the development of pregnancy gingivitis.

Sex Hormone Levels

During pregnancy, hormonal levels rise dramatically (Box 43-1). Progesterone reaches levels of 100 ng/ml, 10 times the peak luteal phase of menses. Estradiol in the plasma may reach 30 times higher levels than during the reproductive cycle. In early pregnancy and during the normal ovarian cycle, the corpus luteum is the major source of estrogen and progesterone. During pregnancy the placenta begins to produce estrogens and progesterone.

Estrogen may regulate cellular proliferation, differentiation, and keratinization, whereas progesterone influences the permeability of the microvasculature,[47,48] alters the rate and pattern of collagen production, and increases the metabolic breakdown of folate (necessary for tissue maintenance).[99] High concentration of sex hormones in gingival tissues, saliva, serum, and GCF also may exaggerate the response.

Regulation of most cellular processes by hormones occurs through the interaction of these products with intracellular receptors. The resulting effects depend on the concentration of unbound hormone diffused through the cell membrane. Vittek et al.[94] have demonstrated specific estrogen and progesterone receptors in gingival tissues, providing direct biochemical evidence that this tissue may function as a target organ for sex hormones. Muramatsu and Takaesu[60] found increasing concentration of sex hormones in saliva from the first month and peaking in the ninth month of gestation, along with increasing percentages of *P. intermedia*. Probing depth, number of gingival sites with bleeding, and redness increased until 1 month postpartum. Also, evidence indicates sex hormone concentration in GCF, providing a growth media for periodontal pathogens.

Other Oral Manifestations of Pregnancy

As previously mentioned, perimylolysis (acid erosion of teeth) may occur if "morning sickness" or esophageal reflux is severe and involves repeated vomiting of the gastric contents. Severe reflux may cause scarring of the esophageal sphincter, and the patient may become a more likely candidate for GERD later in life.

BOX 43-1

Etiology of Gingival Responses to Elevated Estrogen and Progesterone during Pregnancy

Subgingival Plaque Composition

Increase in anaerobic/aerobic ratio
Higher concentrations of *Prevotella intermedia* (substitutes sex hormone for vitamin K–growth factor)
Higher concentrations of *Bacteroides melaninogenicus*
Higher concentrations of *Porphyromonas gingivalis*

Maternal Immunoresponse

Depression of cell-mediated immunity
Decreased neutrophil chemotaxis
Depression of antibody and T-cell responses
Decrease in ratio of peripheral T helper cells to T suppressor-cytotoxic cells (CD4/CD8 ratio)
Cytotoxicity directed against macrophages and B cells may result in diminished immunoresponsiveness.
Decrease in absolute numbers of CD3+, CD4+, and CD19+ cells in peripheral blood during pregnancy versus postpartum
Stimulation of prostaglandin production

Sex Hormone Concentration

Estrogen
Increases cellular proliferation in blood vessels (known in the endometrium).
Decreases keratinization, while increasing epithelial glycogen.
Specific receptors are found in gingival tissues.

Progesterone
Increases vascular dilation, and thus increases permeability (resulting in edema and accumulation of inflammatory cells).
Increases proliferation of newly formed capillaries in gingival tissues (increased bleeding tendency).
Alters rate and pattern of collagen production.
Increased metabolic breakdown of folate (folate deficiency can inhibit tissue repair).
Specific receptors are found in gingival tissues.
Decreases plasminogen activator inhibitor type 2, and thus increases tissue proteolysis.

Estrogen and Progesterone
Affect ground substance of connective tissue by increasing fluidity.
Concentrations increase in saliva and fluid with increased concentrations in serum.

Xerostomia is a frequent complaint among pregnant women. One study found this persistent dryness in 44% of pregnant participants.[21]

A rare finding in pregnancy is *ptyalism,* or *sialorrhea.* This excessive secretion of saliva usually begins at 2 to 3 weeks of gestation and may abate at the end of the first trimester. The etiology of ptyalism has not been identified, but it may result from the inability of nauseated gravid women to swallow normal amounts of saliva, rather than from a true increase in saliva production.[15]

Because pregnancy places the woman in an immunocompromised state, the clinician must be aware of the patient's total health. Gestational diabetes, leukemia, and other medical conditions may appear during pregnancy.

Clinical Management

A thorough medical history is an imperative component of the periodontal examination, especially in the pregnant patient. Because of immunologic alterations, increased blood volume (ruling out mitral valve prolapse and heart murmurs), and fetal interactions, the clinician must diligently and consistently monitor the patient's medical and periodontal stability. Medical history dialog should include pregnancy complications, previous miscarriages, and recent history of cramping, spotting, or pernicious vomiting. The patient's obstetrician should be contacted to discuss her medical status, periodontal or dental needs, and the proposed treatment plan.

Establishing a healthy oral environment and maintaining optimal oral hygiene levels are primary objectives in the pregnant patient. A preventive periodontal program consisting of nutritional counseling and rigorous plaque control measures in the dental office and at home should be reinforced.

Plaque Control. The increased tendency for gingival inflammation during pregnancy should be clearly explained to the patient so that acceptable oral hygiene techniques may be taught, reinforced, and monitored throughout pregnancy. Scaling, polishing, and root planing may be performed whenever necessary during pregnancy. Some practitioners avoid the use of high-alcohol-content antimicrobial rinses in pregnant women and prefer to use non–alcohol-based oral rinses.

Prenatal Fluoride. The prescribing of prenatal fluoride supplements has been an area of controversy. Although two studies have claimed beneficial results,[29,30] others suggest that the clinical efficacy of prenatal fluoride supplements is uncertain, and that the mechanism by which prenatal fluorides might impart cariostasis is unclear.[73]

The American Dental Association (ADA) does not recommend the use of prenatal fluoride because its efficacy has not been demonstrated. The American Academy of Pediatric Dentistry supports this position as well. The American Academy of Pediatrics has no stated position on prescribing prenatal fluorides.

Treatment

Elective Dental Treatment. Other than good plaque control, it is prudent to avoid elective dental care if possible during the first trimester and the last half of the third trimester. The first trimester is the period of organogenesis, when the fetus is highly susceptible to environmental influences. In the last half of the third trimester, a hazard of premature delivery exists because the uterus is very sensitive to external stimuli. Prolonged chair time may need to be avoided because the woman is most uncomfortable at this time. Further, *supine hypotensive syndrome* may occur. In a semireclining or supine position, the great vessels, particularly the inferior vena cava, are compressed by the gravid uterus. By interfering with venous return, this compression will cause maternal hypotension, decreased cardiac output, and eventual loss of consciousness. Supine hypotensive syndrome can usually be reversed by turning the patient on her left side, thereby removing pressure on the vena cava and allowing blood to return from the lower extremities and pelvic area. A preventive 6-inch soft wedge (rolled towel) should be placed on the patient's right side when she is reclined for clinical treatment.

The second trimester is the safest period for providing routine dental care. The emphasis at this time is on controlling active disease and eliminating potential problems that could arise in late pregnancy. Major oral or periodontal surgery should be postponed until after delivery. "Pregnancy tumors" that are painful, interfere with mastication, or continue to bleed or suppurate after mechanical debridement may require excision and biopsy before delivery. The American Academy of Periodontology (www.perio.org) has developed a position statement regarding the need for providing proper periodontal therapy for pregnant patients.

Dental Radiographs. The safety of dental radiography during pregnancy has been well established, provided features such as high-speed film, filtration, collimation, and lead aprons are used. However, it is most desirable not to have *any* irradiation during pregnancy, especially during the first trimester, because the developing fetus is particularly susceptible to radiation damage.[49] When radiographs are needed for diagnosis, the most important aid for the patient is the protective lead apron. Studies have shown that when an apron is used during contemporary dental radiography, gonadal and fetal radiation is virtually immeasurable.[7]

Even with the obvious safety of dental radiography, x-ray films should be taken selectively during pregnancy and only when necessary and appropriate to aid in diagnosis and treatment. In most cases, only bite-wing, panoramic, or selected periapical films are indicated.

Medications. Drug therapy in the pregnant patient is controversial because drugs can affect the fetus by diffusion across the placenta. Prescriptions should be only the duration absolutely essential for the pregnant patient's well-being and only after careful consideration of potential side effects. The classification system established by the U.S. Food and Drug Administration (FDA) in 1979 to rate fetal risk levels associated with many prescription drugs provides safety guidelines (Box 43-2). The prudent practitioner should consult references such as Briggs et al.'s *Drugs in Pregnancy and Lactation*[12] and Olin's *Drug Facts and Comparisons*[68] for information on the FDA pregnancy risk factor associated with prescription drugs. Ideally, no drug should be administered during pregnancy, especially the first trimester.[49] However, it is sometimes impossible to adhere to this rule. Fortunately, therefore, most common drugs in dental

BOX 43-2

FDA Drug Classification System Based on Potential for Causing Birth Defects

A Controlled studies in women fail to demonstrate a risk to the fetus in the first trimester (there is no evidence of a risk in later trimesters), and the possibility of fetal harm appears remote.
B Either animal reproduction studies have not demonstrated a fetal risk but there are no controlled studies in pregnant women, or animal reproduction studies have shown an adverse effect (other than a decrease in fertility) that was not confirmed in controlled studies in women in the first trimester (and there is no evidence of a risk in later trimesters).
C Either studies in animals have revealed adverse effects on the fetus (teratogenic, embryocidal, or other) and there are no controlled studies in women, or studies in women and animals are not available. Drugs should be given only if the potential benefit justifies the potential risk to the fetus.
D There is positive evidence of human fetal risk, but the benefits from use in pregnant women may be acceptable despite the risk (e.g., if the drug is needed in a life-threatening situation or for a serious disease for which safer drugs cannot be used or are ineffective).
X Studies in animals or humans have demonstrated fetal abnormalities, or there is evidence of fetal risk based on human experience, or both, and the risk of using the drug in pregnant women clearly outweighs any possible benefit. The drug is contraindicated in women who are or who may become pregnant.

practice can be given during pregnancy with relative safety, although there are a few important exceptions; Tables 43-1, 43-2, and 43-3 present general guidelines for anesthetic and analgesic, antibiotic, and sedative-hypnotic drugs, respectively.[79,91] In particular, antibiotics are often needed in periodontal therapy. The effect of a particular medication on the fetus depends on the type of antimicrobial, dosage, trimester, and duration of the course of therapy.[69] Research regarding subgingival irrigation and local site delivery in relation to the developing fetus is inadequate at this date.

Breastfeeding. Usually, there is a risk that the drug can enter breast milk and be transferred to the nursing infant, in whom exposure could have adverse effects (Tables 43-4 and 43-5). Unfortunately, there is little conclusive information about drug dosage and effects through breast milk; however, retrospective clinical studies and empiric observations coupled with known pharmacologic pathways allow recommendations to be made.[49] The amount of drug excreted in breast milk is usually not more than 1% to 2% of the maternal dose; therefore it is highly unlikely that most drugs have any pharmacologic significance for the infant.[88,98]

The mother should take prescribed drugs just after breastfeeding and then avoid nursing for 4 hours or more, if possible,[49,88] to decrease the drug concentration in breast milk.

ORAL CONTRACEPTIVES

Women may have responses to oral contraceptives (OCs) similar to those seen in pregnant patients. An exaggerated response to local irritants occurs in gingival tissues. Inflammation ranges from mild edema and erythema to severe inflammation with hemorrhagic or hyperplasic gingival tissues. It has been reported that more exudate is present in inflamed gingival tissues of OC users than in pregnant women.[86,100]

Investigators have suggested several mechanisms for the heightened response in gingival tissues. Kalkwarf[39] reported that the response may be caused by an altered microvasculature, increased gingival permeability, and increasing synthesis of prostaglandin. Prostaglandin E, a potent mediator of inflammation,[24] appears to rise significantly with increasing levels of sex hormones. Jensen et al.[38] found dramatic microbial changes in pregnant and OC groups compared with a nonpregnant group. A 16-fold increase in *Bacteroides* species was noted in the OC group versus the nonpregnant group, despite no statistically significant clinical differences in gingival index or GCF flow. The authors stated that the increased female sex hormones substituting for the naphthaquinone requirement of certain *Bacteroides* species were most likely responsible for this increase.

The OC-associated gingival inflammation may become chronic (vs. that of acute inflammation of pregnancy) because of the extended periods that women are exposed to elevated levels of estrogen and progesterone.[41,72] Some have reported that the inflammation increases with prolonged use of OCs. Kalkawarf[39] did not find that duration of use made a significant difference; however, the brand used resulted in different responses. Further studies need to be performed in relation to dosage, duration, and type of OC used in association with the periodontium. The concentration of female sex hormones in current OCs is significantly less than that of the 1970s, with the same level of contraceptive efficacy.

Salivary composition changed notably in patients taking OCs in studies from the 1970s. A decreased concentration of protein, sialic acid, hexosamine fucose, hydrogen ions, and total electrolytes has been reported. Salivary flow rates were increased in one report[54] and decreased in 30% of subjects in another report.[22]

The dental literature reports that women taking OCs experience a twofold to threefold increase in the incidence of localized osteitis after extraction of mandibular third molars.[89] The higher incidence of osteitis is these patients may be attributed to the effects of OCs (estrogens) on clotting factors. However, a number of studies refute these finding.[14] Evidence thus far is inconclusive on osteitis after third molar extraction and OC use.

Also, a spotty melanotic pigmentation of the skin may occur with OC use. This suggests a relationship between the use of OCs and the occurrence of gingival melanosis,[35] especially in fair-skinned individuals.

TABLE 43-1

Local Anesthetic and Analgesic Administration during Pregnancy

Drug	FDA Category (Prescription Drug)	During Pregnancy
Local Anesthetics*		
Lidocaine	B	Yes
Mepivacaine	C	Use with caution; consult physician.
Prilocaine	B	Yes
Bupivacaine	C	Use with caution; consult physician.
Etidocaine	B	Yes
Procaine	C	Use with caution; consult physician.
Articaine	B	Yes; no blocks
Analgesics		
Aspirin	C/D, third trimester	Caution; avoid in third trimester.
Acetaminophen	B	Yes
Ibuprofen	B/D, third trimester	Caution; avoid in third trimester.
Codeine†	C	Use with caution; consult physician.
Hydrocodone†	B	Use with caution; consult physician.
Oxycodone†	B	Use with caution; consult physician.
Propoxyphene	C	Use with caution; consult physician.

*Can use vasoconstrictors if necessary.
†Avoid prolonged use.
FDA, U.S. Food and Drug Administration.

TABLE 43-2

Antibiotic Administration during Pregnancy

Drug(s)	FDA Category (Prescription Drug)	During Pregnancy	Risks
Penicillins	B	Yes	Diarrhea
Erythromycin	B	Yes; avoid estolate form.	Intrahepatic jaundice in mother
Clindamycin	B	Yes, with caution	Drug concentrated in fetal bone, spleen, lung, and liver
Cephalosporins	B	Yes	Limited information
Tetracycline	D	Avoid.	Depression of bone growth, enamel hypoplasia, gray-brown tooth discoloration
Ciprofloxacin	C	Avoid.	Possible developing cartilage erosion
Metronidazole	B	Avoid; controversial.	Theoretic carcinogenic data in animals
Gentamicin	C	Caution; consult physician.	Limited information Ototoxicity
Vancomycin	C	Caution; consult physician.	Limited information
Clarithromycin	D	Avoid; use only if potential benefit justifies risk to fetus.	Limited information Adverse effects on pregnancy, outcome, and embryo/fetal development in animals

Management

Medical histories should include OCs under the heading of "Medications," and an oral dialog should include questions regarding OCs in women of childbearing age. The patient should be informed of the oral and periodontal side effects of OCs and the need for meticulous home care and compliance with periodontal maintenance.

Treatment of gingival inflammation exaggerated by OCs should include establishing an oral hygiene program and eliminating local predisposing factors. Periodontal surgery may be indicated if resolution after initial therapy (scaling and root planing) is inadequate. It may be advisable to perform extraction of teeth (especially of

TABLE 43-3

Sedative-Hypnotic Drug Administration during Pregnancy

Drug(s)	FDA Category	During Pregnancy
Benzodiazepines	D	Avoid.
Barbiturates	D	Avoid.
Nitrous oxide	Not assigned	Avoid in first trimester; otherwise use with caution; consult physician.

TABLE 43-4

Local Anesthetic and Analgesic Administration during Breastfeeding

Drug	During Breastfeeding
Local Anesthetics	
Lidocaine	Yes
Mepivacaine	Yes
Prilocaine	Yes
Bupivacaine	Yes
Etidocaine	Yes
Procaine	Yes
Analgesics	
Aspirin	Avoid.
Acetaminophen	Yes
Ibuprofen	Yes
Codeine	Yes
Hydrocodone	No data
Oxycodone	Yes
Propoxyphene	Yes

TABLE 43-5

Antibiotic and Sedative-Hypnotic Administration during Breastfeeding

Drug(s)	During Breastfeeding
*Antibiotics**	
Penicillins	Yes
Erythromycin	Yes
Clindamycin	Yes, with caution
Cephalosporins	Yes
Tetracycline	Avoid.
Ciprofloxacin	Avoid.
Metronidazole	Avoid.
Gentamicin	Avoid.
Vancomycin	Avoid.
Sedative-Hypnotics	
Benzodiazepines	Avoid.
Barbiturates	Avoid.
Nitrous oxide	Yes

*Antibiotics have the risk of diarrhea and sensitization in the mother and infant.

third molars) on nonestrogenic days (days 23-28) of the OC cycle to reduce the risk of a postoperative localized osteitis[26]; however, evidence of this association is inconclusive and warrants further investigation.

Although the results from animal studies have demonstrated antibiotic interference adversely affecting contraceptive sex hormone levels, several human studies have failed to support such an interaction.[6,27,61,63] This issue is controversial, and antibiotics possibly could render OCs ineffective in preventing pregnancies. In 1991 an ADA report stated that all women of childbearing age should be informed of possible reduced efficacy of steroid OCs during antibiotic therapy and advised women to use additional forms of contraception during short-term antibiotic therapy.[4] During long-term antibiotic therapy, they should consult their physician about using high-dose OC preparations. Although only research regarding oral manifestations attributed to OCs has been reported in the literature, the same effects presumably could occur with the use of contraceptive implants. Similarly, the remote possibility of reduced efficacy of the contraceptive implant with concurrent antibiotic administration also exists, and woman can adhere to the same precautions as with OC use.

MENOPAUSE

Female life expectancy is 80+ years, so many women will live 40% of their lives in menopause. This cohort represents a large number of the patients that present in clinical practices. Therefore, dental clinicians must be aware of the effects of reduced hormones on the periodontal tissues as well as the systemic changes that may manifest.

Throughout a woman's lifetime, the number of oocytes steadily diminishes. Menopause is associated with symptoms of estrogen deficiency. Estradiol levels fall gradually in the years before menopause. Levels of FSH and LH begin to rise, and levels of sex hormones begin to fluctuate. This stage of "perimenopause" is characterized by increasing ovarian unresponsiveness, and thus sporadic ovulation ensues. Anovulatory cycles indicate low estradiol and progesterone because of absent corpus luteum function.

Oral Changes

It is important for the clinician to recognize the effect of hormonal alterations on the oral cavity as well as systemic and psychologic changes. Oral changes in menopause include thinning of the oral mucosa, oral discomfort ("burning mouth"), gingival recession, xerostomia, altered taste sensation, alveolar bone loss, and alveolar ridge resorption.

Fluctuations of sex hormones during menopause have been implicated as factors in inflammatory changes in the human gingiva, hypertrophy, or atrophy. Estrogen affects cellular proliferation, differentiation, and keratinization of the gingival epithelium. Hormone receptors have been identified in basal and spinous layers of the epithelium and connective tissue,[4] implicating gingiva and other oral tissues as targets to manifest hormone deficiencies. Sex steroids are known to have a direct effect on connective tissue, with estrogens increasing the intracellular fluid content. Estrogen deficiency can lead to a reduction in collagen formation in connective tissues, resulting in a decrease in skin thickness.[97] Alterations in collagen affect tissues such as joints, hair, nails, and glands. Mohammed et al.[58] noted significantly increased recession in postmenopausal patients with low bone density.

Osteopenia and osteoporosis have been associated with the menopausal patient. *Osteopenia* is a reduction in bone mass caused by an imbalance between bone resorption and formation, favoring resorption and resulting in demineralization and osteoporosis. *Osteoporosis* is a disease characterized by low bone mass and fragility and a consequent increase in fracture risk.[95] In most women, peak bone mass occurs between 20 and 30 years of age, then declines. Menopause accelerates declining bone mass.[93] An estimated 25 million Americans have osteoporosis, 80% of whom are female. Ongoing studies are examining the association of postmenopausal primary osteoporosis with mandibular and maxillary bone mineral density, tooth loss, alveolar ridge atrophy, and clinical periodontal attachment loss. The effects of hormone replacement therapy (HRT) or estrogen replacement therapy (ERT) on the oral bone and tooth loss also are under investigation. Evidence indicates a probable association between osteoporosis and tooth loss as well as alveolar bone loss.[37,71,80,81]

Clinical Management

It is the clinician's responsibility to review the patient's medical history and keep information up to date. Because of possible alterations in oral soft and osseous tissues during perimenopause and after menopause, appropriate questioning regarding hormone changes should be performed and documented. The many available therapies for HRT/ERT, from prescriptions to holistic approaches, need to be followed. Many medications may alter clotting times, prolong the effects of other medications, and interfere with absorption or effectiveness of prescription medications.

If gingival and mucosal tissue thinning occurs, soft tissue augmentation may be performed. Brushing with an extrasoft toothbrush using the "toe" or "heel" of the brush may prevent "scrubbing" the thinning gingiva. Dentifrices with minimal abrasive particles should be used. Rinses should have low alcohol concentration. During periodontal maintenance, root surfaces should be debrided gently with minimal soft tissue trauma. Oral pain may result from thinning tissues, xerostomia, inadequate nutritional intake, or hormone depletion. In patients with oral symptoms who receive HRT, symptoms may be significantly reduced.

If the patient is susceptible to osteoporosis (menopausal, Caucasian or Asian, smoker, minimal physical activity, low calcium intake, thin build or low body weight {<58 kg}, systemic disease associated with predisposition, genetic history),[37] the dentist should consult the patient's physician as to the risks versus benefits of HRT/ERT and calcium/vitamin D supplementation for the individual patient. Sodium fluoride, biphosphonates (e.g., alendronate), selective estrogen receptor modulators, and parathyroid hormone may be other therapies for the osteoporotic patient. Close monitoring of the patient's periodontal stability, performing titrated periodontal maintenance, informing the patient about potential risks of hormone depletion on the oral tissues, and consulting the treating physician are advised. The National Institutes of Health (NIH 1994 Conference on Optimal Calcium Intake) recommends 1000 mg of calcium per day for premenopausal women and 1500 mg/day for postmenopausal women (Box 43-3).

BOX 43-3

National Institutes of Health (NIH) Consensus Conference Recommendations for Optimal Calcium Intake

Premenopausal women (25-50 years old):	1000 mg/day
Postmenopausal women (estrogen therapy):	1000 mg/day
Postmenopausal women (no estrogen therapy):	1500 mg/day
Men (25-65 years old):	1000 mg/day
Women and men >65 years old:	1500 mg/day

To date, no data are available regarding success or failure with periodontal regeneration procedures in osteoporotic versus nonosteoporotic individuals. Also, no scientific data are available to contraindicate the use of osseointegrated implants in osteoporotic patients, despite articles stating osteoporosis as a risk factor. Much research is needed to address the increasing number of patients who may present to periodontal practices with osteoporosis or osteopenia, most of whom will be undiagnosed.

CONCLUSION

Clinical periodontal therapy includes an understanding of the clinician's role in the total health and well-being of female patients. Dentists do not treat localized infections without affecting other systems (and fetus or

SCIENCE TRANSFER

Clinicians have a responsibility to master all the specific responses that require additional considerations in the periodontal care of women.

It is well recognized that a patient's response to microbial challenges can change over time and can be influenced by a number of factors. These changes can occur in the inflammatory reaction to the challenge or in the immune response. The episodic changes in host response can result in periods of periodontal tissue breakdown or stability. *Superimposed on these changes, female patients have alternations caused by the hormonal changes that occur throughout their life.*

Hormonal changes in women occur at puberty, monthly, during pregnancy, and at menopause and result in inflammatory and immune-related consequences. Thus, when treating female patients, the clinician must always be aware of exaggerated responses to microbial plaque. This awareness must also be reflected in the treatment plan. Further, it is now clear that periodontal infections can likewise affect the female patient systemically. For example, untreated periodontal disease may be associated with a higher risk for adverse pregnancy outcomes, emphasizing the bidirectionality of periodontal-systemic connections. *This means that all pregnant women should be evaluated for periodontal disease and that appropriate treatment should be given to control periodontal inflammation.*

Understanding the role of gingival tissues as target organs for estrogen and progesterone forms the basis for periodontal care of female patients. In menopause the osteopenic effects make periodontal disease more severe, and these patients require careful long-term management and counseling about dietary calcium. *Clinicians need to take the initiative and become familiar with all these systemic relationships and to initiate treatment coordination with the woman's physician.*

breast-fed infant). Therefore, female patients may present with periodontal and systemic considerations that alter conventional therapy.

The cyclic nature of the female sex hormones often is reflected in the gingival tissues as initial signs and symptoms. Medical histories and dialogs should include thoughtful investigation of the individual patient's problems and needs. Questioning should reflect hormonal stability and medications associated with regulation. Patients should be educated regarding the profound effects the sex hormones may play on periodontal and oral tissues as well as the consistent need for home and office removal of local irritants.

Research regarding female issues and medical/periodontal therapy is in process. In the near future, information regarding specific management and etiology of sex hormone–mediated infections will enhance our ability to provide quality care to our patients.

REFERENCES

1. Aboul-Dahab OM, el-Sherbiny MM, Abdel-Rahman R, et al: Identification of lymphocytes subsets in pregnancy, *Egypt Dent J* 40:653, 1994.
2. American Academy of Periodontology: Position paper: Periodontal disease as a potential risk factor for systemic disease, *J Periodontol* 69:841, 1998.
3. American Dental Association (ADA), Council on Access, Prevention, and Interpersonal Relations: *Women's oral health issues,* Chicago, 1995, ADA.
4. American Dental Association Health Foundation Research Institute, Department of Toxicology: Antibiotic interference with oral contraceptives, *J Am Dent Assoc* 122:79, 1991.
5. Aschkenazi S, Naftolin F, Mor G: Menopause, sex hormones and the immune system, *Menopause Manag* 9:6, 2000.
6. Back DJ, Orme M: Pharmacokinetic drug interactions with oral contraceptives, *Clin Pharmacokinet* 18:472, 1990.
7. Bean LR Jr, Devore WD: The effects of protective aprons in dental roentgenography, *Oral Surg* 28:505, 1969.
8. Bhashkar SN, Jacoway JR: Pyogenic granuloma: clinical features, incidence, histology, and results of treatment report of 242 cases, *J Oral Surg* 24:391, 1966.
9. Bischof P, Lauber K, Girard JP, et al: Circulating levels of pregnancy proteins and depression of lymphoblastogenesis during pregnancy, *J Clin Lab Immunol* 12:93, 1983.
10. Brabin BJ: Epidemiology of infection in pregnancy, *Rev Infect Dis* 7:579, 1985.
11. Brannstrom M, Friden BE, Jasper M, Norman RJ: Variations in peripheral blood levels of immunoreactive tumor necrosis factor alpha throughout the menstrual cycle and secretion of TNF-α from the human corpus luteum, *Curr J Obstet Gynecol Reprod Biol* 83:213, 1999.
12. Briggs GG, Freeman RK, Yaffe SJ: *Drugs in pregnancy and lactation,* ed 4, Baltimore, 1994, Williams & Wilkins.
13. Brown S, Bonifaz DZ: An overview of anorexia and bulimia nervosa and the impact of eating disorders on the oral cavity, *Compend Contin Educ Dent* 14:1594, 1993.
14. Cohen ME, Simecek JW: Effects of gender-related factors on the incidence of localized alveolar osteitis, *Oral Surg Oral Med Oral Pathol* 79:416, 1995.
15. Cruikshank O, Hayes PM: Maternal physiology. In Gabbe S, Niebyl JR, Simpson JL, editors: *Pregnancy in obstetrics: normal and problem pregnancies,* New York, 1986, Churchill Livingstone.
16. Cutolo M, Sulli A, Seriolo B, et al: Estrogens, the immune response and autoimmunity, *Clin Exp Rheumatol* 13:217, 1995.
17. Damare SM, Wells S, Offenbacher S: Eicosanoids in periodontal diseases: potential for systemic involvement, *Adv Exp Med Biol* 433:23, 1997.
18. Dasanayake AP: Poor periodontal health of the pregnant woman as a risk, *Ann Periodontol* 3:206, 1998.
19. Davenport ES, Williams CE, Sterne JA, et al: The East London study of maternal chronic periodontal disease and preterm low birth weight infants: study design and prevalence, *Ann Periodontol* 3:213, 1998.
20. DeLiefde B: The dental care of pregnant women, *NZ Dent J* 80:41, 1984.
21. El-Ashiry G: Comparative study of the influence of pregnancy and oral contraceptives on the gingivae, *Oral Surg* 30:472, 1970.

22. El-Ashiry G, El-Kafrawy AH, Nasr MF, et al: Effects of oral contraceptives on the gingiva, *J Periodontol* 42:273, 1971.
23. El-Attar TM: Prostaglandin F2 in human gingiva in health and disease and its stimulation by female sex steroids, *Prostaglandins* 11:331, 1976.
24. El-Attar TM, Roth GD, Hugoson A: Comparative metabolism of 4-C progesterone in normal and chronically inflamed human gingival tissue, *J Periodontal Res* 8:79, 1973.
25. Ferguson MM, Carter J, Boyle P: An epidemiological study of factors associated with recurrent aphthae in women, *J Oral Med* 39:212, 1984.
26. Fleisher AB Jr, Resnick SD: The effect of antibiotics in the efficacy of oral contraceptives, *Arch Dermatol* 125:1582, 1980.
27. Fraser IS, Jansen RP: Why do inadvertent pregnancies occur in oral contraceptive users? Effectiveness of oral contraceptive regimens and interfering factors, *Contraception* 27:531, 1983.
28. Gibbs RS, Romero R, Hillier SL, et al: A review of premature birth and subclinical infections, *Am J Obstet* 166:1515, 1992.
29. Glenn FB: Immunity conveyed by a fluoride supplement during pregnancy, *J Dent Child* 44:391, 1977.
30. Glenn FB, Glenn WD III, Duncan RC: Fluoride tablet supplementation during pregnancy for caries immunity: a study of the offspring produced, *Am J Obstet Gynecol* 143:560, 1982.
31. Grant D, Stern J, Listgarten M: The epidemiology, etiology, and public health aspects of periodontal disease. In Grant D, Stern J, Listegarten M, editors: *Periodontics,* St Louis, 1988, Mosby.
32. Grossi SG, Jeffcoat MK, Genco RJ: Osteopenia, osteoporosis, and oral disease. In Rose LR, Genco RJ, Cohen DW, et al, editors: *Periodontal medicine,* New York, 2000, BC Decker.
33. Gusberti FA, Mombelli A, Lang NP, et al: Changes in subgingival microbiota during puberty, *J Clin Periodontol* 17:685, 1990.
34. Hanson L, Sobol SM, Abelson T: The otolaryngologic manifestations of pregnancy, *J Fam Pract* 23:151, 1986.
35. Hertz RS, Beckstead PC, Brown WJ: Epithelial melanosis of the gingiva possibly resulting from the use of oral contraceptives, *J Am Dent Assoc* 100:173, 1980.
36. Jeffcoat MK: Osteoporosis: a possible modifying factor in oral bone loss, *Ann Periodontol* 3:312, 1998.
37. Jeffcoat MK, Lewis CE, Reddy MS, et al: Postmenopausal bone loss and its relationship to oral bone loss, *Periodontol 2000* 23:94, 2000.
38. Jensen J, Lilijmack W, Blookquist C: The effect of female sex hormones on subgingival plaque, *J Periodontol* 52:599, 1981.
39. Kalkwarf KL: Effect of oral contraceptive therapy on gingival inflammation in humans, *J Periodontol* 49:560, 1978.
40. Kinnby B, Matsson L, Astedt B: Aggravation of gingival inflammatory symptoms during pregnancy associated with the concentration of activator inhibitor type 2 (PAI-2) in gingival fluid, *J Periodontal Res* 31:271, 1996.
41. Knight GM, Wade AB: The effects of oral contraceptives on the human periodontium, *J Periodontol Res* 9:18, 1974.
42. Kornman K, Loseche JF: Direct interaction of estradiol and progesterone with *Bacteroides melaninogenicus, J Dent Res* 58A:10, 1979.
43. Kornman KS, Loesche WJ: The subgingival flora during pregnancy, *J Periodontol* 15:111, 1980.
44. Lapp CA, Thomas ME, Lewis JB: Modulation by progesterone of interleukin-6 production by gingival fibroblasts, *J Periodontol* 66:279, 1995.
45. Lieff S, Boggess KA, Murtha AP, et al: The oral conditions and pregnancy study: periodontal status of a cohort of pregnant women, *J Periodontol* 75:116, 2004.
46. Levin RP: Pregnancy gingivitis, *Md State Dent Assoc* 30:27, 1987.
47. Lindhe J, Branemark P: Changes in microcirculation after local application of sex hormones, *J Periodontal Res* 2:185, 1967.
48. Lindhe J, Branemark P: Changes in vascular permeability after local application of sex hormones, *J Periodontal Res* 2:259, 1967.
49. Little JW, Falace DA: *Dental management of the medically compromised patient,* ed 4, St Louis, 1993, Mosby.
50. Löe H, Silness J: Periodontal disease in pregnancy. 1. Prevalence and severity, *Acta Odontol Scand* 21:533, 1984.
51. Lopatin DE, Kornman KS, Loesche WJ: Modulation of immunoreactivity to periodontal disease-associated microorganisms during pregnancy, *Infect Immun* 28:713, 1980.
52. Lundgren D, Magnssen B, Lindhe J: Connective tissue alterations in gingiva of rats treated with estrogens and progesterone, *Odontology* 24:49, 1973.
53. Machtei EE, Mahler D, Sanduri H, Peled M: The effect of the menstrual cycle on periodontal health, *J Periodontol* 75:408, 2004.
54. Magnusson T, Ericson T. Hugoson A: The effect of oral contraceptives on some salivary substance in women, *Arch Oral Biol* 20:119, 1975.
55. Mandel L, Kaynar A: Bulimia and parotid swelling: a review and case report, *J Oral Maxillofac Surg* 50:1122, 1992.
56. Miyagi M, Morishita M, Iwamoto Y: Effect of sex hormones on production of prostaglandin E_2 by human peripheral monocytes, *J Periodontol* 64:1075, 1993.
57. Miyagi M, Aoyama H, Morishita M, et al: Effects of sex hormones on chemotaxis of polymorphonuclear leukocytes and monocytes, *J Periodontol* 63:28, 1992.
58. Mohammed AR, Brunsvold M, Bauer R: The strength of association between systemic postmenopausal osteoporosis and periodontal disease, *Int J Prosthet* 9:479, 1996.
59. Mombelli A, Rutar A, Lan NP: Correlation of the periodontal status 6 years after puberty with clinical and microbiological conditions during puberty, *J Clin Periodontol* 22:300, 1995.
60. Muramatsu Y, Takaesu Y: Oral health status related to subgingival bacterial flora and sex hormones in saliva during pregnancy, *Bull Tokyo Dent Coll* 35:139, 1994.
61. Murphy AA, Zacur HA, Charache P, et al: The effect of tetracycline on levels of oral contraceptives, *Am J Obstet Gynecol* 164:28, 1991.
62. Nakagawa S, Fujii H, Machida Y, et al: A longitudinal study from prepuberty to puberty of gingivitis: correlation between the occurrence of *Prevotella intermedia* and sex hormones, *J Clin Periodontol* 21:658, 1994.
63. Neely JL, Abate M, Swinker M, et al: The effect of doxycycline on serum levels on ethinyl estradiol, norethindrone, and endogenous progesterone, *Obstet Gynecol* 77:416, 1991.
64. O'Neil TC: Maternal T-lymphocyte response and gingivitis in pregnancy, *J Periodontol* 50:178, 1979.
65. Offenbacher S, Jared HL, O'Reilly PG, et al: Potential pathogenic mechanisms of periodontitis associated pregnancy complications, *Ann Periodontol* 3:233, 1998.
66. Offenbacher S, Katz V, Fertik G, et al: Periodontal infection as a possible risk factor for preterm low birthweight, *J Periodontol* 67(suppl):1103, 1996.
67. Ojanotko-Harri AO, Harri MP, Hurrita HP, et al: Altered tissue metabolism of progesterone in pregnancy gingivitis and granuloma, *J Clin Periodontol* 18:262, 1991.
68. Olin BR: *Drug facts and comparisons,* St Louis, 1994, Kluwer.

69. Otomo-Corgel J: Systemic considerations for female patients. In *Antibiotic/antimicrobial use in dental practice,* Tokyo, 1990, Quintessence.
70. Pack AR, Thomson ME: Effects of topical and systemic folic acid supplementation on gingivitis in pregnancy, *J Clin Periodontol* 7:402, 1980.
71. Paganini-Hill A: Benefits of estrogen replacement therapy on oral health: the leisure world cohort, *Arch Intern Med* 155:2325, 1995.
72. Pankhurst CL: The influence of oral contraceptive therapy on the periodontium: duration of drug therapy, *J Periodontol* 52:617, 1981.
73. *Pediatric Dentistry* special issue: Reference manual, *Pediatr Dent* 16(7), 1994.
74. Pinard A: Gingivitis in pregnancy, *Dent Register* 31:258, 1877.
75. Pitcarin J: A case of disease of the gums [that] occurred during pregnancy, *Dubing Hosp Rep* 2:309, 1818.
76. Raber-Durlacher JE, van Steenbergen TJ, van der Velden U: Experimental gingivitis during pregnancy and postpartum: clinical, endocrinological and microbiological aspects, *J Clin Periodontol* 21:549, 1994.
77. Raber-Durlacher JE, Leene W, Palmer-Bouva CC, et al: Experimental gingivitis during pregnancy and postpartum: immunohistochemical aspects, *J Periodontol* 64:211, 1993.
78. Raber-Durlacher JE, Zeylemaker WP, Meinesz AA, et al: CD4 to CD8 ratio and in vitro lymphoproliferative responses during experimental gingivitis in pregnancy and postpartum, *J Periodontol* 62:663, 1991.
79. Reese RE, Betts RF: *Handbook of antibiotics,* ed 2, Boston, 1993, Little, Brown.
80. Reinhardt RA, Payne JB, Maze C, et al: Gingival fluid IL-beta in postmenopausal females on supportive periodontal therapy: a longitudinal 2-year study, *J Clin Periodontol* 25:1029, 1998.
81. Reinhardt RA, Payne JB, Maze CA, et al: Influence of estrogen and osteopenia/osteoporosis on clinical periodontitis in postmenopausal women, *J Periodontol* 70:823, 1999.
82. Robb-Nicholson C: PMS: it's real, *Harv Women Health Watch* 1(11):2, 1994.
83. Robb-Nicholson C: Gastroesophageal reflux disease, *Harv Women Health Watch* 4(6):4, 1999.
84. Samant A, Malik CP, Chabra SK, et al: Gingivitis and periodontal disease in pregnancy, *J Periodontol* 47:415, 1976.
85. Schuurs A, Verheul H: Effects of gender and sex steroids on the immune response and autoimmune disease, *J Steroid Biochem* 35:157, 1990.
86. Sooriyamoorthy M, Gower DB: Hormonal influences on gingival tissues: relationship to periodontal disease, *J Clin Periodontol* 16:201, 1989.
87. Sridama V, Pacini F, Yang SL, et al: Decreased levels of helper T cells: a possible cause of immunodeficiency in pregnancy, *N Engl J Med* 307:352, 1982.
88. Steinberg BJ: Sex hormonal alterations. In Rose LD, Kay D, editors: *Internal medicine for dentistry,* ed 2, St Louis, 1990, Mosby.
89. Sweet JB, Butler DP: Increased incidence of postoperative localized osteitis in mandibular 3rd molar surgery associated with patients using oral contraceptives, *Am J Obstet Gynecol* 127:518, 1977.
90. Thomson ME, Pack AR: Effects of extended systemic and topical folate supplementation on gingivitis in pregnancy, *J Clin Periodontol* 9:275, 1982.
91. Turner M, Aziz SR: Management of the pregnant oral and maxillofacial surgery patient, *J Oral Maxillofac Surg* 60:1479, 2002.
92. Valdimarsson H, Mulholland C, Fridriksdottir V, et al: A longitudinal study of leukocyte blood counts and lymphocyte responses in pregnancy: a marked early increase of monocyte-lymphocyte ratio, *Clin Exp Immunol* 53:437, 1983.
93. Vinco L, Prallet B, Chappard D, et al: Contributions of chronological age, age at menarche and menopause and of anthropometric parameters to axial and peripheral bone densities, *Osteoporosis Int* 2:153, 1992.
94. Vittek J, Gordon G, Rappaport C, et al: Specific progesterone receptors in rabbit gingiva, *J Periodontal Res* 17:657, 1982.
95. Wactawski-Wende J, Grossi SG, Trevisan M, et al: The role of osteopenia in oral bone loss and periodontal disease, *J Periodontol* 67:1076, 1996.
96. Whitacre CC, Reingold SC, O'Looney PA: A gender gap in autoimmunity, *Science* 283:1277, 1999.
97. Whitehear MI, Whitcroft SI, Hillard TC: *An atlas of the menopause,* New York, 1993, Parthenon.
98. Wilson JT, Brown RD, Cherek DR, et al: Drug excretion in human breast milk: principles, pharmacokinetics and projects consequences, *Clin Pharmacokinet* 5:1, 1980.
99. Zachariasen RD: Ovarian hormones and oral health: pregnancy gingivitis, *Compend Contin Educ Dent* 10:508, 1989.
100. Zachariasen RD: The effects of elevated ovarian hormones on periodontal health: oral contraceptives and pregnancy, *Women Health* 20(2):21, 1993.
101. Zoeller J: The top 200 drugs, *Am Druggist,* 1999, p 41.

Periodontal Treatment of Medically Compromised Patients

Brian L. Mealey, Perry R. Klokkevold, and Joan Otomo-Corgel

CHAPTER 44

Chapter Outline

Many patients seeking dental care have significant medical conditions that may alter both the course of their oral disease and the therapy provided. The older age of the average periodontal patient increases the likelihood of underlying disease. Therefore the therapeutic responsibility of the clinician includes identification of the patient's medical problems to formulate proper treatment plans. Thorough medical histories are paramount.[67] If significant findings are unveiled, consultation with or referral of the patient to an appropriate physician may be indicated. This ensures correct patient management and provides medicolegal coverage to the clinician.

This chapter covers common medical conditions and associated periodontal management. Review of each topic area is general, and the reader is encouraged to consult other references for more detailed coverage of specific disorders. Understanding these conditions will enable the clinician to treat the total patient, not merely the periodontal reflection of underlying disease.

CARDIOVASCULAR DISEASES

Cardiovascular diseases are the most prevalent category of systemic disease in the United States and many other countries, and they are more common with increasing age.[89] Health histories should be closely scrutinized for cardiovascular problems. These conditions include hypertension, angina pectoris, myocardial infarction, previous cardiac bypass surgery, previous cerebrovascular accident, congestive heart failure, presence of cardiac pacemakers or automatic cardioverter-defibrillators, and infective endocarditis.

In most cases the patient's physician should be consulted, especially if stressful or prolonged treatment is anticipated. Short appointments and a calm, relaxing

SCIENCE TRANSFER

This chapter covers a wide range of systemic conditions that either compromise periodontal treatment or require special precautions before therapy.

Patients will present with a broad array of medical conditions, ranging from undiagnosed to diagnosed conditions and from those at some stage of treatment to those that may have been treated in the past. For this reason, *the clinician needs to be familiar with a large number of diseases and systemic/medical conditions and their consequences.* Likewise, many common medications have either periodontal implications or implications for periodontal therapy.

In many cases, consultation with the patient's physician is indicated. This is consistent with a team approach to treatment and can involve interdisciplinary care. The dental clinician should also remember *that the periodontal-systemic connection works both ways and that either can influence the other.* Current and readily accessible reference materials can be extremely helpful in this regard.

Appropriate emergency drugs and equipment must always be available, and the clinical staff must be trained in their use.

environment help minimize stress and maintain hemodynamic stability.

Hypertension

Hypertension, the most common cardiovascular disease, affects more than 50 million American adults, many of whom are undiagnosed.[31] In 2003 the National Heart, Lung and Blood Institute issued revised guidelines for evaluation and management of hypertension.[11,12,33] These "JNC-7 guidelines"[11] simplified the classification of blood pressure (Table 44-1).

Compared with previous classification schemes,[38,39] the JNC-7 guidelines emphasize the importance of *systolic* blood pressure (BP) greater than 140 mm Hg. Systolic BP greater than 140 mm Hg is considered a greater risk factor for cardiovascular disease than elevated diastolic pressure. JNC-7 also introduced a BP category known as *prehypertension.* People with systolic BP between 120 and 139 mm Hg or diastolic BP between 80 and 89 mm Hg are classified as "prehypertensive." Prehypertension replaces the previous category of "high normal" BP. In addition, "frank" hypertension is now classified into only two categories, versus three under past classification schemes. *Stage 1 hypertension* is defined by systolic pressure of 140 to 159 mm Hg or diastolic pressure of 90 to 99 mm Hg. *Stage 2 hypertension* is defined by a systolic pressure greater than 160 mm Hg or diastolic pressure greater than 100 mm Hg.

Hypertension is not diagnosed on a single elevated BP recording. Rather, classification is usually based on the average value of two or more BP readings taken at two

TABLE 44-1

Classification of Adult Blood Pressure

Classification	Systolic Blood Pressure (mm Hg)	Diastolic Blood Pressure (mm Hg)	Dental Treatment Modifications
Normal	<120	and <80	No changes in dental treatment.
Prehypertension	120-139	or 80-89	No changes in dental treatment; monitor blood pressure (BP) at each appointment.
Stage 1 hypertension	140-159	or 90-99	Inform patient of findings. Routine medical consultation/referral. Monitor BP at each appointment. No changes in dental treatment; minimize stress.
Stage 2 hypertension	≥160	≥100	Inform patient. Medical consultation/referral. Monitor BP at each appointment. If systolic BP is <180 and diastolic is <110, perform selective dental care (routine exam, prophylaxis, restorative nonsurgical endodontics and periodontics); minimize stress. If systolic BP ≥180 or diastolic ≥100, give immediate medical consultation/referral, and perform emergency dental care only (to alleviate pain, bleeding, infection);* minimize stress. Consider stress reduction protocol.

*Risk of providing emergency dental care must outweigh risk of possible hypertensive complications. See references 11, 12, and 32.

or more appointments. The higher value of either the systolic or diastolic pressure determines the patient's classification. Patients with hypertension enter the dental practice every day and are particularly common among the older population seen in most periodontal practices. Evidence from the Framingham Heart Study revealed that people with normal BP at age 55 still have a 90% risk of becoming hypertensive later in life.[90]

Hypertension is divided into primary and secondary types. *Primary* (essential) *hypertension* occurs when no underlying pathologic abnormality can be found to explain the disease. Approximately 95% of all hypertensive patients have primary hypertension. The remaining 5% have *secondary hypertension,* in which an underlying etiology can be found and often treated. Examples of the conditions responsible for secondary hypertension are renal disease, endocrinologic changes, and neurogenic disorders.

In early hypertension the patient may be asymptomatic. If not identified and diagnosed, hypertension may persist and increase in severity, leading eventually to coronary artery disease, angina, myocardial infarction, congestive heart failure, cerebrovascular accident, or kidney failure.[45] The dental office can play a vital role in the detection of hypertension and maintenance care of the patient with hypertensive disease. The first dental office visit should include two BP readings spaced at least 10 minutes apart, which are averaged and used as a baseline. Before the clinician refers a patient to a physician because of elevated BP, readings should be taken at a minimum of two appointments, unless the measurements are extremely high (i.e., systolic pressure >180 mm Hg or diastolic pressure >100 mm Hg). The periodontal recall system is an ideal method for hypertension detection and monitoring. Almost three of every four adult patients with hypertension in the United States do not control their BP well enough to attain the goal of systolic pressure less than 140 mm Hg and diastolic pressure less than 90 mm Hg.[7] Lack of compliance with antihypertensive therapy is the primary reason for this failure. Dentists can help achieve greater success in managing hypertension by taking BP readings at each periodontal recall visit.

Periodontal procedures should not be performed until accurate BP measurements and histories have been taken to identify those patients with significant hypertensive disease. The time of day should be recorded along with the BP reading because blood pressure varies significantly throughout the day.[60] Table 44-1 outlines appropriate medical referral or consultation and dental treatment modifications, depending on the patient's stage of hypertension.

Dental treatment for hypertensive patients is generally safe as long as stress is minimized.[45,51] If a patient is currently receiving antihypertensive therapy, consultation with the physician may be warranted regarding the current medical status, medications, periodontal treatment plan, and patient management. Many physicians are not knowledgeable about the nature of specific periodontal procedures. The dentist must inform the physician regarding the estimated degree of stress, length of the procedures, and complexity of the individualized treatment plan. Morning dental appointments were once suggested for hypertensive patients. However, recent evidence indicates that BP generally increases around awakening and peaks at midmorning.[5,60,82] Lower BP levels occur in the afternoon; therefore, afternoon dental appointments may be preferred.

No routine periodontal treatment should be given to a patient who is hypertensive and not under medical management. For patients with systolic BP greater than 180 mm Hg or diastolic BP greater than 110 mm Hg, treatment should be limited to emergency care until hypertension is controlled. Analgesics are prescribed for pain and antibiotics for infection. Acute infections may require surgical incision and drainage, although the surgical field should be limited because excessive bleeding may be seen with elevated BP.

When treating hypertensive patients, the clinician should not use a local anesthetic containing an epinephrine concentration greater than 1:100,000, nor should a vasopressor be used to control local bleeding. Local anesthesia without epinephrine may be used for short procedures (<30 minutes). In a patient with hypertensive disease, however, it is important to minimize pain by providing profound local anesthesia to avoid an increase in endogenous epinephrine secretion.[45,51] The benefits of the small doses of epinephrine used in dentistry far outweigh the potential for hemodynamic compromise. The smallest possible dose of epinephrine should be used, and aspiration before injection of local anesthetics is critical. Intraligamentary injection is generally contraindicated because hemodynamic changes are similar to intravascular injection.[81] If the hypertensive patient exhibits anxiety, use of conscious sedation in conjunction with periodontal procedures may be warranted.[86]

Beta-adrenergic receptor antagonists, or β-blockers, are typically used to treat hypertension (Table 44-2).

TABLE 44-2

Nonselective and Selective β-Adrenergic Receptor Antagonists (β-Blockers)

Generic Name	Trade Name
Nonselective β-Blockers	
Carvedilol	Coreg
Carteolol hydrochloride	Cartrol
Nadolol	Corgard
Penbutolol sulfate	Levatol
Pindolol	Visken
Propranolol hydrochloride	Inderal; Inderal LA
Timolol maleate	Blocadren
Selective β-Blockers	
Acebutolol hydrochloride	Sectral
Atenolol	Tenormin
Betaxolol hydrochloride	Kerlone
Bisoprolol fumarate	Zebeta
Metoprolol tartrate	Lopressor
Metoprolol succinate	Toprol-XL

β-Blockers are either *cardioselective,* blocking only β-1 cardiac receptors (β_1 receptors), or *nonselective,* blocking both β-1 cardiac receptors and β-2 peripheral receptors (β_2 receptors). Epinephrine, an α-adrenergic and β-adrenergic agonist, produces an increase in heart rate through direct stimulation of cardiac β-1 receptors. Epinephrine also stimulates α-adrenergic receptors, producing vasoconstriction of arteries, as well as β-2 receptors, causing vasodilation of skeletal muscle arterioles. Administration of local anesthetics containing epinephrine to patients taking nonselective β-blockers (e.g., propranolol, nadolol) may cause elevated BP.[96] Epinephrine-induced α-adrenergic stimulation results in vasoconstriction and increased BP. Because the patient's nonselective medication has blocked the β-2 receptors, epinephrine will not stimulate the normal compensatory β-2 receptor–induced vasodilation. This may result in dramatically increased BP, followed by reflex bradycardia mediated by the vagus nerve and carotid baroreceptors. The end result is a patient with severe hypertension and bradycardia, resulting in a dangerous decrease in vascular perfusion and possible death. Because of this potential complication, epinephrine-containing local anesthetics should be used cautiously and only in very small amounts in patients taking nonselective β-blockers, with careful monitoring of vital signs.[45,96]

The clinician should be aware of the many side effects of various antihypertensive medications. *Postural hypotension* is common and can be minimized by slow positional changes in the dental chair.[45] *Depression* is a side effect of which many patients are unaware. Nausea, sedation, oral dryness, lichenoid drug reactions, and gingival overgrowth are associated with certain classes of antihypertensive agents.[51]

Ischemic Heart Diseases

Ischemic heart disease includes disorders such as angina pectoris and myocardial infarction (Figure 44-1). *Angina pectoris* occurs when myocardial oxygen demand exceeds supply, resulting in temporary myocardial ischemia.[33] Patients with a history of *unstable* angina pectoris (angina that occurs irregularly or on multiple occasions without predisposing factors) should be treated only for emergencies and then in consultation with their physician. Patients with *stable* angina (angina that occurs infrequently, is associated with exertion or stress, and is easily controlled with medication and rest) can undergo elective dental procedures. Because stress often induces an acute anginal attack, stress reduction is important. Profound local anesthesia is vital, and conscious sedation may be indicated for anxious patients.[86] Supplemental oxygen delivered by nasal cannula may also help prevent intraoperative anginal attacks.

Patients who treat acute anginal attacks with *nitroglycerin* should be instructed to bring their medication to dental appointments. Nitroglycerin should also be kept in the office emergency medical kit. For particularly stressful procedures, the patient may take a nitroglycerin tablet preoperatively to prevent angina, although this generally is not necessary. The patient's nitroglycerin should be readily accessible on the dental tray in case it is needed during treatment. Because the shelf life of nitroglycerin is relatively short, the expiration date of the patient's nitroglycerin should be noted, as should the expiration date of the nitroglycerin in the office's emergency medical kit. Also, patients with angina may be taking longer-acting forms of nitroglycerin (tablet, patch), β-blockers, or calcium channel blockers (also used in treatment of hypertension) for prevention of angina. Restrictions on use of local anesthetics containing epinephrine are similar to those for the patient with hypertension. In addition, intraosseous injection with epinephrine-containing local anesthetics using special systems (e.g., Stabident, Fairfax Dental) should be done cautiously in patients with ischemic heart disease, because it results in transient increases in heart rate and myocardial oxygen demand.[64]

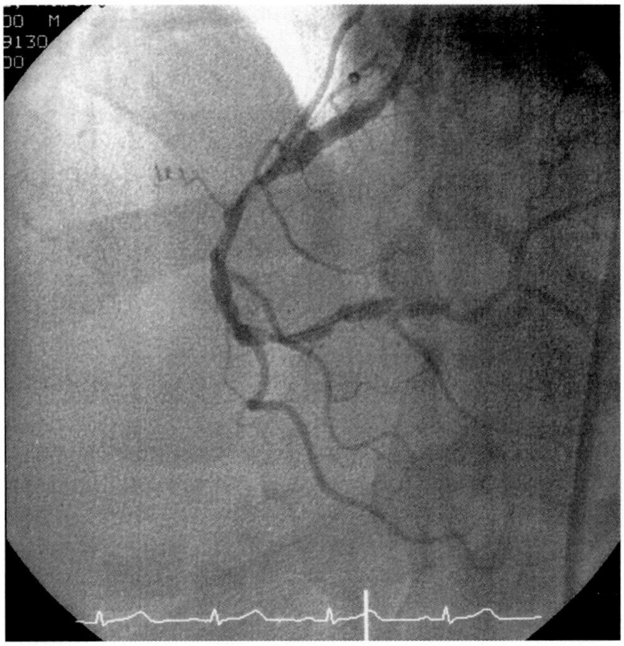

Figure 44-1 Coronary angiogram. Atherosclerosis can result in narrowing of the coronary arteries and onset of signs and symptoms of ischemic heart disease.

If the patient becomes fatigued or uncomfortable or has a sudden change in heart rhythm or rate during a periodontal procedure, the procedure should be discontinued as soon as possible. A patient who has an anginal episode in the dental chair should receive the following emergency medical treatment:

1. Discontinue the periodontal procedure.
2. Administer 1 tablet (0.3-0.6 mg) of nitroglycerin sublingually.
3. Reassure the patient, and loosen restrictive garments.
4. Administer oxygen with the patient in a reclined position.
5. If the signs and symptoms cease within 3 minutes, complete the periodontal procedure if possible, making sure that the patient is comfortable. Terminate the procedure at the earliest convenient time.

6. If the anginal signs and symptoms do not resolve with this treatment within 2 to 3 minutes, administer another dose of nitroglycerin, monitor the patient's vital signs, call the patient's physician, and be ready to accompany the patient to the emergency department.
7. A third nitroglycerin tablet may be given 3 minutes after the second. Chest pain that is not relieved by 3 tablets of nitroglycerin indicates likely myocardial infarction. The patient should be transported to the nearest emergency medical facility immediately.

Myocardial infarction (MI) is the other category of ischemic heart disease encountered in dental practice. Dental treatment is generally deferred for at least 6 months after MI because peak mortality occurs during this time.[25] After 6 months, MI patients can usually be treated using techniques similar to those for the stable angina patient.

Cardiac (aortocoronary) bypass, femoral artery bypass, angioplasty, and endarterectomy have become common surgical procedures in patients with ischemic heart disease. If one of these procedures was performed recently, the physician should be consulted before elective dental therapy to determine the degree of heart damage or arterial occlusive disease, the stability of the patient's condition, and the potential for infective endocarditis or graft rejection. Prophylactic antibiotics are not usually necessary for cardiac bypass patients unless recommended by the cardiologist.

Congestive Heart Failure

Congestive heart failure (CHF) is a condition in which the pump function of the heart is unable to supply sufficient amounts of oxygenated blood to meet the body's needs.[25] CHF usually begins with left ventricular failure caused by a disproportion between the hemodynamic load and the capacity to handle that load. CHF may be caused by a chronic increase in workload (as in hypertension or aortic, mitral, pulmonary, or tricuspid valvular disease), direct damage to the myocardium (as in MI or rheumatic fever), or an increase in the body's oxygen requirements (as in anemia, thyrotoxicosis, or pregnancy).

Patients with poorly controlled or untreated CHF are not candidates for elective dental procedures. These individuals are at risk for sudden death, usually from ventricular arrhythmias.[24] For patients with treated CHF, the clinician should consult with the physician regarding the severity of CHF, underlying etiology, and current medical management. Medical management of CHF may include use of calcium channel blockers, direct vasodilators, diuretics, angiotensin-converting enzyme (ACE) inhibitors, α-receptor blockers, and cardiotonic agents such as digoxin.[22,41] Each of these medications has potential side effects that may have an impact on periodontal therapy. Because of the presence of *orthopnea* (inability to breathe unless in an upright position) in some CHF patients, the dental chair should be adjusted to a comfortable level for the patient rather than being placed in a supine position. Short appointments, stress reduction with profound local anesthesia and possibly conscious sedation, and use of supplemental oxygen should be considered.[25,45]

Cardiac Pacemakers and Implantable Cardioverter-Defibrillators

Cardiac arrhythmias are most often treated with medications; however, some are also treated with implantable pacemakers or automatic cardioverter-defibrillators.[24,45,66] Pacemakers are usually implanted in the chest wall and enter the heart transvenously. Automatic cardioverter-defibrillators are more often implanted subcutaneously near the umbilicus and have electrodes passing into the heart transvenously or directly attached to the epicardium. Consultation with the patient's physician allows determination of the underlying cardiac status, the type of pacemaker or automatic cardioverter-defibrillator, and any precautionary measures to be taken. Older pacemakers were unipolar and could be disrupted by dental equipment that generated electromagnetic fields, such as ultrasonic and electrocautery units. Newer units are bipolar and are generally not affected by dental equipment. Automatic cardioverter-defibrillators activate without warning when certain arrhythmias occur. This may endanger the patient during dental treatment because such activation often causes sudden patient movement. Stabilization of the operating field during periodontal treatment with bite blocks or other devices can prevent unexpected trauma.

Infective Endocarditis

Infective endocarditis (IE) is a disease in which microorganisms colonize the damaged endocardium or heart valves.[27] Although the incidence of IE is low, it is a serious disease with a poor prognosis, despite modern therapy. The term *infective endocarditis* is preferred to the previous term *bacterial endocarditis* because the disease can also be caused by fungi and viruses. The organisms most often encountered in IE are α-hemolytic streptococci (e.g., *Streptococcus viridans*). However, nonstreptococcal organisms often found in the periodontal pocket have been increasingly implicated, including *Eikenella corrodens, Actinobacillus actinomycetemcomitans, Capnocytophaga,* and *Lactobacillus* species.[4]

IE has been divided into acute and subacute forms. The *acute* form involves virulent organisms, generally nonhemolytic streptococci and strains of staphylococci, which invade normal cardiac tissue, produce septic emboli, and cause infections that run a rapid, generally fatal course. The *subacute* form, on the other hand, results from colony formation on damaged endocardium or heart valves by low-grade pathogenic organisms; the classic example is rheumatic carditis consequent to rheumatic fever.

The risk for IE varies with the underlying disorder (Box 44-1).[16,17] The high-risk category includes patients at high risk of developing IE after dental-induced bacteremia and those in whom the resultant IE is associated with high morbidity and mortality. The moderate-risk category includes patients at higher risk for IE than the general population.

BOX 44-1

Heart Conditions Associated with Infective Endocarditis (IE)*

Endocarditis Prophylaxis Recommended

High-risk patients

Previous history of IE

Prosthetic heart valves

Major congenital heart disease

- Tetralogy of Fallot
- Transposition of great arteries
- Single-ventricle states
- Surgically constructed systemic pulmonary shunts or conduits

Moderate-risk patients

Acquired valvular dysfunction (e.g., rheumatic heart disease)

Most other congenital heart malformations

Hypertrophic cardiomyopathy

Mitral valve prolapse with valvular regurgitation, thickened leaflets, or both

Endocarditis Prophylaxis Not Recommended (No Greater Risk than General Population)

Mitral valve prolapse without valvular regurgitation

Previous coronary artery bypass graft surgery

Physiologic, functional, or innocent heart murmurs

Previous rheumatic fever without valvular dysfunction

Cardiac pacemakers and implanted defibrillators

Isolated secundum atrial septal defect

Surgically repaired atrial septal defect, ventricular septal defect, or patent ductus arteriosus

Previous Kawasaki disease without valvular dysfunction

*Recommendations by the American Heart Association.[16,17]

The practice of periodontics is intimately concerned with the prevention of IE. Because dental procedures that involve bleeding may induce a transient bacteremia, the American Heart Association (AHA) recommends antibiotic prophylaxis before procedures "associated with significant bleeding from hard or soft tissues, periodontal surgery, scaling and professional teeth cleaning."[17] However, bacteremia may occur even in the absence of dental procedures, especially in individuals with poor oral hygiene and significant periodontal inflammation. Thus, prevention of periodontal inflammation is paramount. The AHA states that patients who are at risk for IE should "establish and maintain the best possible oral health to reduce potential sources of bacterial seeding." To provide adequate preventive measures for IE, the clinician's major concern should be to reduce the microbial population in the oral cavity so as to minimize soft tissue inflammation and bacteremia.

Preventive measures to reduce the risk of IE should consist of the following:

1. *Define the susceptible patient.* A careful medical history will disclose the previously mentioned susceptible patients. Health questioning should cover history of all potential categories of risk (see Box 44-1). If any doubt exists, the patient's physician should be consulted.
2. *Provide oral hygiene instruction.* Oral hygiene should be practiced with methods that improve gingival health but minimize bacteremia. In patients with significant gingival inflammation, oral hygiene should initially be limited to gentle procedures (i.e., oral rinses and gentle toothbrushing with a soft brush) to minimize bleeding. As gingival health improves, more aggressive oral hygiene may be initiated. Oral irrigators are generally not recommended because their use may induce bacteremia.[55] Susceptible patients should be encouraged to maintain the highest level of oral hygiene once soft tissue inflammation is controlled.
3. *During periodontal treatment, currently recommended antibiotic prophylactic regimens should be practiced with all susceptible patients* (Table 44-3). If any doubt regarding susceptibility exists, the patient's physician should be consulted. In patients who have been receiving continuous oral penicillin for secondary prevention of rheumatic fever, penicillin-resistant α-hemolytic streptococci are occasionally found in the oral cavity. It therefore is recommended that an alternate regimen be followed instead. Likewise, if the periodontal patient is taking a systemic antibiotic as part of periodontal therapy, changes in the IE prophylaxis regimen may be indicated. For example, a patient currently taking a penicillin agent after regenerative therapy may be placed on azithromycin before the next periodontal procedure. Patients with early-onset forms of periodontitis often have high levels of *Actinobacillus actinomycetemcomitans* in the subgingival plaque. This organism has been associated with IE and is often resistant to penicillins. Therefore, in patients with early-onset periodontitis who are also at risk for IE, Slots et al.[80] suggested using tetracycline, 250 mg, four times daily for 14 days to eliminate or reduce *A. actinomycetemcomitans,* followed by the conventional prophylaxis protocol at the time of dental treatment.
4. *Periodontal treatment should be designed for susceptible patients to accommodate their particular degree of periodontal involvement.* The nature of periodontal therapy enhances the problems related to the prophylaxis of subacute IE. Patients are faced with long-term therapy, healing periods that extend beyond a 1-day antibiotic regimen, multiple visits, and procedures that easily elicit gingival bleeding. The following guidelines should aid in the development of periodontal treatment plans for patients susceptible to IE:
   - Periodontal disease is an infection with potentially wide-ranging systemic effects. In patients at risk for IE, every effort should be made to eliminate this infection. Teeth with severe periodontitis and a poor prognosis may require extraction. Teeth with less severe involvement in a motivated patient should be retained, treated, and maintained closely.

TABLE 44-3

Recommended Antibiotic Prophylaxis Regimens for Periodontal Procedures in Adults at Risk for Infective Endocarditis

Regimen	Antibiotic	Dosage
Standard oral regimen	Amoxicillin	2.0 g 1 hour before procedure
Alternate regimen for patients allergic to amoxicillin/penicillin	Clindamycin	600 mg 1 hour before procedure
	or	
	Azithromycin or clarithromycin	500 mg 1 hour before procedure
	or	
	Cephalexin or cefadroxil*	2.0 g 1 hour before procedure
Patients unable to take oral medications	Ampicillin	2.0 g intramuscularly or intravenously within 30 minutes before procedure
Patients unable to take oral medications *and* allergic to penicillin	Clindamycin	600 mg intravenously within 30 minutes before procedure (must be diluted and injected slowly)
	or	
	Cefazolin*	1.0 g intramuscularly or intravenously within 30 minutes before procedure

Children's dosages are lower. See References 16 and 17.
*Cephalosporins should *not* be used in patients with immediate-type hypersensitivity reactions to penicillins (e.g., urticaria, angioedema, anaphylaxis).

- All periodontal treatment procedures (including probing) require antibiotic prophylaxis; gentle oral hygiene methods are excluded. Pretreatment chlorhexidine rinses are recommended before all procedures, including periodontal probing, because these oral rinses significantly reduce the presence of bacteria on mucosal surfaces.[17]
- To reduce the number of visits required and thereby minimize the risk of developing resistant bacteria, numerous procedures may be accomplished at each appointment, depending on the patient's needs and ability to tolerate dental treatment.[45]
- When possible, allow at least 7 days between appointments (preferably 10-14 days). If this is not possible, select an alternative antibiotic regimen for appointments within a 7-day period.
- Evidence does not support or refute a need to place patients at risk for IE on extended antibiotic regimens after treatment.[45] Therefore, patients who have had periodontal surgery are not generally placed on antibiotics for the first week of healing (unless there are specific indications to do so). If patients are placed on such regimens, the dosages are inadequate to prevent endocarditis during ensuing appointments. Therefore the standard prophylactic antibiotic dose is still needed. For example, if a patient was placed on 250 mg of amoxicillin three times a day for 10 days after periodontal surgery and was returning to the office for more treatment on the seventh day, the patient would still require a full 2.0-g dose of amoxicillin before that treatment. Alternatively, clindamycin or azithromycin could be used at the second appointment.
- The need for antibiotic prophylaxis before simple suture removal is controversial; some authors suggest it is needed, whereas others think prophylaxis is unnecessary. When possible, sutures that resorb in a short time, such as chromic gut, may be indicated for patients at risk of IE.
- Regular recall appointments, with an emphasis on oral hygiene reinforcement and maintenance of periodontal health, are extremely important in the IE patient population.

Cerebrovascular Accident

A cerebrovascular accident (CVA), or *stroke,* results from ischemic changes (e.g., cerebral thrombosis caused by an embolus) or hemorrhagic phenomena. Hypertension and atherosclerosis are predisposing factors for CVA and should alert the clinician to evaluate the patient's medical history carefully for the possibility of early cerebrovascular insufficiency and to be aware of symptoms of the disease. A physician's referral should precede periodontal therapy if the signs and symptoms of early cerebrovascular insufficiency are evident.

To prevent a repeat stroke, active infections should be treated aggressively because even minor infection may alter blood coagulation and trigger thrombus formation and ensuing cerebral infarction. The clinician should counsel the patient about the importance of thorough oral hygiene.[68] Poststroke weakness of the facial area or paralysis of extremities may make oral hygiene procedures extremely difficult.[54] The clinician may need to modify oral hygiene instruments for ease of use, perhaps in consultation with an occupational therapist. Long-term chlorhexidine rinses may greatly aid in plaque control.

Dental clinicians should treat post-CVA patients with the following guidelines in mind:

1. No periodontal therapy (unless for an emergency) should be performed for 6 months because of the high risk of recurrence during this period.
2. After 6 months, periodontal therapy may be performed using short appointments with an emphasis on minimizing stress. Profound local anesthesia should be obtained using the minimal effective dose of local anesthetic agents. Concentrations of epinephrine greater than 1:100,000 are contraindicated.
3. Light conscious sedation (inhalation, oral, or parenteral) may be used for anxious patients. Supplemental oxygen is indicated to maintain thorough cerebral oxygenation.
4. Stroke patients are frequently placed on oral anticoagulants. For procedures that entail significant bleeding, such as periodontal surgery or tooth extraction, the anticoagulant regimen may need adjustment, depending on the level of anticoagulation at which the patient is maintained. Changes in anticoagulant regimens for a stroke patient should always be done in consultation with the patient's physician.
5. Blood pressure should be monitored carefully. Recurrence rates for CVAs are high, as are rates of associated functional deficits.

ENDOCRINE DISORDERS

Diabetes

The diabetic patient requires special precautions before periodontal therapy. The two major types of diabetes are *type 1* (formerly known as "insulin-dependent diabetes") and *type 2* (formerly called "non–insulin-dependent diabetes").[47] Over the past decade, the medical management of diabetes has changed significantly in an effort to minimize the debilitating complications associated with this disease.[20,88] Patients are more tightly managing their blood glucose levels (glycemia) through diet, oral agents, and insulin therapy.[46]

If the clinician detects intraoral signs of undiagnosed or poorly controlled diabetes, a thorough history is indicated.[63] The classic signs of diabetes include *polydipsia* (excessive thirst), *polyuria* (excessive urination), and *polyphagia* (excessive hunger, often with unexplained concurrent weight loss). If the patient has any of these signs or symptoms, or if the clinician's index of suspicion is high, further investigation with laboratory studies and physician consultation is indicated. Periodontal therapy has limited success in the presence of undiagnosed or poorly controlled diabetes.

If a patient is suspected of having undiagnosed diabetes, the following procedures should be performed:

1. Consult the patient's physician.
2. Analyze laboratory tests (Box 44-2): fasting blood glucose and casual glucose.[3]

BOX 44-2

Diagnostic Criteria for Diabetes Mellitus

Diabetes mellitus may be diagnosed by any one of three different laboratory methods. Whichever method is used, *it must be confirmed on a subsequent day* by using any one of the three methods.

1. *Symptoms of diabetes plus casual (nonfasting) plasma glucose ≥200 mg/dl.* Casual glucose may be drawn at any time of day without regard to time since the last meal. Classic symptoms of diabetes include polyuria, polydipsia, and unexplained weight loss.
2. *Fasting plasma glucose ≥126 mg/dl.* "Fasting" is defined as no caloric intake for at least 8 hours. (Normal fasting glucose is 70-100 mg/dl.)
3. *Two-hour postprandial glucose ≥200 mg/dl during an oral glucose tolerance test.** The test should be performed using a glucose load containing the equivalent of 75 g of anhydrous glucose dissolved in water. (Normal 2-hour postprandial glucose is <140 mg/dl.)

Data from American Diabetes Association: *Diabetes Care* 26(suppl 1):5, 2003.

*The third method is *not* recommended for routine clinical use.

BOX 44-3

Laboratory Evaluation of Diabetes Control: Glycosylated Hemoglobin Assay (Hb A_{1c})*

4%-6%	Normal
<7%	Good diabetes control
7%-8%	Moderate diabetes control
>8%	Action suggested to improve diabetes control

*American Diabetes Association guidelines.

3. Rule out acute orofacial infection or severe dental infection; if present, provide emergency care immediately.
4. Establish best possible oral health through nonsurgical debridement of plaque and calculus; institute oral hygiene instruction. Limit more advanced care until diagnosis has been established and good glycemic control obtained.

If a patient is known to have diabetes, it is critical that the level of glycemic control be established before initiating periodontal treatment. The fasting glucose and casual glucose tests provide "snapshots" of the blood glucose concentration at the time the blood was drawn; these tests reveal nothing about long-term glycemic control. The primary test used to assess glycemic control in a known diabetic individual is the *glycosylated* (or glycated) *hemoglobin* (Hb) *assay* (Box 44-3). Two different tests are available, the Hb A_1 and the Hb A_{1c} assay; the *Hb A_{1c}*

(also HbA1c) is used more often.[46] This assay reflects blood glucose concentrations over the preceding 6 to 8 weeks and may provide an indication of the potential response to periodontal therapy. Patients with relatively well-controlled diabetes (Hb A_{1c} <8%) usually respond to therapy in a manner similar to nondiabetic individuals.[13,84,94] Poorly controlled patients (Hb A_{1c} >10%) often have a poor response to treatment, with more postoperative complications and less favorable long-term results.[47,84]

As discussed in Chapter 17, periodontal infection may worsen glycemic control and should be managed aggressively. Diabetic patients with periodontitis should receive oral hygiene instructions, mechanical debridement to remove local factors, and regular maintenance. When possible, an Hb A_{1c} of less than 10% should be established before surgical treatment is performed. Systemic antibiotics are not needed routinely, although recent evidence indicates that tetracycline antibiotics in combination with scaling and root planing may positively influence glycemic control. If the patient has poor glycemic control and surgery is absolutely needed, prophylactic antibiotics may be given; penicillins are most often used for this purpose. Frequent reevaluation after active therapy is needed to assess treatment response and prevent recurrence of periodontitis.

Almost all diabetic patients use *glucometers* for immediate blood glucose self-monitoring. These devices use capillary blood from a simple finger stick to provide blood glucose readings in seconds. Diabetic patients should be asked whether they have glucometers and how often they use them. Because these devices provide instantaneous assessment of blood glucose, they are highly beneficial in the dental office environment. The following guidelines should be observed:

1. Patients should be asked to bring their glucometer to the dental office at each appointment.
2. Patients should check their blood glucose before any long procedure to obtain a baseline level. Patients with blood glucose levels at or below the lower end of normal before the procedure may become hypoglycemic intraoperatively. It is advisable to have such a patient consume some carbohydrate before starting treatment. For example, if a 2-hour procedure is planned and the pretreatment glucose level is 70 mg/dl (lower end of normal range), providing 4 oz of juice preoperatively may help prevent hypoglycemia during treatment. If pretreatment glucose levels are excessively high, the clinician should determine whether or not the patient's glycemic control has been poor recently. This can be done by thorough patient questioning and by determining the most recent Hb A_{1c} values. If glycemic control has been poor over the preceding few months, the procedure may need to be postponed until better glycemic control is established. If glycemic control has been good, and the currently high glucometer reading is a fairly isolated event, the surgical procedure may proceed.
3. If the procedure lasts several hours, it is often beneficial to check the glucose level during the procedure to ensure that the patient does not become hypoglycemic.
4. After the procedure, the blood glucose can be checked again to assess fluctuations over time.
5. Any time the patient feels symptoms of hypoglycemia, blood glucose should be checked immediately. This may prevent onset of severe hypoglycemia, a medical emergency.

BOX 44-4

Signs and Symptoms of Hypoglycemia

Shakiness or tremors
Confusion
Agitation and anxiety
Sweating
Tachycardia
Dizziness
Feeling of "impending doom"
Unconsciousness
Seizures

The most common dental office complication seen in diabetic patients taking insulin is symptomatic low blood glucose, or *hypoglycemia* (Box 44-4). Hypoglycemia is also associated with the use of numerous oral agents (Table 44-4). In patients receiving conscious sedation, the warning signs of an impending hypoglycemic episode may be masked, making the patient's glucometer one of the best diagnostic aids. Hypoglycemia does not usually occur until blood glucose levels fall below 60 mg/dl. However, in patients with poor glycemic control who have prolonged *hyperglycemia* (high blood glucose levels), a rapid drop in glucose can precipitate signs and symptoms of hypoglycemia at levels well above 60 mg/dl.

As medical management of diabetes has intensified over the last decade, the incidence of severe hypoglycemia has risen.[21] The clinician should question diabetic patients about past episodes of hypoglycemia. Hypoglycemia is more common in patients with better glycemic control. When planning dental treatment, it is best to schedule appointments before or after periods of peak insulin activity. This requires knowledge of the pharmacodynamics of the drugs being taken by the diabetic patient. Patients taking insulin are at greatest risk, followed by those taking sulfonylurea agents. Metformin and thiazolidinediones generally do not cause hypoglycemia (see Table 44-4).

Insulins are classified as rapid-acting, short-acting, intermediate-acting, or long-acting agents (Table 44-5). The categories vary in their onset, peak, and duration of activity. It is important that the clinician establish exactly which insulins the diabetic patient takes, the amount, the number of times per day, and the time of the last dose. Periodontal treatment often can be timed to avoid peak insulin activity. Many diabetic patients take multiple injections each day, in which case it is difficult, if not impossible, to avoid peak insulin activity. Checking the pretreatment glucose with the patient's glucometer, checking again during long procedures, and checking

TABLE 44-4

Oral Agents Used in Management of Diabetes

Agent	Action	Risk of Hypoglycemia
Sulfonylureas (first generation): Chlorpropamide Tolbutamide Tolazamide	Stimulate pancreatic insulin secretion	++
Sulfonylureas (second generation): Glyburide Glipizide	Stimulate pancreatic insulin secretion	+++
Sulfonylureas (third generation): Glimepiride	Stimulates pancreatic insulin secretion	+
Meglitinides: Repaglinide Nateglinide	Stimulates rapid pancreatic insulin secretion (different mechanism than sulfonylureas)	+
Biguanides: Metformin	Blocks production of glucose by liver; improves tissue sensitivity to insulin	–
Thiazolidinediones: Rosiglitazone Pioglitazone	Improves tissue sensitivity to insulin	–
α-Glucosidase inhibitors: Acarbose Miglitol	Slows absorption of some carbohydrates from gut, decreasing postprandial peaks in glycemia	–
Combination agents	*Combine metformin with either a sulfonylurea or a thiazolidinedione:*	
	Metformin + glyburide	++
	Metformin + glipizide	++
	Metformin + rosiglitazone	–

TABLE 44-5

Types of Insulin

		ACTIVITY		
Type	**Classification**	**Onset**	**Peak**	**Duration**
Lispro/Aspart	Rapid acting	15 minutes	30-90 minutes	<5 hours
Regular	Short acting	30-60 minutes	2-3 hours	4-12 hours
NPH	Intermediate acting	2-4 hours	4-10 hours	14-18 hours
Lente	Intermediate acting	3-4 hours	4-12 hours	16-20 hours
Ultralente	Long acting	6-10 hours	12-16 hours	20-30 hours
Glargine	Long acting	6 to 8 hours	"Peakless" (has no peak in activity)	>24 hours

again at the end of the procedure provide a better understanding of the patient's insulin pharmacodynamics and help prevent hypoglycemia.

If hypoglycemia occurs during dental treatment, therapy should be immediately terminated. If a glucometer is available, the blood glucose level should be checked. Treatment guidelines include the following[46]:

1. Provide approximately 15 g of oral carbohydrate to the patient:
   - 4 to 6 oz of juice or soda
   - 3 or 4 tsp of table sugar
   - Hard candy with 15 g of sugar
2. If the patient is unable to take food or drink by mouth, or if the patient is sedated:
   - Give 25 to 30 ml of 50% dextrose intravenously (which provides 12.5 to 15.0 g of dextrose), *or*
   - Give 1 mg of glucagon intravenously (glucagon results in rapid release of stored glucose from the liver), *or*
   - Give 1 mg of glucagon intramuscularly or subcutaneously (if no intravenous access).

Emergencies resulting from hyperglycemia are rare in the dental office. They generally take days to weeks to develop. However, the glucometer may be used to rule out hyperglycemic emergencies such as diabetic ketoacidosis, a life-threatening event.

Because periodontal therapy may render the patient unable to eat for some time, adjustment in insulin or oral agent dosages may be required. It is absolutely critical that patients eat their normal meal before dental treatment. Taking insulin without eating is the primary cause of hypoglycemia. If the patient is restricted from eating before treatment (e.g., for conscious sedation), normal insulin doses will need to be reduced. As a general guideline, *well-controlled diabetic patients having routine periodontal treatment may take their normal insulin doses as long as they also eat their normal meal.* If the procedures are going to be particularly long, the insulin dose before treatment may need to be reduced. Likewise, if the patient will have dietary restrictions after treatment, insulin or sulfonylurea dosages may need to be reduced.

Consultation with the patient's physician is prudent and allows both practitioners to review the proposed treatment plan and determine any modifications needed. When periodontal surgery is indicated, it is usually best to limit the size of the surgical fields so that the patient will be comfortable enough to resume a normal diet immediately.

Thyroid and Parathyroid Disorders

Periodontal therapy requires minimal alterations in the patient with adequately managed thyroid disease.[59,77] Patients with *thyrotoxicosis* and those with inadequate medical management should not receive periodontal therapy until their conditions are stabilized. Patients with a history of *hyperthyroidism* should be carefully evaluated to determine the level of medical management, and they should be treated in a way that limits stress and infection. Hyperthyroidism may cause tachycardia and other arrhythmias, increased cardiac output, and myocardial ischemia. Medications such as epinephrine and other vasopressor amines should be given with caution in patients with treated hyperthyroidism, although the small amounts used in dental anesthetics rarely cause problems.[77,96] These drugs should not be given to patients with thyrotoxicosis or poorly controlled thyroid disorders. Patients with *hypothyroidism* require careful administration of sedatives and narcotics because of the potential for excessive sedation.

Routine periodontal therapy may be provided to patients with parathyroid disease once that disorder has been identified and the proper medical treatment given. However, patients who have not received medical care may have significant renal disease, uremia, and hypertension. Also, if hypercalcemia or hypocalcemia is present, the patient may be more prone to cardiac arrhythmias.

Adrenal Insufficiency

Acute adrenal insufficiency is associated with significant morbidity and mortality as a result of peripheral vascular collapse and cardiac arrest. Therefore the periodontist should be aware of the clinical manifestations (Box 44-5) and ways of preventing acute adrenal insufficiency in patients with histories of *primary* adrenal insufficiency (Addison's disease) or *secondary* adrenal insufficiency (most often caused by use of exogenous glucocorticosteroids).

BOX 44-5

Manifestations of Acute Adrenal Insufficiency (Adrenal Crisis)

- Mental confusion, fatigue, and weakness
- Nausea and vomiting
- Hypertension
- Syncope
- Intense abdominal pain, lower back pain, and leg pain
- Loss of consciousness
- Coma

The use of systemic corticosteroids is common in patients with allergic, endocrine, respiratory, joint, intestinal, neurologic, renal, liver, skin, and connective tissue disorders. Significant complications associated with corticosteroid use include alterations in glucose metabolism (steroid-induced diabetes), increased risk of infection, altered wound healing, osteoporosis, skin disorders, cataracts, glaucoma, and suppression of the hypothalamic-pituitary-adrenal (HPA) axis.[29,45] In the normal healthy patient, stress activates the HPA axis, stimulating increased endogenous cortisol production by the adrenal glands. Exogenous steroids may suppress the HPA axis and impair the patient's ability to respond to stress with increased endogenous cortisol production, leading to the potential for acute adrenal crisis (see Box 44-5). The degree of adrenal suppression depends on the drugs used, dose, duration of administration, time elapsed since steroid therapy was terminated, and route of administration.

It has been common practice in the past to administer prophylactic systemic steroids before dental treatment for patients who are taking or who recently have taken exogenous steroids. Such steroid supplementation may not be required for many periodontal procedures.[29] In fact, *adrenal crisis* is rare in dentistry, especially when associated with secondary adrenal suppression caused by steroid use.[50] Shapiro et al.[76] found that patients taking 5 to 20 mg/day prednisone maintained at least some adrenal reserve after immediate termination of steroid therapy. Higher doses may suppress the adrenal glands to a greater degree. Although exogenous steroids may suppress normal adrenal cortisol secretion for an extended period, the ability of the adrenal gland to respond to stress may return quickly after termination of steroid therapy.

Despite its rarity, the severe consequences of adrenal crisis suggest caution in patient management. Before providing extensive dental treatment to a patient with a history of recent or current steroid use, physician consultation is indicated to determine whether the patient's periodontal needs and proposed treatment plan suggest a requirement for supplemental steroids. Use of a stress

TABLE 44-6

Equivalent Doses of Corticosteroids

Corticosteroid	Equivalent Dose (mg)
Cortisone	25
Hydrocortisone	20
Prednisone	5
Prednisolone	5
Methyl prednisone	5
Methylprednisolone	4
Triamcinolone	4
Dexamethasone	0.75
Betamethasone	0.6

reduction protocol and profound local anesthesia may help minimize the physical and psychologic stress associated with therapy and reduce the risk of acute adrenal crisis. A rapid assay is available to determine the degree of adrenal reserve by measurement of serum cortisol levels 30 and 60 minutes after intravenous administration of synthetic corticotropin.[76]

There is no set protocol for steroid prophylaxis. Topical corticosteroids generally have minimal HPA effect, and steroid supplementation generally is not required for these patients. For the patient currently receiving systemic steroid therapy, the need for corticosteroid prophylaxis depends on the drug used because of the variance in equivalent therapeutic doses (Table 44-6). Glucocorticosteroid coverage regimens vary, but most provide a twofold to fourfold increase in coverage, depending on the stress produced by the procedure. For patients taking large doses of greater than 20 mg cortisol-equivalent per day and requiring stressful periodontal procedures, doubling or tripling the normal steroid dose 1 hour before the procedure is often recommended. For those patients receiving low doses for short periods (i.e., <1 month), no supplementation is generally warranted. Again, in an emergency situation, increasing the steroid dose before the procedure may decrease the chances of acute adrenal crisis. If emergency treatment is not needed, consultation with the physician before treatment is best.

Management of the patient in an acute adrenal insufficiency crisis is as follows:

1. Terminate periodontal treatment.
2. Summon medical assistance.
3. Give oxygen.
4. Monitor vital signs.
5. Place the patient in a supine position.
6. Administer 100 mg of hydrocortisone sodium succinate (Solu-Cortef) intravenously over 30 seconds or intramuscularly.

RENAL DISEASES

The most common causes of renal failure are glomerulonephritis, pyelonephritis, kidney cystic disease, renovascular disease, drug nephropathy, obstructive uropathy, and hypertension.[30,40] Renal failure may result in severe electrolyte imbalances, cardiac arrhythmias, pulmonary congestion, CHF, and prolonged bleeding.[45] Because the dental management of patients with renal disease may need to be drastically altered, physician consultation is necessary to determine the stage of renal disease, regimen for medical management, and alterations in periodontal therapy. The patient in chronic renal failure has a progressive disease that ultimately may require kidney transplantation or dialysis. It is preferable to treat the patient before, rather than after, transplant or dialysis. The following treatment modifications should be used:

1. Consult the patient's physician.
2. Monitor blood pressure (patients in end-stage renal failure are usually hypertensive).
3. Check laboratory values: *partial thromboplastin time* (PTT), *prothrombin time* (PT), bleeding time, and platelet count; hematocrit; blood urea nitrogen (do not treat if <60 mg/dl); and serum creatinine (do not treat if <1.5 mg/dl).
4. Eliminate areas of oral infection to prevent systemic infection.
   - Good oral hygiene should be established.
   - Periodontal treatment should aim at eliminating inflammation or infection and providing easy maintenance. Questionable teeth should be extracted if medical parameters permit.
   - Frequent recall appointments should be scheduled.
5. Drugs that are nephrotoxic or metabolized by the kidney should not be given (e.g., phenacetin, tetracycline, aminoglycoside antibiotics). Acetaminophen may be used for analgesia and diazepam for sedation. Local anesthetics such as lidocaine are generally safe.[45,65]

The patient who is receiving dialysis requires modifications in treatment planning.[30,40] The three modes of dialysis are intermittent peritoneal dialysis (IPD), chronic ambulatory peritoneal dialysis (CAPD), and hemodialysis. Only hemodialysis patients require special precautions. These patients have a high incidence of viral hepatitis, anemia, and prolonged hemorrhage. The risk for hemorrhage is related to anticoagulation during dialysis, platelet trauma from dialysis, and the uremia that develops with renal failure.[45] Hemodialysis patients have either an internal arteriovenous fistula or an external arteriovenous shunt. This shunt is often located in the arm and must be protected from trauma. Thus, in addition to guidelines for patients with chronic renal disease, the following recommendation are made for those receiving hemodialysis:

1. Screen for hepatitis B and hepatitis C antigens and antibody before any treatment.
2. Provide antibiotic prophylaxis to prevent endarteritis of the arteriovenous fistula or shunt. (IPD and CAPD patients do not generally require prophylactic antibiotics.)
3. Patients receive heparin anticoagulation on the day of hemodialysis. Therefore, provide periodontal treatment on the day *after* dialysis, when the effects of heparinization have subsided. Hemodialysis

treatments are generally performed three or four times a week. (IPD and CAPD patients are not systemically heparinized; therefore they usually do not have the potential bleeding problems associated with hemodialysis.)

4. Be careful to protect the hemodialysis shunt or fistula when the patient is in the dental chair. If the shunt or fistula is placed in the arm, do not cramp the limb; *blood pressure readings should be taken from the other arm.* Do not use the limb for the injection of medication. Patients with leg shunts should avoid sitting with the leg dependent for longer than 1 hour. If appointments last longer, allow the patient to walk about for a few minutes, then resume therapy.
5. Refer the patient to the physician if uremic problems develop, such as uremic stomatitis. To prevent systemic dissemination, refer to the physician if oral infections do not resolve promptly.

The renal transplant patient's greatest foe is infection. Transplant patients take immunosuppressive drugs that greatly reduce resistance to infection.[65] Excessive bleeding may occur during or after periodontal treatment because of drug-induced thrombocytopenia, anticoagulation, or both. A periodontal abscess is a potentially life-threatening situation; therefore a dental team approach should be used *before* transplantation to determine which teeth can be easily maintained. Many organ transplant centers now include dental examination in their standard pretransplant protocol. Teeth with severe bone and attachment loss, furcation invasion, periodontal abscesses, or extensive surgical requirements should be extracted, leaving an easily maintainable dentition. In addition to the recommendations for patients with chronic renal failure, the following should be considered for the renal transplant patient:

1. Hepatitis B and C screening.
2. Determination of level of immune system compromise resulting from antirejection drug therapy.
3. Prophylactic antibiotics (using AHA recommendations). Not all transplant patients require antibiotic coverage, and physician consultation is warranted before prescribing.

LIVER DISEASES

Liver diseases may range from mild conditions to complete liver failure. Major causes of liver disease include drug toxicity, cirrhosis, viral infections (e.g., hepatitis B and C), neoplasms, and biliary tract disorders.[97] Because the liver is the site of production for most of the clotting factors, excessive bleeding during or after periodontal treatment may occur in patients with severe liver disease. Many drugs are metabolized in the liver; thus, liver disease alters normal drug metabolism. Treatment recommendations for patients with liver disease include the following:

1. Consultation with the physician concerning current stage of disease, risk for bleeding, potential drugs to be prescribed during treatment, and required alterations to periodontal therapy.
2. Screening for hepatitis B and C.
3. Check laboratory values for PT and PTT.

PULMONARY DISEASES

The periodontal treatment of a patient with pulmonary disease may require alteration depending on the nature and the severity of the respiratory problem. Pulmonary diseases range from obstructive lung diseases (e.g., asthma, emphysema, bronchitis, acute obstruction) to restrictive ventilatory disorders caused by muscle weakness, scarring, obesity, or any condition that could interfere with effective lung ventilation.[58,69] Combined restrictive-obstructive lung disease may also develop.

The clinician should be aware of the signs and symptoms of pulmonary disease, such as increased respiratory rate, cyanosis, clubbing of the fingers, chronic cough, chest pain, hemoptysis, dyspnea or orthopnea, and wheezing. Patients with these problems should be referred for medical evaluation and treatment. Most patients with chronic lung disease may undergo routine periodontal therapy if they are receiving adequate medical management. Caution should be practiced in relation to any treatment that may depress respiratory function.

Acute respiratory distress may be caused by slight airway obstruction or depression of respiratory function. Because of their limited vital lung capacity, these patients also have decreased cough effectiveness.[69] They must continually deal with the mental anxiety caused by air hunger and alter their position in attempts to improve their ventilatory efficiency.

The following guidelines should be used during periodontal therapy:

1. Identify and refer patients with signs and symptoms of pulmonary disease to their physician.
2. In patients with known pulmonary disease, consult with their physician regarding medications (antibiotics, steroids, chemotherapeutic agents) and the degree and severity of pulmonary disease.
3. Avoid elicitation of respiratory depression or distress:
   - Minimize the stress of a periodontal appointment. The patient with emphysema should be treated in the afternoon, several hours after sleep, to allow for airway clearance.
   - Avoid medications that could cause respiratory depression (e.g., narcotics, sedatives, general anesthetics).
   - Avoid bilateral mandibular block anesthesia, which could cause increased airway obstruction.
   - Position the patient to allow maximal ventilatory efficiency; be careful to prevent physical airway obstruction; keep the patient's throat clear; and avoid excess periodontal packing.
4. In a patient with a history of asthma, especially if asthma attacks are frequent, make sure the patient's medication (inhaler) is available. The inhaler should be readily accessible on the countertop in the dental treatment room.
5. Patients with active fungal or bacterial respiratory diseases should not be treated unless the periodontal procedure is an emergency.

IMMUNOSUPPRESSION AND CHEMOTHERAPY

Immunosuppressed patients have impaired host defenses as a result of an underlying immunodeficiency or drug administration (primarily related to organ transplantation or cancer chemotherapy).[48,74] Because chemotherapy is often cytotoxic to bone marrow, destruction of platelets and red and white blood cells results in thrombocytopenia, anemia, and leukopenia. Immunosuppressed individuals are at greatly increased risk for infection, and even minor periodontal infections can become life threatening if immunosuppression is severe.[61,63] Intraorally, bacterial, viral, and fungal infections may manifest. Patients receiving bone marrow transplantation require special attention because these patients receive extremely high-dose chemotherapy and are particularly susceptible to dissemination of oral infections.

Treatment in these patients should be directed toward the prevention of oral complications that could be life threatening. The greatest potential for infection occurs during periods of extreme immunosuppression; therefore, treatment should be conservative and palliative. It is always preferable to evaluate the patient before initiation of chemotherapy.[48,74] Teeth having a poor prognosis should be extracted, with thorough debridement of remaining teeth to minimize the microbial load. The clinician must teach and emphasize the importance of good oral hygiene. Antimicrobial rinses such as chlorhexidine are recommended, especially for patients with chemotherapy-induced mucositis, to prevent secondary infection.

Chemotherapy is usually performed in cycles, with each cycle lasting several days, followed by intervening periods of myelosuppression and recovery. If periodontal therapy is needed during chemotherapy, it is best done the day *before* chemotherapy is given, when white blood cell counts are relatively high. Coordination with the oncologist is critical. Dental treatment should be done when white cell counts are above 2000/mm^3, with an absolute granulocyte count of 1000 to 1500/mm^3.[45]

RADIATION THERAPY

The use of radiotherapy, alone or in conjunction with surgical resection, is common in the treatment of head and neck tumors. The side effects of ionizing radiation include dramatic perioral changes of significant concern to dental health personnel.[35,49,73] The extent and severity of mucositis, dermatitis, xerostomia, dysphagia, gustatory alteration, radiation caries, vascular changes, trismus, temporomandibular joint degeneration, and periodontal change depend on the type of radiation used, fields of irradiation, number of ports, types of tissues in the fields, and dosage.

Patients scheduled to receive head and neck radiation therapy require dental consultation *at the earliest possible time* to reduce the morbidity of the known perioral side effects.[71] *Preirradiation treatment* depends on the patient's prognosis, compliance, and residual dentition in addition to the fields, ports, dose, and immediacy of radiotherapy. The initial visit should include panoramic and intraoral radiographs, a clinical dental examination, a periodontal evaluation, and a physician consultation. The physician should be asked about the amount of radiation to be administered, extent and location of the lesion, nature of any surgical procedures already performed or to be performed, number of radiation ports, exact fields to be irradiated, mode of radiation therapy, and patient's prognosis (i.e., likelihood of metastasis). Preirradiation treatment should commence immediately after the physician consultation. The first decision should involve possible extractions because radiation can cause side effects that interfere with healing.

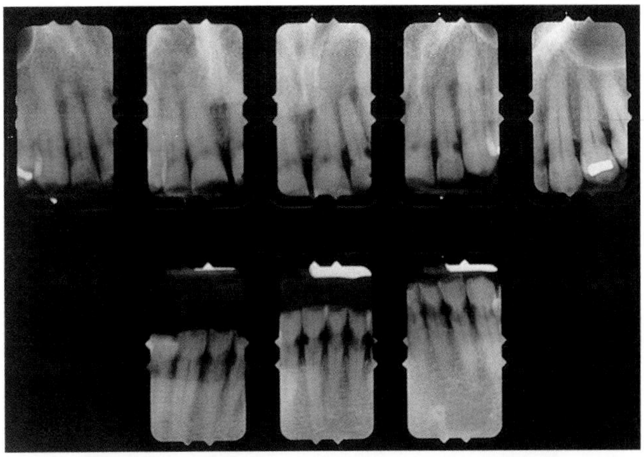

Figure 44-2 Radiographs of anterior teeth of 52-year-old man with postradiation caries. Patient received 6000-cGy radiation treatment to the posterior mandible and base of tongue for squamous cell carcinoma. Radiation caries developed within 1 year after radiation treatment, affecting the cervical areas and incisal edges of the anterior teeth.

For head and neck squamous cell carcinomas, the radiation dose is usually 5000 to 7000 cGy (centigrays; 1 cGy = 1 rad) delivered in a fractionated method (150-200 cGy/day over a 6- to 7-week course).[6,49] This is considered "full-course" radiation treatment, and the degree of perioral side effects depends on which tissues are irradiated, that is, the radiation fields. If this dose is administered to the salivary gland tissues, *xerostomia* will ensue. The parotid is the most radiosensitive of the salivary glands; saliva may become extremely viscous or nonexistent, depending on the dose delivered to the particular gland. Xerostomia causes a decrease in the normal salivary cleansing mechanisms, buffering capacity of saliva, and pH of oral fluids.[49] Oral bacterial populations shift to a preponderance of cariogenic forms (e.g., *Streptococcus mutans, Actinomyces* spp., *Lactobacillus* spp.). Radiation-induced caries may progress rapidly and primarily affects smooth tooth surfaces (Figures 44-2 and 44-3).

High-dose radiation therapy results in hypovascularity of irradiated tissues with a reduction in wound-healing capacity.[54,91,92] Most severe among the resulting oral complications is *osteoradionecrosis* (ORN). Decreased vascularity renders the bone less capable of resolving trauma or infection. Such events may cause severe destruction of bone. The risk of ORN continues for the remainder of the patient's life and does not decrease with time.[44]

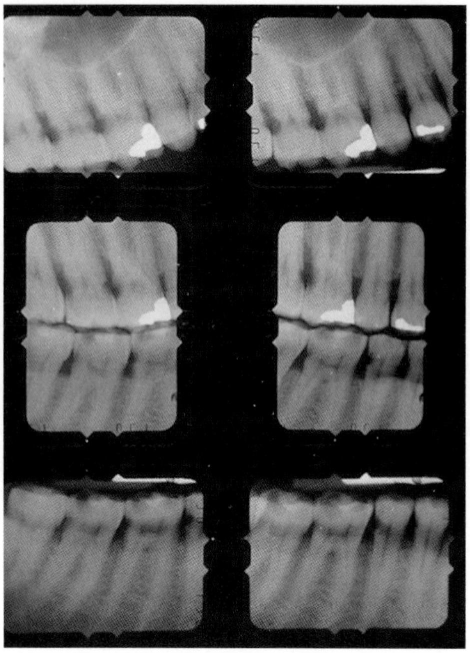

Figure 44-3 Radiographs of posterior sextants of same patient in Figure 44-2. Caries affects the cervical areas and cusp tips of the posterior teeth.

Periodontal disease can be a precipitating factor in ORN.[8,26] Tooth extraction after radiation treatment involves a high risk of developing ORN, and surgical flap procedures are generally discouraged after radiation. For these reasons, it is important that the clinician address the patient's periodontal disease *before* radiation begins, whenever possible. Teeth that are nonrestorable or severely periodontally diseased should be extracted, ideally at least 2 weeks before radiation.[49] Extractions should be performed in a manner that allows primary closure. Mucoperiosteal flaps should be gently elevated; teeth should be extracted in segments; alveolectomy should be performed, allowing no rough bony spicules to remain; and primary closure should be provided without tension. It is unnecessary to extract teeth that can be retained with conservative restorative, endodontic, or periodontal therapy. However, prudence dictates extraction of questionable teeth because periodontal treatment after irradiation may be limited to nonsurgical forms of therapy. Flap surgery or extraction of teeth after radiation may lead to ORN. Management of ORN is often difficult and costly, involving progressively more aggressive treatment if bone does not respond to conservative therapy. Costly hyperbaric oxygen therapy is frequently required for complete resolution.

During radiation therapy, patients should receive weekly prophylaxis, oral hygiene instruction, and professionally applied fluoride treatments, unless mucositis prevents such treatment. Patients should be instructed to brush daily with a 0.4% stannous or 1.0% sodium fluoride gel. Custom gel trays allow optimum fluoride application.[39,91] All remaining teeth should receive thorough debridement (scaling and root planing).

Postirradiation follow-up consists of palliative treatment given as indicated. Viscous lidocaine may be prescribed for painful mucositis, and salivary substitutes may be given for xerostomia. Daily topical fluoride application and oral hygiene are the best means of preventing radiation caries over time. A long-term, 3-month recall interval is ideal.

PROSTHETIC JOINT REPLACEMENT

The main treatment consideration for patients with prosthetic joint replacements relates to the potential need for antibiotic prophylaxis before periodontal therapy. Currently, no scientific evidence indicates that prophylactic antibiotics prevent late prosthetic joint infections, which might occur from transient bacteremia induced by dental treatment.[18,45,75] Furthermore, although dental-induced bacteremia could theoretically cause prosthetic joint infection, scant reports demonstrate dental treatment as a source of joint infection, and none of these actually documents a cause-and-effect relationship.[13,67,87] Thus the American Dental Association, American Academy of Orthopedic Surgeons, American Academy of Oral Medicine, and British Society for Antimicrobial Chemotherapy all agree that routine antibiotic prophylaxis before dental treatment is not indicated for most patients with prosthetic joint replacements.[1,15,23,85] However, prophylaxis is indicated for almost all patients within the first 2 years after joint replacement and for so-called "high-risk" patients, including those with previous prosthetic joint infections, immunosuppression, rheumatoid arthritis, systemic lupus erythematosus, type 1 diabetes, hemophilia, and malnourishment.[1] Importantly, many authors consider patients with severe periodontal disease or other potential dental infections to be "high risk," and antibiotic prophylaxis may be indicated for these patients before dental treatment.[53,85]

Although the evidence demonstrates no need for antibiotic prophylaxis in most patients, many orthopedic surgeons still prefer such treatment,[78] most likely because of the high morbidity and potential mortality associated with prosthetic joint infections. Consultation with the patient's orthopedic surgeon before periodontal treatment is in the patient's best interest and may help assess the risk for joint infection relative to current dental status and type of periodontal treatment planned. Because individuals with significant periodontal disease are considered "high risk," antibiotic prophylaxis before treatment is common in the periodontal practice (Table 44-7).[1]

PREGNANCY

The aim of periodontal therapy for the pregnant patient is to minimize the potential exaggerated inflammatory response related to pregnancy-associated hormonal alterations. Meticulous plaque control, scaling, root planing, and polishing should be the only nonemergency periodontal procedures performed.

The second trimester is the safest time to perform treatment. However, long, stressful appointments and periodontal surgical procedures should be delayed until the postpartum period. As the uterus increases in size

TABLE 44-7

Antibiotic Regimens for Prevention of Prosthetic Joint Infections

Patient Characteristics	Drug Regimen
Patients *not* allergic to penicillins	Cephalexin, cephradine, or amoxicillin: 2 g orally 1 hour before dental procedure
Patients allergic to penicillins	Clindamycin: 600 mg orally 1 hour before dental procedure
Patients *not* allergic to penicillins, but unable to take oral medication	Cefazolin 1 g or ampicillin 2 g intramuscularly or intravenously 1 hour before dental procedure
Patients allergic to penicillins, and unable to take oral medications	Clindamycin 600 mg intravenously 1 hour before dental procedure (must be diluted and injected slowly)

Data from American Dental Association, American Academy of Orthopedic Surgeons: *Am Dent Assoc J* 128:1004, 1997.

during the second and third trimesters, obstruction of the vena cava and aorta may occur if the patient is placed in a supine position. The reduction in return cardiac blood supply may cause *supine hypotensive syndrome,* with decreased placental perfusion.[83] Decreasing blood pressure, syncope, and loss of consciousness may occur. This can be prevented by placing the patient on her left side or simply by elevating the right hip 5 to 6 inches during treatment. Appointments should be short, and the patient should be allowed to change positions frequently. A fully reclined position should be avoided if possible.

Other precautions during pregnancy relate to the potential toxic or teratogenic effects of therapy on the fetus. Ideally, no medications should be prescribed. However, analgesics, antibiotics, local anesthetics, and other drugs may be required during pregnancy, depending on the patient's needs. Before being prescribed, all drugs should be reviewed for potential adverse effects on the fetus.[45,83]

As for all patients, use of dental radiographs during pregnancy should be kept to a minimum. The small amount of radiation exposure during diagnostic dental radiography poses little, if any, risk to the fetus as long as the mother is properly shielded.[2,83] The American Dental Association has stated that "normal radiographic guidelines do not need to be altered because of pregnancy."[2] Use of a properly positioned lead apron is an absolute requirement. (See Chapter 43.)

HEMORRHAGIC DISORDERS

Patients with a history of bleeding problems caused by disease or drugs should be managed to minimize risks of hemorrhage. Identification of these patients through the health history, clinical examination, and clinical laboratory tests is paramount. Health questioning should cover (1) history of bleeding after previous surgery or trauma, (2) past and present drug history, (3) history of bleeding problems among relatives, and (4) illnesses associated with potential bleeding problems.

Clinical examination should detect the presence of jaundice, ecchymosis, spider telangiectasia, hemarthrosis, petechiae, hemorrhagic vesicles, spontaneous gingival bleeding, and gingival hyperplasia. Laboratory tests should include methods to measure the hemostatic, coagulation, or lytic phases of the clotting mechanism, depending on clues regarding which phase is involved (Table 44-8). These tests include bleeding time, tourniquet test, complete blood cell count, PT, PTT, and coagulation time.

Bleeding disorders may be classified as coagulation disorders, thrombocytopenic purpuras, or nonthrombocytopenic purpuras.

Coagulation Disorders

The main inherited coagulation disorders include hemophilias A and B and von Willebrand's disease[63,70] (Table 44-9). *Hemophilia A* results in a deficiency of coagulation factor VIII, and the clinical severity of the disorder depends on the level of factor VIII remaining.[56] Patients with severe hemophilia who have less than 1% of normal factor VIII levels may have severe bleeding on the slightest provocation, whereas those with more moderate hemophilia (1%-5% factor VIII) have less frequent spontaneous hemorrhage but still bleed with minimal trauma.[45] Patients with mild hemophilia (6%-30% factor VIII) rarely bleed spontaneously but may still have hemorrhage after severe trauma or during surgical procedures. The clinician should consult the patient's physician before dental treatment to determine the risk for bleeding and treatment modifications required. To prevent surgical hemorrhage, factor VIII levels of at least 30% are needed.[45,56] Parenteral 1-deamino-8-D-arginine vasopressin (DDAVP, desmopressin) can be used to raise factor VIII levels twofold to threefold in patients with mild or moderate hemophilia. DDAVP has the significant advantage of avoiding the risk of viral disease transmission from factor VIII infusion and is considered the drug of choice in responsive patients. Most patients with moderate and severe hemophilia require infusion of factor VIII concentrate before surgical procedures. Before 1985 the risk of viral disease transmission from these infusions was high. In recent years, virally safe, highly purified monoclonal antibody or recombinant DNA factor VIII products have come into widespread use.

Hemophilia B, or Christmas disease, results in a deficiency of factor IX. The severity of the disorder depends on the relative amount of existing factor IX. Surgical therapy requires a factor IX level of 30% to 50% and is

TABLE 44-8

Laboratory Tests for Bleeding Disorders

Hemostatic Tests			
Vascular	**Platelet**	**Coagulation**	**Lytic**
1. Tourniquet test *N:* 10 petechiae *Abn:* >10 petechiae	1. Platelet count *N:* 150,000-300,000/mm^3 *Abn:* Thrombocytopenia = <100,000/mm^3; clinical bleeding occurs at <80,000/mm^3; spontaneous bleeding occurs at <20,000/mm^3.	1. Prothrombin time (PT; measures extrinsic and common pathways: factors I, II, V, VII, and X) *N:* 11-14 sec (depending on laboratory) measured against control. PT is reported as international normalized ratio (INR): *N:* INR = 1.0 *Abn:* INR >1.5	1. Euglobin clot lysis time *N:* <90 min *Abn:* >90 min
2. Bleeding time *N:* 1-6 min *Abn:* >6 min	2. Bleeding time 3. Clot retraction 4. Complete blood cell count	2. Partial thromboplastin time (PTT; measures intrinsic and common pathways: factors III, IX, XI, and low levels of factors I, II, V, X, and XII) *N:* 25-40 sec (depending on laboratory) measured against control. *Abn:* >1.5 times normal 3. Clotting (coagulation) time *N:* 30-40 min *Abn:* >1 hr	
Clinical Disease Association			
Vascular (capillary) wall defect	Thrombocytopenia		Increase in fibrinolytic activity
Rule out: Thrombocytopenia Purpuras Telangiectasia Aspirin or NSAID therapy Leukemia Renal dialysis	*Rule out:* Vascular wall defect Acute/chronic leukemia Aplastic anemia Liver disease Renal dialysis	*All three tests:* Liver disease Warfarin therapy Aspirin or NSAID therapy Malabsorption syndrome or long-term antibiotic therapy (lack of vitamin K utilization) *Prothrombin time:* Factor VII deficiency *Partial thromboplastin time:* Hemophilia Renal dialysis	

N, Normal; *Abn,* abnormal; *NSAID,* nonsteroidal antiinflammatory drug.

usually achieved by administration of purified prothrombin complex concentrates or factor IX concentrates.[56]

Von Willebrand's disease results from a deficiency of von Willebrand factor, which mediates adhesion of platelets to the injured vessel wall and is required for primary hemostasis. Von Willebrand factor also carries the coagulant portion of factor VIII in the plasma. The disorder has three major subtypes with a wide range of clinical severity. In fact, many cases of von Willebrand's disease go undiagnosed, and bleeding during dental treatment may be the first sign of the underlying disease. More severe forms require preoperative factor VIII concentrate or cryoprecipitate infusion. Patients with milder forms respond favorably to administration of DDAVP before periodontal surgery or tooth extraction.[56,57]

Periodontal treatment may be performed in patients with these coagulation disorders, provided that sufficient precautions are taken. Probing, scaling, and prophylaxis can usually be done without medical modification. More invasive treatment, such as local block anesthesia, root planing, or surgery, dictate prior physician consultation.

During treatment, local measures to ensure clot formation and stability are of major importance. Complete wound closure and application of pressure will reduce

TABLE 44-9

Inherited Coagulation Disorders

Type	Prolonged	Normal	Treatment
Hemophilia A	Partial thromboplastin time	Prothrombin time Bleeding time	DDAVP (desmopressin) Factor VIII concentrate or cryoprecipitate Fresh-frozen plasma Fresh whole blood ε-Aminocaproic acid (EACA) Tranexamic acid
Hemophilia B	Partial thromboplastin time	Prothrombin time Bleeding time	Purified prothrombin complex concentrates Factor IX concentrates Fresh-frozen plasma
Von Willebrand's disease	Bleeding time Partial thromboplastin time Variable factor VIII deficiency	Prothrombin time Platelet count	DDAVP (desmopressin) Factor VIII concentrate or cryoprecipitate

hemorrhage. Antihemostatic agents such as oxidized cellulose or purified bovine collagen may be placed over surgical sites or into extraction sockets. The antifibrinolytic agent *epsilon-aminocaproic acid* (EACA), given orally or intravenously, is a potent inhibitor of initial clot dissolution.[37] *Tranexamic acid* is a more potent antifibrinolytic agent than EACA and has been shown to prevent excessive oral hemorrhage after periodontal surgery and tooth extraction.[62] It is available as an oral rinse and may be used either alone or in combination with systemic tranexamic acid for several days after surgery.[79]

Not all coagulation disorders are hereditary. Liver disease may affect all phases of blood clotting because most coagulation factors are synthesized and removed by the liver. Long-term alcohol abusers or chronic hepatitis patients often demonstrate inadequate coagulation. Coagulation may be impaired by vitamin K deficiency, often caused by malabsorption syndromes, or by prolonged antibiotic administration, which alters the intestinal microflora that produces vitamin K. Dental treatment planning for patients with liver disease should include the following:

1. Physician consultation.
2. Laboratory evaluations: PT, bleeding time, platelet count, and PTT (in patients in later stages of liver disease).
3. Conservative, nonsurgical periodontal therapy, whenever possible.
4. If surgery is required (may require hospitalization):
   - International normalized ratio (INR; PT) should generally be less than 2.0. For simple surgical procedures, INR less than 2.5 is generally safe.[34]
   - Platelet count should be less than 80,000/mm^3.

The most common cause of abnormal coagulation may be drug therapy. Patients with prosthetic heart valves or histories of MI, CVA, or thromboembolism are frequently placed on anticoagulant therapy using coumarin derivatives such as dicumarol and warfarin.[34,43] These drugs are vitamin K antagonists that decrease production of vitamin K–dependent coagulation factors II, VII, IX, and X. The effectiveness of anticoagulation therapy is monitored by the PT. The recommended level of anticoagulation for most patients is an INR of 2.0 to 3.0, with prosthetic heart valve patients generally in the 2.5 to 3.5 range.[34] Periodontal treatment should be altered as follows:

1. Consult the patient's physician to determine the nature of the underlying medical problem and the degree of required anticoagulation.
2. The procedure to be done determines the acceptable INR. Infiltration anesthesia, scaling, and root planing may be done safely in patients with an INR less than 3.0. Block anesthesia, minor periodontal surgery, and simple extractions usually require an INR less than 2.0 to 2.5. Complex surgery or multiple extractions may require an INR less than 1.5 to 2.0.
3. The physician should be consulted about discontinuing or reducing anticoagulant dosage until the desired INR is achieved. The dentist must inform the physician what degree of intraoperative and postoperative bleeding are usually expected with the procedures planned. Discontinuing anticoagulant therapy before dental surgery was common in the past. However, most clinicians no longer recommend discontinuing anticoagulation for many procedures because this has significant potential risks to patient health.[36,72] If the INR is higher than the level at which significant bleeding is likely to accompany a particular procedure, the physician may elect to change anticoagulant therapy. Often, the anticoagulant is discontinued for 2 to 3 days before periodontal treatment (clearance half-life of warfarin is 36-42 hours), and the INR is checked on the day of therapy. If the INR is within the acceptable target range, the procedure is done and the anticoagulant resumed immediately after treatment.
4. Careful technique and complete wound closure are paramount. For all procedures, application of pressure can minimize hemorrhage. Use of oxidized

cellulose, microfibrillar collagen, topical thrombin, and tranexamic acid should be considered for persistent bleeding.

Aspirin interferes with normal platelet aggregation and can result in prolonged bleeding. Because it binds irreversibly to platelets, the effects of aspirin last at least 4 to 7 days. Aspirin is generally used in small doses of 325 mg or less per day, which usually does not alter bleeding time. In general, patients taking low doses of aspirin daily do not need to discontinue aspirin therapy before periodontal procedures.[72] However, higher doses may increase bleeding time and predispose the patient to postoperative bleeding.[45] For patients taking more than 325 mg of aspirin per day, aspirin may need to be discontinued 7 to 10 days before surgical therapy that might result in significant bleeding, in consultation with the physician. *Nonsteroidal antiinflammatory drugs* (NSAIDs) such as ibuprofen also inhibit platelet function. Because NSAIDs bind reversibly, the effect is transitory, lasting only a short time after the last drug dose. The bleeding time is used when questions arise about the potential effect of aspirin or NSAIDs. Aspirin should not be prescribed for patients who are receiving anticoagulation therapy or who have illnesses related to bleeding tendencies.

Heparin is generally used for short-term anticoagulation and is given intravenously (usually in a hospital environment). It is a powerful anticoagulant with a duration of action of 4 to 8 hours. Periodontal treatment is rarely required while a patient is taking heparin.

Thrombocytopenic Purpuras

Thrombocytopenia is defined as a platelet count of less than $100,000/mm^3$. Bleeding caused by thrombocytopenia may be seen with idiopathic thrombocytopenic purpuras, radiation therapy, myelosuppressive drug therapy (e.g., chemotherapy), leukemia, or infections. *Pupuras* are hemorrhagic diseases characterized by extravasation of blood into the tissues under the skin or mucosa, producing spontaneous petechiae (small red patches) or ecchymoses (bruises).

Periodontal therapy for patients with thrombocytopenia should be directed toward reducing inflammation by removing local irritants to avoid the need for more aggressive therapy.[45,56] Oral hygiene instructions and frequent maintenance visits are paramount. Physician referral is indicated for a definitive diagnosis and to determine any alterations in planned therapy. Scaling and root planing are generally safe unless platelet counts are less than $60,000/mm^3$. No surgical procedures should be performed unless the platelet count is greater than $80,000/mm^3$. Platelet transfusion may be required before surgery. Surgical technique should be as atraumatic as possible, and local hemostatic measures should be applied.

Nonthrombocytopenic Purpuras

Nonthrombocytopenic purpuras result from either vascular wall fragility or *thrombasthenia* (impaired platelet aggregation). Vascular wall fragility may result from hypersensitivity reactions, scurvy, infections, chemicals (phenacetin, aspirin), dysproteinemia, and other causes. Thrombasthenia occurs in uremia, Glanzmann's disease, aspirin ingestion, and von Willebrand's disease.[56] Both types of nonthrombocytopenic purpura may result in immediate bleeding after gingival injury. Treatment consists primarily of direct pressure applied for at least 15 minutes. This initial pressure should control the bleeding unless coagulation times are abnormal or reinjury occurs. Surgical therapy should be avoided until the qualitative and quantitative platelet problems are resolved.

BLOOD DYSCRASIAS

Numerous disorders of red and white blood cells may affect the course of periodontal therapy. Alterations in wound healing, bleeding, tissue appearance, and susceptibility to infection may occur. Clinicians should be aware of the clinical signs and symptoms of blood dyscrasias, availability of screening laboratory tests, and need for physician referral.

Leukemia

Altered periodontal treatment for patients with leukemia is based on their enhanced susceptibility to infections, bleeding tendency, and the effects of chemotherapy.[45] The treatment plan for leukemia patients is as follows:

1. Refer the patient for medical evaluation and treatment. Close cooperation with the physician is required.
2. Before chemotherapy, a complete periodontal treatment plan should be developed with a physician (see previous discussion).
   - Monitor hematologic laboratory values daily: bleeding time, coagulation time, PT, and platelet count.
   - Administer antibiotic coverage before any periodontal treatment because infection is a major concern.
   - Extract all hopeless, nonmaintainable, or potentially infectious teeth at least 10 days before the initiation of chemotherapy, if systemic conditions allow.
   - Periodontal debridement (scaling and root planing) should be performed and thorough oral hygiene instructions given if the patient's condition allows. Twice-daily rinsing with 0.12% chlorhexidine gluconate is recommended after oral hygiene procedures. Recognize the potential for bleeding caused by thrombocytopenia. Use pressure and topical hemostatic agents as indicated.
3. During the acute phases of leukemia, patients should receive only emergency periodontal care. Any source of potential infection must be eliminated to prevent systemic dissemination. Antibiotic therapy is frequently the treatment of choice, combined with nonsurgical or surgical debridement as indicated.
4. Oral ulcerations and mucositis are treated palliatively with agents such as viscous lidocaine. Systemic

antibiotics may be indicated to prevent secondary infection.

5. Oral candidiasis is common in the leukemic patient and can be treated with nystatin suspensions (100,000 U/ml four times daily) or clotrimazole vaginal suppositories (10 mg four or five times daily).[49]
6. For patients with chronic leukemia and those in remission, scaling and root planing can be performed without complication, but periodontal surgery should be avoided if possible.
   - Platelet count and bleeding time should be measured on the day of the procedure. If either is low, postpone the appointment and refer the patient to a physician.

Agranulocytosis

Patients with agranulocytosis (cyclic neutropenia and granulocytopenia) have an increased susceptibility to infection. The total white blood cell count is reduced, and granular leukocytes (neutrophils, eosinophils, basophils) are reduced or disappear. These disorders are often marked by early, severe periodontal destruction.[93] When possible, periodontal treatment should be done during periods of disease remission. At such times, treatment should be as conservative as possible while reducing potential sources of systemic infection. After physician consultation, severely affected teeth should be extracted. Oral hygiene instruction should include use of chlorhexidine rinses twice daily. Scaling and root planing should be performed carefully under antibiotic protection.

INFECTIOUS DISEASES

Because many infectious diseases are occult in nature, and because medical histories are often inaccurate or incomplete, all periodontal patients should be treated as though they have an infectious disease.[19] Protection of patients, clinicians, and office staff requires use of universal (standard) precautions for all patients, maximizing prevention of infection and cross-contamination. This section provides a brief discussion of hepatitis, human immunodeficiency virus (HIV) and acquired immunodeficiency syndrome (AIDS), and tuberculosis in relation to the precautions required in periodontal therapy.

Hepatitis

To date, six distinct viruses causing viral hepatitis have been identified: hepatitis A, B, C, D, E, and G viruses.[14,28,42] In addition, a single-stranded deoxyribonucleic acid (DNA) virus known as *transfusion-transmitted virus* has recently been identified in cases of acute and chronic hepatitis[42,95]; its role as an etiologic agent is still undetermined. These forms of viral hepatitis differ in their virology, epidemiology, and prophylaxis (Table 44-10). Because the majority of hepatitis infections are undiagnosed, the clinician must be aware of high-risk groups, such as renal dialysis patients, health care workers, immunosuppressed patients, patients who have received multiple blood transfusions, homosexuals, drug users, and institutionalized patients.

Hepatitis A virus (HAV) and *hepatitis E virus* (HEV) are both self-limiting infections with no associated chronic liver disease. These viruses are primarily transmitted via the fecal-oral route. HAV transmission in the United States usually results from close personal household, sexual, or day care center contact. Conversely, HEV is transmitted mainly through fecally contaminated drinking water and is thus relatively uncommon in the United States. Currently, a vaccination is available to protect against HAV infection but not HEV infection.

Hepatitis B virus (HBV) infection may result in chronic liver disease and a chronic carrier state. Chronic HBV infection develops in about 5% to 10% of infected individuals, with much higher rates among infants and children. Because it is transmitted primarily through a hematogenous route, HBV is a major concern for health care workers; the highest rates of HBV infection are found among dentists and oral surgeons.[28] Percutaneous or permucosal injury with contaminated instruments or needles is the most common route of infection in the dental office. The HBV vaccine is recommended for all health care workers.

Hepatitis D virus (HDV) is a defective virus that requires the presence of HBV for its survival, replication, and infectivity. The HDV genetic material is packaged within the HBV surface antigen coating. Thus, prevention of HDV infection is similar to prevention for HBV and relies strongly on HBV vaccination. Once antibody titers to HBV are elevated to a protective level, the patient is also protected against HDV infection.

Hepatitis C virus (HCV) is probably the most serious of all viral hepatitis infections because of its high chronic infection rate. Only 15% of patients infected with HCV recover completely; 85% develop chronic HCV infection, which dramatically increases the risk for cirrhosis, hepatocellular carcinoma, and liver failure. In fact, HCV infection is the leading cause of liver transplantation in the United States. Unfortunately, no vaccine is available for HCV. Because HCV is transmitted primarily through a percutaneous or permucosal route, health care workers are at risk from injury with contaminated instruments.

Hepatitis G virus (HGV) is a ribonucleic acid (RNA) virus, and its epidemiology and virology are not fully understood. HGV rarely occurs as a solitary infection, usually appearing as a co-infection with hepatitis A, B, or C. HGV is known to be transmitted through the blood and has frequently been associated with transfusions.

Transfusion-transmitted virus (TTV) was first identified in 1997 and is common in the general population.[42,52] The virus is often present in patients with hepatitis and chronic liver disease. Similar to HGV, TTV may not actually cause a specific form of hepatitis. Patients infected with TTV may develop a chronic carrier state without having clinically evident disease, or they may develop frank disease. Evidence indicates that TTV can be transmitted not only by the blood (e.g., transfusions), but also via a fecal-oral route and from mother to child. Also, as with HGV, TTV is often associated with HCV.

The following guidelines are offered for treating hepatitis patients:

1. If the disease, regardless of type, is active, do not provide periodontal therapy unless the situation is an

TABLE 44-10

Comparison of Hepatitis Viruses

	A	B	C	D	E	G	TTV*
Source	Feces	Blood and body fluids	Blood and body fluids	Blood and body fluids	Feces	Blood	Blood, possibly feces
Primary modes of transmission	Fecal-oral	Percutaneous, permucosal; sexual	Percutaneous, permucosal	Percutaneous, permucosal (occurs only after previous infection with HBV or as co-infection with HBV)	Fecal-oral	Percutaneous (usually occurs as co- infection with other hepatitis viruses)	Blood (transfusion), possible fecal-oral
Incubation period	15-50 days	50-160 days	15-150 days	15-150 days	15-60 days	Unknown	Unknown
Risk of chronic infection	No chronic infection	Varies with age: adults 5%-10%; children 25%-50%; infants >85%	Very high (>85%)	5% when acquired as co-infection with HBV; >70% when acquired as a second infection in chronic HBV carrier	No chronic infection	Unknown whether chronic infection occurs	Unclear
Protective immunity after infection?	Yes; anti-HAV antibody	Usually; antibody to core antigen, e antigen, and surface antigen (HBsAg) are produced; anti-HBsAg is most protective; chronic carrier state exists.	No; anti-HCV antibody is produced but is usually not protective.	Because HDV infection requires previous infection or co-infection with HBV, protective immunity is similar to hepatitis B.	Unknown	Unknown	Unknown
Vaccine available?	Yes	Yes	No	Yes (HBV vaccine protects against HDV)	No	No	No

*Transfusion-transmitted virus.

emergency. In an emergency case, follow the protocol for patients positive for *hepatitis B surface antigen* (HBsAg).
2. For patients with a past history of hepatitis, consult the physician to determine the type of hepatitis, course and length of the disease, mode of transmission, and any chronic liver disease or viral carrier state.
3. For recovered HAV or HEV patients, perform routine periodontal care.
4. For recovered HBV and HDV patients, consult with the physician and order HBsAg and anti-HBs (antibody to HBV surface antigen) laboratory tests.
   - If HBsAg and anti-HBs tests are negative but HBV is suspected, order another HBs determination.
   - Patients who are HBsAg positive are probably infective (chronic carriers); the degree of infectivity is measured by an HBsAg determination.
   - Patients who are anti-HBs positive may be treated routinely (they have antibody to HBsAg).
   - Patients who are HBsAg negative may be treated routinely.
5. For HCV patients, consult with the physician to determine the patient's risk for transmissibility and current status of chronic liver disease.
6. If a patient with active hepatitis, positive-HBsAg (HBV carrier) status, or positive-HCV carrier status requires emergency treatment, use the following precautions:
   - Consult the patient's physician regarding status.
   - If bleeding is likely during or after treatment, measure PT and bleeding time. Hepatitis may alter coagulation; change treatment accordingly.
   - All personnel in clinical contact with the patient should use full barrier technique, including masks, gloves, glasses or eye shields, and disposable gowns.
   - Use as many disposable covers as possible, covering light handles, drawer handles, and bracket trays. Headrest covers should also be used.
   - All disposable items (e.g., gauze, floss, saliva ejectors, masks, gowns, gloves) should be placed in one lined wastebasket. After treatment, these items and all disposable covers should be bagged, labeled, and disposed of, following proper guidelines for biohazardous waste.
   - Aseptic technique should be followed at all times. Minimize aerosol production by not using ultrasonic instrumentation, air syringe, or high-speed handpieces; remember that saliva contains a distillate of the virus. Prerinsing with chlorhexidine gluconate for 30 seconds is highly recommended.
   - When the procedure is completed, all equipment should be scrubbed and sterilized. If an item cannot be sterilized or disposed of, it should not be used.

If a percutaneous or permucosal injury occurs during dental treatment of a HBV carrier, current Centers for Disease Control and Prevention (CDC) guidelines recommend administration of *hepatitis B immune globulin* (HBIG).[10] The HBV vaccine should also be administered if the injured individual has not previously received it. Unfortunately, postexposure prophylaxis with immune globulin or antiviral agents is generally ineffective if a percutaneous injury occurs during treatment of a hepatitis C carrier.[9,14]

HIV and AIDS

Since the beginning of the AIDS epidemic, a wide range of oral lesions has been associated with HIV infection; these lesions are discussed in Chapter 34.

As with hepatitis, not all HIV-infected patients know that they are infected when they report for dental treatment. Furthermore, individuals with known HIV infection may not admit their status on the medical history. Therefore, every patient receiving dental treatment should be managed as a potentially infected person, using universal precautions for all therapy.

Extensive periodontal treatment plans must be considered in regard to the patient's systemic health, prognosis, and survival time.[45] Large variations in progression of HIV disease exist among individuals, and selection of an appropriate treatment plan depends on the state of the patient's overall health. Although there appear to be few contraindications to routine dental treatment for many HIV-infected patients, the periodontal treatment plan is influenced by the patient's overall systemic health and coincident oral infections or diseases. An awareness of oral disorders associated with HIV infection may allow the clinician to recognize previously undiagnosed disease or to modify treatment protocols appropriately.

Tuberculosis

The patient with tuberculosis should receive only emergency care, following the guidelines listed in the section on hepatitis. If the patient has completed chemotherapy, the patient's physician should be consulted regarding infectivity and the results of sputum cultures for *Mycobacterium tuberculosis*. When medical clearance has been given and the sputum culture results are negative, these patients may be treated normally. Any patient who gives a history of poor medical follow-up (e.g., lack of yearly chest radiographs) or shows signs or symptoms indicative of tuberculosis should be referred for evaluation. Adequate treatment of tuberculosis requires a minimum of 18 months, and thorough posttreatment follow-up should include chest radiographs, sputum cultures, and a review of the patient's symptoms by the physician at least every 12 months.

REFERENCES

1. American Dental Association, American Academy of Orthopedic Surgeons: Advisory statement: Antibiotic prophylaxis for dental patients with total joint replacements, *J Am Dent Assoc* 128:1004, 1997.
2. American Dental Association Council on Dental Materials, Instruments, and Equipment: Recommendations in radiographic practices: an update, 1988, *J Am Dent Assoc* 118:115, 1989.
3. American Diabetes Association: Report of the Expert Committee on the Diagnosis and Classification of Diabetes Mellitus, *Diabetes Care* 26(suppl 1):5, 2003.

4. Barco CT: Prevention of infective endocarditis: a review of the medical and dental literature, *J Periodontol* 62:510, 1991.
5. Black HR: The coronary artery disease paradox, *Am J Hypertens* 9(4, pt 3):2, 1996.
6. Blaha PJ, Reeve CM: Periodontal treatment for patients with cancer, *Curr Opin Periodontol* 64-70, 1994 (review).
7. Burt VL, Whelton P, Roccella EJ, et al: Prevalence of hypertension in the U.S. adult population: results from the third National Health and Nutrition Examination Survey, 1988–1991, *Hypertension* 25:303, 1995.
8. Carl W: Local radiation and systemic chemotherapy: preventing and managing the oral complications, *J Am Dent Assoc* 124:119, 1993.
9. Centers for Disease Control and Prevention: Recommendations for follow-up of health-care workers after occupational exposure to hepatitis C virus, *MMWR* 46:603, 1997.
10. Centers for Disease Control and Prevention: Immunization of health-care workers: recommendation of the Advisory Committee on Immunization Practices (ACIP) and the Hospital Infection Control Practices Advisory Committee (HICPAC), *MMWR* 46(RR-18):1, 1997.
11. Chobanian AV, Bakris GL, Black HR, et al: National Heart, Lung and Blood Institute Joint National Committee on Prevention, Detection, Evaluation, and Treatment of High Blood Pressure; National High Blood Pressure Education Program Coordinating Committee: The seventh report of the Joint National Committee on Prevention, Detection, Evaluation, and Treatment of High Blood Pressure: the JNC 7 report, *JAMA* 289:2560, 2003.
12. Chobanian AV, Bakris GL, Black HR, et al: National Heart, Lung and Blood Institute Joint National Committee on Prevention, Detection, Evaluation, and Treatment of High Blood Pressure; National Heart, Lung and Blood Institute; National High Blood Pressure Education Program Coordinating Committee: Seventh report of the Joint National Committee on Prevention, Detection, Evaluation, and Treatment of High Blood Pressure, *Hypertension* 42:1206, 2003.
13. Christgau M, Palitzsch KD, Schmalz G, et al: Healing response to non-surgical periodontal therapy in patients with diabetes mellitus: clinical, microbiological, and immunological results, *J Clin Periodontol* 25:112, 1998.
14. Cleveland JL, Gooch BF, Shearer BG, et al: Risk and prevention of hepatitis C virus infection: implications for dentistry, *J Am Dent Assoc* 130:641, 1999.
15. Council on Dental Therapeutics: Management of dental patients with prosthetic joints, *J Am Dent Assoc* 121:537, 1990.
16. Dajani AS, Taubert KA, Wilson W, et al: Prevention of bacterial endocarditis: recommendations by the American Heart Association, *JAMA* 277:1794, 1997.
17. Dajani AS, Taubert KA, Wilson W, et al: Prevention of bacterial endocarditis: recommendations by the American Heart Association, *J Am Dent Assoc* 128:1142, 1997.
18. Deacon JM, Pagliaro AJ, Zelicof SB, et al: Current concepts review: prophylactic use of antibiotics for procedures after total joint replacement, *J Bone Joint Surg* 78A:1755, 1996.
19. DePaola LG: Managing the care of patients infected with bloodborne diseases, *J Am Dent Assoc* 134:350, 2003.
20. Diabetes Control and Complications Trial Research Group: The effect of intensive treatment of diabetes on the development and progression of long-term complications in insulin-dependent diabetes mellitus, *N Engl J Med* 329:977, 1993.
21. Diabetes Control and Complications Trial Research Group: Hypoglycemia in the diabetes control and complications trial, *Diabetes* 46:271, 1997.
22. Eisenberg MJ, Brox A, Bestawros AN: Calcium channel blockers: an update, *Am J Med* 116:35, 2004.
23. Eskinazi D, Rathbun W: Is systemic antimicrobial prophylaxis justified in dental patients with prosthetic joints? *Oral Surg Oral Med Oral Pathol* 66:430, 1988.
24. Estes NA, Weinstock J, Wang PJ, et al: Use of antiarrhythmics and implantable cardioverter-defibrillators in congestive heart failure, *Am J Cardiol* 91(6, suppl 1):45, 2003.
25. Findler M, Garfunkel AA, Galili D: Review of very high-risk patients in the dental setting, *Compend Contin Educ Dent* 15:58, 1994.
26. Galler C, Epstein JB, Guze KA, et al: The development of osteoradionecrosis from sites of periodontal disease activity: report of 3 cases, *J Periodontol* 63:310, 1992.
27. Genco RJ, Offenbacher S, Beck J, et al: Cardiovascular diseases and oral infections. In Rose LF, Genco RJ, Mealey BL, et al, editors: *Periodontal medicine,* Toronto, 1999, BC Decker.
28. Gillchrist JA: Hepatitis viruses A, B, C, D, E and G: implications for dental personnel, *J Am Dent Assoc* 130:509, 1999.
29. Glick M: Glucocorticosteroid replacement therapy: a literature review and suggested replacement therapy, *Oral Surg Oral Med Oral Pathol* 67:614, 1989.
30. Gudapati A, Ahmed P, Rada R: Dental management of patients with renal failure, *Gen Dent* 50:508, 2002.
31. Hajjar I, Kotchen TA: Trends in prevalence, awareness, treatment and control of hypertension in the United States, 1988-2000, *JAMA* 290:199, 2003.
32. Herman WW, Konzelman JL: Angina: an update for dentistry, *J Am Dent Assoc* 127:98, 1996.
33. Herman WW, Konzelman JL Jr, Prisant LM: New national guidelines on hypertension: a summary for dentistry, *J Am Dent Assoc* 135:576, 2004.
34. Herman WW, Konzelman JL, Sutley SH: Current perspectives on dental patients receiving coumarin anticoagulant therapy, *J Am Dent Assoc* 128:327, 1997.
35. Huber MA, Terezhalmy GT: The head and neck radiation oncology patient, *Quintessence Int* 34:693, 2003.
36. Jeske AH, Suchko GD: Lack of a scientific basis for routine discontinuation of oral anticoagulation therapy before dental treatment, *J Am Dent Assoc* 134:1492, 2003.
37. Johnson WT, Leary JM: Management of dental patients with bleeding disorders: review and update, *Oral Surg Oral Med Oral Pathol* 66:297, 1988.
38. Joint National Committee on Prevention, Detection, Evaluation, and Treatment of High Blood Pressure: The fifth report of the Joint National Committee on Prevention, Detection, Evaluation, and Treatment of High Blood Pressure (JNC V), *Arch Intern Med* 153:154, 1993.
39. Joint National Committee on Prevention, Detection, Evaluation, and Treatment of High Blood Pressure: The sixth report of the Joint National Committee on Prevention, Detection, Evaluation, and Treatment of High Blood Pressure (JNC VI), NIH Pub No 98-4080, Bethesda, Md, 1997, National Institutes of Health, National Heart, Lung and Blood Institute.
40. Kerr AR: Update on renal disease for the dental practitioner, *Oral Surg Oral Med Oral Pathol Oral Radiol Endod* 92:9, 2001.
41. Konstam MA: Improving clinical outcomes with drug treatment in heart failure: what have trials taught? *Am J Cardiol* 91(6, suppl 1):9, 2003.
42. Lodi G, Bez C, Porter SR, et al: Infectious hepatitis C, hepatitis G, and TT virus: review and implications for dentists, *Spec Care Dentist* 22:53, 2002.
43. Martinowitz U, Mazar AL, Taicher S, et al: Dental extraction for patients on oral anticoagulant therapy, *Oral Surg Oral Med Oral Pathol* 70:274, 1990.
44. Marx RE, Johnson RP: Studies in the radiobiology of osteoradionecrosis and their clinical significance, *Oral Surg Oral Med Oral Pathol* 64:379, 1987.

45. Mealey BL: Periodontal implications: medically compromised patients, *Ann Periodontol* 1:256, 1996.
46. Mealey BL: Impact of advances in diabetes care on dental treatment of the diabetic patient, *Compend Contin Educ Dent* 19:41, 1998.
47. Mealey BL: Diabetes mellitus. In Rose LF, Genco RJ, Mealey BL, et al, editors: *Periodontal medicine,* Toronto, 1999, BC Decker.
48. Mealey BL, Semba SE, Hallmon WW: Dentistry and the cancer patient. Part 1. Oral manifestations and complications of chemotherapy, *Compend Contin Educ Dent* 15:1252, 1994.
49. Mealey BL, Semba SE, Hallmon WW: The head and neck radiotherapy patient. Part 2. Management of oral complications, *Compend Contin Educ Dent* 15:442, 1994.
50. Miller CS, Little JW, Falace DA: Supplemental corticosteroids for dental patients with adrenal insufficiency: reconsideration of the problem, *J Am Dent Assoc* 132:1570, 2001.
51. Muzyka BC, Glick M: The hypertensive dental patient, *J Am Dent Assoc* 128:1109, 1997.
52. Naoumov NV: TT virus: highly prevalent, but still in search of a disease, *J Hepatol* 33:157, 2000.
53. Norden CW: Antibiotic prophylaxis in orthopedic surgery, *Rev Infect Dis* 13(suppl 10):842, 1991.
54. Ostuni E: Stroke and the dental patient, *J Am Dent Assoc* 125:721, 1994.
55. Pallasch TJ, Slots J: Antibiotic prophylaxis and the medically compromised patient, *Periodontol 2000* 10:107, 1996.
56. Patton LL, Ship JA: Treatment of patients with bleeding disorders, *Dent Clin North Am* 38:465, 1994.
57. Petrover MG, Cohen CI: The use of desmopressin in the management of two patients with von Willebrand's disease undergoing periodontal surgery: 2 case reports, *J Periodontol* 61:239, 1990.
58. Phillips YY, Hnatiuk OW: Diagnosing and monitoring the clinical source of chronic obstructive pulmonary disease, *Respir Care Clin North Am* 4:371, 1998.
59. Pinto A, Glick M: Management of patients with thyroid disease: oral health considerations, *J Am Dent Assoc* 133:849, 2002.
60. Raab FJ, Schaffer EM, Guillaume-Cornelissen G, et al: Interpreting vital sign profiles for maximizing patient safety during dental visits, *J Am Dent Assoc* 129:461, 1998.
61. Raber-Durlacher JE, Epstein JB, Raber J, et al: Periodontal infection in cancer patients treated with high-dose chemotherapy, *Support Care Cancer* 10:466, 2002.
62. Ramstrom G, Sindet-Pedersen S, Hall G, et al: Prevention of postsurgical bleeding in oral surgery using tranexamic acid without dose modification of oral anticoagulants, *J Oral Maxillofac Surg* 51:1211, 1993.
63. Rees TD, Mealey BL: Periodontal treatment of the medically compromised patient. In Rose LF, Mealey BL, Genco RJ, Cohen DW, editors: *Periodontics: medicine, surgery, and implants*, St Louis, 2004, Mosby, Elsevier.
64. Replogle K, Reader A, Nist R, et al: Cardiovascular effects of intraosseous injections of 2 percent lidocaine with 1:100,000 epinephrine and 3 percent mepivacaine, *J Am Dent Assoc* 130:649, 1999.
65. Rhodus NL, Little JW: Dental management of the renal transplant patient, *Compend Contin Educ Dent* 14:518, 1993.
66. Rhodus NL, Little JW: Dental management of the patient with cardiac arrhythmias: an update, *Oral Surg Oral Med Oral Pathol Oral Radiol Endod* 96:659, 2003.
67. Rose LF: Medical evaluation. In Rose LF, Genco RJ, Mealey BL, et al, editors: *Periodontal medicine,* Toronto, 1999, BC Decker.
68. Rose LF, Mealey B, Minsk L, Cohen DW: Oral care for patients with cardiovascular disease and stroke, *J Am Dent Assoc* 133(suppl):7, 2002.
69. Scannapieco FA: Respiratory diseases. In Rose LF, Genco RJ, Mealey BL, et al, editors: *Periodontal medicine,* Toronto, 1999, BC Decker.
70. Schardt-Sacco D: Update on coagulopathies, *Oral Surg Oral Med Oral Pathol Oral Radiol Endod* 90:559, 2000.
71. Schiodt M, Hermund NU: Management of oral disease prior to radiation therapy, *Support Care Cancer* 10:40, 2002.
72. Scully C, Wolff A: Oral surgery in patients on anticoagulant therapy, *Oral Surg Oral Med Oral Pathol Oral Radiol Endod* 94:57, 2002.
73. Semba SE, Mealey BL, Hallmon WW: The head and neck radiotherapy patient. Part 1. Oral manifestations of radiation therapy, *Compend Contin Educ Dent* 15:250, 1994.
74. Semba SE, Mealey BL, Hallmon WW: Dentistry and the cancer patient. Part 2. Oral health management of the chemotherapy patient, *Compend Contin Educ Dent* 15:1378, 1994.
75. Seymour RA, Whitworth JM: Antibiotic prophylaxis for endocarditis, prosthetic joints, and surgery, *Dent Clin North Am* 46:635, 2002.
76. Shapiro R, Carroll PB, Tzakis A, et al: Adrenal reserve in renal transplant recipients with cyclosporine/azathioprine/prednisone immunosuppression, *Transplantation* 49:1011, 1990.
77. Sherman RG, Lasseter DH: Pharmacologic management of patients with diseases of the endocrine system, *Dent Clin North Am* 40:727, 1996.
78. Shrout MK, Scarbrough F, Powell BJ: Dental care and the prosthetic joint patient: a survey of orthopedic surgeons and general dentists, *J Am Dent Assoc* 125:429, 1994.
79. Sindet-Pedersen S, Stenbjerg S, Ingerslev J: Control of gingival hemorrhage in hemophilic patients by inhibition of fibrinolysis with tranexamic acid, *J Periodontal Res* 23:72, 1988.
80. Slots J, Rosling BG, Genco RJ: Suppression of penicillin resistant oral *Actinobacillus actinomycetemcomitans* with tetracycline: considerations in endocarditis prophylaxis, *J Periodontol* 54:193, 1983.
81. Smith GN, Pashley DH: Periodontal ligament injection: evaluation of systemic effects, *Oral Surg Oral Med Oral Pathol* 56:571, 1983.
82. Smolensky MH: Chronobiology and chronotherapeutics: applications to cardiovascular medicine, *Am J Hypertens* 9(4, pt 3):11, 1996.
83. Tarsitano BF, Rollings RE: The pregnant patient: evaluation and management, *Gen Dent* 41:226, 1993.
84. Tervonen T, Karjalainen K: Periodontal disease related to diabetic status: a pilot study of the response to periodontal therapy in type 1 diabetes, *J Clin Periodontol* 24:505, 1997.
85. Thyne GM, Ferguson JW: Antibiotic prophylaxis during dental treatment in patients with prosthetic joints, *J Bone Joint Surg* 73B:191, 1991.
86. Tibbetts LS: Conscious sedation. In Rose LF, Mealey BL, Genco RJ, Cohen DW, editors: *Periodontics: medicine, surgery, and implants*, St Louis, 2004, Mosby, Elsevier.
87. Tong DC, Rothwell BR: Antibiotic prophylaxis in dentistry: a review and practice recommendations, *J Am Dent Assoc* 131:366, 2000.
88. UK Prospective Diabetes Study (UKPDS) Group: Intensive blood glucose control with sulphonylureas or insulin compared with conventional treatment and risk of complications in patients with type 2 diabetes (UKPDS 33), *Lancet* 352:837, 1998.
89. Umino M, Nagao M: Systemic diseases in elderly dental patients, *Int Dent J* 43:213, 1993.
90. Vasan RS, Beiser A, Seshadri S, et al. Residual lifetime risk for developing hypertension in middle aged women and men: the Framingham Heart Study, *JAMA* 287:1003, 2002.

91. Vissink A, Burlage FR, Spijkervet FK, et al: Prevention and treatment of the consequences of head and neck radiotherapy, *Crit Rev Oral Biol Med* 14:213, 2003.
92. Vissink A, Jansma J, Spijkervet FK, et al: Oral sequelae of head and neck radiotherapy, *Crit Rev Oral Biol Med* 14:199, 2003.
93. Watanabe K: Prepubertal periodontitis: a review of diagnostic criteria, pathogenesis, and differential diagnosis, *J Periodontal Res* 25:31, 1990.
94. Westfelt E, Rylander H, Blohme G, et al: The effect of periodontal therapy in diabetics: results after 5 years, *J Clin Periodontol* 23:92, 1996.
95. Winsom C, Siegel MA: Advances on the diagnosis and management of human viral hepatitis, *Dent Clin North Am* 47:431, 2003.
96. Yagiela JA: Adverse drug interactions in dental practice: interactions associated with vasoconstrictors, *J Am Dent Assoc* 130:701, 1999.
97. Ziccardi VB, Abubaker AO, Sotereanos GC, et al: Maxillofacial considerations in orthotopic liver transplantation, *Oral Surg Oral Med Oral Pathol* 71:21, 1991.

Periodontal Treatment for Older Adults

Sue S. Spackman and Janet G. Bauer

45 CHAPTER

CHAPTER OUTLINE

Older adults are expected to compose a larger proportion of the population than in the past. Population growth among long-lived older adults contributes to this increase worldwide. For dentistry, this means that older adults are retaining more of their natural dentition. Currently, almost 70% of older adults in the United States have natural teeth.[17] However, retention of teeth may result in more teeth at risk for periodontal disease, and thus the prevalence of periodontal disease may be associated with aging. This association was addressed by Beck[11] at the 1996 World Workshop on Periodontics: "It may be that risk factors do change as people age or at least the relative importance of risk factors change."

This chapter focuses on the interrelationship between aging and oral health, with an emphasis on periodontal health.

THE AGING PERIODONTIUM

Normal aging of the periodontium is a result of cellular aging. In general, cellular aging is the basis for the intrinsic changes seen in oral tissues over time. The aging process does not affect every tissue in the same way. For example, muscle tissue and nerve tissue undergo minimal renewal, whereas epithelial tissue, which is one of the primary components of the periodontium, always renews itself.

Intrinsic Changes

In epithelium, a progenitor population of cells (stem cells), situated in the basal layer, provides new cells. These cells of the basal layer are the least differentiated cells of the oral epithelium. A small subpopulation of these cells produces basal cells and retains proliferative potential of the tissue. A larger subpopulation of these cells (amplifying cells) produces cells available for subsequent maturation. This maturing population of cells continually undergoes a process of differentiation or maturation.

By definition, this differentiated cell, or epithelial cell, can no longer divide. On the other hand, the basal cell remains as part of the progenitor population of cells, ready to return to the mitotic cycle and again produce both types of cells. Thus there is a constant source of renewal (Figure 45-1). In the aging process, cell renewal takes place at a slower rate and with fewer cells, so the effect is to slow down the regenerative processes. As the progenitor cells wear out and die, there are fewer and fewer of these cells to renew the dead ones. This effect is characteristic of the age-related changes and biologic changes that occur with aging.

By the action of gerontogene(s) or replicative senescence (Hayflick's limit and telomere shortening), the number of progenitor cells decreases. Hayflick, an American microbiologist, observed that fetal cells (i.e., fibroblasts) displayed a consistently greater growth potential (approximately 50 cumulative population doublings) than those derived from adult tissues (20-30 cumulative population doublings). As a result, the decreased cellular component has a concomitant effect to decrease cellular reserves and protein synthesis. This affects the oral epithelium in that the tissue becomes thin, with reduced keratinization.

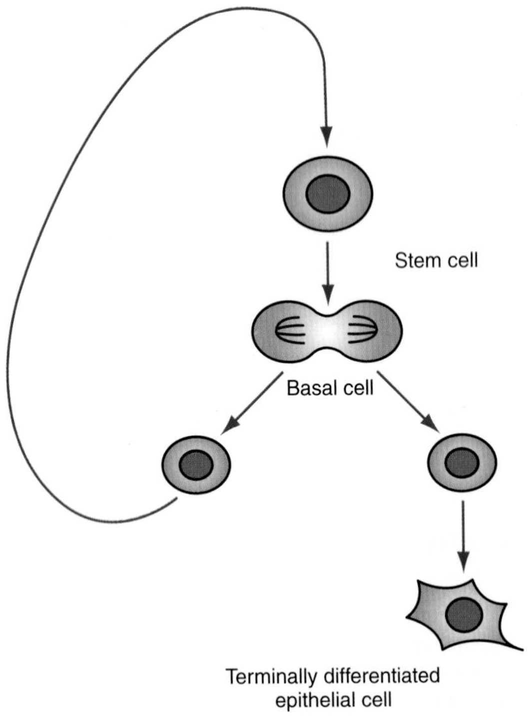

Figure 45-1 Cell renewal cycle in which the basal cell produces the epithelial cell and returns to the progenitor cell population.

Stochastic Changes

Stochastic changes occurring within cells also affect tissue; for example, glycosylation and cross-linking produce morphologic and physiologic changes. Structures become stiffer, with a loss of elasticity and increased mineralization (fossilization). With a loss of regenerative power, structures become less soluble and more thermally stable. Somatic mutations lead to decreased protein synthesis and structurally altered proteins. Free radicals contribute to the accumulation of waste in the cell.

All these changes produce a decline in the physiologic processes of tissue. Most changes are primarily a result of aging, although some are secondary to physiologic deterioration. For example, loss of elasticity and increased resistance of the tissue may lead to decreased permeability, decreased nutrient flow, and the accumulation of wastes in the cell. Thus, vascular peripheral resistance (decreased blood supply) may secondarily decrease cellular function.

Physiologic Changes

In the periodontal ligament, a decrease in the number of collagen fibers leads to a reduction or loss in tissue elasticity. A decrease in vascularity results in decreased production of mucopolysaccharides.

All these types of changes are seen in the alveolar bone. With aging, the alveolar bone shows a decrease in bone density and an increase in bone resorption; a decrease in vascularity also occurs. In contrast, however, cementum shows cemental thickness.

Functional Changes

With aging, the cells of the oral epithelium and periodontal ligament have reduced mitotic activity, and all cells experience a reduction in metabolic rate. These changes also affect the immune system and affect healing in the periodontium. There is a reduction in healing capacity and rate. Inflammation, when present, develops more rapidly and more severely. Individuals are highly susceptible to viral and fungal infections because of abnormalities in T-cell function.

Clinical Changes

Compensatory changes occur as a result of aging or disease. These changes affect the tooth or periodontium that presents the clinical condition. Gingival recession and reductions in bone height are common conditions. Attrition is a compensatory change that acts as a stabilizer between loss of bony support and excessive leveraging from occlusal forces imposed on the teeth. In addition, a reduction in "overjet" of the teeth is seen, manifesting as an increase in the edge-to-edge contact of the anterior teeth. Typically, this is related to the approximal wear of the posterior teeth. An increase is seen in the food table area, with loss of "sluiceways," and in mesial migration.

Functional changes are associated with reduced efficiency of mastication. Although effectiveness of mastication may remain, efficiency is reduced because of missing teeth, loose teeth, poorly fitting prostheses, or noncompliance of the patient, who may refuse to wear prosthetic appliances.

DEMOGRAPHICS

Population Distribution

In 2000, adults 65 years of age and older were 12.0% of the U.S. population, or 35 million people. From 2001 to 2010, this population will grow by 13%. The greatest growth will occur in those age 85 and older (29%) and those 100 and older (65%). By the mid–twenty-first century, the U.S. population is expected to increase by 42%. During this same period, the population age 65 and older is expected to increase by 126%. Of this population, those 85 and older are expected to increase by 316%, with centenarians (age 100+) increasing by 956%.[49]

The increase in the aging population is the result of the dramatic increase in life expectancy during the past and present centuries. Average life expectancy was 75 years in 1990, an increase of 28 years from 1900. In 2000, life expectancy (at birth) was projected to be 77 years. Adults who reached the age of 65 in 1990 could expect to live an average of 17 additional years.[48,49]

Differences in population growth between urban and rural older adults have special significance to oral health. The expected increase in the proportion of older adults will be 3% larger in rural areas. Because rural older adults use dental services less than their urban counterparts, the risk for adverse changes in oral health and self-care may be greater.[53]

SCIENCE TRANSFER

In the United States and throughout the world, the number of older adults is increasing, and these individuals are retaining more of their teeth. This population has unique problems that necessitate alterations in their treatment plans. They also use more medications, many of which can cause problems such as xerostomia and decreased saliva. Thus, aging can significantly alter the host immune response and inflammatory reactions to bacterial plaque and in different ways than in younger populations. In these older adults, education, nutrition counseling, regular dental care, and compensatory home and professional care techniques may be required.

Advances in medical and dental care account for the increasing number of patients over 65 years of age with more remaining teeth. Older patients do not have an increased susceptibility to periodontal disease and respond well to periodontal therapy, including implant surgery. On the other hand, these patients often have increased risk of root caries, dry mouth, and oral cancer. *Clinicians need to focus on the particular oral disease susceptibilities of older patients and emphasize preventive measures, including the increased need for assisting oral hygiene with mechanical devices and antiseptic mouthwashes and applying fluorides when there is evidence of root caries.*

Health Status

Increase life expectancy has changed the way the public and health care policy makers and providers think about "aging." Instead of controlling chronic disease and morbidity, aging is seen in terms of "successful aging" or "healthy aging." This paradigm shift is based on study of what promotes health and longevity. Current research is now examining aging in terms of the physical, mental, and social well-being of older adults, not just disease or morbidity. The MacArthur Studies of Successful Aging asked the fundamental question, "What genetic, biomedical, behavioral, and social factors are crucial to maintaining health and functional capacities in the later years?"[31]

Despite this paradigm shift, the number of older adults with acute and chronic diseases continues to increase.[49] Visual impairments, cataracts, glaucoma, and hearing impairments increase in frequency with advancing age. Almost half of people age 65 and older have arthritis.[51] Most older adults have at least one chronic condition, and many have several chronic conditions. In 1994 the chronic conditions that occurred most often in older adults were arthritis, hypertension, heart disease, hearing impairment, cataract, orthopedic impairment, sinusitis, and diabetes (Table 45-1).[1] Although heart disease remains the leading cause of death among older adults, cancer may become the leader during the twenty-first century. Currently among older adults, approximately 7 in 10 deaths are caused by heart disease, cancer, or stroke.[49]

In the early 1900s, Dr. Ignatz Leo was the first to recognize that older adults had health needs and concerns that set them apart from younger adults.[35] Not until the later half of the twentieth century, however, did *geriatrics* (medicine for older adults) become a discipline in health care. A "geriatric patient" is an older adult who is frail, dependent, or both and who requires health and social

TABLE 45-1

Percentage of Chronic Conditions in Older Adults

Conditions	Percentage
Arthritis	50
Hypertension	36
Heart disease	32
Hearing impairments	29
Cataracts	17
Orthopedic impairments	16
Sinusitis	15
Diabetes	10

Data from Administration on Aging: A profile of older Americans, 1998, http://www.aoa.dhhs.gov.

TABLE 45-2

Functional Categories for Older Adults

Category	Description	Issues	Limitations
Functionally independent	Those who reside in the community and receive little or no assistance.	Majority of older adults fall into this category.	Access and use dental services similar to younger adults in the community.
Frail	Those who reside in the community and maintain some degree of independence with assistance from others.	Include those who are "homebound," or spend most of their time in their homes, and those at risk for being institutionalized.	Need assistance with some activities of daily living and are dependent on another for most instrumental activities of daily living.
Bathing, dressing, and transportation problems were the three limitations that most homebound elderly experienced.			
Functionally dependent	Those who cannot maintain any level of independence and are totally dependent on assistance.	Include those who are institutionalized or are a at highest risk for institutionalization.	Dependent on another for most if not all the instrumental and basic activities of daily living.

support services to attain an optimal level of physical, psychologic, and social functioning. Thus the treatment plan must reflect the professional knowledge to resolve physical and psychologic aspects of health status, as well as being sensitive to an individual's all-encompassing social functioning. This functioning may include aspects of race, ethnicity, culture, personal relationships, esthetics, and social and economic conditions.

The main focus of geriatrics is *frail and functionally dependent older adults*. Functionally independent older adults are included, but only to make them aware of services that they may need if they experience functional deficits that impair their daily activities (Table 45-2). Specialists in geriatric medicine, *geriatricians,* have additional training in health care for frail and functionally dependent older adults. In geriatric medicine, numerous assessment instruments have been developed to assist the geriatrician, and some aspects of these are important to dentists in identifying risks and functional declines. These include activities of daily living (ADLs), Tinetti Balance and Gait Evaluation, geriatric depression scale (GDS), and Mini-Mental State Questionnaire. Each assesses risks to morbidity and mortality in maintaining a patient's optimal health and functional independence.

Care for geriatric patients crosses many disciplines. Thus, an interdisciplinary team is formed to care for and treat geriatric patients and may include the dentist. Including dentistry in the interdisciplinary effort has benefits for the patient; for example, oral care has been incorporated into nursing educational programs and practice for the geriatrician nurse practitioner.[37] Likewise, dieticians have educational content in oral care. The focus is to include oral health as part of *medical nutrition therapy* (MNT) in achieving the patient's total health needs.[5] A "last frontier" for the interdisciplinary team is the community. When geriatric patients require multidisciplinary strategies to improve their conditions at the community level, efforts have been less than satisfactory. Problems have been encountered when coordination is needed for geriatric patients to access multiple providers across a range of health care settings. Shared decision making and patient education are needed to improve access and realize successful outcomes.[22]

Functional Status

In dentistry, prevention of oral diseases and improvements in healthy lifestyles have contributed to older adults keeping and maintaining their dentition. In dentistry for geriatric patients, or *geriatric dentistry,* this has emphasized an interdisciplinary approach to diagnosis, treatment, and prevention of dental and oral diseases.[20] Specialists in geriatric dentistry are *geriatric dentists.* Similar geriatric health and functional instruments used in medicine assist geriatric dentists in assessing risks that compromise oral health.

Functional impairments have a significant impact on oral health and self-care. Sensory impairments and arthritis make it more difficult for older adults to understand dental outcomes, communicate oral health care needs and concerns, and perform effective oral self-care. Functional testing or measuring instruments may become part of the dentist's armamentarium to assess an older adult's ability to perform oral care tasks in achieving and maintaining oral health. The *index of activities of daily oral hygiene* (ADOH) is one such dental assessment instrument that quantifies the functional ability of older adults, specifically frail and functionally dependent older adults, in performing oral self-care tasks.[8] The index of ADOH provides the dentist or dental assistant with the means to determine the functional ability of an older adult to manipulate aids used in daily oral hygiene care. From these findings, strategies may be developed to rehabilitate and then remeasure for improvements in functional deficits. If improvements are not forthcoming, alternative strategies and assistive devices are recommended.

Accommodating dentists in the interdisciplinary team is increasing, including their participation in primary care. For example, edentulism and denture wearing in older adults may be related to poor quality of life and risk for undiagnosed oral disease. They may also indicate other medical comorbidities. Thus, medical and dental geriatricians must incorporate knowledge of comorbidities to identify risks that manifest as reciprocation of disease and poor quality of life.[54,59] In managing periodontal disease, the dental geriatrician is challenged with integrating primary care, oral health, and patient and caregiver education in nontraditional settings, such as residential, institutional, and hospital practice settings.

Although geriatric medicine training programs have grown remarkably over the past three decades, this growth is still not producing the number of geriatricians needed to care for the growing older adult population. Comparatively, the training of dental geriatricians is much less. In response, the geriatric dentistry community has advocated the use of dental geriatricians to train general dentists in the care of geriatric dental patients. Kayak and Brudvik[29] see this type of training essential to "successful aging" and periodontal health care in both dental practice and nontraditional settings. Thus, dental geriatricians as faculty are needed to train practitioners.[54]

Nutritional Status

Whereas "diet" refers to the consumption of types and varieties of food resources, *nutrition* is the process by which food is used to provide energy and sustain, restore, and maintain tissue of living organisms. With aging, there is an increased risk of nutritional deficiencies among older adults. However, the real risk is not malnutrition; among older adults in the United States, the rate of malnutrition is low. The real risk is attributed to *unbalanced diets*.

An older adult's dietary patterns may be associated with numerous factors, including the aging process, diseases and the medications used in their treatment, and social and economic conditions. In general, energy needs and intake in older adults decline with age.

Beyond middle age, body weight and lean body mass decline with age, in part because of primary aging. Age changes in physiologic functioning, including metabolic, hormonal, and neural changes, have been associated with poor-quality diets in older adults.

Older adults do not compensate well, or take in more food, when bodily changes alter their energy levels. For example, a slower metabolic rate accompanied with decreased levels of physical activity explains why older adults have reduced food intake. This is also associated with altered sensations of hunger, thirst, and satiety or fullness. Reductions are seen in fluid intake, uncompensated by increased thirst. The variety of foods eaten is reduced, or characteristic bland diets may result from lowered sensory-specific satiety. In other words, older adults have a lowered enjoyment of foods because of deficits in smell and possibly taste. More than half of people age 65 to 80 have a major olfactory impairment, with 75% of those age 80 and older affected. Thus, food recognition diminishes with age.

All these factors may place the older adult at risk for serious problems. *Anorexia,* or low food intake, increases the risk of nutrition-related illnesses. *Electrolytic imbalances* (e.g., salt and water imbalances) are associated with age-related changes in regulatory systems, such as changes in central nervous system (CNS) receptors that detect changes in the level of sodium in blood. *Dehydration,* which can lead to illness and death, is a common cause of fluid and electrolyte disturbance. *Deconditioning* is an almost complete disturbance of physical functioning. These conditions may present when a frail older adult comes to the dental office seeking care and are seen more often in homebound, hospital, and nursing home residents.

Poor nutrition and low body weight may often precede and predispose older adults to secondary age changes. *Secondary aging changes* are a result of acute and chronic disease and medication use. The most common age-associated chronic diseases are hypertension, hyperlipidemia, atherosclerosis, and diabetes. Compounding effects of secondary aging may include impaired mobility, inability to feed oneself, poor oral health, and the use of dentures, all of which may affect the amount and types of foods consumed. Age-associated decreases in saliva production and swallowing problems may also make eating difficult. In addition, nutrient malabsorption can be caused by altered gastric acid secretion or by interaction with medications. The cumulative effect of these changes may account for taste loss in the older adult.

Economic and social factors have also been linked with significant changes in eating patterns, such as loss of appetite. *Economic factors* include a lower economic status resulting from retirement, failing health, living on a fixed income, or death of a spouse. *Social factors* include isolation, loneliness, and the effects of depression or dementia. All these factors may affect the type and quality of food consumed. For example, socialization at meals may increase the amount of food consumed by older adults.

In addition, *impaired chewing* can cause changes in food selection, such as decreasing the variety in the diet, which may contribute to nutritional problems. Currently, 42% of older adults have no natural teeth. Rehabilitation with complete dentures may restore only 25% of normal chewing effectiveness.[40] Of those with teeth, 60% have tooth decay and 90% have periodontal disease, which may contribute to impaired chewing ability or loss of appetite.

These aging-related disease states and social factors may result in inadequate consumption of nutrient-dense foods or inadequate intake of some vitamins and minerals. Minerals are important to the absorption and utilization of vitamins. Both are important to antibody formation and the immune system in combating infection, foreign substances, and toxins (Table 45-3).[13]

Psychosocial Factors

Dental diseases have their greatest effect on behaviors and mental and social well-being. In other words, dental diseases impact psychologic and social functioning and thus are almost always preventable by behavioral and social means. On average, older adults use fewer dental services, perhaps because of conflicting economic priorities between medical and dental needs. For many older adults, dental services are a discretionary choice and not part of their primary care options. This may result in part from their poorer health status, lack of

TABLE 45-3

Nutrient Effects on the Immune Response

		EFFECT OF INSUFFICIENT INTAKE OF NUTRIENT	
Nutrient	**Component in Biological Processes**	**Increase Function**	**Decrease Function**
Protein energy intake	Energy metabolism Deoxyribonucleic acid and ribonucleic acid (DNA/RNA) synthesis	Bacterial adhesion	Salivary antimicrobial properties Immunoglobulin production Lysozymes Activation of lymphocytes Production of antibodies
Vitamin A	Cellular differentiation and proliferation Integrity of immune system	Bacterial adhesion	Immune cell differentiation Response to antigens Antibody production Immunoglobulin production Production of lymphocytes
Vitamin E	Antioxidant protecting lipid membranes from oxidation	—	Antibody synthesis Response of lymphocytes Phagocytic function
Vitamin C	Antioxidant that reduces free radicals that cause DNA damage to immune cells	—	Phagocytic function of neutrophils and macrophages Antibody response Cytotoxic T-cell activity
Riboflavin, vitamin B_6, and panthothenic acid	Coenzymes in metabolic processes	—	Antibody synthesis Cytotoxic T-cell activity Lymphocyte response
Folic acid and vitamin B_{12}	Involved in DNA/RNA synthesis	—	Production of lymphocytes Cytotoxic T-cell activity Phagocytic function of neutrophils
Zinc	More than 100 enzymes associated with carbohydrate and energy metabolism Protein catabolism and synthesis Nucleic acid synthesis	—	Antibody response Phagocytic function of macrophages B-cell and T-cell proliferation
Iron	Involved in hemoglobin, myoglobin, and cytochrome systems	—	Lymphocyte proliferation Neutrophil cytotoxic activity Antibody response

Data from Boyd LD, Madden TE: *Dent Clin North Am* 47:337, 2003.

dental insurance or coverage by government-sponsored health care programs, or simply their functional status or independence.

Older adults with positive attitudes toward oral health have predictably better dental behaviors that translate into higher utilization rates of dental services. Positive attitudes are highly associated with educational level.[10] The education level of older adults is increasing. In 1995, only 64% of noninstitutionalized older adults completed at least high school, and 13% possessed a bachelor's degree. By 2015, it is estimated that 76% of older adults will have completed at least high school, with 20% obtaining a bachelor's degree. Those with more education were three to four times more likely to have visited a dentist in the past year, indicating that an informed and knowledgeable public provides a culture of healthy behaviors that guide older adults toward the long-term preservation of teeth and function.

Impediments to the utilization of dental services are associated with low income and an associated lack of a regular source of care. Those with higher education tend to be better off financially than those with low education. Poverty is less prevalent today among older adults for all race, gender, and ethnic groups.[49,50] In general, older adults have the highest disposable income of all ages.[57] Thus, higher educational achievement with lower poverty levels is a predictor for an increase in demand for oral health care among older adults.[28]

However, differences in the prevalence of periodontal disease were seen in relation to race. Among dentate non-Hispanic blacks, non-Hispanic whites, and Mexican Americans 50 years of age and older, blacks had higher levels of periodontal disease, even those in higher-income groups. Thus, Borrell et al.,[12] suggest that race and ethnicity are important factors in combating health disparities.

Reciprocally, oral disease may affect behaviors, and behavioral problems may adversely affect oral health. Adverse oral health conditions affect three aspects of daily living: (1) systemic health, (2) quality of life, and (3) economic productivity.

Both systemic health and quality of life are compromised when edentulism, xerostomia, soft tissue lesions, and poorly fitting dentures affect eating and food choices. Conditions such as oral clefts, missing teeth, severe malocclusion, and severe caries are associated with feelings of embarrassment, withdrawal, and anxiety. Oral and facial pain from dentures, temporomandibular joint disorders, and oral infections affect social interaction and daily behaviors.[27]

Behavioral problems may worsen oral conditions. Older adults today grew up during Prohibition or the Great Depression, when alcohol consumption was much lower. Since then, *alcohol consumption* has increased, especially in women, along with alcohol-related health problems. Alcohol-related disorders include alcohol abuse and dependence and alcoholic liver disease, psychoses, cardiomyopathy, gastritis, and polyneuropathy.

A general consensus states that light drinking, or one drink per day, is not harmful as long as the older adult is reasonably healthy and not taking medications that interact with alcohol. However, alcohol may react differently in older than younger adults. A decrease in body water content may produce higher peak serum ethanol levels. In particular, alcohol intake may make older adults vulnerable to changes in the capacity of the liver to metabolize drugs and to symptomatic behaviors such as confusion, depression, and dementia.

The patterns of drinking and alcohol-related problems may not differ between older and younger problem drinkers. However, numerous reports suggest that alcohol as the primary substance of abuse is higher in the older than in the younger adult. A peak onset for alcohol-related problems is 65 to 74 years. Unfortunately, alcohol consumption is directly correlated with clinical attachment loss in periodontal disease.[47]

Periodontal disease may also be exacerbated in those with depression.[3,30] *Depression* is a common public health problem among elderly persons, affecting 15% of adults over age 65 in the United States. The suicide rate for those over 85 is about two times the national rate. Geriatric depression is treatable, so recognition of this disorder is a vital step in the prevention of disability and mortality.[42] However, depression is not easy to recognize. Depression may also accompany a wide variety of physical illnesses, such as fatigue, poor appetite, sleep disturbances, cardiovascular disease, and cancer. It may be the primary cause of somatic complaints, including oral discomfort. The classic signs and symptoms for depression include sadness, decreased appetite, weight loss, confusion, difficulty in decision making, dissatisfaction, and irritability. Many older adults, however, present with a less dramatic level of actual sadness and frequently have apparent cognitive impairment, especially memory deficits, and therefore differentiation from dementia is important. Recognizing the signs of depression can significantly reduce depression, by about 70%, in those over 65 years of age.

Dentate Status

In dentistry the level of illness is measured as "tooth mortality" or tooth loss. Still among the most ubiquitous of human diseases, dental disease places all segments of the population at risk. Older adults are at greatest risk, especially those over 85 years of age. Oral health changes in health and functional well-being (functional disabilities) potentiate risks to oral disease, including dental caries (particularly root caries), periodontal disease, oral cancer, xerostomia (dry mouth), disorders associated with denture wearers, and systemic disease with oral symptoms.

Over a 30-year period, edentulism and partial tooth loss declined substantially.[17] The most current estimates of tooth loss and tooth retention in the U.S. population indicate that 75% of older adults age 65 to 69 and over half of adults age 75 and older are dentate (Table 45-4). By the year 2030, the number of teeth retained by older adults is expected to double, an estimated 800 million increase in tooth retention. It is expected that over the next three decades the average number of retained teeth will increase from the current 20 to 25.9 teeth.[19] Thus the risk of periodontal disease and dental caries is expected to be a major problem of older adults. Because few older adults are covered by dental insurance,[9] payment for treatments will be the responsibility of the geriatric patient. Costs and the inability to afford care will always affect health care utilization, particularly dentistry, which is often considered discretionary.

TABLE 45-4

Percentage of Dentate Older Adults: United States, 1988 to 1991

Age Group	All Older Adults	Male	Female
50-54	88	90	86
55-59	82	82	83
60-64	76	77	76
65-69	74	73	75
70-74	69	71	67
75+	56	53	58

Data from US Census Bureau: U.S. interim projections by age, sex, race and Hispanic origin, 2004, http://www.census.gov/ipc/www/usinterimproj/.

Periodontal Status

The classic periodontal disease model suggested that virtually all older adults would, at some time in their life, become susceptible to severe periodontitis. This result was attributed to an insidious process in which gingivitis slowly progressed into periodontitis, with probable bone and tooth loss. Thus, it was asserted that susceptibility to periodontitis increased with age, resulting in tooth loss seen predominantly after age 35 years.

The current periodontal disease model suggests that only a small proportion of adults have advanced periodontal destruction. Mild gingivitis is common, as is mild to moderate periodontitis. Most adults show some loss of probing attachment while maintaining a functional dentition. In addition, severe periodontal disease is not a part of normal aging and is not the major cause of tooth loss. There may be exceptions to this, but when disease occurs, it is usually in those age 85 and older.

The model asserts that gingivitis does precede periodontitis, but relatively few sites with gingivitis develop periodontitis. The bacterial flora associated with gingivitis and periodontitis shows similarities but does not reciprocate causally. In all, the current model of periodontal disease indicates that the following:

- The prevalence of periodontal disease is low and possibly decreasing.
- The progress of periodontal disease is episodic and infrequent.
- Active and inactive disease sites coexist.
- Most of the reported cases of periodontal disease occur in a small, high-risk population of older adults.
- There is a continued effort to identify risk factors for periodontal disease.

The current risk factors suggested for periodontal disease include age, smoking, diabetes mellitus, and the presence of subgingival *Porphyromonas gingivalis* and *Tannerella forsythia*.

The prevalence of periodontal disease is therefore expected to increase with age[11] as a result of a cumulative disease progression over time, not susceptibility.[7,33] In a 30-year preventive home care study, periodontal findings showed a 75% improvement in the number of healthy periodontal sites in the 51- to 65-year-old age group.[7] Thus, recent data suggest that older adults who maintain optimum oral self-care are less susceptible to periodontitis.[15]

Advanced periodontal disease among older adults is not as common as once thought.[15] Moderate levels of attachment loss are seen in a high proportion of older adults, but severe loss is detected in only a small proportion of older adults (Figure 45-2). The amount of periodontal disease associated with age does not appear to be clinically significant, and it is unclear whether the higher prevalence of periodontal disease is a function of age or time.[33] Figures 45-3 to 45-5 illustrate periodontal disease data from phase I of the third National Health and Nutrition Examination Survey (NHANES III) conducted in the United States from 1988 to 1991.[14] Gingival recession increased with advancing age, with one third (35%) of persons age 55 to 84 and less than half (46%) of persons age 85 and older having 3 mm or more of gingival recession (Figure 45-3). Pocket depth of 6 mm or greater was detected in 7% of persons 45 to 54 years of age, 8% of persons age 55 to 64, and 7% of persons age 65 and older (Figure 45-4). Attachment loss increases with age, although less than half of persons age 65 and older had loss of attachment measuring 5 mm or greater (Figure 45-5).

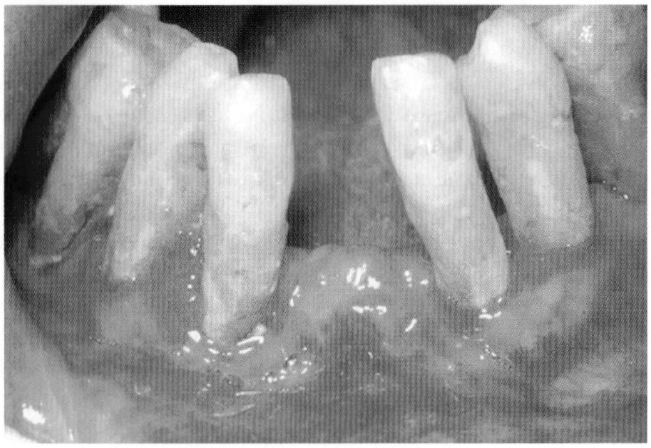

Figure 45-2 Severe periodontal disease with potential danger of tooth aspiration.

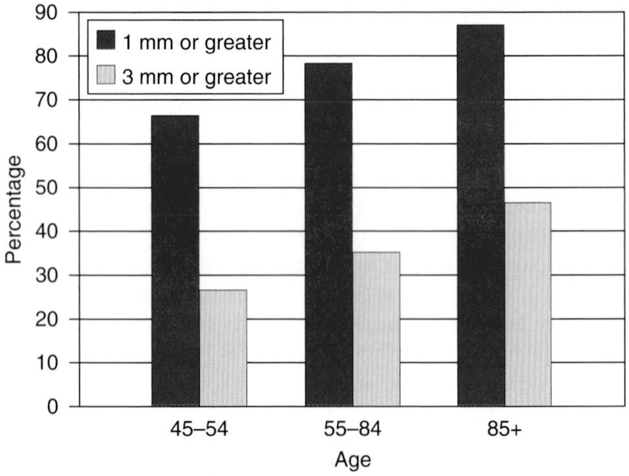

Figure 45-3 Percentage of older persons with gingival recession, 1988 to 1991. (From Brown LJ, Brunelle JA, Kingman A: *J Dent Res* 75:672, 1996.)

Caries Status

Root caries is a disease that has a particular predilection for older adults. Exposed root surfaces in combination with compromised health status and use of multiple medications make older adults at high risk for root caries. Caries examinations from phase I of NHANES III indicate that root caries prevalence increases greatly with age. Decayed or filled root surfaces were detected in 47% of persons age 65 to 74 and in 55.9% of those 75 and older.[63]

The majority of older adults are at low risk for developing root caries, but mediating factors increase this risk, including immune system dysfunction and ineffective oral self-care. With the prospect of older adults retaining more of their teeth through improved access, prevention programs, and personal oral hygiene, it is likely that a sound root surface will remain caries free. Once a lesion is present, however, one-surface and multiple-surface lesions progress aggressively to infect other adjoining tooth surfaces rather than cavitating the infected surface. This natural occurrence in older adults is caused by dentinal sclerosis; caries progression spreads without cavitation. In older adults the active four-surface lesion produces a characteristic "apple coring," or collar of caries extending circumferentially along the cementoenamel junction, below the clinical enamel crown of the tooth. The four-surface lesion becomes chronic, with morphologic loss dependent on the balance of forces during demineralization and remineralization. Loss of the root

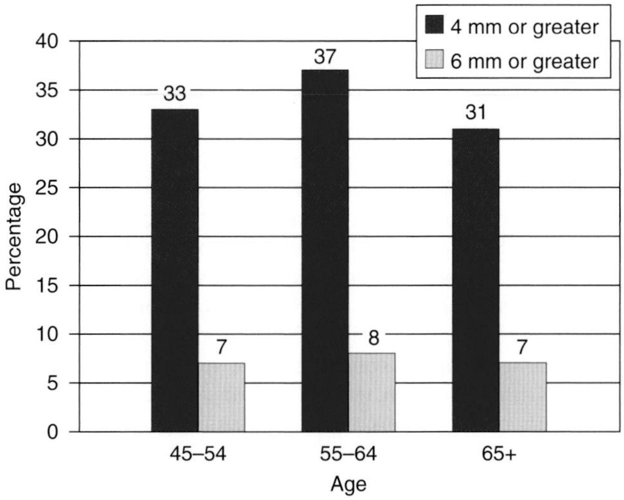

Figure 45-4 Percentage of older persons with pocket depths by age, 1988 to 1991. (From Brown LJ, Brunelle JA, Kingman A: *J Dent Res* 75:672, 1996.)

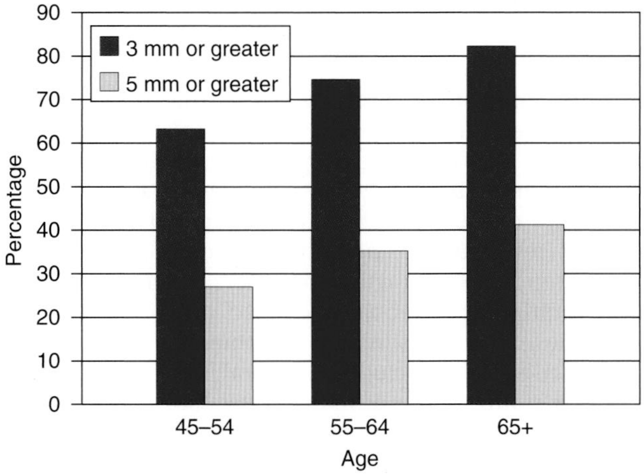

Figure 45-5 Percentage of older persons with loss of attachment by age, 1988 to 1991. (From Brown LJ, Brunelle JA, Kingman A: *J Dent Res* 75:672, 1996.)

structure may be so significant that it undermines the support of the clinical crown. When tooth structure is compromised, the tooth is at a high risk for fracture, and oral or tooth function is impaired (Figure 45-6). The tooth may then be lost because of clinical outcomes that disallow its rehabilitation.

Dental Visits

Fundamentally, dental visits by older adults are correlated with having teeth, not age.[62] Data from the 1995 Behavioral Risk Factor Surveillance System (BRFSS), which is a continuous state-based, random-digit-dialed telephone survey of the U.S. noninstitutionalized population age 18 years and older, indicate that older adults are frequent users of dental services.[16]

Although their total consumption of dental services approximates that of younger adults, older adults make fewer dental visits: 21% to 53% of dentate adults visited the dentist in the last 12 months. Approximately 40% of these older adults utilize these visits for episodic care, indicating a lack of sustained and consistent care. Those least likely to visit a dentist were older adults who were either homebound or institutionalized.

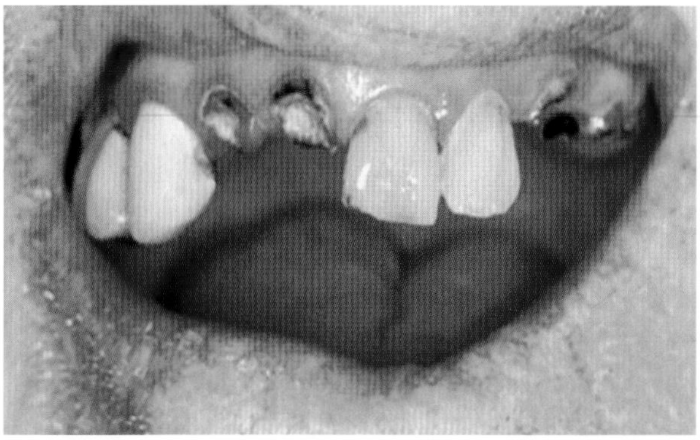

Figure 45-6 Root tips remain after coronal portion of the tooth is lost as a result of root caries, leaving a pathway for infection.

When dentate and edentulous adults express positive attitudes regarding the efficacy of dental care, their care-seeking behaviors translate into use, continuous use, and recent use of dental services. However, the belief among dentate and edentulous older adults that their dental problems are a result of aging prevails. Despite clinically evident disease or problems, beliefs and values of older adults regarding the usefulness of dental care to resolve oral problems are limited. They have difficulty incorporating their perceived need into care-seeking behaviors. In addition, nursing home residents often refuse dental care, even when cost is not a barrier, and believe prevention or treatment would not be efficacious in solving their oral problems.

Recent studies report dramatic increases in dentate older adults accessing dental care, with older adults now using dental services to the same extent as dentate adults between ages 35 and 44. Among adults age 65 and older, 62% of all respondents reported having a dental visit during the previous year, and 75% of those with natural teeth reported a dental visit in the past year.[16]

As the trend for tooth retention in older adults continues, older adults will account for a greater proportion of dental practice income and visits. Even the oldest persons in the elderly population have reversed earlier, negative attitudes and demonstrated increased awareness and concern for oral health.[30,32,60] Dental expenditure data indicate that older adults have a higher cost per visit than younger persons and are willing to make a significant investment in dental care.[57] Despite these trends, older adults in nursing homes seldom access dental services.

Xerostomia

Saliva plays an essential role in maintaining oral health. Besides a loss of acinar cells occurring with aging, many older adults take medications for chronic medical conditions and disorders. When challenged with medications

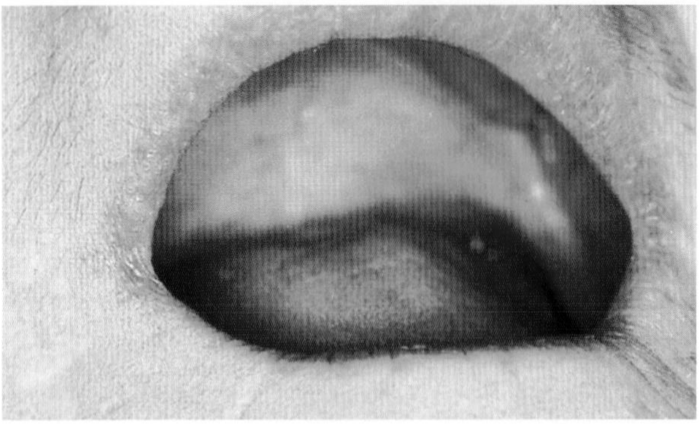

Figure 45-7 Severe xerostomia after radiation therapy when the parotid glands were not spared.

that cause dry mouth, older adults are more adversely affected than younger adults, which supports the secretory reserve hypothesis of salivary function.[25]

More than 500 prescription and over-the-counter medications are associated with decreased saliva, dry mouth, and xerostomia. The medications most often associated with xerostomia and decreased saliva are the tricyclic antidepressants, antihistamines, antihypertensives, and diuretics. Medication use is frequently associated with dry mouth; however, certain medical diseases, disorders, or conditions are also associated with dry mouth, such as radiation treatment for oral, head, neck, and thyroid cancers; Sjögren's syndrome; poorly controlled diabetes; bone marrow transplantation; thyroid disorders; and depression (Figure 45-7).

Symptomatic and corrective therapies have been suggested, such as parotid-sparing radiation therapy. The effect of this treatment has been shown to reduce xerostomia in each of four domains of quality of life: eating, communication, pain, and emotion. Both xerostomia and quality-of-life scores improved significantly over time during the first year after therapy. These results suggest that the efforts to reduce xerostomia using parotid-sparing radiation therapy may improve broad aspects of quality of life.[32]

Medications that induce xerostomia may also be associated with compromised chewing, speaking, tasting, or swallowing and increased risk for caries, periodontal disease, and candidiasis.

Future research directions include (1) gene therapy approaches to direct salivary growth and differentiation or modify remaining tissues to promote secretion, (2) creation of a biocompatible artificial salivary gland, and (3) salivary transplantation. With improved secretagogues, the effects of conditions that result in reduced salivary function and increased caries will be ameliorated.[23]

Candidiasis

Candidiasis is caused by an overproliferation of *Candida albicans*. A pathogenic infection occurs when *C. albicans* infiltrates into the oral mucosal layers. Candidiasis can be both local and systemic.[26]

Any condition compromising a patient's immune system can be considered a risk factor for candidiasis. Oral candidiasis can occur with long-term use of antibiotics, steroid therapies, or chemotherapy. Diabetes mellitus, head and neck radiation therapy, and human immunodeficiency virus (HIV) are risk factors for acute pseudomembranous candidal infection. *Pseudomembranous candidiasis* presents as white lesions that can be wiped away with gauze, leaving an erythematous area.[26]

Chronic atrophic candidiasis presents most often as an erythematous area under a maxillary denture and is associated with poor oral hygiene. In patients without a prosthesis, chronic atrophic candidiasis may present as a generalized redness or even generalized burning of the mouth.[26]

Chronic atrophic candidiasis, or *angular cheilitis,* can also manifest itself in the creases or commissures of the lips. This occurs when a patient has a tendency to pool saliva around the corners of the mouth or constantly lick the lips in some cases.[26]

A new treatment for candidiasis is being investigated using bioadhesive nanoparticles as modulators of adherence to buccal epithelial cells.[36]

DENTAL AND MEDICAL ASSESSMENTS

Review of Dental History

Initially, the patient interview assists the patient in disclosing needs, desires, preferences, and values for dental treatment. The dental history includes dates of the last dental examination and visit, radiographs taken, and the frequency of tooth prophylaxis. Also included is a review of past restorations, endodontic therapies, extractions, oral surgeries, prosthetic appliances (including single and multiple, removable and fixed units), periodontal therapies, and gnathologic treatments. Other useful information may include daily oral self-care regimens, fluoride status of the drinking water (bottled, well, and community sources), and type of toothpaste used (fluoride vs. nonfluoride).

Review of Medical History

The medical history of the older adult should be detailed and should include a careful review of past and current medical and mental conditions, including emergency and hospital visits and any serious illnesses (Box 45-1). The review should focus on a careful evaluation of systemic diseases and disorders, particularly those that influence dental treatment, such as bleeding disorders and use of anticoagulants, diabetes, heart valve problems, certain cardiovascular conditions, stroke, artificial joints, and use of corticosteroids. A consultation with the patient's physician is advisable, especially for older adults with medical problems, or if complicated or invasive procedures are planned. The medical history review should also include medications taken regularly and allergies to medications, metals, and environmental allergens. The social history is reviewed to determine the patient's age, tobacco use (type and pack-years estimate), alcohol use, and caregiver status. Caregiver status indicates the functional level of the patient as functionally independent, frail, or functionally dependent.

Obtaining a complete medical history may take longer in severely compromised older adults. However, the time

BOX 45-1

Dental Patient Interview: Older Adult

Medical (Physical) History

Assess for endocrine and nutritional disorders.

Assess for systemic disease.

Behavior History

Assess *overdependence:* Is the patient demanding, repetitious, or expressing urgency in his or her demands?

Assess *pseudocooperativeness:* Is the patient noncompliant in maintaining daily self-care?

Assess *perfectionism:* Is the patient unrealistic in his or her expectations yet noncompliant in maintaining oral self-care regimens?

Social History

Assess the presence or lack of a support system for the frail and dependent older adult.

spent to disclose conditions will determine if the use of the interdisciplinary team is indicated. Coordinating and managing oral health care in this manner may increase the success of dental outcomes.[44]

Review of Medication Use

Older adults are high users of prescription and over-the-counter (OTC) medications. Table 45-5 lists the top 20 drugs prescribed in the United States in 2003. Many medications used by older adults can have a negative impact on oral health. To obtain a complete list of prescription and OTC medications, ask patients to bring each medication bottle or package to the dental office. This not only helps to obtain a complete medication list, but also provides additional information, such as medication dose and number of physicians prescribing medications.

Extraoral and Intraoral Examinations

The *extraoral examination* provides assessments of the head and neck. The head and neck examination determines if the skull is normal in shape with no traumatic injuries. Also included are assessments of the skin, nodes, and cranial nerves involved in oral function. The temporomandibular joint is also assessed at this time. Findings include changes from normal, apparent lesions, and dysfunction.

The *intraoral examination* provides assessment of soft and hard tissue of the oral cavity (Box 45-2). Assessments help to determine the state of the teeth: past restorations, caries, occlusal dysfunction, and missing teeth. The periodontal examination includes gingival bleeding points and pocket depths. The remaining intraoral examination assesses the lips, cheeks, tongue, gingiva, floor of the mouth, palate, retromolar region, and oropharyngeal area for tissue abnormalities, red or white patches, ulcerations, and swellings. A major focus of these examinations is the assessment for oral and pharyngeal cancer.

BOX 45-2

Dental Examination: Assessments for Older Adult Patients

Oral Epithelium

Assess a decrease in intracellular water content, amount of subcutaneous fat, elasticity and vascularity of tissue, muscle tone, and vertical dimension.

Assess for a thin, waxy appearance of the tissue.

Assess for a hyperkeratosis of keratin areas.

Tongue

Assess for defoliation of papillae, fissures (dorsum side), and varicosities (ventral side).

Assess for alteration in taste.

Assess clinical complaints of the following:

- Smooth, glossy, and painful tongue (may indicate vitamin B_{12} deficiency)
- Geographic tongue (erythema migrans)
- Oral infections (e.g., candidiasis)

Saliva

Assess for xerostomia (altered salivary flow) that produces a decrease in the following:

- Antibacterial activity
- Buffering capacity
- Transport of taste sensors
- Lubrication of the oral cavity
- Digestive function

Note any signs of xerostomia, including the following:

- Intraoral dryness
- Burning sensations
- Altered tongue surface
- Dysphagia
- Cheilosis
- Alterations in taste
- Difficulty with speech
- Root caries

Immune System

Assess for pronounced inflammatory responses of the gingiva to infection.

It can be difficult to differentiate between a benign lesion and either a precancerous or early cancerous lesion. For this reason, a product called OralCDx has been developed; this computer-assisted brush biopsy test can aid in screening for cancer.[18,41]

Oral cancer may appear as an ulceration, a swelling, or a red or white sore that does not heal in 1 to 2 weeks. Other signs of oral cancer may be swollen lymph nodes and difficulty swallowing and speaking.[21] Particularly alarming, oral and pharyngeal cancer lesions may not be painful. Unfortunately, the 5-year survival of patients with oral cancer has not improved.[4]

Xerostomia screening may be done by sialometry or by oral examination. With *sialometry,* depending on the

TABLE 45-5

Top 20 Drugs Prescribed in the United States, 2003

Brand Name	Drug Action	Manufacturer
Hydrocodone w/APAP	Opioid analgesic, antitussive, antipyretic	Various; data for two or more generic manufacturers have been combined.
Lipitor	Lipid-lowering agent used for treating cholesterolemia	Pfizer US Pharmaceuticals
Synthroid	Synthetic human thyroid used for treating hypothyroidism	Abbott
Atenolol	Synthetic, β_1-selective (cardioselective) adrenoreceptor blocking agent	Various; data for two or more generic manufacturers have been combined.
Zithromax	Antibiotic similar to erythromycin	Pfizer US Pharmaceuticals
Amoxicillin	Antibiotic-antibacterial drug	Various; data for two or more generic manufacturers have been combined.
Furosemide	Potent diuretic contained in Lasix	Various; data for two or more generic manufacturers have been combined.
Hydrochlorothiazide	Diuretic Antihypertensive	Various; data for two or more generic manufacturers have been combined.
Norvasc	Long-acting calcium channel blocker	Pfizer US Pharmaceuticals
Lisinopril	Synthetic peptide derivative used as an oral long-acting angiotensin-converting enzyme (ACE) inhibitor	Various; data for two or more generic manufacturers have been combined.
Alprazolam	One of the benzodiazepine class of central nervous system–active compounds used for treating anxiety and contained in Xanax	Various; data for two or more generic manufacturers have been combined.
Zoloft	Selective serotonin reuptake inhibitor (SSRI) used for treating depression	Pfizer US Pharmaceuticals
Albuterol Aerosol	Inhalation aerosol used for treating asthma and contained in Proventil	Various; data for two or more generic manufacturers have been combined.
Toprol-XL	Synthetic, β_1-selective (cardioselective) adrenoreceptor blocking agent	AstraZeneca
Zocor	Lipid-lowering agent used for treating cholesterolemia	MSD
Premarin	Estrogen used for treating menopause: hormone replacement therapy (HRT)	Wyeth Pharmaceuticals
Prevacid	Inhibits gastric acid secretion	Tap Pharmaceuticals
Zyrtec	Selective H_1-receptor antagonist used for treating allergies	Pfizer US Pharmaceuticals
Ibuprofen	Nonsteroidal antiinflammatory agent Analgesic Both contained in Motrin	Various; data for two or more generic manufacturers have been combined.
Levoxyl	Synthetic human thyroid used for treating hypothyroidism	Monarch Pharmaceuticals

Data from RxList: Top 200 prescriptions for 2003 by number of U.S. prescriptions dispensed, http://www.rxlist.com/top200.htm. Feb. 21, 2005.

type of gland, the precise collection of saliva may require 5 to 15 minutes (Table 45-6). Specific screening tools may be required for different gland types. For example, modified Carlson-Crittenden collectors are used to suction saliva from the parotid gland through Stensen's duct, and specialized equipment is used for the submandibular gland (through Wharton's ducts) and the minor salivary glands.

A less quantitative measure of saliva for xerostomia is by oral examination using a tongue blade (Figure 45-8). The saliva collected from either the floor of the mouth or the buccal vestibules is absorbed onto the tongue blade (see Figure 45-8, *A* and *B*). If only the tip of the tongue blade demonstrates wetness rather than a greater portion of the end of the blade, then an abnormal finding is noted (see Figure 45-8, *C*).

TABLE 45-6

Sialometry for Xerostomia Screening: Salivary Flow Rates

Category	Normal	Abnormal
Whole saliva	0.5-1.2 ml/min	0.0-0.2 ml/min
Whole saliva, stimulated	1.0-2.0 ml/min	0.01-0.4 ml/min

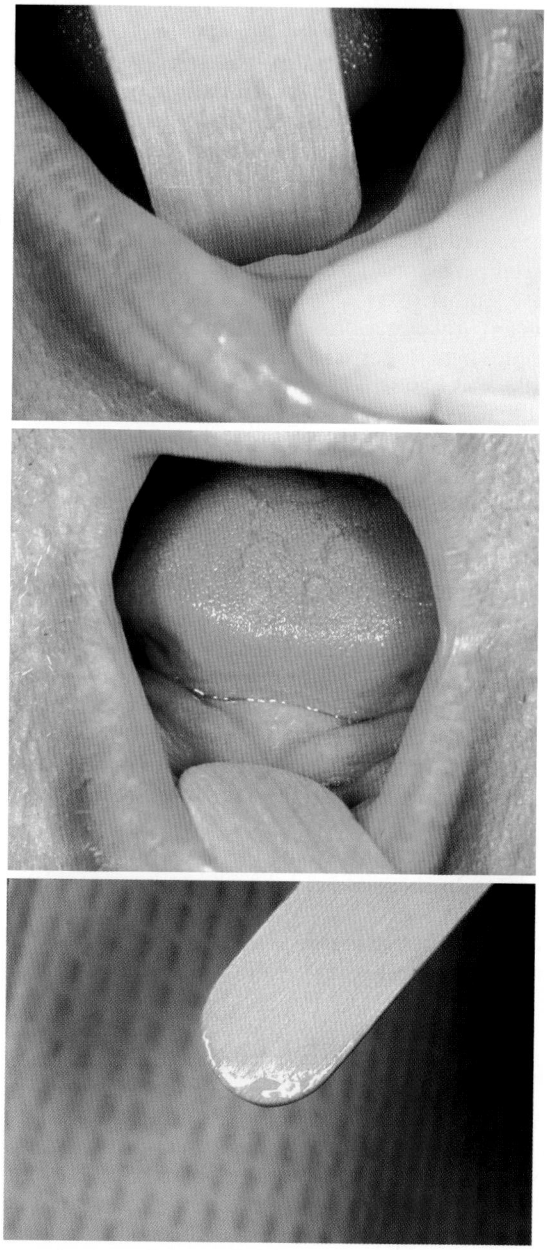

A

B

C

Figure 45-8 Tongue blade screen for saliva testing. **A,** Screening begins by placing the tongue blade in the sublingual area at the mandibular anterior quadrant. **B,** For the saliva screen, wet the tongue blade for about 5 seconds. **C,** Tongue blade screen showing minimal wetness, an indication of xerostomia.

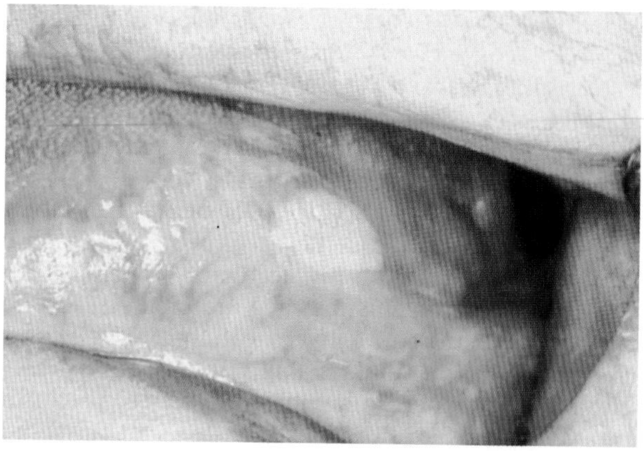

Figure 45-9 Early carcinoma in situ.

Assessment of Risk

Assessment of risk is determined after completion of the patient interview and the extraoral and intraoral examinations. Oral and medical problems may influence the risk for disease, pain, oral dysfunction, and nutritional disorders, both in quality and quantity of foods.[39] Risk assessments may also serve as predictors for successful treatment outcomes, maintenance protocols, and patient compliance. For example, the risk factors that influence periodontal therapy are smoking, genetic susceptibility, compliance, and diabetes.[61]

Assessment tests use genetic markers to demonstrate susceptibility to periodontal disease. Specific genetic markers associated with increased levels of interleukin-1 (IL-1) production indicate a strong susceptibility to severe periodontitis in older adults. When the genotype for polymorphic IL-1 gene cluster was identified, it was correlated with an odds ratio of 18.9, indicating severe periodontitis in nonsmoking adults.

Risk factors for oral and pharyngeal cancer are age, tobacco use, frequent use of alcohol, and exposure to sunlight (lip). Oral cancer is treatable if discovered and treated early. Most dentists can easily identify an early carcinoma in situ (Figure 45-9). At this stage, however, the lesion may have already spread to the lymph nodes. Oral and pharyngeal cancer detected at later stages can cause disfigurement, loss of function, decreased quality of life, and death. Surveillance, Epidemiology, and End Results (SEER) data indicated that more than 50% of tongue and floor of mouth cancers had metastasized to a distant site at the time of diagnosis.[43]

Quality of Life

The conditions predisposing the older patient to disease or changes in oral health status may result from physical or psychologic problems, or both. These problems may be the result of the older person's social conditions. Whatever the cause, these underlying problems must be addressed so that dental outcomes will be positive. This may require the dentist first to address the patient's fears and expectations about treatment outcomes. For example, older adults who are experiencing the loss of teeth and the adjustment to removable appliances or dentures can experience tremendous difficulty in accepting a reduced level of oral functioning. Their coping mechanism may also be stressed because of other socially important factors, such as esthetics and social esteem. Thus the patient's presenting conditions may affect the rendering of the treatment plan.

Many conditions limit an older person's ability to withstand or cope with dental treatment. For example, some older adults with physically or psychologically based behavior problems may require premedication in order for the dentist to deliver treatment. Other conditions may limit the dentist's ability to render treatment. For example, an older patient may not tolerate a reclining chair position for restorative procedures because of a chronic heart ailment or arthritis.

With treatment, there is a concomitant risk for causing problems, referred to as *iatrogenic* effects. Iatrogenic problems arise from side effects of treatment or from treatment procedures and range from drug interactions to medical emergencies.

Under certain conditions, the most appropriate care is to do nothing. In some severely compromised patients, treatment is only rendered if the potential for sepsis is suspected. Otherwise, treatment is withheld. In less serious situations, a dentist may decide not to treat a cracked tooth but to dome it and leave its root intact in tissue. This maintains the bone in the area and allows for a prosthetic appliance to be placed. In general, the dentist uses a determination of the risk/benefit of treatment for patient-related outcomes in deciding whether or not to provide treatment.

In addition, the dentist often may not have the special skills, equipment, or training to meet the needs of poorly functioning or nonfunctioning older adults. This may require the dentist to obtain the additional training and equipment to treat this population, especially in a rural community where access to services is extremely limited. Alternatively, the dentist may need to become familiar with the referral resources to contact clinicians who can treat such patients. One major referral base would be a trained hospital dentist who is capable of managing and treating the patient impaired by dementia or some physical problem or disease.

PERIODONTAL DISEASES IN OLDER ADULTS

Etiology

Periodontal disease in older adults is usually referred to as *chronic periodontitis*.[26,46] Because periodontitis is a chronic disease, much of the ravages of the disease detected in older adults results from an accumulation of the disease over time. Research has shown that the advanced stages of periodontitis are less prevalent than the moderate stages in the older adult population.[14] One theory is that many sites of advanced periodontal disease have resulted in tooth loss earlier in life, suggesting that older age is not a risk factor for periodontal disease.[26,46]

Evidence is limited on whether the risk factors for periodontal disease differ with age.[11] General health status, immune status, diabetes, nutrition, smoking, genetics, medications, mental health status, salivary flow, functional deficits, and finances may modify the relationship between periodontal disease and age.[11,61]

Some frequently prescribed medications for older adults can alter the gingival tissues. *Steroid-induced gingivitis* has been associated with postmenopausal women receiving steroid therapy. *Gingival overgrowth* can be induced by such medications as cyclosporines, calcium channel blockers, and anticonvulsants (e.g., nifedipine, phenytoin) in the presence of poor oral hygiene. This gingival overgrowth further decreases a person's ability to maintain good oral hygiene.[26]

Relationship to Systemic Disease

A review of the literature by Loesche and Lopatin[34] indicates that poor oral health has been associated with medical conditions such as aspiration pneumonia and cardiovascular disease. In particular, periodontal disease can be associated with coronary heart disease and cerebrovascular accident (CVA, stroke). In addition, the Surgeon General's Report on Oral Health emphasizes that animal and population-based studies demonstrate an association between periodontal disease and diabetes, cardiovascular disease, and stroke.[52]

Recent investigations confirm these associations. For example, a periodontal examination may assist cardiovascular risk assessment in hypertensive patients. Angeli et al.[6] reported an association between periodontal disease and left ventricular mass in untreated patients with essential hypertension.

Pneumonia is a common cause of morbidity and mortality in the older adult. Improvements in oral care have greatly reduced the incidence of pneumonia in elderly nursing home patients. Although the mechanism is currently under investigation, it is thought that the cough reflex can be improved by reducing the oropharyngeal microbial pathogens present.[55] Expanding on these findings, studies have been conducted on the prevention of ventilator-associated pneumonia. Providing oral therapy for intensive care patients to reduce bacterial colonization in the mouth and teeth can reduce mortality and morbidity by 42%.[24]

The presence and extent of periodontal disease may be related to increased risk of weight loss in older, well-functioning adults. This association is independent of smoking and diabetes mellitus. Changes in nutrient intake may be related to periodontal disease and a higher systemic inflammatory burden.[60]

PERIODONTAL TREATMENT PLANNING

Generally, periodontal disease in older adults is not a rapidly progressive disease but often presents as long-standing chronic disease. Because periodontal disease has periods of exacerbation and remission, understanding and documenting periods of active disease versus quiescent periods are essential to the formulation of the treatment plan and prognosis.[46]

Periodontal disease must be diagnosed regardless of age. The goal of periodontal treatment for both young and old patients is to preserve function and eliminate or prevent the progression of inflammatory disease.[58]

The goal of clinically managing periodontal disease in older adults is based on specific, individualized care. The major consideration is improving or maintaining function, with an emphasis on quality-of-life issues. Emphasizing care over cure is the cornerstone of any proposed treatment plan. Prevention, comfort, function, esthetics, and ease of maintenance are the criteria for successful management of an older adult, particularly a frail or functionally dependent older patient.

Several factors must be considered during treatment planning for older individuals.[46] It is important first to remember that periodontal healing and recurrence of disease are *not* influenced by age.[11] Factors to consider in the older patient are medical and mental health status, medications, functional status, and lifestyle behaviors that influence periodontal treatment, outcome, or progression of disease.[58] Periodontal disease severity, ability to perform oral hygiene procedures, and ability to tolerate treatment should be evaluated during treatment planning. The risks and benefits of both surgical and nonsurgical therapy should be considered.[46] The amount of remaining periodontal support or past periodontal destruction, tooth type, number of occlusal contacts, and individual patient preferences are also important.[58] Dental implants are a reliable replacement for missing teeth in older adults;[62] age alone is not a contraindication for implant placement.

For older adults, a nonsurgical approach is often the first treatment choice. Depending on the nature and extent of periodontal disease, surgical therapy may be indicated. Surgical technique should minimize the amount of additional root exposure. Individuals responding best to surgical therapy are those who are able to maintain the surgical result. Age alone is not a contraindication to surgery. For individuals who are unable to comply with treatment, who have poor oral hygiene, or who are medically or mentally compromised or functionally impaired, palliative supportive periodontal care instead of surgical periodontal treatment is often the optimal treatment approach.[46,58]

A common goal for all older adults is to decrease bacteria through oral hygiene and mechanical debridement. Clinical trials with older adults show that the development or progression of periodontal disease can be prevented or arrested by the control of plaque. For certain patients, topical antibiotic therapy may complement repeated subgingival instrumentation during supportive care. Oral hygiene maintenance should also focus on root surfaces susceptible to caries.[58]

Decision making for frail and functionally dependent older adults may be challenging to the general dentist. For this reason, dentists, other health care professionals, and other scientists are creating high-quality office-based methods to access evidence-based decision-making programs and accommodating websites to help with complicated oral health care issues.[2,45,56]

PREVENTION OF PERIODONTAL DISEASE AND MAINTENANCE OF PERIODONTAL HEALTH IN OLDER ADULTS

For both younger and older persons, the most important factors determining a successful outcome of periodontal treatment are plaque control and frequency of professional care. Advanced age does not decrease plaque control; however, older adults may have difficulty performing adequate oral hygiene because of compromised health, altered mental status, medications, or altered mobility and dexterity.[58] Older adults may change toothbrush habits because of disabilities such as hemiplegia secondary to CVA, visual difficulties, dementia, and arthritis. The newer, lightweight, electric-powered toothbrushes may be more beneficial than a manual toothbrush for older adults with physical and sensory limitations. The proportion of people who floss their teeth decreases after age 40 years.[57] This may be partly caused by impairment of fine motor skills secondary to disease or injury. Interproximal brushes, shaped wooden toothpicks, and mechanical flossing devices often can be used in place of traditional flossing with satisfactory outcomes.

In addition, multidisciplinary strategies are increasingly becoming part of periodontal health care promotion. Assessments of overall health, functional status, and patient education are fundamental to promoting and maintaining optimum periodontal health. Older adults, their families, and caregivers need to be informed and trained by dentists in the appropriate devices, chemotherapeutic agents, and techniques to provide oral self-care and maintain healthy lifestyles. The outcomes are instrumental in achieving overall health, oral and periodontal health, self-esteem, nutrition, and quality of life. Barriers to achieving these benefits are access and costs. For those older adults who are homebound or institutionalized, these barriers inhibit their achieving and maintaining optimum oral and periodontal health.

Chemotherapeutic Agents

Antiplaque Agents

Patients who are unable to remove plaque adequately secondary to disease or disability may benefit from antiplaque agents such as chlorhexidine, subantimicrobial tetracycline, and Listerine or its generic counterparts.[38,46,58]

Chlorhexidine is a cationic bisbiguanide that has been used as a broad-spectrum antiseptic in medicine since the 1950s. In Europe, a 0.2% concentration of chlorhexidine has been used for years as a preventive and therapeutic agent.[46,57] Chlorhexidine is either bacteriostatic or bactericidal, depending on the dose. Adverse effects of chlorhexidine include an increase in calculus formation, dysgeusia (altered taste), and permanent staining of teeth.[4] Chlorhexidine is a prescription rinse for short-term use (<6 months); long-term use (>6 months) has not been extensively studied.[57] The American Dental Association (ADA) Council on Dental Therapeutics[4] has approved chlorhexidine to help prevent and reduce supragingival plaque and gingivitis. Although chlorhexidine has not been studied in older adults, outcomes in younger persons, including those with disabilities, suggest that it is also effective in older adults. Chlorhexidine may be particularly useful for older adults who have difficulty with plaque removal and those who take phenytoin, calcium channel blockers, or cyclosporines and who are at risk for gingival hyperplasia.[46,57]

Subantimicrobial tetracycline (Periostat) is useful in treating moderate to severe chronic periodontitis. The active ingredient in Periostat is *doxycycline hyclate.* In concert with scaling and root planing, Mohammad et al.[38] have shown this treatment to be effective in institutionalized older adults. Periostat is contraindicated for those patients with an allergy to tetracycline.

Listerine antiseptic and its generic counterparts are approved by the ADA Council on Dental Therapeutics[4] to help prevent and reduce supragingival plaque and gingivitis. The active ingredients in Listerine are *methyl salicylate* and three essential oils (eucalyptol, thymol, and menthol). Listerine has been shown to be effective in reducing plaque and gingivitis compared with placebo rinses in young healthy adults. Listerine may exacerbate xerostomia because of its high alcohol content, ranging from 21.6% to 26.9%. Listerine is generally contraindicated in patients under treatment for alcoholism who take Antabuse (disulfiram). Listerine may benefit patients who do not tolerate the taste or staining of chlorhexidine and who prefer OTC medicaments that are less expensive and easier to obtain.[46,57]

Fluoride

Fluoride, "nature's cavity fighter," is the most effective caries-preventive agent currently available. Fluoride's effects are as follows[46,57]:

1. Reduces enamel solubility.
2. Promotes remineralization of early carious lesions.
3. Is bactericidal to bacterial plaque.

Topical fluorides are recommended for the prevention and treatment of dental caries. OTC fluorides include fluoride dentifrices, rinses, and gels that contain concentrations of 230 to 1500 parts per million (ppm) of fluoride ions. Prescription 1.1% neutral sodium fluoride gels are available with a fluoride concentration of 5000 ppm fluoride ion. Professionally applied fluoride gel, foam, or varnish products are between 9050 and 22,600 ppm fluoride ion.[4]

Saliva Substitutes

Saliva substitutes, which are intended to match the chemical and physical traits of saliva, are available to relieve the symptoms of dry mouth. Their composition is varied; however, they usually contain salt ions, a flavoring agent, paraben (preservative), cellulose derivative or animal mucins, and fluoride. The ADA's seal of approval has been granted for some artificial saliva products (e.g., Saliva Substitute, Salivart).[4] Most saliva substitutes can be used as desired by patients and are dispensed in spray bottle, rinse/swish bottle, or oral swab stick.[4,57] In addition, products such as dry-mouth toothpastes and moisturizing gels are also available. Biotene products are marketed to relieve the symptoms of xerostomia.

Patients with dry mouth may also benefit by stimulating saliva flow with sugarless candies and sugarless gum. Xylitol chewing gum has been shown to have anticariogenic properties in children. Medicated chewing gum with xylitol and chlorhexidine or xylitol alone has the added benefits of reducing oral plaque scores and gingivitis in elderly persons who live in residential facilities.[5]

Salivary substitutes and stimulants are only effective in the short term. Under investigation is acupuncture-like transcutaneous nerve stimulation (Codetron), a method to treat radiation-induced xerostomia. Unlike traditional acupuncture therapy, Codetron does not use invasive needles to achieve stimulation. This method helps the patient to produce their own saliva and reduce symptoms of xerostomia for several months. Acupuncture therapy has demonstrated improvements lasting up to 3 years.[64]

Risk Reduction

Cessation of tobacco use has been primarily an issue of patient compliance. Most smokers (90%) quit "cold turkey." However, nicotine replacement therapy may help strongly addicted patients. The transdermal nicotine patch or nicotine polacrilex (gum) can reduce the symptoms of nicotine withdrawal. For behavioral modification, the four steps to tobacco cessation are as follows:

1. Ask the patient about tobacco.
2. Advise the patient to stop using tobacco.
3. Assist the patient in stopping by selecting a quitting date (usually within the next 4 weeks).
4. Arrange patient follow-up services.

Clinical studies show that all four components, used routinely, result in much higher patient cessation rates than if only two or three are used. Both forms of nicotine replacement have been shown to increase cessation rates when used in combination with behavioral interventions.

Nicotine replacement therapy is intended to be used for a few (6-12) weeks so that patients can learn psychologic and social coping skills without going through nicotine withdrawal at the same time. It is not recommended for use for more than 6 months.

Nicotine replacement therapy should probably *not* be considered for the following persons:

- Individuals who have not previously tried to quit.
- Individuals who use only small amounts of tobacco or who are occasional users.
- Individuals who have tried to quit and have not had significant physical symptoms of nicotine withdrawal.
- Individuals who do not receive behavioral support from clinic staff.

Alcoholism and alcohol abuse are diagnosed using the *Diagnostic and Statistical Manual of Mental Disorders,* third edition, revised *(DSM-IIIR),* and fourth edition *(DSM-IV).* The tests suggested to screen for alcohol abuse are the self-administered questionnaire, the Michigan Alcoholism Screening Test (MAST), and the CAGE (from a series of four questions about drinking: *c*ut down; *a*nnoyed; *g*uilty; and *e*ye-opener) questionnaire, a four-item screening tool (Figure 45-10). A score of 2 in the elderly patient (an affirmative answer to two questions) provides clinical evidence or suspicion of alcohol abuse, with a sensitivity of about 50% and a specificity over 90%. The MAST with a cutoff score of 5 produces sensitivity ranging from 50% to 70% and a specificity above 90%.

The most common treatment for alcoholism is referral to a substance abuse facility. For the older adults, the most effective treatment is a program that emphasizes older adult–specific groups using nonconfrontational therapy and encouraging reminiscence as well as discussion of

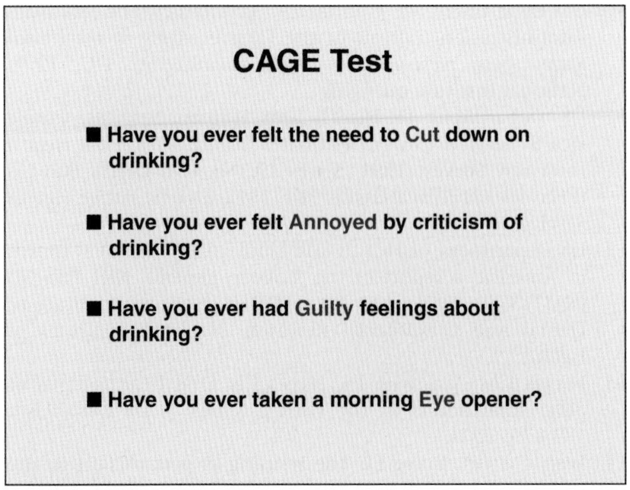
CAGE Test
Have you ever felt the need to Cut down on drinking?
Have you ever felt Annoyed by criticism of drinking?
Have you ever had Guilty feelings about drinking?
Have you ever taken a morning Eye opener?

Figure 45-10 Method of determining alcohol abuse using the modified CAGE test. The acronym CAGE is derived from a series of four questions about drinking: cut down; annoyed; guilty; and eye-opener) test. (From Mallin R: Smoking cessation: integration of behavioral and drug therapies, *Am Fam Physician* 65:1107, 2002.)

current problems. Discussion of current problems is relevant because of the role that stress plays in recent widowhood, recent retirement, or disruption or removal from one's residence.

CONCLUSION

Future oral health care trends will see increased numbers of older adults seeking periodontal therapy. Dental practitioners of the twenty-first century should be comfortable providing comprehensive periodontal care for this segment of the population. Aging dental patients have particular oral and general health conditions that dentists should be familiar with detecting, consulting, and treating. Medical diseases and conditions that occur more often with age may require modification to periodontal preventive tools as well as for the planning and treatment phases of periodontal care.

REFERENCES

1. Administration on Aging: A profile of older Americans, 1998, http://www.aoa.dhhs.gov.
2. Agency for Healthcare Research and Quality: Evidence-based practice, 2005, http://www.ahrq.gov/clinic/epcix.htm.
3. Alliance for Aging Research, Task Force on Aging Research Funding, Washington, DC, 2004, The Alliance.
4. American Dental Association: *Guide to dental therapeutics,* ed 2, Chicago, 2000, ADA.
5. American Dietetic Association: Oral health and nutrition, *J Am Diet Assoc* 103:615, 2003.
6. Angeli F, Verdecchia P, Pellegrino C, et al: Association between periodontal disease and left ventricle mass in essential hypertension, *Hypertension* 41:488, 2003.
7. Axelsson P, Nystrom B, Lindhe J: The long-term effect of a plaque control program on tooth mortality, caries and periodontal disease in adults: results after 30 years of maintenance, *J Clin Periodontol* 31:749, 2004.
8. Bauer JG: The index of ADOH: concept of measuring oral self-care functioning in the elderly, *Spec Care Dent* 21:63, 2001.
9. Bauer JG, Spackman S: Financing dental services in the US: best practice model, *Braz J Oral Sci* 2:187, 2003.
10. Bauer JG, Spackman S, Chiappelli F, et al: Issues in dentistry for patients with Alzheimer-related dementia, *Long-Term Care—Interface* 6:30, 2005.
11. Beck JD: Periodontal implications: older adults, *Ann Periodontol* 1:322, 1996.
12. Borrell LN, Burt BA, Neighbors HW, Taylor GW: Social factors and periodontitis in an older population, *Am J Public Health* 94:748, 2004.
13. Boyd LD, Madden TE: Nutrition, infection, and periodontal disease, *Dent Clin North Am* 47:337, 2003.
14. Brown LJ, Brunelle JA, Kingman A: Periodontal status in the United States, 1988–1991: prevalence, extent, and demographic variation, *J Dent Res* 75:672 1996 (special issue).
15. Burt BA, Eklund SA: *Dentistry, dental practice, and the community,* Philadelphia, 1999, Saunders.
16. Centers for Disease Control and Prevention: Dental service use and dental insurance coverage—United States, Behavioral Risk Factor Surveillance System, 1995, *MMWR* 46:1199, 1997.
17. Centers for Disease Control and Prevention: Public health and aging: retention of natural teeth among older adults—United States, 2002, *MMWR* 52:1226, 2003.
18. Christian DC: Computer-assisted analysis of oral brush biopsies at an oral cancer screening program, *J Am Dent Assoc* 133:357, 2002.
19. Ettinger RL: The unique oral health needs of an aging population, *Dent Clin North Am* 41:633, 1997.
20. Ettinger RL, Mulligan R: The future of dental care for the elderly population, *J Calif Dent Assoc* 27:687, 1999.
21. Fedele DJ, Jones JA, Niessen LC: Oral cancer screening in the elderly, *J Am Geriatr Soc* 39:920, 1991.
22. Fortinsky RH, Iannuzzi-Sucich M, Baker, et al: Fall—risk assessment and management in clinical practice: views from healthcare providers, *J Am Geriatr Soc* 52:1522, 2004.
23. Fox PC: Salivary enhancement therapies, *Caries* 38:241, 2004.
24. Garcia R, Jendresky L, Colbert L: Reduction of microbial colonization in the oropharynx and dental plaque reduces ventilator-associated pneumonia. Poster presented at Association for Professionals in Infection Control (APIC) Conference and Epidemiology Annual Educational Conference and International Meeting, Phoenix, 2004.
25. Ghezzi EM, Ship JA: Aging and secretory reserve capacity of major salivary glands, *J Dent Res* 82:844, 2003.
26. Gibson G, Niessen LC: Aging and the oral cavity. In Cassel CK, Cohen HJ, Larson EB, et al, editors: *Geriatric medicine,* New York, 1997, Springer-Verlag.
27. Hollister MC, Weintraub JA: The association of oral status with systemic health, quality of life, and economic productivity, *J Dent Educ* 57:901, 1993.
28. Jones JA, Fedele DJ, Bolden AJ, et al: Gains in dental care use not shared by minority elders, *J Public Health Dent* 54:39, 1994.
29. Kayak HA, Brudvik J: Dental students' self-assessed competence in geriatric dentistry, *J Dent Educ* 56:728, 1992.
30. Kiecolt-Glaser JK, Glaser R: Depression and immune function: central pathways to morbidity and mortality, *J Psychosom Res* 53:873, 2002.
31. Kiyak HA: Successful aging: implications for oral health, *J Public Health Dent* 60:276, 2000.
32. Lin A, Kim HM, Terrell JE, et al: Quality of life after parotid-sparing IMRT for head and neck cancer: a prospective longitudinal study, *Int J Radiat Oncol Biol Phys* 57:61, 2003.
33. Locker D, Slade GD, Murray H: Epidemiology of periodontal disease among older adults: a review, *Periodontol 2000* 16:16, 1998.

34. Loesche WJ, Lopatin DE: Interaction between periodontal disease, medical disease and immunity in the older individual, *Periodontol 2000* 16:80, 1998.
35. MacFayden D: International geriatric health promotion study/activities. In Abdellah FG, Moore SR, editors: *Proceedings of the Surgeon General's Workshop on Health Promotion and Aging,* Washington, DC, 1988, US Department of Health and Human Services.
36. McCarron PA: Bioadhesive, non-drug-loaded nanoparticles as modulators of candidal adherence to buccal epithelial cells: a potentially novel prophylaxis for candidosis, *Biomaterials* 25: 2399, 2004.
37. Mezey M, Capezuti E, Fulmer T: Care of older adults, *Nurs Clin North Am* 39(3):xiii, 2004.
38. Mohammad AR, Preshaw PM, Hefti AF, et al: Subantimicrobial-dose doxycycline for treatment of periodontitis in an institutionalized geriatric population. Presented at 81st General Session of International Association for Dental Research (IADR), Goteborg, Sweden, 2003.
39. Ritchie CS: Oral health, taste, and olfaction, *Clin Geriatr Med* 18:709, 2002
40. Ritchie CS, Joshipura K, Hung HC, Douglass CW: Nutrition as a mediator in the relation between oral and systemic disease: associations between specific measures of adult oral health and nutrition outcomes, *Crit Rev Oral Biol Med* 13:291, 2002.
41. Sciubba JJ: Improving detection of precancerous and cancerous oral lesions: computer-assisted analysis of the oral brush biopsy, US Collaborative OralCDx Study Group, *J Am Dent Assoc* 130:1445, 1999.
42. Serby M, Yu M: Overview: depression in the elderly, *Mt Sinai J Med* 70:38, 2003.
43. Shiboski CH, Shiboski SC, Silverman S Jr: Trends in oral cancer rates in the United States, 1973–1996, *Community Dent Oral Epidemiol* 28:249, 2000.
44. Ship JA, Duffy V, Jones JA, Langmore S: Geriatric oral health and its impact on eating, *J Am Geriatr Soc* 44:456, 1996.
45. Sutherland SE, Matthews DC: Conducting systemic reviews and creating clinical practice guidelines in dentistry: lessons learned, *J Am Dent Assoc* 135:747, 2004.
46. Suzuki JB, Niessen LC, Fedele DJ: Periodontal diseases in the older adult. In Papas AS, Niessen LC, Chauncey HH, editors: *Geriatric dentistry: aging and oral health,* St Louis, 1991, Mosby.
47. Tezal M, Grossi SG, Ho AW, Genco RJ: Alcohol consumption and periodontal disease: the third National Health and Nutrition Examination Survey, *J Clin Periodontol* 31:484, 2004.
48. US Bureau of the Census: *Statistical abstract of the United States: 1996,* ed 116, Washington, DC, 1996, The Bureau.
49. US Department of Commerce, Bureau of the Census: Census 2000 brief, 2001, http://www.census.gov.
50. US Department of Commerce, Economics and Statistics Administration, Bureau of the Census: *Aging in the United States: past, present, and future,* Washington, DC, 1997, National Institute on Aging.
51. US Department of Health and Human Services, Public Health Service: Current estimates from the National Health Interview Survey, 1991, Series 10, No 184, DHHS Pub No (PHS) 93-1512, Hyattsville, Md, 1992, DHHS, Public Health Service.
52. US Department of Health and Human Services: Oral health in America: a report of the surgeon general, NIH Pub No 00-4713, Rockville, Md, 2000, DHHS, National Institute of Dental and Craniofacial Research, National Institutes of Health.
53. Vargas CM, Yellowitz JA, Hayes KL: Oral health status of older rural adults in the United States, *J Am Dent Assoc* 134:479, 2003.
54. Warshaw GA, Bragg EJ: The training of geriatricians in the United States: three decades of progress, *J Am Geriatr Soc* 51(7 suppl):S338, 2003.
55. Watando A, Ebihara S, Ebihara T, et al: Daily oral care and cough reflex sensitivity in elderly nursing home patients, *Chest* 126:1066, 2004.
56. WebCampus of Dentistry for Seniors: Professional and student learning centers, 2005, http://www.webddsseniors.com/professional/frmhome.html.
57. Wells LM, Kolavic S, Niessen LC, et al: Caring for older adults: maintaining oral health for a lifetime. In Hardin JF, editor: *Clark's clinical dentistry,* vol 1, Philadelphia, 1996, Lippincott.
58. Wennstrom JL: Treatment of periodontal disease in older adults, *Periodontol 2000* 16:106, 1998.
59. Weyant RJ, Pandav RS, Plowman JL: Medical and cognitive correlates of denture wearing in older community-dwelling adults, *J Am Geriatr Soc* 2:596, 2004.
60. Weyant RJ, Newman AB, Kritchevsky SB, et al: Periodontal disease and weight loss in older adults, *J Am Geriatr Soc* 52:547, 2004.
61. Wilson TG: Using risk assessment to customized periodontal treatment, *CDA J* 27:627, 1999.
62. Wilson TG, Higginbottom FL: Periodontal disease and dental implants in older adults, *J Esthet Dent* 10:265, 1998.
63. Winn DM, Brunelle JA, Selwitz RH, et al: Coronal and root caries in the dentition of adults in the United States, 1988–1991, *J Dent Res* 75:642, 1996 (special issue).
64. Wong RK, Jones GW, Sagar SM, et al: Phase I-II study in the use of acupuncture-like transcutaneous nerve stimulation in the treatment of radiation-induced xerostomia in head-and-neck cancer patients treated with radical radiotherapy, *Int J Radiat Oncol Biol Phys* 57:472, 2003.

CHAPTER 46

Treatment of Aggressive and Atypical Forms of Periodontitis

Perry R. Klokkevold and Richard J. Nagy

CHAPTER OUTLINE

The majority of patients with common forms of periodontal disease respond predictably well to conventional therapy, including oral hygiene instruction, nonsurgical debridement, surgery, and supportive periodontal maintenance. However, patients diagnosed with aggressive and some atypical forms of periodontal disease often do not respond as predictably or as favorably to conventional therapy. Fortunately, only a small percentage of patients with periodontal disease are diagnosed with aggressive periodontitis. Patients who are diagnosed with periodontal disease (any type) that is *refractory* to treatment present in small numbers as well. Even fewer patients are diagnosed with necrotizing ulcerative periodontitis. Each of these atypical disease entities poses significant challenges for the clinician not only because they are infrequently encountered, but also because they often do not respond favorably to conventional periodontal therapy.[26,43] Furthermore, the severe loss of periodontal support associated with these cases leaves the clinician faced with uncertainty about treatment outcomes and difficulty in making decisions about whether to save compromised teeth or to extract them.

This chapter outlines important considerations for the treatment of patients diagnosed with aggressive periodontitis and atypical forms of periodontal disease, including refractory cases of periodontitis and necrotizing ulcerative periodontitis.

AGGRESSIVE PERIODONTITIS

Aggressive periodontitis, by definition, causes rapid destruction of the periodontal attachment apparatus and the supporting alveolar bone (see Chapter 33). The responsiveness of aggressive periodontitis to conventional periodontal treatment is unpredictable, and the overall prognosis for these patients is poorer than for patients with chronic periodontitis. Because these patients do not respond "normally" to conventional methods and their disease progresses unusually fast, the logical question is whether there are problems associated with an impaired host immune response that may contribute to such a *different* disease and result in a *limited* response to the usual therapeutic measures. Indeed, defects in polymorphonuclear leukocyte (PMN, neutrophil) function have been identified in some patients with aggressive periodontitis.[33,34] Also, in a small number of cases, a systemic disease such as neutropenia can be identified that clearly explains the unusual severity of the periodontal disease for that individual.[13,14] In most patients with aggressive periodontitis, however, systemic diseases or disorders cannot be identified. In fact, the irony is that these patients are typically quite healthy. Numerous attempts to examine immunologic profiles in patients with aggressive periodontitis have failed to identify any specific etiologic factors common to all patients.

The prognosis for patients with aggressive periodontitis depends on (1) whether the disease is generalized or localized, (2) the degree of destruction present at the time of diagnosis, and (3) the ability to control future progression. *Generalized* aggressive periodontitis rarely undergoes spontaneous remission, whereas *localized* forms of the disease have been known to arrest spontaneously.[31] This unexplained curtailment of disease progression has sometimes been referred to as a "burnout" of the disease. It appears that cases of localized aggressive periodontitis often have a limited period of rapid periodontal attachment and alveolar bone loss, followed by a slower, more chronic phase of disease progression. Overall, patients with generalized aggressive periodontitis tend to have a poorer prognosis because they typically have more teeth affected by the disease and because the disease is less likely to go spontaneously into remission compared with patients with localized forms of aggressive periodontitis.

Therapeutic Modalities

Early detection is critically important in the treatment of aggressive periodontitis (generalized or localized) because preventing further destruction is often more predictable than attempting to regenerate lost supporting tissues. Therefore, at the initial diagnosis, it is helpful to obtain any previously taken radiographs to assess the rate of progression of the disease. Together with future radiographs, this documentation will also facilitate the clinician's assessment of treatment success and control of the disease.

Treatment of aggressive periodontitis must be pursued with a logical and regimented approach. Several aspects of treatment must be particularly considered when managing a patient with aggressive periodontitis. One of the most important aspects of treatment success is to educate the patient about the disease, including the causes and the risk factors for disease, and to stress the importance of the patient's role in the success of treatment.[1] Essential therapeutic considerations for the clinician are to control the infection, arrest disease progression, correct anatomic defects, replace missing teeth, and ultimately help the patient maintain periodontal health with frequent periodontal maintenance care. Educating family members is another important factor because aggressive periodontitis is known to have familial aggregation. Thus, family members, especially younger siblings, of the patient diagnosed with aggressive periodontitis should be examined for signs of disease, educated about preventive measures, and monitored closely. It cannot be stressed enough that early diagnosis, intervention, and, if possible, prevention of disease are more desirable than attempting to reverse the destruction that results from aggressive periodontitis.

Many different treatment approaches have been used to manage patients with aggressive periodontitis, including nonsurgical, surgical, and antimicrobial therapy. Recent advances in our understanding of the role of the host response in disease pathogenesis are leading to new opportunities for treatment. The advantages and limitations of conventional, antimicrobial, and combination therapy for the treatment of aggressive periodontitis as well as restorative considerations are discussed next.

SCIENCE TRANSFER

Some patients present with a large amount of periodontal destruction either early in life or over a relatively short time. Likewise, other patients undergo conventional treatment, but do not respond to the therapy. These groups of patients present a dilemma for clinicians and researchers because no unique characteristics distinguish these patients. Periodontal disease results from a microbiologic challenge in a susceptible host, and no unique bacterial species or obvious immune defects are present; therefore it is likely that other, unknown host response mechanisms are altered. These changes could be at the systemic level, but because of the localized nature of some lesions, the alterations may occur in a specific site around the tooth. Until such alterations can be identified, therapeutic efforts are aimed at frequent recalls and combination mechanical and antimicrobial therapies.

In most patients, aggressive periodontitis can be successfully treated with conventional therapy, and clinicians need to combine a wide range of therapeutic procedures to increase the chances of disease resolution. Initial therapy and surgical therapy focusing on regenerative approaches are combined with systemic antibiotics to change the destructive microbial elements and with host modulation agents to optimize the patient's response. *This all-encompassing approach is necessary and must be followed with a comprehensive maintenance phase.*

Because they often have teeth with advanced bone loss, many patients require tooth extraction, ridge maintenance surgery, and implant placement. These therapies all seem to have a good prognosis in patients with aggressive periodontitis. At present, it is generally not possible to identify the systemic changes responsible for the aggressive forms of periodontitis, and therefore it is not necessary to recommend specific blood analyses for these patients.

Conventional Periodontal Therapy

Conventional periodontal therapy for aggressive periodontitis consists of patient education, oral hygiene improvement, scaling and root planing, and regular (frequent) recall maintenance. It may or may not include periodontal flap surgery.[3,60] Unfortunately, the response of aggressive periodontitis to conventional therapy alone has been limited and unpredictable. Patients who are diagnosed with aggressive periodontitis at an early stage and who are able to enter therapy may have a better outcome than those who are diagnosed at an advanced stage of destruction. In general, the earlier the disease is diagnosed, the more conservative the therapy and the more predictable the outcome.

Teeth with moderate to advanced periodontal attachment loss and bone loss often have a poor prognosis and pose the most difficult challenge. Depending on the condition of the remaining dentition, treatment of these teeth may have a limited prospect for improvement and may even diminish the overall treatment success for the patient. Clearly, some of these teeth should be extracted; however, other teeth may be pivotal to the stability of that individual's dentition, and thus it may be desirable to attempt treatment to maintain them. Treatment options for teeth with deep periodontal pockets and bone loss may be nonsurgical or surgical. Surgery may be purely resective, regenerative, or a combination of these approaches.

Surgical Resective Therapy. Resective periodontal surgery can be effective to reduce or eliminate pocket depth in patients with aggressive periodontitis. However, it may be difficult to accomplish if adjacent teeth are unaffected, as often seen in cases of localized aggressive periodontitis. If a significant height discrepancy exists between the periodontal support of the affected tooth and the adjacent unaffected tooth, the gingival transition (following the bone) will often result in deep probing pocket depth around the affected tooth despite surgical efforts. A less-than-ideal outcome must be taken into consideration before deciding to treat increased pocket depth surgically.

It is important to realize the limitations of surgical therapy and to appreciate the possible risk that surgical therapy may further compromise teeth that are mobile because of extensive loss of periodontal support. For example, in a patient with severe horizontal bone loss, surgical resective therapy may result in increased tooth mobility that is difficult to manage, and a nonsurgical approach may be indicated. Therefore, careful evaluation of the risks versus the benefits of surgery must be considered on a case-by-case basis.

Regenerative Therapy. The concept and application of periodontal regeneration has been established in patients with chronic forms of periodontal disease (see Chapter 67). The use of regenerative materials, including bone grafts, barrier membranes, and wound-healing agents, are well documented and often used. Intrabony defects, particularly vertical defects with multiple osseous walls, are often amenable to regeneration with these techniques. Most of the success and predictability of periodontal regeneration have been achieved in patients with chronic periodontitis; much less evidence is available about the use of periodontal regeneration for patients with aggressive periodontitis.

Periodontal regenerative procedures have been successfully demonstrated in patients with localized aggressive periodontitis in some clinical case reports. Dodson et al.[15] demonstrated the regenerative potential of a severe, localized osseous defect around a mandibular incisor in a healthy, 19-year-old black man diagnosed with localized aggressive periodontitis. The patient presented with severe bone loss localized around one of the mandibular incisors. Using open-flap surgical debridement, root surface conditioning (tetracycline solution), and an allogenic bone graft reconstituted with sterile saline and tetracycline powder, the surgeons reduced the probing pocket depth from 9 to 12 mm down to 1 to 3 mm (3 mm of recession was noted), and significant bone fill of the defect (about 80%) was reported (Figure 46-1). This case illustrates the potential for healing of severe defects in patients with localized aggressive periodontitis, especially when local factors are controlled and sound surgical principles are followed. The authors cited several factors that likely contributed to the success of this case, including a probable transition of disease activity from aggressive to chronic, tooth stabilization before surgery, sound surgical management of hard and soft tissues, and good postoperative care.[15]

It is important to note that although the potential for regeneration in patients with aggressive periodontitis appears to be good, expectations are limited for patients with severe bone loss. Depending on the anatomy of the defect and teeth involved, the potential for bone fill and periodontal regeneration may be poor. This is especially true if the bone loss is horizontal and if it has progressed to involve furcations. The usual criteria of case selection and sound principles of surgical management for regenerative therapy apply equally to cases of aggressive periodontitis. Good clinical judgment must be used to determine whether a particular tooth should be treated with the goal of regeneration.

Recent advances in regenerative therapy have advocated the use of an *enamel matrix protein* (Emdogain) to aid in the regeneration of cementum and new attachment in periodontal defects. A systematic review of the literature concluded that treatment with an enamel matrix protein can improve probing attachment level (mean difference, 1.3 mm) and probing pocket depth (mean difference, 1.0 mm) compared with flap debridement alone in patients with chronic periodontitis.[16] However, no evidence has been reported to suggest significant advantages for the use of enamel matrix proteins in patients with aggressive periodontitis. One recent case report described use of the protein in a 15-year-old patient with localized aggressive periodontitis.[7] No comparative sites were treated, so the effect that may be attributed to enamel matrix protein could not be determined. A recent clinical and radiographic study with a split-mouth design included four patients with aggressive periodontitis and four patients with chronic periodontitis. The authors concluded that enamel matrix proteins offered no advantage over surgical debridement alone in these patients.[62] Although this study attempted to use controls to measure the effect of enamel matrix proteins, there were insufficient patients to appreciate a difference in outcome. At this time, it is unknown whether the use of enamel matrix proteins offers significant advantages for the patient with aggressive periodontitis.

Antimicrobial Therapy

The presence of periodontal pathogens, specifically *Actinobacillus actinomycetemcomitans*, has been implicated as the reason that aggressive periodontitis does not respond to conventional therapy alone. These pathogens are known to remain in the tissues after therapy to reinfect the pocket.[10,58] In the late 1970s and early 1980s, the identification of *A. actinomycetemcomitans* as a major culprit and the discovery that this organism penetrates

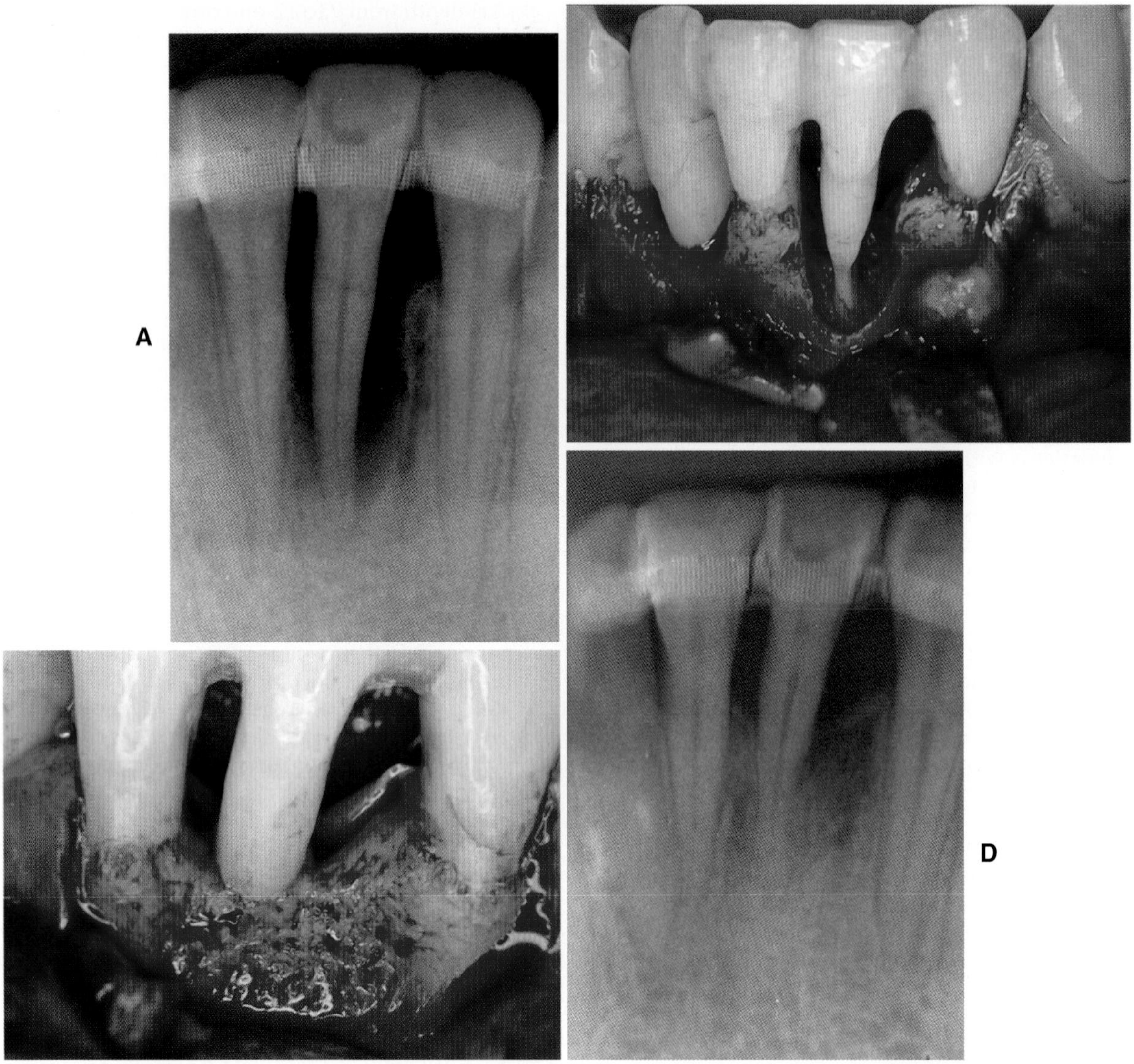

Figure 46-1 Clinical photographs and periapical radiographs demonstrating regenerative success in patient with localized aggressive periodontitis. **A,** Periapical radiograph of the right lateral incisor at the initial diagnosis. Notice the severe, vertical bone loss associated with the right lateral incisor. Tooth has been splinted to adjacent teeth for stability. **B,** Facial view of the circumferential osseous defect around the lower right lateral incisor during open flap surgery. There is complete loss of buccal, lingual, mesial, and distal bone around the lateral incisor, with minimal bone support limited to the apical few millimeters. **C,** Facial view of reentered surgical site 1 year after treatment. Bone fill around all surfaces demonstrates remarkable potential for regeneration of a large osseous defect in young patient with localized aggressive periodontitis. **D,** Periapical radiograph taken 1 year after regenerative therapy. Note the increased radiopacity and bone fill. (From Dodson SA, Takei HH, Carranza FA Jr: *Int J Periodont Restor Dent* 16:455, 1996.)

the tissues offered another perspective to the pathogenesis of aggressive periodontitis and offered new hope for therapeutic success, namely, antibiotics.[10] The use of systemic antibiotics was thought to be necessary to eliminate pathogenic bacteria (especially *A. actinomycetemcomitans*) from the tissues. Indeed, several authors have reported success in the treatment of aggressive periodontitis using antibiotics as adjuncts to standard therapy.[36-38,73]

Systemic Administration Of Antibiotics. There is compelling evidence that adjunctive antibiotic treatment frequently results in a more favorable clinical response than mechanical therapy alone.[67] In a systematic review, Herrera et al.[25] found that systemic antimicrobials in conjunction with scaling and root planing offer benefits over scaling and planing alone in terms of clinical attachment level, probing pocket depth, and reduced risk of additional attachment loss. Patients with deeper, progressive

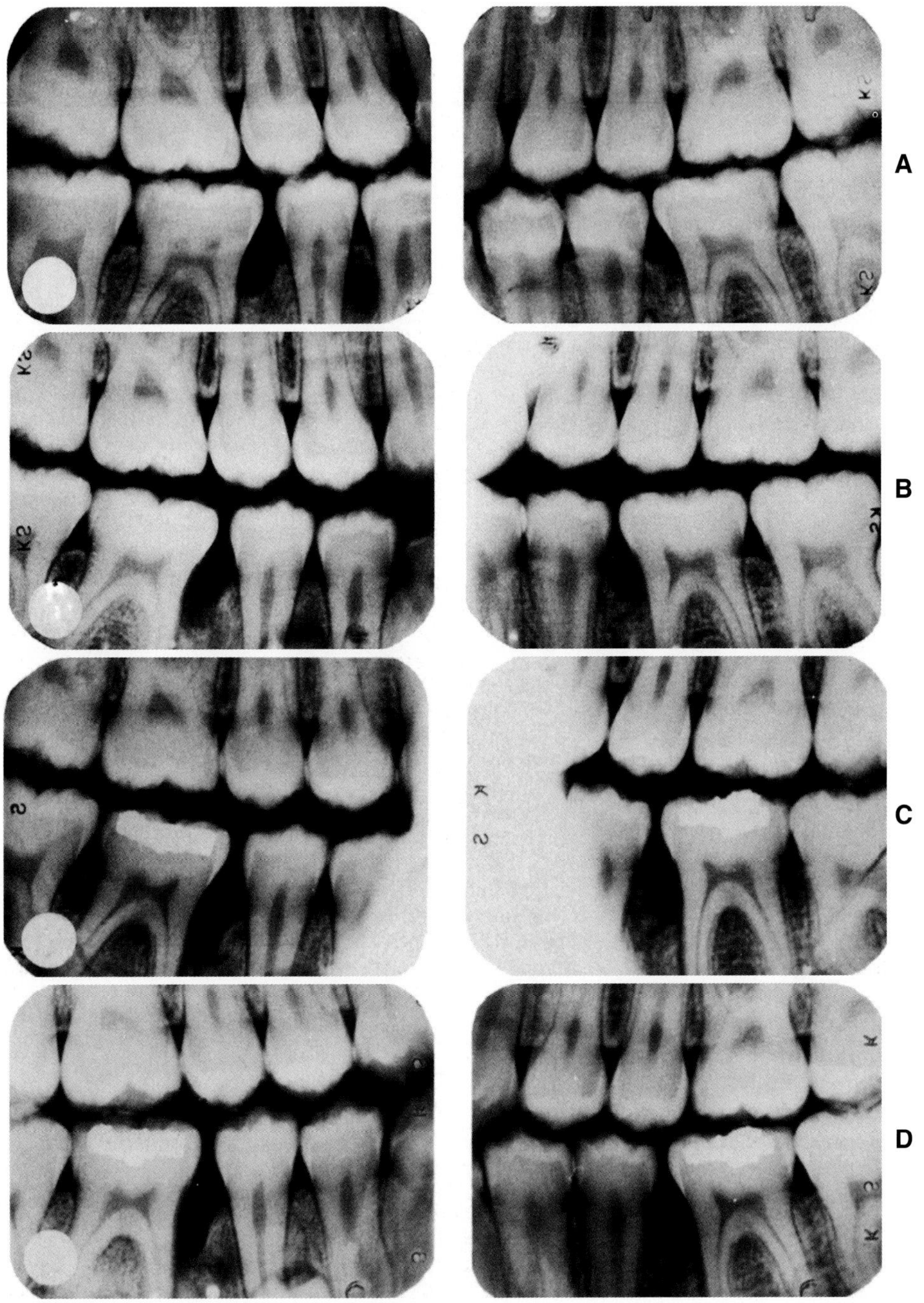

Figure 46-2 Radiographs depicting progression of the osseous lesion in patient with localized aggressive periodontitis (formerly "localized juvenile periodontitis"). **A,** January 29, 1979; **B,** August 16, 1979; **C,** February 22, 1980; **D,** May 15, 1981. Note the progressive deterioration of the osseous level. (From Barnett ML, Baker RL: *J Periodontol* 54:148, 1983.)

pockets seem to benefit the most from systemic administration of adjunctive antibiotics. Many different antibiotic types and regimens were reviewed. Because of limitations in comparing data from different studies, however, definitive recommendations were not possible.

Genco et al.[20] treated *localized* aggressive periodontitis patients with scaling and root planing plus systemic administration of tetracycline (250 mg four times daily for 14 days every 8 weeks). Measurements of vertical defects were made at intervals of up to 18 months after the initiation of therapy. Bone loss had stopped, and one third of the defects demonstrated an increase in bone level, whereas in the control group, bone loss continued.

Liljenberg and Lindhe[36] treated patients with *localized* aggressive periodontitis with systemic administration of tetracycline (250 mg four times daily for 2 weeks), modified Widman flaps, and periodic recall visits (one visit every month for 6 months, then one visit every

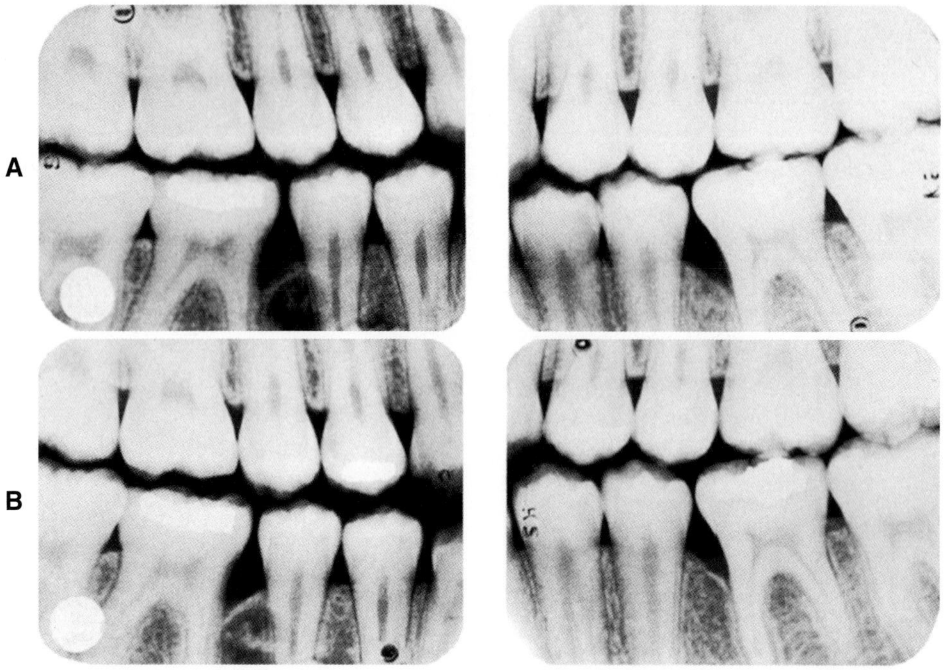

Figure 46-3 Postoperative radiographs of the patient in Figure 46-2. **A,** November 6, 1981; **B,** March 3, 1982. Treatment consisted of oral hygiene instruction, scaling and root planing concurrently with 1 g of tetracycline per day for 2 weeks, and modified Widman flaps. (From Barnett ML, Baker RL: *J Periodontol* 54:148, 1983.)

3 months). The lesions healed more rapidly and more completely than similar lesions in control patients. These investigators reevaluated their results after 5 years and found that the treatment group continued to demonstrate resolution of gingival inflammation, gain of clinical attachment, and refill of bone in angular defects.[37] Figures 46-2 and 46-3 show radiographs of a case with similar treatment and results.[4]

Clearly, numerous studies support the use of adjunctive tetracycline along with mechanical debridement for the treatment of *A. actinomycetemcomitans*–associated aggressive periodontitis (Box 46-1). Given the possible emergence of tetracycline-resistant *A. actinomycetemcomitans*, there is concern that tetracycline may not be effective. In these cases the combination of metronidazole and amoxicillin may be advantageous. Haffajee et al.[24] concluded that a systemically administered combination of antibiotics (amoxicillin and metronidazole) with periodontal therapy (scaling and root planing and/or surgery) provided better disease control in difficult-to-manage periodontitis cases than similar periodontal therapy without antibiotics. In a systematic review of the literature, Haffajee et al.[23] concluded that systemically administered antibiotics with or without scaling and root planing and/or surgery appeared to provide greater clinical improvement in attachment level change than similar periodontal therapy without antibiotics. Similar effects were seen for a variety of antibiotic types. However, as with Herrera's systematic review,[25] a lack of sufficient sample sizes among studies prevented the authors from offering specific recommendations about which antibiotics were most effective.

BOX 46-1

Systemic Tetracycline in Treatment of Aggressive Periodontitis

Systemic tetracycline (250 mg of tetracycline hydrochloride four times daily for at least 1 week) should be given in conjunction with local mechanical therapy. If surgery is indicated, systemic tetracycline should be prescribed and the patient instructed to begin taking the antibiotic approximately 1 hour before surgery. Doxycycline, 100 mg/day, may be used instead of tetracycline. Chlorhexidine rinses should be prescribed and continued for several weeks to enhance plaque control and facilitate healing.

The criteria for selection of antibiotics are not clear. Good clinical and microbiologic responses have been reported with several individual antibiotics and antibiotic combinations (Table 46-1). The optimal antibiotic or combination for any particular infection probably depends on the case. Choices must be made based on patient-related and disease-related factors.

Microbial Testing. Some investigators and clinicians advocate microbial testing as a necessary means of identifying the specific periodontal pathogens responsible for disease and to select an appropriate antibiotic based on sensitivity and resistance. There may be specific cases in which bacterial identification and antibiotic-sensitivity testing is invaluable. For example, in localized aggressive

TABLE 46-1

Antibiotic Therapy for Aggressive Periodontitis

Associated Microflora	Antibiotic of Choice
Gram-positive organisms	Amoxicillin–clavulanate potassium (Augmentin)[11,69]
Gram-negative organisms	Clindamycin[21,22,65,69]
Nonoral gram-negative, facultative rods	Ciprofloxacin[39]
Pseudomonads, staphylococci	
Black-pigmented bacteria and spirochetes	Metronidazole[22,61]
Prevotella intermedia *Porphyromonas gingivalis*	Tetracycline[51]
Actinobacillus actinomycetemcomitans	Metronidazole-amoxicillin[22,61]
	Metronidazole-ciprofloxacin
	Tetracycline[49]
P. gingivalis	Azithromycin[50]

periodontitis cases, tetracycline-resistant *Actinobacillus* species have been suspected. If antibiotic susceptibility tests determine that tetracycline-resistant species exist in the lesion, the clinician may be advised to consider another antibiotic or an antibiotic combination, such as amoxicillin and metronidazole.[17,51,62]

In practice, antibiotics are often used empirically without microbial testing. One study evaluated and compared the results of microbial testing offered by two independent laboratories.[44,59] Two microbiologic cultures, sampled simultaneously from the same sites in 20 patients, were submitted separately to each of the two independent laboratories for bacterial identification and antibiotic-sensitivity testing. The results obtained for the paired samples from different laboratories were quite variable. The reported presence of bacterial species varied from one laboratory to another, as did their antimicrobial recommendations. Interestingly, the combination of amoxicillin and metronidazole yielded the highest level of agreement (80%) between the laboratories for paired samples. The high level of agreement in the recommended use of amoxicillin and metronidazole is likely attributed to the effectiveness of this combination as well as a clinical predisposition to favor a known regimen. These findings suggest that the usefulness of microbial testing may be limited and led the authors to conclude that the empiric use an antibiotics, such as a combination of amoxicillin and metronidazole, may be more clinically sound and cost-effective than bacterial identification and antibiotic-sensitivity testing.[44,59]

Nonetheless, the use of microbial testing should be considered whenever a case of aggressive periodontitis is not responding or if the destruction continues despite good therapeutic efforts. An accurate identification of periodontal pathogens and their antibiotic sensitivities is more important when the disease is not responding to the given antibiotics and periodontal therapy.

Local Delivery. The use of local delivery to administer antibiotics offers a novel approach to the management of periodontal "localized" infections. The primary advantage of local therapy is that smaller total dosages of topical agents can be delivered inside the pocket, avoiding the side effects of systemic antibacterial agents while increasing the exposure of the target microorganisms to higher concentrations, and therefore more therapeutic levels, of the medication. Local delivery agents have been formulated in many different forms, including solutions, gels, fibers, and chips[18,19,29] (see Chapter 52).

Full-Mouth Disinfection

Another approach to antimicrobial therapy in the control of infection associated with periodontitis is the concept of full-mouth disinfection. The concept, described by Quirynen et al.,[52] consists of full-mouth debridement (removal of all plaque and calculus) completed in two appointments within a 24-hour period. In addition to scaling and root planing, the tongue is brushed with a chlorhexidine gel (1%) for 1 minute, the mouth is rinsed with a chlorhexidine solution (0.2%) for 2 minutes, and periodontal pockets are irrigated with a chlorhexidine solution (1%).

In a clinical and microbiologic study, 10 patients with advanced chronic periodontitis were randomly assigned to test or control groups. Test patients were treated as just described while control patients received scaling and root planing by quadrant at 2-week intervals along with oral hygiene instructions. At 1 and 2 months after treatment, the test group showed significantly higher reduction in probing pocket depth, especially for pockets that were initially deep (7-8 mm). Patients in the test group also had significantly lower pathogenic microorganisms after treatment compared with controls. Several follow-up studies by the same center demonstrated similar results for up to 6 months after therapy.[5,6,63] In another study, the same group included a test group who did *not* use chlorhexidine as part of the one-stage full-mouth disinfection.[54] Interestingly, the results of both test groups (with and without chlorhexidine) were similar and were significantly better than for controls. The authors concluded that the beneficial effects of one-stage full-mouth disinfection probably result from the full-mouth debridement within 24 hours rather than the adjunctive chlorhexidine treatment.

A few reports have included patients with aggressive (early-onset) periodontitis in their evaluation of the one-stage full-mouth disinfection protocol.[12,46,53] As with the advanced chronic periodontitis group, De Soete et al.[12] found a significant reduction in probing pocket depth and gain in clinical attachment in patients with aggressive periodontitis up to 8 months after treatment compared with controls (scaling and root planing by quadrant at 2-week intervals). They also found significant reductions in periodontal pathogens up to 8 months after therapy. *Porphyromonas gingivalis* and *Tannerella forsythia* (formerly *Bacteroides forsythus*) were reduced to levels below detection.

Host Modulation

Currently, the influence of the host immune response in the pathogenesis of periodontitis is well known. Variations in host response between individuals are greatly responsible for observed differences in disease severity. This is especially true for individuals with aggressive periodontitis. A better understanding of and appreciation for the role of the host immune response in disease pathogenesis have created the opportunity for new, innovative approaches to treatment.

A novel approach in the treatment of aggressive periodontitis and difficult-to-control forms of periodontal disease is the administration of agents that modulate the host response. Several agents have been used or evaluated to modify the host response to disease (see Chapter 53). The use of *subantimicrobial-dose doxycycline* (SDD) may help to prevent the destruction of the periodontal attachment by controlling the activation of matrix metalloproteinases, primarily collagenase and gelatinase, from both infiltrating cells and resident cells of the periodontium, primarily the neutrophils.[61] SDD as an adjunct to repeated mechanical debridement resulted in clinical improvement in patients with generalized aggressive periodontitis.[32] More than 50% of the patients in this study were smokers. Other agents, such as flurbiprofen, indomethacin, and naproxen, may reduce inflammatory mediator production.[27] Further research needs to be done to substantiate the effects of these agents.

Treatment Planning and Restorative Considerations

Successful management of patients with aggressive periodontitis must include tooth replacement as part of the treatment plan. In some advanced cases of aggressive periodontitis, the overall treatment success for the patient may be enhanced if severely compromised teeth are extracted. The outcome of treatment for these teeth is limited, and more importantly, the retention of severely diseased teeth over time may result in additional bone loss and teeth that are further compromised. The risk of further bone loss is even a greater concern now with the current success and predictability of dental implants and the desire to preserve bone for implant placement. Any additional alveolar bone loss in an area that has already undergone severe bone loss may further compromise residual anatomy and impair the opportunity for tooth replacement with a dental implant. This is especially true for certain areas with poor bone quality or limited bone volume, such as the posterior maxilla. Fortunately, healing of extraction sites is typically uneventful in patients with aggressive periodontitis, and bone augmentation of defect sites is predictable.

In the patient with aggressive periodontitis, the approach to restorative treatment should be made based on a single premise: extract severely compromised teeth early, and plan treatment to accommodate future tooth loss. The teeth with the best prognosis should be identified and considered when planning the restorative treatment. The lower cuspids and first premolars are generally more resistant to loss, probably because of the favorable anatomy (single roots, no furcations) and easier access for patient oral hygiene. As a rule, an extensive fixed prosthesis should be avoided, and removable partial dentures should be planned in such a way as to allow for the addition of teeth.

When hopeless teeth are extracted, they need to be replaced. The desire to replace missing teeth in a permanent manner without preparation of adjacent teeth for a fixed partial denture motivated clinicians to attempt transplantation of teeth from one site to another. Transplantation of developing third molars to the sockets of hopeless first molars has been attempted with limited success.[8,35,42] Clearly, the success and predictability of dental implants have obviated the need for attempting to transplant teeth to edentulous sites.

Use of Dental Implants

Initially, the use of dental implants was suggested and implemented with much caution in patients with aggressive periodontitis because of an unfounded fear of bone loss. However, evidence to the contrary appears to support the use of dental implants in patients with aggressive periodontal disease.[40,45,47,72] Currently, the use of dental implants must be considered in the overall treatment plan for patients with aggressive periodontitis.

Periodontal Maintenance

When patients with aggressive periodontitis are transferred to maintenance care, their periodontal condition must be stable (i.e., no clinical signs of disease and no periodontal pathogens). Each maintenance visit should consist of a medical history review, an inquiry about any recent periodontal problems, a comprehensive periodontal and oral examination, thorough root debridement, and prophylaxis, followed by a review of oral hygiene instructions. If oral hygiene is poor, patients may benefit most from a review of oral hygiene instructions and visualization of plaque in their own mouth before debridement and prophylaxis.

Frequent maintenance visits appear to be one of the most important factors in the control of disease and the success of treatment in patients with aggressive periodontitis.[37,65] In a study of 25 individuals with aggressive (early-onset) periodontitis followed with maintenance every 3 to 6 months for 5 years, it was concluded that patients with aggressive periodontitis could be effectively maintained with clinical and microbiologic improvements after active periodontal therapy.[28] The presence of high bacterial counts (particularly *P. gingivalis* and *Treponema denticola*), number of acute episodes, number of teeth lost, smoking, and stress appear to be significant factors in the small percentage of sites that showed progressive bone loss. In a 5-year follow-up study of 13 patients with aggressive periodontitis, comprehensive mechanical, surgical, and antimicrobial therapy with supportive periodontal maintenance every 3 to 4 months, periodontal disease progression was arrested in 95% of the initially affected lesions. Only 2% to 5% experienced discrete episodes of loss of periodontal support.[9]

A supportive periodontal maintenance program aimed at early detection and treatment of sites that begin to lose attachment should be established. The duration between these recall visits is usually short during the first period after the patient's completion of therapy, generally no longer than 3-month intervals. Acute episodes of gingival inflammation can be detected and managed earlier when the patient is on a frequent monitoring cycle. Monitoring as frequently as every 3 to 4 weeks may be necessary when the disease is thought to be active. If signs of disease activity and progression persist despite therapeutic efforts, frequent visits and good patient compliance, microbial testing may be indicated. The rate of disease progression may be faster in younger individuals, and therefore the clinician should monitor such patients more frequently. Over time the recall maintenance interval can be adjusted (more or less often) to suit the patient's level of oral hygiene and control of disease, as determined by each examination.

Close collaboration between members of the treatment team, including the periodontist, general dentist, dental hygienist, and patient's physician, is required for continuity of care and for patient motivation and encouragement. It is important to monitor and observe the patient's overall physical status as well, because weight loss, depression, and malaise have been reported in patients with generalized aggressive periodontitis. Finally, there is a constant need to reinforce patient education about disease etiology and preventive practices (i.e., oral hygiene and control of risk factors).

PERIODONTITIS REFRACTORY TO TREATMENT

Although refractory periodontitis is not currently considered a separate disease entity (see Chapter 7), patients who fail to respond to conventional therapy are considered to have periodontitis that is "refractory" to treatment. It is possible to characterize any form of periodontal disease (e.g., chronic periodontitis, aggressive periodontitis) as refractory to treatment.

These cases are difficult to manage because the etiology behind their lack of response to therapy is unknown. Initially, because contributing factors may have been overlooked, it is important to evaluate the adequacy of treatment attempts thoroughly and to consider other possible etiologies before concluding that a case truly is *refractory.*

A patient with periodontitis that is refractory to treatment often does not have any distinguishing clinical characteristics on initial examination compared with cases of periodontitis that respond normally. Therefore the initial treatment would follow conventional therapeutic modalities for periodontitis. After treatment, if the patient has not responded as expected, the clinician should rule out the following conditions:

1. *Inadequately treated periodontitis.* Most forms of periodontitis can be treated effectively with currently available modalities if they are performed properly. After treatment, if it is determined that the patient has not responded, the clinician must evaluate whether the therapy was adequately performed. Undetected or inaccessible subgingival calculus may be present in one or more areas. Re-treatment may be the best way to ensure that therapy was adequately performed. All root surfaces must be meticulously inspected.
2. *Periodontitis associated with poor plaque control.* Plaque control is essential to the success of periodontal therapy.[48,56,57] Patients must understand the role of bacterial plaque in their disease process, and they must comply with daily oral hygiene instructions. Thus, patient compliance and the adequacy of their daily plaque control should be assessed before concluding that a case of periodontitis is refractory to treatment.
3. *Endodontic infection.* The presence of nonperiodontal infections in the area can perpetuate periodontal disease activity and prevent a normal healing response to conventional periodontal therapy. Endodontic infection of teeth in the area should be suspected and ruled out before a concluding that a case is refractory to treatment. The clinician should suspect an endodontic etiology especially in those patients with localized recurrent disease.

A case may be considered *refractory* to treatment only when loss of periodontal attachment and bone continues after well-executed treatment in a patient with good oral hygiene and no other infections or etiologic factors.

Clinicians are in a quandary when presented with a patient who is not responding to periodontal therapy. Therapeutic means must be broad in scope and thorough to ensure that all aspects of the host response are addressed. At a minimum, a frequent and intensive recall maintenance and home care program is necessary. Mechanical debridement with scaling and root planing can reduce total supragingival and subgingival bacterial masses, but major periodontal pathogens may persist. Surgical treatment may aid in providing access for debridement and in elimination of bacterial pathogens.[58] In addition, the morphology of the gingival tissues should be modified to facilitate daily plaque removal by the patient.

Systemic antibiotic therapy is administered to reinforce mechanical periodontal treatment and support the host defense system in overcoming the infection by killing subgingival pathogens that remain after conventional mechanical periodontal therapy. Many antibiotics have been used according to the target microflora with various degrees of success[21] (see Table 46-1). For patients with refractory disease who fail to respond to initial antibiotic therapy, subsequent treatment should include microbial testing with bacterial identification and antimicrobial susceptibility.

Antibiotic resistance is a potential problem. Patients with periodontitis that is refractory to treatment often present with a history of previous tetracycline therapy, and thus they may have a microflora that is resistant to this drug.[30,41,67,70] Tetracycline-resistant bacteria have been isolated from patients with periodontitis refractory to treatment.[49] However, some patients with refractory disease may still benefit from the use of tetracycline or one of its derivatives.

Cases of periodontitis (refractory) in which the associated microflora consists primarily of gram-positive microorganisms have been successfully treated with *amoxicillin–clavulanate potassium.* Many efforts have been made to establish the most appropriate regimen of antibiotic therapy for these patients. Similar antimicrobial regimens, consisting of 250 mg of amoxicillin and

125 mg of clavulanate potassium, have been administered three times daily for 14 days, with scaling and root planing, and produced a reduction in attachment loss for at least 12 months. A regimen of 1 capsule containing the same amount of drug every 6 hours for 2 weeks, with intrasulcular full-mouth lavage using a 10% povidone-iodine solution and chlorhexidine oral rinses twice daily, resulted in a reduction in attachment loss that persisted at approximately 34 months.[11] A regimen of 500 mg of metronidazole three times daily for 7 days was shown to be effective in treating periodontitis (refractory) in patients who were culture positive for *T. forsythia* in the absence of *A. actinomycetemcomitans*.[71]

Clindamycin is a potent antibiotic that penetrates well into gingival fluid, although it is not usually effective against *A. actinomycetemcomitans* and *Eikenella corrodens*.[67] However, clindamycin has been effective in controlling the extent and rate of disease progression in refractory cases in patients who have a microflora susceptible to this antibiotic.[22,39,66] A regimen of clindamycin hydrochloride, 150 mg, four times daily for 7 days combined with scaling and root planing produced a decrease in the incidence of disease activity from an annual rate of 8% to an annual rate of 0.5% of sites per patient.[22] Clindamycin should be prescribed with caution because of the potential for pseudomembranous colitis from superinfections with *Clostridium difficile*. Patients should be warned and advised to discontinue the antibiotic if symptoms of diarrhea develop.

Azithromycin may be effective in periodontitis that is refractory to treatment, especially in patients infected with *P. gingivalis*.[50]

Combinations of antibiotic therapy may offer greater promise as adjunctive treatment for the management of refractory periodontitis.[2,11,17,41] The rationale is based on the diversity of putative pathogens[20,62] and no single antibiotic being bactericidal for all known pathogens. Combination antibiotic therapy may help broaden the antimicrobial range of the therapeutic regimen beyond that attained by any single antibiotic. Other advantages include lowering the dose of individual antibiotics by exploiting possible synergy between two drugs against targeted organisms. In addition, combination therapy may prevent or forestall the emergence of bacterial resistance. Many combinations of antibiotics have demonstrated significant improvement in the clinical aspects of the disease.[41] Examples of combinations include amoxicillin-clavulanate[17] or metronidazole-amoxicillin for the treatment of *A. actinomycetemcomitans*–associated periodontitis; metronidazole-doxycycline for the prevention of recurrent periodontitis; metronidazole-ciprofloxacin[55] for the treatment of recurrent cases containing a microflora associated with enteric rods and pseudomonads; and amoxicillin-doxycycline[41] in the treatment of periodontitis associated with *A. actinomycetemcomitans* and *P. gingivalis*.

Some cases of refractory periodontitis may not respond to a given antibiotic regimen. When this occurs, the clinician should consider a different antimicrobial therapy based on microbial susceptibility analysis. At this point in the therapy, strong consideration should be given to consulting with the patient's physician for an evaluation of a possible host immune system deficiency or a metabolic problem such as diabetes.

NECROTIZING ULCERATIVE PERIODONTITIS

Necrotizing ulcerative periodontitis (NUP) is a rare disease, especially in developed countries. Often, NUP is diagnosed in individuals with a compromised host immune response (see Chapter 32). The incidence of NUP in specific populations (e.g., HIV-positive/AIDS patients) has been reported as 0% to 6%. Most patients diagnosed with NUP apparently have diseases or conditions that impair their host immune response. These patients often have an underlying predisposing systemic factor that renders them susceptible to necrotizing ulcerative periodontal disease. For this reason, patients presenting with NUP should be treated in consultation with their physician. A comprehensive medical evaluation and diagnosis of any condition that may be contributing to an altered host immune response should be completed. It is also important to rule out any hematologic disease (e.g., leukemia) before initiating treatment of a case that has a similar presentation to NUP (see Chapter 17 and Figures 17-16 and 17-17).

Treatment can be initiated only after a thorough medical history and examination to identify the existence of any systemic diseases, such as leukemia or other hematologic disorder, that might contribute to the oral presentation. Treatment for NUP includes local debridement of lesions with scaling and root planing, lavage, and instructions for good oral hygiene. It may be necessary to use local anesthesia during the debridement because lesions are frequently painful. The use of ultrasonic instrumentation with profuse irrigation may enhance debridement and flushing of the deep lesions. Home care may be difficult as well until the lesions and associated pain resolve.

Antimicrobial adjuncts such as chlorhexidine added to the oral hygiene regimen may be effective in contributing to the daily reduction of bacterial loads. Patients frequently complain of pain. The use of locally applied topical antimicrobials and systemic antibiotics as well as systemic analgesics should be used as indicated by signs and symptoms.

Patients with NUP often harbor bacteria, fungi, viruses, and other nonoral microorganisms, complicating the selection of antimicrobial therapy. Superinfection or overgrowth of fungi and viruses may be propagated by antibiotic therapy. Antifungal agents can be considered prophylactically against fungal infection or after it is diagnosed. Because oral hygiene for these patients is complicated by the painful lesions, alternative methods should be encouraged. In such patients, irrigation with diluted cleansing and antibacterial agents can be of some benefit.

Ultimately, the successful treatment of NUP may depend in the resolution or treatment of the systemic condition (e.g., immune compromise) that predisposed the individual to the disease. Evaluation and treatment of patients with known systemic conditions, such as human immunodeficiency virus (HIV) infection, should be coordinated with the patient's physician.

CONCLUSION

Aggressive and atypical forms of periodontitis are a challenge for the clinician because they are infrequently encountered and because the predictability of treatment success varies from one patient to another. Clearly, the host immune response plays a significant role in these patients. As a result, these unusual disease entities often do not respond well to conventional therapy. Therapeutic measures must be broad in scope and thorough to ensure that all aspects of the host response are addressed. At a minimum, an intense recall maintenance and home care program is necessary. The best treatment for these patients appears to be a combination of conventional treatment with antimicrobial therapy (systemic and/or local delivery) and close follow-up care.

Many questions remain regarding the selection of antibiotic type, dosage, duration, and route of administration. Antibiotic regimens have been successful in selected cases; common practice continues to be somewhat empiric. Bacterial identification may be of value for patients who continue to progress despite diligent efforts by practitioner and patient. The information can be used to determine the antibiotic susceptibility of suspected pathogens. Adjunctive host modulation, although only an emerging area of interest, may prove to be promising in the treatment of patients with aggressive periodontitis as well as periodontitis that is refractory to treatment.

REFERENCES

1. American Academy of Periodontology: Parameter on aggressive periodontitis, *J Periodontol* 71(suppl):867, 2000.
2. Atiken S, Birek P, Kulkarni GV, et al: Serial doxycycline and metronidazole in prevention of recurrent periodontitis in high-risk patients, *J Periodontol* 63:87, 1993.
3. Baer PN, Socransky SS: Periodontosis: case report with long-term follow-up, *Periodont Case Rep* 1:1, 1979.
4. Barnett ML, Baker RL: The formation and healing of osseous lesions in a patient with localized juvenile periodontitis: case report, *J Periodontol* 4(suppl):148, 1983.
5. Bollen CM, Mongardini C, Papaioannou W, et al: The effect of a one-stage full-mouth disinfection on different intra-oral niches: clinical and microbiological observations, *J Clin Periodontol* 25:56, 1998.
6. Bollen CM, Vandekerckhove BN, Papaioannou W, et al: Full- versus partial-mouth disinfection in the treatment of periodontal infections: a pilot study: long-term microbiological observations, *J Clin Periodontol* 23:960, 1996.
7. Bonta H, Llambes F, Moretti AJ, et al: The use of enamel matrix protein in the treatment of localized aggressive periodontitis: a case report, *Quintessence Int* 34:247, 2003.
8. Borring-Moller G, Frandsen A: Autologous tooth transplantation to replace molars lost in patients with juvenile periodontitis, *J Clin Periodontol* 5:152, 1978.
9. Buchmann R, Nunn ME, Van Dyke TE, Lange DE: Aggressive periodontitis: 5-year follow-up of treatment, *J Periodontol* 73:675, 2002.
10. Carranza FA Jr, Saglie FR, Newman MG, et al: Scanning and transmission electron microscopic study of tissue-invading microorganisms in localized juvenile periodontitis, *J Periodontol* 54:598, 1983.
11. Collins JG, Offenbacher S, Arnold RR: Effects of a combination of therapy to eliminate *Porphyromonas gingivalis* in refractory periodontitis, *J Periodontol* 64:98, 1993.
12. De Soete M, Mongardini C, Peuwels M, et al: One-stage full-mouth disinfection: long-term microbiological results analyzed by checkerboard DNA-DNA hybridization, *J Periodontol* 72:374, 2001.
13. Deas DE, Mackey SA, McDonnell HT: Systemic disease and periodontitis: manifestations of neutrophil dysfunction, *Periodontol 2000* 32:82, 2003.
14. Delcourt-Debruyne EM, Boutigny HR, Hildebrand HF: Features of severe periodontal disease in a teenager with Chédiak-Higashi syndrome, *J Periodontol* 71:816, 2000.
15. Dodson SA, Takei HH, Carranza FA Jr: Clinical success in regeneration: report of a case, *Int J Periodont Restor Dent* 16:455, 1996.
16. Esposito M, Coulthard P, Worthington HV: Enamel matrix derivative (Emdogain) for periodontal tissue regeneration in intrabony defects, *Cochrane Database System Rev* 2, 2003.
17. Flemmig TF, Milian E, Karch H, et al: Differential clinical treatment outcome after systemic metronidazole and amoxicillin in patients harboring *Actinobacillus actinomycetemcomitans* and/or *Porphyromonas gingivalis, J Clin Periodontol* 25:380, 1998.
18. Fourmousis I, Tonetti MS, Mombelli A, et al: Evaluation of tetracycline fiber therapy with digital image analysis, *J Clin Periodontol* 25:737, 1998.
19. Garrett S, Johnson L, Drisko CH, et al: Two multi-center studies evaluating locally delivered doxycycline hyclate, placebo control, oral hygiene, and scaling and root planing in the treatment of periodontitis, *J Periodontol* 70:490, 1999.
20. Genco RJ, Ciancio SC, Rosling B: Treatment of localized juvenile periodontitis, *J Dent Res* 60:527, 1981 (abstract).
21. Gordon JM, Walker CB: Current status of systemic antibiotic usage in destructive periodontal disease, *J Periodontol* 64(suppl):760, 1993.
22. Gordon J, Walker C, Hovliaras C, et al: Efficacy of clindamycin hydrochloride in refractory periodontitis: 24-month results, *J Periodontol* 61:689, 1990.
23. Haffajee AD, Socransky SS, Gunsolley JC: Systemic anti-infective periodontal therapy: a systematic review, *Ann Periodontol* 8:115, 2003.
24. Haffajee AD, Uzel NG, Arguello EI, et al: Clinical and microbiological changes associated with the use of combined antimicrobial therapies to treat "refractory" periodontitis, *J Clin Periodontol* 31:869, 2004.
25. Herrera D, Sanz M, Jepsen S, et al: A systematic review on the effect of systemic antimicrobials as an adjunct to scaling and root planing in periodontitis patients, *J Clin Periodontol* 29(suppl 3):136, 160 (discussion), 2002.
26. Hirschfeld L, Wasserman B: A long-term survey of tooth loss in 600 treated periodontal patients, *J Periodontol* 49:225, 1978.
27. Howell T, Williams R: Pharmacologic blocking of host response as an adjunct in the management of periodontal disease: a research update, Position paper, Chicago, 1992, American Academy of Periodontology.
28. Kamma JJ, Baehni PC: Five-year maintenance follow-up of early-onset periodontitis patients, *J Clin Periodontol* 30:562, 2003.
29. Killoy WJ: The use of locally delivered chlorhexidine in the treatment of periodontitis: clinical results, *J Clin Periodontol* 25:953, 1998.
30. Kornman KS, Karl EH: The effect of long-term, low-dose tetracycline therapy on the subgingival microflora in refractory adult periodontitis, *J Periodontol* 53:604, 1982.
31. Lang N, Bartold PM, Cullinan M, et al: Consensus report: aggressive periodontitis, *Ann Periodontol* 4:53, 1999.

32. Lee HM, Ciancio SG, Tuter G, et al: Subantimicrobial dose doxycycline efficacy as a matrix metalloproteinase inhibitor in chronic periodontitis patients is enhanced when combined with a non-steroidal anti-inflammatory drug, *J Periodontol* 75:453, 2004.
33. Lavine WS, Maderazo EG, Stolman J, et al: Impaired neutrophil chemotaxis in patients with juvenile and rapidly progressing periodontitis, *J Periodontal Res* 14:10, 1979.
34. Leino L, Hurttia H: A potential role of an intracellular signaling defect in neutrophil functional abnormalities and promotion of tissue damage in patients with localized juvenile periodontitis, *Clin Chem Lab Med* 37:215, 1999.
35. Levine RA: Twenty-five month follow-up of an autogenous third molar transplantation in a localized juvenile periodontitis patient: a case report, *Compend Contin Educ Dent* 8:560, 1987.
36. Liljenberg B, Lindhe J: Juvenile periodontitis. Some microbiological, histopathological and clinical characteristics, *J Clin Periodontol* 7:48, 1980.
37. Lindhe J, Liljenberg B: Treatment of localized juvenile periodontitis: results after 5 years, *J Clin Periodontol* 11:399, 1984.
38. Mabry T, Yukna R, Sepe W: Freeze-dried bone allografts with tetracycline in the treatment of juvenile periodontitis, *J Periodontol* 56:74, 1985.
39. Magnusson I, Low SB, McArthur WP, Marks RG, et al: Treatment of subjects with refractory periodontal disease, *J Clin Periodontol* 21:628, 1994.
40. Malmstrom HS, Fritz ME, Timmis DP, Van Dyke TE: Osseointegrated implant treatment of a patient with rapidly progressive periodontitis: a case report, *J Periodontol* 61:300, 1990.
41. Matisko MW, Bissada NF: Short-term sequential administration of amoxicillin/clavulanate potassium and doxycycline in the treatment of recurrent/progressive periodontitis, *J Periodontol* 64:553, 1993.
42. Mattout P, Moskow BS, Fourel J: Repair potential in localized juvenile periodontitis: a case in point, *J Periodontol* 61:653, 1990.
43. McFall WT: Tooth loss in 100 treated patients with periodontal disease in a long-term study, *J Clin Periodontol* 53:539, 1982.
44. Mellado JR, Freedman AL, Salkin LM, et al: The clinical relevance of microbiologic testing: a comparative analysis of microbiologic samples secured from the same sites and cultured in two independent laboratories, *Int J Periodont Restor Dent* 21:232, 2001.
45. Mengel R, Schroder T, Flores-de-Jacoby L: Osseointegrated implants in patients treated for generalized chronic periodontitis and generalized aggressive periodontitis: 3- and 5-year results of a prospective long-term study, *J Periodontol* 72:977, 2001.
46. Mongardini C, van Steenberghe D, Dekeyser C, Quirynen M: One stage full- versus partial-mouth disinfection in the treatment of chronic adult or generalized early-onset periodontitis. I. Long-term clinical observations, *J Periodontol* 70:632, 1999.
47. Nevins M, Langer B: The successful use of osseointegrated implants for the treatment of the recalcitrant periodontal patient, *J Periodontol* 66:150, 1995.
48. Nyman S, Lindhe J, Rosling B: Periodontal surgery in plaque-infected dentitions, *J Clin Periodontol* 4:240, 1977.
49. Olsvik B, Teniver FC: Tetracycline resistance in periodontal pathogens, *Clin Infect Dis* 16(suppl 4):8310, 1993.
50. Pajukanta R: In vitro antimicrobial susceptibility of *Porphyromonas gingivalis* to azithromycin, a novel macrolide, *Oral Microbiol Immunol* 8:325, 1993.
51. Pavicic MJ, van Winkelhoff AJ, Pavivic-Temming YA, et al: Metronidazole susceptibility factors in *Actinobacillus actinomycetemcomitans*, *J Antimicrob Chemother* 35:263, 1995.
52. Quirynen M, Bollen CM, Vandekerckhove BN, et al: Full- vs. partial-mouth disinfection in the treatment of periodontal infections: short-term clinical and microbiological observations, *J Dent Res* 74:1459, 1995.
53. Quirynen M, Mongardini C, Pauwels M, et al: One stage full- versus partial-mouth disinfection in the treatment of chronic adult or generalized early-onset periodontitis. II. Long-term impact on microbial load, *J Periodontol* 70:646, 1999.
54. Quirynen M, Mongardini C, de Soete M, et al: The role of chlorhexidine in the one-stage full-mouth disinfection treatment of patients with advanced adult periodontitis: long-term clinical and microbiological observations. *J Clin Periodontol* 27:578, 2000.
55. Rams TE, Feik D, Slots J: Ciprofloxacin/metronidazole treatment of recurrent adult periodontitis, *J Dent Res* 71:319, 1992 (abstract 1708, special issue).
56. Rosling B, Nyman SF, Lindhe J: The effect of systemic plaque control on bone regeneration in infrabony pockets, *J Clin Periodontol* 3:38, 1976.
57. Rosling B, Nyman SF, Lindhe J, et al: The healing potential of the periodontal tissues following different techniques of periodontal surgery in plaque-free dentitions: a 2-year study, *J Clin Periodontol* 3:233, 1976.
58. Saglie FR, Carranza FA Jr, Newman MG, et al: Identification of tissue invading bacteria in human periodontal disease, *J Periodontal Res* 17:452, 1982.
59. Salkin LM, Freedman AL, Mellado JR, et al: The clinical relevance of microbiologic testing. Part 2. A comparative analysis of microbiologic samples secured simultaneously from the same sites and cultured in the same laboratory, *Int J Periodont Restor Dent* 23(2):121, 2003.
60. Tanner ACR, Socransky SS, Goodson M: Microbiota of periodontal pockets losing crestal alveolar bone, *J Periodontal Res* 19:279, 1984.
61. Thomas JG, Metheny RJ, Karakiozis JM: Long-term subantimicrobial doxycycline (Periostat) as adjunctive management in adult periodontitis: effects on subgingival bacterial population dynamics, *Adv Dent Res* 12:32, 1998.
62. Van Winklehoff AJ, Tijhof CJ, de Graaff: Microbial and clinical results of metronidazole plus amoxicillin therapy in *Actinobacillus actinomycetemcomitans*–associated periodontitis, *J Periodontol* 63:52, 1992.
63. Vandana KL, Shah K, Prakash S: Clinical and radiographic evaluation of Emdogain as a regenerative material in the treatment of interproximal vertical defects in chronic and aggressive periodontitis patients, *Int J Periodont Restor Dent* 24:185, 2004.
64. Vandekerckhove BN, Bollen CM, Dekeyser C, et al: Full- versus partial-mouth disinfection in the treatment of periodontal infections: long-term clinical observations of a pilot study, *J Periodontol* 67:1251, 1996.
65. Waerhaug J: Subgingival plaque and loss of attachment in periodontosis as evaluated on extracted teeth, *J Periodontol* 48:125, 1977.
66. Walker C, Gordon J: The effect of clindamycin on the microbiota associated with refractory periodontitis, *J Periodontol* 61:692, 1990.
67. Walker C, Karpinia K: Rationale for use of antibiotics in periodontics, *J Periodontol* 73:1188, 2002.
68. Walker CB, Gordon JM, Socransky SS: Antibiotic susceptibility testing on subgingival plaque samples, *J Clin Periodontol* 10:422, 1983.
69. Walker CB, Pappas JD, Tyler KZ, Cohen JM: Antibiotic susceptibilities to eight antimicrobial agents, *J Periodontol* 56(suppl):67, 1985.
70. Walker CB, Gordon JM, Magnusson I, et al: A role for antibiotics in the treatment of refractory periodontitis, *J Periodontol* 64:772, 1993.

71. Winkel EG, Van Winkelhoff AJ, Timmerman MF, et al: Effects of metronidazole in patients with "refractory" periodontitis associated with *Bacteroides forsythus, J Clin Periodontol* 24:573, 1997.
72. Yalcin S, Yalcin F, Gunay Y, et al: Treatment of aggressive periodontitis by osseointegrated dental implants: a case report, *J Periodontol* 72:411, 2001.
73. Yukna R, Sepe W: Clinical evaluation of localized periodontosis defects with freeze-dried bone allografts combined with local and systemic tetracyclines, *Int J Periodont Restor Dent* 5:9, 1982.

SECTION ▪ II ▪ Treatment of Periodontal Emergencies

Henry H. Takei

Treatment of Acute Gingival Disease

Phillip T. Marucha

CHAPTER 47

CHAPTER OUTLINE

The treatment of acute gingival disease entails the alleviation of the acute symptoms and elimination of all other periodontal disease, both chronic and acute, throughout the oral cavity. Treatment is not complete if periodontal pathologic changes or factors capable of causing them are still present.

ACUTE NECROTIZING ULCERATIVE GINGIVITIS

Necrotizing ulcerative gingivitis (NUG) results from an impaired host response to a potentially pathogenic microflora. Depending on the degree of immunosuppression, NUG may occur in a mouth essentially free of other gingival involvement or may be superimposed on underlying chronic gingival disease. Treatment should include the alleviation of the acute symptoms and the correction of the underlying chronic gingival disease. The former is the simpler part of the treatment, whereas the latter requires more comprehensive procedures.

The treatment of NUG consists of (1) alleviation of the acute inflammation by reducing the microbial load and removal of necrotic tissue, (2) treatment of chronic disease either underlying the acute involvement or elsewhere in the oral cavity, (3) alleviation of generalized symptoms such as fever and malaise, and (4) correction of systemic conditions or factors that contribute to the initiation or progression of the gingival changes. Chapter 34 provides further information on the management and treatment of NUG in patients with acquired immunodeficiency syndrome (AIDS).

Sequence of Treatment

Treatment of NUG should follow an orderly sequence, according to specific steps at three clinical visits.

First Visit

At the first visit, the clinician should do a complete evaluation of the patient, including a comprehensive medical history with special attention to recent illness, living conditions, dietary background, cigarette smoking, type of employment, hours of rest, risk factors for human immunodeficiency virus (HIV), and psychosocial parameters (e.g., stress, depression). The patient is questioned regarding the history of the acute disease and its onset and duration, as follows:

- Is the disease recurrent?
- Are the recurrences associated with specific factors, such as menstruation, particular foods, exhaustion, or mental stress?
- Has there been any previous treatment? When and for how long?

The clinician should also inquire as to the type of treatment received and the patient's impression regarding its effect.

The examination of the patient should include general appearance, presence of halitosis, presence of skin lesions, vital signs including temperature, and palpation for the presence of enlarged lymph nodes, especially submaxillary and submental nodes.

The oral cavity is examined for the characteristic lesion of NUG (see Chapters 24 and 32), its distribution, and the possible involvement of the oropharyngeal region. Oral hygiene is evaluated, with special attention to the presence of pericoronal flaps, periodontal pockets, and local factors (e.g., poor restorations, distribution of calculus). Periodontal probing of NUG lesions is likely to be very painful and may need to be deferred until after the acute lesions are resolved.

The goals of initial therapy are to reduce the microbial load and remove necrotic tissue to the degree that repair and regeneration of normal tissue barriers are reestablished. Treatment during this initial visit is confined to the acutely involved areas, which are isolated with cotton rolls and dried. A topical anesthetic is applied, and after 2 or 3 minutes the areas are gently swabbed with a moistened cotton pellet to remove the pseudomembrane and nonattached surface debris. Bleeding may be profuse. Each cotton pellet is used in a small area, then discarded; sweeping motions over large areas with a single pellet are not recommended. After the area is cleansed with warm water, the superficial calculus is removed. Ultrasonic scalers are very useful for this purpose because they do not elicit pain, and the water jet and cavitation aid in lavage of the area.

Subgingival scaling and curettage are contraindicated at this time because these procedures may extend the infection into the deeper tissues and may also cause bacteremia. *Unless an emergency exists, procedures such as extractions or periodontal surgery are postponed until the patient has been symptom free for 4 weeks, to minimize the likelihood of exacerbating the acute symptoms.*

Patients with moderate or severe NUG and local lymphadenopathy or other systemic signs or symptoms are placed on an antibiotic regimen of amoxicillin, 500 mg orally every 6 hours for 10 days. For amoxicillin-sensitive patients, other antibiotics are prescribed, such as erythromycin (500 mg every 6 hours) or metronidazole (500 mg twice daily for 7 days). Systemic complications should subside in 1 to 3 days.

Surgical Procedures. Tooth extraction or periodontal surgery should be postponed until 4 weeks after the acute signs and symptoms of NUG have subsided. If emergency surgery is required in the presence of acute symptoms, systemic antibiotics (e.g., amoxicillin) are indicated to prevent worsening or spreading of the acute disease.

Patient Instructions. The patient is discharged with the following instructions:

1. Avoid tobacco, alcohol, and condiments.
2. Rinse with a glassful of an equal mixture of 3% hydrogen peroxide and warm water every 2 hours and/or twice daily with 0.12% chlorhexidine solution.
3. Get adequate rest. Pursue usual activities, but avoid excessive physical exertion or prolonged exposure to the sun, as in golf, tennis, swimming, or sunbathing.
4. Confine toothbrushing to the removal of surface debris with a bland dentifrice and an ultrasoft brush; overzealous brushing and the use of dental floss or interdental cleaners will be painful. Chlorhexidine mouth rinses are also helpful in controlling plaque throughout the mouth.
5. An analgesic, such as a nonsteroidal antiinflammatory drug (NSAID; e.g., ibuprofen), is appropriate for pain relief.

Patients are asked to report back to the clinician in 1 to 2 days. The patient should be advised of the extent of total treatment that the condition requires and warned that treatment is not complete when pain stops. The patient should be informed of the presence of chronic gingival or periodontal disease, which must be eliminated to reduce the likelihood of recurrence of the acute symptoms.

Second Visit

At the second visit, 1 or 2 days after the first visit, the patient is evaluated for amelioration of signs and symptoms. The patient's condition is usually improved; the pain is diminished or no longer present. The gingival margins of the involved areas are erythematous, but without a superficial pseudomembrane.

Scaling is performed if necessary and sensitivity permits. Shrinkage of the gingiva may expose previously covered calculus, which is gently removed. The instructions to the patient are the same as those given previously.

Third Visit

At the next visit, approximately 5 days after the second visit, the patient is evaluated for resolution of symptoms, and a comprehensive plan for the management of the patient's periodontal conditions is formulated. The patient should be essentially symptom free. Some erythema may still be present in the involved areas, and the gingiva may be slightly painful on tactile stimulation (Figure 47-1). The patient is instructed in plaque control procedures (see Chapter 50), which are essential for the success of the treatment and the maintenance of periodontal health. The patient is further counseled on nutrition, smoking cessation, and other conditions or habits associated with a potential recurrence. The hydrogen peroxide rinses are discontinued, but chlorhexidine rinses can be maintained for 2 or 3 weeks. Scaling and root planing are repeated if necessary. Unfortunately, the patient often

A

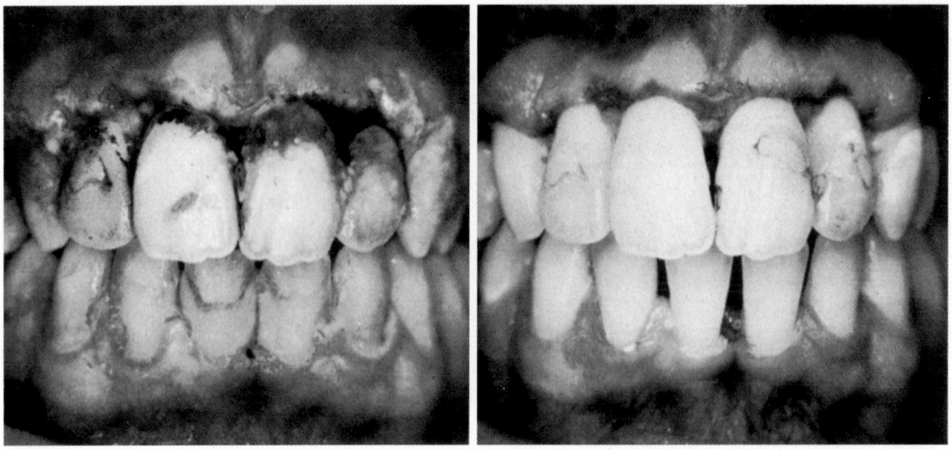

B

Figure 47-1 Initial response to treatment of patient with acute necrotizing ulcerative gingivitis (NUG). **A,** Severe acute NUG. **B,** Third day after treatment. Patient still has some erythema, but the condition is greatly improved.

discontinues treatment because the acute condition has subsided; however, this is when comprehensive treatment of the patient's chronic periodontal problem should start.

Appointments should be scheduled for the treatment of chronic gingivitis, periodontal pockets, and pericoronal flaps, as well as for the elimination of all forms of local irritation. The patient should be reevaluated at 1 month to determine compliance with oral hygiene, health habits, psychosocial factors, the potential need for reconstructive or esthetic surgery, and the interval of subsequent recall visits.

Gingival Changes with Healing

The characteristic lesion of NUG undergoes the following changes in the course of healing in response to treatment:

1. Removal of the surface pseudomembrane exposes the underlying red, hemorrhagic, craterlike depressions in the gingiva, indicating inflammation caused by necrosis and microbial infiltration of tissue that has lost the normal barrier function of the epithelium.
2. In the next stage, the bulk and redness of the crater margins are reduced, indicating a reduction in inflammation and reepithelialization, but the surface remains shiny (see Figure 47-1).
3. This is followed by the early signs of restoration of normal gingival contour and color, indicating reestablishment of the normal barrier function of the epithelium, including keratinization, and further reduction of inflammation.
4. In the final stage, the normal gingival color, consistency, surface texture, and contour may be restored. Portions of the root exposed by the acute disease may be covered by healthy gingiva (Figures 47-2 and 47-3).

A

B

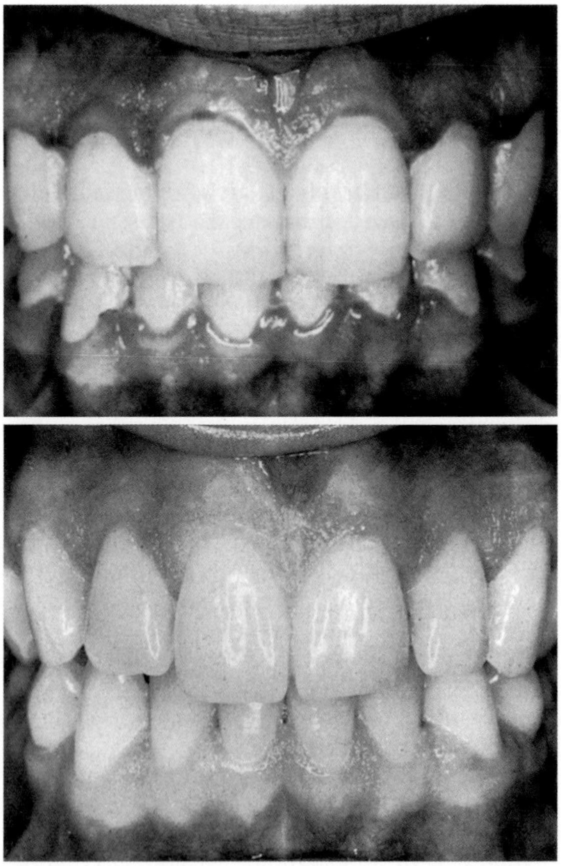

Figure 47-2 Treatment of acute NUG. **A,** Before treatment. Note the characteristic interdental lesions. **B,** After treatment, showing restoration of healthy gingival contour.

Additional Treatment Considerations

Contouring of Gingiva as Adjunctive Procedure. Even in cases of severe gingival necrosis, healing often leads to restoration of the normal gingival contour, although normal architecture of the gingiva may be achieved only after several weeks or months (Figure 47-4). However, if there has been loss of interdental bone, if the teeth are irregularly aligned, or if the entire papilla is lost, healing sometimes results in the formation of a shelflike

A

B

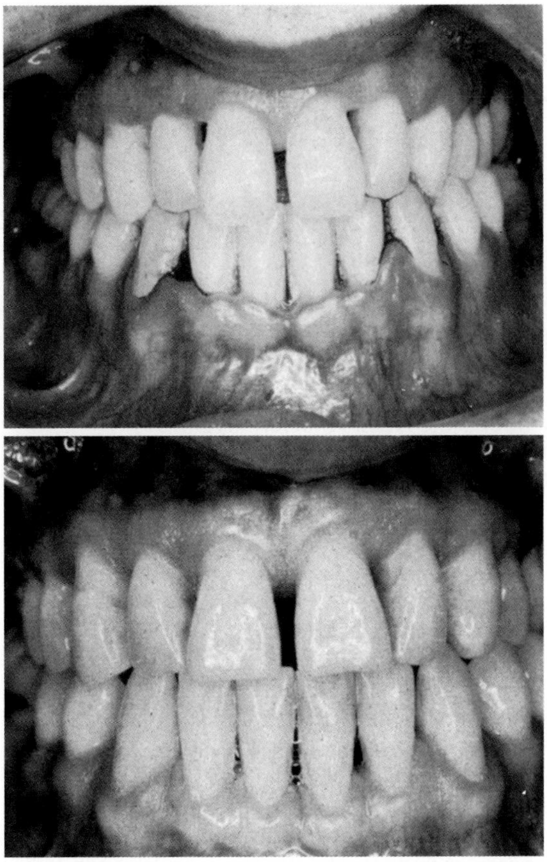

Figure 47-3 Physiologic contour and new attachment of gingiva after treatment of acute NUG. **A,** Acute NUG showing the characteristic punched-out eroded gingival margin with surface pseudomembrane. **B,** After treatment. Note the restoration of physiologic gingival contour and reattachment of the gingiva to the surfaces of the mandibular teeth, which had been exposed by the disease.

gingival margin, which may be an esthetic problem and favors retention of plaque and recurrence of gingival inflammation. This can be corrected by an attempt to restore lost tissue through periodontal plastic procedures or by reshaping the gingiva surgically (Figure 47-5). Effective plaque control by the patient is particularly important to establish and maintain the normal gingival contour in areas of tooth irregularity.

Systemic Antibiotics and Topical Antimicrobials. *Antibiotics are administered systemically only in patients with systemic complications or local adenopathy.* Antibiotics are not recommended in NUG patients who do not have these complications. A large variety of drugs have been used in the treatment of NUG.[3] Topical drug therapy is only an adjunctive measure; *no drug, when used alone, can be considered complete therapy.*

When used, systemic antibiotics also reduce the oral bacterial flora and alleviate the oral symptoms,[11,12] but they are only an adjunct to the complete local treatment that the disease requires. Patients treated by systemic antibiotics alone should be cautioned that the acute painful symptoms may recur after the drug is discontinued.

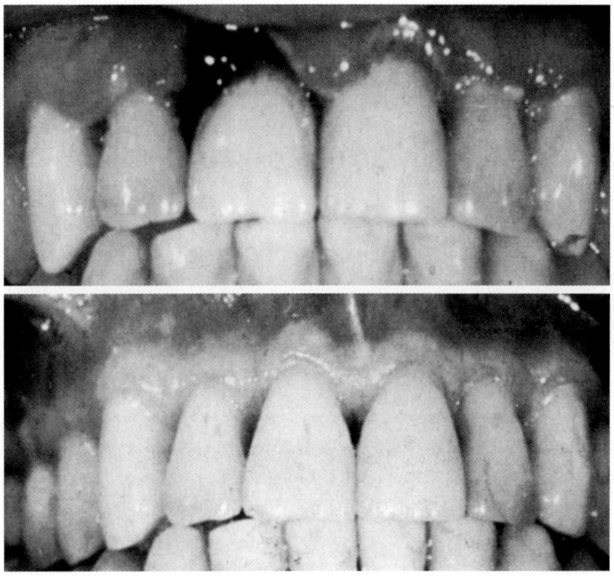

Figure 47-4 Gingival healing after treatment of acute NUG. **A,** Before treatment. Severe acute NUG with crater formation. **B,** After treatment. Note the restored gingival contour.

Supportive Systemic Treatment. In addition to systemic antibiotics, supportive treatment consists of copious fluid consumption and administration of analgesics for relief of pain. Bed rest is necessary for patients with systemic complications such as high fever, malaise, anorexia, and general debility.

Nutritional Supplements. The rationale for nutritional supplements in the treatment of NUG is based on the following:

1. Lesions resembling those of NUG have been produced experimentally in animals with certain nutritional deficiencies (see Chapter 17).
2. Difficulty in chewing raw fruits and vegetables in a painful condition such as NUG could lead to the patient selecting a diet inadequate in vitamins B and C.
3. Isolated clinical studies report fewer recurrences when local treatment of NUG is supplemented with vitamin B or vitamin C.[5,7]

Early during therapy, when eating may be painful, the patient may benefit from the use of liquid medical nutritional supplements. The patient should then be placed on a natural diet with the required nutritional content as soon as the oral condition permits. Nutritional supplements may be discontinued after 2 months.

When the intake of water-soluble vitamins B and C has been severely curtailed because of pain in NUG, nutritional supplements may be indicated along with local treatment to ward off deficiencies of these vitamins. Under such circumstances the patient may be given a standard multivitamin preparation combined with a therapeutic dose of vitamins B and C.

Local procedures are the keystone for the treatment of necrotizing ulcerative gingivitis. Inflammation is a local

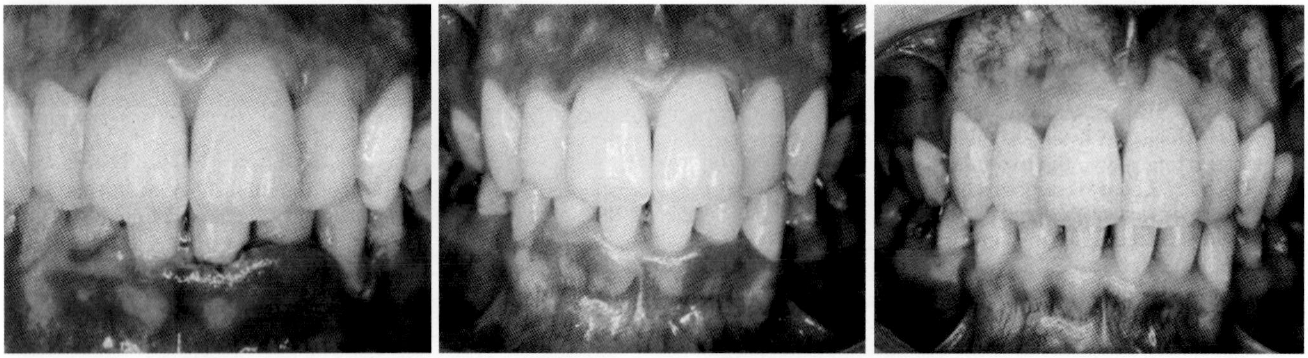
A B C

Figure 47-5 Reshaping the gingiva in the treatment of acute NUG. **A,** Before treatment, showing bulbous gingiva and interdental necrosis in the mandibular anterior area. **B,** After treatment. Gingival contours still undesirable. **C,** Final result. Physiologic contours obtained by reshaping the gingiva.

conditioning factor that impairs the nutrition of the gingiva regardless of the systemic nutritional status. Local irritants should be eliminated to foster normal metabolic and reparative processes in the gingiva. Persistent or recurrent NUG is more likely to be caused by the failure to remove local irritants and by inadequate plaque control than by nutritional deficiency.

Persistent or Recurrent Cases

Adequate local therapy with optimal home care will resolve most cases of NUG. If a case of NUG persists despite therapy or if it recurs, the patient should be reevaluated, with a focus on the following factors:

1. *Reassessment of differential diagnosis to rule out diseases that resemble NUG.* Several diseases and conditions may initially present with a similar appearance as NUG, such as desquamative gingivitis. A renewed search for skin lesions and other sign or symptoms should be undertaken, with a biopsy if warranted NUG (see Chapter 17).
2. *Underlying systemic disease causing immunosuppression.* In particular, HIV infection may frequently present with symptoms of NUG or necrotizing ulcerative periodontitis (NUP). The patient should be reassessed for risk factors and may need counseling about testing for HIV or other suspected underlying systemic diseases (e.g., lymphoproliferative disease). The patient will likely need referral to his or her physician for further evaluation.
3. *Inadequate local therapy.* Too often, treatment is discontinued when the symptoms have subsided, without eliminating the chronic gingival disease and periodontal pockets that remain after the superficial acute condition is relieved. Remaining calculus and other local factors that predispose to gingival inflammation may permit recurrence. Recurrent acute involvement in the mandibular anterior area can be associated with persistent pericoronal inflammation arising from partial eruption and pericoronal inflammation of third molars.[8] The anterior involvement is less likely to recur after the third molar situation is corrected.
4. *Inadequate compliance.* Poor plaque control, heavy use of tobacco, ineffective stress management, and continued malnutrition can also contribute to persistence or recurrence of NUG.

The clinician should evaluate the quality and consistency of plaque control. Further assessment and counseling on tobacco use will also determine the role of tobacco in this patient. If the clinician perceives that psychosocial factors are unresolved and are complicating health behaviors and contributing to immunosuppression, the patient should be referred to the appropriate professional. A reassessment of the patient's nutritional state, with potential dietary analysis or nutritional testing, may be required.

ACUTE PERICORONITIS

The treatment of pericoronitis depends on the severity of the inflammation, the systemic complications, and the advisability of retaining the involved tooth. All pericoronal flaps should be viewed with suspicion. Persistent symptom-free pericoronal flaps should be removed as a preventive measure against subsequent acute involvement.

The treatment of acute pericoronitis consists of (1) gently flushing the area with warm water to remove debris and exudate and (2) swabbing with antiseptic after elevating the flap gently from the tooth with a scaler. The underlying debris is removed, and the area is flushed with warm water (Figure 47-6). The occlusion is evaluated to determine if an opposing tooth is occluding with the pericoronal flap. Removal of soft tissue or occlusal adjustment may be necessary. Antibiotics can be prescribed in severe cases and in patients who may have clinical evidence of diffuse microbial infiltration of the tissue. If the gingival flap is swollen and fluctuant, the clinician uses a #15 blade to make an anteroposterior incision to establish drainage.

After the acute symptoms have subsided, a determination is made about whether to retain or extract the tooth.

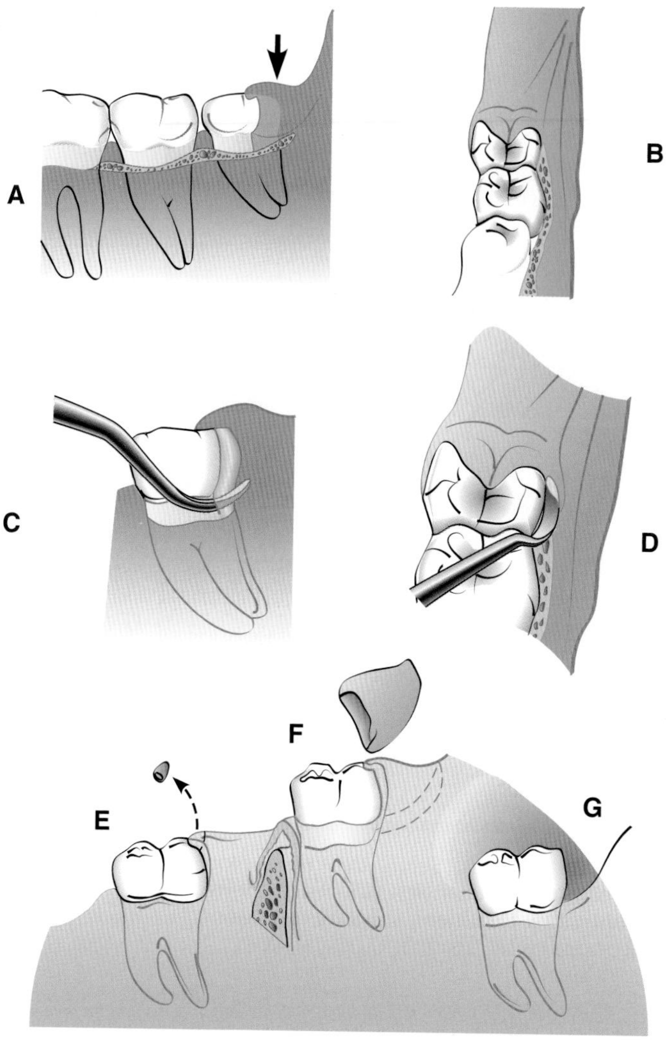

Figure 47-6 Treatment of acute pericoronitis. **A,** Inflamed pericoronal flap *(arrow)* in relation to the mandibular third molar. **B,** Anterior view of third molar and flap. **C,** Lateral view with scaler in position to gently remove debris under flap. **D,** Anterior view of scaler in position. **E,** Incorrect removal of the tip of the flap, permitting the deep pocket to remain distal to the molar. **F,** Removal of section of the gingiva distal to the third molar, after the acute symptoms subsided. The line of incision is indicated by the broken line. **G,** Appearance of the healed area.

The decision is governed by the likelihood of further eruption into a good functional position. Bone loss on the distal surface of the second molars is a hazard after the extraction of partially or completely impacted third molars,[2] and the problem is significantly greater if the third molars are extracted after the roots are formed or in patients older than their early 20s. To reduce the risk of bone loss around second molars, partially or completely impacted third molars should be extracted as early as possible in their development.

If the decision is made to retain the tooth, the pericoronal flap is removed using periodontal knives or electrosurgery (Figure 47-6). It is necessary to remove the tissue distal to the tooth, as well as the flap on the occlusal surface. Incising only the occlusal portion of the flap leaves a deep distal pocket, which invites recurrence of acute pericoronal involvement. It is critical to leave the patient with a cleansable site. On healing, the patient needs appropriate instruction in long-term maintenance.

ACUTE HERPETIC GINGIVOSTOMATITIS

Primary infection with herpes simplex virus in the oral cavity results in a condition known as acute herpetic gingivostomatitis, which is an oral infection often, accompanied by systemic signs and symptoms (see Chapter 24). This infection typically occurs in children, but it can occur in adults as well. It runs a 7- to 10-day course and usually heals without scarring. A recurrent herpetic episode may be precipitated in individuals with a history of herpesvirus infections by dental treatment, respiratory infections, sunlight exposure, fever, trauma, exposure to chemicals, and emotional stress.

Treatment consists of early diagnosis and immediate initiation of antiviral therapy. Until recently, therapy for primary herpetic gingivostomatitis consisted of palliative care. With the development of antiviral therapy, however, the standard of care has changed. In a randomized double-blind placebo-controlled study, Amir et al.[1] demonstrated that antiviral therapy with 15 mg/kg of an acyclovir suspension given five times daily for 7 days substantially changes the course of the disease without significant side effects. Acyclovir reduced symptoms, including fever, from 3 days to 1 day; decreased new extraoral lesions from 5.5 to 0 days; and reduced difficulty with eating from 7 to 4 days. Furthermore, viral shedding stopped at 1 day for the acyclovir group compared with 5 days for the control group. Overall, oral lesions were present for only 4 days in the acyclovir group but for 10 days in the control group. Although no clear clinical evidence indicates that this regimen will reduce recurrences, research data suggest that a greater number of latent virus copies incorporated into ganglia will increase the severity of recurrences.[1] In summary, if primary herpetic gingivostomatitis is diagnosed within 3 days of onset, acyclovir suspension should be prescribed, 15 mg/kg five times daily for 7 days. If diagnosis occurs after 3 days in an immunocompetent patient, acyclovir therapy may have limited value.

All patients, including those presenting more than 3 days after disease onset, may receive palliative care, including removal of plaque and food debris. An NSAID (e.g., ibuprofen) can be given systemically to reduce fever and pain. Patients may use either nutritional supplements or topical anesthetics (e.g., viscous lidocaine) before eating to aid in proper nutrition during the early phases in acute herpetic gingivostomatitis. Periodontal therapy should be postponed until the acute symptoms subside to avoid the possibility of exacerbation (Figure 47-7).

Local or systemic application of antibiotics is sometimes advised to prevent opportunistic infection of ulcerations, especially in the immunocompromised patient. If the condition does not resolve with 2 weeks, the patient should be referred to a physician for medical consultation.[6]

The patient should be informed that herpetic gingivostomatitis is contagious at certain stages, such as

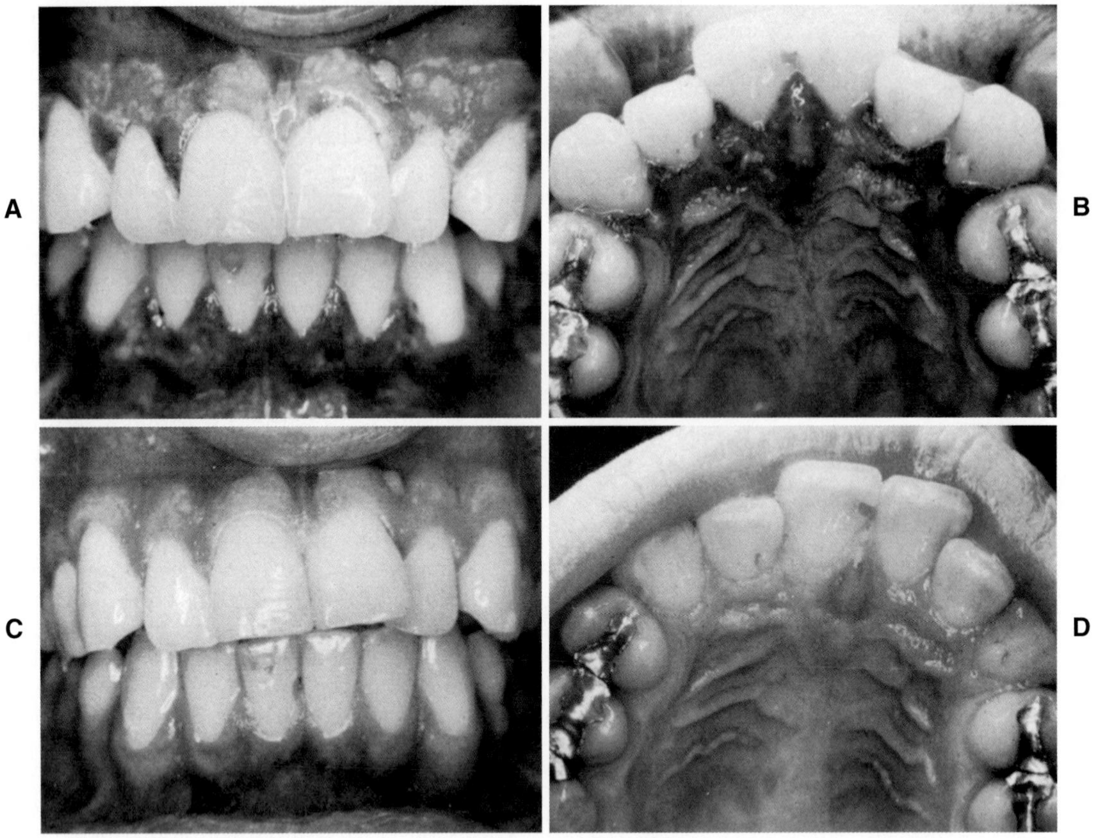

Figure 47-7 Treatment of acute herpetic gingivostomatitis. **A,** Before treatment. Note diffuse erythema and surface vesicles. **B,** Before treatment, palatal view, showing gingival edema and ruptured vesicle on palate. **C,** One month after treatment, showing restoration of normal gingival contour and stippling. **D,** One month after treatment, palatal view.

SCIENCE TRANSFER

Several acute conditions that occur in the oral cavity present with more intense symptoms than generally encountered with periodontal disease. The symptoms can involve extremely painful gingivae, lymphadenopathy, fever, and general malaise. These conditions clearly demonstrate an exaggerated host response to the periodontal infection. Adding to the enigma of these conditions is that some are confined to the gingiva, whereas others involve periodontal tissues. The affected host mechanisms that permit such a reaction are unknown, but one apparent underlying factor is stress. The stress may result from lack of rest or high anxiety and may be combined with poor oral hygiene and smoking. These mechanisms emphasize the multifactorial nature of these acute conditions and the lack of understanding regarding their pathogenesis. In all cases, however, a bacterial or viral etiology is the basis for stimulating the host response, and mechanical and antimicrobial or antiviral therapies are usually highly effective.

Clinicians should be able to diagnose correctly the differences between acute necrotizing ulcerative gingivitis and acute herpetic gingivostomatitis in the early stages, because each has specific treatment needs. Of particular importance is the possibility of transmission of herpetic lesions to other people and the need to consider immunocompromised conditions as part of the etiologic background for acute gingival disease. Acute herpetic gingival lesions may result from periodontal treatment (e.g., flap surgery, root planing) in patients who harbor the herpesvirus after an initial infection.

when vesicles are present (highest viral titer). All individuals exposed to an infected patient should take precautions. Herpetic infection of a clinician's finger, referred to as *herpetic whitlow,* can occur if a seronegative clinician becomes infected with a patient's herpetic lesions.[9,10]

REFERENCES

1. Amir J, Harel L, Smetana Z, Varsano I: Treatment of herpes simplex gingivostomatitis with acyclovir in children: a randomised double-blind placebo-controlled study, *BMJ* 314:1800, 1997.
2. Ash MM Jr, Costich ER, Hayward JR: A study of periodontal hazards of third molars, *J Periodontol* 33:209, 1962.
3. Burket LW: *Oral medicine,* ed 3, Philadelphia, 1946, Lippincott.
4. Glickman I, Johannessen LB: The effect of a six percent solution of chromic acid on the gingiva of the albino rat: a correlated gross, biomicroscopic, and histologic study, *J Am Dent Assoc* 41:674, 1950.
5. King JD: Nutritional and other factors in "trench mouth" with special reference to the nicotinic acid component of the vitamin B_2 complex, *Br Dent J* 74:113, 1943.
6. Langlais RP, Miller CS: *Color atlas of common oral diseases,* ed 2, New York, 1998, Williams & Wilkins.
7. Linghorne WJ, McIntosh WG, Tice JW, et al: The relation of ascorbic acid intake to gingivitis, *J Can Dent Assoc* 12:49, 1946.
8. Mitchell DF, Baker BR: Topical antibiotic control of necrotizing gingivitis, *J Periodontol* 39:81, 1968.
9. Regezi JA, Sciubba JJ: *Oral pathology: clinical-pathologic correlations,* Philadelphia, 1989, Saunders.
10. Snyder ML, Church DH, Rickles NH: Primary herpes infection of right second finger, *Oral Surg* 27:598, 1969.
11. Wade AB, Blake G, Mirza K: Effectiveness of metronidazole in treating the acute phase of ulcerative gingivitis, *Dent Pract* 16:440, 1966.
12. Wade AB, Blake GC, Manson JD, et al: Treatment of the acute phase of ulcerative gingivitis (Vincent's type), *Br Dent J* 115:372, 1963.
13. Williamson RT: Diagnosis and management of recurrent herpes simplex induced by fixed prosthodontic tissue management: a clinical report, *J Prosthet Dent* 82:1, 1999.

Treatment of Periodontal Abscess

Philip R. Melnick and Henry H. Takei

48

CHAPTER

CHAPTER OUTLINE

CLASSIFICATION OF ABSCESSES

The periodontal abscess is a localized purulent inflammation of the periodontal tissues.[6] It has been classified into three diagnostic groups: gingival abscess, periodontal abscess, and pericoronal abscess. The *gingival abscess* involves the marginal gingival and interdental tissues. The *periodontal abscess* is an infection located contiguous to the periodontal pocket and may result in destruction of the periodontal ligament and alveolar bone. The *pericoronal abscess* is associated with the crown of a partially erupted tooth.[22]

Periodontal Abscess

The periodontal abscess is typically found in patients with untreated periodontitis and in association with moderate to deep periodontal pockets.[5,25] Periodontal abscesses often arise as an acute exacerbation of a preexisting pocket[6] (Figure 48-1). Primarily related to incomplete calculus removal, periodontal abscesses have been linked to a number of clinical situations.[8,15,16,24] They have been identified in patients after periodontal surgery,[12] after preventive maintenance (Figure 48-2),[7,10,17,21] after systemic antibiotic therapy,[26] and as the result of recurrent disease.[15,16] Conditions in which periodontal abscess is not related to inflammatory periodontal disease include tooth perforation or fracture[2,24] (Figure 48-3) and foreign body impaction.[1,23] Poorly controlled diabetes mellitus has been considered a predisposing factor for periodontal abscess formation[22] (Figure 48-4). Formation of periodontal abscess has been reported as a major cause of tooth loss.[12-21] However, with proper treatment followed by consistent preventive periodontal maintenance, teeth with significant bone loss may be retained for many years[7] (see Figure 48-10).

Gingival Abscess

The gingival abscess is a localized, acute inflammatory lesion that may arise from a variety of sources, including microbial plaque infection, trauma, and foreign body impaction.[22] Clinical features include a red, smooth, sometimes painful, often fluctuant swelling (Figure 48-5).

Periocoronal Abscess

The pericoronal abscess results from inflammation of the soft tissue operculum, which covers a partially erupted tooth. This situation is most often observed around the mandibular third molars. As with the gingival abscess, the inflammatory lesion may be caused by the retention of microbial plaque, food impaction, or trauma.

SCIENCE TRANSFER

An abscess can occur in the periodontal tissues, the gingiva, or the periocoronal tissues and can be acute or chronic. Different etiologies can account for abscess formation, and in most cases the offending agent or condition is easily identified. Purulence is often observed, indicating an aggressive white blood cell reaction. Severe inflammation is also usually present, indicating localized engorgement of the blood vessels. Thus, although occurring in a predictable sequence, the host inflammatory response is accentuated in a very localized area. This reaction therefore may represent an effective host reaction to a defined etiologic agent or event (e.g., food impaction, fractured tooth). Treatment usually involves dramatic improvement in the tissues and rapid resolution of the abscess.

The differential diagnosis of a periodontal abscess must include periapical abscesses. Therefore, all patients with an abscess should have a radiograph taken of the region, together with a complete history and clinical examination that includes pocket measurements and tooth vitality tests. Periodontal abscesses need to be treated with drainage, usually obtained by curettage of the pocket or by incision through gingival tissue. In cases of cellulitis, fever, lymphadenopathy, or inability to provide drainage, as well as in immunocompromised patients, systemic antibiotics are needed.

Diabetic patients have an increased propensity for periodontal abscesses, and this should be considered if episodes recur. Acute periodontal abscesses can often be treated successfully with a complete restoration of periodontal health. Some patients, however, will require additional therapy after resolution of the acute phase.

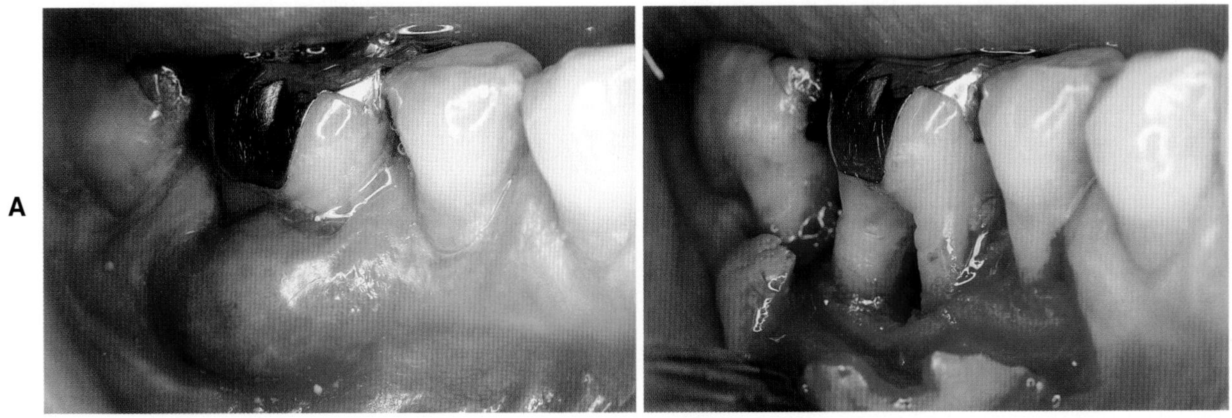

Figure 48-1 **A,** Deep furcation invasions are a common location for the periodontal abscess. **B,** Furcation anatomy often prevents the definitive removal of calculus and microbial plaque.

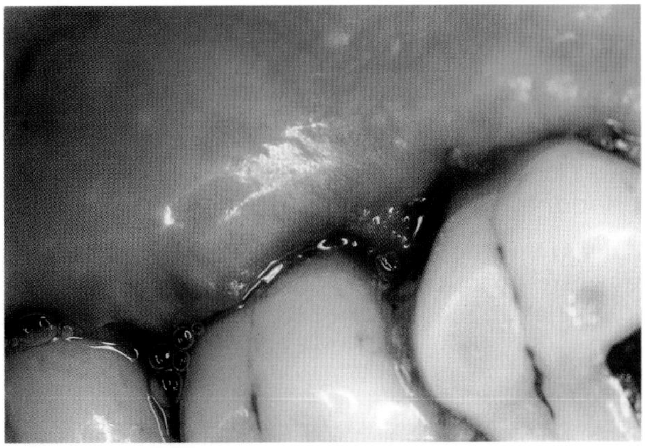

Figure 48-2 Postprophylaxis periodontal abscess resulting from partial healing of a periodontal pocket over residual calculus.

Acute versus Chronic Abscess

Abscesses are categorized as acute or chronic. The *acute abscess* is often an exacerbation of a chronic inflammatory periodontal lesion. Influencing factors include increased number and virulence of bacteria present, combined with lowered tissue resistance and lack of spontaneous drainage.[11,25] The drainage may have been prevented by a deep, tortuous pocket morphology, debris, or closely adapted pocket epithelium blocking the pocket orifice. Acute abscesses are characterized by painful, red, edematous, smooth, ovoid swelling of the gingival tissues.[15,16,25] Exudate may be expressed with gentle pressure; the tooth may be percussion sensitive and feel elevated in the socket (Figure 48-6). Fever and regional lymphadenopathy are occasional findings.[22]

The *chronic abscess* forms after the spreading infection has been controlled by spontaneous drainage, host

A
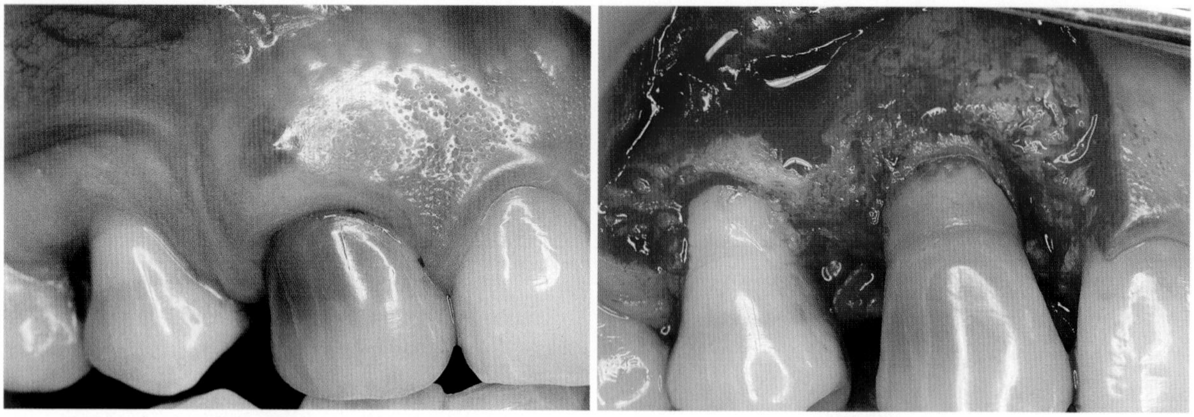
B

Figure 48-3 **A,** Fistula is observed in attached gingiva of maxillary right canine. **B,** Elevated flap shows the cause to be a root fracture.

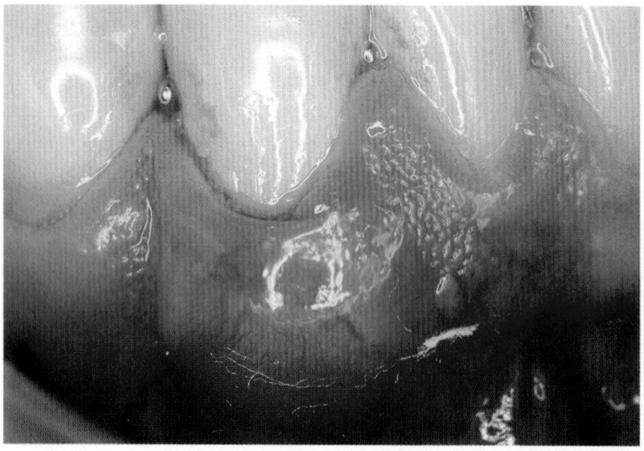

Figure 48-4 Localized periodontal abscess of mandibular right canine of male adult with poorly controlled type 2 diabetes mellitus. For some patients, periodontal abscess formation may be the first sign of the disease.

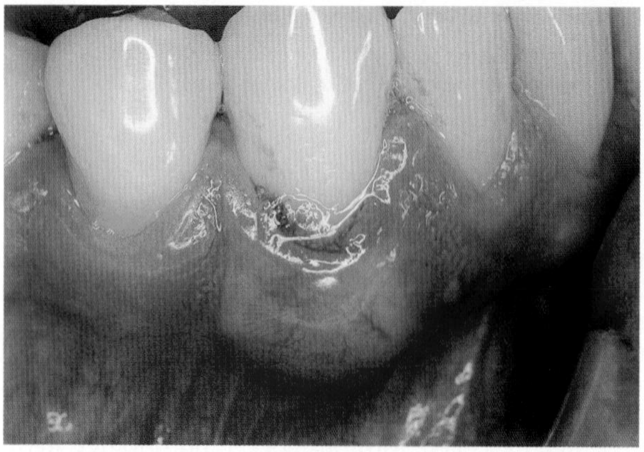

Figure 48-5 Plaque-associated gingival abscess of mandibular right canine.

response, or therapy. Once homeostasis between the host and infection has been reached, the patient may have few or no symptoms.[9] However, dull pain may be associated with the clinical findings of a periodontal pocket, inflammation, and a fistulous tract.[22]

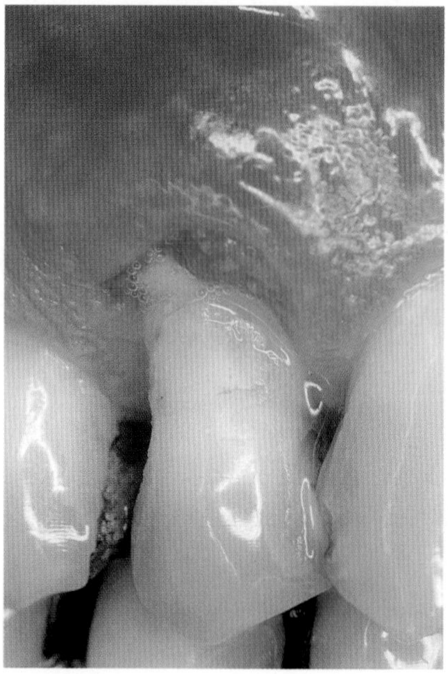

Figure 48-6 Patient presenting with acute abscess complained of dull pain and a sensation of tooth elevation in the socket. Signs of tissue distention and exudation are evident.

Box 48-1 compares the signs and symptoms of the acute and chronic abscess.

Periodontal versus Pulpal Abscess

To determine the cause of an abscess and thus establish a proper treatment plan, it is often necessary to perform a differential diagnosis between a periodontal and pulpal abscess[4] (Box 48-2). (See Figures 48-6 to 48-8.)

SPECIFIC TREATMENT APPROACHES

Treatment of the periodontal abscess includes two phases: resolving the acute lesion, followed by the management of the resulting chronic condition[24] (Box 48-3).

BOX 48-1

Signs and Symptoms of Periodontal Abscess

Acute Abscess

Mild to severe discomfort
Localized red, ovoid swelling
Periodontal pocket
Mobility
Tooth elevation in socket
Tenderness to percussion or biting
Exudation
Elevated temperature*
Regional lymphadenopathy*

Chronic Abscess

No pain or dull pain
Localized inflammatory lesion
Slight tooth elevation
Intermittent exudation
Fistulous tract often associated with a deep pocket
Usually without systemic involvement

Data from Dahlen G: *Periodontol 2000* 28:206, 2002; Meng HX: *Ann Periodontol* 4:79, 1999; and Sanz M, Herrera D, van Winkelhoff AJ: The periodontal abscess. In *Clinical periodontology,* Copenhagen, 2000, Munksgaard.
*May indicate the need for systemic antibiotics.

BOX 48-2

Differential Diagnosis of Periodontal and Pulpal Abscess

Periodontal Abscess

Associated with preexisting periodontal pocket.
Radiographs show periodontal angular bone loss and furcation radiolucency.
Tests show vital pulp.
Swelling usually includes gingival tissue, with occasional fistula.
Pain usually dull and localized.
Sensitivity to percussion may or may not be present.

Pulpal Abscess

Offending tooth may have large restoration.
May have no periodontal pocket, or if present, probes as a narrow defect.
Tests show nonvital pulp.
Swelling often localized to apex, with a fistulous tract.
Pain often severe and difficult to localize.
Sensitivity to percussion.

Modified from Corbet EF: *Periodontol 2000* 34:204, 2004.

A

B

C

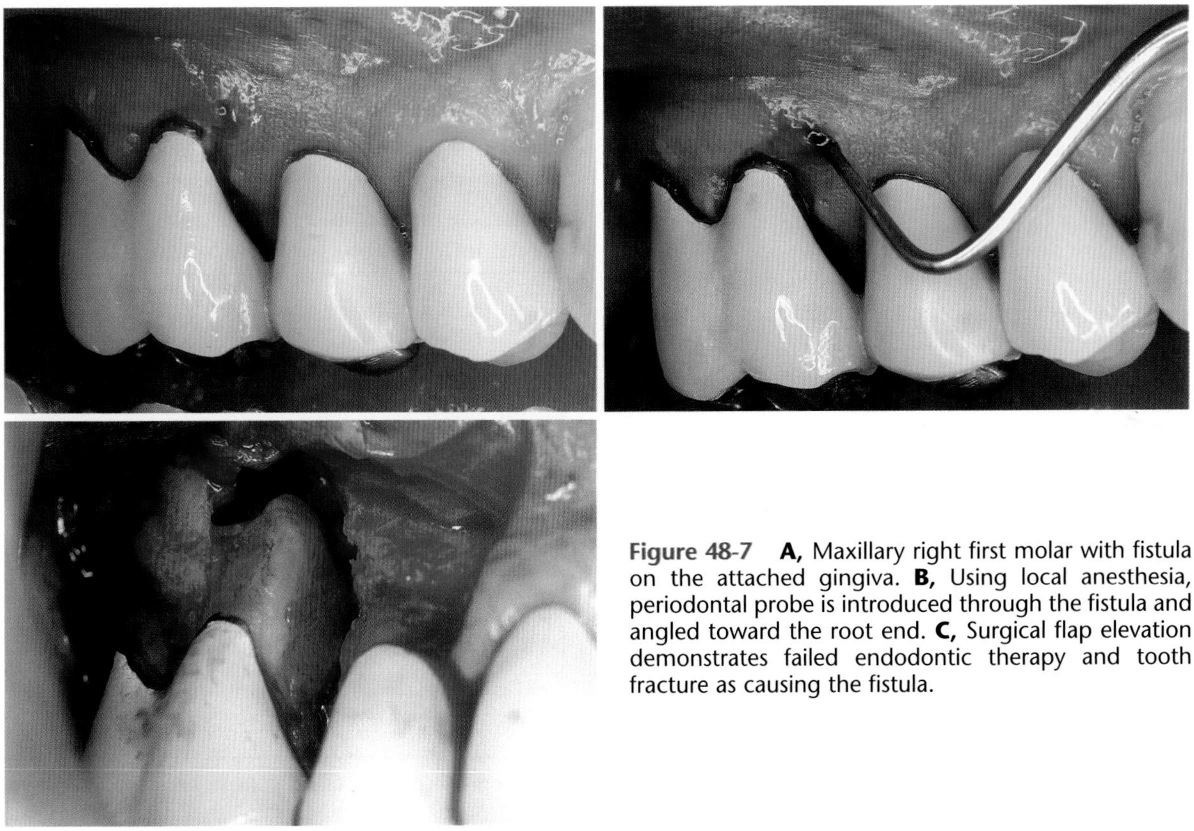

Figure 48-7 **A,** Maxillary right first molar with fistula on the attached gingiva. **B,** Using local anesthesia, periodontal probe is introduced through the fistula and angled toward the root end. **C,** Surgical flap elevation demonstrates failed endodontic therapy and tooth fracture as causing the fistula.

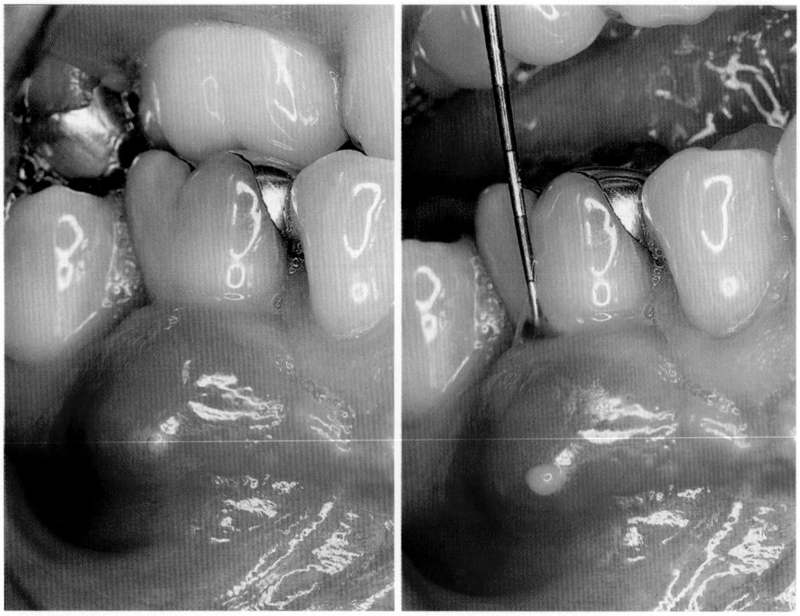

Figure 48-8 **A,** Periodontal abscess of maxillary left first molar. **B,** Periodontal probe is used to retract the pocket wall gently.

BOX 48-3

Treatment Options for Periodontal Abscess

1. Drainage through pocket retraction or incision
2. Scaling and root planing
3. Periodontal surgery
4. Systemic antibiotics
5. Tooth removal

Modified from Sanz M, Herrera D, van Winkelhoff AJ: The periodontal abscess. In *Clinical periodontology,* Copenhagen, 2000, Munksgaard.

BOX 48-4

Indications for Antibiotic Therapy in Patients with Acute Abscess

1. Cellulitis (nonlocalized, spreading infection)
2. Deep, inaccessible pocket
3. Fever
4. Regional lymphadenopathy
5. Immunocompromised patient

Acute Abscess

The acute abscess is treated to alleviate symptoms, control the spread of infection, and establish drainage.[19] Before treatment, the patient's medical history, dental history, and systemic condition are reviewed and evaluated to assist in the diagnosis and to determine the need for systemic antibiotics (Boxes 48-4 and 48-5).

Drainage through Periodontal Pocket. The peripheral area around the abscess is anesthetized with sufficient topical and local anesthetic to ensure comfort. The pocket wall is gently retracted with a periodontal probe or curette in an attempt to initiate drainage through the pocket entrance (see Figure 48-8). Gentle digital pressure and irrigation may be used to express exudates and clear the pocket (Figure 48-9). If the lesion is small and access uncomplicated, debridement in the form of scaling and root planing may be undertaken. If the lesion is large and drainage cannot be established, root debridement by scaling and root planing or surgical

BOX 48-5

Antibiotic Options for Periodontal Infections

Antibiotic of Choice
Amoxicillin, 500 mg

- 1.0-g loading dose, then 500 mg three times a day for 3 days
- Reevaluation after 3 days to determine need for continued or adjusted antibiotic therapy

Penicillin Allergy
Clindamycin

- 600-mg loading dose, then 300 mg four times a day for 3 days

Azithromycin (or clarithromycin)
- 1.0-g loading dose, then 500 mg four times a day for 3 days

Data from American Academy of Periodontology: *J Periodontol* 67:1553, 2004.

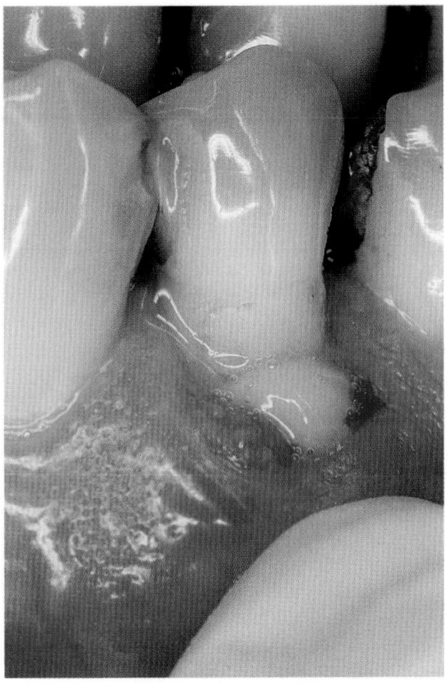

Figure 48-9 Gentle digital pressure may be sufficient to express purulent discharge.

access should be delayed until the major clinical signs have abated.[18] In these patients, use of adjunctive systemic antibiotics[13-16] with short-term high-dose regimens is recommended[20] (see Box 48-5). Antibiotic therapy alone without subsequent drainage and subgingival scaling is contraindicated.[14]

Drainage through External Incision. The abscess is dried and isolated with gauze sponges. Topical anesthetic is applied, followed by local anesthetic injected peripheral to the lesion. A vertical incision through the most fluctuant center of the abscess is made with a #15 surgical blade. The tissue lateral to the incision can be separated with a curette or periosteal elevator. Fluctuant matter is expressed and the wound edges approximated under light digital pressure with a moist gauze pad.

In abscesses presenting with severe swelling and inflammation, aggressive mechanical instrumentation should be delayed in favor of antibiotic therapy so as to avoid damage to healthy contiguous periodontal tissues.[24]

Once bleeding and suppuration have ceased, the patient may be dismissed. For those who do not need systemic antibiotics, posttreatment instructions include frequent rinsing with warm salt water (1 tbsp/8-oz. glass) and periodic application of chlorhexidine gluconate either by rinsing or locally with a cotton-tipped applicator. Reduced exertion and increased fluid intake are often recommended for patients showing systemic involvement. Analgesics may be prescribed for comfort. By the following day, the signs and symptoms have usually subsided. If not, the patient is instructed to continue the previously recommended regimen for an additional 24 hours. This often results in satisfactory healing, and the lesion can be treated as a chronic abscess.[25]

Chronic Abscess

As with a periodontal pocket, the chronic abscess is usually treated with scaling and root planing or surgical therapy. Surgical treatment is suggested when deep vertical or furcation defects are encountered that are beyond the therapeutic capabilities of nonsurgical instrumentation (Figure 48-10). The patient should be advised of the possible postoperative sequelae usually associated with periodontal nonsurgical and surgical procedures. As with the acute abscess, antibiotic therapy may be indicated.[25]

Gingival Abscess

Treatment of the gingival abscess is aimed at reversal of the acute phase and, when applicable, immediate removal of the cause. To ensure procedural comfort, topical or local anesthesia by infiltration is administered. When possible, scaling and root planing are completed to establish drainage and remove microbial deposits. In more acute situations the fluctuant area is incised with a #15 scalpel blade, and exudate may be expressed by gentle digital pressure. Any foreign material (e.g., dental floss, impression material) is removed. The area is irrigated with warm water and covered with moist gauze under light pressure.

Once bleeding has stopped, the patient is dismissed with instructions to rinse with warm salt water every 2 hours for the remainder of the day. After 24 hours the area is reassessed, and if resolution is sufficient, scaling not previously completed is undertaken. If the residual lesion is large or poorly accessible, surgical access may be required.

Pericoronal Abscess

As with the other abscesses of the periodontium, the treatment of the pericoronal abscess is aimed at management of the acute phase, followed by resolution of the chronic condition. The acute pericoronal abscess is properly anesthetized for comfort, and drainage is established by gently lifting the soft tissue operculum with a periodontal probe or curette. If the underlying debris is easily accessible, it may be removed, followed by gentle irrigation with sterile saline. If there is regional swelling, lymphadenopathy, or systemic signs, systemic antibiotics may be prescribed.

The patient is dismissed with instructions to rinse with warm salt water every 2 hours, and the area is reassessed after 24 hours. If discomfort was one of the original complaints, appropriate analgesics should be employed. Once the acute phase has been controlled, the partially erupted tooth may be definitively treated with either surgical excision of the overlying tissue or removal of the offending tooth.

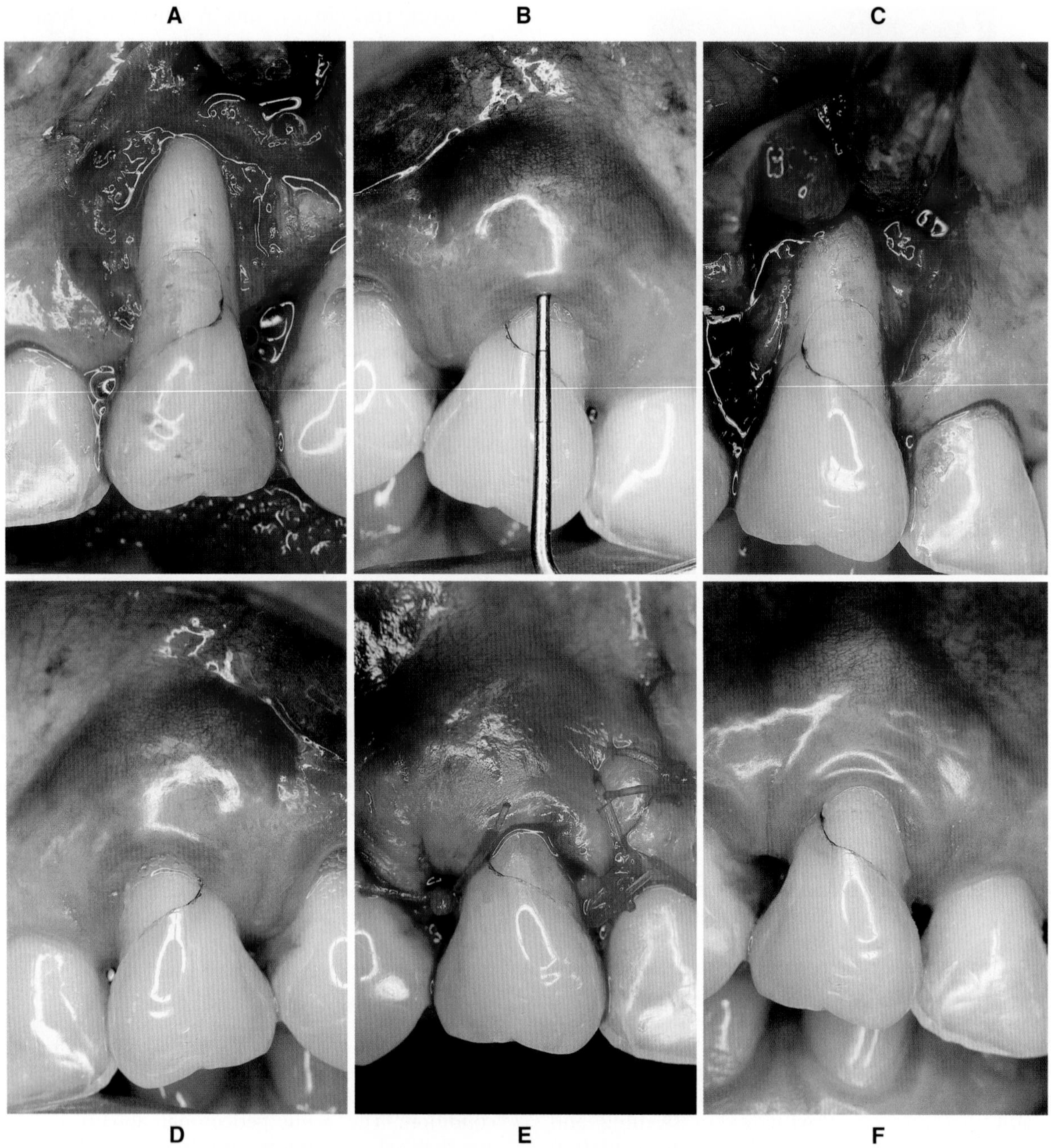

Figure 48-10 **A,** Chronic periodontal abscess of maxillary right canine. **B,** Using local anesthesia, periodontal probe is inserted to determine severity of the lesion. **C,** Using mesial and distal vertical incisions, a full-thickness flap is elevated, exposing severe bone dehiscence, a subgingival restoration, and root calculus. **D,** Root surface has been planed free of calculus and the restoration smoothed. **E,** Full-thickness flap has been replaced to its original position and sutured with absorbable sutures. **F,** At 3 months, gingival tissues are pink, firm, and well adapted to the tooth, with minimal periodontal probing depth.

REFERENCES

1. Abrams H, Kopczyk R: Gingival sequela from a retained piece of dental floss, *J Am Dent Assoc* 106:57, 1983.
2. Abrams H, Cunningham C, Lee S: Periodontal changes following coronal/root perforation and formocresol pulpotomy, *J Endod* 18:399, 1992.
3. American Academy of Periodontology: Position paper: Systemic antibiotics in periodontics, *J Periodontol* 67:1553, 2004.
4. Ammons WF Jr, Harrington GW: The periodontic-endodontic continuum. In Newman MG, Takei HH, Carranza FA, editors: *Carranza's clinical periodontology,* ed 9, Philadelphia, 2002, Saunders.
5. Becker W, Berg L, Becker B: The long-term evaluation of periodontal treatment and maintenance in 95 patients, *Int J Periodont Restor Dent* 2:55, 1984.
6. Carranza FA, Camargo PM: The periodontal pocket. In Newman MG, Takei HH, Carranza FA, editors: *Carranza's clinical periodontology,* ed 9, Philadelphia, 2002, Saunders.
7. Chace R, Low SB: Survival characteristics of periodontally involved teeth: a 40-year study, *J Periodontol* 64:701, 1993.
8. Corbet EF: Diagnosis of acute periodontal lesions, *Periodontol 2000* 34:204, 2004.
9. Dahlen G: Microbiology and treatment of dental abscesses and periodontal-endodontic lesions, *Periodontol 2000* 28:206, 2002.
10. Dello Russo NM: The post-prophylaxis periodontal abscess: etiology and treatment, *Int J Periodont Restor Dent* 5:29, 1985.
11. Epstein S, Scopp IW: Antibiotics and the intraoral abscess, *J Periodontol* 48:236, 1977.
12. Garrett S, Polson A, Stoller N, et al: Comparison of a bioabsorbable GTR barrier to a non-absorbable barrier in treating human class II furcation defects: a multi-center parallel design randomized single-blind study, *J Periodontol* 668:667, 1997.
13. Genco RJ: Using antimicrobials agents to manage periodontal diseases, *J Am Dent Assoc* 122:31, 1991.
14. Hafstrom CA, Wikstrom MB, Renvert SN, Dahlen GG: Effect of treatment on some periodontopathogens and their antibody levels in periodontal abscesses, *J Periodontol* 65:1022, 1994.
15. Herrera D, Roldan S, Sanz M: The periodontal abscess: a review, *J Clin Periodontol* 27:377, 2000.
16. Herrera D, Roldan S, Gonzalez I, Sanz M: The periodontal abscess. I. Clinical and microbiology findings, *J Clin Periodontol* 27:287, 2000.
17. Kaldahl WB, Kalwarf KL, Patil KD, et al: Long-term evaluation of periodontal therapy. I. Response to 4 therapeutic modalities, *J Periodontol* 67:93, 1996.
18. Lewis MA, MacFarlane TW: Short-course high dosage amoxicillin in the treatment of acute dento-alveolar abscess, *Br Dent J* 161:299, 1986.
19. Manson JD: *Periodontics,* ed 3, Philadelphia, 1975, Lea & Febiger.
20. Martin MV, Longman LP, Hill JB, Hardy P: Acute dentoalveolar infections: an investigation of the duration of antibiotic therapy, *Br Dent J* 183:135, 1997.
21. McLeod DE, Lainson PA, Spivey JD: Tooth loss due to periodontal abscess: a retrospective study, *J Periodontol* 68:963, 1997.
22. Meng HX: Periodontal abscess, *Ann Periodontol* 4:79, 1999.
23. O'Leary TJ, Standish SM, Bloomer RS: Severe periodontal destruction following impression procedures, *J Periodontol* 44:43, 1973.
24. Sanz M, Herrera D, van Winkelhoff AJ: The periodontal abscess. In *Clinical periodontology,* Copenhagen, 2000, Munksgaard.
25. Takei HH: Treatment of the periodontal abscess. In Newman MG, Takei HH, Carranza FA, editors: *Carranza's clinical periodontology,* ed 9, Philadelphia, 2002, Saunders.
26. Topoll H, Lange D, Muller R: Multiple periodontal abscesses after systemic antibiotic therapy, *J Clin Periodontol* 17:268, 1990.

Phase I Periodontal Therapy

49

CHAPTER

Dorothy A. Perry, Max O. Schmid, and Henry H. Takei

■ ■ ■

CHAPTER OUTLINE

RATIONALE
TREATMENT SESSIONS
SEQUENCE OF PROCEDURES

RESULTS
HEALING
DECISION TO REFER FOR SPECIALIST TREATMENT

*P*hase I therapy is the first step in the chronologic sequence of procedures that constitute periodontal treatment. The objective of Phase I therapy is to alter or eliminate the microbial etiology and contributing factors for gingival and periodontal diseases. The result is halting the progression of disease and returning the dentition to a state of health and comfort.[1] Phase I therapy is referred to by a number of names, including *initial therapy,*[1] *nonsurgical periodontal therapy,*[10] *cause-related therapy,*[6] and the *etiotropic phase of therapy.*[13] All terms refer to the procedures performed to treat gingival and periodontal infections, up to and including tissue reevaluation.

RATIONALE

Reduction and elimination of etiologic and contributing factors in periodontal treatment are achieved by complete removal of calculus, correction of defective restorations, treatment of carious lesions, and institution of a comprehensive daily plaque control regimen.[3-5,7,12] This initial phase of therapy is provided to all patients with periodontal pockets who later will be evaluated for surgical intervention as well as those with gingivitis or

mild chronic periodontitis who are unlikely to need surgical treatment. The procedures included in Phase I therapy may be the only procedures required to solve the patient's periodontal problems, or they may constitute the preparatory phase for surgical therapy. Figures 49-1 and 49-2 (see also Figure 51-82) show the results of Phase I therapy in two patients with periodontal disease.

Phase I therapy is a critical aspect of periodontal treatment. Data from clinical research indicate that the long-term success of periodontal treatment depends predominantly on maintaining the results achieved with Phase I therapy and much less on any specific surgical procedures. In addition, Phase I therapy provides an opportunity for the dentist to evaluate tissue response and the patient's attitude toward periodontal care, both of which are crucial to the overall success of treatment.

Based on the knowledge that microbial plaque harbors the primary pathogens of gingival inflammation, the specific aim of Phase I therapy for every patient is *effective plaque control*. Plaque control is the key objective of every therapeutic periodontal procedure, but it can be effectively accomplished only if the tooth surfaces are free of rough deposits and irregular contours so that they are readily accessible to oral hygiene aids. Control or

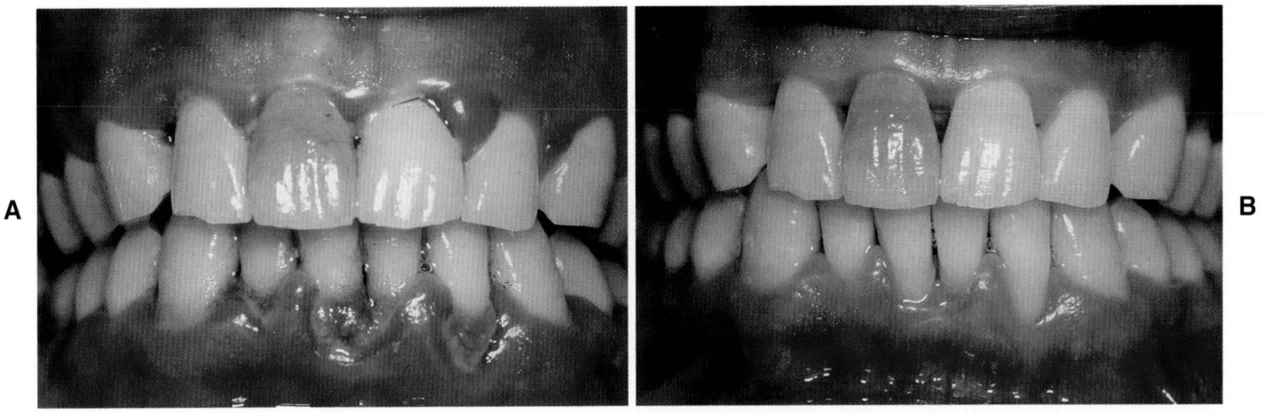

Figure 49-1 Results of Phase I therapy, severe chronic periodontitis. **A,** Patient with deep pockets, bone loss, and severe swelling and redness. **B,** Healing results 3 weeks after elimination of irritants. Tissue has returned to a more normal contour, with redness and swelling dramatically reduced.

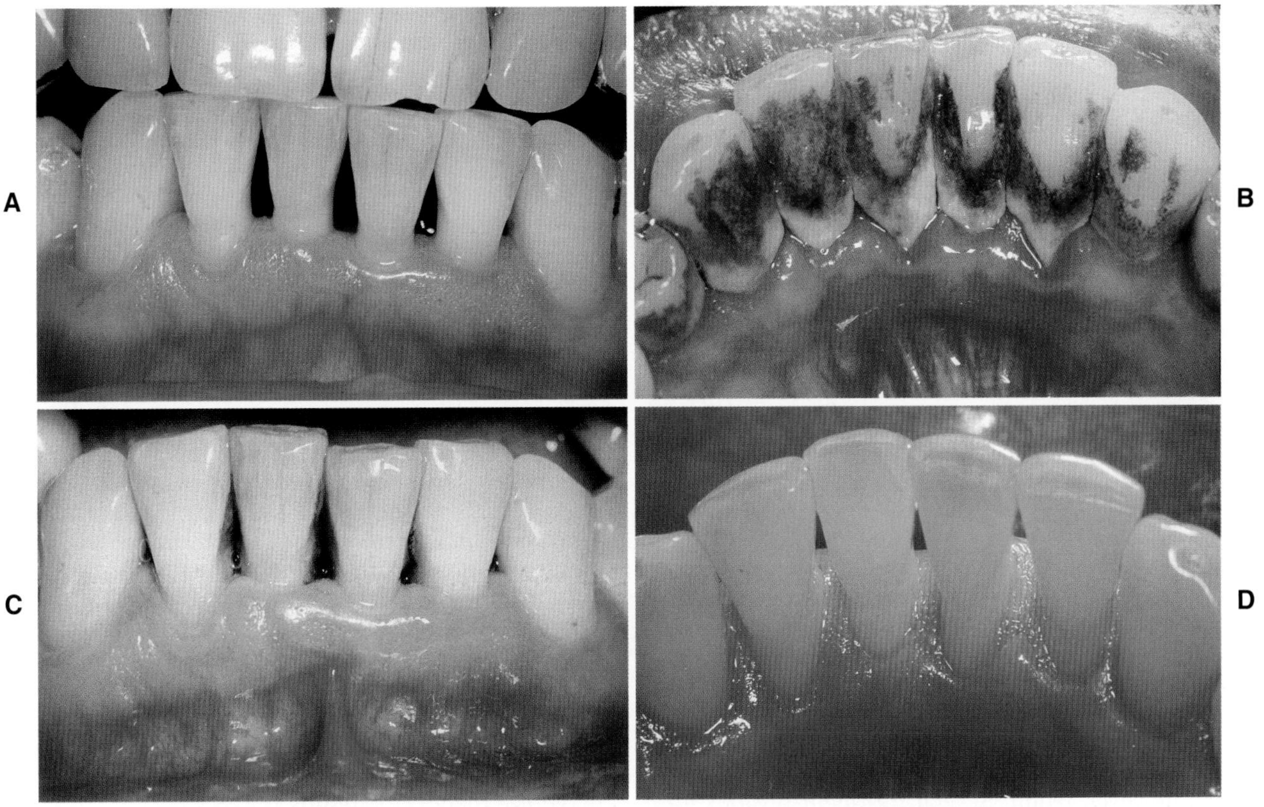

Figure 49-2 Results of Phase I therapy, moderate chronic periodontitis. **A,** Patient with moderate attachment loss, pockets in the 4-mm to 6-mm range. Note that the gingival appears pink because it is fibrotic, and the inflammation is deep in the periodontal pockets. **B,** Lingual view with more visible inflammation and heavy calculus deposits. **C** and **D,** Same areas with significant improvement in gingival health 18 months after scaling, root planing, and plaque control instruction. Patient returned for regular maintenance visits.

elimination of contributing local factors includes the following therapies, as required:

1. Complete removal of calculus (Chapters 51, 54, and 55)
2. Correction or replacement of poorly fitting restorations and prosthetic devices (Chapter 72)
3. Restoration of carious lesions
4. Orthodontic tooth movement (Chapter 57)
5. Treatment of food impaction areas
6. Treatment of occlusal trauma (Chapter 56)
7. Extraction of hopeless teeth

The control of inflammation and pocket reduction by mechanical means may need to be complemented by

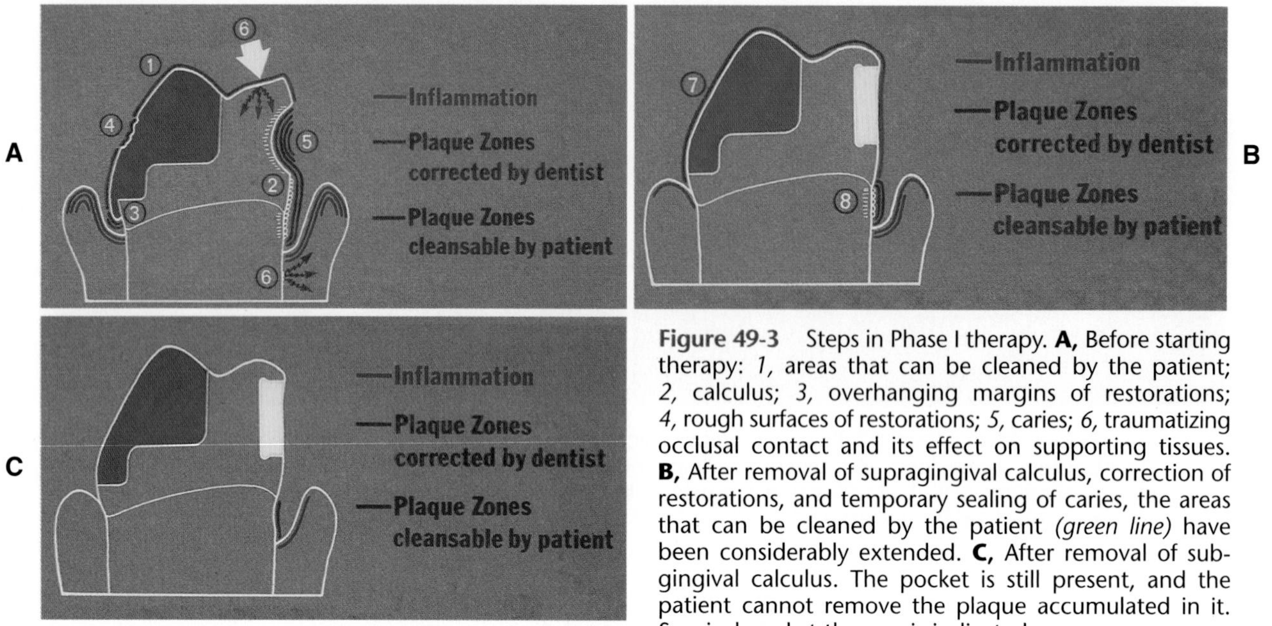

Figure 49-3 Steps in Phase I therapy. **A,** Before starting therapy: *1,* areas that can be cleaned by the patient; *2,* calculus; *3,* overhanging margins of restorations; *4,* rough surfaces of restorations; *5,* caries; *6,* traumatizing occlusal contact and its effect on supporting tissues. **B,** After removal of supragingival calculus, correction of restorations, and temporary sealing of caries, the areas that can be cleaned by the patient *(green line)* have been considerably extended. **C,** After removal of subgingival calculus. The pocket is still present, and the patient cannot remove the plaque accumulated in it. Surgical pocket therapy is indicated.

the appropriate use of antimicrobial agents and devices, including necessary plaque sampling and antibiotic-sensitivity testing (see Chapter 52).

Figure 49-3, *A* and *B,* shows how Phase I therapy extends the area of the tooth that can be cleaned by the patient and reduces or eliminates the inflammatory response. Figure 49-3, *C,* depicts the indication for further therapy when the patient cannot clean plaque out of a pocket.

TREATMENT SESSIONS

After careful analysis of the case and diagnosis of the specific periodontal condition present, the dentist determines the treatment plan for the scaling and root-planing portion of Phase I therapy. This is an estimate of the procedures and number of appointments needed to complete the initial phase of therapy after carious lesions are controlled and inadequate restorations corrected. Patients with small amounts of calculus and relatively healthy tissues can be treated in one appointment. Most patients, however, require several treatment sessions for the dentist to perform a complete debridement of tooth surfaces.

In addition to the amount of calculus visualized, the following conditions must also be considered to plan the Phase I treatment sessions needed[10]:

- General health and tolerance of treatment
- Number of teeth present
- Amount of subgingival calculus
- Probing pocket depths and attachment loss
- Furcation involvements
- Alignment of teeth
- Margins of restorations
- Developmental anomalies
- Physical barriers to access (i.e., limited opening or tendency to gag)
- Patient cooperation and sensitivity (requiring use of anesthesia or analgesia)

The dentist should estimate the number of appointments needed on the basis of the conditions presented by each patient. Also, consideration should be given to the control of infectious organisms during the period of active Phase I treatment. One proposed option consists of scheduling one long appointment or two appointments on consecutive days while the patient is receiving an aggressive prescribed regimen of antimicrobial agents, then scheduling follow-up appointments during healing. This treatment sequence has been referred to as "anti-infective" or "disinfection" treatment.[8,11] Data from these studies indicated that improvements in probing depths and reduction of periodontal pathogens were somewhat greater for the group using antimicrobial adjuncts. As our understanding of the best use of antimicrobial agents increases, treatment plans undoubtedly will evolve to maximize therapeutic results.

SEQUENCE OF PROCEDURES

Step 1: Limited Plaque Control Instruction. This should start in the first treatment appointment and should include only the correct use of the toothbrush on all smooth and regular surfaces of the teeth. The use of dental floss should await the removal of calculus and overhanging restorations.

Step 2. Supragingival Removal of Calculus. This step can be done with scalers, curettes, or ultrasonic instrumentation (see Chapters 51 and 54).

Step 3. Recontouring Defective Restorations and Crowns. This step may require replacing the entire restoration or crown or correcting it with finishing burs or diamond-coated files mounted on a special handpiece. For overhangs located subgingivally, this step may require reflection of a miniflap to facilitate access.

Step 4. Obturation of Carious Lesions. This step involves complete removal of the carious tissue and placement of a final or a temporary restoration. The latter is especially indicated when prognosis of the tooth depends on the result of periodontal therapy. Caries control and treatment of active carious lesions are often-overlooked aspects of Phase I therapy. Caries is now recognized as an infection.[2] As such, carious teeth must be temporized, with removal of the infectious process and improved tooth contours established to maximize the healing achieved during the scaling and root-planing treatment. Frank carious lesions, particularly class V lesions in the cervical areas of teeth and those on root surfaces, provide a reservoir for bacteria and can contribute to the repopulation of the periodontal plaque. The cavities themselves are receptacles where plaque is sheltered from even the most energetic mechanical plaque removal attempts. For these reasons, it is imperative that caries control and at least temporization of carious lesions be completed during Phase I therapy.

Step 5. Comprehensive Plaque Control Instruction. At this stage the patient should learn to remove plaque completely from all supragingival areas, using toothbrush, dental floss, and any other necessary complementary method (see Figure 49-1 and Chapter 50).

Step 6. Subgingival Root Treatment. At this time, complete calculus removal and root planing can be effectively performed and constitute the final step in achieving smooth and regular contours on all tooth surfaces (see Chapter 51).

Step 7. Tissue Reevaluation. The periodontal tissues are reexamined to determine the need for further therapy. Pockets are reprobed, and all related anatomical conditions are carefully evaluated to decide whether surgical treatment is indicated.

Additional improvement through surgery can be expected only if Phase I therapy has been successful. Surgical treatment of periodontal pockets should be attempted only if the patient is exercising effective plaque control and the gingiva is free of overt inflammation.

RESULTS

Phase I therapy involves complex and individualized treatment. It requires detailed analysis of each patient's disease and contributing factors and customized therapy. Treatments common to all Phase I therapy are plaque control, caries control, and scaling and root planing to remove supragingival calculus, subgingival calculus, and plaque deposits. Plaque control performed by the patient at home is complex and requires changing lifelong habits. It is difficult to achieve and varies among patients, but strategies for success exist, as presented in Chapter 50.

Scaling and root-planing therapy has been studied extensively to evaluate its effects on periodontal disease. A review of such studies indicate that the treatment is both effective and reliable.[4] Studies ranging from 1 month to 2 years in length demonstrate up to 80% reduction in bleeding on probing and mean probing depth reduction of 2 to 3 mm. Others have demonstrated that the number of pockets 4 mm in depth or greater was reduced by 52% to 80% (see Figures 49-1 and 49-2).

Additional individual treatments, such as caries control and correction of poorly fitting restorations, only augment the positive results of healing gained through good plaque control and scaling and root planing. Figure 49-4 shows the effects of an overhanging amalgam restoration on the gingiva. Maximal healing from scaling and root planing is not possible when local conditions retain plaque and provide reservoirs for repopulation of periodontal pathogens.

HEALING

Reevaluation of the periodontal case should occur about 4 weeks after completion of the scaling and root-planing procedures. This permits time for both epithelial and connective tissue healing and allows the patient sufficient practice with oral hygiene skills to achieve maximum improvement.

Gingival inflammation is usually substantially reduced or eliminated within 3 to 4 weeks after removal of calculus and local irritants. Healing consists of the formation of a long junctional epithelium rather than new connective tissue attachment to the root surfaces. The attachment epithelium reappears in 1 to 2 weeks. Gradual reductions in inflammatory cell population, crevicular fluid flow, and repair of connective tissue result in decreased clinical signs of inflammation, with less redness and swelling.[4]

Transient root hypersensitivity and recession of the gingival margins frequently accompany the healing process. Patients should be warned of these potential results at the outset of treatment to avoid an unpleasant surprise. These unexpected and uncomfortable consequences may result in distrust and loss of motivation to continue therapy, so patient education is important. (See Chapter 50 for management of tooth hypersensitivity.)

DECISION TO REFER FOR SPECIALIST TREATMENT

The treatment of most periodontal problems is in the hands of the general dentist. However, advanced or complicated cases require specialized treatment. The question remains when to refer a patient for specialist periodontal care. A few patients have disease that is so severe or unusual in presentation that referral to a periodontist is the obvious approach. Many patients are treatable in the general dentist's office and likely to heal sufficiently well after Phase I therapy that no further treatment is required beyond routine maintenance. Any patient who

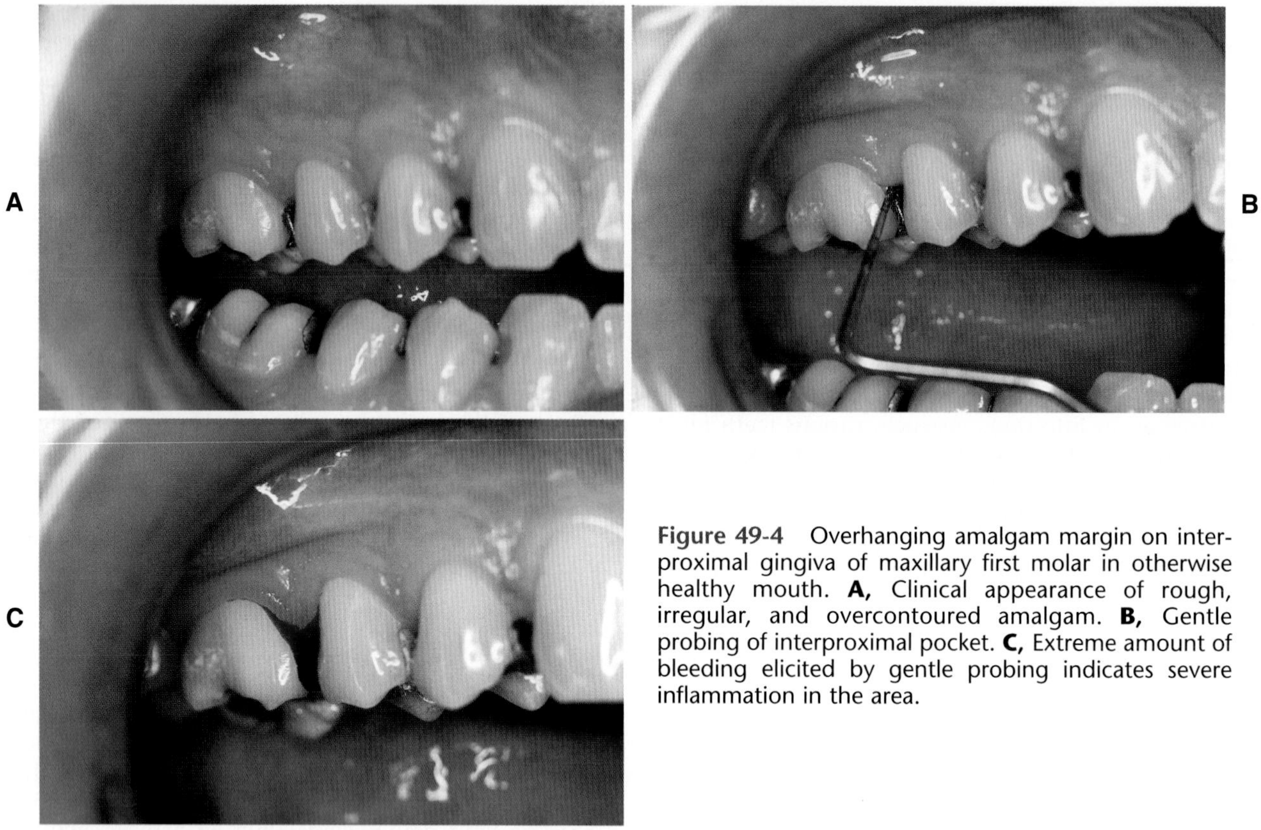

Figure 49-4 Overhanging amalgam margin on interproximal gingiva of maxillary first molar in otherwise healthy mouth. **A,** Clinical appearance of rough, irregular, and overcontoured amalgam. **B,** Gentle probing of interproximal pocket. **C,** Extreme amount of bleeding elicited by gentle probing indicates severe inflammation in the area.

does not clearly fall into either category is called a "candidate for referral."[9]

The *5-mm standard* has been proposed as a guideline for referral. If the patient has loss of attachment (distance between cementoenamel junction and bottom of pocket) of 5 mm or greater at reevaluation, referral should be considered. The 5-mm standard is based on the typical root length being about 13 mm (Figure 49-5). Because the crest of the alveolar bone is about 2 mm apical to the bottom of the pocket, when loss of attachment is 5 mm, only about half the root support remains. Specialist care could help preserve the tooth in these patients by eliminating deep pockets and regenerating support for the tooth.

In addition to the 5-mm standard, the following factors must also be considered in the decision to refer:

1. *Extent of disease,* with generalized or localized involvement. Deep, localized areas of bone loss detected radiographically suggest the need for specialized reconstructive techniques.
2. *Root length.* Short roots are more seriously jeopardized by 5 mm of clinical attachment loss than long roots.
3. *Hypermobility,* which suggests a more guarded prognosis.
4. *Difficulty of scaling and root planing.* The presence of deep pockets and furcations make instrumentation much more difficult.
5. *Restorative work.* Long-term prognosis of the tooth is an important consideration in planning extensive restorative work.

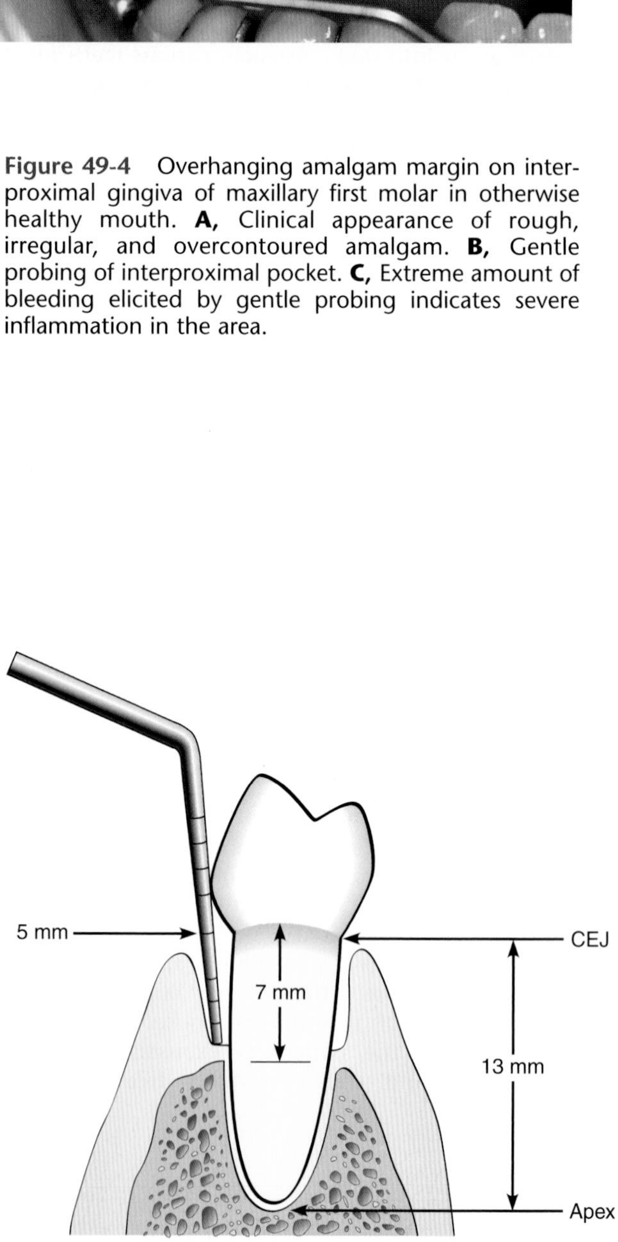

Figure 49-5 The 5-mm standard for referral to a periodontist is based on root length, probing depth, and attachment loss. The standard serves as a reasonable guideline to trigger further analysis of the case and possible need for specialist care. *CEJ,* Cementoenamel junction. (Redrawn from Armitage G, editor: *Periodontal maintenance therapy,* Berkeley, Calif, 1974, Praxis.)

SCIENCE TRANSFER

Phase I care is important for several reasons, *but the ability of the treatment to reduce inflammation is perhaps the most critical reason.* The rationale for this is predominantly twofold. First, most therapy is based on resolving inflammation. Active periodontal disease, as a measure of progressive attachment loss, is difficult to determine at every site and around every tooth; this requires repetitive attachment level measurement to make detection more sensitive over time, which most clinicians do not perform. Second, a lack of bleeding and inflammation is significantly associated with health. However, bleeding and inflammation are not necessarily associated with periodontal disease or its progression.

Thus, Phase I therapy is directed at eliminating inflammation as its major outcome and establishing conditions that are highly correlated with health. In areas where healthy tissue cannot be established, the patient should be referred to a periodontal specialist.

Phase I therapy includes many different procedures with the overall aim of controlling periodontal breakdown and inflammation. Plaque control is central to success, and in some patients with moderate periodontal disease, thorough Phase I therapy will adequately treat their periodontal condition. *A recent suggestion has been to complete root planing visits in 1 or 2 days to control reinfection of treated teeth.*

Phase I therapy is used as a preceding treatment in most patients who require Phase II periodontal surgical therapy because it allows for optimal tissue health and plaque control, which enhance surgical outcomes.

6. *Age of the patient.* The younger the patient with extensive attachment loss, the more aggressive the disease process is likely to be.
7. *Resolution after scaling and planing.* If inflammation persists, further therapy may be necessary.

Treatment of advanced periodontal disease generally is successful in patients with 6-mm to 8-mm probing depths or attachment loss. Specialists have limited success when depths are 9 mm or greater, so early referral of advanced cases is likely to provide the best results.

Each patient is unique, and the decision process for each patient is complex. The considerations presented in this section should provide some guidance in making referral decisions (see Chapter 82).

REFERENCES

1. American Academy of Periodontology, Ad Hoc Committee on the Parameters of Care: Phase I therapy, *J Periodontol* 71(suppl):856, 2000.
2. Anderson MH, Bales DJ, Omnell KA: Modern management of dental caries: the cutting edge is not the dental bur, *J Am Dent Assoc* 124:37, 1993.
3. Axelsson P, Lindhe J: The effect of a preventive programme on dental plaque, gingivitis and caries in school children: results after one and two years, *J Clin Periodontol* 1:126, 1974.
4. Cobb CM: Non-surgical pocket therapy: mechanical, *Ann Periodontol* 1:443, 1996.
5. Lightner LM, O'Leary TJ, Drake RB, et al: Preventive periodontics treatment procedures: results over 46 months, *J Periodontol* 42:555, 1971.
6. Lindhe J: *Textbook of clinical periodontology,* Philadelphia, 1983, Saunders.
7. Lindhe J, Kock G: The effect of supervised oral hygiene on the gingiva of children: progression and inhibition of gingivitis, *J Periodontal Res* 1:260, 1966.
8. Mongardini C, van Steenberghe D, Dekeyser C, et al: One stage full- versus partial-mouth disinfection in the treatment of chronic adult or generalized early-onset periodontitis. I. Long-term clinical observations, *J Periodontol* 70:632, 1999.
9. Parr RW, Pipe P, Watts T: Shall I refer? In Armitage G, editor: *Periodontal maintenance therapy,* ed 2, Berkeley, Calif, 1982, Praxis.
10. Perry DA, Beemsterboer PB, Taggart EJ: Periodontology for the dental hygienist, Philadelphia, 2001, Saunders.
11. Quirynen M, Mongardini C, Pauwels M, et al: One stage full- versus partial-mouth disinfection in the treatment of chronic adult or generalized early-onset periodontitis. II. Long-term impact on microbial load, *J Periodontol* 70:646, 1999.
12. Suomi JD, Greene JC, Vermillion JR, et al: The effect of controlled oral hygiene procedures on the progression of periodontal disease in adults: results after third and final year, *J Periodontol* 42:152, 1971.
13. Wilkins EM: *Clinical practice of the dental hygienist,* Philadelphia, 1989, Lea & Febiger.

Plaque Control for the Periodontal Patient

50

CHAPTER

Dorothy A. Perry

CHAPTER OUTLINE

Plaque control is the regular removal of dental plaque and the prevention of its accumulation on the teeth and adjacent gingival surfaces. Plaque is the major etiology of periodontal diseases and is related to dental caries; therefore, gaining patient cooperation in daily plaque removal is critical to long-term success of all periodontal and dental treatment. The 1998 European Workshop on Mechanical Plaque Control emphasized this view by concluding, "Forty years of experimental research, clinical trials, and demonstration projects in different geographical and social settings have confirmed that effective removal of dental plaque is essential to dental and periodontal health throughout life."[113]

In 1965, Löe et al.[98] conducted the classic study demonstrating the relationship between plaque accumulation and the development of experimental gingivitis in humans. Subjects in the study stopped brushing and other plaque control procedures, resulting in the development of gingivitis in every person within 7 to 21 days. The composition of the plaque bacteria also shifted so that gram-negative organisms predominated in the plaque flora. The study also showed that gingivitis was reversible. Daily removal of dental plaque led to complete resolution of gingival inflammation for all subjects within 1 week.

Good supragingival plaque control has also been shown to affect the growth and composition of subgingival plaque, so that it favors a healthier microflora, and to reduce calculus formation.[128] Carefully performed daily home plaque control, combined with frequent professionally delivered plaque removal, has been demonstrated to reduce supragingival plaque; decrease the total number of microorganisms in moderately deep pockets, including furcation areas; and greatly reduce the number of subgingival sites with *Porphyromonas gingivalis,* a significant periodontal pathogen.[67] Thus, plaque control is an effective way of treating and preventing gingivitis and is a critical part of all the procedures involved in the treatment and prevention of periodontal diseases.[18]

Good plaque control practices are particularly important for periodontal patients because they have active infections or previously treated disease, and they have demonstrated susceptibility to periodontal infections. The role of other risk factors for periodontal infections, such as smoking, genetic predisposition, and systemic disease, also are important but often beyond the control of the clinician. Plaque control and preventive procedures can be relied on to improve periodontal infections; however, the resolution of disease also depends on the type of periodontal infection and the presence of additional risk factors.[49]

The daily use of a toothbrush and other oral hygiene aids is the most dependable way of achieving oral health benefits for all patients. Plaque growth occurs within hours and must be completely removed at least every 48 hours in periodontally healthy subjects to prevent inflammation.[127] Toothbrushing alone is not sufficient to control gingival and periodontal diseases because periodontal lesions are predominantly found in interdental locations.[83] It has been demonstrated in healthy subjects that plaque formation begins on the interproximal surfaces where the toothbrush does not reach. Masses of plaque first develop in the molar and premolar areas, followed by the proximal surfaces of the anterior teeth and the facial surfaces of the molars and premolars. Lingual surfaces accumulate the least amount of plaque. Patients consistently leave more plaque on the posterior teeth than the anterior teeth, with interproximal surfaces retaining the highest amounts of plaque, exactly the places where periodontal infections begin.[127] In addition, periodontal patients often have complex defects in gingival architecture and long, exposed root surfaces to clean, compounding the difficulty of doing a good job.

Plaque control efforts for periodontal patients must focus on improved brushing and cleaning interproximal areas, tasks that require mastering difficult and time-consuming daily oral hygiene habits. Periodontal patients should completely remove plaque from the teeth at least once every 24 hours because of their demonstrated susceptibility to disease. The task is complex and may take up to 30 minutes.[4]

Chemical inhibitors of plaque and calculus that are incorporated in mouthwashes or dentifrices also play important roles in plaque control. Fluorides are essential for caries control. Many products are available as common adjunctive agents to mechanical techniques. These medicaments, as with any drug, should be recommended and prescribed according to the needs of individual patients. Chemical plaque control is a rapidly growing field and will become even more significant for periodontal patients and practices in the future as increasingly effective products become available.

SCIENCE TRANSFER

Periodontal disease is manifested by microbial, plaque-induced inflammation. As such, therapeutic intervention and maintenance therapy are based on plaque removal. Many strategies for plaque removal exist, but the endpoint remains the same: remove as much plaque as possible daily. Although 100% plaque removal is not possible, the tolerance of some inflammation suggests that the host response can effectively handle a degree of inflammation. Under certain conditions that are not evident, however, some periodontal sites undergo tissue destruction and loss. Therefore the patient and therapist must constantly be diligent and persistent in plaque removal. This includes continuing education and motivation using a variety of devices and techniques.

Many manual and powered toothbrushes are available with claims of superiority for a particular design. Many studies have shown that one design is better than another with respect to plaque removal, but the real test is whether this difference results in better periodontal health. The counterrotational oscillatory brush has the best research demonstrating its effectiveness. When measurements of periodontal health are evaluated, only small differences seem to exist among the many toothbrushes. Dental floss of various types and other interdental cleaning instruments also appear to be very similar in their clinical effectiveness.

Chlorhexidine in mouth rinses and triclosan in toothpastes are important agents for plaque reduction and improvements in gingival health. Essential oil mouth rinses may be effective, and almost all other chemical agents for plaque control show wide variation in effectiveness.

Plaque control is one of the key elements of the practice of dentistry. It permits each patient to assume responsibility for his or her own oral health on a daily basis. Without it, optimal oral health through periodontal treatment cannot be attained or preserved. Every patient in every dental practice should be educated about daily plaque control and encouraged to adopt it. Good plaque control facilitates the return to health for patients with gingival and periodontal diseases, prevents tooth decay, and preserves oral health for a lifetime.

THE TOOTHBRUSH

The bristle toothbrush appeared about the year 1600 in China, was first patented in America in 1857, and has undergone little change. Generally, toothbrushes vary in size and design as well as in length, hardness, and arrangement of the bristles[122] (Figure 50-1). Some toothbrush

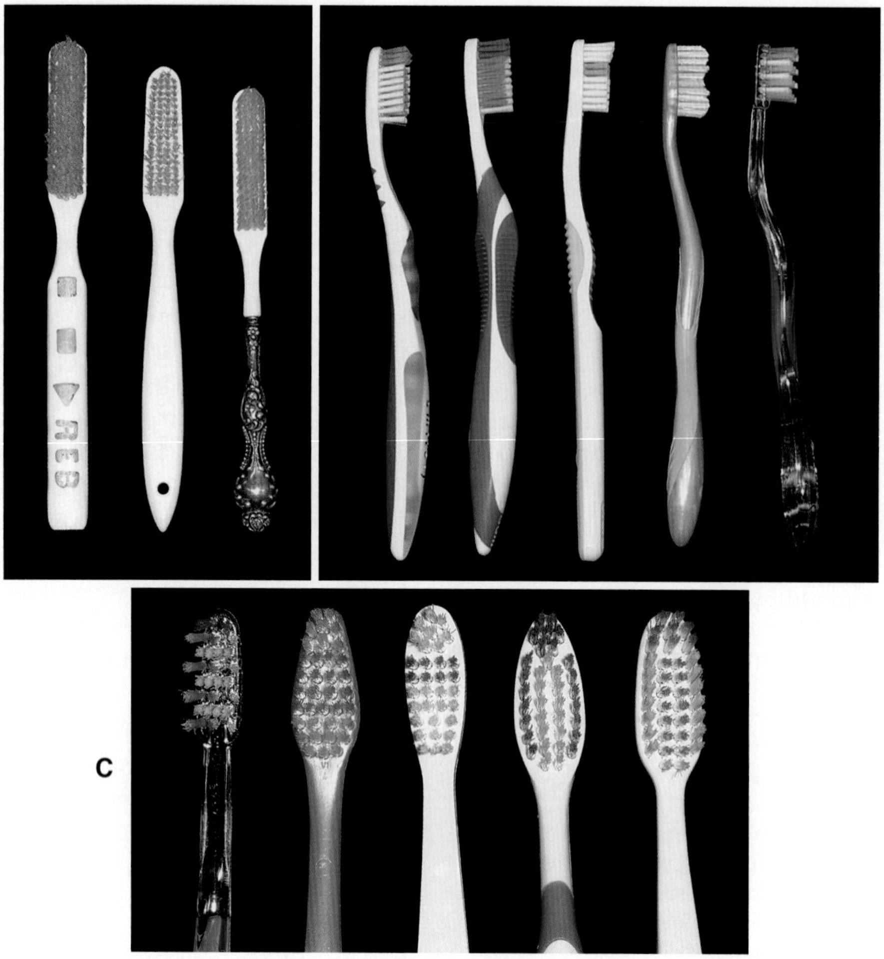

Figure 50-1 Manual toothbrushes. **A,** Toothbrushes from the nineteenth and twentieth centuries, one with an ivory handle from about 1890 *(left)*, one with a composition handle from the 1950s *(center)*, and one with a sterling silver handle from the early twentieth century *(right)*. The ivory-handled brush belonged to a dental student who used the handle to practice cutting preparations and filling the "preps" with amalgam or gold foil. **B,** Various types of toothbrushes are available; note the variation in brush head and handle design. **C,** Brush heads, showing various bristle configurations. (Antique brushes from the UCSF School of Dentistry Historical Collection, courtesy Dean Charles N. Bertolami, San Francisco.)

manufacturers claim superiority of design for such factors as minor modifications of bristle placement, length, and stiffness. These claims are primarily based on plaque removal shown to be significantly superior to comparable toothbrushes in clinical studies. However, the research does not show significant differences in gingivitis scores or bleeding indices, which are the more important measures of improved gingival health. It is questionable whether slight differences in the measurement of plaque removal are clinically significant because no toothbrush and few tooth brushers remove all plaque. In fact, at least one study compared four commercially available toothbrushes for total plaque removal at a single brushing; all four toothbrushes removed plaque equally, and the authors concluded that no one design was superior to others.[28]

When recommending a particular toothbrush, ease of use by the patient as well as the perception that the brush works well are important considerations. The effectiveness of and potential injury from different types of brushes depend to a great degree on how the brushes are used. Data from in vitro studies of abrasion by different manual toothbrushes suggest that brush designs permitting the bristles to carry more toothpaste while brushing contribute to abrasion more than brush bristles themselves.[37] However, all agree that use of hard toothbrushes, vigorous horizontal brushing, and use of extremely abrasive dentifrices may lead to cervical abrasions of teeth and recession of gingiva.[75]

Some novel toothbrush designs intended to make difficult-to-reach areas more accessible have been described. One brush, designed to brush buccal, lingual, and occlusal/incisal surfaces at one time, has curved bristles on both sides of the brush head and shorter bristles running down the center. One study even demonstrated a brush's improved plaque removal ability compared with a conventional brush, but as with other toothbrush studies, absolute differences were slight.[25] The plaque-removing efficacy of another design featuring a U-shaped head with bristles that would also reach buccal, lingual, and occlusal/incisal surfaces at one time is supported by a small clinical trial, but changes in gingival health were not evaluated.[142] The notion of brushing all reachable surfaces of the teeth at one time is attractive, and these inventive brush designs may be useful for some patients to achieve better plaque control. There is no reason to discourage use of any particular device, especially if the patient likes it and uses it more or better than a conventional brush. There may well be a truly better design in the hands of an individual patient that results in better plaque removal and improved gingival health.

Toothbrush Design

Toothbrush bristles are grouped in tufts that are usually arranged in three or four rows. Rounded bristle ends cause fewer scratches on the gingiva than flat-cut bristles with sharp ends.[32,122] Two types of bristle material are used in toothbrushes: natural bristles from hogs and artificial filaments made of nylon. Both types remove plaque, but nylon bristle brushes vastly predominate in the market.[17] Natural bristles fray, break, soften, and lose their elasticity quickly. Patients accustomed to the softness of an older natural bristle brush can easily traumatize the gingiva when using a new brush with comparable vigor.

Bristle hardness is proportional to the square of the diameter and inversely proportional to the square of bristle length.[62] Diameters of common bristles range from 0.007 inch (0.2 mm) for soft brushes to 0.012 inch (0.3 mm) for medium brushes and 0.014 inch (0.4 mm) for hard brushes.[69] Soft bristle brushes of the type described by Bass[11] have gained wide acceptance.

Opinions regarding the merits of hard and soft bristles are based on studies that are not comparable, are often inconclusive, and contradict one another.[70] Softer bristles are more flexible, clean slightly below the gingival margin when used with a sulcular brushing technique,[12] and reach farther onto the proximal surfaces.[51] Use of hard-bristled toothbrushes is associated with more gingival recession, and frequent brushers who use hard bristles have more recession than those who use soft bristles.[81] However, the manner in which a brush is used and the abrasiveness of the dentifrice affect the action and abrasion to a greater degree than the bristle hardness itself.[1,102] Bristle hardness does not significantly affect wear on enamel surfaces.[116]

The amount of force used to brush is not critical for effective plaque removal.[131] Vigorous brushing is not necessary and can lead to gingival recession; bacteremia, especially in patients with pronounced gingivitis; wedge-shaped defects in the cervical area of root surfaces;[50,117] and painful ulceration of the gingiva.[111]

Toothbrushes must also be replaced periodically, although the amount of visible bristle wear does not appear to affect plaque removal for up to 9 weeks.[31] Wear patterns differ widely among individuals, but with regular use, most brushes show signs of wear within a few months. If all the bristles are flattened in a few days, brushing is too vigorous; if the bristles still look new after 6 months, the brush probably has not been used every day.

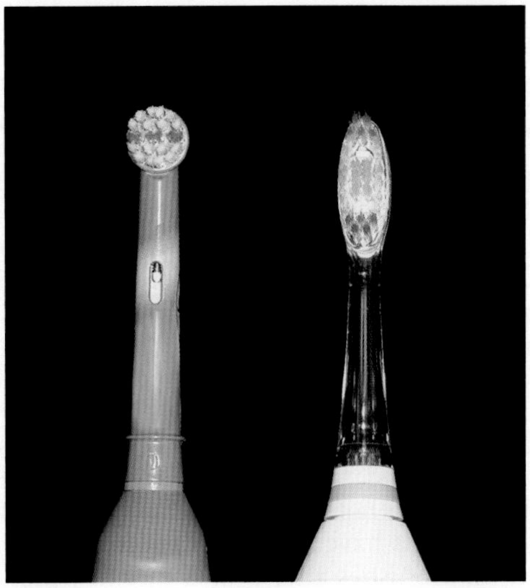

Figure 50-2 Powered toothbrush designs offer options in head shape and size.

The preference of handle characteristics is a matter of individual taste (Figure 50-1). Some clinical evidence supports that slightly bent brush handles improve posterior access for plaque removal under supervised brushing conditions.[75] One study described a toothbrush with a double angulation of the neck of the handle and demonstrated significantly more plaque reduction, especially on the buccal and lingual surfaces of posterior teeth.[82] The clinical significance of these findings has not been determined, but modifications improving access may help some patients to brush more effectively.

Recommendations

- Soft, nylon bristle toothbrushes clean effectively (when used properly), remain effective for a reasonable time, and tend not to traumatize the gingiva or root surfaces.
- Toothbrushes need to be replaced about every 3 months.
- If patients perceive a benefit from a particular brush design, they should use it.

POWERED TOOTHBRUSHES

Electrically powered toothbrushes designed to mimic back-and-forth brushing techniques were invented in 1939. Subsequent models featured circular or elliptic motions, and some with combinations of motions. Currently, powered toothbrushes have oscillating and rotating motions (Figure 50-2), and some brushes use low-frequency acoustic energy to enhance cleaning ability.

Powered toothbrushes rely primarily on mechanical contact between the bristles and the tooth to remove plaque. The addition of low-frequency acoustic energy generates dynamic fluid movement and provides cleaning slightly away from the bristle tips.[48] The vibrations have also been shown to interfere with bacterial adherence to oral surfaces. Neither the sonic vibration nor the mechanical motion of powered toothbrushes has been shown to affect bacterial cell viability.[100] Hydrodynamic shear forces created by these brushes disrupt plaque a short distance from the bristle tips, providing additional interproximal plaque removal.[74]

Typically, comparison studies of powered toothbrushes, manual toothbrushes, or other powered devices demonstrate slightly improved plaque removal for the device of interest in a short-term clinical trial. A distinct overall advantage for any one particular product has not been demonstrated.[104]

Patient acceptance of powered toothbrushes is good. One study reported that 88.9% of patients introduced to a powered toothbrush would continue to use it.[135] However, patients have also been reported to quit using powered toothbrushes after 5 or 6 months, presumably when the novelty is gone.[65] Powered toothbrushes with features that permit slightly better brushing on proximal surfaces and timers to remind patients to brush longer are useful for some patients.[132] Powered toothbrushes have been shown to improve oral health for (1) children and adolescents, (2) children with physical or mental disabilities, (3) hospitalized patients, including older adults who need to have their teeth cleaned by caregivers, and (4) patients with fixed orthodontic appliances. Powered brushes have not been shown to provide benefits routinely for patients with rheumatoid arthritis, children who are well-motivated brushers, or patients with chronic periodontitis.[65]

Many studies have compared powered brushes to manual brushes. A 6-month study of 157 subjects demonstrated findings typical of these comparisons: the powered brush removed slightly but significantly more plaque but did not improve measures of gingival inflammation beyond those achieved by manual brushes.[35] Powered brushes with oscillating, rotating motions demonstrated modestly greater reductions in plaque and gingivitis than manual toothbrushes.[64]

Patients sometimes are reluctant to purchase power toothbrushes because of the relatively high cost compared with manual toothbrushes. Less expensive models are now available, however, and have been shown to be as effective as the higher-priced models.[15]

Recommendations

- Powered toothbrushes remove plaque as well as, if not slightly better than, manual toothbrushes.
- Patients who want to use powered toothbrushes should be encouraged to do so.
- Patients need to be instructed in the proper use of powered devices.
- Patients who are poor brushers, children, and caregivers may particularly benefit from using powered toothbrushes.

DENTIFRICES

Dentifrices aid in cleaning and polishing tooth surfaces. They are used mostly in the form of pastes, although tooth powders and gels are also available. Dentifrices are made up of abrasives (e.g., silicon oxides, aluminum oxides, granular polyvinyl chlorides), water, humectants, soap or detergent, flavoring and sweetening agents, therapeutic agents (e.g., fluorides, pyrophosphates), coloring agents, and preservatives.[63]

Composing 20% to 40% of dentifrices, *abrasives* are insoluble inorganic salts that enhance the abrasive action of toothbrushing as much as 40 times.[102] Tooth powders are much more abrasive than pastes and contain about 95% abrasive materials. The abrasive quality of dentifrices affects enamel only slightly and is a much greater concern for patients with exposed roots. Dentin is abraded 25 times faster and cementum 35 times faster than enamel, so root surfaces are easily worn away, leading to notching and root sensitivity.[126] Hard tissue damage from oral hygiene procedures is mainly caused by abrasive dentifrices, although gingival lesions can be produced by the toothbrush alone[111,116] (Figure 50-3).

Access to buccal surfaces and right-handedness or left-handedness contribute to the abrasion pattern. Typically, more wear occurs on maxillary than mandibular teeth and on the left half than on the right half of the dental arch.[40]

Dentifrices are useful for delivering therapeutic agents to the teeth and gingiva. The pronounced caries-preventive effect of *fluorides* incorporated in dentifrices has been proved beyond question.[125] Fluoride ion must be available in the amount of 1000 to 1100 parts per million (ppm) to achieve caries reduction effects. Toothpaste products that have been tested by the American Dental Association (ADA) and have fluoride ion available

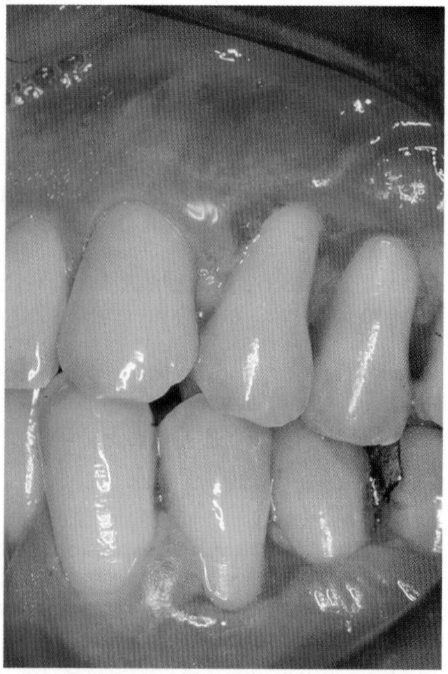

Figure 50-3 Vigorous toothbrushing with an abrasive dentifrice can result in trauma to the gingiva and wearing away of the tooth surfaces, especially root surfaces, and can contribute to gingival recession.

in the appropriate amount carry the ADA seal of approval for caries control and can be relied on to provide caries protection.

"Calculus control toothpastes," also referred to as "tartar control toothpastes," contain *pyrophosphates* and have been shown to reduce the deposition of new calculus on teeth. These ingredients interfere with crystal formation in calculus but do not affect the fluoride ion in the paste or increase tooth sensitivity. Dentifrice with pyrophosphates has been shown to reduce the formation of new supragingival calculus by 30% or more.[77,101,141] Pyrophosphate-containing toothpastes do not affect subgingival calculus formation or gingival inflammation. The inhibitory effect reduces the deposition of new supragingival calculus but will not affect existing calculus deposits. To achieve the greatest effect from calculus control toothpaste, the patient's teeth must be cleaned and completely free of supragingival calculus when starting to use the product daily.

Recommendations

- Dentifrices increase the effectiveness of brushing but should cause a minimum of abrasion to root surfaces.
- Products containing fluorides and antimicrobial agents provide additional benefits for controlling caries and gingivitis.
- Patients who form significant amounts of supragingival calculus benefit from the use of a calculus control dentifrice.

TOOTHBRUSHING METHODS

Many methods for brushing the teeth have been described and promoted as being efficient and effective. These methods can be categorized primarily according to the pattern of motion when brushing and are primarily of historical interest, as follows[75]:

Roll: Roll method[3] or modified Stillman technique[71]
Vibratory: Stillman,[124] Charters,[24] and Bass[12] techniques
Circular: Fones technique[47]
Vertical: Leonard technique[90]
Horizontal: Scrub technique[137]

Controlled studies evaluating the effectiveness of the most common brushing techniques have demonstrated no clear superiority for any method. The *scrub technique* is probably the simplest and most common method of brushing. Patients with periodontal disease are most frequently taught a sulcular brushing technique using a vibratory motion to improve access in the gingival areas. The method most often recommended is the *Bass technique* because it emphasizes sulcular placement of bristles. The basic premise is to adapt the bristles tips to the gingival margin in order to reach the supragingival plaque, using controlled movement to avoid trauma and moving the brush systematically around all the teeth. Clinicians and patients often modify brushing techniques for their own situation. Also, brushing with a powered toothbrush is an equally effective alternative.

Bass Technique[12]

1. Place the head of a soft brush parallel with the occlusal plane, with the brush head covering three to four teeth, beginning at the most distal tooth in the arch.
2. Place the bristles at the gingival margin, pointing at a 45-degree angle to the long axis of the teeth.
3. Exert gentle vibratory pressure, using short, back-and-forth motions without dislodging the tips of the bristles. This motion forces the bristle ends into the gingival sulcus area (Figure 50-4), as well as partly into the interproximal embrasures. The pressure should be firm enough to blanch the gingiva (Figure 50-5).
4. Complete several strokes in the same position. The repetitive motion cleans the tooth surfaces, concentrating on the apical third of the clinical crowns, the gingival sulci, and as far onto the proximal surfaces as the bristles can reach.
5. Lift the brush, move it to the adjacent teeth, and repeat the process for the next three or four teeth.
6. Continue around the arch, brushing about three teeth at a time. Then, use the same method to brush the lingual surfaces.
7. After completing the maxillary arch, move the brush to the mandibular arch, and brush in the same organized way to reach all the teeth.
8. If the brush is too large to reach the lingual surfaces of the anterior teeth, it should be turned vertically to press the end of the brush into the gingival sulcus area.
9. Brush the occlusal surfaces of three or four teeth at a time by pressing the bristles firmly into the pits and fissures and brushing with several short, back-and-forth strokes.

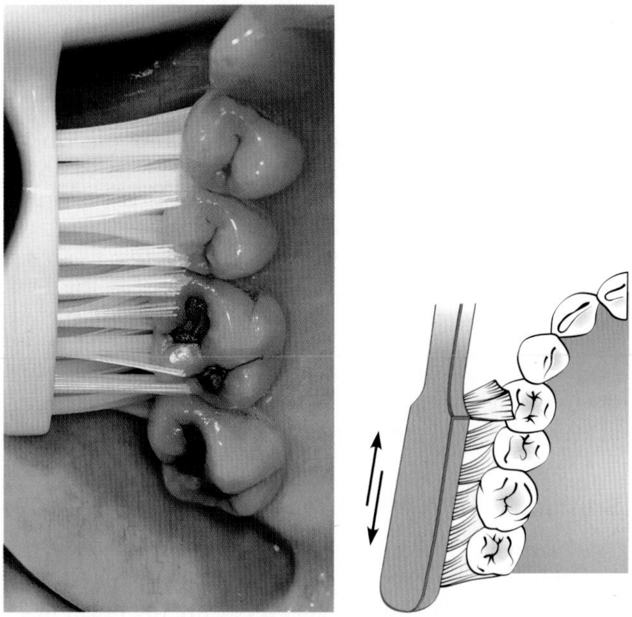

A B

Figure 50-4 Bass method. **A,** Place the toothbrush so that the bristles are angled approximately 45 degrees from the tooth surfaces. **B,** Start at the most distal tooth in the arch, and use a vibrating, back-and-forth motion to brush.

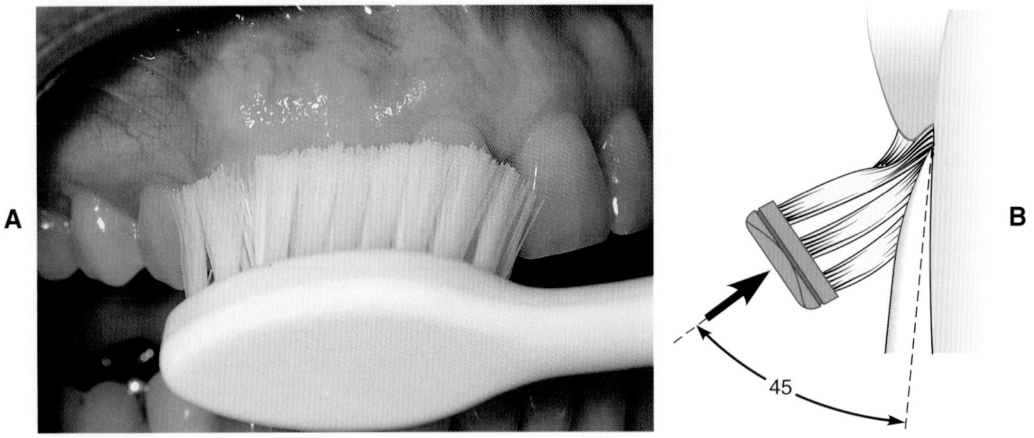

Figure 50-5 Bass method. **A,** Proper position of the brush in the mouth aims the bristle tips toward the gingival margin. **B,** Diagram shows the ideal placement, which permits slight subgingival penetration of the bristle tips.

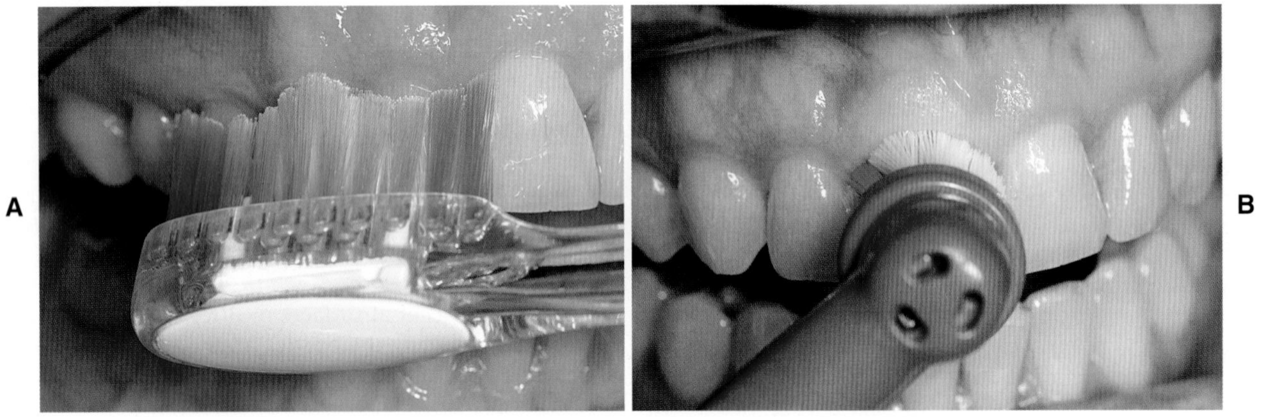

Figure 50-6 Positioning the powered toothbrush head and bristle tips so that they reach the gingival margin is critical to achieving the most effective cleaning results. **A,** Straight-head placement. **B,** Round-head placement.

The Bass technique requires patience and placement of the toothbrush in many different positions to cover the full dentition. Patients need to be instructed to brush in a controlled and systematic sequence.

Other methods of brushing, such as the modified Stillman[71,124] and Charters,[24] are variations of the Bass technique also designed to achieve thorough plaque removal at the gingival margins. They emphasize stimulation of the gingival circulation, which has not been demonstrated to achieve healing results beyond those achieved by good plaque removal.

Brushing with Powered Toothbrushes

The various mechanical motions built into powered toothbrushes do not require special techniques. The patient need only concentrate on placing the brush head next to the teeth at the gingival margin and proceeding systematically around the dentition.[130] Additional placement adjustments can be made to clean difficult areas, such as the distal surfaces of the third molars, furcations, or gingival clefts. A systematic method of brushing all the teeth, similar to the method described for manual brushing, should be used with powered toothbrushes (Figure 50-6).

Recommendations

- The principles of the Bass method have two advantages over other, more complex techniques:
  1. Short, back-and-forth motion is easy to master because it is similar to the scrubbing that most patients normally perform.
  2. Cleaning action is focused on the cervical and interproximal portions of the teeth, where plaque accumulates first.
- Brushing with a powered toothbrush requires a systematic routine to reach all areas, even though the brush head does most of the work.
- Patients will modify any technique to their needs, with the goal of brushing until the teeth are free of plaque.

INTERDENTAL CLEANING AIDS

Any toothbrush, regardless of the brushing method used, does not completely remove interdental plaque. This is true for all brushers, even periodontal patients with wide-open embrasures.[53,119] Daily interdental plaque removal is crucial to augment the effects of toothbrushing because most dental and periodontal diseases originate in interproximal areas.[2]

Tissue destruction associated with periodontal disease often leaves large, open spaces between teeth and long, exposed root surfaces with anatomic concavities and furcations. These areas are both difficult for patients to clean and poorly accessible to the toothbrush.[83]

Patients need to understand that the purpose of interdental cleaning is to remove plaque, not to dislodge food wedged between teeth. Although interdental cleaning does remove food fragments, correcting proximal tooth contacts and plunger cusps is required to stop chronic food impaction.

Many tools are available for interproximal cleaning. They should be recommended based on the patient's interdental architecture (e.g., size of interdental spaces), presence of furcations, tooth alignment, and presence of orthodontic appliances or fixed prostheses. Also, ease of use and patient cooperation are important considerations. Common aids are dental floss and interdental cleaners, such as wooden or plastic tips and interdental brushes.

Dental Floss

Dental floss is the most widely recommended tool for removing plaque from proximal tooth surfaces.[52] Floss is available as a multifilament nylon yarn that is twisted or nontwisted, bonded or nonbonded, waxed or unwaxed, and thick or thin. Some prefer monofilament flosses made of a nonstick material because they are slick and do not fray. Clinical research has demonstrated no significant differences in the ability of the various types of floss to remove dental plaque; they all work equally well.[45,68,79,80] Waxed dental floss was thought to leave a waxy film on proximal surfaces, thus contributing to plaque accumulation and gingivitis. It has been shown, however, that wax is not deposited on tooth surfaces,[112] and that improvement in gingival health is unrelated to the type of floss used.[45] Factors influencing the choice of dental floss include the tightness of tooth contacts, roughness of proximal surfaces, and the patient's manual dexterity, not the superiority of any one product. Therefore, recommendations about type of floss should be based on ease of use and personal preference.

Technique. The floss must contact the proximal surface from line angle to line angle to clean effectively. It must also clean the entire proximal surface, not just be slipped apical into the contact area. The following description is a primer in floss technique:

1. Start with a piece of floss long enough to grasp securely; 12 to 18 inches is usually sufficient. It may be wrapped around the fingers, or the ends may be tied together in a loop.

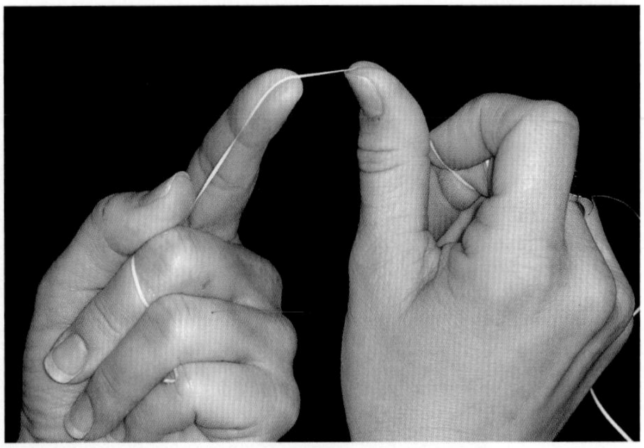

Figure 50-7 Dental floss should be held securely in the fingers or tied in a loop.

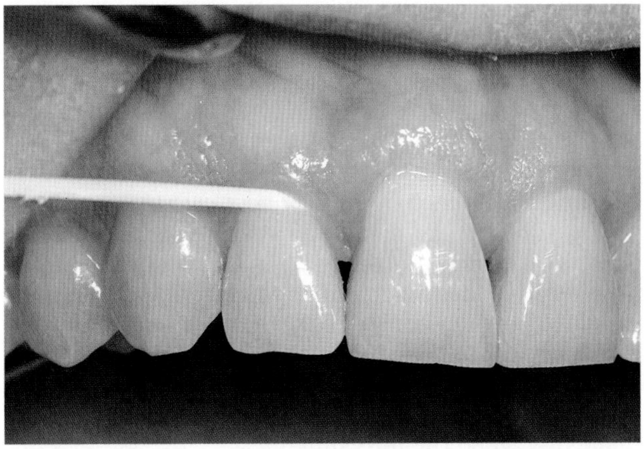

Figure 50-8 Dental floss technique. The floss is slipped between the contact area of the teeth (in this case, teeth #7 and #8), is wrapped around the proximal surface, and removes plaque by using several up-and-down strokes. The process must be repeated for the distal surface of tooth #8.

2. Stretch the floss tightly between the thumb and forefinger (Figure 50-7), or between both forefingers, and pass it gently through each contact area with a firm back-and-forth motion. Do not snap the floss past the contact area because this may injure the interdental gingiva. In fact, zealous snapping of floss through contact areas creates proximal grooves in the gingiva.
3. Once the floss is apical to the contact area between the teeth, wrap the floss around the proximal surface of one tooth, and slip it under the marginal gingiva. Move the floss firmly along the tooth up to the contact area and gently down into the sulcus again, repeating this up-and-down stroke two or three times (Figure 50-8). Then, move the floss across the interdental gingiva, and repeat the procedure on the proximal surface of the adjacent tooth.
4. Continue through the whole dentition, including the distal surface of the last tooth in each quadrant. When the working portion of the floss shreds or becomes dirty, move to a fresh portion of floss.

A 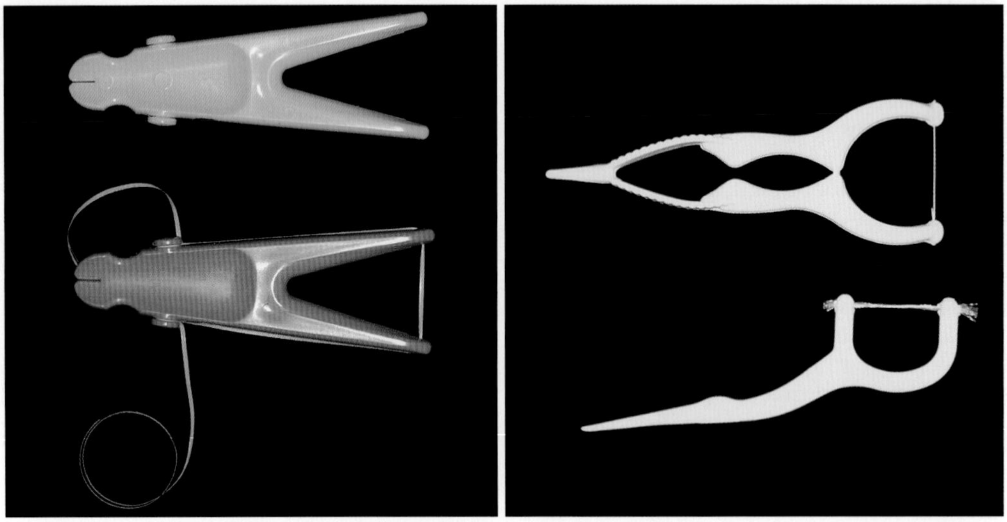 B

Figure 50-9 Floss holders can simplify the manipulation of dental floss. **A,** Reusable floss tools require stringing the floss around a series of knobs and grooves to secure it. **B,** Disposable floss tools have prestrung floss and are easy to use, but the floss may shred and break, requiring several tools to complete flossing the teeth.

Flossing is facilitated by using a *floss holder* (Figure 50-9, *A*). Floss holders are helpful for patients lacking manual dexterity and for caregivers assisting handicapped and hospitalized patients in cleaning their teeth. A floss holder should be rigid enough to keep the floss taut when penetrating into tight contact areas, and it should be simple to string with floss. The disadvantage is that floss tools are time-consuming because they must be rethreaded frequently when the floss shreds.

Disposable, single-use floss holders with prethreaded floss are also available. Short-term clinical studies suggest that plaque reduction and improvement in gingivitis scores are similar for patients using disposable floss devices as for patients who hold the floss with their fingers[21,123] (Figure 50-9, *B*).

Powered flossing devices are also available (Figure 50-10). These devices have a single bristle that moves in a circular motion. The devices have been shown to be safe and effective, but no better at plaque removal than finger flossing.[29,57]

The establishment of a lifelong habit of flossing the teeth is difficult to achieve for both patients and dentists, regardless of whether one uses a tool or flosses with the fingers. In fact, the daily use of floss is universally low. It has been reported that only about 8% of 12- to 16-year olds in Great Britain floss daily,[99] with similar percentages reported for other countries.[83] No information is available about the establishment of long-term flossing habits comparing the various tools to finger flossing. However, the tools may be useful to help some individuals begin flossing or to make flossing possible if patients have limited dexterity.

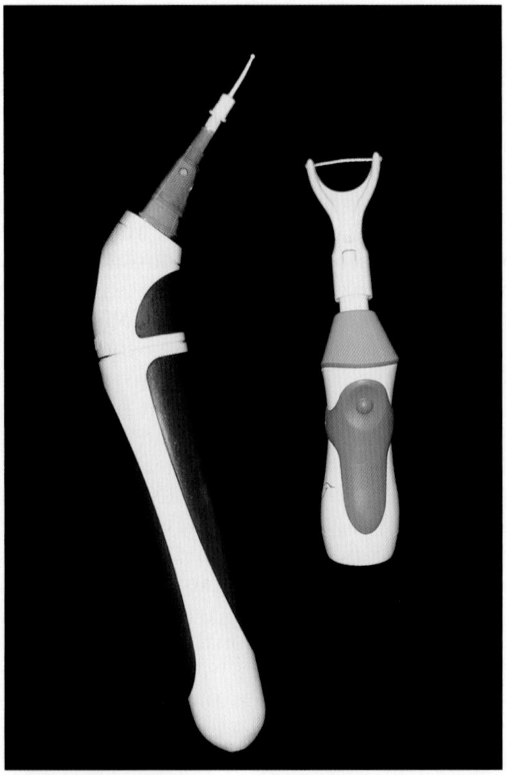

Figure 50-10 Powered flossing devices can be easier for some patients to use than handheld floss. The tip is inserted into the proximal space, and a bristle or wand comes out of the tip and moves in a circular motion when the device is turned on *(left)*. Alternately, the device moves the prestrung floss in short motions to provide interproximal cleaning *(right)*.

Recommendations

- The benefits of interproximal cleaning using dental floss are undisputed.

- Flossing tools work as well as flossing with the traditional method.
- The flossing habit is difficult to establish, so the patient should keep trying.

Interdental Cleaning Devices

Concave root surfaces and furcations that are often present in periodontal patients who have experienced significant attachment loss and recession are not as thoroughly cleaned with dental floss alone. A comparison study of dental floss and interdental brushes used by patients with moderate to severe periodontal disease showed that the interproximal brushes removed slightly more interproximal plaque and that subjects found them easier to use than dental floss. However, no differences were seen in probe depth reductions or bleeding indices.[26] Therefore, interproximal cleaning aids that are easy to handle and adaptable to irregular and long, exposed root surfaces can be recommended for proximal cleaning of teeth when interdental spaces permit access.[83]

Embrasure spaces vary greatly in size and shape. Figure 50-11 provides a representation of the size and anatomy of three types of embrasures and the type of interdental cleaner often recommended for each. As a general rule, the larger the space, the larger should be the device used to clean it. However, some devices are more difficult to assemble and use than others, so a favorite tool of one patient may be impossible for another to use.

A wide variety of interdental cleaning devices are available for removing soft debris from between the teeth (Figure 50-12). The most common types are conical or cylindrical brushes, tapered wooden toothpicks that are round or triangular in cross section, and single-tufted brushes. Many interdental devices can be attached to a handle for convenient manipulation around the teeth and in posterior areas. Clinical research has shown that the devices are effective on lingual and facial tooth surfaces as well as on proximal surfaces.[83,119,133]

Interdental Brushes. Interdental brushes are cone-shaped or cylindrical brushes made of bristles mounted on a handle (Figure 50-12, *C* and *D*), single-tufted brushes (Figure 50-12, *E*), or small cylindrical brushes (Figure 50-12, *F*). Interdental brushes are particularly suitable for cleaning large, irregular, or concave tooth surfaces adjacent to wide interdental spaces.

Technique. Interdental brushes of any style are inserted through interproximal spaces and moved back and forth between the teeth with short strokes. For the most efficient cleaning, the diameter of brush should be slightly larger than the gingival embrasures to be cleaned. This size permits bristles to exert pressure on both proximal tooth surfaces, working their way into concavities on the roots.

Single-tufted brushes provide access to furcation areas, or isolated areas of deep recession, and work well on the lingual surfaces of mandibular molars and premolars. These areas are often missed when using a toothbrush,

Wooden or Rubber Tips. Wooden toothpicks are used either with or without a handle (Figure 50-12, *A* and *B*). Access is easier from the buccal surfaces for tips without handles, primarily in the anterior and bicuspid areas. Wooden toothpicks used on handles improve access to all areas and have been shown to be as effective as dental floss in reducing plaque and bleeding scores in subjects with gingivitis.[93]

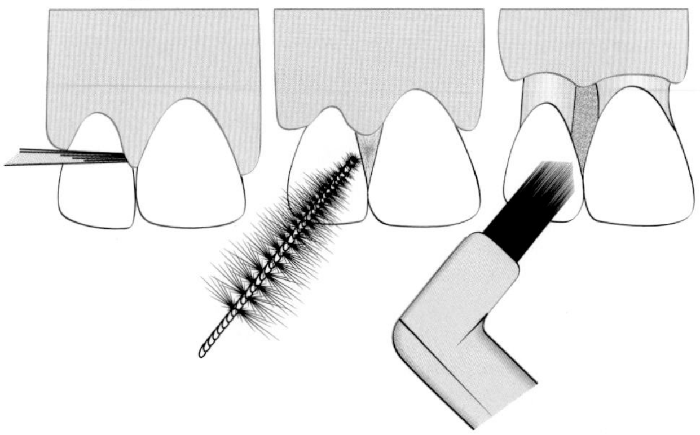

Figure 50-11 Interproximal embrasure spaces vary greatly in patients with periodontal disease. In general, **A,** embrasures with no gingival recession are adequately cleaned using dental floss; **B,** larger spaces with exposed root surfaces require the use of an interproximal brush; and **C,** single-tufted brushes clean efficiently in interproximal spaces with no papillae.

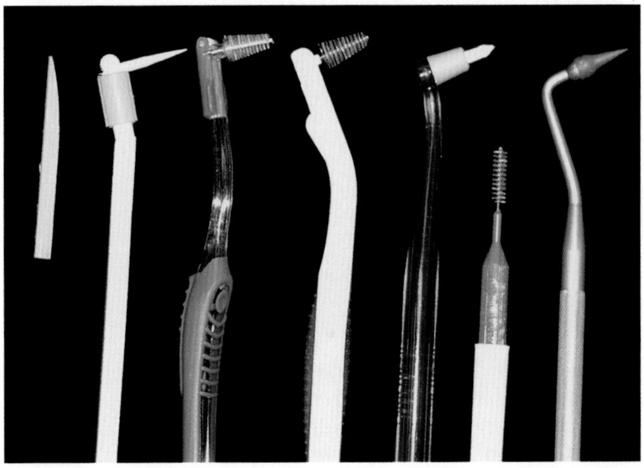

Figure 50-12 Interproximal cleaning devices include wooden tips (**A** and **B**), interproximal brushes (**C** through **F**), and rubber tip stimulators (**G**).

Triangular wooden tips are also available; this design is most useful in the anterior areas when used from the buccal surfaces of the teeth. Rubber tips are conical and are mounted on handles or the ends of toothbrushes; they can be easily adapted to all proximal surfaces in the mouth. Plastic tips that resemble wooden or rubber tips are also available and are used in the same way. Both rubber and plastic tips can be rinsed and reused and are easily carried in a pocket or purse.

Technique. Toothpicks are common devices and readily available in most homes. They can be used around

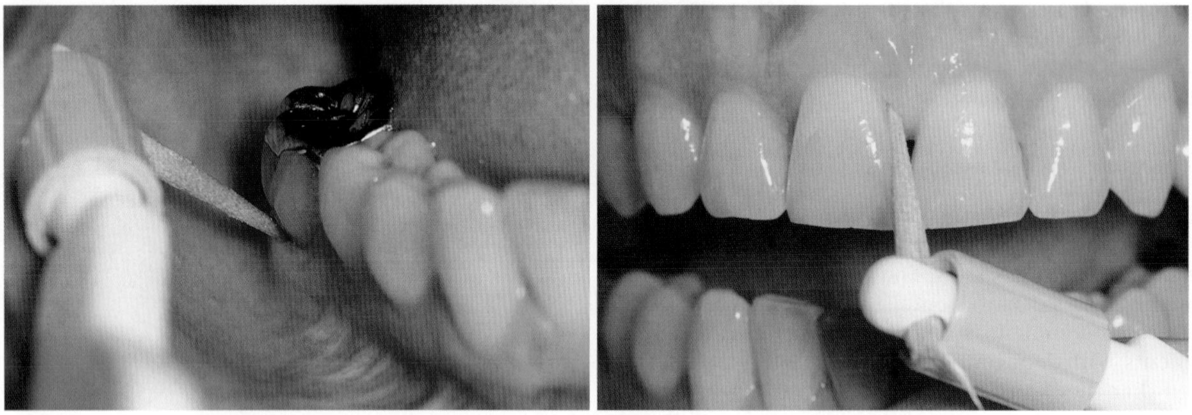

Figure 50-13 Wooden toothpick. **A,** The tip is a common wooden toothpick held in a handle and broken off. It is used to clean subgingivally and reach into periodontal pockets. **B,** The tip can also be used to clean along the gingival margins of the teeth and reach under the gingiva.

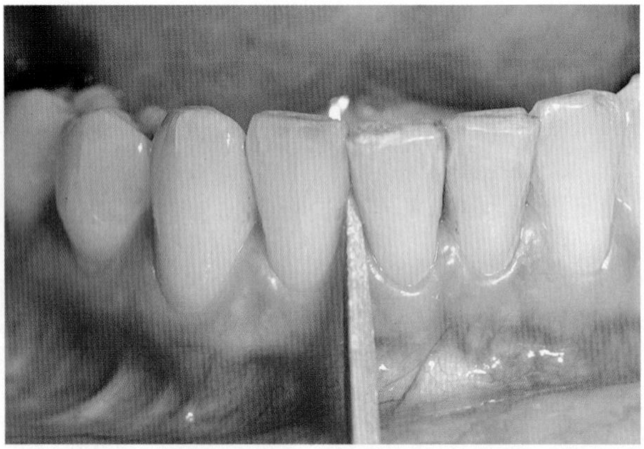

Figure 50-14 Triangular wooden tips are also popular with patients. The tip is inserted between the teeth, with the triangular portion resting on the gingival papilla. The tip is moved in and out to remove plaque; however, it is very difficult to use on posterior teeth and from the lingual aspect of all teeth.

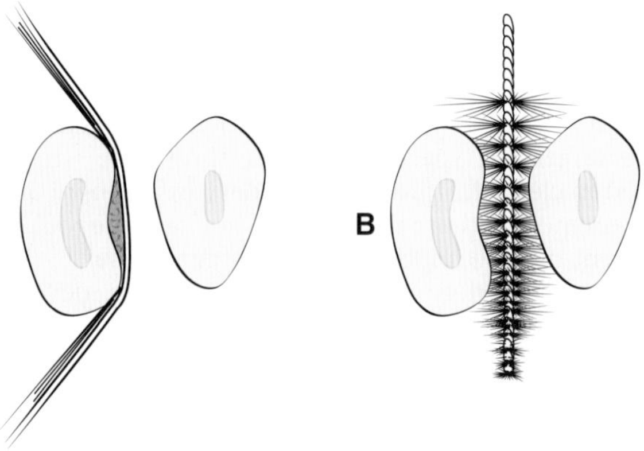

Figure 50-15 Cleaning of concave or irregular proximal tooth surfaces. Dental floss **(A)** may be less effective than an interdental brush **(B)** on long root surfaces with concavities.

all surfaces of the teeth when attached to commercially available handles (Figure 50-12, *B*). Once mounted on the handle, the toothpick is broken off so that it is only 6 or 7 mm long. The tip of the toothpick is used to trace along the gingival margin and into the proximal areas from both the facial and the lingual surface of each tooth (Figure 50-13). Toothpicks mounted on handles are efficient for cleaning along the gingival margin[52] and into periodontal pockets and furcations.

Soft, triangular wooden picks or plastic alternatives are placed in the interdental space with the base of the triangle resting on the gingiva and the sides in contact with the proximal tooth surfaces (Figure 50-14). The pick is then repeatedly moved in and out of the embrasure to remove plaque. The disadvantage of triangular wooden or plastic tips is that they do not reach well into the posterior areas or on the lingual surfaces.

Rubber tips should be placed into the embrasure space and used in a circular motion. They can be applied to interproximal spaces and other defects throughout the mouth and are easily adaptable to lingual surfaces.

Recommendations

- Often a toothbrush and dental floss are not sufficient to clean interdental spaces adequately, so it is extremely important to find an interdental device that the patient likes and will use.
- Many interdental cleaning aids are available for patients. The clinician might need to try several devices before finding one that works for the individual patient.
- In general, the largest brush or device that fits into a space will clean most efficiently (Figure 50-15).

GINGIVAL MASSAGE

Massaging the gingiva with a toothbrush or an interdental cleaning devices produces epithelial thickening, increased keratinization, and increased mitotic activity in the epithelium and connective tissue.[19,22,55] The increased

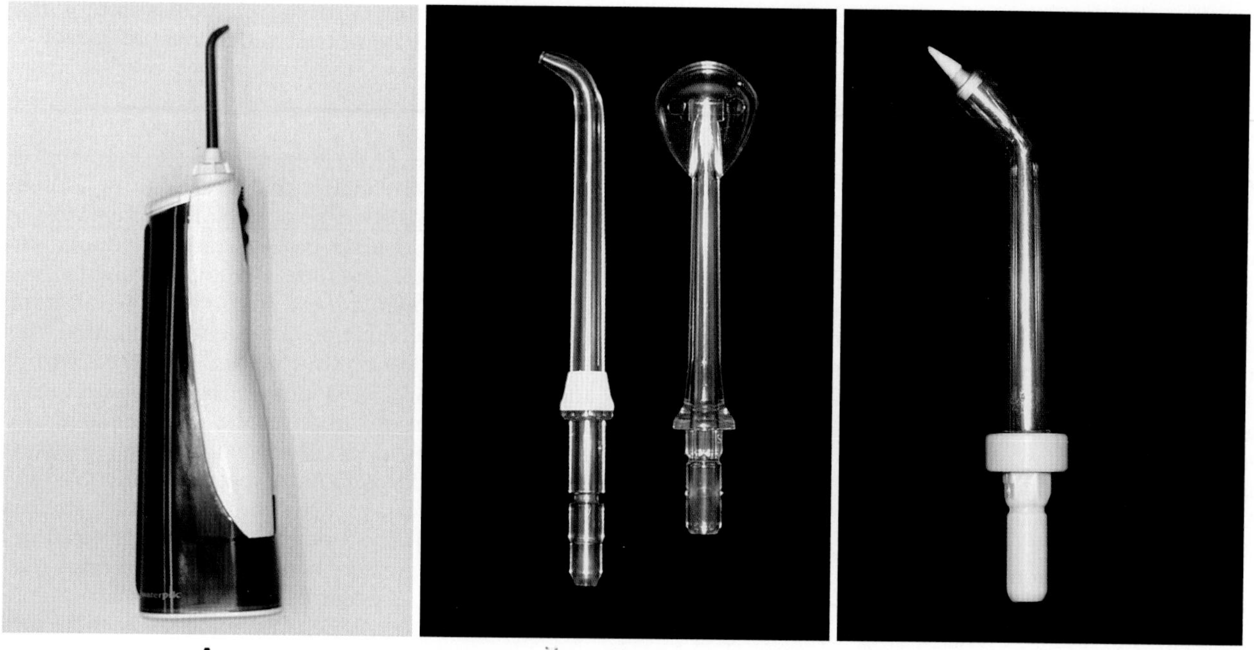

Figure 50-16 Oral irrigation. **A,** The most common oral irrigators have a built-in pump and reservoir. **B,** Conventional plastic tips are used for daily supragingival irrigation at home by the patient. *Left,* Tip for gingival irrigation. *Right,* Tip for cleaning dorsal surface of the tongue **C,** Soft rubber tip is used for daily subgingival irrigation by the patient at home.

keratinization occurs only on the oral gingiva and not on the areas more vulnerable to microbial attack: the sulcular epithelium and the interdental areas where the gingival col is present.

Epithelial thickening, increased keratinization, and increased blood circulation have not been shown to be beneficial for restoring gingival health.[54] Improved gingival health associated with interdental stimulation is much more likely the result of plaque removal than gingival massage. In addition, use of chemotherapeutic mouth rinses containing chlorhexidine have been shown to improve gingival health for short periods in the absence of any mechanical oral hygiene procedure.[97] These data underscore the importance of emphasizing plaque removal rather than stimulating or thickening the keratinized surface in the plaque control program.

ORAL IRRIGATION

Supragingival Irrigation

Oral irrigators for daily home use by patients work by directing a high-pressure, steady or pulsating stream of water through a nozzle to the tooth surfaces. Most often, a device with a built-in pump generates the pressure (Figure 50-16, *A*). Oral irrigators clean nonadherent bacteria and debris from the oral cavity more effectively than toothbrushes and mouth rinses. Irrigators are particularly helpful for removing debris from inaccessible areas around orthodontic appliances and fixed prostheses. When used as adjuncts to toothbrushing, these devices can have a beneficial effect on periodontal health by reducing the accumulation of plaque and calculus[73,95,115] and decreasing inflammation and pocket depth.[20,115]

Oral irrigation has been shown to disrupt and detoxify subgingival plaque and can be useful in delivering antimicrobial agents into periodontal pockets.[106] Irrigation can be supragingival or subgingival. Daily supragingival irrigation with a dilute antiseptic, chlorhexidine, for 6 months resulted in significant reductions in bleeding and gingivitis compared with water irrigation and chlorhexidine rinse controls. Irrigation with water alone also reduced gingivitis significantly, but not as much as the dilute chlorhexidine.[46]

Technique

1. The common home-use irrigator tip is a plastic nozzle with a 90-degree bend at the tip (Figure 50-16, *B*), attached to a pump providing pulsating beads of water at speeds regulated by a dial. Patients should be instructed to aim the pulsating jet across the proximal papilla, hold it there for 10 to 15 seconds, then trace along the gingival margin to the next proximal space, and repeat the procedure.
2. The irrigator should be used from both the buccal and the lingual surface.
3. By the time the patient has irrigated all the proximal spaces in the full dentition, the irrigator reservoir will be empty.
4. Irrigation must be done while leaning across the bathroom sink because water will drip down the patient's arm.
5. Patients with gingival inflammation usually start at lower pressure and then can increase the pressure

comfortably to about medium as tissue health improves. Some individuals like to use the device on the highest pressure setting, with no reported harm. Patient comfort should be the guide for pressure setting.

Subgingival Irrigation

Subgingival irrigation performed both in the dental office and at home by the patient, particularly when antimicrobial agents are used, has been shown to provide some site-specific therapy. It is performed by aiming or placing the irrigation tip into the periodontal pocket, attempting to insert the tip at least 3 mm, using a soft rubber tip[36] (Figure 50-16, *C*). Irrigation performed in the dental office, also called *lavage* or "flushing of the periodontal pocket," as a one-time treatment after scaling and root planing, has not been shown to improve clinical healing, and data do not support its use in improving therapeutic results.[59,120]

Subgingival irrigation performed with an oral irrigator using chlorhexidine diluted to one-third strength, performed regularly at home and after scaling, root planing, and in-office irrigation therapy, has produced significant gingival improvement compared with controls.[59,76,120] Subgingival irrigation has been shown to disrupt more than half the subgingival plaque[72] and reach about half the depth of pockets, up to 7 mm, much further apically than a toothbrush or floss can reach.[38] These data suggest that patients can benefit from daily subgingival irrigation, particularly in difficult sites such as furcations and residual pockets.

Technique. The soft rubber irrigator tip is most useful for subgingival irrigation and can be inserted in pockets (Figure 50-16, *C*). It reduces the pressure and flow of the pulsating jet of water. Effective penetration of irrigant of up to 70% in laboratory simulation has been shown when using the soft rubber tip.[27,72]

The subgingival irrigation tip should be gently inserted into pockets or furcation areas, 3 mm if possible, and each pocket should be flushed for a few seconds.

One caution must be considered. Transient *bacteremia* has been reported after water irrigation in patients with periodontitis[44] and patients receiving periodontal maintenance therapy.[134] However, bacteremia has also been found after toothbrushing[109] and is known to occur in some significant number of patients after scaling alone.[134] Subgingival irrigation at home is not the oral hygiene procedure of choice for patients requiring antibiotic prophylaxis before dental treatment, particularly if extensive inflammation is present.[36] For these patients, supragingival irrigation used in combination with toothbrushing and other interdental cleaning aids is recommended.

Recommendations

- Supragingival irrigation reduces gingival inflammation and is easier for some patients than using mechanical interdental aids.
- Subgingival irrigation with specialized tips for deep pockets and furcation areas is effective when used daily as part of the home care routine.
- Patients requiring antibiotic premedication for dental procedures should not use subgingival irrigation devices.

CARIES CONTROL

Dental caries, particularly root caries, can be a problem for periodontal patients because of attachment loss associated with the disease process and periodontal therapeutic procedures. *Root caries* develops through a process similar to coronal caries, involving the alternating cycle of demineralization and remineralization of the surfaces[136] and other risk factors associated with diet and salivary flow. The demineralization process requires the fermentation of carbohydrates in the plaque by oral bacteria, resulting in loss of mineral from the root surface. *Lactobacillus* and *Streptococcus* species are involved in the root caries process, as with coronal caries.[41] The major difference is that the amount of organic material in the root surfaces is greater than in enamel, so once the demineralization has occurred, the organic matrix—mostly collagen—is exposed. Organic material is then further broken down by bacterial enzymes, resulting in rapid destruction of the root surface.[41]

Fluoride works primarily by topical effects to prevent and reverse the caries process, whether in enamel, cementum, or dentin. Low concentrations of topical fluoride inhibit demineralization, enhance remineralization, and inhibit the enzyme activity in bacteria by acidifying the cells.[42,43]

Adult patients benefit from the prevention and reversal of root caries provided by low-concentration topical fluoride delivered by toothpastes or other topical applications.[42] It also has been demonstrated that the use of fluoride dentifrice containing 5000 ppm of fluoride was more effective in reversing active root caries lesions than the fluoride level of 1100 ppm found in conventional toothpastes.[14]

Recommendations

- All periodontal patients should be encouraged to use a fluoride-containing toothpaste, 1000 to 1100 ppm, daily to reduce demineralization and enhance remineralization of tooth surfaces.
- Patients at high risk for caries, including those with a history of root lesions or active lesions, should use higher-concentration fluoride toothpaste or gels, 5000 ppm, daily until the risk for caries is controlled.
- Other considerations in caries control, such as diet and reduced salivary flow, should be evaluated as with all dental patients.

CHEMICAL PLAQUE CONTROL WITH ORAL RINSES

Improved understanding of the infectious nature of dental diseases has dramatically increased interest in chemical methods of plaque control and holds great promise for advances in disease control and prevention. The ADA Council on Scientific Affairs has adopted a program for acceptance of plaque control agents. The agents must be evaluated in placebo-controlled clinical trials of 6 months or longer that demonstrate significantly improved gingival health compared with controls. To date, the ADA has accepted two agents for treatment of gingivitis: prescription solutions of chlorhexidine digluconate oral rinse and nonprescription essential oil rinse.

Prescription Chlorhexidine Rinse

The agent that has shown the most positive antibacterial results to date is chlorhexidine, a diguanidohexane with pronounced antiseptic properties. Several other clinical investigations confirmed the initial finding that two daily rinses with 10 ml of a 0.2% aqueous solution of chlorhexidine digluconate almost completely inhibited the development of dental plaque, calculus, and gingivitis in the human model for experimental gingivitis.[60] Clinical studies of several months' duration have reported plaque reductions of 45% to 61% and, more importantly, gingivitis reductions of 27% to 67%.[60,87] The 0.12% chlorhexidine digluconate preparation available in the United States for reducing plaque and gingivitis has been shown to be equally effective as the higher-concentration product.[4,78,85]

Localized, reversible side effects to chlorhexidine use may occur, primarily brown staining of the teeth, tongue, and silicate and resin restorations[87] and transient impairment of taste perception.[96] Chlorhexidine has very low systemic toxic activity in humans, has not produced any appreciable resistance of oral microorganisms, and has not been associated with teratogenic alterations.[85] The preparation contains 12% alcohol, which may be of concern to clinicians and patients because regular use of alcohol increases the risk of oropharyngeal cancer. However, an extensive review of the available epidemiologic evidence associating alcohol-containing oral rinse preparations with cancer concluded that existing data do not support this association.[39] Regardless, many patients continue to express this concern or simply do not want to consume alcohol in any form.

Nonprescription Essential Oil Rinse

Essential oil mouth rinses contain thymol, eucalyptol, menthol, and methyl salicylate.[4] These preparations have been evaluated in three long-term clinical studies and demonstrate plaque reductions of 20% to 35% and gingivitis reductions of 25% to 35%.[34,56,84] This type of oral rinse has a long history of daily use and safety since the nineteenth century, and many patients have used the products for decades. These products also contain alcohol (up to 24% depending on the preparation), so some patients and clinicians are concerned about using them. Limited clinical evidence shows that regular use of essential oil mouth rinse may be as effective as flossing for subjects with gingivitis.[7,8] These findings await confirmation.

Other Products

A preparation containing *triclosan* has shown some effectiveness in reducing plaque and gingivitis. It is available in toothpaste form, and the active ingredient is more effective in combination with zinc citrate or a copolymer of methoxyethylene.[61]

Other oral rinse products on the market have shown some evidence of plaque reduction, although long-term improvement in gingival health has not been substantiated. These include stannous fluoride,[92,139] cetylpyridinium chloride (quaternary ammonia compounds),[8,9] and sanguinarine.[103,110] Evidence suggests that these and other available mouth rinse products do not possess the antimicrobial potential of either chlorhexidine products or essential oil preparations.

One type of agent has been marketed as a prebrushing oral rinse to improve the effectiveness of toothbrushing. The active ingredient is sodium benzoate. Research to support its effectiveness is contradictory, but the preponderance of evidence suggests that using a prebrushing rinse is no more effective than brushing alone.[16,17]

Chemical plaque control has been shown to be effective for both plaque reduction and improved wound healing after periodontal surgery.[118] Both chlorhexidine[6] and essential oil[140] mouth rinses have significant positive effects when prescribed for use after periodontal surgery for 1 to 4 weeks.

Recommendations

- Chemical plaque control can augment mechanical plaque control procedures.
- Fluoride preparations are essential for caries control in periodontal patients.
- Antimicrobial oral rinses will reduce gingivitis in periodontal patients.
- Chlorhexidine rinses can be used to augment plaque control during Phase I therapy, for patients with recurrent problems, for ineffective plaque control for any reason, for some uncommon oral mucous membrane diseases, and for use after periodontal or oral surgery.
- Essential oil rinses are effective but to a lesser degree than chlorhexidine. They may be advantageous because they have fewer side effects and are available without a prescription.
- Oral irrigators used with dilute solutions of effective antimicrobial agents reduce gingivitis.
- Oral rinse preparations are also available with no alcohol content, which may be preferable to some clinicians and patients.
- The use of cosmetic oral rinses and prebrushing rinses should not be used to replace proven mechanical and chemical means of plaque removal but can be useful if patients perceive benefits from them.

DISCLOSING AGENTS

Disclosing agents are solutions or wafers capable of staining bacterial deposits on the surfaces of teeth, tongue, and gingiva. These can be used as educational and motivational tools to improve the efficiency of plaque control procedures[7] (Figure 50-17).

Solutions and wafers are available commercially. Solutions are applied to the teeth as concentrates on

A 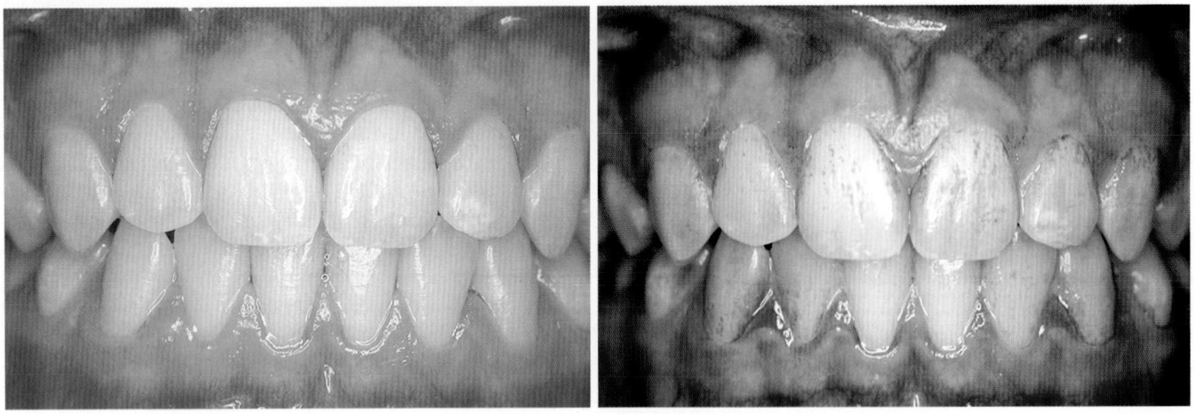 B

Figure 50-17 Effect of a disclosing agent. **A,** Unstained, the teeth look clean, but close inspection shows subtle signs of gingivitis. **B,** Plaque shows as dark-red particulate matter when stained with a disclosing dye. It is useful to demonstrate toothbrushing in the patient's mouth with the teeth disclosed and plaque visible.

cotton swabs or diluted as rinses. They usually produce heavy staining of bacterial plaque, gingiva, tongue, lips, and fingers, as well as the sink. Wafers are crushed between the teeth and swished around the mouth for a few seconds and then spit out. Either form can be used for plaque control instruction in the office and dispensed for home use to aid periodontal patients in evaluating the effectiveness of their oral hygiene routines.

FREQUENCY OF PLAQUE REMOVAL

In the controlled and supervised environment of clinical research, where well-trained individuals remove all visible plaque, gingival health can be maintained by one thorough cleaning with brush, floss, and toothpicks every 24 to 48 hours.[75,83,86] Most patients, however, fall far short of this goal. The average daily home care routine lasts less than 2 minutes and removes only 40% of plaque.[36] It has been reported that improved plaque removal and therefore improved periodontal health is associated with increasing the frequency of brushing to twice per day.[75,105] Cleaning three or more times per day does not appear to further improve periodontal conditions.

Recommendations

- Emphasis should be placed on cleaning the teeth meticulously once daily with all necessary tools.
- If plaque control is not adequate, a second daily brushing will help.

PATIENT MOTIVATION AND EDUCATION

In periodontal therapy, plaque control has two important purposes: to minimize gingival inflammation and to prevent the recurrence or progression of periodontal disease and caries. Daily mechanical removal of plaque by the patient, including the use of appropriate antimicrobial agents, is the only practical means for improving oral health on a long-term basis. The process requires interest on the part of the patient and education and instruction from you, the dentist, followed by encouragement and reinforcement. Keeping records of patient performance facilitates this process. Figure 50-18 provides an example of a plaque control record that permits repeated measures and comparison over time.

Motivation for Effective Plaque Control

Once you and your patient have determined the appropriate regimen, incorporating the new techniques into habits remains a significant challenge. Motivating patients to perform effective plaque control is one of the most critical and difficult elements of long-term success in periodontal therapy. It requires both commitment by the patient to change daily habits and regular return visits for maintenance and reinforcement.

Patients often stop using the prescribed oral hygiene regimens and fail to return for regular visits to the dental office; the scope of this problem is immense. It has been shown that patients stop using interproximal cleaning aids in a very short time. Heasman et al.[66] followed 100 patients who had been treated for moderate to severe periodontal disease. All had been taught to use one or more interdental cleaning aids, but only 20% used the aids after 6 months. Of those who had started using three devices, one third had stopped all interdental cleaning at 6 months; the others used one or two of the aids.[72] The situation is no better when looking at patient willingness to return for office visits. In one study of 1280 patients, most of whom had periodontal surgery in multiple sites after intensive scaling, root planing, and plaque control instruction, 25% never returned for a follow-up visit; only 40% returned regularly.[107] Wilson et al.[138] reported that 67% of periodontal patients were noncompliant with return visits in a 20-year retrospective of a private periodontal practice.

However, adopting new habits and returning for office visits is not an impossible task. To be successful, the patient (1) must be receptive and must understand the concepts of pathogenesis, treatment, and prevention

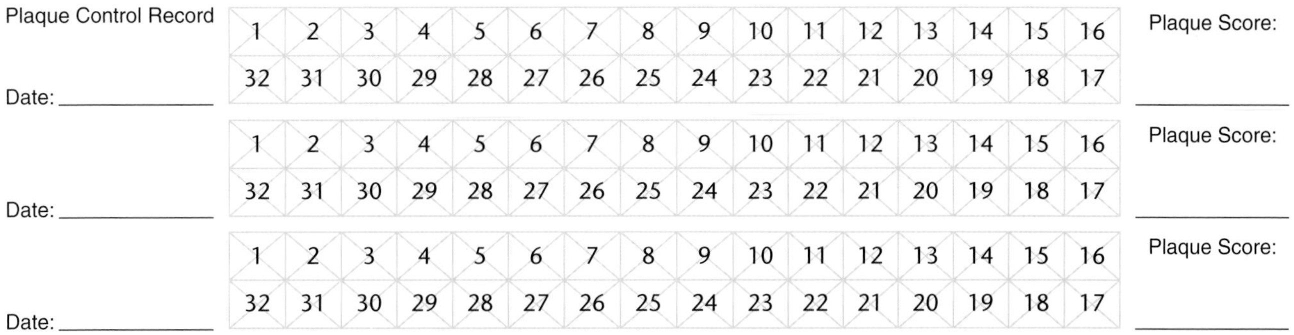
Plaque Control Record
Date:
Date:
Date:
1 2 3 4 5 6 7 8 9 10 11 12 13 14 15 16
32 31 30 29 28 27 26 25 24 23 22 21 20 19 18 17
1 2 3 4 5 6 7 8 9 10 11 12 13 14 15 16
32 31 30 29 28 27 26 25 24 23 22 21 20 19 18 17
1 2 3 4 5 6 7 8 9 10 11 12 13 14 15 16
32 31 30 29 28 27 26 25 24 23 22 21 20 19 18 17
Plaque Score:
Plaque Score:
Plaque Score:

Figure 50-18 The plaque control record can be an effective motivator for patients. This form permits easy comparison of scores over time. (Courtesy Dean Charles N. Bertolami, University of California, San Francisco School of Dentistry, San Francisco.)

of periodontal disease; (2) must be willing to change the habits of a lifetime; and (3) must be able to adjust personal beliefs, practices, and values to accommodate new regimens.

It is your responsibility as the patient's dentist to provide information about periodontal disease, its effects, and the patient's responsibility in achieving and maintaining oral health. Manual skills must be developed and used to establish an effective plaque control regimen. In addition, the patient must understand your role in treating and maintaining periodontal health.[114] If not, long-term success of treatment is much less likely. The process of changing the habits of a lifetime begins by educating the patient about periodontal health and disease, developing an acceptable plaque control strategy, and reinforcing positive changes in behavior.

Education and Scoring Systems

Many patients believe that visits to the dental office for periodontal care will eliminate the disease process. Treatment is not a passive process, however, and it is incumbent on you to educate and reinforce the patient's responsibility for long-term success of therapy and cure. Our health-conscious society is an advantage with regard to patient education. Most patients know what gingivitis is because they have heard about it on television or read about it in magazines or on the Internet. They are willing to spend time and money to try new products such as toothbrushes and mouth rinses. Educating each patient is a process that must be individualized according to need and level of understanding.

Patients must also be informed that periodic assessment and debridement of the teeth in the dental office are required to prevent recurrence of periodontal diseases and identify problems that may arise. These procedures work best when combined with an individualized oral hygiene regimen practiced daily at home. Therefore, time spent in the dental office teaching the patient how to perform plaque control procedures is as central to care as scaling the teeth. The purpose of the recall visit is not to remove plaque, because it forms every day anyway. Patients sometimes have the concept that "cleanings" every few months are sufficient for plaque removal and disease control. Only the combination of regular office visits with conscientious home care significantly reduces gingivitis and loss of supporting periodontal tissues over the long term.[94,128]

Periodontal patients should be shown how periodontal disease has manifested in their own mouth. Stained dental plaque, the bleeding of inflamed gingiva, and demonstrations of the periodontal probe inserted into pockets are impressive demonstrations of the presence of pathogens and symptoms of disease. It also is of educational value to patients to have their oral cleanliness and periodontal condition recorded periodically[10] so that improvements in performance can be used for positive reinforcement. The plaque control record and the bleeding points index are simple indices and useful for patient education and motivation.

Plaque Control Record (O'Leary Index).[108] Have the patient use a disclosing solution or tablet and examine each tooth surface (except occlusal surfaces) for the presence or absence of stained plaque at the dentogingival junction. Plaque is recorded on the appropriate box in a diagram for four surfaces on each tooth. After all teeth have been scored, the index number is calculated for the percentage of surfaces with plaque by dividing the number of surfaces with plaque by the total number of surfaces scored and then multiplying by 100. A reasonable goal for patients is 10% or fewer surfaces with plaque. If plaque is always present in the same areas, provide a tool and instructions to improve performance in those areas. It is extremely difficult to achieve a perfect score of 0, so patients should be rewarded for approaching it.

Some frequently used plaque indices do not require staining the teeth, such as the plaque index of Silness and Löe.[121] These are more convenient to use and possibly more acceptable to patients, but they have some disadvantages for patient education. Identification of plaque is not as quick and easy for the clinician's record making, and because plaque is not stained, it is not highlighted for the patient to see and remove.

Bleeding Points Index.[89] The bleeding points index provides an evaluation of bleeding gingiva around each tooth in the patient's mouth. Retract the cheek, and place the periodontal probe 1 mm into the sulcus or pocket at the distal aspect of the most posterior tooth in the quadrant. Carry the probe lightly across the length of the sulcus to the mesial interproximal area on the facial aspect. Continue along all the teeth in the quadrant from the facial aspect. Wait 30 seconds, and record the presence of bleeding on the distal, facial, and mesial surfaces on the chart. Repeat on the lingual-palatal aspect, recording bleeding only for the direct lingual surface, not for the mesial or distal surfaces. This results in four separate scores for each tooth and does not score the mesial and distal surfaces twice. Repeat the steps for each quadrant. The percentage of the number of bleeding surfaces is calculated by dividing the number of surfaces that bled by the total number of tooth surfaces (four per tooth) and by multiplying by 100 to convert the score to a percentage. This index is designed to demonstrate bleeding gingiva rather than plaque. Again, a goal of 10% or fewer bleeding points is good, but 0 is ideal. If a few bleeding points repeatedly occur in the same areas, plaque control for those areas should be reinforced or modified.

Significance of Plaque Scores and Bleeding Scores. Plaque scores are helpful as indicators of patient compliance and success with daily plaque control procedures. However, plaque levels themselves do not necessarily reflect gingival health or risk of disease progression, even though plaque is highly correlated with the presence of gingivitis.[98] In terms of predicting success in controlling inflammation and reducing the chance of disease progression, *bleeding* is a much better indicator. Although bleeding on probing is not the most specific or sensitive measure of health, it has a strong negative correlation to disease progression. If bleeding is absent at any given site in the mouth, reflecting good plaque control and disease management, it is unlikely that periodontal disease will progress.[88]

Instruction and Demonstration

Patients can reduce the incidence of plaque and gingivitis with repeated instruction and encouragement much more effectively than with self-acquired oral hygiene habits.[58,128] However, instruction in how to clean teeth must be more than a cursory chairside demonstration on the use of a toothbrush. It is a painstaking procedure that requires patient participation, careful supervision with correction of mistakes, and reinforcement during return visits, until the patient demonstrates that he or she has developed the necessary proficiency.[5,91]

Any strategy for introducing plaque control to the periodontal patient includes several elements. At the first instruction visit, the patient should be given a new toothbrush, an interdental cleaner, and a disclosing agent. The patient's plaque should be disclosed because dental plaque otherwise is difficult for the patient to see (see Figure 50-17, *A*). Be sure to have the patient rinse to remove excess dye and stained saliva so that the stained plaque and pellicle can be shown to the patient (see Figure 50-17, *B*). Polished dental restorations do not take up the stain, but the oral mucosa and the lips may retain it for up to several hours. Use petroleum jelly to keep the dye off the patient's lips.

Toothbrushing should be demonstrated in the patient's mouth while the patient observes with a hand mirror. The patient then takes over and repeats the procedures on the teeth with the instructor giving assistance, correction, and positive reinforcement.

Repeat the demonstration and instruction process with dental floss and interdental cleaning aids according to the patient's needs. The teeth can be restained to evaluate the efficiency of plaque removal, but even after vigorous cleaning, some stain usually remains on proximal surfaces.

Teaching videos and pamphlets can be used to augment personalized instruction, but they are not a substitute; reminder pamphlets may be useful for the patient to take home. More importantly, however, the patient should be given the hygiene aids necessary to start the process.

Encourage your patients to clean the teeth thoroughly at least once a day. Be sure to inform them that home care procedures on a full dentition take 5 to 10 minutes, and for complex periodontal maintenance cases, home care procedures may take 30 minutes. The patient should set aside a convenient time and place in the daily schedule to perform the procedures reliably every day. Subsequent instruction visits should be used to reinforce or modify previous instructions, periodically recording the state of gingival health and amount of plaque.

Recommendations

The following list provides some strategies that will assist you in educating and motivating your patients:

- Provide encouragement.
- Demonstrate how devices work, and allow the patient to practice with them.
- Provide samples so that the patient does not have to stop and buy products on the way home; the patient may not follow through with the purchase.
- Show improvements at subsequent appointments, even if they are modest.
- Use positive reinforcement[129]; threats are not effective.

Also, some strategies simply do not work. Waiting until the end of the appointment, for example, when the patient is exhausted and likely anesthetized or when the patient is sore, is not conducive to education and shows insensitivity to the patient. Failing to provide positive reinforcement, handing the patient too many tools, and relying on pamphlets and printed material to provide education are likely to result in an insufficient or ineffective instruction process.

SUMMARY

- All patients require the regular use of a toothbrush, either manual or electric, at least once per day. The brushing method should emphasize access to the gingival margins of all accessible tooth surfaces and extension as far onto the proximal surfaces as possible.
- Dental floss should be used in all interdental spaces that are filled with gingiva. The technique requires

wrapping the floss around the proximal surfaces and inserting the floss into the sulcus, then cleaning with a controlled up-and-down motion. Flossing may be accomplished either with a tool or by using the fingers.
- Interdental aids such as interproximal brushes, wooden tips, rubber tips, or toothpicks should be used in all areas where the toothbrush and floss techniques cannot adequately remove the plaque. This includes large embrasure spaces and furcation areas.
- Caries control requires the daily use of a dentifrice with low-concentration fluoride. Topical oral rinses and gels with higher concentrations of fluoride should be used if the patient demonstrates caries risk.
- Daily at-home subgingival irrigation may be a good choice for reduction of inflammation and maintenance for patients with residual deep pockets and those who struggle with mechanical interproximal cleaning devices. The effectiveness of irrigation is enhanced by the addition of a chlorhexidine or essential oil rinse to the irrigation water.
- Chemical antimicrobial agents such as chlorhexidine and essential oils can be used to disinfect the patient's mouth and control infection. These oral rinses may be continued indefinitely; no specific duration for their use has been recommended, and many patients have used these rinses for years. Staining of teeth and taste alteration are side effects that may limit the use of these products.
- Reinforcement of daily plaque control practices and routine visits to the dental office for maintenance care are essential to successful plaque control and long-term success of therapy.

REFERENCES

1. Abrasivity of current dentifrices. Report of the Council of Dental Therapeutics, *J Am Dent Assoc* 81:1177, 1970.
2. Addy M, Adriaens P: Epidemiology and etiology of periodontal diseases and the role of plaque control in dental caries. In Lang NP, Ättstrom R, Löe H, editors: *Proceedings of the European Workshop on Mechanical Plaque Control,* Chicago, 1998, Quintessence.
3. American Academy of Periodontology, Committee Report: The tooth brush and methods of cleaning the teeth, *Dent Items Int* 42:193, 1920.
4. American Academy of Periodontology: Position paper: Treatment of gingivitis and periodontitis, *J Periodontol* 68:1246, 1997.
5. Anderson JL: Integration of plaque control into the practice of dentistry, *Dent Clin North Am* 16:621, 1972.
6. Anderson L, Sanz M, Newman MG, et al: Clinical effects of a 0.12% chlorhexidine mouthrinse on periodontal surgical wounds without periodontal dressing, *J Dent Res* 67:329, 1988 (abstract 1728).
7. Arnim SS: The use of disclosing agents for measuring tooth cleanliness, *J Periodontol* 34:227, 1963.
8. Ashley FP, Skinner A, Jackson P, et al: The effect of a 0.1% cetylpyridinium chloride mouthrinse on plaque and gingivitis in adult subjects, *Br Dent J* 157:191, 1984.
9. Ashley FP, Skinner A, Jackson PY, et al: Effect of a 0.1% cetylpyridinium chloride mouthrinse on the accumulation and biochemical composition of dental plaque in young adults, *Caries Res* 18:465, 1984.
10. Barrikman R, Penhall O: Graphing indexes reduce plaque, *J Am Dent Assoc* 87:1404, 1973.
11. Bass CC: The optimum characteristics of toothbrushes for personal oral hygiene, *Dent Items Int* 70:697, 1948.
12. Bass CC: An effective method of personal oral hygiene. Part II, *J La State Med Soc* 106:100, 1954.
13. Bauroth K, Charles C, Mankodi S, et al: Essential oil mouthrinses vs. flossing: antiplaque/antigingivitis efficacy, *J Dent Res* 8: 2867, 2002.
14. Baysan A, Lynch E, Ellwood R, et al: Reversal of primary root caries using dentifrices containing 5000 and 1100 ppm fluoride, *Caries Res* 35:41, 2001.
15. Biesbrock AR, Bayuk LM, Santana MV, et al: The clinical effectiveness of a novel power toothbrush and its impact on oral health, *J Contin Dent Pract* 3:1, 2002.
16. Beiswander BB, Mallott MC, Mau MS, et al: The relative plaque removal effect of a prebrushing mouthrinse, *J Am Dent Assoc* 120:190, 1990.
17. Binney A, Addy M, Newcombe RG: The plaque removal effects of single rinsings and brushings, *J Periodontol* 64:181, 1993.
18. Brandtzaeg P: The significance of oral hygiene in the prevention of dental diseases, *Odont T* 72:460, 1964.
19. Cantor MT, Stahl SS: The effects of various interdental stimulators upon the keratinization of the interdental col, *Periodontics* 3:243, 1965.
20. Cantor MT, Stahl SS: Interdental col tissue responses to the use of a water pressure device, *J Periodontol* 40:292, 1969.
21. Carter-Hanson C, Gadbury-Amyot C, Killoy WJ: Comparison of the plaque removal efficacy of a new flossing aid (Quik-Floss) to finger flossing, *J Clin Periodontol* 23:873, 1996.
22. Castenfelt T: *Toothbrushing and massage in periodontal disease: an experimental clinical histologic study,* Stockholm, 1952, Nordisk Rotegravyr.
23. Charles C, Sharma N, Qaaqish J, et al: Antiplaque/antigingivitis efficacy of an essential oil mouthrinse vs. flossing, *J Dent Res* 81:2866, 2002.
24. Charters WJ: Eliminating mouth infections with the toothbrush and other stimulating instruments, *Dent Digest* 38:130, 1932.
25. Chava VK: An evaluation of the efficacy of a curved bristle and conventional toothbrush: a comparative clinical study, *J Periodontol* 71:785, 2000.
26. Christou V, Timmerman MF, van der Velden U, et al: Comparison of different approaches of interdental oral hygiene: interdental brushes versus dental floss, *J Periodontol* 69:759, 1998.
27. Ciancio SC: Clinical benefits of powered subgingival irrigation, *Biol Ther Dent* 8:13, 1992.
28. Claydon N, Addy M: Comparative single-use plaque removal by toothbrushes of different designs, *J Clin Periodontol* 23:1112, 1996.
29. Cronin M, Dembling W: An investigation of the efficacy and safety of a new electric interdental plaque remover for the reduction of interproximal plaque and gingivitis, *J Clin Dent* 7:74, 1996.
30. Dajani AS, Taubert KA, Wilson W, et al: Prevention of bacterial endocarditis: recommendations by the American Heart Association, *J Am Dent Assoc* 128:1142, 1997.
31. Daly CG, Chapple CC, Cameron AC: Effect of toothbrush wear on plaque control, *J Clin Periodontol* 23:45, 1996.
32. Danser MM, Timmerman MF, Ijzerman Y, et al: Evaluation of the incidence of gingival abrasion as a result of toothbrushing, *J Clin Periodontol* 25:701, 1998.
33. De la Rosa MR, Guerra JZ, Johnston DA, et al: Plaque growth and removal with daily toothbrushing, *J Periodontol* 50:661, 1979.

34. De Paola LG, Overholser CD, Meiller TF, et al: Chemotherapeutic reduction of plaque and gingivitis development: a 6 month investigation, *J Dent Res* 65:274, 1986 (abstract 941).
35. Dentino AR, Kerkerian G, Wolf MA, et al: Six-month comparison of powered versus manual toothbrushing for safety and efficacy in the absence of professional instruction in mechanical plaque control, *J Periodontol* 73:770, 2002.
36. Drisko CH: Nonsurgical periodontal therapy: pharmacotherapeutics, *Ann Periodontol* 1:491, 1996.
37. Dyer D, Addy M, Newcombe RG: Studies in vitro of abrasion by different manual toothbrush heads and a standard toothpaste, *J Clin Periodontol* 27:99, 2000.
38. Eakle WS, Ford C, Boyd RL: Depth of penetration in periodontal pockets with oral irrigation, *J Clin Periodontol* 13:39, 1986.
39. Elmore JG, Horwitz JI: Oral cancer and mouthwash use: evaluation of the epidemiologic evidence, *Otolaryngol Head Neck Surg* 113:253, 1995.
40. Ervin JC, Bucher ET: Prevalence of tooth root exposure and abrasion among dental patients, *Dent Items Int* 66:7601, 1944.
41. Featherstone JD: Fluoride, remineralization and root caries, *Am J Dent* 7:271, 1994.
42. Featherstone JD: Prevention and reversal of dental caries: role of low level fluoride, *Community Dent Oral Epidemiol* 27:31, 1999.
43. Featherstone JD: The science and practice of caries prevention, *J Am Dent Assoc* 131:887, 2000.
44. Felix JA, Rosen S, App GR: Detection of bacteremia after the use of an oral irrigation device in subjects with periodontitis, *J Periodontol* 42:785, 1971.
45. Finkelstein P, Grossman E: The effectiveness of dental floss in reducing gingival inflammation, *J Dent Res* 58:1034, 1979.
46. Flemmig TF, Newman MG, Doherty FM, et al: Supragingival irrigation with 0.06% chlorhexidine in naturally occurring gingivitis. I. Six month clinical observations, *J Periodontol* 61:112, 1990.
47. Fones AC: *Mouth hygiene,* ed 4, Philadelphia, 1934, Lea & Febiger.
48. Forgas-Brockmann LB, Carter-Hanson C, Killoy WJ: The effects of an ultrasonic toothbrush on plaque accumulation and gingival inflammation, *J Clin Periodontol* 25:375, 1998.
49. Garmyn P, van Steenberghe D, Quirynen M. In Lang NP, Ättstrom R, Löe H, editors: *Proceedings of the European Workshop on Mechanical Plaque Control,* Chicago, 1998, Quintessence.
50. Gillette WB, van House RL: Ill effects of improper oral hygiene procedures, *J Am Dent Assoc* 101:476, 1980.
51. Gilson CM, Charbeneau GT, Hill HC: A comparison of physical properties of several soft toothbrushes, *J Mich Dent Assoc* 51:347, 1969.
52. Gjermo P, Flotra L: The plaque removing effect of dental floss and toothpicks: A group comparison study, *J Periodontal Res* 4:170, 1969 (abstract).
53. Gjermo P, Flotra L: The effect of different methods of interdental cleaning, *J Periodontal Res* 5:230, 1970.
54. Glickman I, Petralis R, Marks R: The effect of powered toothbrushing plus interdental stimulation upon the severity of gingivitis, *J Periodontol* 35:519, 1964.
55. Glickman I, Petralis R, Marks R: The effect of powered toothbrushing and interdental stimulation upon microscopic inflammation and surface keratinization of the interdental gingiva, *J Periodontol* 36:108, 1965.
56. Gordon JM, Lamster IV, Seiger MC: Efficacy of Listerine antiseptic in inhibiting the development of plaque and gingivitis, *J Clin Periodontol* 12:697, 1985.
57. Gordon JM, Frascella JA, Reardon RC: A clinical study of the safety and efficacy of a novel electric interdental cleaning device, *J Clin Dent* 7:70, 1996.
58. Gravelle HR, Shackelford NF, Lovett JT: The oral hygiene of high school students as affected by three different educational programs, *J Public Health Dent* 27:91, 1967.
59. Greenstein G: Effects of subgingival irrigation on periodontal status, *J Periodontol* 58:827, 1987.
60. Grossman E, Reiter G, Sturzenberger OP, et al: Six-month study of the effects of a chlorhexidine mouthrinse on gingivitis in adults, *J Periodontal Res* 21(suppl):33, 1986.
61. Hancock EP: Prevention, *Ann Periodontol* 1:223, 1996.
62. Harrington JH, Terry IA: Automatic and hand toothbrushing abrasion studies, *J Am Dent Assoc* 68:343, 1964.
63. Harris NO: Dentifrices, mouth rinses, and oral irrigators. In Harris NO, Christen AG, editors: *Primary preventive dentistry,* ed 3, East Norwalk, Conn, 1991, Appleton & Lange.
64. Heanue M, Deacon SA, Deery C, et al: Manual versus powered toothbrushing for oral health, *Cochrane Rev* 2, 2004.
65. Heasman PA, McCracken GI: Powered toothbrushes: a review of clinical trials, *J Clin Periodontol* 26:407, 1999.
66. Heasman PA, Jacobs DJ, Chapple IL: An evaluation of the effectiveness and patient compliance with plaque control methods in the prevention of periodontal disease, *J Clin Prev Dent* 11:24, 1989.
67. Hellstrom MK, Ramberg P, Krok L, et al: The effects of supragingival plaque control on subgingival microflora in human periodontitis, *J Clin Periodontol* 23:934, 1996.
68. Hill HC, Levi PA, Glickman I: The effects of waxed and unwaxed dental floss on interdental plaque accumulation and interdental gingival health, *J Periodontol* 44:411, 1973.
69. Hine MK: Toothbrush, *Int Dent J* 6:15, 1956.
70. Hiniker JJ, Forscher BK: The effect of toothbrush type on gingival health, *J Periodontol* 25:40, 1954.
71. Hirschfeld I: The toothbrush, its use and abuse, *Dent Items Int* 3:833, 1931.
72. Hollander BN, Boyd RL, Eakle WS: Comparison of subgingivally placed cannula oral irrigator tip with a supragingivally placed standard irrigator tip, *J Clin Periodontol* 19:340, 1992.
73. Hoover DR, Robinson HB, Billingsley A: The comparative effectiveness of the Water-Pik in a noninstructed population, *J Periodontol* 39:43, 1968 (abstract).
74. Hope CK, Petrie A, Wilson M: In vitro assessment of the plaque-removing ability of hydrodynamic shear forces produces beyond the bristles by 2 electric toothbrushes, *J Periodontol* 1017, 2003.
75. Jepson S: The role of manual toothbrushes in effective plaque control: advantages and limitations. In Lang NP, Ättstrom R, Löe H, editors: *Proceedings of the European Workshop on Mechanical Plaque Control,* Chicago, 1998, Quintessence.
76. Jolkovsky DL, Waki MY, Newman MN, et al: Clinical and microbiological effects of subgingival and gingival marginal irrigation with chlorhexidine gluconate, *J Periodontol* 61:663, 1990.
77. Kazmierczak M, Mather M, Ciancio S, et al: A clinical evaluation of anticalculus dentifrices, *J Clin Prev Dent* 12:13, 1990.
78. Keijser J, Verkade H, Timmerman M, et al: Comparison of 2 commercially available chlorhexidine mouthrinses, *J Periodontol* 74:214, 2003.
79. Keller SE, Manson-Hing LR: Clearance studies of proximal tooth surfaces. Part II. In vivo removal of interproximal plaque, *Ala J Med Sci* 6:266, 1969.
80. Keller SE, Manson-Hing LR: Clearance studies of proximal tooth surfaces. Parts III and IV. In vivo removal of interproximal plaque, *Ala J Med Sci* 6:399, 1969.

81. Khocht A, Simon G, Person P, et al: Gingival recession in relation to history of hard toothbrush use, *J Periodontol* 64:900, 1993.
82. Kieser J, Groeneveld H: A clinical evaluation of a novel toothbrush design, *J Clin Periodontol* 24:419, 1997.
83. Kinane DF: The role of interdental cleaning in effective plaque control: need for interdental cleaning in primary and secondary prevention. In Lang NP, Ättstrom R, Löe H, editors: *Proceedings of the European Workshop on Mechanical Plaque Control,* Chicago, 1998, Quintessence.
84. Lamster IB, Alfano MC, Seiger MC, et al: The effect of Listerine antiseptic on reduction of existing plaque and gingivitis, *J Clin Prev Dent* 5:12, 1983.
85. Lang NP, Brecx MC: Chlorhexidine digluconate: an agent for chemical plaque control and prevention of gingival inflammation, *J Periodontal Res* 21(suppl):74, 1986.
86. Lang NP, Cumming BR, Löe H: Toothbrushing frequency as it relates to plaque development and gingival health, *J Periodontol* 44:396, 1973.
87. Lang NP, Hotz P, Graf H, et al: Effects of supervised chlorhexidine mouthrinses in children: a longitudinal clinical trial, *J Periodontal Res* 17:101, 1982.
88. Lang NP, Joss A, Orsanic T, et al: Bleeding on probing: a predictor for the progression of periodontal diseases? *J Clin Periodontol* 13:590, 1986.
89. Lenox JA, Kopczyk RA: A clinical system for scoring a patient's oral hygiene performance, *J Am Dent Assoc* 86:849, 1973.
90. Leonard JF: Conservative treatment of periodontoclasia, *J Am Dent Assoc* 26:1308, 1939.
91. Less W: Mechanics of teaching plaque control, *Dent Clin North Am* 16:647, 1972.
92. Leverett DH, McHugh WD, Jensen DE: Effect of daily rinsing with stannous fluoride on plaque and gingivitis: final report, *J Dent Res* 63:1083, 1984.
93. Lewis MW, Holder-Ballard C, Selders RJ Jr, et al: Comparison of the use of a toothpick holder to dental floss in improvement of gingival health in humans, *J Periodontol* 75:551, 2004.
94. Lindhe J, Nyman S: The effect of plaque control and surgical pocket elimination on the establishment and maintenance of periodontal health: a longitudinal study of periodontal therapy in cases of advanced disease, *J Clin Periodontol* 2:67, 1975.
95. Lobene RR: The effect of a pulsed water pressure cleaning device on oral health, *J Periodontol* 40:667, 1969.
96. Löe H: Does chlorhexidine have a place in the prophylaxis of dental disease? *J Periodontal Res* 8(suppl 12):93, 1973.
97. Löe H, Schiott CR: The effect of mouthrinses and topical application of chlorhexidine on the development of dental plaque and gingivitis in man, *J Periodontal Res* 5:79, 1970.
98. Löe H, Theilade E, Jensen SB: Experimental gingivitis in man, *J Periodontol* 36:177, 1965.
99. Macgregor ID, Balding JW, Regis D: Flossing behaviour in English adolescents, *J Clin Periodontol* 25:291, 1998.
100. MacNeill S, Walter DM, Day A, et al: Sonic and mechanical toothbrushes an in vitro study showing altered microbial surface structures but lack of effect on viability, *J Clin Periodontol* 25:988, 1998.
101. Mallatt ME, Beiswanger BB, Stookey GK, et al: Influence of soluble pyrophosphates on calculus formation in adults, *J Dent Res* 64:1159, 1985.
102. Manly RS, Brudevold F: Relative abrasiveness of natural and synthetic toothbrush bristles on cementum and dentin, *J Am Dent Assoc* 55:779, 1957.
103. Mauriello SM, Bader JD: Six-month effects of a sanguinarine dentifrice on plaque and gingivitis, *J Periodontol* 59:238, 1988.
104. McKendrick AJ, Barbenel LM, McHugh WD: A two-year comparison of hand and electric toothbrushes, *J Periodontal Res* 3:224, 1968.
105. McKendrick AJ, Barbenel LM, McHugh WD: The influence of time of examination, eating, smoking, and frequency of brushing on the oral debris index, *J Periodontal Res* 5:205, 1970.
106. Mueller-Joseph LM, Davis C, Jones B: Oral irrigation and antimicrobial plaque control. In Woodall IR, editor: *Comprehensive dental hygiene care,* ed 4, St Louis, 1993, Mosby.
107. Novaes AB, Novaes AB Jr, Moraes N, et al: Compliance with supportive periodontal therapy, *J Periodontol* 67:213, 1996.
108. O'Leary TJ, Drake RB, Naylor JE: The plaque control record, *J Periodontol* 43:38, 1972.
109. O'Leary TJ, Shafer WG, Swenson HM, et al: Possible penetration of crevicular tissue from oral hygiene procedures. II. Use of the toothbrush, *J Periodontol* 41:158, 1970.
110. Parsons LG, Thomas LG, Southard GL, et al: Effect of sanguinaria extract on established plaque and gingivitis when supragingivally delivered as a manual rinse or under pressure in an oral irrigator, *J Clin Periodontol* 14:381, 1987.
111. Pattison GA: Self-inflicted gingival injuries: literature review and case report, *J Periodontol* 54:299, 1983.
112. Perry DA, Pattison G: The investigation of wax residue on tooth surfaces after the use of waxed dental floss, *Dent Hygiene* 60:16, 1986.
113. *Proceedings of the European Workshop on Mechanical Plaque Control,* Chicago, 1998, Quintessence.
114. Renvert S, Glavind L: Individualized instruction and compliance in oral hygiene practices: recommendations and means of delivery. In Lang NP, Ättstrom R, Löe H, editors: *Proceedings of the European Workshop on Mechanical Plaque Control,* Chicago, 1998, Quintessence.
115. Robinson HB, Hoover PR: The comparative effectiveness of a pulsating oral irrigator as an adjunct in maintaining oral health, *J Periodontol* 42:37, 1971.
116. Sangnes G: Traumatization of teeth and gingiva related to habitual tooth cleaning procedures, *J Clin Periodontol* 3:94, 1976.
117. Sangnes G, Gjermo P: Prevalence of oral soft and hard tissue lesions related to mechanical tooth cleaning procedures, *Community Dent Oral Epidemiol* 4:77, 1976.
118. Sanz M, Herrera D: Role of oral hygiene during the healing phase of periodontal therapy. In Lang NP, Ättstrom R, Löe H, editors: *Proceedings of the European Workshop on Mechanical Plaque Control,* Chicago, 1998, Quintessence.
119. Schmid MO, Balmelli O, Saxer UP: The plaque removing effect of a toothbrush, dental floss and a toothpick, *J Clin Periodontol* 3:157, 1976.
120. Shiloah J, Hovious LA: The role of subgingival irrigations in the treatment of periodontitis, *J Periodontol* 64:835, 1993.
121. Silness J, Löe H: Periodontal disease in pregnancy. II. Correlation between oral hygiene and periodontal condition, *Acta Odontol Scand* 22:121, 1964.
122. Silverstone LM, Featherstone MJ: A scanning electron microscope study of the end rounding of bristles in eight toothbrush types, *Quintessence Int* 19:87, 1988.
123. Spolsky VA, Perry DA, Meng Z, et al: Evaluating the efficacy of a new flossing aid, *J Clin Periodontol* 20:490, 1993.
124. Stillman PR: A philosophy of the treatment of periodontal disease, *Dent Digest* 38:314, 1932.
125. Stookey G: Are all fluoride dentifrices the same? In Wei SHY, editor: *Clinical uses of fluorides,* Philadelphia, 1985, Lea & Febiger.
126. Stookey GK, Muhler JC: Laboratory studies concerning the enamel and dentin abrasion properties of common dentifrice polishing agents, *J Dent Res* 47:524, 1968.

127. Straub AM, Salvi GE, Lang NP: Supragingival plaque formation in the human dentition. In Lang NP, Ättstrom R, Löe H, editors: *Proceedings of the European Workshop on Mechanical Plaque Control,* Chicago, 1998, Quintessence.
128. Suomi JD, Green JC, Vermillion JR, et al: The effect of controlled oral hygiene procedures on the progression of periodontal disease in adults: results after two years, *J Periodontol* 40:416, 1969.
129. Tedesco LA, Keffler MA, Davis EL, et al: Effect of a social cognitive intervention on oral health status, behavior reports, and cognition, *J Periodontol* 63:567, 1992.
130. Tritten CB, Armitage GA: Comparison of a sonic and a manual toothbrush for efficacy in supragingival plaque removal and reduction of gingivitis, *J Clin Periodontol* 23:641, 1996.
131. Van der Weijden GA, Timmerman MF, Danser MM, et al: Relationship between the plaque removal efficacy of a natural toothbrush and brushing force, *J Clin Periodontol* 25:413, 1998.
132. Van der Weijden GA, Timmerman MF, Danser MM, et al: The role of electric toothbrushes: advantages and limitations. In Lang NP, Ättstrom R, Löe H, editors: *Proceedings of the European Workshop on Mechanical Plaque Control,* Chicago, 1998, Quintessence.
133. Waerhaug J: The interdental brush and its place in operative and crown and bridge dentistry, *J Oral Rehabil* 3:107, 1976.
134. Waki MY, Jolkovsky DL, Otomo-Corgel J, et al: Effects of subgingival irrigation on bacteremia following scaling and root planing, *J Periodontol* 61:405, 1990.
135. Warren PR, Ray TS, Cugini M, et al: A practice-based study of a power toothbrush: assessment of effectiveness and acceptance, *J Am Dent Assoc* 131:389, 2000.
136. Wefel JS: Root caries histopathology and chemistry, *Am J Dent* 7:261, 1994.
137. Wilkins EM: Oral disease control: toothbrushes and toothbrushing. In *Clinical practice of the dental hygienist,* ed 6, Philadelphia, 1992, Lea & Febiger.
138. Wilson TG Jr, Glover ME, Schoen J, et al: Compliance with maintenance therapy in a private dental practice, *J Periodontol* 55:468, 1984.
139. Yankell SL: Toothbrushing and toothbrushing techniques. In Harris NO, Christen AG, editors: *Primary preventive dentistry,* ed 3, East Norwalk, Conn, 1991, Appleton & Lange.
140. Yukna RA, Broxson AW, Mayer ET, et al: Comparison of Listerine mouthwash and periodontal dressing following periodontal flap surgery, *Clin Prev Dent* 4:14, 1986.
141. Zacheri WA, Pheiffer HJ, Swancar JR: The effect of soluble pyrophosphates on dental calculus in adults, *J Am Dent Assoc* 110:737, 1985.
142. Zimmer S, Didner B, Roulet JF: Clinical study on the plaque-removing ability of a new triple-headed toothbrush, *J Clin Periodontol* 26:281, 1999.

Scaling and Root Planing

Anna M. Pattison and Gordon L. Pattison

51 CHAPTER

CHAPTER OUTLINE

Periodontal instruments are designed for specific purposes, such as removing calculus, planing root surfaces, curetting the gingiva, and removing diseased tissue. On first investigation, the variety of instruments available for similar purposes appears confusing. With experience, however, clinicians select a relatively small set that fulfills all requirements.

CLASSIFICATION OF PERIODONTAL INSTRUMENTS

Periodontal instruments are classified according to the purposes they serve, as follows:

1. *Periodontal probes* are used to locate, measure, and mark pockets, as well as determine their course on individual tooth surfaces.
2. *Explorers* are used to locate calculus deposits and caries.
3. *Scaling, root-planing, and curettage instruments* are used for removal of plaque and calcified deposits from the crown and root of a tooth, removal of altered cementum from the subgingival root surface, and debridement of the soft tissue lining the pocket. Scaling and curettage instruments are classified as follows:
   - *Sickle scalers* are heavy instruments used to remove supragingival calculus.
   - *Curettes* are fine instruments used for subgingival scaling, root planing, and removal of the soft tissue lining the pocket.
   - *Hoe, chisel, and file scalers* are used to remove tenacious subgingival calculus and altered cementum. Their use is limited compared with that of curettes.
   - *Ultrasonic and sonic instruments* are used for scaling and cleansing tooth surfaces and curetting the soft tissue wall of the periodontal pocket.[39,40,58]
4. The *periodontal endoscope* is used to visualize deeply into subgingival pockets and furcations, allowing the detection of deposits.
5. *Cleansing and polishing instruments,* such as rubber cups, brushes, and dental tape, are used to clean and

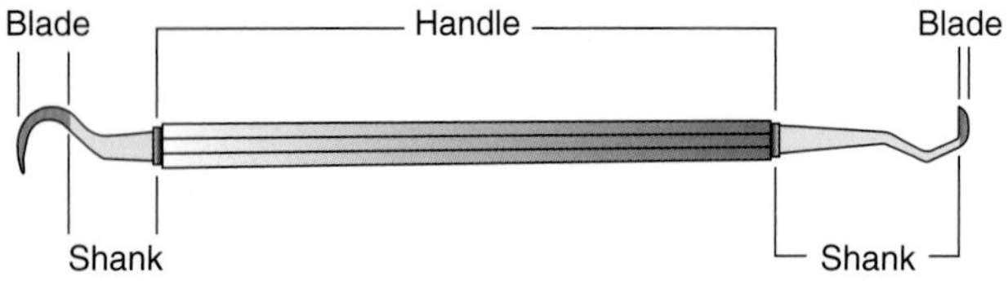

Figure 51-1 Parts of a typical periodontal instrument.

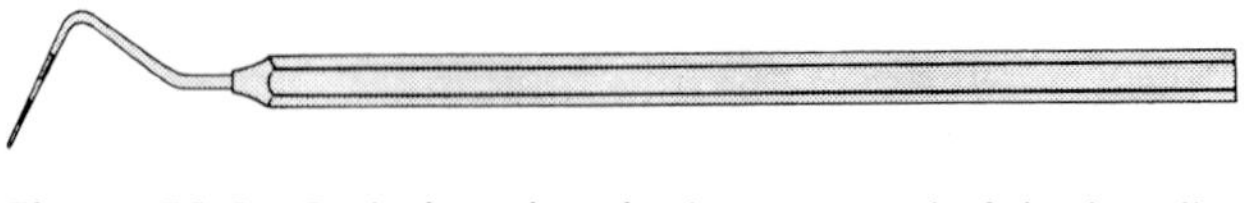

Figure 51-2 Periodontal probe is composed of the handle, shank, and calibrated working end.

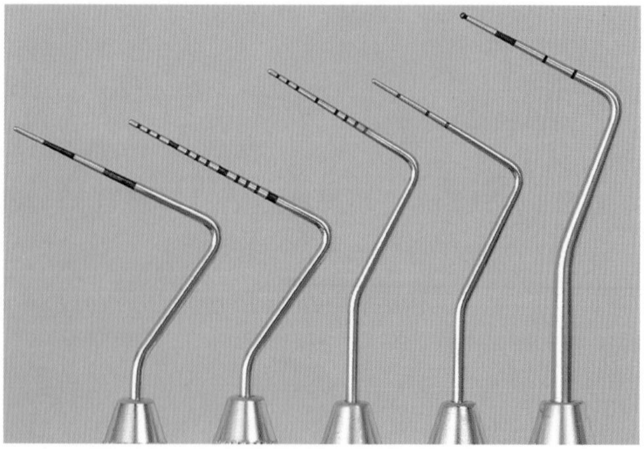

Figure 51-3 Types of periodontal probes. **A,** Marquis color-coded probe. Calibrations are in 3-mm sections. **B,** UNC-15 probe, a 15-mm-long probe with millimeter markings at each millimeter and color coding at the fifth, tenth, and fifteenth millimeters. **C,** University of Michigan "O" probe, with Williams markings (at 1, 2, 3, 5, 7, 8, 9, and 10 mm). **D,** Michigan "O" probe with markings at 3, 6, and 8 mm. **E,** World Health Organization (WHO) probe, which has a 0.5-mm ball at the tip and millimeter markings at 3.5, 8.5, and 11.5 mm and color coding from 3.5 to 5.5 mm.

polish tooth surfaces. Also available are *air-powder abrasive systems* for tooth polishing.

The wearing and cutting qualities of some types of steel used in periodontal instruments have been tested,[82,83,142] but specifications vary among manufacturers.[142] Stainless steel is used most often in instrument manufacture. High-carbon-content steel instruments are also available and are considered by some clinicians to be superior.

Each group of instruments has characteristic features; individual therapists often develop variations with which they operate most effectively. Small instruments are recommended to fit into periodontal pockets without injuring the soft tissues.[105,157]

The parts of each instrument are referred to as the *working end, shank,* and *handle* (Figure 51-1).

Periodontal Probes

Periodontal probes are used to measure the depth of pockets and to determine their configuration. The typical probe is a tapered, rodlike instrument calibrated in millimeters, with a blunt, rounded tip (Figure 51-2). There are several other designs with various millimeter calibrations (Figure 51-3). The World Health Organization (WHO) probe has millimeter markings and a small, round ball at the tip (Figure 51-3, *E*). Ideally, these probes are thin, and the shank is angled to allow easy insertion into the pocket. Furcation areas can best be evaluated with the curved, blunt Nabers probe (Figure 51-4).

When measuring a pocket, the probe is inserted with a firm, gentle pressure to the bottom of the pocket. The shank should be aligned with the long axis of the tooth surface to be probed. Several measurements are made to determine the level of attachment along the surface of the tooth.

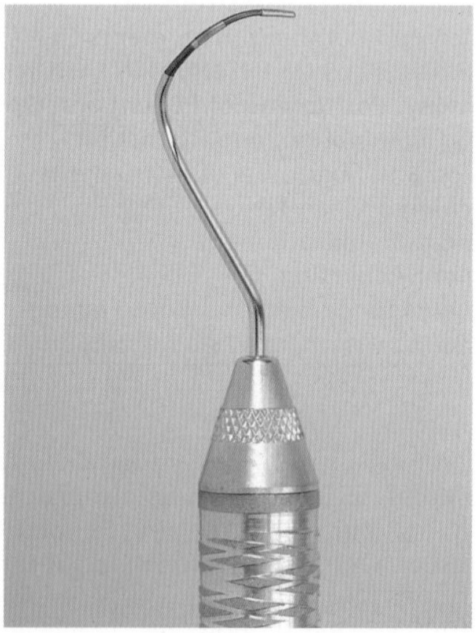

Figure 51-4 Curved #2 Nabers probe for detection of furcation areas, with color-coded markings at 3, 6, 9, and 12 mm.

Explorers

Explorers are used to locate subgingival deposits and carious areas and to check the smoothness of the root surfaces after root planing. Explorers are designed with different shapes and angles, with various uses (Figure 51-5), as well as limitations (Figure 51-6). The periodontal probe can also be useful in the detection of subgingival deposits (Figure 51-6, *D*).

Scaling and Curettage Instruments

Scaling and curettage instruments are illustrated in Figure 51-7.

Sickle Scalers (Supragingival Scalers). Sickle scalers have a flat surface and two cutting edges that

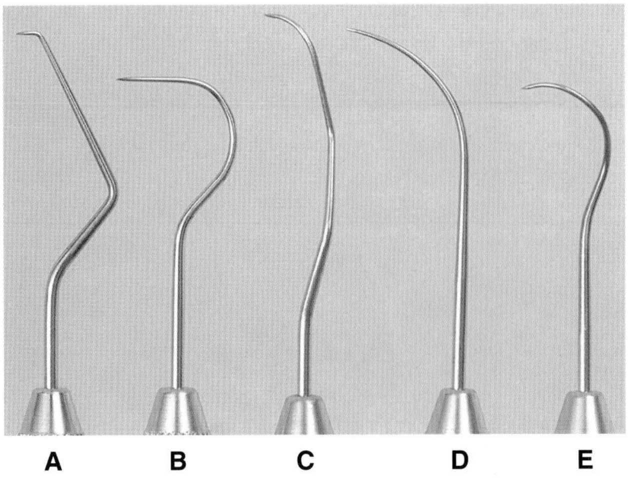

Figure 51-5 Five typical explorers. **A,** #17; **B,** #23; **C,** EXD 11-12; **D,** #3; **E,** #3CH Pigtail.

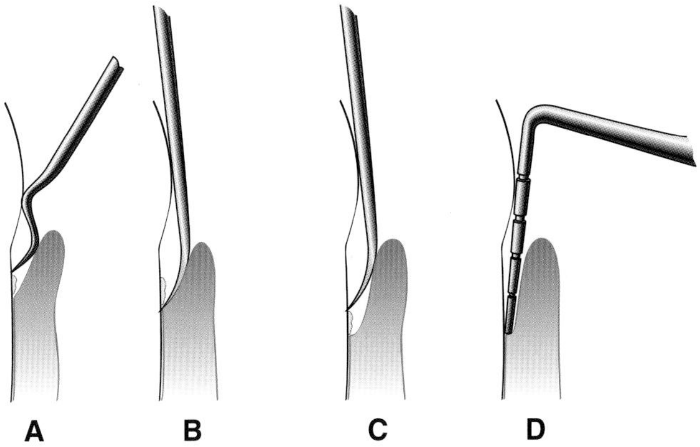

Figure 51-6 Insertion of two types of explorers and a periodontal probe in a pocket for calculus detection. **A,** The limitations of the pigtail explorer in a deep pocket. **B,** Insertion of the #3 explorer. **C,** Limitations of the #3 explorer. **D,** Insertion of the periodontal probe.

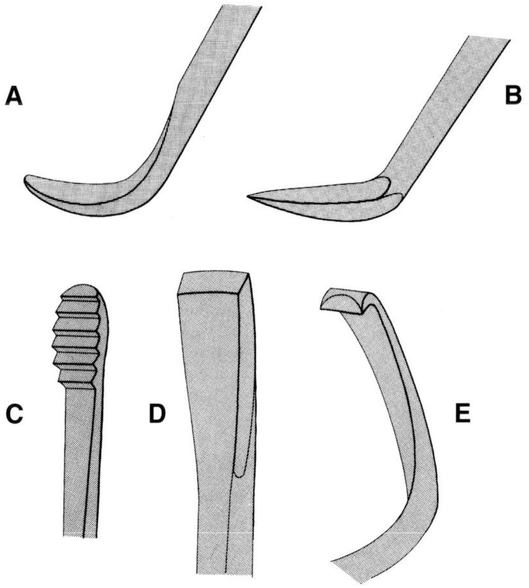

Figure 51-7 The five basic scaling instruments. **A,** Curette; **B,** sickle; **C,** file; **D,** chisel; **E,** hoe.

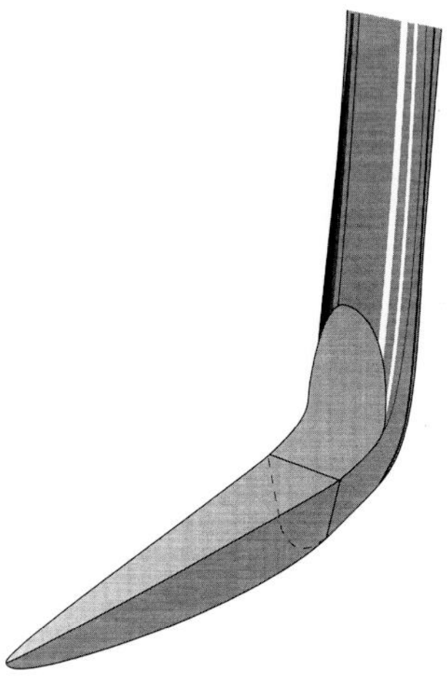

Figure 51-8 Basic characteristics of a sickle scaler: triangular shape, double-cutting edge, and pointed tip.

converge in a sharply pointed tip. The shape of the instrument makes the tip strong so that it will not break off during use (Figure 51-8). The sickle scaler is used primarily to remove supragingival calculus (Figure 51-9). Because of the design of this instrument, it is difficult to insert a large sickle blade under the gingiva without damaging the surrounding gingival tissues (Figure 51-10). Small, curved sickle scaler blades such as the 204SD can be inserted under ledges of calculus a few millimeters below the gingiva. Sickle scalers are used with a pull stroke.

It is important to note that sickle scalers with the same basic design can be obtained with different blade sizes and shank types to adapt to specific uses. The U15/30 (Figure 51-11), Ball, and Indiana University sickle scalers are large. The Jaquette sickle scalers #1, 2, and 3 have medium-size blades. The curved 204 sickle scalers are available with large, medium, or small blades (Figure 51-12). The Nevi 2 posterior sickle scaler is a new design that is thin enough to be inserted several millimeters subgingivally for removal of moderate ledges of calculus. The selection of these instruments should be based on the area to be scaled. Sickle scalers with straight shanks are designed for use on anterior teeth and premolars. Sickle scalers with contra-angled shanks adapt to posterior teeth.

Curettes. The curette is the instrument of choice for removing deep subgingival calculus, root planing altered cementum, and removing the soft tissue lining the periodontal pocket (Figure 51-13). Each working end has a cutting edge on both sides of the blade and a rounded toe. The curette is finer than the sickle scalers and does not have any sharp points or corners other than the cutting edges of the blade (Figure 51-14). Therefore, curettes can be adapted and provide good access to deep pockets, with minimal soft tissue trauma (see Figure

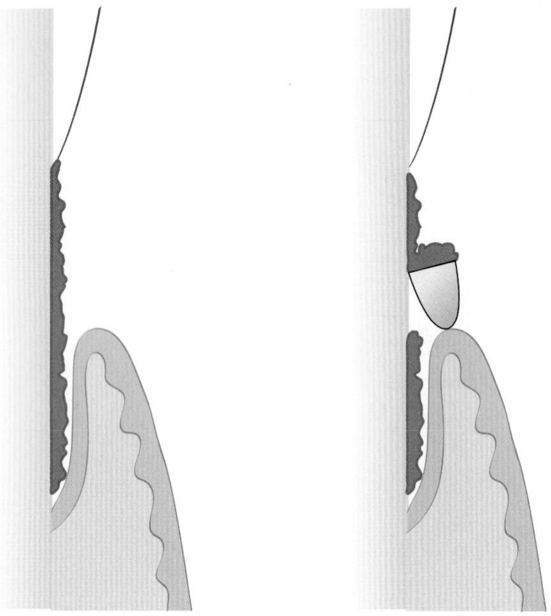

Figure 51-9 Use of a sickle scaler for removal of supragingival calculus.

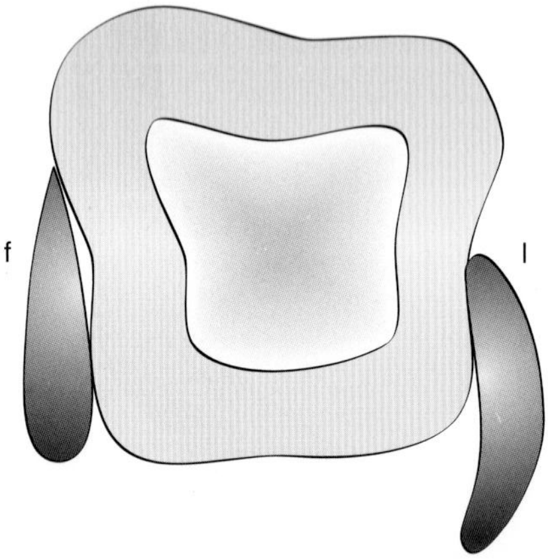

Figure 51-10 Subgingival adaptation around the root is better with the curette than with the sickle; *f,* facial; *l,* lingual.

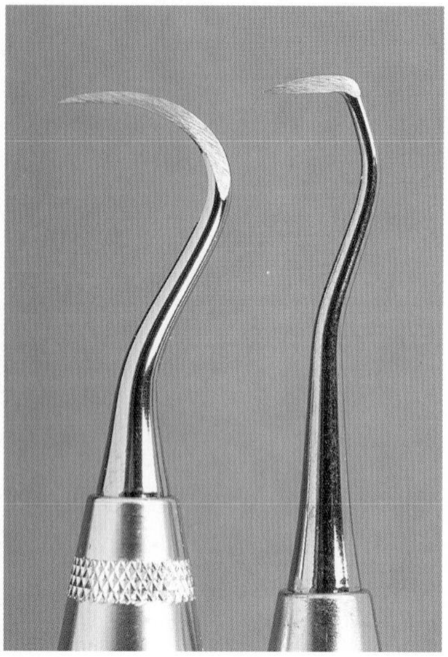

Figure 51-11 Both ends of a U15/30 scaler.

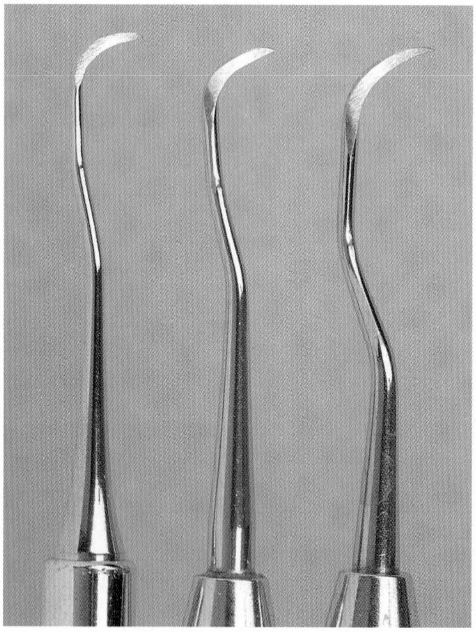

Figure 51-12 Three different sizes of 204 sickle scalers.

51-10). In cross section the blade appears semicircular with a convex base. The lateral border of the convex base forms a cutting edge with the face of the semicircular blade. There are cutting edges on both sides of the blade. Both single-end and double-end curettes may be obtained, depending on the preference of the operator.

As shown in Figure 51-10, the curved blade and rounded toe of the curette allow the blade to adapt better to the root surface, unlike the straight design and pointed end of a sickle scaler, which can cause tissue laceration and trauma. There are two basic types of curettes: universal and area specific.

Universal Curettes. Universal curettes have cutting edges that may be inserted in most areas of the dentition by altering and adapting the finger rest, fulcrum, and hand position of the operator. The blade size and the angle and length of the shank may vary, but the face of the blade of every universal curette is at a 90-degree angle (perpendicular) to the lower shank when seen in cross section from the tip (Figure 51-15, *A*). The blade of the universal curette is curved in one direction from the head of the blade to the toe. The Barnhart curettes #1-2 and 5-6 and the Columbia curettes #13-14, 2R-2L, and 4R-4L (Figures 51-16 and 51-17, *A*) are examples of universal curettes. Other popular universal curettes are the Younger-Good #7-8, the McCall's #17-18, and the Indiana University #17-18 (Figure 51-17, *B*).

Area-Specific Curettes

Gracey Curettes. Gracey curettes are representative of the area-specific curettes, a set of several instruments

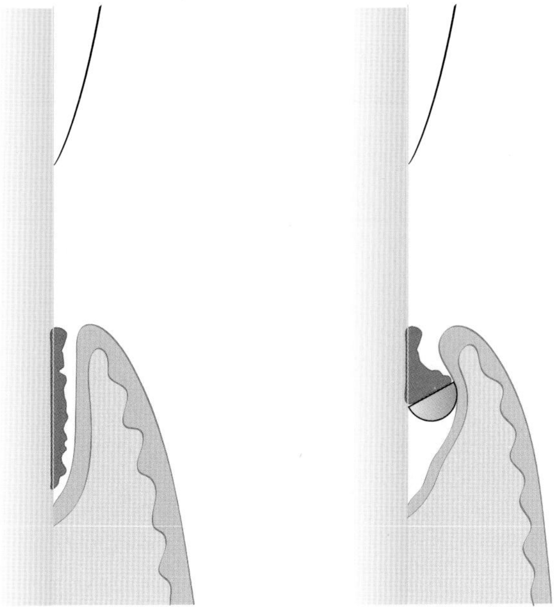

Figure 51-13 The curette is the instrument of choice for subgingival scaling and root planing.

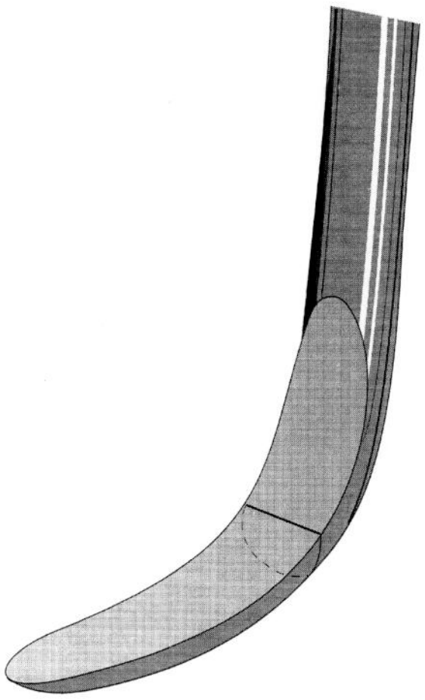

Figure 51-14 Basic characteristics of a curette: spoon-shaped blade and rounded tip.

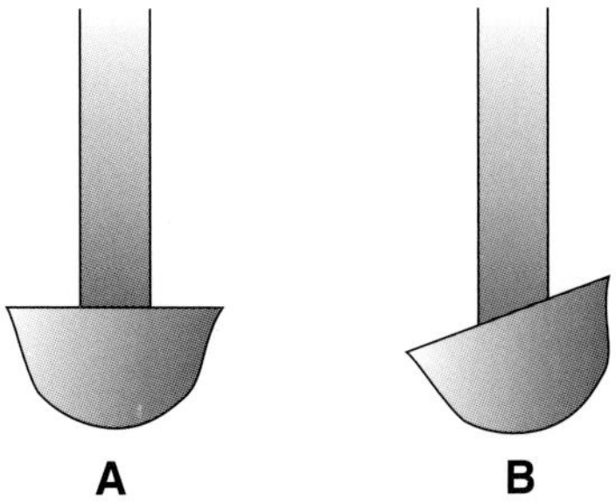

Figure 51-15 Principal types of curettes as seen from the toe of the instrument. **A,** Universal curette. **B,** Gracey curette. Note the offset blade angulation of the Gracey curette.

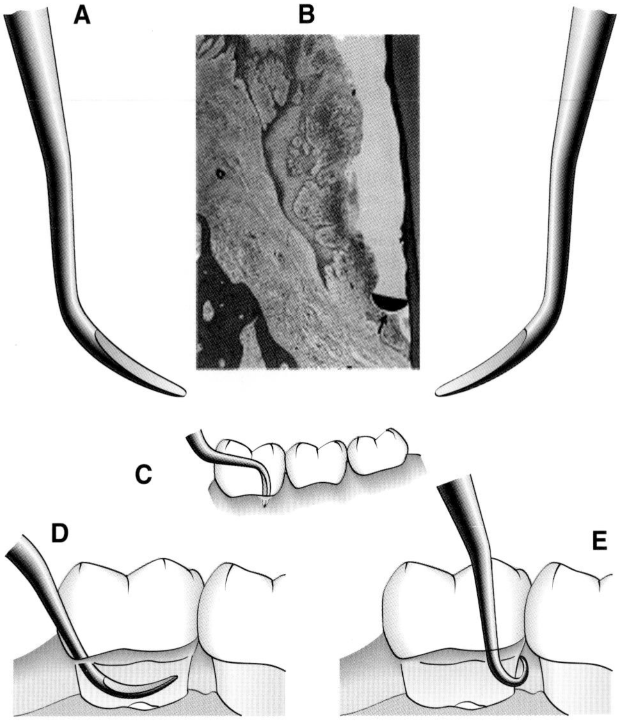

Figure 51-16 **A,** Double-ended curette for the removal of subgingival calculus. **B,** Cross section of the curette blade *(arrow)* against the cemental wall of a deep periodontal pocket. **C,** Curette in position at the base of a periodontal pocket on the facial surface of a mandibular molar. **D,** Curette inserted in a pocket with the tip directed apically. **E,** Curette in position at the base of a pocket on the distal surface of the mandibular molar.

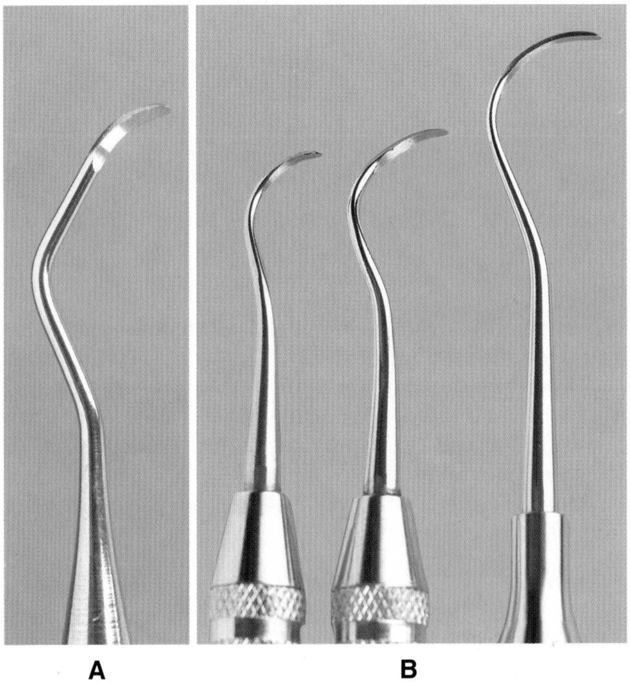

Figure 51-17 **A,** Columbia #4R-4L universal curette. **B,** Younger-Good #7-8, McCall's #17-18, and Indiana University #17-18 universal curettes.

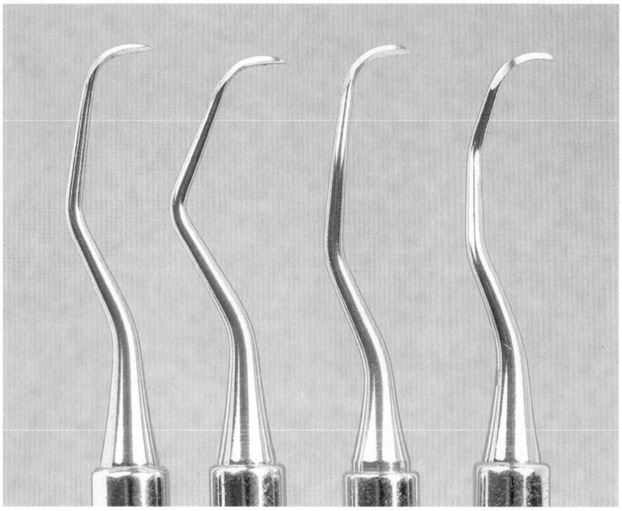

Figure 51-18 Reduced set of Gracey curettes. *From left,* #5-6, #7-8, #11-12, and #13-14.

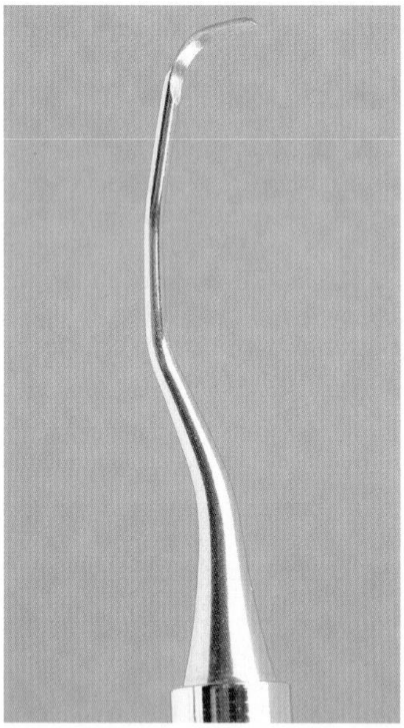

Figure 51-19 Gracey #11-12 curette. Note the double turn of the shank.

designed and angled to adapt to specific anatomic areas of the dentition (Figure 51-18).

These curettes and their modifications are probably the best instruments for subgingival scaling and root planing because they provide the best adaptation to complex root anatomy.

Double-ended Gracey curettes are paired in the following manner:

Gracey #1-2 and 3-4: Anterior teeth
Gracey #5-6: Anterior teeth and premolars
Gracey #7-8 and 9-10: Posterior teeth: facial and lingual
Gracey #11-12: Posterior teeth: mesial (Figure 51-19)
Gracey #13-14: Posterior teeth: distal (Figure 51-20)

Single-ended Gracey curettes can also be obtained; for these curettes a set comprises 14 instruments. Although

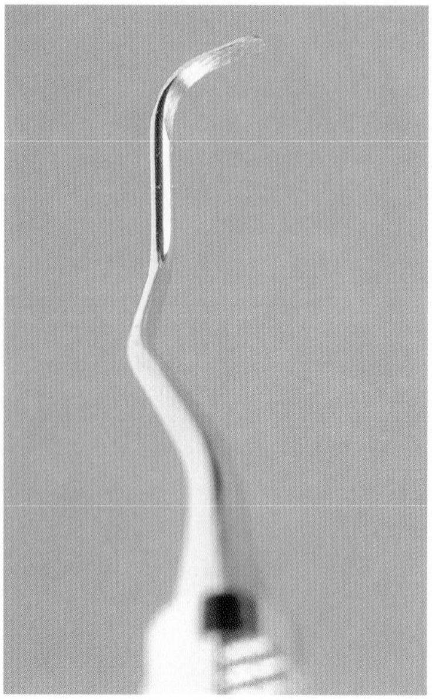

Figure 51-20 Gracey #13-14 curette. Note the acute turn of the blade.

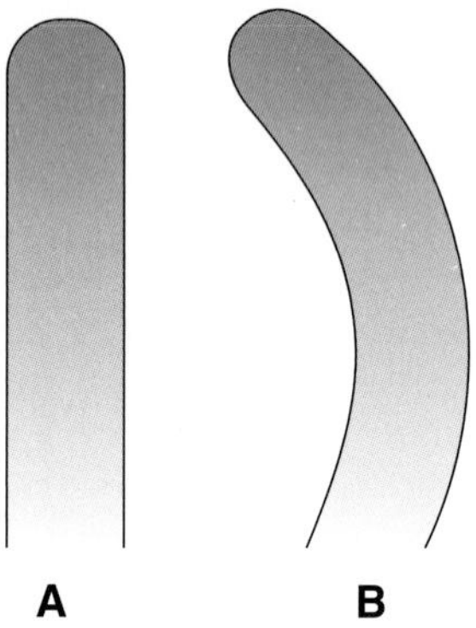

Figure 51-21 **A,** Universal curette as seen from the blade. Note that the blade is straight. **B,** Gracey curette as seen from the blade. The blade is curved; only the convex cutting edge is used.

these curettes are designed to be used in specific areas, an experienced operator can adapt each instrument for use in several different areas by altering the position of his or her hand and the position of the patient.

The Gracey curettes also differ from the universal curettes in that the blade is not at a 90-degree angle to the lower shank. The term *offset blade* is used to describe Gracey curettes, because they are angled approximately 60 to 70 degrees from the lower shank (see Figure 51-15, *B*). This unique angulation allows the blade to be inserted in the precise position necessary for subgingival scaling and root planing, provided that the lower shank is parallel with the long axis of the tooth surface being scaled.

Area-specific curettes also have a curved blade. Whereas the blade of the universal curette is curved in one direction (Figure 51-21, *A*), the Gracey blade is curved from head to toe and also along the side of the cutting

TABLE 51-1

Comparison of Area-Specific (Gracey) and Universal Curettes

	Gracey Curette	Universal Curette
Area of use	Set of many curettes designed for specific areas and surfaces.	One curette designed for all areas and surfaces.
Cutting Edge		
Use	One cutting edge used; work with outer edge only.	Both cutting edges used; work with either outer or inner edge.
Curvature	Curved in two planes; blade curves up and to the side.	Curved in one plane; blade curves up, not to the side.
Blade angle	Offset blade; face of blade beveled at 60 degrees to shank.	Blade not offset; face of blade beveled at 90 degrees to shank.

Modified from Pattison G, Pattison A: *Periodontal instrumentation,* ed 2, Norwalk, Conn, 1992, Appleton & Lange.

edge (Figure 51-21, *B*). Thus, only a pull stroke can be used. Table 51-1 lists some of the major differences between Gracey (area-specific) curettes and universal curettes.

Gracey curettes are available with either a "rigid" or a "finishing" type of shank. The rigid Gracey has a larger, stronger, and less flexible shank and blade than the standard finishing Gracey. The rigid shank allows the removal of moderate to heavy calculus without using a separate set of heavy scalers, such as sickles and hoes. Although some clinicians prefer the enhanced tactile sensitivity that the flexible shank of the finishing Gracey provides, both types of Gracey curettes are suitable for root planing.

Recent additions to the Gracey curette set have been the Gracey #15-16 and 17-18. The Gracey #15-16 is a modification of the standard #11-12 and is designed for the mesial surfaces of posterior teeth (Figure 51-22). It consists of a Gracey #11-12 blade combined with the more acutely angled #13-14 shank. When the clinician is using an intraoral finger rest, it is often difficult to position the lower shank of the Gracey #11-12 so that it is parallel with the mesial surfaces of the posterior teeth, especially on the mandibular molars. The new shank angulation of the Gracey #15-16 allows better adaptation to posterior mesial surfaces from a front position with intraoral rests. If alternative fulcrums such as extraoral or opposite-arch rests are used, the Gracey #11-12 works well, and the new #15-16 is not essential. The Gracey #17-18 is a modification of the #13-14. It has a terminal shank elongated by 3 mm and a more accentuated angulation of the shank to provide complete occlusal clearance and better access to all posterior distal surfaces. The horizontal handle position minimizes interference from opposing arches and allows a more relaxed hand position when scaling distal surfaces. In addition, the blade is 1 mm shorter to allow better adaptation of the blade to distal tooth surfaces.

Extended-Shank Curettes. Extended-shank curettes, such as the *After Five* curettes (Hu-Friedy, Chicago), are modifications of the standard Gracey curette design. The terminal shank is 3 mm longer, allowing extension into deeper periodontal pockets of 5 mm or more (Figures 51-23 and 51-24). Other features of the After Five curette include a thinned blade for smoother subgingival insertion and reduced tissue distention and a large-diameter, tapered shank. All standard Gracey numbers except for the #9-10 (i.e., #1-2, 3-4, 5-6, 7-8, 11-12, 13-14) are available in the After Five series. The After Five curettes are available in finishing or rigid designs. For heavy or tenacious calculus removal, rigid After Five curettes should be used. For light scaling or deplaquing in a periodontal maintenance patient, the thinner, finishing After Five curettes will insert subgingivally more easily.

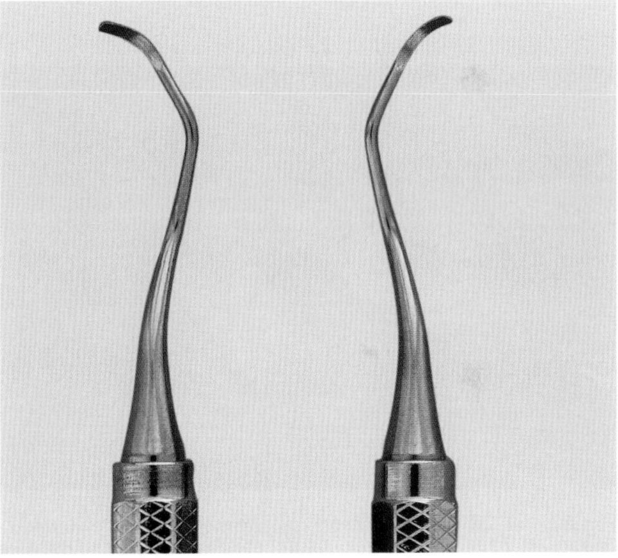

Figure 51-22 Gracey #15-16. New Gracey curette, designed for mesioposterior surfaces, combines a Gracey #11-12 blade with a Gracey #13-14 shank.

Mini-Bladed Curettes. Mini-bladed curettes, such as the Hu-Friedy *Mini Five* curettes, are modifications of the After Five curettes. The Mini Five curettes feature blades that are half the length of the After Five or standard Gracey curettes (Figure 51-25). The shorter blade

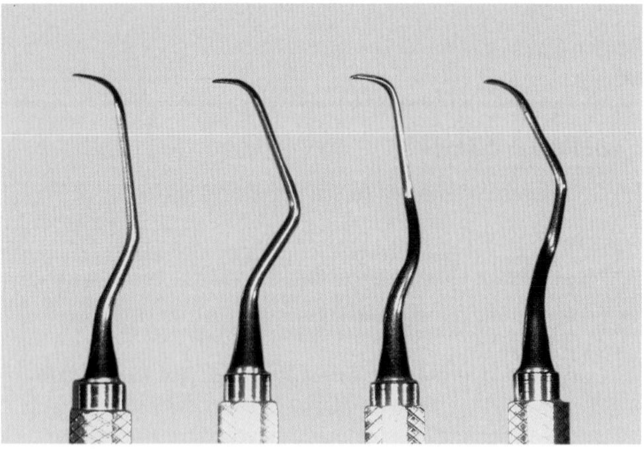

Figure 51-23 After Five curette. Note the extra 3 mm in the terminal shank of the After Five curette compared with the standard Gracey curette. **A,** #5-6; **B,** #7-8; **C,** #11-12; **D,** #13-14.

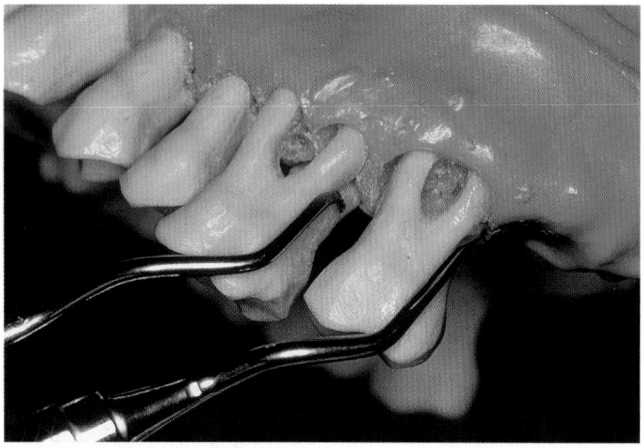

Figure 51-24 Comparison of After Five curette with standard Gracey curette. Rigid Gracey #13-14 adapted to the distal surface of the first molar and rigid After Five #13-14 adapted to the distal surface of the second molar. Notice the extralong shank of the After Five curette, which allows deeper insertion and better access.

allows easier insertion and adaptation in deep, narrow pockets; furcations; developmental grooves; line angles; and deep, tight, facial, lingual, or palatal pockets. In any area where root morphology or tight tissue prevents full insertion of the standard Gracey or After Five blade, the Mini Five curettes can be used with vertical strokes, with reduced tissue distention, and without tissue trauma (Figure 51-26).

In the past the only solution in most of these areas of difficult access was to use the Gracey curettes with a toe-down horizontal stroke. The Mini Five curettes, along with other short-bladed instruments relatively recently introduced, open a new chapter in the history of root instrumentation by allowing access to areas that previously were extremely difficult or impossible to reach with standard instruments. The Mini Five curettes are available in both finishing and rigid designs. Rigid Mini Five curettes are recommended for calculus removal.

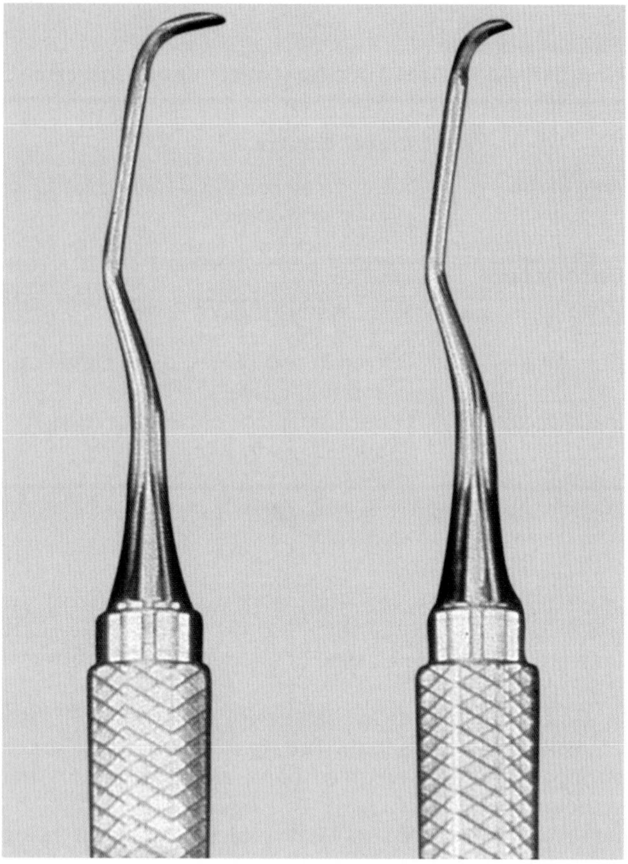

Figure 51-25 Comparison of After Five curette and Mini Five curette. The shorter Mini Five blade (half the length) allows increased access and reduced tissue trauma.

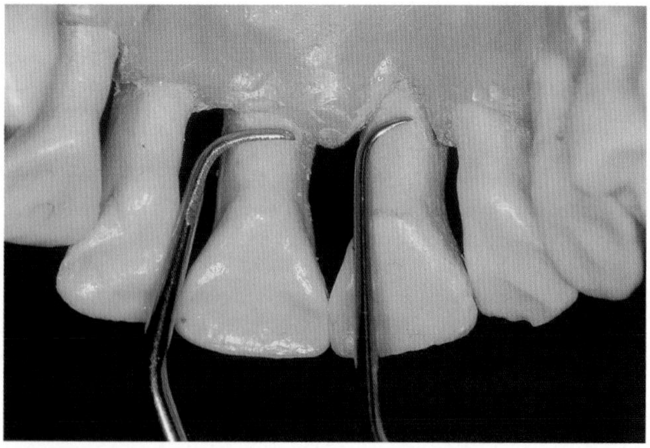

Figure 51-26 Comparison of standard rigid Gracey #5-6 with rigid Mini Five #5-6 on the palatal surfaces of the maxillary central incisors. Mini Five curette can be inserted to the base of these tight anterior pockets and used with a straight vertical stroke. Standard Gracey or After Five curette usually cannot be inserted vertically in this area because the blade is too long.

The more flexible, shanked, finishing Mini Five curettes are appropriate for light scaling and deplaquing in periodontal maintenance patients with tight pockets. As with the After Five series, the Mini Five curettes are available in all standard Gracey numbers, except the #9-10.

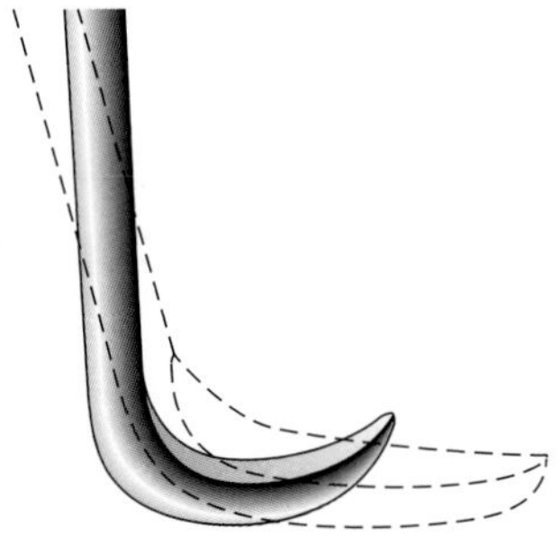

Figure 51-27 Gracey Curvette blade. This diagram shows the 50% shorter blade of the Gracey Curvette superimposed on the standard Gracey curette blade *(dotted lines)*. Notice the upward curvature of the Curvette blade and blade tip. (Redrawn from Pattison G, Pattison A: *Periodontal instrumentation,* ed 2, Norwalk, Conn, 1992, Appleton & Lange.)

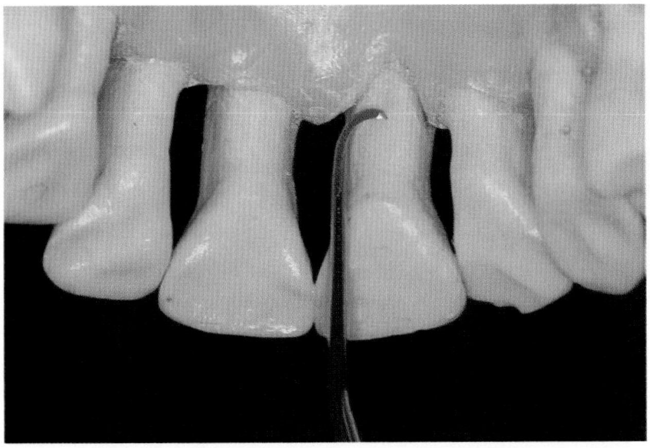

Figure 51-28 Gracey Curvette Sub-0 on the palatal surface of a maxillary central incisor. The long shank and short, curved, and blunted tip make this a superior instrument for deep anterior pockets. This curette provides excellent blade adaptation to the narrow root curvatures of the maxillary and mandibular anterior teeth.

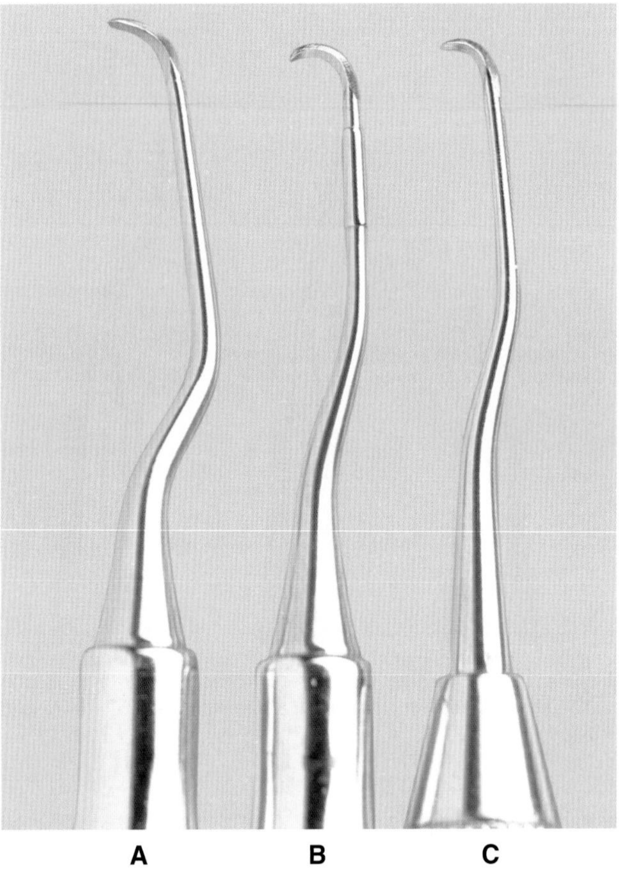

Figure 51-29 Comparison of three different mini-bladed instruments designed for use on the maxillary and mandibular anterior teeth. **A,** Hu-Friedy Mini Five #5-6; **B,** Hu-Friedy Curvette Sub-0; **C,** Hartzell Sub-0.

The *Gracey Curvettes* are another set of four mini-bladed curettes; the Sub-0 and the #1-2 are used for anterior teeth and premolars, the #11-12 is used for posterior mesial surfaces, and the #13-14 for posterior distal surfaces. The blade length of these instruments is 50% shorter than that of the conventional Gracey curette, and the blade has been curved slightly upward (Figure 51-27). This curvature allows the Gracey Curvettes to adapt more closely to the tooth surface than any other curettes, especially on the anterior teeth and on line angles (Figure 51-28). However, this curvature also carries the risk of gouging or "grooving" into the root surfaces on the proximal surfaces of the posterior teeth when the Gracey Curvette #11-12 or 13-14 is used. Additional features that represent improvements on the standard Gracey curettes are a precision-balanced blade tip in direct alignment with the handle, a blade tip perpendicular to the handle, and a shank closer to parallel with the handle.

For many years, the *Morse scaler,* a miniature sickle, was the only mini-bladed instrument available. However, the mini-bladed curettes have largely replaced this instrument (Figure 51-29).

Langer and Mini-Langer Curettes. This set of three curettes combines the shank design of the standard Gracey #5-6, 11-12, and 13-14 curettes with a universal blade honed at 90 degrees rather than the offset blade of the Gracey curette. This marriage of the Gracey and universal curette designs allows the advantages of the area-specific shank to be combined with the versatility of the universal curette blade. The Langer #5-6 curette adapts to the mesial and distal surfaces of anterior teeth; the Langer #1-2 curette (Gracey #11-12 shank) adapts to the mesial and distal surfaces of mandibular posterior teeth; and the Langer #3-4 curette (Gracey #13-14 shank) adapts to the mesial and distal surfaces of maxillary posterior teeth (Figure 51-30). These instruments can be adapted to both mesial and distal tooth surfaces without changing instruments. The standard Langer curette shanks are heavier than a finishing Gracey but less rigid than the rigid Gracey. Langer curettes are also available with either rigid or finishing shanks and can be obtained in the extended-shank (After Five) and mini-bladed (Mini Five) versions.

Schwartz Periotrievers. The Schwartz Periotrievers are a set of two double-ended, highly magnetized instruments designed for the retrieval of broken instrument

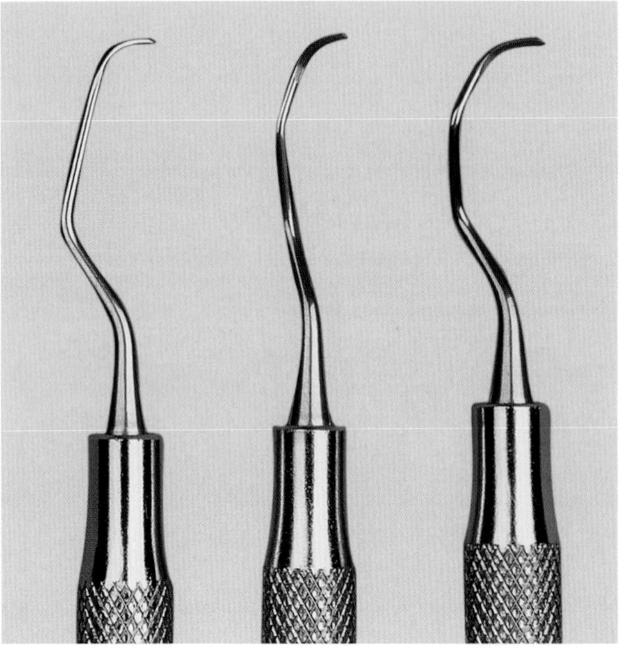

Figure 51-30 Langer curettes combine Gracey-type shanks with universal curette blades. *Left to right,* #5-6, #1-2, and #3-4.

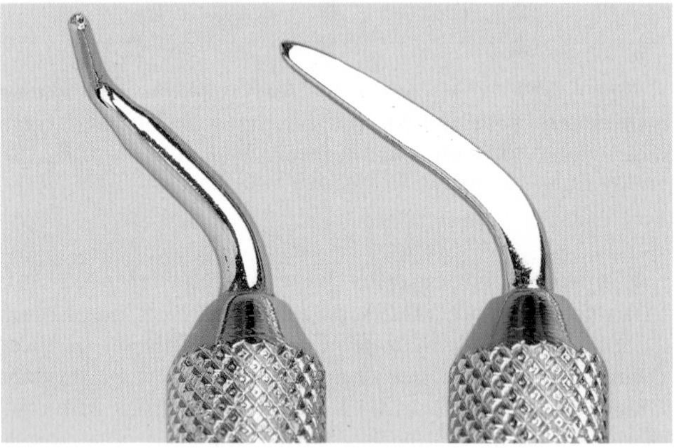

Figure 51-31 Schwartz Periotriever tip designs. The long blade is for general use in pockets, and the contra-angled tip is for use in furcations. (From Pattison G, Pattison A: *Periodontal instrumentation,* ed 2, Norwalk, Conn, 1992, Appleton & Lange.)

tips from the periodontal pocket (Figures 51-31 and 51-32). They are indispensable when the clinician has broken a curette tip in a furcation or deep pocket.[134]

Plastic Instruments for Implants. Several different companies are manufacturing plastic instruments for use on titanium and other implant abutment materials. It is important that plastic rather than metal instruments be used to avoid scarring and permanent damage to the implants* (Figures 51-33 and 51-34).

*References 21, 36, 40, 43, 52, 88, 128.

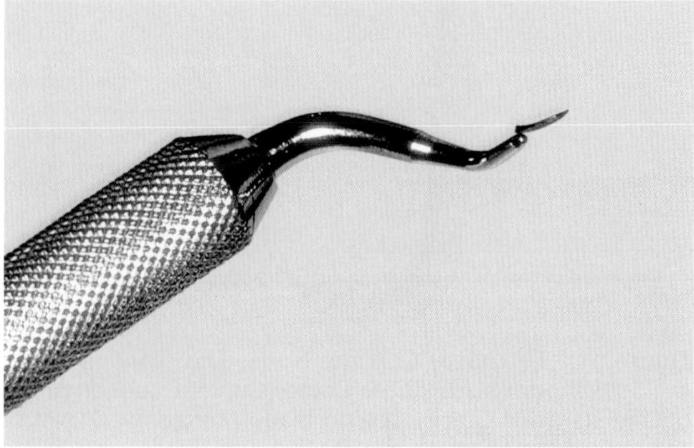

Figure 51-32 Broken instrument tip attached to the magnetic tip of the Schwartz Periotriever. (From Pattison G, Pattison A: Periodontal instrumentation, ed 2, Norwalk, Conn, 1992, Appleton & Lange.)

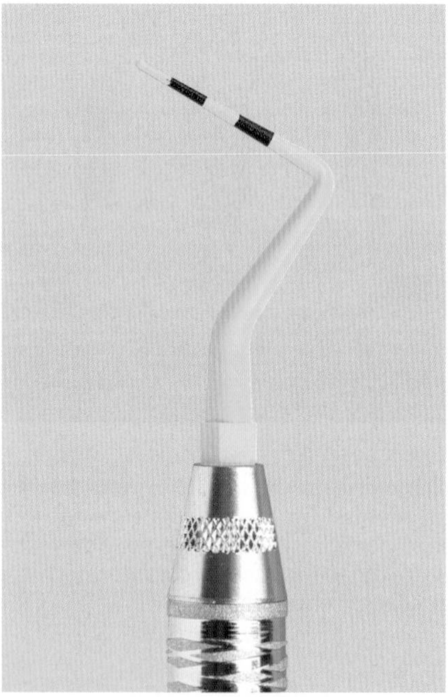

Figure 51-33 Plastic probe: Colorvue (Hu-Friedy, Chicago).

Hoe Scalers. Hoe scalers are used for scaling of ledges or rings of calculus (Figure 51-35). The blade is bent at a 99-degree angle; the cutting edge is formed by the junction of the flattened terminal surface with the inner aspect of the blade. The cutting edge is beveled at 45 degrees. The blade is slightly bowed so that it can maintain contact at two points on a convex surface. The back of the blade is rounded, and the blade has been reduced to minimal thickness to permit access to the roots without interference from the adjacent tissues.

Hoe scalers are used in the following manner:

1. The blade is inserted to the base of the periodontal pocket so that it makes two-point contact with the tooth (Figure 51-35). This stabilizes the instrument and prevents nicking of the root.

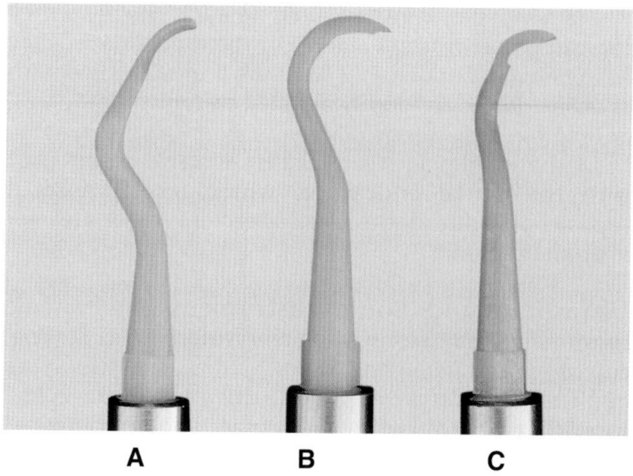

Figure 51-34 Implacare implant instruments (Hu-Friedy). These implant instruments have autoclavable stainless steel handles and three different cone-socket plastic tip designs. **A,** Columbia 4R-4L curette tip; **B,** H6-H7 sickle scaler tip; **C,** 204S sickle scaler tip.

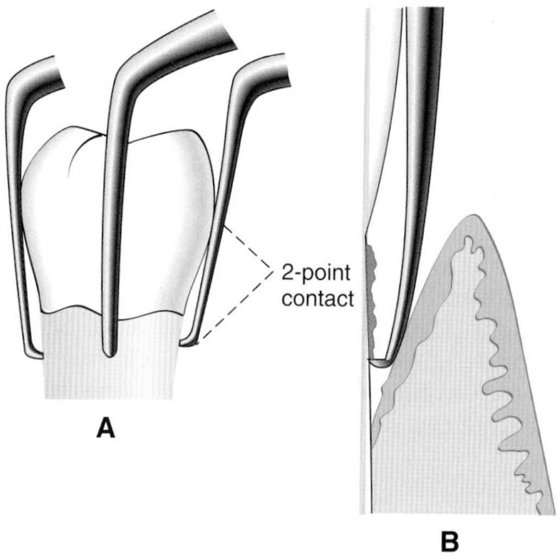

Figure 51-35 **A,** Hoe scalers designed for different tooth surfaces, showing "two-point" contact. **B,** Hoe scaler in a periodontal pocket. The back of the blade is rounded for easier access. The instrument contacts the tooth at two points for stability.

2. The instrument is activated with a firm pull stroke toward the crown, with every effort being made to preserve the two-point contact with the tooth.

McCall's #3, 4, 5, 6, 7, and 8 are a set of six hoe scalers designed to provide access to all tooth surfaces. Each instrument has a different angle between the shank and handle.

Files. Files have a series of blades on a base (Figure 51-36). Their primary function is to fracture or crush large deposits of tenacious calculus or burnished sheets of calculus. Files can easily gouge and roughen root surfaces when used improperly. Therefore, they are not suitable for fine scaling and root planing. Mini-bladed curettes are currently preferred for fine scaling in areas where files were once used. Files are sometimes used for removing overhanging margins of dental restorations.

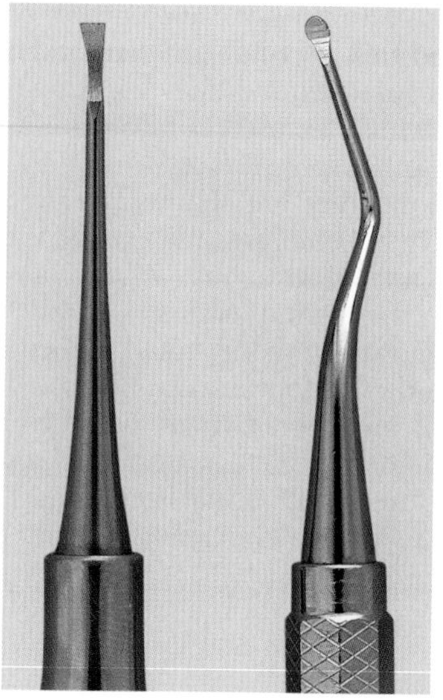

Figure 51-36 Chisel scaler **(A)** and file scaler **(B)**.

Chisel Scalers. The chisel scaler, designed for the proximal surfaces of teeth too closely spaced to permit the use of other scalers, is usually used in the anterior part of the mouth. It is a double-ended instrument with a curved shank at one end and a straight shank at the other (see Figure 51-36); the blades are slightly curved and have a straight cutting edge beveled at 45 degrees.

The chisel is inserted from the facial surface. The slight curve of the blade makes it possible to stabilize it against the proximal surface, whereas the cutting edge engages the calculus without nicking the tooth. The instrument is activated with a push motion while the side of the blade is held firmly against the root.

Quétin Furcation Curettes. The Quétin furcation curettes are actually hoes with a shallow, half-moon radius that fits into the roof or floor of the furcation. The curvature of the tip also fits into developmental depressions on the inner aspects of the roots. The shanks are slightly curved for better access, and the tips are available in two widths (Figure 51-37). The BL1 *(buccal-lingual)* and MD1 *(mesial-distal)* instruments are small and fine, with a 0.9-mm blade width. The BL2 and MD2 instruments are larger and wider, with a 1.3-mm blade width.

These instruments remove burnished calculus from recessed areas of the furcation where curettes, even the mini-bladed curettes, are often too large to gain access. Using mini-bladed Gracey curettes and Gracey Curvettes in the roof or floor of the furcation may unintentionally create gouges and grooves. The Quétin instruments, however, are well suited for this area and lessen the likelihood of root damage.

Diamond-Coated Files. Diamond-coated files are unique instruments used for final finishing of root surfaces. These files do not have cutting edges; instead, they are coated with very-fine-grit diamond (Figure 51-38). The most useful diamond files are the buccal-lingual instruments, which are used in furcations and also adapt well to many other root surfaces.

New diamond files are sharply abrasive and should be used with light, even pressure against the root surface to avoid gouging or grooving. When viewing the root surface with the dental endoscope after all tactilely detectable deposits are gone, small embedded remnants of calculus in the root surface can be observed. Diamond files are used similar to an emery board to remove these minute remnants of calculus from the root, creating a surface that is free of all visible accretions. Diamond files can produce a smooth, even, clean, highly polished root surface.

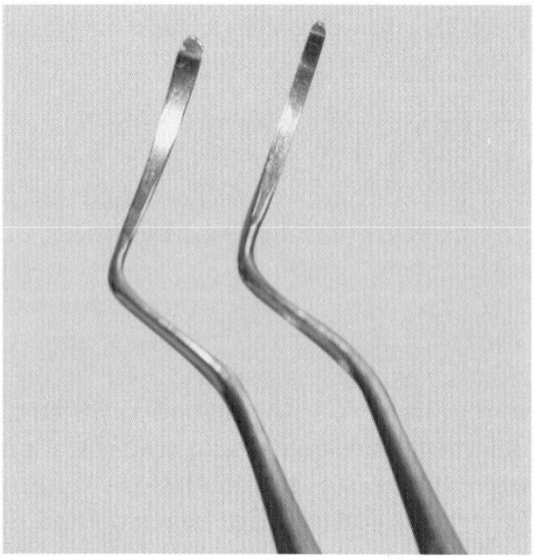

Figure 51-37 Quétin furcation curettes: BL2 (larger) and BL1 (smaller) (Hu-Friedy).

Diamond files must be used carefully because they can cause overinstrumentation of the root surface. They will remove too much root structure if they are used with excessive force, are poorly adapted to root morphology, or used too long in one place.

Diamond files are particularly effective when used with the dental endoscope, which reveals residual deposits and directs the clinician to the exact area for instrumentation.

Ultrasonic and Sonic Instruments. Ultrasonic instruments may be used for removing plaque, scaling, curetting, and removing stain.[39,40,58,126] The two types of ultrasonic units are magnetostrictive and piezoelectric. In both types, alternating electrical current generates oscillations in materials in the handpiece that cause the scaler tip to vibrate. Depending on the manufacturer, these ultrasonic vibrations at the tip of the instruments of both types range from 20,000 to 45,000 cycles per second (cps; also referred to as *Hertz* [Hz]). In *magnetostrictive units* the pattern of vibration of the tip is elliptic, which means that all sides of the tip are active and will work when adapted to the tooth (Figure 51-39). In *piezoelectric units* the pattern of vibration of the tip is linear, or back and forth, meaning that the two sides of the tip are the most active (Figures 51-40 and 51-41).

Sonic units consist of a handpiece that attaches to a compressed-air line and uses a variety of specially designed tips (Figure 51-42). Vibrations at the sonic tip range from 2000 to 6500 cps, which provides less power for calculus removal than ultrasonic units.

Ultrasonic and sonic tips with different shapes are available for scaling, curetting, root planing, and surgical debridement (Figure 51-43). For many years, only large, bulky tips designed for supragingival removal of heavy calculus were available. In recent years, however, thinner, more delicate tips designed for subgingival debridement

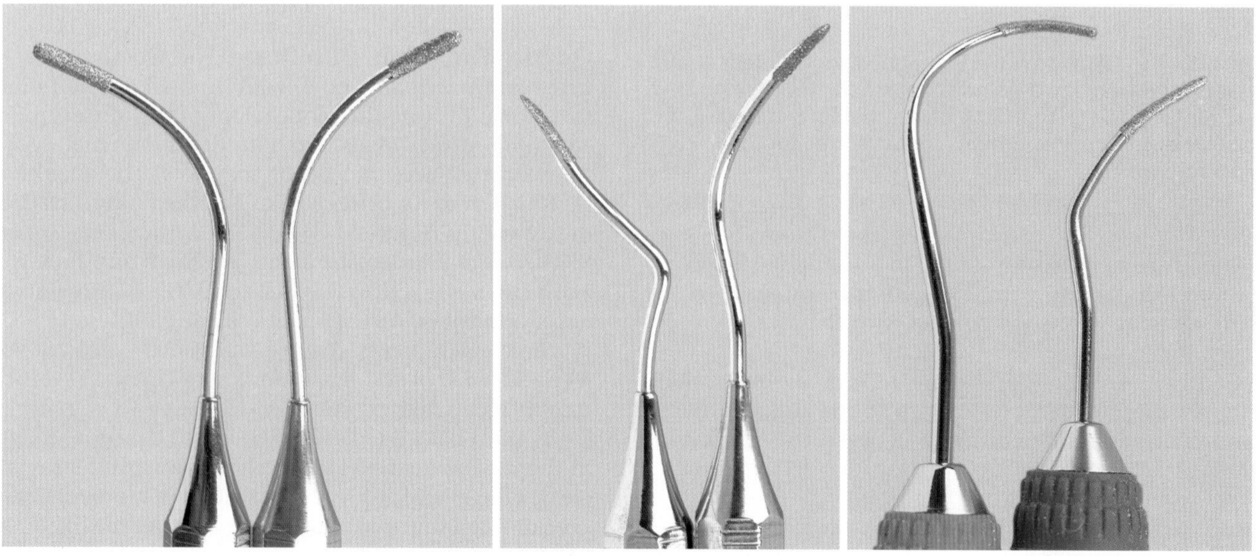

A B C

Figure 51-38 Diamond files. **A,** #1,2; **B,** #3,4 (Brasseler, Savannah, Ga). **C,** SDCN 7, SDCM/D 7 (Hu-Friedy, Chicago).

have become available[58] (Figure 51-44). All tips are designed to operate in a wet field with a water spray directed at the end of the tip. Within the water droplets of this spray mist are tiny vacuum bubbles that quickly collapse, releasing energy in a process known as *cavitation*. The cavitating water spray serves to flush calculus, plaque, and debris dislodged by the vibrating tip from the pocket. Magnetostrictive ultrasonic tips generate heat and require this water for cooling. Sonic and piezoelectric units do not generate this heat but still utilize water for cooling frictional heat and flushing away debris.

Dental Endoscope. A dental endoscope has been introduced recently for use subgingivally in the diagnosis and treatment of periodontal disease (Figure 51-45). The *Perioscopy* system (DentalView, Irvine, Calif) consists of a 0.99-mm-diameter, reusable fiberoptic endoscope over which is fitted a disposable, sterile sheath. The

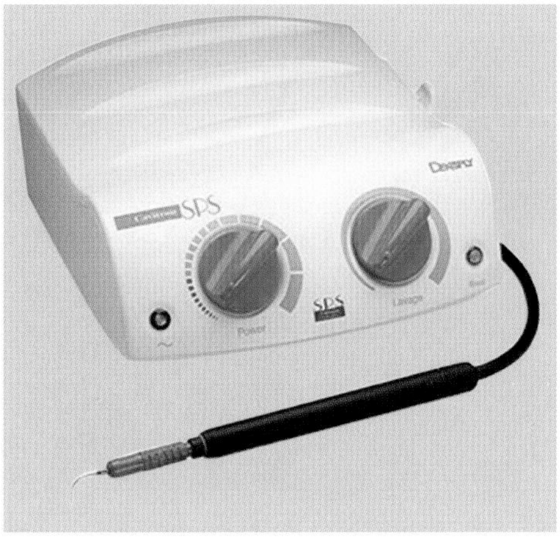

Figure 51-39 Magnetostrictive ultrasonic unit: Cavitron SPS ultrasonic scaler. (Courtesy Dentsply International, York, Pa.)

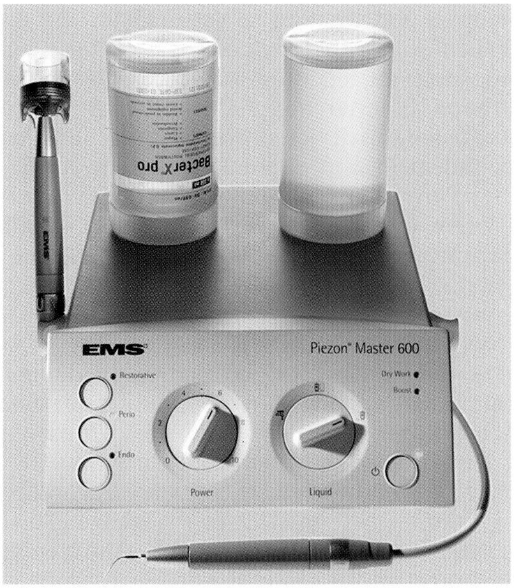

Figure 51-40 Piezoelectric ultrasonic unit: Piezon Master 600. (Courtesy EMS, Electromedical Systems, Dallas.)

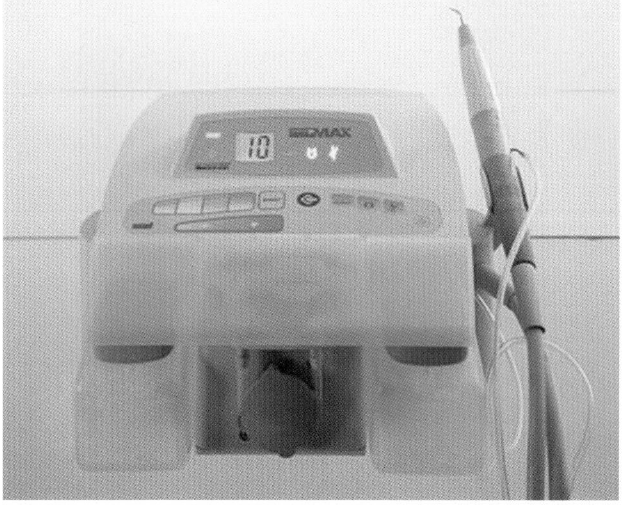

Figure 51-41 Piezoelectric ultrasonic unit: Suprasson P-Max. (Courtesy Satelec/Acteon North America, Mount Laurel, NJ.)

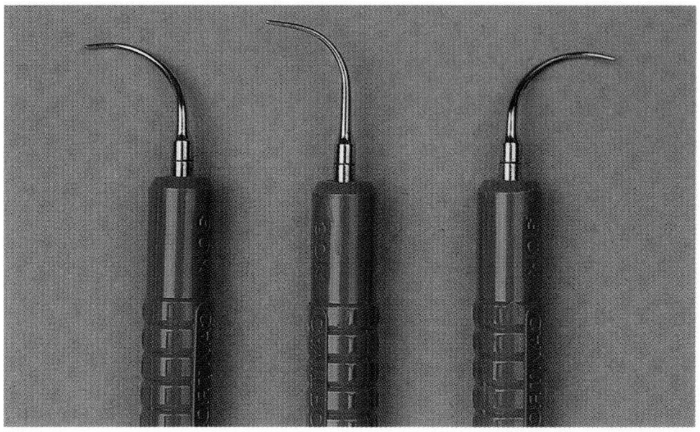

Figure 51-42 Sonic scaler: Titan-S sonic scaler (Star Dental Products, Valley Forge, Pa).

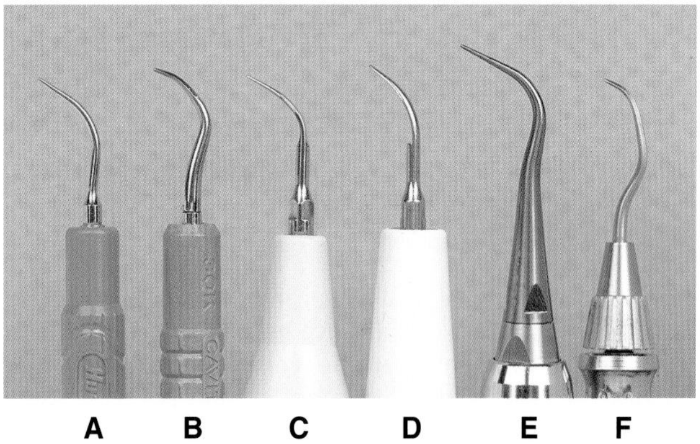

Figure 51-43 Ultrasonic and sonic tips. **A,** #100 insert (Hu-Friedy). **B,** FSI 1000 insert (Dentsply Cavitron). **C,** Piezoelectric "A" insert (EMS). **D,** Piezoelectric #1 insert (Satelec). **E,** Piezoelectric insert (ProDentec). **F,** Sonic insert for Titan-S (Star Dental Products).

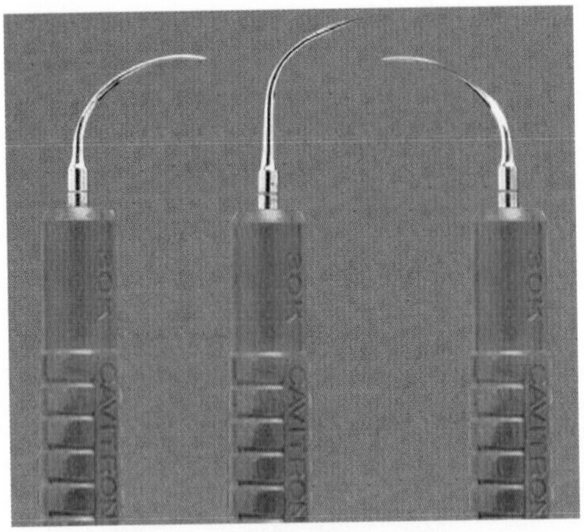

Figure 51-44 Cavitron FSI Slim Line ultrasonic tips. Thin inserts from Dentsply Cavitron allow better insertion into deep periodontal pockets and furcations.

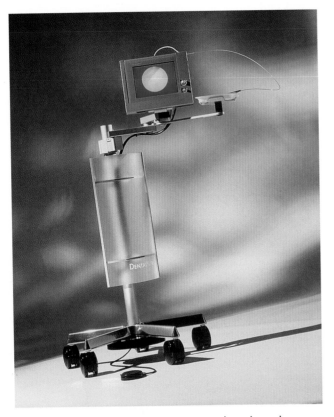

Figure 51-45 Periscopy system, dental endoscope. (Courtesy DentalView, Irvine, Calif.)

fiberoptic endoscope fits onto periodontal probes and ultrasonic instruments that have been designed to accept it (Figure 51-46). The sheath delivers water irrigation that flushes the pocket while the endoscope is being used, keeping the field clear. The fiberoptic endoscope attaches to a medical-grade charged-coupled device (CCD) video camera and light source that produces an image on a flat-panel monitor for viewing during subgingival exploration and instrumentation. This device allows clear visualization deeply into subgingival pockets and

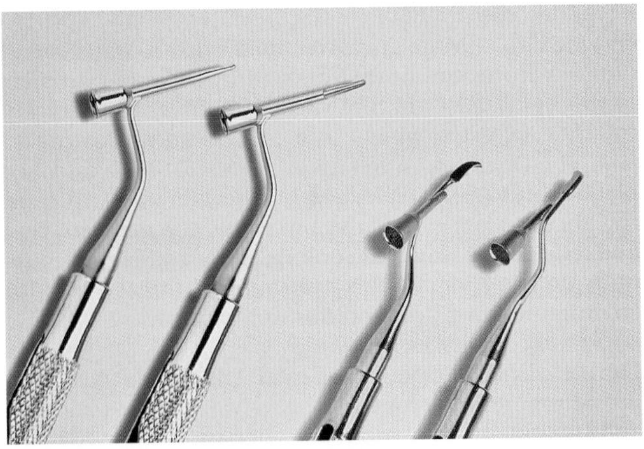

Figure 51-46 Viewing periodontal explorers (left/right/full viewing) for the Perioscopy system. (Courtesy DentalView, Irvine, Calif.)

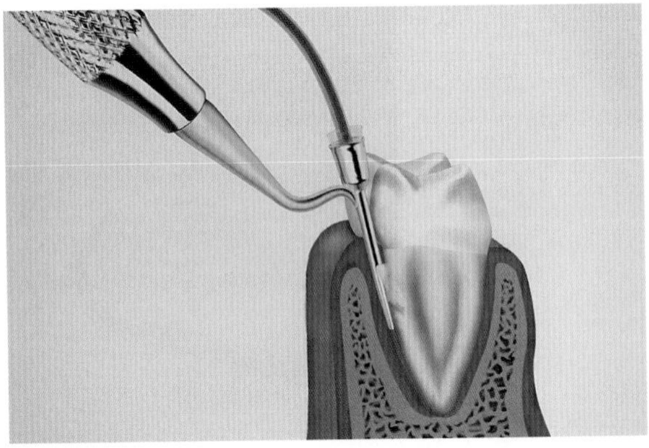

Figure 51-47 Perioscope instrumentation permits deep subgingival visualization in pockets and furcations. (Courtesy DentalView, Irvine, Calif.)

furcations (Figure 51-47). It permits operators to detect the presence and location of subgingival deposits and guides them in the thorough removal of these deposits. Magnification ranges from ×24X to ×46X, enabling visualization of even minute deposits of plaque and calculus. Using this device, operators can achieve levels of root debridement and cleanliness that are much more difficult or impossible to produce without it. The Perioscopy system can also be used to evaluate subgingival areas for caries, defective restorations, root fractures, and resorption.

EVA System. Probably the most efficient and least traumatic instruments for correcting overhanging or overcontoured proximal alloy and resin restorations are the motor-driven diamond files of the EVA prophylaxis instrument. These files, which come in symmetric pairs, are made of aluminum in the shape of a wedge protruding from a shaft; one side of the wedge is diamond coated, and the other side is smooth. The files can be mounted on a special dental handpiece attachment that generates reciprocating strokes of variable frequency. When the unit is activated interproximally with the

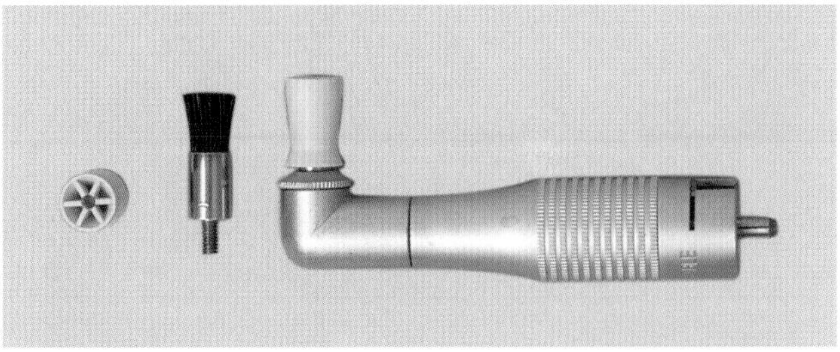

Figure 51-48 Metal prophylaxis angle with rubber cup and brush.

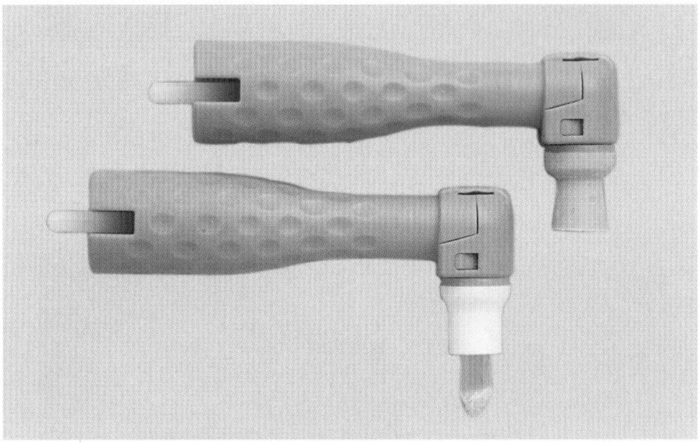

Figure 51-49 Disposable plastic prophylaxis angle with rubber cup and with brush.

diamond-coated side of the file touching the restoration and the smooth side adjacent to the papilla, the oscillating file swiftly planes the contour of the restoration and reduces it to the desired shape.

Cleansing and Polishing Instruments

Rubber Cups. Rubber cups consist of a rubber shell with or without webbed configurations in the hollow interior (Figure 51-48). They are used in the handpiece with a special prophylaxis angle. The handpiece, prophylaxis angle, and rubber cup must be sterilized after each patient use, or a disposable plastic prophylaxis angle and rubber cup may be used and then discarded (Figure 51-49). A good cleansing and polishing paste that contains fluoride should be used and kept moist to minimize frictional heat as the cup revolves. Polishing pastes are available in fine, medium, or coarse grits and are packaged in small, convenient, single-use containers. Aggressive use of the rubber cup with any abrasive may remove the layer of cementum, which is thin in the cervical area.

Bristle Brushes. Bristle brushes are available in wheel and cup shapes (see Figure 51-48). The brush is used in the prophylaxis angle with a polishing paste. Because the bristles are stiff, use of the brush should be confined to the crown to avoid injuring the cementum and the gingiva.

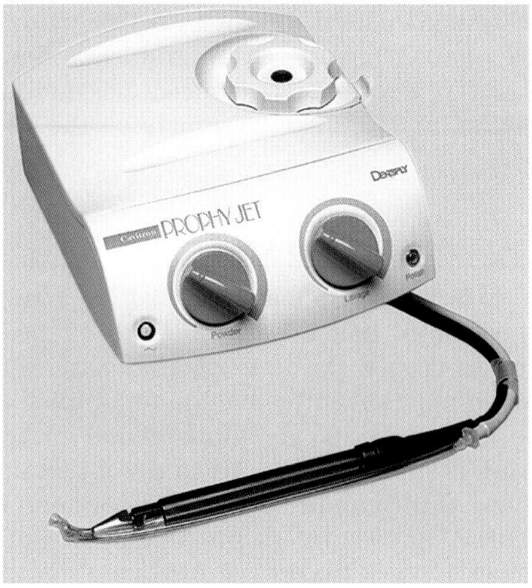

Figure 51-50 Prophy-Jet air-powder polishing device. (Courtesy Dentsply International, York, Pa.)

Dental Tape. Dental tape with polishing paste is used for polishing proximal surfaces that are inaccessible to other polishing instruments. The tape is passed interproximally while being kept at a right angle to the long axis of the tooth and is activated with a firm labiolingual motion. Particular care is taken to avoid injury to the gingiva. The area should be cleansed with warm water to remove all remnants of paste.

Air-Powder Polishing. The first specially designed handpiece to deliver an air-powered slurry of warm water and sodium bicarbonate for polishing was introduced in the early 1980s. This device, called the *Prophy-Jet,* is very effective for the removal of extrinsic stains and soft deposits (Figure 51-50). The slurry removes stains rapidly and efficiently by mechanical abrasion and provides warm water for rinsing and lavage. The flow rate of abrasive cleansing power can be adjusted to increase the amount of powder for heavier stain removal. Currently, many manufacturers produce air-powder polishing systems that use various powder formulas.

The results of studies on the abrasive effect of the air-powder polishing devices using sodium bicarbonate on cementum and dentin show that significant tooth substance can be lost.[4,19,87,114] Damage to gingival tissue is transient and insignificant clinically, but amalgam restorations, composite resins, cements, and other nonmetallic materials can be roughened.[13,41,86,87] For this reason, polishing powders containing aluminum trihydroxide or other substances rather than sodium bicarbonate recently have been introduced.[64,113,159] Air-powder polishing can be used safely on titanium implant surfaces.[71,122]

Patients with medical histories of respiratory illnesses and hemodialysis are not candidates for the use of the air-powder polishing device.[71,114,116] Powders containing sodium bicarbonate should not be used on patients with histories of hypertension, sodium-restricted diets, or medications affecting the electrolyte balance.[97,114,116] Patients with infectious diseases should not be treated with this device because of the large quantity of aerosol created. A preprocedural rinse with 0.12% chlorhexidine gluconate should be used to minimize the microbial content of the aerosol.[17] High-speed evacuation should also be used to eliminate as much of the aerosol as possible.[54]

GENERAL PRINCIPLES OF INSTRUMENTATION

Effective instrumentation is governed by a number of general principles that are common to all periodontal instruments. Proper position of the patient and the operator, illumination and retraction for optimal visibility, and sharp instruments are fundamental prerequisites. A constant awareness of tooth and root morphologic features and of the condition of the periodontal tissues is also essential. Knowledge of instrument design enables the clinician to select the proper instrument for the procedure and the correct area in which it will be performed. In addition to these principles, the basic concepts of grasp, finger rest, adaptation, angulation, and stroke must be understood before clinical instrument-handling skills can be mastered.

Accessibility: Positioning of Patient and Operator

Accessibility facilitates thoroughness of instrumentation. The position of the patient and operator should provide maximal accessibility to the area of operation. Inadequate accessibility impedes thorough instrumentation, prematurely tires the operator, and diminishes his or her effectiveness.

The clinician should be seated on a comfortable operating stool that has been positioned so that the clinician's feet are flat on the floor with the thighs parallel to the floor. The clinician should be able to observe the field of operation while keeping the back straight and the head erect.

The patient should be in a supine position and placed so that the mouth is close to the resting elbow of the clinician. For instrumentation of the maxillary arch, the patient should be asked to raise the chin slightly to provide optimal visibility and accessibility. For instrumentation on the mandibular arch, it may be necessary to raise the back of the chair slightly and request that the patient lower the chin until the mandible is parallel to the floor. This will especially facilitate work on the lingual surfaces of the mandibular anterior teeth.

Visibility, Illumination, and Retraction

Whenever possible, *direct vision* with *direct illumination* from the dental light is most desirable (Figure 51-51). If this is not possible, *indirect vision* may be obtained by using the mouth mirror (Figure 51-52), and *indirect illumination* may be obtained by using the mirror to reflect light to where it is needed (Figure 51-53). Indirect vision and indirect illumination are often used simultaneously (Figure 51-54).

Retraction provides visibility, accessibility, and illumination. Depending on the location of the area of operation, the fingers and/or the mirror are used for retraction. The *mirror* may be used for retraction of the cheeks or

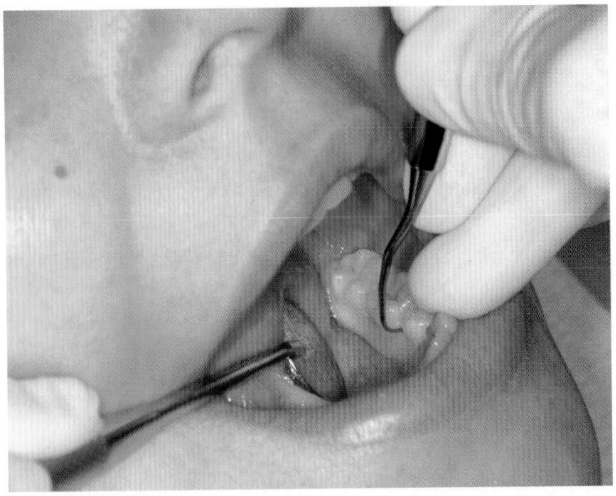

Figure 51-51 Direct vision and direct illumination in the mandibular left premolar area.

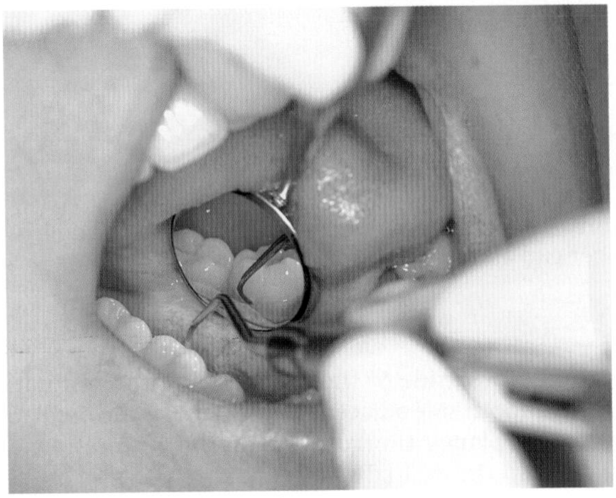

Figure 51-52 Indirect vision using the mirror for the lingual surfaces of the mandibular anterior teeth.

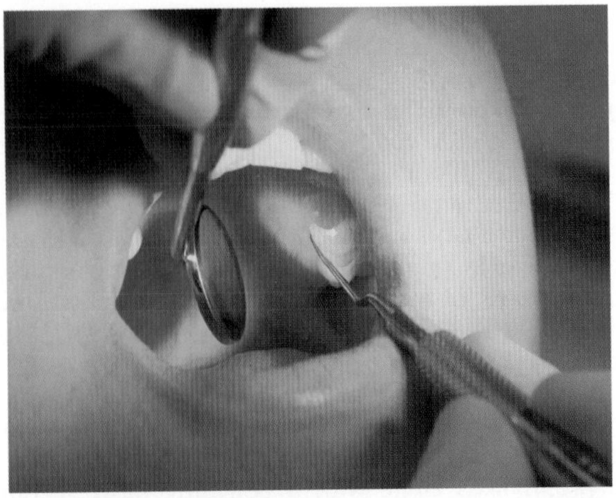

Figure 51-53 Indirect illumination using the mirror to reflect light onto the maxillary left posterior lingual region.

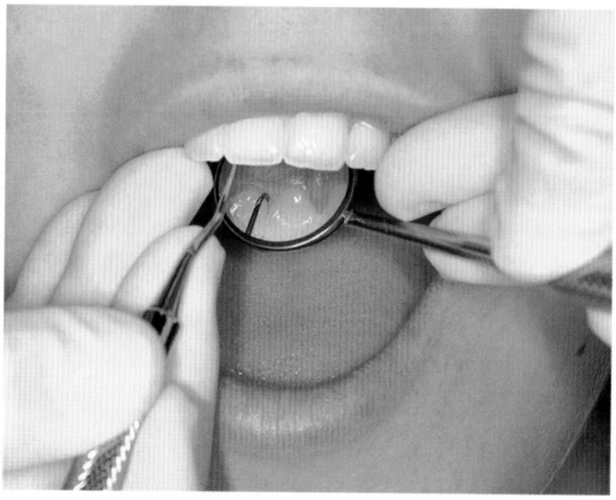

Figure 51-54 Combination of indirect illumination and indirect vision for the lingual surfaces of the maxillary anterior teeth.

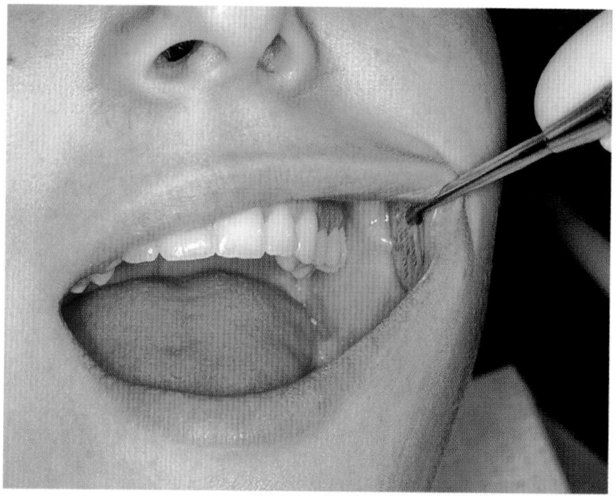

Figure 51-55 Retracting the cheek with the mirror.

the tongue; the *index finger* is used for retraction of the lips or cheeks. The following methods are effective for retraction:

1. Use of the mirror to deflect the cheek while the fingers of the nonoperating hand retract the lips and protect the angle of the mouth from irritation by the mirror handle.
2. Use of the mirror alone to retract the lips and cheek (Figure 51-55).
3. Use of the fingers of the nonoperating hand to retract the lips (Figure 51-56).
4. Use of the mirror to retract the tongue (Figure 51-57).
5. Combinations of the preceding methods.

When retracting, care should be taken to avoid irritation to the angles of the mouth. If the lips and skin are dry, softening the lips with petroleum jelly before instrumentation is a helpful precaution against cracking and bleeding. Careful retraction is especially important for patients with a history of recurrent *herpes labialis,* because these patients may easily develop herpetic lesions after instrumentation.

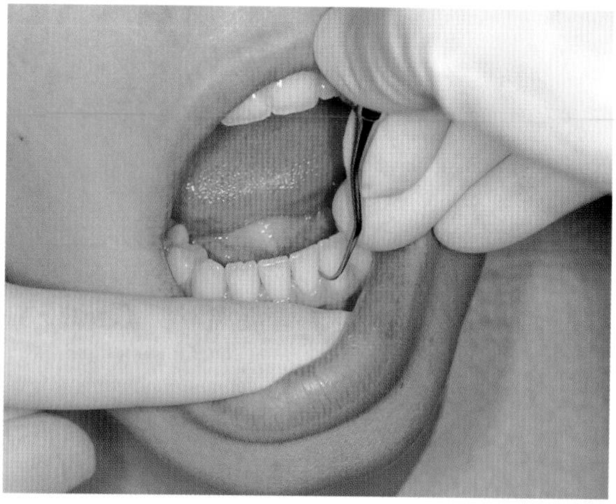

Figure 51-56 Retracting the lip with the index finger of the nonoperating hand.

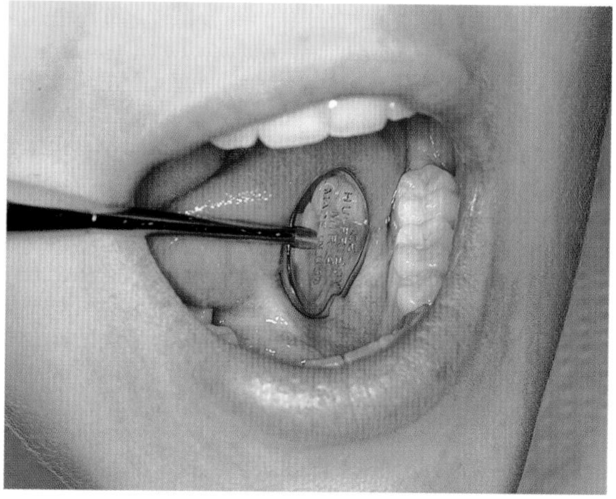

Figure 51-57 Retracting the tongue with the mirror.

Condition and Sharpness of Instruments

Before any instrumentation, all instruments should be inspected to make sure that they are clean, sterile, and in good condition. The working ends of pointed or bladed instruments must be sharp to be effective. Sharp instruments enhance tactile sensitivity and allow the clinician to work more precisely and efficiently (see later discussion). Dull instruments may lead to incomplete calculus removal and unnecessary trauma because of the excess force usually applied to compensate for their ineffectiveness.

Maintaining a Clean Field

Despite good visibility, illumination, and retraction, instrumentation can be hampered if the operative field is obscured by saliva, blood, and debris. The pooling of saliva interferes with visibility during instrumentation and impedes control because a firm finger rest cannot be established on wet, slippery tooth surfaces. Adequate suction is essential and can be achieved with a saliva ejector or, if working with an assistant, an aspirator.

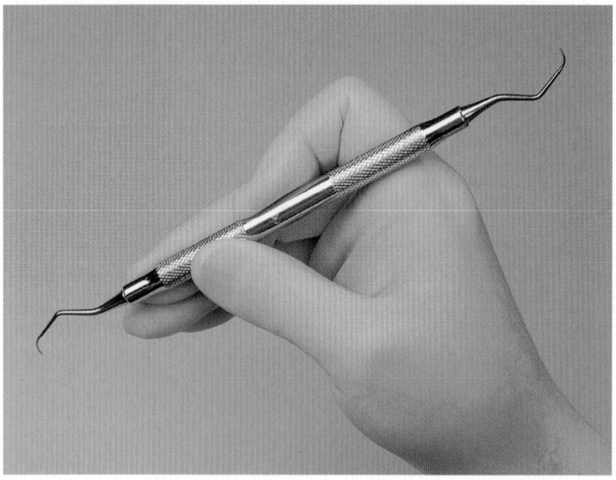

Figure 51-58 Modified pen grasp. The pad of the middle finger rests on the shank.

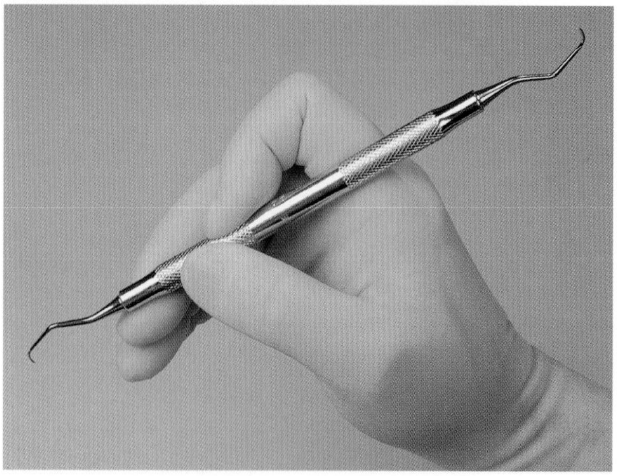

Figure 51-59 Standard pen grasp. The side of the middle finger rests on the shank.

Gingival bleeding is an unavoidable consequence of subgingival instrumentation. In areas of inflammation, bleeding is not necessarily an indication of trauma from incorrect technique, but rather may indicate ulceration of the pocket epithelium. Blood and debris can be removed from the operative field with suction and by wiping or blotting with gauze squares. The operative field should also be flushed occasionally with water.

Compressed air and gauze squares can be used to facilitate visual inspection of tooth surfaces just below the gingival margin during instrumentation. A jet of air directed into the pocket deflects a retractable gingival margin. Retractable tissue can also be deflected away from the tooth by gently packing the edge of a gauze square into the pocket with the back of a curette. Immediately after the gauze is removed, the subgingival area should be clean, dry, and clearly visible for a brief interval.

Instrument Stabilization

Stability of the instrument and the hand is the primary requisite for controlled instrumentation. Stability and control are essential for effective instrumentation and avoidance of injury to the patient or clinician. The two factors of major importance in providing stability are the instrument grasp and the finger rest.

Instrument Grasp. A proper grasp is essential for precise control of movements made during periodontal instrumentation. The most effective and stable grasp for all periodontal instruments is the *modified pen grasp* (Figure 51-58). Although other grasps are possible, this modification of the *standard pen grasp* (Figure 51-59) ensures the greatest control in performing intraoral procedures.

The thumb, index finger, and middle finger are used to hold the instrument as a pen is held, but the middle finger is positioned so that the side of the pad next to the fingernail is resting on the instrument shank. The index finger is bent at the second joint from the fingertip and is positioned well above the middle finger on the same side of the handle.

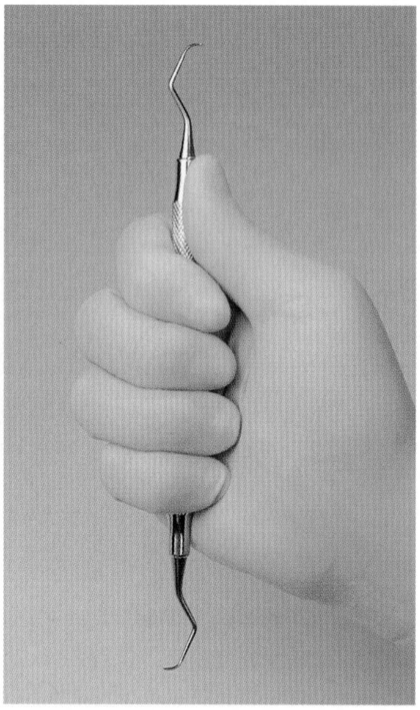

Figure 51-60 Palm and thumb grasp, used for stabilizing instruments during sharpening.

The pad of the thumb is placed midway between the middle and index fingers on the opposite side of the handle. This creates a triangle of forces, or *tripod effect,* that enhances control because it counteracts the tendency of the instrument to turn uncontrollably between the fingers when scaling force is applied to the tooth. This stable modified pen grasp enhances control because it enables the clinician to roll the instrument in precise degrees with the thumb against the index and middle fingers to adapt the blade to the slightest changes in tooth contour. The modified pen grasp also enhances tactile sensitivity, because slight irregularities on the tooth surface are best perceived when the tactile-sensitive pad of the middle finger is placed on the shank of the instrument.

The *palm and thumb grasp* (Figure 51-60) is useful for stabilizing instruments during sharpening and for

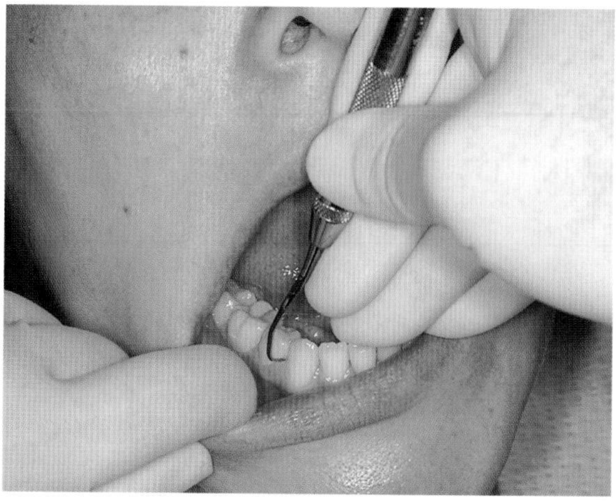

Figure 51-61 Intraoral conventional finger rest. The fourth finger rests on the occlusal surfaces of adjacent teeth.

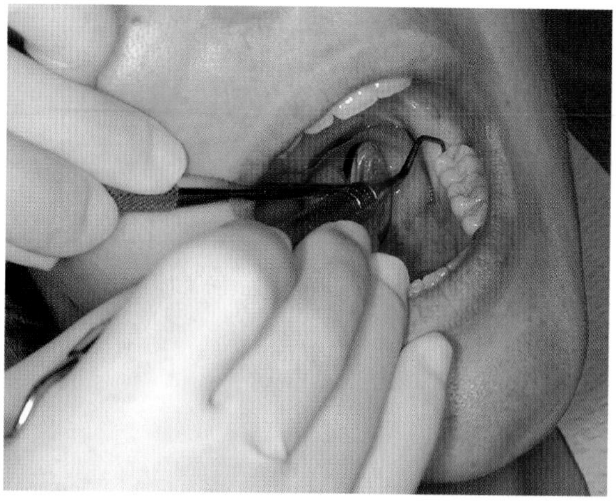

Figure 51-62 Intraoral cross-arch finger rest. The fourth finger rests on the incisal surfaces of teeth on the opposite side of the same arch.

manipulating air and water syringes, but it is not recommended for periodontal instrumentation. Maneuverability and tactile sensitivity are so inhibited by this grasp that it is unsuitable for the precise, controlled movements necessary during periodontal procedures.

Finger Rest. The finger rest serves to stabilize the hand and the instrument by providing a firm fulcrum as movements are made to activate the instrument. A good finger rest prevents injury and laceration of the gingiva and surrounding tissues by poorly controlled instruments. The fourth (ring) finger is preferred by most clinicians for the finger rest. Although it is possible to use the third (middle) finger for the finger rest, this is not recommended, because it restricts the arc of movement during the activation of strokes and severely curtails the use of the middle finger for both control and tactile sensitivity. Maximal control is achieved when the middle finger is kept between the instrument shank and the fourth finger. This "built-up" fulcrum is an integral part of the wrist-forearm action that activates the powerful working stroke for calculus removal. Whenever possible, these two fingers should be kept together to work as a *one-unit fulcrum* during scaling and root planing. Separation of the middle and fourth fingers during scaling strokes results in a loss of power and control because it forces the clinician to rely solely on finger flexing for activation of the instrument.

Finger rests may be generally classified as intraoral finger rests or extraoral fulcrums. *Intraoral finger rests* on tooth surfaces ideally are established close to the working area. Variations of intraoral finger rests and extraoral fulcrums are used whenever good angulation and a sufficient arc of movement cannot be achieved by a finger rest close to the working area. The following examples illustrate the different variations of the intraoral finger rest:

1. *Conventional:* The finger rest is established on tooth surfaces immediately adjacent to the working area (Figure 51-61).

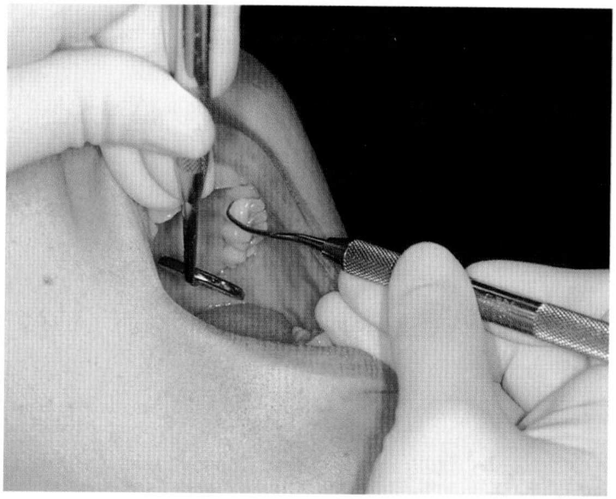

Figure 51-63 Intraoral opposite-arch finger rest. The fourth finger rests on the mandibular teeth while the maxillary posterior teeth are instrumented.

2. *Cross-arch:* The finger rest is established on tooth surfaces on the other side of the same arch (Figure 51-62).
3. *Opposite arch:* The finger rest is established on tooth surfaces on the opposite arch (e.g., mandibular arch finger rest for instrumentation on the maxillary arch) (Figure 51-63).
4. *Finger on finger:* The finger rest is established on the index finger or thumb of the nonoperating hand (Figure 51-64).

Extraoral fulcrums are essential for effective instrumentation of some aspects of the maxillary posterior teeth. When properly established, they allow optimal access and angulation while providing adequate stabilization. Extraoral fulcrums are not "finger rests" in the literal sense, because the tips or pads of the fingers are not used for extraoral fulcrums as they are for intraoral finger rests. Instead, as much of the front or back surface of the fingers as possible is placed on the patient's face to

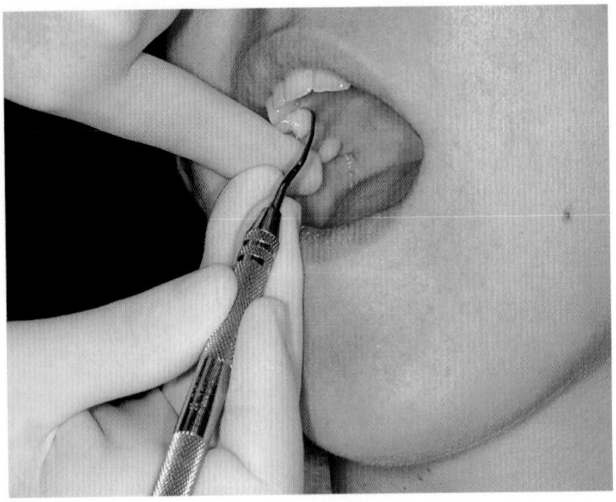

Figure 51-64 Intraoral finger-on-finger rest. The fourth finger rests on the index finger of the nonoperating hand.

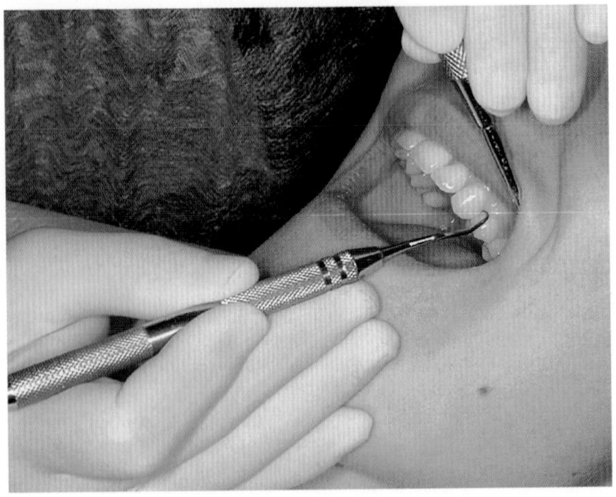

Figure 51-66 Extraoral palm-down fulcrum. The front surfaces of the fingers rest on the left lateral aspect of the mandible while the maxillary left posterior teeth are instrumented.

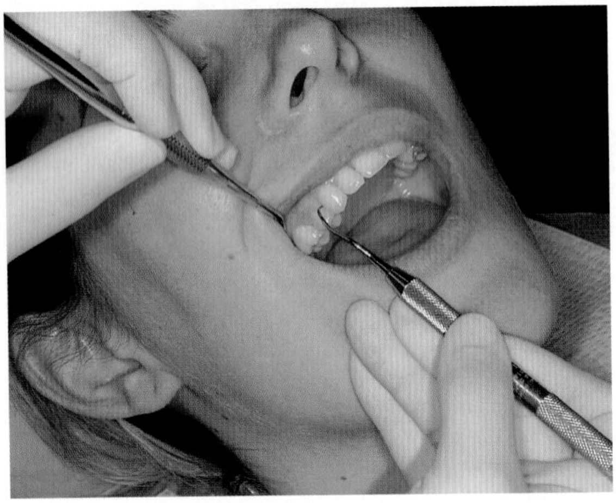

Figure 51-65 Extraoral palm-up fulcrum. The backs of the fingers rest on the right lateral aspect of the mandible while the maxillary right posterior teeth are instrumented.

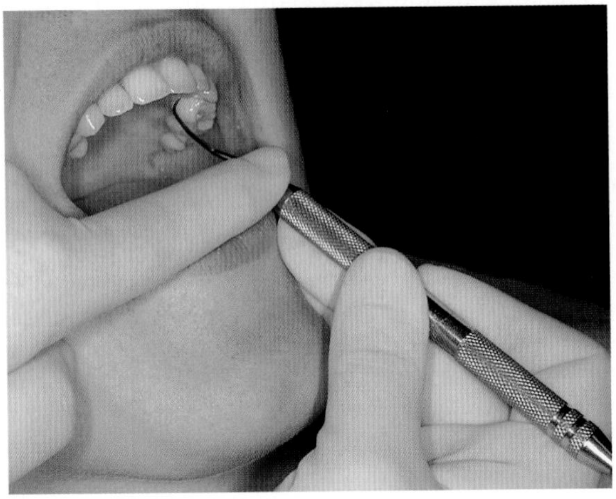

Figure 51-67 Index finger–reinforced rest. The index finger is placed on the shank for pressure and control in the maxillary left posterior lingual region.

provide the greatest degree of stability. The two most common extraoral fulcrums are used as follows:

1. *Palm up:* The palm-up fulcrum is established by resting the backs of the middle and fourth fingers on the skin overlying the lateral aspect of the mandible on the right side of the face (Figure 51-65).
2. *Palm down:* The palm-down fulcrum is established by resting the front surfaces of the middle and fourth fingers on the skin overlying the lateral aspect of the mandible on the left side of the face (Figure 51-66).

Both intraoral finger rests and extraoral fulcrums may be reinforced by applying the index finger or thumb of the nonoperating hand to the handle or shank of the instrument for added control and pressure against the tooth. The reinforcing finger is usually employed for opposite-arch or extraoral fulcrums when precise control and pressure are compromised by the longer distance between the fulcrum and the working end of the instrument. Figure 51-67 shows the index finger–reinforced rest, and Figure 51-68 shows the thumb-reinforced rest.

Instrument Activation

Adaptation. *Adaptation* refers to the manner in which the working end of a periodontal instrument is placed against the surface of a tooth. The objective of adaptation is to make the working end of the instrument conform to the contour of the tooth surface. Precise adaptation must be maintained with all instruments to avoid trauma to the soft tissues and root surfaces and to ensure maximum effectiveness of instrumentation.

Correct adaptation of the probe is quite simple. The tip and side of the probe should be flush against the tooth surface as vertical strokes are activated within the crevice. Bladed instruments (e.g., curettes) and sharp-pointed instruments (e.g., explorers) are more difficult to adapt. The ends of these instruments are sharp and can lacerate

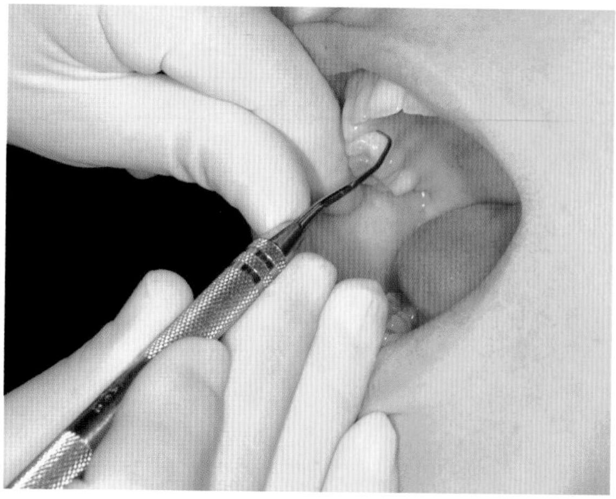

Figure 51-68 Thumb-reinforced rest. The thumb is placed on the handle for control in the maxillary right posterior lingual region.

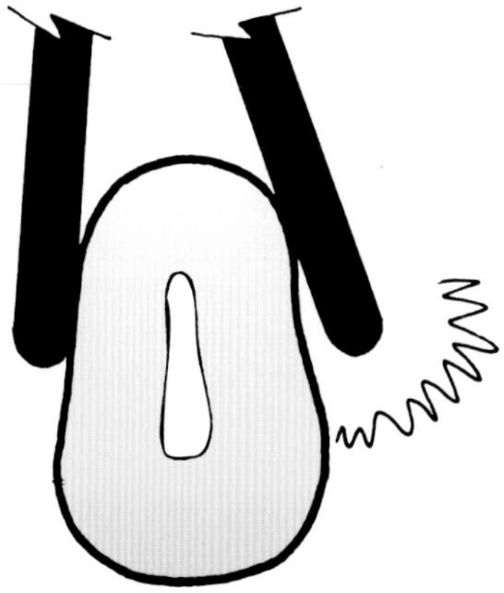

Figure 51-70 Blade adaptation. The curette on the left is properly adapted to the root surface. The curette on the right is incorrectly adapted; the toe juts out, lacerating the soft tissues.

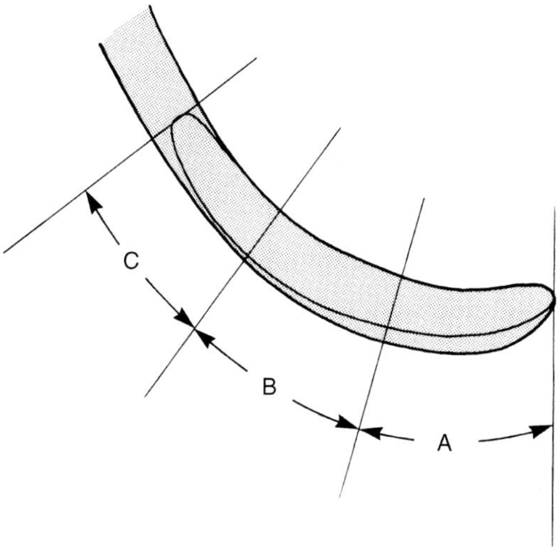

Figure 51-69 Gracey curette blade divided into three segments: *A,* the lower one third of the blade, consisting of the terminal few millimeters adjacent to the toe; *B,* the middle one third; and *C,* the upper one third, which is adjacent to the shank.

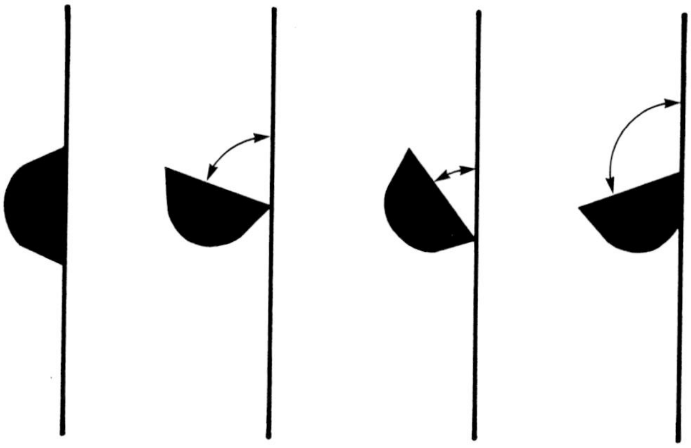

Figure 51-71 Blade angulation. **A,** 0 degrees: correct angulation for blade insertion. **B,** 45 to 90 degrees: correct angulation for scaling and root planing. **C,** Less than 45 degrees: incorrect angulation for scaling and root planing. **D,** More than 90 degrees: incorrect angulation for scaling and root planing, correct angulation for gingival curettage.

tissue, so adaptation in subgingival areas becomes especially important. The lower third of the working end, which is the last few millimeters adjacent to the toe or tip, must be kept in constant contact with the tooth while it is moving over varying tooth contours (Figure 51-69). Precise adaptation is maintained by carefully rolling the handle of the instrument against the index and middle fingers with the thumb. This rotates the instrument in slight degrees so that the toe or tip leads into concavities and around convexities. On convex surfaces such as line angles, it is not possible to adapt more than 1 or 2 mm of the working end against the tooth. Even on what appear to be broader, flatter surfaces, no more than 1 or 2 mm of the working end can be adapted because the tooth surface, although it may seem flat, is actually slightly curved.

If only the middle third of the working end is adapted on a convex surface so that the blade contacts the tooth at a tangent, the toe or sharp tip will jut out into soft tissue, causing trauma and discomfort (Figure 51-70). If the instrument is adapted so that only the toe or tip is in contact, the soft tissue can be distended or compressed by the back of the working end, also causing trauma and discomfort. A curette that is improperly adapted in this manner can be particularly damaging because the toe can gouge or groove the root surface.

Angulation. *Angulation* refers to the angle between the face of a bladed instrument and the tooth surface. It may also be called the *tooth-blade relationship.*

Correct angulation is essential for effective calculus removal. For subgingival insertion of a bladed instrument such as a curette, angulation should be as close to 0 degree as possible (Figure 51-71, *A*). The end of the instrument can be inserted to the base of the pocket more easily with the face of the blade flush against the tooth. During scaling and root planing, optimal angulation is between 45 and 90 degrees (Figure 51-71, *B*). The exact blade angulation depends on the amount and nature of the calculus, the procedure being performed, and the condition of the tissue. Blade angulation is diminished or closed by tilting the lower shank of the instrument toward the tooth. It is increased or opened by tilting the lower shank away from the tooth. During scaling strokes on heavy, tenacious calculus, angulation should be just less than 90 degrees so that the cutting edge "bites" into the calculus. With angulation of less than 45 degrees, the cutting edge will not bite into or engage the calculus properly (Figure 51-71, *C*). Instead, it will slide over the calculus, smoothing or "burnishing" it. If angulation is more than 90 degrees, the lateral surface of the blade, rather than the cutting edge, will be against the tooth, and the calculus will not be removed and may become burnished (Figure 51-71, *D*). After the calculus has been removed, angulation of just less than 90 degrees may be maintained, or the angle may be slightly closed as the root surface is smoothed with light, root-planing strokes.

When gingival curettage is indicated, angulation greater than 90 degrees is deliberately established so that the cutting edge will engage and remove the pocket lining (Figure 51-71, *D*).

Lateral Pressure. *Lateral pressure* refers to the pressure created when force is applied against the surface of a tooth with the cutting edge of a bladed instrument. The exact amount of pressure applied must be varied according to the nature of the calculus and according to whether the stroke is intended for initial scaling to remove calculus or for root planing to smooth the root surface.

Lateral pressure may be firm, moderate, or light. When removing calculus, lateral pressure is initially applied firmly or moderately and is progressively diminished until light lateral pressure is applied for the final root-planing strokes. When insufficient lateral pressure is applied for the removal of heavy calculus, rough ledges or lumps may be shaved to thin, smooth sheets of burnished calculus that are difficult to detect and remove. This burnishing effect often occurs in areas of developmental depressions and along the cementoenamel junction.

Although firm lateral pressure is necessary for the thorough removal of calculus, indiscriminate, unwarranted, or uncontrolled application of heavy forces during instrumentation should be avoided. Repeated application of excessively heavy strokes often nicks or gouges the root surface.

The careful application of varied and controlled amounts of lateral pressure during instrumentation is an integral part of effective scaling and root-planing techniques and is critical to the success of both these procedures.

Strokes. Three basic types of strokes are used during instrumentation: the exploratory stroke, the scaling stroke, and the root-planing stroke. Any of these basic strokes may be activated by a pull or a push motion in a vertical, oblique, or horizontal direction (Figure 51-72). *Vertical* and *oblique* strokes are used most frequently.

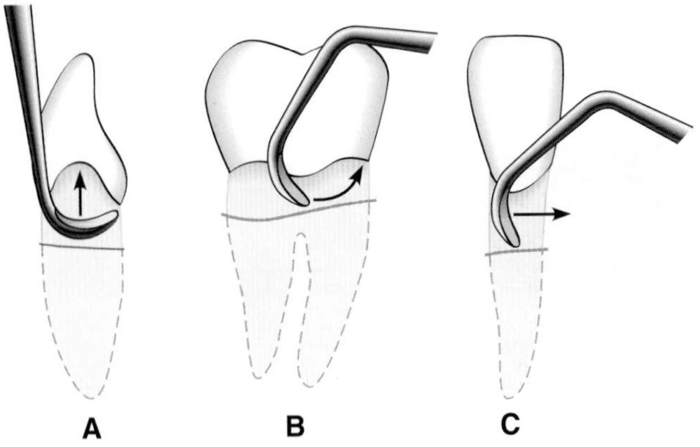

Figure 51-72 Three basic stroke directions. **A,** Vertical; **B,** oblique; **C,** horizontal.

Horizontal strokes are used selectively on line angles or deep pockets that cannot be negotiated with vertical or oblique strokes. The direction, length, pressure, and number of strokes necessary for either scaling or root planing are determined by four major factors: (1) gingival position and tone, (2) pocket depth and shape, (3) tooth contour, and (4) the amount and nature of the calculus or roughness.

The **exploratory stroke** is a light, "feeling" stroke that is used with probes and explorers to evaluate the dimensions of the pocket and to detect calculus and irregularities of the tooth surface. With bladed instruments such as the curette, the exploratory stroke is alternated with scaling and root-planing strokes for these same purposes of evaluation and detection. The instrument is grasped lightly and adapted with light pressure against the tooth to achieve maximal tactile sensitivity.

The **scaling stroke** is a short, powerful pull stroke that is used with bladed instruments for the removal of both supragingival and subgingival calculus. The muscles of the fingers and hands are tensed to establish a secure grasp, and lateral pressure is firmly applied against the tooth surface. The cutting edge engages the apical border of the calculus and dislodges it with a firm movement in a coronal direction. The scaling motion should be initiated in the forearm and transmitted from the wrist to the hand with a slight flexing of the fingers. Rotation of the wrist is synchronized with movement of the forearm. The scaling stroke is not initiated in the wrist or fingers, nor is it carried out independently without the use of the forearm.

It is possible to initiate the scaling motion by rotating the wrist and forearm or by flexing the fingers. The use of wrist and forearm action versus finger motion has long been debated among clinicians. Perhaps the strong opinions on both sides should be the most valid indication that there is a time and a place for each. Neither method can be advocated exclusively, because a careful analysis of effective scaling and root-planing technique reveals that, indeed, both types of stroke activation are necessary for complete instrumentation. The *wrist and forearm motion,* pivoting in an arc on the finger rest, produces a more powerful stroke and is therefore preferred for scaling. *Finger flexing* is indicated for precise control over stroke length in areas such as line angles and when horizontal strokes are used on the lingual or facial aspects of narrow-rooted teeth.

The *push scaling motion* has been advocated by some clinicians. In the push stroke, the instrument engages the lateral or coronal border of the calculus, and the fingers provide a thrust motion that dislodges the deposit. Because the push stroke may force calculus into the supporting tissues, its use, especially in an apical direction, is not recommended.

The **root-planing stroke** is a moderate to light pull stroke that is used for final smoothing and planing of the root surface. Although hoes, files, and ultrasonic instruments have been used for root planing, curettes are widely acknowledged to be the most effective and versatile instruments for this procedure.* The design of the curette, which allows it to be more easily adapted to subgingival tooth contours, makes curettes particularly suitable for root planing in periodontal patients. With a moderately firm grasp, the curette is kept adapted to the tooth with even, lateral pressure. A continuous series of long, overlapping shaving strokes is activated. As the surface becomes smoother and resistance diminishes, lateral pressure is progressively reduced.

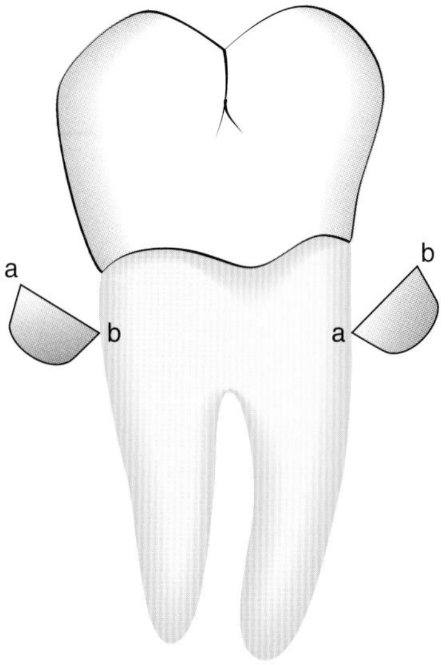

Figure 51-73 Adaptation of the universal curette on a posterior tooth. Cross-sectional representations of the same universal curette blade as its cutting edges (*a* and *b*) are adapted to the mesial and distal surfaces of a posterior tooth.

Instruments for Scaling and Root Planing

Universal Curettes. The working ends of the universal curette are designed in pairs so that all surfaces of the teeth can be treated with one double-ended instrument or a matched pair of single-ended instruments (see Figure 51-16).

In any given quadrant, when approaching the tooth from the facial aspect, one end of the universal curette adapts to the mesial surfaces, and the other end adapts to the distal surfaces. When approaching from the lingual aspect in the same quadrant, the double-ended universal curette must be turned end for end because the blades are mirror images. This means that the end that adapts to the mesial surfaces on the facial aspect also adapts to the distal surfaces on the lingual aspect, and vice versa. Both ends of the universal curette are used for instrumentation of the anterior teeth. On posterior teeth, however, because of the limited access to distal surfaces, a single working end can be used to treat both mesial and distal surfaces by using both its cutting edges. To do this, the instrument is first adapted to the mesial surface with the handle nearly parallel to the mesial surface. Because the face of the universal curette blade is honed at 90 degrees to the lower shank, if the lower shank is positioned so that it is absolutely parallel to the surface being instrumented, the tooth-blade angulation is 90 degrees. To close this angle and thus obtain proper working angulation, the lower shank must be tilted slightly toward the tooth. The distal surface of the same posterior tooth can be instrumented with the opposite cutting edge of the same blade. This cutting edge can be adapted at proper working angulation by positioning the handle so that it is *perpendicular* to the distal surface (Figure 51-73).

When adapting the universal curette blade, as much of the cutting edge as possible should be in contact with the tooth surface, except on narrow convex surfaces such as line angles. Although the entire cutting edge should contact the tooth, pressure should be concentrated on the lower third of the blade during scaling strokes. During root-planing strokes, however, lateral pressure should be distributed evenly along the cutting edge.

The primary advantage of these curettes is that they are designed to be used universally on all tooth surfaces, in all regions of the mouth. However, universal curettes have limited adaptability for the treatment of deep pockets in which apical migration of the attachment has exposed furcations, root convexities, and developmental depressions. For this reason, many clinicians prefer the Gracey curettes and the new modifications of Gracey curettes, which are area specific and specially designed for subgingival scaling and root planing in periodontal patients.

Gracey Curettes. As discussed earlier, Gracey curettes are a set of area-specific instruments that were designed by Dr. Clayton H. Gracey of Michigan in the mid-1930s (see Figure 51-18). Four design features make the Gracey curettes unique: (1) they are area specific, (2) only one cutting edge on each blade is used, (3) the blade is curved in two planes, and (4) the blade is "offset" (see Table 51-1.) Each of these features directly influences the manner in which the Gracey curettes are used, as discussed next.

Area Specificity. There are seven pairs of curettes in the set. The Gracey curettes #1-2 and 3-4 are used on anterior teeth. The Gracey #5-6 may be used on both anterior and premolar teeth. The facial and lingual surfaces of posterior teeth are instrumented with Gracey curettes #7-8 and 9-10. The Gracey #11-12 is designed for

*References 15, 44-46, 48, 67, 105, 131, 133, 152, 160.

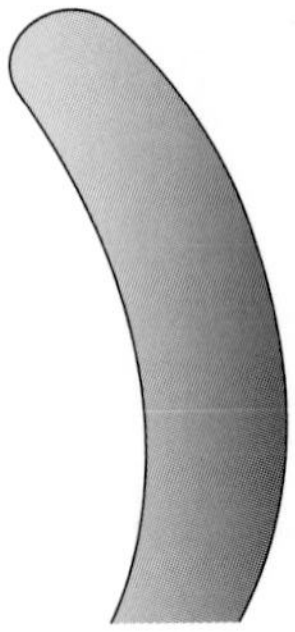

Figure 51-74 Determining the correct cutting edge of a Gracey curette. When viewed from directly above the face of the blade, the correct cutting edge is the one forming the larger, outer curve on the right.

mesial surfaces of posterior teeth, and the #13-14 adapts to the distal surfaces of posterior teeth. Although these guidelines for areas of use were originally established by Dr. Gracey, it is possible to use a Gracey curette in an area of the mouth other than the one for which it was specifically designed if the general principles regarding these curettes are understood and applied. Gracey curettes need not be reserved exclusively for periodontal patients. In fact, many clinicians prefer Gracey curettes for general scaling because of their excellent adaptability.

Single Cutting Edge Used. As with a universal curette, the Gracey curette has a blade with two cutting edges. Unlike the universal curette, however, the Gracey instrument is designed so that only one cutting edge is used. To determine which of the two is the correct cutting edge to adapt to the tooth, the blade should be held face up and parallel to the floor. When viewed from this angle, the blade can be seen to curve to the side. One cutting edge forms a larger outer curve, and the other forms a shorter, small inner curve. The larger outer curve, which has also been described as the "inferior cutting edge" or as the cutting edge farther away from the handle, is the *correct* cutting edge (Figure 51-74).

Blade Curves in Two Planes. As with the toe of the universal curette, the toe of the Gracey curette curves upward. However, the toe of the Gracey curette also curves to the side, as previously mentioned. This unique curvature enhances the blade's adaptation to convexities and concavities as the working end is advanced around the tooth. Only the lower third or half of the Gracey blade is in contact with the tooth during instrumentation. The cutting edge of a universal curette blade, on the other hand, is straight and does not curve to the side, making it less adaptable to root concavities.

Offset Blade. Gracey curette blades are honed at an *offset angle,* which means that the face of the blade is not perpendicular to the lower shank as it is on a universal curette. Instead, Gracey curettes are designed so that the tooth-blade working angulation is 60 to 70 degrees when the lower shank is held parallel to the tooth surface. Gracey curettes were originally designed to be used with *push strokes* and were beveled to provide a tooth-blade angulation of 40 degrees when the lower shank was parallel to the tooth surface; for many years, Gracey curettes were available only in this form. Currently, Gracey curettes are available not only in the original push design but also in a modified version to be used with *pull strokes.* It is important to understand this when purchasing Gracey curettes to avoid obtaining instruments that are not properly designed for pull strokes. If Gracey curettes that are designed to be used with push strokes are used with pull strokes instead, they are likely to burnish calculus rather than completely remove it. The design of the Gracey curette was modified in response to requests from clinicians who liked the shank design and adaptability of the original Gracey instruments but were opposed to the use of push strokes for scaling and root planing. The push stroke is not recommended, especially for the novice clinician, because it is likely to cause undue trauma to the junctional epithelium and to embed fragments of dislodged calculus in the soft tissues.

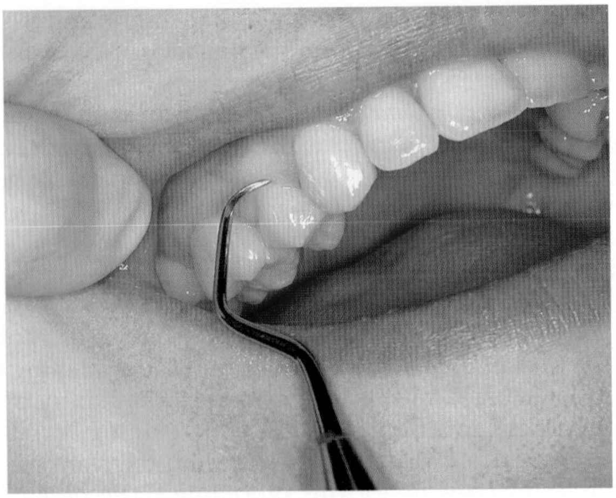

Figure 51-75 Correct cutting edge of a Gracey curette adapted to the tooth.

Principles of Use. The following general principles of use of the Gracey curettes are essentially the same as those for the universal curette; italicized principles apply only to Gracey curettes:

1. *Determine the correct cutting edge.* The correct cutting edge should be determined by visually inspecting the blade and confirmed by lightly adapting the chosen cutting edge to the tooth with the lower shank parallel to the surface of the tooth. With the toe pointed in the direction to be scaled (e.g., mesially with a #7-8 curette), only the back of the blade can be seen if the correct cutting edge has been selected (Figure 51-75). If the wrong cutting edge has been adopted, the flat, shiny face of the blade will be seen instead (Figure 51-76).
2. *Make sure the lower shank is parallel to the surface to be instrumented.* The lower shank of a Gracey curette is that portion of the shank between the blade and the first bend in the shank. Parallelism of the handle or upper shank is not an acceptable guide with Gracey curettes because the angulations of the shanks vary. On anterior teeth the lower shank of the Gracey #1-2, 3-4, or 5-6 should be parallel to the mesial, distal, facial, or lingual surfaces of the teeth (Figure 51-77). On posterior teeth the lower shank of the #7-8 or

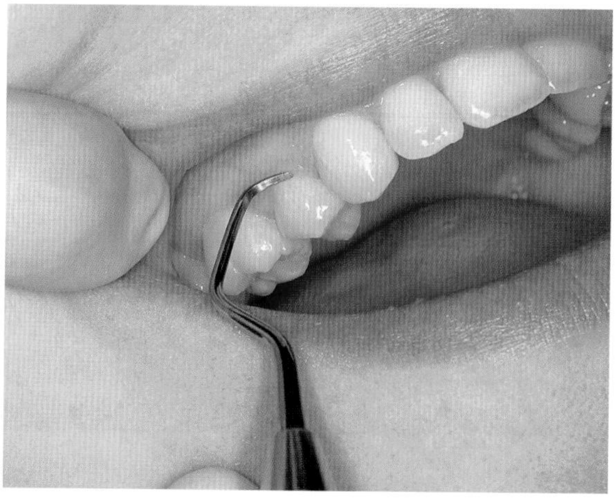

Figure 51-76 Incorrect cutting edge of a Gracey curette adapted to the tooth.

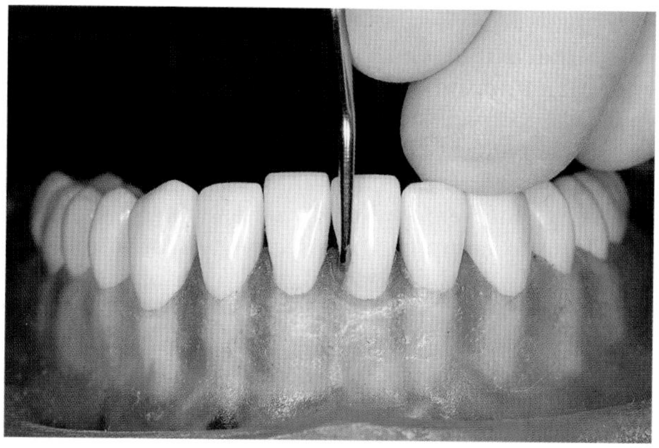

Figure 51-77 Gracey #5-6 curette adapted to an anterior tooth.

9-10 should be parallel to the facial or lingual surfaces of the teeth (Figure 51-78); the lower shank of the #11-12 should be parallel to the mesial surfaces of the teeth (Figure 51-79); and the lower shank of the #13-14 should be parallel to the distal surfaces of the teeth (Figure 51-80).

3. When using intraoral finger rests, keep the fourth and middle fingers together in a built-up fulcrum for maximum control and wrist-arm action.
4. Use extraoral fulcrums or mandibular finger rests for optimal angulation when working on the maxillary posterior teeth.
5. Concentrate on using the lower third of the cutting edge for calculus removal, especially on line angles or when attempting to remove a calculus ledge by breaking it away in sections, beginning at the lateral edge.
6. Allow the wrist and forearm to carry the burden of the stroke, rather than flexing the fingers.
7. Roll the handle slightly between the thumb and fingers to keep the blade adapted as the working end is advanced around line angles and into concavities.
8. Modulate lateral pressure from firm to moderate to light depending on the nature of the calculus, and reduce pressure as the transition is made from scaling to root-planing strokes.

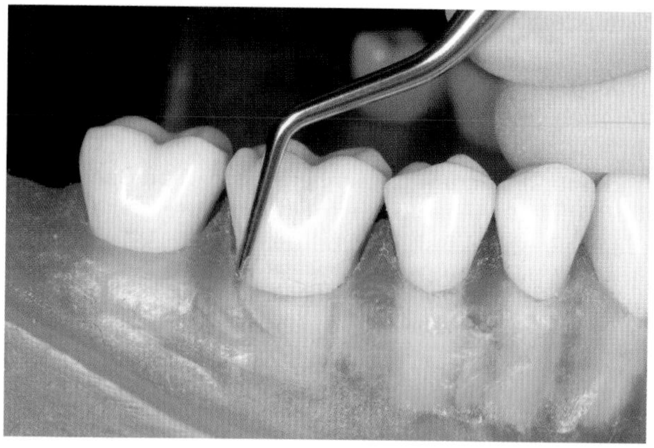

Figure 51-78 Gracey #7-8 curette adapted to the facial surface of a posterior tooth.

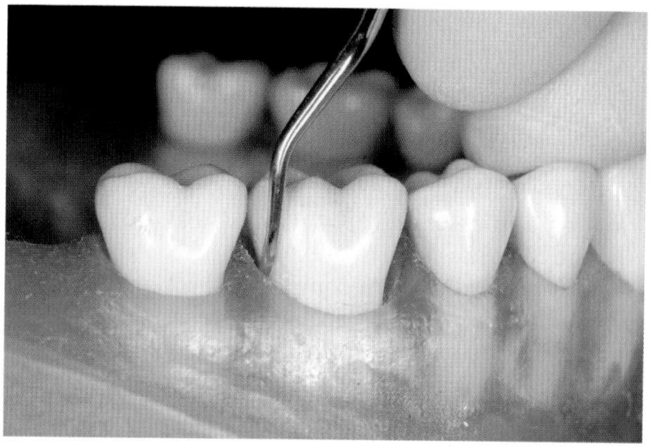

Figure 51-79 Gracey #11-12 curette adapted to the mesial surface of a posterior tooth.

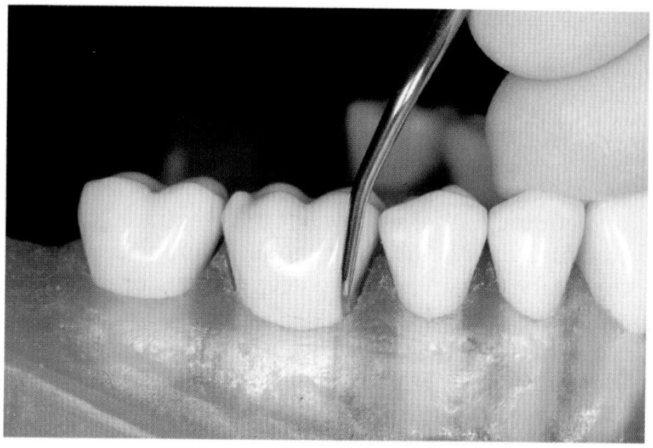

Figure 51-80 Gracey #13-14 curette adapted to the distal surface of a posterior tooth.

Extended-Shank Gracey Curettes. Extended-shank Gracey curettes, such as the After Five curettes, are 3 mm longer in the terminal shank than the standard Gracey curettes but are used with the same technique (see Figure 51-23). They are most useful for deep pockets on maxillary and mandibular posterior teeth, where the longer terminal shank allows better access, especially to deep mesial and distal pockets (see Figure 51-24). Although the longer lower shank makes access easier while using a conventional intraoral finger rest, the use of an extraoral fulcrum allows better access and adaptation to all the maxillary posterior teeth. After Five curettes with rigid shanks should be used for scaling of heavy calculus; those with regular, finishing shanks should be used for periodontal maintenance patients with deep residual pockets.

Mini-Bladed Gracey Curettes. Mini-bladed Gracey curettes, such as the Mini Five curettes and the Gracey Curvettes, have a terminal shank that is 3 mm longer than the standard Gracey curettes and a blade that is 50% shorter (see Figures 51-26 and 51-27). These mini-bladed instruments are generally used in the same manner as the Gracey curettes, except for the following specific differences:

1. Mini-bladed curettes should not be used routinely in place of standard Gracey or After Five curettes. Instead, they should be used to supplement conventional curettes and ultrasonic instruments in areas difficult to access, such as furcations, line angles, and deep, tight, or narrow pockets (see Figure 51-28).
2. Large #4 handles are recommended for any mini-bladed instruments because the larger diameter of the handles allows better control of the small blades.
3. Mini-bladed curettes can be used to scale with the toe directed either mesially or distally. In fact, the Mini Five curettes often adapt more effectively to the root curvatures of many posterior teeth when the blade is inserted with the toe pointed distally and when strokes are activated from the mesial toward the distal line angle (Figure 51-81).
4. Use rigid-shank mini-bladed curettes for calculus removal. Use the thinner, standard-shank mini-bladed curettes for deplaquing during maintenance.
5. When using mini-bladed curettes for calculus removal, use intraoral finger rests close to the working area. When performing light root planing or deplaquing, either intraoral rests or extraoral fulcrums may be used. Extraoral fulcrums are usually necessary to gain access to deep pockets on maxillary second and third molars.
6. Mini Five curettes are generally used with straight, vertical strokes. They may also be used with oblique or horizontal strokes, but because of the shortness of the blade, these strokes might not extend far enough subgingivally unless the tissue is very retractable. Horizontal strokes with the Mini Fives are most effective when used in the cementoenamel junction or in developmental depressions just below it.

When properly used, mini-bladed Gracey curettes allow unprecedented access and effectiveness for both nonsurgical and surgical root debridement. One study showed that Gracey Curvettes performed better than standard Gracey curettes in deep anterior pockets.[73] In areas such as line angles, furcations, and narrow, curved, facial, or palatal root surfaces, these miniature curettes

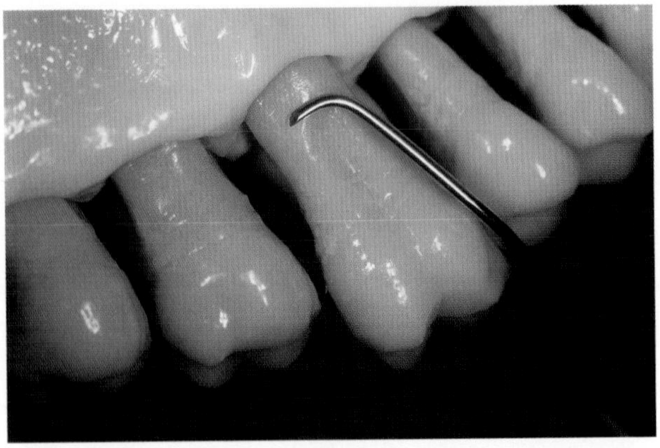

Figure 51-81 Mini Five 13/14 curette adapted to the palatal surface of a maxillary molar with the toe directed distally.

provide excellent adaptation with better tactile sensitivity than modified, slim ultrasonic tips. Studies also demonstrated that Gracey Curvette curettes performed better than ultrasonic slim tips on deep mandibular anterior pockets, furcations, and furcation entrances.[106,107] No comparison of hand instruments and modified, slim ultrasonic tips can be made unless mini-bladed curettes have been fully employed. To date, some research has been done to compare the effectiveness of mini-bladed instruments with the modified, slim ultrasonic tips. More of these studies need to be performed in vivo to guide clinicians in the optimal utilization of these newer types of instruments.[111]

PRINCIPLES OF SCALING AND ROOT PLANING*

Definitions and Rationale

Scaling is the process by which plaque and calculus are removed from both supragingival and subgingival tooth surfaces. No deliberate attempt is made to remove tooth substance along with the calculus. *Root planing* is the process by which residual embedded calculus and portions of cementum are removed from the roots to produce a smooth, hard, clean surface.

The primary objective of scaling and root planing is to restore gingival health by completely removing elements that provoke gingival inflammation (i.e., plaque, calculus, endotoxin) from the tooth surface (Figure 51-82). Instrumentation has been shown to reduce dramatically the numbers of subgingival microorganisms and produce a shift in the composition of subgingival plaque from one with high numbers of gram-negative anaerobes to one dominated by gram-positive facultative bacteria compatible with health.† After thorough scaling and root planing, a profound reduction in spirochetes, motile

*Material in this section modified from Pattison A, Pattison G, Matsuda S: *Periodontal instrumentation,* ed 3, Upper Saddle River, NJ, Prentice-Hall, Pearson Education (in press).

†References 84, 87, 97, 123, 126, 136, 138.

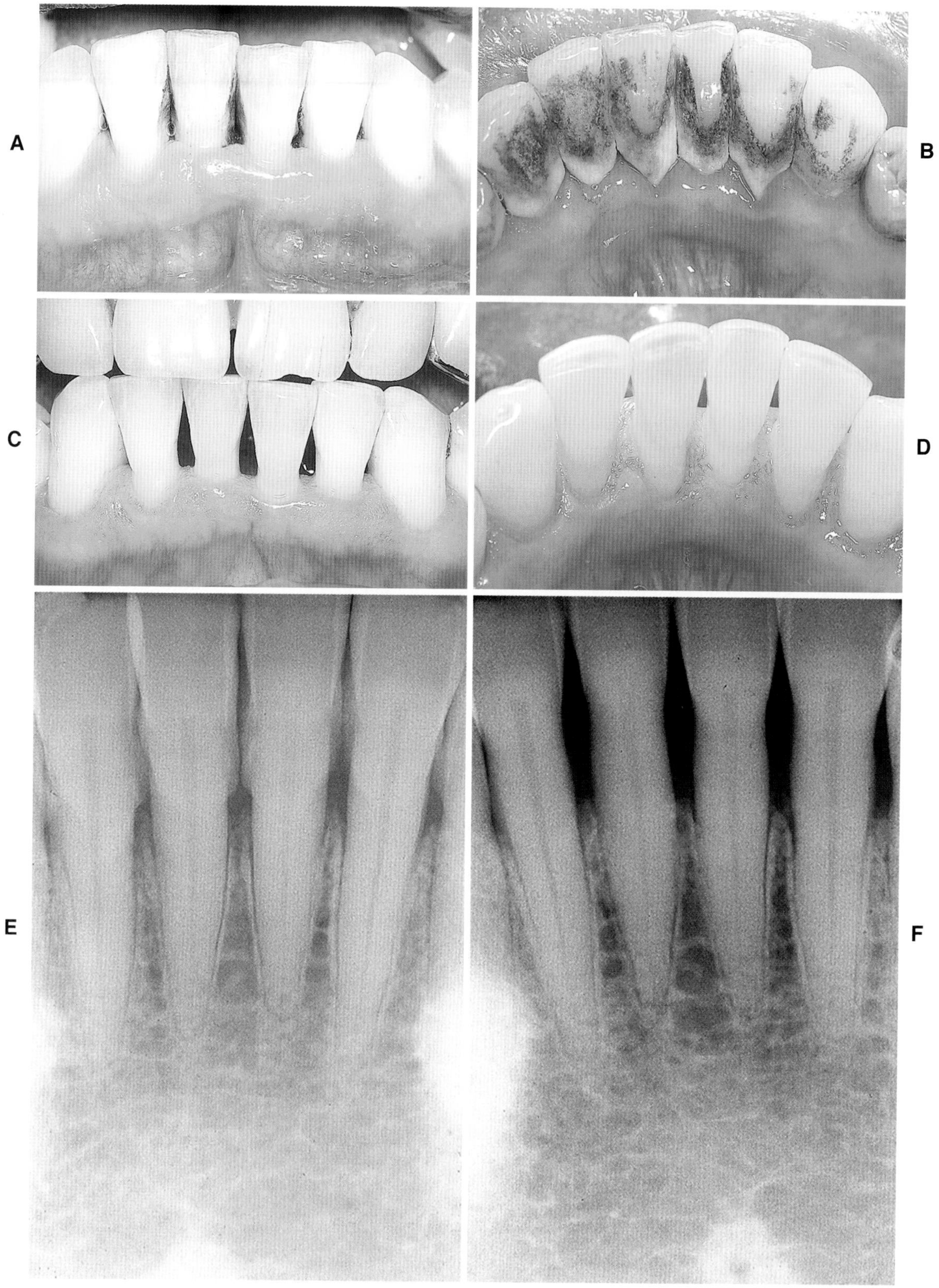

Figure 51-82 Results of Phase I therapy. **A** through **F,** Moderate chronic periodontitis. **A,** Patient presenting with moderate attachment loss and probe depths in the 4- to 6-mm range. Note the gingiva appears pink because it is fibrotic and the inflammation is deep in the periodontal pockets. **B,** Lingual view before treatment, with more visible inflammation and heavy deposits of calculus. **C** and **D,** The same areas with significant improvement in gingival health 18 months after scaling, root planing, and plaque control therapy were provided; the patient returned for regular maintenance visits. **E** and **F,** Presenting radiographs of the lower anterior teeth. Radiograph taken 18 months after Phase I therapy and maintenance shows no increase in bone loss.

rods, and putative pathogens, such as *Actinobacillus actinomycetemcomitans, Porphyromonas gingivalis,* and *Prevotella intermedia,* and an increase in coccoid cells occur.* These changes in the microbiota are accompanied by a reduction or elimination of inflammation clinically.† This positive microbial change must be sustained by the periodic scaling and root planing performed during supportive periodontal therapy.‡

Scaling and root planing are not separate procedures; all the principles of scaling apply equally to root planing. The difference between scaling and root planing is only a matter of *degree.* The nature of the tooth surface determines the degree to which the surface must be scaled or planed.

Plaque and calculus on enamel surfaces provoke gingival inflammation. Unless they are grooved or pitted, enamel surfaces are relatively smooth and uniform. When plaque and calculus form on enamel, the deposits are usually superficially attached to the surface and are not locked into irregularities. Scaling alone is sufficient to remove plaque and calculus completely from enamel, leaving a smooth, clean surface.

Root surfaces exposed to plaque and calculus pose a different problem. *Deposits of calculus on root surfaces are frequently embedded in cemental irregularities.*[1,24,96,132,162] Subgingival calculus is porous and harbors bacteria and endotoxin and therefore should be removed completely.[23,147] When dentin is exposed, plaque bacteria may invade dentinal tubules.[1] Therefore, scaling alone is insufficient to remove them, and a portion of the root surface must be removed to eliminate these deposits. Furthermore, when the root surface is exposed to plaque and the pocket environment, its surface is contaminated by toxic substances, notably endotoxins.[3,4,56] Evidence suggests that these toxic substances are only superficially attached to the root and do not permeate it deeply.§ Removal of extensive amounts of dentin and cementum is not necessary to render the roots free of toxins and should be avoided.[45,85,112] In areas where cementum is thin, however, instrumentation may expose dentin. Although this is not the aim of treatment, such exposure may be unavoidable.[131,152]

Scaling and root planing should not be viewed as separate procedures unrelated to the rest of the treatment plan. These procedures belong in the initial phase of an orderly sequence of treatment. After careful analysis of a case, the number of appointments needed to complete this phase of treatment is estimated. Patients with small amounts of calculus and relatively healthy tissues can be treated in one appointment. Most other patients require several treatment sessions. The dentist should estimate the number of appointments needed on the basis of the number of teeth in the mouth, severity of inflammation, amount and location of calculus, depth and activity of pockets, presence of furcation invasions, patient's comprehension of and compliance with oral hygiene instructions, and need for local anesthesia.

*References 87, 123, 130, 136, 153, 161.
†References 11, 45, 48, 62, 66, 85, 116, 118.
‡References 8, 18, 82, 85, 112, 136, 158.
§References 25, 26, 60, 61, 95, 99, 100, 139.

When the rationale for scaling and root planing is thoroughly understood, it becomes apparent that mastery of these skills is essential to the ultimate success of any course of periodontal therapy. Of all clinical dental procedures, subgingival scaling and root planing in deep pockets are the most difficult and exacting skills to master. It has been argued that such proficiency in instrumentation cannot be attained, and therefore periodontal surgery is necessary to gain access to root surfaces. Others have argued that although proficiency is possible, it need not be developed because access to the roots can be gained more easily with surgery. However, without mastering subgingival scaling and root-planing skills, the clinician will be severely hampered and unable to treat adequately those patients for whom surgery is contraindicated.

Detection Skills

Good visual and tactile detection skills are required for the accurate initial assessment of the extent and nature of deposits and root irregularities before scaling and root planing. Valid evaluation of results of instrumentation depends on these detection skills.

Visual examination of supragingival and subgingival calculus just below the gingival margin is not difficult with good lighting and a clean field. Light deposits of supragingival calculus are often difficult to see when they are wet with saliva. Compressed air may be used to dry supragingival calculus until it is chalky white and readily visible. Air also may be directed into the pocket in a steady stream to deflect the marginal gingiva away from the tooth so that subgingival deposits near the surface can be seen.

Tactile exploration of the tooth surfaces in subgingival areas of pocket depth, furcations, and developmental depressions is much more difficult than visual examination of supragingival areas and requires the skilled use of a fine-pointed explorer or probe. The explorer or probe is held with a light but stable modified pen grasp. This provides maximal tactile sensitivity for detection of subgingival calculus and other irregularities. The pads of the thumb and fingers, especially the middle finger, should perceive the slight vibrations conducted through the instrument shank and handle as irregularities in the tooth surface are encountered.

After a stable finger rest is established, the tip of the instrument is carefully inserted subgingivally to the base of the pocket. Light exploratory strokes are activated vertically on the root surface. When calculus is encountered, the tip of the instrument should be advanced apically over the deposit until the termination of the calculus on the root is felt. The distance between the apical edge of the calculus and the bottom of the pocket usually ranges from 0.2 to 1.0 mm. The tip is adapted closely to the tooth to ensure the greatest degree of tactile sensitivity and avoid tissue trauma. When a proximal surface is being explored, strokes must be extended at least halfway across that surface past the contact area to ensure complete detection of interproximal deposits. When an explorer is used at line angles, convexities, and concavities, the handle of the instrument must be rolled slightly between the thumb and fingers to keep the tip constantly adapted to the changes in tooth contour.

Although exploration technique and good tactile sensitivity are important, *interpreting various degrees of roughness and making clinical judgments based on these interpretations* also require much expertise. The beginning student usually has difficulty detecting fine calculus and altered cementum. Such detection must begin with the recognition of ledges, lumps, or spurs of calculus, then smaller spicules, then slight roughness, and finally a slight graininess that feels like a sticky coating or film covering the tooth surface. Overhanging or deficient margins of dental restorations, caries, decalcification, and root roughness caused by previous instrumentation are all typically found during exploration. These and other irregularities must be recognized and differentiated from subgingival calculus. Because this requires a great deal of experience and a high degree of tactile sensitivity, many clinicians agree that the development of detection skills is as important as the mastery of scaling and root-planing technique.

Supragingival Scaling Technique

Supragingival calculus is generally less tenacious and less calcified than subgingival calculus. Because instrumentation is performed coronal to the gingival margin, scaling strokes are not confined by the surrounding tissues. This makes adaptation and angulation easier. It also allows direct visibility as well as a freedom of movement not possible during subgingival scaling.

Sickles, curettes, and ultrasonic and sonic instruments are most often used for the removal of supragingival calculus; hoes and chisels are less frequently used. To perform supragingival scaling, the sickle or curette is held with a modified pen grasp, and a firm finger rest is established on the teeth adjacent to the working area. The blade is adapted with an angulation of slightly less than 90 degrees to the surface being scaled. The cutting edge should engage the apical margin of the supragingival calculus while short, powerful, overlapping scaling strokes are activated coronally in a vertical or an oblique direction. The sharply pointed tip of the sickle can easily lacerate marginal tissue or gouge exposed root surfaces, so careful adaptation is especially important when this instrument is being used. The tooth surface is instrumented until it is visually and tactilely free of all supragingival deposits. If the tissue is retractable enough to allow easy insertion of the bulky blade, the sickle may be used slightly below the free gingival margin. If the sickle is used in this manner, final scaling and root planing with the curette should always follow.

Subgingival Scaling and Root-Planing Technique

Subgingival scaling and root planing are much more complex and difficult to perform than supragingival scaling. *Subgingival calculus* is usually harder than supragingival calculus and is often locked into root irregularities, making it more tenacious and therefore more difficult to remove.[24,96,131,162] The overlying tissue creates significant problems in subgingival instrumentation. Vision is obscured by the bleeding that inevitably occurs during instrumentation and by the tissue itself. The clinician must rely heavily on tactile sensitivity to detect calculus and irregularities, guide the instrument blade during scaling and root planing, and evaluate the results of instrumentation.

In addition, the adjacent pocket wall limits the direction and length of the strokes. The confines of the soft tissue make careful adaptation to tooth contours imperative to avoid trauma. Such precise adaptation cannot be accomplished without a thorough knowledge of tooth morphologic features. The clinician must form a mental image of the tooth surface to anticipate variations in contour, continually confirming or modifying the image in response to tactile sensations and visual cues, such as the position of the instrument handle and shank. The clinician then must instantaneously adjust the adaptation and angulation of the working end to the tooth. It is this complex and precise coordination of visual, mental, and manual skills that makes subgingival instrumentation one of the most difficult of all dental skills. *The curette is preferred by most clinicians for subgingival scaling and root planing because of the advantages afforded by its design.* Its curved blade, rounded toe, and curved back allow the curette to be inserted to the base of the pocket and adapted to variations in tooth contour with minimal tissue displacement and trauma.

Sickles, hoes, files, and ultrasonic instruments also are used for subgingival scaling of heavy calculus. Some small files (e.g., Hirschfeld file) may be inserted to the base of the pocket to crush or initially fracture tenacious deposits. Larger files, hoes, sickles, and standard ultrasonic tips for supragingival use are too bulky and cannot be inserted easily into deep pockets or areas where tissue is firm and fibrotic. Hoes and files cannot be used to produce as smooth a surface as curettes. Hoes, files, and standard large ultrasonic tips are all more hazardous than the curette in terms of trauma to the root surface and surrounding tissues.[15,105,131] Although thin ultrasonic tips designed for scaling of deep pockets and furcations can be inserted more easily subgingivally, they must be used on low power.[39,40,57] When low-power scaling is performed on heavy calculus or tenacious sheets of calculus, thin ultrasonic tips are likely to burnish the calculus rather than thoroughly remove it. Therefore, ultrasonic scaling should be followed by careful assessment with an explorer and further instrumentation with curettes when necessary.

Subgingival scaling and root planing are accomplished with either universal or area-specific (Gracey) curettes using the following basic procedure. The curette is held with a modified pen grasp, and a stable finger rest is established. The correct cutting edge is slightly adapted to the tooth, with the lower shank kept parallel to the tooth surface. The lower shank is moved toward the tooth so that the face of the blade is nearly flush with the tooth surface. The blade is then inserted under the gingiva and advanced to the base of the pocket by a light exploratory stroke. When the cutting edge reaches the base of the pocket, a working angulation of between 45 and 90 degrees is established, and pressure is applied laterally against the tooth surface. Calculus is removed by a series of controlled, overlapping, short, powerful strokes primarily using wrist-arm motion (Figure 51-83). As calculus is removed, resistance to the passage of the cutting edge diminishes until only a slight roughness remains. Longer, lighter root-planing strokes are then activated with less lateral pressure until the root surface is completely smooth and hard. The instrument handle must be rolled carefully between the thumb and fingers to keep the blade adapted closely to the tooth surface as line angles, developmental depressions, and other changes in tooth contour are followed. Scaling and root-planing strokes should be confined to the portion of the tooth where calculus or altered cementum is found; this area is known as the *instrumentation zone.* Sweeping the instrument over the crown where it is not needed wastes operating time, dulls the instrument, and causes loss of control.

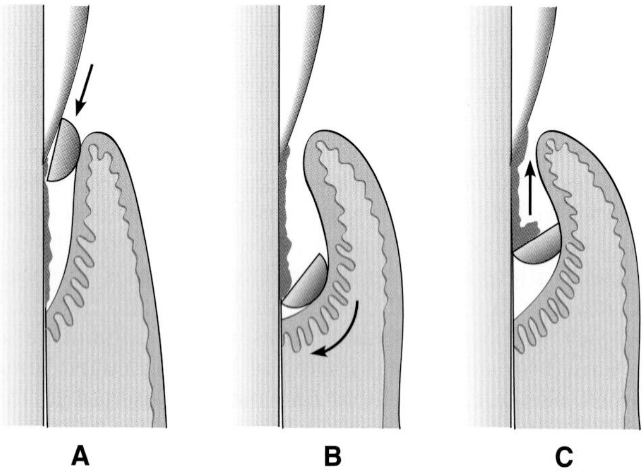

Figure 51-83 Subgingival scaling procedure. **A,** Curette inserted with the face of the blade flush against the tooth. **B,** Working angulation (45-90 degrees) is established at the base of the pocket. **C,** Lateral pressure is applied, and the scaling stroke is activated in the coronal direction.

The amount of lateral pressure applied to the tooth surface depends on the nature of the calculus and whether the strokes are for initial calculus removal or final root planing. If heavy lateral pressure is continued after the bulk of calculus has been removed and the blade is repeatedly readapted with short, choppy strokes, the result will be a root surface roughened by numerous nicks and gouges, resembling the rippled surface of a washboard.[111] If heavy lateral pressure is continued with long, even strokes, the result will be excessive removal of root structure, producing a smooth but "ditched" or "riffled" root surface. To avoid these hazards of over-instrumentation, a deliberate transition from short, powerful scaling strokes to longer, lighter root-planing strokes must be made as soon as the calculus and initial roughness have been eliminated.

When scaling strokes are used to remove calculus, force can be maximized by concentrating lateral pressure onto the lower third of the blade (see Figure 51-69). This small section, the terminal few millimeters of the blade, is positioned slightly apical to the lateral edge of the deposit, and a short vertical or oblique stroke is used to split the calculus from the tooth surface. Without withdrawing the instrument from the pocket, the lower third of the blade is advanced laterally and repositioned to engage the next portion of the remaining deposit. Another vertical or oblique stroke is made, slightly overlapping the previous stroke. This process is repeated in a series of powerful scaling strokes until the entire deposit has been removed. The overlapping of these pathways or "channels" of instrumentation[111] ensures that the entire instrumentation zone is covered (Figure 51-84).

Engaging a large, tenacious ledge or piece of calculus with the entire length of the cutting edge is not recommended because the force is distributed through a longer

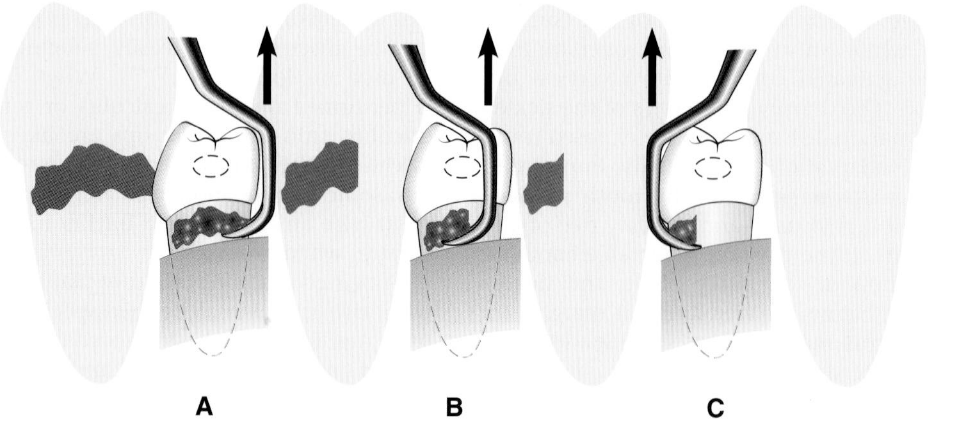

Figure 51-84 Instrumentation for calculus removal. **A,** Calculus is removed by engaging the apical or lateral edge of the deposit with the cutting edge of a scaler; vertical movement of the instrument will remove the fragment of calculus engaged by the instrument, as seen in the shaded drawing. **B,** The instrument is moved laterally and again engages the edge of the calculus, overlapping the previous stroke to some extent; the shaded drawing shows further removal. **C,** The final portion of the deposit is engaged and removed. Note how the procedure is performed in an interdental space by entering facially and lingually.

section of the cutting edge rather than concentrated. Much more lateral pressure is required to dislodge the entire deposit in one stroke. Although some clinicians may possess the strength to remove calculus completely in this manner, the heavier forces required diminish tactile sensitivity and contribute to a loss of control that results in tissue trauma. A single heavy stroke usually is not sufficient to remove calculus entirely. Instead, the blade skips over or skims the surface of the deposit. Subsequent strokes made with the entire cutting edge tend to shave the deposit down layer by layer. When a series of these repeated whittling strokes is applied, the calculus may be reduced to a thin, smooth, burnished sheet that is difficult to distinguish from the surrounding root surface.

A common error in instrumenting proximal surfaces is failing to reach the midproximal region apical to the contact. This area is relatively inaccessible, and the technique requires more skill than instrumentation of buccal or lingual surfaces. It is extremely important to extend strokes at least halfway across the proximal surface so that no calculus or roughness remains in the interproximal area. With properly designed curettes, this can be accomplished by keeping the lower shank of the curette parallel with the long axis of the tooth (Figure 51-85, *A*). With the lower shank parallel to the long axis, the blade of the curette will reach the base of the pocket and the toe will extend beyond the midline as strokes are advanced across the proximal surface. This extension of strokes beyond the midline ensures thorough exploration and instrumentation of these surfaces. If the lower shank is angled or tilted away from the tooth, the toe will move toward the contact area. Because this prevents the blade from reaching the base of the pocket, calculus apical to the contact will not be detected or removed. Strokes will be hampered because the toe tends to become lodged in the contact. If the instrument is angled or tilted too far toward the tooth, the lower shank will hit the tooth or the contact area, preventing extension of strokes to the midproximal region (Figure 51-85, *B* and *C*).

The relationship between the location of the finger rest and the working area is important for two reasons. First, the finger rest or fulcrum must be positioned to allow the lower shank of the instrument to be parallel or nearly parallel to the tooth surface being treated. This parallelism is a fundamental requirement for optimal working angulation. Second, the finger rest must be positioned to enable the operator to use wrist-arm motion to activate strokes. On some aspects of the maxillary posterior teeth, these requirements can be met only with the use of extraoral or opposite-arch fulcrums. When intraoral finger rests are used in other regions of the mouth, the finger rest must be close enough to the working area to fulfill these two requirements. A finger rest that is established too far from the working area forces the clinician to separate the middle finger from the fourth finger in an effort to obtain parallelism and proper angulation. Effective wrist-arm motion is possible only when these two fingers are kept together in a built-up fulcrum. Separation of the fingers commits the clinician to the exclusive use of finger flexing for the activation of strokes.

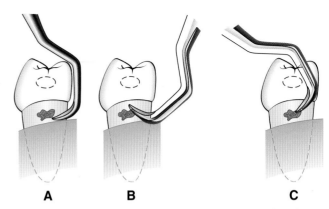

Figure 51-85 Shank position for scaling proximal surfaces. **A,** Correct shank position, parallel with the long axis of the tooth. **B,** Incorrect shank position, tilted away from the tooth. **C,** Incorrect shank position, tilted too far toward the tooth. Sextant: lingual aspect.

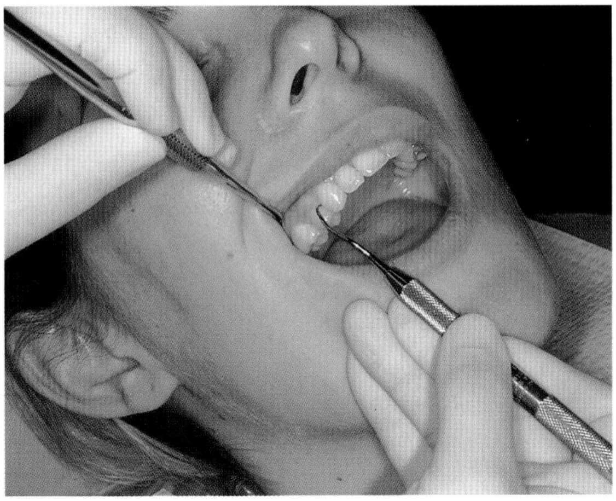

Figure 51-86 Maxillary right posterior sextant: facial aspect.

As instrumentation proceeds from one tooth to the next, the body position of the operator and the location of the finger rest must be frequently adjusted or changed to allow parallelism and wrist-arm motion. Various approaches to instrumentation in different areas of the mouth are illustrated here. The examples shown provide maximal efficiency for the clinician and comfort for the patient. For most areas, more than one approach is presented. Other approaches are possible and are acceptable if they provide equal efficiency and comfort. The following approaches may be used:

Maxillary right posterior sextant: facial aspect (Figure 51-86).
Operator position: Side position.
Illumination: Direct.
Visibility: Direct (indirect for distal surfaces of molars).
Retraction: Mirror or index finger of the nonoperating hand.
Finger rest: Extraoral, palm up. Backs of the middle and fourth fingers on the lateral aspect of the mandible on the right side of the face.

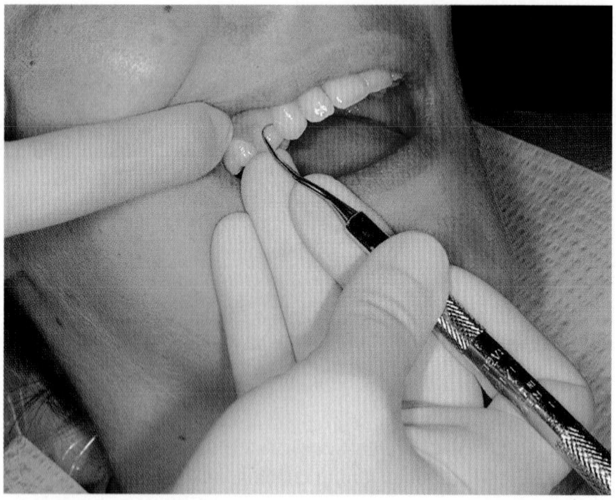

Figure 51-87 Maxillary right posterior sextant, premolar region only: facial aspect.

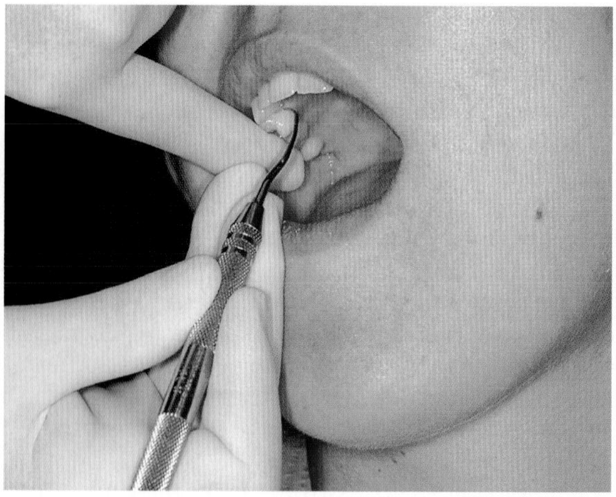

Figure 51-89 Maxillary right posterior sextant: lingual aspect.

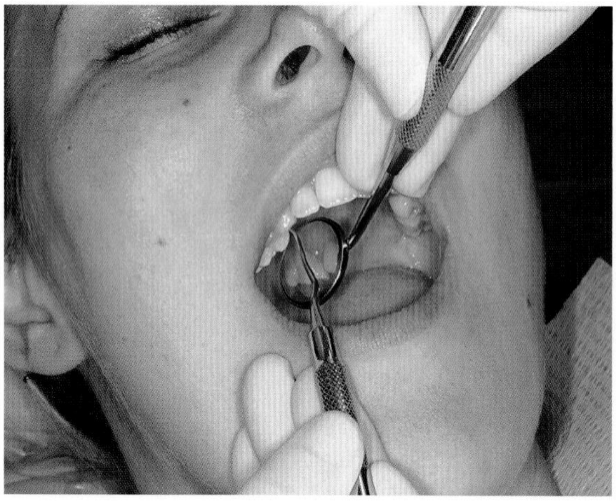

Figure 51-88 Maxillary right posterior sextant: lingual aspect.

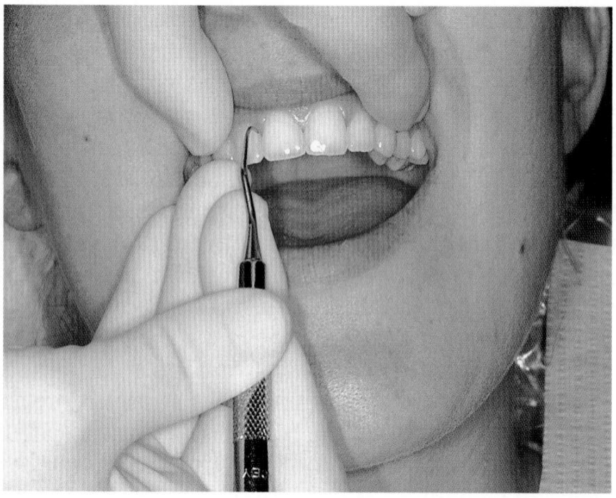

Figure 51-90 Maxillary anterior sextant: facial aspect, surfaces away from the operator.

Maxillary right posterior sextant, premolar region only: facial aspect (Figure 51-87).
Operator position: Side or back position.
Illumination: Direct.
Visibility: Direct.
Retraction: Mirror or index finger of the nonoperating hand.
Finger rest: Intraoral, palm up. Fourth finger on the occlusal surfaces of the adjacent maxillary posterior teeth.

Maxillary right posterior sextant: lingual aspect (Figure 51-88).
Operator position: Side or front position.
Illumination: Direct and indirect.
Visibility: Direct or indirect.
Retraction: None.
Finger rest: Extraoral, palm up. Backs of the middle and fourth fingers on the lateral aspect of the mandible on the right side of the face.

Maxillary right posterior sextant: lingual aspect (Figure 51-89).
Operator position: Front position.
Illumination: Direct.
Visibility: Direct.
Retraction: None.
Finger rest: Intraoral, palm up, finger on finger. Index finger of the nonoperating hand on the occlusal surfaces of the maxillary right posterior teeth; fourth finger of the operating hand or the index finger of the nonoperating hand.

Maxillary anterior sextant: facial aspect, surfaces away from the operator (Figure 51-90).
Operator position: Back position.
Illumination: Direct.
Visibility: Direct.
Retraction: Index finger of the nonoperating hand.
Finger rest: Intraoral, palm up. Fourth finger on the incisal edges or occlusal surfaces of adjacent maxillary teeth.

Maxillary anterior sextant: facial aspect, surfaces toward the operator (Figure 51-91).
Operator position: Front position.

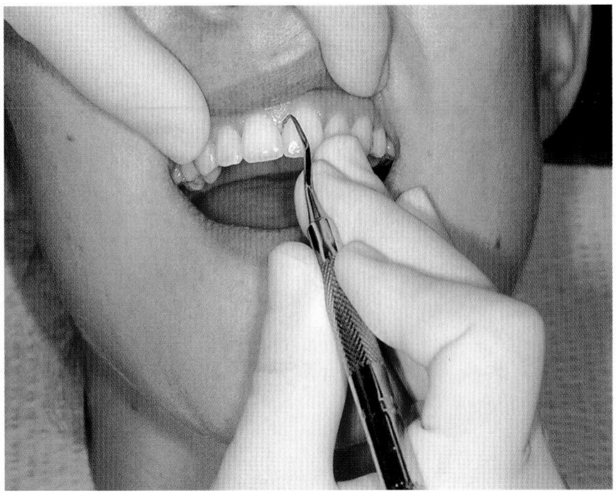

Figure 51-91 Maxillary anterior sextant: facial aspect, surfaces toward the operator.

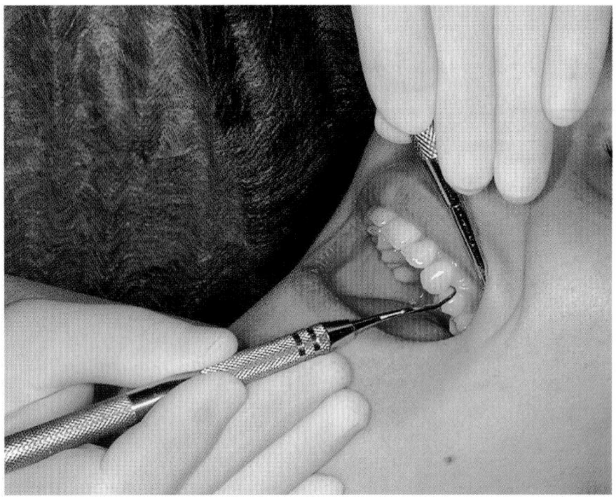

Figure 51-93 Maxillary left posterior sextant: facial aspect.

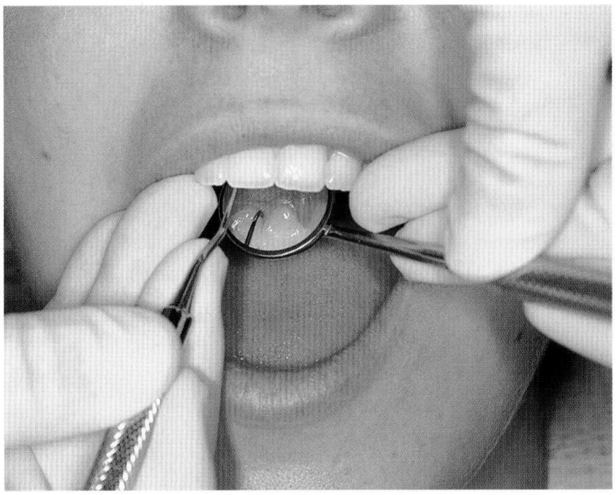

Figure 51-92 Maxillary anterior sextant: lingual aspect, surfaces away from the operator (surfaces toward the operator are scaled from a front position).

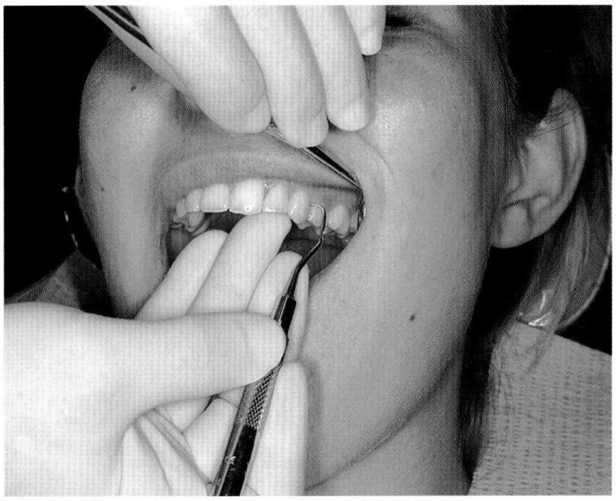

Figure 51-94 Maxillary left posterior sextant: facial aspect.

Illumination: Direct.
Visibility: Direct.
Retraction: Index finger of the nonoperating hand.
Finger rest: Intraoral, palm down. Fourth finger on the incisal edges or the occlusal or facial surfaces of adjacent maxillary teeth.

Maxillary anterior sextant: lingual aspect, surfaces away from the operator (surfaces toward the operator are scaled from a front position) (Figure 51-92).
Operator position: Back position.
Illumination: Indirect.
Visibility: Indirect.
Retraction: None.
Finger rest: Intraoral, palm up. Fourth finger on the incisal edges or the occlusal surfaces of adjacent maxillary teeth.

Maxillary left posterior sextant: facial aspect (Figure 51-93).
Operator position: Side or back position.
Illumination: Direct or indirect.
Visibility: Direct or indirect.
Retraction: Mirror.
Finger rest: Extraoral, palm down. Front surfaces of the middle and fourth fingers on the lateral aspect of the mandible on the left side of the face.

Maxillary left posterior sextant: facial aspect (Figure 51-94).
Operator position: Back or side position.
Illumination: Direct or indirect.
Visibility: Direct or indirect.
Retraction: Mirror.
Finger rest: Intraoral, palm up. Fourth finger on the incisal edges or the occlusal surfaces of adjacent maxillary teeth.

Maxillary left posterior sextant: lingual aspect (Figure 51-95).
Operator position: Front position.
Illumination: Direct.
Visibility: Direct.
Retraction: None.

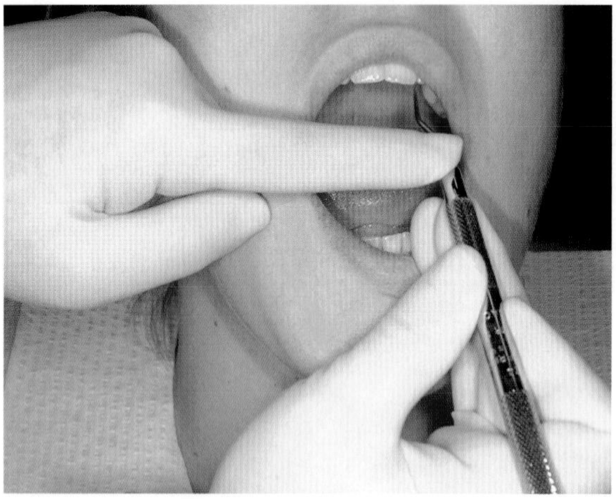

Figure 51-95 Maxillary left posterior sextant: lingual aspect.

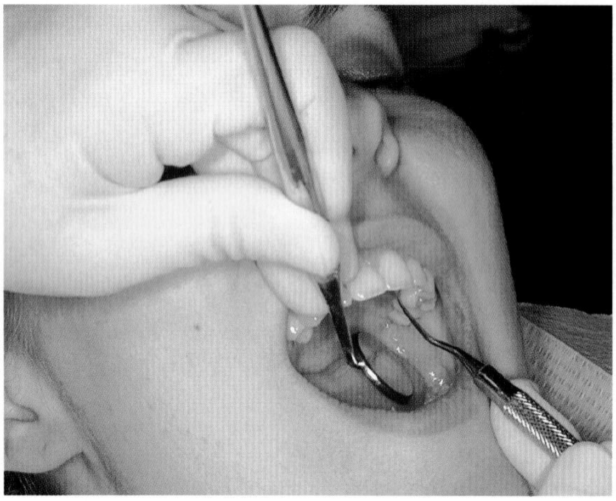

Figure 51-96 Maxillary left posterior sextant: lingual aspect.

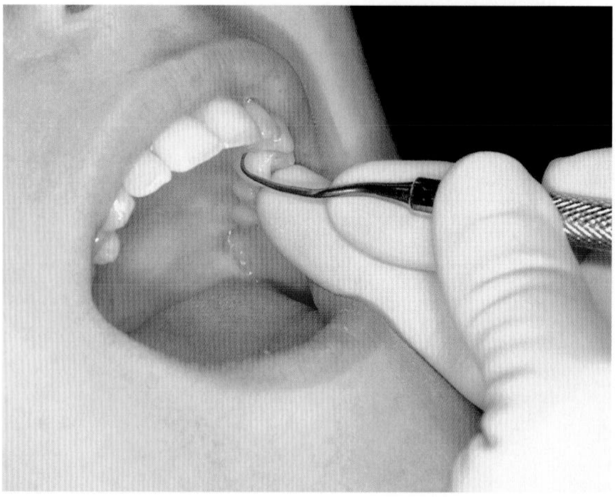

Figure 51-97 Maxillary left posterior sextant: lingual aspect.

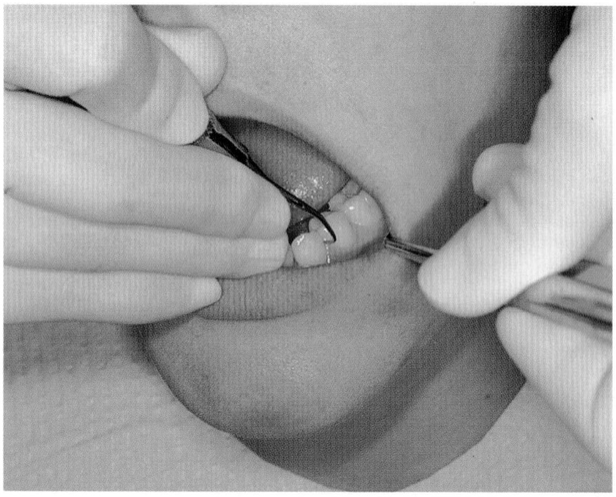

Figure 51-98 Mandibular left posterior sextant: facial aspect.

Finger rest: Intraoral, palm down, opposite arch, reinforced. Fourth finger on the incisal edges of the mandibular anterior teeth or the facial surfaces of the mandibular premolars, reinforced with the index finger of the nonoperating hand.

Maxillary left posterior sextant: lingual aspect (Figure 51-96).
Operator position: Front position.
Illumination: Direct and indirect.
Visibility: Direct and indirect.
Retraction: None.
Finger rest: Extraoral, palm down. Front surfaces of the middle and fourth fingers on the lateral aspect of the mandible on the left side of the face. The nonoperating hand holds the mirror for indirect illumination.

Maxillary left posterior sextant: lingual aspect (Figure 51-97).
Operator position: Side or front position.
Illumination: Direct.
Visibility: Direct.
Retraction: None.
Finger rest: Intraoral, palm up. Fourth finger on the occlusal surfaces of adjacent maxillary teeth.

Mandibular left posterior sextant: facial aspect (Figure 51-98).
Operator position: Side or back position.
Illumination: Direct.
Visibility: Direct or indirect.
Retraction: Index finger or mirror of the nonoperating hand.
Finger rest: Intraoral, palm down. Fourth finger on the incisal edges or the occlusal or facial surfaces of adjacent mandibular teeth.

Mandibular left posterior sextant: lingual aspect (Figure 51-99).
Operator position: Front or side position.
Illumination: Direct and indirect.
Visibility: Direct.
Retraction: Mirror retracts tongue.
Finger rest: Intraoral, palm down. Fourth finger on the incisal edges or the occlusal surfaces of adjacent mandibular teeth.

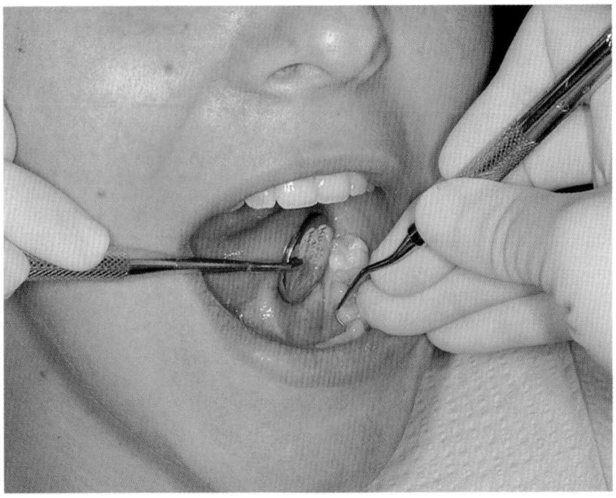

Figure 51-99 Mandibular left posterior sextant: lingual aspect.

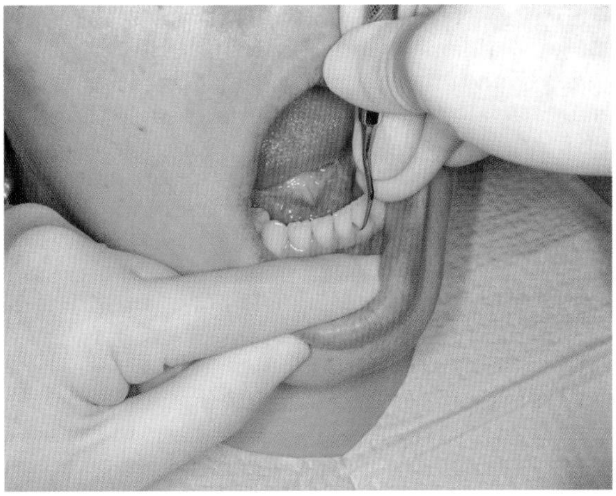

Figure 51-100 Mandibular anterior sextant: facial aspect, surfaces toward the operator.

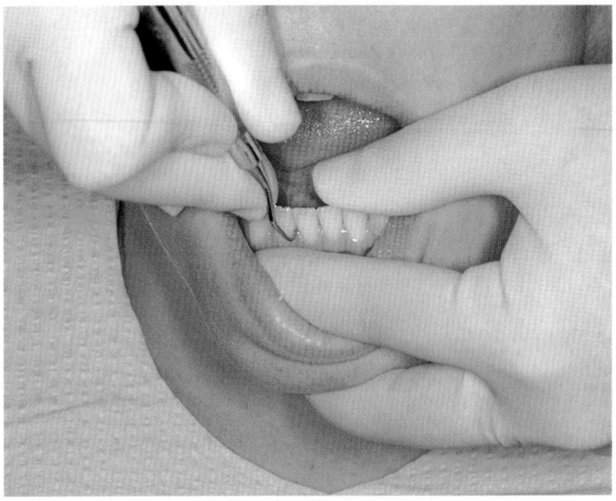

Figure 51-101 Mandibular anterior sextant: facial aspect, surfaces away from the operator.

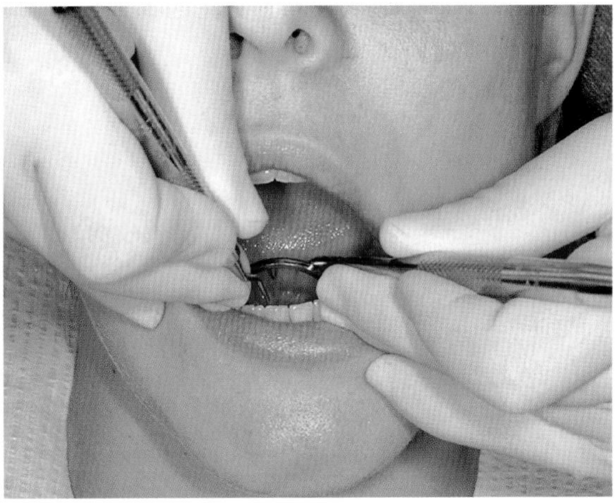

Figure 51-102 Mandibular anterior sextant: lingual aspect, surfaces away from the operator.

Mandibular anterior sextant: facial aspect, surfaces toward the operator (Figure 51-100).
Operator position: Front position.
Illumination: Direct.
Visibility: Direct.
Retraction: Index finger of the nonoperating hand.
Finger rest: Intraoral, palm down. Fourth finger on the incisal edges or the occlusal surfaces of adjacent mandibular teeth.

Mandibular anterior sextant: facial aspect, surfaces away from the operator (Figure 51-101).
Operator position: Back position.
Illumination: Direct.
Visibility: Direct.
Retraction: Index finger or thumb of the nonoperating hand.
Finger rest: Intraoral, palm down. Fourth finger on the incisal edges or the occlusal surfaces of adjacent mandibular teeth.

Mandibular anterior sextant: lingual aspect, surfaces away from the operator (Figure 51-102).
Operator position: Back position.
Illumination: Direct and indirect.
Visibility: Direct and indirect.
Retraction: Mirror retracts tongue.
Finger rest: Intraoral, palm down. Fourth finger on the incisal edges or the occlusal surfaces of adjacent mandibular teeth.

Mandibular anterior sextant: lingual aspect, surfaces toward the operator (Figure 51-103).
Operator position: Front position.
Illumination: Direct and indirect.
Visibility: Direct and indirect.
Retraction: Mirror retracts tongue.
Finger rest: Intraoral, palm down. Fourth finger on the incisal edges or the occlusal surfaces of adjacent mandibular teeth.

Mandibular right posterior sextant: facial aspect (Figure 51-104).
Operator position: Side or front position.
Illumination: Direct.
Visibility: Direct.

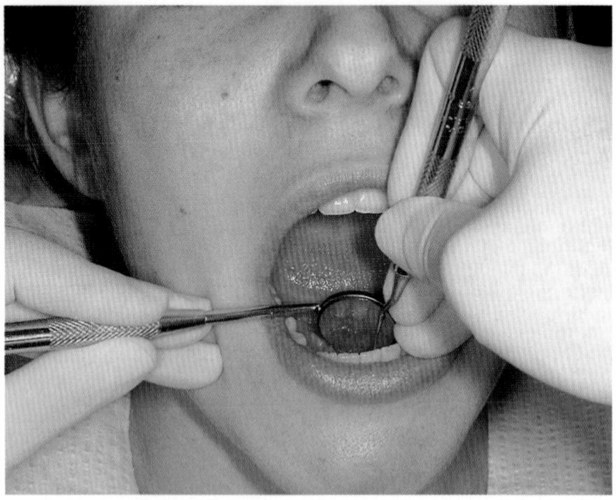

Figure 51-103 Mandibular anterior sextant: lingual aspect, surfaces toward the operator.

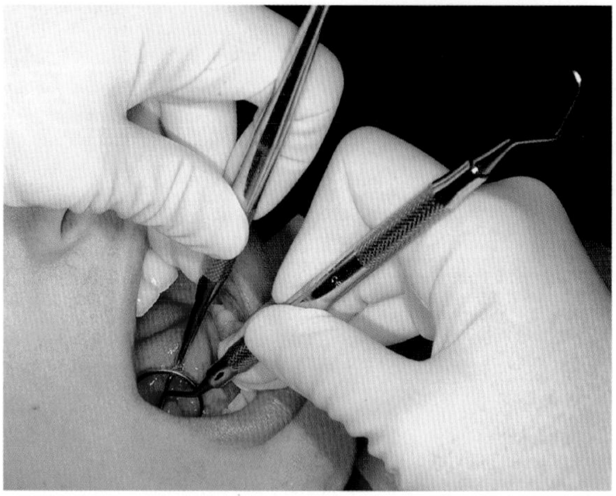

Figure 51-105 Mandibular right posterior sextant: lingual aspect.

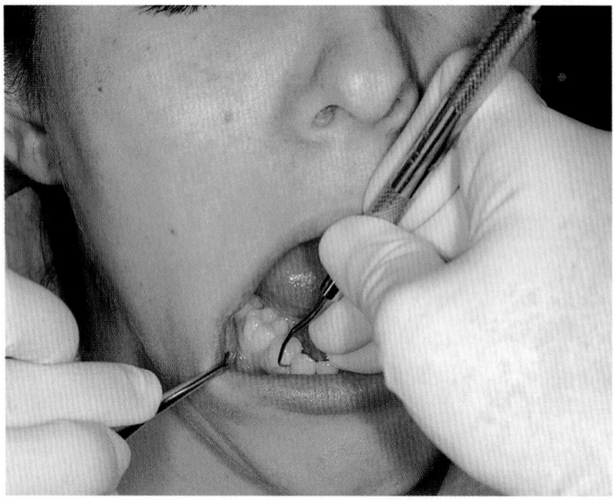

Figure 51-104 Mandibular right posterior sextant: facial aspect.

Retraction: Mirror or index finger of the nonoperating hand.
Finger rest: Intraoral, palm down. Fourth finger on the incisal edges or the occlusal surfaces of adjacent mandibular teeth.

Mandibular right posterior sextant: lingual aspect (Figure 51-105).
Operator position: Front position.
Illumination: Direct and indirect.
Visibility: Direct and indirect.
Retraction: Mirror retracts tongue.
Finger rest: Intraoral, palm down. Fourth finger on the incisal edges or the occlusal surfaces of adjacent mandibular teeth.

Ultrasonic Scaling

Instruments

Ultrasonic instruments have been used as a valuable adjunct to conventional hand instrumentation for many years. Until relatively recently, all ultrasonic tips were large and bulky, making them generally suitable only for supragingival scaling or subgingival scaling where tissue was inflamed and retractable. However, newly designed, thin ultrasonic tips have allowed better access to subgingival areas previously accessible only with hand instruments.[38] It is important to understand this historical perspective when attempting to interpret the literature comparing the effects of hand and ultrasonic instruments on root surfaces. Earlier studies using older tip designs generally showed that ultrasonic instruments left a rougher, more damaged surface than curettes.* More recent studies, especially those using the newer, thinner tips, show that ultrasonic instruments can produce root surfaces as smooth or smoother than those produced by curettes.[38,39,44,124] Whether these relative degrees of smoothness are important has not been clearly established.† It is evident, however, that both methods of instrumentation are able to provide satisfactory clinical results, as measured by removal of plaque and calculus, reduction of bacteria, reduction of inflammation and pocket depth, and gain in clinical attachment.‡

Ultrasonic instruments have been shown to be more effective than hand instruments at reducing spirochetes and motile rods in class II and III furcations.[78] Two in vitro studies found that ultrasonic and sonic scalers do not kill periodontal pathogenic bacteria by vibrational energy, rather suggesting an antimicrobial effect from an increase in temperature.[102,132] Other in vitro studies found that Gracey Curvettes were more effective than slim ultrasonic inserts in debriding root trunks, furcation entrances, and furcation areas of mandibular first molars.[107,108]

The selection of either ultrasonic or hand instrumentation should be determined by the clinician's preference and experience and the needs of each patient. The success of either treatment method is determined by the time devoted to the procedure and the thoroughness of root debridement. In practice, clinicians typically use a combination of both ultrasonic and hand instrumentation to achieve thorough debridement.

*References 5, 29, 45, 47, 63, 67, 145, 152, 160.
†References 45, 57, 68, 77, 101, 133.
‡References 8-12, 35, 48, 83, 103, 116, 145, 149.

The vibrational energy produced by the ultrasonic instrument makes it useful for removing heavy, tenacious deposits of calculus and stain. Such deposits can be removed more quickly and with less effort ultrasonically than manually. When ultrasonic instruments are properly manipulated, less tissue trauma and therefore less postoperative discomfort occur. This makes ultrasonic instrumentation useful for initial debridement in patients with acute painful conditions such as necrotizing ulcerative gingivitis. This same quality can be used to advantage with the new, thin ultrasonic tips for subgingival root debridement and deplaquing in maintenance patients with residual pocket depth. Ultrasonic scaling devices also have been used for gingival curettage and to remove overhangs and excess cement after cementing orthodontic appliances. Opinions differ regarding the effectiveness of ultrasonic instruments for removing stain compared with conventional polishing methods.[7,22]

Some contraindications exist to the use of ultrasonic and sonic scaling devices. These devices have been reported to interfere with the function of older cardiac pacemakers.[163] Patients with newer pacemakers can be treated safely; however, there may be a risk if the patient is medically fragile or if electronically defective ultrasonic devices are used.[90,150,163] Patients with known communicable diseases that can be transmitted by aerosols should not be treated with ultrasonic or sonic scaling devices. The water spray creates a contaminated aerosol that fills the operating area, exposing personnel and surfaces.[74,98] Even when treating patients without known communicable diseases, it is especially important that proper infection control measures be observed (i.e., use of protective clothing, eyewear, masks, and gloves) and proper surface decontamination be performed afterward. Prerinsing for 1 minute with an antimicrobial mouthwash such as 0.12% chlorhexidine significantly reduces the number of bacteria in the aerosol for approximately 1 hour.[154] Patients at risk for respiratory disease should not be treated with ultrasonic or sonic devices, including patients who are immunosuppressed or have chronic pulmonary disorders.[137,146] Finally, metal ultrasonic and sonic inserts are contraindicated for titanium implants, which can be etched or gouged, and for porcelain or bonded restorations, which can be fractured or removed.[20,37,75,120,155] Magnetostrictive and piezoelectric plastic-tipped ultrasonic inserts that do not cause damage to titanium implants are available[72] (Figure 51-106). Also, plastic and Teflon-coated sonic scaler tips have been developed for titanium implants and for deplaquing and subgingival polishing of root surfaces.[69,70,128]

Technique

Ultrasonic instrumentation is accomplished with a light touch and light pressure, keeping the tip parallel to the tooth surface and constantly in motion.[39,57,115] Leaving the tip in one place for too long or using the point of the tip against the tooth can produce gouging and roughening of the root surface or overheating of the tooth.[38] Using a lower-power setting and applying only slight pressure reduce the volume and depth of tooth structure removal.[29,115] The working end of the ultrasonic instrument must come in contact with the calculus deposit to fracture and remove it. As with hand instruments, instrument adaptation to the tooth is critical to success. The working tip must contact all aspects of the root surface to remove plaque and toxins thoroughly. Although as much as 10 mm or more of the length of the ultrasonic tip vibrates, only a small portion of it can be adapted to contact the curved root surface at any one time or point. As with hand instruments, a series of focused, overlapping strokes must be activated to ensure complete root coverage.[57] However, light strokes with a blunt, vibrating working end impair tactile sensitivity, and the constant water spray necessary for the operation of the instrument hampers visibility. For these reasons, during ultrasonic instrumentation, the tooth surface should be frequently examined with an explorer to evaluate the completeness of debridement.

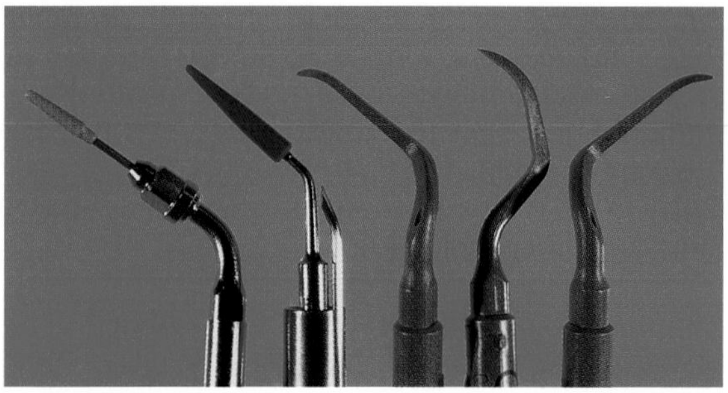

Figure 51-106 Ultrasonic tips for implants. **A,** Plastic Piezon Implant insert (EMS). **B,** Blue plastic magnetostrictive insert (Tony Riso). **C, D,** and **E,** Carbon composite piezoelectric inserts: PH1, PH2R, and PH2L (Satelec).

The aerosol produced by sonic and ultrasonic instrumentation may contain potentially infectious blood-borne and airborne pathogens.* Pneumococci, staphylococci, α-hemolytic streptococci, and *Mycobacterium tuberculosis* are among the bacteria that have been found in dental aerosols.[65,79] Aerosols also subject dental personnel and patients to many viruses, including herpes simplex virus, hepatitis virus, influenza virus, common cold viruses, Epstein-Barr virus, and cytomegalovirus.[27-33,89,148] Of additional concern are pathogens that do not originate from patients but are from the contaminated waterlines of the dental unit or the ultrasonic device.[34,42,109] Putative pathogens such as *Pseudomonas* species and *Legionella pneumophila* have been isolated from dental unit water and can become aerosolized by an ultrasonic scaler.[34,42,49,104] Aerosol from ultrasonic instrumentation always contains blood[13,91] and lingers in the air for 30 minutes or longer in the entire operatory and in areas of the dental office outside the operatory.[74,76,92,93] Unprotected patients may be more susceptible to infection from the aerosol than dental personnel who are wearing protective barriers, such as masks, gloves, eyewear, and clinical clothing.[16,27,137] High-speed evacuation, preprocedural rinsing with chlorhexidine, flushing of the handpiece and waterlines or a self-contained sterile

*References 7, 49-51, 59, 74, 92, 93, 125, 151.

water source, thorough disinfection of environmental surfaces, and adequate ventilation and air filtration units with high-efficiency particulate air (HEPA) filters are all important precautions to minimize the potential hazards of ultrasonic aerosols.[53,54,55,129]

With these points in mind, the ultrasonic device is used in the following manner:

1. Thoroughly wipe the ultrasonic unit with a disinfectant. Use a sterile, autoclavable ultrasonic handpiece, or wipe the handpiece with disinfectant. Cover the ultrasonic unit or control knobs and the handpiece with plastic or latex barriers. Flush the waterlines and handpiece for 2 minutes to decrease the number of microorganisms in the lines.[159] Use waterline filters or sterile water whenever possible.
2. Direct the patient to rinse for 1 minute with an antimicrobial oral rinse such as 0.12% chlorhexidine to reduce the contaminated aerosol.[153,159]
3. The clinician and the assistant should wear protective eyewear and masks and use high-speed evacuation to minimize inhalation of the contaminated aerosol produced during instrumentation.[53,54,55]
4. Turn on the unit, select an insert, place it into the handpiece, and then adjust the water control knob to produce a light mist of water at the working tip. Adequate aspiration is necessary to remove this water as it accumulates in the mouth. The power setting should begin on low and be adjusted no higher than necessary to remove calculus. Medium- to high-power settings have been shown to cause damage to roots when the tip is not parallel to the root surface.
5. The instrument is grasped with a light pen or modified pen grasp, and a finger rest or extraoral fulcrum should be established to allow a featherlike touch. Extraoral hand rests should be used for the maxillary teeth. For the mandibular teeth, either intraoral or extraoral fulcrums may be used.
6. Use short, light, vertical, horizontal, or oblique overlapping strokes. Keep the working tip adapted to the tooth surface as it is passed over the deposit. Heavy lateral pressure is unnecessary because the vibrational energy of the instrument dislodges the calculus. However, the working end must touch the deposit for this to occur.
7. The working end should be kept in constant motion, and the tip should be kept parallel to the tooth surface or at no more than a 15-degree angle to avoid etching or grooving the tooth surface.[159]
8. The instrument should be switched off periodically to allow for aspiration of water, and the tooth surface should be examined frequently with an explorer.
9. Any remaining irregularities of the root surface may be removed with sharp standard or mini-bladed curettes if necessary.

Evaluation

The adequacy of scaling and root planing is evaluated when the procedure is performed and again later, after a period of soft tissue healing.

Immediately after instrumentation, the tooth surfaces should be carefully inspected visually with optimal lighting and the aid of a mouth mirror and compressed air; surfaces also should be examined with a fine explorer or probe. Subgingival surfaces should be hard and smooth. Although complete removal of calculus is definitely necessary for the health of the adjacent soft tissue,[156] little documented evidence of the necessity for root smoothness is available.[45,48,149] Nevertheless, relative smoothness is still the best immediate clinical indication that calculus has been completely removed.[45]

Although smoothness is the criterion by which scaling and root planing are immediately evaluated, the ultimate evaluation is based on *tissue response*.[156] Clinical evaluation of the soft tissue response to scaling and root planing, including probing, should not be conducted earlier than 2 weeks postoperatively. Reepithelialization of the wounds created during instrumentation takes 1 to 2 weeks.[143,144] Until then, gingival bleeding on probing can be expected even when calculus has been completely removed because the soft tissue wound is not epithelialized. Any gingival bleeding on probing noted after this interval is more likely the result of persistent inflammation produced by residual deposits not removed during the initial procedure or inadequate plaque control. Positive clinical changes after instrumentation often continue for weeks or months. Therefore a longer period of evaluation may be indicated before deciding whether to intervene with further instrumentation or surgery.[28]

Occasionally the clinician may find that some slight root roughness remains after scaling and root planing.[67,145,160] If sound principles of instrumentation have been followed, the roughness may not be calculus. Because calculus removal, not root smoothness, has been shown to be necessary for tissue health, it might be more prudent in such a case to stop short of perfect smoothness and reevaluate the patient's tissue response after 2 to 4 weeks or longer. This avoids overinstrumentation and removal of excessive root structure in the pursuit of smoothness for its own sake. If the tissue is healthy after an interval of 2 to 4 weeks or longer, no further root planing is necessary. If the tissue is inflamed, the clinician must determine to what extent this is caused by plaque accumulation or the presence of residual calculus and to what degree further root planing is necessary.

INSTRUMENT SHARPENING

It is impossible to carry out periodontal procedures efficiently with dull instruments. A sharp instrument cuts more precisely and quickly than a dull instrument. To do its job at all, a dull instrument must be held more firmly and pressed harder than a sharp instrument. This reduces tactile sensitivity and increases the possibility that the instrument will inadvertently slip. *Therefore, to avoid wasting time and operating haphazardly, clinicians must be thoroughly familiar with the principles of sharpening and able to apply them to produce a keen cutting edge on the instruments they are using.* Development of this skill requires patience and practice, but clinical excellence cannot be attained without it.

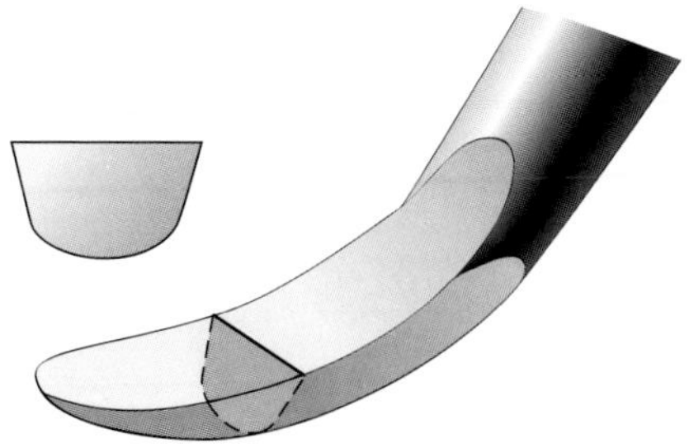

Figure 51-107 The cutting edge of a curette is formed by the angular junction of the face and the lateral surfaces of the instrument. When the instrument is sharp, the cutting edge is a fine line.

Figure 51-108 The cutting edge of a dull curette is rounded.

Evaluation of Sharpness

The *cutting edge* of an instrument is formed by the angular junction of two surfaces of its blade. The cutting edges of a curette, for example, are formed where the face of the blade meets the lateral surfaces (Figure 51-107).

When the instrument is sharp, this junction is a fine line running the length of the cutting edge. As the instrument is used, metal is worn away at the cutting edge, and the junction of the face and lateral surface becomes rounded or dulled[6,81] (Figure 51-108). Thus the cutting edge becomes a rounded surface rather than an acute angle. This is why a dull instrument cuts less efficiently and requires more pressure to do its job.[46]

Sharpness can be evaluated by sight and touch in one of the following ways:

1. When a dull instrument is held under a light, the rounded surface of its cutting edge reflects light back to the observer. It appears as a bright line running the length of the cutting edge (Figure 51-109). The acutely angled cutting edge of a sharp instrument, on the other hand, has no surface area to reflect light. When a sharp instrument is held under a light, no bright line can be observed (see Figure 51-107).
2. Tactile evaluation of sharpness is performed by drawing the instrument lightly across an acrylic rod known as a "sharpening test stick." A dull instrument will slide smoothly, without "biting" into the surface and raising a light shaving as a sharp instrument would.[159]

Objective of Sharpening

The objective of sharpening is to restore the fine, thin, linear cutting edge of the instrument. This is done by grinding the surfaces of the blade until their junction is once again sharply angular rather than rounded. For any given instrument, several sharpening techniques may produce this result. A technique is acceptable if it produces a sharp cutting edge without unduly wearing the instrument or altering its original design. To maintain the original design, the operator must understand the location and course of the cutting edges and the angles between the surfaces that form them. It is important to restore the cutting edge without distorting the original angles of the instrument. When these angles have been altered, the instrument does not function as it was designed to function, which limits its effectiveness.

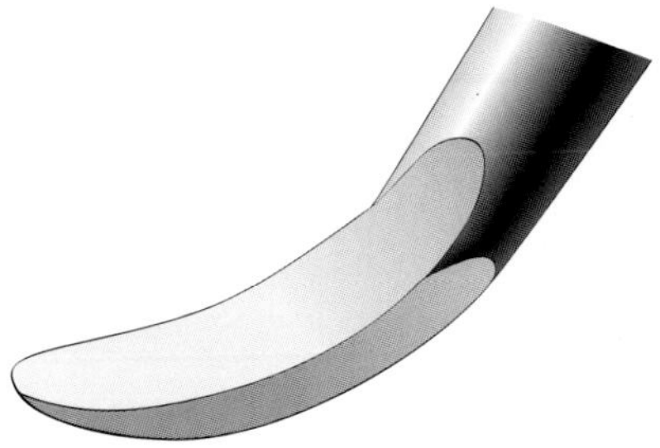

Figure 51-109 Light reflected from the rounded cutting edge of a dull instrument appears as a bright line.

Sharpening Stones

Sharpening stones may be quarried from natural mineral deposits or produced artificially. In either case, the surface of the stone is made up of abrasive crystals that are harder than the metal of the instrument to be sharpened. Coarse stones have larger particles and cut more rapidly; they are used on instruments that are dull. Finer stones with smaller crystals cut more slowly and are reserved for final sharpening to produce a finer edge and for sharpening instruments that are only slightly dull.[127,140] India and Arkansas oilstones are examples of natural abrasive stones. Carborundum, ruby, and ceramic stones are synthetically produced (Figure 51-110).

Sharpening stones can also be categorized by their method of use.

Mounted Rotary Stones. These stones are mounted on a metal mandrel and used in a motor-driven handpiece. They may be cylindrical, conical, or disc shaped. These stones are generally not recommended for routine use because they (1) are difficult to control precisely and can ruin the shape of the instrument, (2) tend to wear down the instrument quickly, and (3) can generate considerable frictional heat, which may affect the temper of the instrument.

Unmounted Stones. Unmounted stones come in a variety of sizes and shapes. Some are rectangular with flat or grooved surfaces, whereas others are cylindrical or cone shaped. Unmounted stones may be used in two ways: the instrument may be stabilized and held stationary while the stone is drawn across it, or the stone may be stabilized and held stationary while the instrument is drawn across it.

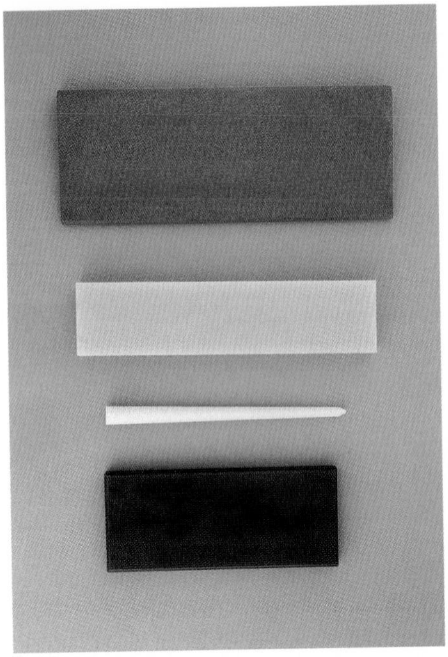

Figure 51-110 Sharpening stones. *Top to bottom,* A flat India stone, a flat Arkansas stone, a cone-shaped Arkansas stone, and a ceramic stone.

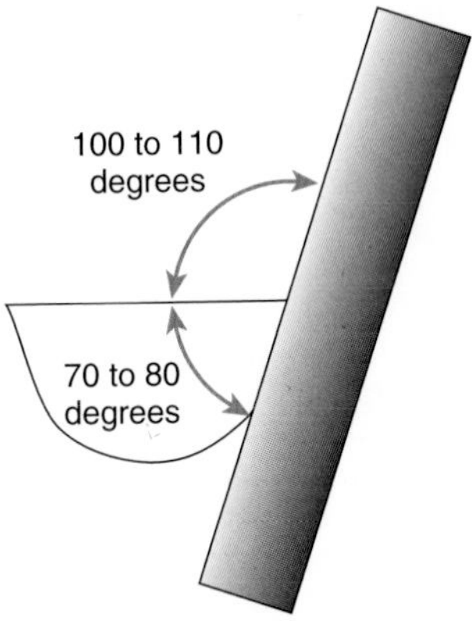

Figure 51-111 When the sharpening stone forms a 100- to 110-degree angle with the face of the blade, the 70- to 80-degree angle between the face and the lateral surface is automatically preserved.

Principles of Sharpening

1. Choose a stone suitable for the instrument to be sharpened—one that is of an appropriate shape and abrasiveness.
2. Use a sterilized sharpening stone if the instrument to be sharpened will not be resterilized before it is used on a patient.
3. Establish the proper angle between the sharpening stone and the surface of the instrument on the basis of an understanding of its design.
4. Maintain a stable, firm grasp of both the instrument and the sharpening stone. This ensures that the proper angulation is maintained throughout the controlled sharpening stroke. In this manner, the entire surface of the instrument can be reduced evenly, and the cutting edge is not improperly beveled.
5. Avoid excessive pressure. Heavy pressure causes the stone to grind the surface of the instrument more quickly and may shorten the instrument's life unnecessarily.
6. Avoid the formation of a "wire edge," characterized by minute filamentous projections of metal extending as a roughened ledge from the sharpened cutting edge.[6,46,110,159] When the instrument is used on root surfaces, these projections produce a grooved surface rather than a smooth surface. A wire edge is produced when the direction of the sharpening stroke is away from, rather than into or toward, the cutting edge.[6,110] When back-and-forth or up-and-down sharpening strokes are used, formation of a wire edge can be avoided by finishing with a down stroke toward the cutting edge.[81]
7. Lubricate the stone during sharpening. This minimizes clogging of the abrasive surface of the sharpening stone with metal particles removed from the instrument.[46,110,159] It also reduces heat produced by friction. Oil should be used for natural stones and water for synthetic stones.
8. Sharpen instruments at the first sign of dullness. A grossly dull instrument is inefficient and requires more pressure when used, which hinders control. Furthermore, sharpening such an instrument requires the removal of a great deal of metal to produce a sharp cutting edge. This shortens the effective life of the instrument.

Sharpening Individual Instruments

Universal Curettes. Several techniques will produce a properly sharpened curette. Regardless of the technique used, the clinician must keep in mind that the angle between the face of the blade and the lateral surface of any curette is 70 to 80 degrees (Figure 51-111). This is the most effective design for removing calculus and root planing (Figure 51-112, *left*). Changing this angle distorts the design of the instrument and makes it less effective. A cutting edge of less than 70 degrees is quite sharp but also thin (Figure 51-112, *center*). It wears down quickly and becomes dull. A cutting edge of 90 degrees or more requires heavy lateral pressure to remove deposits (Figure 51-112, *right*). Calculus removal with such an instrument is often incomplete, and root planing cannot be done effectively.

The following technique is recommended because it enables the clinician to visualize the critical 70- to 80-degree angle easily and thereby consistently restores an effective cutting edge:

Sharpening The Lateral Surface. When a flat, handheld stone is correctly applied to the lateral surface of a curette to maintain the 70- to 80-degree angle, the angle between the face of the blade and the surface of the stone will be 100 to 110 degrees (see Figure 51-111). This can best be visualized by holding the curette so that the face of the blade is parallel with the floor. A palm

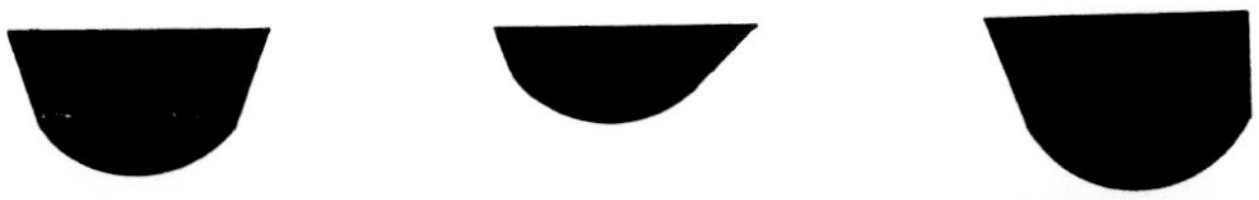

Figure 51-112 *Left,* Properly sharpened curette maintains a 70- to 80-degree angle between its face and lateral surface. *Center,* Curette has been sharpened so that one of its cutting edges is less than 70 degrees. This fine edge is quite sharp but dulls easily. *Right,* One of the cutting edges of the curette has been sharpened to 90 degrees. Heavy lateral pressure must be applied to the tooth to remove deposits with such an instrument.

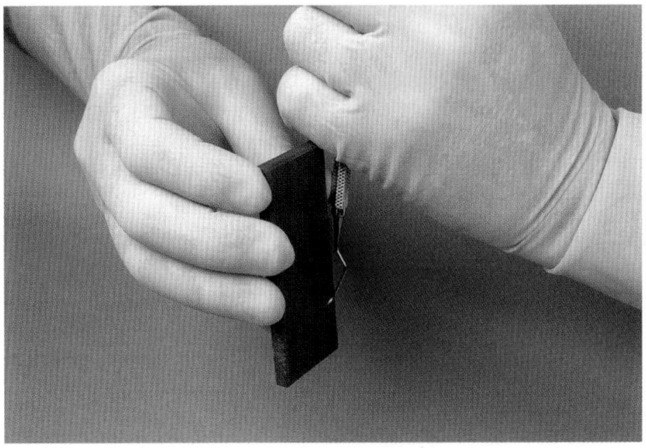

Figure 51-113 Using a palm grasp, operator holds the universal curette so that the face of the blade is parallel to the floor. The stone makes a 100- to 110-degree angle with the face of the blade.

grasp should be used and the upper arm braced against the body for support.

1. Apply the sharpening stone to the lateral surface of the curette so that the angle between the face of the blade and the stone is 100 to 110 degrees (Figure 51-113; see also Figure 51-111).
2. Beginning at the shank end of the cutting edge and working toward the toe, activate the stone with short, up-and-down strokes. Use consistent, light pressure and keep the stone continuously in contact with the blade. Make sure that the 100- to 110-degree angle is constantly maintained (Figure 51-113).
3. Check for sharpness as previously described, and continue sharpening as necessary. To prevent the toe of the curette from becoming pointed, sharpen the entire blade from shank end to toe. When approaching the toe, be sure to sharpen around it to preserve its rounded form (Figure 51-114).
4. As the stone is moved along the cutting edge, finish each section with a down stroke into or toward the cutting edge; this will minimize the formation of a wire edge. Check the cutting edge under a light.
5. Sharpening the curette in this manner tends to flatten the lateral surface. This can be corrected by lightly grinding the lateral surface and the back of the instrument, away from the cutting edge, each time the instrument is sharpened.

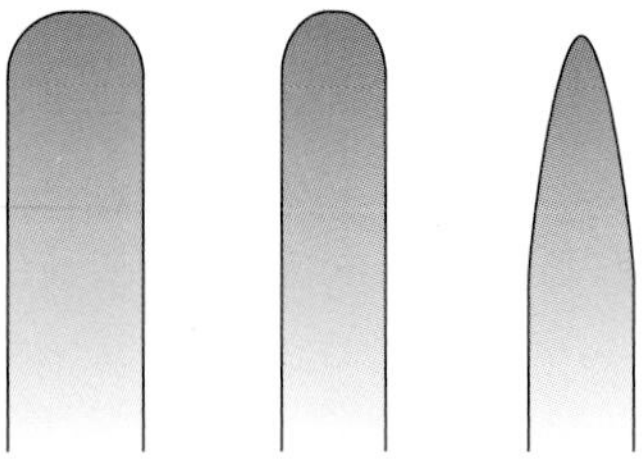

Figure 51-114 *Left,* New, unsharpened curette viewed from directly above the face of the blade. *Center,* Curette has been correctly sharpened to maintain the rounded toe. *Right,* Curette has been incorrectly sharpened, producing a pointed toe.

Figure 51-115 *Left,* Angulation is difficult to control when sharpening the face of the blade and often results in unwanted beveling. *Right,* Sharpening the face also weakens the blade by narrowing it from face to back.

6. When one edge has been properly sharpened, the opposite cutting edge can be sharpened in the same manner.

Sharpening The Face Of The Blade. This may be done by moving a handheld cylindrical or cone-shaped stone back and forth across the face of the blade. A similar stone mounted in a handpiece may also be used by applying it to the face of the blade with the stone rotating toward the toe. These methods are not recommended for routine use for the following reasons:

1. The angulation between the instrument and the stone is difficult to maintain, and therefore the blade may be improperly beveled[6] (Figure 51-115, *left*).
2. Sharpening the face of the blade narrows the working end from face to back. This weakens the blade and makes it likely to bend or break while in use[6,81,110,134] (Figure 51-115, *right*).
3. Sharpening the face of the blade with a handheld stone using a back-and-forth motion produces a wire edge that interferes with the sharpness of the blade.[6]

Area-Specific (Gracey) Curettes. As with a universal curette, a Gracey curette has an angle of 70 to 80 degrees between the face and lateral surface of its blade. Therefore the technique described for sharpening a universal curette can be used to sharpen a Gracey curette. However, several unique design features that distinguish a Gracey from a universal curette must be understood to avoid distorting the design of the instrument while sharpening (see earlier discussion).

As previously noted, Gracey curettes have an offset blade; that is, the face of the blade is not perpendicular to the shank of the instrument, as it is on a universal curette, but is offset at a 70-degree angle (Figure 51-116). A Gracey curette is further distinguished by the curvature of its cutting edges. When viewed from directly above

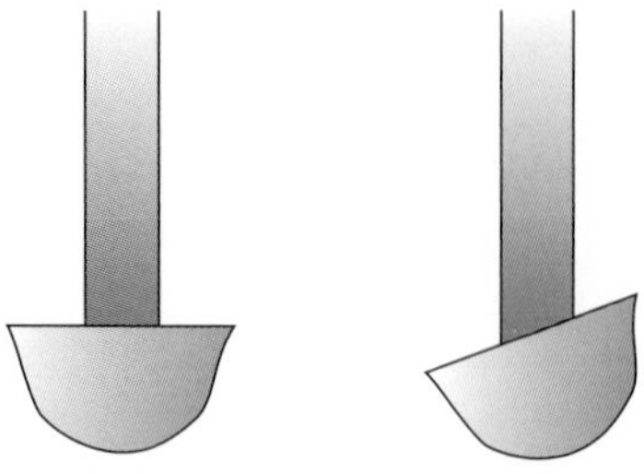

Figure 51-116 **A,** Face of a universal curette is at 90 degrees to its shank. **B,** Face of a Gracey curette is offset, forming a 70-degree angle with its shank.

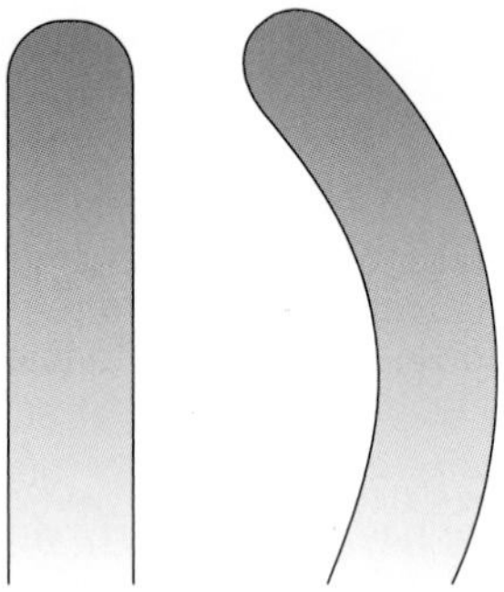

Figure 51-117 Cutting edges of a universal curette extend straight from shank to toe. The cutting edges of a Gracey curette gently curve from shank to toe. Only the larger, outer cutting edge at the right is used for scaling and needs to be sharpened.

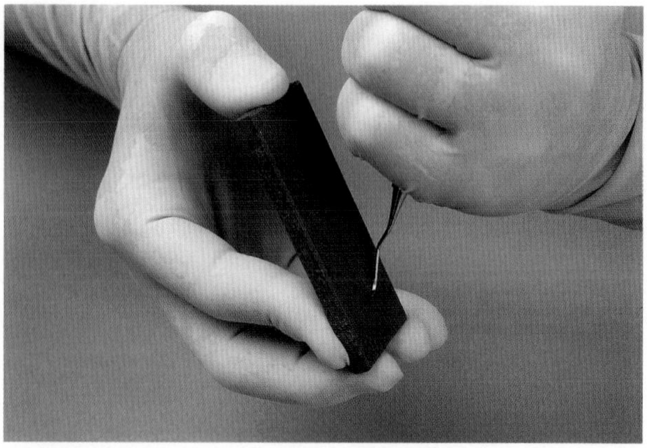

Figure 51-118 Note that when a Gracey curette is held in proper sharpening position, its shank is not perpendicular to the floor because of its offset blade angle. The stone meets the blade at an angle of 100 to 110 degrees. Compare this position with the sharpening position of a universal curette, as shown in Figure 51-113.

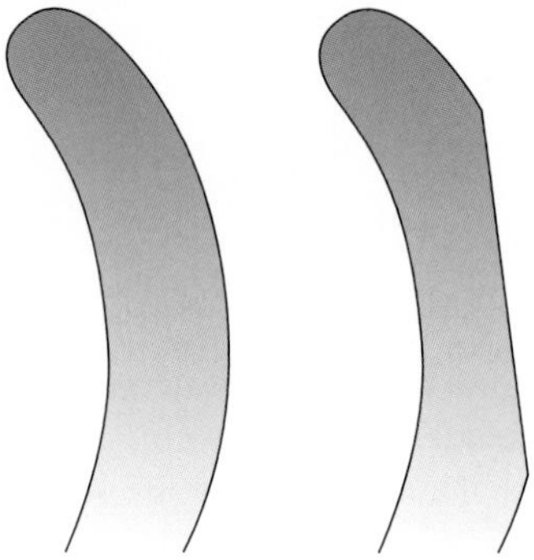

Figure 51-119 Gracey curette on the left has been properly sharpened to maintain a symmetric curve on its outer cutting edge. For the curette on the right, the sharpening stone was activated too long in one place, thereby flattening the blade.

the face of the blade, the cutting edges of a universal curette extend in straight lines from shank to toe; both cutting edges can be used for scaling and root planing. The cutting edges of a Gracey curette, on the other hand, curve gently from shank to toe, and only the larger, outer cutting edge is used for scaling and root planing (Figure 51-117).

With these points in mind, a Gracey curette is sharpened in the following manner:

1. Hold the curette so that the face of the blade is parallel with the floor. Because the blade is offset, the shank of the instrument will not be perpendicular to the floor, as it is with universal curettes (Figure 51-118).
2. Identify the edge to be sharpened. Remember that only one cutting edge is used, so only that edge must be sharpened (Figure 51-119, *left*). Apply the stone to the lateral surface so that the angle between the face of the blade and the stone is 100 to 110 degrees.
3. Activate short, up-and-down strokes, working from the shank end of the blade to the curved toe. Finish with a down stroke.
4. Remember that the cutting edge is curved. Preserve the curve by turning the stone while sharpening from shank to toe. If the stone is kept in one place for too many strokes, the blade will be flattened (Figure 51-119, *right*).
5. Evaluate sharpness as previously described. Continue sharpening as necessary.

Extended-Shank and Mini-Bladed Gracey Curettes. Extended-shank Gracey curettes, such as the After Five curettes, are sharpened in exactly the same manner as the standard Gracey curettes. Although the terminal shank is 3 mm longer, the blade size and shape are very similar, and thus there is no difference in the sharpening technique.

Mini-bladed Gracey curettes, such as the Mini Five curettes or Gracey Curvettes, are also sharpened with the same technique. These blades are only half the length of a standard Gracey blade, but the angle between the face and the lateral surface of the blade is still 70 to 80 degrees. However, sharpening too heavily or too often around the toe of a mini-bladed curette should be avoided to prevent excessive shortening of the blade.

Sickle Scalers. The two types of sickle scalers are the straight sickle and curved sickle. On a straight sickle

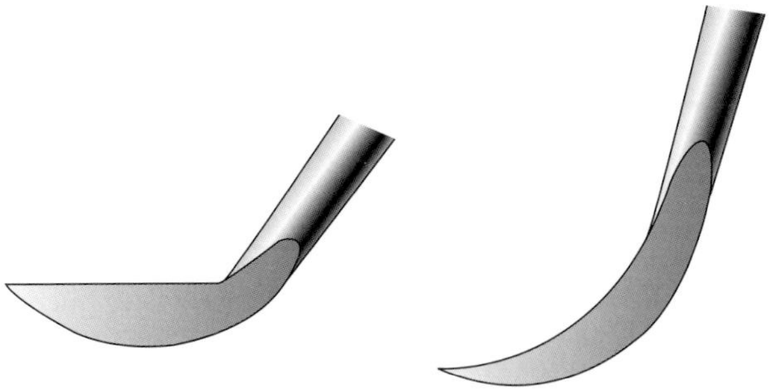

Figure 51-120 Face of the blade on a straight sickle is flat from shank to tip *(left)*, whereas on the curved sickle the blade face forms a gentle arc *(right)*.

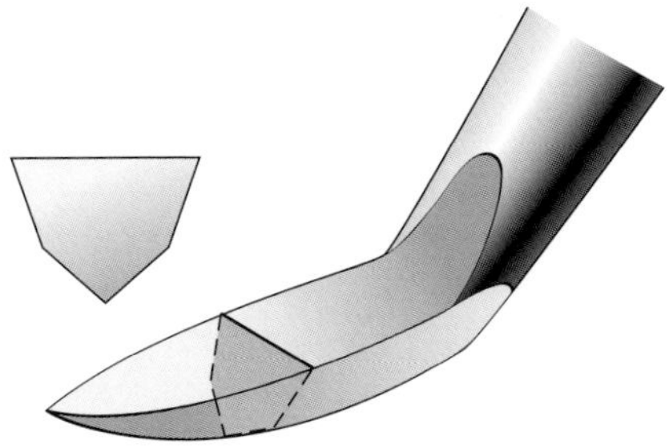

Figure 51-121 As with the curette, the sickle has an angle of 70 to 80 degrees between the face of the blade and the lateral surface.

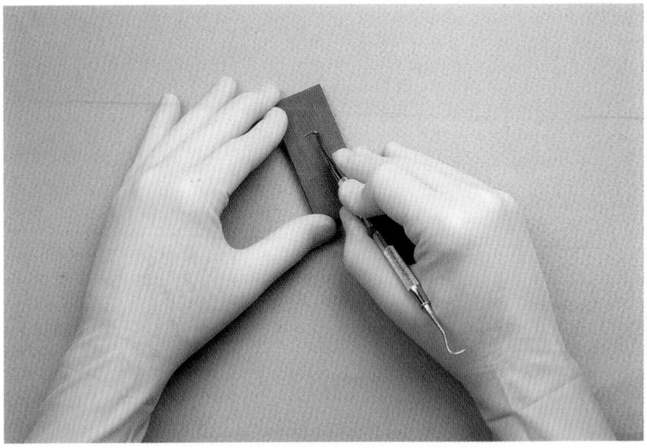

Figure 51-122 Large, flat stone may also be used to sharpen the sickle. The stone is stabilized on a flat surface. The fourth finger of the right hand guides the sharpening stroke as the instrument is pulled across the face of the stone toward the operator.

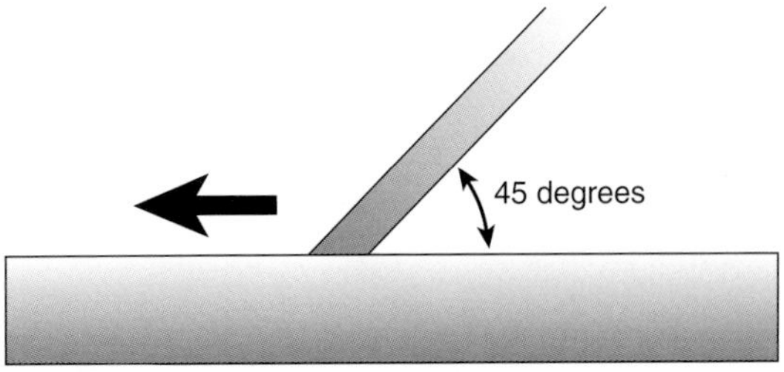

Figure 51-123 When the entire bevel on a chisel contacts the sharpening stone, the angle between the instrument and the stone is 45 degrees. The cutting edge will be properly sharpened if this angle is maintained as the instrument is pushed across the stone.

the face of the blade is flat from shank to tip, whereas on a curved sickle the face of the blade forms a gentle curve (Figure 51-120). However, the straight and curved sickles have similar cross-sectional designs. As in the curette, the angle between the face of the blade and the lateral surface of a sickle is 70 to 80 degrees (Figure 51-121). When a sharpening stone is correctly applied to the lateral surface to preserve this angle, the angle between the face of the blade and the surface of the stone is 100 to 110 degrees. With this in mind, the sickle scaler can be sharpened in a manner similar to that described for the curette, except that the sickle has a sharp, pointed toe that must not be rounded.

A large, flat stone may also be used to sharpen sickles (Figure 51-122). The stone is stabilized on a table or cabinet with the left hand. The sickle is held in the right hand with a modified pen grasp and applied to the stone so that the angle between the face of the blade and the stone is 100 to 110 degrees. The fourth finger is placed on the right-hand edge of the stone to stabilize and guide the sharpening movement. The right hand then pushes and pulls the sickle across the surface of the stone. To avoid a wire edge, the operator finishes with a pull stroke, being sure that the proper angulation is always maintained.

Chisels and Hoes. Chisels have a single, straight cutting edge that is perpendicular to the shank. The face of the blade is continuous with the shank of the instrument, which may be directly in line with the handle or slightly curved. The end of the blade is beveled at 45 degrees to form the cutting edge.

To sharpen a chisel, stabilize a flat sharpening stone on a flat surface. Grasp the instrument with a modified pen grasp. Establish a finger rest with the pads of the third and fourth fingers against the straight edge of the sharpening stone. Apply the flat beveled surface of the chisel to the surface of the stone. If the entire surface of the bevel is contacting the stone, the 45-degree angle between the beveled surface and the face of the blade will be maintained, and the design of the instrument will not be altered (Figures 51-123 and 51-124).

Using moderate, steady pressure, with the hand and arm acting as a unit and the finger resting on the edge of the stone as a guide, push the instrument across the surface of the sharpening stone. Release pressure slightly, and draw the instrument back to its starting point. Repeat the sharpening stroke until a sharp edge has been obtained. Remember to finish with a push stroke to prevent the formation of a wire edge. Check for sharpness as previously described. Examine the instrument carefully to be sure that its design has not been inadvertently altered.

Back-action surgical chisels and hoe scalers are sharpened with exactly the same technique described for

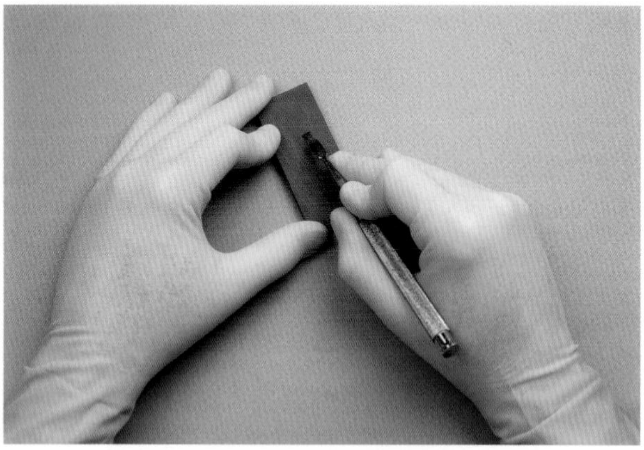

Figure 51-124 Chisel also can be sharpened on a stationary, flat sharpening stone.

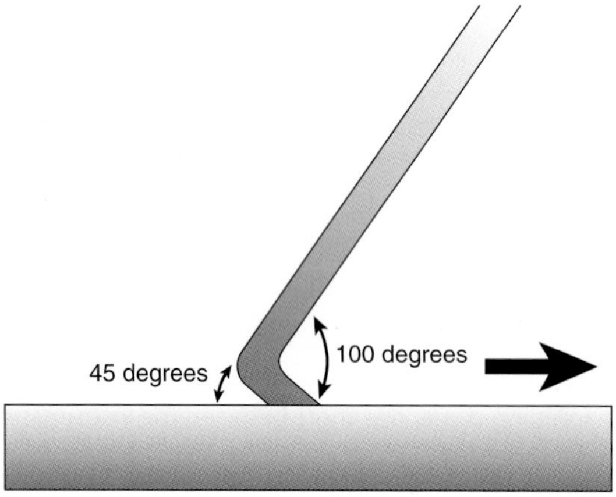

Figure 51-125 Back-action chisels and hoes are sharpened with a pull stroke.

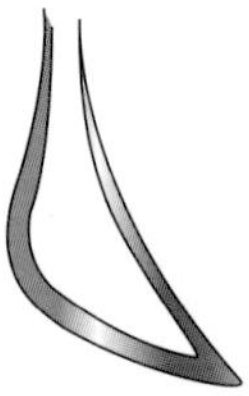

Figure 51-126 Flat-bladed gingivectomy knives such as this Kirkland knife have a cutting edge that extends around the entire blade. The entire cutting edge must be sharpened.

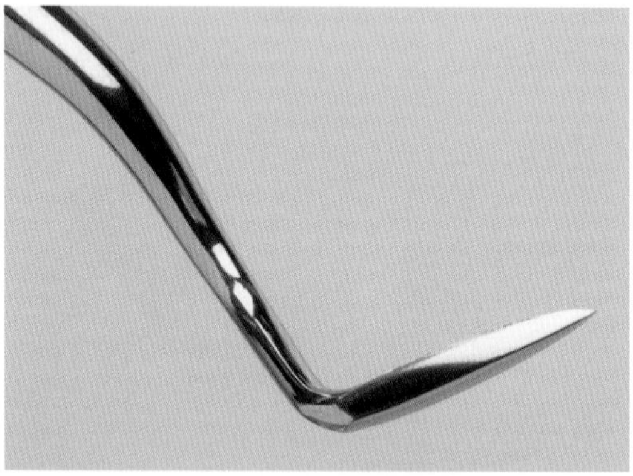

Figure 51-127 The two cutting edges of an interproximal knife are formed by bevels on the front and back surfaces of the blade.

chisels except that a pull stroke is used rather than a push stroke (Figure 51-125).

Periodontal Knives. There are two general types of periodontal knives. The first type includes the disposable scalpel blades that come prepackaged and are presharpened and sterilized by the manufacturer. These knives are not resharpened when they become dull but are discarded and replaced.

The second type of periodontal knife is reusable and must be sharpened when it becomes dull. The most common knives in this group are the flat-bladed gingivectomy knives (e.g., Kirkland knives #15K and 16K) and the narrow, pointed interproximal knives.

Flat-Bladed Gingivectomy Knives. These knives have broad, flat blades that are nearly perpendicular to the lower shank of the instrument. The curved cutting edge extends around the entire outer edge of the blade and is formed by bevels on both the front and the back surface of the blade (Figure 51-126).

When sharpening these instruments, only the bevel on the back surface of the instrument needs to be ground. This can be done by drawing the blade across a stationary, flat sharpening stone or by holding the instrument stationary and drawing the stone across its blade.

Interproximal Knives. The blades of interproximal knives have two long, straight cutting edges that come together at the sharply pointed tip of the instrument. The cutting edges are formed by bevels on the front and back surfaces of the blade. The entire blade is roughly perpendicular to the lower shank of the instrument (Figure 51-127).

As with the flat-bladed gingivectomy knives, only the bevels on the back surface of the interproximal knives need to be sharpened. Again, this can be accomplished by drawing the instrument across a stationary stone or by holding the instrument stationary and moving the stone across it.

Stationary Stone Technique. Stabilize a flat sharpening stone on a flat surface. Grasp the handle of the instrument with a modified pen grasp, and apply the bevel on the back surface of the blade to the flat surface of the sharpening stone. With moderate pressure, pull the instrument toward you (Figures 51-128 and 51-129). Release pressure slightly, and return to the starting point. Begin at one end of the cutting edge, and continue around the blade by rolling the handle of the instrument slightly between the thumb and the first and second fingers. Finish each section of the blade with a pull stroke to prevent formation of a wire edge. Check for sharpness as described previously.

Stationary Instrument Technique. Grasp the instrument with the palm. Apply the flat surface of a handheld

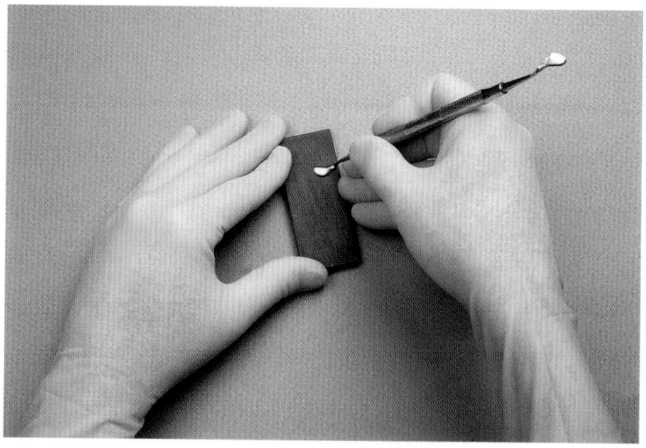

Figure 51-128 Gingivectomy knife may be sharpened on a stationary flat stone. The instrument is held with a modified pen grasp. The fourth finger guides the sharpening stroke as the instrument is rolled between the fingers so that all sections of the blade are sharpened.

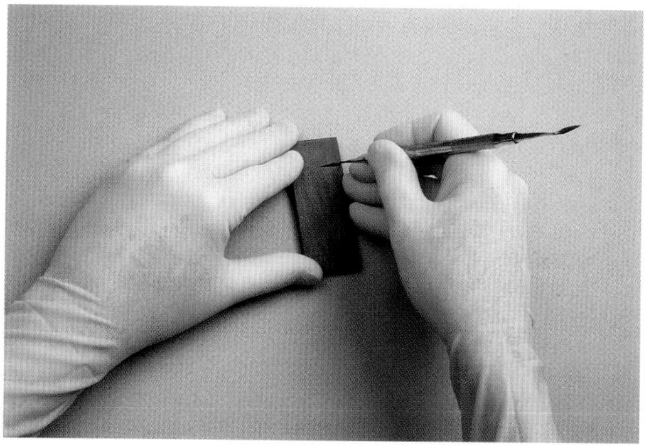

Figure 51-129 Interproximal knife may be sharpened on a flat stationary stone. The blade is drawn toward the operator.

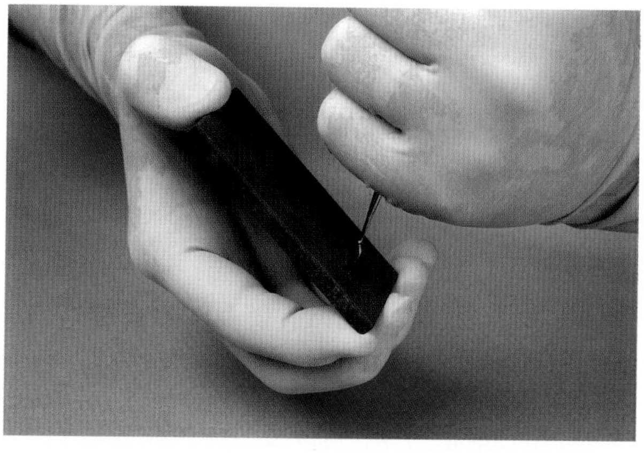

Figure 51-130 Interproximal knife may also be sharpened with a handheld stone. The instrument is held with a palm grasp, and the stone is applied to the entire cutting edge.

SCIENCE TRANSFER

The mechanical removal of plaque and calculus provides the basis for reducing inflammation around the teeth. Elaborate instrumentation and techniques have evolved because of the morphology of the crown and root structures. The ultimate goal of these procedures is to eliminate the instigating cause of the inflammatory and immune host response. The nature of the host response appears to be the critical aspect in determining whether the host can contain the microbial challenge or whether the host is overwhelmed by the challenge, resulting in tissue loss and periodontal disease. It is not known, however, whether it is the quality or the quantity (or a combination) of the microbial challenge that can tip the balance in the host response from protection toward destruction. In either case, the most effective means to reduce the challenge to the host is by meticulous removal of plaque and calculus. This removal is reflected by healthy tissues, and thus the amount of inflammation present is used to determine the effectiveness of periodontal instrumentation and home care by the patient.

Root planing is one of the most demanding procedures to be mastered by clinicians. Experienced clinicians show greater skill in the use of these instruments than novices, because years of practice are needed to refine the associated technical expertise. This chapter provides the detailed bases for clinicians to refine their abilities to treat periodontal problems with nonsurgical instrumentation.

sharpening stone to the bevel on the back surface of the blade (Figure 51-130). Begin at one end of the cutting edge, and with moderate pressure, draw the stone back and forth across the instrument. To prevent the formation of a wire edge, finish each section with a stroke into or toward the cutting edge. Proceed around the entire length of the cutting edge by gradually rotating the instrument and the stone in relation to one another.

REFERENCES

1. Adriaens P, Edwards C, DeBoever J, et al: Ultrastructural observations on bacterial invasion in cementum and radicular dentin of periodontally diseased human teeth, *J Periodontol* 59:493, 1988.
2. Agger MS, Horsted-Bindslev P, Hovgaard O: Abrasiveness of an air-powder polishing system on root surfaces in vitro, *Quintessence Int* 32:407, 2001.
3. Aleo J, DeRenzis F, Farber P: In vitro attachment of human gingival fibroblasts to root surfaces, *J Periodontol* 46:639, 1975.
4. Aleo J, DeRenzis F, Farber P, et al: The presence and biological activity of cementum-bound endotoxin, *J Periodontol* 45:672, 1974.

5. Allen EF, Rhoads RH: Effects of high-speed periodontal instruments on tooth surfaces, *J Periodontol* 34:352, 1963.
6. Antonini CJ, Brady JM, Levin MP, et al: Scanning electron microscope study of scalers, *J Periodontol* 48:45, 1977.
7. Ashimoto A, Chen C, Bakker I, et al: Polymerase chain reaction detection of 8 putative periodontal pathogens in subgingival plaque of gingivitis and advanced periodontitis lesions, *Oral Microbiol Immunol* 11:266, 1996.
8. Axelsson P, Lindhe J: Effect of controlled oral hygiene procedures on caries and periodontal disease in adults: results after 6 years, *J Clin Periodontol* 8:239, 1981.
9. Baderstein A, Nilveus R, Egelberg J: Effect of nonsurgical periodontal therapy. I. Moderately advanced periodontitis, *J Clin Periodontol* 8:57, 1981.
10. Baderstein A, Nilveus R, Egelberg J: 4-year observations of basic periodontal therapy, *J Clin Periodontol* 14:438, 1987.
11. Baderstein A, Nilveus R, Egelberg J: Scores of plaque, bleeding, suppuration, and probing depth to predict probing attachment loss: 5 years of observation following nonsurgical periodontal therapy, *J Clin Periodontol* 17:102, 1990.
12. Baehni P, Thilo P, Chapuis B, et al: Effects of ultrasonic and sonic scalers on dental plaque microflora in vitro and in vivo, *J Clin Periodontol* 19:455, 1992.
13. Barnes C, Hayes E, Leinfelder K: Effects of an air abrasive polishing system on restored surfaces, *Gen Dent* 35:186, 1987.
14. Barnes JB, Harrel SK, Rivera-Hidalgo F: Blood contamination of the aerosols produced by in vivo use of ultrasonic scalers, *J Periodontol* 69:434, 1998.
15. Barnes JE, Schaffer EM: Subgingival root planing: a comparison using files, hoes, and curets, *J Periodontol* 31:300, 1960.
16. Basu MK, Browne RM, Potts AJ, et al: A survey of aerosol-related symptoms in dental hygienists, *J Soc Occup Med* 38:23, 1988.
17. Bay N, Overman P, Krust-Bray K, Cobb C, et al: Effectiveness of antimicrobial mouthrinses on aerosols produced by an air polisher, *J Dent Hyg* 67:312, 1993.
18. Becker W, Berg LE, Becker BE: Long-term evaluation of periodontal treatment and maintenance in 95 patients, *Int J Periodont Restor Dent* 4:54, 1984.
19. Berkstein S, Reiff RL, McKinney JF, et al: Supragingival root surface removal during maintenance procedures utilizing an air-powder abrasive system or hand scaling: an in vitro study, *J Periodontol* 58:327, 1987.
20. Bjornson EJ, Collins DE, Engler WO: Surface alteration of composite resins after curette, ultrasonic and sonic instrumentation: an in vitro study, *Quintessence Int* 21:381, 1990.
21. Brookshire FV, Nagy WW, Dhuru VB, et al: The qualitative effects of various types of hygiene instrumentation on commercially pure titanium and titanium alloy implant abutments: an in vitro and scanning electron microscope study, *J Prosthet Dent* 78:286, 1997.
22. Burman LR, Alderman NE, Ewen SJ: Clinical application of ultrasonic vibrations for supragingival calculus and stain removal, *J Dent Med* 13:156, 1968.
23. Cadosch J, Zimmermann U, Ruppert M, et al: Root surface debridement and endotoxin removal, *J Periodontal Res* 38:229, 2003.
24. Canis MF, Kramer GM, Pameijer CM: Calculus attachment: review of the literature and findings, *J Periodontol* 50:406, 1979.
25. Checchi L, Pelliccioni GA: Hand versus ultrasonic instrumentation in the removal of endotoxin from root surface in vitro, *J Periodontol* 59:398, 1998.
26. Cheetham WA, Wilson M, Kieser JB: Root surface debridement: an in vitro assessment, *J Clin Periodontol* 15:228, 1988.
27. Chen SK, Vesley D, Brosseau LM, et al: Evaluation of single-use masks and respirators for protection of health care workers against mycobacterial aerosols, *Am J Infect Control* 22:65, 1994.
28. Claffey N: Decision making in periodontal therapy: the reevaluation, *J Clin Periodontol* 18:364, 1991.
29. Clark S, Group H, Mabler D: The effect of ultrasonic instrumentation on root surfaces, *J Periodontol* 39:125, 1968.
30. Contreras A, Slots J: Active cytomegalovirus infection in human periodontitis, *Oral Microbiol Immunol* 13:225, 1998.
31. Contreras A, Slots J: Herpesviruses in human periodontal disease, *J Periodontal Res* 35:3, 2000.
32. Contreras A, Slots J: Mammalian viruses in human periodontitis, *Oral Microbiol Immunol* 11:381, 1996.
33. Contreras A, Umeda M, Chen C, et al: Relationship between herpesviruses and adult periodontitis and periodontopathic bacteria, *J Periodontol* 70:478, 1999.
34. Council on Dental Materials, Instruments and Equipment, American Dental Association: Dental units and water retraction, *J Am Dent Assoc* 16:417, 1988.
35. Copulos TA, Low SB, Walker CB, et al: Comparative analysis between a modified ultrasonic tip and hand instruments on clinical parameters of periodontal disease, *J Periodontol* 64:694, 1993.
36. Cross-Poline GN, Shaklee RL, Stach DJ: Effect of implant curets on titanium implant surfaces, *Am J Dent* 10:41, 1997.
37. Cutler BJ, Goldstein GR, Simonelli G: The effect of dental prophylaxis instruments on the surface roughness of metals used for metal ceramic crowns, *J Prosthet Dent* 73:219, 1995.
38. Dragoo MR: A clinical evaluation of hand and ultrasonic instruments on subgingival debridement. Part I. With unmodified and modified ultrasonic inserts, *Int J Periodontol* 12:311, 1992.
39. Drisko CL: Scaling and root planing without overinstrumentation: hand versus power-driven scalers, *Curr Opin Periodontol* 3:78, 1993.
40. Drisko CL, Cochran DL, Blieden T, et al: Position paper: Sonic and ultrasonic scalers in periodontics. Research, Science and Therapy Committee of the American Academy of Periodontology, *J Periodontol* 71:1792, 2000.
41. Eliades GC, Tzoutzas JG, Vougiouklakis GJ: Surface alterations on dental restorative materials subjected to an air-powder abrasive instrument, *J Prosthet Dent* 65:27, 1991.
42. Fitzgibbon EJ, Bartzokas CA, Martin MV, et al: The source, frequency and extent of bacterial contamination of dental unit water systems, *Br Dent J* 157:98, 1984.
43. Fox SC, Moriarty JD, Kusy RP: The effects of scaling a titanium implant surface with metal and plastic instruments: an in vitro study, *J Periodontol* 61:485, 1990.
44. Garnick JJ, Dent J: A scanning electron micrographical study of root surfaces and subgingival bacteria after hand scaling and ultrasonic instrumentation, *J Periodontol* 60:441, 1989.
45. Garrett JS: Effects of nonsurgical periodontal therapy on periodontitis in humans: a review, *J Clin Periodontol* 10:515, 1983.
46. Green E, Ramfjord SR: Tooth roughness after subgingival root planing, *J Periodontol* 37:396, 1966.
47. Green E, Seyer PC: *Sharpening curets and sickle scalers,* ed 2, Berkeley, Calif, 1972, Praxis.
48. Greenstein G: Nonsurgical periodontal therapy in 2000: a literature review, *J Am Dent Assoc* 131:1580, 2000.
49. Gross A, Devine MJ, Cutright DE: Microbial contamination of dental units and ultrasonic scalers, *J Periodontol* 47:670, 1976.

50. Gross KB, Overman PR, Cobb C, et al: Aerosol generation by two ultrasonic scalers and one sonic scaler. A comparative study. *J Dent Hyg* 66:314, 1992.
51. Haffajee AD, Socransky SS: Microbial etiological agents of destructive periodontal diseases, *Periodontol 2000* 5:78, 1994.
52. Hallmon WW, Waldrop TC, Meffert RM, et al: A comparative study of the effects of metallic, nonmetallic, and sonic instrumentation on titanium abutment surfaces, *Int J Oral Maxillofac Implants* 11:96, 1996.
53. Hannan MM, Azadian BS, Gazzard BG, et al: Hospital infection control in an era of HIV infection and multi-drug resistant tuberculosis, *J Hosp Infect* 44:5, 2000.
54. Harrel SK, Barnes JB, Rivera-Hidalgo F: Reduction of aerosols produced by ultrasonic scalers, *J Periodontol* 67:28, 1996.
55. Harrel SK, Barnes JB, Rivera-Hidalgo F: Aerosol and splatter contamination from the operative site during ultrasonic scaling, *J Am Dent Assoc* 129:1241, 1998.
56. Hatfield CG, Baumhammers A: Cytotoxic effects of periodontally involved surfaces of human teeth, *Arch Oral Biol* 16:465, 1971.
57. Holbrook T, Low S: Power-driven scaling and polishing instruments, *Clin Dent* 3:1, 1989.
58. Holbrook T, Low S: Power-driven scaling and polishing instruments. In Hardin JF, editor: *Clarke's clinical dentistry,* Philadelphia, 1991, Lippincott.
59. Holbrook WP, Muir KF, MacPhee IT, et al: Bacteriological investigation of the aerosol from ultrasonic scalers, *Br Dent J* 144:245, 1978.
60. Hughes FJ, Smales FC: Immunohistochemical investigation of the presence and distribution of cementum-associated lipopolysaccharides in periodontal disease, *J Periodont Res* 21:660, 1986.
61. Hughes FJ, Auger DW, Smales FC: Investigation of the distribution of cementum-associated lipopolysaccharides in periodontal disease with scanning electron microscope immunohistochemistry, *J Periodontal Res* 23:100, 1988.
62. Hughes TP, Caffesse RG: Gingival changes following scaling root planing and oral hygiene: a biometric evaluation, *J Periodontol* 49:245, 1978.
63. Johnson WN, Wilson JR: The application of the ultrasonic dental units to scaling procedures, *J Periodontol* 28:24, 1957.
64. Johnson WW, Barnes CM, Covey DA, et al: The effects of a commercial aluminum airpolishing powder on dental restorative materials, *J Prosthodont* 13:166, 2004.
65. Jokit W, editor: *Zinsser's microbiology,* ed 20, Norwalk, Conn, 1992, Appleton & Lange.
66. Kaldahl WB, Kalkwarf KL, Patil KD, et al: Long-term evaluation of periodontal therapy. I. Response to 4 therapeutic modalities, *J Periodontol* 67:93, 1996.
67. Kerry GJ: Roughness of root surfaces after use of ultrasonic instruments and hand curets, *J Periodontol* 38:340, 1967.
68. Khatiblou FA, Ghodssi A: Root surface smoothness or roughness in periodontal treatment: a clinical study, *J Peridontol* 54:365, 1983.
69. Kocher T, Konig J, Hansen P, et al: Subgingival polishing compared to scaling with steel curettes: a clinical pilot study, *J Clin Periodontol* 28:194, 2001.
70. Kocher T, Langenbeck M, Ruhling A, et al: Subgingival polishing with a Teflon-coated sonic scaler insert in comparison to conventional instruments as assessed on extracted teeth. I. Residual deposits, *J Clin Periodontol* 27:243, 2000.
71. Koka S, Han J, Razzoog ME, et al: The effects of two air-powder abrasive prophylaxis systems on the surface of machined titanium: a pilot study, *Implant Dent* 1:259, 1992.
72. Kwan J, Zablotsky MH, Meffert RM: Implant maintenance using a modified ultrasonic instrument, *J Dent Hyg* 64:422, 1990.
73. Landry C, Long B, Singer D, et al: Comparison between a short and a conventional blade periodontal curet: an in vitro study, *J Clin Periodontol* 26:548, 1999.
74. Larato DC, Ruskin PF, Martin A: Effect of an ultrasonic scaler on bacterial counts in air, *J Periodontol* 38:550, 1967.
75. Lee SY, Lai YL, Morgano SM: Effects of ultrasonic scaling and periodontal curettage on surface roughness of porcelain, *J Prothet Dent* 73:227, 1995.
76. Legnani P, Checchi L, Pelliccioni GA, et al: Atmospheric contamination during dental procedures, *Quintessence Int* 25:435, 1994.
77. Leknes KN, Lie T, Wikesjo UM, et al: Influence of tooth instrumentation roughness on subgingival microbial colonization, *J Periodontol* 65:303, 1994.
78. Leon LE, Vogel RI: A comparison of the effectiveness of hand scaling and ultrasonic debridement in furcations as evaluated by differential dark-field microscopy, *J Periodontol* 58:86, 1987.
79. Lever MS, Williams A, Bennett AM: Survival of mycobacterial species in aerosols generated from artificial saliva, *Lett Appl Microbiol* 31:238, 2000.
80. Lindhe J: Evaluation of periodontal scalers. II. Wear following standardized or diagonal cutting tests, *Odontol Rev* 17:121, 1966.
81. Lindhe J, Jacobson L: Evaluation of periodontal scalers. I. Wear following clinical use, *Odontol Rev* 17:1, 1966.
82. Lindhe J, Nyman S: Long-term maintenance of patients treated for advanced periodontal disease, *J Clin Periodontol* 11:504, 1984.
83. Lindhe J, Nyman S, Karring T: Scaling and root planing in shallow pockets, *J Clin Periodontol* 9:415, 1982.
84. Listgarten MA, Lindhe J, Hellden L: Effect of tetracycline and/or scaling on human periodontal disease: clinical microbiological and histological observations, *J Clin Periodontol* 5:246, 1978.
85. Lowenguth RA, Greenstein G: Clinical and microbiological response to nonsurgical mechanical periodontal therapy, *Periodontol 2000* 9:14, 1995.
86. Lubow RM, Cooley RL: Effect of air-powder abrasive instrument on restorative materials, *J Prosthet Dent* 55:462, 1986.
87. Magnusson I, Lindhe J, Yoneyama T, et al: Recolonization of a subgingival microbiota following scaling in deep pockets, *J Clin Periodontol* 11:193, 1984.
88. Mengel R, Buns CE, Mengel C, et al: An in vitro study of the treatment of implant surfaces with different instruments, *Int J Oral Maxillofac Implants* 13:91, 1998.
89. Michalowicz BS, Ronderos M, Camara-Silva R, et al: Human herpesviruses and *Porphyromonas gingivalis* are associated with juvenile periodontitis, *J Periodontol* 71:981, 2000.
90. Miller CS, Leonelli FM, Latham E: Selective interference with pacemaker activity by electrical dental devices, *Oral Surg Oral Med Oral Pathol Oral Radiol Endod* 85:33, 1998.
91. Miller RL: Characteristics of blood-containing aerosols generated by common powered dental instruments, *Am Ind Hyg Assoc J* 56:670, 1995.
92. Miller RL, Micik RE: Air pollution and its control in the dental office, *Dent Clin North Am* 22:453, 1978.
93. Miller RL, Micik RE, Abel C, et al: Studies on dental aerobiology. II. Microbial splatter discharged from the oral cavity of dental patients, *J Dent Res* 50:621, 1971.
94. Mongardini C, van Steenberghe D, Dekeyser C, et al: One stage full- versus partial-mouth disinfection in the treatment of chronic adult or generalized early-onset

periodontitis. I. Long-term clinical observations, *J Periodontol* 70:632, 1999.
95. Moore J, Wilson M, Kieser JB: The distribution of bacterial lipopolysaccharide (endotoxin) in relation to periodontally involved root surfaces, *J Clin Periodontol* 13:748, 1986.
96. Moskow BS: Calculus attachment in cemental separations, *J Periodontol* 40:125, 1969.
97. Mousques T, Listgarten MA, Phillips RW: Effect of scaling and root planing on the composition of human subgingival microbial flora, *J Periodontal Res* 7:199, 1980.
98. Muir KF, Ross PW, MacPhee IT, et al: Reduction of microbial contamination from ultrasonic scalers, *Br Dent J* 145:760, 1978.
99. Nakib NM, Bissada NF, Simmelink JW, et al: Endotoxin penetration into root cementum of periodontally healthy and diseased human teeth, *J Periodontol* 53:368, 1982.
100. Nyman S, Westfelt E, Sarhed G, et al: Role of "diseased" root cementum in healing following treatment of periodontal disease: a clinical study, *J Clin Periodontol* 15:464, 1988.
101. Oberholzer R, Rateitschak KH: Root cleaning or root smoothing: an in vivo study, *J Clin Periodontol* 23:326, 1996.
102. O'Leary R, Sved AM, Davies EH, et al: The bactericidal effects of dental ultrasound on *Actinobacillus actinomycetemcomitans* and *Porphyromonas gingivalis:* an in vitro investigation, *J Clin Periodontol* 24:432, 1997.
103. Oosterwall PJ, Matee MI, Mikx FHM, et al: The effect of subgingival debridement with hand and ultrasonic instruments on subgingival microflora, *J Clin Periodontol* 14:528, 1987.
104. Oppenheim BA, Sefton AM, Gill ON, et al: Widespread *Legionella pneumophila* contamination of dental stations in a dental school without apparent human infection, *Epidemiol Infect* 99:159, 1987.
105. Orban B, Manella V: Macroscopic and microscopic study of instruments designed for root planing, *J Periodontol* 27:120, 1956.
106. Orton GS: Clinical use of an air-powder abrasive system, *Dent Hyg* 75:513, 1987.
107. Otero-Cagide FJ, Long BA: Comparative in vitro effectiveness of closed root debridement with fine instruments on specific areas of mandibular first molar furcations. I. Root trunk and furcation entrance, *J Periodontol* 68:1093, 1997.
108. Otero-Cagide FJ, Long BA: Comparative in vitro effectiveness of closed root debridement with fine instruments on specific areas of mandibular first molar furcations. I. Furcation area, *J Periodontol* 68:1098, 1997.
109. Pankhurst CL, Johnson NW, Woods RG: Microbial contamination of dental unit waterlines: the scientific argument, *Int Dent J* 48:359, 1998.
110. Paquette OE, Levin MP: The sharpening of scaling instruments. I. An examination of principles, *J Periodontol* 48:163, 1977.
111. Parr R, Green E, Madsen L, et al: *Subgingival scaling and root planing,* Berkeley, Calif, 1976, Praxis.
112. Pattison AM: The use of hand instruments in supportive periodontal treatment, *Periodontol 2000* 12:71, 1996.
113. Petersilka GJ, Bell M, Haberlein I, et al: In vitro evaluation of novel low abrasive air polishing powders, *J Clin Periodontol* 30:9, 2003.
114. Petersilka GJ, Bell M, Mehl A, et al: Root defects following air polishing, *J Clin Periodontol* 30:165, 2003.
115. Petersilka GJ, Flemmig TF, Mehl A, et al: Comparison of root substance removal by magnetostrictive and piezoelectric ultrasonic and sonic scalers in vitro, *J Clin Periodontol* 24:864, 1997.
116. Pihlstrom BL, McHugh RB, Oliphant TH, et al: Comparison of surgical and nonsurgical treatment of periodontal disease: a review of current studies and additional results after 6 years, *J Clin Periodontol* 10:524, 1983.
117. Proye M, Caton J, Polson A: Initial healing of periodontal pockets after a single episode of root planing monitored by controlled probing force, *J Periodontol* 53:296, 1982.
118. Quirynen M, Mongardini C, de Soete M, et al: The role of chlorhexidine in the one-stage full-mouth disinfection treatment of patients with advanced adult periodontitis: long-term clinical and microbiological observations, *J Clin Periodontol* 27:578, 2000.
119. Quirynen M, Mongardini C, Pauwels M, et al: One stage full- versus partial-mouth disinfection in the treatment of chronic adult or generalized early-onset periodontitis. II. Long-term impact on microbial load, *J Periodontol* 70:646, 1999.
120. Rajstein J, Tal M: The effects of ultrasonic scaling on the surface of Class V amalgam restorations: a scanning electron microscope study, *J Oral Rehabil* 11:299, 1984.
121. Rawson RD, Nelson BN, Jewell BD, et al: Alkalosis as a potential complication of air polishing systems: a pilot study, *Dent Hyg* 59:500, 1985.
122. Razzoog ME, Koka S: In vitro analysis of the effects of two air-abrasive prophylaxis systems and inlet air pressure on the surface of titanium abutment cylinders, *J Prosthodont* 3:103, 1994.
123. Renvert S, Wikström M, Dahlén G, et al: Effect of root debridement on the elimination of *Actinobacillus actinomycetemcomitans* and *Bacteroides gingivalis* from periodontal pockets, *J Clin Periodontol* 17:345, 1990.
124. Ritz L, Hefti AF, Rateitschak KH: An in vitro investigation on the loss of root substance in scaling with various instruments, *J Clin Peridontol* 18:643, 1991.
125. Rivera-Hidalgo F, Barnes JB, Harrel SK: Aerosol and splatter production by focused spray and standard ultrasonic inserts, *J Periodontol* 70:473, 1999.
126. Rosenberg ES, Evian CI, Listgarten M: The composition of the subgingival microbiota after periodontal therapy, *J Periodontol* 52:435, 1981.
127. Rossi R, Smukler H: A scanning electron microscope study comparing the effectiveness of different types of sharpening stones and curets, *J Peridontol* 66:956, 1995.
128. Ruhling A, Kocher T, Kreusch J, et al: Treatment of subgingival implant surfaces with Teflon-coated sonic and ultrasonic scaler tips and various implant curettes: an in vitro study, *Clin Oral Implants Res* 5:19, 1994.
129. Rutala WA, Jones SM, Worthington JM, et al: Efficacy of portable filtration units in reducing aerosolized particles in the size range of *Mycobacterium tuberculosis, Infect Control Hosp Epidemiol* 16:391, 1995.
130. Sbordone L, Ramaglia L, Guletta E, et al: Recolonization of the subgingival microflora after scaling and root planing in human periodontitis, *J Periodontol* 61:579, 1990.
131. Schaffer EM: Histologic results of root curettage on human teeth, *J Periodontol* 27:269, 1956.
132. Schenk G, Flemmig TF, Lob S, et al: Lack of antimicrobial effect on periodontopathic bacteria by ultrasonic and sonic scalers in vitro, *J Clin Periodontol* 27:116, 2000.
133. Schlageter L, Rateitschak-Pluss EM, Schwarz JP: Root surface smoothness or roughness following open debridement: an in vivo study, *J Clin Periodontol* 23:460, 1996.
134. Schwartz M: The prevention and management of the broken curet, *Compend Contin Educ Dent* 19:418, 1998.
135. Selvig KA: Attachment of plaque and calculus to tooth surfaces, *J Periodontal Res* 5:8, 1970.
136. Shiloah J, Patters M: Repopulation of periodontal pockets by microbial pathogens in the absence of supportive therapy, *J Peridontol* 67:130, 1996.

137. Shreve WB, Hoerman KC, Trautwein CA: Illness in patients following exposure to dental aerosols, *J Public Health Dent* 32:34, 1972.
138. Slots J, Mashimo P, Levine MJ, et al: Periodontal therapy in humans. I. Microbiological and clinical effects of a single course of periodontal scaling and root planing, and of adjunctive tetracycline therapy, *J Periodontol* 50:495, 1979.
139. Smart GJ, Wilson M, Davis EH, et al: The assessment of ultrasonic root surface debridement by determination of residual endotoxin levels, *J Clin Periodontol* 17:174, 1990.
140. Smith BA, Setter MS, Caffesse RG, et al: The effect of sharpening stones upon curette surface roughness, *Quintessence Int* 18:603, 1987.
141. Snyder JA, McVay JT, Brown FH, et al: The effect of air abrasive polishing on blood pH and electrolyte concentrations in healthy mongrel dogs, *J Periodontol* 64:81, 1990.
142. Stach DJ, Cross-Poline GN, Newmand SM, et al: Effect of repeated sterilization and ultrasonic cleaning on curet blades, *J Dent Hyg* 69:31, 1995.
143. Stahl SS, Slavkin HC, Yamada L, et al: Speculations about gingival repair, *J Periodontol* 43:395, 1972.
144. Stahl SS, Weiner JM, Benjamin S, et al: Soft tissue healing following curettage and root planing, *J Periodontol* 42:678, 1971.
145. Stende GW, Schaffer EM: A comparison of ultrasonic and hand scaling, *J Periodontol* 32:312, 1961.
146. Suzuki JB, Delisle AL: Pulmonary actinomycosis of periodontal origin, *J Periodontol* 55:581, 1984.
147. Tan B, Gillam DG, Mordan NJ, Galgut PN: A preliminary investigation into the ultrastructure of dental calculus and associated bacteria, *J Clin Periodontol* 31:364, 2004.
148. Ting M, Contreras A, Slots J: Herpesvirus in localized juvenile periodontitis, *J Periodontal Res* 35:17, 2000.
149. Torfason T, Kiger R, Selvig KA, et al: Clinical improvement of gingival conditions following ultrasonic versus hand instrumentation of periodontal pockets, *J Clin Periodontol* 6:165, 1979.
150. Trenter SC, Walmsley AD: Ultrasonic dental scaler: associated hazards, *J Clin Periodontol* 30:95, 2003.
151. Umeda M, Contreras A, Chen C, et al: The utility of whole saliva to detect the oral presence of periodontopathic bacteria, *J Periodontol* 69:828, 1998.
152. Van Volkinburg J, Green E, Armitage G: The nature of root surfaces after curette, Cavitron, and alpha-sonic instrumentation, *J Periodontal Res* 11:374, 1976.
153. Van Winkelhoff AJ, van der Velden U, de Graaff J: Microbial succession in recolonizing deep periodontal pockets after a single course of supra- and subgingival debridement, *J Clin Periodontol* 15:116, 1988.
154. Veksler AE, Kayrouz GA, Newman MG: Reduction of salivary bacteria by pre-procedural rinses with chlorhexidine 0.12%, *J Periodontol* 62:649, 1991.
155. Vermilyea SG, Prasanna MK, Agar JR: Effect of ultrasonic cleaning and air polishing on porcelain labial margin restorations, *J Prosthet Dent* 71:447, 1994.
156. Waerhaug J: Healing of the dentoepithelial junction following subgingival plaque control, *J Periodontol* 49:1, 1978.
157. Waerhaug J, Arno A, Lovdal A: The dimension of instruments for removal of subgingival calculus, *J Periodontol* 25:281, 1954.
158. Westfelt E, Nyman S, Socransky SS, et al: Significance of frequency of professional tooth cleaning following periodontal surgery, *J Clin Periodontol* 10:148, 1983.
159. Wilkins EM: *Clinical practice of the dental hygienist,* ed 9, Philadelphia, 2005, Lippincott, Williams & Wilkins.
160. Wilkinson RF, Maybury J: Scanning electron microscopy of the root surface following instrumentation, *J Periodontol* 44:559, 1973.
161. Ximenez-Fyvie LA, Haffajee AD, Socransky SS: Comparison of the microbiota of supra- and subgingival plaque in health and periodontitis, *J Clin Periodontol* 27:648, 2000.
162. Zander HA: The attachment of calculus to root surfaces, *J Periodontol* 24:16, 1953.
163. Zappa U, Studer M, Merkle A, et al: Effect of electrically powered dental devices on cardiac parameter function in humans, *Parodontology* 2:299, 1991.

Chemotherapeutic Agents

David L. Jolkovsky and Sebastian Ciancio

52 CHAPTER

CHAPTER OUTLINE

It is well established that the various periodontal diseases are caused by bacterial infection. Bacteria begin reattaching to the crowns of teeth soon after the teeth have been cleaned. Over time, this supragingival plaque becomes more complex, leading to a succession of bacteria that are more pathogenic. Bacteria grow in an apical direction and become subgingival, and eventually, as bone is destroyed, a periodontal pocket is formed. In a periodontal pocket the bacteria form a highly structured and complex *biofilm*. As this process continues, the bacterial biofilm extends so far subgingivally that the patient cannot reach it during oral hygiene efforts. Additionally, this complex biofilm now may offer some protection from the host's immunologic mechanisms in the periodontal pocket, as well as from antibiotics used for treatment. It has been suggested that an antibiotic strength 500 times greater than the usual therapeutic dose may be needed to be effective against bacteria arranged in biofilms.[37]

It is therefore logical to treat periodontal pockets by mechanical removal of local factors (including calculus that harbors bacteria) and also by disruption of the subgingival plaque biofilm itself. Mechanical removal includes manual instrumentation (e.g., scaling and root planing) and machine-driven instrumentation (e.g., ultrasonic scalers), and these procedures can be considered "antiinfective therapy." Many chemotherapeutic agents are now available to clinicians treating periodontal diseases. *Systemic* antiinfective therapy (oral antibiotics) and *local* antiinfective therapy (placing antiinfective agents directly into the periodontal pocket) can reduce the bacterial challenge to the periodontium.

Bacteria and their toxic products cause "direct bone loss." Ultimately, however, the host's own immunologic response to this bacterial infection can cause even more bone destruction ("indirect bone loss") than that caused by pathogenic bacteria and their byproducts. This immunologic response can be influenced by environmental (e.g., tobacco use), acquired (e.g., systemic disease), and genetic risk factors.[62,66] Chemotherapeutic agents can modulate the host's immune response to bacteria and reduce the host's self-destructive immunologic response to bacterial pathogens and thus reduce bone loss. It is also incumbent on health care providers to counsel patients concerning the detrimental effects of systemic factors, including stress and tobacco use.[37]

This chapter reviews the indications and protocols for optimizing the use of chemotherapeutic agents in the treatment of periodontal diseases.

It is important to note that significant work has been performed in a systematic *evidence-based approach* to evaluate the various antiinfective and host modulation therapies (see Chapters 2 and 3). Meta-analysis of similar research studies has given power to statistical analysis for evaluating chemotherapeutic agents in the treatment of periodontal diseases. Unfortunately, a standardized research protocol has not yet been implemented. Therefore, some studies, although relevant, have not been used in the evidence-based approach because of their study design. Further evidence-based and similar research is needed to define protocols more precisely for the use of antiinfective agents in treating periodontal diseases.

DEFINITIONS

Chemotherapeutic agent is a general term for a chemical substance that provides a clinical therapeutic benefit. This term does not specify in what way the agent aids in attaining a clinical benefit. Clinical benefits can be derived through antimicrobial actions or an increase in the host's resistance. An *antiinfective agent* is a chemotherapeutic agent that works by reducing the number of bacteria present. An *antibiotic* is a naturally occurring, semisynthetic, or synthetic type of antiinfective agent that destroys or inhibits the growth of selective microorganisms, generally at low concentrations. An *antiseptic* is a chemical antimicrobial agent applied topically or subgingivally to mucous membranes, wounds, or intact dermal surfaces to destroy microorganisms and inhibit their reproduction or metabolism. In dentistry, antiseptics are widely used as the active ingredient in antiplaque and antigingivitis oral rinses and dentifrices. *Disinfectants,* a subcategory of antiseptics, are antimicrobial agents that are generally applied to inanimate surfaces to destroy microorganisms.[19]

Chemotherapeutic agents can be administered *locally* or *orally.* With either approach, their purpose is to reduce the number of bacteria present in the diseased periodontal pocket. *Systemic administration* of antibiotics may be a necessary adjunct in controlling bacterial infection because bacteria can invade periodontal tissues, making mechanical therapy alone sometimes ineffective.[12,16,65] *Local administration* of antiinfective agents, generally directly in the pocket, has the potential to provide greater concentrations directly to the infected area and reduce possible systemic side effects.

Additionally, a single chemotherapeutic agent can have a dual mechanism of action. For example, tetracyclines (especially doxycycline) are chemotherapeutic agents that can reduce collagen and bone destruction through their ability to inhibit the enzyme collagenase. As antibiotic agents, they also can reduce periodontal pathogens in periodontal tissues.[18,19]

SYSTEMIC ADMINISTRATION OF ANTIBIOTICS

Background and Rationale

The treatment of periodontal diseases is based on the infectious nature of these diseases (Table 52-1). Ideally, the causative microorganism(s) should be identified and the most effective agent selected using antibiotic-sensitivity tests. Although this appears simple, the

TABLE 52-1

Antibiotics Used to Treat Periodontal Diseases

Category	Agent	Major Features
Penicillin*	Amoxicillin	Extended spectrum of antimicrobial activity; excellent oral absorption; used systemically.
	Augmentin†	Effective against penicillinase-producing microorganisms; used systemically.
Tetracyclines	Minocycline	Effective against broad spectrum of microorganisms; used systemically and applied locally (subgingivally).
	Doxycycline	Effective against broad spectrum of microorganisms; used systemically and applied locally (subgingivally). Chemotherapeutically used in subantimicrobial dose for host modulation (Periostat).
	Tetracycline	Effective against broad spectrum of microorganisms.
Quinolone	Ciprofloxacin	Effective against gram-negative rods; promotes health-associated microflora.
Macrolide	Azithromycin	Concentrates at sites of inflammation; used systemically.
Lincomycin derivative	Clindamycin	Used in penicillin-allergic patients; effective against anaerobic bacteria; used systemically.
Nitroimidazole‡	Metronidazole	Effective against anaerobic bacteria; used systemically and applied locally (subgingivally) as gel.

**Indications:* Localized aggressive periodontitis (LAP), generalized aggressive periodontitis (GAP), medically related periodontitis (MRP), refractory periodontitis (RP).

†Amoxicillin and clavulanate potassium.

‡*Indications:* LAP, GAP, MRP, RP, necrotizing ulcerative periodontitis.

TABLE 52-2

Common Antibiotic Regimens Used to Treat Periodontal Diseases*

	Regimen	Dosage/Duration
Single Agent		
Amoxicillin	500 mg	Three times daily for 8 days
Azithromycin	500 mg	Once daily for 4-7 days
Ciprofloxacin	500 mg	Twice daily for 8 days
Clindamycin	300 mg	Three times daily 10 days
Doxycycline or minocycline	100-200 mg	Once daily for 21 days
Metronidazole	500 mg	Three times daily for 8 days
Combination Therapy		
Metronidazole + amoxicillin	250 mg of each	Three times daily for 8 days
Metronidazole + ciprofloxacin	500 mg of each	Twice daily for 8 days

Data from Jorgensen MG, Slots J: *Compend Contin Educ Dent* 21:111, 2000.
*These regimens are prescribed with a review of the patient's medical history, periodontal diagnosis, and antimicrobial testing. Clinicians must consult pharmacology references such as *Mosby's GenRx*[67] or manufacturer's guidelines for warnings, contraindications, and precautions.

difficulty lies primarily in identifying specific etiologic microorganism(s) rather than microorganisms simply associated with various periodontal disorders.[17,18]

An ideal antibiotic for use in prevention and treatment of periodontal diseases should be specific for periodontal pathogens, allogenic and nontoxic, substantive, not in general use for treatment of other diseases, and inexpensive.[29] Currently, an ideal antibiotic for the treatment of periodontal diseases does not exist.[42] Although oral bacteria are susceptible to many antibiotics, no single antibiotic at concentrations achieved in body fluids inhibits all putative periodontal pathogens.[85] Indeed, a combination of antibiotics may be necessary to eliminate all putative pathogens from some periodontal pockets[61] (Table 52-2).

As always, the clinician in concert with the patient must make the final decision on any treatment. Thus the treatment of the individual patient must be based on the patient's clinical status, nature of the colonizing bacteria, and the risks and benefits associated with the proposed treatment plan. The clinician is responsible for choosing the correct antimicrobial agent. Some adverse reactions include allergic/anaphylactic reactions, superinfections of opportunistic bacteria, development of resistant bacteria, interactions with other medications, upset stomach, nausea, and vomiting. Most adverse reactions take the form of gastrointestinal upset.[42] Other concerns include the cost of the medication and the patient's willingness and ability to comply with the proposed therapy.

No consensus exists concerning the magnitude of the risk for developing bacterial resistance. Common and indiscriminate use of antibiotics worldwide has contributed to increasing numbers of resistant bacterial strains over the last 15 to 20 years, and this trend is likely to continue given the widespread use of antibiotics.[84] The overuse, misuse, and widespread prophylactic application of antiinfective drugs are some of the factors that have led to the emergence of resistant microorganisms. Increasing levels of resistance of subgingival microflora to antibiotics has been correlated with the increased use of antibiotics in individual countries.[77] However, researchers have noted that the subgingival microflora tends to revert to similar proportions of antibiotic-resistant isolates 3 months after therapy.[26,38]

Biologic Implications

Systemic antibiotics are released from the pocket wall into the *gingival crevicular fluid* (GCF). The putative periodontal pathogens ("red complex") tend to reside in the section of the biofilm attached to the epithelial surface of the periodontal pocket. The susceptibility of bacteria and their susceptibility to antibiotics may be the key to the efficacy of systemic antibiotics in the treatment of periodontal diseases. A recent systematic review concluded that when a patient uses a systemic antibiotic, it is likely to be of benefit for treatment of the patient's periodontal infection.[38]

Guidelines for use of antibiotics in periodontal therapy include the following:

1. The *clinical diagnosis* and situation dictate the need for possible antibiotic therapy as an adjunct in controlling active periodontal disease (Figure 52-1). The patient's diagnosis can change over time. For example, a patient who presents with generalized, mild chronic periodontitis can return to a diagnosis of periodontal health after initial therapy. However, if this patient has been treated appropriately and continues to have active disease, the diagnosis can change to refractory periodontitis.
2. Continuing disease activity, as measured by continuing attachment loss (pocket probing depth plus recession), purulent exudate, and continuing periodontal pockets of 5 mm or greater[47,48] that bleed

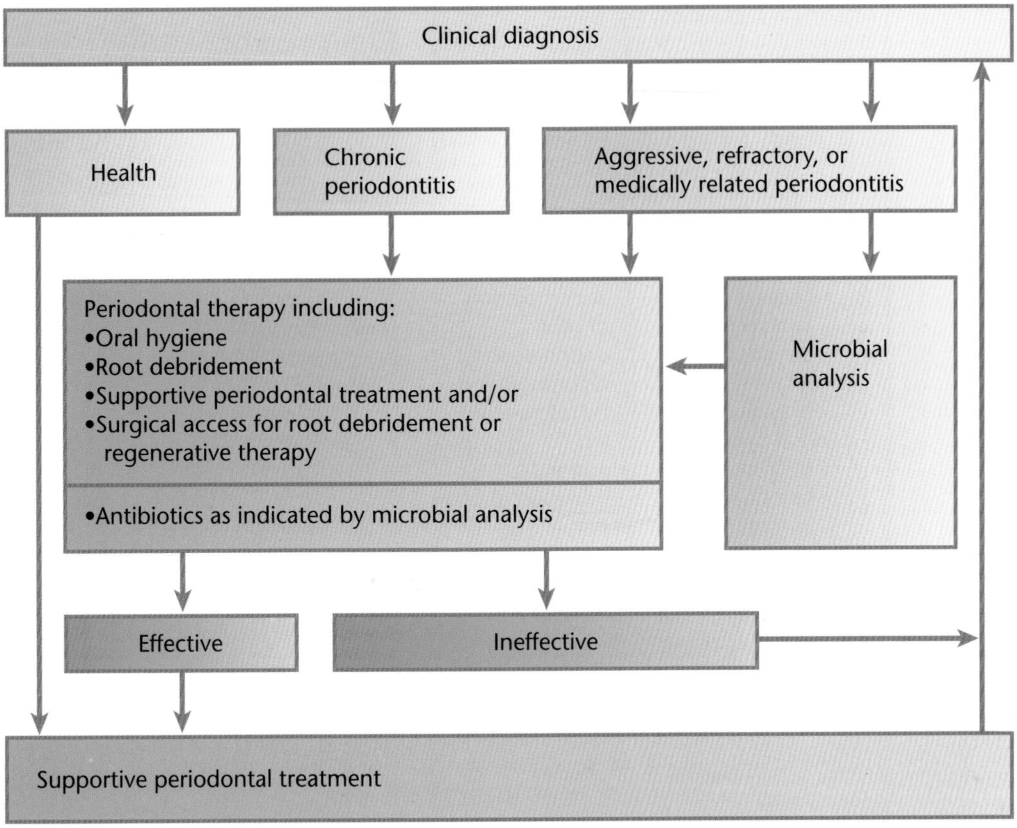

Figure 52-1 Guidelines for use of antimicrobial therapy.

on probing, is an indication for periodontal intervention and possible microbial analysis through plaque sampling. Also, cases of refractory or aggressive periodontitis may indicate the need for antimicrobial therapy.[37]

3. When used to treat periodontal disease, antibiotics are selected based on the patient's medical and dental status, current medications,[42] and results of microbial analysis, if performed.
4. Microbiologic plaque sampling may be performed according to the instructions of the reference laboratory. The samples usually are taken at the beginning of an appointment before instrumentation of the pocket. Supragingival plaque is removed, and an endodontic paper point is inserted subgingivally into the deepest pocket(s) present to absorb bacteria in the loosely associated plaque. This endodontic point is placed in reduced transfer fluid and sent overnight to the laboratory. The laboratory will then send the referring dentist a report that includes the pathogens present and any appropriate antibiotic regimen.
5. Plaque sampling can be performed at the initial examination, root planing, reevaluation, or supportive periodontal therapy appointment. Clinical indications for microbial plaque testing include aggressive forms of periodontal disease, diseases refractory to standard mechanical therapy, and periodontitis associated with systemic conditions (see Figure 52-1).
6. Antibiotics have also been shown to have value in reducing the need for periodontal surgery in patients with chronic periodontitis.[52]
7. Some studies have shown attachment gain with antibiotics given as monotherapy. However, the evidence is insufficient at present to recommend systemic antimicrobial therapy as *monotherapy* (i.e., as stand-alone treatment without scaling and root planing or surgery). Therefore, systemic antimicrobial therapy should be an adjunct to a comprehensive periodontal treatment plan (Figure 52-2). Debridement of root surfaces, optimal oral hygiene, and frequent supportive periodontal therapy are important parts of comprehensive periodontal therapy. As mentioned earlier, an antibiotic strength 500 times greater than the systemic therapeutic dose may be required to be effective against the bacteria arranged in biofilms. It therefore is important to disrupt this biofilm physically so that the antibiotic agents can have access to the periodontal pathogens.[37]

Other chemotherapeutic adjuncts include locally placed subgingival antiinfective agents, chlorhexidine rinse after debridement, and home intraoral irrigation (e.g., Water Pik) with or without chemotherapeutic agents.[42] Chlorhexidine gluconate is effective as an antiplaque rinse to reduce gingivitis, but not as a subgingival irrigant to reduce periodontal pocketing. Chlorhexidine gluconate's antiinfective activity is greatly reduced in the

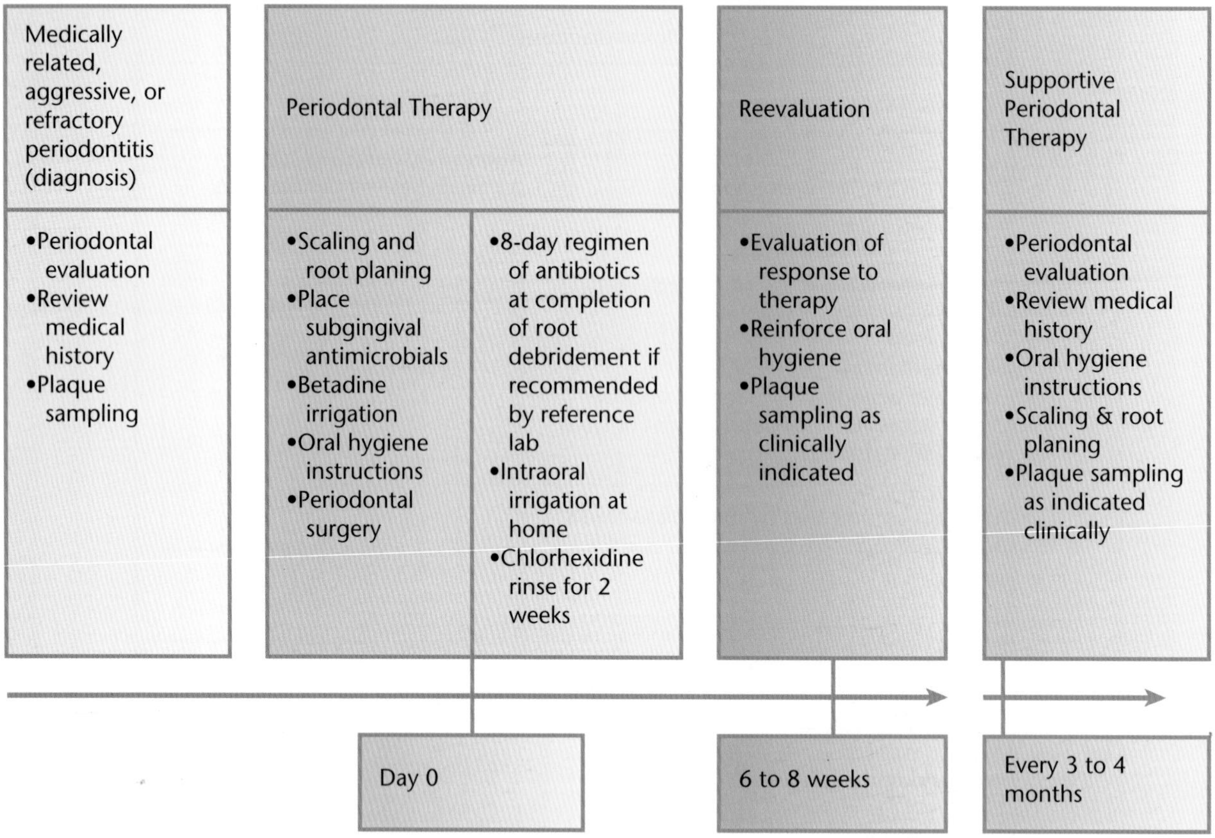

Figure 52-2 Sequencing of antimicrobial agents. (Modified from Jorgensen MG, Slots J: *Compend Contin Educ Dent* 21:111, 2000.)

presence of organic matter in the subgingival periodontal pocket. Some evidence suggests that povidone-iodine (Betadine) may be an effective antibacterial agent when used directly into the periodontal pocket, even at low concentrations, but further studies are needed to substantiate these data.[4,42,64] Povidone-iodine must be used with caution in patients sensitive to iodine, although the sensitization rate is low.[56] It also should be used with caution in patients who are pregnant or lactating.[15]

8. Slots et al.[70] described a series of steps using antiinfective agents for enhancing regenerative healing. They recommend starting antibiotics 1 to 2 days before surgery and continuing for a total of at least 8 days.[42,58] However, the value of this regimen has not been well documented, and further studies are encouraged.
9. Using evidence-based techniques, meta-analysis has shown statistically significant improvements in attachment loss when tetracycline and metronidazole are used as adjuncts to scaling and root planing. Clindamycin and doxycycline also showed statistically significant increases in attachment levels. There was borderline significance using amoxicillin plus metronidazole because of smaller numbers of pooled subjects in the meta-analysis. Spiramycin and penicillin appeared to give the *least* improvement in attachment levels. Improvements in the attachment levels were consistent for chronic and aggressive periodontitis, although aggressive periodontitis patients benefited more from the antibiotics. Haffajee et al.[38] concluded that data support similar effects for most antibiotics. Therefore the selection of an antibiotic must be made based on other factors. The clinician must make the final decision with the patient. Risks and benefits concerning antibiotics as adjuncts to periodontal therapy must be discussed with the patient before antibiotics are used.

The following antiinfective agents have all been used successfully in the treatment of periodontal diseases. Unfortunately, there is no one best choice of antibiotic at present (i.e., no "silver bullet"). Therefore the clinician must integrate history of the patient's disease, clinical signs and symptoms, and results of radiographic examinations and possibly microbiologic sampling to determine the course of periodontal therapy. The clinician must obtain a thorough medical history, including current medications and possible adverse effects of combining these medicines, before prescribing any antibiotic therapy.

Tetracyclines

Tetracyclines have been widely used in the treatment of periodontal diseases. They have been frequently used in treating refractory periodontitis, including *localized aggressive periodontitis* (LAP) (see Table 52-1). Tetracyclines have the ability to concentrate in the periodontal tissues and inhibit the growth of *Actinobacillus actinomycetemcomitans*. In addition, tetracyclines exert an anticollagenase effect that can inhibit tissue destruction and may aid bone regeneration (see Host Modulation).

Pharmacology. The tetracyclines are a group of antibiotics produced naturally from certain species of *Streptomyces* or derived semisynthetically. These antibiotics are bacteriostatic and are effective against rapidly multiplying bacteria. They generally are more effective against gram-positive bacteria than gram-negative bacteria.[89] Tetracyclines are effective in treating periodontal diseases in part because their concentration in the gingival crevice is 2 to 10 times that in serum.[2,6,34] This allows a high drug concentration to be delivered into periodontal pockets. In addition, several studies have demonstrated that tetracyclines at a low GCF concentration (2-4 μg/ml) are very effective against many periodontal pathogens.[7,8,89]

Clinical Use. Tetracyclines have been investigated as adjuncts in the treatment of LAP. *A. actinomycetemcomitans* is a frequent causative microorganism in LAP and is tissue invasive. Therefore, mechanical removal of calculus and plaque from root surfaces may not eliminate this bacterium from the periodontal tissues. Systemic tetracycline can eliminate tissue bacteria and has been shown to arrest bone loss and suppress *A. actinomycetemcomitans* levels in conjunction with scaling and root planing.[73] This combination therapy allows mechanical removal of root surface deposits and elimination of pathogenic bacteria from within the tissues. Increased posttreatment bone levels have been noted using this method.[30,73] Because of increased resistance to tetracyclines, metronidazole or amoxicillin with metronidazole has been found more effective in treating aggressive periodontitis in children. Some investigators believe metronidazole combined with amoxicillin–clavulanic acid is the preferable antibiotic.[81]

Long-term use of low antibacterial doses of tetracyclines has been advocated in the past. One long-term study of patients taking low doses of tetracycline (250 mg/day for 2-7 years) showed persistence of deep pockets that did not bleed on probing. These sites contained high proportions of tetracycline-resistant, gram-negative rods *(Fusobacterium nucleatum)*. After the antibiotic was discontinued, the flora was characteristic of sites with disease.[45] Therefore, it is not advisable to prescribe long-term regimens of tetracyclines because of the possible development of resistant bacterial strains. Although often used in the past as antiinfective agents, especially for LAP and other types of aggressive periodontitis, tetracyclines now tend to be replaced by more effective combination antibiotics.[42,77]

Specific Agents. Tetracycline, minocycline, and doxycycline are semisynthetic members of the tetracycline group that have been used in periodontal therapy.

Tetracycline. Tetracycline requires administration of 250 mg four times daily (qid). It is inexpensive, but compliance may be reduced by having to take four capsules per day.

Minocycline. Minocycline is effective against a broad spectrum of microorganisms. In patients with adult periodontitis, it suppresses spirochetes and motile rods as effectively as scaling and root planing, with suppression evident up to 3 months after therapy. Minocycline can be given twice daily (bid), thus facilitating compliance compared with tetracycline. Although associated with less phototoxicity and renal toxicity than tetracycline, minocycline may cause reversible vertigo. Minocycline administered 200 mg/day for 1 week results in a reduction in total bacterial counts, complete elimination of spirochetes for up to 2 months, and improvement in all clinical parameters.[19]

Doxycycline. Doxycycline has the same spectrum of activity as minocycline and may be equally as effective.[18] Because doxycycline can be given only once daily (qd), however, patients may be more compliant. Compliance is also favored because its absorption from the gastrointestinal (GI) tract is only slightly altered by calcium, metal ions, or antacids, as is absorption of other tetracyclines. The recommended dosage when used as an anti-infective agent is 100 mg bid the first day, then 100 mg qd. To reduce GI upset, 50 mg can be taken bid. When used in a subantimicrobial dose (to inhibit collagenase), doxycycline is recommended in a 20-mg dose twice daily[14] (see Host Modulation, below). Periostat (Collagenex Pharmaceutical Inc) and generic forms are currently available in a dose of 20 mg of doxycycline.

Metronidazole

Pharmacology. Metronidazole is a nitroimidazole compound developed in France to treat protozoal infections. It is bactericidal to anaerobic organisms and is believed to disrupt bacterial deoxyribonucleic acid (DNA) synthesis in conditions with a low reduction potential. Metronidazole is not the drug of choice for treating *A. actinomycetemcomitans* infections, but it may be effective at therapeutic levels because of its hydroxy metabolite. However, metronidazole is effective against *A. actinomycetemcomitans* when used in combination with other antibiotics.[60,61] Metronidazole is also effective against anaerobes such as *Porphyromonas gingivalis* and *Prevotella intermedia*.[36]

Clinical Use. Metronidazole has been used clinically to treat gingivitis, acute necrotizing ulcerative gingivitis (NUG), chronic periodontitis, and aggressive periodontitis. It has been used as monotherapy and also in combination with both root planing and surgery or with other antibiotics. Metronidazole has been used successfully to treat NUG.[53]

Studies in humans have demonstrated the efficacy of metronidazole in the treatment of gingivitis and periodontitis.[51,52] A single dose of metronidazole (250 mg orally) appears in both serum and GCF in sufficient quantities to inhibit a wide range of suspected periodontal pathogens. Administered systemically (750-1000 mg/day for 2 weeks), metronidazole reduces the growth of anaerobic flora, including spirochetes, and decreases the clinical and histopathologic signs of periodontitis.[51] The most common regimen is 250 mg three times daily (tid) for 7 days.[53]

Loesche et al.[52] found that 250 mg of metronidazole tid for 1 week was of benefit to patients with a diagnosed anaerobic periodontal infection. In this study an infection was considered "anaerobic" when spirochetes composed 20% or more of the total microbial count. Metronidazole used as a supplement to rigorous scaling and root planing resulted in a significantly reduced need for surgery compared with root planing alone. The bacteriologic data of this study showed that only the spirochete count was significantly reduced. Currently, the critical level of spirochetes needed to diagnose an anaerobic infection, the appropriate time to give metronidazole, and the ideal dosage or duration of therapy are unknown.[36]

As monotherapy (no concurrent root planing), metronidazole is inferior and at best only equivalent to root planing. Therefore, if used, metronidazole should not be administered as monotherapy.

Metronidazole offers some benefit in the treatment of refractory periodontitis, particularly when used in combination with amoxicillin. The existence of refractory periodontitis as a diagnostic category indicates that some patients do not respond to conventional therapy, including root planing, surgery, or both. Soder et al.[71] showed that metronidazole was more effective than placebo in the management of sites unresponsive to root planing. Nevertheless, many patients still had sites that bled on probing despite metronidazole therapy.

Studies have suggested that when combined with amoxicillin or amoxicillin–clavulanate potassium (Augmentin), metronidazole may be of value in the management of patients with LAP or refractory periodontitis (see later discussion).

Side Effects. Metronidazole has an Antabuse effect when alcohol is ingested. The response is generally proportional to the amount ingested and can result in severe cramps, nausea, and vomiting. Products containing alcohol should be avoided during therapy and for at least 1 day after therapy is discontinued. Metronidazole also inhibits warfarin metabolism. Patients undergoing anticoagulant therapy should avoid metronidazole because it prolongs prothrombin time.[37] It also should be avoided in patients who are taking lithium.

Penicillins

Pharmacology. Penicillins are the drugs of choice for the treatment of many serious infections in humans and are the most widely used antibiotics. Penicillins are natural and semisynthetic derivatives of broth cultures of the *Penicillium* mold. They inhibit bacterial cell wall production and therefore are bactericidal.

Clinical Use. Penicillins other than amoxicillin and amoxicillin–clavulanate potassium (Augmentin) have not been shown to increase periodontal attachment levels, and their use in periodontal therapy does not appear to be justified.[88]

Side Effects. Penicillins may induce allergic reactions and bacterial resistance; up to 10% of patients may be allergic to penicillin.

Amoxicillin. Amoxicillin is a semisynthetic penicillin with an extended antiinfective spectrum that includes gram-positive and gram-negative bacteria. It demonstrates excellent absorption after oral administration. Amoxicillin is susceptible to penicillinase, a β-lactamase produced by certain bacteria that breaks the penicillin ring structure and thus renders penicillins ineffective.[88]

Amoxicillin may be useful in the management of patients with aggressive periodontitis, in both localized and generalized forms. Recommended dosage is 500 mg tid for 8 days.[42,43]

Amoxicillin–Clavulanate Potassium. The combination of amoxicillin with clavulanate potassium makes this antiinfective agent resistant to penicillinase enzymes produced by some bacteria. Amoxicillin with clavulanate (Augmentin) may be useful in the management of patients with LAP or refractory periodontitis.[60] Bueno et al.[11] reported that Augmentin halted alveolar bone loss in patients with periodontal disease that was refractory to treatment with other antibiotics, including tetracycline, metronidazole, and clindamycin.

Cephalosporins

Pharmacology. The family of β-lactams known as cephalosporins is similar in action and structure to penicillins. They are frequently used in medicine and are resistant to a number of β-lactamases normally active against penicillin.

Clinical Use. Cephalosporins are generally not used to treat dental-related infections. The penicillins are superior to cephalosporins in their range of action against periodontal pathogenic bacteria.

Side Effects. Patients allergic to penicillins must be considered allergic to all β-lactam products. Rashes, urticaria, fever, and GI upset have been associated with cephalosporins.[83]

Clindamycin

Pharmacology. Clindamycin is effective against anaerobic bacteria.[76] It is effective in situations in which the patient is allergic to penicillin.

Clinical Use. Clindamycin has shown efficacy in patients with periodontitis refractory to tetracycline therapy. Walker et al.[87] showed that clindamycin assisted in stabilizing refractory patients; dosage was 150 mg qid for 10 days. Jorgensen and Slots[43] recommend a regimen of 300 mg bid for 8 days.

Side Effects. Clindamycin has been associated with pseudomembranous colitis, but the incidence is higher with cephalosporins and ampicillin. When needed, however, clindamycin can be used with caution, but it is not indicated in patients with a history of colitis. Diarrhea or cramping that develops during clindamycin therapy may be indicative of colitis, and clindamycin should be discontinued. If symptoms persist, the patient should be referred to an internist.

Ciprofloxacin

Pharmacology. Ciprofloxacin is a quinolone active against gram-negative rods, including all facultative and some anaerobic putative periodontal pathogens.

Clinical Use. Because it demonstrates minimal effect on *Streptococcus* species, which are associated with periodontal health, ciprofloxacin therapy may facilitate the establishment of a microflora associated with periodontal health. At present, ciprofloxacin is the only antibiotic in periodontal therapy to which all strains of *A. actinomycetemcomitans* are susceptible. It also has been used in combination with metronidazole.[61]

Side Effects. Nausea, headache, metallic taste in the mouth, and abdominal discomfort have been associated with ciprofloxacin. Quinolones inhibit the metabolism of theophylline, and caffeine and concurrent administration can produce toxicity. Quinolones have also been reported to enhance the effect of warfarin and other anticoagulants.[83]

Macrolides

Pharmacology. Macrolide antibiotics contain a many-membered lactone ring to which one or more deoxy sugars are attached. They inhibit protein synthesis by binding to the 50S ribosomal subunits of sensitive microorganisms. Macrolides can be bacteriostatic or bactericidal, depending on the concentration of the drug and the nature of the microorganism. The macrolide antibiotics used for periodontal treatment include erythromycin, spiramycin, and azithromycin.

Clinical Use. **Erythromycin** does not concentrate in GCF, and it is not effective against most putative periodontal pathogens. For these reasons, erythromycin is not recommended as an adjunct to periodontal therapy.

Spiramycin is active against gram-positive organisms; it is excreted in high concentrations in saliva. It is used as an adjunct to periodontal treatment in Canada and Europe but is not available in the United States. Spiramycin has minimal effect on increasing attachment levels.

Azithromycin is a member of the azalide class of macrolides. It is effective against anaerobes and gram-negative bacilli. After an oral dosage of 500 mg qd for 3 days, significant levels of azithromycin can be detected in most tissues for 7 to 10 days.[9] The concentration of azithromycin in tissue specimens from periodontal lesions is significantly higher than that of normal gingiva.[54] It has been proposed that azithromycin penetrates fibroblasts and phagocytes in concentrations 100 to 200 times greater than that of the extracellular compartment. The azithromycin is actively transported to sites of inflammation by phagocytes, then released directly into the sites of inflammation as the phagocytes rupture during phagocytosis.[30,42] Therapeutic use requires a single dose of 250 mg/day for 5 days after an initial loading dose of 500 mg.[83]

SERIAL AND COMBINATION ANTIBIOTIC THERAPY

Rationale

Because periodontal infections may contain a wide diversity of bacteria, no single antibiotic is effective against all putative pathogens. Indeed, differences exist in the microbial flora associated with the various periodontal disease syndromes.[87] These "mixed" infections can include a variety of aerobic, microaerophilic, and anaerobic bacteria, both gram negative and gram positive. In these cases it may be necessary to use more than one antibiotic, either serially or in combination.[60] Before combinations of antibiotics are used, however, the periodontal pathogen(s) being treated must be identified and antibiotic-susceptibility testing performed.

Clinical Use

Antibiotics that are *bacteriostatic* (e.g., tetracycline) generally require rapidly dividing microorganisms to be effective. They do not function well if a *bactericidal* antibiotic (e.g., amoxicillin) is given concurrently. *When both types of drugs are required, they are best given serially, not in combination.*

Rams and Slots[60] reviewed combination therapy using systemic metronidazole along with amoxicillin, amoxicillin-clavulanate (Augmentin), or ciprofloxacin. The metronidazole-amoxicillin and metronidazole-Augmentin combinations provided excellent elimination of many organisms in adult and localized aggressive periodontitis that had been treated unsuccessfully with tetracyclines and mechanical debridement. These drugs have an additive effect regarding suppression of *A. actinomycetemcomitans.* Tinoco et al.[74] found metronidazole and amoxicillin to be clinically effective in treating LAP, although 50% of patients harbored *A. actinomycetemcomitans* 1 year later. Metronidazole ciprofloxacin combination is effective against *A. actinomycetemcomitans;* metronidazole targets obligate anaerobes, and ciprofloxacin targets facultative anaerobes. This is a powerful combination against mixed infections. Studies of this drug combination in the treatment of refractory periodontitis have documented marked clinical improvement. This combination may provide a *therapeutic benefit* by reducing or eliminating pathogenic organisms and a *prophylactic benefit* by giving rise to a predominantly streptococcal microflora.[61]

Systemic antibiotic therapy combined with mechanical therapy appears valuable in the treatment of recalcitrant periodontal infections and LAP infections involving *A. actinomycetemcomitans.* Antibiotic treatment should be reserved for specific subsets of periodontal patients who do not respond to conventional therapy. Selection of specific agents should be guided by the results of cultures and sensitivity tests for subgingival plaque microorganisms.

SCIENCE TRANSFER

The inflammation found in the periodontal diseases is initiated by microbial plaque and bacterial infection. Therapeutic approaches have therefore focused on limiting the bacterial insult. Typically, the predominant approach is periodically to remove the bacteria mechanically, either manually or with electronic instrumentation. Another approach is to use chemotherapeutic agents systemically or locally to limit the bacterial insult, either as adjunctive therapy or as monotherapy. Although some improvement in clinical outcome is usually achieved, the rationale of this second approach in a disease characterized by a bacteria-host relationship can be questioned. That is, simply limiting bacterial growth for a brief time or even removing bacteria without altering the host or the anatomy of the defect results in a regrowth of bacteria in a relatively short period. Thus the benefits of a therapy aimed solely at the bacteria (i.e., chemotherapeutics) may be short term. *Recent emphasis on the host response indicates that more effective therapeutic approaches to treating periodontal disease will involve both aspects of the disease: the bacteria and the host.*

Many of the systemic chemotherapeutic agents, including antibiotics and host modulation agents, have resulted in a statistical improvement in periodontal measurements such as pocket depth attachment level and bleeding on probing. However, the amount of improvement over conventional initial therapy in general is minimal, often less than 1 mm, and so it would be difficult for practicing clinicians to detect such benefits in many of their patients. A similar relationship exists with the locally applied agents reviewed in this chapter. *Thus, at present, these approaches should be used as supportive measures to conventional therapy to gain small, additional benefits for patients or, in some cases, to stabilize the patient's periodontal status.*

Many regenerative surgical procedures result in improvements in attachment levels and pocket depth of 3 to 4 mm. Therefore, practitioners can see more dramatic results when these procedures are used for treating advanced periodontal disease.

HOST MODULATION (See Chapters 15 and 53)

Doxycycline Hyclate

Now approved by the U.S. Food and Drug Administration (FDA) for the adjunctive treatment of periodontitis, doxycycline hyclate is available as a 20-mg capsule for use by patients twice daily. The mechanism of action is by suppression of the activity of collagenase, particularly that produced by polymorphonuclear leukocytes (PMNs). Although in the antibiotic family, doxycycline hyclate does not produce antibacterial effects because the dose of 20 mg bid is too low to affect bacteria. As a result, resistance to this medication has not been seen.

Figure 52-3 provides a schematic diagram of the progression of periodontal disease and the role of matrix metalloproteinases, of which doxycycline is an inhibitor.

Four double-blind, multicenter clinical studies of more than 650 patients have demonstrated that doxycycline hyclate improves the effectiveness of professional periodontal care and slows the progression of the disease process. The results of the first three studies showed that doxycycline hyclate resulted in approximately a 50% improvement in clinical attachment levels in pockets with probing depths of 4 to 6 mm and a 34% improvement in pockets with probing depths of 7 mm or greater. Also, attachment loss was prevented in sites with normal probing depths (0-3 mm), whereas the placebo groups lost 0.13 mm at 12 months ($p = 0.05$).[13,23]

Caton et al.[14] showed statistically significant reductions in probing depths and increases in clinical attachment levels with adjunctive doxycycline hyclate in conjunction with root planing at 3-, 6-, and 9-month evaluations compared with placebo groups undergoing root planing alone. Although statistically significant, the net changes were considered limited alterations in patients with moderate to severe chronic periodontitis.[4]

Results of safety studies showed that doxycycline hyclate (20 mg bid) with or without mechanical therapy (scaling and root planing) did not exert an anti-infective effect on the periodontal microflora and did not result in a detrimental shift in the normal flora. The colonization or overgrowth of the periodontal pocket by bacteria resistant to doxycycline, tetracycline, minocycline, amoxicillin, erythromycin, or clindamycin has not been observed. In addition, no evidence of a tendency toward the acquisition of multiantibiotic resistance was found.[23,86] Periostat (Collagenex Pharmaceutical Inc.) and generic forms are currently available in a dose of 20 mg of doxycycline.

Nonsteroidal Antiinflammatory Drugs

The role of the host's inflammatory system in periodontal disease only relatively recently has begun to be understood. Following activation of inflammatory cells in the periodontium by bacteria, phospholipids in the plasma membranes of cells are acted on by phospholipase. This leads to the liberation of free arachidonic acid, which then can be metabolized into prostaglandins, thromboxanes, and prostacycline by the enzyme cyclooxygenase. The lipoxygenase pathway can produce leukotrienes and hydroxyeicosatetraenoic acids from arachidonic acid. Strong evidence suggests that cyclooxygenase pathway products (e.g., prostaglandins) may be important mediators of some pathologic events occurring in periodontal disease.[63] Therefore, modulation of the host's inflammatory response to bacteria may alter the incidence and severity of periodontal disease.

Nonsteroidal antiinflammatory drugs (NSAIDs) may be of therapeutic value in treating periodontal disease

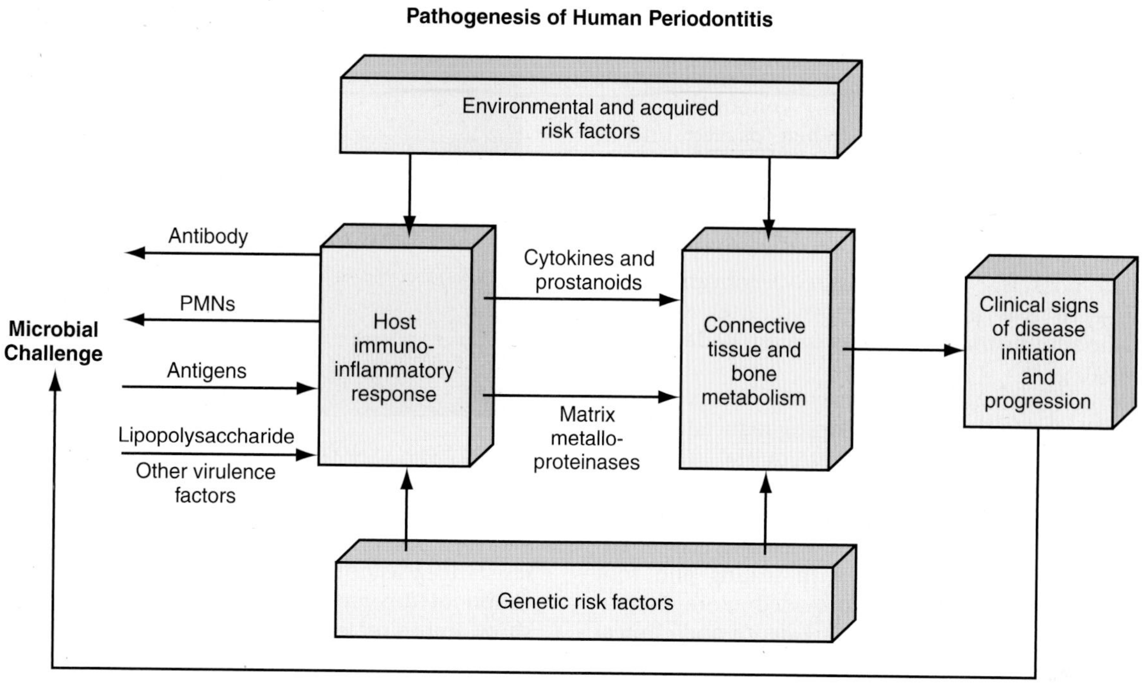

Figure 52-3 Pathogenesis of periodontitis. *PMNs,* Polymorphonuclear leukocytes. (From Page RC, Kornman KS: The pathogenesis of human periodontitis: an introduction, *Periodontol 2000* 14:9, 1997.)

TABLE 52-3

Currently Available or Investigational, Locally Delivered Antimicrobials for Periodontal Therapy

Antimicrobial Agent	FDA Clearance	Dosage Form
2% Minocycline microspheres	Yes	Biodegradable powder in syringe
10% Doxycycline gel	Yes	Biodegradable mixture in syringe
25% Metronidazole gel	No	Biodegradable mixture in syringe
Chlorhexidine (2.5 mg) in gelatin matrix	Yes	Biodegradable device

FDA, U.S. Food and Drug Administration.

because of their ability to interfere with arachidonic acid metabolism and thereby inhibit the inflammatory process. This expectation has been validated in studies in both animals and humans.[25,59,80,92,94] Some NSAIDs have been shown to affect the response of PMNs to inflammation not related to prostaglandin inhibition.[26,44] Beneficial effects of NSAIDs have also been found after topical application.[39,79,91] Drugs such as flurbiprofen, ibuprofen, mefenamic acid, and naproxen have been studied.[90]

Flurbiprofen appears to be an NSAID worthy of further investigation. It inhibits PMN migration, reduces vascular permeability, and inhibits platelet aggregation by inhibiting cyclooxygenase.[39] In a 3-year study, Williams et al.[91] reported that flurbiprofen significantly inhibited radiographic alveolar bone loss when compared with placebo. Unfortunately, by 24 months, the difference in the rate of bone loss had disappeared. This group also reported a return to baseline in the rate of bone loss after treatment with flurbiprofen was discontinued.[93]

A recent study suggests that concomitant administration of doxycycline and flurbiprofen may result in enhancement of the anticollagenase effects of doxycycline and deserves further investigation.[50]

LOCAL DELIVERY OF ANTIBIOTICS

The limitations of mouth rinsing and irrigation have prompted research for the development of alternative delivery systems. Recently, advances in delivery technology have resulted in the controlled release of drugs (Table 52-3). The requirements for treating periodontal disease include a means for targeting an antiinfective agent to infection sites and sustaining its localized concentration at effective levels for a sufficient time while concurrently evoking minimal or no side effects.

Tetracycline-Containing Fibers

The first local delivery product available in the United States was extensively studied, an ethylene/vinyl acetate copolymer fiber (diameter, 0.5 mm) containing tetracycline, 12.7 mg per 9 inches. When packed into a periodontal pocket, it was well tolerated by oral tissues, and for 10 days it sustained tetracycline concentrations exceeding 1300 μg/ml, well beyond the 32 to 64 μg/ml required to inhibit the growth of pathogens isolated from periodontal pockets.[75,86] In contrast, GCF concentrations of only 4 to 8 μg/ml were reported after systemic tetracycline administration, 250 mg qid for 10 days (total oral dose, 10 g).[34]

Studies demonstrated that tetracycline fibers applied with or without scaling and root planing reduced probing depth, bleeding on probing, and periodontal pathogens and provided gains in clinical attachment level. Such effects were significantly better than those attained with scaling and root planing alone or with placebo fibers. In a 2-month study, compared with scaling and root planing, the fibers used alone provided more than a 60% greater improvement in probing depth and clinical attachment level than scaling alone.[31]

No change in antibiotic resistance to tetracycline was found after tetracycline fiber therapy among the tested putative periodontal pathogens.[31] Disadvantages of the fiber included the length of time required for placement (≥10 minutes per tooth), the considerable learning curve required to gain proficiency at placement, and the need for a second patient appointment 10 days after placement for fiber removal. Also, placement of fibers around 12 or more teeth resulted in oral candidiasis in a few patients.

Another study suggested that rinsing with 0.12% chlorhexidine after fiber placement had a synergistic effect, enhancing the reduction of bacterial pathogens.[55] Evaluation of the effect of tetracycline fibers on root surfaces, using fluorescent light and scanning electron microscopy, showed superficial penetration of tetracycline, with minor penetration into dental tubules, and a few areas of demineralized root surface. Microscopy also revealed reductions in the subgingival microbial flora on the root surfaces of teeth treated with the fibers versus the control specimens.[55]

Subgingival Doxycycline

The FDA approved 10% doxycycline in a gel system using a syringe (Atridox) (Figure 52-4). It is the only local delivery system accepted by the American Dental Association and is available in the United States and a number of other countries.

In a 9-month multicenter study of 180 patients, treatment with 10% doxycycline gel alone was more effective than the other treatments at all time periods, with the exception of the 3-month clinical attachment level value. For the 10% doxycycline gel group, the reduction in clinical attachment level at 9 months showed a gain of 0.4 mm compared with vehicle control; the reduction in probing depth was 0.6 mm greater than vehicle control; and the reduction of bleeding on probing was 0.2 units greater than vehicle control. The differences were clinically small but statistically significant. Although

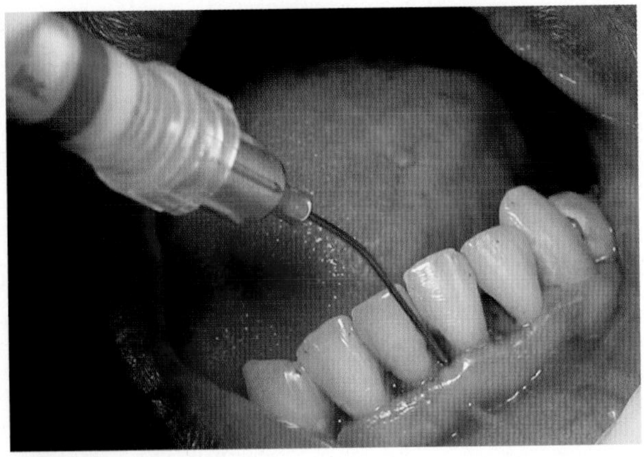

Figure 52-4 Placement of 10% doxycycline (Atridox) gel.

resistance was not evaluated in this study, the local application of doxycycline has previously been reported to show transient increases in resistance in oral microbes and no overgrowth of foreign pathogens.[49]

Two multicenter clinical trials each studied 411 patients with moderate to severe periodontitis.[27] At baseline, patients were randomized to one of four treatment groups: 10% doxycycline gel, vehicle control, oral hygiene only, and scaling and root planing. Sites with probing depth of 5 mm or greater that bled on probing were treated at baseline and then again with the same treatment at 4 months. Clinical assessments were made for 9 months, measuring clinical attachment level, probing depth, and bleeding on probing. All treatment groups in both studies showed clinical improvements from baseline over the 9-month period. The results for all parameters measured were significantly better in the 10% doxycycline gel group compared with vehicle control and oral hygiene only. Compared with scaling and root planing, the effects of 10% doxycycline gel as monotherapy on clinical attachment level gain and probing depth reduction were equivalent (see also Chapter 53).

Subgingival Minocycline

The FDA recently approved a new, locally delivered, sustained-release form of minocycline microspheres (Arestin) for subgingival placement as an adjunct to scaling and root planing (Figure 52-5). The 2% minocycline is encapsulated into bioresorbable microspheres in a gel carrier. When compared to controls (scaling and root planing with nonactive vehicle as subgingival irrigant), there was a statistically significant increase in clinical attachment levels in patients who presented with pockets of 6 mm or greater probing depth.[20]

In a four-center, double-blind, randomized trial, patients with periodontal pockets at least 5 mm deep were selected, and either 2% minocycline gel or vehicle were applied once every 2 weeks for four applications after initial scaling and root planing.[77] A total of 343 teeth (976 sites) were included in the minocycline group, with 299 teeth (810 sites) in the control group. Reductions in *P. gingivalis* and *P. intermedia* at weeks 2, 4, 6, and

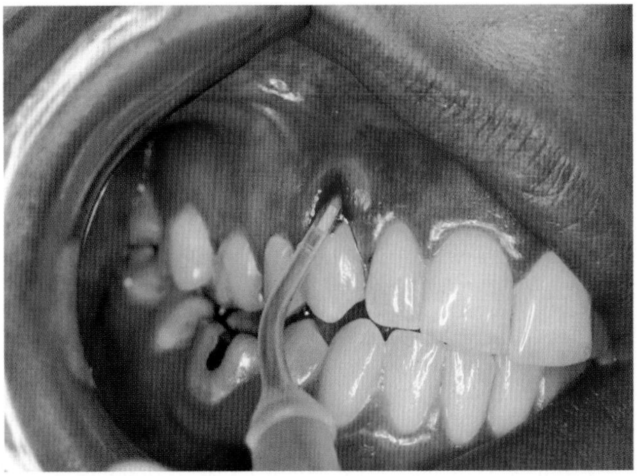

Figure 52-5 Placement of minocycline microspheres (Arestin).

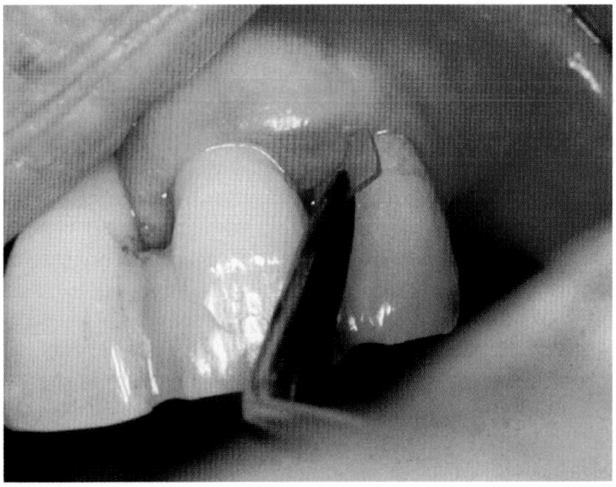

Figure 52-6 Placement of chlorhexidine gluconate chip (PerioChip).

12 and at weeks 6 and 12 for *A. actinomycetemcomitans* were statistically significant. These results demonstrated the advantages of supplementing standard subgingival debridement with minocycline gel application. The three primary clinical efficacy variables in this study were probing depth, clinical attachment level, and bleeding index. There was a trend toward clinical improvement in both treatment groups for all three measures, and the reduction in probing depth was significantly greater with minocycline gel. When sites with probing depth of at least 7 mm and significant bleeding at baseline were considered, the improvements were greater than with 5-mm pockets. The improvements with minocycline were statistically significantly better than the control group.

Applications of 2% minocycline were also evaluated in a 3-month study in 30 patients.[35] Active or placebo gel was placed subgingivally at planed sites in each subject according to a double-blind protocol, immediately after scaling and root planing and 2 and 4 weeks later. Differences between groups in mean probing depth did not reach statistical significance at any visit, but mean clinical attachment levels favored the minocycline group ($p < 0.05$) at both reassessments. The number of sites that bled after deep probing at 12 weeks also favored the minocycline group ($p < 0.05$). This product (2% minocycline) is not available in the United States.

Subgingival Metronidazole

A topical medication containing an oil-based metronidazole 25% dental gel (glyceryl mono-oleate and sesame oil) has been tested in a number of studies.[1] This product is not available in the United States. It is applied in viscous consistency to the pocket, where it is liquidized by the body heat and then hardens again, forming crystals in contact with water. As a precursor, the preparation contains metronidazole-benzoate, which is converted into the active substance by esterases in GCF. Two 25% gel applications at a 1-week interval have been used.[45]

Studies have shown that metronidazole gel is equivalent to scaling and root planing but have not shown adjunctive benefits with scaling and root planing. In a 6-month study of 30 patients, treatment consisted of two applications of the dental gel in two randomly selected quadrants at 1-week intervals, as well as simultaneous subgingival scaling of the remaining quadrants.[73] Oral hygiene instructions were given on day 21. Statistical analyses showed that both treatments were effective in reducing probing depth and bleeding on probing over the 6-month period. At the end of the follow-up period, the mean reduction in probing depth was 1.3 mm after gel treatment and 1.5 mm after subgingival scaling. Bleeding on probing was reduced by 35% and 42%, respectively. No significant differences between the two treatments were detected. Dark-field microscopy showed a shift toward a seemingly healthier microflora for both treatment modalities; this effect persisted throughout the 6-month period.

A large, multicenter study of 206 subjects investigated two applications of metronidazole gel in two randomly selected quadrants versus two quadrants of scaling.[1] Probing depths were reduced by 1.2 mm in the gel and 1.5 mm in the scaling group. At 6 months, the differences between treatments were statistically but not clinically significant. Also, bleeding on probing was reduced by 88% for both treatment groups.

LOCAL DELIVERY OF ANTISEPTIC AGENT

A resorbable delivery system has been tested for the subgingival placement of chlorhexidine gluconate with positive clinical results (Figure 52-6). PerioChip is a small chip (4.0 × 5.0 × 0.35 mm) composed of a biodegradable hydrolyzed gelatin matrix, cross-linked with glutaraldehyde and also containing glycerin and water, into which 2.5 mg of chlorhexidine gluconate has been incorporated per chip. This delivery system releases chlorhexidine and maintains drug concentrations in the GCF greater than 100 μg/ml for at least 7 days,[72] concentrations well above the tolerance of most oral bacteria.[10] Because the chip biodegrades in 7 to 10 days, a second appointment for removal is not needed.

Two multicenter, randomized, double-blind, parallel-group, controlled clinical trials of this chip were conducted in the United States with a total of 447 patients in 10 centers.[41] In these studies, patients received a supragingival prophylaxis for up to 1 hour, followed by scaling and root planing for 1 hour. Chips were placed in target sites with probing depth of 5 to 8 mm at baseline that bled on probing and again at 3 and 6 months if probing depth remained at 5 mm or greater. Sites in control subjects received either a placebo chip (inactive) with scaling and root planing or scaling and root planing alone. Sites in test subjects received either a chlorhexidine chip (active) with scaling and root planing or scaling and root planing alone. Examinations were performed at baseline and again at 3, 6, and 9 months. At 9 months, significant decreases in probing depth from baseline favoring the active chip compared with controls were observed: chlorhexidine chip with scaling and root planing, –0.95 ± 0.05 mm; placebo chip with scaling and root planing, –0.69 ± 0.05 mm (p = 0.001); scaling and root planing alone, –0.65 ± 0.05 mm (p = 0.00001). Although statistically significant, the net clinical changes were limited. The proportion of pocket sites with a probing depth reduction of 2 mm or more was increased in the chlorhexidine chip group (30%) compared with scaling and root planing alone (16%), a statistically significant difference on a per-patient basis ($p < 0.0001$).

No signs of staining were noted in any of the previous three studies as a result of the chlorhexidine chip treatment, as measured by a stain index. Adverse effects were minimal, with a few patients who complained of slight pain and swelling in the first 24 hours after chip placement.

CONCLUSION

Scaling and root planing alone are effective in reducing pocket depths, gaining increases in periodontal attachment levels, and decreasing inflammation levels (bleeding on probing). When scaling and root planing are combined with the subgingival placement of sustained-release vehicles (e.g., minocycline gel, microencapsulated minocycline), however, additional clinical benefits are possible, including further reduction in pocket depths, additional gain in clinical attachment level, and further decrease in inflammation. Improvement in clinical attachment levels also occurs with the chlorhexidine chip and doxycycline gel. Evidence indicates that some antibiotics provide additional improvement in attachment levels when used as adjuncts to scaling and root planing. Use of chemotherapeutic treatment adjuncts does not result in significant patient-centered adverse effects.

REFERENCES

1. Ainamo J, Lie T, Ellingsen BH, et al: Clinical responses to subgingival application of a metronidazole 25% gel compared to the effect of subgingival scaling in adult periodontitis, *J Clin Periodontol* 19(pt II):723, 1992.
2. Alger FA, Solt CW, Vuddhankanok S, et al: The histologic evaluation of new attachment in periodontally diseased human roots treated with tetracycline hydrochloride and fibronectin, *J Periodontol* 61:447, 1990.
3. American Academy of Periodontology: Parameters of care, *J Periodontol* 71(suppl):847, 2000.
4. American Academy of Periodontology, Research, Science and Therapy Committee: Systemic antibiotics in periodontics, *J Periodontol* 75:1553, 2004.
5. American Dental Association, Council on Scientific Affairs: Combating antibiotic resistance, *J Am Dent Assoc* 135:484, 2004.
6. Bader HI, Goldhaber P: The passage of intravenously administered tetracycline into the gingival sulcus of dogs, *J Oral Ther Pharmacol* 2:324, 1968.
7. Baker PJ, Evans RT, Slots J, et al: Antibiotic susceptibility of anaerobic bacteria from the oral cavity, *J Dent Res* 65:1233, 1985.
8. Baker PJ, Evans RT, Slots J, et al: Susceptibility of human oral anaerobic bacteria to antibiotics suitable for topical use, *J Clin Periodontol* 12:201, 1985.
9. Blandizzi C, Tecla M, Lupetti A, et al: Periodontal tissue disposition of azithromycin in patients affected by chronic inflammatory periodontal diseases, *J Periodontol* 70:960, 1999.
10. Briner WW, Kayrouz GA, Chanak MX: Comparative antimicrobial effectiveness of a substantive (0.12% chlorhexidine) and a nonsubstantive (phenolic) mouthrinse in vivo and in vitro, *Compend Contin Educ Dent* 15:1158, 1994.
11. Bueno L, Walker C, van Ness W, et al: Effect of Augmentin on microbiota associated with refractory periodontitis, *J Dent Res* 67:246, 1988 (abstract 1064).
12. Carranza FA Jr, Saglie R, Newman MG, et al: Scanning and transmission electron microscopic study of tissue-invading microorganisms in localized juvenile periodontitis, *J Periodontol* 54:598, 1983.
13. Caton J, Bleiden T, Adams D, et al: Subantimicrobial doxycycline therapy for periodontitis, *J Dent Res* 76:1307, 1997 (abstract).
14. Caton JG, Ciancio SG, Blieden TM, et al: Treatment with subantimicrobial dose doxycycline improves the efficacy of scaling and root planing in patients with adult periodontitis, *J Periodontol* 71:521, 2000.
15. Chanoine, J, Boulvain M, Bourdoux, D, et al: Increased recall rate at screening for congenital hypothyroidism in breast fed infants born to iodine overloaded mothers, *Arch Dis Child* 63:1207, 1988.
16. Christersson LA, Slots J, Rosling BG, et al: Microbiological and clinical effects of surgical treatment of localized juvenile periodontitis, *J Clin Periodontol* 12:465, 1985.
17. Ciancio SG: Use of antibiotics in periodontal therapy. In Newman MG, Goodman A, editors: *Antibiotics in dentistry,* Chicago, 1983, Quintessence.
18. Ciancio SG: Antibiotics in periodontal therapy. In Newman MG, Kornman K, editors: *Antibiotic/antimicrobial use in dental practice,* Chicago, 1990, Quintessence.
19. Ciancio SG: Antiseptics and antibiotics as chemotherapeutic agents for periodontitis management, *Compend Contin Educ Dent* 21:59, 2000.
20. Ciancio SG, editor: FDA approves Arestin marketing. In *Biological therapies in dentistry,* 17(suppl 1):s1, Hamilton, Ontario, Canada, 2001, BC Decker (newsletter).
21. Ciancio SG, Adams D, Blieden T, et al: Subantimicrobial dose doxycycline: a new adjunctive therapy for adult periodontitis. Presented at Annual Meeting of American Academy of Periodontology, Boston, 1998.
22. Ciancio SG, Slots J, Reynolds HS, et al: The effect of short-term administration of minocycline HCl administration on gingival inflammation and subgingival microflora, *J Periodontol* 53:557, 1982.
23. Crout R, Adams D, Blieden T, et al: Safety of doxycycline hyclate 20 mg bid in patients with adult periodontitis.

Presented at Annual Meeting of American Academy of Periodontology, Boston, 1998.
24. Edelson H, Kaplan H, Korchak H: Differing effects of nonsteroidal anti-inflammatory agents on neutrophil functions, *Clin Res* 30:469A, 1982.
25. Feldman R, Szeto B, Chauncey H, et al: Nonsteroidal anti-inflammatory drugs in the reduction of human alveolar bone loss, *J Clin Periodontol* 10:131, 1983.
26. Feres M, Haffajee AD, Allard K, et al: Antibiotic resistance of subgingival species during and after periodontal therapy, *J Clin Periodontol* 28:12, 2002.
27. Garrett S, Adams D, Bandt C, et al: Two multicenter clinical trials of subgingival doxycycline in the treatment of periodontitis, *J Dent Res* 76:153, 1997 (abstract 1113).
28. Genco RJ, Cianciola JJ, Rosling H: Treatment of localized juvenile periodontitis, *J Dent Res* 60:527, 1981 (abstract 872).
29. Gibson W: Antibiotics and periodontal disease: a selective review of the literature, *J Am Dent Assoc* 104:213, 1982.
30. Gladue RP, Snyder ME: Intracellular accumulation of azithromycin by cultured human fibroblasts, *Antimicrob Agents Chemother* 34:1056, 1990.
31. Goodson JM, Tanner A: Antibiotic resistance of the subgingival microbiota following local tetracycline therapy, *Oral Microbiol Immunol* 7:113, 1992.
32. Goodson JM, Cugini M, Kent RL, et al: Multicenter evaluation of tetracycline fiber therapy. II. Clinical response, *J Periodontal Res* 26:371, 1991.
33. Gordon JM, Walker CB, Murphy JC: Concentration of tetracycline in human gingival fluid after single doses, *J Clin Periodontol* 8:117, 1981.
34. Gordon JM, Walker CB, Murphy CJ, et al: Tetracycline: levels achievable in gingival crevice fluid and in vitro effect on subgingival organisms. Part I. Concentrations in crevicular fluid after repeated doses, *J Periodontol* 52:609, 1981.
35. Grace MA, Watts TL, Wilson RF, et al: A randomized controlled trial of a 2% minocycline gel as an adjunct to nonsurgical periodontal treatment, using a design with multiple matching criteria, *J Clin Periodontol* 24:249, 1997.
36. Greenstein G: The role of metronidazole in the treatment of periodontal diseases, *J Periodontol* 64:1, 1993.
37. Greenstein G: Changing periodontal concepts: treatment considerations, *Compend Contin Educ Dent* 26:81, 2005.
38. Haffajee AD, Socransky SS, Gunsolley JC: Systemic anti-infective periodontal therapy: a systematic review, *Ann Periodontol* 8:115, 2003.
39. Heasam PA, Benn DK, Kelly PJ, et al: The use of topical flurbiprofen as an adjunct to non-surgical management of periodontal disease, *J Clin Periodontol* 20:457, 1993.
40. Hoepelman IM, Schneider MM: Azithromycin: the first of the tissue-selective azalides, *Int J Antimicrob Agents* 5:145, 1995.
41. Jeffcoat M, Bray KS, Ciancio SG, et al: Adjunctive use of a subgingival controlled-release chlorhexidine chip reduces probing depth and improves attachment level compared with scaling and root planing alone, *J Periodontol* 69:989, 1998.
42. Jorgensen MG, Slots J: Practical antimicrobial periodontal therapy, *Compend Contin Educ Dent* 21:111, 2000.
43. Jorgensen MG, Slots J: Responsible use of antimicrobials in periodontics, *J Cal Dent Assoc* 28:185, 2000.
44. Kaplan H, Edelson H, Korchak H, et al: Effects of nonsteroidal anti-inflammatory agents on neutrophil functions in vitro and in vivo, *Biochem Pharmacol* 33:371, 1984.
45. Klinge B, Attström R, Karring T, et al: Three regimens of topical metronidazole compared with subgingival scaling on periodontal pathology in adults, *J Clin Periodontol* 19(pt II):708, 1992.
46. Kornman KS, Karl EH: The effect of long-term low-dose tetracycline therapy on the subgingival microflora in refractory adult periodontitis, *J Periodontol* 53:604, 1982.
47. Lang NP, Adler R, Joss A, et al: The absence of bleeding on probing: an indicator of periodontal stability, *J Clin Periodontol* 17:714, 1990.
48. Lang NP, Joss A, Orsanic T, et al: Bleeding on probing: a predictor for the progression of periodontal disease? *J Clin Periodontol* 13:590, 1986.
49. Larsen T: Occurrence of doxycycline-resistant bacteria in the oral cavity after local administration of doxycycline in patients with periodontal disease, *Scand J Infect Dis* 23:89, 1991.
50. Lee HM, Ciancio SG, Tuter G, et al: Subantimicrobial dose doxycycline efficacy as a matrix metalloproteinase inhibitor in chronic periodontitis is enhanced when combined with a non-steroidal anti-inflammatory drug, *J Periodontol* 75:453, 2004.
51. Lekovic V, Kenney EB, Carranza FA Jr, et al: Effect of metronidazole on human periodontal disease: a clinical and microbiologic study, *J Periodontol* 54:476, 1983.
52. Loesche WJ, Giordano JR, Hujoel P, et al: Metronidazole in periodontitis: reduced need for surgery, *J Clin Periodontol* 19:103, 1992.
53. Lozdan J, Sheiham A, Pearlman BA, et al: The use of nitrimidazine in the treatment of acute ulcerative gingivitis: a double-blind controlled trial, *Br Dent J* 130:294, 1971.
54. Malizia T, Tejada MR, Ghelardi E, et al: Periodontal tissue disposition of azithromycin, *J Periodontol* 68:1206, 1997.
55. Morrison SL, Cobb CM, Kazakos GM, et al: Root surface characteristics associated with subgingival placement of monolithic tetracycline-impregnated fibers, *J Periodontol* 63:137, 1992.
56. Neidner R: Cytotoxicity and sensitization of povidone-iodine and other frequently used anti-infective agents, *Dermatology* 195(suppl):89, 1997.
57. Niederman R, Holborow D, Tonetti M, et al: Reinfection of periodontal sites following tetracycline fiber therapy, *J Dent Res* 69:277, 1990 (abstract 1345).
58. Nowzari H, McDonald ES, Flynn J, et al: The dynamics of microbial colonization of barrier membranes for guided tissue regeneration, *J Periodontol* 67:694, 1996.
59. Offenbacher S, Braswell L, Loos A, et al: Effects of flurbiprophen on the progression of periodontitis in *Macaca mulatta, J Periodontal Res* 22:473, 1987.
60. Rams TE, Slots J: Antibiotics in periodontal therapy: an update, *Compend Contin Educ Dent* 13:1130, 1992.
61. Rams TE, Feik D, Slots J: Ciprofloxacin/metronidazole treatment of recurrent adult periodontitis, *J Dent Res* 71:319, 1992 (abstract).
62. Reddy MS, Geurs NC, Gunsolley JC: Periodontal host modulation with antiproteinase, anti-inflammatory, and bone sparing agents: a systematic review, *Ann Periodontol* 8:12, 2003.
63. Research, Science and Therapy Committee: Pharmacologic blocking of host responses as an adjunct in the management of periodontal diseases: a research update, Chicago, 1992, American Academy of Periodontology.
64. Rosling BG, Slots J, Christersson LA, et al: Topical antimicrobial therapy and diagnosis of subgingival bacteria in the management of inflammatory periodontal disease, *J Clin Periodontol* 13:975, 1986.
65. Saglie FR, Carranza FA Jr, Newman MG, et al: Identification of tissue invading bacteria in human periodontal disease, *J Periodontal Res* 17:452, 1982.
66. Salvi GE, Lawrence HP, Offenbacher S, Beck JD: Influence of risk factors on the pathogenesis of periodontal disease, *Periodontol 2000* 14:173, 1997.
67. Schrefer J, publisher: *Mosby's GenRx,* ed 10, St Louis, 2001, Mosby.

68. Slots J, Rams TE: Antibiotics and periodontal therapy: advantages and disadvantages, *J Clin Periodontol* 17:479, 1990.
69. Slots J, Rosling BG: Suppression of periodontopathic microflora in localized juvenile periodontitis by systemic tetracycline, *J Clin Periodontol* 10:465, 1983.
70. Slots J, McDonald ES, Nowzari H: Infectious aspects of periodontal regeneration, *Periodontol 2000* 19:164, 1999.
71. Soder P, Frithiof L, Wikner S, et al: The effects of systemic metronidazole after non-surgical treatment in moderate and advanced periodontitis in young adults, *J Periodontol* 61:281, 1990.
72. Soskolne WA, Heasman PA, Stabholz A, et al: Sustained local delivery of chlorhexidine in the treatment of periodontitis: a multi-center study, *J Periodontol* 68:32, 1997.
73. Stelzel M, Flores-De-Jacoby L: Topical metronidazole application compared with subgingival scaling: a clinical and microbiological study on recall patients, *J Clin Periodontol* 23:24, 1996.
74. Tinoco EM, Beldi M, Campedelli F, et al: Clinical and microbiologic effects of adjunctive antibiotics in treatment of localized aggressive periodontitis: a controlled clinical study, *J Periodontol* 69:1355, 1998.
75. Tonetti M, Cugini AM, Goodson JM: Zero order delivery with periodontal placement of tetracycline loaded ethylene vinyl acetate fibers, *J Periodontal Res* 25:243, 1990.
76. Tyler K, Walker CB, Gordon J, et al: Evaluation of clindamycin in adult refractory periodontitis: antimicrobial susceptibilities, *J Dent Res* 64:360, 1985 (special issue; abstract 1667).
77. Van Steenberghe D, Bercy P, Kohl J: Subgingival minocycline hydrochloride ointment in moderate to severe chronic adult periodontitis: a randomized, double-blind, vehicle-controlled, multicenter study, *J Periodontol* 64:637, 1993.
78. Van Winkelhoff AJ, Gonzales DH, Winkel EG, et al: Antimicrobial resistance in the subgingival microflora in patients with adult periodontitis: a comparison between the Netherlands and Spain, *J Clin Periodontol* 27:79, 2000.
79. Vogel R, Schneider L, Goteinter D: The effects of a topical nonsteroidal anti-inflammatory drug on ligature induced periodontal disease in the squirrel monkey, *J Clin Periodontol* 12:139, 1986.
80. Waite I, Saxon C, Young A, et al: The periodontal status of subjects receiving nonsteroidal anti-inflammatory drugs, *J Periodontal Res* 16:100, 1981.
81. Walker C, Karpinia K: Rationale for use of antibiotics in periodontics, *J Periodontol* 73:1188, 2002.
82. Walker C, Thomas J: The effect of subantimicrobial doses of doxycycline on the microbial flora and antibiotic resistance in patients with adult periodontitis. Presented at Annual Meeting of American Academy of Periodontology, Boston, 1998.
83. Walker CB: Selected antimicrobial agents: mechanisms of action, side effects and drug interactions, *Periodontol 2000* 10:12, 1996.
84. Walker CB: The acquisition of resistance of antibiotic resistance in the periodontal microflora, *Periodontol 2000* 10:79, 1996.
85. Walker CB, Gordon JM, Socransky SS: Antibiotic susceptibility testing of subgingival plaque samples, *J Clin Periodontol* 10:422, 1983.
86. Walker CB, Gordon JM, Mcquilkin SJ, et al: Tetracycline: levels achievable in gingival crevice fluid and in vitro effect on subgingival organisms. Part II. Susceptibilities of periodontal bacteria, *J Periodontol* 52:613, 1981.
87. Walker CB, Gordon JM, Magnusson I, et al: A role for antibiotics in the treatment of refractory periodontitis, *J Periodontol* 64:772, 1993.
88. Weinstein L: Antimicrobial agents: penicillins and cephalosporins. In Goodman LS, Gilman A, editors: *The pharmacological basis of therapeutics,* ed 5, New York, 1975, Macmillan.
89. Weinstein L: Antimicrobial agents: tetracyclines and chloramphenicol. In Goodman LS, Gilman A, editors: *The pharmacological basis of therapeutics,* ed 5, New York, 1975, Macmillan.
90. Williams RC, Jeffcoat MK, Howell T, et al: Altering the progression of human alveolar bone loss with the nonsteroidal anti-inflammatory drug flurbiprofen, *J Periodontol* 60:485, 1989.
91. Williams RC, Jeffcoat MK, Howell T, et al: Ibuprofen: an inhibitor of alveolar bone resorption in beagles, *J Periodontal Res* 23:225, 1988.
92. Williams RC, Jeffcoat MK, Howell T, et al: Indomethacin or flurbiprofen treatment of periodontitis in beagles: comparison of effect on bone loss, *J Periodontal Res* 22:403, 1987.
93. Williams RC, Jeffcoat MK, Howell T, et al: Three year trial of flurbiprofen treatment in humans: post-treatment period, *J Dent Res* 70:448, 1991 (abstract 1617).
94. Williams RC, Jeffcoat MK, Wechter WJ, et al: Flurbiprofen: a potent inhibitor of alveolar bone resorption in beagles, *Science* 227:640, 1985.

53 CHAPTER

Host Modulation Agents

Philip M. Preshaw, Maria Emanuel Ryan, and William V. Giannobile

Chapter Outline

Periodontists previously believed that periodontal disease was an inevitable consequence of aging and was uniformly distributed in the population. They thought that disease severity was directly correlated with plaque levels (i.e., the worse the oral hygiene, the worse the periodontal disease) and that disease progression occurred in a continuous, linear manner throughout life.

Now, as a result of better epidemiologic data, there has been a paradigm shift in how periodontists view the prevalence and progression of this common disease. It is now apparent that although gingivitis and mild periodontitis (pockets of 4-5 mm) are common, possibly affecting a majority of the population, severe periodontitis (pockets ≥6 mm) is much less prevalent, affecting approximately 8% to 15% of adult populations in Western countries. It has been well established that periodontal disease is not a natural consequence of aging and that disease severity is not correlated with plaque levels. Anecdotally, any dentist will be able to identify patients with abundant plaque and calculus deposits with widespread gingivitis and shallow pocketing, but with minimal deep pocketing. By contrast, other patients, despite maintaining a high standard of plaque control, succumb to aggressive forms of periodontitis, with deep pocketing, tooth mobility, and early tooth loss. The former group of patients is *periodontal disease resistant,* whereas the latter group is *periodontal disease susceptible.* Clearly, the response of the periodontal tissues to plaque is different in these two types of patients, and certain patients undergo advanced periodontal breakdown even though they achieve a high standard of oral hygiene.

HOST RESPONSE

The previous observations led researchers to realize that the *host response* to the bacterial challenge presented by subgingival plaque is *the* important determinant of disease severity. Although plaque bacteria are capable of causing direct damage to the periodontal tissues (e.g., by release of H_2S, butyric acid, and other enzymes and mediators), it is now recognized that the great majority of the destructive events occurring in the periodontal tissues result from activation of destructive processes that occur as part of the host immune-inflammatory response to plaque bacteria. The host response is essentially protective by intent but paradoxically can also result in tissue damage, including breakdown of connective tissue fibers in the periodontal ligament and resorption of alveolar bone.

The nature of the host response to the presence of plaque is modified by genetic factors (helping to explain why aggressive periodontitis tends to have a familial aggregation) and systemic and environmental factors (e.g., smoking, diabetes, stress). Periodontal disease is a multifactorial, complex disease, and an upregulated or maladapted immune-inflammatory response to bacterial plaque predisposes patients to periodontal breakdown. The importance of the host response as a determinant of disease susceptibility is now driving researchers to identify genetic traits that characterize individuals as disease resistant or disease susceptible (see Chapter 11). Researchers are also investigating *host modulatory therapies* (HMTs), which aim to modify or reduce destructive aspects of the host response so that the immune-inflammatory response to plaque is less damaging to the periodontal tissues. A range of pharmaceuticals will likely be developed, HMTs targeting different aspects of the host response as adjunctive treatments for periodontal disease.

This chapter discusses the HMTs researched to date, use of HMTs in clinical practice, and what the future might hold for HMTs.

HOST MODULATORY THERAPY

Definition and Rationale

Host modulatory therapy (HMT) is a treatment concept that aims to reduce tissue destruction and stabilize or even regenerate the periodontium by modifying or downregulating destructive aspects of the host response and upregulating protective or regenerative responses. HMTs are systemically or locally delivered pharmaceuticals that are prescribed as part of periodontal therapy and are used as adjuncts to conventional periodontal treatments, such as scaling and root planing (SRP) and surgery. Interest in the potential application of HMTs in treating periodontitis has been driven by improved understanding of periodontal pathogenesis and awareness of the importance of the host response in disease susceptibility and progression.

HMTs offer the potential to move periodontal treatment strategies to a new level. Historically, treatment has focused on reducing the bacterial challenge by the use of SRP, improved oral hygiene, and periodontal surgery. However, the outcomes after conventional treatment of this chronic disease are not always predictable or stable. Periodontal disease and health can be seen as a balance between (1) a persisting bacterial burden and proinflammatory destructive events in the tissues and (2) resolution of inflammation and downregulation of destructive processes (see Figure 16-2). Removal of plaque by SRP targets one aspect of the pathogenic process by reducing the bacterial burden and therefore the antigenic challenge that drives the inflammatory response in the host tissues. However, the bacterial challenge is never completely eliminated after SRP, and recolonization by bacterial species occurs. HMTs offer the potential for downregulating destructive aspects and upregulating protective aspects of the host response so that, in combination with conventional treatments to reduce the bacterial burden, the balance between health (resolution of inflammation and wound healing) and disease progression (continued proinflammatory events) is tipped in the direction of a healing response.

HMT is a *means of treating the host side of the host-bacteria interaction*. The host response is responsible for most of the tissue breakdown that occurs, leading to the clinical signs of periodontitis. HMTs offer the opportunity for modulating or reducing this destruction by *treating* aspects of the chronic inflammatory response. HMTs do not "switch off" normal defense mechanisms or inflammation; instead, they ameliorate excessive or pathologically elevated inflammatory processes to enhance the opportunities for wound healing and periodontal stability.

A variety of different drug classes have been evaluated as host modulation agents, including the nonsteroidal antiinflammatory drugs (NSAIDs), bisphosphonates, tetracyclines, enamel matrix proteins, growth factors, and bone morphogenetic proteins.

Systemically Administered Agents

Nonsteroidal Antiinflammatory Drugs

NSAIDs inhibit the formation of prostaglandins, including *prostaglandin E_2* (PGE_2), which is produced by neutrophils, macrophages, fibroblasts, and gingival epithelial cells in response to the presence of *lipopolysaccharide* (LPS), a component of the cell wall of gram-negative bacteria. PGE_2 has been extensively studied in periodontal disease because it upregulates bone resorption by osteoclasts,[30,44] and levels of PGE_2 have been shown to be elevated in patients with periodontal disease compared with healthy patients.[26,44] PGE_2 also inhibits fibroblast function and has inhibitory and modulatory effects on the immune response.[27]

NSAIDs inhibit prostaglandins and therefore reduce tissue inflammation. They are used to treat pain, acute inflammation, and a variety of chronic inflammatory conditions. NSAIDs include the salicylates (e.g., aspirin), indomethacin, and the propionic acid derivatives (e.g., ibuprofen, flurbiprofen, naproxen). The ability of NSAIDs to block PGE_2 production, thereby reducing inflammation and inhibiting osteoclast activity in the periodontal tissues, has been investigated in patients with periodontitis. Studies have shown that systemic NSAIDs such as indomethacin,[64] flurbiprofen,[65] and naproxen[31] administered daily for up to 3 years significantly slowed the rate of alveolar bone loss compared with placebo.

However, the NSAIDs have some serious disadvantages when considered for use as adjunctive treatment for periodontitis. Daily administration for extended periods is necessary for periodontal benefits to become apparent, and NSAIDs are associated with significant side effects, including gastrointestinal problems, hemorrhage (from decreased platelet aggregation), and renal and hepatic impairment. Furthermore, research shows that the periodontal benefits of taking long-term NSAIDs are lost when patients stop taking the drugs, with a return to, or even an acceleration of, the rate of bone loss seen before NSAID therapy, often referred to as a "rebound effect."[66] For these reasons, the long-term use of NSAIDs as an adjunctive treatment for periodontitis has never really developed beyond research studies.

It was previously anticipated that the selective COX-2 inhibitors may offer promise as adjunctive treatments in the management of periodontitis. The enzyme cyclooxygenase, which converts arachidonic acid to prostaglandins, exists in two functionally distinct isoforms,

COX-1 and COX-2. COX-1 is constitutively expressed and has antithrombogenic and cytoprotective functions. Therefore, inhibition of COX-1 by nonselective NSAIDs causes side effects such as gastrointestinal ulceration and impaired hemostasis. COX-2 is induced after stimulation by various cytokines, growth factors, and LPS, and results in the production of elevated quantities of prostaglandins. Inhibition of COX-2 by selective COX-2 inhibitors results in reduction of inflammation. Researchers considered that the use of selective COX-2 inhibitors offered the prospect for reducing periodontal inflammation without the side effects typically observed after long-term (nonselective) NSAID therapy, and preliminary studies identified that selective COX-2 inhibitors slowed alveolar bone loss in animal models[4,29] and modified prostaglandin production in human periodontal tissues.[59] However, the selective COX-2 inhibitors were later identified to be associated with significant and life-threatening adverse effects, resulting in some drugs being withdrawn.

In summary, NSAIDs (including the selective cyclooxygenase-2 (COX-2) specific inhibitors) are presently not indicated as adjunctive HMTs in the treatment of periodontal disease.

Bisphosphonates

The bisphosphonates are bone-seeking agents that inhibit bone resorption by disrupting osteoclast activity. Their precise mechanism of action is unclear, but research has shown that bisphosphonates interfere with osteoblast metabolism and secretion of lysosomal enzymes.[63] More recent evidence has suggested that bisphosphonates also possess anticollagenase properties.[42] The ability of bisphosphonates to modulate osteoclast activity clearly may be useful in the treatment of periodontitis. Research is at an early stage, but in naturally occurring periodontitis in beagles, treatment with the bisphosphonate alendronate significantly increased bone density compared with placebo.[49] In animal models of experimentally induced periodontitis, bisphosphonates reduced alveolar bone resorption.[54,63] In human studies, these agents resulted in enhanced alveolar bone status and density.[12,50]

Some bisphosphonates have the unwanted effects of inhibiting bone calcification and inducing changes in white blood cell counts. Also, there have been recent reports of avascular necrosis of the jaws following bisphosphonate therapy, with the resultant risk of bone necrosis following dental extractions.[7] As with NSAIDs, at present there are no bisphosphonate drugs that are approved and indicated for treatment of periodontal disease.

Subantimicrobial-Dose Doxycycline

Subantimicrobial-dose doxycycline (SDD) is a 20-mg dose of doxycycline (Periostat) that is approved and indicated as an adjunct to SRP in the treatment of chronic periodontitis. It is taken twice daily for 3 months, up to a maximum of 9 months of continuous dosing. The 20-mg dose exerts its therapeutic effect by enzyme, cytokine, and osteoclast inhibition rather than by any antibiotic effect. Research studies have found no detectable antimicrobial effect on the oral flora or the bacterial flora in other regions of the body and have identified clinical benefit when used as an adjunct to SRP. At present, SDD is the only HMT specifically indicated for the treatment of chronic periodontitis that is approved by the U.S. Food and Drug Administration (FDA) and accepted by the American Dental Association (ADA) (see Chapter 52).

Locally Administered Agents

Nonsteroidal Antiinflammatory Drugs

Topical NSAIDs have shown benefit in the treatment of periodontitis. One study of 55 patients with chronic periodontitis who received topical ketorolac mouth rinse reported that gingival crevicular fluid levels of PGE_2 were reduced by approximately half over 6 months and that bone loss was halted.[33] In addition, locally administered ketoprofen has been investigated. To date, topically administered NSAIDs have not been approved as local HMTs for the management of periodontitis.

Enamel Matrix Proteins, Growth Factors, and Bone Morphogenetic Proteins

A number of local host modulation agents have been investigated for potential use as adjuncts to surgical procedures, not only to improve wound healing but also to stimulate regeneration of lost bone, periodontal ligament, and cementum, restoring the complete periodontal attachment apparatus. These have included enamel matrix proteins (Emdogain), bone morphogenetic proteins (BMP-2, BMP-7), growth factors (platelet-derived growth factor, insulin-like growth factor), and tetracyclines. The only local host modulation agent currently approved by the FDA for adjunctive use during surgery is Emdogain (see Chapter 67).

The remainder of this chapter focuses on the clinical utility of host modulation for nonsurgical procedures in clinical practice and the use of SDD (Periostat) in clinical practice.

HOST MODULATION AND COMPREHENSIVE PERIODONTAL MANAGEMENT

The term *periodontal management* suggests a much broader concept of periodontal care than the term *periodontal treatment*. Management includes history and examination (including special tests such as radiographs), assessment of risk factors, diagnosis, development of a treatment strategy, initial and definitive treatment planning, review of treatment outcomes and reevaluation, long-term supportive periodontal therapy (maintenance care), and assessment of prognosis. Controlling the bacteria that cause periodontal infections remains a central focus of effective periodontal treatment. Understanding the importance of the host response and the impact of risk factors now allows clinicians to provide different but complementary treatment strategies simultaneously for their patients.

If the decision is made to use an HMT, this must be discussed with the patient and the rationale for treatment thoroughly explained. This takes time at the chairside, but it is time well spent; patients become increasingly interested in their periodontal status and are more likely to develop ownership of their management,

SCIENCE TRANSFER

In the past, elimination of the microbial etiology was the focus and main tenet of periodontal therapy. Currently, however, many therapeutic approaches are focusing on how the host response can be manipulated in favor of controlling excessive inflammatory responses locally. Many aspects of the host response can be affected, including modification of proteolytic enzymes such as matrix metalloproteinases, stimulation of cellular activity, and alteration of the extracellular matrix; all these aspects can be considered as *host modulation.* It is likely in the future that more effective therapeutic approaches will include multiple, synergistic host modulation therapies combined with treatments that target the microbial etiology. This new awareness has resulted in the recognition of periodontal etiology as being a chronic microbial challenge in a susceptible host.

Host modulatory therapy (HMT) has been tested using various systemic and local agents, as follows:

- Subantimicrobial-dose (formerly low-dose) doxycycline (SDD) therapy extending at least 3 months has shown beneficial results when combined with nonsurgical root planing, with minimal adverse effects.
- Bisphosphonates provide only minor changes in periodontal parameters, and their long-term use has recently been questioned because of the increased risk of bone necrosis of large parts of the alveolus after tooth extractions.
- The use of systemic or topical nonsteroidal anti-inflammatory drugs (NSAIDs) has *not* had significant clinical application because of the small magnitude of improvement and the need for prolonged therapy, with the concomitant risk of adverse side effects.

thereby enhancing compliance with plaque control and treatment protocols. Compliance with an HMT is greatly facilitated if the rationale for prescribing is clearly explained. The need for compliance with the prescribed drug regimen is important because with SDD, for example, a tablet must be taken twice daily (once in the morning and once in the evening) and should not be taken with calcium supplements. It should be emphasized to the patient that the use of HMT is not a substitute for excellent plaque control (just as it is not a substitute for excellent root surface instrumentation by the treating clinician). To achieve the best results, patients must be interested and well informed about their condition so that compliance is maximized. Furthermore, they must also be convinced that comprehensive and frequent recall appointments are absolutely necessary in the maintenance phase of periodontal care.

In addition to patient motivation, oral hygiene instruction, and SRP to reduce the bacterial challenge, a key treatment strategy when managing periodontitis patients is *risk factor modification.* The harmful effects of smoking on the periodontal tissues are well documented,[34] and successful smoking cessation therapy will likely be of major benefit to patients with periodontitis. Smoking cessation counseling can be undertaken in the dental office (if staff are appropriately trained) or through collaboration with the patient's physician or specialized clinics. Given the evidence that smokers have worse periodontal disease than nonsmokers,[55,67] and that the magnitude and predictability of clinical improvements after treatment are significantly reduced in smokers,[1,46] smoking cessation counseling should form a major part of treatment for smokers with periodontitis. Patients with poorly controlled diabetes are also at increased risk for periodontitis,[40] and periodontal therapy may have an impact on diabetic control.[27] Collaboration with medical colleagues when treating diabetic patients with periodontitis is warranted to ascertain the degree of diabetic control.[16] Other possible risks for periodontitis include nonmodifiable factors such as genetics, gender, and race. As the relevance of different risk factors is established through epidemiologic research, clinicians must remain aware of their responsibilities for informing and changing patients' behaviors in relation to modifiable risks.

The management of patients with periodontitis can therefore involve the following complementary treatment strategies:

- Patient education and motivation, including oral hygiene instruction, use of antiseptic rinses, and explanation of the rationale for any adjunctive treatments.
- Reduction of the bacterial burden by high-quality SRP.
- Site-specific antibacterial treatment with local delivery systems.
- Host response modulation by HMT.
- Risk factor modification and risk reduction.
- Periodontal surgery.

It is the responsibility of the dentist to select and provide appropriate treatments on an individual basis, following discussion and informed decision making by the patient. Good communication and showing an interest in the patient's condition are essential to maximize compliance and modify risk factors. The best chance for clinical improvement may come from a combination of targeted treatment approaches for each patient (Figure 53-1).

SUBANTIMICROBIAL-DOSE DOXYCYCLINE

As previously discussed, SDD is currently the only FDA-approved, systemically administered HMT indicated specifically in the treatment of periodontitis. SDD is used as an adjunct to SRP and must not be used as a stand-alone therapy (monotherapy). Because SDD, previously called "low-dose doxycycline" (LDD) and currently marketed as Periostat, is based on subantimicrobial dosage of doxycycline, a member of the tetracycline family of compounds, the use of tetracyclines for the management of periodontal diseases must be put in perspective.

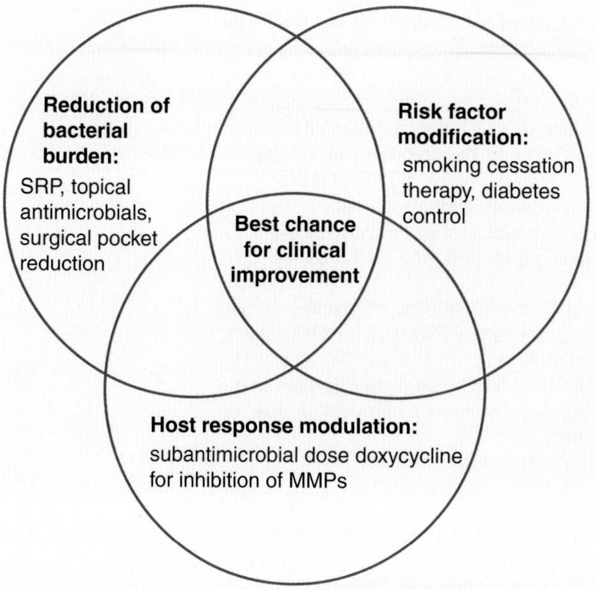

Figure 53-1 Complementary treatment strategies in periodontitis. The best chance for clinical improvement may come from implementing complementary treatment strategies that target different aspects of the periodontal balance. Reduction of the bacterial burden by scaling and root planing *(SRP)* is the cornerstone of treatment and can be augmented by the use of topical antimicrobials and surgical pocket therapy. In addition to this antibacterial treatment approach, the host response can be treated by the use of host modulatory therapy, such as subantimicrobial-dose doxycycline for the inhibition of matrix metalloproteinases *(MMPs)*. Risk factor assessment and modification must form a key part of any periodontal treatment strategy, including smoking cessation counseling. These different but complementary treatment strategies can be used together as part of a comprehensive management approach.

In regard to incorporation of a medical pharmacologic approach into the management of a disease in the dental practice setting, no class of drugs has made more of an impact on periodontal therapy than the tetracyclines. They have been used in conjunction with SRP, the "gold standard" of nonsurgical therapy, as well as with both resective and regenerative surgical procedures. The tetracyclines have been used locally and systemically as antimicrobial agents and, more recently, systemically as a host modulation agent (Periostat). The tetracyclines have been prescribed not only to address chronic periodontitis but also to manage specific and often more aggressive types of periodontitis. Most recently, the tetracyclines have been advocated for the management of patients with systemic diseases such as diabetes; doxycycline has led to improvements in both the periodontal health of compromised diabetic patients and long-term markers of glycemic control (e.g., glycated hemoglobin).[28] As an adjunct to mechanical therapies, the goal of tetracycline therapy has been to enhance reattachment or even to stimulate new attachment of the supporting apparatus and osseous formation.

This section concentrates on the use of these pleiotropic compounds for modulation of the host response in the treatment of periodontitis.

Mechanisms of Action

In addition to its antibiotic properties, doxycycline (as well as the other members of the tetracycline family) has the ability to downregulate *matrix metalloproteinases* (MMPs), a family of zinc-dependant enzymes that are capable of degrading extracellular matrix molecules, including collagen.[5,51] MMPs are secreted by the major cell types in the periodontal tissues (fibroblasts, keratinocytes, macrophages, PMNs, endothelial cells) and play a key role in periodontitis. Excessive quantities of MMPs are released in inflamed periodontal tissues, resulting in breakdown of the connective tissue matrix. The predominant MMPs in periodontitis, particularly MMP-8 and MMP-9, derive from polymorphonuclear leukocytes (PMNs)[22] and are extremely effective in degrading type I collagen, the most abundant collagen type in gingiva and periodontal ligament.[39] Levels of PMN-type MMPs have been shown to increase with severity of periodontal disease and decrease after therapy.[17,22] The release of large quantities of MMPs in the periodontium leads to significant anatomic disruption and breakdown of the connective tissues, contributing to the clinical signs of periodontitis.

The rationale for using SDD as an HMT in the treatment of periodontitis is that doxycycline downregulates the activity of MMPs by a variety of synergistic mechanisms, including reductions in cytokine levels, and stimulates osteoblastic activity and new bone formation by upregulating collagen production (Figure 53-2).

Clinical Research Data and Patient Populations

Tetracyclines work well as host modulation agents because of their pleiotropic effects on multiple components of the host response (see Figure 16-3). The only enzyme (MMP) inhibitors that have been tested for the treatment of periodontitis are members of the tetracycline family of compounds. In an early study using these different tetracyclines, Golub et al.[23] reported that the semisynthetic compounds (e.g., doxycycline) were more effective than tetracycline in reducing excessive collagenase activity in the gingival crevicular fluid (GCF) of chronic periodontitis patients. Because doxycycline was found to be a more effective inhibitor of collagenase than either minocycline or tetracycline,[6,18] and because of its safety profile, pharmacokinetic properties, and ready systemic absorption, recent clinical trials have focused on this compound. In an effort to eliminate the side effects of long-term tetracycline therapy, especially the emergence of tetracycline-resistant organisms, SDD capsules were prepared and tested.[22] Each capsule contained 20 mg of doxycycline, versus the commercially available 50 mg and 100 mg, antimicrobially effective, capsules. Multiple clinical studies using subantimicrobial doses of doxycycline have shown no difference in the composition or resistance level of the oral flora.[57,62] More recent studies also demonstrate no appreciable differences in either fecal

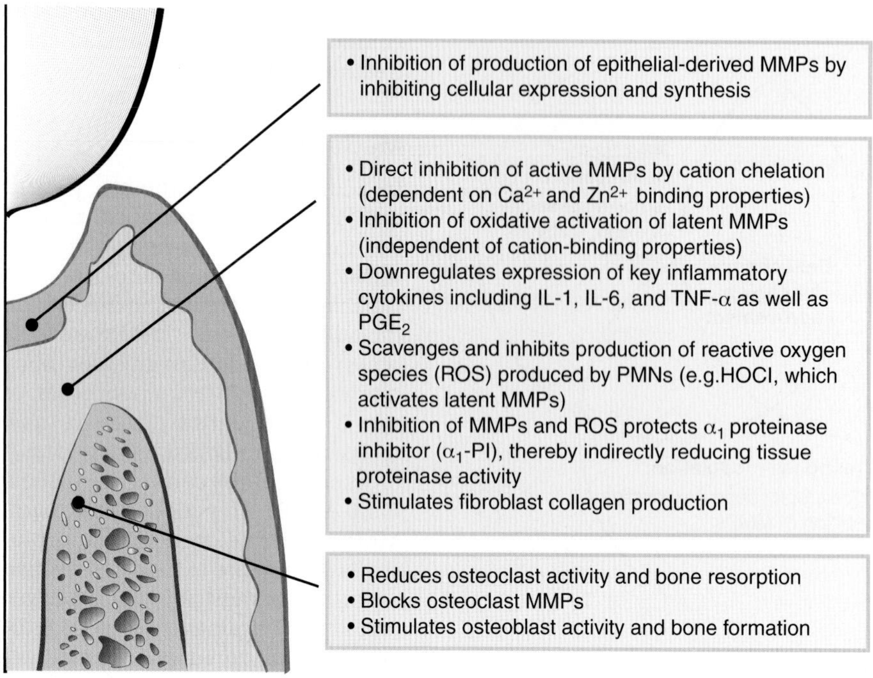

• Inhibition of production of epithelial-derived MMPs by inhibiting cellular expression and synthesis
• Direct inhibition of active MMPs by cation chelation (dependent on Ca^{2+} and Zn^{2+} binding properties)
• Inhibition of oxidative activation of latent MMPs (independent of cation-binding properties)
• Downregulates expression of key inflammatory cytokines including IL-1, IL-6, and TNF-α as well as PGE_2
• Scavenges and inhibits production of reactive oxygen species (ROS) produced by PMNs (e.g.HOCl, which activates latent MMPs)
• Inhibition of MMPs and ROS protects α_1 proteinase inhibitor (α_1-PI), thereby indirectly reducing tissue proteinase activity
• Stimulates fibroblast collagen production
• Reduces osteoclast activity and bone resorption
• Blocks osteoclast MMPs
• Stimulates osteoblast activity and bone formation

Figure 53-2 Schematic of periodontal pocket indicating the pleiotropic mechanisms by which doxycycline inhibits connective tissue breakdown. Downregulation of destructive events occurring in the periodontal tissues by doxycycline results from modulation of a variety of different proinflammatory pathways. (From Golub LM, Lee HM, Ryan ME, et al: *Adv Dent Res* 12:12, 1998.)

or vaginal microflora samples.[61] In addition, these studies have shown no overgrowth of opportunistic pathogens such as *Candida* in the oral cavity, gastrointestinal system, or genitourinary system.

With regard to MMP inhibition, Golub et al.[17] reported that a 2-week regimen of SDD reduced collagenase in GCF and in the adjacent gingival tissues surgically excised for therapeutic purposes. Subsequent studies using SDD therapy adjunctive to routine scaling and prophylaxis indicated continued reductions in the excessive levels of collagenase in the GCF after 1 month of treatment. After cessation of SDD administration, however, there was a rapid rebound of collagenase activity to placebo levels, suggesting that a 1-month treatment regimen with this host modulation agent was insufficient to produce a long-term benefit.[3] In contrast, during the same study, a 3-month regimen produced a prolonged drug effect without a rebound in collagenase levels to baseline during the no-treatment phase of the study. The mean levels of GCF collagenase were significantly reduced (47.3% from baseline levels) in the SDD group versus the placebo group, who received scaling and prophylaxis alone (29.1% reduction from baseline levels). Accompanying these reductions in collagenase levels were gains in the relative attachment levels in the SDD group.[3,21] Continuous drug therapy over several months appears to be necessary for maintaining collagenase levels near normal over prolonged periods. However, it is reasonable to speculate that levels of these MMPs will eventually increase again in the more susceptible patients, and those individuals having the most risk factors and the greatest microbial challenge will require more frequent HMT than other patients.

General Patient Populations

Data from clinical trials of SDD are summarized in Table 53-1. A series of double-blind, placebo-controlled studies of 3, 6, and 9 months' duration all showed clinical efficacy based on reductions in probing depth and gains in clinical attachment as well as biochemical efficacy, based on the inhibition of collagenase activity and protection of serum α_1-antitrypsin (a naturally occurring protective mediator) from collagenase attack in the periodontal pocket.[10,18,35] Golub et al.[19] showed that a 2-month regimen of SDD significantly decreased both the level of bone-type collagen breakdown products (ICTP; carboxy terminal peptide, a pyridinoline-containing cross-linked peptide of type I collagen) and MMP-8 and MMP-13 enzyme levels (neutrophil and bone-type collagenase) in chronic periodontitis subjects (Figure 53-3).

A 9-month, randomized, double-blind, placebo-controlled trial conducted at five dental centers demonstrated clinical efficacy and safety of SDD versus placebo as an adjunct to SRP. The benefits of HMT as an adjunct to mechanical therapy were again seen, with statistically significant reductions in probing depths and gains in clinical attachment levels as well as the prevention of disease progression.[8] When SDD administration was discontinued after 9 months of continuous therapy, the incremental improvements demonstrated in the SDD group were maintained for at least 3 months. There was no rebound effect in either the pocket depth reductions

TABLE 53-1

Summary of Data Reported in Clinical Trials of Subantimicrobial-Dose Doxycycline (SDD)

					MEAN CAL CHANGE (mm)		MEAN PD REDUCTION (mm)		% SITES WITH CAL GAIN†		% SITES WITH PD REDUCTION†	
Study (Year)	**Disease**	**Duration**	**Study groups**	***N***	**4-6 mm pockets**	**7+ mm pockets**	**4-6 mm pockets**	**7+ mm pockets**	**≥ 2 mm**	**≥ 3 mm**	**≥ 2 mm**	**≥ 3 mm**
Caton et al. (2000)[8]	Chronic periodontitis	9 months	SRP + SDD	90	1.03*	1.55*	0.95**	1.68**	46	22	47*	22*
			SRP + placebo	93	0.86	1.17	0.69	1.20	38	16	35	13
Golub et al. (2001)[21]	Chronic periodontitis	36 weeks	SRP + SDD‡	27	–0.15*							
			SRP + placebo	39	–0.80							
Novak et al. (2002)[43]	Severe generalized periodontitis	9 months	SRP + SDD	10	1.00	1.78	1.20	3.02	29	15	48	26**
			SRP + placebo	10	0.56	1.24	0.97	1.42	21	11	21	6
Preshaw et al. (2004)[48]	Chronic periodontitis	9 months	SRP + SDD	107	1.27**	2.09*	1.29**	2.31**	58*	33**	62**	37**
			SRP + placebo	102	0.94	1.60	0.96	1.77	44	20	45	21
Preshaw et al. (2005)[47]	Chronic periodontitis§	9 months	SRP + SDD#	66	1.29**	2.12*	1.33**	2.35**	63*	37**	66*	42**
			SRP + placebo#	76	1.01	1.55	1.00	1.75	45	20	47	22
			SRP + SDD##	41	1.19*	2.02	1.19	2.25	50	27	59*	28
			SRP + placebo##	26	0.85	1.88	0.93	1.89	42	20	39	18

*$p < 0.05$ compared with placebo.

**$p < 0.01$ compared with placebo.

†Percentage of sites with CAL gain and PD reduction ≥2 mm and ≥3 mm calculated for all sites that had 6+ mm probing depths at baseline.

‡SDD for two cycles of 12 weeks, with SRP at the beginning of each cycle, separated by a 12-week period of no drug.

§Same study population as Preshaw et al. (2004),[48] stratified by smoking status: # = non-smokers, ## = smokers

N, Number of subjects; *SRP,* scaling and root planing; *CAL,* clinical attachment level; CAL change can be positive (CAL gain) or negative (CAL loss); *PD,* probing depth.

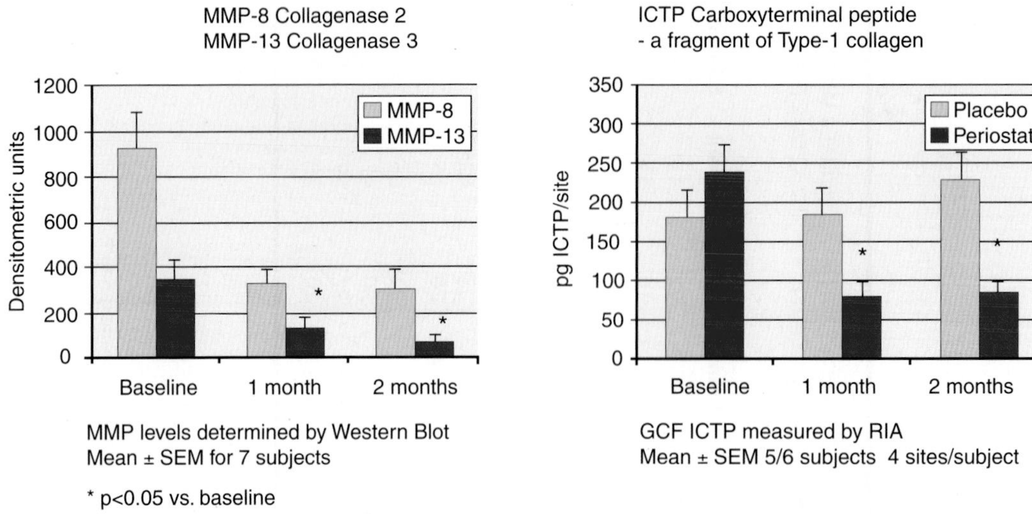

Figure 53-3 Effect of subantimicrobial-dose doxycycline (SDD) on gingival crevicular fluid *(GCF)* collagenase (MMP-8, MMP-13) and ICTP. A 2-month regimen of SDD significantly decreased levels of matrix metalloproteinases (MMP-8 and MMP-13, neutrophil and bone-type collagenases, respectively) and ICTP compared with placebo in GCF samples of adult periodontitis patients. Decreased levels of GCF bone-type collagen breakdown products (ICTP, pyridinoline-containing cross-linked peptide of type I collagen) in the SDD group versus the placebo group provides biochemical evidence of a reduction in bone resorption. *RIA,* Radioimmunoassay. (From Golub LM, Lee HM, Greenwald RA, et al: *Inflamm Res* 46:310, 1997.)

or the clinical attachment level gains; in fact, there appeared to be slight continued improvement in both these clinical parameters, presumably because of the enhanced clinical status of the patients who had benefited from adjunctive SDD, and possibly also because of the known persistence of doxycycline in the bone and soft tissue of the periodontium. The clinical relevance of such findings confirms the utility of an MMP inhibitor in the management of chronic periodontitis.

Special Patient Populations

More recent phase IV (i.e., post-licensing) clinical studies have revealed success using SDD in particular populations of susceptible individuals. Much interest has focused on genetic susceptibility to periodontal disease, and particularly whether a specific variation in the genes that regulate the cytokine interleukin-1 (IL-1) confers increased susceptibility to disease. This polymorphism is known as the *periodontitis-associated genotype* (PAG), the presence of which can be characterized using a commercially available screening test, the PST genetic susceptibility test. Investigation of patients who possess this gene polymorphism has been driven by the assumption that local phenotypic differences exist in chronic periodontitis associated with this genotype (e.g., that PAG-positive patients produce more IL-1 cytokines for a given bacterial challenge, resulting in increased tissue damage and more extensive periodontal disease). However, few studies exist of the impact of cytokine gene polymorphism on tissue IL-1 cytokine levels in periodontal disease to support this, although IL-1β levels in shallow periodontal pockets have been reported to be higher in patients with the genotype than those without.[14] The studies that have investigated associations between PAG and periodontal disease status have thus far generated conflicting data (as reviewed by Taylor et al.).[56] A reasonable assumption currently is that there are genetic associations between polymorphisms in the IL-1 gene cluster and periodontal disease, but that unambiguous results are not yet apparent because of the heterogeneity of the disease and/or the variable design of the reported studies. Cullinan et al. concluded that IL-1 genotype is a contributory, but nonessential, risk factor for periodontal disease progression.[11]

A 5-month preliminary investigation by Ryan et al.[52] was designed to evaluate the impact of treatment on IL-1 and MMP levels in PST-positive patients who presented with elevated levels of these biochemical markers in their GCF. These patients were initially treated with SRP, resulting in no change in the levels of these biochemical markers after 1 month. Al-Shammari et al.[2] reported similar findings, with no changes in GCF levels of IL-1β and ICTP before and after SRP in patients who had not been genotyped. When the genotype-positive patients received SDD and these biochemical markers were monitored at 2 and 4 months, a significant decrease (50%-61%) in the IL-1β and MMP-9 levels was noted after treatment with SDD. Correspondingly, gains in clinical attachment and reduced probing depths were also observed. The study concluded that a subantimicrobial dose of doxycycline may provide PST-positive patients with a therapeutic strategy that specifically addresses their exaggerated host response.

Another recent study was conducted in susceptible patients with severe generalized periodontitis using host modulation (SDD) as an adjunct to repeated subgingival debridement.[43] Seventy percent of the patients who completed this 9-month double-blind, placebo-controlled study were smokers. SDD as an adjunct to mechanical therapy versus mechanical therapy alone resulted in significantly greater mean probing depth reductions in pockets of 7 mm or greater at baseline as early as 1 month after therapy (2.52 mm vs. 1.25 mm, respectively). These improvements in the SDD group compared with the group receiving mechanical therapy only were maintained during the 5.25 months of therapy (2.85 mm vs. 1.48 mm, respectively) and even at 3 months after stopping drug therapy (3.02 mm vs. 1.41 mm), demonstrating that no rebound effect occurred. Because of the beneficial effects of HMT in susceptible patients, multicenter studies are using SDD in other susceptible populations, including diabetic, osteoporotic, and institutionalized patients, as well as smokers.

High-Risk Patients: Smokers. The harmful effects of cigarette smoking and the reduced response to periodontal treatment in smokers compared with nonsmokers are well established.[34] A recent meta-analysis of two randomized clinical trials of SDD used as an adjunct to SRP revealed a benefit when using SDD in smokers with periodontitis[47] (Table 53-1). A hierarchic treatment response was observed such that nonsmokers who received SDD demonstrated the best clinical improvements, and smokers who received placebo had the poorest treatment response. The responses of the smokers who received SDD and the nonsmokers who received placebo were intermediate to the two extremes and were broadly identical. This suggests that even patients traditionally considered resistant to periodontal treatment (i.e., smokers) can benefit from SDD, with a treatment response similar to that expected if treating a *nonsmoker by scaling and root planing alone.*

Suggested Uses and Other Considerations

Until relatively recently, treatment options for periodontal disease have focused solely on reducing the bacterial challenge by nonsurgical therapy, surgery, and systemic or local antimicrobial therapy. The development of SDD as an HMT, driven by research into the pathogenesis of periodontal disease, is a great example of how basic science research can lead to new treatments. By better understanding the biochemical processes that are important in periodontal disease, a pharmacologic principle (doxycycline downregulates MMP activity) has been used in the development of a new drug treatment. Data presented from research studies show the clinical benefits of adjunctive SDD, and the science behind SDD has been transferred into clinical practice. In other words, dentists now have the opportunity to use SDD for patient care, with the aim being to enhance the treatment response to conventional therapy.

Candidate Patients

When deciding whether to use SDD as an adjunct to SRP, first consider the patient's motivation toward periodontal care, the medical history, and the patient's willingness to take a systemic drug treatment. SDD is contraindicated in any patient with a history of allergy or hypersensitivity to tetracyclines. It should not be given to pregnant or lactating women or children less than 12 years old (because of the potential for discoloration of the developing dentition). Doxycycline may reduce the efficacy of oral contraceptives, and therefore alternative forms of birth control should be discussed, if necessary. There is a risk of increased sensitivity to sunlight (manifested by an exaggerated sunburn) seen with higher doses of doxycycline, although this has not been reported in the clinical trials using the subantimicrobial dose.

The rationale for using SDD must be clearly explained to the patient. By discussing the etiology of periodontal disease, the available treatment options, and the anticipated outcomes, patients become more interested in their periodontal management, are more likely to comply with treatment, and take more responsibility for managing their disease. Therefore the anticipated compliance and likely commitment to treatment must also be gauged when considering SDD therapy. Patients who show little enthusiasm for complying with the treatment plan or with oral hygiene practices are less likely to be good candidates for systemic drug therapy.

Treatable Periodontal Conditions

SDD is indicated in the management of chronic periodontitis, and studies to date have focused on chronic and aggressive forms of periodontitis.[8,13,43,48] SDD should not be used in conditions such as gingivitis and periodontal abscess or when an antibiotic is indicated. SDD can be used in patients with aggressive periodontitis who are being treated nonsurgically. Furthermore, emerging studies have supported efficacy of SDD as an adjunct to periodontal surgery.[15] SDD may also be of benefit in cases that are refractory to treatment, as well as in patients with risk factors such as smoking or diabetes, in whom the treatment response might be limited.

Side Effects

Doxycycline at antibiotic doses (≥100 mg) is associated with adverse effects, including photosensitivity, hypersensitivity reactions, nausea, vomiting, and esophageal irritation. In the clinical trials of SDD (20-mg dose), the drug was well tolerated, however, and the profile of unwanted effects was virtually identical in the SDD and placebo groups.[8,13,43,48] The types of adverse events did not differ significantly between treatment groups, and the typical side effects of the tetracycline class were not observed.[8,48] Furthermore, there was no evidence of adverse events that could be attributed to antimicrobial effects of treatment and no evidence of developing antibiotic resistance of the microflora.[8,57,58,62] Therefore the drug appears to be well tolerated, with a very low incidence of adverse effects.

Sequencing Prescription with Periodontal Treatment

Again, SDD is indicated as an adjunct to mechanical periodontal therapy and should not be used as a standalone therapy. SDD should be prescribed to coincide with the first episode of SRP and is prescribed for 3 months, up to a maximum of 9 months of continuous dosing. Modification of any risk factors, such as smoking, nutrition, stress, contributing medications, faulty restorations, poor oral hygiene, and poor diabetic control, can also be addressed at this time. A patient's refusal or inability to modify contributing risk factors is an important consideration for treatment planning and evaluation of therapeutic responses.

After initial periodontal treatment, the patient is enrolled into an intensive periodontal maintenance program. This involves regular monitoring of probing depths, reinforcement of oral hygiene, and remotivation of the patient, with further SRP to disrupt the plaque biofilm and remove re-forming calculus deposits. The 3-month prescription of SDD fits in well with the typical maintenance recall interval of 3 months, which in turn is based on the duration reported for recolonization of treated periodontal pockets.[37]

Thus, SDD therapy is commenced at the start of initial periodontal therapy and continues for 3 months until the first maintenance appointment. At maintenance appointments, the need for further prescription of SDD can be assessed. For patients demonstrating a good treatment response with significant reductions in probing depths, further SDD may not be necessary. Periodontal maintenance care must continue, with an emphasis on plaque control, monitoring, and prophylaxis. In other patients the treatment response after completion of initial therapy may be less favorable. Sites with persisting or progressing pockets may require additional instrumentation, and the prescription of SDD may be extended for an additional 3 months.

Figure 53-4 shows proposed treatment algorithms for incorporating SDD into periodontal practice, depending on the outcomes of treatment. Remember that periodontitis is a chronic disease, and the treatment (whether SDD is used or not) is long term. The patient must be regularly reevaluated to determine disease stability or progression.

Therefore, patients may cycle between phases of "active" treatment (SRP + SDD) and long-term periodontal maintenance. The success of the maintenance phase of treatment will be affected by many factors, including the following:

- Compliance with the maintenance regimen.
- Compliance with oral hygiene instruction.
- Presence of risk factors, such as smoking, poorly controlled diabetes, or stress.
- Extent (i.e., number) and severity (i.e., depth) of residual deep pockets.

Maintenance therapy is more likely to be successful in patients with good compliance, good oral hygiene, minimal or no systemic risk factors, and minimal residual deep pocketing. The patient who enters the maintenance program may have periodontal stability for months or years. However, plaque control may deteriorate, the patient may develop or acquire new risk factors, and disease progression (i.e., further loss of attachment) may become apparent, indicating that a further course of treatment is required. A further course of SRP will then be undertaken together with adjunctive SDD to restore periodontal stability.

Combining with Periodontal Surgery or Local Delivery Systems

Most clinical research to date has focused on using SDD as an adjunct to nonsurgical periodontal treatment. However, emerging data in which SDD was used as an adjunct to access flap surgery in 24 patients revealed better probing depth reductions in surgically treated sites greater than 6 mm compared with surgically treated sites in patients given placebo.[15] Furthermore, the SDD group demonstrated greater reductions in ICTP (carboxyterminal peptide, a breakdown product of collagen) than the placebo group, indicating that collagenolytic activity was reduced in the patients taking SDD.

SDD treatment can also be combined with the local delivery of antibiotics into the periodontal pocket through sustained-delivery systems. The two treatment approaches target different aspects of the pathogenic process: local delivery systems deliver antimicrobial concentrations of an antibacterial agent directly into the site of the pocket, whereas SDD is a systemic host response modulator. Thus, combining these two complementary treatment strategies is another example of how antibacterial therapy (SRP + local antibiotics) can be combined with HMT (SDD) to maximize the clinical benefit for patients. Preliminary results from a 6-month, 180-patient clinical trial designed to evaluate the safety and efficacy of SDD combined with a locally applied antimicrobial (Atridox) and SRP versus SRP alone demonstrated that patients receiving the combination of treatments experienced more than a 2-mm improvement in mean attachment gains and probing depth reductions ($p < 0.0001$) compared with SRP alone.

Monitoring Benefits of Therapy

To improve the ability of dentists to make appropriate treatment decisions for patients undergoing periodontal therapy, it would be extremely useful if they had access to the types of diagnostic tests available to their medical colleagues. Such tests might be used, for example, to distinguish between active and inactive lesions. Studies have shown that SRP alone, although effective for improving clinical parameters such as probing depths, may not be sufficient to reduce excessive levels of many underlying destructive mediators, particularly in more susceptible patients. It would be valuable, therefore, if it were possible to monitor the levels of such inflammatory mediators as treatment progresses. SDD results in downregulation of MMP activity in inflamed periodontal tissues.[17,19] Therefore, in theory, MMP levels could be monitored before, during, and after SRP plus SDD treatment. Published data support a concomitant reduction in MMP levels in GCF[9,13] and improvements in clinical parameters when combining SDD and SRP.[13] Although chairside tests for MMPs have been developed,[38] they are not in widespread use because of concerns about their specificity or sensitivity.

In the absence of new chairside tests or a centralized diagnostic facility for monitoring the inflammatory status of the tissues, dentists must rely on clinical periodontal monitoring to assess the outcomes of treatment. In addition to the reductions in probing depths and gains in attachment that may be observed after SRP plus SDD, the quality of the periodontal tissues also tends to improve after treatment with SDD. The tissues are pinker, firmer, and more resilient and appear less inflamed (Figure 53-5). In addition, with more sensitive radiographic techniques, assessments of bone density and bone height

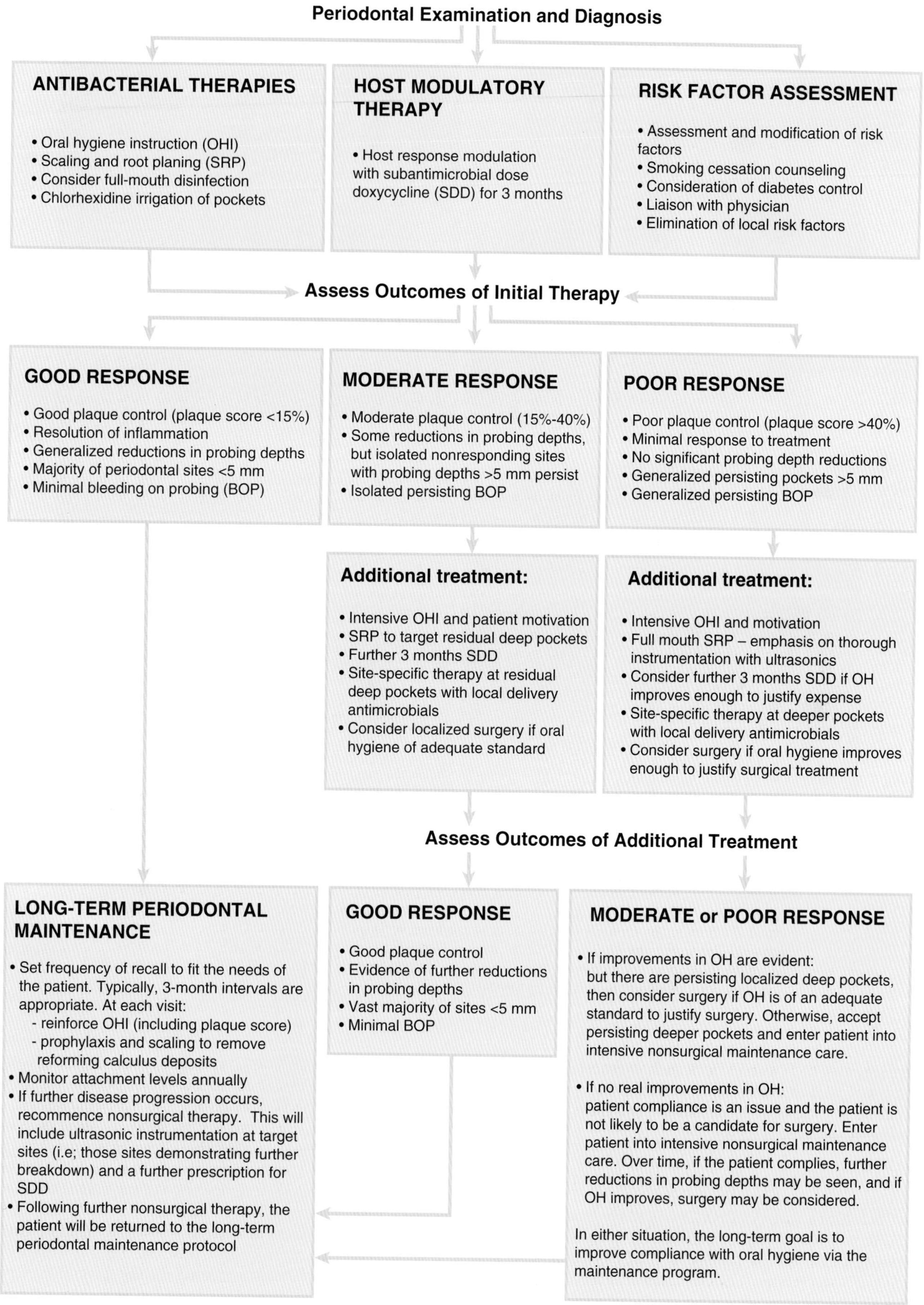

Periodontal Examination and Diagnosis
ANTIBACTERIAL THERAPIES
• Oral hygiene instruction (OHI)
• Scaling and root planing (SRP)
• Consider full-mouth disinfection
• Chlorhexidine irrigation of pockets
HOST MODULATORY THERAPY
• Host response modulation with subantimicrobial dose doxycycline (SDD) for 3 months
RISK FACTOR ASSESSMENT
• Assessment and modification of risk factors
• Smoking cessation counseling
• Consideration of diabetes control
• Liaison with physician
• Elimination of local risk factors
Assess Outcomes of Initial Therapy
GOOD RESPONSE
• Good plaque control (plaque score <15%)
• Resolution of inflammation
• Generalized reductions in probing depths
• Majority of periodontal sites <5 mm
• Minimal bleeding on probing (BOP)
MODERATE RESPONSE
• Moderate plaque control (15%-40%)
• Some reductions in probing depths, but isolated nonresponding sites with probing depths >5 mm persist
• Isolated persisting BOP
POOR RESPONSE
• Poor plaque control (plaque score >40%)
• Minimal response to treatment
• No significant probing depth reductions
• Generalized persisting pockets >5 mm
• Generalized persisting BOP
Additional treatment:
• Intensive OHI and patient motivation
• SRP to target residual deep pockets
• Further 3 months SDD
• Site-specific therapy at residual deep pockets with local delivery antimicrobials
• Consider localized surgery if oral hygiene of adequate standard
Additional treatment:
• Intensive OHI and motivation
• Full mouth SRP – emphasis on thorough instrumentation with ultrasonics
• Consider further 3 months SDD if OH improves enough to justify expense
• Site-specific therapy at deeper pockets with local delivery antimicrobials
• Consider surgery if oral hygiene improves enough to justify surgical treatment
Assess Outcomes of Additional Treatment
LONG-TERM PERIODONTAL MAINTENANCE
• Set frequency of recall to fit the needs of the patient. Typically, 3-month intervals are appropriate. At each visit:
- reinforce OHI (including plaque score)
- prophylaxis and scaling to remove reforming calculus deposits
• Monitor attachment levels annually
• If further disease progression occurs, recommence nonsurgical therapy. This will include ultrasonic instrumentation at target sites (i.e; those sites demonstrating further breakdown) and a further prescription for SDD
• Following further nonsurgical therapy, the patient will be returned to the long-term periodontal maintenance protocol
GOOD RESPONSE
• Good plaque control
• Evidence of further reductions in probing depths
• Vast majority of sites <5 mm
• Minimal BOP
MODERATE or POOR RESPONSE
• If improvements in OH are evident: but there are persisting localized deep pockets, then consider surgery if OH is of an adequate standard to justify surgery. Otherwise, accept persisting deeper pockets and enter patient into intensive nonsurgical maintenance care.
• If no real improvements in OH: patient compliance is an issue and the patient is not likely to be a candidate for surgery. Enter patient into intensive nonsurgical maintenance care. Over time, if the patient complies, further reductions in probing depths may be seen, and if OH improves, surgery may be considered.
In either situation, the long-term goal is to improve compliance with oral hygiene via the maintenance program.

Figure 53-4 Algorithm for incorporating host modulatory therapy with subantimicrobial-dose doxycycline into periodontal management protocols.

A B
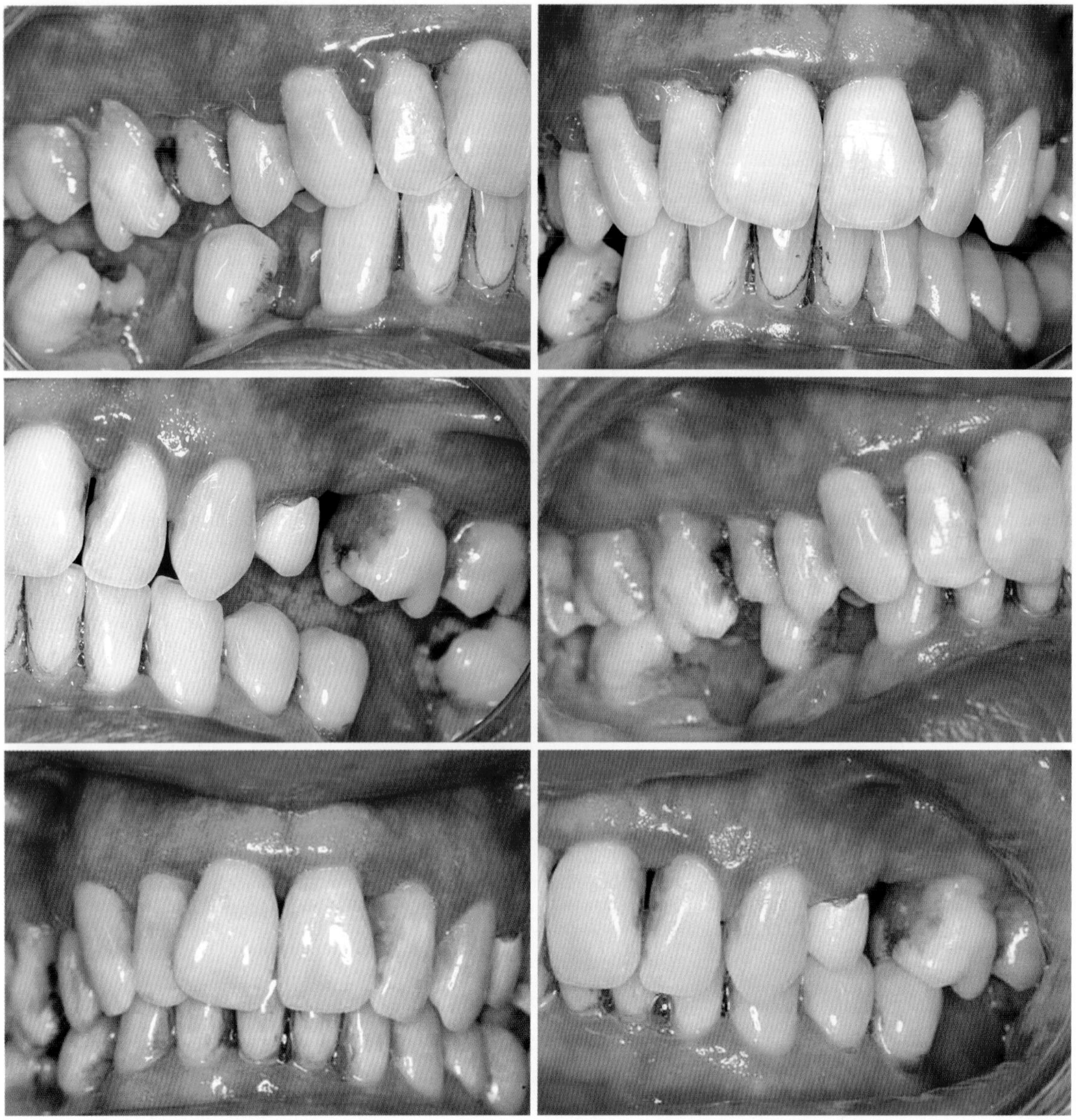
C D
E F

Figure 53-5 Patient treated by scaling and root planing (SRP) plus subantimicrobial-dose doxycycline (SDD). **A, B,** and **C,** Initial presentation of 35-year-old smoker (male) with chronic periodontitis manifested by generalized pocketing of 5 to 8 mm. **D, E,** and **F,** Same patient 3 months after full-mouth SRP and a 3-month course of SDD. Note the reduction of inflammation in the tissues, gingival shrinkage, and improved tissue quality. The patient continued to smoke throughout treatment.

changes may be possible. Until such diagnostic techniques are made widely available, however, clinicians must rely on clinical judgment to determine the most appropriate course of therapy.

EMERGING HOST MODULATORY THERAPIES

In the future a variety of HMTs will likely be developed as adjunctive treatments for periodontitis. One of the most promising groups of potential HMTs is the *chemically modified tetracyclines* (CMTs). These nonantibiotic tetracycline analogs are tetracycline molecules that have been modified to remove all antibiotic properties, but which retain host modulatory, anticollagenolytic effects. The CMTs are also designed to be more potent inhibitors of proinflammatory mediators and can increase levels of antiinflammatory mediators such as interleukin-10 (IL-10). This would enable the clinician to increase the dose for patients with more risk factors and who might be more difficult to manage. CMTs such as CMT-3 and CMT-8 (both of which lack antibiotic activity but retain anti-MMP activity) have been shown to inhibit osteoclastic bone resorption and promote bone formation,[53] enhance wound healing,[45] and inhibit proteinases produced by periodontal pathogens.[26] CMTs also are being studied for other effects, such as inhibition of tumor

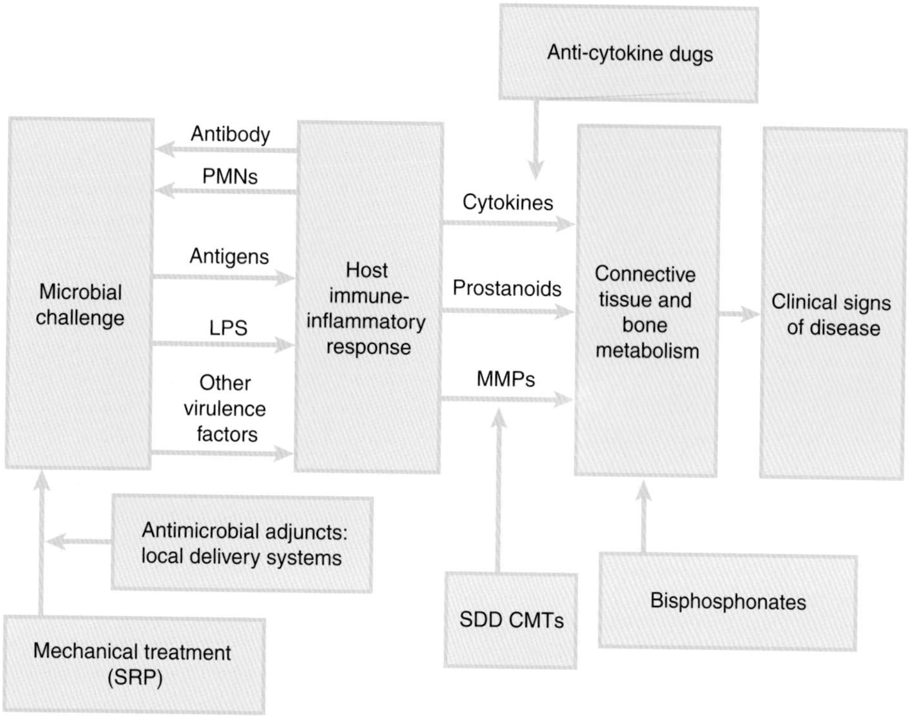

Figure 53-6 Host modulatory therapies (HMTs) as treatment for periodontitis. Schematic illustration of the pathogenesis of periodontitis, including targets and potential targets for adjunctive therapies. Scaling and root planing *(SRP)* is undertaken to disrupt the plaque biofilm physically, and local delivery of antimicrobial systems may be used to reduce further the bacterial challenge. Subantimicrobial-dose doxycycline *(SDD)* and chemically modified tetracyclines *(CMTs)* would inhibit the elevated production of matrix metalloproteinases *(MMPs)*. Anticytokine drugs could be used to target the elevated release of cytokines, such as interleukins and tumor necrosis factor-α, in the periodontal tissues. Bisphosphonates, which inhibit osteoclastic activity, could be used to reduce alveolar bone destruction. *Note:* As yet, only SDD is licensed and indicated as an HMT in the treatment of periodontitis.

cell invasion[36] and attenuation of intimal thickening after arterial injury.[32] CMTs will likely emerge as drugs that have beneficial effects in a variety of disease states because of their host modulation capabilities.

Other potential HMTs include the novel *anticytokine drugs* developed for the management of rheumatoid arthritis, a disease with a pathobiology similar to that of periodontitis.[41] Cytokines such as tumor necrosis factor-α (TNF-α) have been targeted by TNF-α antagonists (e.g., Infliximab, Etanercept), which have been shown to be effective in treating rheumatoid arthritis.[60] As yet, such drugs have not been evaluated in the treatment of periodontal disease, but they could offer potential benefits given the importance of inflammatory cytokines such as TNF-α in periodontal pathogenesis. In addition, drugs designed to increase the levels of antiinflammatory or protective mediators, such as IL-1 receptor antagonists, can perform similar functions.

Figure 53-6 presents the potential applications of existing and emerging HMTs for adjunctive treatment of periodontitis. In addition, evidence is emerging to support the benefits of combining HMTs that target different aspects of the disease processes. For example, the combination of SDD with bisphosphonates has also showed synergy in animal models of bone loss.

SUMMARY

The concept of *periodontal medicine* is emerging, in which the dentist treats not only the bacterial challenge (e.g., by SRP) but also the host side of the host-bacterial interactions. The use of HMTs such as SDD offers the opportunity to improve the treatment outcomes that can be anticipated following SRP alone. Patients must be encouraged and motivated so that they become an active participant in the management of their condition.

HMTs are an emerging treatment concept in the management of periodontitis. Subantimicrobial-dose doxycycline (SDD) is the only HMT currently approved and indicated as an adjunct to SRP for treating periodontitis. Clinical trials have demonstrated a clear treatment benefit when using SDD versus SRP alone. SDD should be used as part of a comprehensive treatment strategy that includes antibacterial treatments (SRP, plaque control, oral hygiene instruction, local antimicrobials, periodontal surgery), host response modulation (SDD), and assessment and management of periodontal risk factors. In the future a range of HMTs targeting different aspects of the destructive cascade of breakdown events in the periodontal tissues are likely to be developed as adjunctive treatments for periodontitis. The further development of these agents will permit dentists to treat specific aspects of the underlying biochemical basis for periodontal disease. The goal is to maximize the treatment response by reducing inflammation and inhibiting destructive processes in the tissues, which will result in enhanced periodontal stability after conventional periodontal treatments such as SRP. The dentist is now in the exciting position to be able to combine established treatment strategies with new systemic and local drug treatments for this common, chronic disease.

REFERENCES

1. Ah MK, Johnson GK, Kaldahl WB, et al: The effect of smoking on the response to periodontal therapy, *J Clin Periodontol* 21:91, 1994.
2. Al-Shammari KF, Giannobile WV, Aldredge WA, et al: Effect of non-surgical periodontal therapy on C-telopeptide pyridinoline cross-links (ICTP) and interleukin-1 levels, *J Periodontol* 72:1045, 2001.
3. Ashley RA: Clinical trials of a matrix metalloproteinase inhibitor in human periodontal disease. SDD Clinical Research Team, *Ann NY Acad Sci* 878:335, 1999.
4. Bezerra MM, de Lima V, Alencar VB, et al: Selective cyclooxygenase-2 inhibition prevents alveolar bone loss in experimental periodontitis in rats, *J Periodontol* 71:1009, 2000.
5. Birkedal-Hansen H: Role of matrix metalloproteinases in human periodontal diseases, *J Periodontol* 64:474, 1993.
6. Burns FR, Stack MS, Gray RD, Paterson CA: Inhibition of purified collagenase from alkali-burned rabbit corneas, *Invest Ophthalmol Vis Sci* 30:1569, 1989.
7. Carter G, Goss AN, Doecke C: Bisphosphonates and avascular necrosis of the jaw: a possible association, *Med J Aust* 182:8, 413.
8. Caton JG, Ciancio SG, Blieden TM, et al: Treatment with subantimicrobial dose doxycycline improves the efficacy of scaling and root planing in patients with adult periodontitis, *J Periodontol* 71:521, 2000.
9. Choi DH, Moon IS, Choi BK, et al: Effects of subantimicrobial dose doxycycline therapy on crevicular fluid MMP-8, and gingival tissue MMP-9, TIMP-1 and IL-6 levels in chronic periodontitis, *J Periodontal Res* 39:20, 2004.
10. Crout RJ, Lee HM, Schroeder K, et al: The "cyclic" regimen of low-dose doxycycline for adult periodontitis: a preliminary study, *J Periodontol* 67:506, 1996.
11. Cullinan MP, Westerman B, Hamlet SM, et al: A longitudinal study of interleukin-1 gene polymorphisms and periodontal disease in a general adult population, *J Clin Periodontol* 28:1137, 2001.
12. El-Shinnawi UM, El-Tantawy SI: The effect of alendronate sodium on alveolar bone loss in periodontitis (clinical trial), *J Int Acad Periodontol* 5:5, 2003.
13. Emingil G, Atilla G, Sorsa T, et al: The effect of adjunctive low-dose doxycycline therapy on clinical parameters and gingival crevicular fluid matrix metalloproteinase-8 levels in chronic periodontitis, *J Periodontol* 75:106, 2004.
14. Engebretson SP, Lamster IB, Herrera-Abreu M, et al: The influence of interleukin gene polymorphism on expression of interleukin-1beta and tumor necrosis factor-alpha in periodontal tissue and gingival crevicular fluid, *J Periodontol* 70:567, 1999.
15. Gapski R, Barr JL, Sarment DP, et al: Effect of systemic matrix metalloproteinase inhibition on periodontal wound repair: a proof of concept trial, *J Periodontol* 75:441, 2004.
16. Genco RJ: Current view of risk factors for periodontal diseases, *J Periodontol* 67:1041, 1996.
17. Golub LM, Ciancio S, Ramamurthy NS, et al: Low-dose doxycycline therapy: effect on gingival and crevicular fluid collagenase activity in humans, *J Periodontal Res* 25:321, 1990.
18. Golub LM, Evans RT, McNamara TF, et al: A non-antimicrobial tetracycline inhibits gingival matrix metalloproteinases and bone loss in *Porphyromonas gingivalis*–induced periodontitis in rats, *Ann NY Acad Sci* 732:96, 1994.
19. Golub LM, Lee HM, Greenwald RA, et al: A matrix metalloproteinase inhibitor reduces bone-type collagen degradation fragments and specific collagenases in gingival crevicular fluid during adult periodontitis, *Inflamm Res* 46:310, 1997.
20. Golub LM, Lee HM, Ryan ME, et al: Tetracyclines inhibit connective tissue breakdown by multiple non-antimicrobial actions, *Adv Dent Res* 12:12, 1998.
21. Golub LM, McNamara TF, Ryan ME, et al: Adjunctive treatment with subantimicrobial doses of doxycycline: effects on gingival fluid collagenase activity and attachment loss in adult periodontitis, *J Clin Periodontol* 28:146, 2001.
22. Golub LM, Sorsa T, Lee HM, et al: Doxycycline inhibits neutrophil (PMN)-type matrix metalloproteinases in human adult periodontitis gingiva, *J Clin Periodontol* 22:100, 1995.
23. Golub LM, Wolff M, Lee HM, et al: Further evidence that tetracyclines inhibit collagenase activity in human crevicular fluid and from other mammalian sources, *J Periodont Res* 20:12, 1985.
24. Goodson JM, Dewhirst FE, Brunetti A: Prostaglandin E_2 levels and human periodontal disease, *Prostaglandins* 6:81, 1974.
25. Goodwin JS, Webb DR: Regulation of the immune response by prostaglandins, *Clin Immunol Immunopathol* 15:106, 1980.
26. Grenier D, Plamondon P, Sorsa T, et al: Inhibition of proteolytic, serpinolytic, and progelatinase-b activation activities of periodontopathogens by doxycycline and the non-antimicrobial chemically modified tetracycline derivatives, *J Periodontol* 73:79, 2002.
27. Grossi SG, Genco RJ: Periodontal disease and diabetes mellitus: a two-way relationship, *Ann Periodontol* 3:51, 1998.
28. Grossi SG, Skrepcinski FB, DeCaro T, et al: Treatment of periodontal disease in diabetics reduces glycated hemoglobin, *J Periodontol* 68:713, 1997.
29. Holzhausen M, Rossa C Jr, Marcantonio E Jr, et al: Effect of selective cyclooxygenase-2 inhibition on the development of ligature-induced periodontitis in rats, *J Periodontol* 73:1030, 2002.
30. Howell TH, Williams RC: Non-steroidal anti-inflammatory drugs as inhibitors of periodontal disease progression, *Crit Rev Oral Biol Med* 4:177, 1993.
31. Howell TH, Jeffcoat MK, Goldhaber P, et al: Inhibition of alveolar bone loss in beagles with the NSAID naproxen, *J Periodontal Res* 26:498, 1991.
32. Islam MM, Franco CD, Courtman DW, Bendeck MP: A non-antibiotic chemically modified tetracycline (CMT-3) inhibits intimal thickening, *Am J Pathol* 163:1557, 2003.
33. Jeffcoat MK, Reddy MS, Haigh S, et al: A comparison of topical ketorolac, systemic flurbiprofen, and placebo for the inhibition of bone loss in adult periodontitis, *J Periodontol* 66:329, 1995.
34. Kinane DF, Chestnutt IG: Smoking and periodontal disease, *Crit Rev Oral Biol Med* 11:356, 2000.
35. Lee HM, Golub LM, Chan D, et al: α_1-Proteinase inhibitor in gingival crevicular fluid of humans with adult periodontitis: serpinolytic inhibition by doxycycline, *J Periodontal Res* 32:9, 1997.
36. Lokeshwar BL, Escatel E, Zhu B: Cytotoxic activity and inhibition of tumor cell invasion by derivatives of a chemically modified tetracycline CMT-3 (COL-3), *Curr Med Chem* 8:271, 2001.
37. Magnusson I, Lindhe J, Yoneyama T, Liljenberg B: Recolonization of a subgingival microbiota following scaling in deep pockets, *J Clin Periodontol* 11:193, 1984.

38. Mantyla P, Stenman M, Kinane DF, et al: Gingival crevicular fluid collagenase-2 (MMP-8) test stick for chair-side monitoring of periodontitis, *J Periodontal Res* 38:436, 2003.
39. Mariotti A: The extracellular matrix of the periodontium: dynamic and interactive tissues, *Periodontol 2000* 3:39, 1993.
40. Mealey B: Diabetes and periodontal diseases, *J Periodontol* 71:664, 2000.
41. Mercado FB, Marshall RI, Bartold PM: Inter-relationships between rheumatoid arthritis and periodontal disease: a review, *J Clin Periodontol* 30:761, 2003.
42. Nakaya H, Osawa G, Iwasaki N, et al: Effects of bisphosphonate on matrix metalloproteinase enzymes in human periodontal ligament cells, *J Periodontol* 71:1158, 2000.
43. Novak MJ, Johns LP, Miller RC, Bradshaw MH: Adjunctive benefits of subantimicrobial dose doxycycline in the management of severe, generalized, chronic periodontitis, *J Periodontol* 73:762, 2002.
44. Offenbacher S, Heasman PA, Collins JG: Modulation of host PGE2 secretion as a determinant of periodontal disease expression, *J Periodontol* 64:432, 1993.
45. Pirila E, Ramamurthy N, Maisi P, et al: Wound healing in ovariectomized rats: effects of chemically modified tetracycline (CMT-8) and estrogen on matrix metalloproteinases -8, -13 and type I collagen expression, *Curr Med Chem* 8:281, 2001.
46. Preber H, Bergstrom J: Effect of cigarette smoking on periodontal healing following surgical therapy, *J Clin Periodontol* 17:324, 1990.
47. Preshaw PM, Hefti AF, Bradshaw MH: Adjunctive subantimicrobial dose doxycycline in smokers and non-smokers with chronic periodontitis, *J Clin Periodontol* 32:610, 2005.
48. Preshaw PM, Hefti AF, Novak MJ, et al: Subantimicrobial dose doxycycline enhances the efficacy of scaling and root planing in chronic periodontitis: a multi-center trial, *J Periodontol* 75:1068, 2004.
49. Reddy MS, Weatherford TW, Smith CA, et al: Alendronate treatment of naturally-occurring periodontitis in beagle dogs, *J Periodontol* 66:211, 1995.
50. Rocha M, Nava LE, Vazquez de la Torre C, et al: Clinical and radiological improvement of periodontal disease in patients with type 2 diabetes mellitus treated with alendronate: a randomized, placebo-controlled trial, *J Periodontol* 72:204, 2001.
51. Ryan ME, Ramamurthy NS, Golub LM: Matrix metalloproteinases and their inhibition in periodontal treatment, *Curr Opin Periodontol* 3:85, 1996.
52. Ryan ME, Lee HM, Bookbinder MK, et al: Treatment of genetically susceptible patients with a subantimicrobial dose of doxycycline, *J Dent Res* 79:608, 2000 (abstract 3719).
53. Sasaki T, Ohyori N, Debari K, et al: Effects of chemically modified tetracycline, CMT-8, on bone loss and osteoclast structure and function in osteoporotic states, *Ann NY Acad Sci* 878:347, 1999.
54. Shoji K, Horiuchi H, Shinoda H: Inhibitory effects of a bisphosphonate (risedronate) on experimental periodontitis in rats, *J Periodont Res* 30:277, 1995.
55. Stoltenberg JL, Osborn JB, Pihlstrom BL, et al: Association between cigarette smoking, bacterial pathogens and periodontal status, *J Periodontol* 64:1225, 1993.
56. Taylor JJ, Preshaw PM, Donaldson PT, Cytokine gene polymorphism and immunoregulation in periodontal disease, *Periodontol 2000* 35:158, 2004.
57. Thomas J, Walker C, Bradshaw M: Long-term use of subantimicrobial dose doxycycline does not lead to changes in antimicrobial susceptibility, *J Periodontol* 71:1472, 2000.
58. Thomas JG, Metheny RJ, Karakiozis JM, et al: Long-term sub-antimicrobial doxycycline (Periostat) as adjunctive management in adult periodontitis: effects on subgingival bacterial population dynamics, *Adv Dent Res* 12:32, 1998.
59. Vardar S, Baylas H, Huseyinov A: Effects of selective cyclooxygenase-2 inhibition on gingival tissue levels of prostaglandin E_2 and prostaglandin F_{2a} and clinical parameters of chronic periodontitis, *J Periodontol* 74:57, 2003.
60. Vilcek J, Feldmann M: Historical review: cytokines as therapeutics and targets of therapeutics, *Trends Pharmacol Sci* 25:201, 2004.
61. Walker C, Preshaw PM, Novak J, et al: Long-term treatment with subantimicrobial dose doxycycline has no antibacterial effect on intestinal flora, *J Clin Periodontol* 32:1163, 2005.
62. Walker C, Thomas J, Nango S, et al: Long-term treatment with subantimicrobial dose doxycycline exerts no antibacterial effect on the subgingival microflora associated with adult periodontitis, *J Periodontol* 71:1465, 2000.
63. Weinreb M, Quartuccio H, Seedor JG, et al: Histomorphometrical analysis of the effects of the bisphosphonate alendronate on bone loss caused by experimental periodontitis in monkeys, *J Periodontal Res* 29:35, 1994.
64. Williams RC, Jeffcoat MK, Howell TH, et al: Indomethacin or flurbiprofen treatment of periodontitis in beagles: comparison of effect on bone loss, *J Periodontal Res* 22:403, 1987.
65. Williams RC, Jeffcoat MK, Howell TH, et al: Altering the progression of human alveolar bone loss with the nonsteroidal anti-inflammatory drug flurbiprofen, *J Periodontol* 60:485, 1989.
66. Williams RC, Jeffcoat MK, Howell TH, et al: Three year trial of flurbiprofen treatment in humans: post-treatment period, *J Dent Res* 70:468, 1991 (abstract 1617).
67. Wouters FR, Salonen LE, Frithiof L, Hellden LB: Significance of some variables on interproximal alveolar bone height based on cross-sectional epidemiological data, *J Clin Periodontol* 20:199, 1993.

Sonic and Ultrasonic Instrumentation

Carol A. Jahn

54

CHAPTER

CHAPTER OUTLINE

For many years, clinicians performed scaling and root planing with hand instruments such as curettes. This procedure proved technically demanding, time-consuming, and tiring. As a result, numerous power-driven scalers have been developed over the years. Until recently, their use was mostly limited to supragingival debridement because of their bulky working tips. However, technologic advances and new designs of ultrasonic and sonic scalers have now transformed the role of power-driven oscillating instruments in periodontal therapy. The availability of slender instruments with probelike tips allow efficient instrumentation of deep periodontal pockets with less operator fatigue.[11,13,58] Consequently, power-driven instrumentation has now become an accepted treatment modality for the removal of subgingival biofilm and calculus.

MECHANISM OF ACTION

Various physical factors play a role in the mechanism of action of power scalers. These factors include frequency, stroke, and water flow. In addition to rate of flow, the physiologic effects of water may play a role in the efficacy of power instrument.

Frequency

Frequency is defined as the number of times per second an insert tip moves back and forth during one cycle in an orbital, elliptic, or linear stroke path. For example, a frequency of 25,000 (25K) equates to the tip moving 25,000 times per second, and a 30,000 (30K) frequency equates to the tip moving 30,000 times per second. Frequency is important because it determines the area of the insert tip that is considered active. Only the active portion of the insert can remove hard and soft debris. A higher frequency results in a smaller active area of an insert tip. An insert working in the frequency of 30K would have an active tip area of 4.2 mm, and a 25K tip has a working area of 4.3 mm. The working area of a sonic scaler tip has not been determined.

SCIENCE TRANSFER

Techniques to reduce the microbial challenge to the host have improved over the years with the advent of powered instrumentation. As sophistication of these power-driven instruments has increased, their applicability has broadened. As such, powered instrumentation is used in virtually all aspects of clinical therapy and in supragingival and subgingival areas, including furcation areas. Speed and reduction in operator fatigue are prominent advantages. In any periodontal case, however, the essence of the therapy is to reduce the microbial challenge to the host, and optional future therapeutic approaches will likely include host modulation for high-risk, periodontally susceptible patients.

Power scalers can be either sonic or ultrasonic. Sonic scalers are air driven in a handpiece at a frequency of 2000 to 6500 cycles per second (cps). Ultrasonic scalers are powered by piezoelectric effect or magnetostriction and have a frequency of 18,000 to 50,000 cps. Power scalers have been shown to be as effective as hand instruments. Also, although they produce a slightly rougher surface, power scalers require less time and are effective in difficult-to-reach areas such as narrow furcations. *These power instruments are mainly used in nonsurgical therapy, but they also are valuable during surgery to remove residual calculus and granulation tissue and to provide instrumentation in areas with difficult access.*

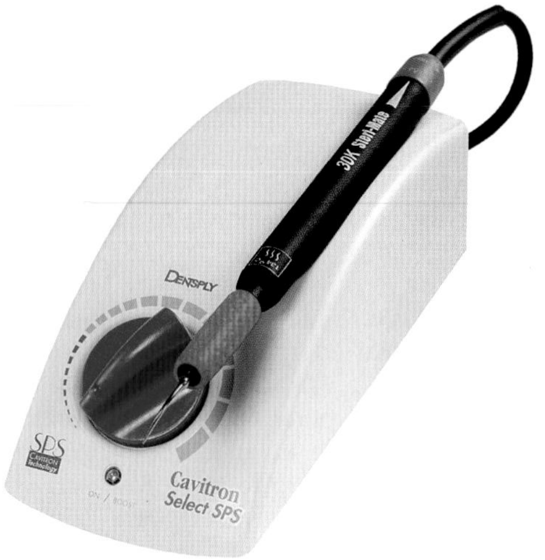

Figure 54-1 Magnetostrictive ultrasonic device with tuning knob for power and water.

Stroke

Stroke is the maximum distance the insert tip travels during one cycle or stoke path. *Amplitude* is equal to one-half the distance of the stroke. The power knob on an ultrasonic unit controls the stroke length of the insert during one cycle. Increasing the power knob increases the distance the tip travels while the frequency remains constant. High power settings produce a longer stroke pattern, and lower power settings provide a shorter stroke pattern.

Water Flow

Ultrasonic scalers may be designed as manually or automatically tuned devices (Figure 54-1). Both types of technology contain a water knob; this controls the volume of water being delivered to the insert tip. Manual-tuned units have three control knobs on the front panel labeled *water, tuning,* and *power.* Manual technology allows the clinician to control the frequency of the unit by adjusting the tuning knob. Auto-tuned units have two control knobs, water and power, and maintain a stable frequency. These units work through feedback that constantly adjusts the insert to ensure it is vibrating at the predetermined frequency level.

Water contributes to three physiologic effects that enhance the efficacy of power scalers: acoustic streaming, acoustic turbulence, and cavitation. *Acoustic streaming* is the unidirectional fluid flow caused by ultrasound waves. *Acoustic turbulence* is created when the movement of the tip causes the coolant to accelerate, producing an intensified swirling effect. This turbulence continues until cavitation occurs. *Cavitation* is the formation of bubbles in water caused by the high turbulence. The bubbles implode and produce shock waves in the liquid, creating further shock waves throughout the water. In vitro, the combination of acoustic streaming, acoustic turbulence, and cavitation has been shown to disrupt microflora.[26,59-61]

TYPES OF POWER INSTRUMENTS

Power scalers fall into two categories: sonic and ultrasonic. *Sonic* units attach to a dental unit because they need compressed air; they work at a frequency of 2000 to 6500 cycles per second (cps). *Ultrasonic* devices are generally freestanding units with an electric generator. The two main types of ultrasonic devices are magnetostrictive and piezoelectric; both work in a frequency range of 18,000 to 50,000 cps.

Sonic Scalers

Sonic scalers are air-driven scalers in which frequency produces a vibration of the insert tip. They use a high-speed or low-speed air source from the dental unit. Water is delivered through the same tubing used to deliver water to a dental handpiece. Sonic scaler tips are large in diameter and universal in design. The stroke pattern in which a sonic scaler tip travels is elliptic to orbital in shape. This stroke pattern allows the instrument to be adapted to all tooth surfaces.

Ultrasonic Scalers

Piezoelectric. Ceramic discs located in the handpiece power piezoelectric technology. They change in dimension as electrical energy is applied to the tip. Piezoelectric tips move in a linear pattern, giving the tip two active surfaces. A variety of insert tip designs and shapes are available for use. Using a wrench to screw the tip into the handpiece changes tips.

Magnetostrictive. Metal stacks that changes dimension when electrical energy is applied power magnetostrictive technology. Vibrations travel from the metal stack to a connecting body, causing the vibration of the working tip. Tips move in an elliptic or orbital stroke pattern; this allows the tip to have four active working surfaces. Magnetostrictive inserts are seated into a handpiece.

EFFICACY AND CLINICAL OUTCOMES

Numerous clinical outcomes have been evaluated from the use of power-driven instruments. A systematic review of the literature on the efficacy of machine-driven and manual subgingival debridement in the treatment of chronic periodontitis found no difference in the efficacy of subgingival debridement using ultrasonic/sonic scalers versus hand instruments in the treatment of single-rooted teeth. A benefit for multirooted teeth could not be determined because of a lack of clinical data.[58] Likewise, a review by the American Academy of Periodontology found no differences in outcomes among sonic, magnetostrictive, and piezoelectric scalers.[14] Also, the use of power-driven or hand instruments resulted in similar reductions in probing depth and bleeding on probing compared with hand instrumentation.

Plaque and Calculus

Traditionally, power-driven instruments were employed to remove heavy subgingival calculus. With the advent of new designs and thinner tips, both deplaquing of root surfaces and subgingival scaling may be effectively accomplished by power-driven instruments.* Clifford et al.[11] found that both traditional ultrasonic and microultrasonic inserts were effective in disrupting the apical plaque border. Although not significant, a trend was shown for the microultrasonic tip to disrupt the apical plaque border better in pockets greater than 7 mm. Likewise, Gagnot et al.[16] found that ultrasonic mini-inserts were more effective in the apical plaque zone than curettes. Garnick and Dent[17] showed that both hand and ultrasonic instrumentation removed plaque equally well.

Thorough calculus removal is integral to effective scaling and root planing. Fortunately, a glassy-smooth root surface is no longer necessary, and it now appears that some root roughness may even be tolerable. Both sonic and ultrasonic instruments have been shown to be effective in removing calculus similar to hand instrumentation.* Busslinger et al.[8] found that hand and ultrasonic instrumentation with either a magnetostrictive or a piezoelectric insert were equally effective in calculus removal. Similarly, Patterson et al.[39] found sonic and ultrasonic scalers removed similar amounts of calculus. Whether power-driven instruments remove more calculus than hand instruments has not been confirmed. Studies have shown that neither type of instrumentation is capable of removing all calculus.† Some studies indicate that hand instruments produce a smoother root surface.[17,46,62] Whether smoothness makes a difference in wound healing has not been determined, however, because clinical outcomes for scaling using either a hand or a power scaler are similar.[14,58]

Bacterial Reduction and Endotoxin/Cementum Removal

Thirty years ago, the periodontal community espoused the "nonspecific bacteria hypothesis" and believed that a glassy-smooth root surface was necessary to remove endotoxins. This paradigm is now reversed. Specific pathogenic bacteria have been identified as risk factors for periodontal disease, and gentle washing to remove endotoxins and preserve the cementum is the prevailing practice. The use of power-driven instruments with lavage action plays an important role in achieving these objectives.

It is well established that power-driven instruments remove biofilms, bacteria, and calculus through mechanical action. Ultrasonic instruments using high-speed action produce cavitational activity and acoustic microstreaming that may facilitate the disruption of the bacteria in subgingival biofilms. Some in vitro studies have shown that cavitational activity and acoustic microstreaming may enhance cleaning efficacy and increase plaque reduction.[26,59-62]

Two groups studied the antimicrobial activity of ultrasonic scaling on gram-negative pathogens in vitro. O'Leary et al.[37] found that up to 5 minutes of ultrasonic activation resulted in significant killing of *Actinobacillus actinomycetemcomitans* and *Porphyromonas gingivalis*. However, the investigators acknowledged that increased temperature caused by "sonication" may have contributed to the reduction. Conversely, Schenk et al.[46] found that neither sonic nor ultrasonic scaling was capable of killing *A. actinomycetemcomitans* or *P. gingivalis*.

In vivo studies have generally shown that hand, sonic, and ultrasonic scaling equally reduce bacteria.[4,7,38,42] One exception is Leon and Vogel,[30] who found that ultrasonic instrumentation in class II and class III furcations was more effective in reducing bacteria and keeping bacterial at a healthy level longer than hand instrumentation. Renvert et al.[42] demonstrated that neither root debridement with ultrasonic scaling nor osseous flap surgery eliminated *A. actinomycetemcomitans*. Oosterwaal et al.[38] studied subgingival plaque samples after scaling using ultrasonic or hand instruments and found that both

*References 1-4, 6-8, 11-13, 16, 17, 22, 25, 28, 29, 31-33, 36, 38, 39, 55, 56, 60, 62.

*References 7, 8, 13, 16, 22, 25, 28, -29, 31, 39, 40, 49, 50, 62.
†References 7, 16, 22, 31, 50, 62.

reduced subgingival microbiota to a level consistent with periodontal health.

Some researchers have used chlorhexidine for the coolant and lavage and found that it did not reduce subgingival pathogens better than water.[43,54] Similarly, Grossi et al.[19] compared water, chlorhexidine, and povidone-iodine and found all produced similar results (see Chapter 52).

Several in vitro studies investigated the removal of endotoxins from root surfaces with ultrasonic instruments.[9,10,35,51] Most found ultrasonic devices to be effective in reducing root surface endotoxin.[9,10,51] Smart et al.[51] and Chiew et al.[10] found that using light pressure with an ultrasonic instrument effectively removed endotoxin while conserving root structure. Checchi and Pelliccioni[9] compared ultrasonic and hand instrumentation and found both were capable of detoxifying the root surface. Conversely, Nishimine and O'Leary[35] found that hand instruments were more effective than an ultrasonic scaler in reducing root endotoxin.

Studies on which type of instrumentation leaves the smoothest root surface have reported mixed results.* Ritz et al.[44] measured tooth substance loss on mandibular incisors after 12 working strokes over an apicocoronal distance of 6 mm by an ultrasonic scaler, sonic scaler, hand instrument, and fine-grit diamond bur. Results showed that the ultrasonic scaler removed the least substance, 11.6 μm, versus 93.5 μm for the sonic scaler, 108.9 μm for hand instrumentation, and 118.7 μm for the diamond burr. Similarly, Jacobsen et al.[24] showed that both hand and sonic instrumentation produced large grooves, whereas an ultrasonic scaler did not; Jotikasthira et al.[25] also found that a sonic scaler left more roughness than an ultrasonic scaler. Conversely, Schlageter et al.[47] found that hand instruments produced a smoother surface than either sonic or ultrasonic instruments; Hunter et al.[22] reported similar findings. One investigator found no difference in root topography between hand and power scalers.[17] Whether root surface roughness has any relevant clinical implications is debatable; studies show that sonic, ultrasonic, and hand scalers produce similar reductions in clinical parameters.[14,58]

Bleeding on Probing, Probing Depth, and Clinical Attachment

The primary expected clinical outcomes from scaling and root planing are a reduction in bleeding and probing depth and a gain in clinical attachment. In comparing power scalers to hand instruments, both types demonstrate similar outcomes for reductions in bleeding on probing and probing depth and gains in clinical attachment.† Badersten et al.[2,3] found that both hand and ultrasonic instruments reduced bleeding and pocket depth in individuals with moderately advanced (4-7 mm) and severely advanced (up to 12 mm) periodontitis. Likewise, Boretti et al.[6] observed similar gains in clinical attachment with both hand and ultrasonic scaling. Sonic scalers also have been shown to be as effective as hand instruments; Kocher et al.[28] found that both types of instrumentation comparably reduced bleeding on probing and pocket depth. Similarly, in two separate studies, Loos et al.[32,33] found that both sonic and ultrasonic instruments were effective in reducing traditional clinical parameters of bleeding and probing depth[32] up to 2 years later.[33]

*References 17, 22, 24, 25, 31, 44, 47, 48, 62.
†References 2, 3, 6, 12, 27, 28, 32, 33, 36, 38, 49, 56.

Furcation Access

Furcations present one of the greatest challenges to scaling. In many cases the opening of the furcation is narrower than the access achievable by the conventional hand instrument. Therefore, power scalers have been recommended as a means to improve access when scaling furcations. Leon et al.[30] demonstrated that ultrasonic scalers were equal to hand scalers in reducing the bacteria in class I furcations but more effective in class II and III furcations. In two separate studies, Sugaya et al.[52,53] found that an ultrasonic tip specifically designed for furcations was more effective in debriding either class II furcations or furcations with a horizontal probing depth greater than 2 mm. Patterson et al.[39] found that both ultrasonic and sonic tips were similar in their ability to remove calculus in furcations. Diamond-coated sonic tips have also been shown to be effective in furcation debridement[1,27] but are generally recommended for open debridement.

EFFICIENCY

Sonic and ultrasonic instrumentation has the potential to make scaling and root planing less demanding, more time efficient, and more "ergonomically friendly." Modified tip designs allow for improved access in many areas, including furcations. These newer, slimmer designs operate effectively at lower power settings, thus improving patient comfort. Sonic and ultrasonic tips can reduce the time needed for scaling and root planing.

Tip Designs

In the past, ultrasonic tips had the reputation of being bulky, difficult to adapt, and most efficient for heavy supragingival calculus. Current tips are smaller and designed to be both site specific and job specific. There are tips to meet every need, from removing heavy supragingival calculus to definitive debridement of periodontal pockets. Large-diameter tips are created in a universal design and are indicated for the removal of large, tenacious deposits (Figure 54-2); a high power setting is generally recommended. Thinner-diameter tips may have a site-specific design. The straight-tip design is ideal for treating patients with gingivitis and for deplaquing maintenance patients (Figure 54-3). The right and left contra-angled instruments allow for greater access and adaptation to root morphology (Figures 54-4 and 54-5). These inserts are designed to work at a low power setting and may even be used for exploration. The amount of water delivered for lavage can be controlled through the selection of either traditional flow or focused, tip delivery

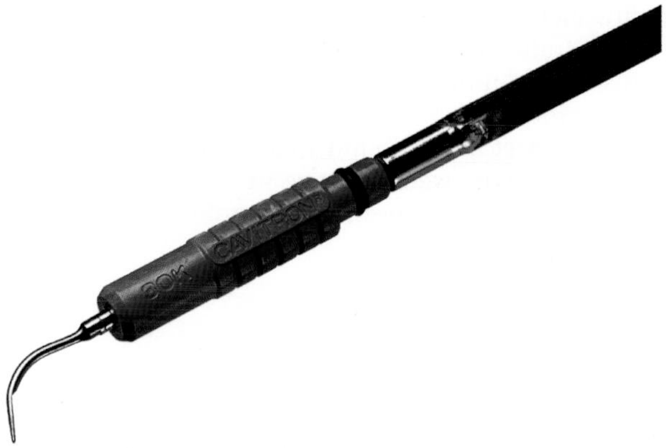

Figure 54-2 Ultrasonic insert with universal design.

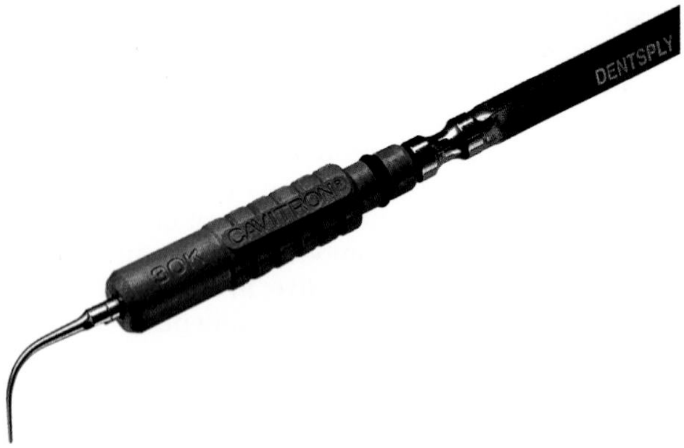

Figure 54-3 Microultrasonic insert with straight-tip design.

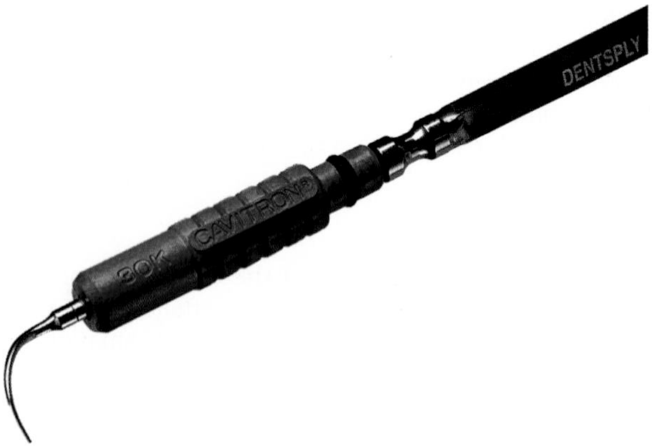

Figure 54-4 Microultrasonic insert with site-specific design (right contra-angle).

flow. Contra-angled designs and larger grips enhance comfort and ergonomics (Figure 54-6).

Studies have demonstrated that the new, thinner inserts are as clinically effective as hand instrumentation.[11,12,13,16] Some studies have found that these types of inserts provide greater apical access.[11,16] Tips specially designed for furcations may enhance debridement in

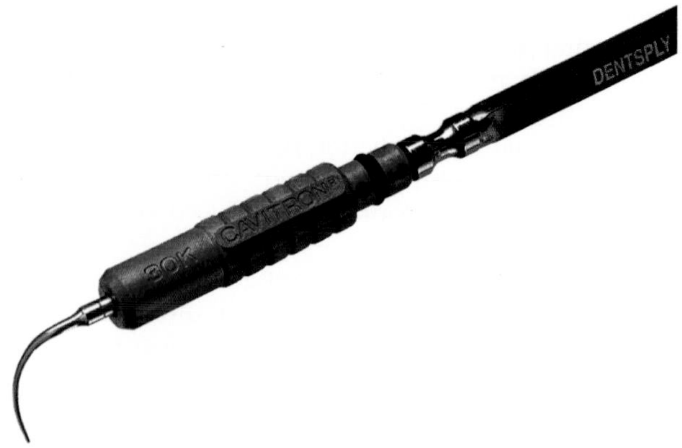

Figure 54-5 Microultrasonic insert with site-specific design (left contra-angle).

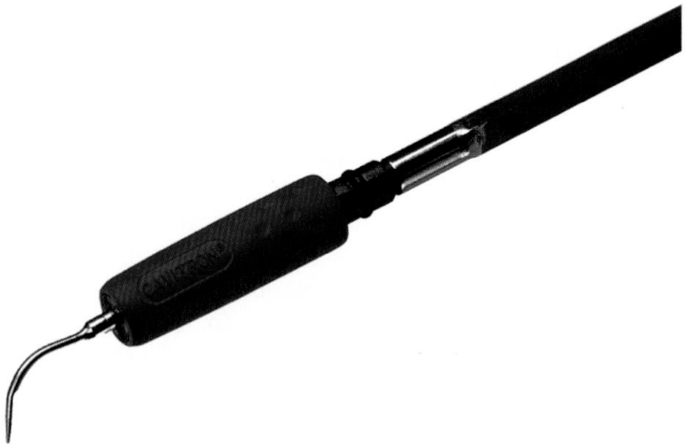

Figure 54-6 Ultrasonic insert with large, comfort grip.

class II and III furcations.[30,52,53] Diamond-coated tips have been shown to remove more calculus in moderate to deep pockets.[62]

Time

One of the advantages of using ultrasonic instruments is the potential to reduce the amount of time needed for scaling and root planing, a benefit for both the practitioner and the patient. Several researchers have found that sonic and ultrasonic scalers require less time than hand scaling.* Copulos et al.[12] found that instrumentation time per tooth with an ultrasonic scaler was 3.9 minutes versus 5.9 minutes for hand instruments. Kocher and Plagmann[27] found that a diamond-coated sonic scaler used to debride furcations during flap surgery reduced treatment time by 50% over hand instrumentation. Comparing sonic and ultrasonic scalers, Jotikasthira et al.[25] found that a sonic scaler required less time than an ultrasonic scaler, whereas Loos et al.[32] found the ultrasonic scaler to be faster.

*References 2, 3, 12, 13, 27, 29, 31, 56, 62.

SPECIAL CONSIDERATIONS

Speculation surrounds the potential hazards of using power scalers. Concerns include aerosol production contaminated with blood, neurologic disturbances of the hand caused by vibration, hearing loss, and interference with cardiac pacemakers.[57] Studies into neurologic and hearing damage from using power scalers are limited and not specific to sonic/ultrasonic use; therefore, no direct proof exists that the use of power scalers causes these conditions. Aerosol contamination is a hazard, and it is recommended that patients with infectious disease be treated only with hand scalers. Magnetostrictive scalers may pose some problems to patients with cardiac pacemakers, and their use should be avoided in this group of patients.

Aerosol Production

Barnes et al.[5] demonstrated that the aerosol produced by the in vivo use of an ultrasonic scaler on periodontally involved teeth was contaminated with blood and that the contamination occurred regardless of the level of inflammation. Gross et al.[18] compared sonic, magnetostrictive, and piezoelectric ultrasonic scalers and found no significant differences in the amount of aerosols generated. Similarly, Rivera-Hidalgo et al.[45] compared focused-spray and standard-spray ultrasonic inserts and found that each produced an equal amount of aerosol contamination. Studying the extent of this aerosol contamination, Huntley et al.[23] found a greater amount of aerosol contamination on the sleeves and chest of scrub jackets with sonic and ultrasonic scalers than with hand scalers.

Universal infection control procedures can help minimize the amount of aerosol produced. Harrel and Molinari[20] recommend three levels of defense in the reduction of dental aerosols: (1) personal protective barriers, such as a mask, gloves, and safety glasses; (2) routine use of a preprocedural antiseptic rinse; and (3) use of a high-speed evacuation device by a dental assistant or attached to the instrument being used. With all patients, clinicians should adhere to the Centers for Disease Control and Prevention (CDC) guidelines for infection control.

High-speed evacuation, aerosol reduction devices attached to the ultrasonic scaler, and antiseptic rinsing have all been shown to reduce aerosol contamination.[15,20,45] Harrel et al.[21] found that a high-speed evacuator significantly reduced aerosol contamination. Rivera-Hidalgo et al.[45] demonstrated a similar outcome with an aerosol reduction device that attaches to an ultrasonic handpiece. Fine et al.[15] showed that preprocedural rinsing with an antiseptic mouthwash can significantly reduce the number of viable bacteria in dental aerosol.

Cardiac Pacemakers

Newer models of cardiac pacemakers often have bipolar titanium insulation that shields the units from the effects of sonic-type devices.[41] However, Miller et al.[34] found atrial and ventricular pacing was inhibited by electromagnetic interference produced by a magnetostrictive ultrasonic scaler. A sonic scaler was also tested but did not produce the same effect.

PRINCIPLES OF INSTRUMENTATION

Ultrasonic technique is different from instrumentation with hand scalers. A modified pen grasp is used with an ultrasonic scaler, together with an extraoral fulcrum. The extraoral fulcrum allows the operator to maintain a light grasp and easier access physically and visually to the oral cavity. Alternate fulcrums using cross-arch or opposite-arch finger rests are acceptable alternatives.

Light pressure is needed with a power instrument. The tip is traveling at a set frequency in a set stroke pattern. Increased pressure by the clinician on the tip causes decreased clinical efficacy.

Sonic/ultrasonic instrumentation requires removal from the coronal to the apical portion of the deposit. This stroke pattern allows the insert to work at its optimal stroke pattern and frequency for quick, effective removal of deposits. A deplaquing stroke should be used when the focus is removal of biofilm and soft debris for the resolution of gingival inflammation. This stroke entails accessing every square millimeter of the tooth surface during ultrasonic deplaquing because of the limited lateral dispersion of the lavage subgingivally.

SUMMARY

Power scalers have emerged from being adjuncts for removing heavy supragingival calculus to a tool that may be used for all aspects of scaling: deplaquing, supragingival scaling, and subgingival scaling. The clinical outcomes achieved are similar to those for hand instrumentation. The advantages from using power instruments are greater access subgingivally and in furcation areas and increased efficiency in time needed for scaling. Power scalers may produce more aerosols than hand instruments, but appropriate universal precautions minimize the risk to the patient and clinician.

ACKNOWLEDGMENT

I thank Donna Radjenovich, RDH, with SunStar Butler for her editorial assistance with the manuscript.

REFERENCES

1. Auplish G, Needleman IG, Moles DR, Newman HN: Diamond-coated sonic tips are more efficient for open debridement of molar furcations: a comparative manikin study, *J Clin Periodontol* 27:302, 2000.
2. Badersten A, Nilveus R, Egelberg J: Effect of nonsurgical periodontal therapy. I. Moderately advanced periodontitis, *J Clin Periodontol* 8:57, 1981.
3. Badersten A, Nilveus R, Egelberg J: Effect of nonsurgical periodontal therapy. II. Severely advanced periodontitis, *J Clin Periodontol* 11:63, 1984.
4. Baehni P, Thilo B, Chapuis B, Pernet D: Effects of ultrasonic and sonic scalers on dental plaque microflora in vitro and in vivo, *J Clin Periodontol* 19:455, 1992.

5. Barnes JB, Harrel SK, Rivera-Hidalgo F: Blood contamination of the aerosols produced by an in vivo use of ultrasonic scalers, *J Periodontol* 69:434, 1998.
6. Boretti G, Zappa U, Graf H, Case D: Short-term effects of Phase I therapy on crevicular cell populations, *J Periodontol* 66:235, 1995.
7. Breininger DR, O'Leary TJ, Blumenshine RV: Comparative effectiveness of ultrasonic and hand scaling for the removal of subgingival calculus, *J Periodontol* 58:9, 1987.
8. Busslinger A, Lampe K, Beuchat M, Lehmann B: A comparative in vitro study of a magnetostrictive and a piezoelectric ultrasonic scaling instrument, *J Clin Periodontol* 28:642, 2001.
9. Checci L, Pelliccioni GA: Hand versus ultrasonic instrumentation in the removal of endotoxins from root surfaces in vitro, *J Periodontol* 59:398, 1988.
10. Chiew SY, Wilson M, Davies EH, Kieser JB: Assessment of ultrasonic debridement of calculus-associated periodontally involved root surfaces by the limulus ameobocyte lysate assay: an in vitro study, *J Clin Periodontol* 18:240, 1991.
11. Clifford LR, Needleman IG, Chan YK: Comparison of periodontal pocket penetration by conventional and microultrasonic inserts, *J Clin Periodontol* 26:124, 1996.
12. Copulos TA, Low SB, Walker CB et al: Comparative analysis between a modified ultrasonic tip and hand instruments on clinical parameters of periodontal disease, *J Periodontol* 64:694, 1993.
13. Dragoo M: A clinical evaluation of hand and ultrasonic instruments on subgingival debridement. I. With unmodified and modified ultrasonic inserts, *Int J Periodont Restor Dent* 12:311, 1992.
14. Drisko C: American Academy of Periodontology report: Sonic and ultrasonic scalers in periodontics, *J Periodontol* 71:1792, 2000.
15. Fine DH, Yip J, Furgang D, et al: Reducing bacteria in dental aerosols: preprocedural use of an antiseptic mouthrinse, *J Am Dent Assoc* 124:56, 1993.
16. Gagnot G, Mora F, Poblete MG, et al: Comparative study of manual and ultrasonic instrumentation of cementum surfaces: influence of lateral pressure, *Int J Periodont Restor Dent* 24:137, 2004.
17. Garnick JJ, Dent J: A scanning electron micrographical study of root surfaces and subgingival bacteria after hand and ultrasonic instrumentation, *J Periodontol* 60:441, 1989.
18. Gross KB, Overman PR, Cobb C, Brockmann S: Aerosol generation by two ultrasonic scalers and one sonic scaler: a comparative study, *J Dent Hyg* 66:314, 1992.
19. Grossi SG, Skrepcinski FB, DeCaro T, et al: Treatment of periodontal disease in diabetics reduces glycated hemoglobin, *J Periodontol* 68:713, 1997.
20. Harrel SK, Molinari J: Aerosols and splatter in dentistry: a brief review of the literature and infection control implications, *J Am Dent Assoc* 135:429, 2004.
21. Harrel SK, Barnes JB, Rivera-Hidalgo F: Reduction of aerosols produced by ultrasonic scalers, *J Periodontol* 67:28, 1996.
22. Hunter RK, O'Leary TJ, Kafrawy AH: The effectiveness of hand versus ultrasonic instrumentation in open flap root planing, *J Periodontol* 55:697, 1984.
23. Huntley DE, Campbell J: Bacterial contamination of scrub jackets during dental hygiene procedures, *J Dent Hyg* 72:19, 1998.
24. Jacobsen L, Blomlof J, Lindskog S: Root surface texture after different scaling modalities, *Scand J Dent Res* 102:156, 1994.
25. Jotikasthira NE, Lie T, Leknes KN: Comparative in vitro studies of sonic, ultrasonic, and reciprocating scaling instruments, *J Clin Periodontol* 19:560, 1992.
26. Khambay BS, Walmsley AD: Acoustic microstreaming: detection and measurement around ultrasonic scalers, *J Periodontol* 70:626, 1999.
27. Kocher T, Plagmann HC: Root debridement of molars with furcations involvement using diamond-coated sonic scaler inserts during flap surgery: a pilot study, *J Clin Periodontol* 26:525, 1999.
28. Kocher T, Konig J, Hansen P, Ruhling A: Subgingival polishing compared to scaling with steel curettes: a clinical pilot study, *J Clin Periodontol* 28:194, 2001.
29. Kocher T, Ruhling A, Momsen H, Plagmann HC: Effectiveness of subgingival instrumentation with power driven instruments in the hands of experienced and inexperienced operators: a study on manikins, *J Clin Periodontol* 24:498, 1997.
30. Leon LE, Vogel RI: A comparison of the effectiveness of hand scaling and ultrasonic debridement in furcations as evaluated by differential dark-field microscopy, *J Periodontol* 58:86, 1987.
31. Lie T, Leknes KN: Evaluation of the effect on root surfaces of air turbine scalers and ultrasonic instrumentation, *J Periodontol* 56:522, 1985.
32. Loos B, Kiger R, Egelberg J: An evaluation of basic periodontal therapy using sonic and ultrasonic scalers, *J Clin Periodontol* 14:29, 1987.
33. Loos B, Nylund K, Claffey N, Engelberg J: Clinical effects of root debridement in molar and non-molar teeth: a 2-year follow-up, *J Clin Periodontol* 16:498, 1989.
34. Miller CS, Leonelli FM, Latham E: Selective interference with pacemaker activity by electrical dental devices, *Oral Surg Oral Med Oral Pathol Oral Radiol Endod* 85:33, 1998.
35. Nishimine D, O'Leary T: Hand instrumentation versus ultrasonics in the removal of endotoxins from root surfaces, *J Periodontol* 50:345, 1979.
36. Obeid PR, D'Hoore W, Bercy P: Comparative clinical responses related to the use of various periodontal instrumentation, *J Clin Periodontol* 31:193, 2004.
37. O'Leary R, Sved AM, Davies EH, et al: The bactericidal effects of dental ultrasound on *Actinobacillus actinomycetemcomitans* and *Porphyromonas gingivalis, J Clin Periodontol* 24:432, 1997.
38. Oosterwaal PJ, Matee MI, Mikx FH, et al: The effect of subgingival debridement with hand and ultrasonic instruments on the subgingival microflora, *J Clin Periodontol* 14:528, 1987.
39. Patterson M, Eick JD, Eberhart AB, et al: The effectiveness of two sonic and two ultrasonic scaler tips in furcations, *J Periodontol* 60:325, 1989.
40. Petersilka GJ, Draenert M, Mehl A, et al: Safety and efficiency of novel sonic scaler tips in vitro, *J Clin Periodontol* 30:551, 2003.
41. Rees T: American Academy of Periodontology report: Periodontal management of patients with cardiovascular diseases, *J Periodontol* 73:954, 2002.
42. Renvert S, Wikstrom M, Dahlen G, et al: On the inability of root debridement and periodontal surgery to eliminate *Actinobacillus actinomycetemcomitans* from periodontal pockets, *J Clin Periodontol* 17:351, 1990.
43. Reynolds MA, Lavigne CK, Minah GE, Suzuki JB: Clinical effects of simultaneous ultrasonic scaling and subgingival irrigation with chlorhexidine: mediating influence of periodontal probing depth, *J Clin Periodontol* 19:595, 1992.
44. Ritz L, Hefti AF, Rateischak KH: An in vitro investigation on the loss of root substance in scaling with various instruments, *J Clin Peirodontol* 18:643, 1991.
45. Rivera-Hidalgo F, Barnes JB, Harrel SK: Aerosol and splatter production by focused spray and standard ultrasonic inserts, *J Periodontol* 70:473, 1999.
46. Schenk G, Flemmig TF, Lob S, et al: Lack of antimicrobial effect on periodontopathic bacteria by ultrasonic and sonic scalers in vitro, *J Clin Periodontol* 27:116, 2000.

47. Schlageter L, Rateitschak-Pluss EM, Schwarz JP: Root surface smoothness or roughness following open debridement: an in vivo study, *J Clin Periodontol* 23:460, 1996.
48. Schmidlin PR, Beuchat M, Busslinger A, et al: Tooth substance loss resulting from mechanical, sonic and ultrasonic root instrumentation assessed by liquid scintillation, *J Clin Periodontol* 28:1058, 2001.
49. Sculean A, Schwarz F, Berakdar M, et al: Non-surgical periodontal treatment with a new ultrasonic device (Vector ultrasonic system) or hand instruments: a prospective, controlled clinical study, *J Clin Periodontol* 31:428, 2004.
50. Sherman PR, Hutchens LH, Jewson LG, et al: The effectiveness of subgingival scaling and root planing. I. Clinical detection of residual calculus, *J Periodontol* 61:65, 1990.
51. Smart GJ, Wilson M, Davies EH, Kieser JB: The assessment of ultrasonic root surface debridement by determination of residual endotoxin levels, *J Clin Periodontol* 17:174, 1990.
52. Sugaya T, Kawanami M, Kato H: Accessibility of an ultrasonic furcation tip to furcation areas of mandibular first and second molars, *J Int Acad Periodontol* 4:132, 2002.
53. Sugaya T, Kawanami M, Kato H: Effects of debridement with an ultrasonic furcation tip in degree II furcation involvement of mandibular molars, *J Int Acad Periodontol* 4:138, 2002.
54. Taggart JA, Palmer RM, Wilson RF: A clinical and microbiological comparison of the effects of water and 0.02% chlorhexidine as coolants during ultrasonic scaling and root planing, *J Clin Periodontol* 17:32, 1990.
55. Thornton S, Garnick J: Comparison of ultrasonic to hand instruments in the removal of subgingival plaque, *J Periodontol* 53:35, 1982.
56. Torfason T, Kiger R, Selvig A, et al: Clinical improvement of gingival conditions following ultrasonic versus hand instrumentation of periodontal pockets, *J Clin Periodontol* 6:165, 1979.
57. Trenter SC, Walmsley AD: Ultrasonic dental scaler: associated hazards, *J Clin Periodontol* 30:95, 2003.
58. Tunkel J, Heinecke A, Flemmig TF: A systematic review of efficacy of machine-driven and manual subgingival debridement in the treatment of chronic periodontitis, *J Clin Periodontol* 29(suppl 3):72, 2002.
59. Walmsley AD, Laird WR, Williams AR: A model system to demonstrate the role of cavitational activity in ultrasonic scaling, *J Dent Res* 63:62, 1984.
60. Walmsley AD, Laird WR, Williams AR: Dental plaque removal by cavitational activity during ultrasonic scaling, *J Clin Periodontol* 15:539, 1988.
61. Walmsley AD, Walsh TF, Laird WR, Williams AR: Effects of cavitational activity on the root surface of teeth during ultrasonic scaling, *J Clin Periodontol* 17:306, 1990.
62. Yukna RA, Scott JB, Aichelmann-Reidy ME, et al: Clinical evaluation of the speed and effectiveness of subgingival calculus removal on single-rooted teeth with diamond-coated ultrasonic tips, *J Clin Periodontol* 68:436, 1997.

Supragingival and Subgingival Irrigation

Carol A. Jahn

55

CHAPTER

■ ■ ■

CHAPTER OUTLINE

PROFESSIONALLY DELIVERED IRRIGATION
 Efficacy
 Clinical Outcomes
HOME (SELF-APPLIED) IRRIGATION
 Mechanism of Action
 Safety
CLINICAL OUTCOMES

 Plaque Removal and Calculus Reduction
 Gingivitis, Bleeding on Probing, and Probing Depth
 Reductions
 Periodontal Pathogens and Inflammatory Mediators
 Patients with Special Considerations
SUMMARY

*I*n patients with periodontal diseases, irrigation has been used in two distinct ways. In the therapy phase, irrigation with an antimicrobial may be delivered in the office setting by a dental professional, generally as an adjunct to scaling and root planing. In the maintenance phase, daily home irrigation with water or an antimicrobial agent may be added to routine oral hygiene (brushing and flossing). The decision to incorporate these different treatment modalities is supported by separate and distinct bodies of evidence. The addition of chairside or professionally delivered irrigation to enhance the outcome of scaling and root planing has been shown to be limited.[28] Conversely, the body of evidence for home or self-applied irrigation demonstrates a clear ability to improve oral health.[19]

PROFESSIONALLY DELIVERED IRRIGATION

Irrigation at chairside with an antimicrobial agent gained favor with the understanding that mechanical debridement of deep pockets is often incomplete. It has been well documented that residual subgingival biofilm and calculus often remain in the pocket.[11,51] The rationale for adding irrigation with an antimicrobial agent at chairside after scaling and root planing is based on the assumption that bacteria left behind during mechanical debridement could be eradicated by an antimicrobial solution applied

into the pocket. Further, it was believed that if additional bacteria could be eliminated, a better outcome could be achieved.

Efficacy

Three factors play a role in the efficacy of professionally delivered irrigation: penetration, concentration, and duration. Initially, the agent must be able to penetrate to the base of the pocket in order to reach the periodontal infection. The agent used must be of a sufficient concentration to be bacteriostatic or bactericidal. Importantly, the agent must maintain this concentration for a sufficient duration to be effective against biofilm.[29]

To penetrate the pocket, professionally delivered irrigation is accomplished with a blunt cannula using a hand syringe or mechanized device placed 1 to 3 mm into the pocket.[30,39] (Figure 55-1). Penetration of the solution through this mechanism ranges from 70%[6] to 95%[30] of the depth of the pocket. Both side-port and end-port cannulas can achieve the same level of penetration; however, side-port cannulas have the lowest ejection site pressure[39] (Figure 55-2). The presence of calculus deposits may impair the subgingival penetration into deep pockets of 7 to 10 mm.[39]

Concentrations of agents that kill planktonic cells may not be effective on cells in a biofilm. The biofilm

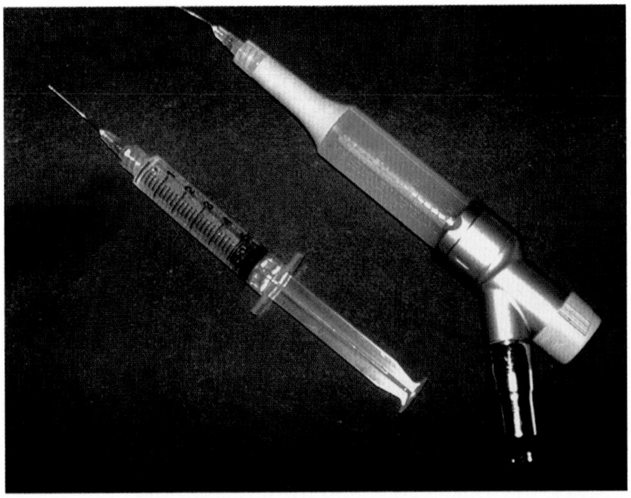

Figure 55-1 Devices for in-office irrigation using a cannula.

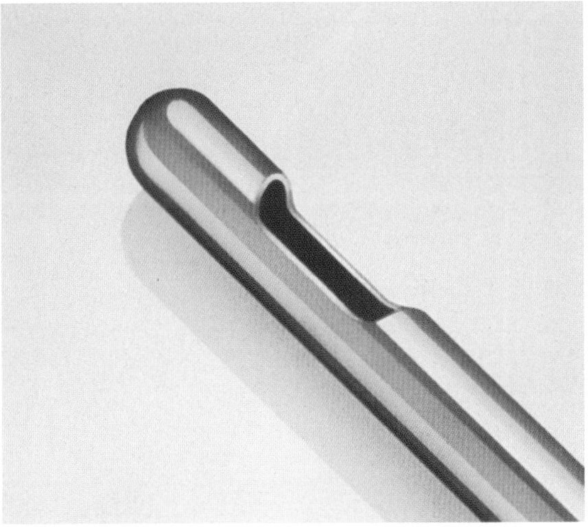

Figure 55-2 Cannula with side-port exit.

structure of subgingival plaque[56] may affect the activity of antimicrobial agents, potentially limiting the efficacy of agents. For example, when planktonic *Streptococcus sanguis* was exposed to either 0.2% chlorhexidine digluconate or 0.05% cetylpyridinium chloride, no viable bacteria were detected after an exposure time of 5 minutes. However, the same bacterium was shown to survive in biofilms even after exposure to chlorhexidine digluconate or cetylpyridinium chloride for 4 hours.[63] Additionally, it has been shown that 50 to 5000 times higher concentrations of antimicrobials are needed to kill bacteria that are embedded in a biofilm compared with planktonic bacteria.[36,45] Also, the effectiveness of chlorhexidine may be greatly reduced or even inactivated when in contact with blood components in the periodontal pocket.[48]

The duration of a solution irrigated into a pocket is affected by the flushing action of the gingival crevicular fluid (GCF). The greater outward flow of GCF causes solutions that are put into the periodontal pocket to be rapidly washed out.[27] Because of this phenomena, antimicrobial agents irrigated subgingivally may not be in contact with the subgingival microflora for a sufficient duration to be effective. The half-life of solutions delivered subgingivally has been shown to be approximately 13 minutes.[47] To compensate for this, other delivery vehicles that prolong duration have been developed (see Chapter 52).

Clinical Outcomes

There is little evidence that the addition of professionally delivered antimicrobial irrigation to scaling and root planing improves clinical outcomes over scaling and root planing alone. A variety of agents with a range of concentrations, including chlorhexidine, tetracycline, stannous fluoride, and povidone-iodine, have been used. In most cases, regardless of the agent used, either no or minimal improvements over scaling and root planing have been demonstrated.[28] For example, a study by Quinyren et al.[50] found that a process that included disinfecting multiple niches of the oral cavity with 0.2% chlorhexidine, including three chairside irrigation applications within 10 minutes, did not provide better results than scaling and root planing alone. However, they did find that those who received the chlorhexidine disinfection process had shorter healing times and reported less pain from the procedure.

HOME (SELF-APPLIED) IRRIGATION

A dentist and his patient, an engineer, developed the home oral irrigator in the 1960s. The new product was enthusiastically embraced by many dentists at its introduction and in the early years but fell out of favor when clinical trials indicated a limited ability to reduce plaque.* Interestingly, despite findings related to the plaque index, the body of evidence on home irrigation has consistently shown reductions in gingivitis, bleeding on probing, and periodontal pathogens, often significantly greater than that achieved by brushing and flossing alone.† These oral health improvements have been demonstrated with the use of water or an antimicrobial agent. Although this may seem paradoxic, emerging evidence indicates that home irrigation stimulates a *host modulation* effect, thus helping explain the previous incongruous findings.[1,17]

Mechanism of Action

The mechanism of action of irrigation occurs through the direct application of a pulsed or steady stream of water or other solution. Studies by Bhaskar et al.[4,5] and Selting et al.[55] have found pulsation and pressure to be critical components of an irrigation device. Pulsating devices are three times as effective as continuous-stream irrigating syringes.[55] Pulsation provides for a compression and decompression phase, which may account for expedient clearing of bacteria from the pocket.[4] A pulsating device

*References 7, 14, 18, 25, 26, 40, 43, 54, 60.

†References 1, 2, 7, 9, 10, 12, 15-17, 20, 23-26, 32, 33, 35, 38, 40, 43, 44, 49, 60, 64.

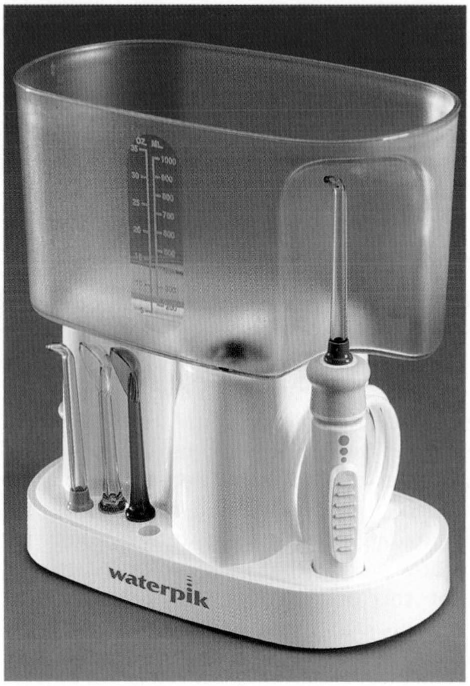

Figure 55-3 Oral irrigator (Waterpik Family Dental Water Jet) with 1200 pulsations per minute and pressure setting ranging from 20 to 90 pounds per square inch (psi).

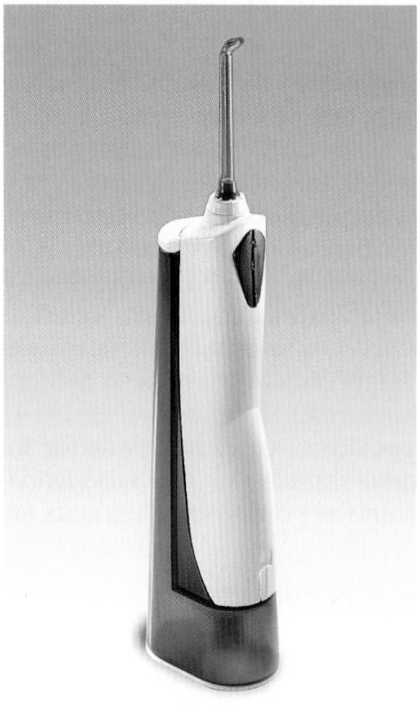

Figure 55-4 Portable oral irrigator (Waterpik Cordless Dental Water Jet) with 1200 pulsations per minute and pressure range from 40 to 60 psi.

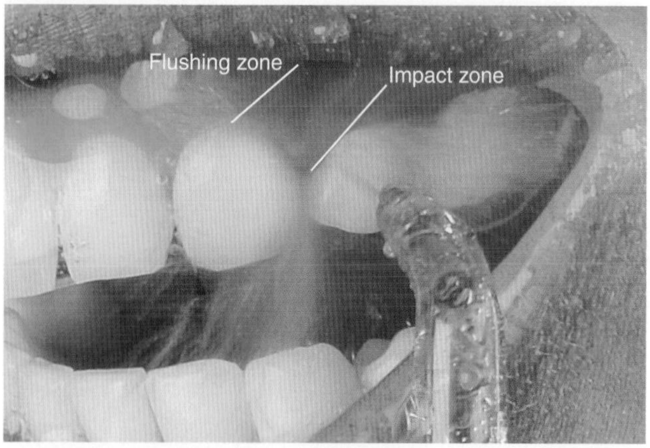

Figure 55-5 Pulsation creates two zones of hydrokinetic activity: the impact zone and the flushing zone.

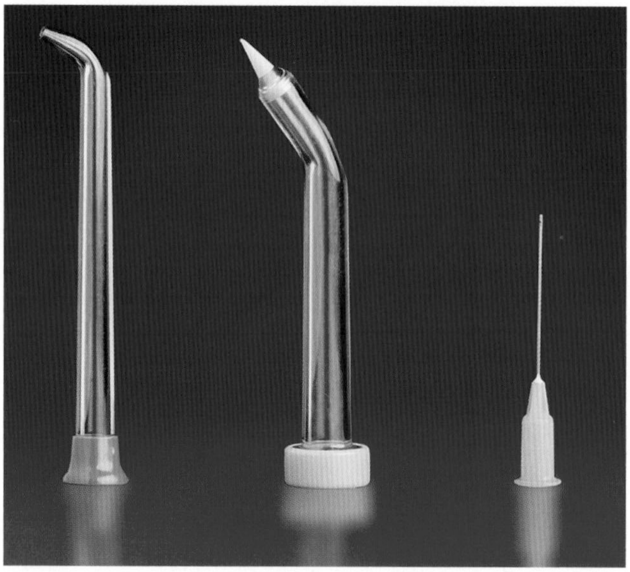

Figure 55-6 Three types of tips that will fit on an oral irrigator. *Left to right,* Standard jet tip, Pik Pocket subgingival irrigation tip, and cannula.

also allows for control of the pressure rate. The majority of studies on home irrigation showing clinical efficacy have been done using an oral irrigator with 1200 pulsations per minute set on a medium to high pressure setting (50-90 psi)[4,5,55] (Figures 55-3 and 55-4). Oral irrigators with varying pulsation and pressure are available, but as with other self-care products, research from one product brand should not extrapolated to other brands because they may have used settings at a different rate.

A pulsation rate of 1200 per minute has been shown to creates two zones of hydrokinetic activity.[16] The *impact zone* is where the solution initially contacts the area, and the *flushing zone* is where solution reaches into the subgingival sulcus (Figure 55-5). The outcome of hydrokinetic activity is subgingival penetration. Home irrigation has been demonstrated to penetrate subgingivally with both a standard jet tip and with a soft, site-specific, subgingival tip (Pik Pocket subgingival irrigation tip, Waterpik Technologies, Fort Collins, Colo)[8,21] (Figure 55-6). Other tips, including cannulas, have been promoted to enhance subgingival penetration, but none has documented evidence to substantiate the claim.

Irrigation with a standard jet tip is generally called *supragingival irrigation;* this refers to the placement of

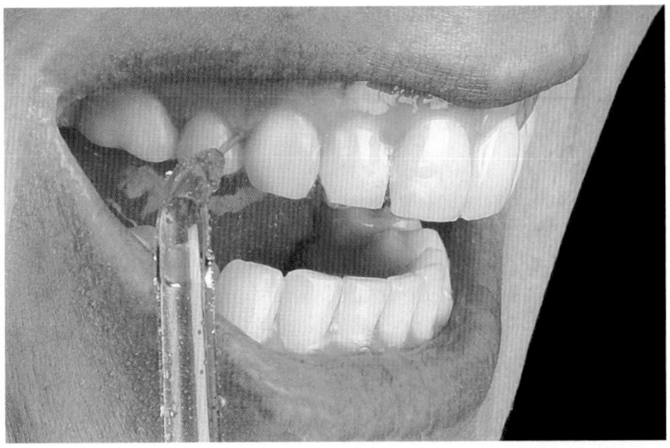

Figure 55-7 The jet tip is placed at a 90-degree angle.

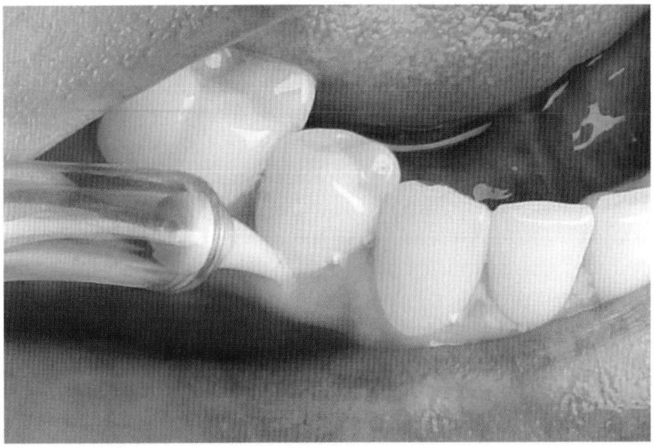

Figure 55-9 The Pik Pocket tip is gently placed slightly subgingivally.

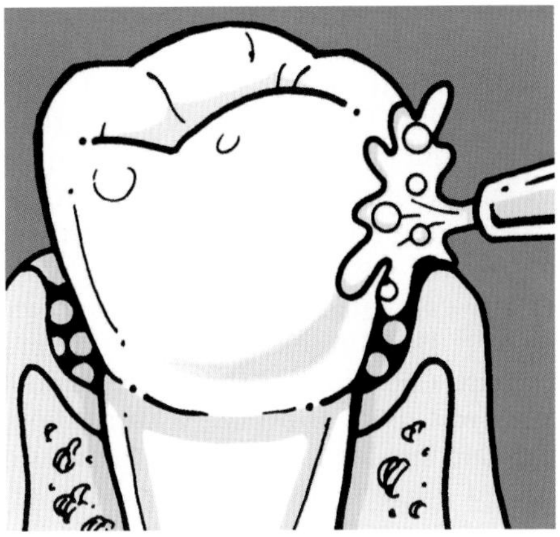

Figure 55-8 Irrigation with a standard jet tip will reach approximately 50% of the depth of the sulcus or pocket.

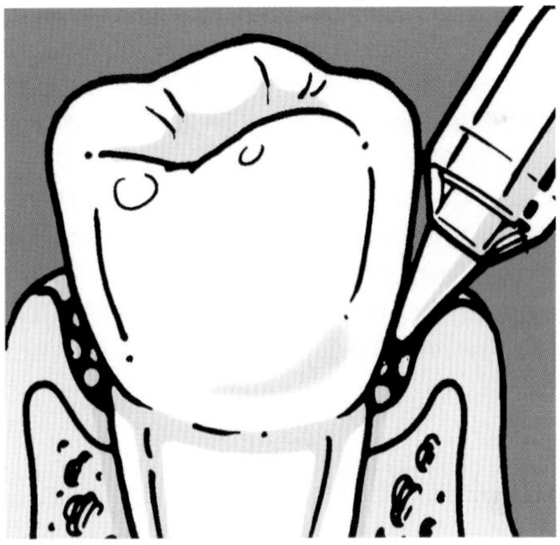

Figure 55-10 Irrigation with the Pik Pocket tip will reach up to 90% of the depth of a 6-mm pocket and 64% of the depth of a pocket 7 mm or greater.

the jet tip (Figure 55-7). The point of delivery of this tip is at or coronal to the gingival margin, resulting in penetration of a solution into the subgingival sulcus to approximately 50%[6,21] (Figure 55-8). The standard jet tip is generally used for full-mouth irrigation. Irrigation with the soft, site-specific tip is often called *subgingival irrigation;* this also refers to the placement of tip, which is placed slightly below the gingival margin (Figure 55-9). The subgingival tip is generally used for the localized irrigation of a specific site, such as a deep pocket, furcation, implant, or crown and bridge. Studies with this site-specific, subgingival tip show that it can deliver a solution into a pocket of 6 mm or less up to 90% of its depth.[8] In pockets greater than 6 mm, the depth of penetration has been shown to be 64%[8] (Figure 55-10).

Safety

Concerns have been expressed about the safety of oral irrigation with regard to soft tissue damage and penetration of bacteria into the pocket, but no scientific evidence exists to support these claims. Several investigators have evaluated the soft tissue and found no trauma or adverse reaction from using a pulsating oral irrigator.* In a study on the safety for soft tissue, researchers examined untreated, chronic periodontal pockets immediately after oral irrigation with a pulsating device at medium-high pressure. Examination of specimens under a scanning electron microscope showed no observable differences between the irrigated and nonirrigated specimens in regard to epithelial topography, cavitations, microulcerations, spatial relationships, and individual cell appearance.[16] This study concurs with early work by Krajewski et al.[37] who found less inflammation, better connective tissue organization, and an increased thickness in the keratin layer in individuals who irrigated twice daily compared with those who did not irrigate. Similarly, Cantor and Stahl[12] found less inflammation in the col area, but no change in keritinzation.

Various researchers have examined the issue of whether irrigation can cause deeper penetration of bacteria into the pocket. Investigators in two studies[42,46] stained tissue with ink and evaluated for penetration of carbon

*References 2, 8, 14, 16, 21, 25, 31, 38, 40, 49.

particles, and both found some penetration of carbon into the crevicular epithelium. O'Leary et al.[46] found that penetration was not influenced by water pressure because both a medium and a high setting had the same degree of penetration. Manhold et al.[42] found that nonirrigated areas also had carbon penetration, leading to speculation that the blade of a knife may drag in particles during the biopsy. Other researchers have found that irrigation reduces the amount of bacteria in the gingival crevice or periodontal pocket.* Specifically, Cobb et al.[16] and Drisko et al.[20] found that bacteria were reduced up to 6 mm.

The advisability of recommending oral irrigation for an individual at risk for infective endocarditis has been debated, with no clear answer.[3,22,53,57,59] The incidence of bacteremia from oral irrigation ranges from 7% in patients with gingivitis[53] up to 50% in those with periodontitis.[22] These percentages of bacteremia are similar to those found with other self-hygiene devices.[13,52,61] Toothbrushing alone has been shown to cause a bacteremia in 38.5% of cases.[52] No bacteremia was found in patients who flossed daily, but it did occur in 86% of those who delayed flossing for 1 to 4 days.[13] Wank et al.[61] found similar rates of bacteremia (10%-14%) for brushing, flossing, and use of the Perio-Aid.

Therefore, before recommending oral irrigation, practitioners need to consider both the overall medical status and the oral health status of the patient. A consultation with the patient's physician may be necessary to assess the patient's overall risk and determine the best clinical judgment.

CLINICAL OUTCOMES

Home irrigation is intended for use with routine or traditional (brushing and flossing) oral hygiene. The body of evidence on home irrigation includes more than 45 research studies conducted in more than 25 independent or university-based research settings. Evaluated outcomes include removal of plaque and reductions in calculus, gingivitis, bleeding on probing, probing depth, periodontal pathogens, and inflammatory mediators.† Home irrigation is applicable for most patients because it has been found to be safe and effective in those with gingivitis,‡ in periodontal maintenance patients,§ and in those with implants,[23] crown and bridge,[37] orthodontic appliances,[10,33] intermaxillary fixation,[49] and diabetes.[1]

Plaque Removal and Calculus Reduction

For the plaque index, the addition of home irrigation to routine oral hygiene has had mixed results compared to routine oral hygiene alone. When the primary agent used was water, some have found additional plaque reductions from adjunctively using irrigation, whereas others have not a reduction.# When an antimicrobial agent such as chlorhexidine was used as the irrigant, statistically significant plaque reductions over routine or traditional oral hygiene were generally demonstrated.*

The correlation between reduction in the plaque index and gingivitis or bleeding reduction is often not substantiated in home irrigation studies. Several investigators have found that despite a lack of reduction in the plaque index, significant reductions in gingivitis and bleeding on probing occurred.† One reason for this may be that current plaque indices only provide a *quantitative* measure of plaque mass as opposed to a *qualitative* evaluation of the biofilm. Even when concurrent plaque, gingivitis, and bleeding on probing reductions occur, a correlation among the measures sometimes cannot be found.[17] These perplexing findings have led researchers to speculate that other factors play a role in the mechanism of action of irrigation, such as reductions in pathogenic bacteria and immunoregulatory agents.[9,12,14,26,43]

Early studies found that irrigation with water lead to a reduction in calculus[31,40] up to as much as 50% over brushing alone.[40] Felo et al.,[23] employing 0.06% chlorhexidine and a soft rubber subgingival tip, found a decrease in calculus formation over rinsing with 0.12% chlorhexidine. Some researchers believe that an irrigator with magnetic polarity can enhance calculus reduction. Two studies using an oral irrigator with a magnetic component found greater calculus reductions on lower anterior teeth compared with the same device minus its magnet.[34,62] These results must be interpreted with caution because a novel index that measured both plaque and calculus was used. However, a correlation between plaque and calculus reductions and gingivitis could not be established because the irrigator with or without magnetic polarity equally reduced gingivitis.[34]

Gingivitis, Bleeding on Probing, and Probing Depth Reductions

As early as the 1960s, Lobene[40] found that that oral irrigation with water added to toothbrushing reduced gingivitis by 52% versus a 30% reduction for toothbrushing alone. Throughout the years, other researchers have found concurring results with the use of plain water.‡ Newman et al.[43] observed that periodontal maintenance patients with residual bleeding and 5-mm pocketing who added daily water irrigation to routine oral hygiene reduced gingivitis and bleeding better than those who only brushed and flossed.[43] Flemmig et al.[25] demonstrated a 50% greater reduction in bleeding on probing in maintenance patients over traditional oral hygiene. Barnes et al.[2a] showed that when a dental water jet was added to either a manual or power toothbrush routine, it was as effective at reducing plaque, bleeding, and gingivitis as a manual toothbrush and floss. In some instances it was superior for the reduction of bleeding and gingivitis.

The use of an antimicrobial agent, such as diluted chlorhexidine or an essential oil, generally enhances

*References 9, 14-16, 20, 24, 33, 35, 44.
†References 1, 2, 7, 9, 10, 14-18, 20, 23-26, 31-35, 38, 40, 43, 44, 49, 54, 60, 62, 64.
‡References 9, 14, 15, 26, 31, 32, 34, 40.
§References 2, 17, 24, 25, 35, 43, 64.
#References 9, 14, 25, 26, 31, 32, 40, 43, 49, 60.

*References 2, 9, 14, 15, 23, 26, 60.
†References 9, 14, 25, 26, 40, 43.
‡References 1, 14, 17, 25, 26, 31, 32, 40, 43.

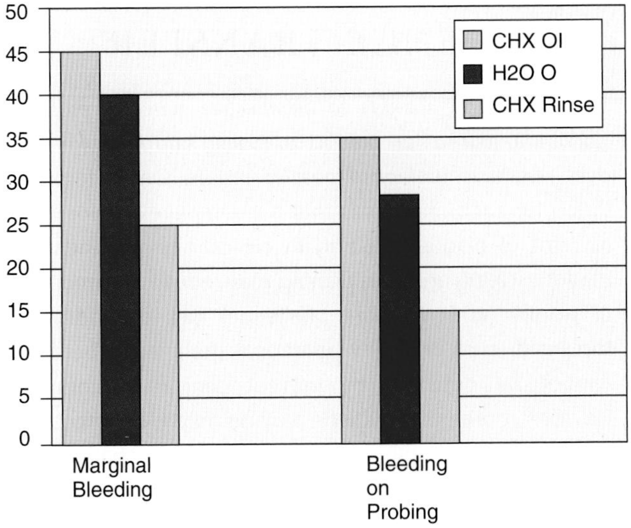

Figure 55-11 Study results showing *irrigation* with chlorhexidine *(CHX)* or water was better than *rinsing* with chlorhexidine in reducing marginal bleeding and bleeding on probing. (From Flemmig TF, Newman MG, Doherty FM, et al: *J Periodontol* 61:112, 1990.)

reductions in gingivitis and bleeding.* Chaves et al.[14] and Brownstein et al.[9] observed that either 0.04% or 0.06% chlorhexidine irrigation with a jet tip was superior to 0.12% chlorhexidine rinsing, whereas Felo et al.[23] demonstrated superiority over 0.12% chlorhexidine rinsing with site-specific subgingival tip and 0.06% chlorhexidine. Flemmig et al.[26] found that when 0.06% chlorhexidine irrigation, water irrigation, and 0.12% chlorhexidine rinsing were compared, 0.6% chlorhexidine (46.5%, 35.4%) was superior to water (39.6%, 24%), but water was better than 0.12% chlorhexidine rinsing (26.4%, 15%) at reducing the percentage of marginal bleeding sites and bleeding on probing, respectively (Figure 55-11). Ciancio et al.[15] showed that essential oil irrigation was more effective than irrigation with a placebo.

Several investigators have examined the impact of home irrigation on probing depth reduction. Most have demonstrated statistically but not clinically significant reductions, generally ranging from 0.1 to 0.4 mm.† This evidence lends support to the safety of irrigation as well as its potential for helping periodontal maintenance patients maintain stability.

Periodontal Pathogens and Inflammatory Mediators

Without a correlation to reductions in the plaque index, some researchers have suggested that the corresponding gingivitis and bleeding reductions may result from reductions in either periodontal pathogens or inflammatory mediators.[9,12,14,26,43] Multiple studies have evaluated the effect of oral irrigation on subgingival pathogens and found that irrigation produces both a quantitative and a qualitative decrease in bacteria, including periodontal pathogens.* Cobb et al.[16] observed changes in putative pathogens up to 6 mm after irrigation with water at a medium-high pressure. Others have observed effectiveness with diluted chlorhexidine or essential oil.† Chaves et al.[14] found that when toothbrushing, 0.12% chlorhexidine rinsing, 0.04% chlorhexidine irrigation, and water irrigation were compared, only the irrigation groups reduced subgingival pathogens.

Emerging evidence indicates that home irrigation may play a role in modulating the host response, particularly the inflammatory mediators associated with clinical attachment loss and alveolar bone loss.[1,17] Cutler et al.[17] demonstrated that over 14 days, daily irrigation with water reduced the inflammatory mediators interleukin-1β (IL-1β) and prostaglandin E_2 (PGE_2), increased the anti-inflammatory mediator IL-10, and kept interferon-γ (IFN-γ) stable, in addition to reducing traditional clinical indices. The authors also found that even though a reduction in plaque occurred, it did not correlate to a corresponding reduction in bleeding on probing. Instead, a reduction in IL-1β was shown to correlate to the reduction in bleeding on probing. It is important to note that GCF measures of inflammatory mediators were taken at least 8 hours after irrigation, thus eliminating a dilution effect.[17] Likewise, in a 12-week study, Al-Mubarek et al.[1] found that twice-daily oral irrigation with water using a site-specific subgingival tip significantly reduced traditional clinical indices as well serum measures of IL-1β, PGE_2, and reactive oxygen species in diabetic patients.

Patients with Special Considerations

Many clinical trials conducted on oral irrigation have studied a population group with gingivitis, a group receiving periodontal maintenance, or both groups. Some have focused on groups with special oral or medical health needs. In adults undergoing orthodontic therapy, Burch et al.[10] found an enhanced benefit in reducing gingivitis and bleeding from the addition of daily oral irrigation to either power or manual toothbrushing.[10] Hurst and Madonia[33] found that oral irrigation was 80% more effective in reducing total aerobic flora and 60% more effective in reducing the lactobacillus count than brushing and rinsing in adolescents with orthodontic appliances. Similarly, Phelps-Sandall and Oxford[49] observed that daily oral irrigation in patients with maxillary fixation had less inflammation than those who used either Proxy Brush or Perio-Aid. Krajewski et al.[37] found that individuals with bridgework or crowns had significant reductions in inflammation from irrigation with water. For patients with implants, a soft, site-specific subgingival tip used with 0.06% chlorhexidine improved oral health better than rinsing with 0.12% chlorhexidine[23] (Figure 55-12). Of note, although many recommend it, the jet tip has not been studied for safety and efficacy on patients with implants. For patients with

*References 2, 9, 14, 15, 24, 26, 35, 60.
†References 7, 10, 15, 17, 25, 26, 35, 43, 60.

*References 9, 12, 14-16, 20, 24, 33, 35, 44, 64.
†References 9, 14, 15, 24, 35, 43.

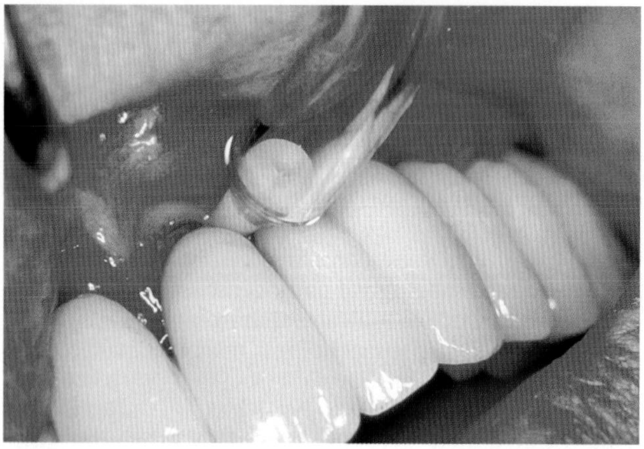

Figure 55-12 Use of the Pik Pocket tip around an implant.

TABLE 55-1

Chlorhexidine Dilutions* Shown Effective in Clinical Trials

Concentration	Water	Chlorhexidine
0.02%[2,60]	5 parts	1 part
0.04%[14,24]	2 parts	1 part
0.06%[9,23,26,44]	1 part	1 part

*Based on 0.12% concentration.

special medical considerations, home irrigation has been studied and shown safe and effective in a group of individuals with either type 1 or type 2 diabetes.[1]

Compliance is a major consideration when recommending any self-care device. Several investigators have observed that individuals like and regularly use an oral irrigator.[2,7,24-26,31,38] Flemmig et al. found a 91.5% compliance rate with oral irrigation.[26] When Lainson et al.[38] followed up with subjects 1 year after the completion of participation in an oral irrigation study, they found two thirds of the subjects were still using the pulsating oral irrigation. Importantly, those using the oral irrigator had significant reductions in gingivitis compared with those who stopped using the oral irrigator.

The use of an antimicrobial agent may also affect compliance. Plain water,* diluted chlorhexidine† (Table 55-1), and full-strength essential oil[15,24] all have evidence to support their use. Most irrigation units will tolerate any type of mouth rinse, except bleach, which may be corrosive to the units. Some clinicians have promoted 0.5% sodium hypochlorite (household bleach) or povidone-iodine as daily irrigants. There is minimal evidence to demonstrate the superiority of bleach over other irrigants, including water.[41] Likewise, only one home irrigation study has employed iodine as an irrigant.[64]

*References 1, 2, 10, 12, 14, 16, 17, 25, 26, 31-33, 37, 38, 40, 43, 49, 58.
†References 2, 9, 14, 23, 26, 35, 44, 60.

SCIENCE TRANSFER

Home irrigation appears to be effective, whereas professional irrigation as an adjunct to scaling and root planing does not have prolonged positive results. One interpretation for such findings is that a *threshold* exists for the amount of plaque resulting in clinical signs of inflammation; scaling and root planing may reduce the amount of plaque (and microbial challenge) well beyond this threshold, such that any additional therapeutic benefit cannot be detected by current clinical outcomes. However, home oral hygiene may be much less effective at removing plaque (and the microbial challenge) compared with professional scaling and root planing and thus may not reach the threshold of plaque reduction required to observe a clinical outcome. Home irrigation in combination with other home oral hygiene measures may provide enough additional benefit (plaque/microbial challenge reduction) to reach the threshold where the clinical outcome is then affected. Current clinical outcomes may not be sensitive enough to detect relatively subtle changes in plaque and bacterial reduction and thus decreases in gingival inflammation.

The use of irrigation by therapists at chairside does not seem to have much effect on periodontal disease status, even when antimicrobial agents such as chlorhexidine are used. However, when combined with routine brushing, the use of pulsating water jet devices by the patient for daily oral hygiene can lead to improvements in periodontal health. The addition of chlorhexidine or essential oils adds to the effectiveness, whereas povidone-iodine and sodium hypochlorite have not been shown to have significant longer-term benefits.

Although povidone-iodine appears safe for many individuals in the short term, the potential side effects from long-term use (e.g., daily irrigation) have not been evaluated.

SUMMARY

Oral irrigation is a generic term that covers two separate treatment modalities—professionally delivered (chairside) irrigation and home (self-applied) irrigation—for the prevention and treatment of periodontal disease. Professional irrigation appears to be of limited value, regardless of agent used, in enhancing the outcomes of scaling and root planing. Use of chlorhexidine may reduce pain and shorten healing time.

Home irrigation has a stronger body of supportive evidence than professional irrigation and is safe and effective for a wide range of patients, including those receiving periodontal maintenance and those with calculus buildup, gingivitis, orthodontic appliances, maxillary fixation, crown and bridge, implants, and diabetes. Clinical outcomes include the reduction of plaque, calculus, gingivitis, bleeding on probing, probing depth, periodontal pathogens, and inflammatory mediators.

REFERENCES

1. Al-Mubarek S, Ciancio, S, Aljada A et al: Comparative evaluation of adjunctive oral irrigation in diabetics, *J Clin Periodontol* 29:295, 2002.
2. Aziz-Gandour IA, Newman HN: The effects of simplified oral hygiene regimen plus supragingival irrigation with chlorhexidine or metronidazole on chronic inflammatory periodontal disease, *J Clin Periodontol* 13:228, 1986.

2a. Barnes CM, Russell CM, Reinhardt RA, et al: Comparison of irrigation to floss as an adjunct to toothbrushing: effect on bleeding, gingivitis, and supragingival plaque, *J Clin Dent* 16:71, 2005.

3. Berger SA, Weitzman S, Edberg SC, Casey JI: Bacteremia after the use of an oral irrigation device, *Ann Intern Med* 80:510, 1974.
4. Bhaskar SN, Cutright DE, Frisch J: Effect of high-pressure water jet on oral mucosa of varied density, *J Periodontol* 40:593, 1969.
5. Bhaskar SN, Cutright DE, Gross A, et al: Water jet devices in dental practice, *J Periodontol* 42:593, 1971.
6. Boyd RL, Hollander BN, Eakle WS: Comparison of a subgingivally placed cannula oral irrigator tip with a supragingivally placed standard irrigator tip, *J Clin Periodontol* 19:340, 1992.
7. Boyd RL, Leggott R, Quinn S, et al: Effect of self-administrated daily irrigation with 0.03% SnF_2 on periodontal disease activity, *J Clin Periodontol* 12:420, 1985.
8. Braun RE, Ciancio SG: Subgingival delivery by an oral irrigation device, *J Periodontol* 63:469, 1992.
9. Brownstein CN, Briggs SD, Schweitzer KL, et al: Irrigation with chlorhexidine to resolve naturally occurring gingivitis: a methodologic study, *J Clin Periodontol* 17:588, 1990.
10. Burch JG, Lanese R, Ngan P: A two-month study of the effects of oral irrigation and automatic toothbrush use in an adult orthodontic population with fixed appliances, *Am J Orthod Dentofac Orthop* 106:121, 1994.
11. Caffesse RG, Sweeny PL, Smith BA: Scaling and root planing with and without periodontal flap surgery, *J Clin Periodontol* 13:205, 1986.
12. Cantor MT, Stahl SS: Interdental col tissue responses to the use of water pressure cleansing device, *J Periodontol* 40:292, 1969.
13. Carroll GC, Sebor RJ: Dental flossing and its relationship to transient bacteremia, *J Periodontol* 51:691, 1980.
14. Chaves ES, Kornman KS, Manwell MA, et al: Mechanism of irrigation effects on gingivitis, *J Periodontol* 65:1016, 1994.
15. Ciancio SG, Mather ML, Zambon JJ, Reynolds HS: Effect of a chemotherapeutic agent delivered by an oral irrigation device on plaque, gingivitis, and subgingival microflora, *J Periodontol* 60:310, 1989.
16. Cobb CM, Rodgers RL, Killoy WJ: Ultrastructural examination of human periodontal pockets following the use of an oral irrigation device in vivo, *J Periodontol* 59:155, 1988.
17. Cutler CW, Stanford TW, Cederberg A, et al: Clinical benefits of oral irrigation for periodontitis are related to reduction of pro-inflammatory cytokine levels and plaque, *J Clin Periodontol* 27:134, 2000.
18. Derdivanis JP, Bushmaker S, Dagenais F: Effects of a mouthwash in an irrigating device on accumulation and maturation of dental plaque, *J Periodontol* 49: 49:81, 1978.
19. Drisko CH: Non-surgical pocket therapy: pharmacotherapeutics, *Ann Periodontol* 1: 491, 1996.
20. Drisko C, White C, Killoy W, Mayberry W: Comparison of dark-field microscopy and a flagella stain for monitoring the effect of a Water Pik on bacterial motility, *J Periodontol* 58:381, 1987.
21. Eakle WS, Ford C, Boyd RL: Depth of penetration in periodontal pockets with oral irrigation, *J Clin Periodontol* 13:39, 1986.
22. Felix JE, Rosen S, App GR: Detection of bacteremia after the use of an oral irrigation device in subjects with periodontitis, *J Periodontol* 42:785, 1971.
23. Felo A, Shibly O, Ciancio SG, et al: Effects of subgingival chlorhexidine irrigation on perio-implant maintenance, *Am J Dent* 10:107, 1997.
24. Fine JB, Harper S, Gordon JM, et al: Short-term microbiological and clinical effects of subgingival irrigation with an antimicrobial mouthrinse, *J Periodontol* 65:30, 1994.
25. Flemmig TF, Epp B, Funkenhauser Z, et al: Adjunctive supragingival irrigation with acetylsalicylic acid in periodontal supportive therapy, *J Clin Periodontol* 22:427, 1995.
26. Flemmig TF, Newman MG, Doherty FM, et al: Supragingival irrigation with 0.06% chlorhexidine in naturally occurring gingivitis. I. 6-month clinical observations, *J Periodontol* 61:112, 1990.
27. Goodsen JM: Gingival crevice fluid flow, *Periodontol 2000* 31:43, 2003.
28. Greenstein G: Supragingival and subgingival irrigation: practical application in the treatment of periodontal diseases, *Compend Contin Educ Dent* 12:1098, 1992.
29. Greenstein G, Polson A: The role of local drug delivery in the management of periodontal diseases: a comprehensive review, *J Periodontol* 69:507, 1998.
30. Hardy JH, Newman HN, Strhan JD: Direct irrigation and subgingival plaque, *J Clin Periodontol* 9:52, 1982.
31. Hoover DR, Robinson HB: The comparative effectiveness of a pulsating oral irrigator as an adjunct in maintaining oral health, *J Periodontol* 42:37, 1971.
32. Hugoson A: Effect of the Water Pik device on plaque accumulation and development of gingivitis, *J Clin Periodontol* 5:95, 1978.
33. Hurst JE, Madonia JV: The effect of an oral irrigating device on the oral hygiene of orthodontic patients, *J Am Dent Assoc* 81: 678, 1970.
34. Johnson KE, Sanders JJ, Gellin RG, et al: The effectiveness of magnetized water oral irrigator (Hydro Floss) on plaque, calculus, and gingival health, *J Clin Periodontol* 25:316, 1998.
35. Jolkovsky DL, Waki M, Newman MG, et al: Clinical and microbiological effects of subgingival and gingival marginal irrigation with chlorhexidine gluconate, *J Periodontol* 61: 663, 1990.
36. Khoury AE, Lam K, Ellis B, et al: Prevention and control of bacterial infections associated with medical devices, *Am Soc Artif Intern Organs* 38:M174, 1992.
37. Krajewski J, Giblin J, Gargiulo AW: Evaluation of a water pressure-cleansing device as an adjunct to periodontal treatment, *Periodontics* 1964; 2:76.
38. Lainson PA, Bergquist JJ, Fraleigh CM: A longitudinal study of pulsating water pressure cleansing devices, *J Periodontol* 43:444, 1972.
39. Larner JR, Greenstein G: Effect of calculus and irrigator tip design on depth of subgingival irrigation, *Int J Periodont Restor Dent* 13:288, 1993.
40. Lobene RR: The effect of a pulsed water pressure–cleansing device on oral health, *J Periodontol* 40:51, 1969.
41. Lobene RR, Soparkar PM, Hein JW, Quigley GA: A study of the effects of antiseptic agents and a pulsating irrigating device on plaque and gingivitis, *J Periodontol* 43:464, 1972.

42. Manhold JH, Vogel RI, Manhold EA: Carbon penetration of gingival tissue by oral irrigating devices, *J Prev Dent* 5:3, 1978.
43. Newman MG, Cattabriga M, Etienne D, et al: Effectiveness of adjunctive irrigation in early periodontitis: multi-center evaluation, *J Periodontol* 65:224, 1994.
44. Newman MG, Flemmig TF, Nachnani S, et al: Irrigation with 0.06% chlorhexidine in naturally occurring gingivitis. II. 6 months microbiological observations, *J Periodontol* 61:427, 1990.
45. Nickel JC, Ruseka I, Wright JB, et al: Tobramycin resistance of *Pseudomonas aeruginosa* cells growing in a biofilm on urinary catheter material, *Antimicrob Agents Chemother* 27:619, 1985.
46. O'Leary TJ, Shafer WG, Swenson M, et al: Possible penetration of crevicular tissue from oral hygiene procedures. I. Use of oral irrigating devices, *J Periodontol* 41:158, 1970.
47. Oosterwaal PJ, Mikx FH, Renggli HH: Clearance of a topically applied fluorescein gel from periodontal pockets, *J Clin Periodontol* 17:613, 1990.
48. Oosterwaal PJ, Mikx FH, van den Brink ME, et al: Bactericidal concentrations of chlorhexidine-digluconate, amine fluoride gel and stannous fluoride gel for subgingival bacteria tested in serum at short contact times, *J Periodont Res* 24:155, 1989.
49. Phelps-Sandall BA, Oxford SJ: Effectiveness of oral hygiene techniques on plaque and gingivitis in patients placed in intermaxillary fixation, *Oral Surg Oral Med Oral Pathol* 56:487, 1983.
50. Quirynen M, Mongardini C, De Soete M, et al: The role of chlorhexidine in the one-stage full-mouth disinfection treatment of patients with advanced adult periodontitis: long-term clinical and microbiological observations, *J Clin Periodontol* 27:578, 2000.
51. Rabbani GM, Ash MM, Caffesse RG: The effectiveness of subgingival scaling and root planing in calculus removal, *J Periodontol* 52:119, 1981.
52. Roberts GJ, Holzel HS, Sury MR, et al: Dental bacteremia in children, *Pediatr Cardiol* 18:24, 1997.
53. Roman AR, App GR: Bacteremia, a result from oral irrigation in subjects with gingivitis, *J Periodontol* 42:757, 1971.
54. Sanders PC, Linden GJ, Newman HN: The effects of a simplified mechanical oral hygiene regime plus supragingival irrigation with chlorhexidine or metronidazole on subgingival plaque, *J Clin Periodontol* 13:237, 1986.
55. Selting WJ, Bhaskar SN, Mueller RP: Water jet direction and periodontal pocket debridement, *J Periodontol* 43:569, 1972.
56. Singleton S, Treloar R, Warren P: Methods for microscopic characterization of oral biofilms: analysis of colonization, microstructure, and molecular transport phenomena, *Adv Dent Res* 11:133, 1997.
57. Tamimi GA, Thomassen PR, Moser EH: Bacteremia study using a water irrigation device, *J Periodontol* 40:4, 1969.
58. Tempel TR, Marcil JF, Seibert JS: Comparison of water irrigation and oral rinsing on clearance of soluble and particulate materials from the oral cavity, *J Periodontol* 46:391, 1975.
59. Waki MY, Jolkovsky DL, Otomo-Corgel J, et al: Effects of subgingival irrigation on bacteremia following scaling and root planing, *J Periodontol* 61:405, 1990.
60. Walsh TF, Glenwright HD, Hull PS: Clinical effects of pulsed oral irrigation with 0.0% chlorhexidine digluconate in patients with adult periodontitis, *J Clin Periodontol* 19:245, 1992.
61. Wank HA, Levison ME, Rose LF, Cohen DW: Quantitative measurement of bacteremia and its relationship to plaque control, *J Periodontol* 47:683, 1976.
62. Watt DL, Rosenfelder C, Sutton CD: The effect of oral irrigation with a magnetic water treatment device on plaque and calculus, *J Clin Periodontol* 20:314, 1993.
63. Wilson M, Patel H, Fletcher J: Susceptibility of biofilms of *Streptococcus sanguis* to chlorhexidine gluconate and cetylpyridinium chloride, *Oral Microbiol Immunol* 11:188, 1996.
64. Wolff LF, Bakdash MB, Pihlstrom BL, et al: The effect of professional and home subgingival irrigation with antimicrobial agents on gingivitis and early periodontitis, *J Dent Hyg* 63:224, 1989.

56

CHAPTER

Occlusal Evaluation and Therapy

Michael J. McDevitt and Carol A. Bibb

CHAPTER OUTLINE

An understanding of the principles of occlusion and the relationship to oral health and disease is necessary for all dental clinicians. Historically, occlusal relationships have been considered largely from a morphologic rather than a biologic perspective. Our growing understanding of the uniqueness of each individual's susceptibility to periodontitis challenges the clinician to differentiate among many factors that may influence or modify a patient's periodontal disease experience. The functional demands of the occlusion may fall well within or may exceed the tolerances and the adaptability of the periodontium (see Chapter 29) and the entire masticatory system (see Chapter 30). The clinician's responsibility is to assess and interpret an individual patient's occlusion in light of the patient's unique susceptibility so that the most appropriate response can be offered.

The current resurgence of interest in occlusion[28,30,41] coincides with the Institute of Medicine's recommendation that the dental profession make use of scientific evidence, outcomes research, and formal consensus processes when devising practice guidelines.[16] Application of this approach to the field of occlusion is already having, and will likely continue to have, a significant impact on clinical practice and an improved standard of patient care, including the care of patients undergoing periodontal therapy.[21,30,31]

Contemporary definitions of occlusion reflect the importance of structure-function relationships in biologic systems. For example, McNeill[44] defines *occlusion* as the functional relationship between the components of the masticatory system, including the teeth, supporting tissues, neuromuscular system, temporomandibular joints, and craniofacial skeleton. An important corollary of this definition is that the occlusion is a *dynamic* relationship and must be defined physiologically as well as morphologically. The clinical application of this definition is that the occlusion cannot be evaluated or treated in isolation. Instead, each component of the masticatory system must be fully understood according to its potential for adaptation and pathophysiology as well as interactions with the other components.

This chapter presents a biologic rationale and practical guidelines for evaluating jaw function status and occlusion in the context of defining each patient's susceptibility to periodontitis and the management of the patient's periodontal disease.

TERMINOLOGY

The complexity surrounding occlusal concepts has been compounded by an abundance of heterogeneous terminology requiring definition and clarification. The key descriptive terms used in this chapter, along with common synonyms, are defined as follows:

Maximum intercuspation: The position of the mandible when there is maximal interdigitation and occlusal contacts between the maxillary and mandibular teeth; also called *centric occlusion* and *intercuspal position* (ICP).
Centric relation: The position of the mandible when both condyle-disc assemblies are in their most superior positioning the glenoid fossa and against the slope of the articular eminence of the temporal bone. (See Chapter 30.)
Initial contact in centric relation: The first occlusal contact in the centric-relation closure arc.
Excursive movement: Any movement of the mandible away from maximum intercuspation.
Laterotrusion: Movement of the mandible laterally to the right or the left from maximum intercuspation.
Working side: The side of either dental arch corresponding to the side of the mandible moving away from the midline.
Nonworking side: The side of either dental arch corresponding to the side of the mandible moving toward the midline; also called *balancing side.*
Protrusion: Movement of the mandible anteriorly from maximum intercuspation.
Retrusion: Movement of the mandible posteriorly.
Guidance: Pattern of opposing tooth contact during excursive movements of the mandible. The teeth making such contact cause separation of the other teeth, which is called *disclusion.*
Interference: Any contact, in the centric-relation closure arc, in maximum intercuspation, or in excursions, that prevents the remaining occlusal surfaces from achieving stable contact; also called *supracontact.*

FUNCTIONAL ANATOMY OF MASTICATORY SYSTEM

An understanding of the biologic basis of occlusal function requires that the teeth, temporomandibular joints (TMJs), and muscles of mastication be considered as a functional unit (Figure 56-1). These structures developed together during embryogenesis and postnatal growth, and perturbations to one component in the system would be expected to influence other components to undergo either adaptive or pathologic changes. Therefore the clinician must recognize that it is inappropriate to consider any component in isolation; instead, all components of the system and their functional interactions must be included as part of any evaluation.

BIOLOGIC BASIS OF OCCLUSAL FUNCTION

The ideal occlusal relationships depicted in textbook diagrams and on typodont models, which have served as the primary focus of traditional dental education, are relatively uncommon in natural dentitions.[2,27,33,53,67] In addition, it is now recognized that the occlusion is a dynamic relationship reflecting an equilibrium between the various components of the masticatory system.[46] Therefore the functional status of an individual's occlusion is more clinically significant than its morphology.

A widely accepted physiologic classification of occlusion is as follows:

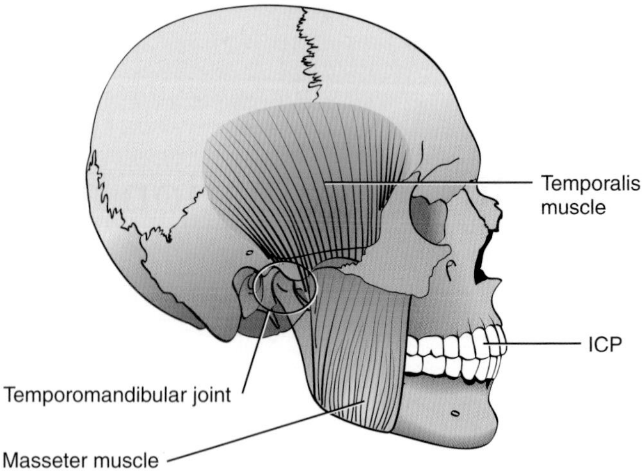

Figure 56-1 Functional anatomy of the masticatory system shown in sagittal view: temporomandibular joint *(circled),* masseter and temporalis muscles, and dental occlusion in maximum intercuspation (*ICP,* intercuspal position).

A **physiologic occlusion** is present when no signs of dysfunction or disease are present and no treatment is indicated.
A **nonphysiologic** (or **traumatic**) **occlusion** is associated with dysfunction or disease caused by tissue injury, and treatment may be indicated. In this text the term *trauma from occlusion* is applied to periodontal tissue injury resulting from occlusal forces.
A **therapeutic occlusion** is the result of specific interventions designed to treat dysfunction or disease.

Maintenance of a physiologic occlusion requires favorable structure-function relationships and optimal tissue adaptation throughout the masticatory system. The anatomic features that contribute to a physiologic occlusion and that should be the goal in a therapeutic occlusion[45] include (1) a stable endpoint of mandibular closure, (2) bilateral distribution of occlusal forces across many posterior teeth, and (3) axial loading of these teeth. When occlusal forces are distributed optimally, the occlusion will be stable by objective criteria and is likely to be subjectively comfortable for the patient.

The signs and symptoms of a nonphysiologic occlusion include damaged teeth and restorations, abnormal mobility, fremitus, a widened periodontal ligament, pain, and a subjective sense of bite discomfort. As emphasized in Chapter 29, the criterion that determines if an occlusion is traumatic is whether it produces periodontal injury, not how the teeth occlude. Alternatively, many so-called malocclusions do not produce discomfort or injury and therefore are not "traumatic occlusions" by definition.

Parafunctional habits such as bruxism are another potential source of occlusal trauma for periodontitis-susceptible patients when they experience increased frequency, intensity, and duration of occlusal loading of teeth. *Bruxism* is defined as diurnal or nocturnal parafunctional activity that includes clenching, bracing, gnashing, and grinding of the teeth. Although no causative association exists between bruxism and gingival inflammation[7] or periodontitis,[22,24] bruxism can cause tooth mobility, tooth wear and fracture, and periodontal and muscle pain[7,51] and may contribute to masticatory system disorders (see Chapter 30). No significant evidence indicates that malocclusions or interferences are causal factors in bruxism.[11] The selective serotonin reuptake inhibitor (SSRI) medications have been reported to encourage bruxism.[19] A maxillary or a mandibular stabilization appliance is generally considered the most effective means of managing bruxism.[8]

Chapter 29 provides a detailed description of the response of the periodontium to occlusal forces and discusses the relationship of trauma from occlusion to the etiology and progression of periodontal disease. The literature on this topic includes numerous experimental animal model studies in which the challenge is to make clinically relevant extrapolations to human periodontal disease.* Human investigations have provided mixed messages and may have provoked some controversy or confusion and lack of consensus in the past.† A variety of occlusal schemes, including chronic excursive interferences, may be clinically acceptable in young individuals, who characteristically have little, if any, periodontal disease experience.[1,48,49,62] The evidenced-based approach facilitates clinical decision making most favorably when the populations studied closely resemble the periodontal disease status of the patient receiving care.

When defined as a risk factor for the progression of periodontitis, trauma from occlusion has the potential to alter disease severity and prognosis. Degree of susceptibility to periodontitis is *patient specific,* whereas occlusal trauma is *tooth specific.* Until recently, human clinical studies have been unable to separate statistically the experience of individual teeth with regard to periodontitis and any influence of the occlusion. In patients experiencing moderate to severe periodontitis, Nunn and Harrell[50] were able to identify significantly increased loss of attachment for specific teeth with occlusal discrepancies when compared to teeth without occlusal discrepancies. Evidence supports the expectation that occlusal therapy will positively influence the outcome of both nonsurgical and surgical therapy for patients affected by moderate to severe periodontitis.[6] There is even evidence indicating that "no intervention" with traumatic occlusion allows periodontitis to progress more readily.[23] The medical model of clinical research that compares an intervention with a placebo (or no intervention) parallels these two studies and validates the application of their findings to the rationale for therapeutic intervention in a periodontitis-susceptible patient with traumatic occlusion. However, the therapeutic priority is to control inflammation, and this must be successful for healing of the periodontal tissues to occur.* It is generally recommended that occlusal therapy be deferred until inflammation is controlled and reevaluation determines that any residual mobility is the result of adverse tooth loading rather than decreased support.[17,30,31]

*References 14, 15, 36-38, 46, 56, 57, 67.

†References 6, 17, 20, 26, 29, 52, 59, 65.

*References 21, 46, 47, 54, 55, 67.

BOX 56-1

Temporomandibular Disorder (TMD) Screening Evaluation

1. Maximal interincisal opening
2. Opening/closing pathway
3. Auscultation for TMJ sounds
4. Palpation for TMJ tenderness
5. Palpation for muscle tenderness

TMJ, Temporomandibular joint.

CLINICAL EVALUATION PROCEDURES

The current standard of care requires that a screening evaluation for masticatory system disorders or *temporomandibular disorders* (TMDs) be included in all routine dental examinations.[41] Clinical evaluation of the entire masticatory system as described in Chapter 30 should be an integral part of each patient's initial comprehensive examination. The screening physical evaluation of the patient then becomes part of each subsequent examination to identify any developing disorder and to help ensure that treatment procedures will not have an adverse impact on preexisting TMDs. In addition, a valid examination of the occlusion requires that the patient's jaw function status be within normal limits.

Temporomandibular Disorder Screening Examination

The recommended screening examination includes health history questions focused on jaw function status, a brief patient history, and a cursory examination expected to take approximately 5 minutes. The generally accepted components of the TMD screening examination[41] are described next (Box 56-1; see also Chapter 30).

Interincisal Opening. The patient is instructed to "open as wide as possible" while a millimeter ruler is placed on the lower incisors. The interincisal distance is recorded in millimeters (mm).

Opening/Closing Pathway. The opening/closing pathway is observed, and any deviations from a midline path are diagrammed.

Temporomandibular Joint Sounds. Light finger pressure is applied bilaterally over the TMJs while the patient is asked to open and close to discern any deflection of tissue. Joint sounds heard through a stethoscope or Doppler instrument are classified as "discrete clicks" or "diffuse grating sounds," termed *crepitus*. The location of the sound in the opening/closing cycle and any associated pain or mechanical disruption should be documented.

Temporomandibular Joint Tenderness. Light bilateral palpation over the lateral aspect of the condyles is used to elicit TMJ tenderness if present. It should be recorded as mild, moderate, or severe. The patient should be asked to compare right and left sides for calibration purposes. Loading of TMJs offers further discrimination of joint status (see Chapter 30).

Muscle Tenderness. The masseter (origin and insertion), pterygoid, and temporalis (anterior and middle) muscles are examined bilaterally using moderate finger pressure. Sites of muscle pain should be localized and described as mild, moderate, and severe on an appropriate anatomic diagram. A common error is to apply insufficient pressure, so the patient should be advised to expect some discomfort and instructed to differentiate pressure from pain. It is also helpful to ask the patient to compare right and left sides for calibration purposes.

Intraoral Evaluation of Occlusion

In addition to collecting standard data on static occlusal relationships, a functional evaluation of the occlusion should be done (Box 56-2). This includes an assessment of stability in maximum intercuspation, the quality of mandibular movements, and tooth mobility and wear. Mobile teeth can be difficult to identify with marking papers and wax because they may move rather than being marked or indenting the wax.

Maximum Intercuspation or Intercuspal Position. The patient should be able to close into maximum intercuspal position consistently without searching for a stable or comfortable bite. An efficient way to locate zones of occlusal contact is to place Mylar strips between the teeth and ask the patient to "close and hold" and then attempt to remove the strip from between apparently occluding teeth to feel how firm a contact exists. The presence or absence of contacts should be documented for the molars, premolars, canines, and incisors. More detailed information on the specific sites of occlusal contacts can be obtained by using occlusal indicator wax or marking ribbon.

BOX 56-2

Intraoral Occlusal Evaluation

1. Identification of occlusal contacts in maximum intercuspation
2. Guidance in excursive movements
3. Initial contact in centric-relation closure arc
4. Tooth mobility
5. Attrition

Excursive Movements. The quality of tooth contact patterns during mandibular movements out of maximum intercuspation are observed by asking the patient to move into right and left excursions and to move toward maximum protrusion. Mylar strips are useful for verifying tooth contact patterns during excursions. Individual deflective occlusal contacts or interferences to closure or to unobstructed mandibular movement should be noted, along with any mobility of teeth.

Initial Contact in Centric-Relation Closure Arc. Guidance of the patient's mandible will allow the first occlusal contact in the centric-relation closure arc to be identified with minimal masticatory muscle recruitment,[25] and any discrepancy with maximum intercuspation can be documented. If tooth-to-tooth contact occurs before maximum intercuspation is acquired, deflection of the mandible or movement of the teeth (if mobile) occurs. If teeth move to permit the greater interdigitation of the dentition, this "permissive intercuspation" of these teeth may prohibit accurate identification of contacts.

Tooth Mobility. Mobility is recorded as part of the initial occlusal evaluation and to monitor any changes over time; Chapter 35 explains the basis for evaluating tooth mobility and presents a means of measurement. Mobility also can be assessed with the teeth loaded. After initial light contact in the closure arc, the patient can squeeze or clench the teeth, and the dentist can observe visually and use tactile detection of movement to determine mobility. Patients can also move in all excursions while individual and groups of teeth are being loading by opposing teeth, and assessment can be made of deflection of individual teeth. Involving patients through watching and touching their own teeth during the discovery of mobility can be effective patient education.

Attrition. Attrition is defined as wear caused by tooth-to-tooth contact. A certain amount of physiologic attrition is normal. However, accelerated attrition should be noted, including the location of significant wear facets, which may indicate ongoing occlusal parafunction with potential for increasing occlusal trauma due to enlargement of occluding surfaces. Significant attrition of the teeth is often indicative of a meaningful chronic occlusal habit, bruxism. Wear of this type may be more moderate for patients who experience a clenching type of parafunction, resulting in overloading the teeth at or near maximum intercuspation. It is likely, however, that clenching the teeth is the most damaging form of occlusal parafunction to the periodontium where the constant "pumping" of the major muscles of mastication intrudes and rocks the teeth within the alveolus.[7,12]

Role of Articulated Casts

Articulated dental casts are not absolutely necessary for a functional evaluation of the occlusion, but they can be critical to the identification of occlusal contacts that can deflect the mandible, deflect mobile teeth, or cause trauma to specific teeth and to the periodontium. The rationale for accurately mounted diagnostic models is presented in Chapter 30 and reinforced in Chapter 72. In specific cases, these models may be required for pretreatment documentation of occlusal relationships, localization of wear facets, trial occlusal adjustments, and monitoring of the progression of occlusal changes.

INTERPRETATION AND TREATMENT PLANNING

Temporomandibular Disorder Screening

The goal of the comprehensive clinical evaluation of the masticatory system and subsequent TMD screening examinations is to determine whether jaw function status is sufficiently within the normal range to permit examination procedures and treatment to proceed without provoking or exacerbating symptoms. Therefore the clinical significance of the findings is considered in this context.

A suggested practical approach is to use the screening examination findings to place the patient in one of the following three categories:

1. The jaw function status is determined to be within normal limits; there are no contraindications to proceeding with further examination and treatment procedures. A patient in this category will have no complaints or significant history of jaw pain or dysfunction, an interincisal opening of at least 40 mm, no significant joint or muscle tenderness, and minimal joint sounds.
2. Certain findings should alert the clinician to the potential for aggravating benign problems, especially with wide opening during long appointments. Examples include a history of jaw problems after long appointments, several sites of mild to moderate muscle tenderness, or a previously benign TMJ click. These patients should be advised of the need to notify the clinician if symptoms develop or progress. Use of a bite block, shortened appointments, and longer intervals between appointments may also be indicated.
3. Significant findings indicate the need for a more comprehensive evaluation or referral before any nonemergency treatment. (Chapter 30 can assist the clinician in determination of an appropriate course of diagnosis.) Examples include a restricted interincisal opening, significant pain on jaw use, severe joint or muscle pain, and progressive locking episodes, such as after wide opening. It should be obvious that continuing with nonemergency treatment would be difficult and likely to exacerbate these problems. Furthermore, evaluation of the occlusion will not be valid unless the patient's jaw function status is determined to be within normal limits.

Although the prevalence of TMD signs and symptoms in adult subjects ranges from 28% to 86% in various studies,[58] only an estimated 5% to 7% are in need of TMD treatment.[60] In triaging patients as described previously, significant pain or dysfunction and progression of symptoms are the key determinants, but the ultimate decision in favor of therapy is based on each patient's condition and the goals for health and comfort. Clinicians treating older adults should be aware that a high prevalence of crepitus and jaw opening of less than 40 mm has been reported in older individuals compared with young adults.[5] These signs were not associated with pain or disability and do not contraindicate treatment. However, they may have an impact on providing dental care to this age group.

Occlusal Evaluation

The findings from the occlusal examination should be reviewed in the context of the definitions of physiologic and nonphysiologic occlusions. The most significant concern is whether the occlusion meets the requirements for occlusal stability (Box 56-3). Although not an absolute requirement, it is very desirable for bilateral simultaneous contact to occur in the centric-relation closure arc, because unilateral contact requires muscle, joint (see Chapter 30), or tooth/periodontal accommodation. This relationship also represents a desired end point for restorative treatment (see Chapter 72). Specific requirements for stability of posterior teeth in maximum intercuspation are illustrated in Figure 56-2. Tooth-by-tooth analysis of the presence or the absence of occlusal interferences and condition of the periodontium may give the clinician insight into site specific susceptibility of individual teeth and into treatment options for affected teeth.[23,50] In effect, each patient, by virtue of overall susceptibility to periodontitis, represents his or her own control for any site-specific susceptibility. Periodontal deterioration much greater than that expected from the bacterially mediated challenge to the periodontium may reflect occlusal trauma directed at that individual tooth.

Diagnostic Interocclusal Appliance

A maxillary or mandibular interocclusal appliance can serve an important diagnostic role within the scope of comprehensive periodontal therapy. Any perceived instability of either or both TMJs related to muscle dysfunction often has occlusal disharmony as a contributing

BOX 56-3

Requirements for Occlusal Stability

1. Maximum intercuspation (see Figure 56-2)
   - Light or absent anterior contacts
   - Well-distributed posterior contacts
   - Coupled contacts between opposing teeth
   - Cross-tooth stabilization
   - Forces directed along long axis of each tooth
2. Smooth excursive movements without interferences
3. No trauma from occlusion
4. Favorable subjective response to occlusal form and function

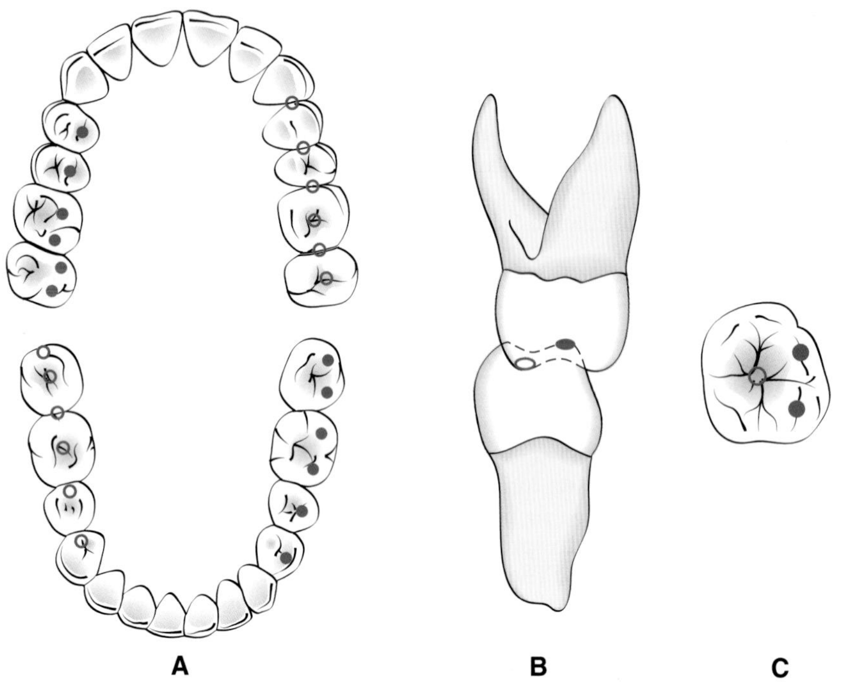

Figure 56-2 **A,** Sites of occlusal contact in maximum intercuspation on supporting cusps *(solid circles)* and corresponding vertical stops *(open circles)*. Cross-tooth stabilization is shown on proximal **(B)** and occlusal **(C)** views. Note the direction of occlusal forces along the long axis of the teeth shown in **B.**

factor. A well-adjusted interocclusal appliance frequently permits less-strained muscular activity[3,13] and may allow for more consistent identification of centric relation and other occlusal references to determine if intervention is appropriate.[35] Such an appliance can encourage tightening of teeth by orthopedically splinting mobile teeth while protecting them from deflective occlusal contacts. When the teeth have tightened to the degree that the condition and quantity of the periodontium permits, the presence or absence of occlusal discrepancies can be determined before making any decision about an irreversible change, such as occlusal adjustment or restorative dentistry.

OCCLUSAL THERAPY

The sequence of occlusal therapy in the overall treatment plan still depends on the unique experience of each patient and how his or her susceptibility to periodontitis manifests itself. Because an inflamed periodontium can contribute to mobility, it can affect the accuracy of clinical assessment of a patient's occlusion. The ideal approach would therefore include at least the development of a therapeutic level of home care and completion of appropriate nonsurgical therapy, including comprehensive scaling and root planing. Persistent or residual mobility of individual teeth would then need to be interpreted to distinguish between occlusal trauma and nonpathologic mobility. If the clinician concludes that specific occlusal discrepancies were responsible for the apparent occlusal trauma, interocclusal appliance therapy or occlusal adjustment could be prescribed. Although evidence indicates that occlusal adjustment can favorably influence the outcome of scaling and root planing,[6] prudence and patient acceptance of the rationale for treatment suggest the ideal approach, addressing the inflammation first, is usually the safest and most effective.

The purpose of occlusal therapy is to establish stable functional relationships favorable to the patient's oral health, including the periodontium. A variety of procedures can contribute to this objective: interocclusal appliance therapy, occlusal adjustment, both provisional and final restorative procedures, orthodontic tooth movement, and orthognathic surgery.

The following guidelines apply to occlusal therapy in general:

1. A sound biologic rationale should exist for the intervention. Has the patient's susceptibility to periodontitis been confirmed?
2. Occlusal interventions should be considered an adjunct to periodontal therapy. Is there clinical evidence that the periodontal disease experience of certain teeth has been negatively influenced by occlusal trauma?
3. Significant, irreversible occlusal changes should be considered in the context of the restorative care planned for the patient.
4. Thorough, informed consent must be provided to the patient; it is critical that the patient understands the goals, limitations, and consequences of the occlusal intervention. The occlusal therapy deemed appropriate is then anticipated by the patient and clinician as probably increasing stability and comfort and possibly enhancing the benefits of periodontal therapy,[6,23] while not treating the periodontal disease itself.

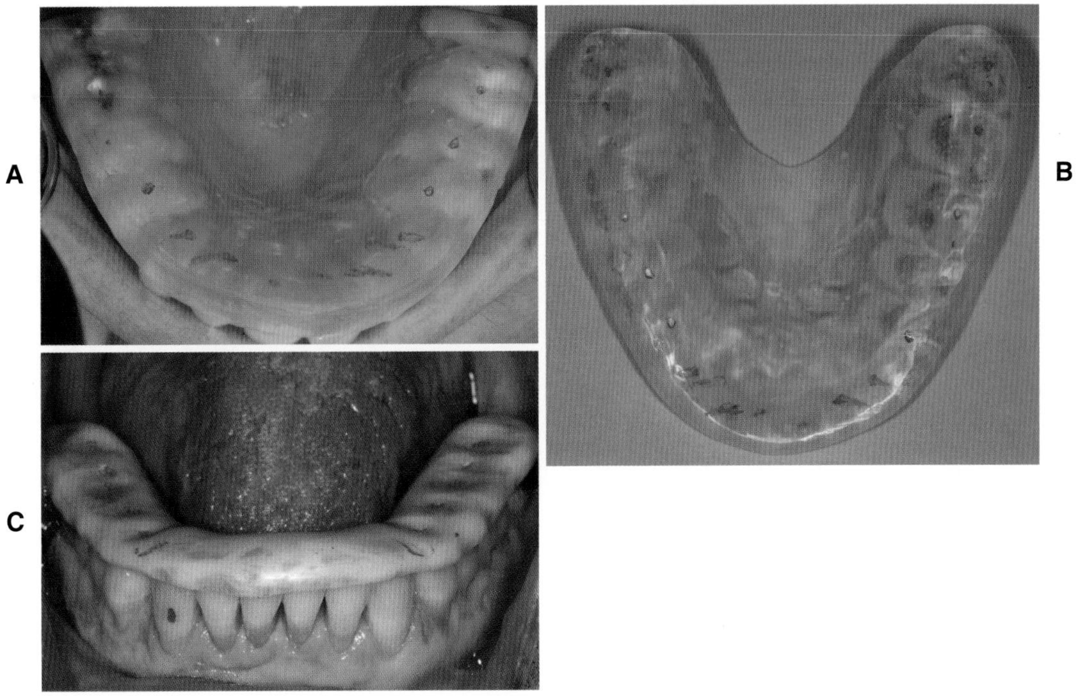

Figure 56-3 **A,** Maxillary interocclusal appliance with intimate palatal contact and maximum comfortable coverage for optimal stabilizing influence on any mobile teeth. **B,** Maxillary interocclusal appliance with marks created by opposing dentition, demonstrating bilateral simultaneous contact in centric relation and immediate disclusion of opposing posterior teeth in all excursions. **C,** Mandibular interocclusal appliance fabricated before surgery, providing stabilizing influence for the incisors in particular.

The contributions of restorative dentistry and orthodontic tooth movement to the management of the periodontal patient are covered in other chapters (e.g., see Chapters 71 and 72). The specific management of masticatory disorders, including the different manifestations of orofacial pain, are beyond the scope of this text; many, varied treatment modalities have been shown to address symptoms effectively.* Therefore the roles of interocclusal appliance therapy and occlusal adjustment in the treatment of patients susceptible to periodontitis are the primary focus of this discussion.

Interocclusal Appliance Therapy

Interocclusal appliances, generally fabricated of hard acrylic or composite resin, have the advantage of providing a reversible means of redistributing occlusal forces and minimizing excessive force on individual teeth. A full-coverage, maxillary or mandibular stabilization appliance is particularly useful in providing physical stability to mobile teeth, especially the maxillary appliance with nearly full palatal contact and coverage (Figure 56-3, *A*). The increased amount of surface area of the firm palatal gingiva in contact dramatically influences the ability of the appliance to encourage tightening of mobile teeth compared with an appliance that covers only the occlusal surfaces of the teeth. The teeth opposing the appliance are favorably influenced by the design of the occluding surface. Specific factors of occlusal stability should include (1) bilateral simultaneous contact in centric relation, (2) immediate disclusion of posterior teeth sustained in all excursions, and (3) guidance responsibility distributed on anterior teeth without stress in any excursive movement (Figure 56-3, *B*).

Mobile teeth in the arch opposing the interocclusal appliance frequently tighten when the appliance is carefully fabricated and the occlusion is meticulously refined. The decision on which arch to address with the appliance is most often determined by the number of teeth and the degree of mobility; both factors usually have greater weight for maxillary teeth. Generally, if either maxillary cuspid is mobile, or if the maxillary incisors as a group are mobile, the clear choice is a maxillary appliance. The mandibular appliance is particularly helpful if the mandibular incisors are mobile (Figure 56-3, *C*) or if the patient thinks a maxillary appliance would be difficult to wear. Both designs are effective in managing bruxism and to a more limited degree, clenching, as part of a comprehensive treatment plan for the patient. Providing such an appliance to the periodontal patient will likely contribute to an overall sense of bite comfort, in addition to minimizing the destructive consequences of occlusal parafunction, and may improve overall prognosis.[40]

In light of increasing concern about occlusal overloading of implants, interocclusal appliances may play an important protective role for implants as well as for teeth with a compromised periodontium,[18,34] especially

*References 6, 18, 34, 41, 1, 61, 64, 66.

when sleep bruxism is suspected.[63] Acceptance and initial accommodation to an appliance can be facilitated when patients have experienced guidance in evaluation of their own persistent mobility and parafunction or when they perceive the value in protecting the teeth, the periodontium, their restorations, and their implants. Appliances are most often worn during sleep, when occlusal experience cannot be monitored by the patient and when they would not interfere with daily activities.

The provider of the occlusal appliance as an adjunct to periodontal therapy should always recognize that muscular and skeletal elements of the masticatory system may also be affected. Because stabilization appliance therapy is considered one of the most appropriate interventions for masticatory system disorders, there is greater likelihood of a positive or neutral muscle or joint response than a negative one. Here, again, the value of the baseline references acquired during initial evaluation of the masticatory system cannot be overstated. Discontinuation of appliance use provides the opportunity for virtually reversible intervention with the occlusion, implying safety when prescribed.[39]

Common characteristics of effective interocclusal appliance design include the following (Figure 56-4):

1. Fabrication on accurately mounted diagnostic casts.
2. Centric stops for all opposing posterior teeth; some designs have light contact with the incisal edge.
3. Immediate disclusion of all posterior teeth sustained in all excursions.
4. Smooth, relatively flat anterior guidance, sufficient to achieve disclusion of posterior teeth without imposing stress on any anterior teeth.
5. Relined to fit the teeth in the arch for which it is fabricated, to maximize appliance stabilityand act as a stabilizing influence on the teeth. Intimate contact between the appliance and as much of the palate as accepted by the patient substantially increases the orthopedic stabilization of maxillary teeth.
6. Subject to multiple adjustments in anticipation of reduced mobility of teeth and functional changes in musculature and in joint relationships.
7. May or may not be followed by occlusal adjustment, depending on individual patient needs.

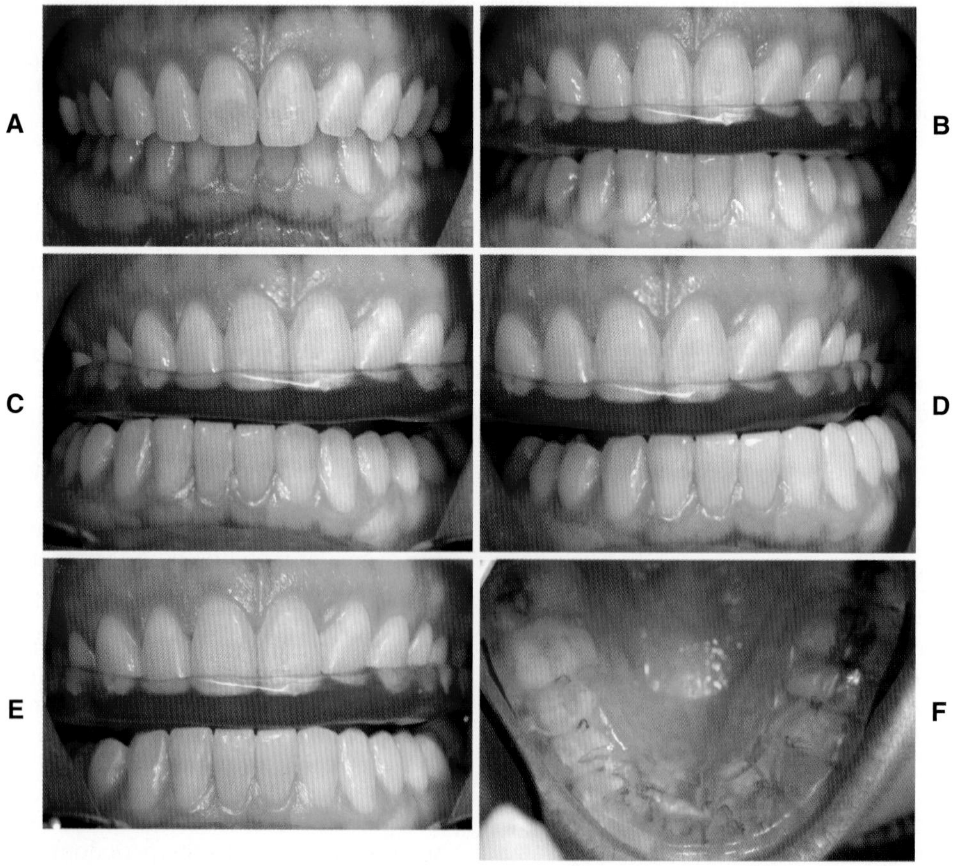

Figure 56-4 Patient with class II occlusal scheme. **A,** Maxillary interocclusal appliance fabricated to enhance axial loading of opposing mandibular teeth **(B).** Bilateral simultaneous contact of cuspids and all posterior teeth in centric relation **(B),** and smooth, relatively flat anterior guidance with immediate and sustained disclusion of all posterior teeth in both lateral excursions (**C** and **D**) and in protrusion **(E). F,** Occlusal surface of appliance shows marks created in centric relations and in all excursions by the opposing cusp tips or incisal edges by articulating paper.

Occlusal Adjustment

Occlusal adjustment, also called *occlusal equilibration* or *coronoplasty,* is the selective reshaping of occlusal surfaces with the goal of establishing a stable, nontraumatic occlusion. The resulting occlusion should meet the requirements for occlusal stability described previously (see Box 56-3) and is termed a *therapeutic occlusion.* Many categories of occlusal adjustment exist, ranging from the altering of contours of a single tooth to major full-mouth equilibration to the degree that maximum intercuspation is coincident with centric relation.

Because occlusal adjustment is an irreversible intervention, the prudent clinician should carefully weigh the scientific and clinical evidence in support of such therapy. In the case of TMD, the evidence leads to the conclusion that occlusal adjustment should rarely be considered as a primary component of TMD treatment and never as a preventive measure.[41] Similarly, there is no evidence that occlusal adjustment is useful in the management of bruxism.[3,32,64]

The role of occlusal adjustment in the management of periodontal disease is more complex because both periodontitis and trauma from occlusion can lead to tooth mobility. In a randomized clinical trial with 2-year follow-up, Burgett et al.[6] concluded that occlusal adjustment adjunctive to either scaling and root planing or modified Widman flap therapy resulted in a more favorable attachment level but no differences in reduction of mobility or pocket depth. Recent evidence showing the benefits of occlusal adjustments adjunctive to periodontal therapy was comparable on an individual tooth basis with teeth not presenting occlusal disharmony in patients susceptible to moderate to severe periodontitis. When occlusal therapy was not selected by patients with periodontitis and occlusal disharmonies, the progression of attachment loss was significantly greater than for patients who did not need occlusal therapy or for those choosing occlusal therapy. Patient self-selection in this research addressed the ethical issues in the study of disease progression.[23] Both these studies seemed to draw reasonable conclusions to support the application of scientific evidence to clinical practice.[6,23] When patients with periodontitis experienced the occlusal adjustment determined to be appropriate for them, the outcome of the periodontal therapy was favorably influenced. The stated goals of occlusal adjustment included the requirements for occlusal stability listed in Box 56-3 and added the objective of minimal difference between initial contact in the centric-relation closure arc and maximum intercuspation.

It is generally recommended that occlusal adjustment be deferred until inflammation is controlled, time is allowed for tissue healing, and reevaluation determines that any residual mobility is the result of adverse tooth loading rather than decreased support.[17,30,31] Exceptions to this recommendation include the need to address pain or dysfunction clearly determined to be the result of occlusal trauma. Occlusal appliance therapy can also be used to address acute occlusal issues, with the advantage of reversibility, and often facilitates the decision making and process involved in an occlusal adjustment.

A major consideration before occlusal adjustment is the restorative needs of the patient. For example, the benefits of placing provisional restorations with optimal contours and well-adjusted occlusal surfaces should not be overlooked. This approach offers the opportunity to restore occlusal stability by distributing forces, as well as to evaluate the response of the periodontium to the anticipated restoration of the patient's dentition.

When occlusal adjustment is determined to be the best approach, the procedure must be preceded by good informed consent.[10] Trial adjustment on accurately mounted diagnostic casts is recommended to determine the extent of alteration required to meet the goals of occlusal stability and elimination of interferences. When any teeth subject to the occlusal equilibration are mobile, multiple appointments are necessary to address changes resulting from the progressive tightening of individual teeth and the recognition of interferences to harmonious occlusal function that the tighter teeth create. If equilibration follows accommodation to an occlusal appliance

SCIENCE TRANSFER

The relationship between periodontal disease and occlusion has long been debated. This debate also extends to the role of occlusal therapy and the treatment of periodontal disease. Occlusal trauma is difficult to diagnose and is usually functionally defined. *It is generally accepted that the inflammatory aspects of the periodontal case should be addressed first and resolved before any occlusal considerations.* The rationale is that resolution of inflammation will change the tooth-tissue relationships, including the relationship of the teeth to the opposing dentition. After resolution of inflammation, the occlusion can be evaluated and any negative consequences addressed. As noted, few individuals have ideal occlusal relationships, but they experience few adverse events. These findings attest to remarkable adaptability of the masticatory system, including the teeth, the periodontal ligament, and the skeletal, muscular, and neurologic systems.

Occlusal therapy can be used to reduce the loading of teeth that have lost bone to periodontal disease. This will help to control trauma and improve the results of conventional periodontal therapy. Clinicians should develop the skills to diagnose occlusal status, use splints for occlusal stability, and develop the techniques of occlusal adjustment. Of particular significance is the development of a stable centric relation and a pattern of disclusion of posterior teeth in protrusive movements. Occlusal therapy on periodontally involved teeth must produce an occlusal pattern that differentially loads individual teeth according to each tooth's periodontal bone support.

(a strongly recommended sequence), having the patient wear the appliance before the appointment for equilibration (e.g., overnight and until seated in the operatory) will encourage the teeth to be as tight as possible. As with the diagnostic interocclusal appliance, decreased masticatory muscle recruitment and tighter teeth can increase the accuracy of identifying occlusal interferences. Clark et al.,[10] McNeill,[43] and Dawson[12] provide detailed practical protocols for occlusal adjustment procedures, with Dr. Dawson offering the most current resource for guidance through this process in his newly published text, *Functional Occlusions* (July 2006).

SUMMARY

Evaluation and management of the periodontal patient must include a thorough examination of the masticatory system (Chapter 30) and functional evaluation of the occlusion. Occlusal interventions should be considered an adjunct to periodontal therapy, reversible when possible, and planned in the context of the patient's restorative needs consistent with goals and expectations.

REFERENCES

1. Agerberg G, Sandstrom R: Frequency of occlusal interferences: a clinical study in teenagers and young adults, *J Prosthet Dent* 59:212, 1988.
2. Anderson JR, Myers GE: Natural contacts in centric occlusion in 32 adults, *J Dent Res* 50:7, 1971.
3. Bailey JO Jr, Rugh JD: Effect of occlusal adjustment on bruxism as monitored by nocturnal EMG recordings, *J Dent Res* 59:317, 1980 (abstract 199).
4. Becker I, Tarantola G, Zambrano J, et al: Effect of a prefabricated anterior bite stop on electromyographic activity of masticatory muscles, *J Prosthet Dent* 82:22, 1999.
5. Bibb CA, Atchison KA, Pullinger AG, et al: Jaw function status in an elderly community sample, *Community Dent Oral Epidemiol* 23:303, 1995.
6. Burgett FG, Ramfjord SP, Nissle RR, et al: A randomized trial of occlusal adjustment in the treatment of periodontitis patients, *J Clin Periodontol* 19:381, 1992.
7. Christensen GJ: Abnormal occlusal conditions: a forgotten part of dentistry, *J Am Dent Assoc* 126:1667, 1995.
8. Clark GT: Interocclusal appliance therapy. In Mohl ND, Zarb GA, Carlsson GE, et al, editors: *A textbook of occlusion,* Chicago, 1988, Quintessence.
9. Clark GT, Love R: The effect of gingival inflammation on nocturnal masseter muscle activity, *J Am Dent Assoc* 102:319, 1981.
10. Clark GT, Mohl ND, Riggs RR: Occlusal adjustment therapy. In Mohl ND, Zarb GA, Carlsson GE, et al, editors: *A textbook of occlusion,* Chicago, 1988, Quintessence.
11. Clark GT, Tsukiyama Y, Baba K, et al: Sixty-eight years of experimental interference studies: what have we learned? *J Prosthet Dent* 82:704, 1999.
12. Dawson PE: *Evaluation, diagnosis, and treatment of occlusal problems,* ed 2, St Louis, 1989, Mosby.
13. Emshoff R, Bertram S: The short-term effect of stabilization-type splints on local cross-sectional dimensions of muscles of the head and neck, *J Prosthet Dent* 80:457, 1998.
14. Ericsson I, Lindhe J: Lack of effect of trauma from occlusion on the recurrence of experimental periodontitis, *J Clin Periodontol* 4:115, 1977.
15. Ericsson I, Giargia M, Lindhe J, et al: Progression of periodontal tissue destruction at splinted/non-splinted teeth: an experimental study in the dog, *J Clin Periodontol* 10:693, 1993.
16. Field MJ, editor: *Dental education at the crossroads,* Washington, DC, 1995, National Academy Press.
17. Fleszar TJ, Knowles JW, Morrison EC, et al: Tooth mobility and periodontal therapy, *J Clin Periodontol* 7:495, 1980.
18. Forssell H, Kalso E, Koskela P, et al: Occlusal treatments in temporomandibular disorders: a qualitative systemic review of randomized controlled trials, *Pain* 83:549, 1999.
19. Gerber PE, Lynd LD: Selective serotonin reuptake inhibitor induced movement disorders, *Ann Pharmacother* 32:692, 1998.
20. Gher ME: Non-surgical pocket therapy: dental occlusion, *Ann Periodontol* 1:567, 1996.
21. Gher ME: Changing concepts: the effect of occlusion on periodontitis, *Dent Clin North Am* 2:285, 1998.
22. Hanamura H, Houston F, Rylander H, et al: Periodontal status and bruxism: a comparative study of patients with periodontal disease and occlusal parafunctions, *J Periodontol* 58:173, 1987.
23. Harrel SK, Nunn ME: The effect of occlusal discrepancies on periodontitis. II. Relationship of occlusal treatment to the progression of periodontal disease, *J Periodontol* 72:495, 2001.
24. Hellsing G: Functional adaptation to changes in vertical dimension, *J Prosthet Dent* 52:867, 1984.
25. Hickman DM, Cramer R: The effect of different condylar positions on the masticatory muscle electromyographic activity in humans, *Oral Surg Oral Med Oral Pathol Oral Radiol Endod* 85:18, 1998.
26. Hoag PM: Occlusal treatment. In *Proceedings of the World Workshop in Clinical Periodontics,* Chicago, 1989, American Academy of Periodontology.
27. Hochman N, Ehrlich J: Tooth contact location in intercuspal position, *Quintessence Int* 18:193, 1987.
28. *J Calif Dent Assoc* 28, 2000 (entire issue).
29. Jin L, Cao C: Clinical diagnosis of trauma from occlusion and its relation with severity of periodontitis, *J Clin Periodontol* 19:92, 1992.
30. Kao RT: The role of occlusion in periodontal disease. In: McNeill C, editor: *Science and practice of occlusion,* Chicago, 1997, Quintessence.
31. Kao RT, Chu R, Curtis D: Occlusal considerations in determining treatment prognosis, *J Calif Dent Assoc* 28:760, 2000.
32. Kardachi BJ, Bailey JO Jr, Ash MM Jr: A comparison of biofeedback and occlusal adjustment on bruxism, *J Periodontol* 49:367, 1978.
33. Korioth TW: Number and location of occlusal contacts in intercuspal position, *J Prosthet Dent* 64:206, 1990.
34. Kreiner M, Betancor E, Clark GT: Occlusal stabilization appliances evidence of their efficacy, *J Am Dent Assoc* 132:770, 2001.
35. Kurita H, Ikeda K, Kurashina K: Evaluation of the effect of a stabilization splint on occlusal force in patients with masticatory muscles disorders, *J Oral Rehabil* 27:79, 2000.
36. Lindhe J, Ericsson I: Effect of longstanding jiggling on experimental marginal periodontitis in the beagle dog, *J Clin Periodontol* 9:497, 1982.
37. Lindhe J, Ericsson I: The effect of elimination of jiggling forces on periodontally exposed teeth in the dog, *J Periodontol* 53:562, 1982.
38. Lindhe J, Svanberg G: Influence of trauma from occlusion on progression of experimental periodontitis in the beagle dog, *J Clin Periodontol* 1:3, 1974.
39. McDevitt MJ, Russell CM, Schmid MJ, Reinhardt RA: Impact of increased occlusal contact, interleukin-1 genotype, and periodontitis severity on gingival crevicular fluid IL-1β levels, *J Periodontol* 74:1302, 2003.

40. McGuire MK, Nunn ME: Prognosis versus actual outcome. II. The effectiveness of clinical parameters in developing an accurate prognosis, *J Periodontol* 67:658, 1996.
41. McNeill C, editor: *Temporomandibular disorders: Guidelines for classification, assessment, and management,* Chicago, 1993, Quintessence.
42. McNeill C, editor: *Science and practice of occlusion,* Chicago, 1997, Quintessence.
43. McNeill C: Selective tooth grinding and equilibration. In McNeill C, editor: *Science and practice of occlusion,* Chicago, 1997, Quintessence.
44. McNeill C: Management of temporomandibular disorders: concepts and controversies, *J Prosthet Dent* 77:510, 1997.
45. McNeill C: Occlusion: what it is and what it is not, *J Calif Dent Assoc* 28:748, 2000.
46. Meitner S: Co-destructive factors of marginal periodontitis and repetitive mechanical injury, *J Dent Res* 54:78, 1975.
47. Miyata T, Kobayashi Y, Araki H, et al: The influence of controlled occlusal overload on peri-implant tissue, *Int J Oral Maxillofac Implants* 13:677, 1998.
48. Nilner M: Prevalence of functional disturbances and diseases of the stomatognathic system in 15–18 year-olds, *Swed Dent J* 5:189, 1981.
49. Nilner M, Lassing SA: Prevalence of functional disturbances and diseases of the stomatognathic system in 7–14 year-olds, *Swed Dent J* 5:173, 1981.
50. Nunn ME, Harrel SK: The effect of occlusal discrepancies on periodontitis. I. Relationship of initial occlusal discrepancies on initial clinical parameters, *J Periodontol* 72:485, 2001.
51. Pavone BW: Bruxism and its effect on the natural teeth, *J Prosthet Dent* 53:692, 1985.
52. Pihlstrom B, Anderson KA, Aeppli D, Schaffer EM: Association between signs of trauma from occlusion and periodontitis, *J Periodontol* 57:1, 1986.
53. Plasmans PJ, Knipers L, Vollenbrock HR, et al: The occlusal status of molars, *J Prosthet Dent* 60:500, 1988.
54. Polson AM: The relative importance of plaque and occlusion in periodontal disease, *J Clin Periodontol* 13:923, 1986.
55. Polson AM, Adams RA, Zander HA: Osseous repair in the presence of active tooth hypermobility, *J Clin Periodontol* 10:370, 1983.
56. Polson AM, Meitner SW, Zander HA: Trauma and progression of marginal periodontitis in squirrel monkeys. III. Adaptation of interproximal alveolar bone to repetitive injury, *J Periodontal Res* 11:279, 1976.
57. Polson AM, Meitner SW, Zander HA: Trauma and progression of marginal periodontitis in squirrel monkeys. IV. Reversibility of bone loss due to trauma alone and trauma superimposed upon periodontitis, *J Periodontal Res* 11:290, 1976.
58. Rugh JD, Solberg WK: Oral health status in the United States: temporomandibular disorders, *J Dent Educ* 49:398, 1985.
59. Shefter GL, McFall WT: Occlusal relations and periodontal status in human adults, *J Periodontol* 55:368, 1984.
60. Solberg WK: Epidemiology, incidence, and prevalence of temporomandibular disorders: a review. Presented at President's Conference on the Examination, Diagnosis, and Management of Temporomandibular Disorders, Chicago, 1983, American Dental Association.
61. Tarantola GJ, Becker IM, Gremillion H, Pink F: The effectiveness of equilibration in the improvement of signs and symptoms in the stomatognathic system, *Int J Periodont Restor Dent* 18:595, 1998.
62. Tipton RT, Rinchuse DJ: The relationship between static occlusion and functional occlusion in a dental school population, *Angle Orthodont* 61:57, 1991.
63. Tosun T, Karabuda C, Cuhadaroglu C: Evaluation of sleep bruxism by polysomnographic analysis in patients with dental implants, *Oral Maxillofac Implants* 18:286, 2003.
64. Tsukiyama Y, Baba K, Clark GT: An evidence-based assessment of occlusal adjustment as a treatment for temporomandibular disorders, *J Prosthetic Dent* 86:57, 2001.
65. Wang H, Frederick G, Burgett F, et al: The influence of molar furcation involvement and mobility on future clinical periodontal attachment loss, *J Periodontol* 65:25, 1994.
66. Wright EF, Schiffman EL: Treatment alternatives for patients with masticatory myofascial pain, *J Am Dent Assoc* 126:1030, 1995.
67. Zander HA, Polson AM: Present status of occlusion and occlusal therapy in periodontics, *J Periodontol* 48:540, 1977.

CHAPTER 57

Adjunctive Role of Orthodontic Therapy

Vincent G. Kokich

CHAPTER OUTLINE

Orthodontic tooth movement may be a substantial benefit to the adult periorestorative patient. Many adults who seek routine restorative dentistry have problems with tooth malposition that compromise their ability to clean and maintain their dentitions. If these individuals also are susceptible to periodontal disease, tooth malposition may be an exacerbating factor that could cause premature loss of specific teeth.

Orthodontic appliances have become smaller, less noticeable, and easier to maintain during orthodontic therapy. Many adults are taking advantage of the opportunity to have their teeth aligned to improve the esthetics of their smiles. If these individuals also have underlying gingival or osseous periodontal defects, these defects often can be improved during orthodontic therapy if the orthodontist is aware of the situation and designs the appropriate tooth movement. In addition, implants have become a major part of the treatment plan for many adults with missing teeth. If adjacent teeth have drifted into edentulous spaces, orthodontic therapy is often helpful to provide the ideal amount of space for implants and subsequent restorations.

This chapter shows the ways in which adjunctive orthodontic therapy can enhance the periodontal health and restorability of teeth.

BENEFITS OF ORTHODONTIC THERAPY

Orthodontic therapy can provide several benefits to the adult periodontal patient. The following six factors should be considered:

1. Aligning crowded or malposed maxillary or mandibular anterior teeth permits the adult patient better access to clean all surfaces of their teeth adequately. This could be a tremendous advantage for patients who are susceptible to periodontal bone loss or do not have the dexterity to maintain their oral hygiene.
2. Vertical orthodontic tooth repositioning can improve certain types of osseous defects in periodontal patients. Often the tooth movement eliminates the need for resective osseous surgery.
3. Orthodontic treatment can improve the esthetic relationship of the maxillary gingival margin levels

before restorative dentistry. Aligning the gingival margins orthodontically avoids gingival recontouring, which could require bone removal and exposure of the roots of the teeth.

4. Orthodontic therapy also benefits the patient with a severe fracture of a maxillary anterior tooth that requires forced eruption to permit adequate restoration of the root. Erupting the root allows the crown preparation to have sufficient resistance form and retention for the final restoration.
5. Orthodontic treatment allows open gingival embrasures to be corrected to regain lost papilla. If these open gingival embrasures are located in the maxillary anterior region, they can be unesthetic. In most patients, these areas can be corrected with a combination of orthodontic root movement, tooth reshaping, and restoration.
6. Orthodontic treatment could improve adjacent tooth position before implant placement or tooth replacement. This is especially true for the patient who has been missing teeth for several years and has drifting and tipping of the adjacent dentition.

PREORTHODONTIC OSSEOUS SURGERY

The extent of the osseous surgery depends on the type of defect (e.g., crater, hemiseptal defect, three-wall defect, furcation lesion). The prudent clinician knows which defects can be improved with orthodontic treatment and which defects require preorthodontic, periodontal, surgical intervention.

Osseous Craters

An osseous crater is an interproximal, two-wall defect that does not improve with orthodontic treatment. Some shallow craters (4- to 5-mm pocket) may be maintainable nonsurgically during orthodontic treatment. However, if surgical correction is necessary, this type of osseous lesion can easily be eliminated by reshaping the defect[12,15] and reducing the pocket depth (Figure 57-1) (see Chapter 66). This in turn enhances the ability to maintain these interproximal areas during orthodontic treatment. The need for surgery is based on the patient's response to initial root planing, the patient's periodontal resistance, the location of the defect, and the predictability of

A

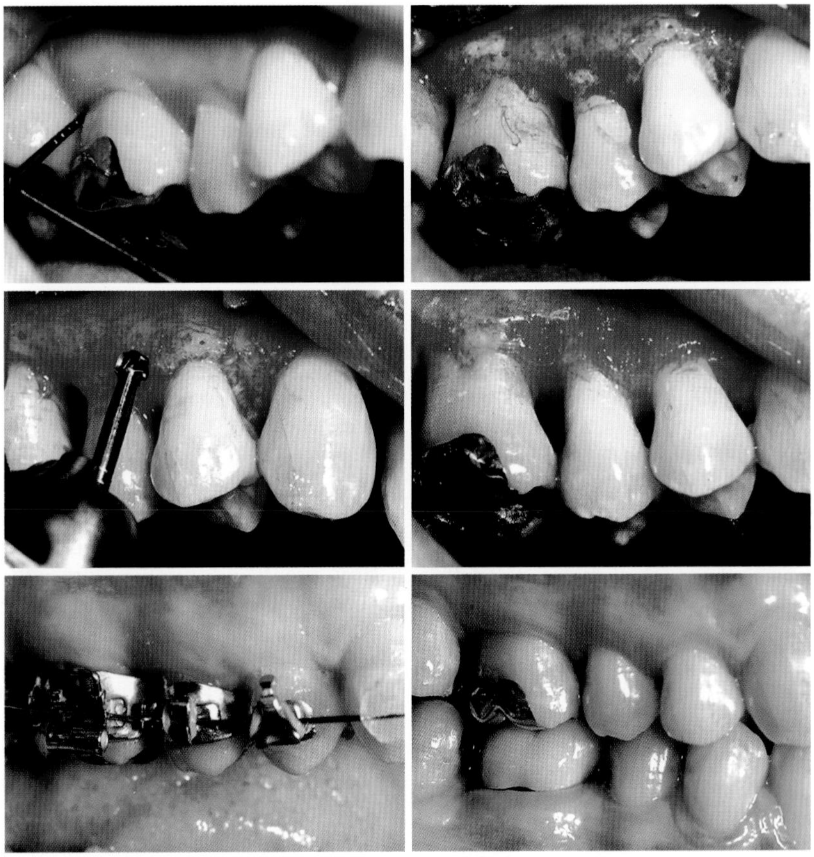

B

C

D

E

F

Figure 57-1 This patient had a 6-mm probing defect distal to the maxillary right first molar **(A).** When this area was flapped **(B),** a cratering defect was apparent. Osseous surgery was used to alter the bony architecture on the buccal and lingual surfaces to eliminate the defect (**C** and **D**). After 6 weeks the probing pocket defect had been reduced to 3 mm, and orthodontic appliances were placed on the teeth **(E).** By eliminating the crater before orthodontic therapy, the patient could maintain the area during and after orthodontic treatment **(F).**

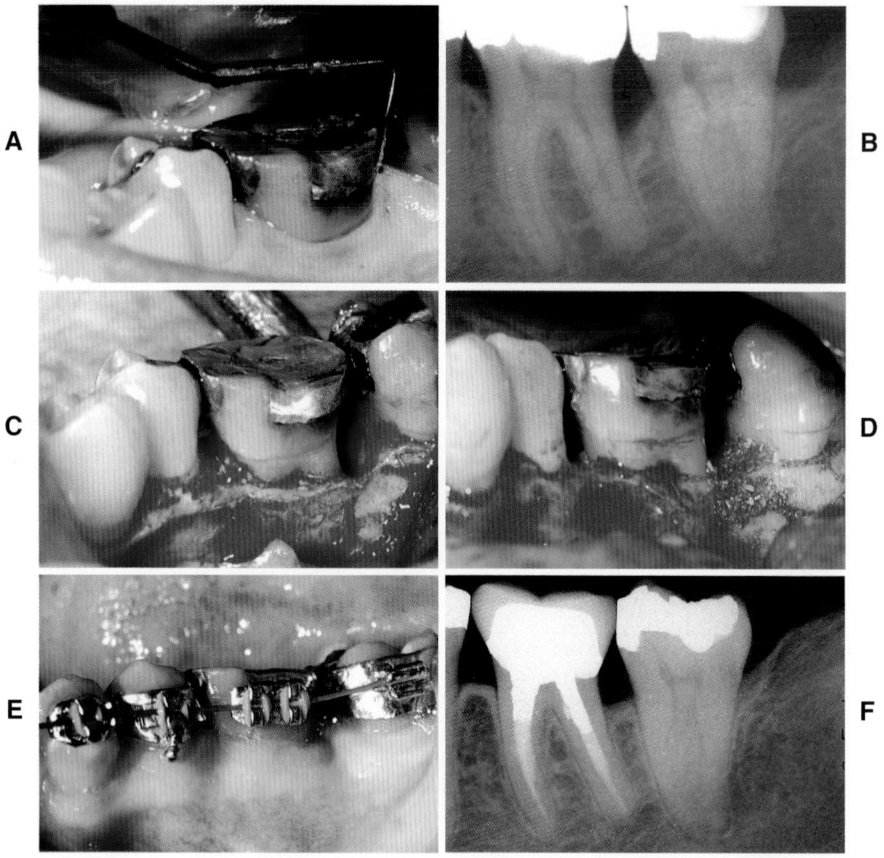

Figure 57-2 This patient had a significant periodontal pocket **(A)** distal to the mandibular right first molar. Periapical radiograph **(B)** confirmed the osseous defect. A flap was elevated **(C),** revealing a deep, three-wall osseous defect. Freeze-dried bone **(D)** was placed in the defect. Six months after the bone graft, orthodontic treatment was initiated **(E).** The final periapical radiograph shows that the preorthodontic bone graft helped regenerate bone and eliminate the defect distal to the molar **(F).**

maintaining defects nonsurgically while the patient is wearing orthodontic appliances.

Three-Wall Intrabony Defects

Three-wall defects are amenable to pocket reduction with regenerative periodontal therapy.[1] Bone grafts using either autogenous bone from the surgical site or allografts along with the use of resorbable membranes have been successful in filling three-wall defects.[14] If the result of periodontal therapy is stable 3 to 6 months after periodontal surgery (Figure 57-2), orthodontic treatment may be initiated.

ORTHODONTIC TREATMENT OF OSSEOUS DEFECTS

Hemiseptal Defects

Hemiseptal defects are one- or two-wall osseous defects that often are found around mesially tipped teeth (Figure 57-3) or teeth that have supererupted (Figure 57-4). Usually, these defects can be eliminated with the appropriate orthodontic treatment. In the case of the tipped tooth, uprighting[2,5] and eruption of the tooth levels the bony defect. If the tooth is supererupted, intrusion and leveling of the adjacent cementoenamel junctions can help level the osseous defect.

It is imperative that periodontal inflammation be controlled before orthodontic treatment. This usually can be achieved with initial debridement and rarely requires any preorthodontic surgery. After the completion of orthodontic treatment, these teeth should be stabilized for at least 6 months and reassessed periodontally. Often, the pocket has been reduced or eliminated, and no further periodontal treatment is needed. It would be injudicious to perform preorthodontic osseous corrective surgery in such lesions if orthodontics is part of the overall treatment plan.

In the periodontally healthy patient, orthodontic brackets are positioned on the posterior teeth relative to the marginal ridges and cusps. However, some adult patients may have marginal ridge discrepancies caused by uneven tooth eruption. When marginal ridge discrepancies are encountered, the decision as to where to place the bracket or band is not determined by the anatomy of the tooth. In these patients, it is important to assess these teeth radiographically to determine the interproximal bone level.

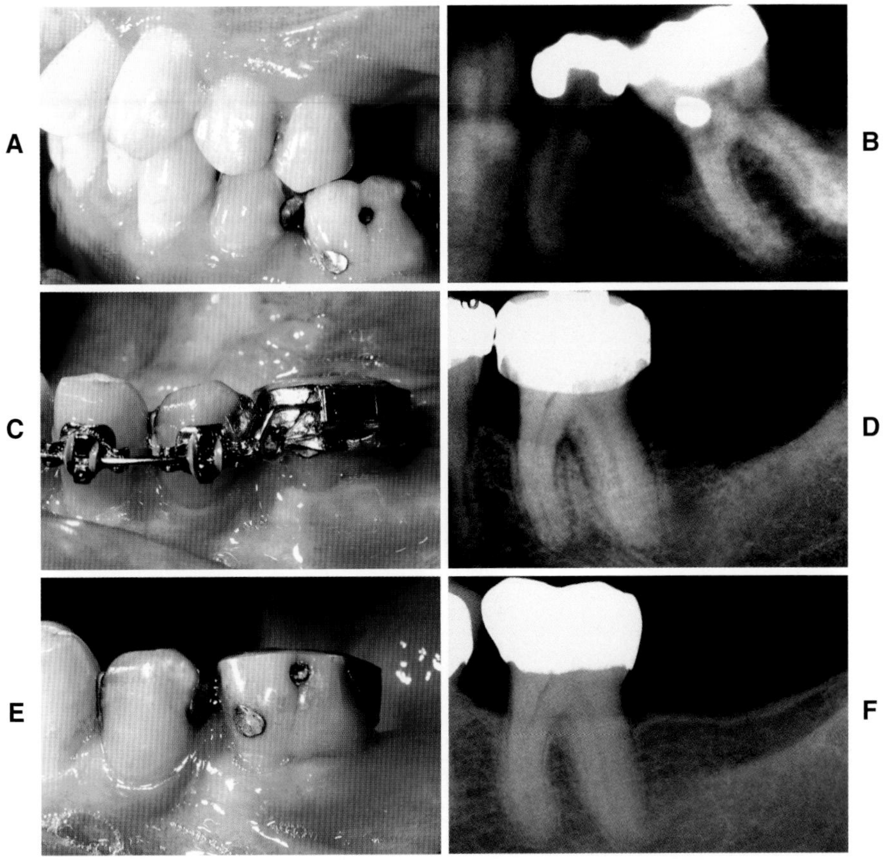

Figure 57-3 This patient was missing the mandibular left second premolar, and the first molar had tipped mesially **(A).** Pretreatment periapical radiograph **(B)** revealed a significant hemiseptal osseous defect on the mesial of the molar. To eliminate the defect, the molar was erupted, and the occlusal surface was equilibrated **(C).** The eruption was stopped when the bone defect was leveled **(D).** The posttreatment intraoral photograph **(E)** and periapical radiograph **(F)** show that the periodontal health had been improved by correcting the hemiseptal defect orthodontically.

If the bone level is oriented in the same direction as the marginal ridge discrepancy, leveling the marginal ridges will level the bone. However, if the bone level is flat between adjacent teeth (see Figure 57-4) and the marginal ridges are at significantly different levels, correction of the marginal ridge discrepancy orthodontically produces a hemiseptal defect in the bone. This could cause a periodontal pocket between the two teeth.

If the bone is flat and a marginal ridge discrepancy is present, the orthodontist should not level the marginal ridges orthodontically. In these situations, it may be necessary to equilibrate the crown of the tooth (see Figure 57-4). For some patients, the latter technique may require endodontic therapy and restoration of the tooth because of the required amount of reduction of the length of the crown. This approach is acceptable if the treatment results in a more favorable bone contour between the teeth.

Some patients have a discrepancy between both the marginal ridges and the bony levels between two teeth. However, these discrepancies may not be of equal magnitude; orthodontic leveling of the bone may still leave a discrepancy in the marginal ridges (Figure 57-5). In these patients the crowns of the teeth should not be used as a guide for completing orthodontic therapy. The bone should be leveled orthodontically, and any remaining discrepancies between the marginal ridges should be equilibrated. This method produces the best occlusal result and improves the patient's periodontal health.

During orthodontic treatment, when teeth are being extruded to level hemiseptal defects, the patient should be monitored regularly. Initially, the hemiseptal defect has a greater sulcular depth and is more difficult for the patient to clean. As the defect is ameliorated through tooth extrusion, interproximal cleaning becomes easier. The patient should be recalled every 2 to 3 months during the leveling process to control inflammation in the interproximal region.

Advanced Horizontal Bone Loss

After orthodontic treatment has been planned, one of the most important factors that determine the outcome of orthodontic therapy is the location of the bands and brackets on the teeth. In a periodontally healthy individual, the position of the brackets is usually determined

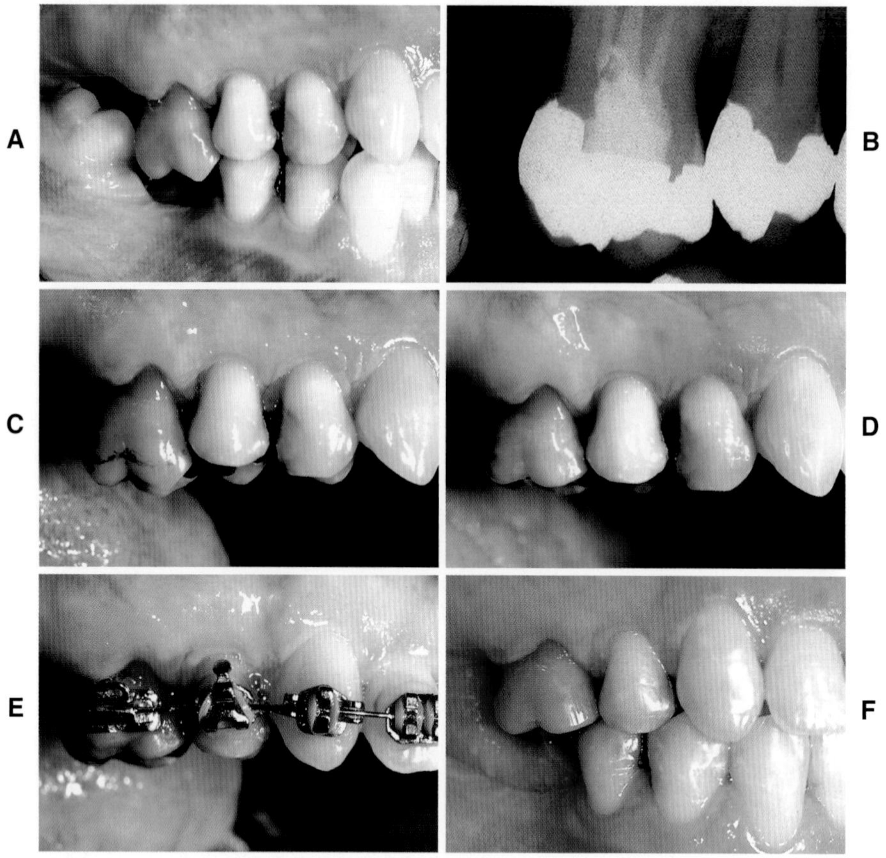

Figure 57-4 This patient showed overeruption of the maxillary right first molar and a marginal ridge defect between the second premolar and first molar **(A).** Pretreatment periapical radiograph **(B)** showed that the interproximal bone was flat. To avoid creating a hemiseptal defect, the occlusal surface of the first molar was equilibrated (**C** and **D**), and the malocclusion was corrected orthodontically (**E** and **F**).

by the anatomy of the crowns of the teeth. Anterior brackets should be positioned relative to the incisal edges. Posterior bands or brackets are positioned relative to the marginal ridges. If the incisal edges and marginal ridges are at the correct level, the cementoenamel junction (CEJ) will also be at the same level. This relationship creates a flat, bony contour between the teeth. However, if a patient has underlying periodontal problems and significant alveolar bone loss around certain teeth, using the anatomy of the crown to determine bracket placement is not appropriate (Figure 57-6).

In a patient with advanced horizontal bone loss, the bone level may have receded several millimeters from the CEJ. As this occurs, the crown-to-root ratio becomes less favorable. By aligning the crowns of the teeth, the clinician may perpetuate tooth mobility by maintaining an unfavorable crown-to-root ratio. In addition, by aligning the crowns of the teeth and disregarding the bone level, significant bone discrepancies occur between healthy and periodontally diseased roots. This could require periodontal surgery to ameliorate the discrepancies.

Many of these problems can be corrected by using the bone level as a guide to position the brackets on the teeth (see Figure 57-6). In these situations the crowns of the teeth may require considerable equilibration. If the tooth is vital, the equilibration should be performed gradually to allow the pulp to form secondary dentin and insulate the tooth during the equilibration process. The goal of equilibration and creative bracket placement is to provide a more favorable bony architecture as well as a more favorable crown-to-root ratio. In some of these patients, the periodontal defects that were apparent initially may not require periodontal surgery after orthodontic treatment.

Furcation Defects

Furcation defects can be classified as *incipient* (class I), *moderate* (class II), or *advanced* (class III). These lesions require special attention in the patient undergoing orthodontic treatment. Often the molars require bands with tubes and other attachments that impede the patient's access to the buccal furcation for home care and instrumentation at the time of recall.

Furcation lesions require special consideration because they are the most difficult lesions to maintain and can worsen during orthodontic therapy. These patients need to be maintained on a 2- to 3-month recall schedule. Detailed instrumentation of these furcations helps minimize further periodontal breakdown.

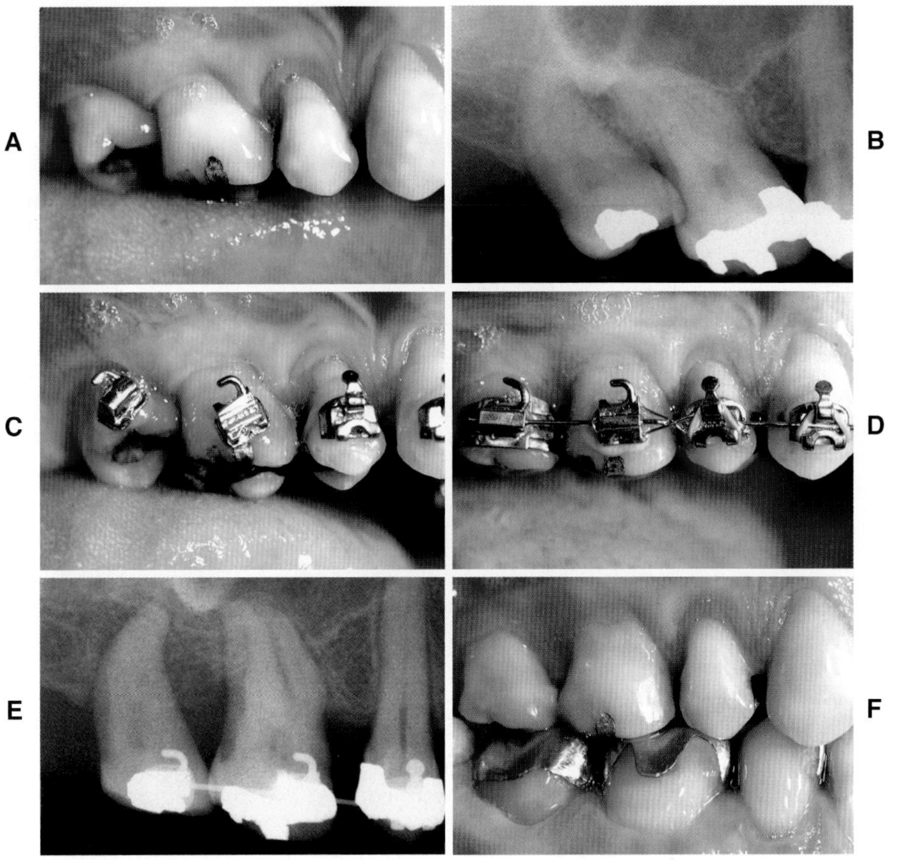

Figure 57-5 Before orthodontic treatment, this patient had significant mesial tipping of the maxillary right first and second molars, causing marginal ridge discrepancies **(A).** The tipping produced root proximity between the molars **(B).** To eliminate the root proximity, the brackets were placed perpendicular to the long axis of the teeth **(C).** This method of bracket placement facilitated root alignment and elimination of the root proximity, as well as leveling of the marginal ridge discrepancies (**D, E,** and **F**).

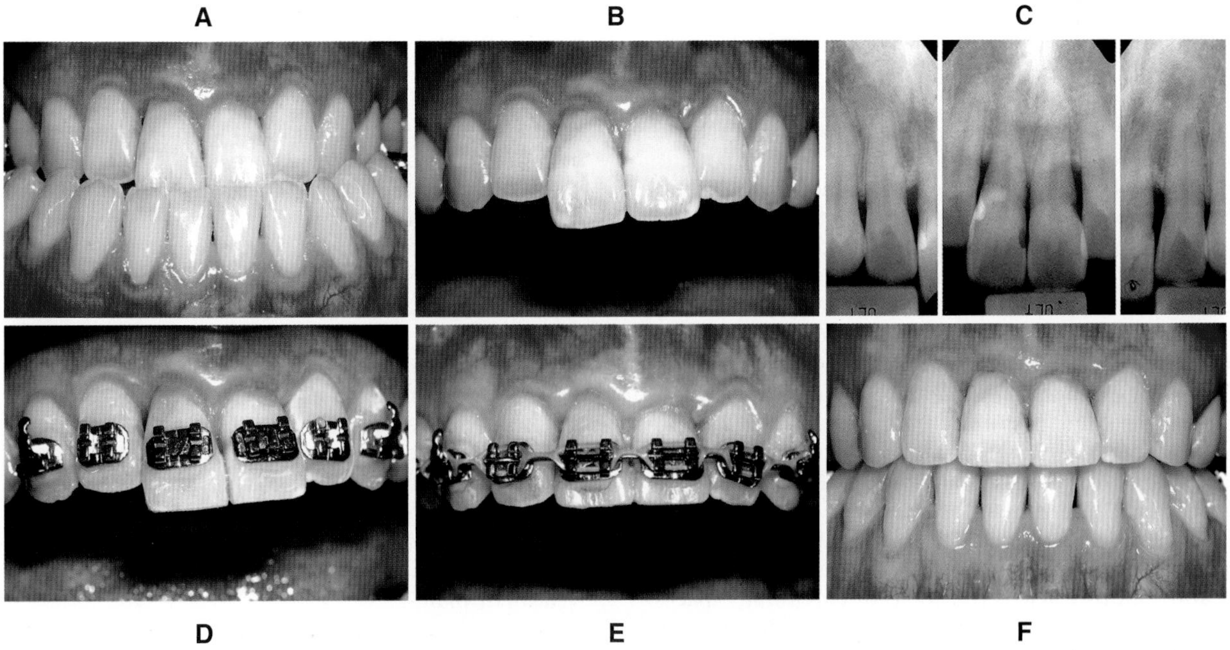

Figure 57-6 Before orthodontic treatment, this patient had a significant class III malocclusion **(A).** The maxillary central incisors had overerupted **(B)** relative to the occlusal plane. Pretreatment periapical radiograph **(C)** showed that significant horizontal bone loss had occurred. To avoid creating a vertical periodontal defect by intruding the central incisors, the brackets were placed to maintain the bone height **(D).** The incisal edges of the centrals were equilibrated **(E),** and the orthodontic treatment was completed without intruding the incisors **(F).**

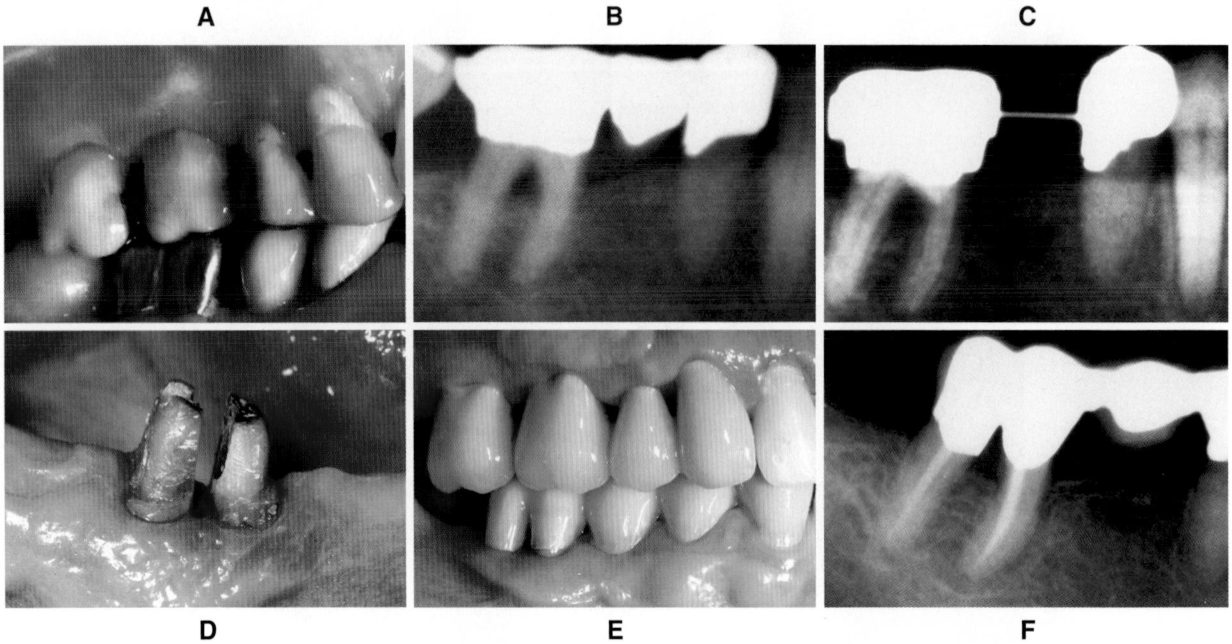

Figure 57-7 This patient had a class III furcation defect before orthodontic treatment (**A** and **B**). Orthodontic treatment was performed **(C)**, and the furcation defect was maintained by the periodontist on 2-month recalls until after orthodontic treatment. After appliance removal, the tooth was hemisected **(D)**, and the roots were restored and splinted together **(E)**. The final periapical radiograph **(F)** shows that the furcation defect has been eliminated by hemisecting and restoring the two root fragments.

If a patient with a class III furcation defect will be undergoing orthodontic treatment, a possible method for treating the furcation is to eliminate it by hemisecting the crown and root of the tooth (Figure 57-7). However, this procedure requires endodontic, periodontal, and restorative treatment. If the patient will be undergoing orthodontic treatment, it is advisable to perform the orthodontic treatment first. This is especially true if the roots of the teeth will not be moved apart. In these patients the molar to be hemisected remains intact during orthodontics. This patient would require 2- or 3-month recall visits to ensure that the furcation defect does not lose bone during orthodontic treatment. Keeping the tooth intact during the orthodontic therapy simplifies the concentration of tooth movement for the orthodontist. After orthodontic treatment, endodontic therapy is required (followed by periodontal surgery) to divide the tooth.

In some patients requiring hemisection of a mandibular molar with a class III furcation, pushing the roots apart during orthodontic treatment may be advantageous (Figure 57-8). If the hemisected molar will be used as an abutment for a bridge after orthodontics, moving the roots apart orthodontically permits a favorable restoration and splinting across the adjacent edentulous spaces. In these patients, hemisection, endodontic therapy, and periodontal surgery must be completed before the start of orthodontic treatment. After completion of these procedures, bands or brackets can be placed on the root fragments and coil springs used to separate the roots. The amount of separation is determined by the size of the adjacent edentulous spaces and the occlusion in the opposing arch. About 7 or 8 mm may be created between the roots of the hemisected molar. This process eliminates the original furcation problem and allows the patient to clean the area with greater efficiency.

In some molars with class III furcation defects, the tooth may have short roots, advanced bone loss, fused roots, or other problems that prevent hemisection and crowning of the remaining roots. In these patients, extracting the root with a furcation defect and placing an implant may be more advisable[11] (Figure 57-9). If this type of plan has been adopted, the timing of the extraction and placement of the implant can occur at any time relative to the orthodontic treatment. In some patients the implant can be used as an anchor to facilitate prerestorative orthodontic treatment.

The implant must remain embedded in bone for 4 to 6 months after placement before it can be loaded as an orthodontic anchor. It must be placed precisely so that it not only provides an anchor for tooth movement, but also may be used an eventual abutment for a crown or fixed bridge. If the implant will not be used as an anchor for orthodontic movement, it may be placed after the orthodontic treatment has been completed. Considerations regarding timing are determined by the restorative treatment plan.

Root Proximity

When roots of posterior teeth are close together, the ability to maintain periodontal health and accessibility for restoration of adjacent teeth may be compromised.[4] However, for the patient undergoing orthodontic therapy, the roots can be moved apart, and bone will form

A B C

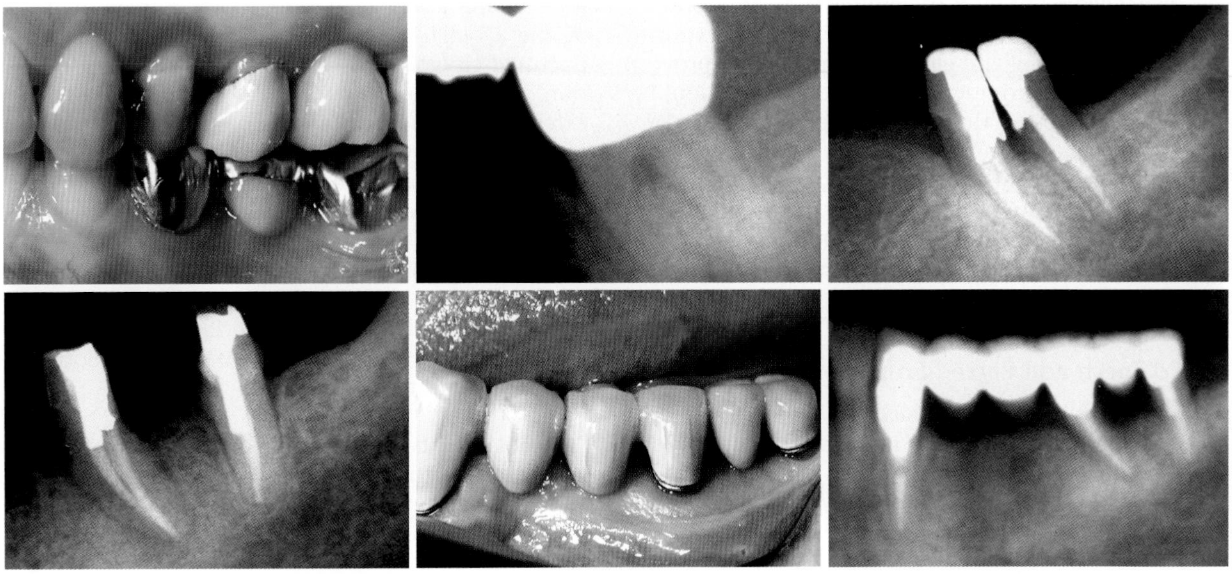

D E F

Figure 57-8 Before orthodontic treatment, this patient had a class III furcation defect in the mandibular left second molar (**A** and **B**). Because the patient had an edentulous space mesial to the molar, the tooth was hemisected **(C),** and the root fragments were separated orthodontically **(D).** After orthodontic treatment, the root fragments were used as abutments to stabilize a multiunit posterior bridge (**E** and **F**).

A B C

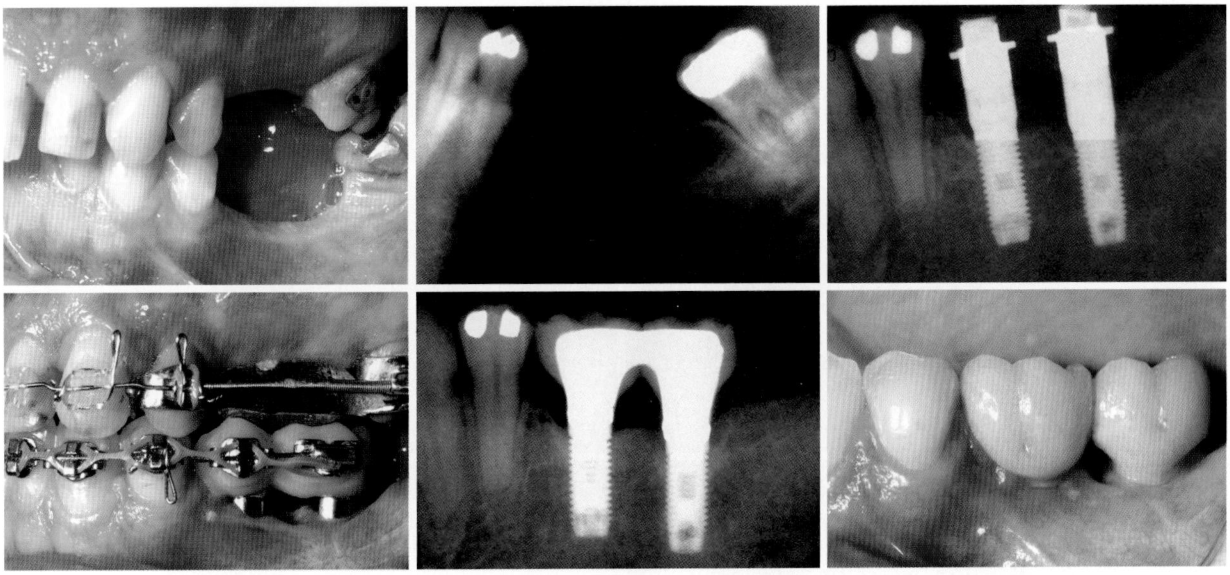

D E F

Figure 57-9 This patient was missing several teeth in the mandibular left posterior quadrant **(A).** The mandibular left third molar had a class III furcation defect and short roots **(B).** The third molar was extracted, and two implants were placed in the mandibular left posterior quadrant **(C).** The implants were used as anchors to facilitate orthodontic treatment **(D)** and help reestablish the left posterior occlusion (**E** and **F**).

between the adjacent roots (see Figure 57-5). This opens the embrasure beneath the tooth contact, provides additional bone support, and enhances the patient's access to the interproximal region for hygiene. This approach generally improves the periodontal health of this area.

If orthodontic treatment will be used to move roots apart, this plan must be known before bracket placement. It is advantageous to place the brackets so that the orthodontic movement to separate the roots will begin with the initial archwires (see Figure 57-5). Therefore, brackets must be placed obliquely to facilitate this process. Radiographs are needed to monitor the progress of orthodontic root separation. Generally, 2 to 3 mm of root separation provides adequate bone and embrasure space to improve periodontal health. During this time, the patient should be maintained to ensure that a favorable bone response occurs as the roots are moved apart. In addition, these patients need occasional occlusal adjustment to recontour the crown because the roots are moving apart. As this occurs, the crowns may develop an unusual occlusal contact with the opposing arch. This should be equilibrated to improve the occlusion.

Fractured Teeth and Forced Eruption

Occasionally, children and adolescents may fall and injure their anterior teeth. If the injuries are minor and result in small fractures of enamel, these can be restored with light-cured composite or porcelain veneers. In some patients, however, the fracture may extend beneath the level of the gingival margin and terminate at the level of the alveolar ridge (Figure 57-10); restoration of the fractured crown is impossible because the tooth preparation would extend to the level of the bone. This overextension of the crown margin could result in an invasion of the biologic width of the tooth and cause persistent inflammation of the marginal gingiva. It may be beneficial in such cases to erupt the fractured root out of the bone and move the fracture margin coronally so that it can be properly restored.[10] However, if the fracture extends too far apically, it may be better to extract the tooth and replace it with an implant or bridge. The following six criteria are used to determine whether the tooth should be forcibly erupted or extracted:

1. *Root length.* Is the root long enough so that a one-to-one crown/root ratio will be preserved after the root has been erupted? To answer this question, the

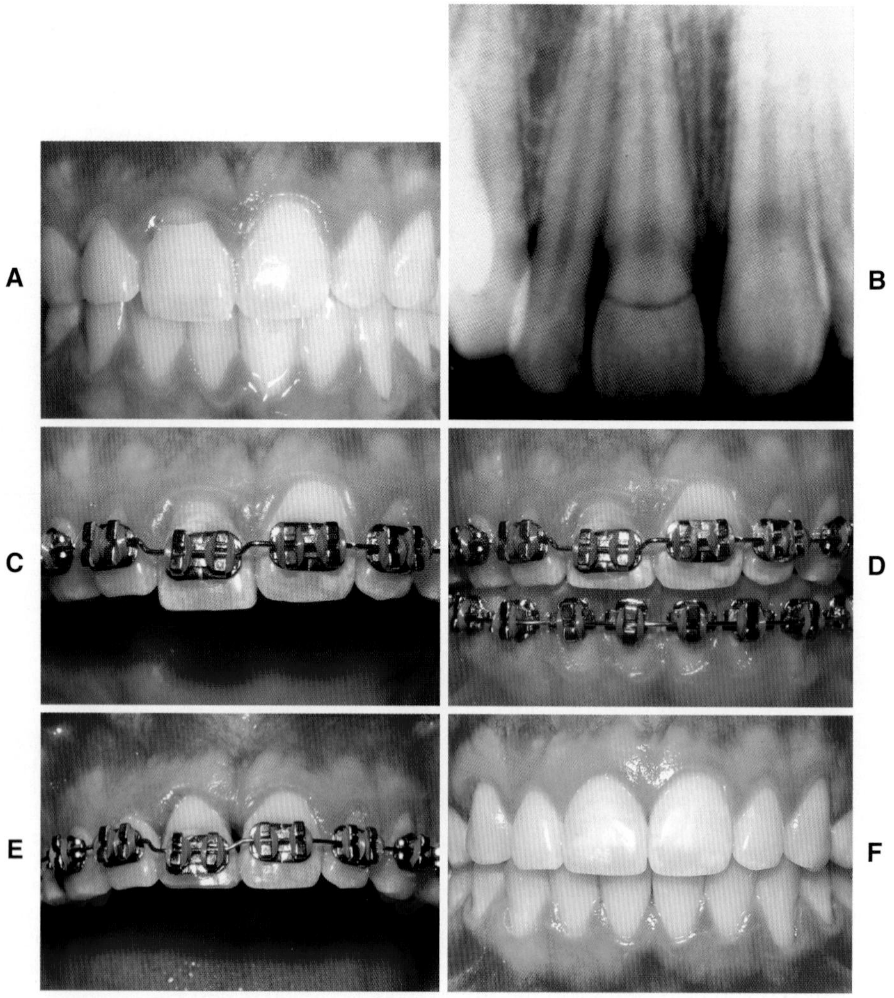

Figure 57-10 This patient had a severe fracture of the maxillary right central incisor **(A)** that extended apical to the level of the alveolar crest on the lingual side **(B)**. To restore the tooth adequately and avoid impinging on the periodontium, the fractured root was extruded 4 mm **(C)**. As the tooth erupted, the gingival margin followed the tooth **(D)**. Gingival surgery was required to lengthen the crown of the central incisor **(E)** so that the final restoration had sufficient ferrule for resistance and retention and the appropriate gingival margin relationship with the adjacent central incisor **(F)**.

clinician must know how far to erupt the root. If a tooth fracture extends to the level of the bone, it must be erupted 4 mm. The first 2.5 mm moves the fracture margin far enough away from the bone to prevent a biologic width problem. The other 1.5 mm provides the proper amount of ferrule for adequate resistance form of the crown preparation. Therefore, if the root is fractured to the bone level and must be erupted 4 mm, the periapical radiograph must be evaluated (see Figure 57-10, *B*) and 4 mm subtracted from the end of the fractured tooth root. The length of the residual root should be compared with the length of the eventual crown on this tooth. The root/crown ratio should be about 1:1. If the root/crown ratio is less than this amount, there may be too little root remaining in the bone for stability. In the latter situation, it may be prudent to extract the root and place a bridge or implant.

2. *Root form.* The shape of the root should be broad and nontapering rather than thin and tapered. A thin, tapered root provides a narrower cervical region after the tooth has been erupted 4 mm. This could compromise the esthetic appearance of the final restoration. The internal root form is also important. If the root canal is wide, the distance between the external root surface and root canal filling will be narrow. In these patients the walls of the crown preparation are thin, which could result in early fracture of the restored root. The root canal should not be more than one third of the overall width of the root. In this way, the root could still provide adequate strength for the final restoration.
3. *Level of the fracture.* If the entire crown is fractured 2 to 3 mm apical to the level of the alveolar bone, it is difficult, if not impossible, to attach to the root to erupt it.
4. *Relative importance of the tooth.* If the patient is 70 years of age and both adjacent teeth have prosthetic crowns, it would be more prudent to construct a fixed bridge. However, if the patient is 15 years of age and the adjacent teeth are unrestored, forced eruption would be much more conservative and appropriate.
5. *Esthetics.* If the patient has a high lip line and displays 2 to 3 mm of gingiva when smiling, any type of restoration in this area will be more obvious. Keeping the patient's own tooth would be much more esthetic than any type of implant or prosthetic replacement.
6. *Endodontic/periodontal prognosis.* If the tooth has a significant periodontal defect, it may not be possible to retain the root. In addition, if the tooth root has a vertical fracture, the prognosis would be poor, and extraction of the tooth would be the proper course of therapy.

If all these factors are favorable, forced eruption of the fractured root is indicated. The orthodontic mechanics necessary to erupt the tooth can vary from elastic traction to orthodontic banding and bracketing. If a large portion of the tooth is still present, orthodontic bracketing is necessary. If the entire crown has fractured, leaving only the root, elastic traction from a bonded bar may be possible. The root may be erupted rapidly or slowly. If the movement is performed rapidly, the alveolar bone will be left behind temporarily, and a circumferential fiberotomy may be performed to prevent bone from following the erupted root. However, if the root is erupted slowly, the bone follows the tooth. In this situation the erupted root requires crown lengthening to expose the correct amount of tooth to create the proper ferrule, resistance form, and retention for the final restoration.

After the tooth root has been erupted, it must be stabilized to prevent it from intruding back into the alveolus. The reason for *reintrusion* is the orientation of the principal fibers of the periodontium. During forced eruption, the periodontal fibers become oriented obliquely and stretched as the root moves coronally. These fibers eventually reorient themselves after about 6 months. Before this occurs, the root can reintrude significantly. Therefore, if this type of treatment is performed, an adequate period of stabilization is necessary to avoid significant relapse and reintrusion of the root.

As the root erupts, the gingiva moves coronally with the tooth. As a result, the clinical crown length becomes shorter after extrusion (see Figure 57-10). In addition, the gingival margin may be positioned more incisally than the adjacent teeth. In these patients, gingival surgery is necessary to create ideal gingival margin heights. The type of surgery varies depending on whether bone removal is necessary. If bone has followed the root during eruption, a flap is elevated, and the appropriate amount of bone is removed to match the bone height of the adjacent teeth. If the bone level is flat between adjacent teeth, a simple excisional gingivectomy corrects the gingival margin discrepancy.

After gingival surgery, an open gingival embrasure may exist between the erupted root and adjacent teeth (see Figure 57-10). The space occurs because the narrower root portion of the erupted tooth has been moved into the oral cavity. This space may be closed in two ways: (1) overcontouring of the replacement restoration and (2) reshaping of the crown of the tooth and movement of the root to close the space. The second method often helps improve the overall shape of the final crown on the restored tooth.

Hopeless Teeth Maintained for Orthodontic Anchorage

Patients with advanced periodontal disease may have specific teeth diagnosed as hopeless, which would be extracted before orthodontic therapy (Figure 57-11). However, these teeth can be useful for orthodontic anchorage if the periodontal inflammation can be controlled. In moderate to advanced cases, some periodontal surgery may be indicated around a hopeless tooth. Flaps are reflected for debridement of the roots to control inflammation around the hopeless tooth during the orthodontic process. The important factor is to maintain the health of the bone around the adjacent teeth. Periodontal recall is imperative during the process.

After orthodontic treatment, there is a 6-month period of stabilization before reevaluating the periodontal status.

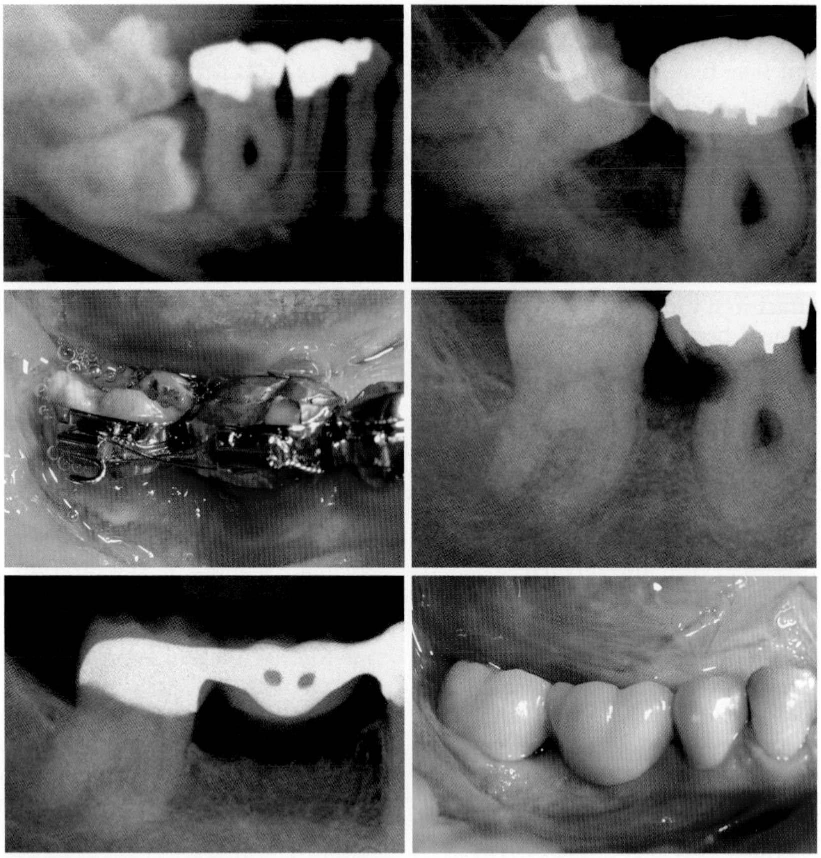

Figure 57-11 This patient had an impacted mandibular right second molar **(A).** The mandibular right first molar was periodontally hopeless because of an advanced class III furcation defect. The impacted second molar was extracted, but the first molar was maintained as an anchor to help upright the third molar orthodontically (**B, C,** and **D**). After orthodontic uprighting of the third molar, the first molar was extracted and a bridge was placed to restore the edentulous space (**E** and **F**).

Occasionally the hopeless tooth may be so improved after orthodontic treatment that it is retained. In most cases, however, the hopeless tooth requires extraction, especially if other restorations are planned in the segment. Again, these decisions require reevaluation by the clinician.

ORTHODONTIC TREATMENT OF GINGIVAL DISCREPANCIES

Uneven Gingival Margins

The relationship of the gingival margins of the six maxillary anterior teeth plays an important role in the esthetic appearance of the crowns. The following four factors contribute to ideal gingival form:

1. The gingival margins of the two central incisors should be at the same level.
2. The gingival margins of the central incisors should be positioned more apically than the lateral incisors and at the same level as the canines.[13]
3. The contour of the labial gingival margins should mimic the CEJs of the teeth.
4. A papilla should exist between each tooth, and the height of the tip of the papilla is usually halfway between the incisal edge and the labial gingival height of contour over the center of each anterior tooth. Therefore the gingival papilla occupies half of the interproximal contact, and the adjacent teeth form the other half of the contact.

However, some patients may have gingival margin discrepancies between adjacent teeth (Figure 57-12). These discrepancies may be caused by abrasion of the incisal edges or delayed migration of the gingival margins. When gingival margin discrepancies are present, the proper solution for the problem must be determined: orthodontic movement to reposition the gingival margins or surgical correction of gingival margin discrepancies.

To make the correct decision, it is necessary to evaluate four criteria. First, the relationship between the gingival margin of the maxillary central incisors and the patient's lip line should be assessed when the patient smiles. If a gingival margin discrepancy is present but the discrepancy is not exposed, it does not require correction.

If a gingival margin discrepancy is apparent, the second step is to evaluate the labial sulcular depth over the two

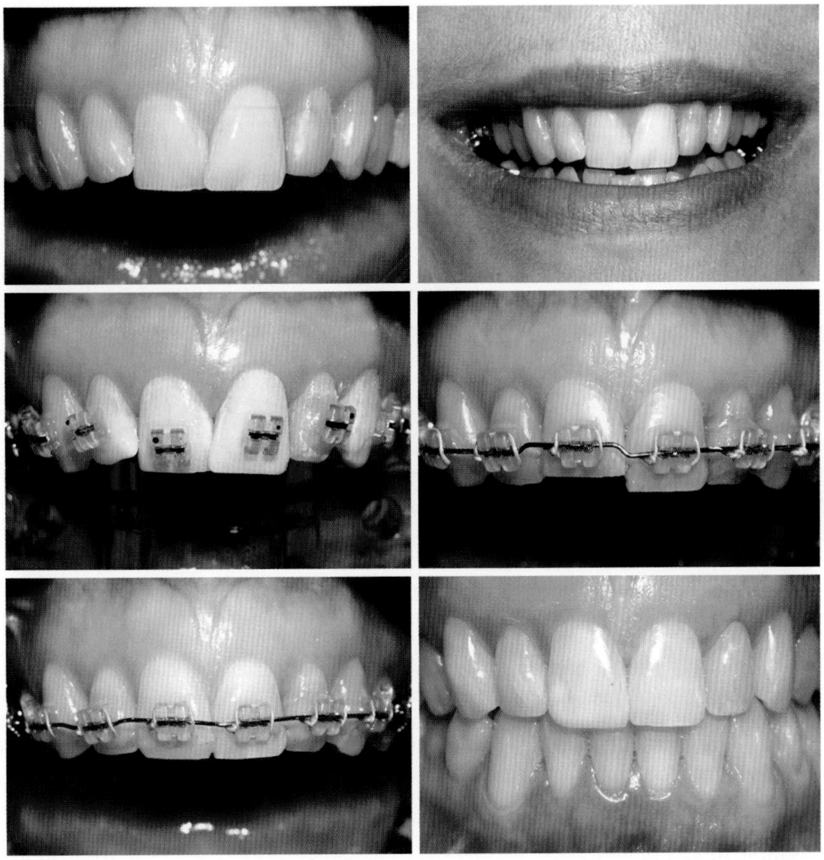

Figure 57-12 This patient had a protrusive bruxing habit that had resulted in abrasion and overeruption of the maxillary right central incisor **(A).** The objective was to level the gingival margins during orthodontic therapy. Although gingival surgery was a possibility, the labial sulcular depth of the maxillary right central incisor was only 1 mm, and the cementoenamel junction was located at the bottom of the sulcus. Therefore the best solution involved positioning the orthodontic brackets to facilitate intrusion of the right central incisor (**B, C,** and **D**). This permitted the restorative dentist to restore the portion of the tooth that the patient had abraded **(E),** resulting in the correct gingival margin levels and crown lengths at the end of treatment **(F).**

central incisors. If the shorter tooth has a deeper sulcus, excisional gingivectomy may be appropriate to move the gingival margin of the shorter tooth apically. However, if the sulcular depths of the short and long incisors are equivalent, gingival surgery does not correct the problem.

The third step is to evaluate the relationship between the shortest central incisor and the adjacent lateral incisors. If the shortest central incisor is still *longer* than the lateral incisors, the other possibility is to extrude the longer central incisor and equilibrate the incisal edge. This moves the gingival margin coronally and eliminates the gingival margin discrepancy. However, if the shortest central incisor is *shorter* than the lateral incisors, this technique would produce an unesthetic relationship between the gingival margins of the central and lateral incisors.

The fourth step is to determine whether the incisal edges have been abraded. This is best accomplished by evaluating the teeth from an incisal perspective. If one incisal edge is thicker labiolingually than the adjacent tooth, this may indicate that it has been abraded and the tooth has overerupted. In such cases, the best method of correcting the gingival margin discrepancy is to intrude the short central incisor (see Figure 57-12). This method moves the gingival margin apically and permits restoration of the incisal edges.[3,6-9] The intrusion should be accomplished at least 6 months before appliance removal. This allows reorientation of the principal fibers of the periodontium and avoids reextrusion of the central incisor(s) after appliance removal.

Significant Abrasion and Overeruption

Occasionally, patients have destructive dental habits, such as a protrusive bruxing habit, that can result in significant wear of the maxillary and mandibular incisors and compensatory overeruption of these teeth (Figure 57-13). The restoration of these abraded teeth is often impossible because of the lack of crown length to achieve adequate retention and resistance form for the crown preparations. Two options are available. One option is extensive crown lengthening by elevating a flap, removing sufficient bone, and apically positioning the flap to expose adequate tooth length for crown preparation. However,

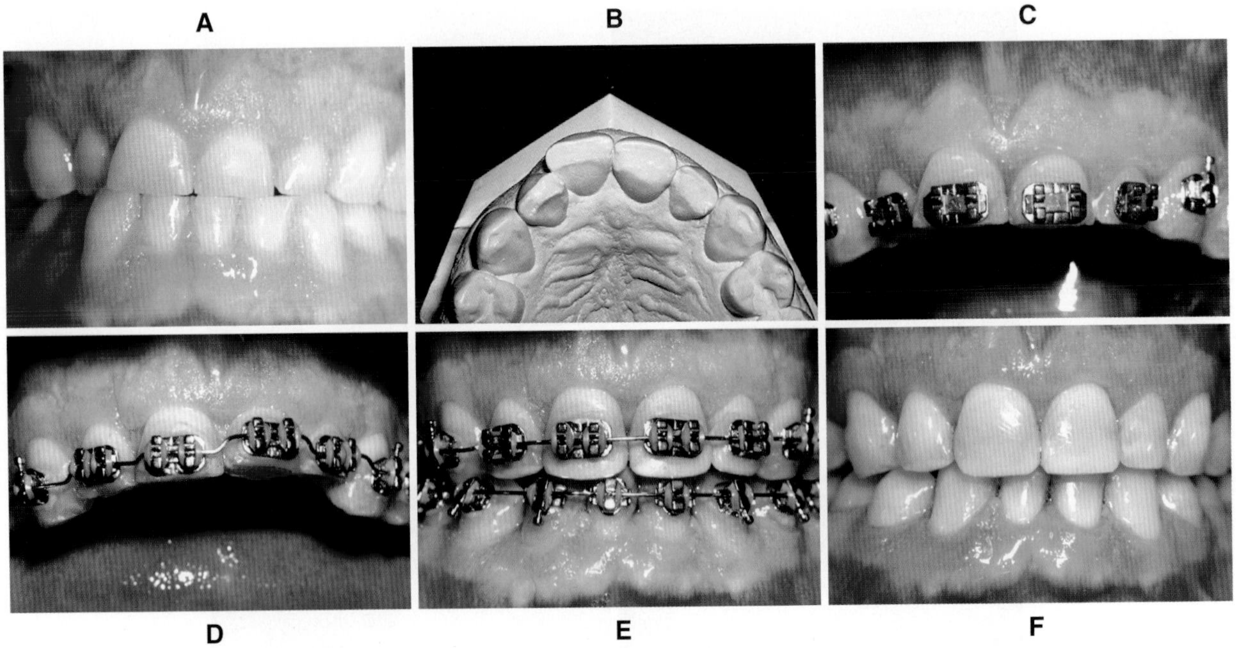

Figure 57-13 This patient had a protrusive bruxing habit that had caused severe abrasion of the maxillary anterior teeth, resulting in the loss of over half of the crown length of the incisors (**A** and **B**). Two possible options existed for gaining crown length to restore the incisors. One possibility was an apically positioned flap with osseous recontouring, which would expose the roots of the teeth. The less destructive option was to intrude the four incisors orthodontically, level the gingival margins (**C** and **D**), and allow the dentist to restore the abraded incisal edges (**E** and **F**). The orthodontic option was clearly successful and desirable in this patient.

this type of procedure is contraindicated in the patient with short, tapered roots because it could adversely affect the final root/crown ratio and potentially open gingival embrasures between the anterior teeth.

The other option for improving the restorability of these short abraded teeth is to intrude the teeth orthodontically and move the gingival margins apically (see Figure 57-13). It is possible to intrude up to four maxillary incisors by using the posterior teeth as anchorage during the intrusion process. This process is accomplished by placing the orthodontic brackets as close to the incisal edges of the maxillary incisors as possible. The brackets are placed in their normal position on the canines and remaining posterior teeth. The patient's posterior occlusion resists the eruption of the posterior teeth, and the incisors gradually intrude and move the gingival margins and the crowns apically. This creates the restorative space necessary to restore the incisal edges of these teeth temporarily and then eventually place the final crowns.

When abraded teeth are significantly intruded, it is necessary to hold these teeth for at least 6 months in the intruded position with orthodontic brackets or archwires (or both), or some type of bonded retainer. The principal fibers of the periodontium must accommodate to the new intruded position, a process that could take a minimum of 6 months in most adult patients. Orthodontic intrusion of severely abraded and overerupted teeth is usually a distinct advantage over periodontal crown lengthening, unless the patient has extremely long and broad roots or has had extensive horizontal periodontal bone loss.

Open Gingival Embrasures

The presence of a papilla between the maxillary central incisors is a key esthetic factor in any individual. Occasionally, adults have open gingival embrasures or lack gingival papillae between their central incisors. These unesthetic areas are often difficult to resolve with periodontal therapy. However, orthodontic treatment can correct many of these open gingival embrasures. This open space is usually caused by (1) tooth shape, (2) root angulation, or (3) periodontal bone loss.[9]

The interproximal contact between the maxillary central incisors consists of two parts: the tooth contact and the papilla. The papilla/contact ratio is 1:1. Half the space is occupied by papilla, and half is formed by the tooth contact. If the patient has an open embrasure, the first aspect that must be evaluated is whether the problem is caused by the papilla or the tooth contact. If the papilla is the problem, the cause is usually a lack of bone support because of an underlying periodontal problem.

In some situations, a deficient papilla can be improved with orthodontic treatment. By closing open contacts, the interproximal gingiva can be squeezed and moved incisally. This type of movement may help create a more esthetic papilla between two teeth despite alveolar bone loss. Another possibility is to erupt adjacent teeth when the interproximal bone level is positioned apically.

Most open embrasures between the central incisors are caused by problems with tooth contact. The first step in the diagnosis of this problem is to evaluate a periapical radiograph of the central incisors. If the root angulation

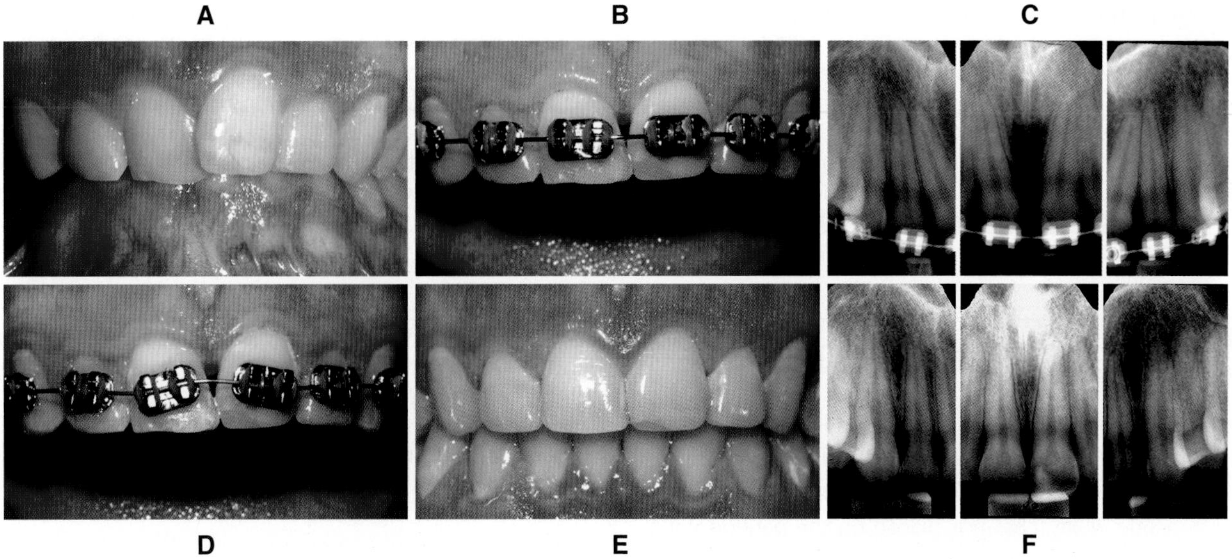

Figure 57-14 This patient initially had overlapped maxillary central incisors **(A),** and after initial orthodontic alignment of the teeth, an open gingival embrasure appeared between the centrals **(B).** Radiograph showed that the open embrasure was caused by divergence of the central incisor roots **(C).** To correct the problem, the central incisor brackets were repositioned **(D),** and the roots were moved together. This required restoration of the incisal edges after orthodontic therapy **(E)** because these teeth had worn unevenly before therapy. As the roots were paralleled **(F),** the tooth contact moved gingivally and the papilla moved incisally, resulting in the elimination of the open gingival embrasure.

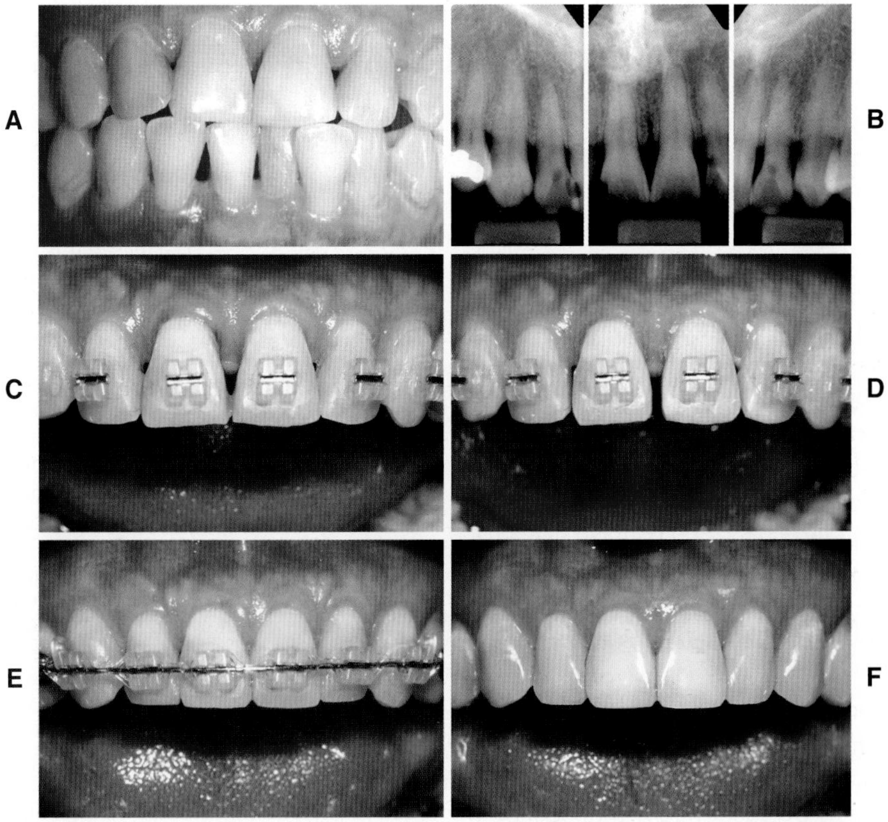

Figure 57-15 This patient initially had triangular-shaped central incisors (**A** and **B**), which produced an open gingival embrasure after orthodontic alignment **(C).** Because the roots of the central incisors were parallel with one another, the appropriate solution for the open gingival embrasure was to recontour the mesial surfaces of the central incisors **(D).** As the diastema was closed **(E),** the tooth contact moved gingivally and the papilla moved incisally, resulting in the elimination of the open gingival embrasure **(F).**

is divergent, the brackets should be repositioned so that the root position can be corrected (Figure 57-14). In these patients the incisal edges may be uneven and require restoration with either composite or porcelain restorations. If the periapical radiograph shows that the roots are in their correct relationship, the open gingival embrasure is caused by a triangular tooth shape (Figure 57-15).

If the shape of the tooth is the problem, two solutions are possible: (1) restore the open gingival embrasure or (2) reshape the tooth by flattening the incisal contact and closing the space (see Figure 57-15). This second option results in lengthening of the contact until it meets the papilla. In addition, if the embrasure space is large, closing the space squeezes the papilla between the central incisors. This helps create a 1:1 ratio between the contact and papilla and restores uniformity to the heights between the midline and adjacent papillae.

SCIENCE TRANSFER

Orthodontic therapy can be used to resolve some types of periodontal osseous defects. As the tooth moves, pressure is placed on the periodontal ligament on the compression side while tension is placed on the periodontal ligament on the opposite side. This results in bone resorption and bone formation, respectively. Interestingly, the periodontal ligament dimensions after the movement are maintained. Thus, sustained tension on the periodontal ligament results in bone formation, and sustained lack of tension results in bone resorption. There appears to be a physiologic equilibrium of forces (or balance of forces) in which bone formation and bone resorption are balanced. This occurs at the same time the periodontal ligament physiologically turns over at a high rate (which likewise could play an important role in the balance of bone formation and resorption). Sustained tension through Sharpey's fibers appears to stimulate osteoblast cell activation or decrease osteoclastic activity; the converse occurs on the opposite side. The exact mechanisms for these processes are not known. However, the periodontal response to orthodontic tooth movement represents an exquisitely controlled tissue response.

Orthodontic movement can enhance the results of periodontal therapy by optimizing tooth positions, and in some hemiseptal defects, extrusion can eliminate the defect. Extrusion may be used to solve problems of short crowns, and if teeth are slowly erupted, bone and gingival margins move coronally with the tooth. With fast, forced eruption, bone remains stable, and a short crown can be moved coronally to improve any biologic width problems. When periodontally involved teeth are being moved orthodontically, it is essential that (1) all calculus be removed by root planing and (2) plaque levels be kept low throughout treatment, with frequent recall appointments. Otherwise, significant bone loss can accompany the orthodontic therapy. Occasionally, a preorthodontic periodontal surgical procedure is necessary to ensure roots are free of calculus.

SUMMARY

There are many benefits to integrating orthodontics and periodontics in the management of adult patients with underlying periodontal defects. The key to treating these patients is communication and proper diagnosis before orthodontic therapy, as well as continued dialog during orthodontic treatment. Not all periodontal problems are treated in the same way. This chapter provides a framework for the integration of orthodontics to solve periodontal problems.

REFERENCES

1. Becker W, Becker BE: Treatment of mandibular 3-wall intrabony defects by flap debridement and expanded polytetrafluoroethylene barrier membranes: long-term evaluation of 32 treated patients, *J Periodontol* 64:1138, 1993.
2. Brown IA: The effect of orthodontic therapy on certain types of periodontal defects. I. Clinical findings, *J Periodontol* 44:742, 1973.
3. Chiche G, Kokich V, Caudill R: Diagnosis and treatment planning of esthetic problems. In Pinault A, Chiche G, editors: *Esthetics in fixed prosthodontics,* Chicago, 1994, Quintessence.
4. Gould MS, Picton DC: The relation between irregularities of the teeth and periodontal disease, *Br Dent J* 121:21, 1966.
5. Ingber J: Forced eruption. Part I. A method of treating isolated one and two wall infrabony osseous defects: rationale and case report, *J Periodontol* 45:199, 1974.
6. Kokich V: Enhancing restorative, esthetic and periodontal results with orthodontic therapy. In Schluger S, Youdelis R, Page R, et al, editors: *Periodontal therapy,* Philadelphia, 1990, Lea & Febiger.
7. Kokich V: Anterior dental esthetics: an orthodontic perspective. I. Crown length, *J Esthet Dent* 5:19, 1993.
8. Kokich V: Esthetics: the orthodontic-periodontic-restorative connection, *Semin Orthod* 2:21, 1996.
9. Kokich V: Esthetics and vertical tooth position: the orthodontic possibilities, *Compend Contin Educ Dent* 1997; 18:1225.
10. Kokich V, Nappen D, Shapiro P: Gingival contour and clinical crown length: their effects on the esthetic appearance of maxillary anterior teeth, *Am J Orthod* 86:89, 1984.
11. Kramer GM: Surgical alternatives in regenerative therapy of the periodontium. *Int J Periodont Restor Dent* 12:11, 1992.
12. Ochsenbein C, Ross S: A re-evaluation of osseous surgery, *Dent Clin North Am* 13:87, 1969.
13. Rufenacht C: Structural esthetic rules. In Rufenacht C, editor: *Fundamental of esthetics,* Chicago, 1990, Quintessence.
14. Schallhorn R, McClain P: Combined osseous composite grafting, root conditioning and guided tissue regeneration, *Int J Periodont Restor Dent* 8:9, 1988.
15. Schluger S: Osseous resection: a basic principle in periodontal surgery, *Oral Surg* 2:316, 1949.

The Periodontic–Endodontic Continuum

William F. Ammons, Jr., and Gerald W. Harrington

58

CHAPTER

CHAPTER OUTLINE

The simultaneous existence of pulpal problems and inflammatory periodontal disease can complicate diagnosis and treatment planning and affect the sequence of care to be performed. This is particularly true for the patient with advanced periodontitis, tooth loss, and pulpal disease.

PULPAL DISEASE

Etiologic Factors

The major causes of pulpal inflammation are (1) instrumentation during periodontal, restorative, or prosthetic dentistry; (2) the progression of dental caries; and (3) direct, local trauma such as tooth fracture. The extent of inflammation of the pulp and the signs and symptoms that result vary with the severity of the insult and the ability of the host to ameliorate the inflammation that results.

Of these, dental caries is the most common cause of pulpal disease. Bacteria are present in carious enamel and dentin. Although the numbers of bacteria may diminish in the deepest layers of the dentin, the ability of microorganisms and their byproducts to penetrate through the dentinal tubules and to provoke pulpal inflammation is well documented.[6,7] Direct exposure of the pulp by caries[21] or sealing infected pulps may alter the process of infection if the pulp is unable to eliminate the bacteria.[6,20] The dynamics of the pulpal reaction is dictated by the virulence of the bacteria, the host response, the effectiveness of pulpal circulation, and the degree of vascular and lymphatic drainage.[41]

Pulpal infection is a polymicrobial process. Although a correlation between causation and any species of bacteria is not currently possible,[2] studies based on culturing suggest that a mean of five bacterial strains may be cultured from infected root canals.[3] The organisms cultured are predominantly gram-negative anaerobes.[2,3,10,13,38] As the infective process proceeds, the proportion of strict anaerobic-to-facultative organisms and the total number of bacteria increase. Table 58-1 lists the most common organisms associated with pulpitis.

Classification

The correlation between the histology of pulpal disease and the patient's symptoms is poor. Therefore, pulpal disease is generally classified based on clinical signs and symptoms rather than on histologic changes[20,41] (Box 58-1).

TABLE 58-1

Bacteria Associated with Pulpitis

Genus of Bacteria	Number of Strains	Gram Stain
Eubacterium	59	Gram positive, nonmotile
Peptostreptococcus	54	Gram positive, nonmotile
Fusobacterium	50	Gram negative, nonmotile
Porphyromonas	32	Gram negative, nonmotile
Prevotella	45	Gram negative, nonmotile
Streptococcus	28	Gram positive, nonmotile
Lactobacillus	24	Gram positive, nonmotile
Wolinella	18	Gram negative, motile
Actinomyces	14	Gram-positive rod, nonmotile

Modified from Sundqvist G, Johansson E, Sjogren U: *J Endodont* 15:13, 1989; and Baumgartner JC, Falkler WA: *J Endodont* 17:380, 1991.

BOX 58-1

Classification of Pulpal Disease

Reversible pulpitis
Irreversible pulpitis
Hyperplastic pulpitis
Pulpal necrosis

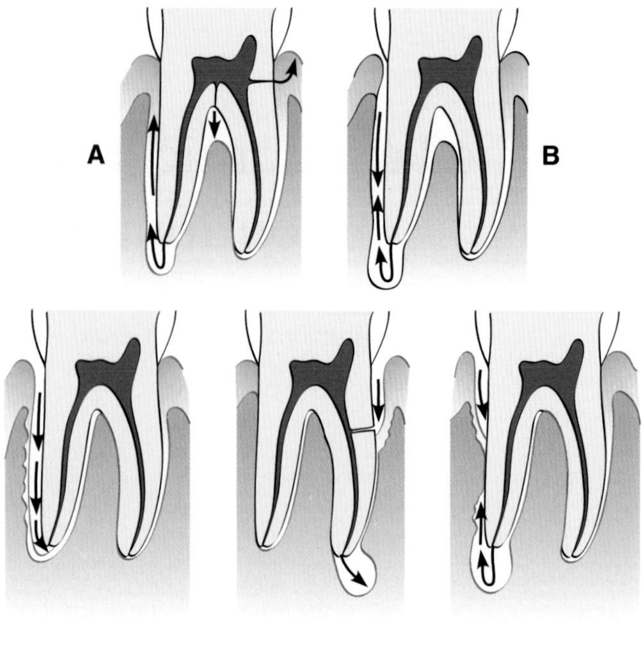

Figure 58-1 Diagrammatic representation of different types of endoperiodontal problems. **A,** Originally an endodontic problem, with fistulization from the apex and along the root to the gingiva. Pulpal infection can also spread through accessory canals to the gingiva or the furcation. **B,** Long-standing periapical lesion draining through the periodontal ligament can become secondarily complicated, leading to a *retrograde periodontitis.* **C,** Periodontal pocket can deepen to the apex and secondarily involve the pulp. **D,** Periodontal pocket can infect the pulp through a lateral canal, which in turn can result in a periapical lesion. **E,** Two independent lesions, periapical and marginal, can coexist and eventually fuse with each other. (Redrawn and modified from Simon JH, Glick DH, Frank AL: *J Periodontol* 43:202, 1972.)

Minor injury such as periodontal root planing or the conservative preparation of a tooth for a restoration may lead to pulpal symptoms. A transient hypersensitivity to thermal stimuli is the most common symptom noted. The application of a thermal stimulus results in a brief, painful response that varies in intensity from mild to severe. The response rapidly disappears after removal of the stimulus. Although permanent pulpal damage may not occur, a transient inflammatory response can lead to the deposition of reparative dentin if odontoblasts are destroyed. The reversibility of inflammation and symptoms, without permanent pulpal damage, has led to a classification of this condition as *reversible pulpitis.*

If the pulp is affected to the point that the inflammatory lesion cannot be resolved, even though the source of the trauma is eliminated, a progressive degeneration of the pulp results. This progression has been described as *irreversible pulpitis;* the patient may have no symptoms or may have intermittent or continuous episodes of spontaneous pain. The application of heat to a tooth with irreversible pulpitis can lead to an immediate painful response that can persist for a prolonged period. Cold may also provoke such a response, although occasionally the application of cold may provide relief from the pain. A reduced responsiveness of teeth with irreversible pulpitis to thermal stimuli has been claimed, but Mumford[26] found similar pain thresholds in both inflamed and noninflamed pulps.

Irreversible pulpitis ultimately leads to loss of pulpal vitality (necrosis). Necrosis usually results from the same factors that induced the irreversible pulpitis and may lead to an alteration in the patient's symptoms. Not all nonvital teeth display signs and symptoms of pulpal disease, and necrotic pulps are often asymptomatic. When present, symptoms may manifest as episodes of spontaneous pain. Testing the pulp with heat may be inconclusive, and a response to cold stimuli is rare.

Effects on the Periodontium

Pulpal tissue may be significantly inflamed and yet exert little or no effect on the periodontium. As long as the pulp remains vital, it is unlikely that significant changes will occur in the periodontium. Necrosis of the pulp, however, can result in bone resorption and the production of radiolucency at the apex of the tooth, in the furcation, or at points along the root[25,34,39,42] (Figure 58-1). Dental radiographs usually document the presence of apical or lateral lesions.

The resulting lesion may be an acute apical lesion or abscess, a more chronic periradicular lesion (cyst or

BOX 58-2

Classification of Periradicular Lesions

Acute apical periodontitis
Chronic apical periodontitis
Condensing osteitis
Acute apical abscess
Chronic apical abscess

granuloma), or a lesion associated with a lateral or accessory canal. The lesion may remain small, or it can expand sufficiently to destroy a substantial amount of the attachment of the tooth and communicate with a lesion of periodontitis. Box 58-2 provides a classification of periradicular lesions.

The histopathologic structure of the periapical inflammatory lesion is usually a highly vascularized granulation tissue infiltrated to varying degrees by inflammatory cells. Neutrophils may be present near the apical foramen, whereas plasma cells, macrophages, lymphocytes, and fibroblasts are increased in the periphery of the lesion.[6,28,43,44] This cellular infiltrate may vary with the nature and intensity of the irritants to the tissues.

Similar lesions may develop adjacent to accessory or lateral canals. These canals form when the epithelial root sheath breaks down before root formation or when anastomoses between the dental papilla and the dental sac persist. Although many of the anastomoses are blocked or reduced by the formation of dentin or the depositing of cementum, some of the communications between the pulp and periodontium may remain patent in the adult dentition. Lateral canals are usually not visible on x-ray films and are most often identified only when the root and lateral canal has been filled with a radiopaque material during endodontic therapy.

The incidence of accessory and lateral canals has been reported as ranging from 2% to 27%, but the true incidence is unknown.[9,12,42] The majority of these canals occur in the apical portion of the root, with decreased numbers in the furcation area. They are more common in posterior teeth and in the apical portion of the root.[9,22,33] The prevalence of lateral canals in the middle and cervical areas of the root and the prevalence of endodontic-derived lesions in the marginal periodontium through lateral or accessory canals are low. The clinical significance of accessory or lateral canals in spreading infection from the necrotic pulp to the periodontium is therefore unclear. Necrotic pulps apparently exert no effect through the dentinal tubules on the cementum.[1]

EFFECT OF PERIODONTITIS ON THE DENTAL PULP

Although the effects of pulpal disease on the periodontium are well documented, a clear-cut relationship between periodontitis and pulpal involvement is less evident. One may postulate that bacteria and the inflammatory products of periodontitis could gain access to the pulp through accessory canals, apical foramina, or dentinal tubules. This process, the reverse of the effects of a necrotic pulp on the periodontal ligament, has been referred to as *retrograde pulpitis*.[31,35]

However, although inflammatory changes have been reported adjacent to accessory canals exposed by periodontitis, periodontitis rarely produces significant changes in the dental pulp. Neither irreversible pulpitis nor pulpal necrosis has been consistently found in histologic studies of teeth extracted because of severe periodontal disease.[8,20,40] It has been suggested that the presence of an intact layer of cementum may protect the pulp from injurious elements produced by plaque microbiota.[1] Severe breakdown of the pulp apparently does not occur until periodontitis has reached a terminal state, that is, when bacterial plaque has involved the main apical foramina.[20] The pulp has a good capacity for defense as long as the blood supply through the apical foramina is intact. Therefore, retrograde periodontitis, if it occurs, is exceedingly rare.[14,15,40]

DIFFERENTIATION BETWEEN PERIODONTAL AND PULPAL LESIONS

Signs and Symptoms of Periodontitis

The signs and symptoms of periodontitis are described in Chapters 31 to 33. Periodontitis is a chronic inflammatory lesion that begins in the marginal gingiva and extends apically, causing attachment loss and periodontal pocket formation. In general, the progression rate of attachment loss is slow, unless an acute event such as a periodontal abscess occurs.

Teeth with chronic periodontal lesions are typically free of acute symptoms. The patient may be unaware of the condition, except for bleeding on brushing and flossing or bad breath, until sufficient attachment is lost, resulting in increased tooth mobility. The pocket may be tender to probing, and extensive deposits may be present on the root(s) of the tooth (teeth). Probing is usually accompanied by bleeding and in deeper pockets with suppuration. However, significant discomfort is not elicited by percussion or thermal stimuli. Increased tooth mobility may occur if sufficient attachment has been lost. Dental radiographs usually disclose the extent of attachment loss, which should correlate with clinical probing data.

Signs and Symptoms of Pulpal Disease

The pulp has the ability to respond to stimulation through enamel or dentin or directly to the pulp. Higher nerve centers interpret these sensations as pain. Some evidence indicates that the pulp may also sense temperature and touch,[27] although the ability to discriminate between hot and cold may be affected by age.[19] The character of the pain may vary with its source. Initiation of pulpal sensation by stimulating dentin is usually fast, sharp, and severe and is mediated by A-delta myelinated fibers. Sensation from the core of the pulp is initiated by smaller, unmyelinated C fibers. This pain has been described as being slower, duller, and more diffuse.[27]

The only symptom a patient with reversible pulpitis may report is a sensitivity to hot or cold fluids. The period of discomfort is usually brief. Teeth in which the inflammation is confined to the pulp chamber respond normally to percussion and palpation. Thermal stimuli or percussion applied to teeth with irreversible pulpitis can provoke severe pain. This pain may be intense and is often described as "bright" or "throbbing." When provoked, a significant period may elapse and medications may be required before the pain is ameliorated. The progression of inflammation alters the response of the tooth to pulp testing. If the inflammatory process extends to involve the periodontal ligament, the affected tooth can become tender to pressure, biting, or light tapping with an instrument. Necrosis of the pulp can result in bony resorption. Thus, pulp death may result in radiolucency at the apex of the tooth, in the furcation,[15,39] or at points along the root (see Figure 58-1).

The ability of inflammatory periodontal disease to affect the pulp is much less certain.[8,40] Dental radiographs usually document the presence of apical or lateral lesions. However, the clinician should remember that some inflamed and necrotic pulps are asymptomatic and that the patient is unaware of their existence.

DIFFERENTIATION BETWEEN PULPAL AND PERIODONTAL ABSCESSES

Periodontal abscesses usually are not severely painful lesions (see Chapter 48). They occur in the pocket or sulcus at the level of the connective tissue attachment, so there is little or no elevation of the periosteum to cause significant pain. The patient becomes aware of a sore or tender area in the gingiva and may notice swelling of the tissues to form a lump. This area may be sensitive to touch, mastication, or toothbrushing and flossing; any stimulus to the site can be painful. The formation of a fistula is less common than with apical periodontitis. If a fistula does form, it may be found in both the gingiva and the mucosa. The path of the sinus tract can be determined by carefully placing a fine gutta percha point into the fistula and then making a radiograph. The point communicates with and stops within the periodontal pocket. Careful probing confirms the presence of the pocket, and dilation of the sulcus usually results in drainage.

Acute apical abscesses typically communicate directly with the external soft tissue surface by a sinus tract and a stoma through the oral mucosa or gingiva. Before the completion of the tract, the patient often experiences acutely painful symptoms as a result of the involvement of the periodontal ligament. The tract may exit through the periodontium and dissect along the root to empty into the gingival sulcus and the interfurcal area. It then goes through the periodontal ligament of an adjacent tooth or into an existing periodontal pocket (see Figure 58-1). When the latter occurs, the resulting defect is a true *combined lesion*.[14,31,35]

Acute apical abscesses can extend to involve the adjacent periodontium. The sinus tract that forms usually extends from the apex of the tooth to the buccal side; thus the mandible and maxillary curvature results in thin plates of bone at these sites. Although palatal or lingual tracts do form, they occur at a much lower frequency than buccal tracts. During formation of a sinus tract, the patient may experience extreme pain because of involvement of the periodontal ligament and elevation of the periosteum. Perforation of the plate is accompanied by swelling, pus formation, and pus collection under the periosteum. The swelling can lead to substantial alterations in facial appearance because substantial volumes of pus may be confined in the lesion. Ultimately, drainage is established through a stoma. As long as the sinus remains open and drainage occurs, the symptoms and signs may be diminished. The acute inflammatory response may then take on the characteristics of a chronic lesion.

The endodontic sinus tract is usually a narrow, constricted lesion directed from the apex of the tooth laterally. In the absence of inflammatory periodontal disease, a tract emptying into the sulcus exerts little effect on the remainder of the sulcus. Prichard and Simon[31] stated that the "pulpal lesion does not change its character and become marginal periodontitis when it reaches the bony crest or gingival margin, and the pulp does not immediately or inevitably become infected when bone resorption from marginal periodontitis reaches the apex." Both endodontic and periodontal lesions may, however, result in attachment loss that affects the furcation[15,31] or the apex of the tooth.[25]

THERAPEUTIC MANAGEMENT OF PULPAL AND PERIODONTAL DISEASE

Patients with pulpal disease may have a healthy periodontium, gingivitis, or varying amounts of attachment loss (periodontitis) on the affected or adjacent teeth. A host of other dental problems may also exist. Therefore, appropriate treatment varies with the presence, nature, and extent of involvement of the diseases.

Primary Endodontic Lesion

Patients with pulpal disease present only diagnostic and treatment decisions relative to the endodontic lesion. Debridement of the pulp chamber and canal, as well as the completion of appropriate endodontic therapy, are sufficient to result in healing of the lesion (Figure 58-2). Pulpal abscesses and apical lesions generally resolve with conventional therapy, although apical surgery may be required in certain cases. Periodontal treatment is not required in the absence of any periodontal involvement.

Occasionally an abscess of pulpal origin, through an apical or lateral canal, may establish drainage through the periodontal ligament and erupt into the furcation or the gingival sulcus.[12,15,31,34] The signs and symptoms of this process are identical to the initial signs and symptoms of abscesses establishing a path in a more horizontal direction, except that a fistula is not evident. Therefore, it becomes necessary to separate the signs and symptoms of pulpal disease from those associated with a periodontal abscess. The patient's history, periodontal probing, radiographs, and pulpal testing should be consistent with pulpal disease. Root canal treatment resolves any tract or stoma that is present.

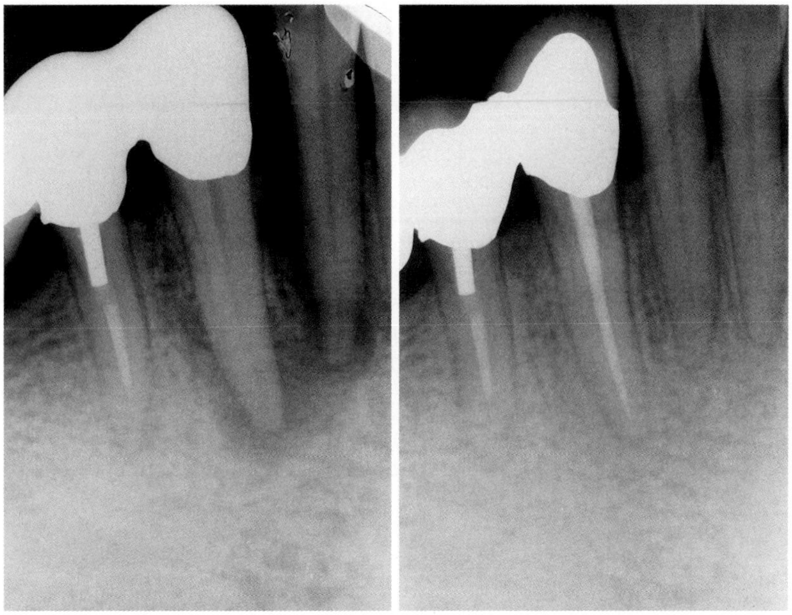

Figure 58-2 Radiographs of suspected combined lesion (periodontal-endodontic lesion) on a mandibular cuspid and lateral incisor. **A,** Note the advanced bone loss on the distal surface of the lateral incisor and the possible extension of the apical lesion to involve the maxillary canine. **B,** Posttreatment response. This canine was treated only by a root canal procedure. The lesion was of pulpal origin, and repair occurred after pulp extirpation and treatment.

Independent Periodontal and Endodontic Lesions

Patients with pulpal disease may also present with inflammatory periodontal disease. Gingivitis or early periodontitis, other than tenderness, bleeding on brushing, or with probing, usually results in little discomfort. Pulpal disease, however, is associated with more noticeable signs and symptoms. The progress of periodontitis is slow, with the exception of acute disease, such as periodontal abscesses or necrotizing ulcerative gingivitis. Therefore the prompt management of the pulpal lesion is the primary concern. Pulpal extirpation and filling of the canals represent the proper course of therapy because extirpation usually eliminates the patient's acute symptoms. Although residual sensitivity to percussion or movement of the tooth may persist for a period, therapy for gingivitis or early periodontitis may be delayed until the acute symptoms of pulpal disease are alleviated.

A different scenario may result if a patient with chronic periodontitis experiences a loss of pulpal vitality. This patient may simultaneously have the clinical signs and symptoms of both periodontitis and apical periodontitis. The extent to which each can affect the tooth is both independent and variable. The involvement of the apical periodontium by a pulpal lesion may obscure the symptoms of periodontitis. Therefore the ability to determine the independence of the two lesions on any tooth or area is a key consideration in the sequence of therapy. In most cases the lesions are independent and do not communicate (Figure 58-3).

Rarely, a patient may present with abscesses of both pulpal and periodontal origin (Figure 58-4). Because the apical lesion tends to be the most painful lesion, endodontic therapy is normally initiated before or during the appointment when the periodontal abscess is drained. Again, the patient's history and thorough probing allow a determination of the extent of each problem and the independence of the two defects. Endodontic therapy results in the resolution of the endodontic lesionbut has little or no effect on the periodontal pocket (see Figure 58-4, *C*), and appropriate periodontal therapy is required for a successful result.[16,17,31]

Combined Periodontal and Endodontic Lesions

The true combined lesion results from the development and extension of an endodontic lesion into an existing periodontal lesion (pocket).[14,31] Such lesions may present with the characteristics of both diseases, which may complicate diagnosis and treatment sequencing (Figure 58-5). A thorough history and careful clinical and radiographic examinations are required to identify and accurately assess the contribution of each lesion to the patient's dental problems and to derive a treatment sequence that is likely to produce an optimal therapeutic result. Usually the developing periapical lesion extends coronally to connect with a preexisting, chronic, wide-based periodontal pocket. On rare occasions a developing periodontal lesion, associated with a developmental groove, may extend apically to connect with an apical or lateral endodontic lesion. Also, if periodontitis progresses to involve a lateral canal or the apex of a tooth, some suggest that a secondary pulpal infection may be induced, referred to as *retrograde pulpitis*. If it exists, retrograde pulpitis is quite rare.[8,14,15,35,40]

A

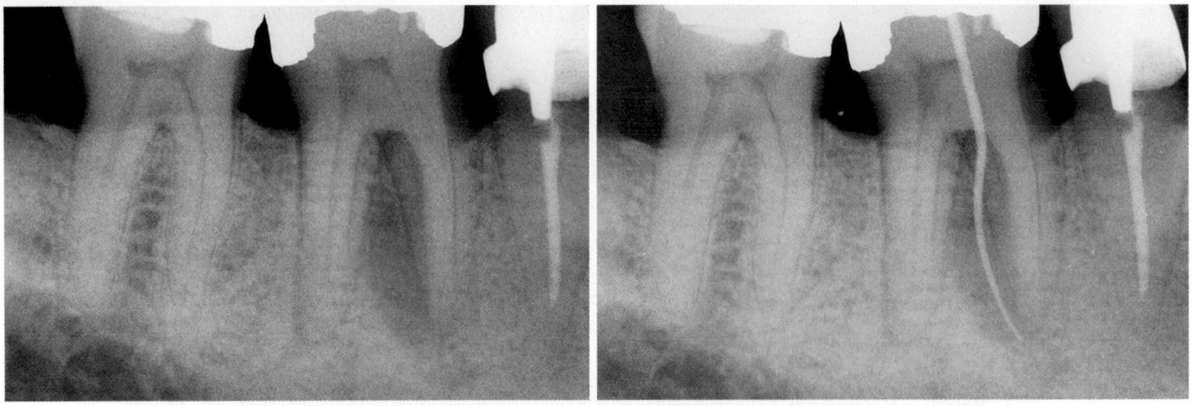

B

Figure 58-3 Independent periodontal and endodontic lesions. **A,** Radiograph of the mandibular left molars. Note the radiographic appearance of bone loss on the first and second molars, a possible cervical enamel projection on the first molar, and a large interradicular area of reduced bone density. **B,** Note the gutta percha point enters the furcation defect and extends to the apex of the mesial root of the molar. Although the molar displays signs consistent with periodontitis, the interradicular defect is purely of endodontic origin.

A

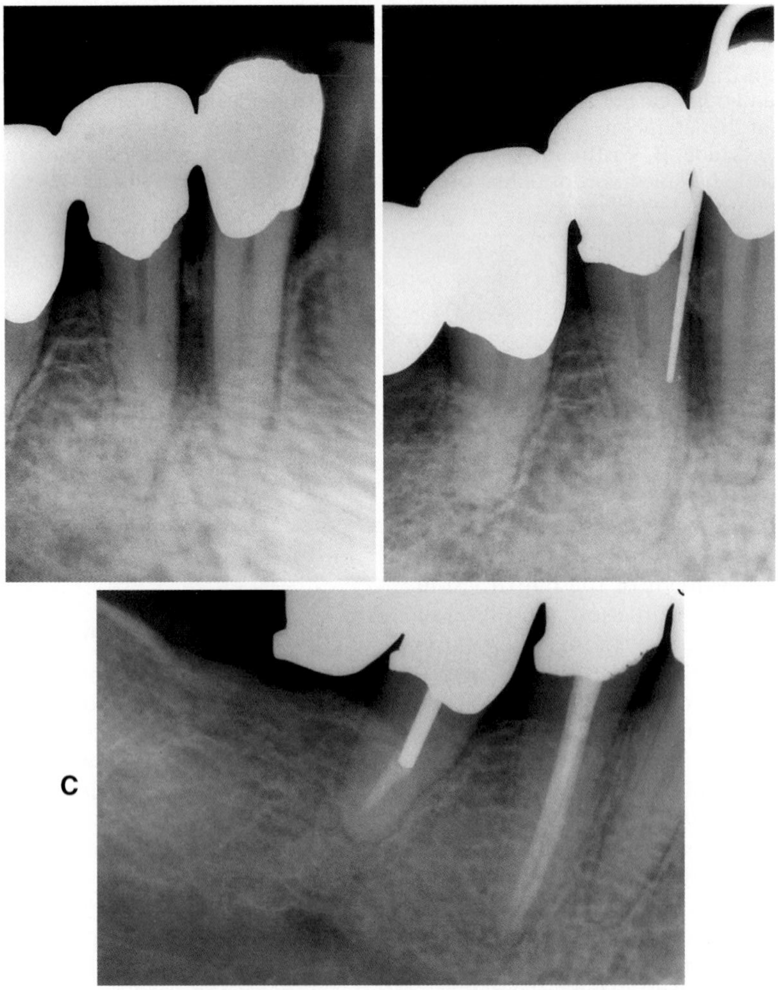

B

C

Figure 58-4 Independent periodontal and endodontic abscesses. **A,** Radiograph of a mandibular left cuspid-bicuspid area. The patient presented with a large abscess involving all three teeth. Note the signs of marginal bone loss on the teeth, along with the area of decreased bone density at the mesial surface of the mandibular left first bicuspid and the apparent calcification of the pulp canals. **B,** Radiograph with periodontal probe inserted into the mesiolingual sulcus. There was, however, no communication with the mesial radiolucent area. **C,** Radiograph taken 6 months after endodontic treatment. Note the resolution of the mesial radiolucent area. The periodontal abscess was debrided, but the residual bony deformities remain.

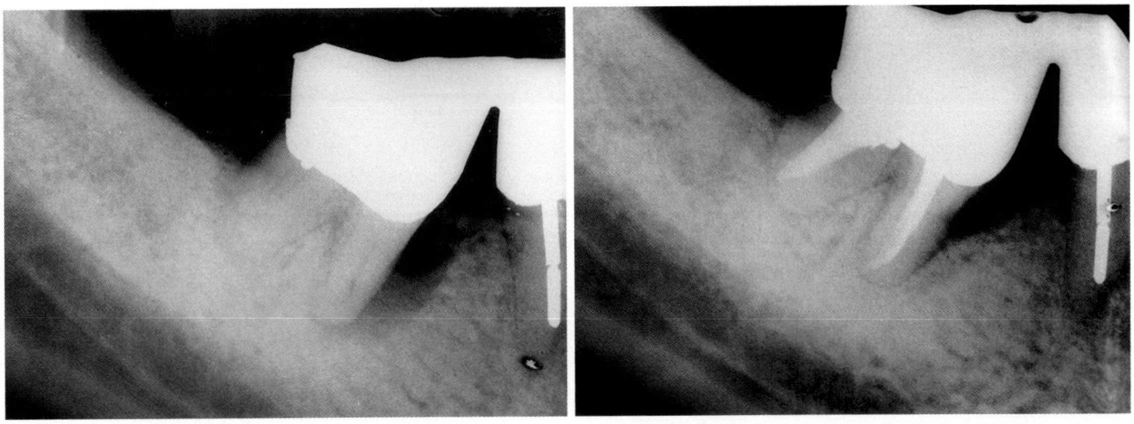

Figure 58-5 Periodontal–endodontic lesion on a mandibular second molar. **A,** Pretreatment radiograph of a deep, combination one-walled and two-walled bony defect on the mesial root of the second molar. Note the apparent involvement of the apex of the mesial root. **B,** After endodontic therapy. Performance of the root canal has resulted in repair of the endodontic component of the defect. Periodontal component of the defect shows little change. Residual bony defect will require periodontal therapy. This is a "true" periodontal–endodontic ("perio–endo") lesion.

The pain from the loss of pulpal vitality is the most common presenting complaint of patients with combined lesions. The symptoms reported are those most often found with pulpal disease. Thermal pulp testing provides information relative to the status of the pulp, and dental radiographs can confirm the presence of apical changes and the extent of bone loss. Careful probing confirms the presence and morphology of any periodontal pocket and permits the location of the communication with the apical lesion. The periodontal portion of the defect usually has plaque, calculus, or root roughness as a finding.[31] This contaminated root surface and the associated osseous defect constitute the major complication to treatment of combined lesions.

The extent to which the periodontal lesion contributes to the loss of bone is a key consideration in diagnosis and treatment planning. Endodontic treatment is highly predictable,[36] and when appropriately performed, the alterations in radiographic appearance and clinical probing disappear (see Figure 58-2). The periodontal component of a combined lesion is a more difficult problem; it cannot resolve as long as the endodontic lesion is present, but effective endodontic treatment cannot eliminate the periodontal pocket. Even with periodontal treatment, the periodontal defect typically does not resolve to the same extent as the endodontic lesion (see Figure 58-5). The ability to eliminate the periodontal component of the defect ultimately dictates treatment of the tooth. If the majority of the bony support has been lost from periodontitis, regardless of the predictability of endodontic therapy, the tooth may have a hopeless prognosis.

Once the decision to retain the tooth is made, endodontic therapy should precede attempts at periodontal pocket elimination.[14] After successful endodontic treatment, the residual periodontal pocket that remains can be more predictably treated. The periodontal therapeutic objectives vary with the extent and configuration of the residual periodontal lesion. The elimination of etiologic factors, alterations in the depth and configuration of the pocket, and facilitation of restorative dentistry may all be legitimate objectives. Thus, periodontal treatment may include scaling and root planing, as well as various surgical treatments. If the endodontic lesion requires apical surgery, the surgical treatment of both apical and periodontal lesions may be accomplished simultaneously.

Prognosis for Combined Lesions

With proper treatment, the healing of an endodontic lesion is highly predictable. However, the prognosis for teeth with combined lesions varies with the extent that each lesion contributes to the loss of attachment. Lesions resulting from pulpal disease tend to resolve with endodontic therapy, whereas the repair or regeneration of attachment loss from periodontitis is less predictable. The long-term prognosis for a tooth with a combined lesion is therefore closely related to the extent and configuration of the periodontal attachment loss. With advanced horizontal attachment loss, even an optimal endodontic result may not be sufficient to retain the tooth as a functioning member of the dentition. If the periodontal lesion is an advanced, multiwalled bony defect, the success of therapy likely depends on the ability to fill or regenerate attachment to obliterate the defect.

Therefore the decision to treat and retain teeth with combined periodontal and endodontic lesions should be carefully considered in regard to the overall dental treatment plan, because the time and cost of combined defect treatment may be considerable.

SPECIAL ISSUES IN ENDODONTIC THERAPY

Potential Complications

As with any therapeutic modality, complications may arise during endodontic treatment. Some are iatrogenic,

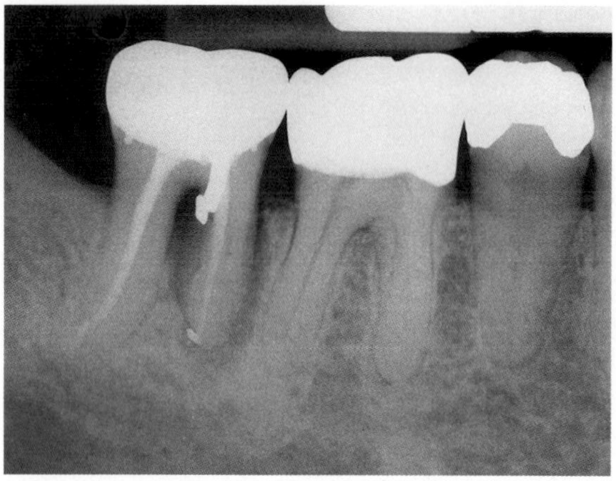

Figure 58-6 Radiograph of mandibular right molar area. Endodontic perforation into the furcation area on the mesial root of a mandibular second molar. The curvature and deep distal fluting on the mesial root of mandibular molars increase the risk of inadvertent root perforation.

such as *perforations* of the floor of the pulp chamber or the root during access, canal instrumentation, or post preparation (Figure 58-6). These accidents may result in periodontal defects, and treatment should be instituted as soon as the perforation occurs. The healing of the lesion occurring in the periodontium depends on whether bacterial infection can be excluded from the wound area by obturation of the perforation site.[4,29] If the perforation occurs in the cervical area of the tooth, a surgical flap approach may provide sufficient access to expose the perforation and allow a successful seal. However, because of the difficulty in sealing a lateral perforation of the root, the prognosis is guarded for such a tooth.

Additional problems are root resorption and vertical root fracture. *Resorption* may be of an internal or external nature. External resorption may follow impact injuries such as luxation or tooth avulsion and is most often seen after reimplantation.

Vertical root fractures are fractures oriented more or less longitudinally toward the apex of the tooth. The cause and prevalence of such fractures are not clearly established. However, vertical root fractures may result during canal obturation, pin or post placement, or cementation of intracoronal restorations.[23,24] These fractures appear to occur spontaneously in some cases and more often in endodontically treated than nonendodontically treated teeth. It has been postulated that endodontic treatment may result in the teeth becoming more brittle and less resistant to forces of mastication.

Vertical root fractures may occur years after endodontic treatment[23] and are not readily visible in radiographs unless the fragments are separated (Figure 58-7). Studies suggest that a thin, halolike apical radiolucency is an indication of vertical root fracture[30] (Figure 58-8). Fractures are often inferred from symptoms of pain or tenderness on mastication or the development of a localized periodontal defect or sinus tract that cannot be explained by other clinical findings. Application of an iodine stain or plaque-disclosing solution and indirect illumination are also useful diagnostic measures. However, surgical exposure and direct visual examination are sometimes required to confirm the fracture. Vertical root fracture generally results in a hopeless prognosis for the affected root.

A

B

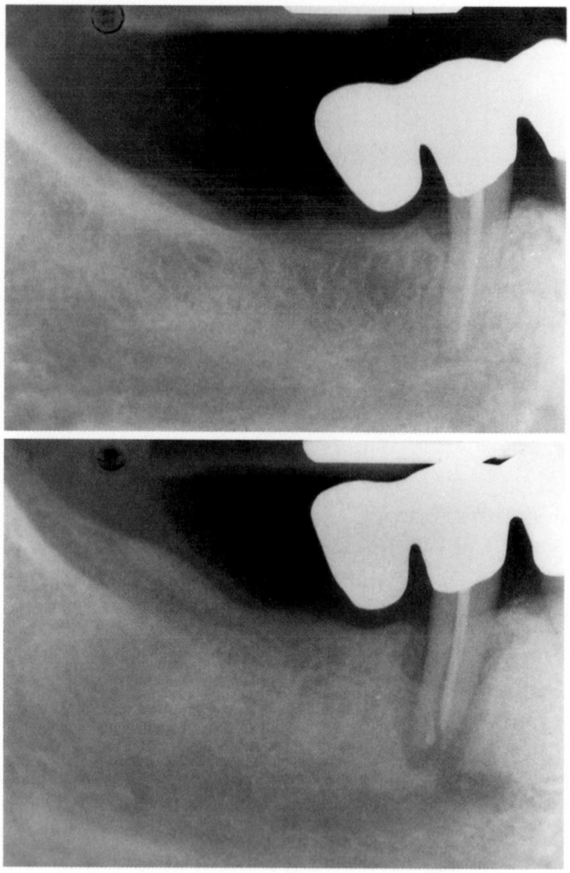

Figure 58-7 Vertical root fractures. **A,** Radiograph of mandibular left second bicuspid with a cantilevered pontic. This tooth shows evidence of periodontal attachment loss at the mesial and distal surfaces and an apparent widening of the periodontal ligament space. **B,** Radiograph of the same bicuspid 6 months later. Note the advanced loss of attachment and the radiographic signs of a vertical root fracture (separation of fragments). Sectioning of the bridge and removal of the tooth were required.

Restorative Implications

Ultimately, most root canal–treated teeth require restorations. Although the initial success rate for endodontic therapy is quite high,[36] long-term retention and function depend greatly on the ability to restore the tooth adequately. Restoration is complicated by the extent of crown loss from caries, fracture, and the size and placement of the access to the pulp chamber.[18] Additional factors are type of restoration used, configuration and number of pulp canals, root form, and need for a post and core.[7,11,24,32,37] Although severely decayed and fractured teeth can often be successfully treated endodontically, such teeth may require periodontal surgery and still may be difficult or impossible to restore. Complex

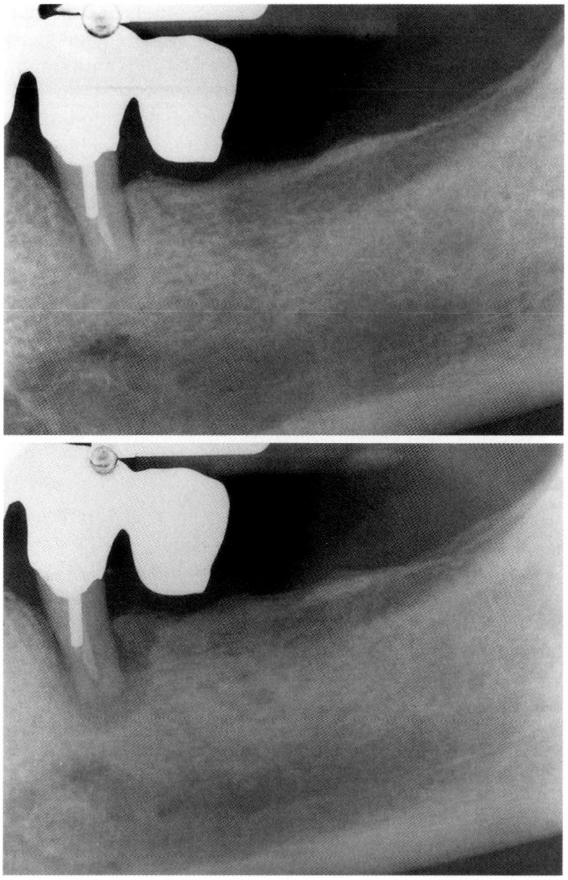

A

B

Figure 58-8 Vertical root fracture. **A,** Radiograph of the mandibular right second bicuspid in same patient as in Figure 58-7. The bicuspid, supporting a cantilevered pontic, has an endodontic post in the root. It also has radiographic evidence of loss of periodontal attachment and widening of the periodontal ligament space. Note the halolike apical radiolucency. **B,** Radiograph of tooth #29 taken 10 months later, showing advanced attachment loss around the apical area of the root and evidence of vertical root fracture. This tooth also required extraction.

interdisciplinary treatment should be confined to teeth that are of critical importance to the overall treatment plan after due consideration of alternate treatment methods.

SCIENCE TRANSFER

In patents with a dental abscess, the differential diagnosis between periodontal and endodontic origin can usually be established by the history, clinical examination, and radiographs. Acute pain is often associated with endodontic lesions and rarely if ever with periodontal lesions. A draining sinus tract most often indicates an endodontic etiology. Radiographic evaluation will show periapical bone loss with endodontic lesions, and use of a diagnostic gutta percha point with the x-ray film will often point to the location of the abscess. Pulp vitality tests are useful to rule out endodontic lesions.

In combined endodontic–periodontic lesions, it is generally wise to treat the endodontic component first, because in many cases this will lead to complete resolution of the problem.

Pulpal and periodontal diseases are related in that both involve an inflammatory process. Also, such inflammation is caused by microbial infection and thus by the two major dental diseases: caries and periodontal disease. The difference between pulpal and periodontal disease essentially involves the route and location of the inflammation. The severity of the inflammatory reaction is also important. With pulpal disease, the body can tolerate inflammation up to a certain point, and then a reversible process occurs. This is analogous to gingivitis, which involves a reversible inflammatory reaction in the marginal tissues of the periodontium. More severe inflammation is not reversible and leads to more serious conditions, such as pulpal necrosis, and thus loss of pulpal vitality. Irreversible inflammation in the periodontium leads to tissue loss and thus periodontal disease.

Therefore the major dental diseases, caries and periodontitis, are related because both involve inflammation. Similarly, the location and severity of the inflammation result in a characteristic degree of tissue involvement, which in turn helps the clinician select the appropriate therapeutic approach.

REFERENCES

1. Armitage GC, Ryder MI, Wilcox SE: Cemental changes in teeth with heavily infected root canals, *J Endodont* 9:127, 1983.
2. Baumgartner JC: Endodontic microbiology. In Walton RE, Torabinejad M, editors: *Principles and practice of endodontics,* ed 3, Philadelphia, 2002, Saunders.
3. Baumgartner JC, Falkler WA: Bacteria in the apical 5 mm of infected root canals, *J Endodont* 17:380, 1991.
4. Beavers RA, Bergenholtz G, Cox CF: Periodontal wound healing following intentional root perforation in permanent teeth of *Macaca mulatta, Int J Endodont* 19:36, 1986.
5. Bergenholtz G, Lindhe J: Effect of soluble plaque factors on inflammatory reaction in the dental pulp, *Scand J Dent Res* 83:153, 1975.
6. Bergenholtz G, Lekholm U, Liljenberg B, et al: Morphometric analysis of chronic inflammatory periapical lesions in root-filled teeth, *Oral Surg Oral Med Oral Pathol* 55:295, 1983.
7. Brannstrom M, Lind PO: Pulpal response to early dental caries, *J Dent Res* 44:1045, 1965.
8. Czarnecki R, Schilder H: A histological evaluation of the human pulp in teeth with varying degrees of periodontal disease, *J Endodont* 5:242, 1979.
9. DeDeus QD: Frequency, location, and direction of the lateral, secondary and accessory canals, *J Endodont* 1:361, 1975.
10. Gharbia S, Haapasalo M, Shah HN, et al: Characterization of *Prevotella intermedia* and *Prevotella nigrescens* isolates from periodontal and endodontic lesions, *J Periodontol* 65:56, 1994.

11. Gutmann JL: Preparation of endodontically treated teeth to receive a post-core restoration, *J Prosthet Dent* 38:413, 1977.
12. Gutmann JL: Prevalence, location and patency of accessory canals in the furcation region of permanent molars, *J Periodontol* 49:21, 1978.
13. Haapasalo M: *Bacteroides* spp in dental root canal infections, *Endodont Dent Traumatol* 5:1, 1989.
14. Harrington GW: The perio-endo question: differential diagnosis, *Dent Clin North Am* 23:673, 1979.
15. Harrington G, Steiner D: Endodontic and periodontal interrelationships. In Walton RE, Torabinejad M, editors: *Principles and practice of endodontics,* ed 3, Philadelphia, 2002, Saunders.
16. Hiatt W: Periodontal pocket elimination by combined endodontic-periodontic therapy, *Periodontics* 1:152, 1963.
17. Hiatt WH, Amen C: Periodontal pocket elimination by combined therapy, *Dent Clin North Am* 9:133, 1964.
18. Johnson J, Schwartz H, Blackwell R: Evaluation and restoration of endodontically treated posterior teeth, *J Am Dent Assoc* 93:597, 1976.
19. Kollman W, Mijatovic E: Age dependent changes in thermoperception in human anterior teeth, *Arch Oral Biol* 30:711, 1985.
20. Langeland K, Rodriques H, Dowden W: Periodontal disease, bacteria and pulpal histopathology, *Oral Surg Oral Med Oral Pathol* 37:257, 1974.
21. Lin LB, Langeland K: Light and electron microscopic study of teeth with carious pulp exposures, *Oral Surg Oral Med Oral Pathol* 51:292, 1981.
22. Lowman JV, Burke RS, Pelleu GB: Patent accessory canals: incidence in moral furcation region, *Oral Surg Oral Med Oral Pathol* 36:580, 1973.
23. Meister F, Lommel TJ, Gerstein H: Diagnosis and possible causes of vertical root fracture, *Oral Surg Oral Med Oral Pathol* 49:243, 1980.
24. Milot P, Stein R: Root fracture in endodontically treated teeth related to post selection and crown design, *J Prosthet Dent* 68:428, 1992.
25. Moller AJ, Fabricius L, Dahlen G, et al: Influence on periapical tissues of indigenous oral bacteria and necrotic pulp tissue in monkeys, *Scand J Dent Res* 89:475, 1981.
26. Mumford JM: Pain perception threshold on stimulating human teeth and the histological condition of the pulp, *Br Dent J* 123:427, 1967.
27. Nahri MV: The characteristics of interdental sensory units and their responses to stimulation, *J Dent Res* 54:654, 1985.
28. Nilsen R, Johannessen AC, Skaug N, et al: In situ characterization of mononuclear cells in human dental periapical inflammatory lesions using monoclonal antibodies, *Oral Surg Oral Med Oral Pathol* 58:160, 1984.
29. Petersson K, Hasselgren G, Tronstad L: Endodontic treatment of experimental root perforations in dog teeth, *Endod Dent Traumatol* 1:22, 1986.
30. Pitts DL, Natkin E: Diagnosis and treatment of vertical root fractures, *J Endodont* 9:338, 1983.
31. Prichard JF, Simon P: Combined periodontal pulpal problems. In Prichard JF, editor: *The diagnosis and treatment of periodontal disease in general dental practice,* Philadelphia, 1979, Saunders.
32. Ross R, Nicholls J, Harrington G: A comparison of strains generated during placement of five endodontic posts, *J Endodont* 17:450, 1991.
33. Seltzer S, Bender IB, Ziontz M: Interrelationship of the pulp and periodontal disease, *Oral Surg Oral Med Oral Pathol* 16:1474, 1963.
34. Simon JH, Glick DH, Frank AL: The relationship of endodontic-periodontic lesions, *J Periodontol* 43:202, 1972.
35. Simring M, Goldberg M: The pulpal pocket approach: retrograde periodontitis, *J Periodontol* 35:22, 1964.
36. Sjogren U, Hagglund B, Sundqvist G, et al: Factors affecting the long-term results of endodontic treatment, *J Endodont* 16:498, 1990.
37. Sorenson J, Englemen M: Ferrule design and fracture resistance of endodontically treated teeth, *J Prosthet Dent* 63:529, 1990.
38. Sundqvist G, Johansson E, Sjogren U: Prevalence of black pigmented *Bacteroides* species in root canal infections, *J Endodont* 15:13, 1989.
39. Torabinejad M: Pulp and periradicular pathosis. In Walton RE, Torabinejad M, editors: *Principles and practice of endodontics,* ed 3, Philadelphia, 2002, Saunders.
40. Torabinejad M, Kiger RD: A histologic evaluation of dental pulp tissue of a patient with periodontal disease, *Oral Surg Oral Med Oral Pathol* 59:198, 1985.
41 Van Hassel HJ: Physiology of the human dental pulp, *Oral Surg Oral Med Oral Pathol* 32:126, 1971.
42. Vertucci TJ, Williams RG: Furcation canals in the human mandibular first molar, *Oral Surg Oral Med Oral Pathol* 38:308, 1974.
43. Walton RE, Garnick JT: The histology of periapical inflammatory lesions in permanent molars in monkeys, *J Endodont* 12:49, 1986.
44. Yanagisawa S: Pathologic study of periapical lesions. I. Periapical granulomas: clinical histopathologic and immunohistopathologic studies, *J Oral Pathol* 9:288, 1980.

SECTION · IV ·

Surgical Therapy

Henry H. Takei

Phase II Periodontal Therapy

Fermin A. Carranza and Henry H. Takei

59

CHAPTER

CHAPTER OUTLINE

Although in a strict sense, all instrumental therapy can be considered surgical, this chapter refers only to those techniques that include the intentional severing or incising of gingival tissue* with the following purposes:

- Controlling or eliminating periodontal disease.
- Correcting anatomic conditions that may favor periodontal disease, impair esthetics, or impede placement of the correct prosthetic appliances.
- Placing implants to replace lost teeth and improving the environment for their placement and function.

*Scaling and root planing are not included because these procedures are not used *intentionally* to act on the gingival tissue.

OBJECTIVES OF THE SURGICAL PHASE

The surgical phase of periodontal therapy has the following main objectives:

1. Improvement of the prognosis of teeth and their replacements.
2. Improvement of esthetics.

The surgical phase consists of techniques performed for pocket therapy and for the correction of related morphologic problems, namely, mucogingival defects. In many cases, procedures are combined so that one surgical intervention fulfills both objectives.

The purpose of surgical pocket therapy is to eliminate the pathologic changes in the pocket walls; to create a stable, easily maintainable state; and, if possible, to promote periodontal regeneration. To fulfill these objectives, surgical techniques (1) increase accessibility to the root surface, making it possible to remove all irritants;

BOX 59-1

Periodontal Surgery

Pocket Reduction Surgery

Resective (gingivectomy, apically displaced flap and undisplaced flap with or without osseous resection)
Regenerative (flaps with grafts, membranes, etc.)

Correction of Anatomic/Morphologic Defects

Plastic surgery techniques to widen attached gingiva (free gingival grafts, and other techniques, etc.)
Esthetic surgery (root coverage, recreation of gingival papillae)
Preprosthetic techniques (crown lengthening, ridge augmentation, vestibular deepening)
Placement of dental implants, including techniques for site development for implants (guided bone regeneration, sinus grafts)

SCIENCE TRANSFER

Many techniques are used in periodontal surgical therapy. In all cases, it is essential that the surgeon pay particular attention to removing all root surface deposits and to root planing, because these provide a unique opportunity to visualize and gain access to previously inaccessible root surfaces. Patients must demonstrate adequate plaque control before any surgical intervention; otherwise, the outcome is uncertain.

In the esthetic zone, most surgical procedures involving the labial tissues will compromise the appearance of the gingival margins and papillae. Therefore, nonsurgical techniques are the procedure of choice, either alone or in combination with palatal flap surgery.

(2) reduce or eliminate pocket depth, making it possible for the patient to maintain the root surfaces free of plaque; and (3) reshape soft and hard tissues to attain a harmonious topography. Pocket reduction surgery seeks to reduce pocket depth by either resective or regenerative means or often by a combination of both methods (Box 59-1). Chapters 64 to 68 describe the different techniques used for these purposes.

The second objective of the surgical phase of periodontal therapy is the correction of anatomic morphologic defects that may favor plaque accumulation and pocket recurrence or impair esthetics. It is important to understand that these procedures are not directed to treat disease but aim to alter the gingival and mucosal tissues to correct defects that may predispose to disease. They are performed on noninflamed tissues and in the absence of periodontal pockets. Three types of techniques fall into this category, as follows (see Box 59-1):

- *Plastic surgery techniques* are used to create or widen the attached gingiva by placing grafts of various types.
- *Esthetic surgery techniques* are used to cover denuded roots and to recreate lost papillae.
- *Preprosthetic techniques* are used to adapt the periodontal and neighboring tissues to receive prosthetic replacements; these include crown lengthening, ridge augmentation, and vestibular deepening.

The plastic and esthetic surgery techniques are presented in Chapter 69 and the preprosthetic techniques in Chapter 71.

In addition, periodontal surgical techniques for the placement of dental implants are available. These involve not only the implant placement techniques but also a variety of surgical procedures to adapt the neighboring tissues, such as the sinus floor or the mandibular nerve canal, for subsequent placement of the implant (see Box 59-1). These methods are discussed in Chapters 76 and 77.

Surgical Pocket Therapy

Surgical pocket therapy can be directed toward (1) access surgery to ensure the removal of irritants from the tooth surface or (2) elimination of, or reduction of the depth of, the periodontal pocket.

The effectiveness of periodontal therapy is predicated on success in completely eliminating calculus, plaque, and diseased cementum from the tooth surface. Numerous investigations have shown that the difficulty of this task increases as the pocket becomes deeper.[2,5] The presence of irregularities on the root surface also increase the difficulty of the procedure. As the pocket becomes deeper, the surface to be scaled increases, more irregularities appear on the root surface, and accessibility is impaired[11,15]; the presence of furcation involvements sometimes creates insurmountable problems (see Chapter 68).

All these problems can be reduced by resecting or displacing the soft tissue wall of the pocket, thereby increasing the visibility and accessibility of the root surface.[3] The flap approach and the gingivectomy technique attain this result.

The need to eliminate or reduce the depth of the pocket is another important consideration. Pocket elimination consists of reducing the depth of periodontal pockets to that of a physiologic sulcus to enable cleansing by the patient. By proper case selection, both resective techniques and regenerative techniques can be used to accomplish this goal. The presence of a pocket produces areas that are impossible for the patient to keep clean, which establishes the vicious cycle depicted in Figure 59-1.

Results of Pocket Therapy

A periodontal pocket can be in an active state or a period of inactivity or quiescence. In an *active* pocket, underlying bone is being lost (Figure 59-2, *top left*). It often can be diagnosed clinically by bleeding, either spontaneously or on probing. After Phase I therapy the inflammatory changes in the pocket wall subside, rendering the pocket inactive and reducing its depth (Figure 59-2, *top center*).

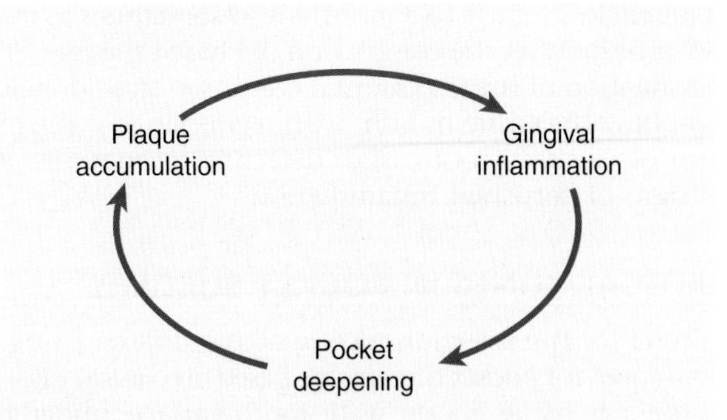

Figure 59-1 Accumulation of plaque leads to gingival inflammation and pocket deepening, which in turn increases the area of plaque accumulation.

The extent of this reduction depends on the depth before treatment and the degree to which the depth is the result of the edematous and inflammatory component of the pocket wall.

Whether the pocket remains inactive depends on its depth and the individual characteristics of the plaque components and the host response. Recurrence of the initial activity is likely.

Inactive pockets can sometimes heal with a long junctional epithelium (Figure 59-2, *top right*). However, this condition also may be unstable, and the chance of recurrence and re-formation of the original pocket is always present because the epithelial union to the tooth is weak. However, one study in monkeys has shown that the long junctional epithelial union may be as resistant to plaque infection as a normal connective tissue attachment.[9]

Studies have shown that inactive pockets can be maintained for long periods with little loss of attachment by means of frequent scaling and root-planing procedures.[6,10,12] A more reliable and stable result is obtained, however, by transforming the pocket into a healthy sulcus. The bottom of the healthy sulcus can be located either where the bottom of the pocket was localized or coronal to it. In the first case, there is no gain of attachment (Figure 59-2, *bottom left*), and the area of the root that was previously the tooth wall of the pocket becomes exposed. This does not mean that the periodontal treatment has caused recession, but rather that it has uncovered the recession previously induced by the disease.

The healthy sulcus can also be located coronal to the bottom of the preexisting pocket (Figure 59-2, *bottom center and right*). This is conducive to a restored marginal periodontium; the result is a sulcus of normal depth with gain of attachment. The creation of a healthy sulcus and a restored periodontium entails a total restoration of the status that existed before periodontal disease began, which is the ideal result of treatment.

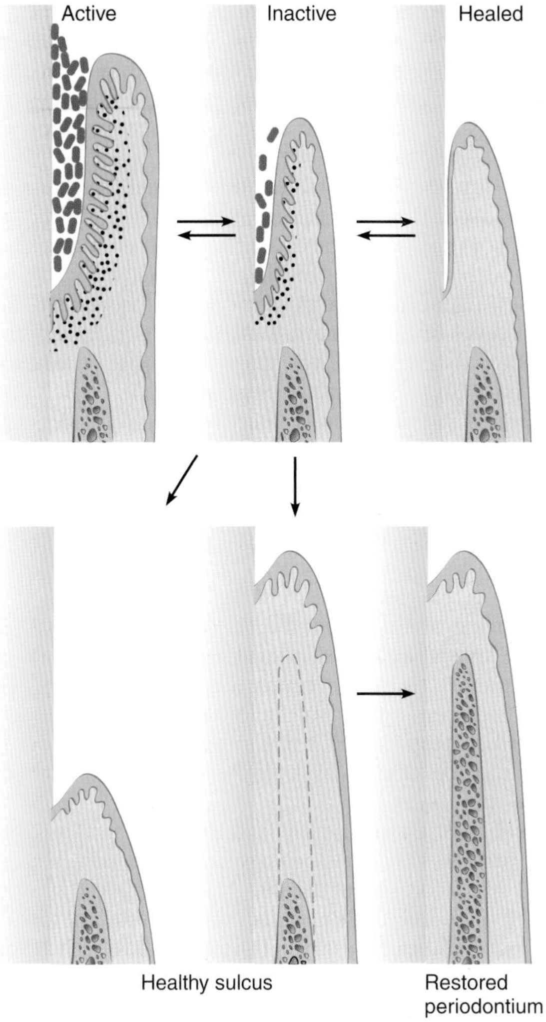

Figure 59-2 Possible results of pocket therapy. An active pocket can become inactive and heal by means of a long junctional epithelium. Surgical pocket therapy can result in a healthy sulcus, with or without gain of attachment. Improved gingival attachment promotes restoration of bone height, with re-formation of periodontal ligament fibers and layers of cementum.

POCKET ELIMINATION VERSUS POCKET MAINTENANCE

Pocket elimination (depth reduction to gingival sulcus levels) has traditionally been considered one of the main goals of periodontal therapy. It was considered vital because of the need to improve accessibility to root surfaces for the therapist during treatment and for the patient after healing. The prevalent opinion now is that although in general the presence of deep pockets after therapy represents a greater risk of disease progression than shallow sites, individual probing depths are not good predictors of future clinical attachment loss. The absence of deep pockets in treated patients, on the other hand, is an excellent predictor of a stable periodontium.[5]

Longitudinal studies of different therapeutic modalities over the last 30 years have given somewhat conflicting results,[7,16] probably because of inherent problems created by the "split-mouth" design. In general, however, after surgical therapy, pockets that rebound to a shallow or moderate depth can be maintained in a healthy state and without radiographic evidence of advancing bone loss by maintenance visits consisting of scaling and root planing, with oral hygiene reinforcement performed at regular intervals of 3 months or less. In these patients the residual pocket can be examined with a thin periodontal probe, but no pain, exudate, or bleeding results; this appears to indicate that no plaque has formed on the subgingival root surfaces.

These findings do not alter the indications for periodontal surgery because the results are based on surgical exposure of the root surfaces for thorough elimination of irritants. However, these findings emphasize the importance of the maintenance phase and the close monitoring of both level of attachment and pocket depth, together with the other clinical variables (bleeding, exudation, tooth mobility). *The transformation of the initial deep, active pocket into a shallower, inactive, maintainable pocket requires some form of definitive pocket therapy and constant supervision thereafter.*

Pocket depth is an extremely useful and widely employed clinical determination, but it must be evaluated together with level of attachment and the presence of bleeding, exudation, and pain. The most important variable for evaluating whether a pocket (or deep sulcus) is progressive is the *level of attachment,* which is measured in millimeters from the cementoenamel junction. The apical displacement of the level of attachment places the tooth in jeopardy, not the increase in pocket depth, which may be caused by coronal displacement of the gingival margin.

Pocket depth remains an important clinical variable that contributes to decisions about treatment selection. Lindhe et al. compared the effect of root planing alone and with a modified Widman flap on the resultant level of attachment and in relation to initial pocket depth.[8] They reported that scaling and root-planing procedures induce loss of attachment if performed in pockets shallower than 2.9 mm, whereas gain of attachment occurs in deeper pockets. The modified Widman flap induces loss of attachment if done in pockets shallower than 4.2 mm but results in a greater gain of attachment than root planing in pockets deeper than 4.2 mm. The loss is a *true* loss of connective tissue attachment, whereas the gain can be considered a *false* gain because of reduced penetrability of connective tissues apical to the bottom of the pocket after treatment.[9,17]

Furthermore, probing depths established after active therapy and healing (approximately 6 months after treatment) can be maintained unchanged or reduced even further during a maintenance period involving careful prophylaxis once every 3 months.[8]

Ramfjord[12] and Rosling[13] and their colleagues showed that, regardless of the surgical technique used for pocket therapy, a certain pocket depth recurs. *Therefore, maintenance of this depth without any further loss of attachment becomes the goal.*

REEVALUATION AFTER PHASE I THERAPY

Longitudinal studies have noted that all patients should be treated initially with scaling and root planing and that a final decision on the need for periodontal surgery should be made only after a thorough evaluation of the effects of Phase I therapy.[5] The assessment is generally made no less than 1 to 3 months and sometimes as much as 9 months after the completion of Phase I therapy.[1] This reevaluation of the periodontal condition should include reprobing the entire mouth, with rechecking for the presence of calculus, root caries, defective restorations, and all signs of persistent inflammation.

CRITICAL ZONES IN POCKET SURGERY

Criteria for the selection of one of the different surgical techniques for pocket therapy are based on clinical findings in the soft tissue pocket wall, tooth surface, underlying bone, and attached gingiva.

Zone 1: Soft Tissue Pocket Wall

The clinician should determine the morphologic features, thickness, and topography of the soft tissue pocket wall and persistence of inflammatory changes in the wall.

Zone 2: Tooth Surface

The clinician should identify the presence of deposits and alterations on the cementum surface and determine the accessibility of the root surface to instrumentation. Phase I therapy should have solved many, if not all, of the problems on the tooth surface. Evaluation of the results of Phase I therapy should determine the need for further therapy and the method to be used.

Zone 3: Underlying Bone

The clinician should establish the shape and height of the alveolar bone next to the pocket wall through careful probing and clinical and radiographic examinations. Bony craters, horizontal or angular bone losses, and other bone deformities are important criteria in selection of the treatment technique.

Zone 4: Attached Gingiva

The clinician should consider the presence or absence of an adequate band of attached gingiva when selecting the pocket treatment method. Diagnostic techniques for mucogingival problems are described in Chapter 69. An inadequate attached gingiva may be caused by a high frenum attachment, marked gingival recession, or a deep pocket that reaches the level of the mucogingival junction. All these possible conditions should be explored and their influence on pocket therapy determined.

INDICATIONS FOR PERIODONTAL SURGERY

The following findings may indicate the need for a surgical phase of therapy:

1. Areas with irregular bony contours, deep craters, and other defects usually require surgical approach.
2. Pockets on teeth in which a complete removal of root irritants is not considered clinically possible may call for surgery. This occurs frequently in molar and premolar areas.

3. In cases of furcation involvement of grade II or III, a surgical approach ensures the removal of irritants; any necessary root resection or hemisection also requires surgical intervention.
4. Intrabony pockets on distal areas of last molars, frequently complicated by mucogingival problems, are usually unresponsive to nonsurgical methods.
5. Persistent inflammation in areas with moderate to deep pockets may require a surgical approach. In areas with shallow pockets or normal sulci, persistent inflammation may point to the presence of a mucogingival problem that needs a surgical solution.

METHODS OF POCKET THERAPY

The methods for pocket therapy can be classified under the following three main headings:

1. **New attachment techniques** offer the ideal result because they eliminate pocket depth by reuniting the gingiva to the tooth at a position coronal to the bottom of the preexisting pocket. New attachment is usually associated with filling in of bone and regeneration of periodontal ligament and cementum.
2. **Removal of the pocket wall** is the most common method. The wall of the pocket consists of soft tissue and may also include bone in the case of intrabony pockets. It can be removed by the following:
   - *Retraction or shrinkage,* in which scaling and root-planing procedures resolve the inflammatory process, and the gingiva therefore shrinks, reducing the pocket depth.
   - *Surgical removal* performed by the gingivectomy technique or by means of an undisplaced flap.
   - *Apical displacement* with an apically displaced flap.
3. **Removal of the tooth side of the pocket,** which is accomplished by tooth extraction or by partial tooth extraction (hemisection or root resection).

The techniques, what they accomplish, and the factors governing their selection are presented in Chapters 62 to 68.

Criteria for Method Selection

Scientific criteria to establish the indications for each technique are difficult to determine. Longitudinal studies following a significant number of cases over a number of years, standardizing multiple factors and many variables, would be needed. Clinical experience, however, has suggested the criteria for selecting the method to treat the pocket. The selection of a technique for treatment of a particular periodontal lesion is based on the following considerations.

1. Characteristics of the pocket: depth, relation to bone, and configuration.
2. Accessibility to instrumentation, including presence of furcation involvements.
3. Existence of mucogingival problems.
4. Response to Phase I therapy.
5. Patient cooperation, including ability to perform effective oral hygiene and, for smokers, willingness to stop their habit at least temporarily (i.e., a few weeks).
6. Age and general health of the patient.
7. Overall diagnosis of the case: various types of gingival enlargement and types of periodontitis (e.g., chronic marginal periodontitis, localized aggressive periodontitis, generalized aggressive periodontitis).
8. Esthetic considerations.
9. Previous periodontal treatments.

Each of these variables is analyzed in relation to the pocket therapy techniques available, and a specific technique is selected. Of the many techniques, the one that would most successfully solve the problems with the fewest undesirable effects should be chosen. *Clinicians who adhere to one technique to solve all problems do not use to the advantage of the patient the wide repertoire of techniques at their disposal.*

Approaches to Specific Pocket Problems

Therapy for Gingival Pockets. Two factors are taken into consideration: (1) the character of the pocket wall and (2) the accessibility of the pocket. The pocket wall can be either edematous or fibrotic. *Edematous* tissue shrinks after the elimination of local factors, thereby reducing or totally eliminating pocket depth. Therefore, scaling and root planing are the technique of choice in these cases.

Pockets with a *fibrotic* wall are not appreciably reduced in depth after scaling and root planing; therefore they are eliminated surgically. Until recently, gingivectomy was the only technique available; it solves the problem successfully, but in cases of marked gingival enlargement (e.g., severe phenytoin enlargement), it may leave a large wound that goes through a painful and prolonged healing process. In these patients, a modified flap technique can adequately solve the problem with fewer postoperative problems (see Chapter 63).

Therapy for Slight Periodontitis. In slight or incipient periodontitis, a small degree of bone loss has occurred, and pockets are shallow to moderate. In these patients, a conservative approach and adequate oral hygiene generally suffice to control the disease. Incipient periodontitis that recurs in previously treated sites may require a thorough analysis of the causes for the recurrence and, occasionally, a surgical approach to correct them.

Therapy for Moderate to Severe Periodontitis in Anterior Sector. The anterior teeth are important esthetically; therefore the techniques that induce the least amount of visual root exposure should be considered first. However, the importance of esthetics may be different for different patients, and nonelimination of the pocket may place the tooth in jeopardy. The final decision may have to be a compromise between health and esthetics, not attaining ideal results in either respect.

Anterior teeth offer two main advantages to a conservative approach: (1) they are all single rooted and easily accessible, and (2) patient compliance and thoroughness in plaque control are easier to attain. *Therefore, scaling and root planing are the technique of choice for the anterior teeth.*

Sometimes, however, a surgical technique may be necessary because of the need for improved accessibility for root planing or regenerative surgery of osseous defects. The *papilla preservation flap* can be used for both purposes and also offers a better postoperative result, with less recession and reduced soft tissue crater formation interproximally.[14] *The papilla preservation flap is the first choice when a surgical approach is needed.*

When the teeth are too close interproximally, the papilla preservation technique may not be feasible, and a technique that splits the papilla must be used. The *sulcular incision flap* offers good esthetic results and is the next choice.

When esthetics are not the primary consideration, the *modified Widman flap* can be chosen. This technique uses an internal bevel incision about 1 to 2 mm from the gingival margin without thinning the flap and may result in some minor recession.

Infrequently, bone contouring may be needed despite the resultant root exposure. The technique of choice is the *apically displaced flap with bone contouring.*

Therapy for Moderate to Severe Periodontitis in Posterior Area. Treatment for premolars and molars usually poses no esthetic problem but frequently involves difficult accessibility. Bone defects occur more often in the posterior than the anterior sector, and root morphologic features, particularly in relation to furcations, may offer unsurmountable problems for instrumentation in a close field. Therefore, surgery is frequently indicated in the posterior region.

The purpose of surgery in the posterior area is either enhanced accessibility or the need for definitive pocket reduction requiring osseous surgery. Accessibility can be obtained by either the undisplaced or the apically displaced flap.

Most patients with moderate to severe periodontitis have developed osseous defects that require some degree of osseous remodeling or reconstructive procedures. When osseous defects amenable to reconstruction are present, the *papilla preservation flap is the technique of choice* because it better protects the interproximal areas where defects are frequently present. *Second and third choices are the sulcular flap and the modified Widman flap,* maintaining as much of the papilla as possible.

When osseous defects with no possibility of reconstruction are present, such as interdental craters, the technique of choice is the *flap with osseous contouring.*

Surgical Techniques for Correction of Morphologic Defects. The objectives and rationale for the techniques performed to correct morphologic defects (mucogingival, esthetic, and preprosthetic) are given in Chapter 69.

Surgical Techniques for Implant Placement and Related Problems. The objectives and rationale for these techniques are described in Chapter 76.

REFERENCES

1. Badersten A, Nilveus R, Egelberg J: Effect of nonsurgical periodontal therapy. II. Severely advanced periodontitis, *J Clin Periodontol* 11:63, 1984.
2. Bower RC: Furcation morphology relative to periodontal treatment: furcation root surface anatomy, *J Periodontol* 50:366, 1979.
3. Caffesse RG, Sweeney PL, Smith BA: Scaling and root planing with and without periodontal flap surgery, *J Clin Periodontol* 11:205, 1986.
4. Gher ME, Vernino AR: Root morphology: clinical significance in pathogenesis and treatment of periodontal disease, *J Am Dent Assoc* 101:627, 1980.
5. Greensteifl G: Contemporary interpretation of probing depth assessment: diagnostic and therapeutic implications: a literature review, *J Periodontol* 68:1194, 1997.
6. Hill RW, Ramfjord SP, Morrison GC, et al: Four types of periodontal treatment compared over two years, *J Periodontol* 52:655, 1981.
7. Kaldahl WB, Kalkwarf KL, Patil KD: A review of longitudinal studies that compared periodontal therapies, *J Periodontol* 64:243, 1993.
8. Lindhe J, Socransky SS, Nyman S, et al: Critical probing depths in periodontal therapy, *J Clin Periodontol* 9:323, 1982.
9. Magnusson I, Runstad L, Nyman S, et al: A long junctional epithelium: a locus minoris resistentiae in plaque infection, *J Clin Periodontol* 10:333, 1983.
10. Pihlstrom BL, Ortiz Campos C, McHugh RB: A randomized four-year study of periodontal therapy, *J Periodontol* 52:227, 1981.
11. Rabbani GM, Ash MM, Caffesse RG: The effectiveness of subgingival scaling and root planing in calculus removal, *J Periodontol* 52:119, 1981.
12. Ramfjord SP, Knowles JW, Nissle RR, et al: Results following three modalities of periodontal therapy, *J Periodontol* 12:522, 1975.
13. Rosling B, Nyman S, Lindhe J, et al: The healing potential of the periodontal tissues following different techniques of periodontal surgery in plaque-free dentitions: a 2-year clinical study, *J Clin Periodontol* 3:233, 1976.
14. Takei HH, Han TJ, Carranza FA Jr, et al: Flap technique for periodontal bone implants: the papilla preservation technique, *J Periodontol* 56:204, 1985.
15. Waerhaug J: Healing of the dentoepithelial junction following subgingival plaque control. II. As observed on extracted teeth, *J Periodontol* 40:119, 1978.
16. Weeks PR: Pros and cons of periodontal pocket elimination procedures, *J West Soc Periodontol* 28:4, 1980.
17. Westfelt E, Bragd L, Socransky SS, et al: Improved periodontal conditions following therapy, *J Clin Periodontol* 12:283, 1985.

General Principles of Periodontal Surgery

Perry R. Klokkevold, Henry H. Takei, and Fermin A. Carranza

60 CHAPTER

CHAPTER OUTLINE

All surgical procedures should be carefully planned. The patient should be adequately prepared medically, psychologically, and practically for all aspects of the intervention. This chapter covers the preparation of the patient and the general considerations common to all periodontal surgical techniques. Complications that may occur during or after surgery are also discussed.

Surgical periodontal procedures are usually performed in the dental office. Hospital periodontal surgery is discussed later in this chapter, followed by a review of common surgical instruments.

OUTPATIENT SURGERY

Patient Preparation

Reevaluation after Phase I Therapy. Almost every patient undergoes the so-called initial or preparatory phase of therapy, which basically consists of thorough scaling and root planing and removing all irritants responsible for the periodontal inflammation. These procedures (1) eliminate some lesions entirely; (2) render the tissues more firm and consistent, thus permitting a more accurate and delicate surgery; and (3) acquaint the patient with the office and the operator and assistants, thereby reducing the patient's apprehension and fear.

The reevaluation phase consists of reprobing and reexamining all the pertinent findings that previously indicated the need for the surgical procedure. Persistence of these findings confirms the indication for surgery. The number of surgical procedures, expected outcome, and postoperative care necessary are all decided before therapy. These are discussed with the patient, and a final decision is made, incorporating any necessary adjustments to the original plan.

Premedication.* For patients who are not medically compromised, the value of administering antibiotics

*Precautions to be taken with medically compromised patients are discussed in Chapter 44.

routinely for periodontal surgery has not been clearly demonstrated.[29] However, some studies have reported reduced postoperative complications, including reduced pain and swelling, when antibiotics are given before periodontal surgery and continued for 4 to 7 days after surgery.[4,12,21,32]

The prophylactic use of antibiotics in patients who are otherwise healthy has been advocated for bone-grafting procedures and purported to enhance the chances of new attachment. Although the rationale for such use appears logical, no research evidence is available to support it. In any case, the risks inherent in the administration of antibiotics should be evaluated together with the potential benefits.

Other presurgical medications include administration of a nonsteroidal antiinflammatory drug (NSAID) such as ibuprofen (Motrin) 1 hour before the procedure and one oral rinse with 0.12% chlorhexidine gluconate (Peridex, PerioGard).[38]

Smoking. The deleterious effect of smoking on healing of periodontal wounds has been amply documented[20,33,43] (see also Chapter 14). Patients should be clearly informed of this fact and requested to quit or stop smoking for a minimum of 3 to 4 weeks after the procedure. For patients who are unwilling to follow this advice, an alternate treatment plan that does not include more sophisticated techniques (e.g., regenerative, mucogingival, esthetic) should be considered.

Informed Consent. The patient should be informed at the initial visit about the diagnosis, prognosis, different possible treatments, with their expected results and all pros and cons of each approach. At surgery the patient should again be informed, verbally and in writing, of the procedure to be performed, and he or she should indicate agreement by signing the consent form.

Emergency Equipment

The operator, all assistants, and office personnel should be trained to handle all the possible emergencies that may arise. Drugs and equipment for emergency use should be readily available at all times.

The most common emergency is *syncope,* or a transient loss of consciousness caused by a reduction in cerebral blood flow. The most common cause is fear and anxiety. Syncope is usually preceded by a feeling of weakness, and then the patient develops pallor, sweating, coldness of the extremities, dizziness, and slowing of the pulse. The patient should be placed in a supine position with the legs elevated; tight clothes should be loosened and a wide-open airway ensured. Administration of oxygen is also useful. Unconsciousness persists for a few minutes. A history of previous syncopal attacks during dental appointments should be explored before treatment is begun, and if these are reported, extra efforts to relieve the patient's fear and anxiety should be made. The reader is referred to other texts for a complete analysis of this important topic.[3]

Measures to Prevent Transmission of Infection

The danger of transmitting infections to the dental team or other patients has become apparent in recent years, particularly with the threat of acquired immunodeficiency syndrome (AIDS) and hepatitis B virus (HBV) infection. Universal precautions, including protective attire, and barrier techniques are strongly recommended and often required by law. These include the use of disposable sterile gloves, surgical masks, and protective eyewear. All surfaces possibly contaminated with blood or saliva that cannot be sterilized (e.g., light handles, unit syringes) must be covered with aluminum foil or plastic wrap. Aerosol-producing devices (e.g., Cavitron) should not be used on patients with suspected infections, and their use should be kept to a minimum in all other patients. Special care should be taken when using and disposing of sharp items such as needles and scalpel blades.

Sedation and Anesthesia

Periodontal surgery should be performed painlessly. The patient should be assured of this at the outset and throughout the procedure. The most reliable means of providing painless surgery is the effective administration of local anesthesia. The area to be treated should be thoroughly anesthetized by means of regional block and local infiltration injections. Injections directly into the interdental papillae may also be helpful.

Apprehensive and neurotic patients require special management with antianxiety or sedative-hypnotic agents. Modalities for the administration of these agents include inhalation, oral, intramuscular, and intravenous routes. The specific agents and modality of administration are based on the desired level of sedation, anticipated length of the procedure, and overall condition of the patient. Specifically, the patient's medical history and physical and emotional status should be considered when selecting agents and techniques.

Perhaps the simplest, least invasive method to alleviate anxiety in the dental office is *nitrous oxide and oxygen inhalation sedation*. For many individuals, this is quite effective. Advantages include a quick onset of action, the ability to adjust the level of sedation throughout the procedure, a rapid recovery, and little or no concern for postoperative impairment of sensory or motor function. One disadvantage is that a small percentage of patients will not achieve the desired effect. This is especially true for the mentally impaired individual because nitrous oxide and oxygen sedation requires some level of patient cooperation. Overall, inhalation sedation with nitrous oxide and oxygen is a safe, effective, and reliable means of reducing mild anxiety.

For individuals with mild to moderate anxiety, oral administration of a *benzodiazepine* can be effective in decreasing anxiety and producing a level of relaxation. Oral administration of a sedative agent can be more effective than inhalation anesthesia because the level of sedation achieved may be more profound. Disadvantages of oral sedative administration include incomplete recovery, an inability to control the level of sedation, and

TABLE 60-1

Oral Benzodiazepine Agents for Perioperative Antianxiety and Sedation

Generic (Brand)	Adult Dose (mg)	Onset (Hours)	Half-Life (Hours)
Alprazolam (Xanax)	0.25-0.5	1-2	12-15
Diazepam (Valium)	2-10	0.5-2	30-70
Lorazepam (Ativan)	1-4	1-6	10-18
Triazolam (Halcion)	0.125-0.5	1-2	1.5-5.5

a prolonged period of impaired sensory and motor skills. A variety of benzodiazepine agents are available for oral administration. Table 60-1 provides a brief description of common benzodiazepines, including dosage, onset of action, and duration of effect (half-life).

Intravenous (IV) administration of a benzodiazepine, alone or in combination with other agents, can be used to achieve a greater level of sedation in individuals with moderate to severe levels of anxiety. Furthermore, the onset of action of IV sedation is almost immediate, and the level of sedation can be titrated on an individual basis to the desired effect. The recovery period depends on the half-life of the agent used and the amount given. The operator should receive formal training in the techniques of sedation; this often is required by law. A thorough understanding of the indications, contraindications, and risks of these agents is required.[3] The reader is referred to other texts for a more detailed discussion of conscious sedation techniques.[26]

Tissue Management

1. *Operate gently and carefully.* In addition to being most considerate to the patient, this is also the most effective way to operate. Tissue manipulation should be precise, deliberate, and gentle. Thoroughness is essential, but roughness must be avoided because it produces excessive tissue injury, causes postoperative discomfort, and delays healing.
2. *Observe the patient at all times.* It is essential to pay careful attention to the patient's reactions. Facial expressions, pallor, and perspiration are distinct signs that may indicate the patient is experiencing pain, anxiety, or fear. The physician's responsiveness to these signs can be the difference between success and failure.
3. *Be certain the instruments are sharp.* Instruments must be sharp to be effective; successful treatment is not possible without sharp instruments. Dull instruments inflict unnecessary trauma because of poor cutting and excessive force applied to compensate for their ineffectiveness. A sterile sharpening stone should be available on the operating table at all times.

Scaling and Root Planing

Although scaling and root planing have been performed previously as part of Phase I therapy, all exposed root surfaces should be carefully explored and planed as needed as part of the surgical procedure. In particular, areas of difficult access, such as furcations or deep pockets, often have rough areas or even calculus that was undetected during the preparatory sessions. The assistant who is retracting the tissues and using the aspirator should also check for the presence of calculus and the smoothness of each surface from a different angle.

Hemostasis

Hemostasis is an important aspect of periodontal surgery because good intraoperative control of bleeding permits an accurate visualization of the extent of disease, pattern of bone destruction, and anatomy and condition of the root surfaces. It provides the operator with a clear view of the surgical site, which is essential for wound debridement and scaling and root planing. In addition, good hemostasis also prevents excessive loss of blood into the mouth, oropharynx, and stomach.

Periodontal surgery can produce profuse bleeding, especially during the initial incisions and flap reflection. After flap reflection and removal of granulation tissue, bleeding disappears or is considerably reduced. Typically, control of intraoperative bleeding can be managed with aspiration. Continuous suctioning of the surgical site with an aspirator is indispensable for performing periodontal surgery. Application of pressure to the surgical wound with moist gauze can be a helpful adjunct to control site-specific bleeding. Intraoperative bleeding that is not controlled with these simple methods may indicate a more serious problem and require additional control measures.

Excessive hemorrhaging after initial incisions and flap reflection may be caused by laceration of venules, arterioles, or larger vessels. Fortunately, the laceration of medium or large vessels is rare because incisions near highly vascular anatomic areas such as the posterior mandible (lingual and inferior alveolar arteries) and the posterior, midpalatal regions (greater palatine arteries) are avoided in incision and flap design. Proper design of the flaps, taking into consideration these areas, avoids accidents (see Chapter 61). However, even when all anatomic precautions are taken, it is possible to cause bleeding from medium or large vessels because anatomic variations do occur and may result in inadvertent laceration. If a medium or large vessel is lacerated, a suture around the bleeding end may be necessary to control hemorrhage.

Pressure should be applied through the tissue to determine the location that will stop blood flow in the severed vessel. Then a suture can be passed through the tissue and tied to restrict blood flow.

Excessive bleeding from a surgical wound also may result from incisions across a capillary plexus. Minor areas of persistent bleeding from capillaries can be stopped by applying cold pressure to the site with moist gauze (soaked in sterile ice water) for several minutes. The use of a local anesthetic with a vasoconstrictor may also be useful in controlling minor bleeding from the periodontal flap. Both these methods act through vasoconstriction, thus reducing the flow of blood through incised small vessels and capillaries. This action is relatively short lived and should not be relied on for long-term hemostasis. It is important to avoid the use of vasoconstrictors to control bleeding before sending a patient home. If a more serious bleeding problem exists or a firm blood clot is not established, bleeding is likely to recur when the vasoconstrictor has metabolized and the patient is no longer in the office.

For slow, constant blood flow and oozing, hemostasis may be achieved with hemostatic agents. Absorbable gelatin sponge (Gelfoam), oxidized cellulose (Oxycel), oxidized regenerated cellulose (Surgicel Absorbable Hemostat), and microfibrillar collagen hemostat (Collacote, Collatape, Collaplug) are useful hemostatic agents for the control of bleeding in capillaries, small blood vessels, and deep wounds (Table 60-2).

Absorbable gelatin sponge is a porous matrix prepared from pork skin that helps stabilize a normal blood clot. The sponge can be cut to the desired dimensions and either sutured in place or positioned within the wound (e.g., extraction socket). It is absorbed in 4 to 6 weeks.

Oxidized cellulose is a chemically modified form of surgical gauze that forms an artificial clot. The material is friable and can be difficult to keep in place. It absorbs in 1 to 6 weeks.

Oxidized regenerated cellulose is prepared from cellulose by reaction with alkali to form a chemically pure, more uniform structure than oxidized cellulose. The material is prepared in a cloth or thin gauze form that can be cut to the desired size and sutured or layered on the bleeding surface. It can be used as a surface dressing because it does not impair epithelialization, and it is bactericidal against many gram-negative and gram-positive microorganisms, both aerobic and anaerobic. Caution should be used when wounds are infected or have an increased potential to becoming infected (e.g., immunocompromised patients) because the absorbable hemostatic agents can serve as a nidus for infection.

Thrombin is a drug capable of hastening the process of blood clotting. It is intended for topical use only because is applied as a liquid or powder. Thrombin should never be injected into tissues because it can cause serious, even fatal intravascular coagulation. Also, because thrombin is a bovine-derived material, caution should be used for any patient with known allergic reaction to bovine products.

TABLE 60-2

Absorbable Hemostatic Agents

Generic (Brand)	Directions	Adverse Effects	Precautions
Absorbable gelatin sponge (Gelfoam)	May be cut into various sizes and applied to bleeding surfaces.	May form nidus for infection or abscess.	Should not be overpacked into extraction site or wound—may interfere with healing.
Oxidized cellulose (Oxycel)	Most effective when applied to wound dry as opposed to moistened.	May cause foreign body reaction.	Extremely friable and difficult to place; should not be used adjacent to bone—impairs bone regeneration; should not be used as a surface dressing—inhibits epithelialization.
Oxidized regenerated cellulose (Surgicel Absorbable Hemostat)	May be cut to various shapes and positioned over bleeding sites; thick or excessive amounts should not be used.	Encapsulation, cyst formation, and foreign body reaction possible.	Should not be placed in deep wounds—may physically interfere with wound healing and bone formation.
Microfibrillar collagen hemostat (Collacote, Collatape, Collaplug)	May be cut to shape and applied to bleeding surface.	May potentiate abscess formation, hematoma, and wound dehiscence; possible allergic reaction or foreign body reaction.	May interfere with wound healing; placement in extraction sockets has been associated with increased pain.
Thrombin (Thrombostat)	May be applied topically to bleeding surface.	Allergic reaction can occur in patients with known sensitivity to bovine materials.	Must not be injected into tissues or vasculature—can cause s evere (possibly fatal) clotting.

Finally, it is imperative to recognize that excessive bleeding may be caused by systemic disorders, including (but not limited to) platelet deficiencies, coagulation defects, medications, and hypertension. As a precaution, all surgical patients should be asked about current medications that may contribute to bleeding, any family history of bleeding disorders, and hypertension. *All* patients, regardless of health history, should have their blood pressure evaluated before surgery, and anyone diagnosed with hypertension must be advised to see a physician before surgery. Patients with known or suspected bleeding deficiencies or disorders must be carefully evaluated before any surgical procedure. A consultation with the patient's physician is recommended, and laboratory tests should be done to assess the risk of bleeding. It may be necessary to refer the patient to a hematologist for a comprehensive workup.

Periodontal Dressings (Periodontal Packs)

In most cases, after the surgical periodontal procedures are completed, the area is covered with a surgical pack. In general, dressings have no curative properties; they assist healing by protecting the tissue rather than providing "healing factors." The pack minimizes the likelihood of postoperative infection and hemorrhage, facilitates healing by preventing surface trauma during mastication, and protects against pain induced by contact of the wound with food or the tongue during mastication. (For a complete literature review on this subject, see Sachs et al.[37])

Zinc Oxide–Eugenol Packs. Packs based on the reaction of zinc oxide and eugenol include the Wondr-Pak developed by Ward[46] in 1923 and several other packs that use modified forms of Ward's original formula. The addition of accelerators such as zinc acetate gives the dressing a better working time.

Zinc oxide–eugenol dressings are supplied as a liquid and a powder that are mixed before use. Eugenol in this type of pack may induce an allergic reaction that produces reddening of the area and burning pain in some patients.

Noneugenol Packs. The reaction between a metallic oxide and fatty acids is the basis for Coe-Pak, which is the most widely used dressing in the United States. This is supplied in two tubes, the contents of which are mixed immediately before use until a uniform color is obtained. One tube contains zinc oxide, an oil (for plasticity), a gum (for cohesiveness), and lorothidol (a fungicide); the other tube contains liquid coconut fatty acids thickened with colophony resin (or rosin) and chlorothymol (a bacteriostatic agent).[37,40] This dressing does not contain asbestos or eugenol, thereby avoiding the problems associated with these substances.

Other noneugenol packs include cyanoacrylates[6,19,24] and tissue conditioners (methacrylate gels).[2] However, these are not in common use.

Retention of Packs. Periodontal dressings are usually kept in place mechanically by interlocking in interdental spaces and joining the lingual and facial portions of the pack.

In isolated teeth or when several teeth in an arch are missing, retention of the pack may be difficult. Numerous reinforcements and splints and stents for this purpose have been described.[17,18,47] Placement of dental floss tied loosely around the teeth enhances retention of the pack.

Antibacterial Properties of Packs. Improved healing and patient comfort with less odor and taste[6] have been obtained by incorporating antibiotics in the pack. Bacitracin,[5] oxytetracycline (Terramycin),[13] neomycin, and nitrofurazone have been tried, but all may produce hypersensitivity reactions. The emergence of resistant organisms and opportunistic infection has been reported.[35]

Incorporation of tetracycline powder in Coe-Pak is generally recommended, particularly when long and traumatic surgeries are performed.

Allergy. Contact allergy to eugenol and rosin has been reported.[34]

Preparation and Application of Dressing. Zinc oxide packs are mixed with eugenol or noneugenol liquids on a wax paper pad with a wooden tongue depressor. The powder is gradually incorporated with the liquid until a thick paste is formed.

Coe-Pak is prepared by mixing equal lengths of paste from tubes containing the accelerator and the base until the resulting paste is a uniform color (Figure 60-1, *A-C*). A capsule of tetracycline powder can be added at this time. The pack is then placed in a cup of water at room temperature (Figure 60-1, *D*). In 2 to 3 minutes the paste loses its tackiness and can be handled and molded; it remains workable for 15 to 20 minutes. Working time can be shortened by adding a small amount of zinc oxide to the accelerator (pink paste) before spatulating.

The pack is then rolled into two strips approximately the length of the treated area. The end of one strip is bent into a hook shape and fitted around the distal surface of the last tooth, approaching it from the distal surface (Figure 60-2, *A*). The remainder of the strip is brought forward along the facial surface to the midline and gently pressed into place along the gingival margin and interproximally. The second strip is applied from the lingual surface. It is joined to the pack at the distal surface of the last tooth, then brought forward along the gingival margin to the midline (Figure 60-2, *B*). The strips are joined interproximally by applying gentle pressure on the facial and lingual surfaces of the pack (Figure 60-2, *C*). For isolated teeth separated by edentulous spaces, the pack should be made continuous from tooth to tooth, covering the edentulous areas (Figure 60-3).

When split flaps have been performed, the area should be covered with tin foil to protect the sutures before placing the pack (see Chapter 64).

The pack should cover the gingiva, but overextension onto uninvolved mucosa should be avoided. *Excess pack irritates the mucobuccal fold and floor of the mouth and interferes with the tongue.* Overextension also jeopardizes

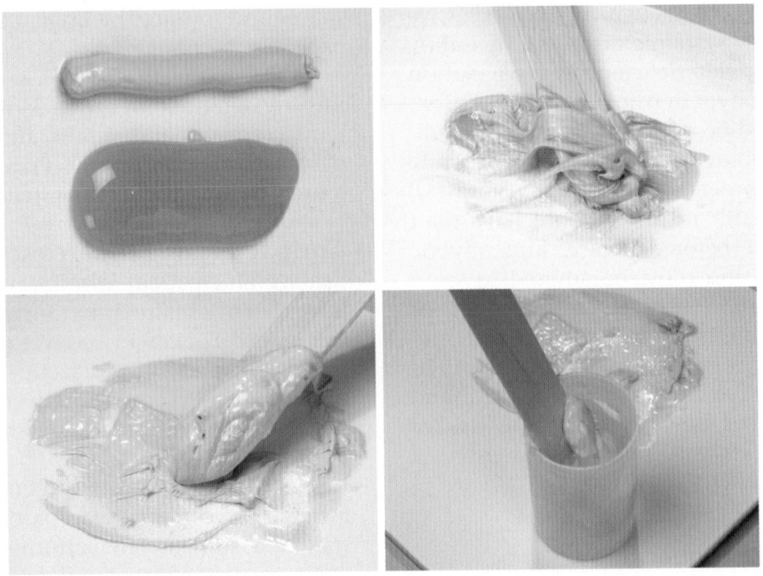

Figure 60-1 Preparing the surgical pack (Coe-Pak). **A,** Equal lengths of the two pastes are placed on a paper pad. **B,** Pastes are mixed with a wooden tongue depressor for 2 or 3 minutes until the paste loses its tackiness **(C)**. **D,** Paste is placed in a paper cup of water at room temperature. With lubricated fingers, it is then rolled into cylinders and placed on the surgical wound.

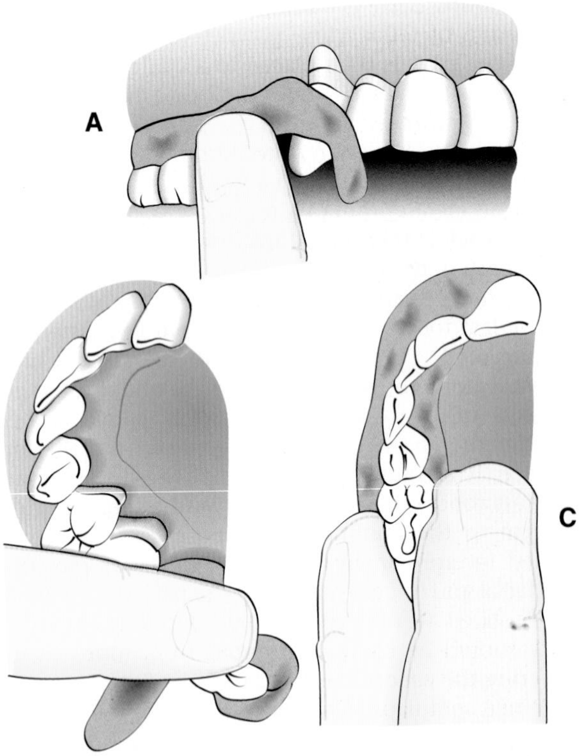

Figure 60-2 Inserting the periodontal pack. **A,** Strip of pack is hooked around the last molar and pressed into place anteriorly. **B,** Lingual pack is joined to the facial strip at the distal surface of the last molar and fitted into place anteriorly. **C,** Gentle pressure on the facial and lingual surfaces joins the pack interproximally.

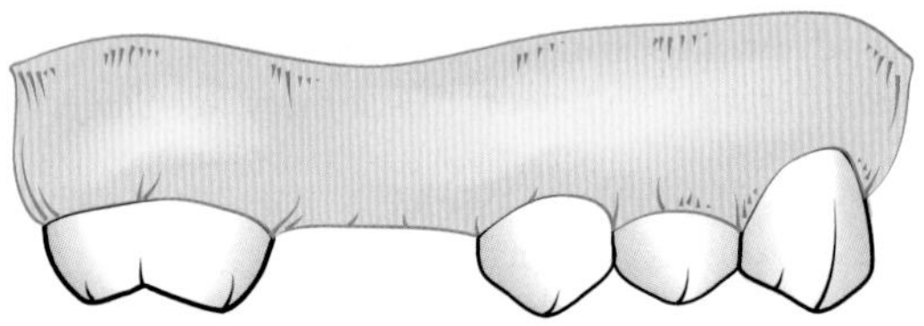

Figure 60-3 Continuous pack covers the edentulous space.

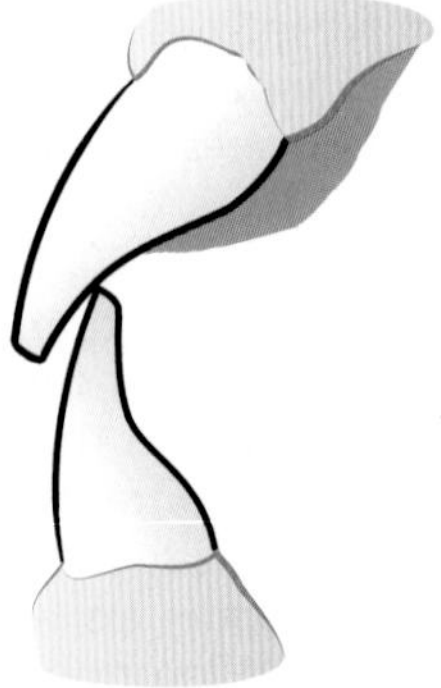

Figure 60-4 Periodontal pack should not interfere with the occlusion.

the remainder of the pack because the excess tends to break off, taking pack from the operated area with it. *Pack that interferes with the occlusion should be trimmed away before the patient is dismissed* (Figure 60-4). Failure to do this causes discomfort and jeopardizes retention of the pack.

The operator should ask the patient to move the tongue forcibly out and to each side, and the cheek and

BOX 60-1

Patient Instructions after Periodontal Surgery

Instructions for ___________ (Patient's Name)

The following information on your gum operation has been prepared to answer questions you may have about how to take care of your mouth. Please read the instructions carefully; our patients have found them very helpful.

Although there will be little or no discomfort when the anesthesia wears off, you should take two acetaminophen (Tylenol) tablets every 6 hours for the first 24 hours. After that, take the same medication if you have some discomfort. Do not take aspirin because this may increase bleeding.

We have placed a periodontal pack over your gums to protect them from irritation. The pack prevents pain, aids healing, and enables you to carry on most of your usual activities in comfort. The pack will harden in a few hours, after which it can withstand most of the forces of chewing without breaking off. It may take a little while to become accustomed to it.

The pack should remain in place until it is removed in the office at the next appointment. If particles of the pack chip off during the week, do not be concerned as long as you do not have pain. If a piece of the pack breaks off and you are in pain, or if a rough edge irritates your tongue or cheek, please call the office. The problem can be easily remedied by replacing the pack.

For the first 3 hours after the operation, avoid hot foods to permit the pack to harden. It is also convenient to avoid hot liquids during the first 24 hours. You can eat anything you can manage, but try to chew on the nonoperated side of your mouth. Semisolid or finely minced foods are suggested. Avoid citrus fruits or fruit juices, highly spiced foods, and alcoholic beverages; these will cause pain. Food supplements or vitamins are generally not necessary.

Do not smoke. The heat and smoke will irritate your gums, and the immunologic effects of nicotine will delay healing and prevent a completely successful outcome of the procedure performed. If possible, use this opportunity to give up smoking. In addition to all other well-known health risks, smokers have more gum disease than nonsmokers.

Do not brush over the pack. Brush and floss the areas of the mouth not covered by the pack as you normally do. Use chlorhexidine (Peridex, PerioGard) oral rinses after brushing (the prescription for this rinse has been given to you).

During the first day, apply ice intermittently on the face over the operated area. It is also beneficial to suck on ice chips intermittently during the first 24 hours. These methods will keep tissues cool and reduce inflammation and swelling.

You may experience a slight feeling of weakness or chills during the first 24 hours. This should not be cause for alarm but should be reported at the next visit. *Follow your regular daily activities, but avoid excessive exertion of any type.* Golf, tennis, skiing, bowling, swimming, or sunbathing should be postponed for a few days after the operation.

Swelling is not unusual, particularly in areas that required extensive surgical procedures. The swelling generally begins 1 to 2 days after the operation and subsides gradually in 3 or 4 days. If this occurs, apply moist heat over the operated area. If the swelling is painful or appears to become worse, please call the office.

Occasionally, blood may be seen in the saliva for the first 4 or 5 hours after the operation. This is not unusual and will correct itself. If there is considerable bleeding beyond this, take a piece of gauze, form it into the shape of a U, hold it in the thumb and index finger, apply it to both sides of the pack, and hold it there under pressure for 20 minutes. Do not remove it during this period to examine it. If the bleeding does not stop at the end of 20 minutes, please contact the office. *Do not try to stop bleeding by rinsing.*

After the pack is removed, the gums most likely will bleed more than they did before the operation. This is perfectly normal in the early stage of healing and will gradually subside. Do not stop cleaning because of it.

If any other problems arise, please call the office.

lips should be displaced in all directions to mold the pack while it is still soft. After the pack has set, it should be trimmed to eliminate all excess.

As a general rule, the pack is kept on for 1 week after surgery. This guideline is based on the usual timetable of healing and clinical experience. It is not a rigid requirement; the period may be extended, or the area may be repacked for an additional week.

Fragments of the surface of the pack may come off during the week, but this presents no problem. If a portion of the pack is lost from the operated area and the patient is uncomfortable, it is usually best to repack the area. The clinician should remove the remaining pack, wash the area with warm water, and apply a topical anesthetic before replacing the pack, which is then retained for 1 week. Again, the patient may develop pain from an overextended margin that irritates the vestibule, floor of the mouth, or tongue. The excess pack should be trimmed away, making sure that the new margin is not rough, before the patient is dismissed.

Postoperative Instructions

After the pack is placed, printed instructions are given to the patient to be read before he or she leaves the chair (Box 60-1).

First Postoperative Week

Properly performed, periodontal surgery presents no serious postoperative problems. Patients should be told to rinse with 0.12% chlorhexidine gluconate (Peridex, PerioGard) immediately after the surgical procedure and twice daily thereafter until normal plaque control technique can be resumed.[30,38,45] The following complications may arise in the first postoperative week, although they are the exception rather than the rule:

1. *Persistent bleeding after surgery.* The pack is removed, the bleeding points are located, and the bleeding is stopped with pressure, electrosurgery, or electrocautery. After the bleeding is stopped, the area is repacked.
2. *Sensitivity to percussion.* Extension of inflammation into the periodontal ligament may cause sensitivity to percussion. The patient should be questioned regarding the progress of the symptoms. Gradually diminishing severity is a favorable sign. The pack should be removed and the gingiva checked for localized areas of infection or irritation, which should be cleaned or incised to provide drainage. Particles of calculus that may have been overlooked should be removed. Relieving the occlusion is usually helpful. Sensitivity to percussion may also be caused by excess pack, which interferes with the occlusion. Removal of the excess usually corrects the condition.
3. *Swelling.* In the first 2 postoperative days, some patients may report a soft, painless swelling of the cheek in the surgical area. Lymph node enlargement may occur, and the temperature may be slightly elevated. The area of operation itself is usually symptom free. This type of involvement results from a localized inflammatory reaction to the procedure. It generally subsides by the fourth postoperative day, without necessitating removal of the pack. If swelling persists, becomes worse, or is associated with increased pain, amoxicillin (500 mg) should be taken every 8 hours for 1 week, and the patient should also be instructed to apply moist heat intermittently over the area. The antibiotic should also be used as a prophylactic measure after the next procedure, starting before the surgical appointment.
4. *Feeling of weakness.* Occasionally, patients report having experienced a "washed-out," weakened feeling for about 24 hours after surgery. This represents a systemic reaction to a transient bacteremia induced by the procedure. This reaction is prevented by premedication with amoxicillin (500 mg) every 8 hours, beginning 24 hours before the next procedure and continuing for 5 days postoperatively.

Removal of Pack and Return Visit

When the patient returns after 1 week, the periodontal pack is taken off by inserting a surgical hoe along the margin and exerting gentle lateral pressure. Pieces of pack retained interproximally and particles adhering to the tooth surfaces are removed with scalers. Particles may be enmeshed in the cut surface and should be carefully picked off with fine cotton pliers. The entire area is rinsed with peroxide to remove superficial debris.

Findings at Pack Removal. The following are usual findings when the pack is removed:

- If a *gingivectomy* has been performed, the cut surface is covered with a friable meshwork of new epithelium, which should not be disturbed. If calculus has not been completely removed, red, beadlike protuberances of granulation tissue will persist. The granulation tissue must be removed with a curette, exposing the calculus so that it can be removed and the root can be planed. Removal of the granulation tissue without removal of calculus is followed by recurrence.
- After a *flap operation,* the areas corresponding to the incisions are epithelialized but may bleed readily when touched; they should not be disturbed. Pockets should not be probed.
- The facial and lingual mucosa may be covered with a grayish yellow or white granular layer of food debris that has seeped under the pack. This is easily removed with a moist cotton pellet. The root surfaces may be sensitive to a probe or to thermal changes, and the teeth may be stained.
- *Fragments of calculus delay healing.* Each root surface should be rechecked visually to be certain that no calculus is present. Sometimes the color of the calculus is similar to that of the root. The grooves on proximal root surfaces and the furcations are areas where calculus is likely to be overlooked.

Repacking. After the pack is removed, it is usually not necessary to replace it. However, repacking for an additional week is advised for patients with (1) a low pain threshold who are particularly uncomfortable when the pack is removed, (2) unusually extensive periodontal involvement, or (3) slow healing. Clinical judgment helps in deciding whether to repack the area or leave the initial pack on longer than 1 week.

Tooth Mobility. Tooth mobility is increased immediately after surgery,[8] but it diminishes below the pretreatment level by the fourth week.[25]

Mouth Care between Procedures

Care of the mouth by the patient between the treatment of the first and the final areas, as well as after surgery is completed, is extremely important.[48] These measures should begin after the pack is removed from the first surgery. The patient has been through a presurgical period of instructed plaque control and should be reinstructed at this time.

Vigorous brushing is not feasible during the first week after the pack is removed. However, the patient is informed that plaque and food accumulation impair healing and is advised to try to keep the area as clean as possible by the gentle use of soft toothbrushes and light water irrigation. Rinsing with a chlorhexidine mouthwash or its topical application with cotton-tipped applicators is indicated for the first few postoperative weeks, particularly in advanced cases. Brushing is introduced when healing of the tissues permits it; the vigor of the overall hygiene regimen is increased as healing progresses. Patients should be told that (1) more gingival bleeding will most likely occur than was present before the procedure, (2) this bleeding is perfectly normal and will subside as healing progresses, and (3) it should not deter them from following their oral hygiene regimen.

Management of Postoperative Pain

Periodontal surgery that follows the basic principles outlined here should produce only minor pain and discomfort.[41] One study of 304 consecutive periodontal surgical interventions revealed that 51.3% of the patients reported minimal or no postoperative pain, and only 4.6% reported severe pain. Of these, only 20.1% took five or more doses of analgesic.[11] The same study showed that mucogingival procedures result in six times more discomfort and osseous surgery in 3.5 times more discomfort than plastic gingival surgery. In the few patients who may have severe pain, its control then becomes an important part of patient management.[29]

A common source of postoperative pain is overextension of the periodontal pack onto the soft tissue beyond the mucogingival junction or onto the frena. Overextended packs cause localized areas of edema, usually noticed 1 to 2 days after surgery. Removal of excess pack is followed by resolution in about 24 hours. Extensive and excessively prolonged exposure and dryness of bone also induce severe pain.

For most healthy patients, a preoperative dose of ibuprofen (600-800 mg) followed by one tablet every 8 hours for 24 to 48 hours is very effective in reducing discomfort after periodontal therapy. Patients are advised to continue taking ibuprofen or change to acetaminophen if needed thereafter. If pain persists, acetaminophen plus codeine (Tylenol #3) can be prescribed.

Caution should be used in prescribing or dispensing ibuprofen to patients with hypertension controlled by medications because it can interfere with the effectiveness of the medication.

When severe postoperative pain is present, the patient should be seen at the office on an emergency basis. The area is anesthetized by infiltration or topically, the pack is removed, and the wound is examined. Postoperative pain related to infection is accompanied by localized lymphadenopathy and a slight elevation in temperature. It should be treated with systemic antibiotics and analgesics.

Treatment of Sensitive Roots. Root hypersensitivity is a relatively common problem in periodontal practice. It may occur spontaneously when the root becomes exposed as a result of gingival recession or pocket formation, or it may appear after scaling and root planing and surgical procedures (see Curro[10] for literature review). It is manifested as pain induced by cold or hot temperature more often cold), by citrus fruits or sweets, or by contact with a toothbrush or a dental instrument.

Root sensitivity occurs more frequently in the cervical area of the root, where the cementum is extremely thin. Scaling and root-planing procedures remove this thin cementum, inducing the hypersensitivity.

Transmission of stimuli from the surface of the dentin to the nerve endings located in the dental pulp or in the pulpal region of the dentin could result from the odontoblastic process or from a hydrodynamic mechanism (displacement of dentinal fluid). The latter process seems more likely and would explain the importance of burnishing desensitizing agents to obturate the dentinal tubule.

An important factor for reducing or eliminating hypersensitivity is adequate plaque control. However, hypersensitivity may prevent plaque control, and therefore a vicious cycle of escalating hypersensitivity and plaque accumulation may be created.

Desensitizing Agents. A number of agents have been proposed to control root hypersensitivity. Clinical evaluation of the many agents proposed is difficult because (1) measuring and comparing pain between different persons is difficult, (2) hypersensitivity disappears by itself after a time, and (3) desensitizing agents usually take a few weeks to act.

The patient should be informed about the possibility of root hypersensitivity before treatment is undertaken. The following information on how to cope with the problem should also be given to the patient:

1. Hypersensitivity appears as a result of the exposure of dentin, which is inevitable if calculus and plaque and their products, buried in the root, are to be removed.
2. Hypersensitivity slowly disappears over a few weeks.
3. Plaque control is important for the reduction of hypersensitivity.
4. Desensitizing agents do not produce immediate relief and must be used for several days or even weeks to produce results.

Desensitizing agents can be applied by the patient at home or by the dentist or hygienist in the dental office. The most likely mechanism of action is the reduction in the diameter of the dentinal tubules so as to limit the displacement of fluid in them. According to Trowbridge and Silver,[44] this can be attained by (1) formation of a smear layer produced by burnishing the exposed surface, (2) topical application of agents that form insoluble precipitates within the tubules, (3) impregnation of tubules with plastic resins, or (4) sealing of the tubules with plastic resins.

Agents Used by the Patient. The most common agents used by the patient for oral hygiene are dentifrices. Although many dentifrice products contain fluoride, additional active ingredients for desensitization are strontium chloride, potassium nitrate, and sodium citrate. The American Dental Association (ADA) has approved the following dentifrices for desensitizing purposes: Sensodyne, and Thermodent, which contain strontium chloride[7,9,36]; Crest Sensitivity Protection, Denquel, and Promise, which contain potassium nitrate[1,9]; and Protect, which contains sodium citrate. Fluoride rinsing solutions and gels can also be used after the usual plaque control procedures.[42]

Patients should be aware that several factors must be considered in the treatment of tooth hypersensitivity, including the history and severity of the problem as well as the physical findings of the tooth or teeth involved. A proper diagnosis is required before any treatment can be initiated so that pathologic causes of pain (e.g., caries, cracked tooth, pulpitis) can be ruled out before attempting to treat hypersensitivity. Desensitizing agents act through the precipitation of crystalline salts on the dentin surface, which block dentinal tubules. Patients must be aware that their use will not prove to be effective unless used continuously for at least 2 weeks.

BOX 60-2

Office Treatments for Dentinal Hypersensitivity

- Cavity varnishes
- Antiinflammatory agents
- Treatments that partially obturate dentinal tubules
  - Burnishing of dentin
  - Silver nitrate
  - Zinc chloride–potassium ferrocyanide
  - Formalin
  - Calcium compounds
    - Calcium hydroxide
    - Dibasic calcium phosphate
  - Fluoride compounds
    - Sodium fluoride
    - Stannous fluoride
  - Iontophoresis
  - Strontium chloride
  - Potassium oxalate
  - Restorative resins
  - Dentin bonding agents

From Trowbridge HO, Silver DR: *Dent Clin North Am* 34:566, 1990.

SCIENCE TRANSFER

Performing surgery is a critical aspect of periodontal therapy. The host response to surgical wounding provides the basis of wound repair and tissue healing of the periodontium. Thus the cardinal signs of inflammation and the molecular cascades in the wound-healing process are initiated literally from the time of the first incision. Osseous repair around the tooth is initiated by creation of acute wounds into the bone by making small penetrations with a round bur, usually in a high-speed handpiece. This stimulates bleeding and the release of chemotactic and proinflammatory proteins. These in turn stimulate cell recruitment into the wound clot. Many events occur in concert, including cell proliferation, differentiation, matrix deposition, and clot degradation. The periodontal surgical procedure allows these events to occur in an environment with minimal bacterial insult, thus creating an opportunity to repair or regenerate the periodontal tissues.

Periodontal surgery requires an organized, step-by-step, gentle approach to each procedure that results in minimal tissue trauma and expedites completion of the surgery in the least time. The clinician must take responsibility for ensuring this approach is used; a patient-centered effort by the office staff is also required. Patient anxieties should be given high consideration.

Although many challenging and different procedures are part of each surgery, all surgeries must include complete removal of calculus and the planing of roots to optimize the treatment outcomes and reduce postoperative complications. Even after careful presurgical root curettage, there will be residual calculus on many regions that can be removed only with the visual access obtained at surgery.

Agents Used in the Dental Office. Box 60-2 lists various office treatments for the desensitization of hypersensitive dentin. These products and treatments aim to decrease hypersensitivity by blocking dentinal tubules with either a crystalline salt precipitation or an applied coating (varnish or bonding agent) on the root surface.[44]

Several agents have been used to precipitate crystalline salts on the dentin surface in an attempt to occlude the dentinal tubules. *Fluoride solutions* and pastes historically have been the agents of choice. In addition to their antisensitivity properties, fluoride agents have the advantage of anticaries activity, which is particularly important for patients with a tendency to develop root caries. Certain agents, however, such as chlorhexidine, decrease the ability of fluoride to bind with calcium on the root surfaces.[1] Thus, it is important to advise patients not to rinse or eat for 1 hour after a desensitizing treatment. Currently, potassium oxalate (Protect) and ferric oxalate (Sensodyne Sealant) solutions are the preferred agents; special applicators have been developed for their use. These agents form insoluble calcium oxalate crystals that occlude the dentinal tubules.[27,30]

A newer method of treatment for hypersensitive dentin is the use of varnishes or bonding agents to occlude dentinal tubules. Newer restorative materials, such as glass-ionomer cements and the dentin bonding agents, are still under investigation, but when the tooth needs recontouring or difficult cases do not respond to other treatments, the dentist may choose to use a restorative material. Resin primers alone could be promising, but the effects are not permanent, and investigations are ongoing.[14]

Despite some successes in decreasing dentin hypersensitivity, it is important to note that these "dental office" treatments have not been a predictable means of solving hypersensitivity, and the success achieved is often short lived. The crystalline salts and varnishes and the sealants can be washed away over time, and hypersensitivity may return. When this occurs, patients can have sensitive root surfaces treated again.

Recently, attempts have been made to improve the success and longevity of these treatments using *lasers.* Low-level laser "melting" of the dentin surface appears to seal dentinal tubules without damage to the pulp.[15,22] In a combined treatment modality, the Nd:YAG laser has been used to congeal fluoride varnish on root surfaces. This in vitro study demonstrated that the laser-treated fluoride varnish resisted removal by electric toothbrushing, with 90% of tubules remaining blocked, whereas in the controls (no laser treatment) the fluoride varnish was almost completely brushed away.[23] Despite these convincing preliminary results, more research is needed before laser treatment can be considered an effective and predictable means of desensitization (see Chapter 70).

HOSPITAL PERIODONTAL SURGERY

Ordinarily, periodontal surgery is an office procedure performed in quadrants or sextants, usually at biweekly or longer intervals. Under certain circumstances, however, it is in the best interest of the patient to treat the mouth at one surgery with the patient in a hospital operating room under general anesthesia.

Indications

Indications for hospital periodontal surgery include optimal control and management of apprehension, convenience for individuals who cannot endure multiple visits to complete surgical treatment, and patient protection.

Patient Apprehension. Gentleness, understanding, and preoperative sedation usually suffice to calm the fears of most patients. For some patients, however, the prospect of a series of surgical procedures is sufficiently stressful to trigger disturbances that jeopardize their well-being and hamper treatment. Explaining that the treatment at the hospital will be performed painlessly and that it will be accomplished by a level of anesthesia that is neither practical nor safe for patients in a dental office is an important step in allaying their fears. The thought of completing the necessary surgical procedures in one session rather than in repeated visits is an added comfort to the patient because it eliminates the prospect of repeated anxiety in anticipation of each treatment.

Patient Convenience. With complete mouth surgery, there is less stress for the patient and less time involved in postoperative care. For patients whose occupation entails considerable contact with the public, surgery performed at biweekly intervals sometimes presents a special problem. It means that for several weeks, some area of the mouth will be covered by a periodontal pack. With the complete mouth technique, the pack is usually retained for only 1 week. Patients find this an acceptable alternative to several weeks of discomfort in different areas of the mouth and multiple dressing applications. For a variety of other reasons, patients may desire to attend to their surgical needs in one session under optimal conditions.

Patient Protection. Some patients have systemic conditions that are not severe enough to contraindicate elective surgery but may require special precautions best provided in a hospital setting. This group includes some patients with cardiovascular disease, abnormal bleeding tendencies, or hyperthyroidism; those undergoing prolonged steroid therapy; and those with a history of rheumatic fever.

The purpose of hospitalization is to protect patients by anticipating their special needs, not to perform periodontal surgery when it is contraindicated by the patient's general condition. For some patients, elective surgery is contraindicated regardless of whether it is performed in the dental office or hospital. When consultation with the patient's physician leads to this decision, palliative periodontal therapy, in the form of scaling and root planing if permissible, is the necessary compromise.

Patient Preparation

Premedication. Patients should be given a sedative the night before surgery. Benzodiazepines work well for most patients, allowing the patient to sleep well the night before surgery. If the patient is extremely nervous about the procedure, it is also helpful to advise them to take a benzodiazepine on the morning of surgery. This ensures that they will be rested and as relaxed as possible before surgery.

Patients with systemic problems (e.g., history of rheumatic fever, cardiovascular problems) are premedicated as needed (see Chapter 44).

Anesthesia. Local or general anesthesia[26] may be used. *Local anesthesia* is the method of choice, except for especially apprehensive patients. It permits unhampered movement of the head, which is necessary for optimal visibility and accessibility to the various root surfaces. Local anesthesia is used in the same manner as for routine periodontal surgery.

When *general anesthesia* is indicated, it is administered by an anesthesiologist. It is important that the patient also receive local anesthesia, administered as for routine periodontal surgery, to ensure comfort for the patient and reduced bleeding during the procedure. The judicious use of local anesthetics to block regional nerves allows the level of sedation or general anesthesia to be lighter. Hence the entire operation is performed with a wider margin of safety.

Positioning and Periodontal Dressing. Surgery in the operating room is performed on the operating table with the patient lying down and the table either positioned flat or with the head inclined up to 30 degrees. Some operating rooms are equipped with dental chairs that can be used either flat or up to 30 degrees.

When general anesthesia is used, it is advisable to delay placing the periodontal dressing until the patient has recovered sufficiently to have a demonstrable cough reflex. Periodontal dressings placed before the end of general anesthesia can be displaced during the recovery period and pose serious risks of blocking the airway.

Postoperative Instructions

After a full recovery from general anesthesia, most patients can be discharged home with a responsible adult. The effects of general anesthesia and sedative agents make the patient drowsy for hours, and adult supervision at home is recommended for up to 24 hours after surgery. The typical postoperative instructions should be given to the responsible adult and the patient scheduled for a postoperative visit in 1 week.

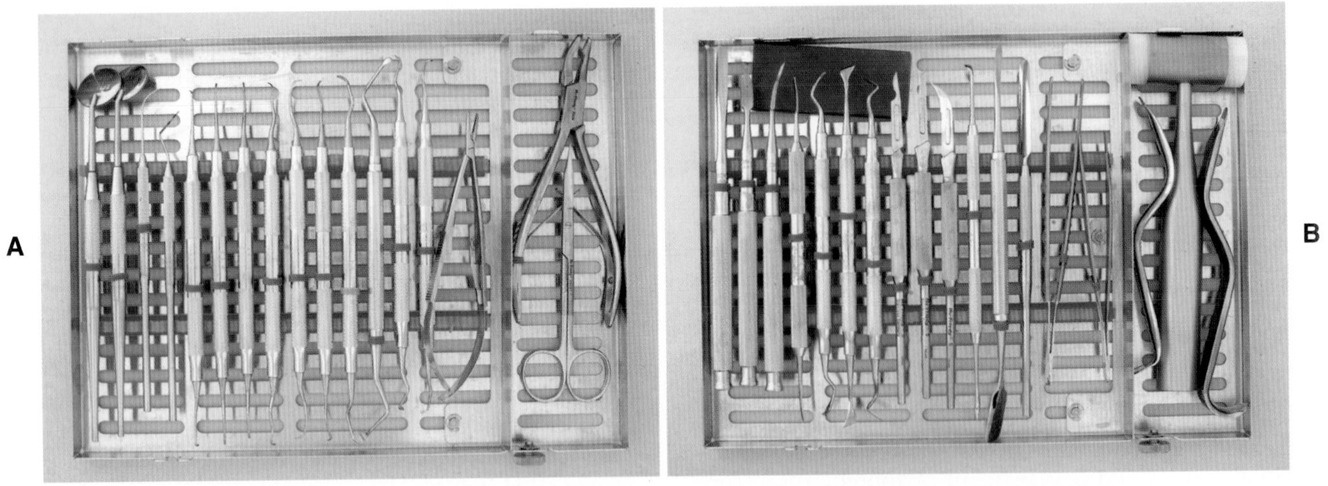

Figure 60-5 Typical series of periodontal surgical instruments, divided into two cassettes. **A,** *From left,* Mirrors, explorer, probe, series of curettes, needleholder, rongeurs, scissors. **B,** *From left,* Series of chisels, Kirkland knife, Orban knife, scalpel handles with surgical blades (#15C, 15, 12D), periosteal elevators, spatula, tissue forceps, cheek retractors, mallet, sharpening stone. (**A** Courtesy Hu-Friedy, Chicago. **B** Courtesy G. Hartzell & Son, Concord, Calif.)

SURGICAL INSTRUMENTS

Periodontal surgery is accomplished with numerous instruments; Figure 60-5 shows a typical surgical cassette. Periodontal surgical instruments are classified as follows:

1. Excisional and incisional instruments
2. Surgical curettes and sickles
3. Periosteal elevators
4. Surgical chisels
5. Surgical files
6. Scissors
7. Hemostats and tissue forceps

Excisional and Incisional Instruments

Periodontal Knives (Gingivectomy Knives). The Kirkland knife is representative of knives typically used for gingivectomy. These knives can be obtained as either double-ended or single-ended instruments. The entire periphery of these kidney-shaped knives is the cutting edge (Figure 60-6, *A*).

Interdental Knives. The Orban knife #1-2 (Figure 60-6, *B*) and the Merrifield knife #1, 2, 3, and 4 are examples of knives used for interdental areas. These spear-shaped knives have cutting edges on both sides of the blade and are designed with either double-ended or single-ended blades.

Surgical Blades. Scalpel blades of different shapes and sizes are used in periodontal surgery. The most common blades are #12D, 15, and 15C (Figure 60-7). The #12D blade is a beak-shaped blade with cutting edges on both sides, allowing the operator to engage narrow, restricted areas with both pushing and pulling cutting motions. The #15 blade is used for thinning flaps and general purposes. The #15C blade, a narrower version of the #15 blade, is useful for making the initial, scalloping-type incision. The slim design of this blade allows for incising into the narrow interdental portion of the flap. All these blades are discarded after one use.

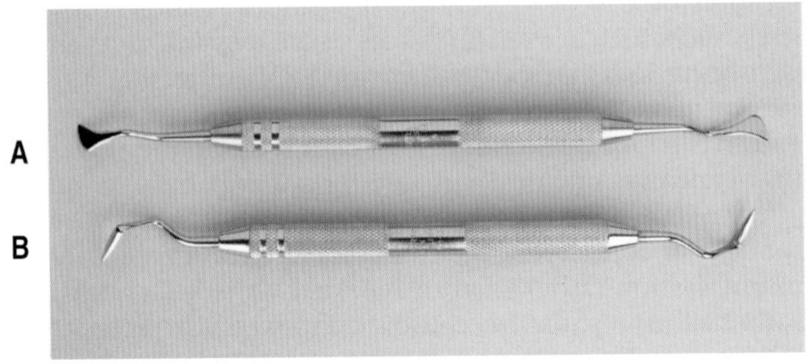

Figure 60-6 Gingivectomy knives. **A,** Kirkland knife. **B,** Orban interdental knife.

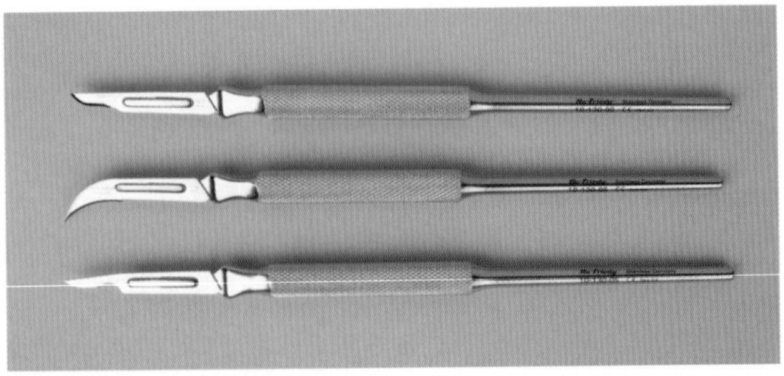

Figure 60-7 Surgical blades. *Top to bottom,* #15, #12D, #15C. These blades are disposable.

Electrosurgery (Radiosurgery) Techniques and Instrumentation. The term *electrosurgery* or *radiosurgery*[39] is currently used to identify surgical techniques performed on soft tissue using controlled, high-frequency electrical (radio) currents in the range of 1.5 to 7.5 million cycles per second, or megahertz. There are three classes of active electrodes: single-wire electrodes for incising or excising; loop electrodes for planing tissue; and heavy, bulkier electrodes for coagulation procedures.[16,28]

The four basic types of electrosurgical techniques are electrosection, electrocoagulation, electrofulguration, and electrodesiccation.

Electrosection, also referred to as *electrotomy* or *acusection,* is used for incisions, excisions, and tissue planing. Incisions and excisions are performed with single-wire active electrodes that can be bent or adapted to accomplish any type of cutting procedure.

Electrocoagulation provides a wide range of coagulation or hemorrhage control by using the electrocoagulation current. Electrocoagulation can prevent bleeding or hemorrhage at the initial entry into soft tissue, but it cannot stop bleeding after blood is present. All forms of hemorrhage must be stopped first by some form of direct pressure (e.g., air, compress, hemostat). After bleeding has momentarily stopped, final sealing of the capillaries or large vessels can be accomplished by a short application of the electrocoagulation current. The active electrodes used for coagulation are much bulkier than the fine tungsten wire used for electrosection.

Electrosection and electrocoagulation are the procedures most often used in all areas of dentistry. The two monoterminal techniques, electrofulguration and electrodesiccation, are not in general use in dentistry.

The most important basic rule of electrosurgery is: *always keep the tip moving.* Prolonged or repeated application of current to tissue induces heat accumulation and undesired tissue destruction, whereas interrupted application at intervals adequate for tissue cooling (5-10 seconds) reduces or eliminates heat buildup. Electrosurgery is not intended to destroy tissue; it is a controllable means of sculpturing or modifying oral soft tissue with little discomfort and hemorrhage for the patient.

The indications for electrosurgery in periodontal therapy and a description of wound healing after electrosurgery are presented in Chapter 62. Electrosurgery is contraindicated for patients who have noncompatible or poorly shielded cardiac pacemakers.

Surgical Curettes and Sickles

Larger and heavier curettes and sickles are often needed during surgery for the removal of granulation tissue, fibrous interdental tissues, and tenacious subgingival deposits. The Prichard curette (Figure 60-8) and the Kirkland surgical instruments are heavy curettes, whereas the Ball scaler #B2-B3 is a popular heavy sickle. The wider, heavier blades of these instruments make them suitable for surgical procedures.

Periosteal Elevators

The periosteal elevators are needed to reflect and move the flap after the incision has been made for flap surgery. The Woodson and Prichard elevators are well-designed periosteal instruments (Figure 60-9).

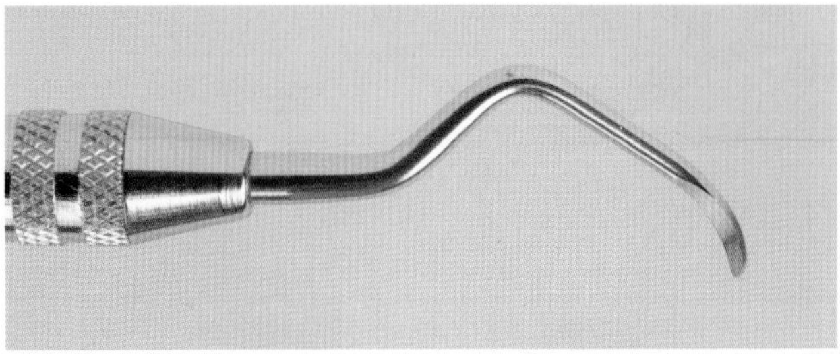

Figure 60-8 Prichard surgical curette. Curettes used in surgery have wider blades than those used for conventional scaling and root planing.

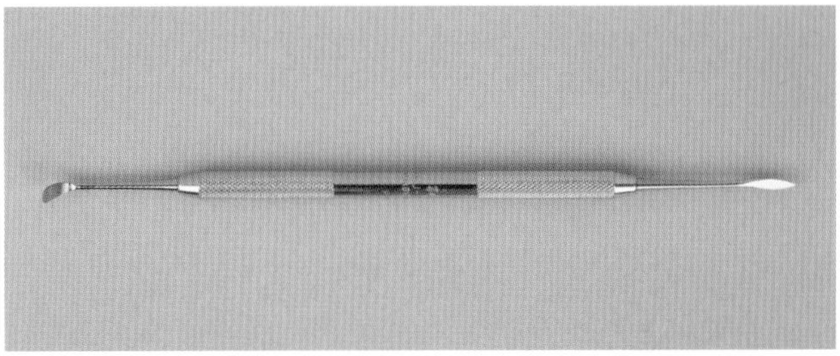

Figure 60-9 Woodson periosteal elevator.

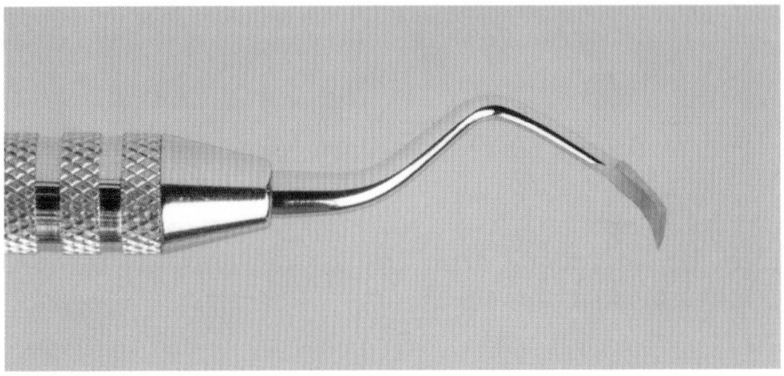

Figure 60-10 Back-action chisel.

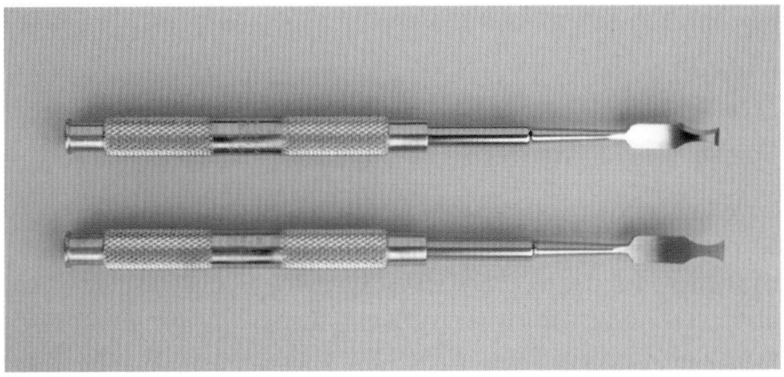

Figure 60-11 Ochsenbein chisels are paired, with the cutting edges in opposite directions.

Surgical Chisels

The back-action chisel is used with a pull motion Figure 60-10, whereas the straight chisel (e.g., Wiedelstadt, Ochsenbein #1-2) is used with a push motion (Figure 60-11). The Ochsenbein chisel is a useful chisel with a semicircular indentation on both sides of the shank that allows the instrument to engage around the tooth and

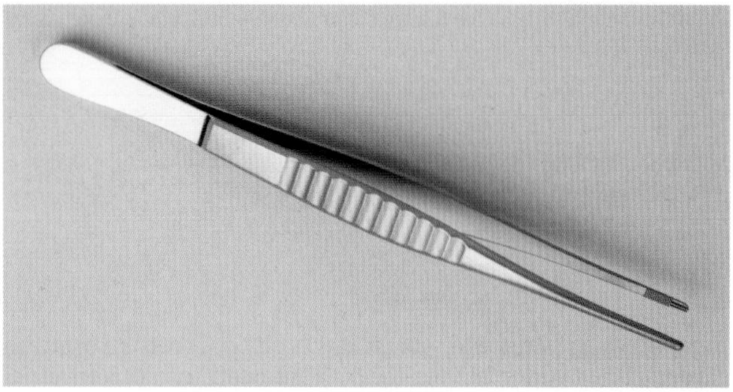

Figure 60-12 DeBakey tissue forceps.

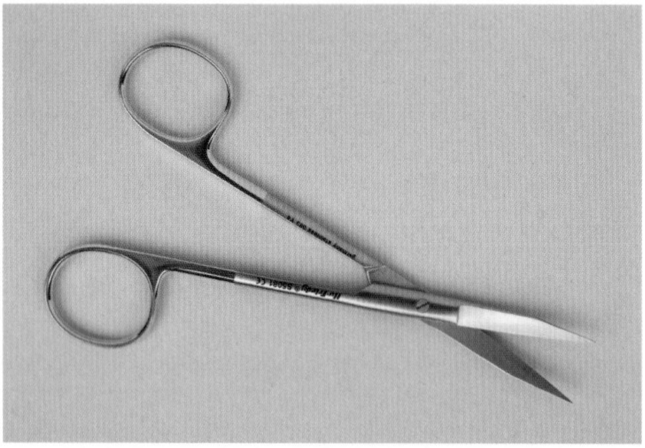

Figure 60-13 Goldman-Fox scissors.

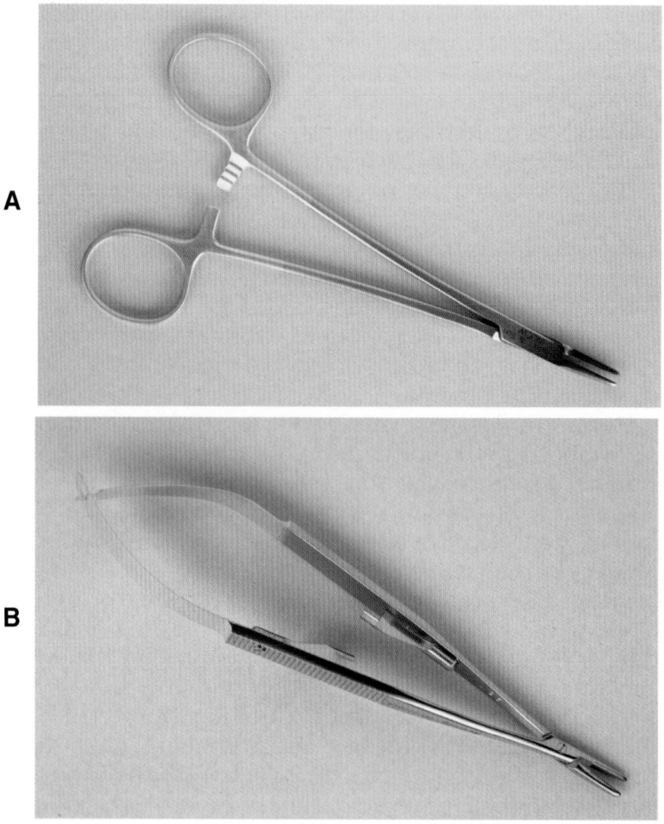

Figure 60-14 **A,** Conventional needleholder. **B,** Castroviejo needleholder.

into the interdental area. The Rhodes chisel is another popular back-action chisel.

Tissue Forceps

The tissue forceps is used to hold the flap during suturing. It is also used to position and displace the flap after the flap has been reflected. The DeBakey forcep is an extremely efficient instrument (Figure 60-12).

Scissors and Nippers

Scissors and nippers are used in periodontal surgery to remove tabs of tissue during gingivectomy, trim the margins of flaps, enlarge incisions in periodontal abscesses, and remove muscle attachments in mucogingival surgery. Many types are available, and individual preference determines the choice. The Goldman-Fox #16 scissors has a curved, beveled blade with serrations (Figure 60-13).

Needleholders

Needleholders are used to suture the flap at the desired position after the surgical procedure has been completed. In addition to the regular types of needleholder (Figure 60-14, A), the Castroviejo needleholder is used for delicate, precise techniques that require quick and easy release and grasp of the suture (Figure 60-14, *B*).

REFERENCES

1. *ADA guide to dental therapeutics,* Chicago, 1998, American Dental Association.
2. Addy M, Douglas WH: A chlorhexidine-containing methacrylic gel as a periodontal dressing, *J Periodontol* 46:465, 1975.
3. Allen GD: *Dental anesthesia and analgesia (local and general),* ed 3, Baltimore, 1984, Williams & Wilkins.
4. Ariaudo AA: The efficacy of antibiotics in periodontal surgery, *J Periodontol* 40:150, 1969.
5. Baer PN, Goldman HM, Scigliano J: Studies on a bacitracin periodontal dressing, *Oral Surg* 11:712, 1958.
6. Baer PN, Summer CF III, Miller G: Periodontal dressings, *Dent Clin North Am* 13:181, 1969.
7. Blitzer B: A consideration of the possible causes of dental hypersensitivity: treatment by a strontium ion dentifrice, *Periodontics* 5:318, 1967.
8. Burch J, Conroy CW, Ferris RT: Tooth mobility following gingivectomy: a study of gingival support of the teeth, *Periodontics* 6:90, 1960.
9. Collins JF, Gingold J, Stanley H, et al: Reducing dentinal hypersensitivity with strontium chloride and potassium nitrate, *Gen Dent* 32:40, 1984.
10. Curro FA: Tooth hypersensitivity, *Dent Clin North Am* 34:403, 1990.
11. Curtis JW Jr, McLain JB, Hutchinson RA: The incidence and severity of complications and pain following periodontal surgery, *J Periodontol* 56:597, 1985.
12. Dal Pra DJ, Strahan JD: A clinical evaluation of the benefits of a course of oral penicillin following periodontal surgery, *Aust Dent J* 17:219, 1972.

13. Fraleigh CM: An evaluation of topical Terramycin in postgingivectomy pack, *J Periodontol* 27:201, 1956.
14. Gangarosa LP Sr: Current strategies for dentist-applied treatment in the management of hypersensitive dentine, *Arch Oral Biol* 39(suppl):101S, 1994.
15. Gerschman JA, Ruben J, Gebart-Eaglemont J: Low-level laser therapy for dentinal tooth hypersensitivity, *Aust Dent J* 39:353, 1994.
16. Gnanasekhar JD, al-Duwairi YS: Electrosurgery in dentistry, *Quintessence Int* 29:649, 1998.
17. Hirschfeld AS, Wassermen BH: Retention of periodontal packs, *J Periodontol* 29:199 1958.
18. Holmes CH: Periodontal pack on single tooth retained by acrylic splint, *J Am Dent Assoc* 64:831, 1962.
19. Javelet J, Torabinejad M, Danforth A: Isobutyl cyanoacrylate: a clinical and histological comparison with sutures in closing mucosal incisions in monkeys, *Oral Surg* 59:91, 1985.
20. Jones JK, Triplett RG: The relationship of cigarette smoking to impaired intraoral wound healing: a review of evidence and implications for patient care, *J Oral Maxillofac Surg* 50:237, 1992.
21. Kidd EA, Wade AB: Penicillin control of swelling and pain after periodontal osseous surgery, *J Clin Periodontol* 1:52, 1974.
22. Lan WH, Liu HC: Treatment of dentin hypersensitivity by Nd:YAG laser, *J Clin Laser Med Surg* 14:89, 1996.
23. Lan WH, Liu HC, Lin CP: The combined occluding effect of sodium fluoride varnish and Nd:YAG laser irradiation on human dentinal tubules, *J Endodont* 25:424, 1999.
24. Levin MP, Cutright DE, Bhaskar SN: Cyanoacrylate as a periodontal dressing, *J Oral Med* 30:40, 1975.
25. Majewski I, Sponholz H: Ergebnisse nach parodonal therapeutischen Massnahmen unter besonderer Berucksichtigung der Zahnbeweglichkeitssung mit dem Makroperiodontometer nach Muhlemann, *Zahnaerztl Rundsch* 75:57, 1966.
26. Malamed SF: *Sedation: a guide to patient management,* ed 3, St Louis, 1995, Mosby.
27. Miller JT, Shannon KL, Kilyore WG, et al: Use of water-free stannous fluoride–containing gel in the control of dental hypersensitivity, *J Periodontol* 40:490, 1969.
28. Moore DA: Electrosurgery in dentistry: past and present, *Gen Dent* 43:460, 1995.
29. Murphy NC, DeMarco TJ: Controlling pain in periodontal patients, *Dent Surv* 55:46, 1979.
30. Newman MG, Sanz M, Nachnani S, et al: Effect of 0.12% chlorhexidine on bacterial recolonization after periodontal surgery, *J Periodontol* 60:577, 1989.
31. Pack PO, Haber J: The incidence of clinical infection after periodontal surgery: a retrospective study, *J Periodontol* 54:441, 1983.
32. Pendrill K, Reddy J: The use of prophylactic penicillin in periodontal surgery, *J Periodontol* 51:44, 1980.
33. Preber H, Bergstrom J: Effect of cigarette smoking on periodontal healing following surgical therapy, *J Clin Periodontol* 17:324, 1990.
34. Romanow I: Allergic reactions to periodontal pack, *J Periodontol* 28:151, 1957.
35. Romanow I: Relationship of moniliasis to the presence of antibiotics in periodontal packs, *Periodontics* 2:298, 1964.
36. Ross MR: Hypersensitive teeth: effect of strontium chloride in a compatible dentifrice, *J Periodontol* 32:49, 1961.
37. Sachs HA, Fanroush A, Checchi L, et al: Current status of periodontal dressings, *J Periodontol* 55:689, 1984.
38. Sanz M, Newman MG, Anderson L, et al: Clinical enhancement of post-periodontal surgical therapy by 0.12 per cent chlorhexidine gluconate mouthrinse, *J Periodontol* 60:570, 1989.
39. Sherman JA: *Oral radiosurgery: an illustrated clinical guide,* ed 2, London, 1997, Martin Dunitz.
40. Smith DC: A materialistic look at periodontal packs, *Dent Pract Dent Rec* 20:273, 1970.
41. Strahan JD, Glenwright HD: Pain experience in periodontal surgery, *J Periodontal Res* 1:163, 1967.
42. Tarbet WJ, Silverman G, Stolman JW, et al: A clinical evaluation of a new treatment for dentinal hypersensitivity, *J Periodontol* 51:535, 1980.
43. Tonetti MS, Pini Prato G, Cortellini P: Effect of cigarette smoking on periodontal healing following GTR in infrabony pockets: a preliminary retrospective study, *J Clin Periodontol* 22:229, 1995.
44. Trowbridge HO, Silver DR: A review of current approaches to in-office management of tooth hypersensitivity, *Dent Clin North Am* 34:583, 1990.
45. Vaughan ME, Garnick JJ: The effect of 0.125 per cent chlorhexidine rinse on inflammation after periodontal surgery, *J Periodontol* 60:704, 1989.
46. Ward AW: Inharmonious cusp relation as a factor in periodontoclasia, *J Am Dent Assoc* 10:471, 1923.
47. Watts TA, Combe EC: Adhesion of periodontal dressings to enamel in vitro, *J Clin Periodontol* 7:62, 1980.
48. Westfelt E, Nyman S, Socransky SS: Significance of frequency of professional cleaning for healing following periodontal surgery, *J Clin Periodontol* 10:148, 1983.

Surgical Anatomy of the Periodontium and Related Structures

CHAPTER 61

Fermin A. Carranza

CHAPTER OUTLINE

MANDIBLE
MAXILLA
MUSCLES
ANATOMIC SPACES

A sound knowledge of the anatomy of the periodontium and the surrounding hard and soft structures is essential to determine the scope and possibilities of surgical periodontal procedures and to minimize their risks. Bones, muscles, blood vessels, and nerves, as well as the anatomic spaces located in the vicinity of the periodontal surgical field, are particularly important. Only those features of periodontal relevance are mentioned in this chapter; the reader is referred to books on oral anatomy for a more comprehensive description of these structures.[3,4]

MANDIBLE

The mandible is a horseshoe-shaped bone connected to the skull by the temporomandibular joints. It presents several landmarks of great surgical importance.

The *mandibular canal,* occupied by the inferior alveolar nerve and vessels, begins at the mandibular foramen on the medial surface of the mandibular ramus and curves downward and forward, becoming horizontal below the apices of the molars (Figure 61-1). The distance from the canal to the apices of the molars is shorter in the third molar area and increases as it goes forward. In the premolar area the canal divides in two: the *incisive canal,* which continues horizontally to the midline, and the *mental canal,* which turns upward and opens in the mental foramen.

The *mental foramen,* from which the mental nerve and vessels emerge, is located on the buccal surface of the mandible below the apices of the premolars, sometimes closer to the second premolar and usually halfway between the lower border of the mandible and the alveolar margin (Figure 61-2). The opening of the mental foramen faces upward and distally, with its posterosuperior border slanting gradually to the bone surface. As it emerges, the *mental nerve* divides into three branches. One branch of the nerve turns forward and downward to supply the skin of the chin. The other two branches course anteriorly and upward to supply the skin and mucous membrane of the lower lip and the mucosa of the labial alveolar surface.

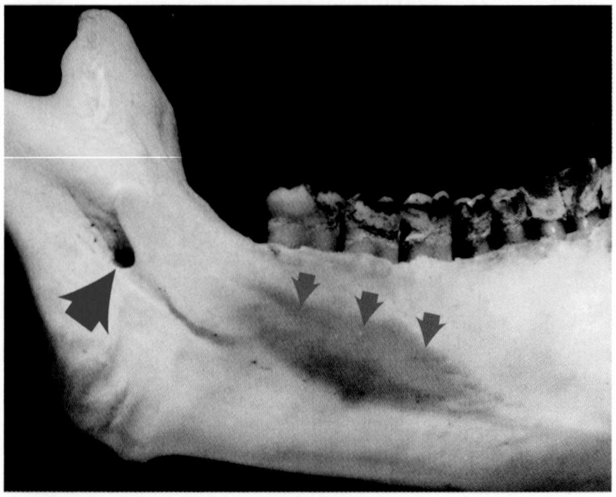

Figure 61-1 Mandible, lingual surface view. Note the lingual, or mandibular, foramen *(blue arrow),* where the inferior alveolar nerve enters the mandibular canal, and the mylohyoid ridge *(red arrows).*

Surgical trauma to the mental nerve can produce paresthesia of the lip, which recovers slowly. Familiarity with the location and appearance of the mental nerve reduces the likelihood of injury (Figure 61-3).

In partially or totally edentulous jaws, the disappearance of the alveolar portion of the mandible brings the mandibular canal closer to the superior border. When these patients are evaluated for placement of implants, the distance between the canal and the superior surface of the bone must be carefully determined to avoid surgical injury to the nerve.

The *lingual nerve,* along with the inferior alveolar nerve, is a branch of the posterior division of the mandibular nerve and descends along the mandibular ramus medial to and in front of the inferior alveolar nerve. The lingual nerve lies close to the surface of the oral mucosa in the third molar area and goes deeper as it goes forward (Figure 61-4; see also Fig. 61-17). It can be damaged during anesthetic injections and during oral surgery procedures such as third molar extractions.[7] Less often, the lingual nerve may be injured when a periodontal partial-thickness flap is raised in the third molar region or when releasing incisions are made.

The *alveolar process,* which provides the supporting bone to the teeth, has a narrower distal curvature than the body of the mandible (Figure 61-5), creating a flat surface in the posterior area between the teeth and the anterior border of the ramus. This results in the formation of the *external oblique ridge,* which runs downward and forward to the region of the second or first molar (Figure 61-6), creating a shelflike bony area. Resective osseous therapy may be difficult or impossible in this area because of the amount of bone that would have to be removed.

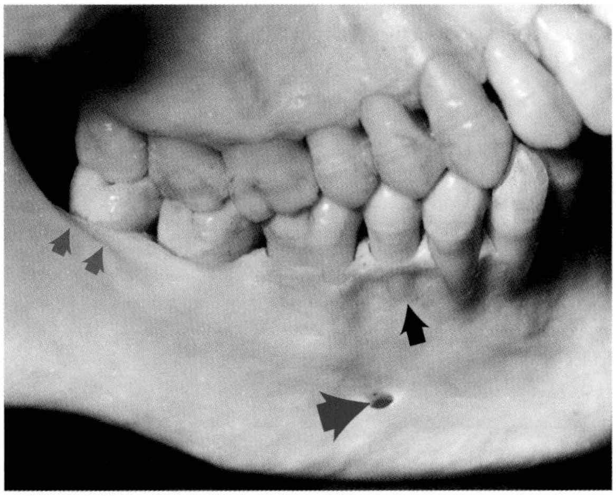

Figure 61-2 Mandible, facial surface view. Note the location of the mental foramen *(blue arrow),* slightly distal and apical to the apex of the second premolar, and the shelflike area in the region of the molars *(red arrows),* created by the external oblique ridge. Note also the fenestration present in the second premolar *(black arrow).*

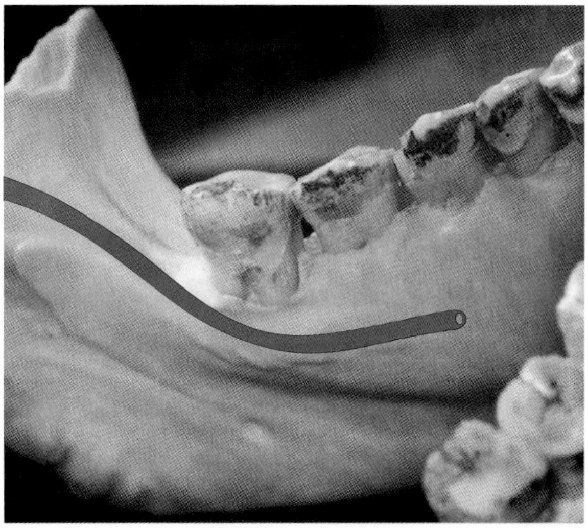

Figure 61-4 Lingual view of mandible showing the pathway of the lingual nerve, which goes near the gingiva in the third molar area and then continues forward, going deeper and medially.

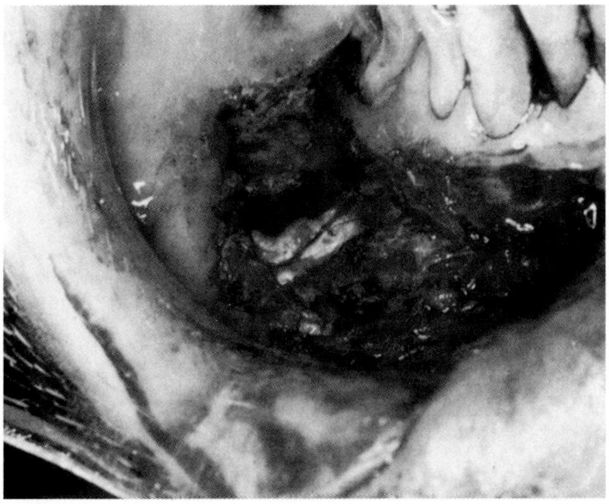

Figure 61-3 Mental nerve emerging from the foramen in the premolar area.

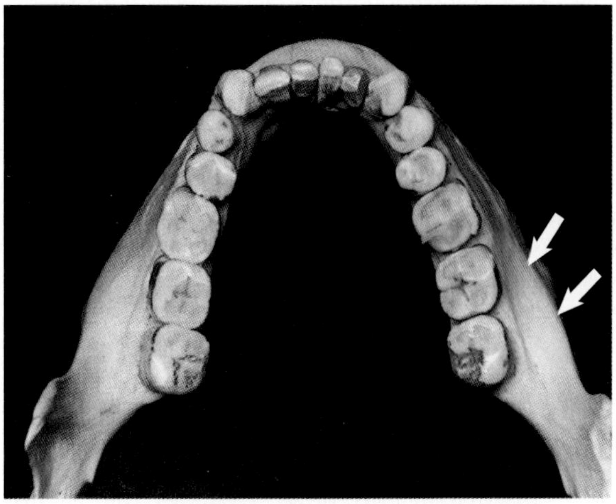

Figure 61-5 Occlusal view of mandible. Note the shelf created in the facial molar areas by the external oblique ridge. Arrows show the attachment of the buccinator muscle.

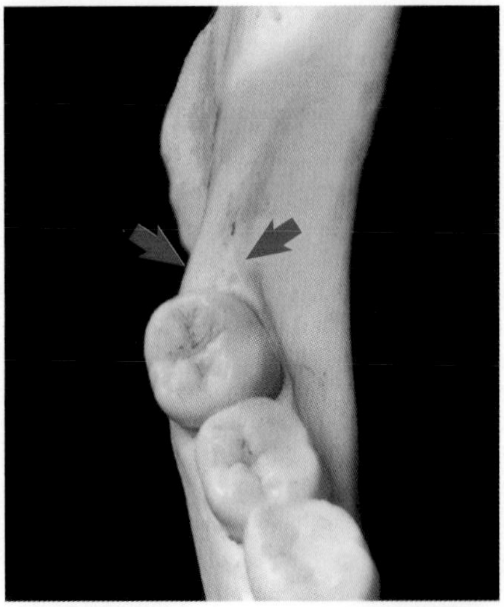

Figure 61-6 Mandible, occlusal view of ramus and molars. Note the retromolar triangle area distal to the third molar *(arrows).*

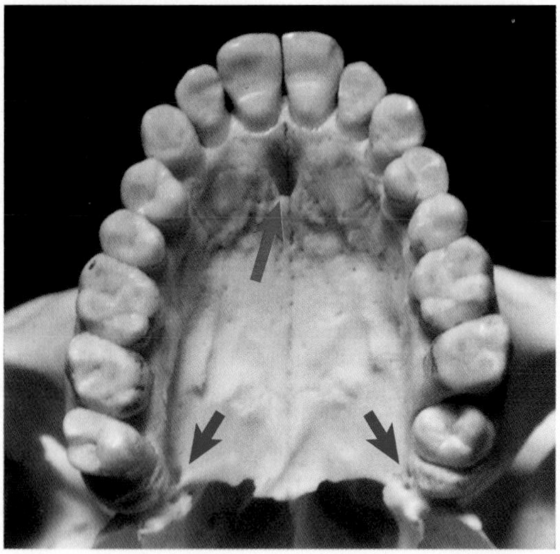

Figure 61-8 Occlusal view of maxilla and palatine bone. Note the opening of the incisive canal or anterior palatine foramen *(red arrow)* and the greater palatine foramen *(blue arrows).*

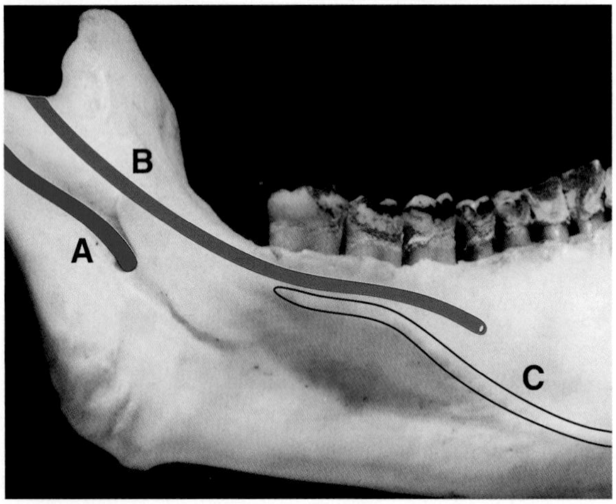

Figure 61-7 Lingual view of mandible showing the inferior alveolar nerve entering the mandibular canal *(A),* the lingual nerve traversing near the lingual surface of the third molar *(B),* and inferiorly, the attachment of the mylohyoid muscle *(C).*

Distal to the third molar, the external oblique ridge circumscribes the *retromolar triangle* (Figure 61-6). This region is occupied by glandular and adipose tissue covered by unattached, nonkeratinized mucosa. If sufficient space exists distal to the last molar, a band of attached gingiva may be present; only in such a case can a distal wedge procedure be performed.

The inner side of the body of the mandible is traversed obliquely by the *mylohyoid ridge,* which starts close to the alveolar margin in the third molar area and continues anteriorly, increasing its distance from the osseous margin as it goes forward (Figure 61-7). The *mylohyoid muscle,* inserted at this ridge, separates the *sublingual space,* located more anteriorly and superiorly, from the *submandibular space,* located more posteriorly and inferiorly (see Figure 61-17).

MAXILLA

The maxilla is a paired bone that is hollowed out by the maxillary sinus. The maxilla has the following four processes:

- The *alveolar process* contains the sockets for the upper teeth.
- The *palatine process* extends horizontally to meet its counterpart from the other maxilla at the midline intermaxillary suture, and it extends posteriorly with the horizontal plate of the palatine bone to form the hard palate.
- The *zygomatic process* extends laterally from the area of the first molar and determines the depth of the vestibular fornix.
- The *frontal process* extends in an ascending direction and articulates with the frontal bone at the frontomaxillary suture.

The terminal branches of the nasopalatine nerve and vessels pass through the incisive canal, which opens in the midline anterior area of the palate (Figure 61-8). The mucosa overlying the incisive canal presents a slight protuberance called the *incisive papilla.* Vessels emerging through the incisive canal are of small caliber, and their surgical interference is of little consequence.

The *greater palatine foramen* opens 3 to 4 mm anterior to the posterior border of the hard palate (Figure 61-9). The greater palatine nerve and vessels emerge through this foramen and run anteriorly in the submucosa of the palate, between the palatal and alveolar processes (Figure 61-10). Palatal flaps and donor sites for gingival grafts should be carefully performed and selected to avoid invading these areas because profuse hemorrhages may ensue, particularly if vessels are damaged at the palatine foramen.

The mucous membrane covering the hard palate is firmly attached to the underlying bone. The submucous

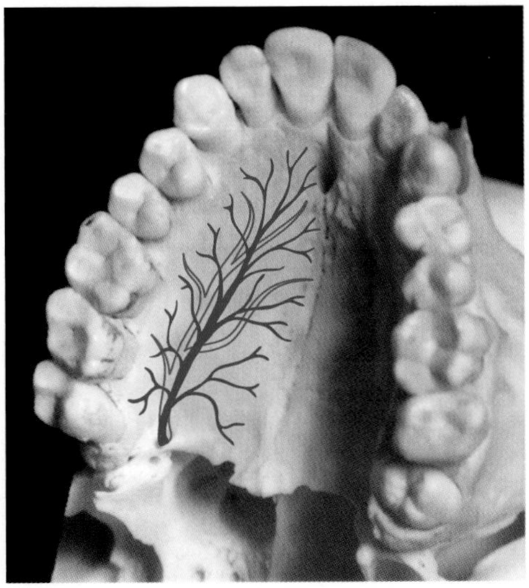

Figure 61-9 Occlusolateral view of palate showing nerves (*red*) and vessels (*blue*) emerging from the greater palatine foramen and continuing anteriorly on the palate.

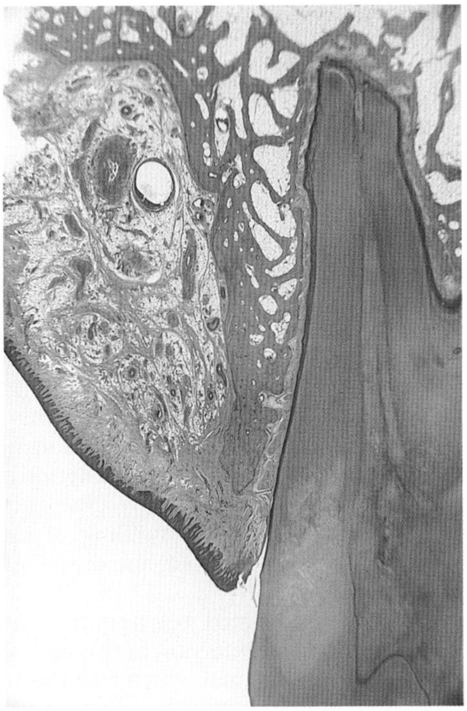

Figure 61-10 Histologic frontal section of human palate at the level of the first molar, showing the location of vessels and nerve, surrounded by adipose and glandular tissue.

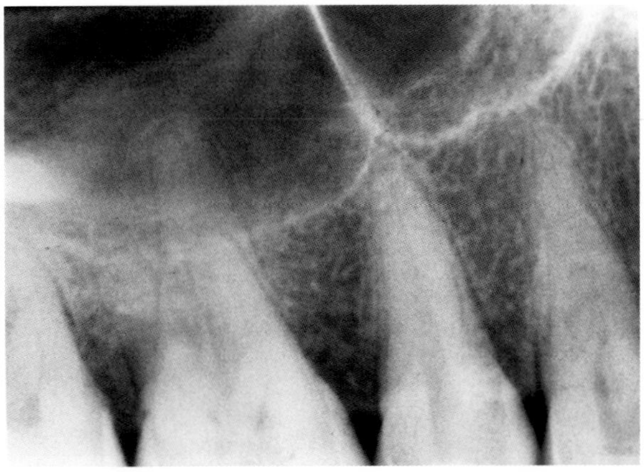

Figure 61-11 Radiograph of upper molars and premolars, with the maxillary sinus apparently near the apices.

layer of the palate posterior to the first molars contains the *palatal glands,* which are more compact in the soft palate and extend anteriorly, filling the gap between the mucosal connective tissue and the periosteum and protecting the underlying vessels and nerve (see Figure 61-16).

The area distal to the last molar is called the *maxillary tuberosity* and consists of the posteroinferior angle of the infratemporal surface of the maxilla; medially it articulates with the pyramidal process of the palatine bone. It is covered by fibrous connective tissue and contains the terminal branches of the middle and posterior palatine nerves. Excision of the area for distal wedge surgery may reach medially to the tensor palati muscle, which comes from the greater wing of the sphenoid bone and ends in a tendon that forms the palatine aponeurosis, which expands, fanlike, to attach to the posterior border of the hard palate.

The body of the maxilla is occupied by the *maxillary sinus,* or *maxillary antrum,* which is a hollow pyramidal area, measuring on the average 30 mm anteroposteriorly and vertically and 25 mm faciomedially, with its base toward the nose and lined by respiratory epithelium (ciliated columnar epithelium). The four walls making up the sinus are the inferior portion, consisting of the alveolar process, and the facial, orbital, and infratemporal walls. The maxillary sinus opens superiorly into the middle nasal fossa and anteriorly in the sinus.[4,11]

Blood supply to the sinus is provided by the anterior and posterior superior alveolar artery and the sphenopalatine artery, all branches from the maxillary artery. The inferior wall of the maxillary sinus is frequently separated from the apices and roots of the maxillary posterior teeth by a thin, bony plate (Figure 61-11). In edentulous posterior areas the maxillary sinus bony wall may be only a thin plate in intimate contact with the alveolar mucosa (Figure 61-12). Adequate determination of the extension of the maxillary sinus into the surgical site is important to avoid creating an oroantral communication, particularly in relation to the placement of implants. In edentulous jaws, determining the amount of available bone in the anterior area, below the floor of the nasal cavity, is also critical (see Chapter 78).

Both the maxilla and the mandible may have *exostoses* or *tori,* which are considered to be within the normal range of anatomic variation. Sometimes these structures may hinder the removal of plaque by the patient and may have to be removed to improve the prognosis of neighboring teeth. The most common location of a mandibular torus is in the lingual area of canine and premolars, above the mylohyoid muscle (Figure 61-13). Maxillary tori are usually located in the midline of

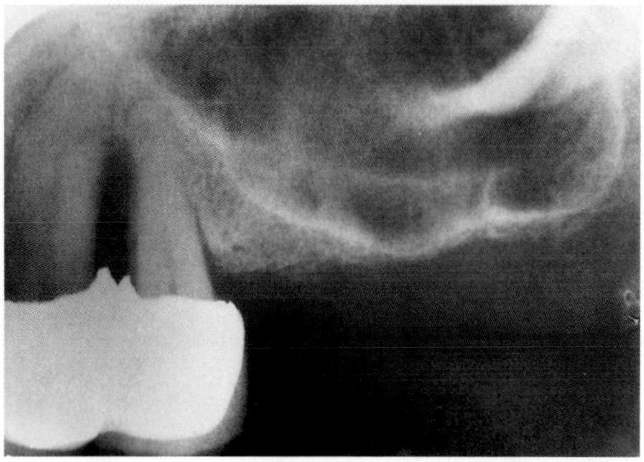

Figure 61-12 Radiograph of edentulous molar maxillary area, with the sinus very close to the surface.

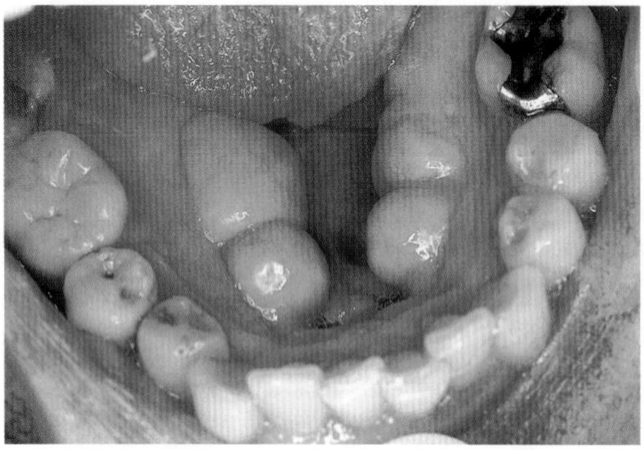

Figure 61-13 Clinical photograph of mandibular torus.

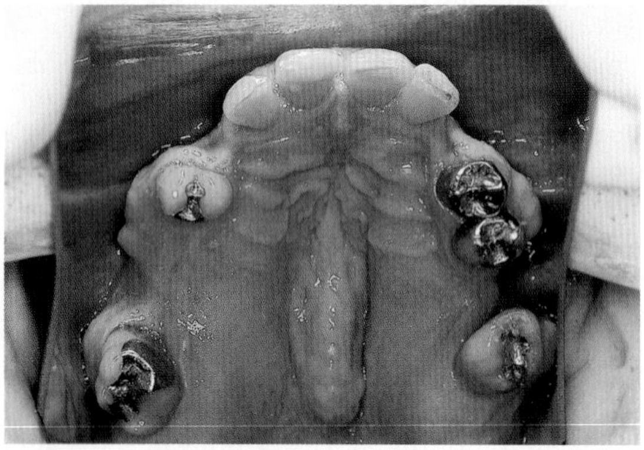

Figure 61-14 Clinical photograph of palatal torus, located in the midline of the palate.

the hard palate (Figure 61-14); smaller tori may be seen over the palatal roots of the molars.

MUSCLES

Several muscles may be encountered when performing periodontal flaps, particularly in mucogingival surgery. These are the mentalis, incisivus labii inferioris, depressor labii inferioris, depressor anguli oris (triangularis), incisivus labii superioris, and buccinator muscles. Their bony attachment is shown in Figure 61-15, and these muscles provide mobility to the lips and cheeks.

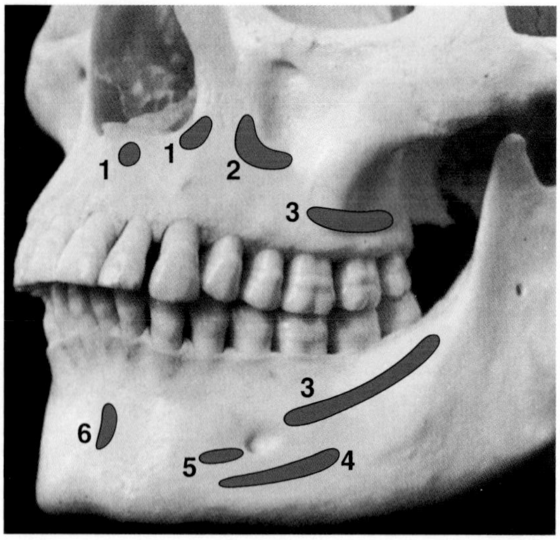

Figure 61-15 Muscle attachments that may be encountered in mucogingival surgery. *1,* Nasalis; *2,* levator anguli oris; *3,* buccinator; *4,* depressor anguli oris; *5,* depressor labii inferioris; *6,* mentalis.

ANATOMIC SPACES

Several anatomic spaces or *compartments* are found close to the operative field of periodontal surgery. These spaces contain loose connective tissue but can be easily distended by inflammatory fluid and infection.

Surgical invasion of these areas may result in dangerous infections and should be carefully avoided. Some of these spaces are briefly described here. For further information, the reader is referred to other sources.[2,5,6,9,10]

The *canine fossa* contains varying amounts of connective tissue and fat and is bounded superiorly by the quadratus labii superioris muscle, anteriorly by the orbicularis oris, and posteriorly by the buccinator. Infection of this area results in swelling of the upper lip, obliterating the nasolabial fold, and of the upper and lower eyelids, closing the eye.

The *buccal space* is located between the buccinator and the masseter muscles. Infection of this area results in swelling of the cheek but may extend to the temporal space or the submandibular space, with which the buccal space communicates.

The *mental,* or *mentalis, space* is located in the region of the mental symphysis, where the mental muscle, depressor muscle of the lower lip, and depressor muscle of the corner of the mouth are attached. Infection of this area results in large swelling of the chin, extending downward.

The *masticator space* contains the masseter muscle, pterygoid muscles, tendon of insertion of the temporalis muscle, and mandibular ramus and posterior part of the body of the mandible. Infection of this area results in swelling of the face and severe trismus and pain. If the abscess occupies the deepest part of this compartment, facial swelling may not be obvious, but the patient may

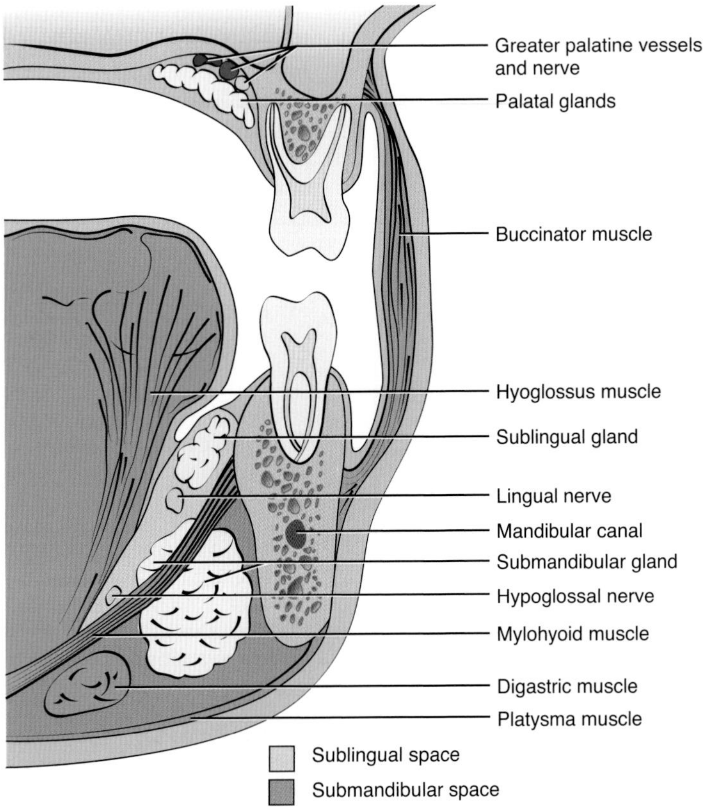

Figure 61-16 Diagram of a frontal section of the human head at the level of the first molars, depicting the most important structures in relation to periodontal surgery. Note the location of the sublingual space, submandibular space, and greater palatine nerve and vessels.

complain of pain and trismus. Patients may also have difficulty and discomfort when moving the tongue and swallowing.

The *sublingual space* is located below the oral mucosa in the anterior part of the floor of the mouth and contains the sublingual gland and its excretory duct, the submandibular or Wharton's duct, and is traversed by the lingual nerve and vessels and hypoglossal nerve (Figure 61-16). Its boundaries are the geniohyoid and genioglossus muscles medially and the lingual surface of the mandible and below the mylohyoid muscle laterally and anteriorly (Figure 61-17). Infection of this area raises the floor of the mouth and displaces the tongue, resulting in pain and difficulty in swallowing but little facial swelling.

The *submental space* is found between the mylohyoid muscle superiorly and the platysma inferiorly. It is bounded laterally by the mandible and posteriorly by the hyoid bone, and it is traversed by the anterior belly of the digastric muscle. Infections of this area arise from the region of the mandibular anterior teeth and result in swelling of the submental region; infections become more dangerous as they proceed posteriorly.

The *submandibular space* is found external to the sublingual space, below the mylohyoid and hyoglossus muscles (see Figures 61-16 and 61-17). This space contains the submandibular gland, which extends partially above

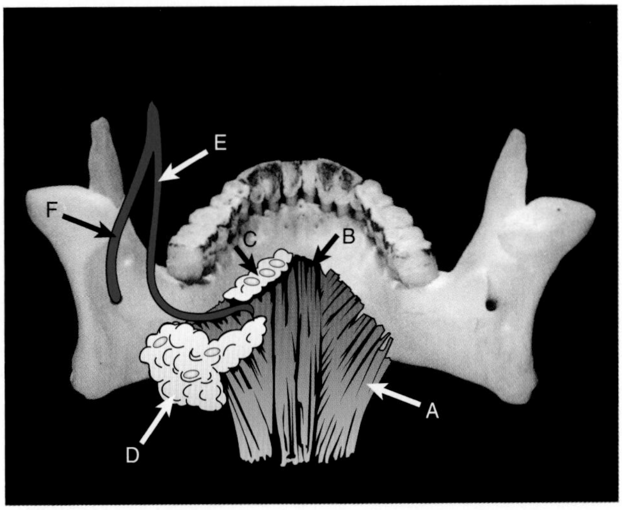

Figure 61-17 Posterior view of mandible, showing the attachment of the mylohyoid muscles *(A)*; geniohyoid muscles *(B)*; sublingual gland *(C)*; submandibular gland *(D)*, which extends below and also to some extent above the mylohyoid muscle; and sublingual *(E)* and inferior alveolar *(F)* nerves.

SCIENCE TRANSFER

In the *mandible* the position of the mandibular nerve must be ascertained before implant placement so that there is no risk of damage. In general, at least a 2-mm space should be present between the coronal border of the nerve and the apex of the implant. The mental nerve must be considered during implant placement and also during mucogingival surgery because damage to this nerve results in debilitating paresthesia. The lingual nerve is most susceptible to damage when it is close to a third molar that will be extracted.

In the *maxilla* the nasopalatine nerves and vessels are of little importance if they are included in the surgical field. However, involvement of the greater palatine artery should be avoided because significant hemorrhage can occur if it is severed. Radiographic evaluation of the position and extent of the maxillary sinus is essential during treatment planning for dental implants.

the mylohyoid muscle, thus communicating with the sublingual space, and numerous lymph nodes. Infections of this area originate in the molar or premolar area and result in swelling that obliterates the submandibular line and in pain when swallowing. *Ludwig's angina* is a severe form of infection of the submandibular space that may extend to the sublingual and submental spaces; it results in hardening of the floor of the mouth and may lead to asphyxiation from edema of the neck and glottis. Although the bacteriology of these infections has not been completely determined, they are presumed to be mixed infections with an important anaerobic component.[1,8]

REFERENCES

1. Bartlett JG, Gorbach SL: Anaerobic infections of the head and neck, *Otolaryngol Clin North Am* 9:655, 1976.
2. Clarke MA, Bueltmann KW: Anatomical considerations in periodontal surgery, *J Periodontol* 42:610, 1971.
3. Dixon AD: *Anatomy for students of dentistry,* ed 5, New York, 1986, Churchill Livingstone.
4. DuBrul EL: *Sicher and DuBrul's oral anatomy,* ed 8, St Louis, 1988, Ishiyaku EuroAmerica.
5. Gregg JM: Surgical anatomy. In Laskin DM: *Oral and maxillofacial surgery,* vol 1, St Louis, 1980, Mosby.
6. Hollinshead WH: *Anatomy for surgeons,* vol 1. The head and neck, New York, 1954, Hoeber-Harper.
7. Kiesselbach JE, Chamberlain JG: Clinical and anatomic observations on the relationship of the lingual nerve to the mandibular third molar region, *J Oral Maxillofac Surg* 42:565, 1984.
8. Mulligan ME: Ear, nose, throat, and head and neck infections. In Finegold SM, George WL, editors: *Anaerobic infections in humans,* San Diego, 1989, Academic Press.
9. Spilka CJ: Pathways of dental infections, *J Oral Surg* 24:111, 1966.
10. Topazian RG, Goldberg MH: *Oral and maxillofacial infections,* ed 3, Philadelphia, 1994, Saunders.
11. Woelfel J: *Dental anatomy: its relevance in dentistry,* ed 4, Philadelphia, 1990, Lea & Febiger.

Gingival Surgical Techniques

Henry H. Takei and Fermin A. Carranza

62

CHAPTER

CHAPTER OUTLINE

Periodontal pocket reduction surgery limited to the gingival tissues only and not involving the underlying osseous structures, without the use of flap surgery, can be classified as **gingival curettage** and **gingivectomy.** Current understanding of disease etiology and therapy limits the use of both techniques, but their place in surgical therapy is essential.

GINGIVAL CURETTAGE

The word *curettage* is used in periodontics to mean the scraping of the gingival wall of a periodontal pocket to separate diseased soft tissue. *Scaling* refers to the removal of deposits from the root surface, whereas *planing* means smoothing the root to remove infected and necrotic tooth substance. Scaling and root planing may inadvertently include various degrees of curettage. However, they are different procedures, with different rationales and indications, and should be considered separate parts of periodontal treatment.

A differentiation has been made between gingival and subgingival curettage (Figure 62-1). *Gingival curettage* consists of the removal of the inflamed soft tissue lateral to the pocket wall, whereas *subgingival curettage* refers to the procedure that is performed apical to the epithelial attachment, severing the connective tissue attachment down to the osseous crest.

It should also be understood that some degree of curettage is done unintentionally when scaling and root planing are performed; this is called *inadvertent curettage.* This chapter refers to the purposeful curettage performed during the same visit as scaling and root planing, or as a separate procedure, to reduce pocket depth by enhancing gingival shrinkage, new connective tissue attachment, or both.

Rationale

Curettage accomplishes the removal of the chronically inflamed granulation tissue that forms in the lateral wall of the periodontal pocket. This tissue, in addition to the usual components of granulation tissues (fibroblastic and angioblastic proliferation), contains areas of chronic inflammation and may also have pieces of dislodged calculus and bacterial colonies. The latter may perpetuate the pathologic features of the tissue and hinder healing.

This inflamed granulation tissue is lined by epithelium, and deep strands of epithelium penetrate into the tissue. The presence of this epithelium is construed as a barrier to the attachment of new fibers in the area.

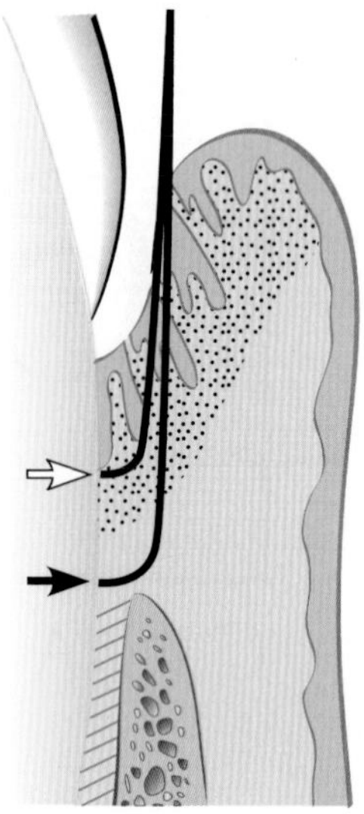

Figure 62-1 Extent of gingival curettage *(white arrow)* and subgingival curettage *(black arrow).*

When the root is thoroughly planed, the major source of bacteria disappears, and the pocket pathologic changes resolve with no need to eliminate the inflamed granulation tissue by curettage. The existing granulation tissue is slowly resorbed; the bacteria present, in the absence of replenishment of their numbers by the pocket plaque, are destroyed by the defense mechanisms of the host. *Therefore the need for curettage only to eliminate the inflamed granulation tissue appears questionable.** It has been shown that scaling and root planing with additional curettage do not improve the condition of the periodontal tissues beyond the improvement resulting from scaling and root planing alone.

Curettage may also eliminate all or most of the epithelium that lines the pocket wall and the underlying junctional epithelium. This purpose of curettage is still valid, particularly when an attempt is made at new attachment, as occurs in intrabony pockets. However, opinions differ regarding whether scaling and curettage consistently remove the pocket lining and the junctional epithelium. Some investigators report that scaling and root planing tear the epithelial lining of the pocket without removing either it or the junctional epithelium,[33] but that both epithelial structures,[6,7,32] sometimes including underlying inflamed connective tissue,[34] are removed by curettage. Other investigators report that the removal of the pocket lining and junctional epithelium by curettage is not complete.[51,54,57]

Curettage and Esthetics

The awareness of esthetics in periodontal therapy has become an integral part of care in the modern practice of periodontics. In the past, pocket elimination was the primary goal of therapy, and little regard was given to the esthetic result. Maximal, rapid shrinkage of gingival tissue was the aim to eliminate the pocket. Currently, esthetics is a major consideration of therapy, particularly in the anterior maxilla (teeth #6-11), and requires preservation of the interdental papilla.

When reconstructive therapy is not possible, every effort should be made to minimize shrinkage or loss of the interdental papilla. A compromise therapy that is feasible in the anterior maxilla, where access is not difficult, consists of thorough subgingival root planing, attempting not to detach the connective tissue beneath the pocket and *avoiding gingival curettage*. The granulation tissue in the lateral wall of the pocket, in an environment free of plaque and calculus, becomes connective tissue, thereby minimizing shrinkage. Thus, although complete pocket elimination is not accomplished, the inflammatory changes are reduced or eliminated while the interdental papilla and the esthetic appearance of the area are preserved.

Surgical techniques specially designed to preserve the interdental papilla, such as the papilla preservation technique (see Chapter 64), result in better esthetic appearance of the anterior maxilla than do aggressive scaling and curettage of the area.

Another important precaution involves root planing apical to the base of the pocket. The removal of the junctional epithelium and disruption of the connective tissue attachment expose the nondiseased portion of the cementum. Root planing in this area of nondiseased cementum may result in excessive shrinkage of the gingiva, increasing recession or requiring "new attachment" where no disease previously existed.

Indications

Indications for curettage are very limited. It can be used after scaling and root planing for the following purposes:

1. Curettage can be performed as part of new attachment attempts in moderately deep intrabony pockets located in accessible areas where a type of "closed" surgery is deemed advisable. However, technical difficulties and inadequate accessibility frequently contraindicate such surgery.
2. Curettage can be done as a nondefinitive procedure to reduce inflammation before pocket elimination using other methods or when more aggressive surgical techniques (e.g., flaps) are contraindicated in patients because of their age, systemic problems, psychologic problems, or other factors. It should be understood that in these patients, the goal of pocket elimination is compromised and prognosis is impaired. The clinician should resort to this approach only when the indicated surgical techniques cannot be performed, and both the clinician and the patient must have a clear understanding of its limitations.
3. Curettage is also frequently performed on recall visits[45] as a method of maintenance treatment for areas of recurrent inflammation and pocket depth,

*This should not be confused with elimination of granulation tissue during flap surgery. The reason for the latter is to remove the bleeding tissue that obstructs the view and prevents the necessary examination of the root surface and the bone morphology. Thus, removal of granulation tissue during surgery is done for technical rather than biologic reasons.

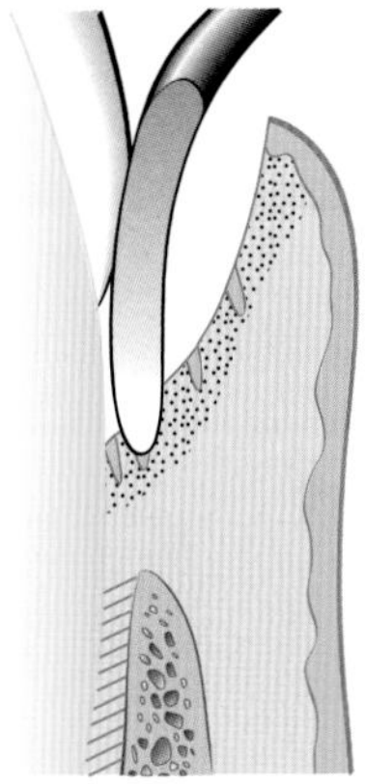

Figure 62-2 Gingival curettage performed with a horizontal stroke of the curette.

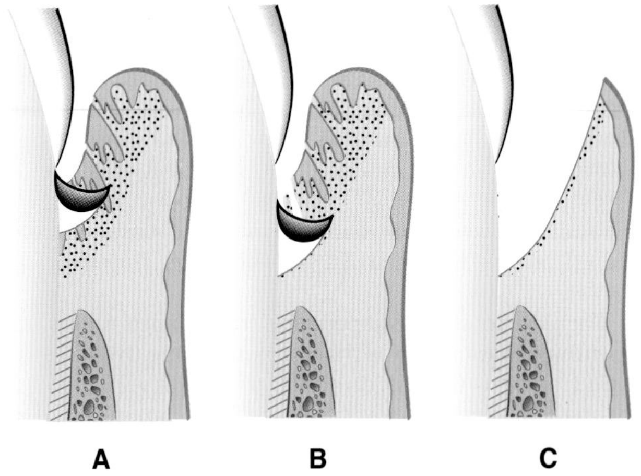

Figure 62-3 Subgingival curettage. **A,** Elimination of pocket lining. **B,** Elimination of junctional epithelium and granulation tissue. **C,** Procedure completed.

particularly where pocket reduction surgery has previously been performed. Careful probing should establish the extent of the required root planing and curettage to avoid unnecessary shrinkage, pocket formation, or both.

Procedure

Basic Technique

Curettage does not eliminate the causes of inflammation (i.e., bacterial plaque and deposits). *Therefore, curettage should always be preceded by scaling and root planing,* the basic periodontal therapy procedure (see Chapter 51). The use of local infiltrative anesthesia for scaling and root planing is optional. However, gingival curettage always requires some type of local anesthesia.

The curette is selected so that the cutting edge will be against the tissue (e.g., Gracey #13-14 for mesial surfaces, Gracey #11-12 for distal surfaces). Curettage can also be performed with a 4R-4L Columbia Universal curette. The instrument is inserted so as to engage the inner lining of the pocket wall and is carried along the soft tissue, usually in a horizontal stroke (Figure 62-2). The pocket wall may be supported by gentle finger pressure on the external surface. The curette is then placed under the cut edge of the junctional epithelium to undermine it.

In subgingival curettage, the tissues attached between the bottom of the pocket and the alveolar crest are removed with a scooping motion of the curette to the tooth surface (Figure 62-3). The area is flushed to remove debris, and the tissue is partly adapted to the tooth by gentle finger pressure. In some cases, suturing of separated papillae and application of a periodontal pack may be indicated.

Other Techniques

Other techniques for gingival curettage include the excisional new attachment procedure, ultrasonic curettage, and the use of caustic drugs:

Excisional New Attachment Procedure (ENAP). ENAP has been developed and used by the U.S. Naval Dental Corps.[40,62,63] It is a definitive subgingival curettage procedure performed with a knife. The technique is as follows:

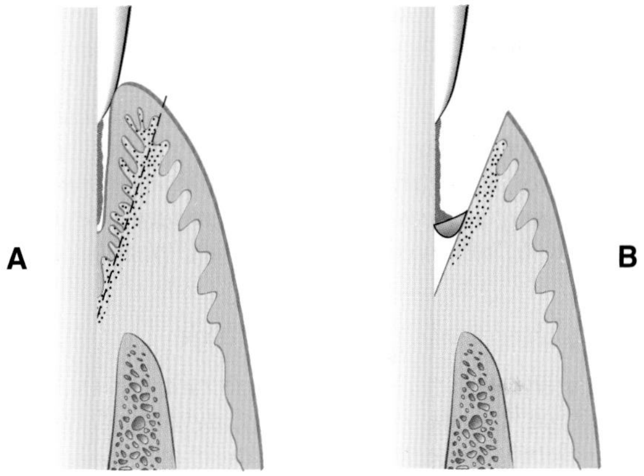

Figure 62-4 Excisional new attachment procedure. **A,** Internal bevel incision to point below bottom of pocket. **B,** After excision of tissue, scaling and root planing are performed.

1. After adequate anesthesia, make an internal bevel incision from the margin of the free gingiva apically to a point below the bottom of the pocket (Figure 62-4). Carry the incision interproximally on both the facial and the lingual side, attempting to retain as much interproximal tissue as possible. The intention is to cut the inner portion of the soft tissue wall of the pocket, all around the tooth.
2. Remove the excised tissue with a curette, and carefully perform root planing on all exposed cementum to achieve a smooth, hard consistency. Preserve all connective tissue fibers that remain attached to the root surface.
3. Approximate the wound edges; if they do not meet passively, recontour the bone until good adaptation of the wound edges is achieved. Place sutures and a periodontal dressing.

Ultrasonic Curettage. The use of ultrasonic devices has been recommended for gingival curettage.[35] When applied to the gingiva of experimental animals, ultrasonic vibrations disrupt tissue continuity, lift off epithelium, dismember collagen bundles, and alter the morphologic features of fibroblast nuclei.[20] Ultrasound is effective for debriding the epithelial lining of periodontal pockets; it results in a narrow band of necrotic tissue (microcauterization), which strips off the inner lining of the pocket.

The Morse scaler-shaped and rod-shaped ultrasonic instruments are used for this purpose. Some investigators found ultrasonic instruments to be as effective as manual instruments for curettage[35,50,64] but resulted in less inflammation and less removal of underlying connective tissue. The gingiva can be made more rigid for ultrasonic curettage by injecting anesthetic solution directly into it.[10]

Caustic Drugs. Since early in the development of periodontal procedures,[53,61] the use of caustic drugs has been recommended to induce a chemical curettage of the lateral wall of the pocket or even the selective elimination of the epithelium. Drugs such as sodium sulfide, alkaline sodium hypochlorite solution (Antiformin),[8,24,26] and phenol[4,9] have been proposed and then discarded after studies showed their ineffectiveness.[5,18,26] The extent of tissue destruction with these drugs cannot be controlled, and they may increase rather than reduce the amount of tissue to be removed by enzymes and phagocytes.

Healing after Scaling and Curettage

Immediately after curettage, a blood clot fills the pocket area, which is totally or partially devoid of epithelial lining. Hemorrhage is also present in the tissues with dilated capillaries, and abundant polymorphonuclear leukocytes (PMNs) appear shortly thereafter on the wound surface. This is followed by a rapid proliferation of granulation tissue, with a decrease in the number of small blood vessels as the tissue matures.

Restoration and epithelialization of the sulcus generally require 2 to 7 days,[27,34,37,57] and restoration of the junctional epithelium occurs in animals as early as 5 days after treatment. Immature collagen fibers appear within 21 days. Healthy gingival fibers inadvertently severed from the tooth and tears in the epithelium[33,46] are repaired in the healing process. Several investigators have reported that in monkeys[11,62] and humans[58] treated by scaling procedures and curettage, healing results in the formation of a long, thin junctional epithelium with no new connective tissue attachment. In some cases, this long epithelium is interrupted by "windows" of connective tissue attachment.[11]

Clinical Appearance after Scaling and Curettage

Immediately after scaling and curettage, the gingiva appears hemorrhagic and bright red.

After 1 week, the gingiva appears reduced in height because of an apical shift in the position of the gingival margin. The gingiva is also slightly redder than normal, but much less so than on previous days.

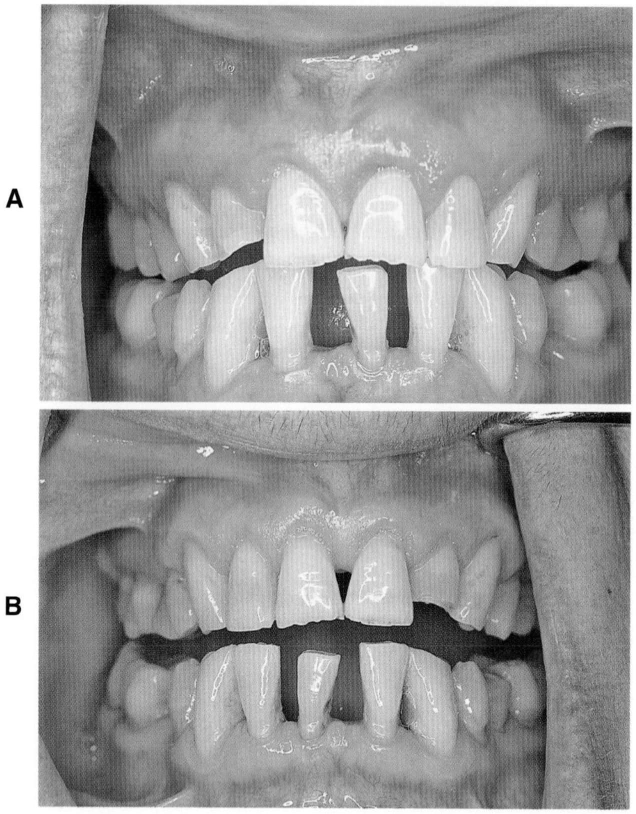

Figure 62-5 Results obtained by treating a suprabony pocket with gingivectomy. **A,** Before treatment. **B,** After treatment.

After 2 weeks, and with proper oral hygiene by the patient, the normal color, consistency, surface texture, and contour of the gingiva are attained, and the gingival margin is well adapted to the tooth.

GINGIVECTOMY

Gingivectomy means excision of the gingiva. By removing the pocket wall, gingivectomy provides visibility and accessibility for complete calculus removal and thorough smoothing of the roots (Figure 62-5), creating a favorable environment for gingival healing and restoration of a physiologic gingival contour.

The gingivectomy technique was widely performed in the past. Improved understanding of healing mechanisms and the development of more sophisticated flap methods have relegated the gingivectomy to a lesser role in the current repertoire of available techniques. However, it remains an effective form of treatment when indicated (see Figure 62-5).

Indications and Contraindications

The gingivectomy technique may be performed for the following indications[16]:

1. Elimination of suprabony pockets, regardless of their depth, if the pocket wall is fibrous and firm.

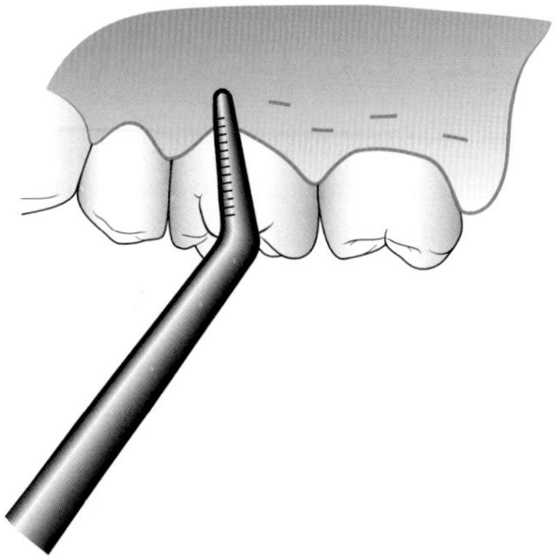

Figure 62-6 Pocket marker makes pinpoint perforations that indicate pocket depth.

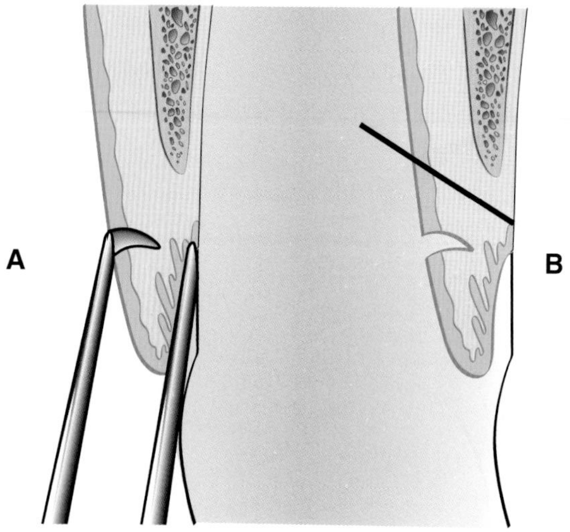

Figure 62-7 Marking the depth of suprabony pocket. **A,** Pocket marker in position. **B,** Beveled incision extends apical to the perforation made by the pocket marker.

2. Elimination of gingival enlargements.
3. Elimination of suprabony periodontal abscesses.

Contraindications to gingivectomy include the following:

1. The need for bone surgery or examination of the bone shape and morphology.
2. Situations in which the bottom of the pocket is apical to the mucogingival junction.
3. Esthetic considerations, particularly in the anterior maxilla.

The gingivectomy technique may be performed by means of scalpels, electrodes, lasers, or chemicals. All these techniques are reviewed here, although the surgical method is the only technique recommended.

Surgical Gingivectomy

Step 1. The pockets on each surface are explored with a periodontal probe and marked with a pocket marker (Figures 62-6 and 62-7). Each pocket is marked in several areas to outline its course on each surface.

Step 2. Periodontal knives (e.g., Kirkland knives) are used for incisions on the facial and lingual surfaces and those distal to the terminal tooth in the arch. Orban periodontal knives are used for supplemental interdental incisions, if necessary, and Bard-Parker knives #11 and #12 and scissors are used as auxiliary instruments.

The incision is started apical to the points marking the course of the pockets[48,56] and is directed coronally to a point between the base of the pocket and the crest of the bone. It should be as close as possible to the bone without exposing it, to remove the soft tissue coronal to the bone. Exposure of bone is undesirable. If it occurs, healing usually presents no problem if the area is adequately covered by the periodontal pack.

Discontinuous or continuous incisions may be used (Figure 62-8). The incision should be beveled at approximately 45 degrees to the tooth surface and should recreate, as far as possible, the normal festooned pattern of the gingiva. Failure to bevel leaves a broad, fibrous plateau that takes more time than usually required to develop a physiologic contour. In the interim, plaque and food accumulation may lead to recurrence of pockets.

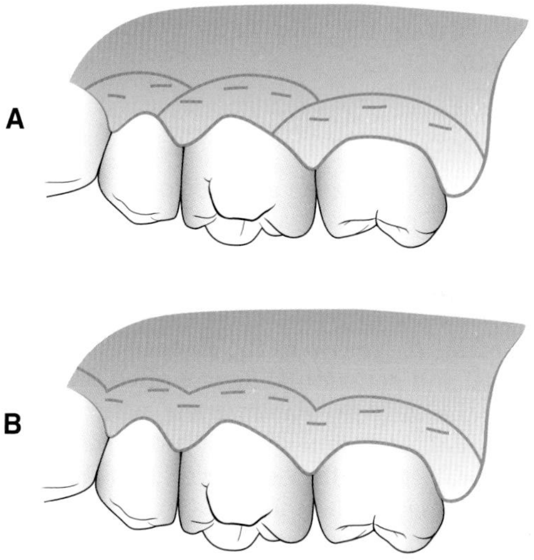

Figure 62-8 **A,** Discontinuous incision apical to bottom of the pocket indicated by pinpoint markings. **B,** Continuous incision begins on the molar and extends anteriorly without interruption.

Step 3. Remove the excised pocket wall, clean the area, and closely examine the root surface. The most apical zone consists of a bandlike light zone where the tissues were attached, and coronally to it some calculus remnants, root caries, or root resorption may be found. Granulation tissue may be seen on the excised soft tissue (Figure 62-9).

Step 4. Carefully curette the granulation tissue, and remove any remaining calculus and necrotic cementum so as to leave a smooth and clean surface.

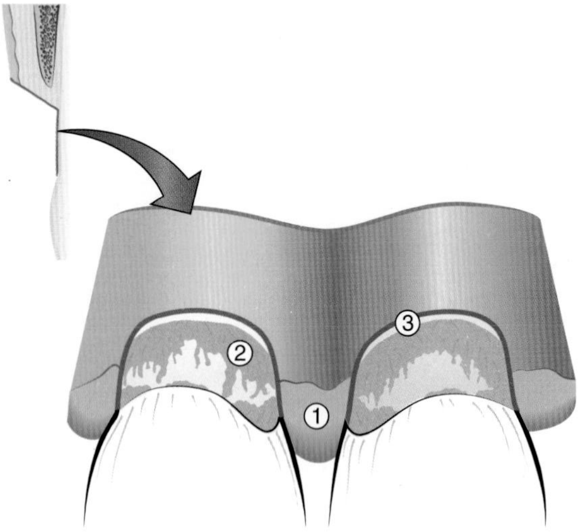

Figure 62-9 Field of operation immediately after removing pocket wall. *1,* Granulation tissue; *2,* calculus and other root deposits; *3,* clear space where junctional epithelium was attached.

Step 5. Cover the area with a surgical pack (see Chapter 60).

Gingivoplasty

Gingivoplasty is similar to gingivectomy, but its purpose is different. Gingivectomy is performed to eliminate periodontal pockets and includes reshaping as part of the technique. Gingivoplasty is a reshaping of the gingiva to create physiologic gingival contours, with the sole purpose of *recontouring the gingiva* in the absence of pockets.

Gingival and periodontal disease often produce deformities in the gingiva that interfere with normal food excursion, collect plaque and food debris, and prolong and aggravate the disease process. Such deformities include (1) gingival clefts and craters, (2) shelflike interdental papillae caused by acute necrotizing ulcerative gingivitis, and (3) gingival enlargements.

Gingivoplasty may be done with a periodontal knife, a scalpel, rotary coarse diamond stones,[44] or electrodes.[13] It consists of procedures that resemble those performed in festooning artificial dentures: tapering the gingival margin, creating a scalloped marginal outline, thinning the attached gingiva, and creating vertical interdental grooves and shaping the interdental papillae to provide sluiceways for the passage of food.

Healing after Surgical Gingivectomy

The *initial response* after gingivectomy is the formation of a protective surface clot; the underlying tissue becomes acutely inflamed, with some necrosis. The clot is then replaced by granulation tissue. *By 24 hours,* there is an increase in new connective tissue cells, mainly angioblasts, just beneath the surface layer of inflammation and necrosis; *by the third day,* numerous young fibroblasts are located in the area.[47] The highly vascular granulation tissue grows coronally, creating a new, free gingival margin and sulcus.[41] Capillaries derived from blood vessels of the periodontal ligament migrate into the granulation tissue, and *within 2 weeks,* they connect with gingival vessels.[59]

After 12 to 24 hours, epithelial cells at the margins of the wound start to migrate over the granulation tissue, separating it from the contaminated surface layer of the clot. Epithelial activity at the margins reaches a peak in 24 to 36 hours.[13] The new epithelial cells arise from the basal and deeper spinous layers of the wound edge epithelium and migrate over the wound over a fibrin layer that is later resorbed and replaced by a connective tissue bed.[25] The epithelial cells advance by a tumbling action, with the cells becoming fixed to the substrate by hemidesmosomes and a new basement lamina.[28]

After 5 to 14 days, surface epithelialization is generally complete. During the first 4 weeks after gingivectomy, keratinization is less than it was before surgery. Complete epithelial repair takes about 1 month.[52] Vasodilation and vascularity begin to decrease after the fourth day of healing and appear to be almost normal by the sixteenth day.[36] Complete repair of the connective tissue takes about 7 weeks.[52]

SCIENCE TRANSFER

The need for curettage only to eliminate the inflamed granulation tissue appears questionable. It is critical to appreciate how this chapter can make this important statement. If this statement were changed to a hypothesis, an experiment could be designed to test if it is true. The experiment would have two groups: patients treated with scaling and root planing only and patients treated with scaling and root planing plus curettage. The primary outcome variable would be soft tissue healing response, which would ideally involve histologic examination of the healed tissues and evaluation by a masked examiner (or two) for the presence or absence of granulation tissue. When this examination reveals that no significant difference exists in the histologic soft tissue healing between the two groups in the study (given that enough different patients are treated in each group), it can then be concluded that the extra treatment, the curettage, had no effect; that is, curettage was not necessary.

Curettage is used with local anesthesia in patients when more surgically oriented procedures are contraindicated. Gingivectomy has only a minor role in the treatment of periodontal pockets because flap techniques offer significant advantages. Gingivoplasty techniques can be of value in some patients requiring crown lengthening, when this can be accomplished without the need for osseous surgery to establish adequate biologic width.

The flow of gingival fluid in humans is initially increased after gingivectomy and diminishes as healing progresses.[1,49] Maximal flow is reached after 1 week, coinciding with the time of maximal inflammation.

Although the tissue changes that occur in post-gingivectomy healing are the same in all individuals, the time required for complete healing varies considerably, depending on the area of the cut surface and interference from local irritation and infection. In patients with physiologic gingival melanosis, the pigmentation is diminished in the healed gingiva.

Gingivectomy by Electrosurgery

Advantages

Electrosurgery permits an adequate contouring of the tissue and controls hemorrhage[17,39]

Disadvantages

Electrosurgery cannot be used in patients who have noncompatible or poorly shielded cardiac pacemakers. The treatment causes an unpleasant odor. If the electrosurgery point touches the bone, irreparable damage can be done.[2,17,22,44] Furthermore, the heat generated by injudicious use can cause tissue damage and loss of periodontal support when the electrode is used close to bone. When the electrode touches the root, areas of cementum burn are produced.[60] *Therefore the use of electrosurgery should be limited to superficial procedures such as removal of gingival enlargements, gingivoplasty, relocation of frenum and muscle attachments, and incision of periodontal abscesses and pericoronal flaps;* extreme care should be exercised to avoid contacting the tooth surface. *Electrosurgery should not be used for procedures that involve proximity to the bone, such as flap operations, or for mucogingival surgery.*

Technique

The removal of gingival enlargements and gingivoplasty[39] is performed with the needle electrode, supplemented by the small, ovoid loop or the diamond-shaped electrodes for festooning. A blended cutting and coagulating (fully rectified) current is used. In all reshaping procedures, the electrode is activated and moved in a concise "shaving" motion.

In the treatment of acute periodontal abscesses, the incision to establish drainage can be made with the needle electrode without exerting painful pressure. The incision remains open because the edges are sealed by the current. After the acute symptoms subside, the regular procedure for the treatment of the periodontal abscess is followed (see Chapter 48).

For hemostasis, the ball electrode is used. Hemorrhage must be controlled by direct pressure (using air, compress, or hemostat) first; then the surface is lightly touched with a coagulating current. Electrosurgery is helpful for the control of isolated bleeding points. Bleeding areas located interproximally are reached with a thin, bar-shaped electrode.

Frenum and muscle attachments can be relocated to facilitate pocket elimination using a loop electrode. For this purpose, the frenum or muscle is stretched and sectioned with the loop electrode and a coagulating current. For cases of acute pericoronitis, drainage may be obtained by incising the flap with a bent-needle electrode. A loop electrode is used to remove the flap after the acute symptoms subside.

Healing after Electrosurgery

Some investigators report no significant differences in gingival healing after resection by electrosurgery and resection with periodontal knives.[14,31] Other researchers find delayed healing, greater reduction in gingival height, and more bone injury after electrosurgery.[44] There appears to be little difference in the results obtained after shallow gingival resection with electrosurgery and that with periodontal knives. *However, when used for deep resections close to bone, electrosurgery can produce gingival recession, bone necrosis and sequestration, loss of bone height, furcation exposure, and tooth mobility, which do not occur with the use of periodontal knives.*[2,17]

Laser Gingivectomy

The lasers most often used in dentistry are the carbon dioxide (CO_2) and the neodymium:yttrium-aluminum-garnet (Nd:YAG), which have wavelengths of 10,600 nm and 1064 nm, respectively, both in the infrared range; they must be combined with other types of visible lasers for the beam to be seen and aimed.

The CO_2 laser has been used for the excision of gingival growths,[3,42] although healing is delayed compared with healing after conventional scalpel gingivectomy.[21,30,43] The use of a laser for oral surgery requires precautionary measures to avoid reflecting the beam on instrument surfaces, which could result in injury to neighboring tissues and the eyes of the operator. (See Chapter 70 for further information on laser therapy.)

Gingivectomy by Chemosurgery

Techniques to remove the gingiva using chemicals, such as 5% paraformaldehyde[38] or potassium hydroxide,[29] have been described in the past but are not currently used. They are presented here to provide a historical perspective.

The chemical gingivectomy has the following disadvantages:

- The depth of action cannot be controlled, and therefore healthy attached tissue underlying the pocket may be injured.
- Gingival remodeling cannot be accomplished effectively.
- Epithelialization and re-formation of the junctional epithelium and reestablishment of the alveolar crest fiber system occur more slowly in chemically treated gingival wounds than in those produced by a scalpel.[55]

The use of chemical methods therefore is not recommended.

Summary

The gingivectomy surgical technique has a long history of use in periodontal surgery. This technique has been attempted using scalpels, electrosurgery, laser, and chemical cautery. Even though this technique may have some use for the minimal reduction of redundant gingival tissue, many limiting factors must be considered. Current periodontal surgery must consider the (1) conservation of keratinized gingiva, (2) minimal gingival tissue loss to maintain esthetics, (3) adequate access to the osseous defects for definitive defect correction, and (4) minimal postsurgical discomfort and bleeding by attempting surgical procedures that will allow primary closure. The gingivectomy surgical technique has limited use in current surgical therapy because it does not satisfy these considerations in periodontal therapy. The clinician must carefully evaluate each case as to the proper application of this surgical procedure used in different ways.

REFERENCES

1. Arnold R. Lunstad G, Bissada N, et al: Alterations in crevicular fluid flow during healing following gingival surgery, *J Periodontal Res* 1:303, 1966.
2. Azzi R, Kenney EB, Tsao TF, et al: The effect of electrosurgery upon alveolar bone, *J Periodontol* 54:96, 1983.
3. Barak S, Kaplan H: The CO_2 laser in the surgical excision of gingival hyperplasia caused by nifedipine, *J Clin Periodontol* 15:633, 1988.
4. Barkann A: A conservative technique for the eradication of a pyorrhea product, *J Am Dent Assoc* 26:61, 1939.
5. Beube FE: An experimental study of the use of sodium sulphide solution in treatment of periodontal pockets, *J Periodontol* 10:49, 1939.
6. Beube FE: Treatment methods for marginal gingivitis and periodontitis, *Texas Dent J* 71:427, 1953.
7. Blass JL, Lite T: Gingival healing following surgical curettage: a histopathologic study, *NY Dent J* 25:127, 1959.
8. Box KF: Periodontal disease and treatment, *J Ontario Dent Assoc* 29:194, 1952.
9. Bunting RW: The control and treatment of pyorrhea by subgingival surgery, *J Am Dent Assoc* 15:119, 1928.
10. Burman LR, Alderman LE, Ewen SJ: Clinical application of ultrasonic vibrations for supragingival calculus and stain removal, *J Dent Med* 13:156, 1958.
11. Caton JC, Zander HA: The attachment between tooth and gingival tissues after periodic root planing and soft tissue curettage, *J Periodontol* 50:462, 1979.
12. Eisenmann D, Malone WF, Kusek J: Electron microscopic evaluation of electrosurgery, *Oral Surg* 29:660, 1970.
13. Engler WO, Ramfjord S, Hiniker JJ: Healing following simple gingivectomy: a tritiated thymidine radioautographic study. I. Epithelialization, *J Periodontol* 37:289, 1966.
14. Fisher SE, Frame JW, Browne RM, et al: A comparative histological study of wound healing following CO_2 laser and conventional surgical excision of the buccal mucosa, *Arch Oral Biol* 28:287, 1983.
15. Flocken JE: Electrosurgical management of soft tissues and restoration dentistry, *Dent Clin North Am* 24:247, 1980.
16. Glickman I: The results obtained with the unembellished gingivectomy technique in a clinical study in humans, *J Periodontol* 27:247, 1956.
17. Glickman I, Imber LR: Comparison of gingival resection with electrosurgery and periodontal knives: biometric and histologic study, *J Periodontol* 41:242, 1970.
18. Glickman J, Patur B: Histologic study of the effect of Antiformin on the soft tissue wall of periodontal pockets in humans, *J Am Dent Assoc* 51:420, 1955.
19. Goldman HM: The development of physiologic gingival contours by gingivoplasty, *Oral Surg* 3:879, 1950.
20. Goldman HM: Histologic assay of healing following ultrasonic curettage versus hand instrument curettage, *Oral Med Oral Pathol* 14:925, 1961.
21. Gottsegen R, Ammons WF Jr: Position paper: Research in lasers in periodontics, Chicago, 1992, American Academy of Periodontology.
22. Henning F: Healing of gingivectomy wounds in the rat: reestablishment of the epithelial seal, *J Periodontol* 39:265, 1968.
23. Henning F: Epithelial mitotic activity after gingivectomy: relationship to reattachment, *J Periodontal Res* 4:319, 1969.
24. Hunter HA: A study of tissues treated with Antiformin citric acid, *J Can Dent Assoc* 21:344, 1955.
25. Innes PB: An electron microscopic study of the regeneration of gingival epithelium following gingivectomy in the dog, *J Periodontal Res* 5:196, 1970.
26. Johnson RW, Waerhaug J: Effect of Antiformin on gingival tissue, *J Periodontol* 27:24, 1956.
27. Kon S, Novaes AB, Ruben MP, et al: Visualization of microvascularization of the healing periodontal wound. II. Curettage, *J Periodontol* 40:96, 1969.
28. Krawczyk WS: A pattern of epithelial cell migration during wound healing, *J Cell Biol* 49:247, 1971.
29. Löe H: Chemical gingivectomy: effect of potassium hydroxide on periodontal tissues, *Acta Odontol Scand* 19:517, 1961.
30. Loumanen M: A comparative study of healing of laser and scalpel incision wounds in rat oral mucosa, *Scand J Dent Res* 95:65, 1987.
31. Malone WF, Eisenmann D, Kusck J: Interceptive periodontics with electrosurgery, *J Prosthet Dent* 22:555, 1969.
32. Morris ML: The removal of the pocket and attachment epithelium in humans: a histological study, *J Periodontol* 25:7, 1954.
33. Moskow BS: The response of the gingival sulcus to instrumentation: a histologic investigation. I. The scaling procedure, *J Periodontol* 33:282, 1962.
34. Moskow BS: The response of the gingival sulcus to instrumentation: a histologic investigation. II. Gingival curettage, *J Periodontol* 35:112, 1964.
35. Nadler H: Removal of crevicular epithelium by ultrasonic curettes, *J Periodontol* 33:220, 1962.
36. Novaes AB, Kon S, Ruben MP, et al: Visualization of the microvascularization of the healing periodontal wound. III. Gingivectomy, *J Periodontol* 40:359, 1969.
37. O'Bannon JY: The gingival tissues before and after scaling the teeth, *J Periodontol* 35:69, 1964.
38. Orban B: New methods in periodontal treatment, *Bur* 42:116, 1942.
39. Oringer MJ: Electrosurgery for definitive conservative modern periodontal therapy, *Dent Clin North Am* 13:53, 1969.
40. Periodontics syllabus: NAVED P5110, 1975, US Naval Dental Corps, p 113.
41. Persson PA: The healing process in the marginal periodontium after gingivectomy with special regard to the regeneration of epithelium (an experimental study on dogs), *Odontol T* 67:593, 1959.
42. Pick RM, Pecaro BC, Silberman CJ: The laser gingivectomy: the use of CO_2 laser for the removal of phenytoin hyperplasia, *J Periodontol* 56:492, 1985.
43. Pogrel MA, Yen CK, Hanser LS: A comparison of carbon dioxide laser, liquid nitrogen cryosurgery and scalpel wound in healing, *Oral Surg Med Pathol* 69:269, 1990.
44. Pope JW, Gargiulo AW, Staffileno H, et al: Effects of electrosurgery on wound healing in dogs, *Periodontics* 6:30, 1968.
45. Ramfjord SP, Ash MM Jr: *Periodontology and periodontics,* Philadelphia, 1979, Saunders.

46. Ramfjord SP, Kiester G: The gingival sulcus and the periodontal pocket immediately following scaling of the teeth, *J Periodontol* 25:167, 1954.
47. Ramfjord SP, Engler WD, Hiniker JJ: A radiographic study of healing following simple gingivectomy. II. The connective tissue, *J Periodontol* 37:179, 1966.
48. Ritchey B, Orban B: The periodontal pocket, *J Periodontol* 23:199, 1952.
49. Sandalli P, Wade AB: Alterations in crevicular fluid flow during healing following gingivectomy and flap procedures, *J Periodontal Res* 4:314, 1969.
50. Sanderson AD: Gingival curettage by hand and ultrasonic instruments: a histologic comparison, *J Periodontol* 37:279, 1966.
51. Sato M: Histopathological study of the healing process after surgical treatment for alveolar pyorrhea, *Bull Tokyo Dent College* 1:71, 1960.
52. Stanton G, Levy M, Stahl SS: Collagen restoration in healing human gingiva, *J Dent Res* 48:27, 1969.
53. Stewart H: Partial removal of cementum and decalcification of tooth in the treatment of pyorrhea alveolaris, *Dent Cosmos* 41:617, 1899.
54. Stone S, Ramfjord SP, Waldron J: Scaling and gingival curettage: a radioautographic study, *J Periodontol* 37:415, 1966.
55. Tonna E, Stahl SS: A polarized light microscopic study of rat periodontal ligament following surgical and chemical gingival trauma, *Helv Odontol Acta* 11:90, 1967.
56. Waerhaug J: Depth of incision in gingivectomy, *Oral Surg* 8:707, 1955.
57. Waerhaug J: Microscopic demonstration of tissue reaction incident to removal of subgingival calculus, *J Periodontol* 26:26, 1955.
58. Waerhaug J: Healing of the dentoepithelial junction following subgingival plaque control. I. As observed in human biopsy material, *J Periodontol* 49:1, 1978.
59. Watanabe Y, Suzuki S: An experimental study in capillary vascularization in the periodontal tissue following gingivectomy or flap operation, *J Dent Res* 42:758, 1963.
60. Wilhelmsen NR, Ramfjord SP, Blankenship JR: Effects of electrosurgery on the gingival attachment in rhesus monkeys, *J Periodontol* 47:160, 1976.
61. Younger WJ: Some of the latest phases in implantations and other procedures, *Dent Cosmos* 35:102, 1893.
62. Yukna RA: A clinical and histological study of healing following the excisional new attachment procedure in rhesus monkeys, *J Periodontol* 47:701, 1976.
63. Yukna RA, Bowers GM, Lawrence JJ, et al: A clinical study of healing in humans following the excisional new attachment procedure, *J Periodontol* 47:696, 1976.
64. Zach L, Cohen G: The histologic response to ultrasonic curettage, *J Dent Res* 40:751, 1961.

Treatment of Gingival Enlargement

Paulo M. Camargo, Fermin A. Carranza, and Henry H. Takei

CHAPTER 63

CHAPTER OUTLINE

Treatment of gingival enlargement is based on an understanding of the cause and underlying pathologic changes (see Chapter 23). Gingival enlargements are of special concern to the patient and the dentist because they pose problems in plaque control, function (including mastication, tooth eruption, and speech), and esthetics. Because gingival enlargements differ in cause, treatment of each type is best considered individually.

CHRONIC INFLAMMATORY ENLARGEMENT

Chronic inflammatory enlargements, which are soft and discolored and are caused principally by edema and cellular infiltration, are treated by *scaling and root planing,* provided the size of the enlargement does not interfere with complete removal of deposits from the involved tooth surfaces.

When chronic inflammatory gingival enlargements include a significant fibrotic component that does not undergo shrinkage after scaling and root planing or are of such size that they obscure deposits on the tooth surfaces and interfere with access to them, *surgical removal* is the treatment of choice. Two techniques are available for this purpose: gingivectomy and flap operation.

Selection of the appropriate technique depends on the size of the enlargement and character of the tissue. When the enlarged gingiva remains soft and friable even after scaling and root planing, a *gingivectomy* is used to remove it because a flap requires a firmer tissue to perform the incisions and other steps in the technique (Figure 63-1). However, if the gingivectomy incision removes all the attached gingiva, creating a mucogingival problem, then a *flap operation* is indicated.

Tumorlike inflammatory enlargements are treated by gingivectomy as follows. With the patient under local anesthesia, the tooth surfaces beneath the mass are scaled to remove calculus and other debris. The lesion is separated from the mucosa at its base with a #12 Bard-Parker blade. If the lesion extends interproximally, the interdental gingiva is included in the incision to ensure exposure of irritating root deposits. After the lesion is removed, the involved root surfaces are scaled and planed, and the area is cleansed with warm water. A periodontal pack is applied and removed after a week, at which time the patient is instructed in plaque control (Figure 63-2).

For the flap operation, see Chapters 64 and 65 and the following discussion of the flap technique for drug-induced enlargements.

PERIODONTAL AND GINGIVAL ABSCESSES

The reader is referred to Chapter 48 for a complete discussion of abscess treatment.

A

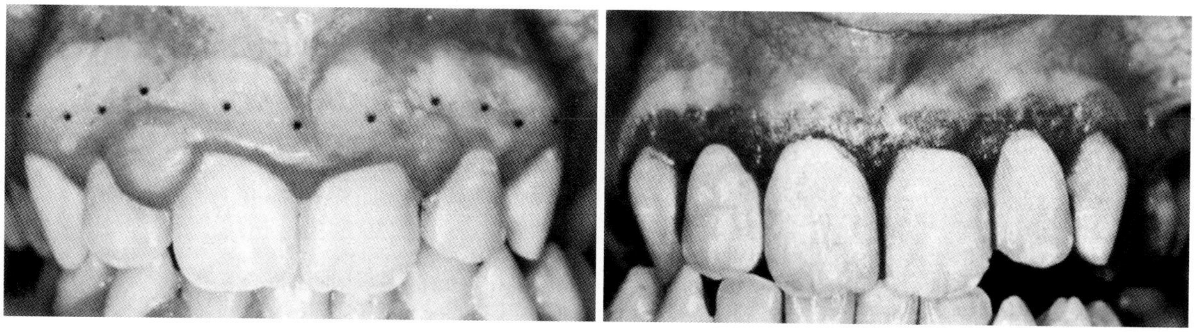

B

Figure 63-1 Gingivectomy incision for gingival enlargement. **A,** Chronic inflammatory gingival enlargement with tumorlike area. Pinpoint markings outline the extent of the enlargement. Note the amount of attached gingiva remaining. **B,** Enlarged gingiva removed. Note the beveled incision.

A

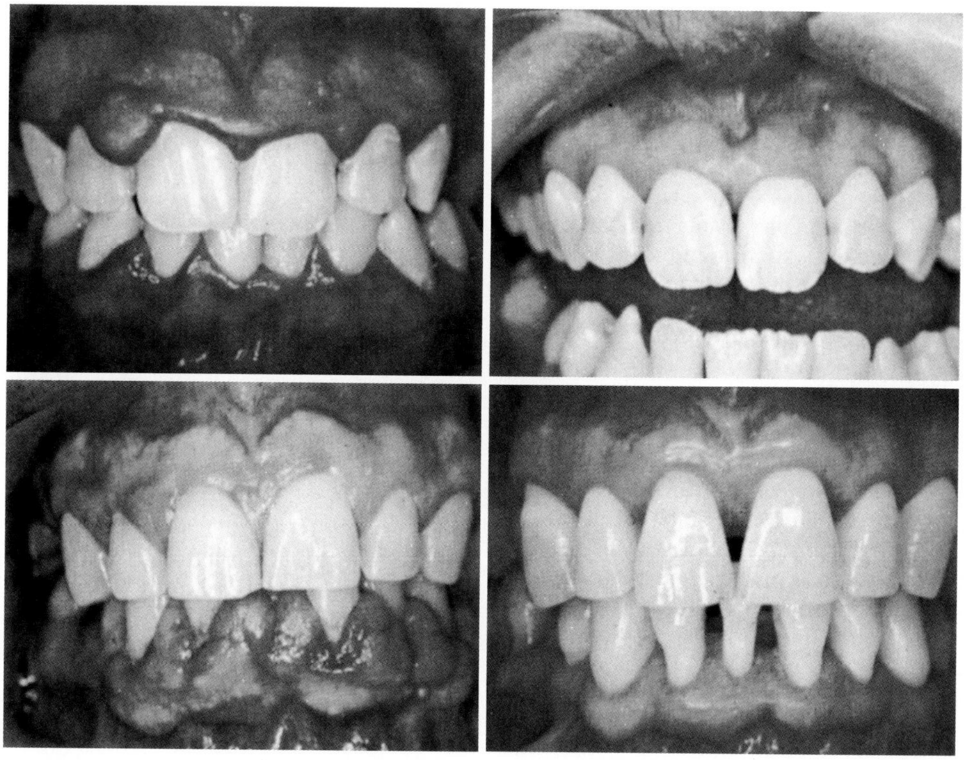

B

Figure 63-2 **A,** Before treatment. Chronic inflammatory gingival enlargement associated with mouth breathing *(top and bottom).* **B,** Appearance after treatment *(top and bottom).*

DRUG-ASSOCIATED GINGIVAL ENLARGEMENT

Gingival enlargement has been associated with the administration of three different types of drugs: anticonvulsants, calcium channel blockers, and the immunosuppressant cyclosporine. Chapter 23 provides a comprehensive review of the clinical and microscopic features and pathogenesis of gingival enlargement induced by these drugs.

Examination of cases of drug-induced gingival enlargement reveals the overgrown tissues to have two components: *fibrotic,* caused by the drug, and *inflammatory,* induced by bacterial plaque. Although the fibrotic and inflammatory components present in the enlarged gingiva are the result of distinct pathologic processes, they almost always are observed in combination. The role of bacterial plaque in the overall pathogenesis of drug-induced gingival enlargement is not clear. Some studies indicate that plaque is a prerequisite for gingival enlargement,[9] whereas others suggest that the presence of plaque is a consequence of its accumulation caused by the enlarged gingiva.

Treatment Options

Treatment of drug-induced gingival enlargement should be based on the medication being used and the clinical features of the case.

First, consideration should be given to the possibility of discontinuing the drug[7,10] or changing medication. These possibilities should be examined with the patient's physician. Simple discontinuation of the offending drug is usually not practical, but its substitution with another medication might be an option. If any drug substitution is attempted, it is important to allow for a 6- to 12-month period to elapse between discontinuation of the offending drug and the possible resolution of gingival enlargement before a decision to implement surgical treatment is made.

Alternative medications to the anticonvulsant *phenytoin* include carbamazepine[6] and valproic acid, both of which have been reported to have a lesser effect in inducing gingival enlargement.

For patients taking *nifedipine,* which has a reported prevalence of gingival enlargement of up to 44%, other calcium channel blockers such as diltiazem or verapamil may be viable alternatives, and their reported prevalence of inducing gingival enlargement is 20% and 4%, respectively.[3,8,12] Also, consideration may be given to the use of another class of antihypertensive medications rather than calcium channel blockers, none of which is known to induce gingival enlargement.

Drug substitutions for *cyclosporine* are more limited. It has been shown that cyclosporine-induced gingival enlargement can spontaneously resolve if tacrolimus is substituted.[11] Preliminary evidence also indicates that the antibiotic azithromycin may aid in decreasing the severity of cyclosporine-induced gingival enlargement.[18]

Second, the clinician should emphasize plaque control as the first step in the treatment of drug-induced gingival enlargement. Although the exact role played by bacterial plaque is not well understood, evidence suggests that good oral hygiene and frequent professional removal of plaque decrease the degree of gingival enlargement and improves overall gingival health.[7,9,17] The presence of drug-induced enlargement is associated with pseudopocket formation, frequently with abundant plaque accumulation, which may lead to development of periodontitis; meticulous plaque control therefore helps maintain attachment levels. Also, adequate plaque control may aid in preventing the recurrence of gingival enlargement in surgically treated cases.

Third, in some patients, gingival enlargement persists after careful consideration of the previous approaches. These patients may require surgery, either gingivectomy or the periodontal flap.

Figure 63-3 presents a decision tree outlining the sequence of events and options in the treatment of drug-induced gingival enlargement.

Gingivectomy. Gingivectomy has the advantage of simplicity and quickness but presents the disadvantages of more postoperative discomfort and increased chance of postoperative bleeding. It also sacrifices keratinized tissue and does not allow for osseous recontouring. The clinician's decision between the two surgical techniques available must consider the extension of the area to be operated, the presence of periodontitis and osseous defects, and the location of the base of the pockets in relation to the mucogingival junction.

In general, small areas (up to six teeth) of drug-induced gingival enlargement with no evidence of attachment loss (and therefore no anticipated need for osseous surgery) can be effectively treated with the gingivectomy technique. An important consideration is the amount of keratinized tissue present, remembering that at least 3 mm in the apicocoronal direction should remain after the surgery is completed.

Chapter 62 describes the gingivectomy technique in detail. Figure 63-4 depicts the procedure diagrammatically, and Figure 63-5 illustrates a case of cyclosporine-induced gingival enlargement treated with the gingivectomy technique.

Gingivectomy or gingivoplasty can also be performed with electrosurgery or a laser device (see Chapter 62).

Flap Technique. Larger areas of gingival enlargement (more than six teeth) or areas where attachment loss and osseous defects are present should be treated by the flap technique, as should any situation in which the gingivectomy technique may create a mucogingival problem.

The periodontal flap technique used for the treatment of gingival enlargements is a simple variation of the one used to treat periodontitis, described in Chapters 64 and 65. Figure 63-6 shows the basic steps in the technique, described as follows:

1. After anesthetizing the area, sounding of the underlying alveolar bone is performed with a periodontal probe to determine the presence and extent of osseous defects.
2. With a #15 Bard-Parker blade, the initial scalloped internal bevel incision is made at least 3 mm coronal to the mucogingival junction, including the creation of new interdental papillae.
3. The same blade is used to thin the gingival tissues in a buccolingual direction to the mucogingival junction. At this point the blade establishes contact with the alveolar bone, and a full-thickness or a split-thickness flap is elevated.
4. Using an Orban knife, the base of each papilla connecting the facial and the lingual incisions is incised.
5. The excised marginal and interdental tissues are removed with curettes.
6. Tissue tabs are removed, the roots are thoroughly scaled and planed, and the bone is recontoured as needed.
7. The flap is replaced and, if necessary, trimmed to reach the bone-tooth junction exactly. The flap is then sutured with an interrupted or a continuous mattress technique, and the area is covered with a periodontal dressing.

Sutures and pack are removed after 1 week, and the patient is instructed to start plaque control methods. Usually it is convenient for the patient to use chlorhexidine oral rinses once or twice daily for 2 to 4 weeks. Figure 63-7 illustrates a patient treated with the flap technique.

Recurrence of drug-induced gingival enlargement is a reality in surgically treated cases.[15] As stated previously, meticulous home care,[5,13] chlorhexidine gluconate

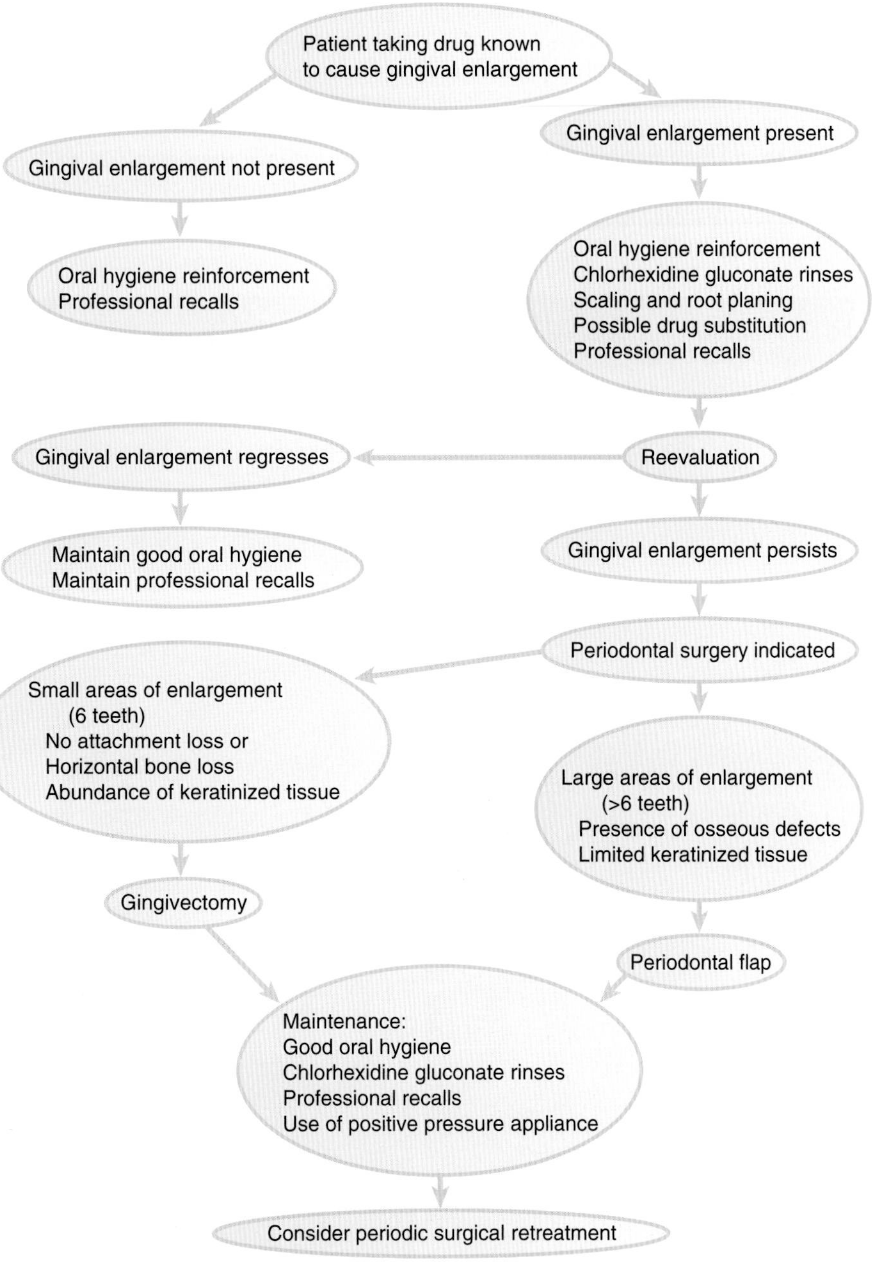

Figure 63-3 Decision tree for treatment of drug-induced gingival enlargements.

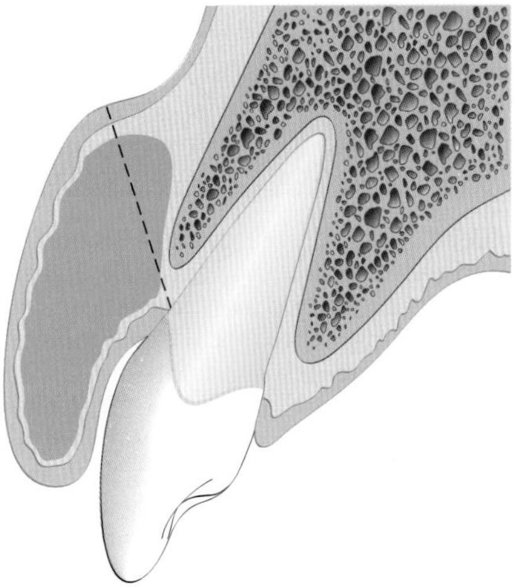

Figure 63-4 Gingivectomy technique as used in treating patients with drug-induced gingival enlargement. The dotted line represents the external bevel incision, and the shaded area corresponds to the tissue to be excised. Gingivectomy incision may not remove the entire hyperplastic tissue *(shaded area)* and may leave a wide wound of exposed connective tissue.

rinses,[16] and professional cleanings can decrease the speed and the degree to which recurrence occurs. A hard, natural rubber, fitted bite guard worn at night may help to control recurrence.[1,2]

Even though the periodontal flap approach may be technically more difficult than the gingivectomy procedure, as indicated earlier, the postsurgical healing of the flap technique presents less discomfort and alleviates hemorrhagic problems. The primary closure of the surgical site with the flap procedure is a great advantage over the secondary open wound resulting from the gingivectomy technique. Also, postsurgical home care can be instituted earlier with the periodontal flap.[4]

Recurrence may occur as early as 3 to 6 months after surgical treatment, but in general, surgical results are maintained for at least 12 months. In one study, 6-month

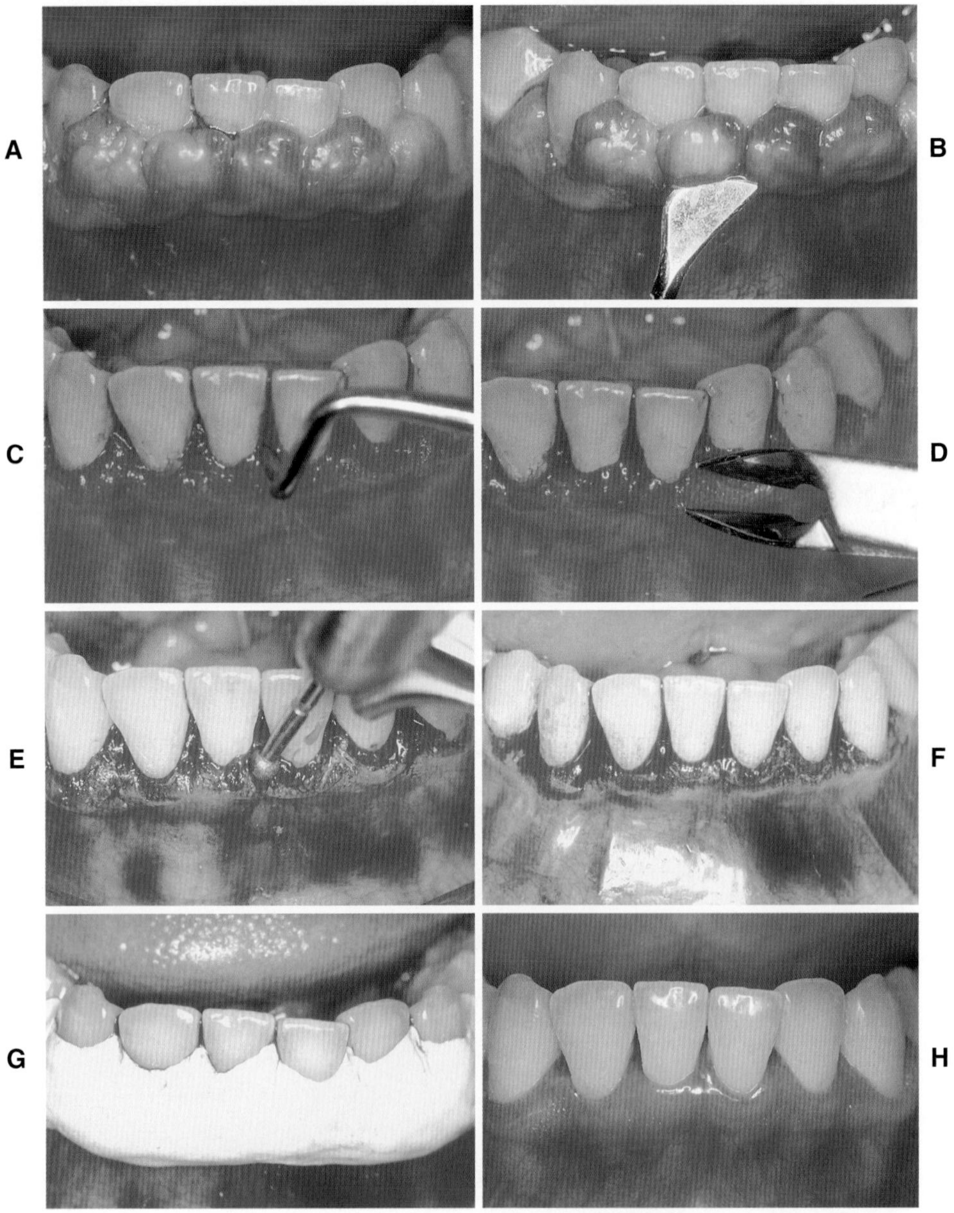

Figure 63-5 Surgical treatment of cyclosporin-induced gingival enlargement using the gingivectomy technique on a 16-year-old girl who had received a kidney allograft 2 years earlier. **A,** Presence of enlarged gingival tissues and pseudopocket formation; no attachment loss or evidence of vertical bone loss existed. **B,** Initial external bevel incision performed with a Kirkland knife. **C,** Interproximal tissue release achieved with an Orban knife. **D** and **E,** Gingivoplasty performed with tissue nippers and a round diamond at high speed with abundant refrigeration. **F,** Aspect of the surgical wound at conclusion of the surgical procedure. **G,** Placement of noneugenol periodontal dressing. **H,** Surgical area 3 months postoperatively. Note the successful elimination of enlarged gingival tissue, restoration of a physiologic gingival contour, and maintenance of an adequate band of keratinized tissue.

postsurgical examination of the recurrence of cyclosporine-induced gingival enlargement after periodontal flap surgery or gingivectomy determined that return of increased pocket depth was slower with the flap.[14] Recurrence of increased thickness of periodontal tissue, however, has not been objectively evaluated.

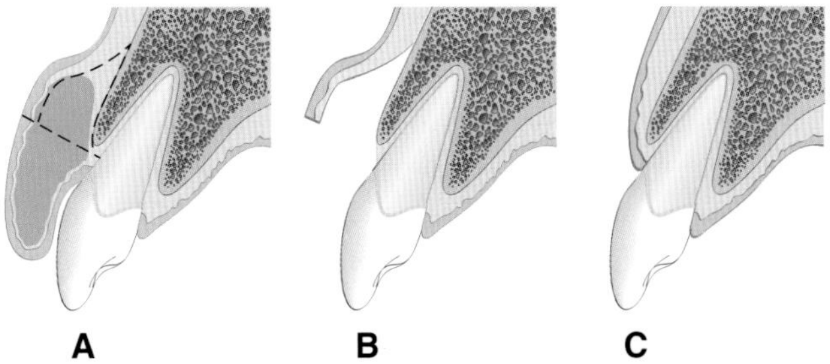

Figure 63-6 Diagram of periodontal flap treatment for drug-induced gingival enlargement. **A,** Initial reverse bevel incision followed by thinning of the enlarged gingival tissue; dotted lines represent incisions, and the shaded area represents the tissue portion to be excised. **B,** After flap elevation, enlarged portion of the gingival tissue is removed. **C,** The flap is placed on top of the alveolar bone and sutured.

LEUKEMIC GINGIVAL ENLARGEMENT

Leukemic enlargement occurs in acute or subacute leukemia and is uncommon in the chronic leukemic state. The medical care of leukemic patients is often complicated by gingival enlargement and superimposed painful acute necrotizing ulcerative gingivitis, which interferes with eating and creates toxic systemic reactions. The patient's bleeding and clotting times and platelet count should be checked and the hematologist consulted before periodontal treatment is instituted (see Chapter 44).

Treatment of acute gingival involvement is described in Chapter 47. After acute symptoms subside, attention is directed to correction of the gingival enlargement. The rationale is to remove the local irritating factors to control the inflammatory component of the enlargement.

The enlargement is treated by scaling and root planing carried out in stages under topical anesthesia. The initial treatment consists of gently removing all loose accumulations with cotton pellets, performing superficial scaling, and instructing the patient in oral hygiene for plaque control, which should include, at least initially, daily use of chlorhexidine mouthwashes. Oral hygiene procedures are extremely important in these patients and should be performed by the nurse if necessary.

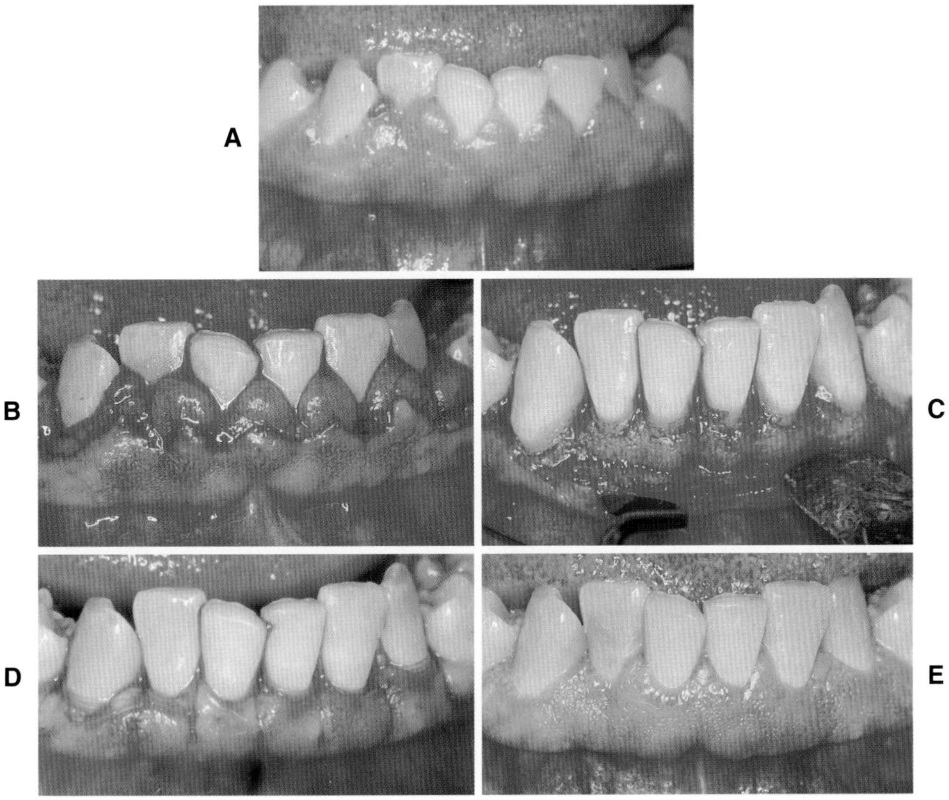

Figure 63-7 Treatment of combined cyclosporin and nifedipine–induced gingival enlargement with a periodontal flap on a 35-year-old female who had received a kidney allograft 3 years earlier. **A,** Presurgical clinical aspect of the lower anterior teeth, showing severe gingival enlargement. **B,** Initial scalloped reverse bevel incision, including maintenance of keratinized tissue and creation of surgical papillae. **C,** Elevation of a full-thickness flap and removal of the inner portion of the previously thinned gingival tissue. After scaling and root planing, osseous recontouring can be performed if necessary. **D,** The flap is positioned on top of the alveolar crest. **E,** Postsurgical aspect of the treated area at 12 months. Note the reduction of enlarged tissue volume and acceptable gingival health.

Progressively deeper scaling is carried out at subsequent visits. Treatments are confined to a small area of the mouth to facilitate control of bleeding. Antibiotics are administered systemically the evening before and for 48 hours after each treatment to reduce the risk of infection.

GINGIVAL ENLARGEMENT IN PREGNANCY

Treatment requires elimination of all local irritants responsible for precipitating the gingival changes in pregnancy. Elimination of local irritants early in pregnancy is a preventive measure against gingival disease, which is preferable to treatment of gingival enlargement after it occurs. Marginal and interdental gingival inflammation and enlargement are treated by scaling and curettage (see Chapters 51 and 62). Treatment of tumorlike gingival enlargements consists of surgical excision and scaling and planing of the tooth surface. The enlargement recurs unless all irritants are removed. Food impaction is frequently an inciting factor.

Timing of Treatment and Indications

Gingival lesions in pregnancy should be treated as soon as they are detected, although not necessarily by surgical means. Scaling and root-planing procedures and adequate oral hygiene measures may reduce the size of the enlargement. Gingival enlargements do shrink after pregnancy, but they usually do not disappear. After pregnancy, the entire mouth should be reevaluated, a full set of radiographs taken, and the necessary treatment undertaken.

Lesions should be removed surgically during pregnancy only if they interfere with mastication or produce an esthetic disfigurement that the patient wants removed.

In pregnancy the emphasis should be on (1) preventing gingival disease before it occurs and (2) treating existing gingival disease before it worsens. All patients should be seen as early as possible in pregnancy. Those without gingival disease should be checked for potential sources of local irritation and should be instructed in plaque control procedures. Those with gingival disease should be treated promptly, before the conditioning effect of pregnancy on the gingiva becomes manifest. Chapter 43 presents the necessary precautions for periodontal treatment of pregnant women.

Every pregnant patient should be scheduled for periodic dental visits, the importance of which in the prevention of serious periodontal disturbances should be stressed.

GINGIVAL ENLARGEMENT IN PUBERTY

Gingival enlargement in puberty is treated by performing scaling and curettage, removing all sources of irritation, and controlling plaque. Surgical removal may be required in severe cases. The problem in these patients is recurrence caused by poor oral hygiene.

SCIENCE TRANSFER

The treatment of gingival enlargement depends on the type of clinical enlargement encountered. The enlargement can be inflammatory, fibrotic, or a combination of both. *It appears that plaque and calculus are major stimulatory factors, even with drug-associated or systemic hormonal enlargements.*

Gingival enlargement is not seen in all patients taking a certain medication, suggesting that some patients are more susceptible to enlargements than others. The cause of this susceptibility is unknown but could be related to the gingival cells possessing either unique receptors on their cell surface or more receptors than other cells. Special subpopulations of cells may also exist in these susceptible individuals. Alternatively, cells may possess specific internal pathways that respond to medications or hormones in a unique way in affected patients.

Plaque-induced inflammation appears to be a general stimulating effect regardless of the mechanism of gingival enlargement.

In recent years, flap procedures have been used more often to treat gingival enlargement than gingivectomy. Flap technique not only gives better postoperative results but also allows for treatment of any osseous defects that may occur with gingival enlargement. In all cases, gingival enlargement may recur multiple times after surgery, so surgical procedures should be timed with as long an interval between them as possible. In some patients, therefore, postsurgical pocket depths are managed with nonsurgical techniques, and further surgery is postponed until indicated by esthetic concerns or pain on chewing.

RECURRENCE OF GINGIVAL ENLARGEMENT

Recurrence after treatment is the most common problem in the management of gingival enlargement. Residual local irritation and systemic or hereditary conditions causing noninflammatory gingival hyperplasia are the responsible factors.

Recurrence of chronic inflammatory enlargement immediately after treatment indicates that all irritants have not been removed. Contributory local conditions, such as food impaction and overhanging margins of restorations, are often overlooked. If the enlargement recurs after healing is complete and normal contour is attained, inadequate plaque control by the patient is the most common cause.

Recurrence during the healing period is manifested as red, beadlike, granulomatous masses that bleed on slight provocation. This is a proliferative vascular inflammatory response to local irritation, usually a fragment of calculus on the root. The condition is corrected by removing the granulation tissue and scaling and planing the root surface.

Familial, hereditary, or idiopathic gingival enlargement recurs after surgical removal even if all local irritants have been removed. The enlargement can be maintained at minimal size by preventing secondary inflammatory involvement.

The use of *escharotic drugs* has been recommended in the past for the removal of gingival enlargements, but their use is currently *not* recommended. The destructive action of the drugs is difficult to control; injury to healthy tissue and root surfaces, delayed healing, and excessive postoperative pain are complications that can be avoided when the gingiva is removed with periodontal knives and scalpels or by electrosurgery.

REFERENCES

1. Aiman R: The use of positive pressure mouthpiece as a new therapy for Dilantin gingival hyperplasia, *Chron Omaha Dent Soc* 131:244, 1968.
2. Babcock JR: The successful use of a new therapy for Dilantin gingival hyperplasia, *Periodontics* 3:196, 1965.
3. Barclay S, Thomason JM, Idle JR, et al: The incidence and severity of nifedipine-induced gingival overgrowth, *J Clin Periodontol* 19:311, 1992.
4. Camargo P, Melnick P, Pirih F, et al: Treatment of drug-induced gingival enlargement: aesthetic and functional considerations, *Periodontol 2000* 27:131, 2001.
5. Ciancio SG, Yaffe SJ, Catz CC: Gingival hyperplasia and diphenylhydantoin, *J Periodontol* 43:411, 1972.
6. Dahilof G, Preber H, Eliasson S, et al: Periodontal condition of epileptic adults treated with phenytoin or carbamazepine, *Epilepsia* 34:960, 1993.
7. Dongari A, O'Donnell HT, Langlais RP: Drug-induced gingival overgrowth, *Oral Surg Oral Med Oral Pathol* 76:543, 1993.
8. Fattore L, Stablein M, Bredfelt G, et al: Gingival hyperplasia: a side effect of nifedipine and diltiazem, *Spec Care Dent* 11:107, 1991.
9. Hall WB: Dilantin hyperplasia: a preventable lesion, *J Periodontal Res* 4:36, 1969.
10. Harel-Raviv M, Eckler M, Lalani K, et al: Nifedipine-induced gingival hyperplasia: a comprehensive review and analysis, *Oral Surg Oral Med Oral Pathol Oral Radiol Endod* 79:115, 1995.
11. Hernandez G, Arriba L, Lucas M, et al: Reduction of severe gingival overgrowth in a kidney transplant patient by replacing cyclosporin A with tacrolimus, *J Periodontol* 71:1630, 2000.
12. Nery EB, Edson RG, Lee KK, et al: Prevalence of nifedipine-induced gingival hyperplasia, *J Periodontol* 66:572, 1995.
13. Nishikawa S, Tada H, Hamasaki A, et al: Nifedipine-induced gingival hyperplasia: a clinical and in vitro study, *J Periodontol* 62:30, 1991.
14. Pilloni A, Camargo PM, Carere M, et al: Surgical treatment of cyclosporine A- and nifedipine-induced gingival enlargement, *J Periodontol* 69:791, 1998.
15. Rees TD, Levine RA: Systemic drugs as a risk factor for periodontal disease initiation and progression, *Compend Contin Educ Dent* 16:20, 1995.
16. Saravia ME, Svirsky JA, Friedman R: Chlorhexidine as an oral hygiene adjunct for cyclosporine-induced gingival hyperplasia, *J Dent Child* 57:366, 1990.
17. Seymour RA, Jacobs DJ: Cyclosporin and the gingival tissues, *J Clin Periodontol* 19:1, 1992.
18. Wahlstrom E, Zamora JU, Teichman S: Improvement in cyclosporin-associated gingival hyperplasia with azithromycin therapy, *N Engl J Med* 332:753, 1995.

The Periodontal Flap

Henry H. Takei and Fermin A. Carranza

64
CHAPTER

CHAPTER OUTLINE

A periodontal flap is a section of gingiva and/or mucosa surgically separated from the underlying tissues to provide visibility of and access to the bone and root surface. The flap also allows the gingiva to be displaced to a different location in patients with mucogingival involvement.

CLASSIFICATION OF FLAPS

Periodontal flaps can be classified based on the following:

- Bone exposure after flap reflection
- Placement of the flap after surgery
- Management of the papilla

Based on bone exposure after reflection, the flaps are classified as either full-thickness (mucoperiosteal) or partial-thickness (mucosal) flaps (Figure 64-1).

In *full-thickness flaps,* all the soft tissue, including the periosteum, is reflected to expose the underlying bone. This complete exposure of, and access to, the underlying bone is indicated when resective osseous surgery is contemplated.

The *partial-thickness flap* includes only the epithelium and a layer of the underlying connective tissue. The bone remains covered by a layer of connective tissue, including the periosteum. This type of flap is also called the *split-thickness flap.* The partial-thickness flap is indicated when the flap is to be positioned apically or when the operator does not want to expose bone.

Conflicting data surround the advisability of uncovering the bone when this is not actually needed. When bone is stripped of its periosteum, a loss of marginal bone occurs, and this loss is prevented when the periosteum is left on the bone.[4] Although usually not clinically significant,[7] the differences may be significant in some cases (Figure 64-2). The partial-thickness flap may be necessary when the crestal bone margin is thin and is exposed with an apically placed flap, or when dehiscences or fenestrations are present. The periosteum left on the bone may also be used for suturing the flap when it is displaced apically.

Based on flap placement after surgery, flaps are classified as (1) *nondisplaced flaps,* when the flap is returned and sutured in its original position, or (2) *displaced flaps,* which are placed apically, coronally, or laterally to their original position. Both full-thickness and partial-thickness flaps can be displaced, but to do so, the attached gingiva must be totally separated from the underlying bone, thereby enabling the unattached portion of the gingiva to be movable. However, palatal flaps cannot be displaced because of the absence of unattached gingiva.

Apically displaced flaps have the important advantage of preserving the outer portion of the pocket wall and

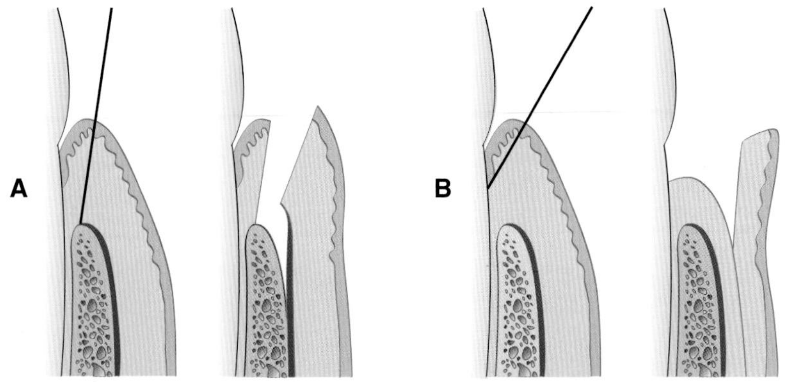

Figure 64-1 **A,** Diagram of the internal bevel incision (first incision) to reflect a full-thickness (mucoperiosteal) flap. Note that the incision ends on the bone to allow for the reflection of the entire flap. **B,** Diagram of the internal bevel incision to reflect a partial-thickness flap. Note that the incision ends on the root surface to preserve the periosteum on the bone.

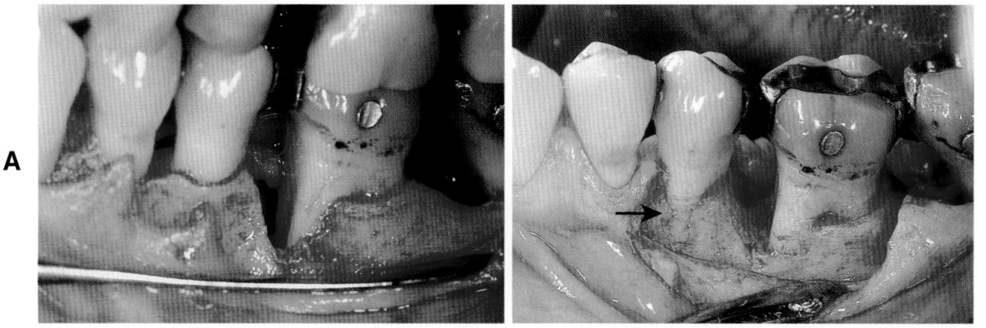

Figure 64-2 Loss of marginal bone as a result of uncovering the osseous crest. **A,** Mucoperiosteal flap elevated as part of a clinical study. **B,** Reentry performed 6 months later reveals loss of marginal bone facial to second premolar *(arrow)*. (Courtesy Dr. Silvia Oreamuno, San Jose, Costa Rica.)

transforming it into attached gingiva. Therefore these flaps accomplish the double objective of eliminating the pocket and increasing the width of the attached gingiva.

Based on management of the papilla, flaps can be conventional or papilla preservation flaps. In the *conventional flap* the interdental papilla is split beneath the contact point of the two approximating teeth to allow reflection of buccal and lingual flaps. The incision is usually scalloped to maintain gingival morphology with as much papilla as possible. The conventional flap is used (1) when the interdental spaces are too narrow, thereby precluding the possibility of preserving the papilla, and (2) when the flap is to be displaced.

Conventional flaps include the modified Widman flap, the undisplaced flap, the apically displaced flap, and the flap for reconstructive procedures. These techniques are described in detail in Chapter 65.

The *papilla preservation flap* incorporates the entire papilla in one of the flaps by means of crevicular interdental incisions to sever the connective tissue attachment and a horizontal incision at the base of the papilla, leaving it connected to one of the flaps.

FLAP DESIGN

The design of the flap is dictated by the surgical judgment of the operator and may depend on the objectives of the procedure. The necessary degree of access to the underlying bone and root surfaces and the final position of the flap must be considered in designing the flap. Preservation of good blood supply to the flap is an important consideration.

Two basic flap designs are used. Depending on how the interdental papilla is dealt with, flaps can either split the papilla (conventional flap) or preserve it (papilla preservation flap).

In the conventional flap procedure, the incisions for the facial and the lingual or palatal flap reach the tip of the interdental papilla or its vicinity, thereby splitting the papilla into a facial half and a lingual or palatal half (Figures 64-3 and 64-4).

The entire surgical procedure should be planned in every detail before the intervention is begun. This should include the type of flap, exact location and type of incisions, management of the underlying bone, and final closure of the flap and sutures. Although some details

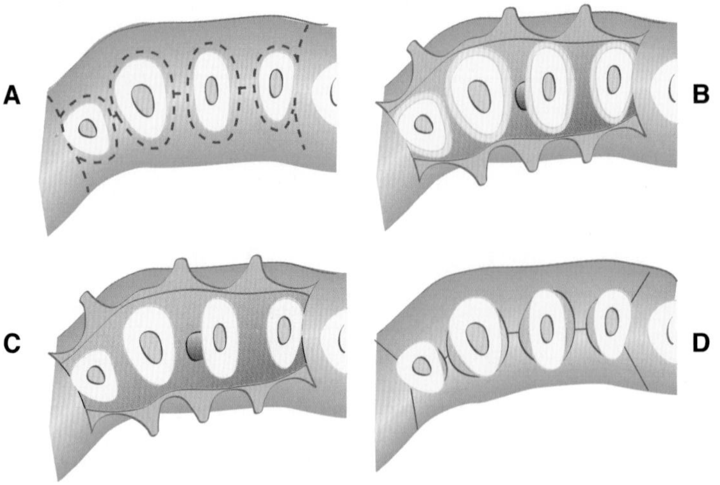

Figure 64-3 Flap design for conventional or traditional flap technique. **A,** Design of incisions: internal bevel incision, splitting the papilla, and vertical incisions are drawn in interrupted lines. **B,** The flap has been elevated, and the wedge of tissue next to the tooth is still in place. **C,** All marginal tissue has been removed, exposing the underlying bone (see defect in one space). **D,** Tissue returned to its original position. Proximal areas are not totally covered.

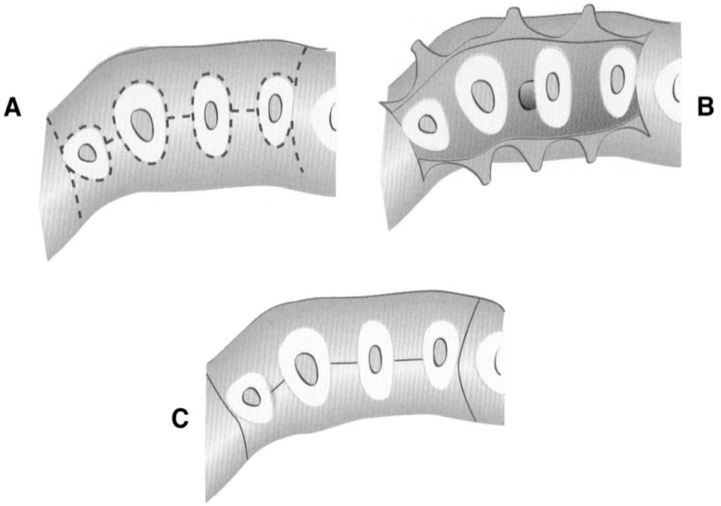

Figure 64-4 Flap design for sulcular incision flap. **A,** Design of incisions: sulcular incisions and vertical incisions are depicted by interrupted lines. **B,** The flap has been elevated, exposing the underlying bone (see defect in one space). **C,** Tissue returned to its original position covers the entire interdental spaces.

may be modified during the actual performance of the procedure, detailed planning allows for a better clinical result.

INCISIONS

Periodontal flaps use horizontal and vertical incisions.

Horizontal Incisions

Horizontal incisions are directed along the margin of the gingiva in a mesial or a distal direction. Two types of horizontal incisions have been recommended: the internal bevel incision,[6] which starts at a distance from the gingival margin and is aimed at the bone crest, and the crevicular incision, which starts at the bottom of the pocket and is directed to the bone margin. In addition, the interdental incision is performed after the flap is elevated.

The *internal bevel incision* is basic to most periodontal flap procedures. It is the incision from which the flap is reflected to expose the underlying bone and root. The internal bevel incision accomplishes three important objectives: (1) it removes the pocket lining; (2) it conserves the relatively uninvolved outer surface of the gingiva, which, if apically positioned, becomes attached gingiva; and (3) it produces a sharp, thin flap margin for adaptation to the bone-tooth junction. This incision

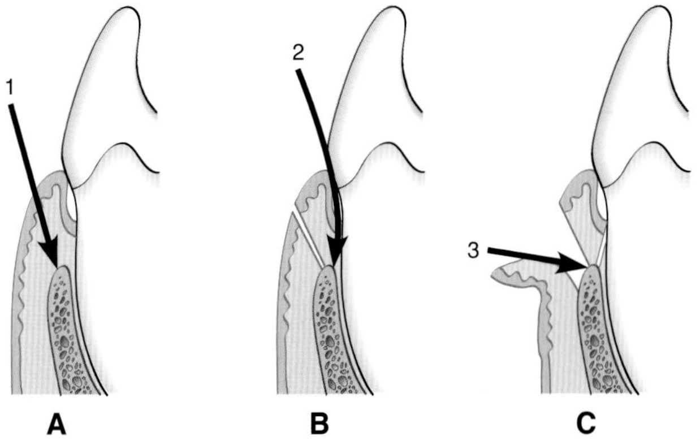

Figure 64-5 Three incisions necessary for flap surgery: **A,** first (internal bevel) incision; **B,** second (crevicular) incision; **C,** third (interdental) incision.

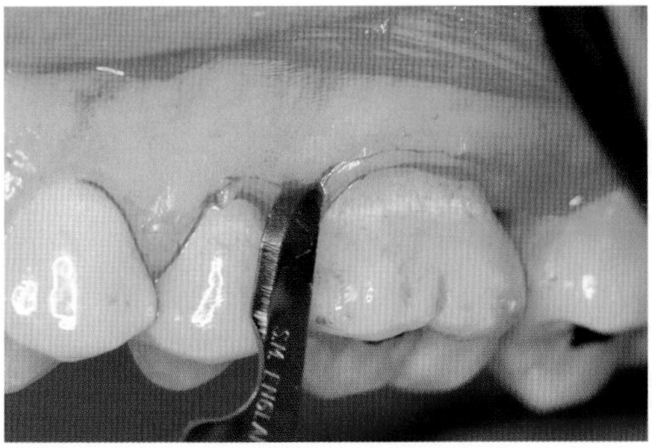

Figure 64-6 Position of knife in performing internal bevel incision.

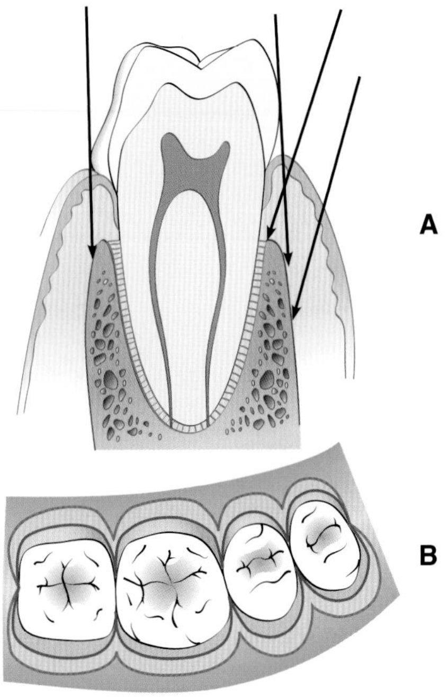

Figure 64-7 **A,** Internal bevel (first) incision can be made at varying locations and angles according to the different anatomic and pocket situations. **B,** Occlusal view of the different locations where the internal bevel incision can be made. Note the scalloped shape of the incisions.

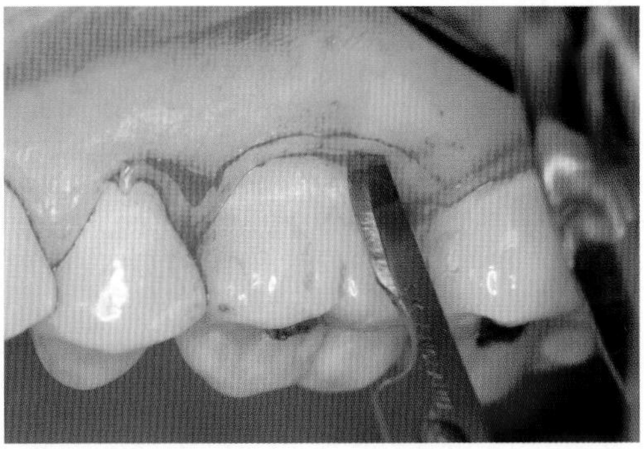

Figure 64-8 Position of knife in performing crevicular (second) incision.

has also been termed the *first incision* because it is the initial incision in the reflection of a periodontal flap, and the *reverse bevel incision* because its bevel is in reverse direction from that of the gingivectomy incision. The #11 or #15 surgical scalpel is used most often to make this incision. That portion of the gingiva left around the tooth contains the epithelium of the pocket lining and the adjacent granulomatous tissue. It is discarded after the crevicular (second) and interdental (third) incisions are performed (Figure 64-5).

The internal bevel incision starts from a designated area on the gingiva and is directed to an area at or near the crest of the bone (Figure 64-6). The starting point on the gingiva is determined by whether the flap is apically displaced or not displaced (Figure 64-7).

The *crevicular incision,* also termed the *second incision,* is made from the base of the pocket to the crest of the bone (Figure 64-8). This incision, together with the initial reverse bevel incision, forms a V-shaped wedge ending at or near the crest of bone; this wedge of tissue contains most of the inflamed and granulomatous areas that constitute the lateral wall of the pocket, as well as the junctional epithelium and the connective tissue fibers that still persist between the bottom of the pocket and the crest of the bone. The incision is carried around the entire tooth. The beak-shaped #12D blade is usually used for this incision.

A periosteal elevator is inserted into the initial internal bevel incision, and the flap is separated from the bone. The most apical end of the internal bevel incision is more exposed and visible. With this access, the surgeon is able to make the *third incision,* or *interdental incision,* to separate the collar of gingiva that is left around the tooth. The Orban knife is usually used for this incision. The incision is made not only around the facial and lingual radicular area but also interdentally, connecting the facial and lingual segments, to free the gingiva completely around the tooth (Figure 64-9; see also Figure 64-5).

These three incisions allow the removal of the gingiva around the tooth (i.e., the pocket epithelium and the adjacent granulomatous tissue). A curette or a large scaler (U15/30) can be used for this purpose. After removal of the large pieces of tissue, the remaining connective tissue

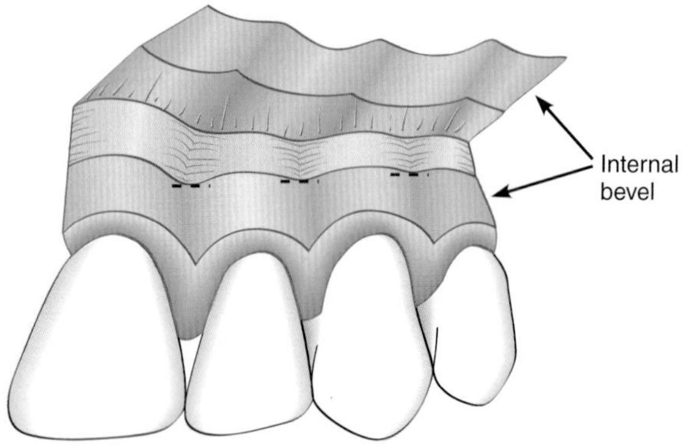

Figure 64-9 After the flap has been elevated, a wedge of tissue remains on the teeth, attached by the base of the papillae. An interdental (third) incision along the horizontal lines seen in the interdental spaces will sever these connections.

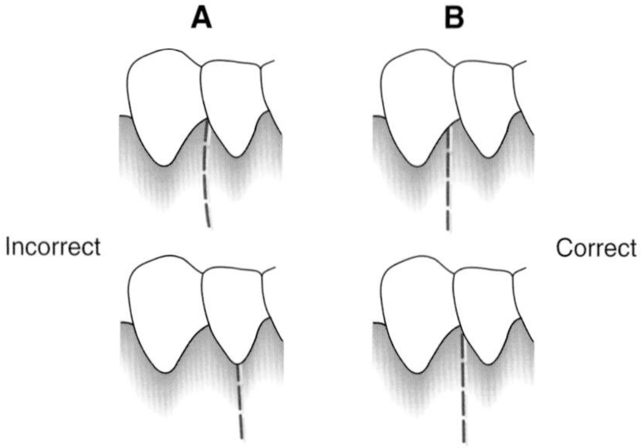

Figure 64-10 Incorrect **(A)** and correct **(B)** locations of a vertical incision. This incision should be made at the line angles to prevent splitting of a papilla or incising directly over a radicular surface.

in the osseous lesion should be carefully curetted so that the entire root and the bone surface adjacent to the teeth can be observed.

Flaps can be reflected using only the horizontal incision if sufficient access can be obtained in this way and if apical, lateral, or coronal displacement of the flap is not anticipated. If no vertical incisions are made, the flap is called an *envelope flap*.

Vertical Incisions

Vertical or oblique releasing incisions can be used on one or both ends of the horizontal incision, depending on the design and purpose of the flap. Vertical incisions at both ends are necessary if the flap is to be apically displaced. Vertical incisions must extend beyond the mucogingival line, reaching the alveolar mucosa, to allow for the release of the flap to be displaced (see Chapter 65).

In general, vertical incisions in the lingual and palatal areas are avoided. Facial vertical incisions should not be made in the center of an interdental papilla or over the radicular surface of a tooth. Incisions should be made at the line angles of a tooth either to include the papilla in the flap or to avoid it completely (Figure 64-10). The vertical incision should also be designed so as to avoid short flaps (mesiodistal) with long, apically directed horizontal incisions because these could jeopardize the blood supply to the flap.

Several investigators proposed the *interdental denudation procedure,* which consists of horizontal, internal bevel, nonscalloped incisions to remove the gingival papillae and denude the interdental space.[1,2,11,12] This technique completely eliminates the inflamed interdental areas, which heal by secondary intention, and results in excellent gingival contour. It is contraindicated when bone grafts are used.

ELEVATION OF THE FLAP

When a full-thickness flap is desired, reflection of the flap is accomplished by blunt dissection. A periosteal elevator is used to separate the mucoperiosteum from the bone

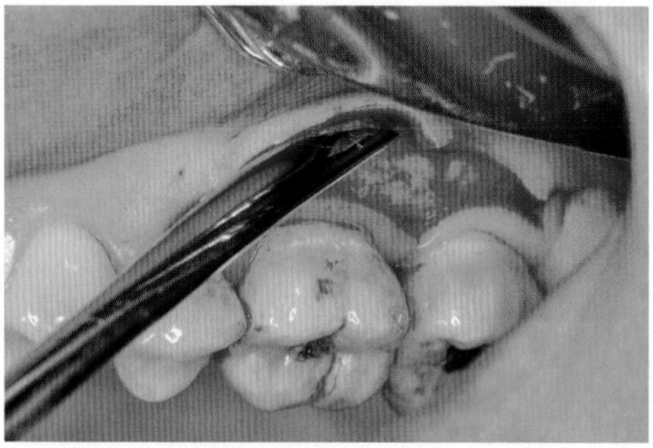

Figure 64-11 Elevation of the flap with a periosteal elevator to obtain a full-thickness flap.

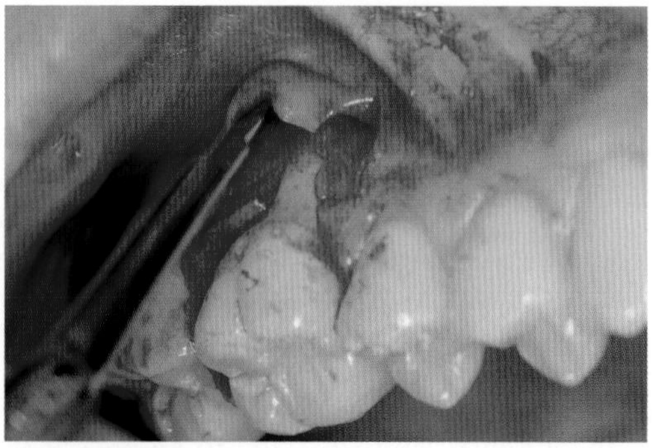

Figure 64-12 Elevation of the flap with a Bard-Parker knife to obtain a split-thickness flap.

by moving it mesially, distally, and apically until the desired reflection is accomplished (Figure 64-11).

Sharp dissection is necessary to reflect a partial-thickness flap. A surgical scalpel (#11 or #15) is used (Figure 64-12).

A combination of full-thickness and partial-thickness flaps often may be indicated to obtain the advantages of both. The flap is started as a full-thickness procedure, then a partial-thickness flap is made at the apical portion. In this way the coronal portion of the bone, which may be subject to osseous remodeling, is exposed while the remaining bone remains protected by its periosteum.

BOX 64-1

Sutures for Periodontal Flaps

Nonabsorbable (Nonresorbable)
Silk: braided
Nylon: monofilament (Ethilon)
ePTFE: monofilament (Gore-Tex)
Polyester: braided (Ethibond)

Absorbable (Resorbable)
Surgical: gut
Plain gut: monofilament (30 days)
Chromic gut: monofilament (45-60 days)

Synthetic
Polyglycolic: braided (16-20 days)
Vicryl (Ethicon)
Dexon (Davis & Geck)
Polyglecaprone: monofilament (90-120 days)
Monocryl (Ethicon)
Polyglyconate: monofilament (Maxon)

SUTURING TECHNIQUES

After all the necessary procedures are completed, the area is reexamined and cleansed, and the flap is placed in the desired position, where it should remain without tension. It is convenient to keep it in place with light pressure using a piece of gauze so that a blood clot can form. The purpose of suturing is to maintain the flap in the desired position until healing has progressed to the point where sutures are no longer needed.

There are many types of sutures, suture needles, and materials.[5,10] Suture materials may be either *nonresorbable* or *resorbable,* and they may be further categorized as *braided* or *monofilament* (Box 64-1). The resorbable sutures have gained popularity because they enhance patient comfort and eliminate suture removal appointments. The monofilament type of suture alleviates the "wicking effect" of braided sutures that may allow bacteria from the oral cavity to be drawn through the suture to the deeper areas of the wound.

The braided silk suture was the most common nonresorbable suture used in the past because of its ease of use and low cost. The expanded polytetrafluoroethylene synthetic monofilament is an excellent nonresorbable suture widely used today.

The most common resorbable sutures are the natural, plain gut and the chromic gut. Both are monofilaments and are processed from purified collagen of either sheep or cattle intestines. The chromic suture is a plain gut suture processed with chromic salts to make it resistant to enzymatic resorption, thereby increasing the resorption time. The synthetic resorbable sutures are also often used.

Technique

The needle is held with the needle holder and should enter the tissues at right angles and no less than 2 to 3 mm from the incision. The needle is then carried through the tissue, following the needle's curvature. The knot should not be placed over the incision.

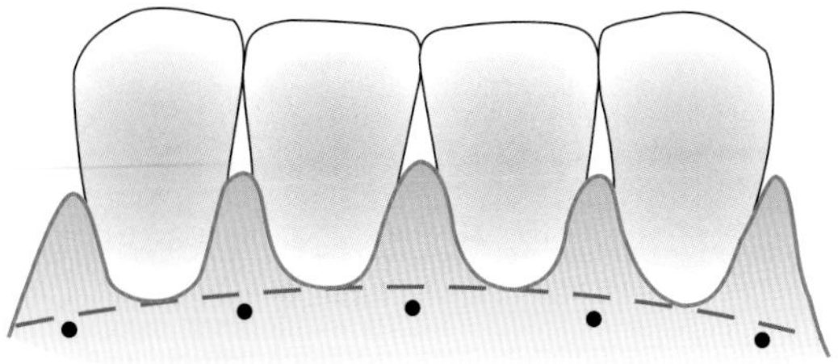

Figure 64-13 Placement of suture in the interdental space below the base of an imaginary triangle in the papilla.

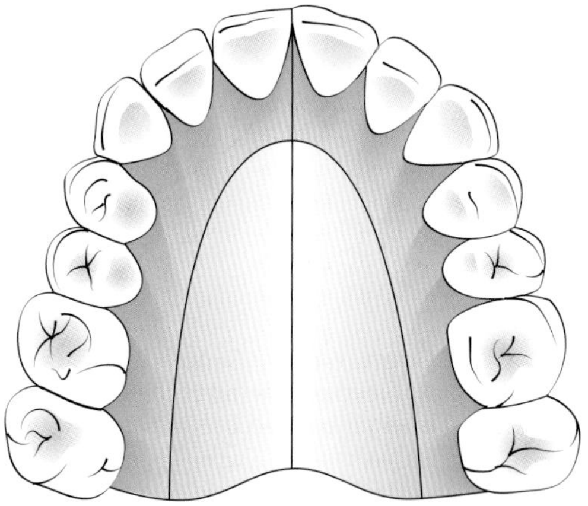

Figure 64-14 Placement of sutures for closing a palatal flap. For slightly or moderately elevated flaps, the sutures are placed in the shaded areas. For more substantial elevation of the flap, the sutures are placed in the central (unshaded) areas of the palate.

The periodontal flap is closed either with independent sutures or with continuous, independent sling sutures. The latter method eliminates the pulling of the buccal and lingual or palatal flaps together and instead uses the teeth as an anchor for the flaps. The flaps are less likely to buckle, and the forces on the flaps are better distributed.

Sutures of any type placed in the interdental papillae should enter and exit the tissue at a point located below the imaginary line that forms the base of the triangle of the interdental papilla (Figure 64-13). The location of sutures for closure of a palatal flap depends on the extent of flap elevation that has been performed. The flap is divided in four quadrants, as depicted in Figure 64-14. If the elevation of the flap is slight or moderate, the sutures can be placed in the quadrant closest to the teeth. If the flap elevation is substantial, the sutures should be placed in the central quadrants of the palate.

The clinician may or may not use periodontal dressings. When the flaps are not apically displaced, it is not necessary to use dressings other than for patient comfort.

Ligation

Interdental Ligation. Two types of interdental ligation can be used: the direct loop suture (Figure 64-15) and

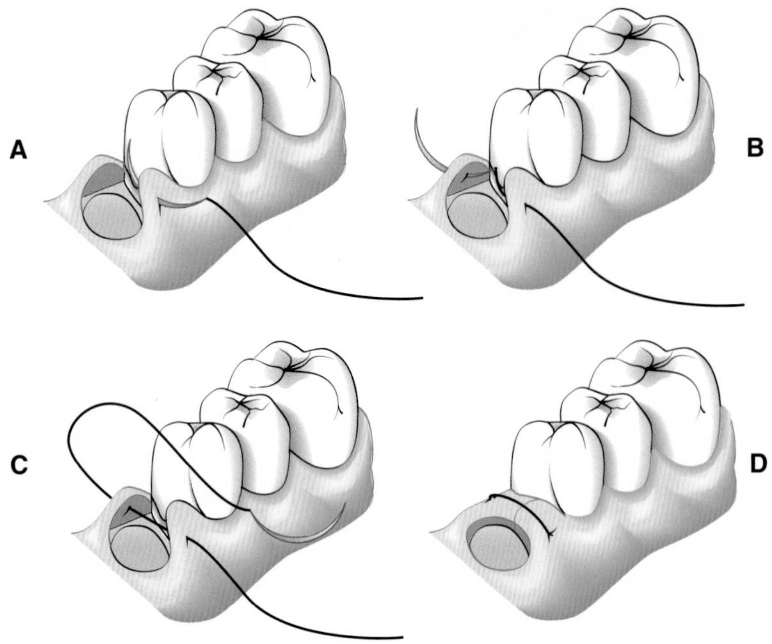

Figure 64-15 Simple loop suture is used to approximate the buccal and lingual flaps. **A,** Needle penetrates the outer surface of the first flap. **B,** Undersurface of the opposite flap is engaged, and the suture is brought back to the initial side **(C)**, where the knot is tied **(D).**

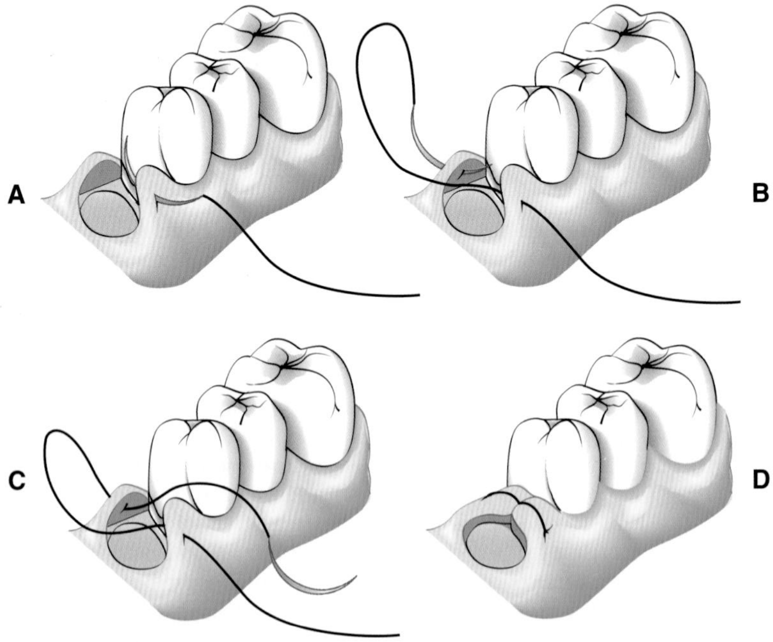

Figure 64-16 Interrupted figure-eight suture is used to approximate the buccal and lingual flaps. The needle penetrates the outer surface of the first flap **(A)** and the outer surface of the opposite flap **(B).** The suture is brought back to the first flap **(C),** and the knot is tied **(D).**

the figure-eight suture (Figure 64-16). In the figure-eight suture, there is thread between the two flaps. This suture is therefore used when the flaps are not in close apposition because of apical flap position or nonscalloped incisions. It is simpler to perform than the direct ligation. The direct suture permits a better closure of the interdental papilla and should be performed when bone grafts are used or when close apposition of the scalloped incision is required.

Sling Ligation. The sling ligation can be used for a flap on one surface of a tooth that involves two interdental spaces (Figure 64-17).

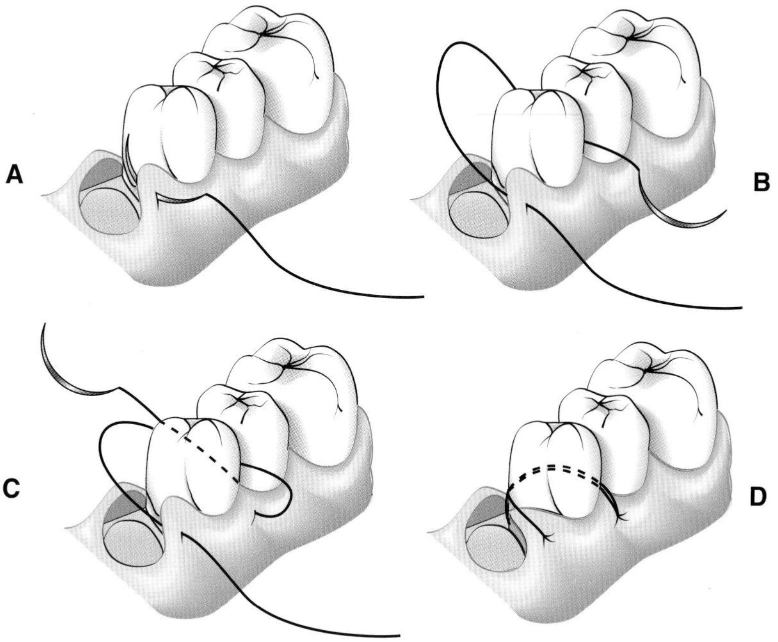

Figure 64-17 Single, interrupted sling suture is used to adapt the flap around the tooth. **A,** Needle engages the outer surface of the flap and encircles the tooth **(B)**. **C,** Outer surface of the same flap of the adjacent interdental area is engaged. **D,** Suture is returned to the initial site and the knot tied.

Types of Sutures

Horizontal Mattress Suture. This suture is often used for the interproximal areas of diastemata or for wide interdental spaces to adapt the interproximal papilla properly against the bone. Two sutures are often necessary. The horizontal mattress suture can be incorporated with continuous, independent sling sutures, as shown in Figure 64-18.

The penetration of the needle is performed in such a way that the mesial and distal edges of the papilla lie snugly against the bone. The needle enters the outer surface of the gingiva and crosses the undersurface of the gingiva horizontally. The mattress sutures should not be close together at the midpoint of the base of the papilla. The needle reappears on the outer surface at the other base of the papilla and continues around the tooth with the sling sutures.

Continuous, Independent Sling Suture. This suture is used when there is both a facial and a lingual flap involving many teeth. The continuous, independent sling suture is initiated on the facial papilla closest to the midline, because this is the easiest place to position the final knot (Figure 64-19). A continuous sling suture is laced for each papilla on the facial surface. When the last tooth is reached, the suture is anchored around it to prevent any pulling of the facial sutures when the lingual flap is sutured around the teeth in a similar manner. The suture is again anchored around the last tooth before tying the final knot.

This type of suture does not produce a pull on the lingual flap when this flap is sutured. The facial and lingual flaps are completely independent of each other because of the anchoring around both the initial and the final tooth. The flaps are tied to the teeth and not to each other because of the sling sutures.

Continuous, independent sling suturing is especially appropriate for the maxillary arch because the palatal gingiva is attached and fibrous, whereas the facial tissue is thinner and mobile.

Anchor Suture. The closing of a flap mesial or distal to a tooth, as in the mesial or distal wedge procedures, is best accomplished by the anchor suture. This suture closes the facial and lingual flaps and adapts them tightly against the tooth. The needle is placed at the line-angle area of the facial or lingual flap adjacent to the tooth, anchored around the tooth, passed beneath the opposite flap, and tied. The anchor suture can be repeated for each area that requires it (Figure 64-20).

Closed Anchor Suture. Another technique to close a flap located in an edentulous area mesial or distal to a tooth consists of tying a direct suture that closes the proximal flap, carrying one of the threads around the tooth to anchor the tissue against the tooth, and then tying the two threads (Figure 64-21).

Periosteal Suture. This type of suture is used to hold in place apically displaced partial-thickness flaps. There are two types of periosteal sutures: the holding suture and the closing suture. The holding suture is a horizontal mattress suture placed at the base of the displaced flap to secure it into the new position. Closing sutures are used to secure the flap edges to the periosteum. Both types of periosteal sutures are shown in Figure 64-22.

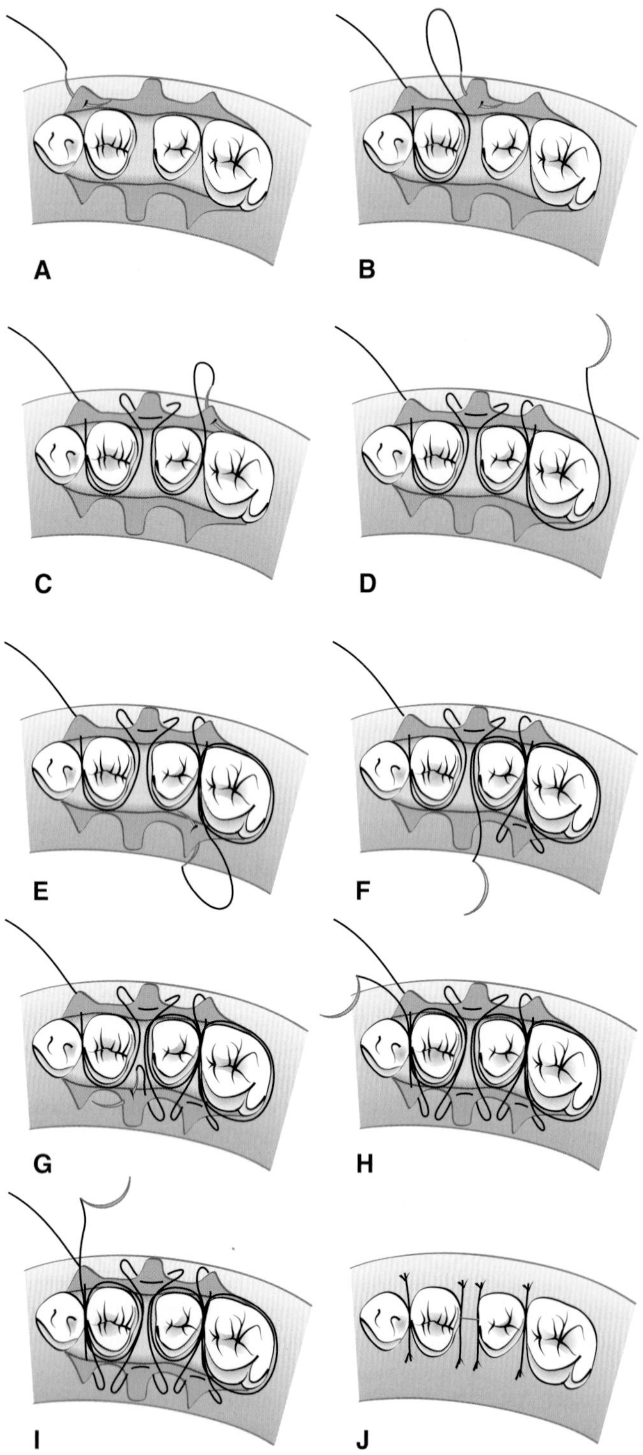

Figure 64-18 **A,** Continuous, independent sling suture using a horizontal mattress suture around diastemata or wide interdental areas (**B** and **C**). This mattress suture is used on both the buccal **(D)** and the lingual (**E** and **F**) surface. Continuation of suture on lingual surfaces (**G, H,** and **I**) and completed suture **(J).**

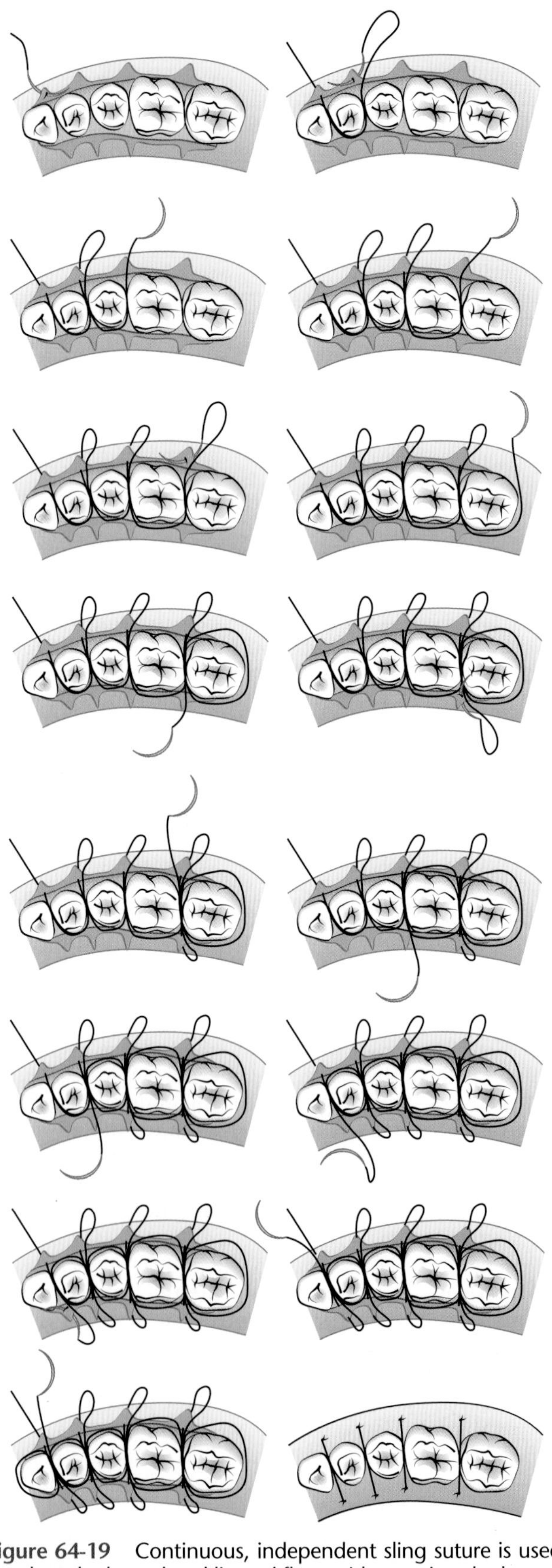

Figure 64-19 Continuous, independent sling suture is used to adapt the buccal and lingual flaps without tying the buccal flap to the lingual flap. The teeth are used to suspend each flap against the bone. It is important to anchor the suture on the two teeth at the beginning and end of the flap so that the suture will not pull the buccal flap to the lingual flap.

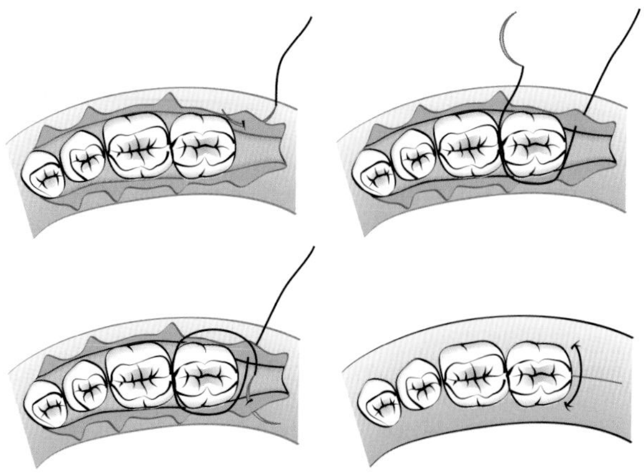

Figure 64-20 Distal wedge suture. This anchor suture is also used to close flaps that are mesial or distal to a lone-standing tooth.

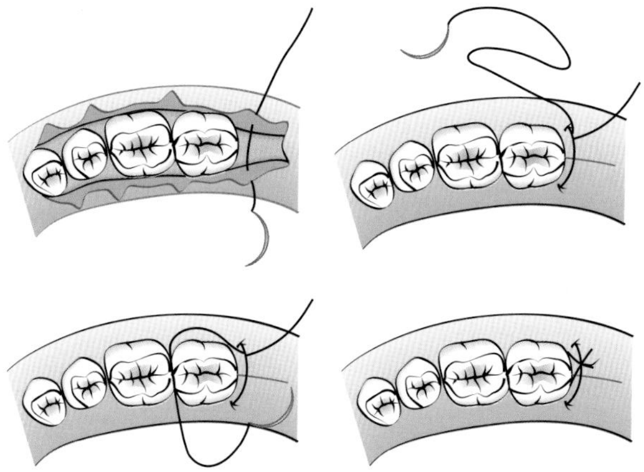

Figure 64-21 The closed anchor suture, another technique to suture distal wedges.

HEALING AFTER FLAP SURGERY

Immediately after suturing (up to 24 hours), a connection between the flap and the tooth or bone surface is established by a blood clot, which consists of a fibrin reticulum with many polymorphonuclear leukocytes, erythrocytes, debris of injured cells, and capillaries at the edge of the wound.[3] A bacteria and an exudate or transudate also result from tissue injury.

One to 3 days after flap surgery, the space between the flap and the tooth or bone is thinner, and epithelial cells migrate over the border of the flap, usually contacting the tooth at this time. When the flap is closely adapted to the alveolar process, there is only a minimal inflammatory response.[3]

One week after surgery, an epithelial attachment to the root has been established by means of hemidesmosomes and a basal lamina. The blood clot is replaced by granulation tissue derived from the gingival connective tissue, the bone marrow, and the periodontal ligament.

Two weeks after surgery, collagen fibers begin to appear parallel to the tooth surface.[3] Union of the flap to the tooth is still weak because of the presence of immature

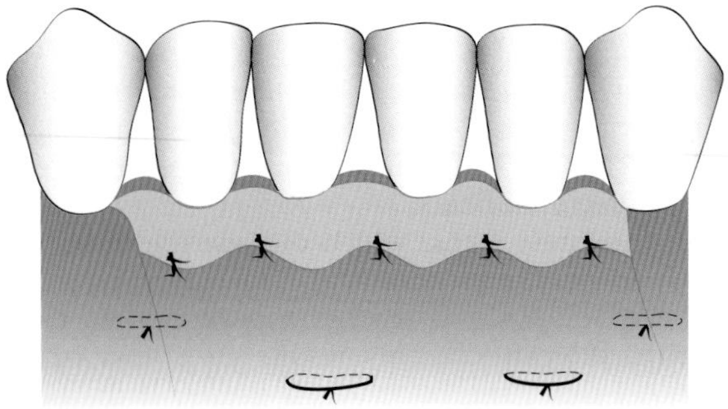

Figure 64-22 Periosteal sutures for an apically displaced flap. Holding sutures, shown at the bottom, are done first, followed by the closing sutures, shown at the coronal edge of the flap.

SCIENCE TRANSFER

The periodontal flap can be made in many different ways depending on the desired outcome. The flap can involve attached and nonattached tissues and involve removing all the tissues from the bone and teeth (full thickness) or incising the tissues and leaving connective tissues overlying the bone (partial thickness). Interestingly, the periodontal tissues have a remarkable ability for physiologic remodeling. For example, when the entire junctional epithelial complex is surgically removed, it will completely reform from the remaining oral epithelium. Similarly, when a full-thickness flap is elevated and replaced, attached tissue is reformed between the remaining periosteum on the flap and the superficial bone. Thus the body has a tremendous physiologic tendency to form the periodontal structures during the wound-healing process after surgical incision. This type of wound healing and outcome allows the surgeon the ability to choose and utilize a variety of flaps and incision designs.

Clinicians need to design flap incisions, flap elevation procedures, bone surgical techniques, and precise suturing approaches for each surgical procedure with great specificity. This means that a wide range of procedures is part of each clinician's armamentarium. *Highly technical skills in tissue management need to be combined with biologic understanding of surgical planning as well as patient management skills.* This combination of talents will be continually enhanced as clinical experience builds on an awareness of the need to improve surgical skills over the clinician's lifetime.

collagen fibers, although the clinical aspect may be almost normal.

One month after surgery, a fully epithelialized gingival crevice with a well-defined epithelial attachment is present. There is a beginning functional arrangement of the supracrestal fibers.

Full-thickness flaps, which denude the bone, result in a superficial bone necrosis at 1 to 3 days; osteoclastic resorption follows and reaches a peak at 4 to 6 days, declining thereafter.[13] This results in a loss of bone of about 1 mm^3; the bone loss is greater if the bone is thin.[14,15]

Osteoplasty (thinning of the buccal bone) using diamond burs, included as part of the surgical technique, results in areas of bone necrosis with reduction in bone height, which is later remodeled by new bone formation. Therefore the final shape of the crest is determined more by osseous remodeling than by surgical reshaping.[8] This may not be the case when osseous remodeling does not include excessive thinning of the radicular bone.[9] Bone repair reaches its peak at 3 to 4 weeks.[15]

Loss of bone occurs in the initial healing stages both in radicular bone and in interdental bone areas. However, in interdental areas, which have cancellous bone, the subsequent repair stage results in total restitution without any loss of bone, whereas in radicular bone, particularly if thin and unsupported by cancellous bone, bone repair results in loss of marginal bone.[15]

REFERENCES

1. Barkann L: A conservative surgical technique for the eradication of pyorrhea pockets, *J Am Dent Assoc* 26:61, 1939.
2. Beube FE: Interdental tissue resection: an experimental study of a surgical technique which aids in repair of the periodontal tissues to their original contour and function, *Oral Surg* 33:497, 1947.
3. Caffesse RG, Ramfjord SP, Nasjleti CE: Reverse bevel periodontal flaps in monkeys, *J Periodontol* 39:219, 1968.
4. Carranza FA Jr, Carraro JJ: Effect of removal of periosteum on postoperative result of mucogingival surgery, *J Periodontol* 34:223, 1963.
5. Dahlberg WH: Incisions and suturing: some basic considerations about each in periodontal flap surgery, *Dent Clin North Am* 113:149, 1969.
6. Friedman N: Mucogingival surgery: the apically repositioned flap, *J Periodontol* 33:328, 1962.
7. Hoag PM, Wood DL, Donnenfeld OW, et al: Alveolar crest reduction following full and partial thickness flaps, *J Periodontol* 43:141, 1972.
8. Lobene RR, Glickman I: The response of alveolar bone to grinding with rotary stones, *J Periodontol* 34:105, 1963.
9. Matherson DG: An evaluation of healing following periodontal osseous surgery in monkeys, *Int J Periodont Restor Dent* 8:9, 1988.
10. Morris ML: Suturing techniques in periodontal surgery, *Periodontics* 3:84, 1965.
11. Prichard JF: Present state of the interdental denudation procedure, *J Periodontol* 48:566, 1977.
12. Ratcliff PA, Raust GT: Interproximal denudation: a conservative approach to osseous surgery, *Dent Clin North Am* 8:121, 1964.
13. Staffileno H, Wentz FE, Orban BJ: Histologic study of healing of split thickness flap surgery in dogs, *J Periodontol* 33:56, 1962.
14. Wilderman MN: Exposure of bone in periodontal surgery, *Dent Clin North Am* 8:23, 1964.
15. Wilderman MN, Pennel BM, King K, et al: Histogenesis of repair following osseous surgery, *J Periodontol* 41:551, 1970.

The Flap Technique for Pocket Therapy

Fermin A. Carranza and Henry H. Takei

65

CHAPTER

CHAPTER OUTLINE

Several techniques can be used for the treatment of periodontal pockets. The periodontal flap is one of the most frequently employed procedures, particularly for moderate and deep pockets in posterior areas (see Chapter 59).

OVERVIEW

Flaps are used for pocket therapy to accomplish the following:

1. Increase accessibility to root deposits.
2. Eliminate or reduce pocket depth by resection of the pocket wall.
3. Expose the area to perform regenerative methods.

To fulfill these purposes, several flap techniques are available and in current use.

Techniques for Access and Pocket Depth Reduction/Elimination

The modified Widman flap facilitates instrumentation but does not attempt to reduce pocket depth. The reduction or elimination of pocket depth is the main purpose of two flap techniques: the undisplaced flap and the apically displaced flap. The decision of which to perform depends on two important anatomic landmarks: pocket depth and location of the mucogingival junction. These landmarks establish the presence and width of the attached gingiva, which is the basis for the decision.

The *modified Widman flap* has been described for exposing the root surfaces for meticulous instrumentation and for removal of the pocket lining.[6] Again, it is not intended to eliminate or reduce pocket depth, except for the reduction that occurs in healing by tissue shrinkage.

The *undisplaced (unrepositioned) flap,* in addition to improving accessibility for instrumentation, removes the pocket wall, thereby reducing or eliminating the pocket. This is essentially an excisional procedure of the gingiva.

The *apically displaced flap* also improves accessibility and eliminates the pocket, but it does the latter by apically positioning the soft tissue wall of the pocket.[2] Therefore, it preserves or increases the width of the attached gingiva by transforming the previously unattached keratinized pocket wall into attached tissue. This increase in width of the band of attached gingiva is supposedly based on an apical shift of the mucogingival junction, which includes apical displacement of the muscle attachments. A study made before and 18 years after apically displaced flaps failed to show a permanent relocation of the mucogingival junction.[1]

Incisions

All three flap techniques just discussed use the basic incisions described in Chapter 64: the internal bevel incision, the crevicular incision, and the interdental incision. However, there are important variations in the way these incisions are performed for the different types of flaps (Figures 65-1 and 65-2).

The modified Widman flap does not intend to remove the pocket wall, but it does eliminate the pocket lining. Therefore the internal bevel incision starts close, no more than 1 to 2 mm apically, to the gingival margin and follows the normal scalloping of the gingival margin (see Figure 65-1).

For the apically displaced flap, the pocket wall also must be preserved to be positioned apically while its lining is removed. The purpose of this surgical technique is to preserve the maximum amount of keratinized gingiva of the pocket wall to displace it apically and transform it into attached gingiva. For this reason, the internal bevel incision should be made as close to the tooth as possible, 0.5 to 1.0 mm (see Figure 65-1). There is no need to determine where the bottom of the pocket is in relation to the incision for the apically displaced flap, as one would for the undisplaced flap; the flap is placed approximately at the tooth-bone junction by apically displacing the flap. Its final position is not determined by the placement of this first incision.

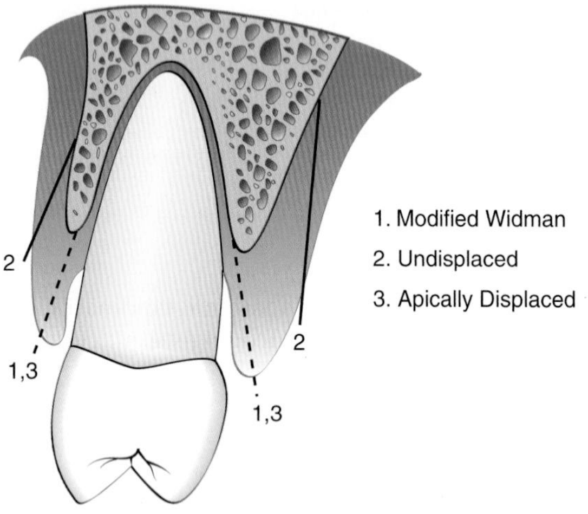

Figure 65-1 Locations of the internal bevel incisions for the different types of flaps.

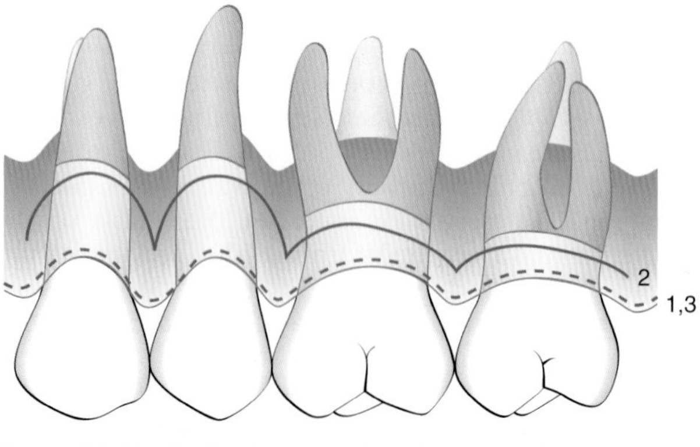

Figure 65-2 Scallopings required for the different types of flaps (see Figure 65-1).

For an undisplaced flap, however, the internal bevel incision is initiated at or near a point just coronal to the projection of the bottom of the pocket on the outer surface of the gingiva (see Figure 65-1). This incision can be accomplished only if sufficient attached gingiva remains apical to the incision. Therefore the two anatomic landmarks, pocket depth and location of the mucogingival junction, must be considered to evaluate the amount of attached gingiva that remains. Because the pocket wall is not displaced apically, the initial incision should also eliminate the pocket wall. If the incision is made too close to the tooth, it will not eliminate the pocket wall and may result in the recreation of a soft tissue pocket. If the tissue is thick, it should also be thinned by the initial incision to cover the bone properly during flap closure. Proper placement of the flap during closure is essential to prevent either recurrence of pockets or bone exposure; placement is determined by where this first incision is placed. The internal bevel incision should be scalloped to preserve, as much as possible, the interdental papilla (see Figure 65-2). This allows better coverage of the bone at both the radicular and the interdental areas.

If the surgeon contemplates osseous surgery, the first incision should be placed in such a way as to compensate for the removal of bone tissue so that the flap ends at the tooth-bone junction.

Reconstructive Techniques

The techniques used for reconstructive and regenerative purposes are the *papilla preservation flap*[8] and the *conventional flap* using only crevicular or pocket incisions, to retain the maximum amount of gingival tissue, including the papilla, for graft or membrane coverage.

MODIFIED WIDMAN FLAP

In 1965, Morris[4] revived a technique described early in the twentieth century in the periodontal literature; he called it the "unrepositioned mucoperiosteal flap." Essentially, the same procedure was presented in 1974 by Ramfjord and Nissle,[6] who called it the "modified Widman flap" (Figure 65-3). This technique offers the possibility of establishing an intimate postoperative adaptation of healthy collagenous connective tissue to tooth surfaces[5,6] and provides access for adequate instrumentation of the root surfaces and immediate closure of the area. The following steps outline the modified Widman flap technique:

Step 1: The initial incision is an internal bevel incision to the alveolar crest starting 0.5 to 1 mm away from the gingival margin (Figure 65-3, *C*). Scalloping follows the gingival margin. Care should be taken to insert the blade in such a way that the papilla is left with a thickness similar to that of the remaining facial flap. Vertical relaxing incisions are usually not needed.

Step 2: The gingiva is reflected with a periosteal elevator (Figure 65-3, *D*).

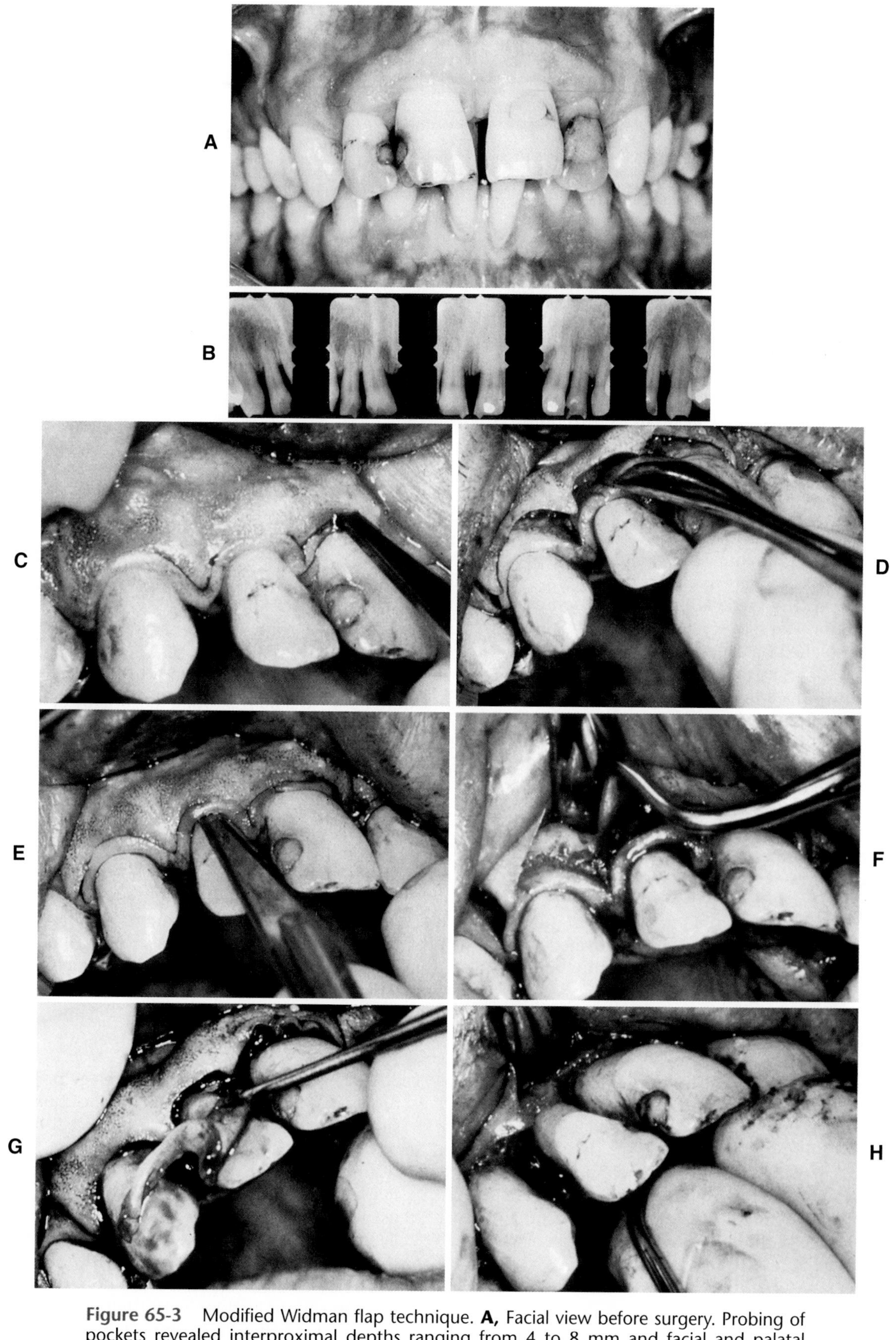

Figure 65-3 Modified Widman flap technique. **A,** Facial view before surgery. Probing of pockets revealed interproximal depths ranging from 4 to 8 mm and facial and palatal depths of 2 to 5 mm. **B,** Radiographic survey of area. Note generalized horizontal bone loss. **C,** Internal bevel incision. **D,** Elevation of the flap, leaving a wedge of tissue still attached by its base. **E,** Crevicular incision. **F,** Interdental incision sectioning the base of the papilla. **G,** Removal of tissue. **H,** Exposure of root surfaces and marginal bone; root planing and removal of remaining calculus.

Continued

I

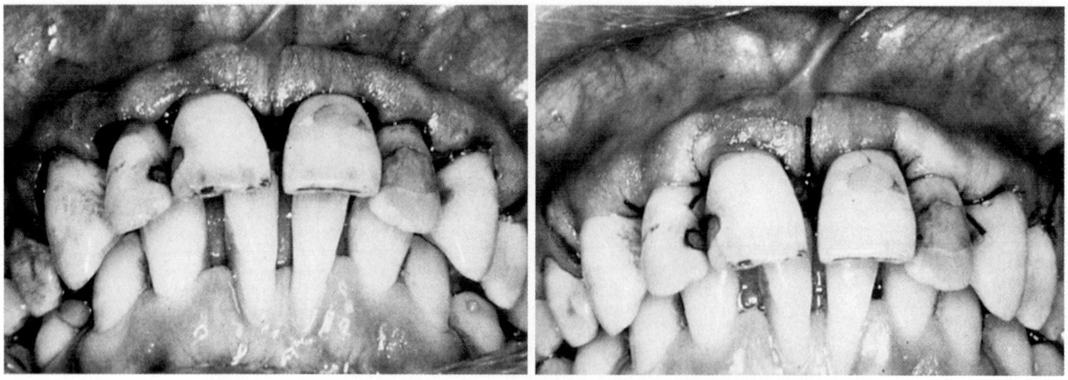

J

Figure 65-3, cont'd Modified Widman flap technique. **I,** Replacement of flap in its original position. **J,** Interdental sutures in place. (Courtesy Dr. Raul G. Caffesse, Houston.)

Step 3: A crevicular incision is made from the bottom of the pocket to the bone, circumscribing the triangular wedge of tissue containing the pocket lining (Figure 65-3, *E*).

Step 4: After the flap is reflected, a third incision is made in the interdental spaces coronal to the bone with a curette or an interproximal knife, and the gingival collar is removed (Figure 65-3, *F* and *G*).

Step 5: Tissue tags and granulation tissue are removed with a curette. The root surfaces are checked, then scaled and planed if needed (Figure 65-3, *H*). Residual periodontal fibers attached to the tooth surface should not be disturbed.

Step 6: Bone architecture is not corrected except if it prevents good tissue adaptation to the necks of the teeth. Every effort is made to adapt the facial and lingual interproximal tissue adjacent to each other in such a way that no interproximal bone remains exposed at the time of suturing (Figure 65-3, *I*). The flaps may be thinned to allow for close adaptation of the gingiva around the entire circumference of the tooth and to each other interproximally.

Step 7: Interrupted direct sutures are placed in each interdental space (Figure 65-3, *J*) and covered with tetracycline (Achromycin) ointment and with a periodontal surgical pack.

Ramfjord and Nissle[6] performed an extensive longitudinal study comparing the Widman procedure, as modified by them, with the curettage technique and the pocket elimination methods that include bone contouring when needed. The patients were assigned randomly to one of the techniques, and results were analyzed yearly up to 7 years after therapy. They reported approximately similar results with the three methods tested. Pocket depth was initially similar for all methods but was maintained at shallower levels with the Widman flap; the attachment level remained higher with the Widman flap.

UNDISPLACED FLAP

Currently, the undisplaced flap may be the most frequently performed type of periodontal surgery. It differs from the modified Widman flap in that the soft tissue pocket wall is removed with the initial incision; thus it may be considered an "internal bevel gingivectomy." The undisplaced flap and the gingivectomy are the two techniques that surgically remove the pocket wall. To perform this technique without creating a mucogingival problem, the clinician should determine that enough attached gingiva will remain after removal of the pocket wall. The following steps outline the undisplaced flap technique:

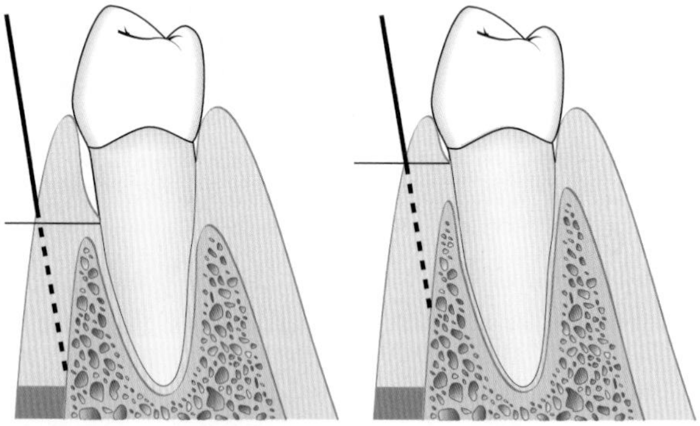

Figure 65-4 Diagram showing the location of two different areas where the internal bevel incision is made in an undisplaced flap. The incision is made at the level of the pocket to discard the tissue coronal to the pocket if there is sufficient remaining attached gingiva.

Step 1: The pockets are measured with the periodontal probe, and a bleeding point is produced on the outer surface of the gingiva to mark the pocket bottom.

Step 2: The initial, or internal bevel, incision is made (Figure 65-4) after the scalloping of the bleeding marks on the gingiva (Figure 65-5). The incision is usually carried to a point apical to the alveolar crest, depending on the thickness of the tissue. The thicker the tissue, the more apical is the ending point of the incision (see Figure 65-4). In addition, thinning of the flap should be done with the initial incision because it is easier to accomplish at this time than later, with a loose, reflected flap that is difficult to manage. (Use of this technique in palatal areas is considered in the following discussion.)

A B C D E F G H I J K L

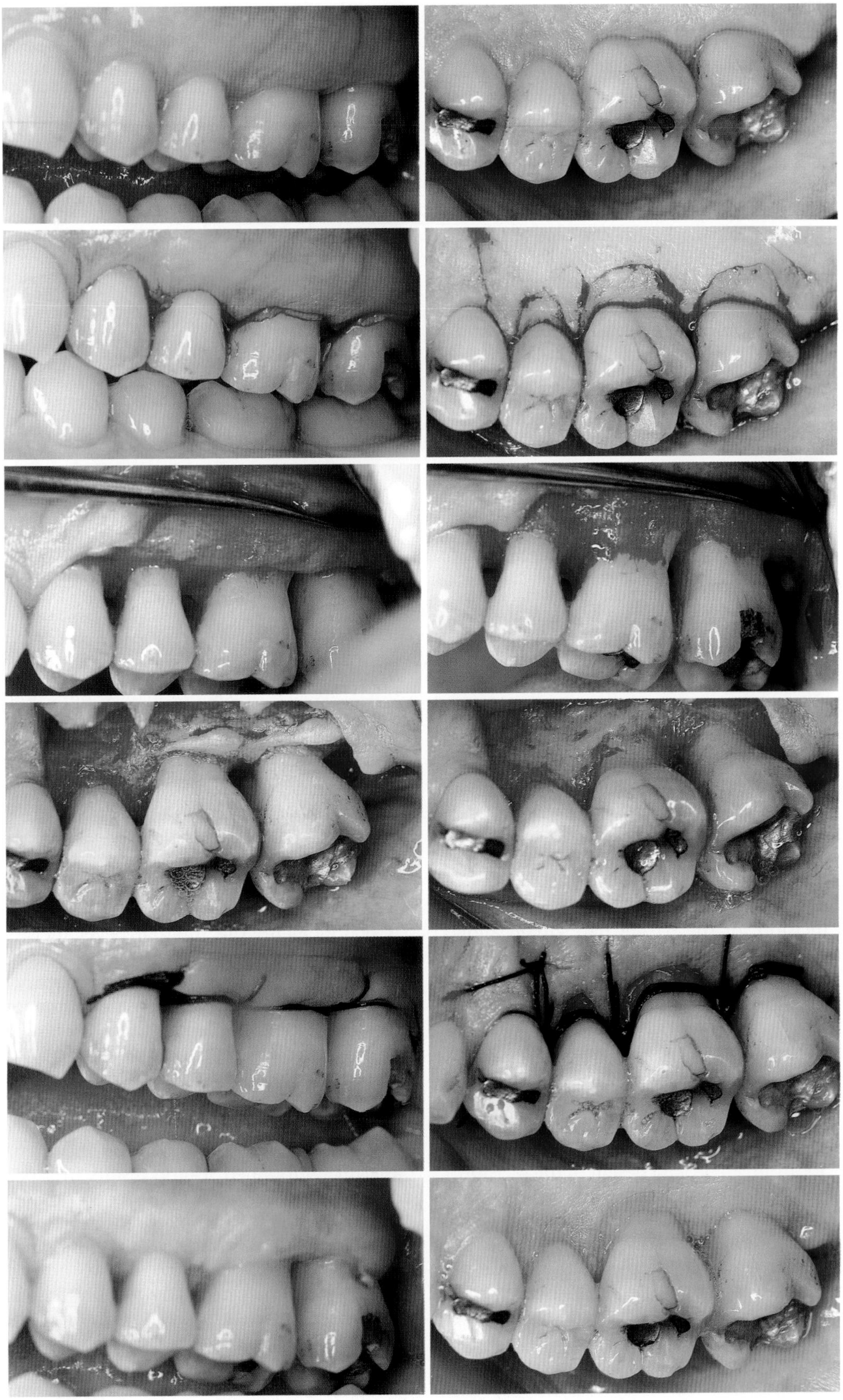

Figure 65-5 Undisplaced flap. **A** and **B,** Preoperative facial and palatal views. **C** and **D,** Internal bevel incisions in the facial and palatal aspects. Note the deeper scalloping palatally for the replaced flap. **E** and **F,** Flap elevated showing osseous defects. **G** and **H,** Osseous surgery has been performed. **I** and **J,** Flaps have been placed in their original site and sutured. **K** and **L,** Postoperative results. (Courtesy Dr. Paulo Camargo, University of California, Los Angeles.)

Step 3: The second, or crevicular, incision is made from the bottom of the pocket to the bone to detach the connective tissue from the bone.

Step 4: The flap is reflected with a periosteal elevator (blunt dissection) from the internal bevel incision. Usually there is no need for vertical incisions because the flap is not displaced apically.

Step 5: The third, or interdental, incision is made with an interdental knife, separating the connective tissue from the bone.

Step 6: The triangular wedge of tissue created by the three incisions is removed with a curette.

Step 7: The area is debrided, removing all tissue tags and granulation tissue using sharp curettes.

Step 8: After the necessary scaling and root planing, the flap edge should rest on the root-bone junction. If this is not the case, because of improper location of the initial incision or the unexpected need for osseous surgery, the edge of the flap is rescalloped and trimmed to allow the flap edge to end at the root-bone junction.

Step 9: A continuous sling suture is used to secure the facial and the lingual or palatal flaps. This type of suture, using the tooth as an anchor, is advantageous to position and hold the flap edges at the root-bone junction. The area is covered with a periodontal pack.

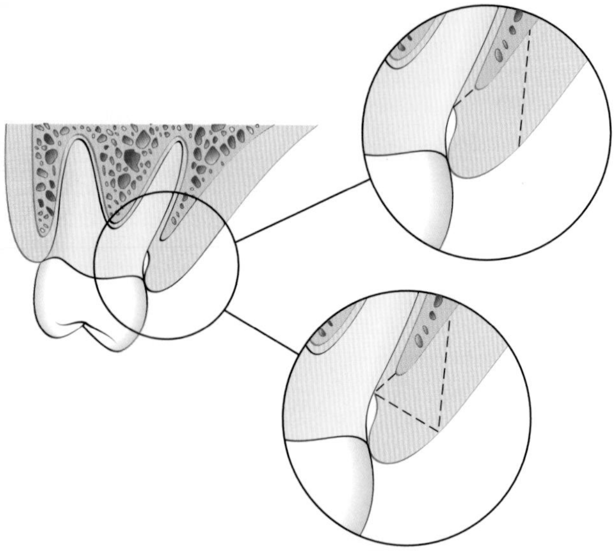

Figure 65-6 Examples of two methods for eliminating a palatal pocket. One incision is an internal bevel incision made at the area of the apical extent of the pocket. The other procedure uses a gingivectomy incision, which is followed by an internal bevel incision.

Palatal Flap

The surgical approach to the palatal area differs from that for other areas because of the character of the palatal tissue and the anatomy of the area. The palatal tissue is all attached, keratinized tissue and has none of the elastic properties associated with other gingival tissues. Therefore the palatal tissue cannot be apically displaced, and a partial-thickness (split-thickness) flap cannot be accomplished.

The initial incision for the palatal flap should allow the flap, when sutured, to be precisely adapted at the root-bone junction. The flap cannot be moved apically or coronally to adapt to the root-bone junction, as can be done with the flaps in other areas. Therefore the location of the initial incision is important for the final placement of the flap.

The palatal tissue may be thin or thick, it may or may not have osseous defects, and the palatal vault may be high or low. These anatomic variations may require changes in the location, angle, and design of the incision.

The initial incision for a flap varies with the anatomic situation. As shown in Figure 65-6, the initial incision may be the usual internal bevel incision, followed by crevicular and interdental incisions. If the tissue is thick, a horizontal gingivectomy incision may be made, followed by an internal bevel incision that starts at the edge of this incision and ends on the lateral surface of the underlying bone. The placement of the internal bevel incision must be done in such a way that the flap fits around the tooth without exposing the bone.

Before the flap is reflected to the final position for scaling and management of the osseous lesions, its thickness must be checked. Flaps should be thin to adapt to the underlying osseous tissue and provide a thin, knifelike gingival margin. Flaps, particularly palatal flaps, often are too thick; they may have a propensity to separate from the tooth and may delay and complicate healing. It is best to thin the flaps before their complete reflection because a free, mobile flap is difficult to hold for thinning (Figure 65-7). A sharp, thin papilla positioned properly around the interdental areas at the tooth-bone junction is essential to prevent recurrence of soft tissue pockets.

The purpose of the palatal flap should be considered before the incision is made. If the intent of the surgery is debridement, the internal bevel incision is planned so that the flap adapts at the root-bone junction when sutured. If osseous resection is necessary, the incision should be planned to compensate for the lowered level of the bone when the flap is closed. Probing and sounding of the osseous level and the depth of the intrabony pocket should be used to determine the position of the incision.

The apical portion of the scalloping should be narrower than the line-angle area because the palatal root tapers apically. A rounded scallop results in a palatal flap that does not fit snugly around the root. This procedure should be done before the complete reflection of the palatal flap, as a loose flap is difficult to grasp and stabilize for dissection.

It is sometimes necessary to thin the palatal flap after it has been reflected. This can be accomplished by holding the inner portion of the flap with a mosquito hemostat or Adson forceps as the inner connective tissue is carefully dissected away with a sharp #15 scalpel blade. Care must be taken not to perforate or overthin the flap. The edge of the flap should be thinner than the base; therefore the blade should be angled toward the lateral surface of the palatal bone. The dissected inner connective tissue is removed with a hemostat. As with any flap, the triangular

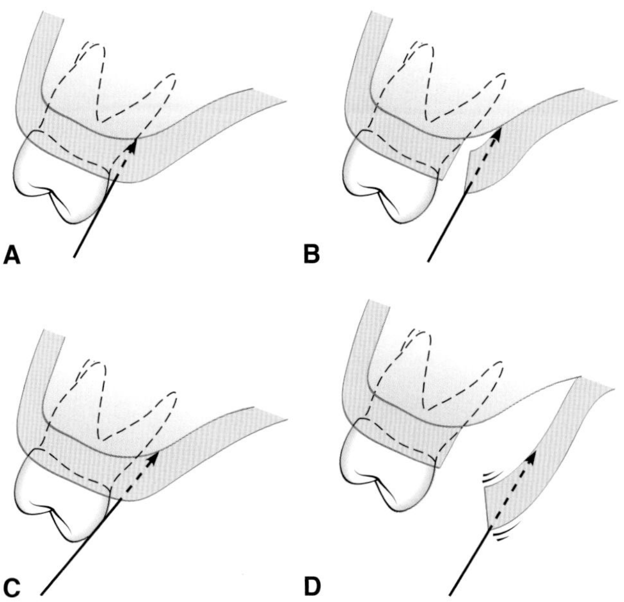

Figure 65-7 Diagrams illustrating the angle of the internal bevel incision in the palate and the different ways to thin the flap. **A,** Usual angle and direction of the incision. **B,** Thinning of the flap after it has been slightly reflected with a second internal incision. **C,** Beveling and thinning of the flap with the initial incision if the position and contour of the tooth allow. **D,** The problem encountered in thinning the flap once it has been reflected. The flap is too loose and free for proper positioning and incision.

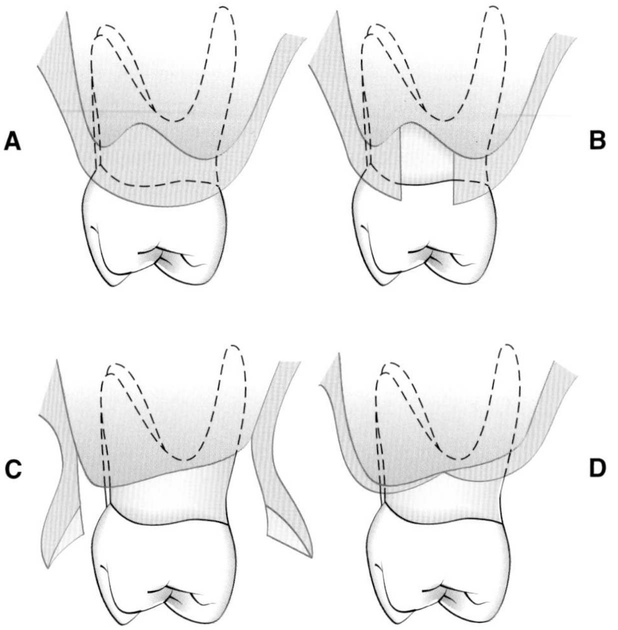

Figure 65-8 **A,** Distal view of incisions made to eliminate a pocket distal to the maxillary second molar. **B,** Two parallel incisions and the removal of the intervening tissue. **C,** Thinning of the flap and contouring of the bone. **D,** Approximation of the buccal and palatal flaps.

papilla portion should be thin enough to fit snugly against the bone and into the interdental area (Figure 65-8).

The principles for the use of vertical releasing incisions are similar to those for using other incisions. Care must be exercised so that the length of the incision is minimal to avoid the numerous vessels located in the palate.

APICALLY DISPLACED FLAP

With some variants, the apically displaced flap technique can be used for (1) pocket eradication and/or (2) widening the zone of attached gingiva. Depending on the purpose, it can be a full-thickness (mucoperiosteal) or a split-thickness (mucosal) flap. The split-thickness flap requires more precision and time, as well as a gingival tissue thick enough to split, but it can be more accurately positioned and sutured in an apical position using a periosteal suturing technique, as follows:

Step 1: An internal bevel incision is made (Figure 65-9). To preserve as much of the keratinized and attached gingiva as possible, it should be no more than about 1 mm from the crest of the gingiva and directed to the crest of the bone (see Figure 65-1). The incision is made after the existing scalloping, and there is no need to mark the bottom of the pocket in the external gingival surface because the incision is unrelated to pocket depth. It is also not necessary to accentuate the scallop interdentally because the flap is displaced apically and not placed interdentally.

Step 2: Crevicular incisions are made, followed by initial elevation of the flap; then interdental incisions are performed, and the wedge of tissue that contains the pocket wall is removed.

Step 3: Vertical incisions are made extending beyond the mucogingival junction. If the objective is a full-thickness flap, it is elevated by blunt dissection with a periosteal elevator. If a split-thickness flap is required, it is elevated using sharp dissection with a Bard-Parker knife to split it, leaving a layer of connective tissue, including the periosteum, on the bone.

Step 4: After removal of all granulation tissue, scaling and root planing, and osseous surgery if needed, the flap is displaced apically. It is important that the vertical incisions, and therefore the flap elevation, reach past the mucogingival junction to provide adequate mobility to the flap for its apical displacement.

Step 5: If a full-thickness flap was performed, a sling suture around the tooth prevents the flap from sliding to a position more apical than that desired, and the periodontal dressing can avoid its movement in a coronal direction. A partial-thickness flap is sutured to the periosteum using a direct loop suture or a combination of loop and anchor suture. A dry foil is placed over the flap before covering it with the dressing to prevent the introduction of pack under the flap.

After 1 week, dressings and sutures are removed. The area is usually repacked for another week, after which the patient is instructed to use chlorhexidine mouth rinse or to apply chlorhexidine topically with cotton-tipped applicators for another 2 or 3 weeks.

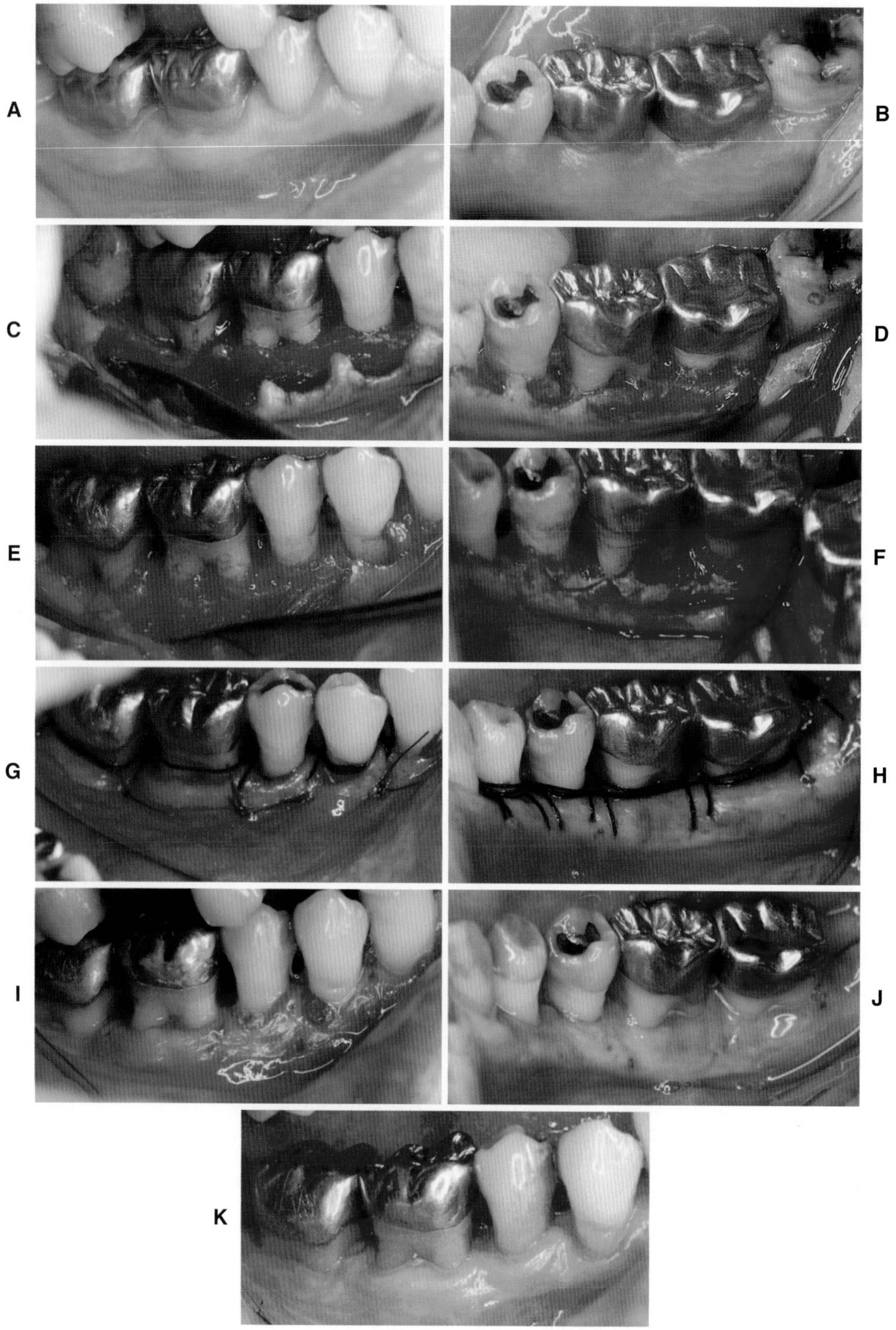

Figure 65-9 Apically displaced flap. **A** and **B,** Facial and lingual preoperative views. **C** and **D,** Facial and lingual flaps elevated. **E** and **F,** After debridement of the areas. **G** and **H,** Sutures in place. **I** and **J,** Healing after 1 week. **K,** Healing after 2 months. Note the preservation of attached gingiva displaced to a more apical position.

FLAPS FOR RECONSTRUCTIVE SURGERY

In current reconstructive therapy, bone grafts, membranes, or a combination of these, with or without other agents, are used for a successful outcome (see Chapter 67). The flap design should therefore be set up so that the maximum amount of gingival tissue and papilla are retained to cover the material(s) placed in the pocket.

Two flap designs are available for reconstructive surgery: the papilla preservation flap and the conventional flap with only crevicular incisions. *The flap design of choice is the papilla preservation flap,* which retains the entire papilla covering the lesion. However, to use this flap, there must be adequate interdental space to allow the intact papilla to be reflected with the facial or lingual/palatal flap. When the interdental space is very narrow, making it impossible to perform a papilla preservation flap, a conventional flap with only crevicular incisions is made.

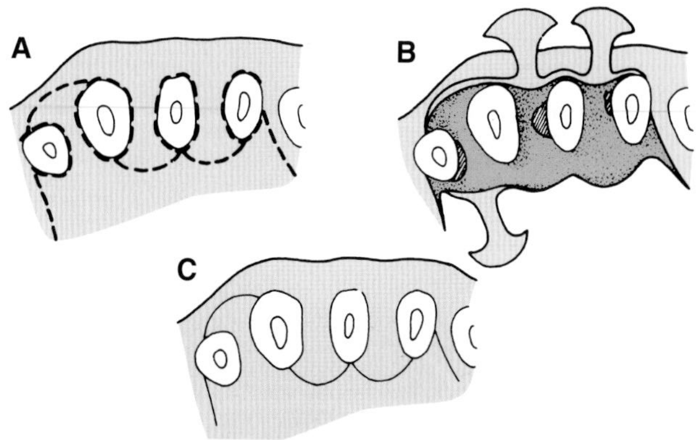

Figure 65-10 Flap design for a papilla preservation flap. **A,** Incisions for this type of flap are depicted by interrupted lines. The preserved papilla can be incorporated into the facial or the lingual-palatal flap. **B,** Reflected flap exposes the underlying bone. Several osseous defects are seen. **C,** Flap returned to its original position, covering the entire interdental spaces.

Papilla Preservation Flap

The technique for employing a papilla preservation flap is as follows (Figures 65-10 and 65-11):

Step 1: A crevicular incision is made around each tooth with no incisions across the interdental papilla.

Step 2: The preserved papilla can be incorporated into the facial or lingual/palatal flap, although it is most often integrated into the facial flap. In these cases the lingual or palatal incision consists of a semilunar incision across the interdental papilla in its palatal or lingual aspect; this incision dips apically from the line angles of the tooth so that the papillary incision is at least 5 mm from the crest of the papilla.

Step 3: An Orban knife is then introduced into this incision to sever half to two-thirds the base of the interdental papilla. The papilla is then dissected from the lingual or palatal aspect and elevated intact with the facial flap.

Step 4: The flap is reflected without thinning the tissue.

Conventional Flap

The technique for employing a conventional flap for reconstructive surgery is as follows:

Step 1: Using a #12 blade, incise the tissue at the bottom of the pocket and to the crest of the bone, splitting the papilla below the contact point. Every effort should be made to retain as much tissue as possible to protect the area subsequently.

Step 2: Reflect the flap, maintaining it as thick as possible, not attempting to thin it as is done for resective surgery. The maintenance of a thick flap is necessary to prevent exposure of the graft or the membrane resulting from necrosis of the flap margins.

DISTAL MOLAR SURGERY

Treatment of periodontal pockets on the distal surface of terminal molars is often complicated by the presence of bulbous fibrous tissue over the maxillary tuberosity or prominent retromolar pads in the mandible. Deep vertical defects are also often present in conjunction with the redundant fibrous tissue. Some of these osseous lesions may result from incomplete repair after the extraction of impacted third molars (Figure 65-12).

The gingivectomy incision is the most direct approach in treating distal pockets that have adequate attached gingiva and no osseous lesions. However, the flap approach is less traumatic postsurgically, because it produces a primary closure wound rather than the open secondary wound left by a gingivectomy incision. In addition, it results in attached gingiva and provides access for examination and, if needed, correction of the osseous defect. Procedures for this purpose were described by Robinson[7] and Braden[2] and modified by several other investigators. Some representative procedures are discussed here.

Maxillary Molars

The treatment of distal pockets on the maxillary arch is usually simpler than the treatment of a similar lesion on the mandibular arch because the tuberosity presents a greater amount of fibrous attached gingiva than does the area of the retromolar pad. In addition, the anatomy of the tuberosity extending distally is more adaptable to pocket elimination than is that of the mandibular molar arch, where the tissue extends coronally. However, the lack of a broad area of attached gingiva and the abruptly ascending tuberosity sometimes complicate therapy (Figure 65-13).

The following considerations determine the location of the incision for distal molar surgery: accessibility, amount of attached gingiva, pocket depth, and available distance from the distal aspect of the tooth to the end of the tuberosity or retromolar pad.

Technique. Two parallel incisions, beginning at the distal portion of the tooth and extending to the mucogingival junction distal to the tuberosity or retromolar

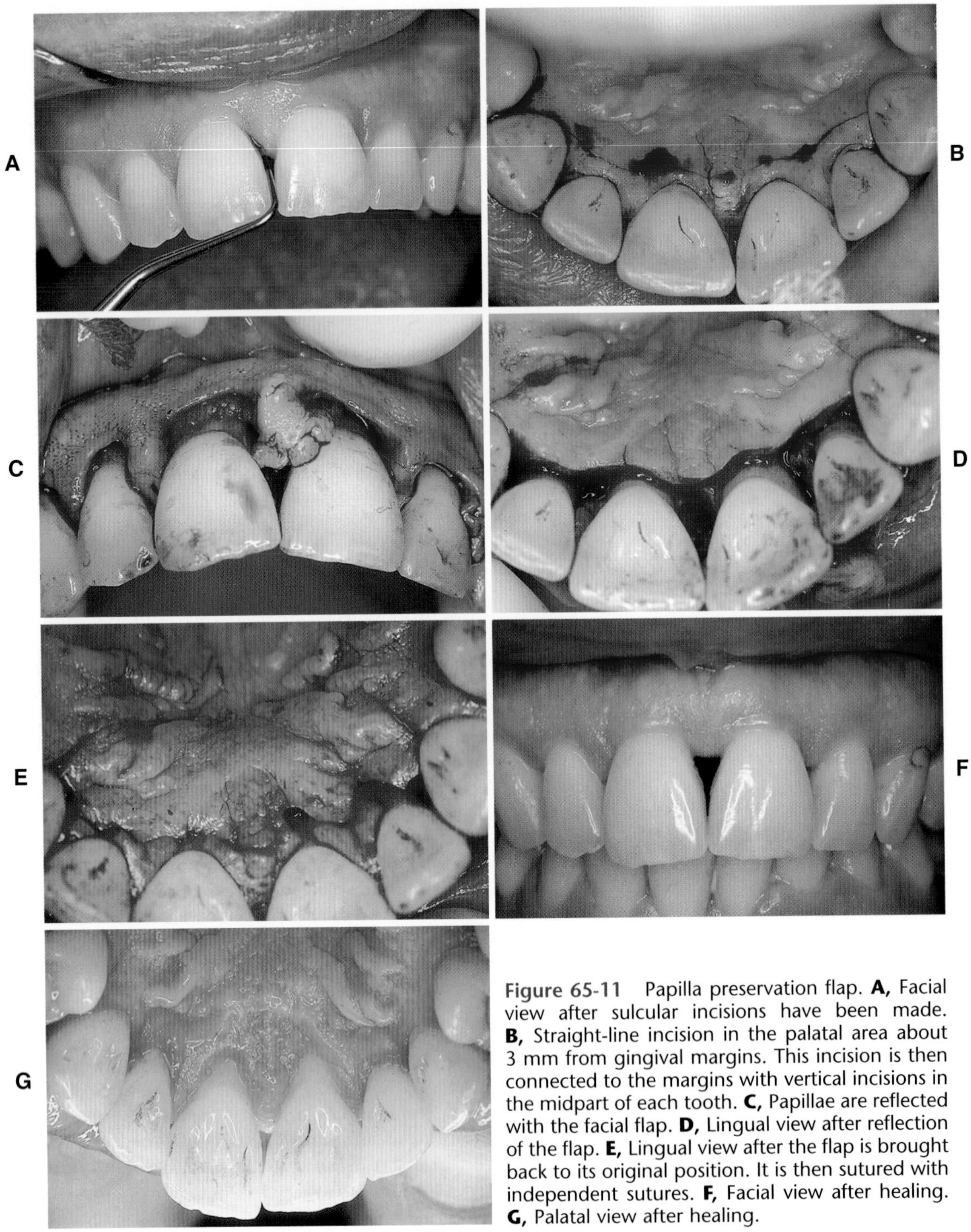

Figure 65-11 Papilla preservation flap. **A,** Facial view after sulcular incisions have been made. **B,** Straight-line incision in the palatal area about 3 mm from gingival margins. This incision is then connected to the margins with vertical incisions in the midpart of each tooth. **C,** Papillae are reflected with the facial flap. **D,** Lingual view after reflection of the flap. **E,** Lingual view after the flap is brought back to its original position. It is then sutured with independent sutures. **F,** Facial view after healing. **G,** Palatal view after healing.

pad, are made (Figure 65-14). The faciolingual distance between these two incisions depends on the depth of the pocket and the amount of fibrous tissue involved. The deeper the pocket, the greater is the distance between the two parallel incisions. Importantly, when the tissue between the two incisions is removed and the flaps are thinned, the two flap edges must approximate each other at a new apical position without overlapping.

When the depth of the pocket cannot be easily estimated, it is better to err on the conservative side, leaving overlapping flaps rather than flaps that are too short and result in exposure of bone. When the two flaps overlap after the surgery is completed, they should be placed one over the other, and the overlapping portion of one of them is grabbed with a hemostat. A sharp knife or scissors is then used to cut the excess.

A transversal incision is made at the distal end of the two parallel incisions so that a long, rectangular piece of tissue can be removed. These incisions are usually interconnected with the incisions for the remainder of

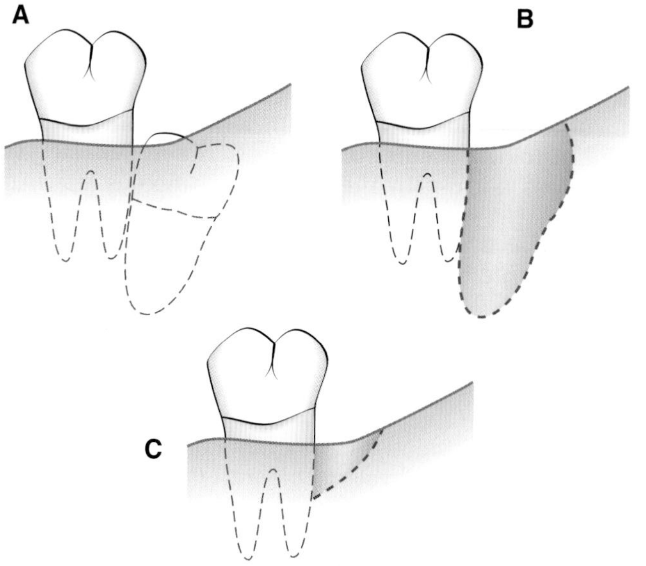

Figure 65-12 **A,** Impaction of a third molar distal to a second molar with little or no interdental bone between the two teeth. **B,** Removal of the third molar creates a pocket with little or no bone distal to the second molar. This often leads to a vertical osseous defect distal to the second molar **(C)**.

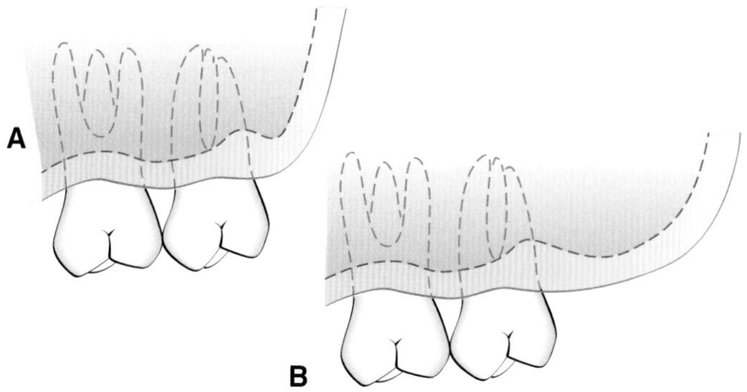

Figure 65-13 **A,** Removal of a pocket distal to the maxillary second molar may be difficult if there is minimal attached gingiva. If the bone ascends acutely apically, the removal of this bone may make the procedure easier. **B,** Long distal tuberosity with abundant attached gingiva is an ideal anatomic situation for distal pocket eradication.

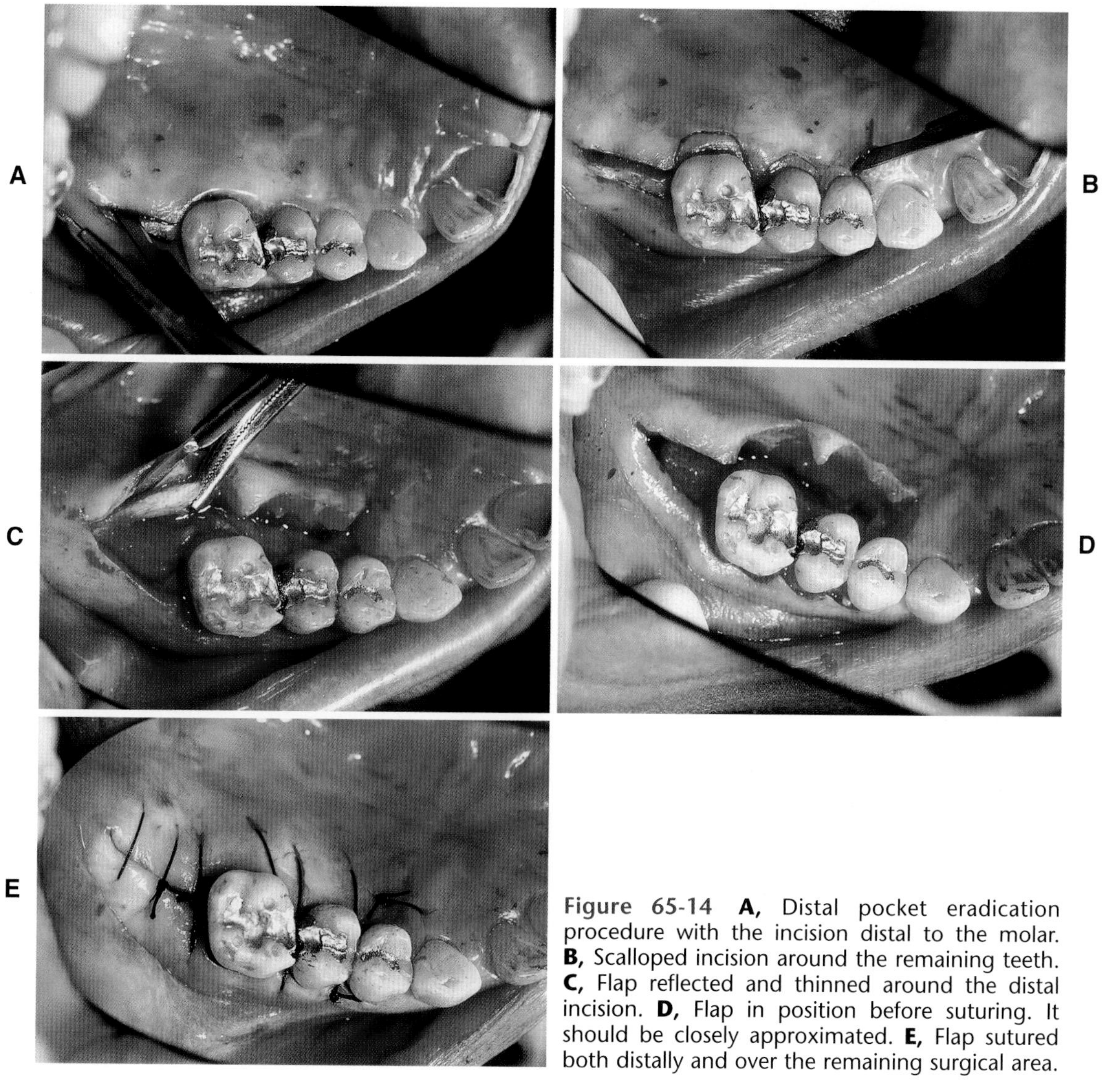

Figure 65-14 **A,** Distal pocket eradication procedure with the incision distal to the molar. **B,** Scalloped incision around the remaining teeth. **C,** Flap reflected and thinned around the distal incision. **D,** Flap in position before suturing. It should be closely approximated. **E,** Flap sutured both distally and over the remaining surgical area.

the surgery in the quadrant involved. The parallel distal incisions should be confined to the attached gingiva because bleeding and flap management become problems when the incision is extended into the alveolar mucosa. If access is difficult, especially if the distance from the distal aspect of the tooth to the mucogingival junction is short, a vertical incision can be made at the end of the parallel incisions.

In treating the tuberosity area, the two distal incisions are usually made at the midline of the tuberosity (Figure 65-15). In most cases, no attempt is made to undermine the underlying tissue at this time. These incisions are made straight down into the underlying bone where access is difficult. A #12B blade is generally used. It is easier to dissect out the underlying redundant tissue when the flap is partially reflected. When the distal flaps are placed back on the bone, the two flap margins should closely approximate each other.

Mandibular Molars

Incisions for the mandibular arch differ from those used for the tuberosity because of differences in the anatomy and histologic features of the areas. The retromolar pad area does not usually present as much fibrous attached gingiva. The keratinized gingiva, if present, may not be found directly distal to the molar. The greatest amount may be distolingual or distofacial and may not be over the bony crest. The ascending ramus of the mandible may also create a short, horizontal area distal to the terminal molar (Figure 65-16). The shorter this area, the more difficult it is to treat any deep distal lesion around the terminal molar.

The two incisions distal to the molar should follow the area with the greatest amount of attached gingiva (Figure 65-17). Therefore the incisions could be directed distolingually or distofacially, depending on which area

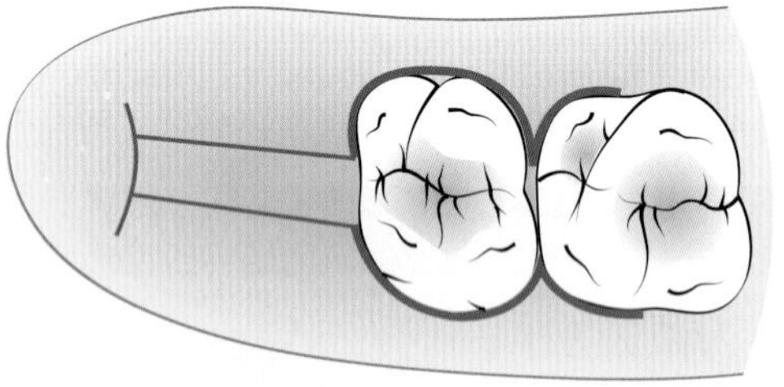

Figure 65-15 Typical incision design for a surgical procedure distal to the maxillary second molar.

A

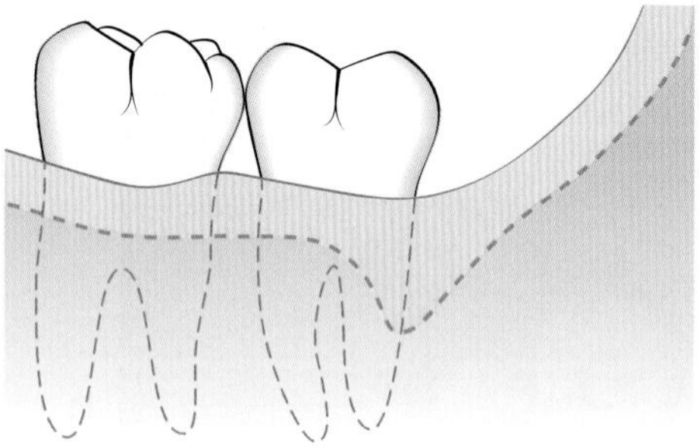

B

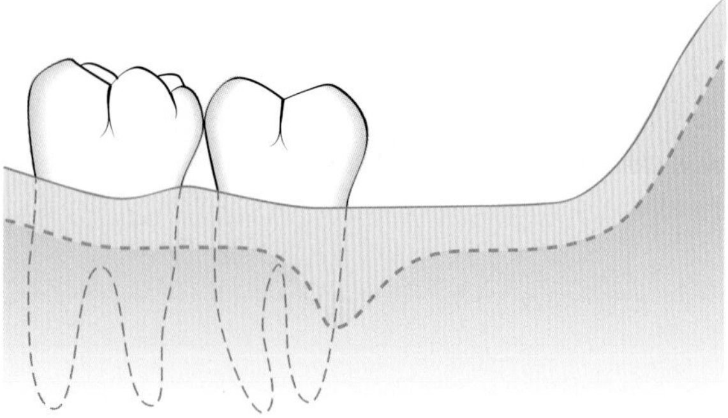

Figure 65-16 **A,** Pocket eradication distal to a mandibular second molar with minimal attached gingiva and a close ascending ramus is anatomically difficult. **B,** For surgical procedures distal to a mandibular second molar, abundant attached gingiva and distal space are ideal.

SCIENCE TRANSFER

Many options exist in the surgical technique used to address moderate to severe periodontal pocketing with or without osseous defects that require therapy. The technique chosen will depend on the objectives of the surgical procedure. One major consequence of all the surgical periodontal therapies is to change the composition of the microbial flora. Although not often considered a goal of surgical therapy, this result may be the most significant outcome achieved. For example, pocket formation encourages a more anaerobic and thus a more pathogenic insult. With all flap therapy, the microbial alteration is always to a more aerobic and thus a less pathogenic result. In addition, the long-term tissue outcomes of different techniques may be similar, likely because of the physiologic remodeling that occurs to reestablish a biologic width around the tooth. This remodeling consists of a junctional epithelium and connective tissue attachment coronal to the periodontal ligament.

A variety of choices in flap design are available in surgical procedures to treat advanced periodontal disease. All flaps result in some postoperative gingival recession and bone resorption. The papilla preservation technique minimizes these postoperative sequelae. In patients for whom pocket reduction is achieved by apical positioning of the entire periodontal attachment apparatus, gingival recession is a goal; therefore, reverse bevel incisions, osseous surgery, and apically displaced flaps are used. *In esthetic regions, flap surgery for treatment of periodontal bone loss may be contraindicated because of the inevitable postoperative gingival recession.*

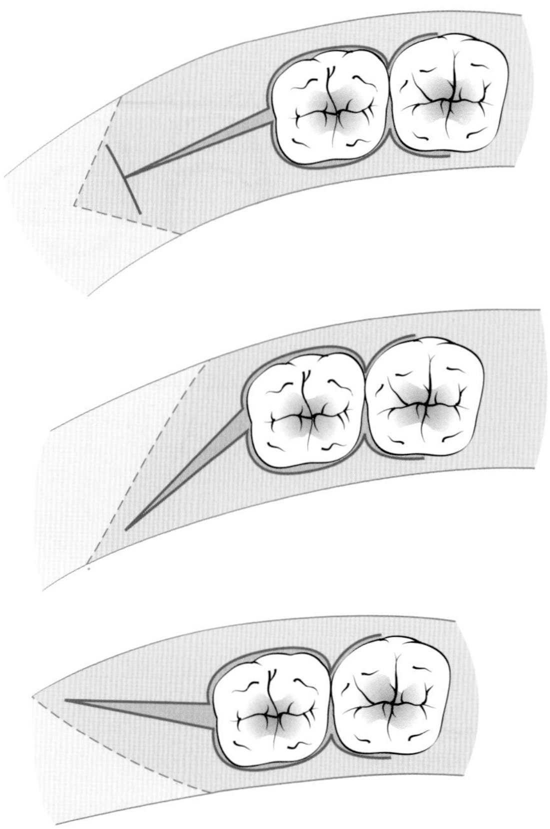

Figure 65-17 Incision designs for surgical procedures distal to the mandibular second molar. The incision should follow the areas of greatest attached gingiva and underlying bone.

has more attached gingiva. Before the flap is completely reflected, it is thinned with a #15 blade. It is easier to thin the flap before it is completely free and mobile. After the reflection of the flap and the removal of the redundant fibrous tissue, any necessary osseous surgery is performed. The flaps are approximated similarly to those in the maxillary tuberosity area.

REFERENCES

1. Ainamo A, Bergenholtz A, Hugoson A, et al: Location of the mucogingival junction 18 years after apically repositioned flap surgery, *J Clin Periodontol* 19:49, 1992.
2. Braden BE: Deep distal pockets adjacent to terminal teeth, *Dent Clin North Am* 13:161, 1969.
3. Matelski DE, Hurt WC: The corrective phase: the modified Widman flap. In Hurt WC, editor: *Periodontics in general practice,* Springfield, Ill, 1976, Charles C Thomas.
4. Morris ML: The unrepositioned mucoperiosteal flap, *Periodontics* 3:147, 1965.
5. Ramfjord SP: Present status of the modified Widman flap procedure, *J Periodontol* 48:558, 1977.
6. Ramfjord SP, Nissle RR: The modified Widman flap, *J Periodontol* 45:601, 1974.
7. Robinson RE: The distal wedge operation, *Periodontics* 4:256, 1966.
8. Takei HH, Han TJ, Carranza FA, et al: Flap technique for periodontal bone implants: papilla preservation technique, *J Periodontol* 56:204, 1985.

CHAPTER 66

Resective Osseous Surgery

Thomas N. Sims and Williams Ammons, Jr.

CHAPTER OUTLINE

The damage resulting from periodontal disease manifests in variable destruction of the tooth-supporting bone. Generally, bony deformities are not uniform; they are not indicative of the alveolar housing of the tooth before the disease process and do not reflect the overlying gingival architecture. Bone loss has been classified as either "horizontal" or "vertical," but in fact, bone loss is most often a combination of horizontal and vertical loss. Horizontal bone loss generally results in a relative thickening of the marginal alveolar bone, because bone tapers as it approaches its most coronal margin.

The effects of this thickening and the development of vertical defects leave the alveolar bone with countless combinations of bony shapes. If these various topographic changes are to be altered to provide a more physiologic bone pattern, a method for osseous recontouring must be followed.

Osseous surgery may be defined as the procedure by which changes in the alveolar bone can be accomplished to rid it of deformities induced by the periodontal disease process or other related factors, such as exostosis and tooth supraeruption.

Osseous surgery can be either additive or subtractive in nature. *Additive osseous surgery* includes procedures directed at restoring the alveolar bone to its original level, whereas *subtractive osseous surgery* is designed to restore the form of preexisting alveolar bone to the level present at the time of surgery or slightly more apical to this level (Figure 66-1).

Additive osseous surgery brings about the ideal result of periodontal therapy; it implies regeneration of lost bone and reestablishment of the periodontal ligament, gingival fibers, and junctional epithelium at a more coronal level. This type of osseous surgery is discussed in Chapter 67.

Subtractive osseous surgery procedures provide an alternative to additive methods and should be used when additive procedures are not feasible. These subtractive procedures are discussed in this chapter.

SELECTION OF TREATMENT TECHNIQUE

The morphology of the osseous defect largely determines the treatment technique to be used. *One-wall angular defects* usually need to be recontoured surgically. *Three-wall defects,* particularly if they are narrow and deep, can be successfully treated with techniques that strive for new attachment and bone reconstruction. *Two-wall angular defects* can be treated with either method, depending on

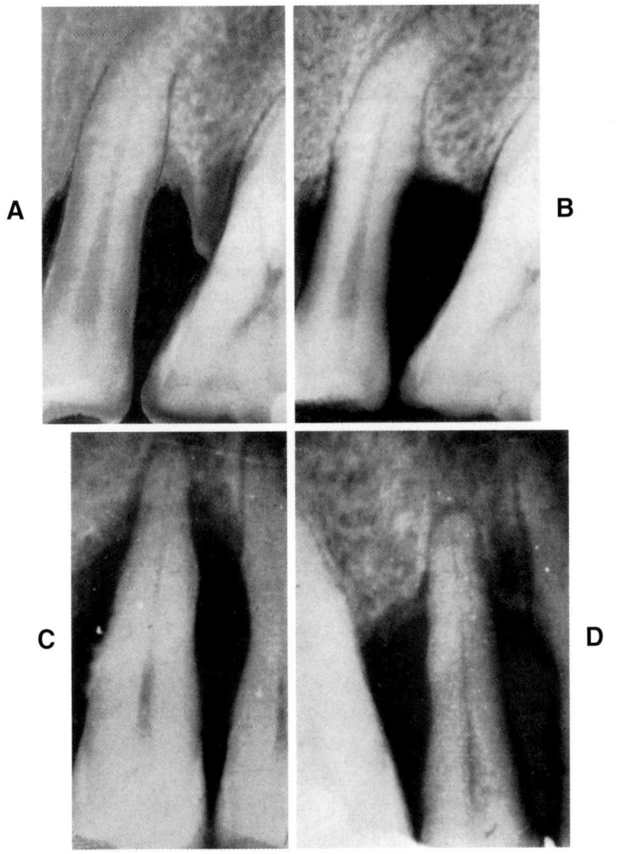

Figure 66-1 Additive and subtractive osseous surgery. **A,** Before, and **B,** immediately after subtractive osseous surgery; the osseous wall of the two adjoining infrabony pockets has been removed. **C,** Before, and **D,** 1 year after additive osseous surgery; the area has been flapped and thoroughly instrumented, resulting in reconstruction of the interdental and periapical bone. (Courtesy Drs. E.A. Albano and B.O. Barletta, Buenos Aires, Argentina.)

their depth, width, and general configuration. Therefore, except for one-wall defects and wide, shallow two-wall defects, along with interdental craters, osseous defects are treated with the objective of obtaining optimal repair by natural healing processes.

RATIONALE

Osseous resective surgery necessitates following a series of strict guidelines for proper contouring of alveolar bone and subsequent management of the overlying gingival soft tissues. The specifics of these techniques are discussed later in this chapter. The techniques discussed here for osseous resective surgery have limited applicability in deep intrabony or hemiseptal defects, which could be treated with a different surgical approach (see Chapter 67). Osseous surgery provides the purest and surest method for reducing pockets with bony discrepancies that are not overly vertical and also remains one of the principal periodontal modalities because of its long-term success and predictability.

Osseous resective surgery is the most predictable pocket reduction technique.[10-12] However, more than any other surgical technique, osseous resective surgery is performed at the expense of bony tissue and attachment level.[1,2,8] Thus its value as a surgical approach is limited by the presence, quantity, and shape of the bony tissues and by the amount of attachment loss that is acceptable.

The major rationale for osseous resective surgery is based on the tenet that discrepancies in level and shapes of the bone and gingiva predispose patients to the recurrence of pocket depth postsurgically.[6] Although this concept is not universally accepted,[3,5] and despite that the procedure induces loss of radicular bone in the healing phase, recontouring of bone is the only logical treatment choice in some cases. The goal of osseous resective therapy is to reshape the marginal bone to resemble that of the alveolar process undamaged by periodontal disease. The technique is performed in combination with apically positioned flaps, and the procedure eliminates periodontal pocket depth and improves tissue contour to provide a more easily maintainable environment. The relative merits of pocket reduction procedures are discussed in Chapters 40 and 59; this chapter discusses the osseous resective technique and how and where it may be accomplished.

It is proposed that the conversion of the periodontal pocket to a shallow gingival sulcus enhances the patient's ability to remove plaque and oral debris from the dentition. Likewise, the ability of dental professionals to maintain the periodontium in a state free of gingivitis and periodontitis is more predictable in the presence of shallow sulci. The more effective the periodontal maintenance therapy, the greater is the longitudinal stability of the surgical result. The efficacy of osseous surgery therefore depends on its ability to affect pocket depth and to promote periodontal maintenance.[11,22,23] The merits of resection versus other treatment procedures are discussed in Chapter 59.

NORMAL ALVEOLAR BONE MORPHOLOGY

Knowledge of the morphology of the bony periodontium in a state of health is required to perform resective osseous surgery correctly (Figure 66-2). The characteristics of a normal bony form are as follows:

1. The interproximal bone is more coronal in position than the labial or lingual/palatal bone and pyramidal in form.
2. The form of the interdental bone is a function of the tooth form and the embrasure width. The more tapered the tooth, the more pyramidal is the bony form. The wider the embrasure, the more flattened is the interdental bone mesiodistally and buccolingually.
3. The position of the bony margin mimics the contours of the cementoenamel junction. The distance from the facial bony margin of the tooth to the interproximal bony crest is more flat in the posterior than the anterior areas. This "scalloping" of the bone on the facial surfaces and lingual/palatal surfaces is related to tooth and root form, as well as tooth position, within the alveolus. Teeth with prominent roots or those displaced to the facial or

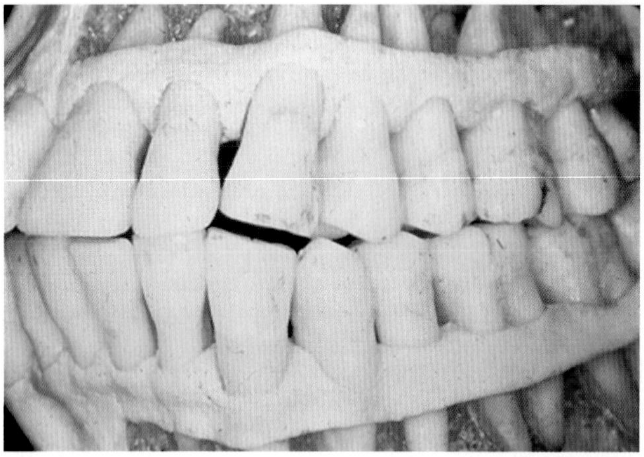

Figure 66-2 Photograph of a healthy bony periodontium in a skull. Although a slight amount of attachment may have been lost, this skull demonstrates the characteristics of normal form.

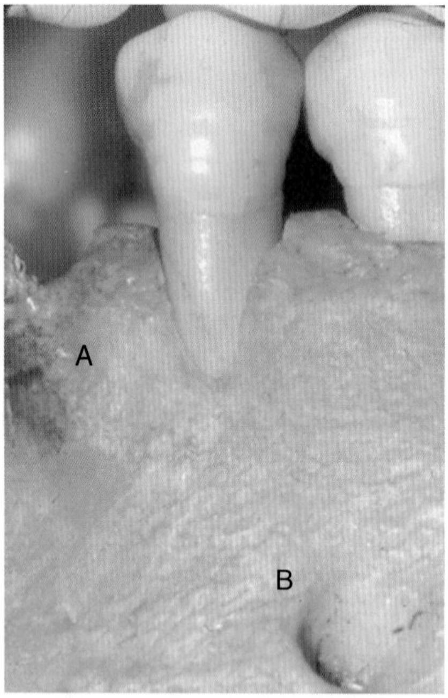

Figure 66-3 Effects of tooth position on facial bony contours. Bony fenestration **(A).** Bony dehiscence **(B).** These deformities can and should be detected by palpation, probing, and sounding before flap surgery.

lingual side may also have fenestrations or dehiscences (Figure 66-3). The molar teeth have less scalloping and a more flat profile than bicuspids and incisors.

Although these general observations apply to all patients, the bony architecture may vary from patient to patient in the extent of contour, configuration, and thickness. These variations may be both normal and healthy.

TERMINOLOGY

Numerous terms have been developed to describe the topography of the alveolar housing, the procedure for its removal, and the resulting correction. These terms should be clearly defined.

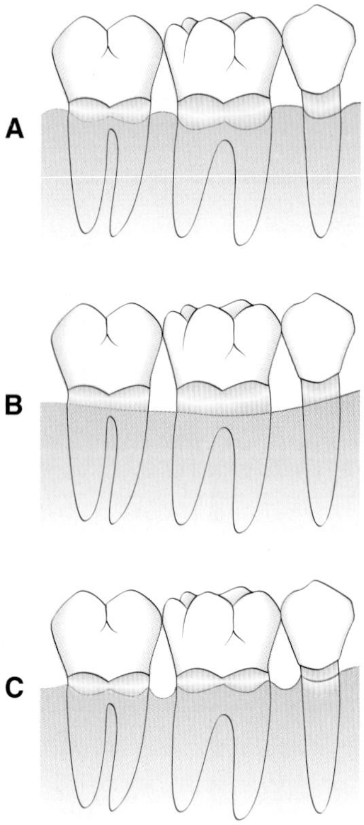

Figure 66-4 Diagram of types of bony architecture. **A,** Positive bony architecture. **B,** Flat bony architecture. **C,** Reversed, or negative, bony form.

Procedures used to correct osseous defects have been classified in two groups: osteoplasty and ostectomy.[7] *Osteoplasty* refers to reshaping the bone without removing tooth-supporting bone. *Ostectomy* (or *osteoectomy*) includes the removal of tooth-supporting bone. One or both of these procedures may be necessary to produce the desired result.

Terms that describe the bone form after reshaping can refer to morphologic features or to the thoroughness of the reshaping performed. Examples of morphologically descriptive terms include *negative, positive, flat,* and *ideal.* These terms all relate to a preconceived standard of ideal osseous form.

Positive architecture and *negative architecture* refer to the relative position of interdental bone to radicular bone (Figure 66-4). The architecture is said to be "positive" if the radicular bone is apical to the interdental bone. The bone is said to have "negative" architecture if the interdental bone is more apical than the radicular bone. *Flat architecture* is the reduction of the interdental bone to the same height as the radicular bone.

Osseous form is considered to be "ideal" when the bone is consistently more coronal on the interproximal surfaces than on the facial and lingual surfaces. The ideal form of the marginal bone has similar interdental height, with gradual, curved slopes between interdental peaks (Figure 66-5).

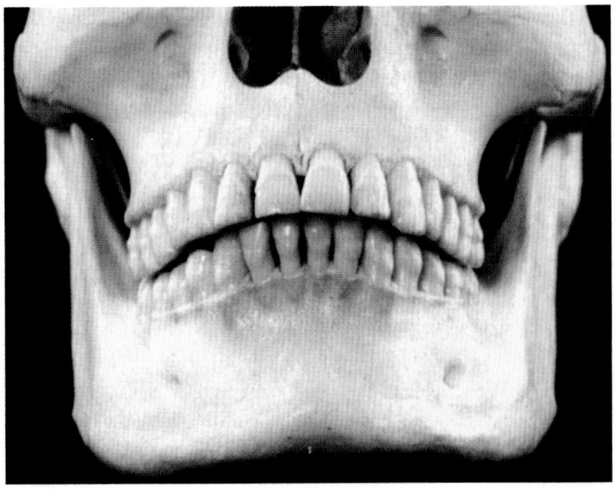

Figure 66-5 Skull photograph of healthy periodontium. Note the shape of the alveolar bone housing. This bone is considered to have ideal form. It is more coronal in the interproximal areas, with a gradual slope around and away from the tooth.

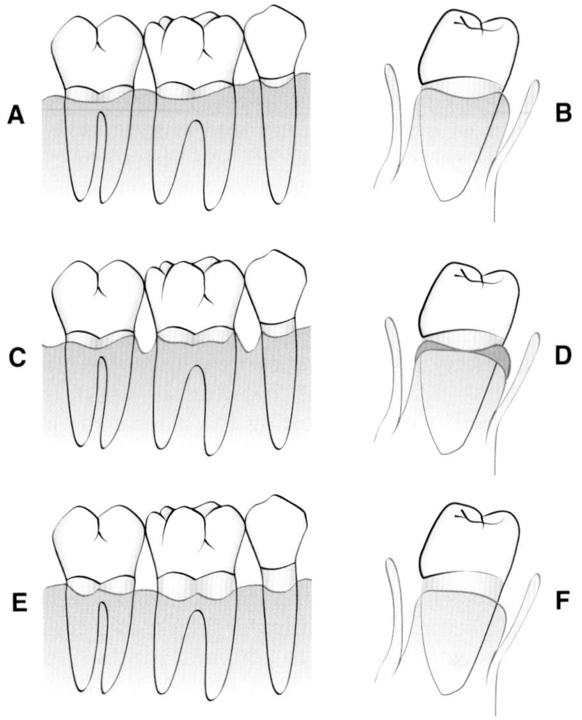

Figure 66-6 Effect of correction of craters. **A** and **B,** Diagram of facial and interproximal bony contours after flap reflection. Note the loss of some interproximal bone and cratering. **C** and **D,** Line angles; this is only osteoplasty and has resulted in a reversed architecture. **E** and **F,** Ostectomy on the facial and lingual bone and the removal of the residual widow's peaks to produce a positive bony architecture.

Terms that relate to the thoroughness of the osseous reshaping techniques include "definitive" and "compromise." *Definitive osseous reshaping* implies that further osseous reshaping would not improve the overall result. *Compromise osseous reshaping* indicates a bone pattern that cannot be improved without significant osseous removal that would be detrimental to the overall result. References to compromise and definitive osseous architecture can be useful to the clinician, not as description of morphologic feature, but as terms that express the expected therapeutic result.

FACTORS IN SELECTION OF RESECTIVE OSSEOUS SURGERY

The relationship between the depth and configuration of the bony lesion(s) to root morphology and the adjacent teeth determines the extent that bone and attachment is removed during resection. Bony lesions have been classified according to their configuration and number of bony walls.[9] The technique of ostectomy is best applied to patients with early to moderate bone loss (2-3 mm) with moderate-length root trunks[18] that have bony defects with one or two walls. These shallow to moderate bony defects can be effectively managed by osteoplasty and osteoectomy. Patients with advanced attachment loss and deep intrabony defects are not candidates for resection to produce a positive contour. To simulate a normal architectural form, so much bone would have to be removed that the survival of the teeth could be compromised.

Two-walled defects, or craters, occur at the expense of the interseptal bone. As a result, they have buccal and lingual/palatal walls that extend from one tooth to the adjacent tooth. The interdental loss of bone exposes the proximal aspects of both adjacent teeth. The buccal-lingual interproximal contour that results is opposite to the contour of the cementoenamel junction of the teeth (Figure 66-6, *A* and *B*). *Two-walled defects (craters) are the most common bony defects found in patients with periodontitis.*[14,20] If the facial and lingual plates of this bone are resected, the resultant interproximal contour would become more flattened or ovate (Figure 66-6, *C* and *D*). However, confining resection only to ledges and the interproximal lesion results in a facial and lingual bone form in which the interproximal bone is located more apically than the bone on the facial or lingual aspects of the tooth. This resulting anatomic form is *reversed,* or *negative,* architecture[17,18,22] (Figure 66-6, *C* and *D*).

Although the production of a reversed architecture minimizes the amount of ostectomy that is performed, it is not without consequences.[5] Peaks of bone typically remain at the facial and lingual/palatal line angles of the teeth *(widow's peaks)*. During healing, the soft tissue tends to bridge the embrasure from the most coronal height of the bone on one tooth to the most coronal heights on the adjacent teeth. The result is therefore the tendency to replicate the attachment contour on the tooth. The interproximal soft tissues invest these peaks of bone, which may subsequently resorb with a tendency to rebound without gain in attachment over time. Inter-proximal pocket depth can recur.[22,24]

Ostectomy to a positive architecture requires the removal of the line-angle inconsistencies (widow's peaks), as well as some of the facial, lingual, and palatal and interproximal bone. The result is a loss of some attachment on the facial and lingual root surfaces but a topography that more closely resembles normal bone form before disease (Figure 66-6, *E* and *F*). Proponents of osseous resection to create a positive contour believe that this architecture, devoid of sharp angles and spines, is conducive to the formation of a more uniform and reduced soft tissue dimension postoperatively.[17,21] The therapeutic result is less pocket depth and increased ease of periodontal maintenance by the patient, dental hygienist, or dentist.

The amount of attachment lost from the use of ostectomy varies with the depth and configuration of the treated osseous defects. Osseous resection applied to two-wall intrabony defects (craters), the most common osseous defects, results in attachment loss at the proximal line angles and the facial and lingual aspects of the affected teeth without affecting the base of the pocket. The extent of attachment loss during resection to a positive architecture has been measured. When the technique is properly applied to appropriate patients, the mean reduction in attachment circumferentially around the tooth has been determined to be 0.6 mm at six probing sites.[22] In practical terms, this means that the technique is best applied to interproximal lesions 1 to 3 mm deep in patients with moderate to long root trunks.[17] Patients with deep, multiwalled defects are not candidates for resective osseous surgery. They are better treated with regenerative therapies or by combining osteoplasty to reduce bony ledges and to facilitate flap closure with new attachment and regeneration procedures.

EXAMINATION AND TREATMENT PLANNING

The potential for the use of resective osseous surgery is usually identified during a comprehensive periodontal examination. Suitable patients display the signs and symptoms of periodontitis (see Chapter 35). The gingiva may be inflamed, and deposits of plaque, calculus, and oral debris may be present. An increased flow of crevicular fluid may be detected, and bleeding on probing and exudation are often observed.

Periodontal probing and exploration are key aspects of the examination. Careful probing reveals the presence of (1) pocket depth greater than that of a normal gingival sulcus, (2) the location of the base of the pocket relative to the mucogingival junction and attachment level on adjacent teeth, (3) the number of bony walls, and (4) the presence of furcation defects. *Transgingival probing,* or *sounding,* under local anesthesia confirms the extent and configuration of the intrabony component of the pocket and of furcation defects.[6,16]

Routine dental radiographs do not identify the presence of periodontitis and do not accurately document the extent of bony defects. Radiographs cannot accurately document the number of bony walls and the presence or extent of bony lesions on the facial/buccal or lingual/palatal walls. Well-made radiographs provide useful information about the extent of interproximal bone loss, the presence of angular bone loss, caries, root trunk length, and root morphology. Films also facilitate the identification of other dental pathoses that require treatment. In addition, a radiographic survey serves as a means of evaluating the success of therapy and documenting the patient's longitudinal stability.[19]

Treatment planning should provide solutions for active periodontal diseases and correction of deformities that result from periodontitis. Planning should also facilitate the performance of other dental procedures included in a comprehensive dental treatment plan. The extent of periodontal involvement can vary significantly from tooth to tooth in the same patient. The response to therapy from patient to patient may also vary, as may the treatment objectives for the patients. Therefore a treatment plan may encompass a number of steps and combinations of procedures in the same surgical area.

After oral hygiene instruction and scaling and root planing, along with other disease control procedures, the response of the patient to these treatment procedures is evaluated by reexamination and recording the changes in the periodontium. Because the extent of periodontal involvement can vary significantly from tooth to tooth in the same patient, the local response to therapy is also variable. The resolution of inflammation and decrease in edema and swelling may have resulted in a return to normal depth and configuration of some pockets, and additional therapy beyond periodic maintenance may not be required.

The patient with moderate to advanced periodontitis and bony defects, although the overt signs of periodontitis may be reduced, may display a persistence of pocket depth bleeding on probing and suppuration. These signs may indicate the presence of residual plaque and calculus, attributable to the difficulty of achieving instrumentation in these deep pockets or the patient's inability or unwillingness to perform adequate oral hygiene in these sites. Patients with inadequate oral hygiene are not good candidates for periodontal surgery. If the supragingival plaque control is good and the residual pocket depths are 5 mm or more, patients with such areas may be candidates for periodontal surgery.[13]

Resective osseous surgery is also used to facilitate certain restorative and prosthetic dental procedures. Dental caries can be exposed for restoration; fractured roots of abutment teeth can be exposed for removal; and bony exostoses and ridge deformities can be altered in contour to improve the performance of removable or fixed prostheses (Figure 66-7). Severely decayed teeth or teeth with short anatomic crowns can be lengthened by resection or by a combination of orthodontic tooth extrusion and osseous resection. Such procedures allow the therapist to expose more tooth for restoration, prevent an invasion of the biologic width of attachment, and create a periodontal attachment of normal dimension.[8,15] Resection can also provide a means of producing optimal crown length for cosmetic purposes.

METHODS OF RESECTIVE OSSEOUS SURGERY

The reshaping process is fundamentally an attempt to gradualize the bone sufficiently to allow soft tissue structures to follow the contour of the bone. The soft tissue predictably attaches to the bone within certain specific dimensions. The length and quality of connective tissue and junctional epithelium that reform in the surgical site depend on numerous factors, including the health of the tissue, condition and topography of the root surface,

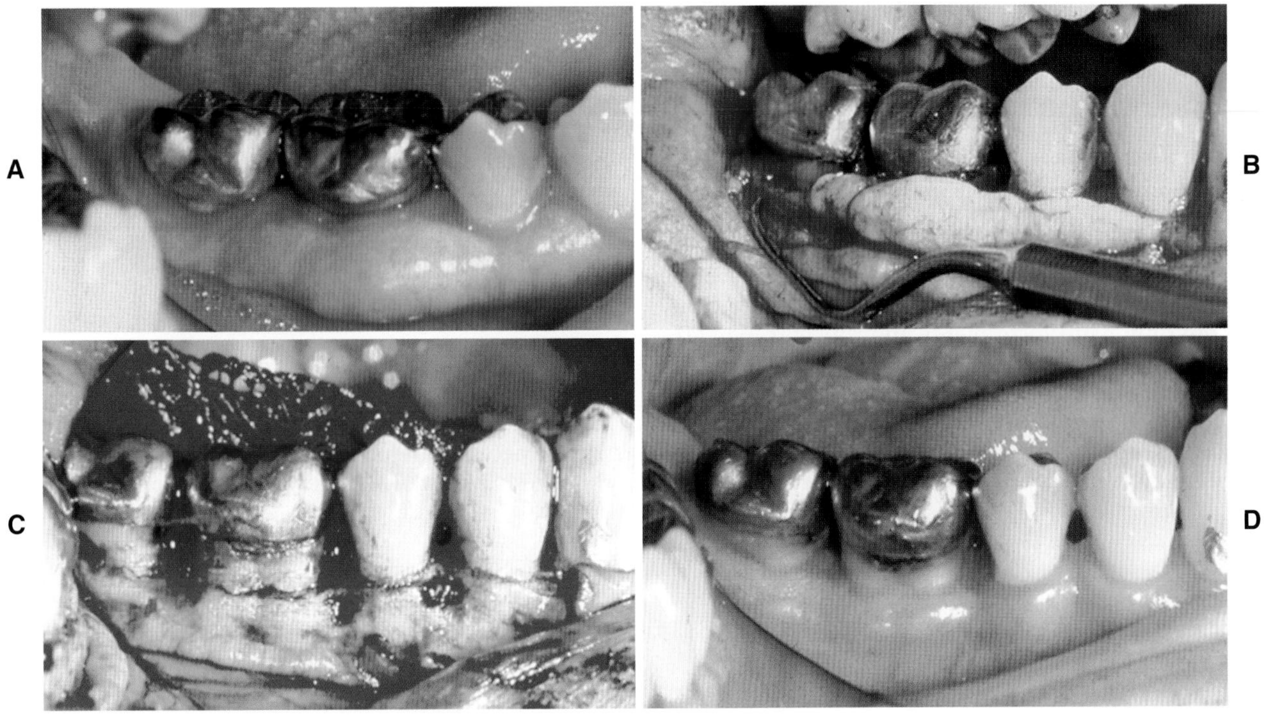

Figure 66-7 Reduction of bony ledges and exposure of caries by osteoplasty. **A,** Buccal preoperative photograph showing two crowns, exostoses, and caries. **B,** Flap reflected to reveal caries on both molars at the restoration margins, interdental cratering, and a facial exostosis. **C,** After osseous surgery; the bulk of the bony removal was by osteoplasty, with minor ostectomy between the two molars. The caries is now exposed, and the crowns are lengthened for restoration. **D,** Postoperative photograph at 6 weeks. The plaque control is deficient, but the teeth should be readily restorable at this time. (Courtesy Dr. Joseph Schwartz, Portland, Ore.)

and proximity of the bone surrounding the tooth. Each of these factors must be controlled to the best of the clinician's ability to obtain the optimal result, making osseous resective surgery an extremely precise technique.

It is assumed in this chapter that the gingival tissue has been reflected by the apically positioned flap described in Chapter 64. Reshaping of the bone may necessitate selective changes in gingival height. These changes must be calculated and accounted for in the initial flap design. For this reason, it is important for the clinician to know about the underlying bone tissue before flap reflection. The clinician must gain as much indirect knowledge as possible from soft tissue palpation, radiographic assessment, and transgingival probing (sounding).

Radiographic examination can reveal the existence of angular bone loss in the interdental spaces; these areas usually coincide with intrabony pockets. The radiograph does not show the number of bony walls of the defect or document with any accuracy the presence of angular cone defects on facial or lingual surfaces. Clinical examination and probing are used to determine the presence and depth of periodontal pockets on any surface of any tooth and can also provide a general sense of the bony topography, although intrabony pockets can go undetected by probing. Both clinical and radiographic examinations can indicate the presence of intrabony pockets when the clinician finds (1) angular bone loss, (2) irregular bone loss, or (3) pockets of irregular depth in adjacent areas of the same tooth or adjacent teeth.

The experienced clinician can use transgingival probing to predict many features of the underlying bony topography. The information thus obtained can change the treatment plan. For example, an area that had been selected for osseous resective surgery may be found to have a narrow defect that was unnoticed in the initial probing and radiographic assessment and is ideal for augmentation procedures. Such findings can and do change the flap design, osseous procedure, and results expected from the surgical intervention. Transgingival probing is extremely useful just before flap reflection. It is necessary to anesthetize the tissue locally before inserting the probe. The probe should be "walked" along the tissue-tooth interface so that the operator can feel the bony topography. The probe may also be passed horizontally through the tissue to provide three-dimensional information regarding bony contours (i.e., thickness, height, and shape of the underlying base). It must be remembered, however, that this information is still "blind," and although it is undoubtedly better than probing alone, it has significant limitations. Nevertheless, this step is recommended immediately before the surgical intervention.

The situations that can be encountered after periodontal flap reflection vary greatly. When all soft tissue is removed around the teeth, there may be larger exotoses, ledges, troughs, craters, vertical defects, or combinations of these defects. Therefore, each osseous situation presents uniquely challenging problems, especially if reshaping to the optimal level is contemplated.

OSSEOUS RESECTION TECHNIQUE

Instrumentation

A number of hand and rotary instruments have been used for osseous resective surgery. Some excellent clinicians use only hand instruments and rongeurs, whereas others prefer a combination of hand and rotary instruments. Rotary instruments are useful for the osteoplastic steps outlined previously, whereas hand instruments provide the most precise and safe results with ostectomy procedures. Nevertheless, care and precision are required for each step of the procedure to prevent excessive bone removal or root damage, both of which are irreversible. Figure 66-8 illustrates some of the instruments commonly used for osseous resection techniques.

To address the many clinical situations, the following sequential steps are suggested for resective osseous surgery (Figure 66-9, *A* to *D*):

1. Vertical grooving
2. Radicular blending
3. Flattening interproximal bone
4. Gradualizing marginal bone

Not all steps are necessary in every case, but the sequencing of the steps in the order given is necessary to expedite the reshaping procedure, as well as to minimize the unnecessary removal of bone. Figure 66-10 illustrates bone reshaping in flap surgery for specific anatomic defects.

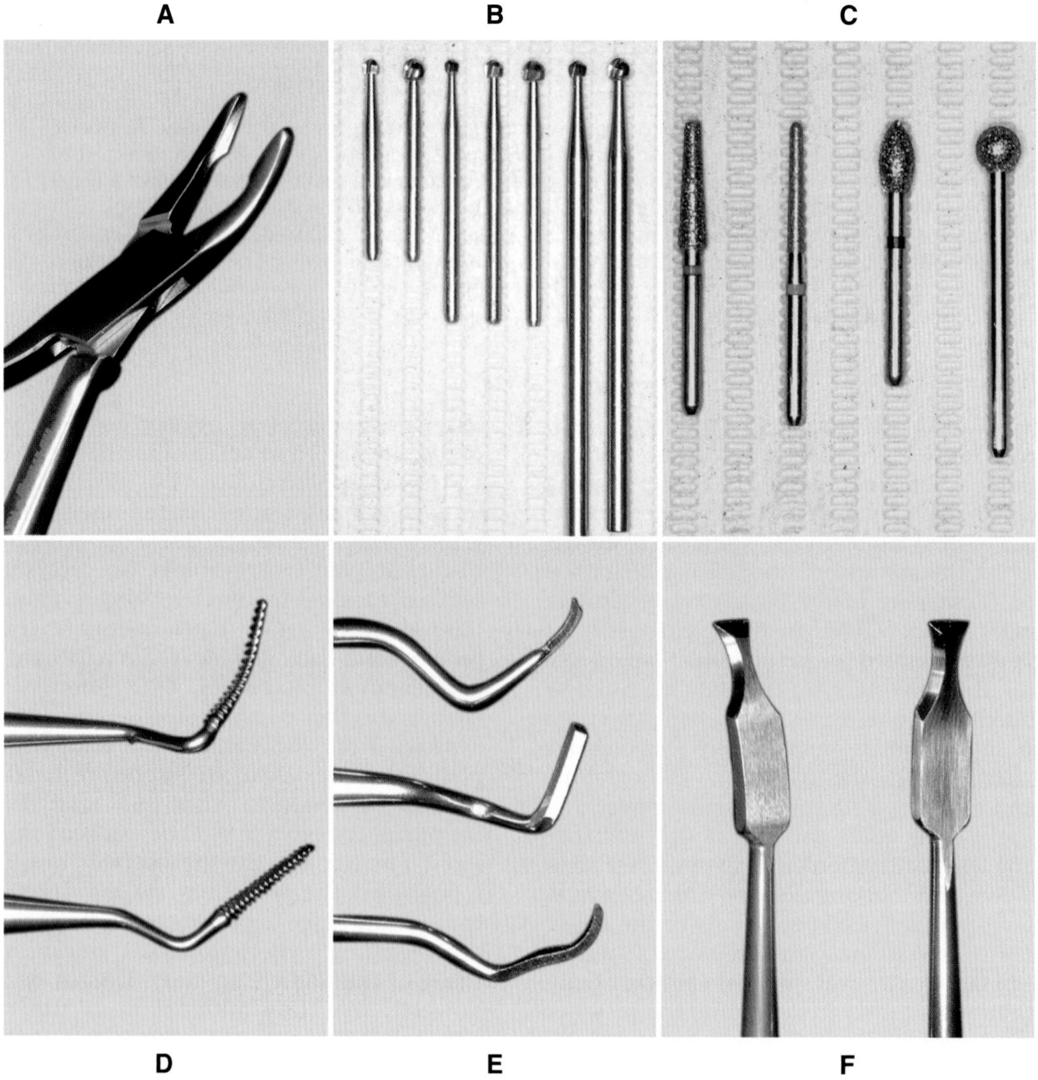

Figure 66-8 Instruments often used in osseous surgery. **A,** Rongeurs: Friedman *(top)* and 90-degree Blumenthal *(bottom)*. **B,** Carbide round burs. *Left to right,* Friction grip, surgical-length friction grip, and slow-speed handpiece. **C,** Diamond burs. **D,** Interproximal files: Schluger and Sugarman. **E,** Back-action chisels. **F,** Ochsenbein chisels.

Vertical Grooving

Vertical grooving is designed to reduce the thickness of the alveolar housing and to provide relative prominence to the radicular aspects of the teeth (see Figure 66-9, *B*). It also provides continuity from the interproximal surface onto the radicular surface. It is the first step of the resective process because it can define the general thickness and subsequent form of the alveolar housing. This step is usually performed with rotary instruments, such as round carbide burs or diamonds. The advantages of vertical grooving are most apparent with thick bony margins, shallow crater formations, or other areas that require maximal osteoplasty and minimal ostectomy. Vertical grooving is contraindicated in areas with close roots or thin alveolar housing.

Radicular Blending

Radicular blending, the second step of the osseous reshaping technique, is an extension of vertical grooving (see Figure 66-9, *C*). Conceptually, it is an attempt to gradualize the bone over the entire radicular surface to provide the best results from vertical grooving. This provides a smooth, blended surface for good flap adaptation. The indications are the same as for vertical grooving (i.e., thick ledges of bone on the radicular surface, where selective surgical resection is desired). Naturally, this step is not necessary if vertical grooving is very minor or if the radicular bone is thin or fenestrated. Both vertical grooving and radicular blending are purely osteoplastic techniques that do not remove supporting bone. In most situations, these two procedures compose the bulk of resective osseous surgery. Classically, shallow crater formations, thick osseous ledges of bone on the radicular surfaces, and class I and early class II furcation involvements are treated almost entirely with these two steps.

Flattening Interproximal Bone

Flattening of the interdental bone requires the removal of very small amounts of supporting bone (Figure 66-11). It is indicated when interproximal bone levels vary horizontally. By definition, most of the indications for this step are one-walled interproximal defects or *hemiseptal* defects. The omission of flattening in such cases results in increased pocket depth on the most apical side of the bone loss. This step is typically not necessary with interproximal crater formations or flat interproximal defects. It is best used in defects that have a coronally placed, one-walled edge of a predominantly three-walled angular defect, and it can be helpful in obtaining good flap closure and improved healing in the three-walled defect. The limitation of this step, as with resective osseous surgical therapy in general, is in the treatment of advanced lesions. Large hemiseptal defects would require removal of inordinate amounts of bone to provide a flattened architecture, and the procedure would be too costly in terms of bony support. Compromised osseous architecture is the only logical solution (Figure 66-12).

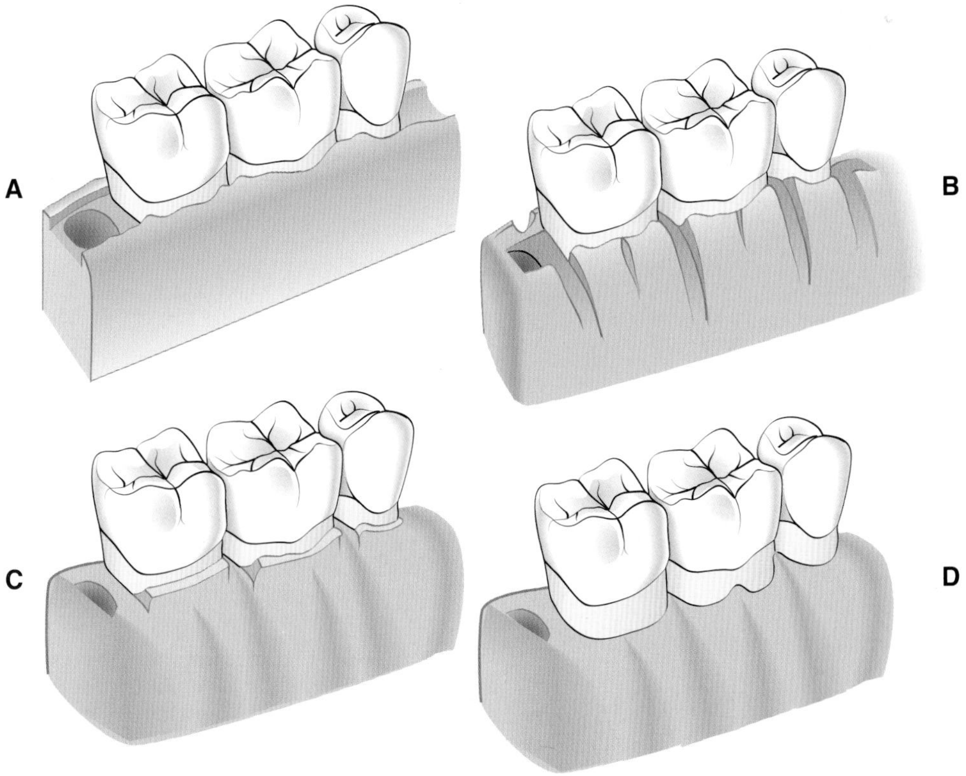

Figure 66-9 **A,** Drawing of bony topography in moderate periodontitis with interdental craters. **B,** Vertical grooving, the first step in correction by osseous reshaping. **C,** Radicular blending and flattening of interproximal bone. **D,** Gradualizing the marginal bone. Note the area of the furcation on the first molar where the bone is preserved.

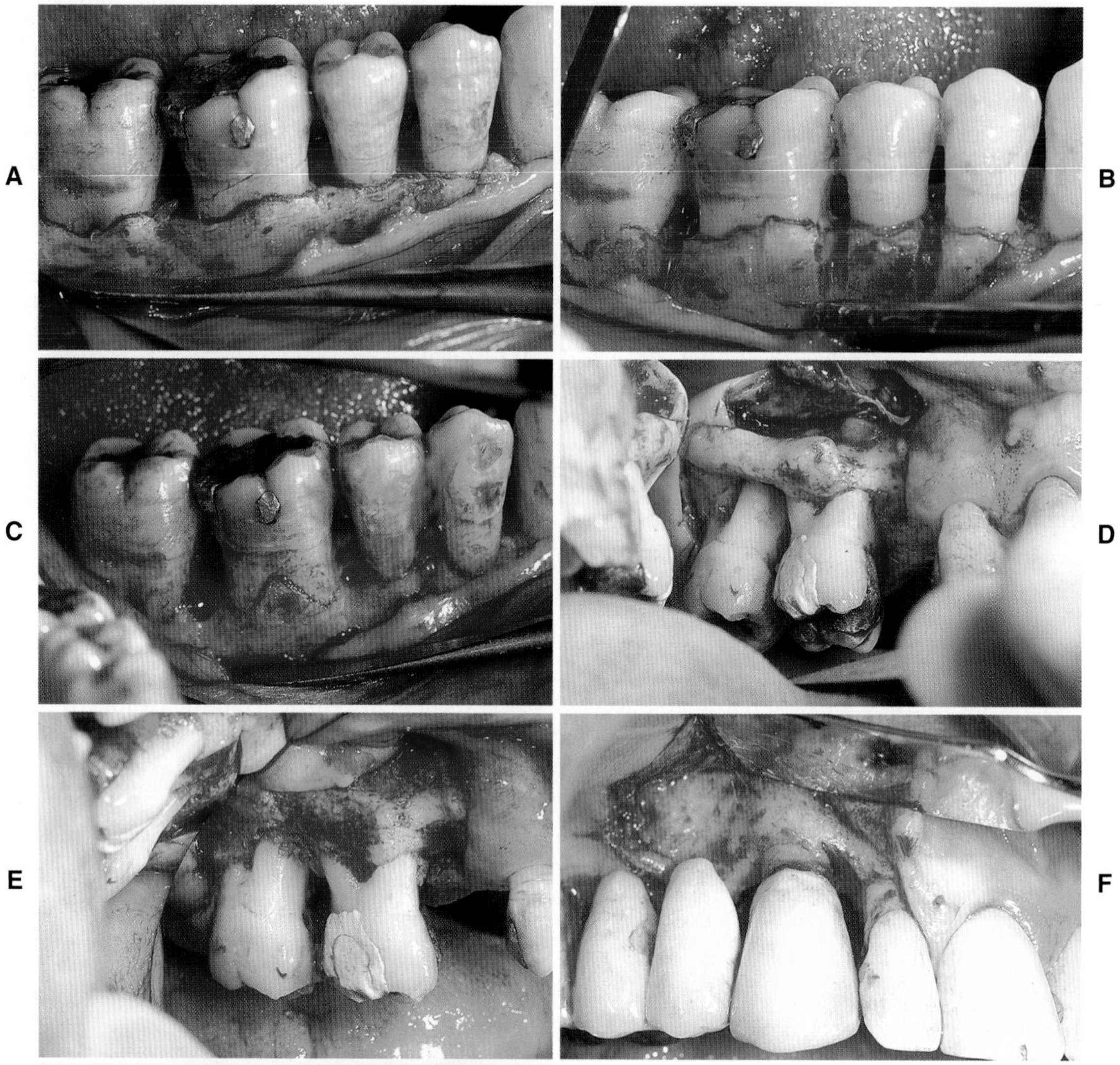

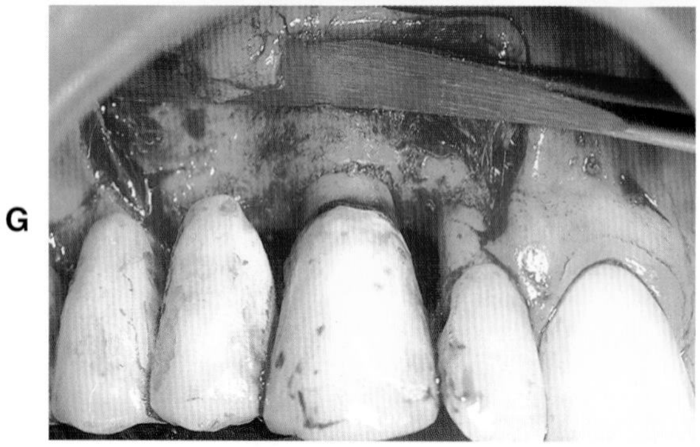

Figure 66-10 Bone contouring in flap surgery. **A, B,** and **C,** Bone contouring in interdental craters. **D** and **E,** Bone contouring in exotoses. **F** and **G,** Bone contouring in one-wall vertical defect.

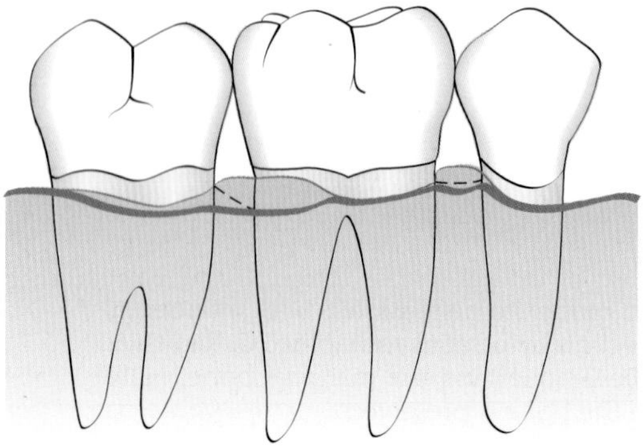

Figure 66-11 Diagrammatic representation of bone irregularities in periodontal disease. The thick line is the proposed correction of the defect. Note the flattening of the interproximal bone between the molars and the protection of the furcal bone on the first molar. Facial crest height is reduced in both interproximal areas to the depth of the defect.

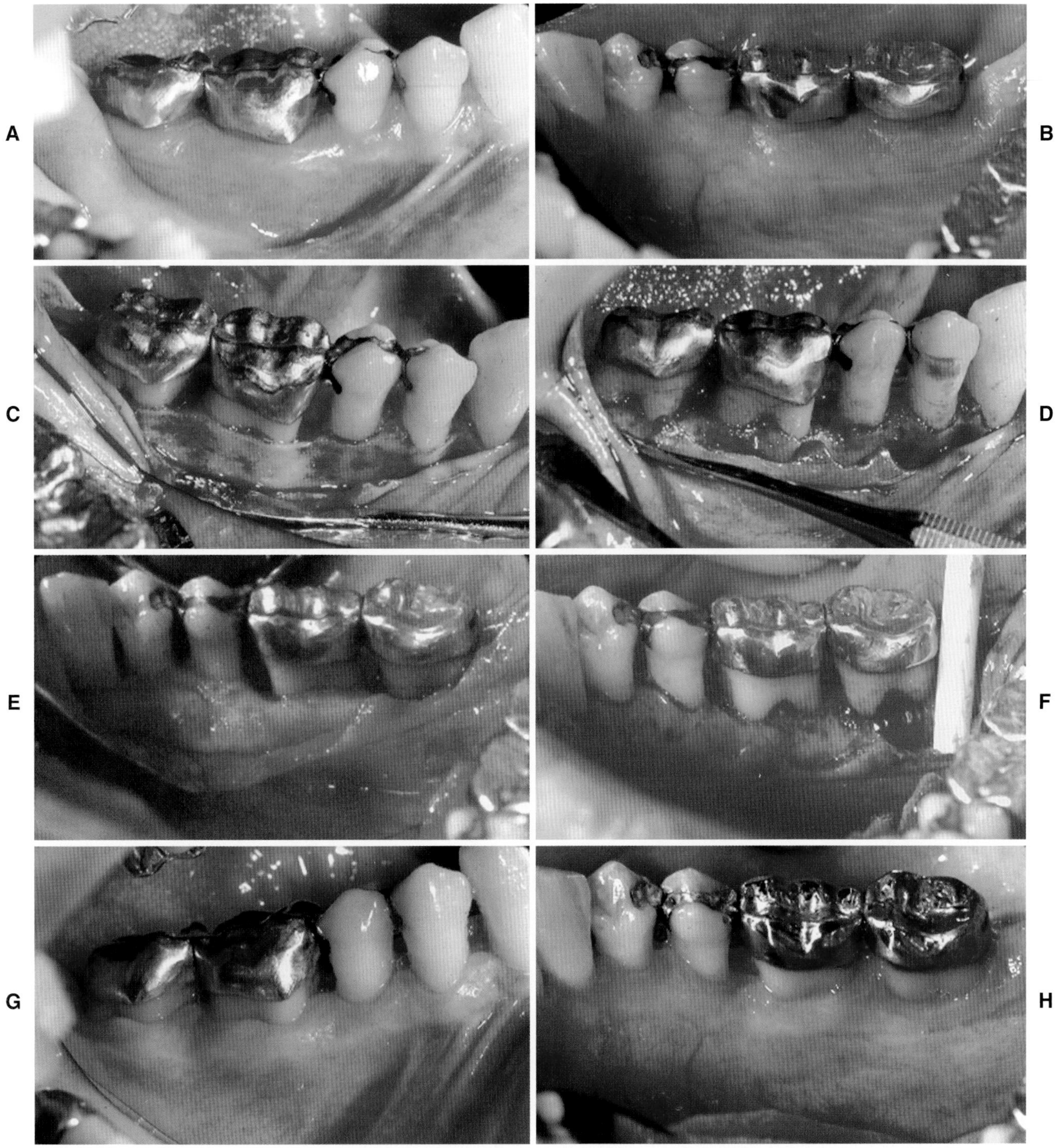

Figure 66-12 Compromise osseous surgery. **A** and **B,** Preoperative views of the buccal and lingual surfaces. **C** and **D,** Preoperative and postoperative views of the buccal osseous recontouring of class I buccal furcation defects, a moderate crater between the two molars, and a deep 1-2-3–walled defect at the mesial of the first involvements. **D,** Buccal aspects of these lesions were corrected with osteoplasty and a small amount of ostectomy. **E** and **F,** Preoperative and postoperative views of the lingual osseous management. **E,** Notice the combination 1-2-3–walled defect between the second bicuspid and first molar, as well as the irregular pattern of bone loss with ledging. **F,** These defects were corrected by osteoplasty and ostectomy, except for the deep defect at the mesial surface of the molar. This area was resected until the residual defect was of two and three walls only and left to repair. **G** and **H,** Buccal and lingual 5-year postoperative views of tissue configuration. Note the residual soft tissue defect between the bicuspid and first molar.

Gradualizing Marginal Bone

The final step in the osseous resection technique is also an ostectomy process. Bone removal is minimal but necessary to provide a sound, regular base for the gingival tissue to follow. Failure to remove small bony discrepancies on the gingival line angles (widow's peaks) allows the tissue to rise to a higher level than the base of the bone loss in the interdental area (see Figure 66-9, *C* and *D*). This may make the process of selective recession and subsequent pocket reduction incomplete. This step of the procedure also requires gradualization and blending on the radicular surface (see Figures 66-10, *C*, and 66-11). The two ostectomy steps should be performed with great care so as not to produce nicks or grooves on the roots. When the radicular bone is thin, it is extremely easy to overdo this step, to the detriment of the entire surgical effort. For this reason, various hand instruments, such as chisels and curettes, are preferable to rotary instruments for gradualizing marginal bone.

FLAP PLACEMENT AND CLOSURE

After performing resection, the clinician positions and sutures the flaps. Flaps may be replaced to their original position, to cover the new bony margin, or they may be apically positioned. Replacing the flap in areas that previously had deep pockets may result initially in greater postoperative pocket depth, although a selective recession may diminish the depth over time. Positioning the flap apically to expose marginal bone is one method of altering the width of the gingiva *(denudation)*. However, such flap placement results in more postsurgical resorption of bone and patient discomfort than if the newly created bony margin were covered by the flap. Positioning the flap to cover the new margin minimizes postoperative complications and results in optimal postsurgical pocket depths (Figure 66-13).

Suturing may be accomplished using a variety of different suture materials and suture knots[4] (see Chapter 64). The sutures should be placed with minimal tension to coapt the flaps, prevent their separation, and maintain the position of the flaps. Sutures placed with excessive tension rapidly pull through the tissues.

POSTOPERATIVE MAINTENANCE

Sutures may be removed at various times after placement. Nonresorbable sutures such as silk are usually removed after 1 week of healing, although some of the newer synthetic materials may be left for up to 3 weeks or longer without adverse consequences. Resorbable sutures maintain wound approximation for varying periods of 1 to 3 weeks or more, depending on the type of suture material. At the suture removal appointment the periodontal dressing, if present, is removed, and the surgical site is gently cleansed of debris with a cotton pellet dampened with saline. Nonresorbable sutures are then cut and removed. If sutures of a resorbable material were used, the area should be inspected carefully to ensure that no suture fragments remain. Suture removal should be accomplished without dragging contaminated portions of the suture through the periodontal tissues. This may be accomplished by lightly compressing the soft tissue immediately adjacent to the suture. This exposes (extrudes) a portion of the suture that was previously under the gingival tissues and less likely to be contaminated by plaque. The suture is then cut at the gingival surface. Removal of the pressure from the site results in the cut surface being slightly submerged in the tissue. The sutures are then removed with cotton pliers by pulling the suture from its contaminated end.

After suture removal the surgical site is examined carefully, and any excessive granulation tissue is removed with a sharp curette. The patient is provided with postsurgical maintenance instructions and the instruments needed to maintain the surgical site in a plaque-free state. These instruments should not produce additional trauma to the healing tissues. Many therapists find the use of a plaque-suppressive agent such as chlorhexidine digluconate to be a valuable adjunct to postsurgical maintenance. A second postoperative visit is often performed at the second or third week, and the surgical site is lightly debrided for optimal results. Professional prophylaxis for complete plaque removal should be done every 2 weeks until healing is complete or the patient is maintaining appropriate levels of plaque control.

Healing should proceed uneventfully, with the attachment of the flap to the underlying bone completed in 14 to 21 days. Maturation and remodeling can continue for up to 6 months. It is usually advisable to wait at least 6 weeks after completion of healing of the last surgical area before beginning dental restorations. For those patients with a major cosmetic concern, it is wise to wait as long as possible to achieve a postoperative soft tissue position and a stable sulcus.

SPECIFIC OSSEOUS RESHAPING SITUATIONS

The osseous corrective procedure previously described is classically applied to shallow craters with heavy faciolingual ledges (Figure 66-14). The correction of other osseous defects is also possible; however, careful case selection for definitive osseous surgery is extremely important.

Correction of one-walled hemiseptal defects requires that the bone be reduced to the level of the most apical portion of the defect. Therefore, great care should be taken to select the appropriate case. If one-walled defects occur next to an edentulous space, the edentulous ridge is reduced to the level of the osseous defect (Figure 66-15).

Other situations that complicate osseous correction are exostoses (Figure 66-16; see also Figure 66-10, *D* and *E*), malpositioned teeth, and supraerupted teeth. Following the four steps previously outlined best controls each of these situations. In most situations the unique feature of the bony profile is well managed by prudently applying the same principles (Figure 66-17; see also Figure 66-10). However, some situations require deviation from the definitive osseous reshaping technique; examples include dilacerated roots, root proximity, and furcations that would be compromised by osseous surgery.

In the absence of ledges or exostoses, the elimination of the bony lesion begins with reduction of the interdental walls of craters, the one-walled component of

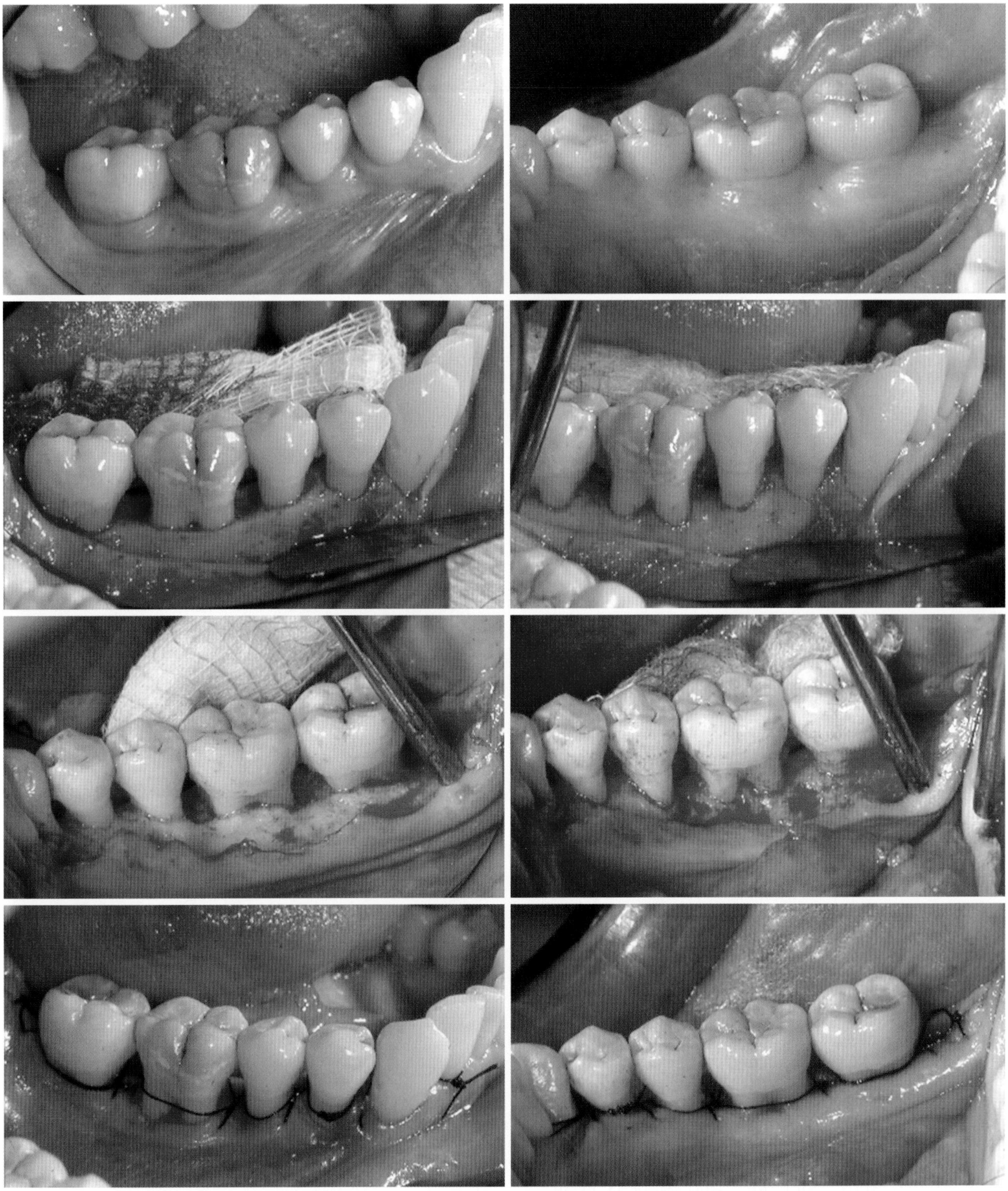

A B C D E F G H

Figure 66-13 Ostectomy and osteoplasty to a positive contour with flap placement at the newly created bony crest for minimal pocket depth. **A** and **B,** Buccal and lingual preoperative views. **C** and **D,** Buccal preoperative view and postoperative correction. Osteoplasty and ostectomy were used to produce a positive contour. Note the osteoplasty into the buccal furcation of the first molar. This is about the extent of craters that can be corrected to a positive contour in teeth with moderate root trunk length. **E** and **F,** Lingual preoperative view and postoperative correction. Osteoplasty and ostectomy were done to produce a positive contour. Note the lingual ledge, which was reduced. Such ledges are common in this area. **G** and **H,** Buccal and lingual flaps sutured with continuous sling sutures to allow placement of the flaps to cover the bony margins. Ostectomy and osteoplasty performed to a positive contour, with flap placement at the newly created bony crest for minimal pocket depth.

Continued

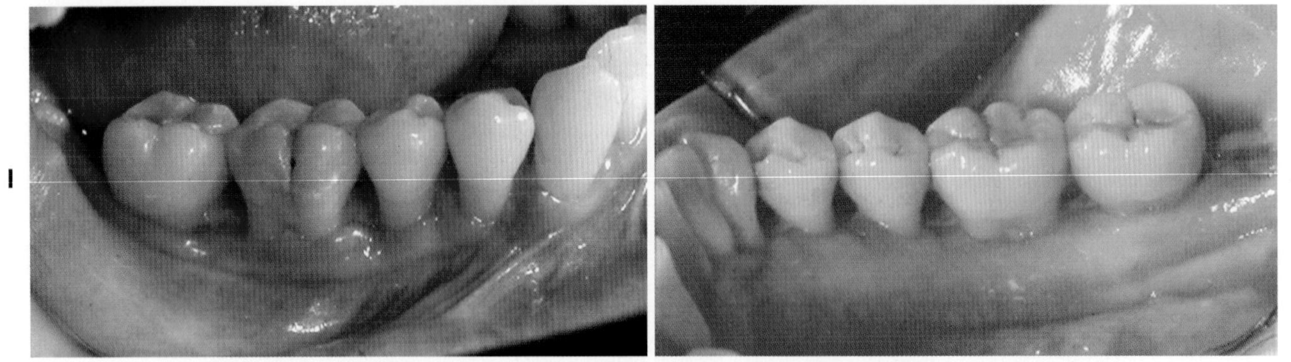

Figure 66-13, cont'd Ostectomy and osteoplasty to a positive contour with flap placement at the newly created bony crest for minimal pocket depth. **I** and **J,** Buccal and lingual postoperative views at 1 week. Soft tissue thickness is minimal, and the interdental areas are granulating in over the positive bony form. Minimal pocket depth results from such management.

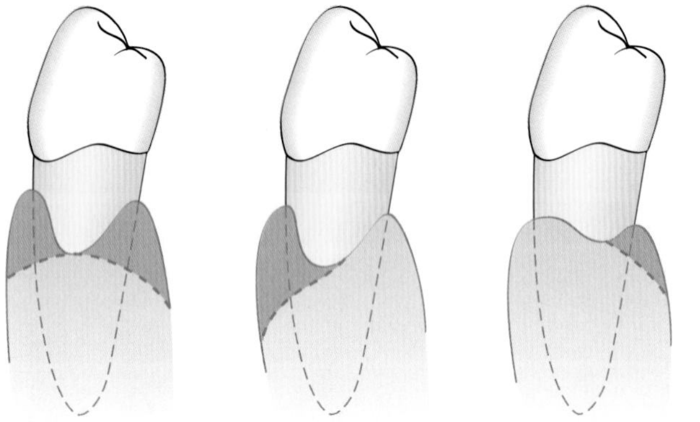

Figure 66-14 Interproximal craters. The shaded areas illustrate different techniques for the management of such defects. The technique that reduces the least amount of supporting bone is preferable.

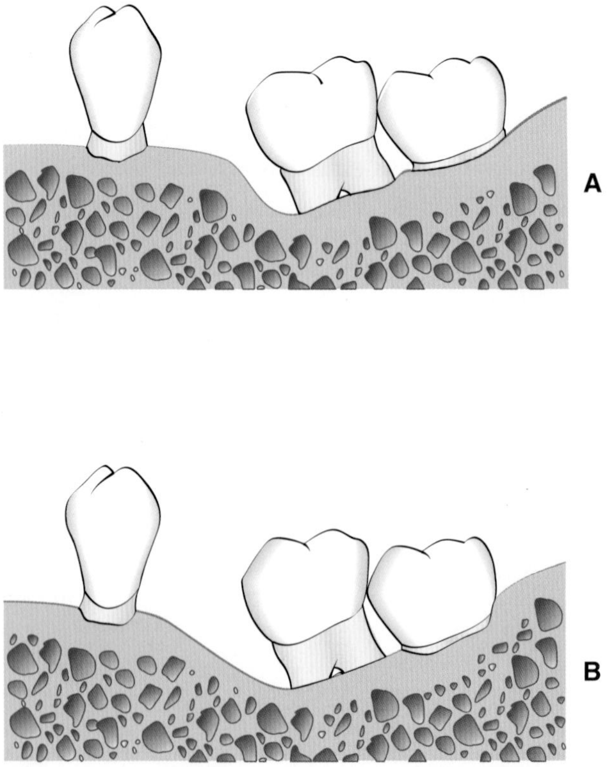

Figure 66-15 Reduction of a one-wall angular defect. **A,** Angular bone defect mesial to the tilted molar. **B,** Defect reduced by "ramping" angular bone.

angular defects, and wells (moats) and grooving into sites of early involvement.[10] The walls of the crater may be reduced at the expense of the buccal, lingual, or both walls (Figure 66-18). The reduction should be made to remove the least amount of alveolar bone required to (1) produce a satisfactory form, (2) prevent the therapeutic invasion of furcations, and (3) blend the contours with the adjacent teeth. The selective reduction of bony defects by "ramping" the bone to the palatal or lingual to avoid involvement of the furcations has been advocated by Ochsenbein and Bohannan[18] and Tibbetts et al.[23] (Figure 66-19).

In the presence of heavy ledges of bone, it is usually wise to do osteoplasty first to eliminate any exostoses or reduce the buccal/lingual bulk of the bone (Figure 62-20). It is common practice to incorporate a degree of vertical grooving during the reduction of bony ledges, because this facilitates the process of blending the radicular bone into the interproximal areas at the next step.

One-walled or hemiseptal defects usually require the removal of some bone from the tooth with the greatest coronal bony height. This removal of bone may result in a significant reduction in attachment on relatively unaffected adjacent teeth to eliminate the defect (see Figure 66-17, *A* and *B*). However, if a tooth in the surgical field has one-walled defects on both its mesial and its distal surface and this is recognized during examination, the severely affected tooth may be extruded by orthodontic therapy during disease control treatment to minimize

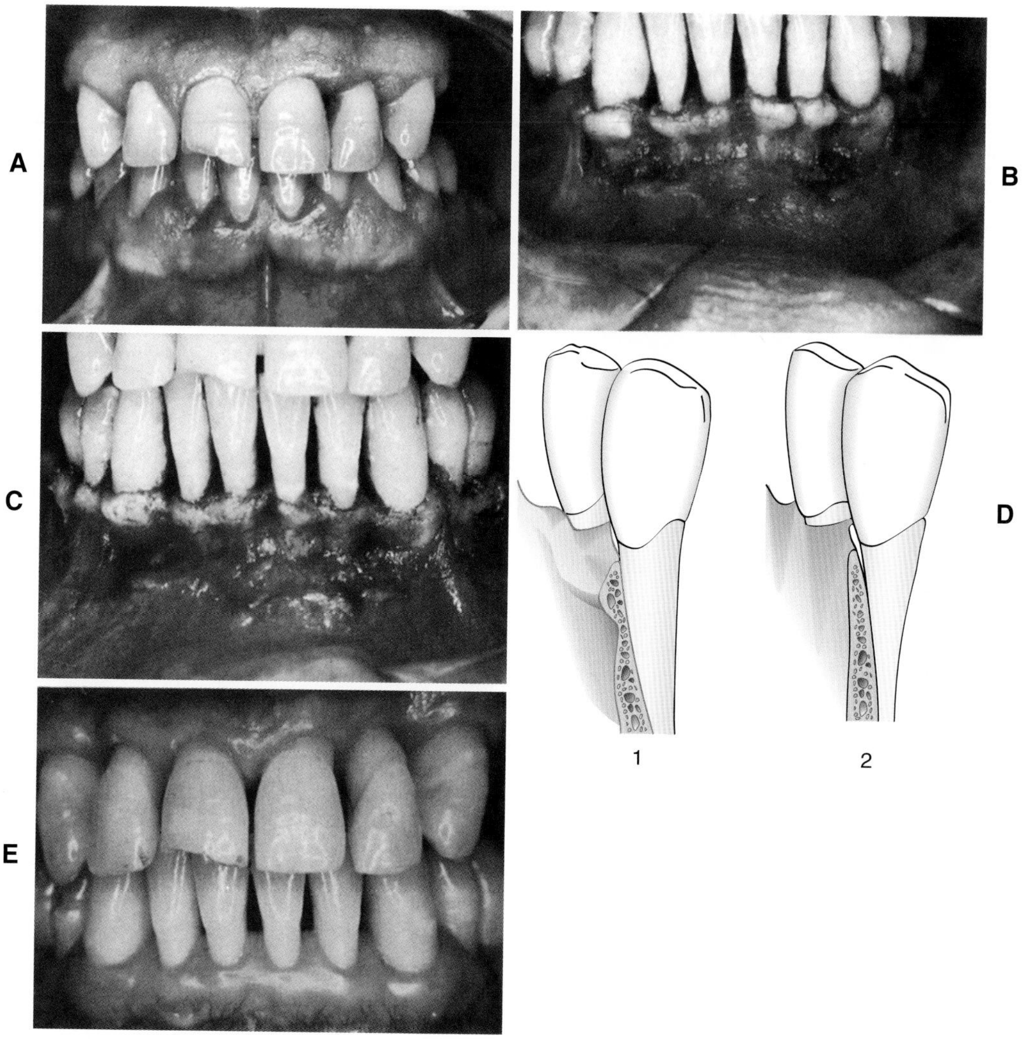

Figure 66-16 Correction of exotoses by osseous surgery. **A,** Periodontal disease in a patient with bulbous gingival contour in the mandible. **B,** Reflected flap reveals exostoses. **C,** Exostoses reduced, interdental grooves established, and interdental bone tapered inward and toward the crest. **D:** *1,* Lateral view, showing exostosis; *2,* exostosis reduced and bone recontoured to provide interdental grooves. **E,** After 10 weeks, pockets are eliminated, and physiologic gingival contour is restored. Compare with *A.* (Courtesy Dr. Charles A. Palioca, Homosassa, Fla.)

or eliminate the need for resection of bone from the adjacent teeth.

SUMMARY

Although osseous surgical techniques cannot be applied to every bony abnormality or topographic modification, it has been clearly demonstrated that properly used osseous surgery can eliminate and modify defects, as well as gradualize excessive bony ledges, irregular alveolar bone, early furcation involvement, excessive bony exostosis, and circumferential defects. When properly performed, resective osseous surgery achieves a physiologic architecture of marginal alveolar bone conducive to gingival flap adaptation with minimal probing depth. The advantages of this surgical modality include a predictable amount of pocket reduction that can enhance oral hygiene and periodic maintenance. It also preserves the width of the attached tissue while removing granulomatous tissue and providing access for debridement of the radicular surfaces. In addition, the osseous resection technique permits recontouring of bony abnormalities, including hemiseptal defects, tori, and ledges. Its substantial benefits include proper assessment for restorative procedures (e.g., crown lengthening) and assessment of restorative overhangs and tooth abnormalities (e.g., enamel projections, enamel pearls, perforations, fractures). Therefore, resective osseous surgery can be an important technique in the armamentarium necessary to provide a maintainable periodontium for periodontal patients.

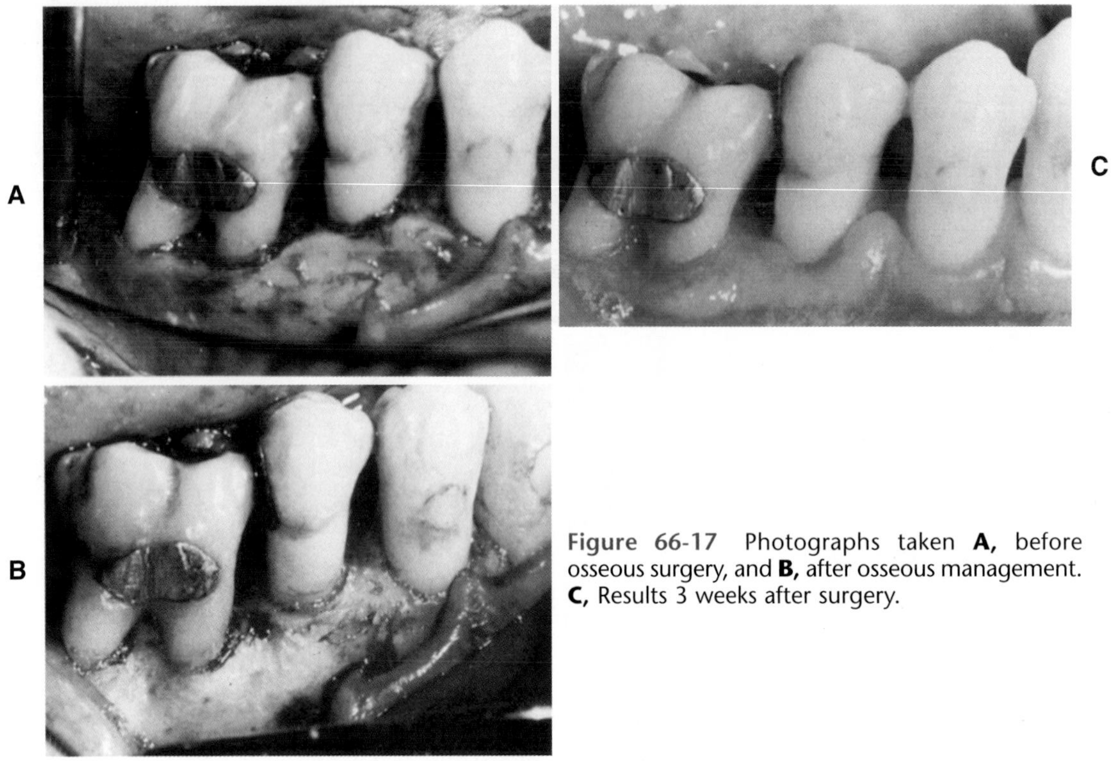

Figure 66-17 Photographs taken **A,** before osseous surgery, and **B,** after osseous management. **C,** Results 3 weeks after surgery.

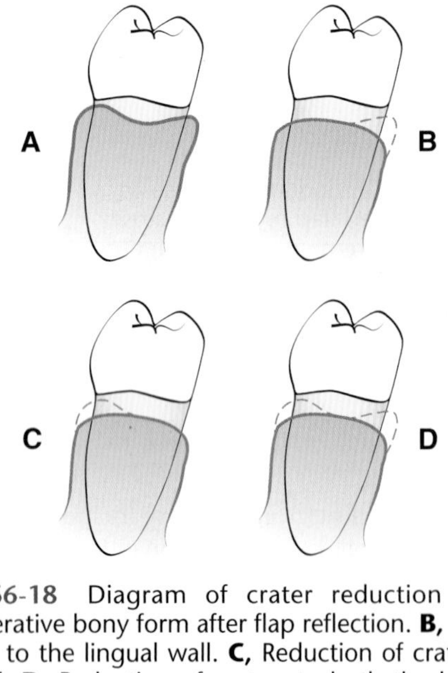

Figure 66-18 Diagram of crater reduction patterns. **A,** Preoperative bony form after flap reflection. **B,** Reduction of craters to the lingual wall. **C,** Reduction of craters to the facial wall. **D,** Reduction of craters to both the buccal and the lingual wall.

SCIENCE TRANSFER

The use of osseous surgery represents a balance between removing existing tissue and maintaining the remaining tissue. *The goal is to establish contours that existed naturally (physiologically), with the assumption that this will facilitate hygiene and long-term maintenance.* If the contours are nonphysiologic and the dimensions of the epithelium and connective tissue are not of biologic width, the host will remodel, or the relationships will allow for potential plaque accumulation and further pathology. For these reasons, judicious use of ostectomy is combined with osteoplasty.

Osseous surgery is a specific approach to recontouring bone used in conjunction with apical flap positioning that requires precise surgical techniques. It is limited to the treatment of moderate bone loss in teeth with adequate residual root in relation to bone volume. Osseous surgery results in the formation of a healthy periodontal attachment apparatus in an apical position to the presurgical level, and thus it has esthetic limitations. Resective osseous surgery is most successful in interproximal bony craters 1 to 2 mm in depth, early furcation defects, and cases with thick alveolar bone surrounding the teeth. Long-term data show that resective osseous surgery is extremely effective in reducing pocket depth, but with an associated loss of attachment and gingival recession.

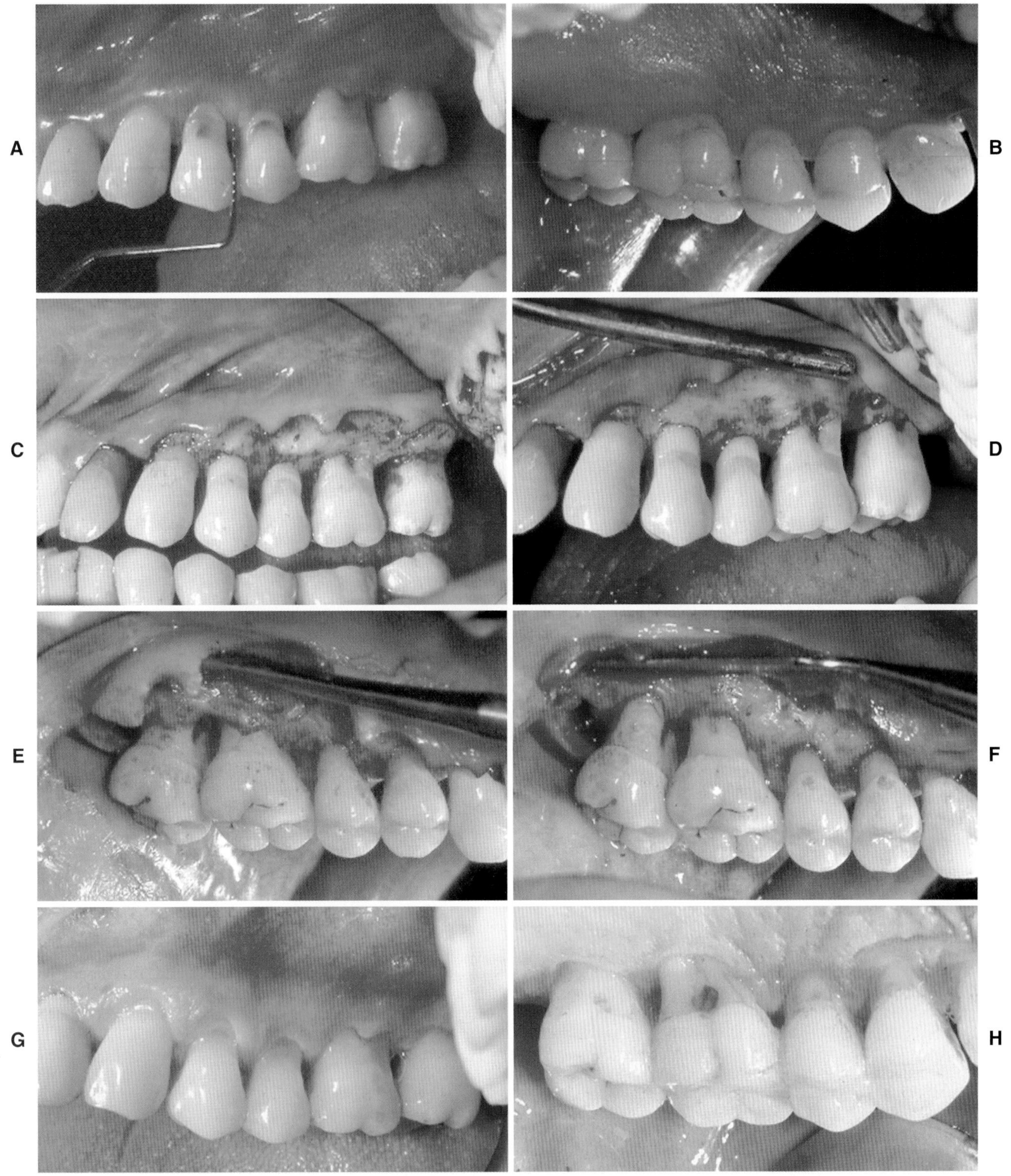

Figure 66-19 Correction of osseous defects largely to the palatal wall. **A** and **B,** Buccal and palatal preoperative views, 6 weeks after completion of scaling and root planing. **C** and **D,** Buccal preoperative and postoperative views. **C,** Note the ledging on the facial wall of molars and the one-wall defects on both molars. **D,** Postoperative view shows the elimination of these defects by osteoplasty on the ledges and ostectomy of the one-wall defects to produce a positive buccal architecture. **E** and **F,** Palatal preoperative and postoperative views. **E,** Note the pattern of bony loss, which is more severe on the palatal wall. In addition to the facial one-wall defects, there is an incipient furcation defect at the mesial wall of the first molar and a class II furcation at the mesial wall of the second molar. **F,** Configuration of the defects was such that ostectomy was performed on the palatal roots of both molars to produce a compromise architecture. **G** and **H,** Ten-year postoperative views of the buccal and palatal areas, showing the pattern of soft tissue adaptation to the surgically produced bony form.

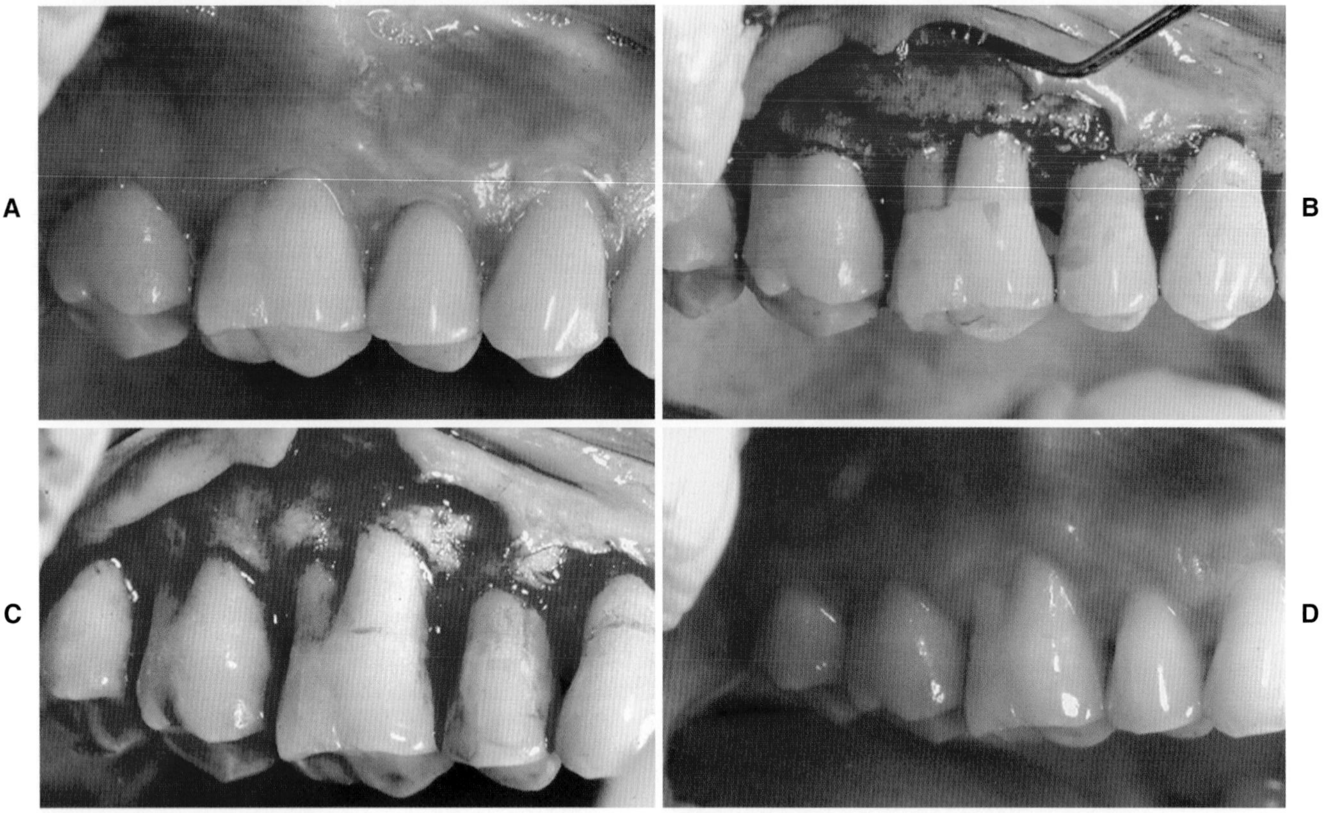

Figure 66-20 Reduction of bony ledges by osteoplasty before correction of interdental defects. **A,** Buccal preoperative view. **B,** Buccal flap reflection. Note the buccal ledge and the class II buccal furcation. **C,** Buccal correction largely by osteoplasty with minor ostectomy over the root prominence to produce a positive architecture. **D,** Ten-year postoperative view of soft tissue form. Minimal pocket depth is present.

REFERENCES

1. Black GV: Surgical treatment of pockets. In Black AD: *Special dental pathology,* ed 3, Chicago, 1917, Medico Dental.
2. Carranza FA, Carranza FA Jr: The management of the alveolar bone in the treatment of the periodontal pocket, *J Periodontol* 27:29, 1956.
3. Caton J, Nyman S: Histometric evaluation of periodontal surgery. III. The effect of bone resection on the connective tissue attachment level, *J Periodontol* 52:405, 1981.
4. Dahlberg WH: Incisions and suturing: some basic considerations about each in periodontal surgery, *Dent Clin North Am* 13:149, 1969.
5. Donnenfeld OW, Hoag PM, Weissman DP: A clinical study of the effects of osteoplasty, *J Periodontol* 32:131, 1961.
6. Easley J: Methods of determining alveolar osseous form, *J Periodontol* 38:112, 1967.
7. Friedman N: Periodontal osseous surgery: osteoplasty and osteoectomy, *J Periodontol* 26:257, 1955.
8. Garguilo AW, Wentz FM, Orban B: Dimensions and relations of the dentogingival junction in humans, *J Periodontol* 32:261, 1961.
9. Goldman HM, Cohen DW: The infrabony pocket: classification and treatment, *J Periodontol* 29:272, 1958.
10. Kaldahl WB, Kalkwarf KL, Patil KD, et al: Evaluation of four modalities of periodontal therapy: mean probing depth, probing attachment level and recession changes, *J Periodontol* 59:783, 1988.
11. Kaldahl WB, Kalkwarf KL, Patil KD, et al: Long-term evaluation of periodontal therapy. I. Response to four therapeutic modalities, *J Periodontol* 67:93, 1996.
12. Knowles J, Burgett F, Nissle R, et al: Results of periodontal treatment related to pocket depth and attachment level: eight years, *J Periodontol* 50:225, 1979.
13. Lindhe J, Socransky S, Nyman S, et al: Critical probing depths in periodontal therapy, *J Clin Periodontol* 9:323, 1982.
14. Manson JD, Nicholson K: The distribution of bone defects in chronic periodontitis, *J Periodontol* 45:88, 1974.
15. Maynard JG, Wilson RD: Physiologic dimensions of the periodontium significant to the restorative dentist, *J Periodontol* 50:170, 1979.
16. Mealey BL, Beybayer MF, Butzin CA, et al: Use of furcal bone sounding to improve the accuracy of furcation diagnosis, *J Periodontol* 65:649, 1994.
17. Ochsenbein C: A primer for osseous surgery, *Int J Periodont Restor Dent* 6:9, 1986.
18. Ochsenbein C, Bohannan HM: The palatal approach to osseous surgery. II. Clinical application, *J Periodontol* 35:54, 1964.
19. Prichard JF: The roentgenographic depiction of periodontal disease, *Periodontics* 3(2), 1973.
20. Schluger S: Osseous resection: a basic principle in periodontal surgery, *Oral Surg Oral Med Oral Pathol* 2:316, 1949.
21. Schluger S, Yuodelis RA, Page RC, et al: Resective periodontal surgery in pocket elimination. In *Periodontal diseases,* Philadelphia, 1990, Lea & Febiger.

22. Selipsky HS: Osseous surgery: how much need we compromise? *Dent Clin North Am* 20:79, 1976.
23. Tibbetts L, Ochsenbein C, Loughlin D: The lingual approach to osseous surgery, *J Periodontol* 20:61, 1976.
24. Townsend-Olsen C, Ammons WF, Van Belle C: A longitudinal study comparing apically repositioned flaps, with and without osseous surgery, *Int J Periodont Restor Dent* 5:11, 1985.

Reconstructive Periodontal Surgery

Fermin A. Carranza, Henry H. Takei, and David L. Cochran

67

CHAPTER

CHAPTER OUTLINE

New attachment with periodontal regeneration is the ideal outcome of therapy because it results in obliteration of the pocket and reconstruction of the periodontium (Figure 67-1). However, the techniques available are not totally dependable, and other therapeutic results may be seen (Figure 67-2), as follows:

1. Healing with a long junctional epithelium, which can result even if filling of bone has occurred.
2. Ankylosis of bone and tooth with resultant root resorption.
3. Recession.
4. Recurrence of the pocket.
5. Any combination of these results.

EVALUATION OF NEW ATTACHMENT AND PERIODONTAL RECONSTRUCTION

It is sometimes difficult in clinical and experimental situations to determine whether new attachment has occurred and the extent to which it has occurred. Evidence of reconstruction of the marginal periodontium can be obtained by clinical, radiographic, surgical reentry, or histologic procedures.[30,107] All these methods have advantages and shortcomings that should be well understood and considered in individual cases and when critically evaluating the literature.

Clinical Methods

Clinical methods to evaluate periodontal reconstruction consist of comparisons between pretreatment and post-treatment pocket probings and determinations of clinical gingival findings. The probe can be used to determine pocket depth, attachment level, and bone level (Figure 67-3). Clinical determinations of attachment level are more useful than probing pocket depths because the latter may change as a result of displacement of the gingival margin (see Chapter 35).

Several studies have determined that the depth of penetration of a probe in a periodontal pocket varies according to the degree of inflammatory involvement of the tissues immediately beneath the bottom of the pocket (Figure 67-4). Therefore, even though the forces used may be standardized with pressure-sensitive probes, there is an inherent margin of error in this method that is difficult to overcome. Fowler et al.[59] have calculated this error to be 1.2 mm, but it is even greater when furcations are probed.[125]

Bone probing performed with the patient under anesthesia is not subject to this error and has been found to be as accurate as bone height measurements made on surgical reentry.[76,153,195]

Measurements of the defect should be made before and after treatment from the same point within the defect and with the same angulation of the probe. This

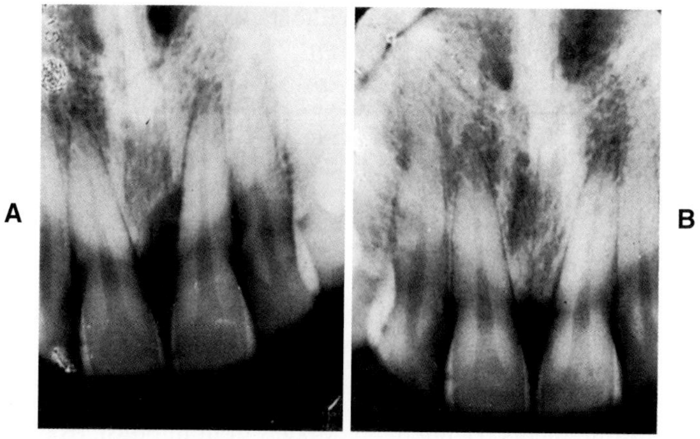

Figure 67-1 Bone regeneration after closed scaling, root planing, and curettage. Before **(A)** and after **(B)** radiographs are shown. (From Carranza FA Sr: *J Periodontol* 25:272, 1954.)

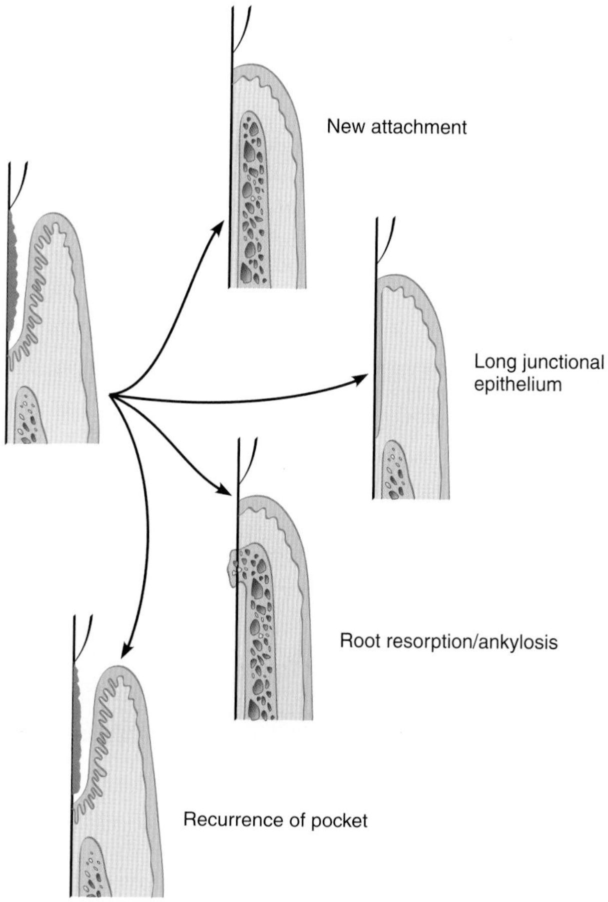

Figure 67-2 Possible outcomes of reconstructive periodontal therapy.

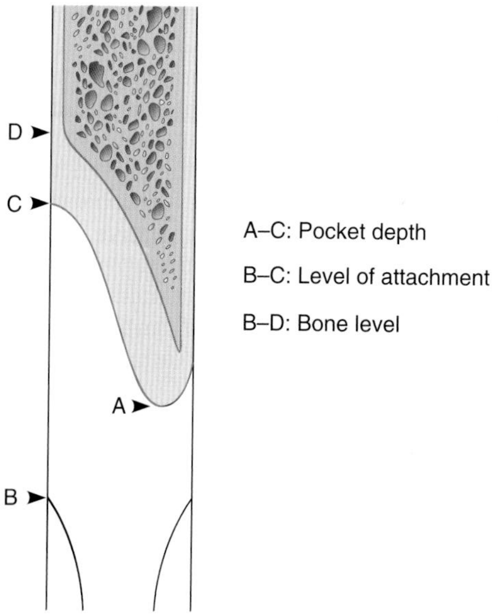

Figure 67-3 Different types of probings in an interdental space.

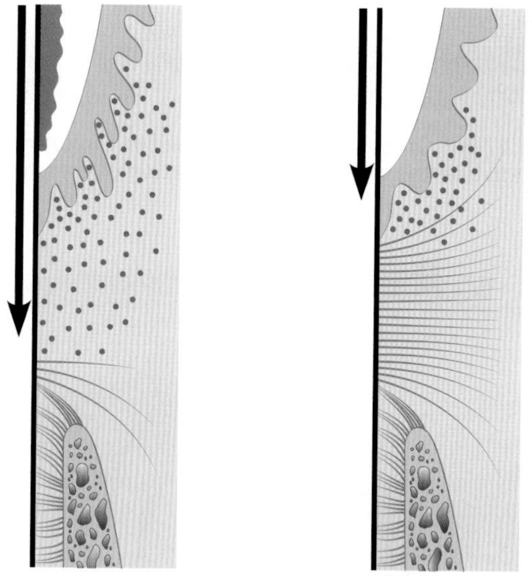

Figure 67-4 *Left,* Arrow pointing downward depicts penetration of a probe in an untreated periodontal pocket. The probe tip goes past the junctional epithelium and the inflamed tissue and is stopped by the first intact, attached collagen fibers. *Right,* After thorough scaling and root planing, the location of the bottom of the pocket has not changed, but the probe penetrates to only about one-third the length of the junctional epithelium (see Chapter 35). *The reduction in probing depth may not reflect a change in attachment level.*

reproducibility of probe placement is difficult and may be facilitated in part by using a grooved stent to guide the introduction of the probe (Figure 67-5). Preoperative and postoperative comparability of probing measurements that do not use this standardized method may be open to question.

Radiographic Methods

Radiographic evaluation of periodontal regeneration allows assessment of the bone tissue adjacent to the tooth. This technique also requires carefully standardized techniques for reproducible positioning of the film and the tube.[136,156] Even with standardized techniques (see Chapters 36 and 37), the radiograph does not show the entire topography of the area before or after treatment. Furthermore, thin bone trabeculae may exist before treatment and go undetected radiographically because a certain minimal amount of mineralized tissue must be present to register on the radiograph. Several studies have demonstrated that radiographs, even those taken with standardized methods, are less reliable than clinical probing techniques.[100,187] A comparative study of pre-treatment bone levels and posttherapy bone fill with 12-month reentry bone measurements showed that linear radiographic analysis significantly underestimates pretreatment bone loss and posttreatment bone fill.[188]

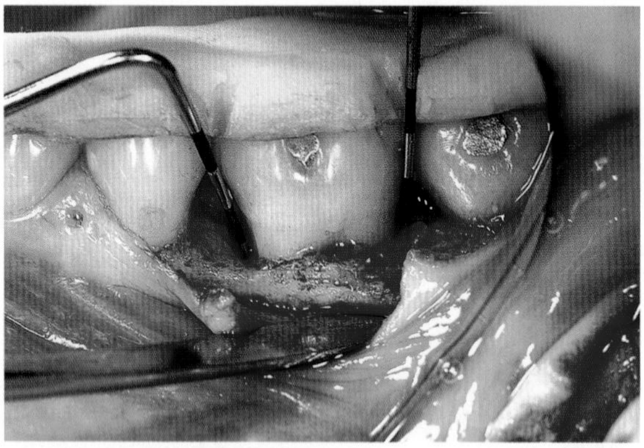

Figure 67-5 Grooved acrylic stent used in clinical research to standardize the direction of introduction of the probe.

Studies with subtraction radiography have enhanced the usefulness of radiographic evaluation.[48,49,198] A comparative study of linear measurement, computer-assisted densitometric image analysis (CADIA; see Chapter 37), and a method combining the two reported that the linear-CADIA method offers the highest level of accuracy.[190]

Surgical Reentry

The surgical reentry of a treated defect after a period of healing can provide a good view of the state of the bone crest that can be compared with the view taken during the initial surgical intervention and can also be subject to measurements (Figure 67-6). Models from impressions of the bone taken at the initial surgery and later at reentry can be used to assess the results of therapy.

This method is very useful but has two shortcomings: it requires a frequently unnecessary second procedure, and it does not show the type of attachment that exists (i.e., new attachment or long junctional epithelium[31]) (Figure 67-7).

Histologic Methods

The type of attachment can be determined only by histologic analysis of tissue blocks obtained from the healed area. Although this method can offer clear evidence of a new attachment apparatus, it is not without problems. The need to remove a tooth with its periodontium after

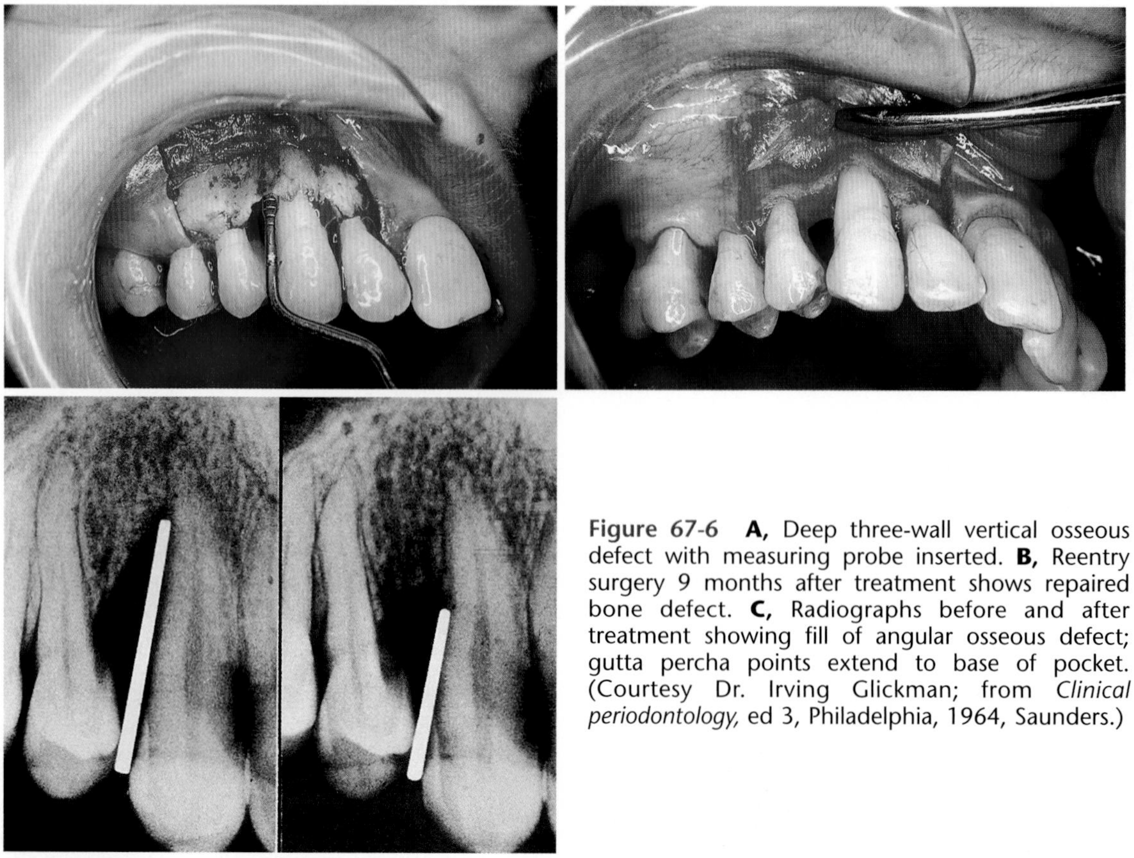

Figure 67-6 **A,** Deep three-wall vertical osseous defect with measuring probe inserted. **B,** Reentry surgery 9 months after treatment shows repaired bone defect. **C,** Radiographs before and after treatment showing fill of angular osseous defect; gutta percha points extend to base of pocket. (Courtesy Dr. Irving Glickman; from *Clinical periodontology,* ed 3, Philadelphia, 1964, Saunders.)

successful treatment limits this method to volunteers who need the extraction for prosthetic or other reasons and who agree to the procedure.

Animal studies can be used to clarify some aspects of the tissue response to different materials. However, species differences should always be remembered when extrapolations to humans are attempted.

Studies of the reconstruction of periodontal structures have been performed in rodents, dogs, monkeys, baboons, and pigs. Because it is difficult to find naturally occurring periodontal osseous defects that would be adequate for a study, experimentally induced bone defects must be used. Surgically produced defects can simulate the shape of osseous periodontal lesions but lack their chronicity and self-sustaining features. These defects can be allowed to become chronically infected, and then their similarity to chronic natural lesions improves, but they are never identical.[199] However, these studies are useful to establish healing sequences and mechanisms.

In addition, the exact location of the bottom of the pocket must be determined before the procedure because the surgical technique opens tissues beyond the bottom of the pocket, and healing below this point does not constitute new attachment. Notches on the root surface must be used to indicate this important point. Because the exact coronal point of the junctional epithelium is lost when surgically opening the area, a decision must be made as to whether to place the notch at the bottom of the calculus or on the crest of the alveolar bone (Figure 67-8). The former is slightly coronal and the latter slightly apical to the actual bottom of the pocket. The bottom of the calculus is a better landmark, but obviously the presence of calculus is required.

Numerous pitfalls are therefore inherent to histologic studies, and their accuracy and reliability should always be carefully considered.

RECONSTRUCTIVE SURGICAL TECHNIQUES

Reconstructive techniques can be subdivided into two major types: non–bone graft–associated new attachment and bone graft–associated new attachment. Many procedures combine both approaches.

All recommended techniques include careful and complete removal of all irritants. Although this can be done in some cases as a closed procedure, in the great majority of cases it should be done after exposure of the area with a flap. Flap design and incisions should follow the description given in Chapter 65 for flaps used in reconstructive surgery. Trauma from occlusion, as well as other factors, may impair posttreatment healing of the supporting periodontal tissues, reducing the likelihood of new attachment. Occlusal adjustment, if needed, is therefore indicated.

Systemic antibiotics are generally used after reconstructive periodontal therapy, although definitive information on the advisability of this measure is still lacking. Case reports have shown extensive reconstruction of periodontal lesions after scaling, root planing, and curettage, with systemic and local treatment using penicillin or tetracycline, in combination with other forms of therapy.[27,127]

Non–Bone Graft–Associated Procedures

Periodontal reconstruction can be attained without the use of bone grafts in meticulously treated three-wall defects (intrabony defects) and in periodontal and endodontal abscesses.[27,85,146] New attachment is more likely to occur when the destructive process has occurred rapidly, such as after treatment of pockets complicated by acute periodontal abscesses and after treatment of acute necrotizing ulcerative lesions.[130]

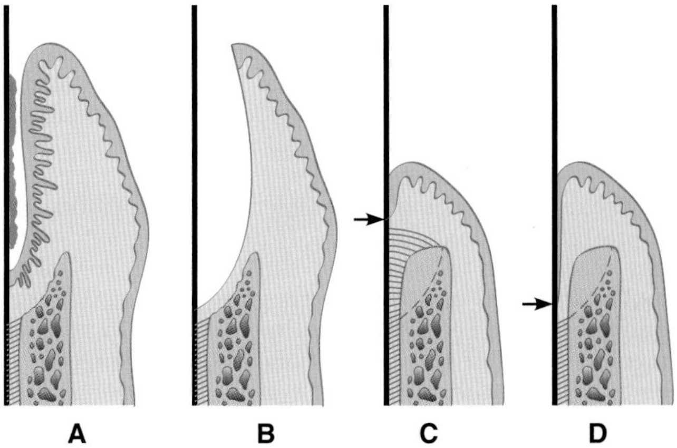

Figure 67-7 **A,** Periodontal pocket preoperatively. **B,** Periodontal pocket immediately after scaling, root planing, and curettage. **C,** New attachment. The arrow indicates the most apical part of the junctional epithelium. Note regeneration of bone and periodontal ligament. **D,** Healing by long junctional epithelium. Again, the arrow indicates the most apical part of the junctional epithelium. Note that the bone is new but the periodontal ligament is not.

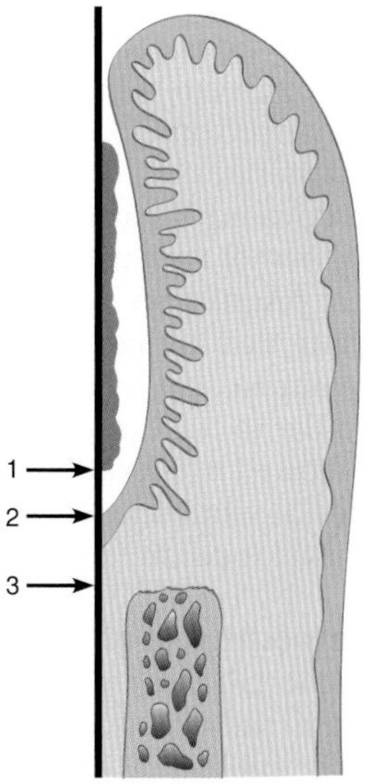

Figure 67-8 For future histologic reference, notches can be placed clinically at the most apical part of the calculus *(1)* or at the level of the osseous crest *(3)*. However, the real landmark that determines whether new attachment has taken place is the base of the pocket *(2)*.

The following sections discuss the rationale and technique for the removal of the junctional and pocket epithelium and the prevention of their migration into the healing area after therapy. The "bio-conditioning" of the root surface and the use of growth factors and enamel matrix proteins to enhance or direct healing are also discussed.

Removal of Junctional and Pocket Epithelium.

Since the earliest attempts at periodontal new attachment, the presence of junctional and pocket epithelium has been perceived as a barrier to successful therapy because its presence interferes with the direct apposition of connective tissue and cementum, thus limiting the height to which periodontal fibers can insert to the cementum.[82,126,149,201]

Several methods have been recommended to remove junctional and pocket epithelia. These include curettage, chemical agents, ultrasonic methods, lasers, and surgical techniques.

Curettage. Results of removal of epithelium by means of curettage vary from complete removal to persistence of as much as 50%.[174] Therefore, curettage is not a reliable procedure. Ultrasonic methods, lasers, and rotary abrasive stones have also been used, but their effects cannot be controlled because of the clinician's lack of vision and lack of tactile sense when using these methods.

Chemical Agents. Chemical agents have also been used to remove pocket epithelium, usually in conjunction with curettage. The drugs used most often have been sodium sulfide, phenol camphor, Antiformin, and sodium hypochlorite. However, the effect of these agents is not limited to the epithelium, and their depth of penetration cannot be controlled. These drugs are mentioned here for their historical interest.

Surgical Techniques. Surgical techniques have been recommended to eliminate the pocket and junctional epithelia. The excisional new attachment procedure consists of an internal bevel incision performed with a surgical knife, followed by removal of the excised tissue.[202] No attempt is made to elevate a flap. After careful scaling and root planing, interproximal sutures are used to close the wound (see Chapter 62).

Glickman[70] and Prichard[145] have advocated performing a *gingivectomy to the crest of the alveolar bone* and debriding the defect. Excellent results have been obtained with this technique in uncontrolled human studies.[8,146]

The modified Widman flap, as described by Ramfjord and Nissle,[150] is similar to the excisional new attachment procedure but is followed by elevation of a flap for better exposure of the area. It eliminates the pocket epithelium with the internal bevel incision (see Chapter 65).

Prevention or Impeding of Epithelial Migration.

Elimination of junctional and pocket epithelia may not be sufficient because the epithelium from the excised margin may rapidly proliferate to become interposed between the healing connective tissue and the cementum.

Several investigators have analyzed in animals and humans the effect of excluding the epithelium by amputating the crown of the tooth and covering the root with the flap ("root submergence").[12,13,17] This experimental technique not only excludes the epithelium but also prevents microbial contamination of the wound during the reparative stages. Successful repair of osseous lesions in the submerged environment was reported, but obviously this method has little or no clinical application.

Two other methods have been proposed to prevent or impede the migration of the epithelium. One consists of total removal of the interdental papilla covering the defect and its replacement with a free autogenous graft obtained from the palate.[51] During healing the graft epithelium necroses and is slowly replaced by proliferating epithelium from the gingival surface. This method has not been widely used.

The second approach is the use of *coronally displaced flaps,* which increase the distance between the epithelium and the healing area. This technique is particularly suitable for the treatment of lower molar furcations and has been used mostly in conjunction with citric acid treatment of the roots.[66,110] Periodontal regeneration after the use of this technique has been demonstrated histologically in humans.[180]

Guided Tissue Regeneration. The method for the prevention of epithelial migration along the cemental wall of the pocket that has gained wide attention is guided tissue regeneration (GTR). This method derives from the classic studies of Nyman, Lindhe, Karring, and Gottlow and is based on the assumption that only the periodontal ligament cells have the potential for regeneration of the attachment apparatus of the tooth.[73,74,133,134] GTR consists of placing barriers of different types to cover the bone and periodontal ligament, thus temporarily separating them from the gingival epithelium. Excluding the epithelium and the gingival connective tissue from the root surface during the postsurgical healing phase not only prevents epithelial migration into the wound, but also favors repopulation of the area by cells from the periodontal ligament and the bone (see Chapter 42).

Initial animal experiments using Millipore filters and Teflon membranes resulted in regeneration of cementum and alveolar bone and a functional periodontal ligament.[31,33,36,124] Clinical case reports showed GTR results in a gain in attachment level that is not necessarily associated with a buildup of alveolar bone.[9,10] Histologic studies in humans provided evidence of periodontal reconstruction in most cases, even with horizontal bone loss.[74,179,183]

The use of polytetrafluoroethylene (PTFE) membranes (Gore-Tex periodontal material, Gore-Tex, Flagstaff, Ariz) has been tested in controlled clinical studies in lower molar furcations and has shown statistically significant decreases in pocket depths and improvement in attachment levels after 6 months; bone level measurements have been inconclusive.[103,144] A study on upper molar furcations did not result in significant gain in attachment or bone levels.[123]

The initial membranes developed were nonresorbable and therefore required a second, although frequently simple, procedure to remove it. This second procedure was done after the initial stages of healing, usually 3 to 6 weeks after the first intervention. The second procedure was a significant obstacle in the utilization of this GTR technique, and therefore resorbable membranes were developed.[197]

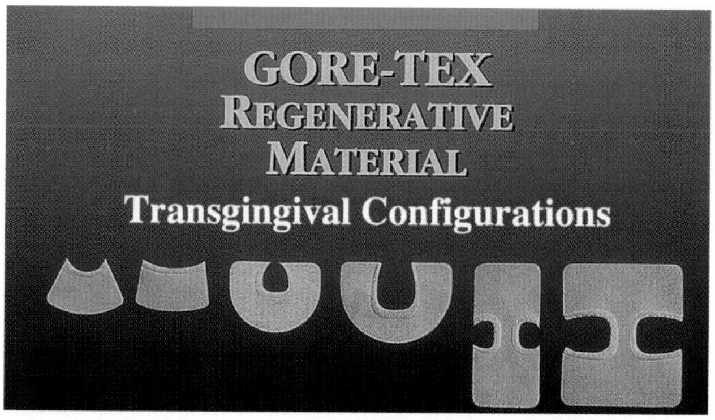

Figure 67-9 Different shapes and sizes of expanded polytetrafluoroethylene membranes marketed by Gore-Tex (Flagstaff, Ariz).

The expanded polytetrafluoroethylene (ePTFE) membrane (nonresorbable) can be obtained in different shapes and sizes to suit proximal spaces and facial/lingual surfaces of furcations (Figure 67-9). The technique for its use is as follows:

1. Raise a mucoperiosteal flap with vertical incisions, extending a minimum of two teeth anteriorly and one tooth distally to the tooth being treated.
2. Debride the osseous defect and thoroughly plane the roots.
3. Trim the membrane with sharp scissors to the approximate size of the area being treated. The apical border of the material should extend 3 to 4 mm apical to the margin of the defect and laterally 2 to 3 mm beyond the defect; the occlusal border of the membrane should be placed 2 mm apical to the cementoenamel junction.[10]
4. Suture the membrane tightly around the tooth with a sling suture.
5. Suture the flap back in its original position or slightly coronal to it, using independent sutures interdentally and in the vertical incisions. The flap should cover the membrane completely.
6. The use of periodontal dressings is optional, and the patient receives antibiotic therapy for 1 week.

After 4 to 6 weeks, the margin of the membrane becomes exposed. The membrane is removed with a gentle tug 5 weeks after the procedure. If it cannot be removed easily, the tissues are anesthetized, and the material is surgically removed using a miniflap.

The results obtained with the GTR technique are enhanced when the technique is combined with grafts placed in the defects (see Combined Techniques).

Biodegradable Membranes. The search for resorbable membranes included tests with rat, bovine or porcine collagen, Cargile membrane derived from the cecum of an ox, polylactic acid, Vicryl (polyglactin 910), synthetic skin (Biobrane), and freeze-dried dura mater.* Clinical studies with a mixture of copolymers derived from polylactic acid and acetyl tributylcitrate resorbable membranes (Guidor membrane, no longer on the market) and a poly-D,L-lactide-co-glycolide (Resolut membrane, also no longer on the market) have shown significant gains in clinical attachment and bone fill.[40,65,189]

Resorbable membranes marketed in the United States include *OsseoQuest* (Gore), a combination of polyglycolic acid, polylactic acid, and trimethylene carbonate that resorbs at 6 to 14 months; *BioGuide* (OsteoHealth), a bilayer porcine-derived collagen; *Atrisorb* (Block Drug), a polylactic acid gel; and *BioMend* (Calcitech), a bovine Achilles tendon collagen that resorbs in 4 to 18 weeks. Of these, BioGuide is easier to use and generally preferred.

The use of membranes is usually combined with autogenous bone from adjacent areas or other graft materials and root biomodifiers. These combined techniques are discussed at the end of this chapter

The potential of using autogenous periosteum as a membrane and also to stimulate periodontal regeneration has been explored in two controlled clinical studies, one of grade II furcation involvements in lower molars and another of interdental defects.[99,102] The periosteum was obtained from the patient's palate by means of a window flap. Both studies reported that autogenous periosteal grafts can be used in GTR and result in significant gains in clinical attachment and osseous defect fill.

Clot Stabilization, Wound Protection, and Space Creation. Some investigators have attributed the successful results reported with graft materials, barrier membranes, and coronally displaced flaps to the fact that these techniques protect the wound and create a space for undisturbed and stable maturation of the clot.[67,80,81] This hypothesis suggests that preservation of the root surface–fibrin clot interface prevents apical migration of the gingival epithelium and allows for connective tissue attachment during the early wound-healing period.[67,199]

The importance of space creation for bone repair has long been recognized in orthopedic and maxillofacial surgery. Transference of this concept to periodontal therapy has been explored for treatment of periodontal and periimplant osseous defects and for root coverage. The space can be created by using a titanium-reinforced ePTFE membrane to prevent its collapse. For the study of reconstructive techniques, these membranes were placed over experimentally created supraalveolar bone defects in dogs, and considerable bone reconstruction was reported.[173]

Biomodification of Root Surface. Changes in the tooth surface wall of periodontal pockets (e.g., degeneration of remnants of Sharpey's fibers, accumulation of bacteria and their products, disintegration of cementum and dentin) interfere with new attachment. Although these obstacles to new attachment can be eliminated by thorough root planing, the root surface of the pocket can be treated to improve its chances of accepting the new attachment of gingival tissues.

Several substances have been proposed for this purpose, including citric acid, fibronectin, and tetracycline.

Citric Acid. Studies by Urist showed that the implantation of demineralized bone, enamel, and dentin matrix

*References 14, 15, 35, 57, 58, 108, 109, 139-141, 197, 204.

into muscle tissue in animals induced mesenchymal cells to differentiate into osteoblasts and started an osteogenic process.[192-194] Following up on this concept, a series of studies applied citric acid to the roots to demineralize the surface, attempting to induce cementogenesis and attachment of collagen fibers.

The following actions of citric acid have been reported:

1. Accelerated healing and new cementum formation occur after surgical detachment of the gingival tissues and demineralization of the root surface by means of citric acid.[151]
2. Topically applied citric acid on periodontally diseased root surfaces has no effect on nonplaned roots, but after root planing, the acid produces a 4-μm-deep demineralized zone with exposed collagen fibers.[69]
3. Root-planed, non–citric acid–treated roots are left with a surface smear layer of microcrystalline debris; citric acid application not only removes the smear layer, exposing the dentinal tubules, but also makes the tubules appear wider and with funnel-shaped orifices.[143]
4. Citric acid has also been shown in vitro to eliminate endotoxins and bacteria from the diseased tooth surface.[44,56]
5. An early fibrin linkage to collagen fibers exposed by the citric acid treatment prevents the epithelium from migrating over treated roots.[142]

This technique using citric acid has been extensively investigated in animals and humans. Studies in dogs have shown encouraging results, especially for the treatment of furcation lesions, but the results in humans have been contradictory.[42,132,151,152,177]

The recommended citric acid technique is as follows:

1. Raise a mucoperiosteal flap and thoroughly instrument the root surface, removing calculus and underlying cementum.
2. Apply cotton pledgets soaked in a saturated solution of citric acid (pH of 1.0) for 2 to 5 minutes.
3. Remove pledgets, and irrigate root surface profusely with water.
4. Replace the flap and suture.

The use of citric acid has also been recommended in conjunction with coverage of denuded roots using free gingival grafts (see Chapter 69).

Fibronectin. Fibronectin is the glycoprotein that fibroblasts require to attach to root surfaces. The addition of fibronectin to the root surface may promote new attachment.[25,55,185] However, increasing fibronectin above plasma levels produces no obvious advantages. Adding fibronectin and citric acid to lesions treated with GTR in dogs did not improve the results.[24,175]

Tetracycline. In vitro treatment of the dentin surfaces with tetracycline increases binding of fibronectin, which in turn stimulates fibroblast attachment and growth while suppressing epithelial cell attachment and migration.[186] Tetracycline also removes an amorphous surface layer and exposes the dentin tubules. In vivo studies, however, have not shown favorable results.[200] A human study showed a trend for greater connective tissue attachment after tetracycline treatment of roots; tetracycline gave better results when used alone than when combined with fibronectin.[2]

Biologic Mediators. Although periodontal regeneration involves the formation of several different tissues, regenerative therapies have generally been directed at the production of one tissue type in the periodontium. For example, periodontal bone defects are treated with some type of bone-grafting material, with the expectation that bone, cementum, and periodontal ligament will all be formed.

A critical aspect of periodontal regeneration is the stimulation of a series of events and cascades at some point, which can result in the coordination and completion of integrated tissue formation.[37] Many approaches have been used involving polypeptide growth and differentiation factors, extracellular matrix proteins, and attachment factors and proteins involved in bone metabolism. These materials are largely physiologic molecules or molecules released by cells, or derivatives of such molecules, that regulate events in wound healing. These molecules can function in either an autocrine or a paracrine mechanism; that is, they can regulate the same cells that produced the molecule, or they can regulate other cells, respectively. Alternatively, these molecules, in addition to acting locally, may systemically act to affect the growth and function of distant cells and tissues.

These growth factors, primarily secreted by macrophages, endothelial cells, fibroblasts, and platelets, include platelet-derived growth factor (PDGF), insulin-like growth factor (IGF), basic fibroblast growth factor (bFGF), bone morphogenetic protein (BMP), and transforming growth factor (TGF). These biologic mediators have been used to stimulate periodontal wound healing (e.g., promoting migration and proliferation of fibroblasts for periodontal ligament formation) or to promote the differentiation of cells to become osteoblasts, thereby favoring bone formation.[75]

The addition of PDGF, for example, has been shown to enhance bone formation in periodontal osseous defects. In a two-center, prospective, randomized, double-masked human trial, 38 patients with bilateral defects were treated in a split-mouth design. Control subjects received conventional periodontal flap surgery and similar surgery, including vehicle. No local or systemic safety issues were noted, and no patients developed antibodies to the recombinant human growth factors. Two PDGF doses were tested, and the results demonstrated significant bone fill increases in defects treated with the larger amount. Such trials indicate current attempts to deliver growth factors to periodontal defects in order to stimulate a cascade that results in periodontal tissue formation. Many questions remain about the best vehicle or carrier material, application of the growth factors, and the release kinetics of the material.

Enamel Matrix Proteins. Enamel matrix proteins, mainly *amelogenin,* are secreted by Hertwig's epithelial root sheath during tooth development and induce acellular cementum formation. Based on these observations, these proteins are believed to favor periodontal regeneration.[78]

One enamel matrix protein derivative obtained from developing porcine teeth has been approved by the U.S. Food and Drug Administration (FDA) and marketed under the trade name *Emdogain*. The material is a viscous gel consisting of enamel-derived proteins from tooth buds in a polypropylene liquid; 1 ml of a vehicle solution is mixed with a powder and delivered by syringe to the defect site. Ninety percent of the protein in this mixture is amelogenin, with the rest primarily proline-rich non-amelogenins, tuftelin, tuft protein, serum proteins, ameloblastin, and amelin.[20,34,98]

The technique using enamel protein derivatives, as described by Mellonig,[117] is as follows (Figure 67-10):

1. Raise a flap for reconstructive purposes (see Chapter 65).
2. Remove all granulation tissue and tissue tags, exposing the underlying bone, and remove all root deposits by hand, ultrasonic scaling, or both.
3. Completely control bleeding within the defect.
4. Demineralize the root surface with citric acid (pH of 1.0), or preferably with 24% ethylenediaminetetraacetic acid (EDTA Biora) (pH of 6.7) for 15 seconds. This removes the smear layer and facilitates adherence of the Emdogain.
5. Rinse the wound with saline, and apply the gel to cover the exposed root surface completely. Avoid contamination with blood or saliva.
6. Close the wound with sutures. Perfect abutment of the flaps is necessary; if this cannot be obtained, correct the scalloping of the gingival margin or perform a slight osteoplasty. Although placement of the dressing is optional, it may protect the wound.

Systemic antibiotic coverage for 10 to 21 days is recommended (doxycycline, 100 mg daily).

Heijl et al.[84] compared the use of enamel matrix derivatives with a placebo in 33 patients with 34 paired test and control sites, mostly one-wall and two-wall defects, followed for 3 years. They found a statistically significant radiographic bone gain of 2.6 mm. Froum et al.[65] reported that use of Emdogain resulted in a reduction in probing depth of 4.94 mm, increase in attachment level of 4.26 mm, and bone fill of 3.83 mm (74% of defects).

In a histologic study of 10 defects in eight patients, Yukna and Mellonig[205] reported evidence of regeneration (new cementum, bone, and periodontal ligament) in three specimens, new attachment (connective tissue attachment, adhesion only) in three specimens, and a long junctional epithelium in four specimens. No evidence of root resorption or ankylosis was found.

Other studies suggest that enamel matrix proteins have characteristics that could enhance periodontal regeneration. For example, the enamel matrix proteins promote bone cell attachment and cell spreading[88] and enhance the proliferation of more immature bone cells while stimulating the differentiation of more mature bone cells.[169] An in vitro wound-healing model demonstrated that the enamel matrix derivative enhanced human

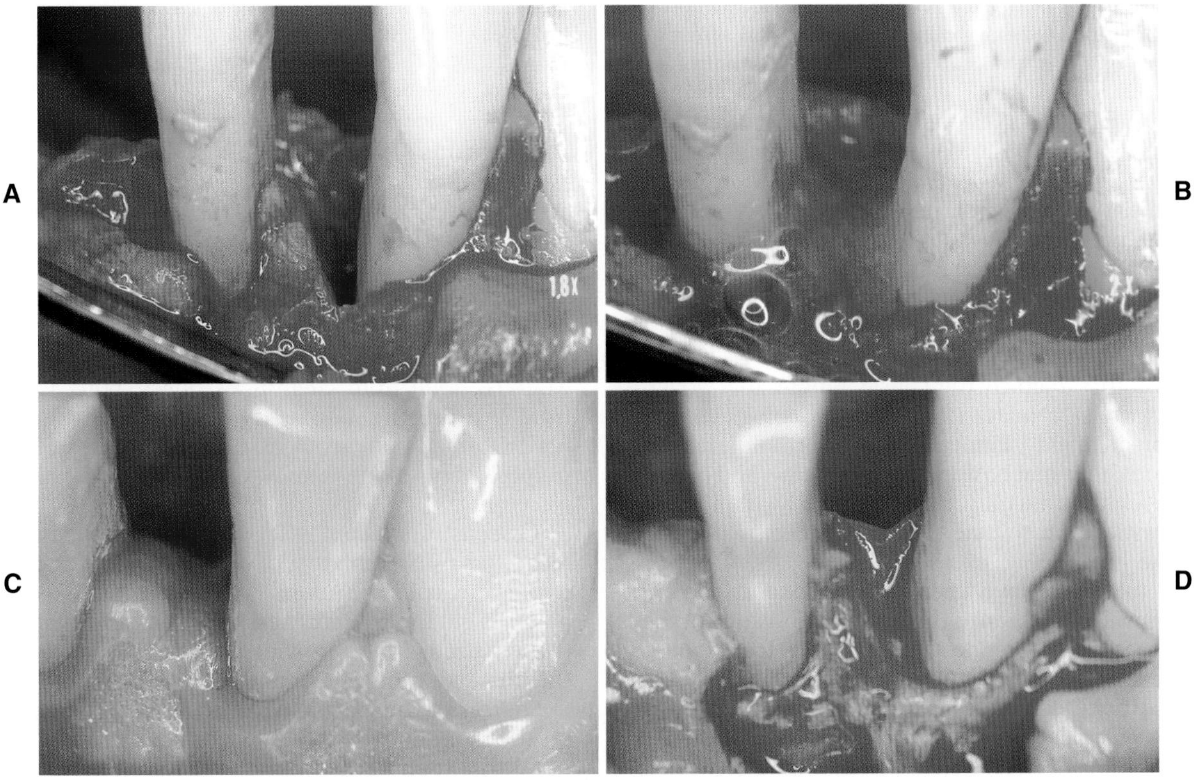

Figure 67-10 **A,** Deep vertical bone loss distal to lower left central incisor. **B,** Area flapped, root prepared, and defect filled with enamel matrix protein (Emdogain). **C,** Postoperative photo 6 months later. **D,** Reentry surgery showing extensive bone fill. (Courtesy Dr. Marco Orsini, Aquila, Italy.)

periodontal ligament fibroblast cell wound healing.[89] Additionally, the enamel matrix derivative is not osteoinductive, but it is "osteopromotive" in that it stimulates bone formation when combined with demineralized freeze-dried bone allograft.[19]

As mentioned earlier, the type of attachment achieved during periodontal reconstructive therapy can only be determined histologically. In two studies involving baboons, the use of enamel matrix derivative alone or in combination with autogenous bone grafting resulted in significantly enhanced histologic periodontal reconstruction. This stimulated tissue response occurred in one-wall periodontal defects ranging from 1 to 6 mm. These data and the results from many other studies support the clinical use of enamel matrix derivatives to stimulate periodontal tissue reconstruction around teeth.

Graft Materials and Procedures

Numerous therapeutic grafting modalities for restoring periodontal osseous defects have been investigated. Material to be grafted can be obtained from the same individual (autografts), from a different individual of the same species (allografts), or from a different species (xenografts).

Bone graft materials are generally evaluated based on their osteogenic, osteoinductive, or osteoconductive potential. *Osteogenesis* refers to the formation or development of new bone by cells contained in the graft. *Osteoinduction* is a chemical process by which molecules contained in the graft (bone morphogenetic proteins) convert the neighboring cells into osteoblasts, which in turn form bone. *Osteoconduction* is a physical effect by which the matrix of the graft forms a scaffold that favors outside cells to penetrate the graft and form new bone.

Periodontal defects as sites for transplantation differ from osseous cavities surrounded by bony walls. Saliva and bacteria may easily penetrate along the root surface, and epithelial cells may proliferate into the defect, resulting in contamination and possible exfoliation of the grafts. Therefore the principles established to govern transplantation of bone or other materials into closed osseous cavities are not fully applicable to transplantation of bone into periodontal defects.[50]

Schallhorn[165] defined the considerations that govern the selection of a material as follows: biologic acceptability, predictability, clinical feasibility, minimal operative hazards, minimal postoperative sequelae, and patient acceptance. It is difficult to find a material with all these characteristics, and to date there is no ideal material or technique.

Graft materials have been developed and tried in many forms. To familiarize the reader with various types of graft material, as defined by either the technique or the material used, a brief discussion of each is provided.

All grafting techniques require presurgical scaling, occlusal adjustment as needed, and exposure of the defect with a full-thickness flap. The flap technique best suited for grafting purposes is the *papilla preservation flap* because it provides complete coverage of the interdental area after suturing (see Chapter 65). The use of antibiotics after the procedure is generally recommended.

A

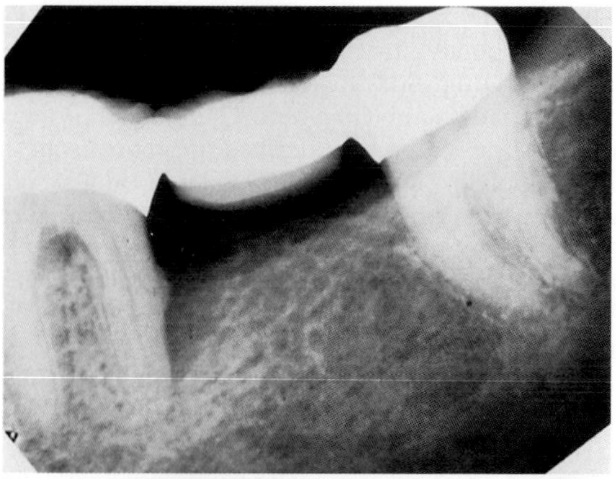

B

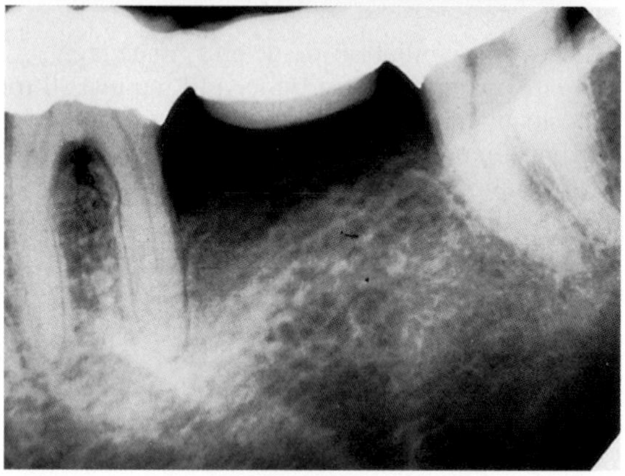

Figure 67-11 Bone defect on the distal root of a first molar treated with osseous coagulum implants. **A,** Before treatment. **B,** One year after treatment, showing bone repair. (Courtesy Dr. R. Earl Robinson.)

Autogenous Bone Grafts

Bone from Intraoral Sites. In 1923, Hegedüs[83] attempted to use bone grafts for the reconstruction of bone defects produced by periodontal disease. The method was revived by Nabers and O'Leary[129] in 1965, and numerous efforts have been made since that time to define its indications and technique.

Sources of bone include bone from healing extraction wounds, bone from edentulous ridges, bone trephined from within the jaw without damaging the roots, newly formed bone in wounds especially created for the purpose, and bone removed during osteoplasty and ostectomy.[29,77,85,86,155]

Osseous Coagulum. R. Earl Robinson described a technique using a mixture of bone dust and blood that he termed "osseous coagulum."[155] The technique uses small particles ground from cortical bone. The advantage of the particle size is that it provides additional surface area for the interaction of cellular and vascular elements.

Sources of the graft material include the lingual ridge on the mandible, exostoses, edentulous ridges, the bone distal to a terminal tooth, bone removed by osteoplasty or ostectomy, and the lingual surface of the mandible or maxilla at least 5 mm from the roots. Bone is removed with a carbide bur #6 or #8 at speeds between 5000 and 30,000 rpm, placed in a sterile dappen dish or amalgam

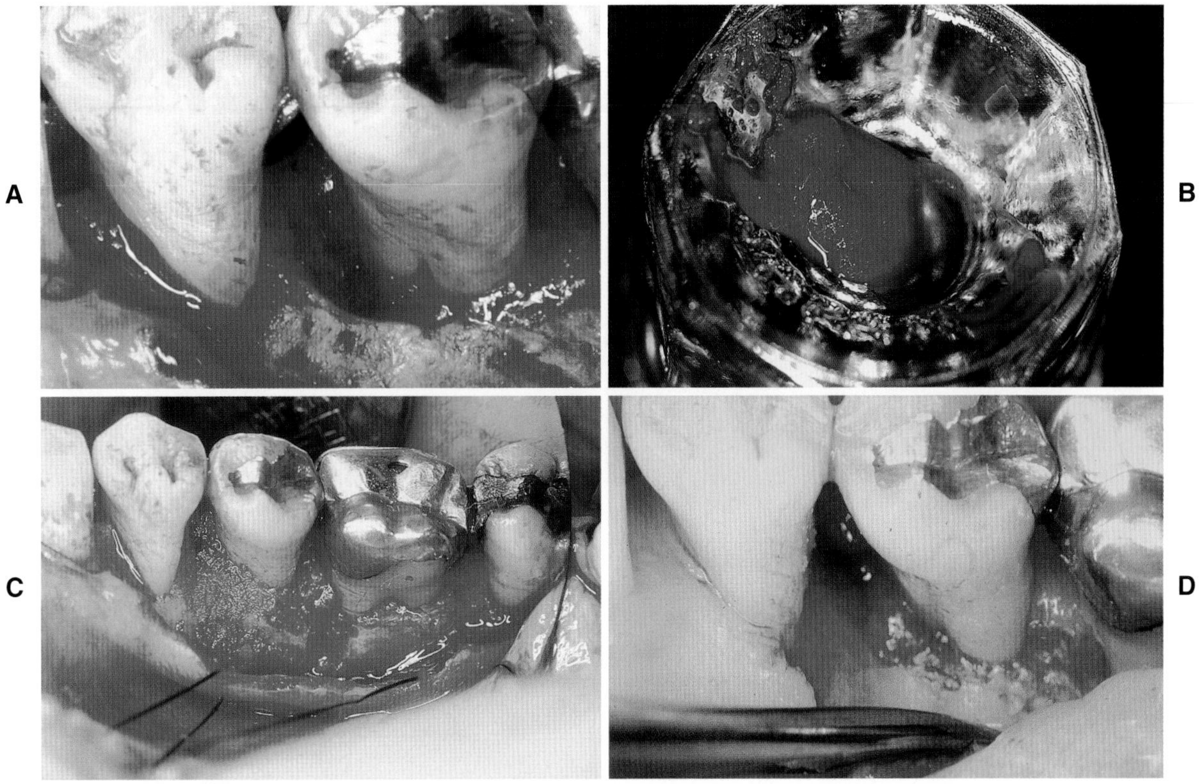

Figure 67-12 **A,** Osseous defect mesial to a second premolar. **B,** Graft material placed in dappen dish before transfer to the graft site. **C,** Material in place. **D,** Reentry 6 months later. (Courtesy Dr. E. Earl Robinson).

cloth, and used to fill the defect (Figure 67-11). The obvious advantage of this technique is the ease of obtaining bone from already-exposed surgical sites; its disadvantages are its relatively low predictability and the inability to procure adequate material for large defects.[60] Although notable success has been reported by many individuals (Figure 67-12), studies documenting the efficacy of the technique are still inconclusive.[41,61,63,154]

Bone Blend. Some disadvantages of osseous coagulum derive from the inability to use aspiration during accumulation of the coagulum; another problem is the unknown quantity and quality of the bone fragments in the collected material. To overcome these problems, the "bone blend technique" has been proposed.[45]

The bone blend technique uses an autoclaved plastic capsule and pestle. Bone is removed from a predetermined site, triturated in the capsule to a workable, plastic-like mass, and packed into bony defects. Froum et al.[61-63] have found osseous coagulum–bone blend procedures to be at least as effective as iliac autografts and open curettage.

Cancellous Bone Marrow Transplants. Cancellous bone can be obtained from the maxillary tuberosity, edentulous areas, and healing sockets.[86] The maxillary tuberosity frequently contains a good amount of cancellous bone, particularly if the third molars are not present; also, foci of red marrow are occasionally observed. After a ridge incision is made distally from the last molar, bone is removed with a curved and cutting rongeur. Care should be taken not to extend the incision too far distally to avoid sectioning the tendons of the palatine muscle; also, the location of the maxillary sinus must be analyzed on the radiograph to avoid cutting into it.

Edentulous ridges can be approached with a flap, and cancellous bone and marrow are removed with curettes, back-action chisels (Figure 67-13), or trephine (Figure 67-14). Sockets are allowed to heal for 8 to 12 weeks, and the apical portion is used as donor material. The particles are reduced to small pieces.

Bone Swaging. This technique requires an edentulous area adjacent to the defect, from which the bone is pushed into con-tact with the root surface without fracturing the bone at its base.[53,157] Bone swaging is technically difficult, and its usefulness is limited.

Bone From Extraoral Sites.

In 1923, Hegedüs also pioneered the use of extraoral sites as a source of bone for grafting into periodontal osseous defects, using bone from the tibia. Schallhorn and Hiatt revived this approach in the 1960s (see following discussion).

Iliac Autografts. The use of fresh or preserved iliac cancellous marrow bone has been extensively investigated. This material has been used by orthopedic surgeons for years. Data from human and animal studies support its use, and the technique has proved successful in bony defects with various numbers of walls, in furcations, and even supracrestally to some extent.* However, because of

*References 11, 22, 43, 46, 47, 162, 163, 168.

A B

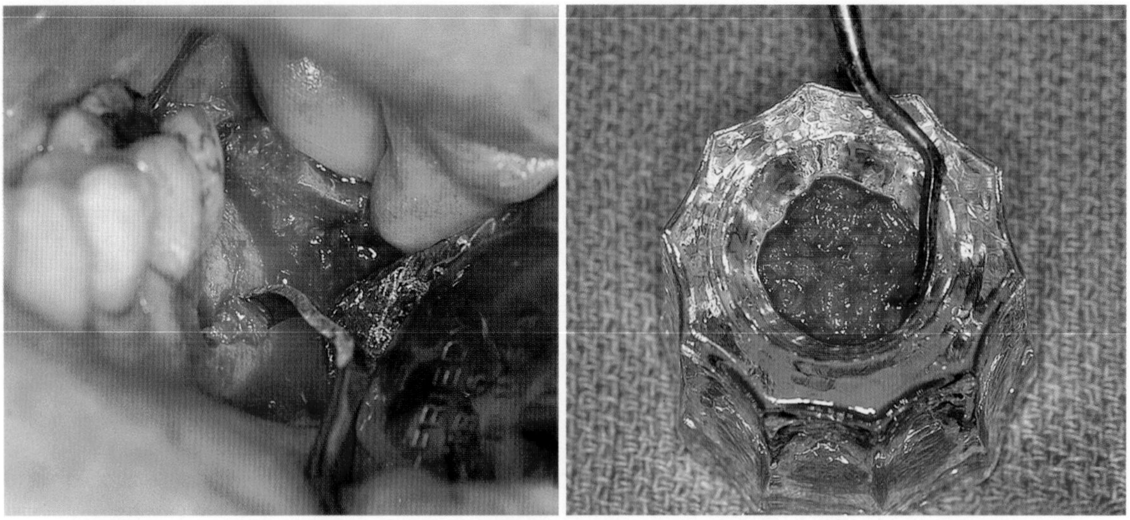

Figure 67-13 **A,** Bone particles obtained by use of back-action chisel, and **B,** placed in dappen dish.

A B C D

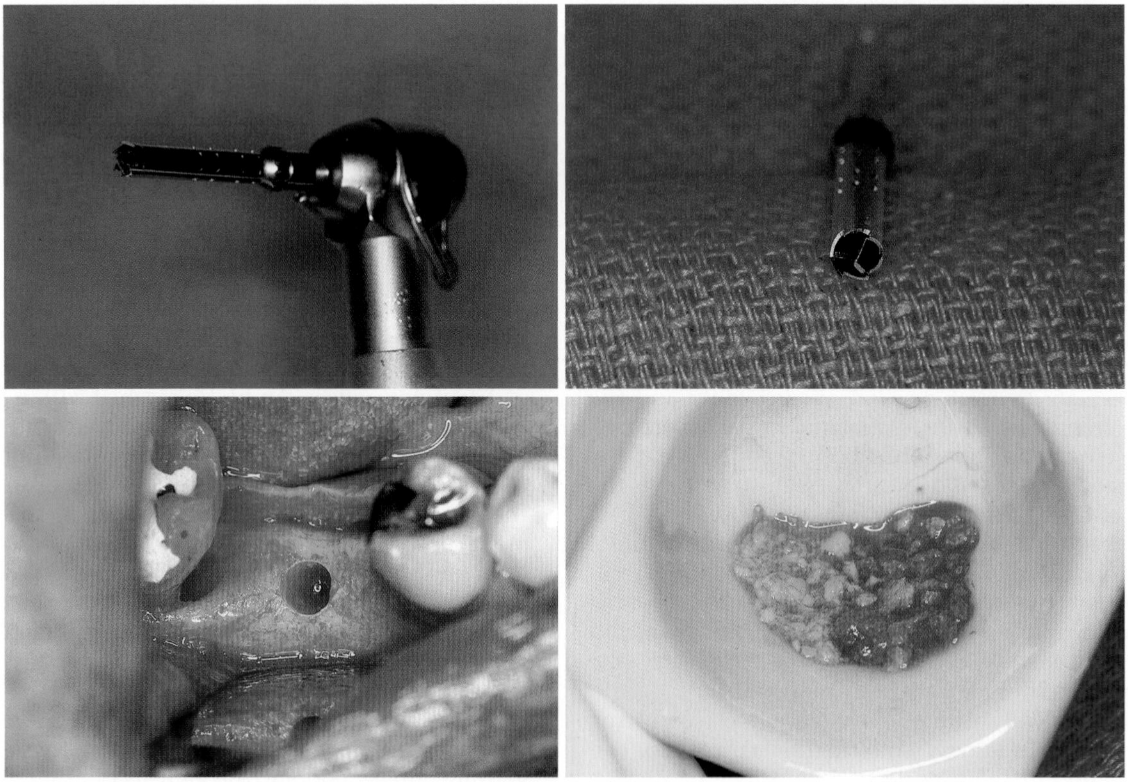

Figure 67-14 **A**, Trephine used for obtaining bone from adjoining jaw area. **B**, Frontal view of trephine. **C**, Donor site after harvesting. **D**, Harvested material placed in dappen dish.

problems associated with its use, such as postoperative infection, exfoliation, and sequestration; varying rates of healing; root resorption; and rapid recurrence of the defect (Figure 67-15), in addition to increased patient expense and difficulty in procuring the donor material, the technique is no longer in use.[22,47,164,165]

Allografts

Obtaining donor material for autograft purposes necessitates inflicting surgical trauma on another part of the patient's body. Obviously, it would be to the patient's and therapist's advantage if a suitable substitute could be used for grafting purposes that would offer similar

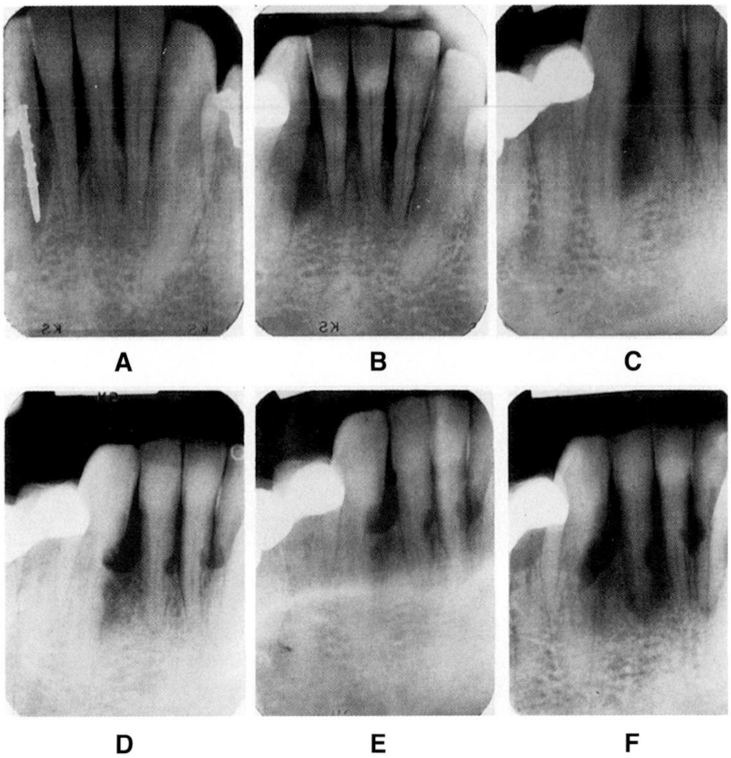

Figure 67-15 **A,** November 1973. Radiograph of a patient immediately before placement of a fresh iliac autograft. **B,** Two months later, bone repair is evident. Note the early radiolucent areas on the mesial aspect of the canine. **C,** After 7 months, "bone fill" is occurring, but obvious root resorption is present. **D,** April 1975. Root resorption is apparent on all grafted teeth. Note the obvious degree of fill of the original bone defects. **E,** February 1976. Further involvement. **F,** October 1977. Four years later, root resorption has progressed into the pulp of the lateral incisor, causing a periosteal-endosteal complication.

potential for repair and not require the additional surgical removal of donor material from the patient. However, both allografts and xenografts are foreign to the organism and therefore have the potential to provoke an immune response. Attempts have been made to suppress the antigenic potential of allografts and xenografts by radiation, freezing, and chemical treatment.[21]

Bone allografts are commercially available from tissue banks. They are obtained from cortical bone within 12 hours of the death of the donor, defatted, cut in pieces, washed in absolute alcohol, and deep-frozen. The material may then be demineralized, and subsequently ground and sieved to a particle size of 250 to 750 μm and freeze-dried. Finally, it is vacuum-sealed in glass vials.

Numerous steps are also taken to eliminate viral infectivity. These include exclusion of donors from known high-risk groups and various tests on the cadaver tissues to exclude individuals with any type of infection or malignant disease. The material is then treated with chemical agents or strong acids to inactivate the virus, if still present. The risk of human immunodeficiency virus (HIV) infection has been calculated as 1 in 1 to 8 million and is therefore characterized as highly remote.[122]

Undecalcified Freeze-Dried Bone Allograft. Several clinical studies by Mellonig, Bowers, and co-workers reported bone fill exceeding 50% in 67% of the defects grafted with freeze-dried bone allograft (FDBA) and in 78% of the defects grafted with FDBA plus autogenous bone.[129,158,171] FDBA, however, is considered an osteoconductive material, whereas decalcified FDBA (DFDBA) is considered an osteoinductive graft. Laboratory studies have found that DFDBA has a higher osteogenic potential than FDBA and is therefore preferred.[116,119,120]

Decalcified Freeze-Dried Bone Allograft. Experiments by Urist[192,193] have established the osteogenic potential of DFDBA. Demineralization in cold, diluted hydro-chloric acid exposes the components of bone matrix, which are closely associated with collagen fibrils and have been termed *bone morphogenetic proteins* (BMPs).[194]

In 1975, Libin et al.[106] reported three patients with 4 to 10 mm of bone regeneration in periodontal osseous defects. Subsequent clinical studies were made with cancellous DFDBA and cortical DFDBA.[137,147] The latter resulted in more desirable results (2.4 mm vs. 1.38 mm of bone fill).

Bowers et al.,[17] in a histologic study in humans, showed new attachment and periodontal regeneration in defects grafted with DFDBA. Mellonig et al.[119,120] tested DFDBA against autogenous materials in the calvaria of guinea pigs and showed it to have similar osteogenic potential.

These studies provided strong evidence that DFDBA in periodontal defects results in significant probing depth

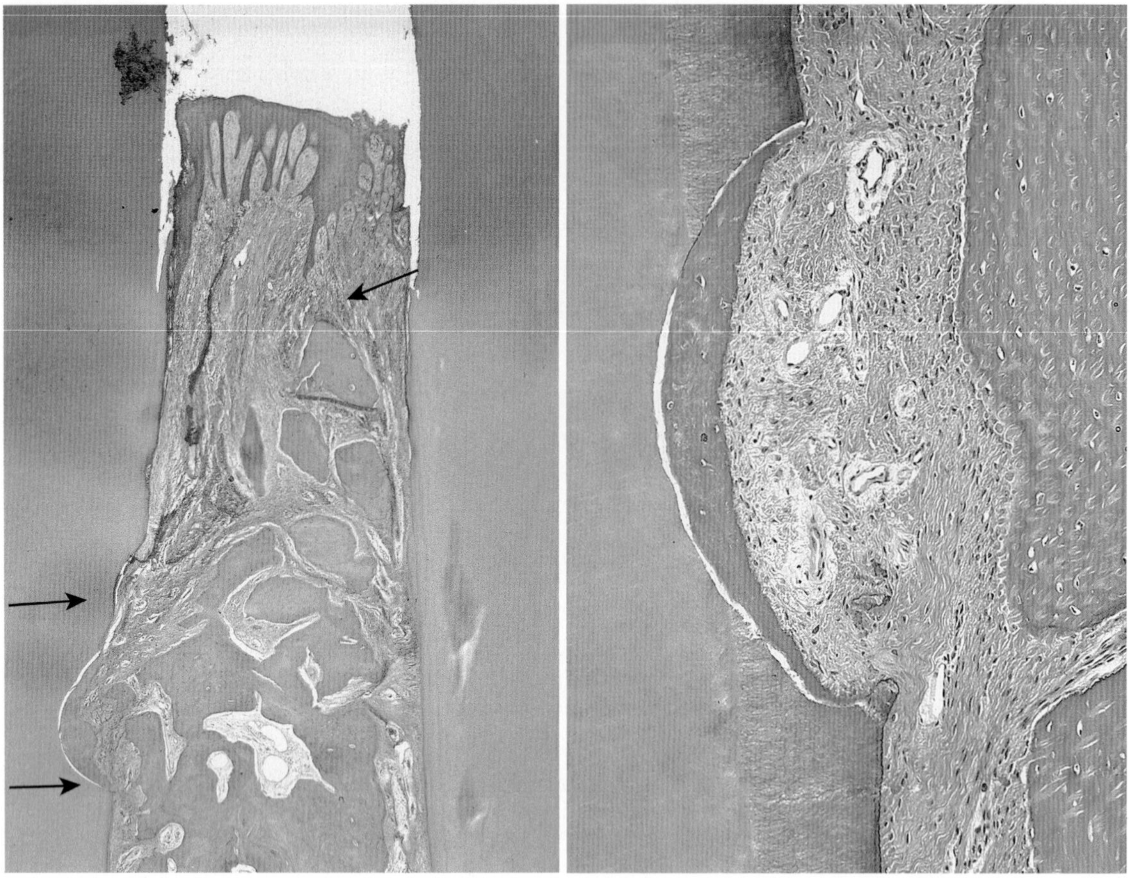

Figure 67-16 **A,** Six-month postoperative histologic block section of experimental site grafted with decalcified freeze-dried bone, depicting osseous regeneration coronal to the crestal bone notch. **B,** Higher magnification of reference notch through calculus at base of defect, showing new cementum (artifactual split during histologic preparation), new bone, and new periodontal ligament. (Courtesy Dr. Gerald Bowers, University of Maryland, College Park, Md.)

reduction, attachment level gain, and osseous regeneration (Figure 67-16); the combination of DFDBA and GTR has also proved to be very successful.[6,166] However, limitations of the use of DFDBA include the possible, although remote, potential of disease transfer from the cadaver.

A bone-inductive protein isolated from the extracellular matrix of human bones, termed *osteogenin* or BMP3, has been tested in human periodontal defects and seems to enhance osseous regeneration.[18]

Xenografts

Calf bone (Boplant), treated by detergent extraction, sterilized, and freeze-dried, has been used for the treatment of osseous defects.[7,170] Kiel bone is calf or ox bone denatured with 20% hydrogen peroxide, dried with acetone, and sterilized with ethylene oxide. Anorganic bone is ox bone from which the organic material has been extracted by means of ethylenediamine; it is then sterilized by autoclaving.[115] These materials have been tried and discarded for various reasons; they are mentioned here to provide a historical perspective.

Currently, an anorganic, bovine-derived bone marketed under the brand name Bio-Oss (OsteoHealth) has been successfully used both for periodontal defects and in implant surgery. It is an osteoconductive, porous bone mineral matrix from bovine cancellous or cortical bone. The organic components of the bone are removed, but the trabecular architecture and porosity are retained.[26,118] The physical features permit clot stabilization and revascularization to allow for migration of osteoblasts, leading to osteogenesis. Bio-Oss is biocompatible with the adjacent tissues, eliciting no systemic immune response.

Several studies have reported successful bone regeneration and new attachment with Bio-Oss in periodontal defects,[26,118] as well as regeneration around implants and sinus grafting (Figure 67-17) (see Chapter 77).

Periodontally, Bio-Oss has been used as a graft material covered with a resorbable membrane (Bio-Guide). The membrane prevents the migration of fibroblasts and connective tissues into the pores and between the granules of the graft. Histologic studies of this technique have shown significant osseous regeneration and cementum formation.

Yukna et al.[208] have used Bio-Oss in combination with a cell-binding polypeptide (P-15) that is a synthetic analog of a 15–amino acid sequence of type I collagen. Marketed as Pepgen P-15 (Dentsply/Ceramed), this

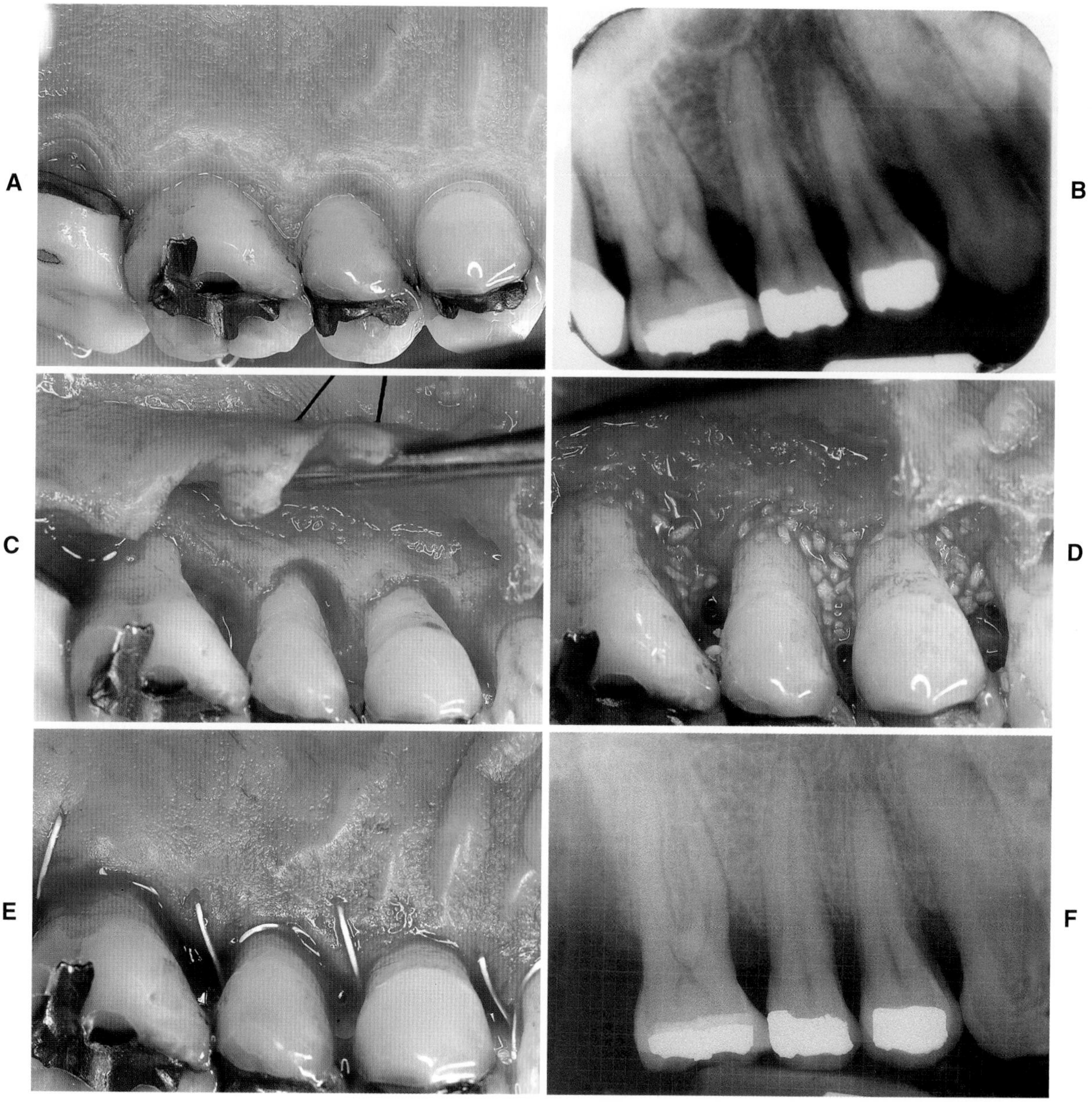

Figure 67-17 **A,** Palatal view of premolar and molar area. **B,** Radiographs show bone loss mesially to first molar and first and second premolars. **C,** After raising a flap, areas of periodontal bone loss are clearly seen. **D,** Teeth undergo careful root planing, and Bio-Oss graft is placed in the defects. **E,** Area is sutured. **F,** Postoperative radiograph at 9 months shows bone repair. (Courtesy Dr. Philip Melnick, Los Angeles.)

combination seems to enhance the bone-regenerative results of the matrix alone in periodontal defects.

Nonbone Graft Materials

In addition to bone graft materials, many nonbone graft materials have been tried for restoration of the periodontium. These include sclera, dura, cartilage, cementum, dentin, plaster of Paris, plastic materials, ceramics, and coral-derived materials.* None offers a reliable substitute to bone graft materials; some of these materials are briefly presented here to offer a complete picture of the many attempts that have been made to solve the crucial problem of periodontal regeneration.

Sclera. Sclera was originally used in periodontal procedures because it is a dense, fibrous connective tissue with poor vascularity and minimal cellularity.[95-97] This affords a low incidence of antigenicity and other untoward reactions.[91] In addition, sclera may provide a barrier to apical migration of the junctional epithelium and serve to protect the blood clot during the initial healing period.

Although some studies show that sclera is well accepted by the host and is sometimes invaded by host

*References 23, 52, 104, 105, 131, 160.

cells and capillaries and replaced by dense connective tissue, it does not appear to induce osteogenesis or cementogenesis.[54,128,135,191] The available scientific research does not warrant the routine use of sclera in periodontal therapy.

Cartilage. Cartilage has been used for repair studies in monkeys and treatment of periodontal defects in humans.[159-161] It can serve as a scaffolding; when so used, new attachment was obtained in 60 of 70 case studies.[161] However, cartilage has received only limited evaluation.

Plaster Of Paris. Plaster of Paris (calcium sulfate) is biocompatible and porous, thereby allowing fluid exchange, which prevents flap necrosis. Plaster of Paris resorbs completely in 1 to 2 weeks. One study in surgically created three-wall defects in dogs showed significant regeneration of bone and cementum.[94] Plaster of Paris was found to be useful in one uncontrolled clinical study, but other investigators have reported that it does not induce bone formation.[1,172] One report suggested its use in combination with DFDBA and a Gore-Tex membrane.[176] Its usefulness in human cases, however, has not been proved.

Plastic Materials. HTR polymer is a nonresorbable, microporous, biocompatible composite of polymethylmethacrylate and polyhydroxyethylmethacrylate. A clinical 6-month study showed significant defect fill and improved attachment level. Histologically, this material is encapsulated by connective tissue fibers, with no evidence of new attachment.[203]

Calcium Phosphate Biomaterials. Several calcium phosphate biomaterials have been tested since the mid-1970s and are currently available for clinical use. Calcium phosphate biomaterials have excellent tissue compatibility and do not elicit any inflammation or foreign body response. These materials are osteoconductive, not osteoinductive, meaning that they will induce bone formation when placed next to viable bone but not when surrounded by non–bone-forming tissue such as skin.

Two types of calcium phosphate ceramics have been used, as follows:

1. Hydroxyapatite (HA) has a calcium-to-phosphate ratio of 1.67, similar to that found in bone material. HA is generally nonbioresorbable.
2. Tricalcium phosphate (TCP), with a calcium-to-phosphate ratio of 1.5, is mineralogically B-whitlockite. TCP is at least partially bioresorbable.

Case reports and uncontrolled human studies have shown that calcium phosphate bioceramic materials are well tolerated and can result in clinical repair of periodontal lesions. Several controlled studies were conducted on the use of Periograf and Calcitite; clinical results were good, but histologically these materials appeared to be encapsulated by collagen.[64,113,148,206]

Bioactive Glass. Bioactive glass consists of sodium and calcium salts, phosphates, and silicon dioxide; for its dental applications, it is used in the form of irregular particles measuring 90 to 170 µm (PerioGlas, Block Drug, Jersey City, NJ) or 300 to 355 µm (BioGran, Ortho Vita, Malvern, Pa). When this material comes into contact with tissue fluids, the surface of the particles becomes coated with hydroxycarbonate apatite, incorporates organic ground proteins such as chondroitin sulfate and glycosaminoglycans, and attracts osteoblasts that rapidly form bone.[5]

These bioactive glass materials also appear to be encapsulated by collagen.

Coral-Derived Materials. Two different coralline materials have been used in clinical periodontics: natural coral and coral-derived porous hydroxyapatite. Both are biocompatible, but whereas natural coral is resorbed slowly (several months), porous hydroxyapatite is not resorbed or takes years for resorption.

Clinical studies on these materials showed pocket reduction, attachment gain, and bone level gain.[87,92,93] Coral-derived materials have also been studied in conjunction with membranes, with good results.[101,181] Both materials have demonstrated microscopic cementum and bone formation, but their slow resorbability or lack of resorption has hindered clinical success in practice.[28,178]

Combined Techniques

Several clinicians have proposed a combination of several of the techniques previously described in an attempt to enhance their results.*

A classic paper published by Schallhorn and McClain[166] in 1988 described a combination technique using graft material, root conditioning with citric acid, and coverage with a nonresorbable membrane (the only available one at the time).[167] More recently, with the advent of osteopromotive agents, such as the enamel matrix derivative (Emdogain) and osteoconductive bovine-derived anorganic bone (Bio-Oss) graft materials, other combination techniques have been advocated.[104] The combined use of these products, along with autogenous bone with resorbable membrane coverage, has resulted in an increased percentage of cases with successful new attachment and periodontal reconstruction (Figures 67-18 and 67-19).

Froum et al.[65] have analyzed the criteria that should guide the choice of treatment technique. They believe that clinical results depend on (1) the dimension and morphology of the defect (deeper lesions result in greater bone fill than shallower defects), (2) the number of walls in the defect[71] (three-wall defects have greater potential to fill than two-wall or one-wall defects), (3) the amount of root surface exposed and the ability to obtain adequate flap coverage,[86,180] and (4) the angle of the defect to the long axis of the tooth[184] (the smaller the angle, the better chance of success). On the basis of these criteria, Froum et al.[61] established the following clinical decision tree:

For Deep, Well-Contained Defects
Use EMD alone,
with a coronally advanced flap (if necessary).

For Moderate to Deep, Noncontained defects
Use EMD + graft,
with a coronally advanced flap (if necessary).

*References 6, 79, 101, 112, 115, 196.

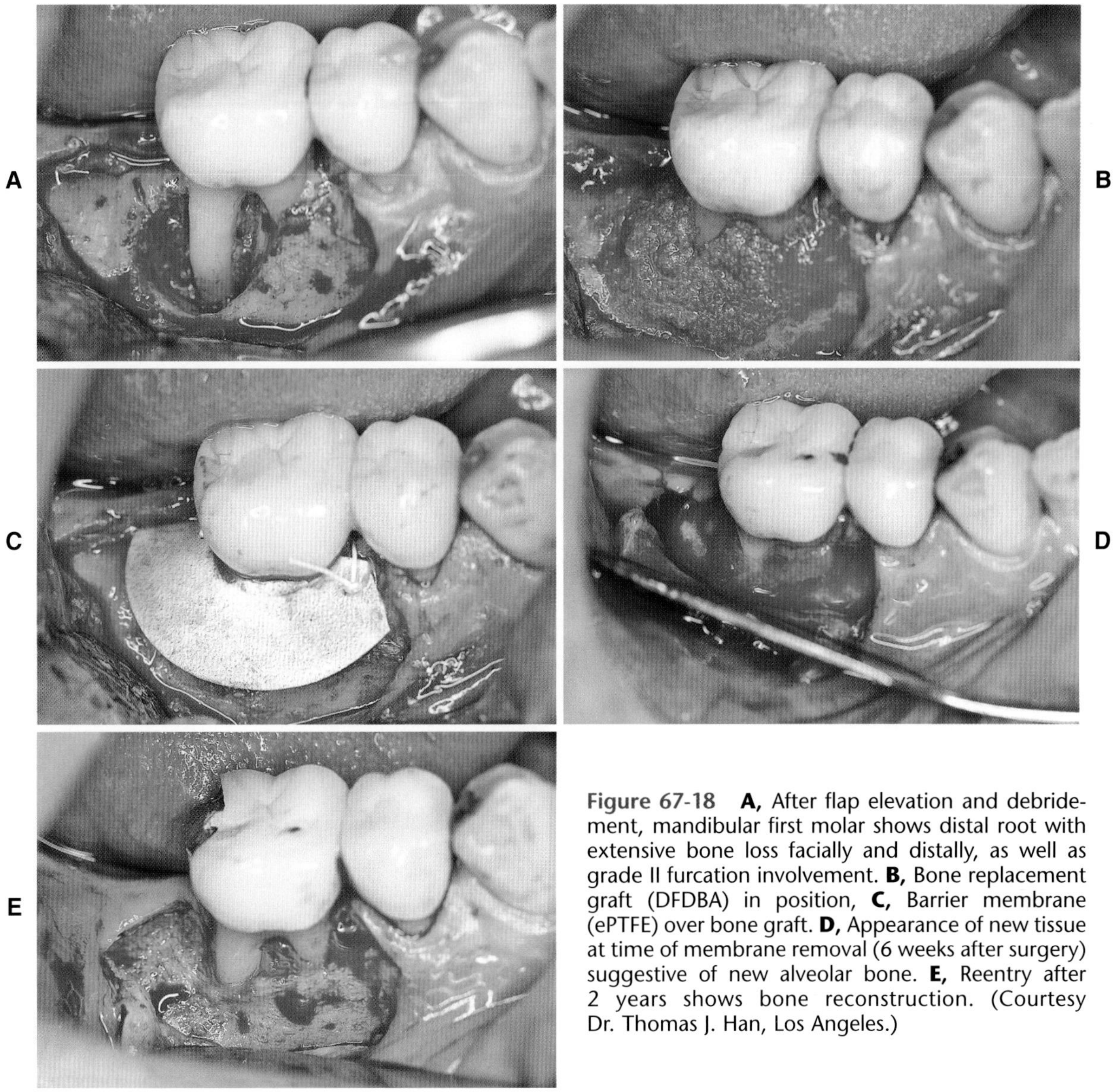

Figure 67-18 **A,** After flap elevation and debridement, mandibular first molar shows distal root with extensive bone loss facially and distally, as well as grade II furcation involvement. **B,** Bone replacement graft (DFDBA) in position, **C,** Barrier membrane (ePTFE) over bone graft. **D,** Appearance of new tissue at time of membrane removal (6 weeks after surgery) suggestive of new alveolar bone. **E,** Reentry after 2 years shows bone reconstruction. (Courtesy Dr. Thomas J. Han, Los Angeles.)

For Supracrestal Defects with a Shallow Vertical Defect
Use EMD + graft + barrier membrane, with a coronally advanced flap.

From Froum S, Lemler J, Horowitz R, Davidson B: *Int J Periodont Restor Dent* 21:437, 2001, and Froum SJ, Weinberg MA, Rosenberg E, Tarnow D: *J Periodontol* 72:25, 2001.
EMD, Enamel matrix derivative.

SUMMARY

Based on available information, a clinically significant reconstruction of human supporting periodontal tissues is possible in select sites and patients with the use of autogenous bone grafts, demineralized freeze-dried bone allografts, and enamel matrix proteins. The advantage of covering the area in all cases with barrier membranes is not yet conclusive.

The future of periodontal reconstruction techniques will depend on the emergence of new products, which will lead to a predictable positive outcome when used in proper combination in select defects. The clinician should attempt to differentiate between techniques that have been studied in depth and with acceptable results and those that are still experimental, although promising. Research papers must be critically evaluated for adequacy of controls, selection of cases, methods of evaluation, and long-term postoperative results. In addition, the clinician should remember that he or she is seeking "clinical" success, which is not always similar to "statistical" success. A gain in clinical attachment of half a millimeter may be statistically significant but not clinically significant.

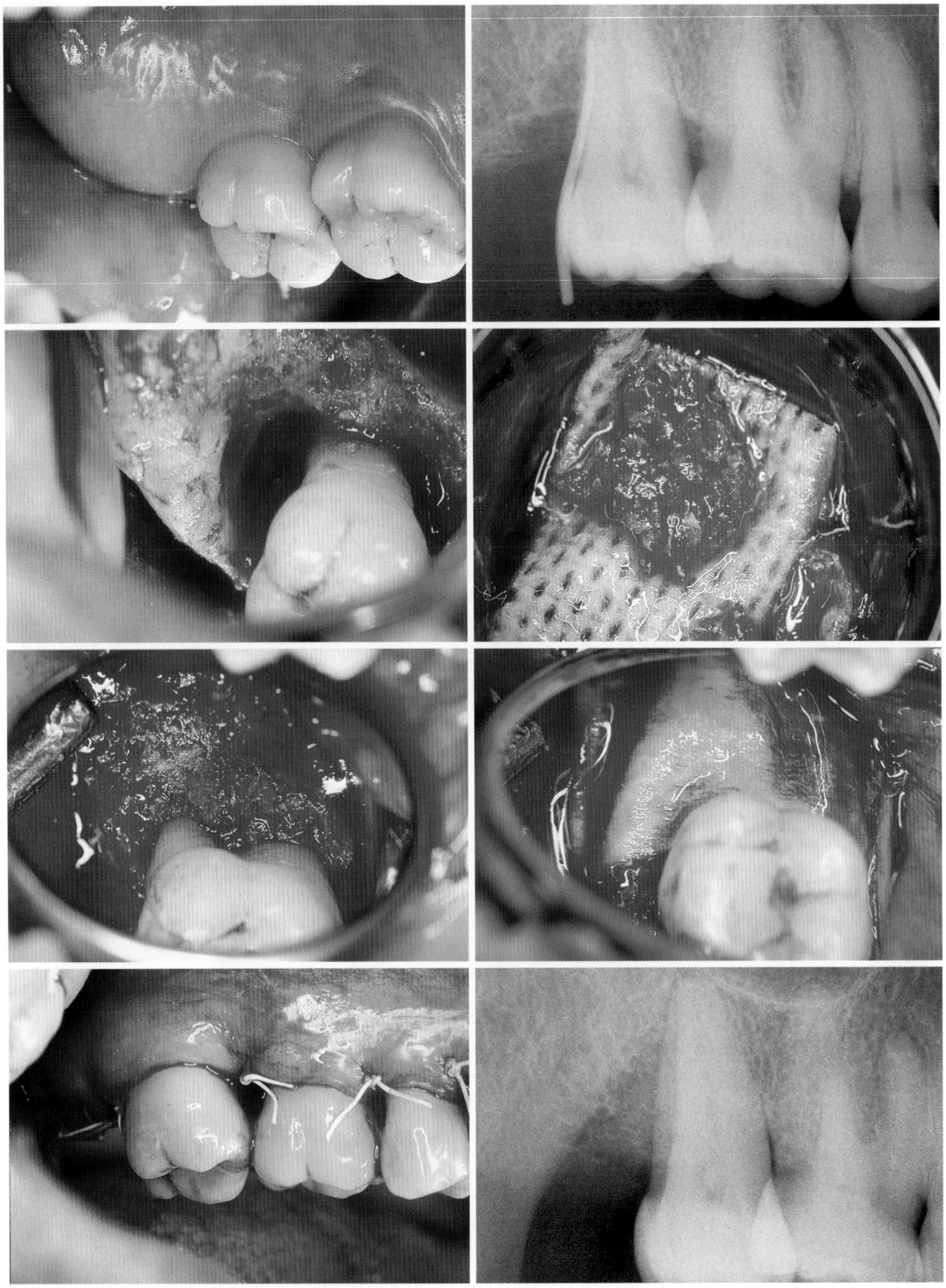

Figure 67-19 **A,** Preoperative view of maxillary first and second molar area. **B,** Preoperative radiograph of second molar showing deep, distal vertical bone loss with a radiopaque pointer to indicate pocket depth. **C,** Clinical view of three-wall osseous defect distal to second molar. **D,** Autogenous bone procured from adjacent area undergoing resective osseous surgery placed in defect. **E,** Autogenous bone placed in defect after scaling and root planing. **F,** Bioresorbable membrane placed over graft to protect it. **G,** Area sutured. **H,** Postoperative radiograph at 6 months showing defect fill.

SCIENCE TRANSFER

Reconstructive periodontal surgical procedures provide the most dramatic improvement in the treatment of intrabony defects of all currently available modalities. Many well-controlled studies of interdental lesions show pocket depth reductions of up to 4 mm, with associated similar attachment level gains and fill of osseous defects. Reconstructive surgical treatment of furcation lesions has a more moderate result but still is superior to other surgical and nonsurgical therapies. Reports also show that these initial postsurgical gains are maintained for 3 to 5 years in patients who comply with normal maintenance schedules. A wide variety of materials have provided similar results, including decalcified freeze-dried bone, porous calcium phosphate, and hydroxyapatite materials, including those from bovine bone, autogenous bone, and enamel matrix proteins. Combinations of some of these materials with resorbable membranes, platelet-enriched plasma, and platelet-derived growth factors seem to provide additional benefits.

Although many different materials have been used to fill intrabony periodontal defects,the results are that the material (1) disappears over time, (2) becomes encapsulated by fibrous tissue, or (3) becomes surrounded by bone. The amount of the defect that is filled by bone (and presumably periodontal ligament and cementum) varies but in optimal cases is 70% to 75% fill. Because many materials result in 50% to 75% bone fill, the material may not be as critical as *how the wound healing occurs and how the material supports the wound healing.* For example, better results might occur when the graft material provides stability for the wound clot and adhesion for the proteins in the clot. If the proteins cannot adhere well to the graft material, the outcome of the procedure may be compromised. Similarly, if the graft material is not stabilized or is remodeling or dissolving over time, again the outcome may be compromised.

Another critical component of the wound-healing process may be the *timing* of cellular invasion and binding within the wound clot and of proteolytic events that must occur during the process. All these events are difficult to study and have not been addressed systematically. Future advancements in periodontal regeneration may require an understanding of such factors.

REFERENCES

1. Alderman NE: Sterile plaster of Paris as an implant in the infrabony environment: a preliminary study, *J Periodontol* 40:11, 1969.
2. Alger FA, Solt CW, Vuddahanok S, et al: The histologic evaluation of new attachment in periodontally diseased human roots treated with tetracycline hydrochloride and fibronectin, *J Periodontol* 61:447, 1990.
3. American Academy of Periodontology: *Glossary of periodontal terms,* ed 3, Chicago, 1992, The Academy.
4. American Dental Association, Council on Scientific Affairs: Products designed to regenerate periodontal tissues: acceptance program guidelines, 1997.
5. Andereeg CR, Alexander DC, Freidman M: A bioactive glass particulate in the treatment of molar furcations, *J Periodontol* 70:384, 1999.
6. Andereeg CR, Martin SJ, Gray JL, et al: Clinical evaluation of the use of decalcified freeze-dried bone allograft with guided tissue regeneration in the treatment of molar furcation invasions, *J Periodontol* 62:264, 1991.
7. Arrocha R, Wittwer J, Gargiulo A: Tissue response to heterogenous bone implantation in dogs, *J Periodontol* 39:162, 1968.
8. Becker W, Becker BE, Berg L, et al: Clinical and volumetric analysis of three-wall intrabony defects following open flap debridement, *J Periodontol* 57:277, 1986.
9. Becker W, Becker BE, Berg L, et al: New attachment after treatment with root isolation procedures: report for treated class III and class II furcations and vertical osseous defects, *Int J Periodont Restor Dent* 8(3):9, 1988.
10. Becker W, Becker BE, Prichard JF, et al: Root isolation for new attachment procedures: a surgical and suturing method: three case reports, *J Periodontol* 58:819, 1987.
11. Bierly JA, Sottosanti JS, Costley JM, et al: An evaluation of the osteogenic potential of marrow, *J Periodontol* 46:277, 1975.
12. Bjorn H: Experimental studies on reattachment, *Dent Pract* 11:351, 1961.
13. Bjorn H, Hollender L, Lindhe J: Tissue regeneration in patients with periodontal disease, *Odont Rev* 16:317, 1965.
14. Blumenthal NM: The use of collagen materials in bone grafted defects to enhance guided tissue regeneration, *Periodont Case Rep* 9:16, 1987.
15. Blumenthal NM: The use of collagen membranes to guide regeneration of new connective tissue attachment in dogs, *J Periodontol* 59:830, 1988.
16. Blumenthal NM, Steinberg J: The use of collagen membrane barriers in conjunction with combined demineralized bone-collagen gel implants in human infrabony defects, *J Periodontol* 61:319, 1990.
17. Bowers GM, Chadroff B, Carnevale R, et al: Histologic evaluation of new attachment apparatus formation in humans. Part III, *J Periodontol* 60:683, 1989.
18. Bowers G, Felton F, Middleton F, et al: Histologic comparison of regeneration in human intrabony pockets when osteogenin is combined with demineralized freeze-dried bone allograft and with purified bovine collagen, *J Periodontol* 62:690, 1991.
19. Boyan BD, Weesner TC, Lohmann CH et al: Porcine fetal enamel matrix derivative enhances bone formation induced by demineralized freeze-dried bone allograft in vivo, *J Periodontol* 71:1278, 2000.
20. Brookes SJ, Robinson C, Kirkham J, Bonass WA: Biochemistry and molecular biology of amelogenin proteins of developing dental enamel, *Arch Oral Biol* 40:1, 1995.
21. Buring K, Urist MR: Effects of ionizing radiation on the bone induction principle in the matrix of bone implants, *Clin Orthop* 55:225, 1967.

22. Burnette WE: Fate of the iliac crest graft, *J Periodontol* 43:88, 1972.
23. Busschopp J, De Boever J: Clinical and histological characteristics of lyophilized allogenic dura mater in periodontal bony defects in humans, *J Clin Periodontol* 10:399, 1983.
24. Caffesse RG, Nasjleti CE, Anderson GB, et al: Periodontal healing following guided tissue regeneration with citric acid and fibronectin application, *J Periodontol* 62:21, 1991.
25. Caffesse RG, Smith BA, Nasjleti CE, et al: Cell proliferation after flap surgery, root conditioning and fibronectin application, *J Periodontol* 58:661, 1987.
26. Carmelo M, Nevins M, Schenk R, et al: Clinical, radiographic and histologic evaluation of human periodontal defects treated with Bio-Oss and Bio-Guide, *Int J Periodont Restor Dent* 18:321, 1998.
27. Carranza FA Sr: A technic for reattachment, *J Periodontol* 25:272, 1954.
28. Carranza FA Jr, Kenney EB, Lekovic V, et al: Histologic study of healing of human periodontal defects after placement of porous hydroxyapatite implants, *J Periodontol* 58:682, 1987.
29. Carraro JJ, Sznajder N, Alonso CA: Intraoral cancellous bone autografts in treatment of infrabony pockets, *J Clin Periodontol* 3:104, 1976.
30. Caton JC: Overview of clinical trials on periodontal regeneration, *Ann Periodontol* 2:215, 1987.
31. Caton J, Zander H: Osseous repair of an infrabony pocket without new attachment of connective tissue, *J Clin Periodontol* 3:54, 1976.
32. Caton JG, DeFuria EL, Polson AM, et al: Periodontal regeneration via selective cell repopulation, *J Periodontol* 58:546, 1987.
33. Caton J, Wagener C, Polson A, et al: Guided tissue regeneration in interproximal defects in monkeys, *Int J Periodont Restor Dent* 12:267, 1992.
34. Cerny R, Slaby I, Hammarstrom L, Wurtz T: A novel gene expressed in a rat ameloblasts codes for proteins with cell binding domains, *J Bone Miner Res* 11:883, 1995.
35. Chung KM, Salkin LM, Stein MD, et al: Clinical evaluation of a biodegradable collagen membrane in guided tissue regeneration, *J Periodontol* 61:732, 1990.
36. Claffey N, Hahn R, Egelberg J: Effect of placement of occlusive membranes on root resorption and bone regeneration during healing of circumferential periodontal defects in dogs, *J Clin Periodontol* 14:371, 1989.
37. Cochran DL, Wozney JM: Biological mediators for periodontal regeneration, *Periodontol 2000* 19:40, 1999.
38. Cochran DL, Wennström JL, Funakoshi E, Heijl L: *Biomimetics in periodontal regeneration,* Carol Stream, Ill, 2003, Quintessence.
39. Cortellini G, Tonetti MS: Focus on intrabony defects: guided tissue regeneration, *Periodontol 2000* 22:104, 2000.
40. Cortellini P, Pini Prato G, Tonetti M: Periodontal regeneration of human infrabony defects with bioresorbable membranes: a controlled clinical study, *J Periodontol* 67:217, 1996.
41. Coverly L, Toto P, Gargiulo A: Osseous coagulum: a histologic evaluation, *J Periodontol* 46:596, 1975.
42. Crigger M, Bogle G, Nilvéus R, et al: Effect of topical citric acid application in the healing of experimental furcation defects in dogs, *J Periodontal Res* 13:538, 1978.
43. Cushing M: Autogenous red marrow grafts: potential for induction of osteogenesis, *J Periodontol* 40:492, 1969.
44. Daly CG: Antibacterial effect of citric acid treatment of periodontally diseased root surface "in vitro," *J Clin Periodontol* 9:386, 1982.
45. Diem CR, Bowers GM, Moffitt WC: Bone blending: a technique for osseous implants, *J Periodontol* 43:295, 1972.
46. Dragoo MR, Irwin RK: A method of procuring cancellous iliac bone utilizing a trephine needle, *J Periodontol* 43:82, 1972.
47. Dragoo MR, Sullivan HC: A clinical and histologic evaluation of autogenous iliac bone grafts in humans. Part II. External root resorption, *J Periodontol* 44:614, 1973.
48. Eickholz P, Hausmann E: Evidence for healing of class II and III furcations after GTR therapy: digital subtraction and clinical measurements, *J Periodontol* 68:636, 1997.
49. Eickholz P, Hausmann E: Evidence for healing of interproximal intrabony defects after conventional and regenerative therapy: digital radiography and clinical measurements, *J Periodontal Res* 33:156, 1998.
50. Ellegaard B: Bone grafts in periodontal attachment procedures, *J Clin Periodontol* 3:5, 1976.
51. Ellegaard B, Karring T, Löe H: Retardation of epithelial migration in new attachment attempts in intrabony defects in monkeys, *J Clin Periodontol* 3:23, 1976.
52. Ellegaard B, Nielsen IM, Karring T: Lyodura grafts in new attachment procedures, *J Dent Res* 55(special issue B):304, 1976.
53. Ewen SJ: Bone swaging, *J Periodontol* 36:57, 1965.
54. Feingold JP, Chasens AI, Doyle J, et al: Preserved scleral allografts on periodontal defects in man. II. Histologic evaluation, *J Periodontol* 48:4, 1977.
55. Fernyhough W, Page RC: Attachment, growth and synthesis of human gingival fibroblasts on demineralized or fibronectin-treated normal and diseased tooth roots, *J Periodontol* 54:133, 1983.
56. Fine DH, Morris ML, Tabak L, et al: Preliminary characterization of material eluted from the roots of periodontally diseased teeth, *J Periodontal Res* 15:10, 1980.
57. Flanary DB, Twohey SM, Gray JL, et al: The use of a synthetic skin substitute as a physical barrier to enhance healing in human periodontal furcation defects: a follow-up report, *J Periodontol* 62:684, 1991.
58. Fleisher N, Waal H, Bloom A: Regeneration of lost attachment apparatus in the dog using Vicryl absorbable mesh (polyglactin 910), *Int J Periodont Restor Dent* 8(2):45, 1988.
59. Fowler C, Garrett S, Crigger M, et al: Histologic probe position in treated and untreated human periodontal tissues, *J Clin Periodontol* 9:373, 1982.
60. Freeman E, Turnbull RS: The value of osseous coagulum as a graft material, *J Periodontal Res* 8:299, 1973.
61. Froum S, Lemler J, Horowitz R, Davidson B: The use of enamel matrix derivative in the treatment of periodontal osseous defects: a clinical decision tree based on biologic principles of regeneration, *Int J Periodont Restor Dent* 21:437, 2001.
62. Froum SJ, Thaler R, Scoop IW, et al: Osseous autografts. I. Clinical responses to bone blend or hip marrow grafts, *J Periodontol* 46:515, 1975.
63. Froum SJ, Thaler R, Scoop IW, et al: Osseous autografts. II. Histologic responses to osseous coagulum-bone blend grafts, *J Periodontol* 46:656, 1975.
64. Froum SJ, Kushner L, Scoop IW, et al: Human clinical and histologic responses to Durapatite implants in intraosseous lesions, *J Periodontol* 53:719, 1982.
65. Froum SJ, Weinberg MA, Rosenberg E, Tarnow D: A comparative study utilizing open flap debridement with and without enamel matrix derivative in the treatment of periodontal intrabony defects: a 12-month re-entry study, *J Periodontol* 72:25, 2001.
66. Gantes BG, Garrett S: Coronally displaced flaps in reconstructive periodontal therapy, *Reconstr Periodont* 35:495, 1991.
67. Garrett S: Early wound healing stability and its importance in periodontal regeneration. In Polson AM, editor:

Periodontal regeneration: current status and directions, Chicago, 1994, Quintessence.
68. Garrett S: Periodontal regeneration around natural teeth. In Proceedings of the 1996 World Workshop in Periodontology, *Ann Periodontol* 7:621, 1996.
69. Garrett S, Crigger M, Egelberg J: Effects of citric acid on diseased root surfaces, *J Periodontal Res* 13:155, 1978.
70. Glickman I: *Clinical periodontology,* Philadelphia, 1953, Saunders.
71. Goldman H, Cohen DW: The intrabony pocket: classification and treatment, *J Periodontol* 29:272, 1958.
72. Gottlow J: Guided tissue regeneration using bioresorbable and non-resorbable devices: initial healing and long-term results, *J Periodontol* 64:1157, 1993.
73. Gottlow J, Nyman S, Lindhe J, et al: New attachment formation as a result of controlled tissue regeneration, *J Clin Periodontol* 11:494, 1984.
74. Gottlow J, Nyman S, Lindhe J, et al: New attachment formation in human periodontium by guided tissue regeneration, *J Clin Periodontol* 13:604, 1986.
75. Graves DT, Cochran DL: Mesenchymal cell growth factors, *Crit Rev Oral Biol* 1:17, 1990.
76. Greenberg J, Laster L, Listgarten MA: Transgingival probing as a potential estimation of alveolar bone level, *J Periodontol* 47:514, 1976.
77. Halliday DG: The grafting of newly formed autogenous bone in the treatment of osseous defects, *J Periodontol* 40:511, 1969.
78. Hammarstrom L: Enamel matrix, cementum development and regeneration, *J Clin Periodontol* 4:658, 1997.
79. Hancock EB: Regenerative procedures. In *Proceedings of the World Workshop in Clinical Periodontics,* Chicago, 1989, American Academy of Periodontology.
80. Haney JM, Nilvéus RE, McMillan PJ, et al: Periodontal repair in dogs: expanded polytetrafluoroethylene barrier membranes support wound stabilization and enhance bone regeneration, *J Periodontol* 64:883, 1993.
81. Hardwick R, Hayes BK, Flynn C: Devices for dentoalveolar regeneration: an up-to-date literature review, *J Periodontol* 55:495, 1995.
82. Hecker F: *Pyorrhea alveolaris,* St Louis, 1913, Mosby.
83. Hegedüs Z: The rebuilding of the alveolar process by bone transplantation, *Dent Cosmos* 65:736, 1923.
84. Heijl L, Heden G, Svardstrom G, et al: Enamel matrix derivative in the treatment of intrabony periodontal defects, *J Clin Periodontol* 24:705, 1997.
85. Hiatt WH: Periodontal pocket elimination by combined endodontic-periodontic therapy, *J Periodontol* 1:153, 1963.
86. Hiatt WH, Schallhorn RG: Intraoral transplants of cancellous bone and marrow in periodontal lesions, *J Periodontol* 44:194, 1973.
87. Hippolyte MP, Fabre D, Peyrol S: Corail et regeneration tissulaire guidée: aspects histologiques, *J Parodontol* 10:279, 1991.
88. Hoang AM, Oates TW, Cochran DL: In vitro wound healing responses to enamel matrix derivative, *J Periodontol* 71:1270, 2000.
89. Hoang AM, Kleb RJ, Steffensen R, et al: Amelogenin is a cell adhesion protein, *J Dent Res* 81:497, 2002.
90. Howell TH, Fiorellini JP, Paquette DW, et al: A Phase I/II clinical trial to evaluate a combination of recombinant human platelet-derived growth factor-BB and recombinant human insulin-like growth factor-I in patients with periodontal disease, *J Periodontol* 68:1186, 1997.
91. Johnson W, Parkhill EM, Grindlay JH: Transplantation of homografts of sclera: experimental study, *Am J Ophthalmol* 54:1019, 1962.
92. Kenney EB, Lekovic V, Han T, et al: The use of a porous hydroxylapatite implant in periodontal defects. I. Clinical results after six months, *J Periodontol* 56:82, 1985.
93. Kenney EB, Lekovic V, Elbaz JJ et al: The use of a porous hydroxylapatite implant in periodontal defects. II. Treatment of class II furcation lesions in lower molars, *J Periodontol* 59:67, 1988.
94. Kim CK, Kim HY, Chai JK, et al: Effect of a calcium sulfate implant with calcium sulfate barrier on periodontal healing in 3-wall intrabony defects in dogs, *J Periodontol* 69:982, 1998.
95. Klingsberg J: Preserved sclera in periodontal surgery, *J Periodontol* 43:634, 1972.
96. Klingsberg J: Scleral allografts in the repair of periodontal osseous defects, *NY State Dent J* 38:418, 1972.
97. Klingsberg J: Periodontal scleral grafts and combined grafts of sclera and bone: two-year appraisal, *J Periodontol* 45:262, 1974.
98. Krebsbach PH, Lee SK, Matsuki Y, et al: Full length sequence, localization, and chromosomal mapping of ameloblastin, *J Biol Chem* 271:4431, 1996.
99. Kwan SK, Lekovic V, Camargo PM, et al: The use of autogenous periosteal grafts as barriers for the treatment of intrabony defects in humans, *J Periodontol* 69:1203, 1998.
100. Lang NP, Hill RW: Radiographs in periodontics, *J Clin Periodontol* 4:16, 1976.
101. Lekovic V, Kenney EB, Carranza FA Jr, et al: Treatment of class II furcation defects using porous hydroxyapatite in conjunction with a polytetrafluoroethylene membrane, *J Periodontol* 61:575, 1990.
102. Lekovic V, Kenney EB, Carranza FA Jr, et al: The use of autogenous periosteal grafts as barriers for the treatment of grade II furcation involvements in lower molars, *J Periodontol* 62:775, 1991.
103. Lekovic V, Kenney EB, Kovacevic K, et al: Evaluation of guided tissue regeneration in class II furcation defects: a clinical study, *J Periodontol* 60:694, 1989.
104. Lekovic V, Camargo P, Weinlander M, et al: A comparison between enamel matrix protein used alone or in combination with bovine porous bone mineral in the treatment of intrabony periodontal defects in humans, *J Periodontol* 71:1110, 2000.
105. Levin MP, Getter L, Adrian J, et al: Healing of periodontal defects with ceramic implants, *J Clin Periodontol* 1:197, 1974.
106. Libin BM, Ward HL, Fishman LL: Decalcified lyophilized bone allografts for use in human periodontal defects, *J Periodontol* 46:51, 1975.
107. Machtei EE: Outcome variables for the study of periodontal regeneration, *Ann Periodontol* 2:229, 1997.
108. Magnusson I, Batich C, Collins BR: New attachment formation following controlled tissue regeneration using biodegradable membranes, *J Periodontol* 59:1, 1988.
109. Magnusson I, Stenberg WV, Batich C, et al: Connective tissue repair in circumferential periodontal defects in dogs following use of a biodegradable membrane, *J Clin Periodontol* 17:243, 1990.
110. Martin M, Gantes B, Garrett S, et al: Treatment of periodontal furcation defects. I. Review of the literature and description of a regenerative surgical technique, *J Clin Periodontol* 15:227, 1988.
111. McClain PK, Schallhorn RG: Long-term assessment of combined osseous composite grafting, root conditioning and guided tissue regeneration, *Int J Periodont Restor Dent* 13:9, 1993.
112. McClain PK, Schallhorn RG: The use of combined periodontal regenerative techniques, *J Periodontol* 70:102, 1999 (editorial).

113. Meffert RM, Thomas JR, Hamilton KM, et al: Hydroxylapatite as an alloplastic graft in the treatment of human periodontal osseous defects, *J Periodontol* 56:63, 1985.
114. Melcher AH: The use of heterogenous anorganic bone as an implant material in oral procedures, *Oral Surg* 15:996, 1962.
115. Mellado JR, Salkin LM, Freedman AL, et al: A comparative study of ePTFE membranes with and without decalcified freeze-dried bone allografts for the regeneration of interproximal intraosseous defects, *J Periodontol* 66:751, 1995.
116. Mellonig JT: Freeze-dried bone allografts in periodontal reconstructive surgery, *Dent Clin North Am* 35:505, 1991.
117. Mellonig JT: Enamel matrix derivative for periodontal reconstructive surgery: technique and clinical and histologic case report, *Int J Periodont Restor Dent* 19:9, 1999.
118. Mellonig JT: Human histologic evaluation of a bovine-derived bone xenograft in the treatment of periodontal osseous defects, *Int J Periodont Restor Dent* 20:19, 2000.
119. Mellonig JT, Bowers GM, Bailey RC: Comparison of bone graft materials. Part I. New bone formation with autografts and allografts determined by strontium-85, *J Periodontol* 52:291, 1981.
120. Mellonig JT, Bowers GM, Bailey RC: Comparison of bone graft materials. Part II. New bone formation with autografts and allografts: a histological evaluation, *J Periodontol* 52:297, 1981.
121. Mellonig JT, Bowers GM, Bright RW, et al: Clinical evaluation of freeze-dried bone allografts in periodontal osseous defects, *J Periodontol* 47:125, 1976.
122. Mellonig JT, Prewett AB, Moyer MP: HIV inactivation in a bone allograft, *J Periodontol* 63:979, 1992.
123. Metzler DG, Seamoons BC, Mellonig JT, et al: Clinical evaluation of guided tissue regeneration in the treatment of maxillary class II molar furcation invasions, *J Periodontol* 62:353, 1991.
124. Minabe M: A critical review of the biologic rationale for guided tissue regeneration, *J Periodontol* 62:171, 1991.
125. Moriarty JD, Hutchens LH, Scheitler LE: Histological evaluation of periodontal probe penetration in untreated facial molar furcations, *J Periodontol* 16:21, 1989.
126. Morris ML: Reattachment of periodontal tissue: a critical study, *Oral Surg* 2:1194, 1949.
127. Moskow BS, Tannenbaum P: Enhanced repair and regeneration of periodontal lesions in tetracycline-treated patients: case reports, *J Periodontol* 62:341, 1991.
128. Moskow BS, Gold SI, Gottsegen R: Effects of scleral collagen upon the healing of experimental osseous wounds, *J Periodontol* 47:596, 1976.
129. Nabers CL, O'Leary TJ: Autogenous bone transplants in the treatment of osseous defects, *J Periodontol* 36:5, 1965.
130. Nabers JM, Meador HL, Nabers CL, et al: Chronology, an important factor in the repair of osseous defects, *Periodontics* 2:304, 1964.
131. Nery EB, Lynch KL: Preliminary clinical studies of bioceramic in periodontal osseous defects, *J Periodontol* 49:523, 1978.
132. Nilvéus R, Bogle G, Crigger M, et al: Effect of topical citric acid application in the healing of experimental furcation defects in dogs. 2. Healing after repeated surgery, *J Periodontal Res* 15:544, 1980.
133. Nyman S, Gottlow J, Karring T, et al: The regenerative potential of the periodontal ligament: an experimental study in the monkey, *J Clin Periodontol* 9:257, 1982.
134. Nyman S, Lindhe J, Karring T, et al: New attachment following surgical treatment of human periodontal disease, *J Clin Periodontol* 9:290, 1982.
135. Passell MS, Bissada NF: Histomorphologic evaluation of scleral grafts in experimental bony defects, *J Periodontol* 46:629, 1975.
136. Patur B, Glickman I: Clinical and roentgenographic evaluation of the post-treatment healing of infrabony pockets, *J Periodontol* 33:164, 1962.
137. Pearson GE, Rosen S, Deporter DA: Preliminary observations on the usefulness of a decalcified freeze-dried cancellous bone allograft material in periodontal surgery, *J Periodontol* 52:55, 1981.
138. Pini Prato G, Clauser C, Cortellini P: Augmentation of periodontal regeneration response using biologic mediators. In Polson A: *Periodontal regeneration: current status and directions,* Chicago, 1994, Quintessence.
139. Pitaru S, Tal H, Soldinger M, et al: Collagen membranes prevent the apical migration of epithelium during periodontal wound healing, *J Periodontal Res* 22:331, 1987.
140. Pitaru S, Tal H, Soldinger M, et al: Partial regeneration of periodontal tissues using collagen barriers: initial observations in the canine, *J Periodontol* 59:380, 1988.
141. Pitaru S, Tal H, Soldinger M, et al: Collagen membranes prevent apical migration of epithelium and support new connective tissue attachment during periodontal wound healing in dogs, *J Periodontal Res* 24:2467, 1989.
142. Polson AM, Proye MP: Fibrin linkage: a precursor for new attachment, *J Periodontol* 54:141, 1983.
143. Polson AM, Frederick GT, Ladenhein S, et al: The production of a root surface smear by instrumentation and its removal by citric acid, *J Periodontol* 55:443, 1984.
144. Pontoriero R, Lindhe J, Nyman S, et al: Guided tissue regeneration in degree II furcation-involved mandibular molars: a clinical study, *J Clin Periodontol* 15:247, 1988.
145. Prichard JF: The intrabony technique as a predictable procedure, *J Periodontol* 28:202, 1957.
146. Proceedings of the 1996 World Workshop in Periodontology, Consensus Report: Periodontal regeneration around natural teeth, *Ann Periodontol* 7:667, 1996.
147. Quintero G, Mellonig JT, Gambill VM, et al: A six-month clinical evaluation of decalcified freeze-dried bone allografts in periodontal osseous defects, *J Periodontol* 53:726, 1982.
148. Rabalais ML, Yukna RA, Mayer ET: Evaluation of Durapatite ceramic as an alloplastic implant in periodontal osseous defects, *J Periodontol* 52:680, 1981.
149. Ramfjord SP: Experimental periodontal reattachment in rhesus monkeys, *J Periodontol* 22:67, 1951.
150. Ramfjord SP, Nissle RR: The modified Widman flap, *J Periodontol* 45:601, 1974.
151. Register AA, Burdick FA: Accelerated reattachment with cementogenesis to dentin, demineralized in situ. II. Defect repair, *J Periodontol* 47:497, 1976.
152. Renvert S, Egelberg J: Healing after treatment of periodontal intraosseous defects. II. Effect of citric acid conditioning of the root surface, *J Clin Periodontol* 8:459, 1981.
153. Renvert S, Badersten A, Nilvéus R, et al: Healing after treatment of periodontal osseous defects. I. Comparative study of clinical methods, *J Clin Periodontol* 8:387, 1981.
154. Rivault AF, Toto PD, Levy S, et al: Autogenous bone grafts: osseous coagulum and osseous retrograde procedures in primates, *J Periodontol* 42:787, 1971.
155. Robinson RE: Osseous coagulum for bone induction, *J Periodontol* 40:503, 1969.
156. Rosling B, Hollender L, Nyman S, et al: A radiographic method for assessing changes in alveolar bone height following periodontal therapy, *J Clin Periodontol* 2:211, 1975.
157. Ross SE, Malamed EH, Amsterdam M: The contiguous autogenous transplant: its rationale, indications and technique, *Periodontics* 4:246, 1966.
158. Sanders J, Sepe W, Bowers G, et al: Clinical evaluation of freeze-dried bone allografts in periodontal osseous defects.

III. Composite freeze-dried bone allograft with and without autogenous bone, *J Periodontol* 54:1, 1983.
159. Schaffer EM: Cartilage transplants into periodontium of rhesus monkeys, *Oral Surg* 11:1233, 1956.
160. Schaffer EM: Cementum and dentine implants in a dog and a rhesus monkey, *J Periodontol* 28:125, 1957.
161. Schaffer EM: Cartilage grafts in human periodontal pockets, *J Periodontol* 29:176, 1958.
162. Schallhorn RG: The use of autogenous hip marrow biopsy implants for bony crater defects, *J Periodontol* 39:145, 1968.
163. Schallhorn RG: Postoperative problems associated with iliac transplants, *J Periodontol* 43:3, 1972.
164. Schallhorn RG: Osseous grafts in the treatment of periodontal osseous defects. In Stahl SS, editor: *Periodontal surgery: biologic basis and technique,* Springfield, Ill, 1976, Charles C Thomas.
165. Schallhorn RG: Present status of osseous grafting procedures, *J Periodontol* 48:570, 1977.
166. Schallhorn RG, McClain PK: Combined osseous composite grafting, root conditioning, and guided tissue regeneration, *Int J Periodont Restor Dent* 8:8, 1988.
167. Schallhorn RG, McClain PK: Clinical and radiographic pattern observations with combined regenerative technique, *Int J Periodont Restor Dent* 14:391, 1994.
168. Schallhorn RG, Hiatt WH, Boyce W: Iliac transplants in periodontal therapy, *J Periodontol* 41:566, 1970.
169. Schwartz Z, Carnes DL Jr, Pulliam R, et al: Porcine fetal enamel matrix derivative stimulates proliferation but not differentiation of pre-osteoblastic 2T9 cells, inhibits proliferation and stimulates differentiation of osteoblast-like MG63 cells, and increases proliferation and differentiation of normal human osteoblast NHOst cells, *J Periodontol* 71:1287, 2000.
170. Scoop IW, Morgan FH, Dooner JJ, et al: Bovine bone (Boplant) implants for infrabony oral lesions (clinical trials in humans), *Periodontics* 4:169, 1966.
171. Sepe W, Bowers G, Lawrence J, et al: Clinical evaluation of freeze-dried bone allograft in periodontal osseous defects. Part II, *J Periodontol* 49:9, 1978.
172. Shaffer CD, App GR: The use of plaster of Paris in treating infrabony periodontal defects in humans, *J Periodontol* 42:685, 1971.
173. Sigurdsson TJ, Hardwick R, Bogle GC, et al: Periodontal repair in dogs: space provision by reinforced ePTFE membranes enhances bone and cementum regeneration in large supraalveolar defects, *J Periodontol* 65:350, 1994.
174. Smith BA, Echeverri M: The removal of pocket epithelium: a review, *J West Soc Periodontol* 32:45, 1984.
175. Smith BA, Smith JS, Caffesse RG, et al: Effect of citric acid and various concentrations of fibronectin on healing following periodontal flap surgery in dogs, *J Periodontol* 58:667, 1987.
176. Sottosanti J: Calcium phosphate: an aid to periodontal, implant and restorative therapy, *J Calif Dent Assoc* 20:45, 1992.
177. Stahl SS, Froum SJ: Human clinical and histologic repair responses following the use of citric acid in periodontal therapy, *J Periodontol* 48:261, 1977.
178. Stahl SS, Froum SJ: Histological and clinical responses to porous hydroxylapatite implants in human periodontal defects three to twelve months post-implantation, *J Periodontol* 58:689, 1987.
179. Stahl SS, Froum SJ: Histologic healing responses in human vertical lesions following the use of osseous allografts and barrier membranes, *J Clin Periodontol* 18:149, 1991.
180. Stahl SS, Froum SJ: Human suprabony healing responses following root demineralization and coronal flap anchorage, *J Clin Periodontol* 18:685, 1991.
181. Stahl SS, Froum SJ: Human intrabony lesion response to debridement, porous hydroxylapatite implants and Teflon barrier membranes, *J Clin Periodontol* 18:605, 1991.
182. Stahl SS, Froum SJ, Tarnow D: Human clinical and histologic responses to the placement of HTR polymer particles in 11 intrabony lesions, *J Periodontol* 61:269, 1990.
183. Stahl SS, Froum SJ, Tarnow D: Human histologic responses to guided tissue regenerative techniques in intrabony lesions, *J Clin Periodontol* 17:191, 1990.
184. Steffensen B, Weber HP: Relationship between the radiographic periodontal defect angle and healing after treatment, *J Periodontol* 60:248, 1989.
185. Terranova VP, Martin GR: Molecular factors determining gingival tissue interaction with tooth structure, *J Periodontal Res* 17:530, 1982.
186. Terranova VP, Franzetti LC, Hic S, et al: A biochemical approach to periodontal regeneration: tetracycline treatment of dentin promotes fibroblast adhesion and growth, *J Periodontal Res* 21:330, 1986.
187. Theilade J: An evaluation of the reliability of radiographs in the measurement of bone loss in periodontal disease, *J Periodontol* 31:143, 1960.
188. Tonetti M, Pini Prato GP, Williams R, et al: Periodontal regeneration of human infrabony defects. III. Diagnostic strategies to detect bone gain, *J Periodontol* 64:269, 1993.
189. Tonetti MS, Cortellini P, Suvan JE, et al: Generalizability of the added benefits of guided tissue regeneration in the treatment of deep intrabony defects: evaluation in a multi-center randomized controlled clinical trial, *J Periodontol* 69:1183, 1998.
190. Topback GA, Brunsvold MA, Nummikoski PV, et al: The accuracy of radiographic methods in assessing the outcome of periodontal regenerative therapy, *J Periodontol* 70:1479, 1999.
191. Turnbull RS, Freeman E, Melcher AH: Histological evaluation of the osteogenic capacity of sclera, *J Dent Res* 55:972, 1976.
192. Urist MR: Bone formation by autoinduction, *Science* 150:893, 1965.
193. Urist MR: Bone histogenesis and morphogenesis in implants of demineralized enamel and dentin, *Oral Surg* 29:38, 1971.
194. Urist MR, Strates BS: Bone morphogenetic protein, *J Dent Res* 50:1392, 1971.
195. Ursell MJ: Relationships between alveolar bone levels measured at surgery, estimated by transgingival probing and clinical attachment level measurements, *J Clin Periodontol* 1989; 16:81.
196. Wallace SC, Gellin RG, Miller MC, et al: Guided tissue regeneration with and without decalcified freeze-dried bone in mandibular class II furcation invasions, *J Periodontol* 65:244, 1994.
197. Wang HL, McNeil RL: Guided tissue regeneration: absorbable barriers, *Dent Clin North Am* 42:505, 1998.
198. Wenzel A, Warrer K, Karring T: Digital subtraction radiography in assessing bone changes in periodontal defects following guided tissue regeneration, *J Clin Periodontol* 19:208, 1992.
199. Wikesjö UM, Nilvéus R: Periodontal repair in dogs: effects of wound stabilization in healing, *J Periodontol* 61:719, 1990.
200. Wikesjö UM, Claffey N, Christersson LA, et al: Repair of periodontal furcation defects in beagle dogs following reconstructive surgery including root surface demineralization with tetracycline hydrochloride and topical fibronectin application, *J Clin Periodontol* 15:73, 1988.
201. Younger WJ: Some of the latest phases in implantations and other operations, *Dent Cosmos* 25:102, 1893.

202. Yukna RA: A clinical and histological study of healing following the excisional new attachment procedure in rhesus monkeys, *J Periodontol* 47:701, 1976.
203. Yukna RA: HTR polymer graft in human periodontal osseous defects. I. 6-month clinical results, *J Periodontol* 61:633, 1990.
204. Yukna RA: Clinical human comparison of expanded polytetrafluoroethylene barrier membrane and freeze-dried dura mater allografts for guided tissue regeneration of lost periodontal support. I. Mandibular molar class II furcations, *J Periodontol* 63:431, 1992.
205. Yukna RA, Mellonig JT: Histologic evaluation of periodontal healing in humans following regenerative therapy with enamel matrix derivative: a 10-case series, *J Periodontol* 71:752, 2000.
206. Yukna RA, Mayer ET, Brite DV: Longitudinal evaluation of Durapatite ceramic as an alloplastic implant in periodontal osseous defects after three years, *J Periodontol* 55:633, 1984.
207. Yukna R, Salinas T, Gara R: Periodontal regeneration following use of ABM/P-15: a case report, *Int J Periodont Restor Dent* 22:147, 2002.
208. Yukna RA, Krauser JT, Callan DP, et al: Multi-center clinical comparison of combination anorganic bovine-derived hydroxyapatite matrix (ABM)/cell binding peptide (P-15) and ABM in human periodontal osseous defects: 6-month results, *J Periodontol* 71:1671, 2000.

Furcation: Involvement and Treatment

William F. Ammons, Jr., and Gerald W. Harrington

68

CHAPTER

CHAPTER OUTLINE

The progress of inflammatory periodontal disease, if unabated, ultimately results in attachment loss sufficient enough to affect the bifurcation or trifurcation of multirooted teeth. The **furcation** is an area of complex anatomic morphology[5,6,10] that may be difficult or impossible to debride by routine periodontal instrumentation.[28,33] Routine home care methods may not keep the furcation area free of plaque.[16,22]

The presence of furcation involvement is one clinical finding that can lead to a diagnosis of advanced periodontitis and potentially to a less favorable prognosis for the affected tooth or teeth. Furcation involvement therefore presents both diagnostic and therapeutic dilemmas.

ETIOLOGIC FACTORS

The primary etiologic factor in the development of furcation defects is *bacterial plaque* and the inflammatory consequences that result from its long-term presence. The extent of attachment loss required to produce a furcation defect is variable and related to local anatomic factors (e.g., root trunk length, root morphology)[11,26] and local developmental anomalies (e.g., cervical enamel projections).[21,26] Local factors may affect the rate of plaque deposition or complicate the performance of oral hygiene procedures, thereby contributing to the development of periodontitis and attachment loss. Studies indicate that prevalence and severity of furcation involvement increase with age.[20,21,33] Dental caries and pulpal death may also affect a tooth with furcation involvement or even the area of the furcation. All these factors should be considered during the diagnosis, treatment planning, and therapy of the patient with furcation defects.

DIAGNOSIS AND CLASSIFICATION OF FURCATION DEFECTS

A thorough clinical examination is the key to diagnosis and treatment planning. Careful probing is required to determine the presence and extent of furcation involvement, the position of the attachment relative to the furca, and the extent and configuration of the furcation defect.[35] Transgingival sounding may further define the anatomy of the furcation defect.[28] The goal of this examination is to identify and classify the extent of furcation involvement and to identify factors that may have contributed to the development of the furcation defect or that could affect treatment outcome. These factors include (1) the morphology of the affected tooth, (2) the position of the tooth relative to adjacent teeth, (3) the local anatomy of the alveolar bone, (4) the configuration of any bony defects, and (5) the presence and extent of other dental diseases (e.g., caries, pulpal necrosis).

The dimension of the furcation entrance is variable but usually quite small; 81% of furcations have an orifice of 1 mm or less, and 58% are 0.75 mm or less.[5,6] The clinician should consider these dimensions, along with the local anatomy of the furcation area,[10-12] when selecting instruments for probing. A probe of small cross section is required if the clinician is to detect early furcation involvement.

Indices of Furcation Involvement

The extent and configuration of the furcation defect are factors in both diagnosis and treatment planning. This has led to the development of a number of indices to record furcation involvement. These indices are based on the horizontal measurement of attachment loss in the furcation,[13,16] on a combination of horizontal and vertical measurements,[34] or a combination of these findings with the localized configuration of the bony deformity.[9] Glickman[13] classified furcation involvement into four grades (Figure 68-1).

Grade I. A grade I furcation involvement is the incipient or early stage of furcation involvement (Figure 68-1, *A*). The pocket is suprabony and primarily affects the soft tissues. Early bone loss may have occurred with an increase in probing depth, but radiographic changes are not usually found.

Grade II. Grade II furcation can affect one or more of the furcations of the same tooth. The furcation lesion is essentially a cul-de-sac (Figure 68-1, *B*) with a definite horizontal component. If multiple defects are present, they do not communicate with each other because a portion of the alveolar bone remains attached to the tooth. The extent of the horizontal probing of the furcation determines whether the defect is early or advanced. Vertical bone loss may be present and represents a therapeutic complication. Radiographs may or may not depict the furcation involvement, particularly with

A B C D
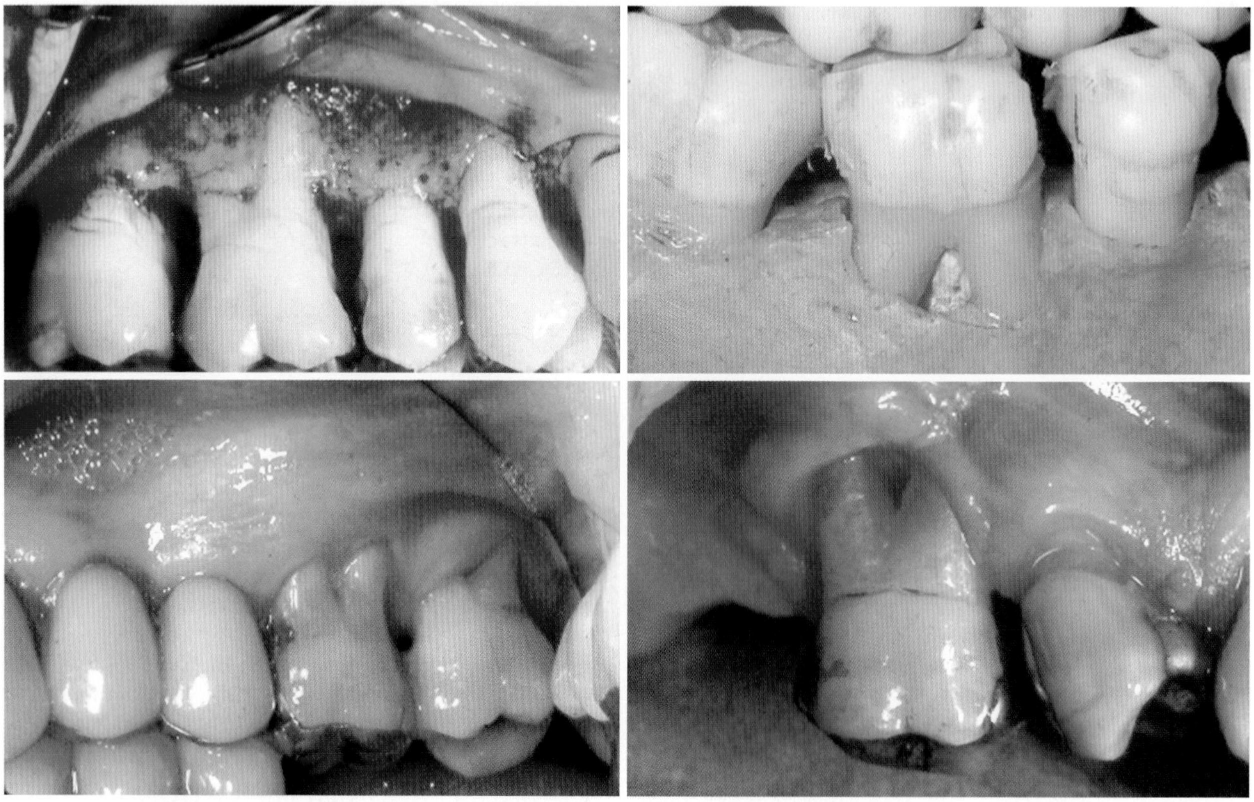

Figure 68-1 Glickman's classification of furcation involvement. **A,** Grade I furcation involvement. Although a space is visible at the entrance to the furcation, no horizontal component of the furcation is evident on probing. **B,** Grade II furcation in a dried skull. Note both the horizontal and the vertical component of this cul-de-sac. **C,** Grade III furcations on maxillary molars. Probing confirms that the buccal furcation connects with the distal furcation of both these molars, yet the furcation is filled with soft tissue. **D,** Grade IV furcation. The soft tissues have receded sufficiently to allow direct vision into the furcation of this maxillary molar.

maxillary molars because of the radiographic overlap of the roots. In some views, however, the presence of furcation "arrows" indicates possible furcation involvement (see Chapter 36).

Grade III. In grade III furcations the bone is not attached to the dome of the furcation. In early grade III involvement the opening may be filled with soft tissue and may not be visible. The clinician may not even be able to pass a periodontal probe completely through the furcation because of interference with the bifurcational ridges or facial/lingual bony margins. However, if the clinician adds the buccal and lingual probing dimensions and obtains a cumulative probing measurement that is equal to or greater than the buccal/lingual dimension of the tooth at the furcation orifice, the clinician must conclude that a grade III furcation exists (Figure 68-1, *C*). Properly exposed and angled radiographs of early class III furcations display the defect as a radiolucent area in the crotch of the tooth (see Chapter 36).

Grade IV. In grade IV furcations the interdental bone is destroyed, and the soft tissues have receded apically so that the furcation opening is clinically visible. A tunnel therefore exists between the roots of such an affected tooth. Thus the periodontal probe passes readily from one aspect of the tooth to another (Figure 68-1, *D*).

Other Classification Indices. Hamp et al.[16] modified a three-stage classification system by attaching a millimeter measurement to separate the extent of horizontal involvement. Easley and Drennan[9] and Tarnow and Fletcher[34] have described classification systems that consider both horizontal and vertical attachment loss in classifying the extent of furcation involvement. Consideration of defect configuration and the vertical component of the defect provides additional information that may be useful in planning therapy.

LOCAL ANATOMIC FACTORS

Clinical examination of the patient should allow the therapist to identify not only furcation defects but also many of the local anatomic factors that may affect the result of therapy (prognosis). Well-made dental radiographs, although not allowing a definitive classification of furcation involvement, provide additional information vital for treatment planning (Figure 68-2). Important local factors include anatomic features of the affected teeth, as described next.

Root Trunk Length

This is a key factor in both the development and the treatment of furcation involvement. The distance from the cementoenamel junction to the entrance of the furcation can vary extensively. Teeth may have very short root trunks, moderate root trunk length, or roots that may be fused to a point near the apex (Figure 68-3). The combination of root trunk length with the number and configuration of the roots affects the ease and success of therapy. The shorter the root trunk, the less attachment

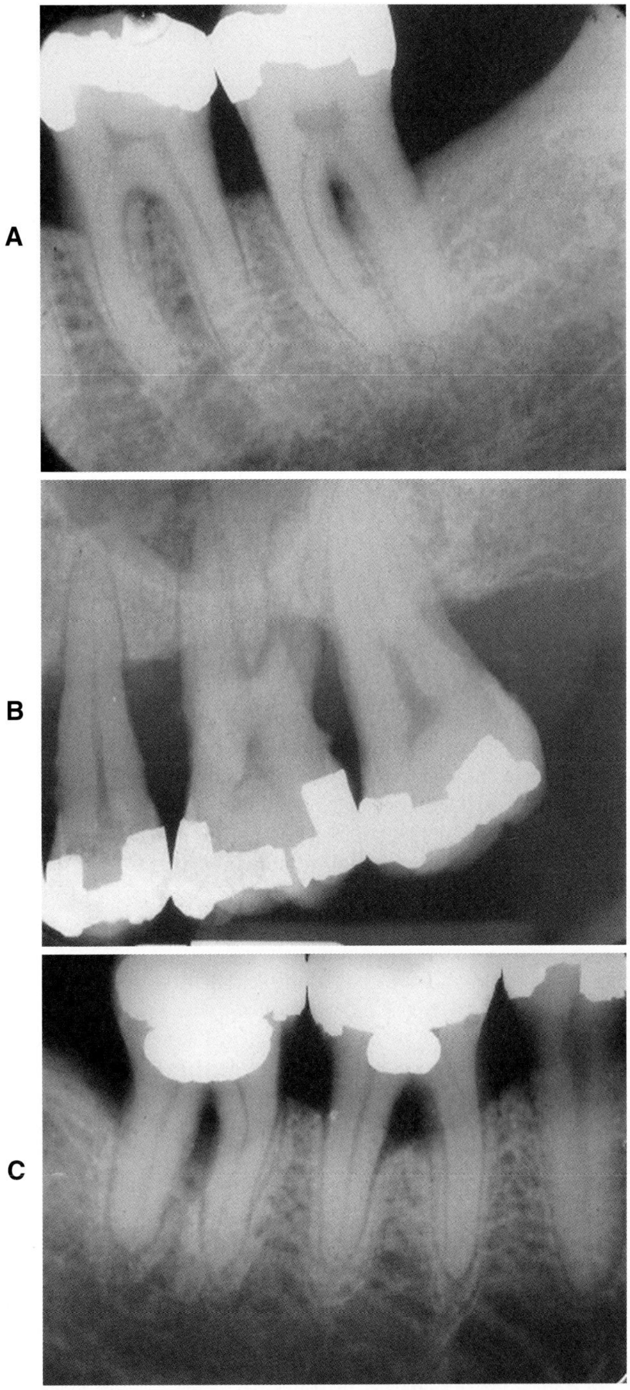

Figure 68-2 Different degrees of furcation involvement in radiographs. **A,** Grade I furcation on the mandibular first molar and a grade III furcation on the mandibular second molar. The root approximation on the second molar may be sufficient to impede accurate probing of this defect. **B,** Multiple furcation defects on a maxillary first molar. Grade I buccal furcation involvement and grade II mesiopalatal and distopalatal furcations are present. Deep developmental grooves on the maxillary second molar simulate furcation involvement in this molar with fused roots. **C,** Grade III and IV furcations on mandibular molars.

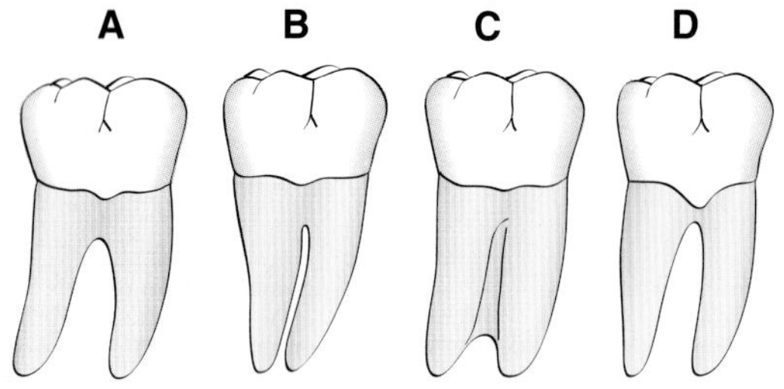

Figure 68-3 Different anatomic features that may be important in prognosis and treatment of furcation involvement. **A,** Widely separated roots. **B,** Roots are separated but close. **C,** Fused roots separated only in their apical portion. **D,** Presence of enamel projection that may be conducive to early furcation involvement.

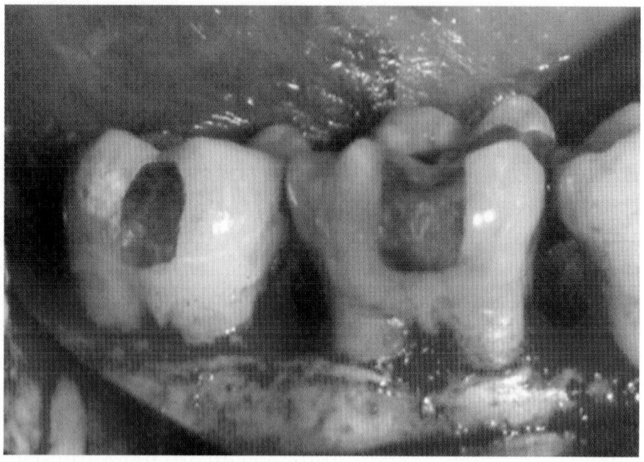

Figure 68-4 Furcation involvement by grade III cervical enamel projections.

needs to be lost before the furcation is involved. Once the furcation is exposed, teeth with short root trunks may be more accessible to maintenance procedures, and the short root trunks may facilitate some surgical procedures. Alternatively, teeth with unusually long root trunks or fused roots may not be appropriate candidates for treatment once the furcation has been affected.

Root Length

Root length is directly related to the quantity of attachment supporting the tooth. Teeth with long root trunks and short roots may have lost a majority of their support by the time that the furcation becomes affected.[12,19] Teeth with long roots and short to moderate root trunk length are more readily treated because sufficient attachment remains to meet functional demands.

Root Form

The mesial root of most mandibular first and second molars and the mesiofacial root of the maxillary first molar are typically curved to the distal side in the apical third. In addition, the distal aspect of this root is usually heavily fluted. The curvature and fluting may increase the potential for root perforation during endodontic therapy or complicate post placement during restoration.[1,24] These anatomic features may also result in an increased incidence of vertical root fracture. The size of the mesial radicular pulp may result in removal of most of this portion of the tooth during preparation.

Interradicular Dimension

The degree of separation of the roots is also an important factor in treatment planning. Closely approximated or fused roots can preclude adequate instrumentation during scaling, root planing, and surgery. Teeth with widely separated roots present more treatment options and are more readily treated.

Anatomy of Furcation

The anatomy of the furcation is complex. The presence of bifurcational ridges, a concavity in the dome,[10] and possible accessory canals[15] complicates not only scaling, root planing, and surgical therapy,[27] but also periodontal maintenance. Odontoplasty to reduce or eliminate these ridges may be required during surgical therapy for an optimal result.

BOX 68-1

Classification of Cervical Enamel Projections

Grade I: The enamel projection extends from the cementoenamel junction of the tooth toward the furcation entrance.
Grade II: The enamel projection approaches the entrance to the furcation. It does not enter the furcation, and therefore no horizontal component is present.
Grade III: The enamel projection extends horizontally into the furcation.

From Masters DH, Hoskins SW: *J Periodontol* 35:49, 1964.

Cervical Enamel Projections

Cervical enamel projections (CEPs) are reported to occur on 8.6% to 28.6% of molars.[25,26,32] The prevalence is highest for mandibular and maxillary second molars. The extent of CEPs was classified by Masters and Hoskins[27] in 1964 (Box 68-1); Figure 68-4 provides an example of a grade III CEP. These projections can affect plaque removal, can complicate scaling and root planing, and may be a local factor in the development of gingivitis and periodontitis. CEPs should be removed to facilitate maintenance.

ANATOMY OF THE BONY LESIONS

Pattern of Attachment Loss

The form of the bony lesions associated with the furcation can vary significantly. Horizontal bone loss can

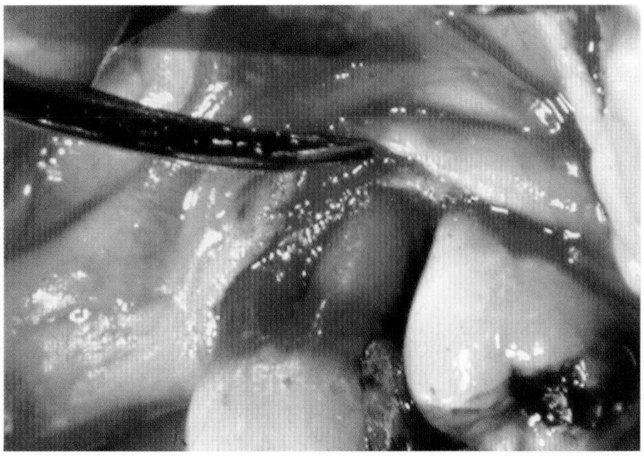

Figure 68-5 Advanced bone loss, furcation involvement, and root approximation. Note the buccal furcation, which communicates with the distal furcation of a maxillary first molar that also displays advanced attachment loss on the distal root and approximation with the mesial root of the maxillary second molar. The patient with such teeth may benefit from root resection of the distobuccal root of the first molar or extraction of the molar.

expose the furcation as thin facial/lingual plates of bone that may be totally lost during resorption. Alternatively, areas with thickened bony ledges may persist and predispose to the development of furcations with deep vertical components. The pattern of bone loss on other surfaces of the affected tooth and adjacent teeth must also be considered during treatment planning. The treatment response in deep, multiwalled bony defects is different from that in areas of horizontal bone loss. Complex multiwalled defects with deep, interradicular vertical components may be candidates for regenerative therapies. Alternatively, molars with advanced attachment loss on only one root may be treated by resective procedures.

Other Dental Findings

The dental and periodontal condition of the adjacent teeth must be considered during treatment planning for furcation involvement. The combination of furcation involvement and root approximation with an adjacent tooth represents the same problem that exists in furcations without adequate root separation. Such a finding may dictate the removal of the most severely affected tooth or the removal of a root or roots (Figure 68-5).

The presence of an adequate band of gingiva and a moderate to deep vestibule will facilitate the performance of a surgical procedure, if indicated.

TREATMENT

The objectives of furcation therapy are to (1) facilitate maintenance, (2) prevent further attachment loss, and (3) obliterate the furcation defects as a periodontal maintenance problem. The selection of therapeutic mode varies with the class of furcation involvement, the extent and configuration of bone loss, and other anatomic factors.

Therapeutic Classes of Furcation Defects

Class I: Early Defects. Incipient or early furcation defects (class I) are amenable to conservative periodontal therapy. Because the pocket is suprabony and has not entered the furcation, oral hygiene, scaling, and root planing are effective.[15] Any thick overhanging margins of restorations, facial grooves, or CEPs should be eliminated by odontoplasty, recontouring, or replacement. The resolution of inflammation and subsequent repair of the periodontal ligament and bone are usually sufficient to restore periodontal health.

Class II. Once a horizontal component to the furcation has developed (class II), therapy becomes more complicated. Shallow horizontal involvement without significant vertical bone loss usually responds favorably to localized flap procedures with odontoplasty and osteoplasty. Isolated deep class II furcations may respond to flap procedures with osteoplasty and odontoplasty (Figure 68-6). This reduces the dome of the furcation and alters gingival contours to facilitate the patient's plaque removal.

Classes II to IV: Advanced Defects. The development of a significant horizontal component to one or more furcations of a multirooted tooth (late class II, class III or IV[13]) or the development of a deep vertical component to the furca poses additional problems. Nonsurgical treatment is usually ineffective because the ability to instrument the tooth surfaces adequately is compromised.[30,36] Periodontal surgery, endodontic therapy, and restoration of the tooth may be required to retain the tooth.

SURGICAL THERAPY

Root Resection

Root resection may be indicated in multirooted teeth with grade II to IV furcation involvements. Root resection may be performed on vital teeth[18] or endodontically treated teeth. It is preferable, however, to have endodontic therapy completed before resection of a root(s).[17] If this is not possible, the pulp should be removed, the patency of the canals determined, and the pulp chamber medicated before resection. It is distressing for both patient and clinician to perform a vital root resection and subsequently have an untoward event occur, such as perforation, fracture of the root, or an inability to instrument the canal.

The indications and contraindications for root resection were well summarized by Bassaraba.[1] In general, teeth planned for root resection include the following:

1. Teeth that are of critical importance to the overall dental treatment plan.[4] Examples are teeth serving as abutments for fixed or removable restorations for which loss of the tooth would result in loss of the prosthesis and entail major prosthetic re-treatment.
2. Teeth that have sufficient attachment remaining for function. Molars with advanced bone loss in the interproximal and interradicular zones, unless the

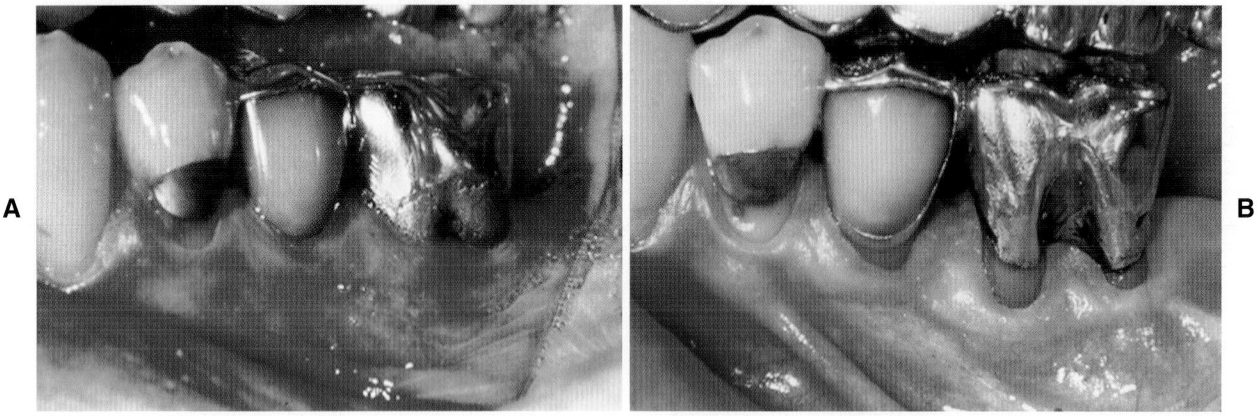

Figure 68-6 Treatment of a grade II furcation by osteoplasty and odontoplasty. **A,** This mandibular first molar has been treated endodontically and an area of caries in the furcation repaired. A class II furcation is present. **B,** Results of flap debridement, osteoplasty, and severe odontoplasty 5 years postoperatively. Note the adaptation of the gingiva into the furcation area. (Courtesy Dr. Ronald Rott, Sacramento, Calif.)

lesions have three bony walls, are not candidates for root amputation.

3. Teeth for which a more predictable or cost-effective method of therapy is not available. Examples are teeth with furcation defects that have been treated successfully with endodontics but now present with a vertical root fracture, advanced bone loss, or caries on bone root.
4. Teeth in patients with good oral hygiene and low activity for caries are suitable for root resection. Patients unable or unwilling to perform good oral hygiene and preventive measures are not suitable candidates for root resection or hemisection. Root-resected teeth require endodontic treatment[17] and usually cast restorations.

These therapies can represent a sizable financial investment by the patient in an effort to save the tooth. Alternative therapies and their impact on the overall treatment plan should always be considered and presented to the patient.

Which Root to Remove

A tooth with an isolated furcation defect in an otherwise intact dental segment may present few diagnostic problems. However, the existence of multiple furcation defects of varying severity combined with generalized advanced periodontitis can be a challenge to treatment planning. Careful diagnosis usually allows the therapist to determine the feasibility of root resection and the identification of which root to remove before surgery (Figure 68-7).

The following is a guide to determining which root should be removed in these cases:

1. Remove the root(s) that will eliminate the furcation and allow the production of a maintainable architecture on the remaining roots.
2. Remove the root with the greatest amount of bone and attachment loss. Sufficient periodontal attachment must remain after surgery for the tooth to withstand the functional demands placed on it. Teeth with uniform advanced horizontal bone loss are not suitable for root resection.
3. Remove the root that best contributes to the elimination of periodontal problems on adjacent teeth. For example, a maxillary first molar with a class III buccal-to-distal furcation is adjacent to a maxillary second molar with a two-walled intrabony defect between the molars and an early class II furcation on the mesial furcation of the second molar. There may or may not be local anatomic factors affecting the teeth. The removal of the distobuccal root of the first molar allows the elimination of the furcation and management of the two-walled intrabony lesion and also facilitates access for instrumentation and maintenance of the second molar (Figure 68-8).
4. Remove the root with the greatest number of anatomic problems, such as severe curvature, developmental grooves, root flutings, or accessory and multiple root canals.
5. Remove the root that least complicates future periodontal maintenance.

Hemisection

Hemisection is the splitting of a two-rooted tooth into two separate portions. This process has been called *bicuspidization* or *separation* because it changes the molar into two separate roots. Hemisection is most likely to be performed on mandibular molars with buccal and lingual class II or III furcation involvements. As with root resection, molars with advanced bone loss in the interproximal and interradicular zones are not good candidates for hemisection. After sectioning of the teeth, one or both roots can be retained. This decision is based on the extent and pattern of bony loss, root trunk and root length, ability to eliminate the osseous defect, and endodontic and restorative considerations. The anatomy of the mesial roots of mandibular molars often leads to their extraction and the retention of the distal root to facilitate both endodontic and restorative therapy.

A B C D E F

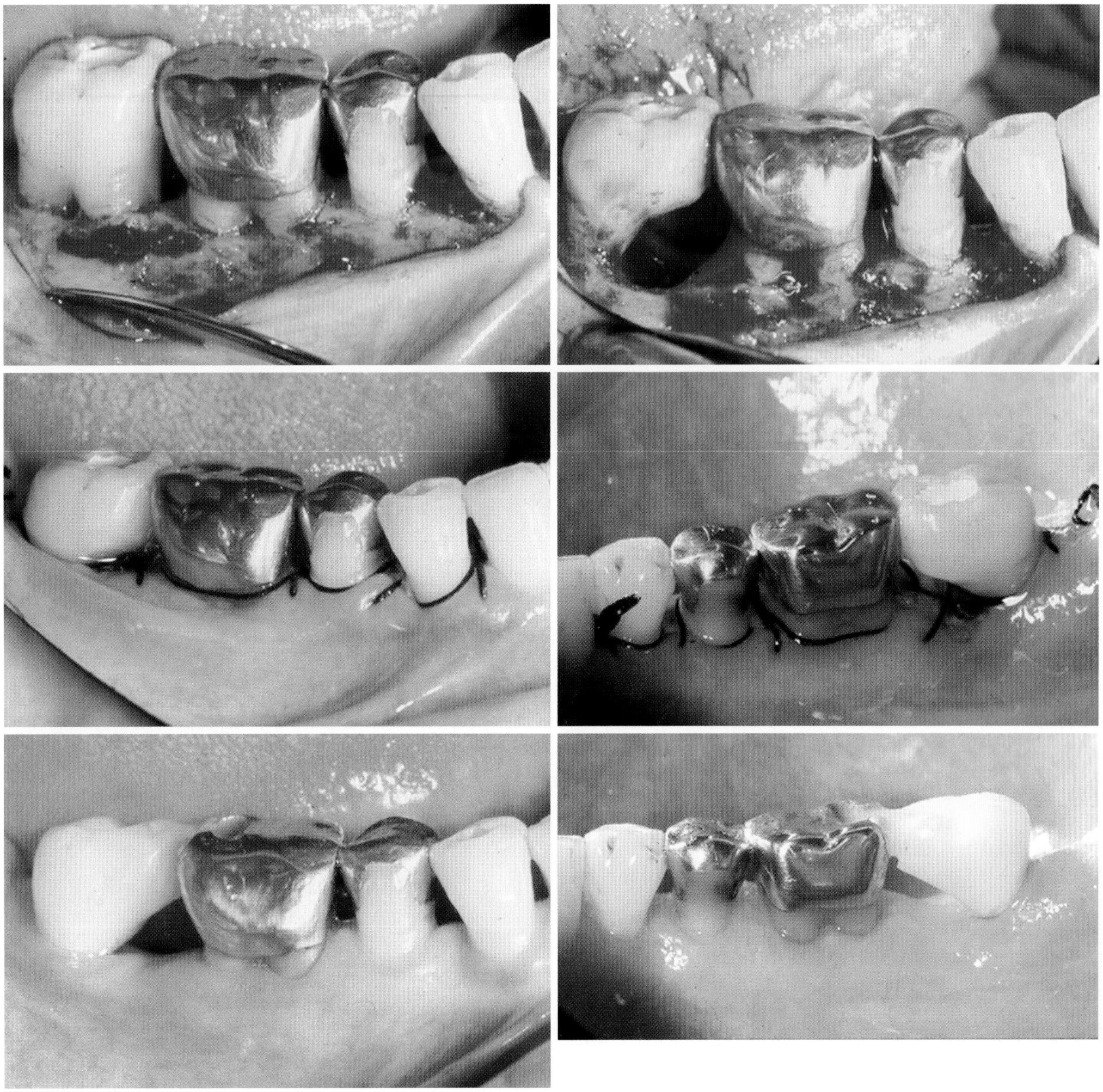

Figure 68-7 Resection of a root with advanced bone loss. **A,** Facial osseous contours. There is an early grade II furcation on the facial aspect of the mandibular first molar and a class III furcation on the mandibular second molar. **B,** Resection of the mesial root. The mesial portion of the crown was retained to prevent mesial drift of the distal root during healing. The grade II furcations were treated by osteoplasty. **C,** Buccal flaps adapted and sutured. **D,** Lingual flaps adapted and sutured. **E,** Three-month postoperative view of the buccal aspect of this resection. New restorations were subsequently placed. **F,** Three-month postoperative view of the lingual aspect of this resection.

The interradicular dimension between the two roots of a tooth to be hemisected is also important. Narrow interradicular zones can complicate the surgical procedure. The retention of both molar roots can complicate the restoration of the tooth, since it may be virtually impossible to finish margins or to provide an adequate embrasure between the two roots for effective oral hygiene and maintenance (Figure 68-9). Therefore, orthodontic separation of the roots is often required to allow restoration with adequate embrasure form (Figure 68-10). The result can be the need for multiple procedures and extensive interdisciplinary therapy. In such patients the availability of other treatment alternatives should be considered, such as guided tissue/guided bone regeneration or replacement by osseointegrated dental implants.

Root Resection/Hemisection Procedure

The most common root resection involves the distobuccal root of the maxillary first molar,[2,25] as diagrammed in Figure 68-11. After appropriate local anesthesia, a full-thickness mucoperiosteal flap is elevated. Root resection

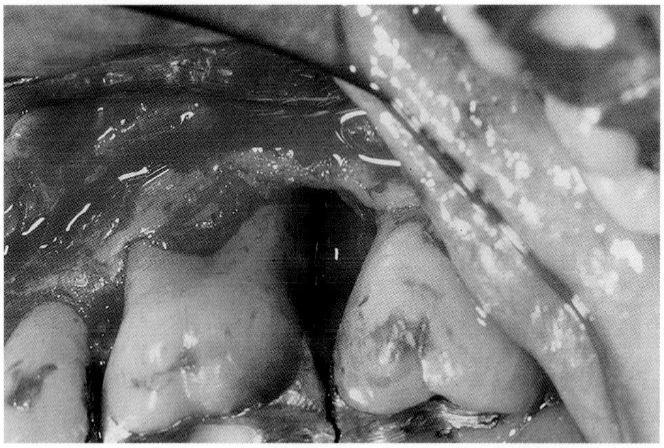

Figure 68-8 Advanced bone loss on one root with furcation involvement. The majority of the attachment has been lost on the distal surface of this maxillary first molar. A buccal grade I and a deep grade II distal furcation defect is present. A shallow two-walled defect, correctable by osteoplasty and osteoectomy, is present at the mesial aspect of the second molar. Treatment options are root amputation or extraction.

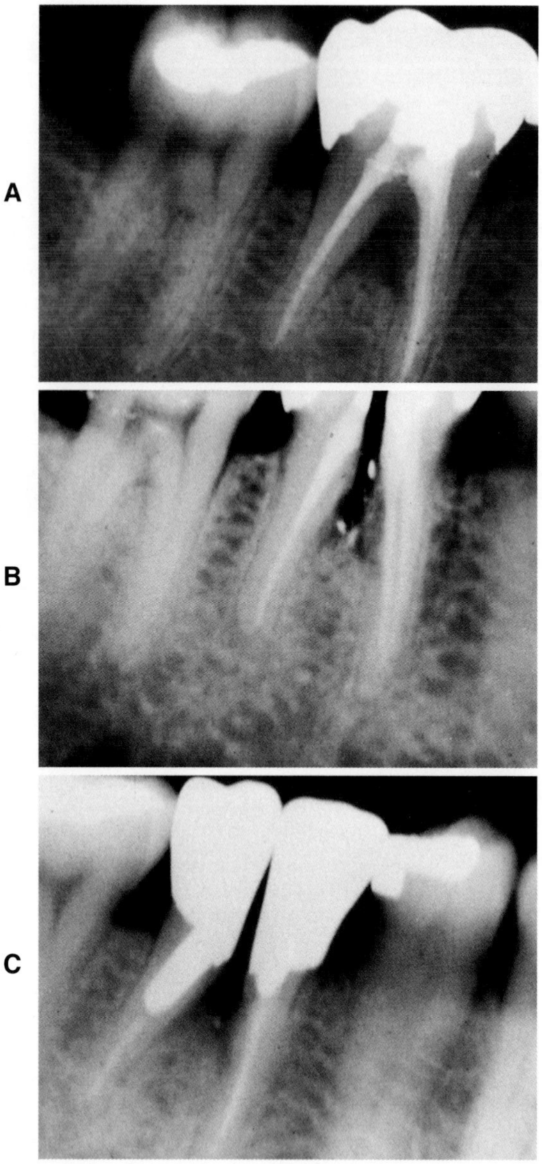

Figure 68-9 **A,** Grade III furcation lesion. **B,** Hemisection to divide the tooth into mesial and distal portions. **C,** Postoperative view of a hemisected mandibular with new crowns for both roots.

or hemisection of teeth with advanced attachment loss usually requires opening both facial and lingual/palatal flaps (see Chapter 64). Typically, a root cannot be resected without elevating a flap. The flap should provide adequate access for visualization and instrumentation and minimize surgical trauma.

After debridement, resection of the root begins with the exposure of the furcation on the root to be removed (Figure 68-11, *A*). The removal of a small amount of facial or palatal bone may be required to provide access for elevation and facilitate root removal (Figure 68-11, *B*). A cut is then directed from just apical to the contact point of the tooth, through the tooth, and to the facial and distal orifices of the furcation (Figure 68-11, *C*). This cut is made with a high-speed, surgical-length fissure or cross-cut fissure carbide bur. The placement of a curved periodontal probe into or through the furcation aids in orienting the angle of the resection. For hemisection, a vertically oriented cut is made faciolingually through the buccal and lingual developmental grooves of the tooth, through the pulp chamber, and through the furcation. If the sectioning cut passes through a metallic restoration, the metallic portion of the cut should be made before flap elevation. This prevents contamination of the surgical field with metallic particles.

If a vital root resection is to be performed, a more horizontal cut through the root is advisable (Figure 68-11, *D*). An oblique cut exposes a large surface area of the radicular pulp and/or dental pulp chamber. This can lead to postoperative pain and can complicate endodontic therapy. A horizontal cut, although it may complicate root removal, has less postoperative complications. This root stump can be removed by odontoplasty after the completion of endodontic therapy or at the time of tooth preparation.

After sectioning, the root is elevated from its socket (Figure 68-11, *E*). Care should be taken not to traumatize bone on the remaining roots or to damage an adjacent tooth. Removal of the root provides visibility to the furcation aspects of the remaining roots and simplifies the debridement of the furcation with hand, rotary, or ultrasonic instruments. If necessary, odontoplasty is performed to remove portions of the developmental ridges and prepare a furcation that is free of any deformity that would enhance plaque retention or adversely affect plaque removal (Figure 68-11, *F*).

Patients with advanced periodontitis often have root resection performed in conjunction with other surgical procedures. Figure 68-12 provides an example of combining root resection and periodontal osseous surgery. The bony lesions that may be present on adjacent teeth are then treated using resective or regenerative therapies. After resection, the flaps are then approximated to cover any grafted tissues or slightly cover the bony margins around the tooth. Sutures are then placed to maintain the

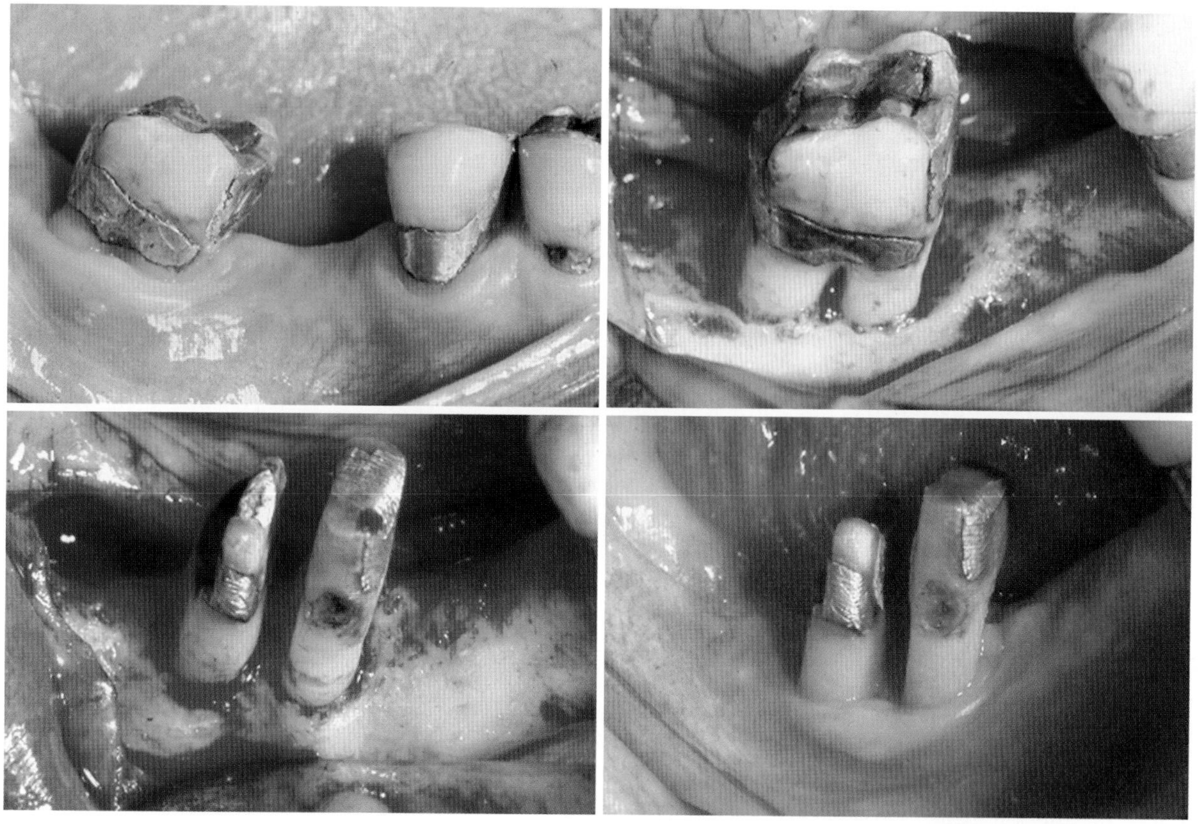

Figure 68-10 Hemisection and interradicular dimension. **A,** Buccal preoperative view of a mandibular right second molar with a deep grade II buccal furcation and root approximation. **B,** Buccal view of bony lesions with flaps. Note the mesial and distal one-wall bony defects. The lingual furcation was similarly affected. **C,** The molar has been hemisected and partially prepared for temporary crowns. Observe the minimal dimension between the two roots. **D,** Buccal view 3 weeks postoperatively. Because the embrasure space is minimal, these roots will be separated with orthodontic therapy to facilitate restoration. (Courtesy Dr. Louis Cuccia, Roseville, Calif.)

position of the flaps. The area may or may not be covered with a surgical dressing.

The removal of a root alters the distribution of occlusal forces on the remaining roots. Therefore it is wise to evaluate the occlusion of teeth from which roots have been resected and, if necessary, adjust the occlusion. Centric holds should be maintained, but eccentric forces should be eliminated from the area over the root that was removed. Patients with advanced attachment loss may benefit from temporary stabilization of the resected tooth to prevent movement (Figure 68-13).

Reconstruction

The periodontal literature has well-documented therapeutic efforts designed to induce new attachment and reconstruction on molars with furcation defects. Many surgical procedures using a variety of grafting materials have been tested on teeth with different classes of furcation involvement. Some investigators have reported clinical success with these techniques,[23] whereas others have suggested that the use of these materials in class II, III, or IV furcations offers little advantage compared with surgical controls.[3,8,29]

Furcation defects with deep two-walled or significant three-walled components, however may be suitable for reconstruction procedures. These vertical bony deformities respond favorably to a variety of other surgical procedures, including debridement with or without membranes and bone grafts. Therapies designed to induce new attachment or reattachment are addressed in Chapter 67.

Extraction

The extraction of teeth with through-and-through furcation defects (classes III and IV) and advanced attachment loss may be the most appropriate therapy for some patients. This is particularly true for individuals who cannot or will not perform adequate plaque control, who have a high level of caries activity, who will not commit to a suitable maintenance program, or who have socioeconomic factors that may preclude more complex therapies. Some patients are reluctant to accept periodontal surgery or even allow the removal of a tooth with advanced furcation involvement, even though the long-term prognosis is poor. The patient may elect to forego therapy, opt to treat the area with scaling and root planing or site-specific antibacterial therapies, and

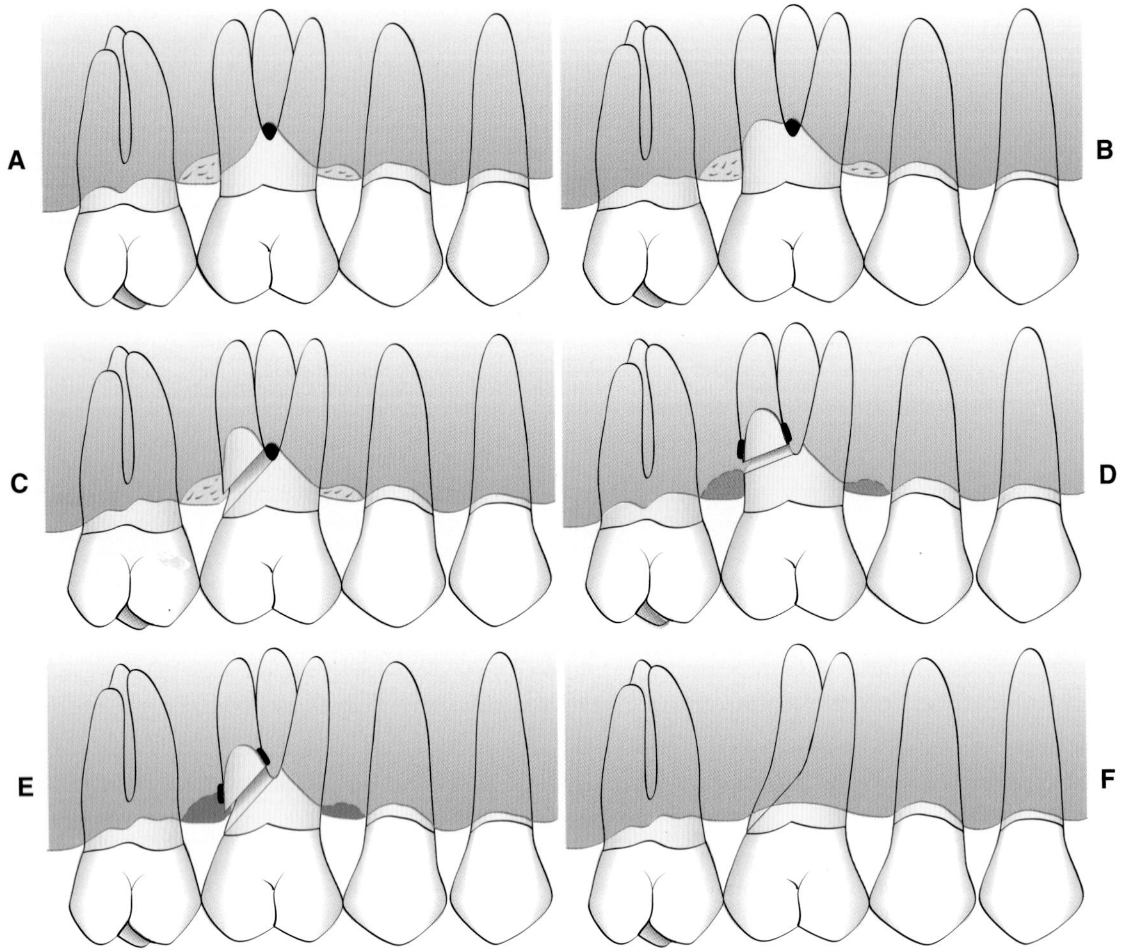

Figure 68-11 Diagrams of distobuccal root resection of maxillary first molar. **A,** Preoperative bony contours with grade II buccal furcation and a crater between the first and second molar. **B,** Removal of bone from the facial side of the distobuccal root and exposure of the furcation for instrumentation. **C,** Oblique section that separates the distal root from the mesial and palatal roots of the molar. **D,** More horizontal section that may be used on a vital root amputation because it exposes less of the pulp of the tooth. **E,** Areas of application of instruments to elevate the sectioned root. **F,** Final contours of the resection.

SCIENCE TRANSFER

Furcation involvement in periodontic therapy is thought to have a strong negative effect on prognosis. However, *all grade I furcations, most grade II furcations, and early grade III furcations have been shown to have a good prognosis if treated appropriately.* Even in some of these cases, when case selection is optimized and furcation involvement is treated with root resection, data show good long-term results. *Once a furcation is grade III or IV, or if there is advanced bone loss in a grade II lesion, the clinician must consider extraction and use of a dental implant to replace the tooth.*

The loss of periodontal structures in the furcations of teeth is problematic because of the anatomy of the area and the inability to gain access for therapeutic intervention or regular maintenance by the patient or professional. A major complication in the treatment of furcations is that much of the area is bounded by tooth structure, and thus less area is available to provide blood supply to new tissue formation. Angiogenesis (process in which new blood vessels are formed) is required for any tissue formation, and with so much area unavailable as a source of angiogenesis, less opportunity exists for new tissue formation. In many patients, therefore, furcation therapy results in achieving and maintaining health with limited tissue regeneration.

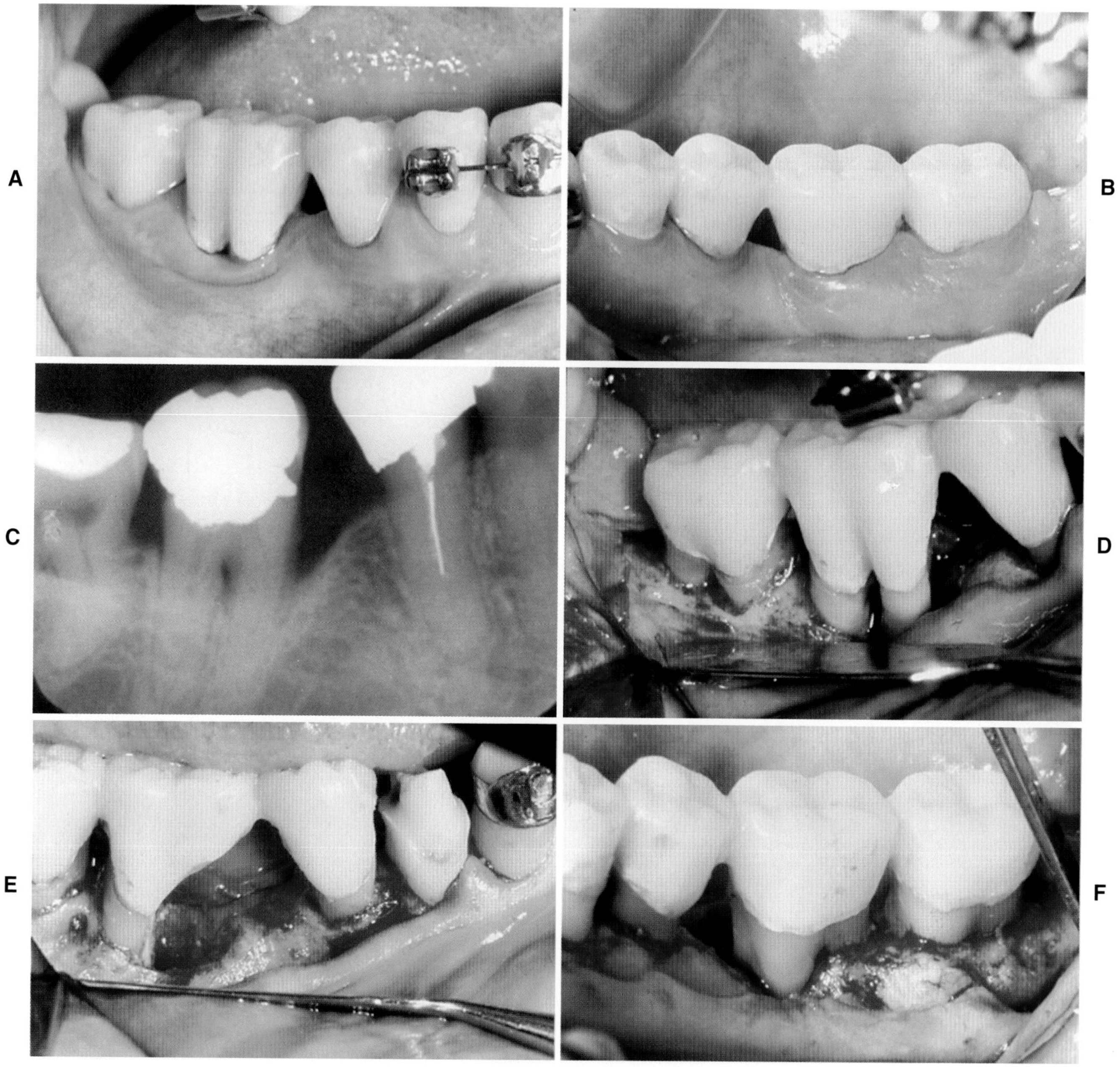

Figure 68-12 Hemisection combined with osseous surgery to treat furcation defects. **A,** Buccal preoperative view with provisional bridge. **B,** Lingual view with provisional bridge in place. **C,** Radiograph of bony defects. Note the deep mesial bony defect, largely of one wall, and the radiolucent area in the furcation of the first molar, indicating a grade II defect. **D,** Buccal view before osseous surgery. In addition to the furcation involvement, a root separation problem exists between the two roots of the first molar. Class II furcations are present on the second molar. **E,** Buccal view after osseous surgery. Mesial root hemisected and removed. The other defects were treated by osteoplasty and ostectomy. **F,** Lingual preoperative view. Note the heavy bony ledging at the lingual surface of these first and second molars. (Courtesy Dr. Louis Cuccia, Roseville, Calif.)

Continued

delay extraction until the tooth becomes symptomatic. Although additional attachment loss may occur, such teeth may survive a significant number of years.[20,31]

The advent of osseointegrated dental implants as an alternative abutment source has had a major impact on the retention of teeth with advanced furcation problems. The high level of predictability of osseointegration may motivate the therapist and patient to consider removal of teeth with a guarded or poor prognosis and to seek an implant-supported prosthetic treatment plan.

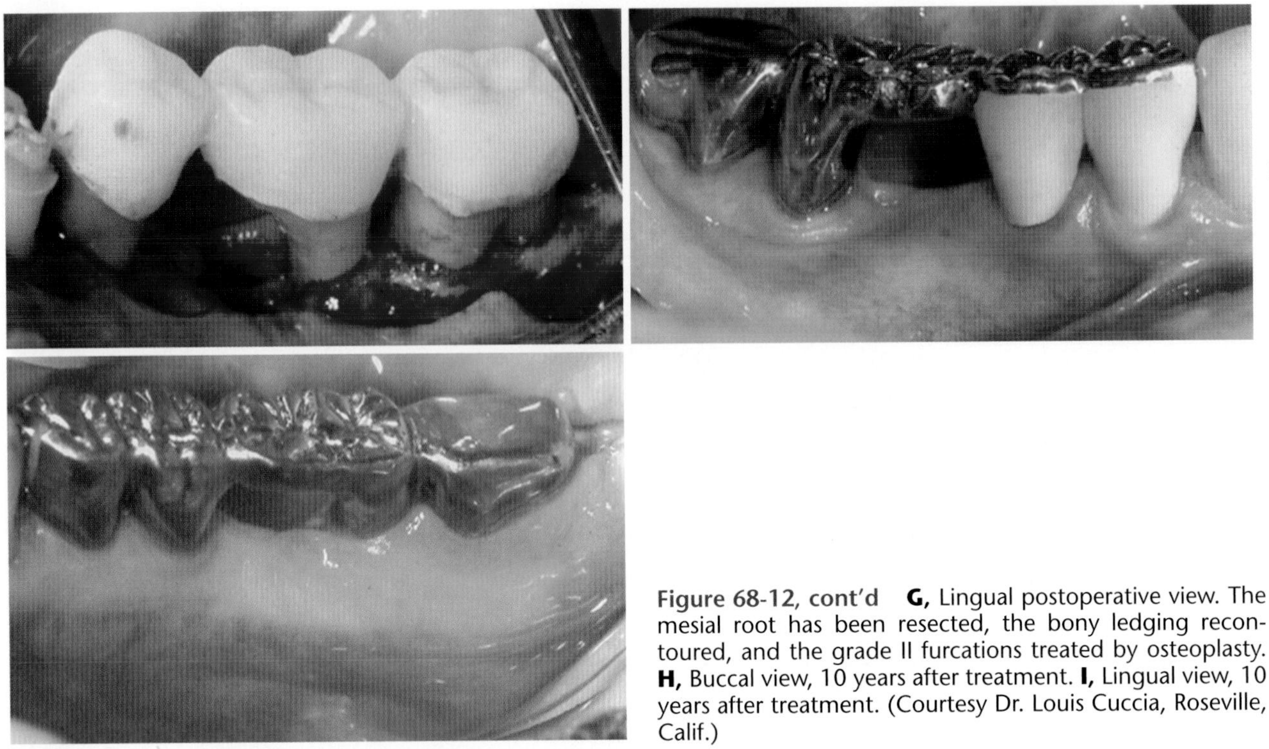

Figure 68-12, cont'd **G,** Lingual postoperative view. The mesial root has been resected, the bony ledging recontoured, and the grade II furcations treated by osteoplasty. **H,** Buccal view, 10 years after treatment. **I,** Lingual view, 10 years after treatment. (Courtesy Dr. Louis Cuccia, Roseville, Calif.)

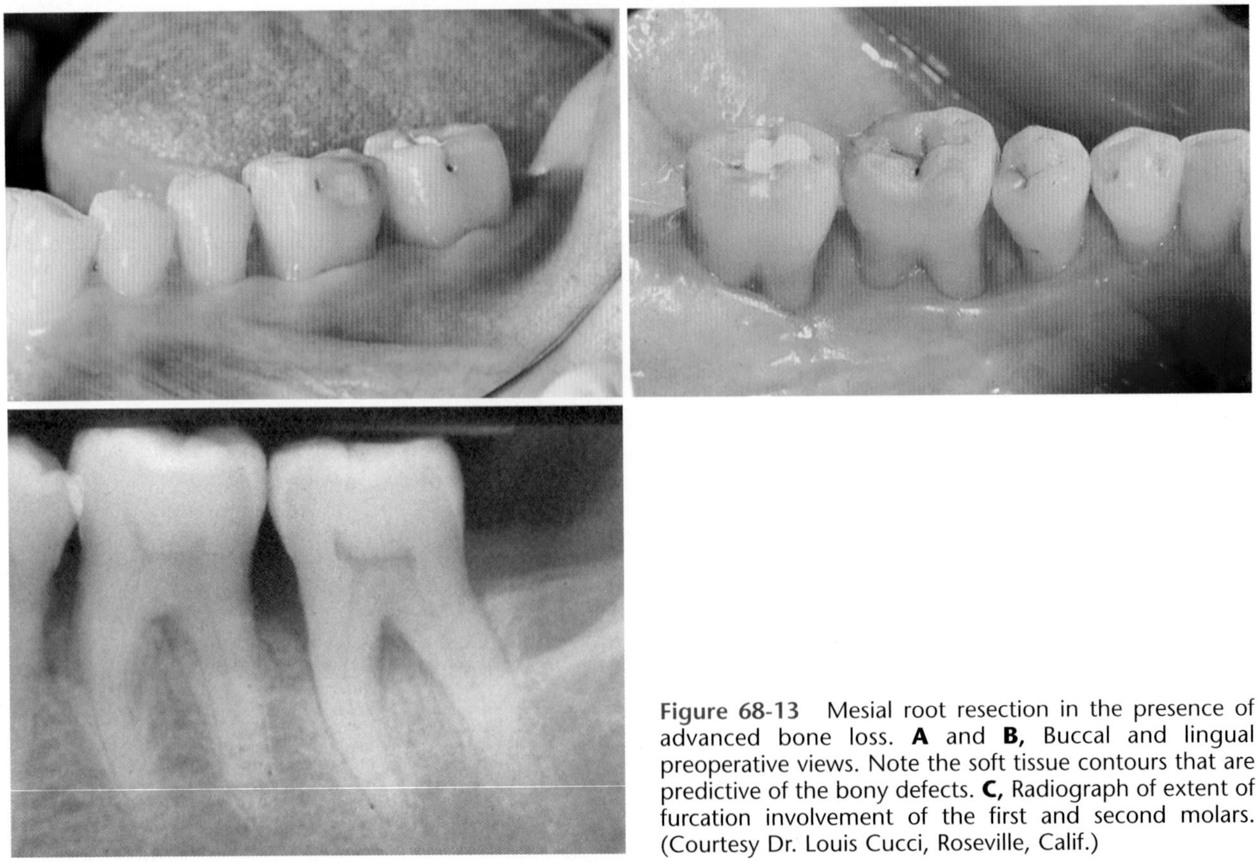

Figure 68-13 Mesial root resection in the presence of advanced bone loss. **A** and **B,** Buccal and lingual preoperative views. Note the soft tissue contours that are predictive of the bony defects. **C,** Radiograph of extent of furcation involvement of the first and second molars. (Courtesy Dr. Louis Cucci, Roseville, Calif.)

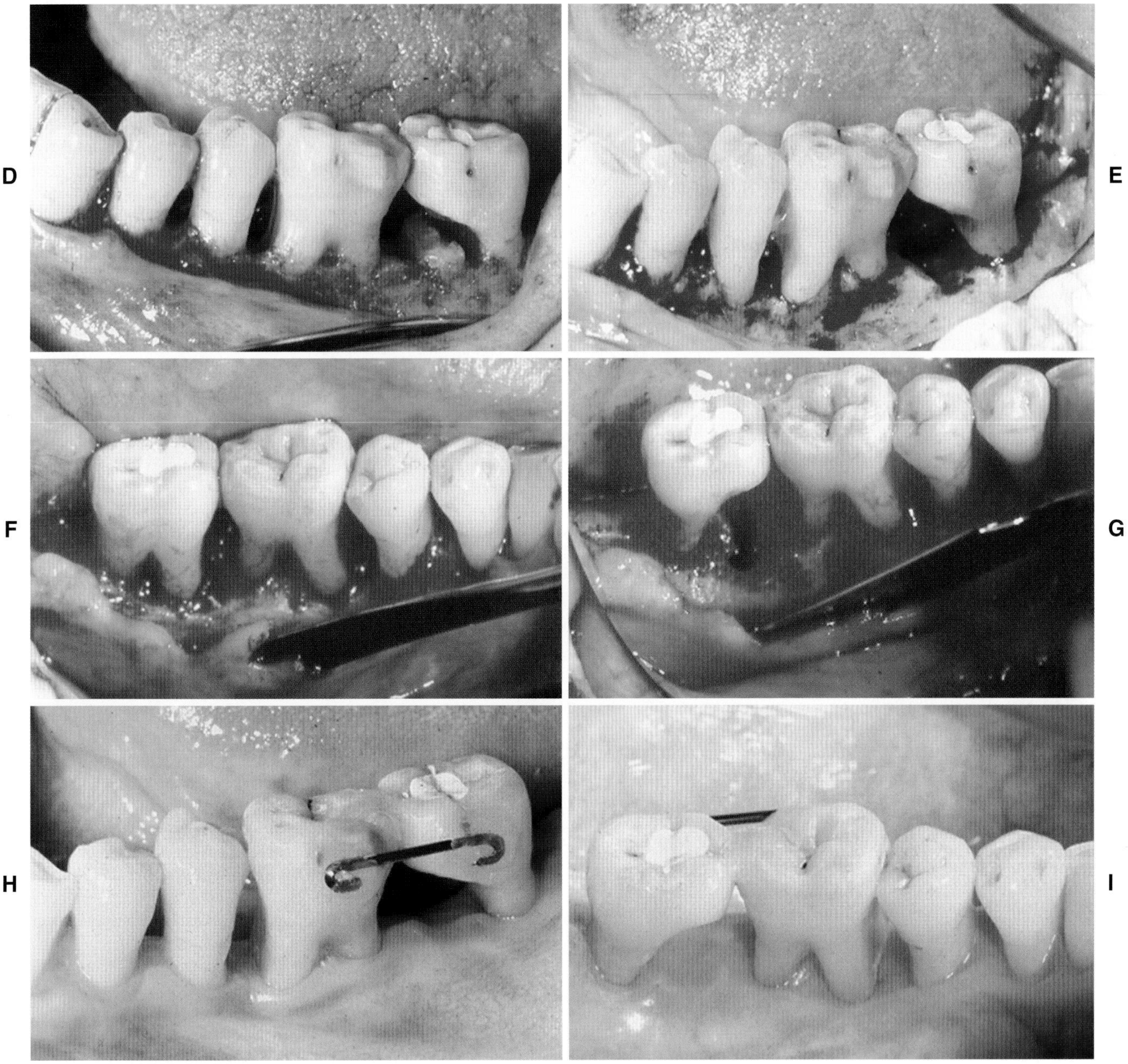

Figure 68-13, cont'd **D** and **E,** Buccal preoperative and postoperative views. The mesial root of the second molar was resected and the interproximal craters treated by osteoplasty and minor ostectomy. **F** and **G,** Lingual preresection and postresection views. The heavy ledges and horizontal bone loss on the lingual surface was managed by osteoplasty. **H** and **I,** Buccal and lingual views 6 weeks postoperatively. A temporary wire splint has been bonded to the molars to prevent tipping of the distal root of the mandibular second molar. (Courtesy Dr. Louis Cucci, Roseville, Calif.)

PROGNOSIS

For many years the presence of significant furcation involvement meant a hopeless long-term prognosis for the tooth. Clinical research, however, has indicated that furcation problems are not as severe a complication as originally suspected if one can prevent the development of caries in the furcation. Relatively simple periodontal therapy is sufficient to maintain these teeth in function for long periods.[20,31] Other investigators have defined the reasons for clinical failure of root-resected or hemisected teeth.[2,24] Their data indicate that recurrent periodontal disease is not a major cause of the failure of these teeth. Investigations of root-resected or hemisected teeth have shown that such teeth can function successfully for long periods.[2,7,24] The keys to long-term success appear to be (1) thorough diagnosis, (2) selection of patients with good oral hygiene, and (3) careful surgical and restorative management.

REFERENCES

1. Bassaraba N: Root amputation and tooth hemisection, *Dent Clin North Am* 13:121, 1969.
2. Basten CH, Ammons WF, Persson R: Long-term evaluation of root resected molars: a retrospective study, *Int J Periodont Restor Dent* 16(3):207, 1996.
3. Becker W, Becker BE, Berg L, et al: New attachment after treatment with root isolation procedures: report for treated class III and class II furcations and vertical osseous defects, *Int J Periodont Restor Dent* 8(3):9, 1988.
4. Black GV: *The American system of dentistry,* Philadelphia, 1886, Lea Brothers.
5. Bower RC: Furcation morphology relative to periodontal treatment: furcation root surface anatomy, *J Periodontol* 50:366, 1979.
6. Bower RC: Furcation morphology relative to periodontal treatment: furcation entrance architecture, *J Periodontol* 50:23, 1979.
7. Carnevale G, DiFebo G, Toyelli MP, et al: A retrospective analysis of the periodontal-prosthodontic treatment of molars with interradicular lesions, *Int J Periodont Restor Dent* 11:188, 1991.
8. Demolon IA, Person GR, Ammons WF, et al: Effects of antibiotic treatment on clinical conditions with guided tissue regeneration: one-year results, *J Periodontol* 65:713, 1994.
9. Easley JR, Drennan GA: Morphological classification of the furca, *J Can Dent Assoc* 35:104, 1969.
10. Everett F, Jump E, Holder T, et al: The intermediate bifurcational ridge: a study of the morphology of the bifurcation of the lower molar, *J Dent Res* 37:162, 1958.
11. Gher ME, Vernino AR: Root morphology: clinical significance in pathogenesis and treatment of periodontal disease, *J Am Dent Assoc* 101:627, 1980.
12. Gher ME Jr, Dunlap RW: Linear variation of the root surface area of the maxillary first molar, *J Periodontol* 56:39, 1985.
13. Glickman I: *Clinical periodontology,* Philadelphia, 1953, Saunders.
14. Goldman HM: Therapy of the incipient bifurcation involvement, *J Periodontol* 29:112, 1958.
15. Gutmann JL: Prevalence, location and patency of accessory canals in the furcation region of permanent molars, *J Periodontol* 49:21, 1978.
16. Hamp SE, Nyman S, Lindhe J: Periodontal treatment of multirooted teeth. Results after 5 years, *J Clin Periodontol* 2:126, 1975.
17. Harrington GW: The perio-endo question: differential diagnosis, *Dent Clin North Am* 23:673, 1979.
18. Haskell EW, Stanley HR: A review of vital root resection, *Int J Periodont Restor Dent* 2(6):29, 1982.
19. Hermann DW, Gher ME Jr, Dumlap RM, et al: The potential attachment area of the maxillary first molar, *J Periodontol* 54:431, 1983.
20. Hirschfeld L, Wasserman B: A long-term survey of tooth loss in 600 treated periodontal patients, *J Periodontol* 49:225, 1978.
21. Hou GL, Tasai CC: Relationship between periodontal furcation involvement and molar cervical enamel projection, *J Periodontol* 58:715, 1978.
22. Kalkwarf K, Kaldahl W, Patil K, et al: Evaluation of furcation region response to periodontal therapy, *J Periodontol* 59:794, 1988.
23. Kenney EB, Lekovic V, Elbaz JJ, et al: The use of porous hydroxylapatite implants in periodontal defects. II. Treatment of class II furcation lesions in lower molars, *J Periodontol* 59:67, 1988.
24. Langer B, Stein SD, Wagenberg B: An evaluation of root resections: a ten-year study, *J Periodontol* 52:719, 1981.
25. Larato DC: Some anatomical factors related to furcation involvement, *J Periodontol* 46:608, 1975.
26. Masters DH, Hoskins SW: Projection of cervical enamel into molar furcations, *J Periodontol* 35:49, 1964.
27. Matia JB, Bissada NF, Maybury JE, et al: Efficiency of scaling of the molar furcation area with and without surgical access, *Int J Periodont Restor Dent* 6(6):25, 1986.
28. Mealy BL, Beybayer MF, Butzin CA, et al: Use of furcal bone sounding to improve accuracy of furcation diagnosis, *J Periodontol* 65:649, 1994.
29. Metzler DG, Seamons BC, Mellonig JT, et al: Clinical evaluation of guided tissue regeneration in the treatment of maxillary class II molar furcation, *J Periodontol* 62:353, 1991.
30. Parashis AO, Anognou-Vareltzides A, Demetrious N: Calculus removal from multirooted teeth with and without surgical access. I. Efficacy on external and furcation surfaces in relation to probing depth, *J Clin Periodontol* 20:63, 1993.
31. Ross I, Thompson RH: A long-term study of root retention of maxillary molars with furcation involvement, *J Periodontol* 49:238, 1978.
32. Tal H: Furcal bony defects in dry mandibles. I. Biometric study, *J Periodontol* 53:360, 1982.
33. Tal H, Lemmer J: Furcal defects in dry mandibles. II. Severity of furcal defects, *J Periodontol* 53:364, 1982.
34. Tarnow D, Fletcher P: Classification of the vertical component of furcation involvement, *J Periodontol* 55:283, 1984.
35. Tibbetts LF: Use of diagnostic probes for detection of periodontal disease, *J Am Dent Assoc* 78:549, 1969.
36. Wylam JM, Mealey B, Mills MP, et al: The clinical effectiveness of open versus closed scaling and root planing on multi-rooted teeth, *J Periodontol* 64:1023, 1993.

Periodontal Plastic and Esthetic Surgery

Henry H. Takei, Robert R. Azzi, and Thomas J. Han

69

CHAPTER

CHAPTER OUTLINE

TERMINOLOGY

The term *mucogingival surgery* was initially introduced in the literature by Friedman[30] to describe surgical procedures for the correction of relationships between the gingiva and the oral mucous membrane with reference to three specific problem areas: attached gingiva, shallow vestibules, and a frenum interfering with the marginal gingiva. With the advancement of periodontal surgical techniques, the scope of nonpocket surgical procedures has increased, now encompassing a multitude of areas that were not addressed in the past. Recognizing this, the 1996 World Workshop in Clinical Periodontics renamed mucogingival surgery as "periodontal plastic surgery,"[2] a term originally proposed by Miller in 1993 and broadened to include the following areas[1,2]:

- Periodontal-prosthetic corrections
- Crown lengthening
- Ridge augmentation
- Esthetic surgical corrections
- Coverage of the denuded root surface
- Reconstruction of papillae
- Esthetic surgical correction around implants
- Surgical exposure of unerupted teeth for orthodontics

Periodontal plastic surgery is defined as the surgical procedures performed to correct or eliminate anatomic, developmental, or traumatic deformities of the gingiva or alveolar mucosa.[1,2] *Mucogingival therapy* is a broader term that includes nonsurgical procedures such as papilla reconstruction by means of orthodontic or restorative therapy. Periodontal plastic surgery includes only the *surgical* procedures of mucogingival therapy.

This chapter discusses the periodontal plastic surgical techniques included in the traditional definition of mucogingival surgery: widening of attached gingiva, deepening of shallow vestibules, and resection of aberrant frena. Other aspects of periodontal plastic surgery, such as periodontal-prosthetic surgery, esthetic surgery around implants, and surgical exposure of teeth for orthodontic therapy, are covered in Chapters 57, 71, and 76.

OBJECTIVES

The three objectives of periodontal plastic surgery addressed in this chapter are as follows:

1. Problems associated with attached gingiva
2. Problems associated with a shallow vestibule
3. Problems associated with an aberrant frenum

Problems Associated with Attached Gingiva

The ultimate goal of mucogingival surgical procedures is the creation or widening of attached gingiva around teeth and implants.[2] The width of the attached gingiva varies in different individuals and on different teeth of the same individual (see Chapter 36). Attached gingiva is not synonymous with "keratinized gingiva" because the latter also includes the free gingival margin.

The width of the attached gingiva is determined by subtracting the depth of the sulcus or pocket from the distance between the crest of the gingival margin and the mucogingival junction.

The original rationale for mucogingival surgery was predicated on the assumption that a minimal width of attached gingiva was required to maintain optimal gingival health. However, several studies have challenged the view that a wide attached gingiva is more protective against the accumulation of plaque than a narrow or a nonexistent zone. No minimum width of attached gingiva has been established as a standard necessary for gingival health. Persons who practice excellent oral hygiene may maintain healthy areas with almost no attached gingiva.

However, those individuals whose oral hygiene practices are less than optimal can be helped by the presence of keratinized gingiva and vestibular depth, which provide room for easier placement of the toothbrush and help to avoid brushing on mucosal tissue. To improve esthetics, the objective is the coverage of the denuded root surface. The maxillary anterior area, especially the facial aspect of the canine, often presents extensive recession. In an individual with a high smile line, this recession may create an esthetic defect. The coverage of the denuded root for esthetic purposes also widens the zone of attached gingiva. A wider zone of attached gingiva is also needed around teeth that serve as abutments for fixed or removable partial dentures, as well as in ridge areas in relation to dentures. Teeth with subgingival restorations and narrow zones of keratinized gingiva have higher gingival inflammation scores than teeth with similar restorations and wide zones of attached gingiva.[68] Therefore, in such cases, techniques for widening the attached gingiva are considered *preprosthetic* periodontal surgical procedures.

Widening the attached gingiva accomplishes the following three objectives:

1. Enhances plaque removal around the gingival margin.
2. Improves esthetics.
3. Reduces inflammation around restored teeth.

Problems Associated with Shallow Vestibule

Another objective of periodontal plastic surgery is the creation of some vestibular depth when this is lacking. Gingival recession displaces the gingival margin apically, thus reducing vestibular depth, which is measured from the gingival margin to the bottom of the vestibule. With minimal vestibular depth, proper hygiene procedures are jeopardized. The sulcular brushing technique requires the placement of the toothbrush at the gingival margin, which may not be possible with reduced vestibular depth.

Minimal attached gingiva with adequate vestibular depth may not require surgical correction if proper atraumatic hygiene is practiced with a soft brush. Minimal amounts of keratinized attached gingiva with no vestibular depth usually benefit from mucogingival correction. Adequate vestibular depth may also be necessary for proper placement of removable prostheses.

Problems Associated with Aberrant Frenum

The final objective of periodontal plastic surgery is to correct frenal or muscle attachments. If adequate gingiva is present coronal to the frenum, there is usually no need to remove it surgically. A frenum that encroaches on the margin of the gingiva may interfere with plaque removal, and tension on this frenum may tend to open the sulcus. In these cases, surgical removal of the frenum is indicated.

ETIOLOGY OF MARGINAL TISSUE RECESSION

The most common cause of the defects just described is abrasive and traumatic toothbrushing habits. Teeth positioned buccally tend to have greater recession. Recession of the gingival tissue and bone exposes the cemental surface, which allows abrasion and "ditching" of the cervical area.

Periodontal inflammation and the resultant loss of attachment results in reduced attached gingiva. Advanced periodontal involvement in areas of minimal attached gingiva result in the base of the pocket extending close to, or apical to, the mucogingival junction.

Frenal and muscle attachments that encroach on the marginal gingiva distend the gingival sulcus, fostering plaque accumulation, increasing the rate of progression of periodontal recession, and causing their recurrence after treatment (Figure 69-1). The problem is more common on facial surfaces, but it may also occur on the lingual surface.[4]

Orthodontic tooth movement through a thin buccal osseous plate leading to a dehiscence beneath a thin gingival tissue margin can cause recession and/or loss of the gingiva[36,80] (Figure 69-2).

FACTORS THAT AFFECT SURGICAL OUTCOME

Irregularity of Teeth

Abnormal tooth alignment is an important cause of gingival deformities that require corrective surgery and also an important factor in determining the outcome

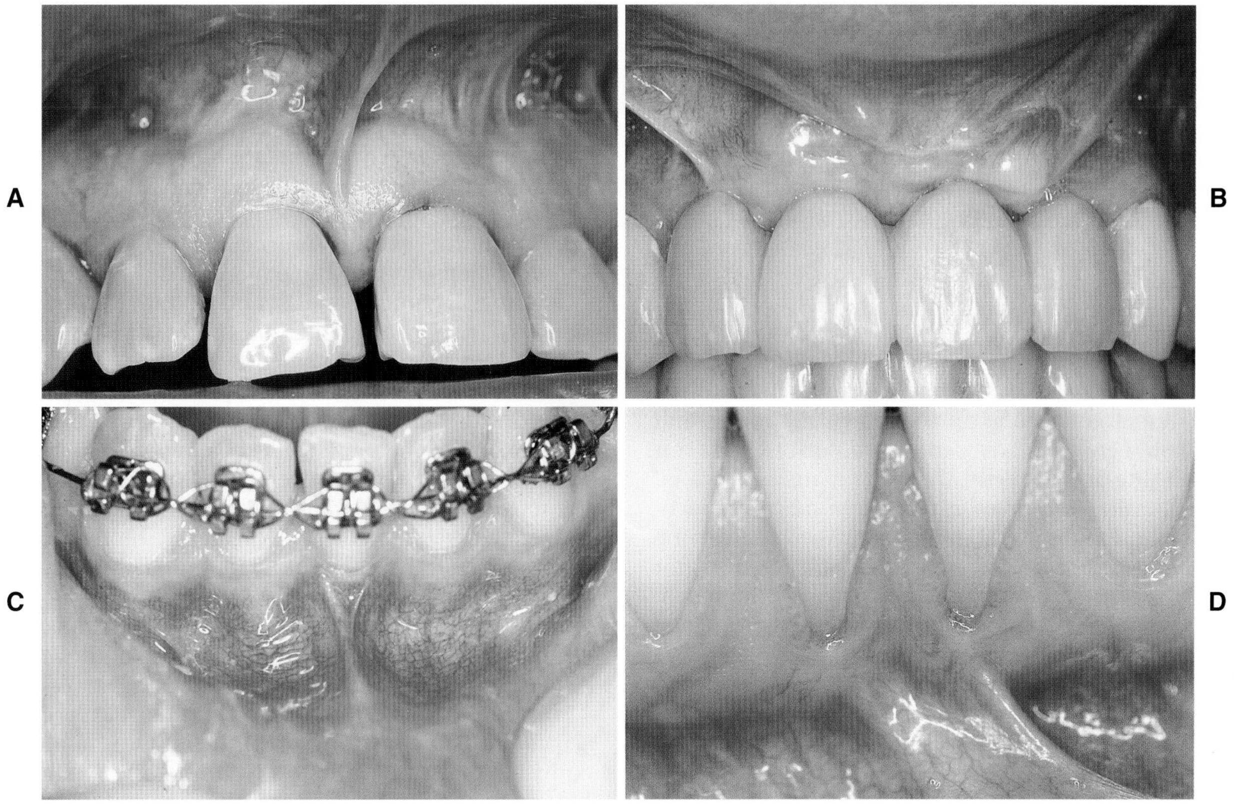

Figure 69-1 High frenum attachments. **A,** Frenum between maxillary central incisors. **B,** Frenum attached to facial surface of maxillary lateral incisors. **C,** Frenum attached to facial surface of mandibular incisor. **D,** Frenum attached to facial surface of an incisor.

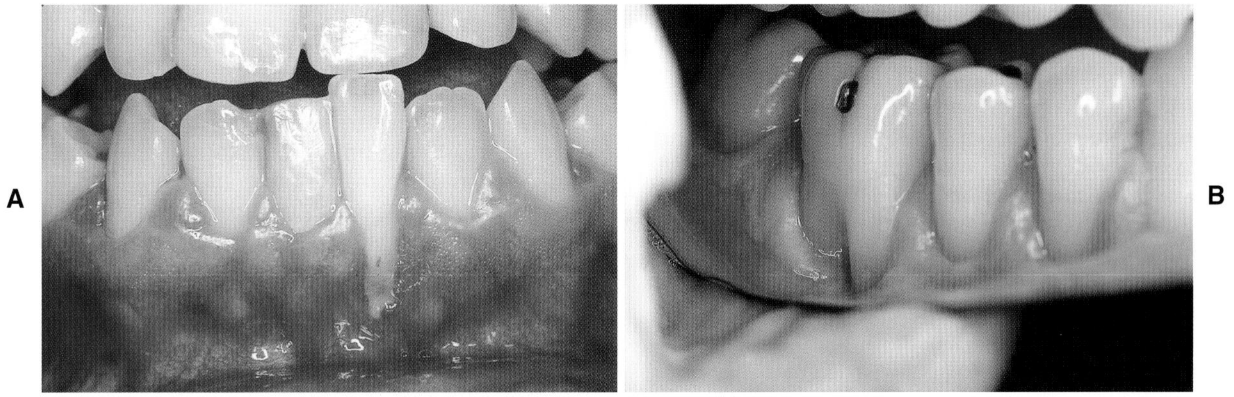

Figure 69-2 **A,** Gingival recession and extreme inflammation around a lower central incisor. **B,** Advanced recession of mesial root of a first lower molar.

of treatment. The location of the gingival margin, width of the attached gingiva, and alveolar bone height and thickness are all affected by tooth alignment. On teeth that are tilted or rotated labially, the labial bony plate is thinner and located farther apically than on the adjacent teeth; therefore the gingiva is recessed so that the root is exposed.[80] On the lingual surface of such teeth, the gingiva is bulbous, and the bone margins are closer to the cementoenamel junction (CEJ). The level of gingival attachment on root surfaces and the width of the attached gingiva after mucogingival surgery are affected as much by tooth alignment as by variations in treatment procedures.

Orthodontic correction is indicated when mucogingival surgery is performed on malposed teeth in an attempt to widen the attached gingiva or to restore the gingiva over denuded roots. If orthodontic treatment is not feasible, the prominent tooth should be reduced to within the borders of the alveolar bone, with special care taken to avoid pulp injury.

Roots covered with thin bony plates present a hazard in mucogingival surgery. Even the most protective type of flap, a partial-thickness flap, creates the risk of bone resorption on the periosteal surface.[38] Resorption in amounts that ordinarily are not significant may cause loss of bone height when the bone plate is thin or tapered at the crest.

Mucogingival Line (Junction)

Normally, the mucogingival line in the incisor and canine areas is located approximately 3 mm apical to the crest of the alveolar bone on the radicular surfaces and 5 mm interdentally.[69] In periodontal disease and on malposed disease-free teeth, the bone margin is located farther apically and may extend beyond the mucogingival line. The distance between the mucogingival line and the CEJ before and after periodontal surgery is not necessarily constant. After inflammation is eliminated, the tissue tends to contract and draw the mucogingival line in the direction of the crown.[23]

TECHNIQUES TO INCREASE ATTACHED GINGIVA

To simplify and better understand the techniques and the result of the surgery, the following classifications are presented:

- *Gingival augmentation* apical *to the area of recession.* A graft, either pedicle or free, is placed on a recipient bed apical to the recessed gingival margin. No attempt is made to cover the denuded root surface where there is gingival and bone recession.
- *Gingival augmentation* coronal *to the recession (root coverage).* A graft (either pedicle or free) is placed covering the denuded root surface. Both the apical and the coronal widening of attached gingiva enhance oral hygiene procedures, but only the latter can correct an esthetic problem. For preprosthetic purposes, the combination of widening keratinized gingiva apical and coronal to the recession would satisfy this objective. Consideration of the objectives as apical, coronal, or both provides a better understanding of the techniques required to achieve the goals.

Widening of the keratinized attached gingiva (apical or coronal to the area of recession) can be accomplished by numerous techniques, such as the free gingival autograft, free connective tissue autograft, and lateral pedicle flap, which can be used for either objective.

Gingival Augmentation Apical to Recession

Techniques for gingival augmentation *apical* to the area of recession include free gingival autograft, free connective tissue autograft,[3] and apically positioned flap.

Free Gingival Autografts

Free gingival grafts are used to create a widened zone of attached gingiva. They were initially described by Bjorn[5] in 1963 and have been extensively investigated since that time (Figure 69-3).

THE CLASSIC TECHNIQUE

Step 1: Prepare the Recipient Site. The purpose of this step is to prepare a firm connective tissue bed to receive the graft. The recipient site can be prepared by incising at the existing mucogingival junction with a #15 blade to the desired depth, blending the incision on both ends with the existing mucogingival line. Periosteum should be left covering the bone.

Another technique consists of outlining the recipient site with two vertical incisions from the cut gingival margin into the alveolar mucosa.

Extend the incisions to approximately twice the desired width of the attached gingiva, allowing for 50% contraction of the graft when healing is complete. The amount of contraction depends on the extent to which the recipient site penetrates the muscle attachments. The deeper the recipient site, the greater is the tendency for the muscles to elevate the graft and reduce the final width of the attached gingiva. The periosteum along the apical border of the graft is sometimes penetrated in an effort to prevent postoperative narrowing of the attached gingiva.

Insert a #15 blade along the cut gingival margin and separate a flap consisting of epithelium and underlying connective tissue without disturbing the periosteum. Extend the flap to the depth of the vertical incisions.

If a narrow band of attached gingiva remains after the pockets are eliminated, it should be left intact, and the recipient site should be started by inserting the blade at the mucogingival junction instead of at the cut gingival margin.

Suture the flap where the apical portion of the free graft will be located. Three to four independent gut sutures are placed. The needle is first passed as a superficial mattress suture perpendicular to the incision and then on the periosteum parallel to the incision (Figure 69-4).

Make an aluminum foil template of the recipient site to be used as a pattern for the graft.

Grafts can also be placed directly on bone tissue. For this technique, the flap should be separated by blunt dissection with a periosteal elevator. Reported advantages of this variant are less postoperative mobility of the graft, less swelling, better hemostasis,[24] and 1.5 to 2 times less shrinkage.[41,42] However, a healing lag is observed for the first 2 weeks.[14,15,28]

Step 2: Obtain the Graft from the Donor Site. The classic or conventional-free gingival graft technique consists of transferring a piece of keratinized gingiva approximately the size of the recipient site. To avoid the large wound that this procedure sometimes leaves in the donor site, some alternative methods have been proposed. The original technique is described first, followed by several of the most common variants. For the classic technique, a partial-thickness graft is used. The palate is the usual site from which donor tissue is removed. The graft should consist of epithelium and a thin layer of underlying connective tissue. Place the template over the donor site, and make a shallow incision around it with a #15 blade. Insert the blade to the desired thickness at one edge of the graft. Elevate the edge and

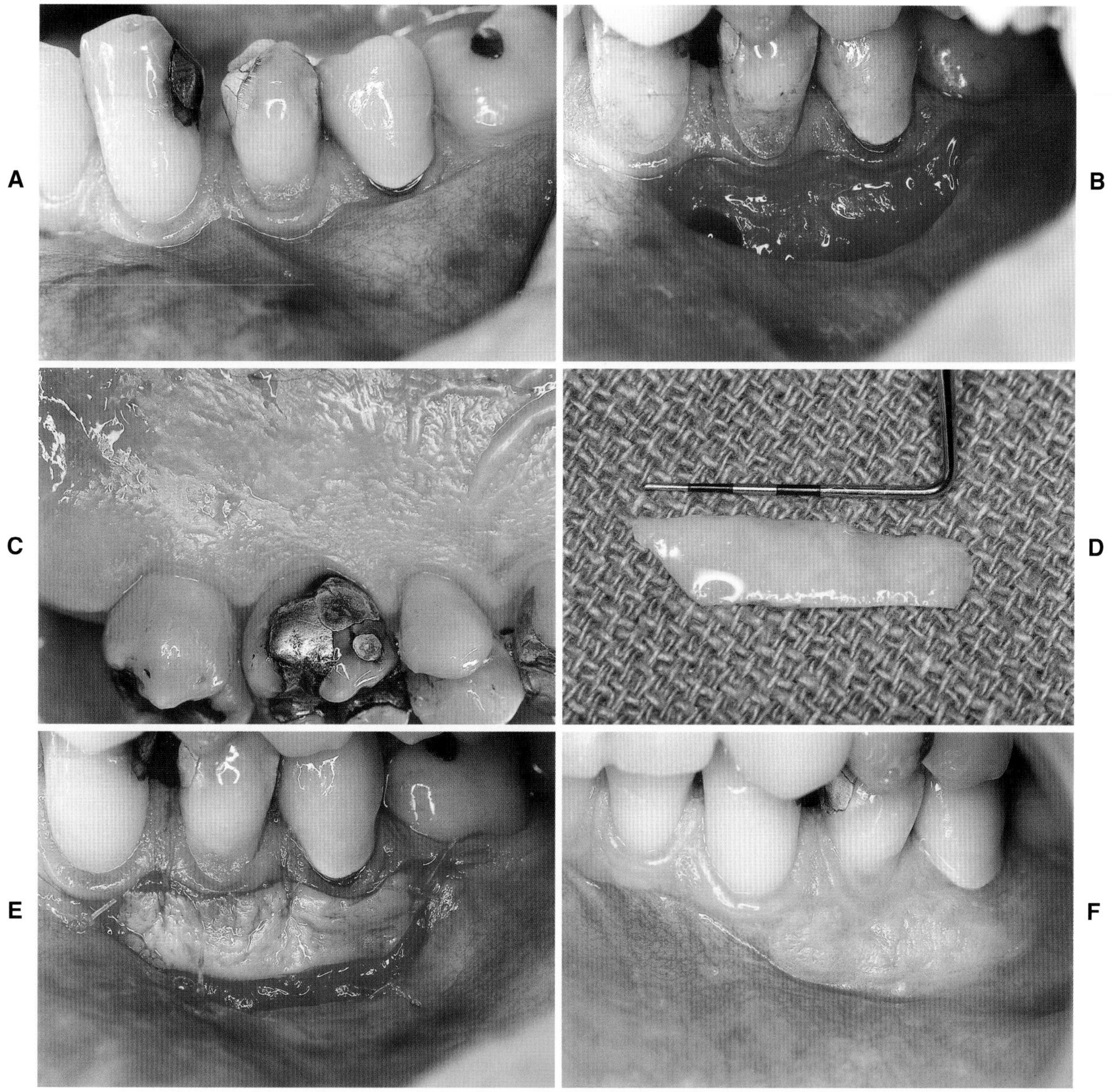

Figure 69-3 Free gingival graft. **A,** Before treatment; minimal keratinized gingiva. **B,** Recipient site prepared for free gingival graft. **C,** Palate will be donor site. **D,** Free graft. **E,** Graft transferred to recipient site. **F,** At 6 months, showing widened zone of attached gingiva. (Courtesy Dr. Perry Klokkevold, Los Angeles.)

hold it with tissue forceps. Continue to separate the graft with the blade, lifting it gently as separation progresses to provide visibility. Placing sutures at the margins of the graft helps control it during separation and transfer and simplifies placement and suturing to the recipient site.[3]

Proper thickness is important for survival of the graft. It should be thin enough to permit ready diffusion of nutritive fluid from the recipient site, which is essential in the immediate posttransplant period. A graft that is too thin may necrose and expose the recipient site.[53,57] If the graft is too thick, its peripheral layer is jeopardized because of the excessive tissue that separates it from new circulation and nutrients. Thick grafts may also create a deeper wound at the donor site, with the possibility of injuring major palatal arteries.[77] The ideal thickness of a graft is between 1.0 and 1.5 mm.[53,57] After the graft is separated, remove loose tissue tabs from the undersurface. Thin the edge to avoid bulbous marginal and interdental contours. Special precautions must be taken with grafts from the palate.

The submucosa in the posterior region is thick and fatty and should be trimmed so that it will not interfere with vascularization. Grafts tend to reestablish their original epithelial structure, so mucous glands may occur in grafts obtained from the palate.

A thick graft can be thinned by holding it between two wet wooden tongue depressors and slicing it longitudinally with a sharp #15 blade.

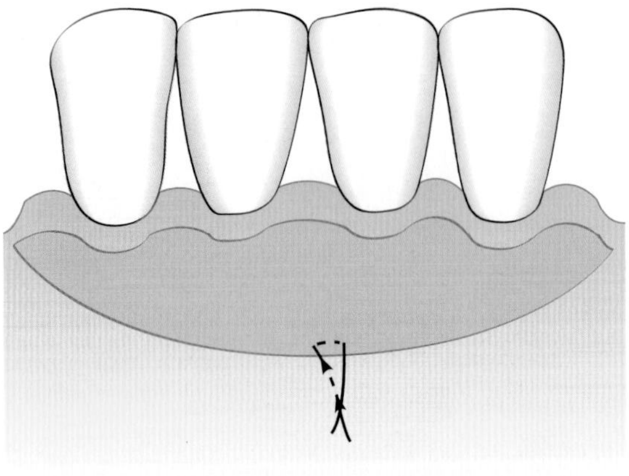

Figure 69-4 Diagram of graft bed suture.

Step 3: Transfer and Immobilize the Graft. Remove the sponge from the recipient site; reapply it, with pressure if necessary, until bleeding is stopped. Remove the excess clot. A thick clot interferes with vascularization of the graft.[54]

Position the graft and adapt it firmly to the recipient site. A space between the graft and the underlying tissue (dead space) impairs vascularization and jeopardizes the graft. Suture the graft at the lateral borders and to the periosteum to secure it in position. Before suturing is completed, elevate the unsutured portion and cleanse the recipient bed beneath it with an aspirator to remove clots or loose tissue fragments. Press the graft back into position and complete the sutures. The graft must be immobilized. Any movement interferes with healing. Avoid excessive tension, which can distort the graft from the underlying surface. Every precaution should be taken to avoid trauma to the graft. Tissue forceps should be used delicately and a minimum number of sutures used to avoid unnecessary tissue perforation.

Step 4: Protect the Donor Site. Cover the donor site with a periodontal pack for 1 week, and repeat if necessary. Retention of the pack on the donor site can be a problem. If facial attached gingiva was used, the pack may be retained by locking it through the interproximal spaces onto the lingual surface. If there are no open interdental spaces, the pack can be covered by a plastic stent wired to the teeth. A modified Hawley retainer is useful to cover the pack on the palate and over edentulous ridges.

VARIANT TECHNIQUES. Variants to the classic technique include the accordion technique, strip technique, and combination of both. All are modifications of the free grafts:

The **accordion technique,** described by Rateitschak et al.,[61] attains expansion of the graft by alternate incisions in opposite sides of the graft.

The **strip technique,** developed by Han et al.,[37] consists of obtaining two or three strips of gingival donor tissue about 3 to 5 mm wide and long enough to cover the entire length of the recipient site (Figure 69-5). These strips are placed side by side to form one donor tissue and sutured on the recipient site. The area is then covered with aluminum foil and surgical pack. The advantages of this technique are the rapid healing of the donor site. The epithelial migration of the close wound edges (3-5 mm) allows rapid epithelialization of the open wound. The donor site usually does not require suturing and heals uneventfully in 1 week.

In some cases, a **combination technique** can be performed as follows. Remove a strip of tissue from the palate about 3 to 4 mm thick, place it between two wet tongue depressors, and split it longitudinally with a sharp #15 blade. Both will be used as free grafts. The superficial portion consists of epithelium and connective tissue, and the deeper portion consists only of connective tissue. These donor tissues are placed on the recipient site as in the strip technique. The minimal donor site wound by obtaining two donor tissues from one site is the advantage of this technique.

HEALING OF THE GRAFT. The success of the graft depends on survival of the connective tissue. Sloughing of the epithelium occurs in most cases, but the extent to which the connective tissue withstands the transfer to the new location determines the fate of the graft. Fibrous organization of the interface between the graft and the recipient bed occurs within 2 to several days.[67]

The graft is initially maintained by a diffusion of fluid from the host bed, adjacent gingiva, and alveolar mucosa.[32] The fluid is a transudate from the host vessels and provides nutrition and hydration essential for the initial survival of the transplanted tissues. During the first day, the connective tissue becomes edematous and disorganized and undergoes degeneration and lysis of some of its elements. As healing progresses, the edema is resolved, and degenerated connective tissue is replaced by new granulation tissue.

Revascularization of the graft starts by the second[6] or third[43] day. Capillaries from the recipient bed proliferate into the graft to form a network of new capillaries and anastomose with preexisting vessels.[43]

Many of the graft vessels degenerate and are replaced by new ones, and some participate in the new circulation. The central section of the surface is the last to vascularize, but this is complete by the tenth day.

The epithelium undergoes degeneration and sloughing, with complete necrosis occurring in some areas.[13,56] It is replaced by new epithelium from the borders of the recipient site. A thin layer of new epithelium is present by the fourth day, with rete pegs developing by the seventh day.

Heterotopically placed grafts maintain their structure (keratinized epithelium), even after the grafted epithelium has become necrotic and has been replaced by neighboring areas of nonkeratinized epithelium, which suggests that a genetic predetermination of the specific character of the oral mucosa exists that depends on stimuli originating in the connective tissue.[44] This is the basis for the technique that uses grafts composed only of connective tissue obtained from areas where it is covered by keratinized epithelium.[10,22,28]

As seen microscopically, healing of a graft of intermediate thickness (0.75 mm) is complete by 10.5 weeks; thicker grafts (1.75 mm) may require 16 weeks or longer.[33] The gross appearance of the graft reflects the tissue changes within it. At transplantation the graft vessels are empty and the graft is pale. The pallor changes to an ischemic grayish white during the first 2 days until vascularization begins and a pink color appears. The plasmatic circulation accumulates and causes softening and swelling of the graft, which are reduced when the edema is removed from the recipient site by the new blood vessels. Loss of epithelium leaves the graft smooth and shiny. New epithelium creates a thin, gray, veil-like surface that develops normal features as the epithelium matures.

Functional integration of the graft occurs by the seventeenth day, but the graft is morphologically distinguishable from the surrounding tissue for months. The graft eventually blends with adjacent tissues, but sometimes, although pink, firm, and healthy, it is somewhat bulbous. This usually presents no problem, but if the graft traps plaque or is esthetically unacceptable, thinning of the graft may be necessary. Thinning the surface of the grafted tissue does reduce the bulbous condition because the surface epithelium tends to proliferate again. The graft should be thinned by making the necessary incisions to elevate it from the periosteum, removing tissue from its undersurface, and suturing it back in place.

ACCOMPLISHMENTS. Free gingival grafts effectively widen the attached gingiva. Several biometric studies have analyzed the width of the attached gingiva after the placement of a free gingival graft.[12,38,41] After 24 weeks, grafts placed on denuded bone shrink 25%, whereas grafts placed on periosteum shrink 50%.[49] The greatest amount of shrinkage occurs within the first 6 weeks.

The placement of a gingival graft does not "improve" the status of the gingiva.[26,27,75] Therefore the indication

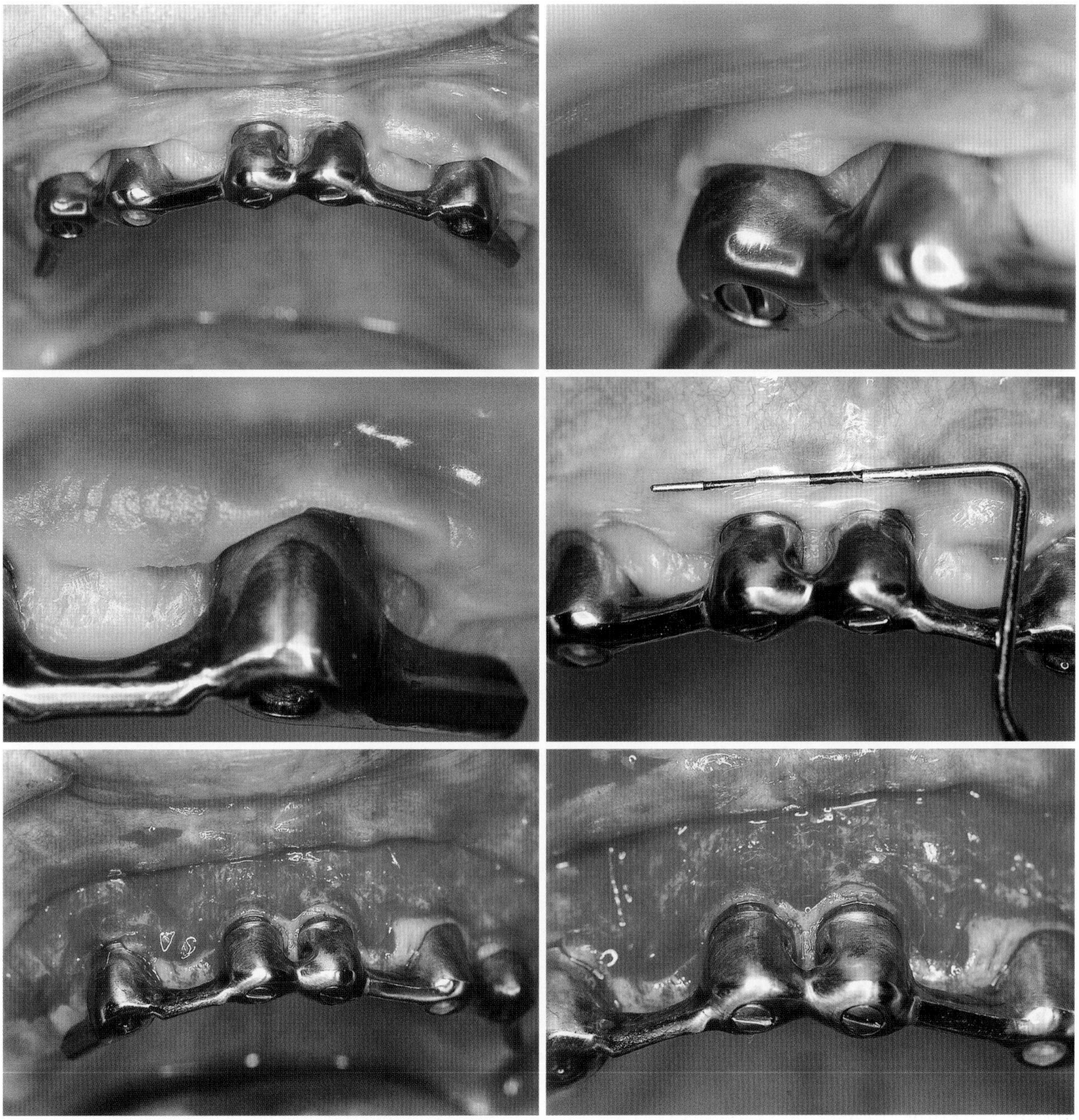

Figure 69-5 Free gingival graft: strip technique. **A** to **D,** Mucosal tissue around implants. **E** and **F,** Recipient site prepared.

Continued

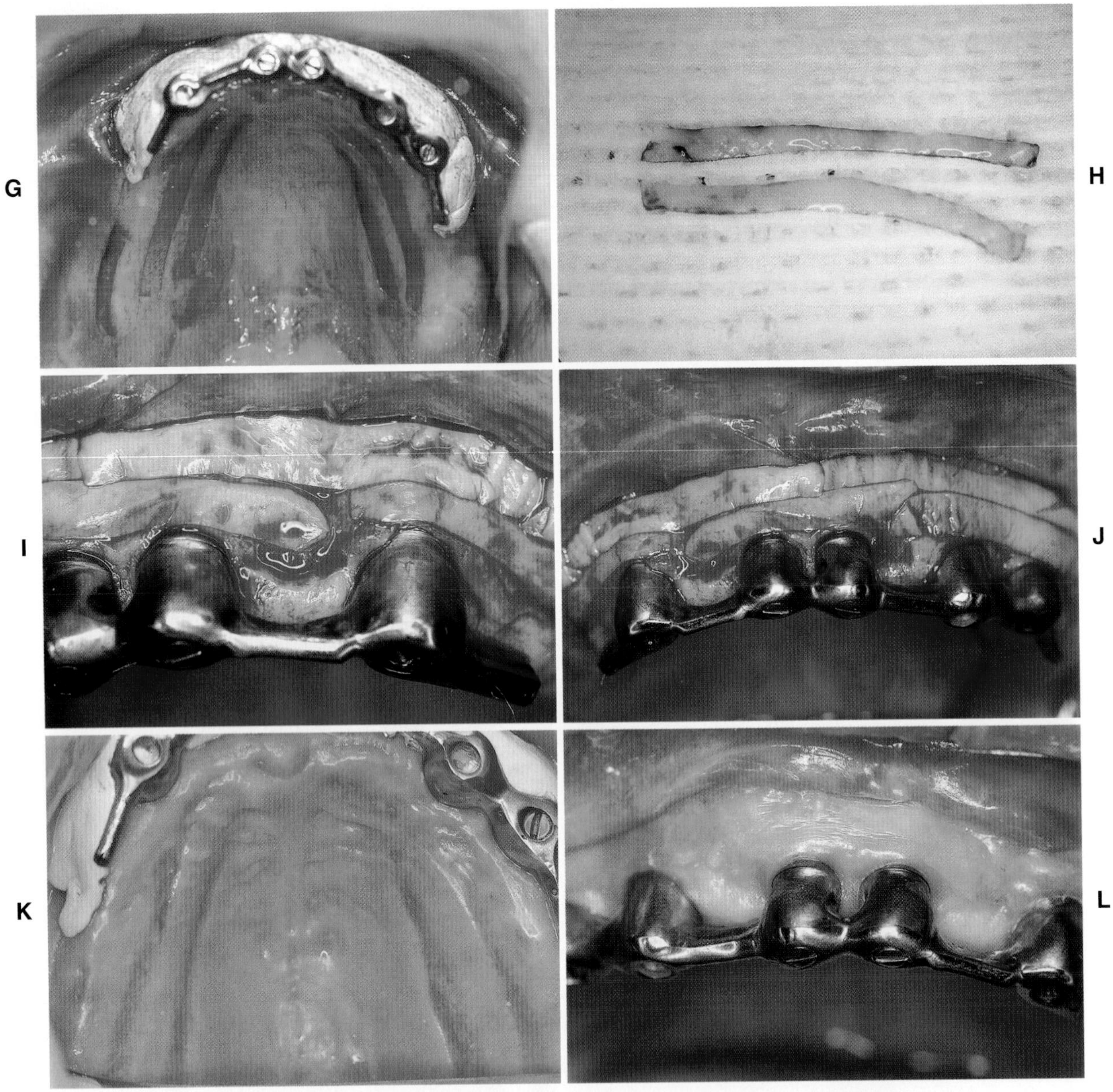

Figure 69-5, cont'd **G,** Donor site with strips of free graft removed. **H,** Donor strips of free graft. **I** and **J,** Strips placed side by side on recipient site. **K,** Donor area 1 week after graft removal. **L,** Healing of recipient site after 3 months. Note good, keratinized, attached gingiva.

for a free gingival graft should be based on the presence of progressive gingival recession and inflammation. When recession continues to progress after a few months with good plaque control, a graft can be placed to prevent further recession and loss of attached gingiva.

Other materials have been used to replace gingival tissue in gingival extension procedures. Attempts with lyophilized dura mater[66] and sclera[50] have not been satisfactory. The use of irradiated free gingival allografts showed satisfactory results,[64] but further research is necessary before they can be considered for clinical use.

Free autogenous gingival grafts have been found to be useful for covering nonpathologic dehiscences and fenestrations. *Nonpathologic* refers to openings of the bone through the tooth surface not previously exposed to the oral environment and found in the course of flap surgery.[25]

The use of free gingival autografts to cover denuded roots is described in the section on gingival augmentation coronal to the recession.

Free Connective Tissue Autografts

The connective tissue autograft technique was originally described by Edel[28] and is based on the fact that the connective tissue carries the genetic message for the overlying epithelium to become keratinized. Therefore, only connective tissue from a keratinized zone can be used as a graft (Figure 69-6).

The advantage of this technique is that the donor tissue is obtained from the undersurface of the palatal

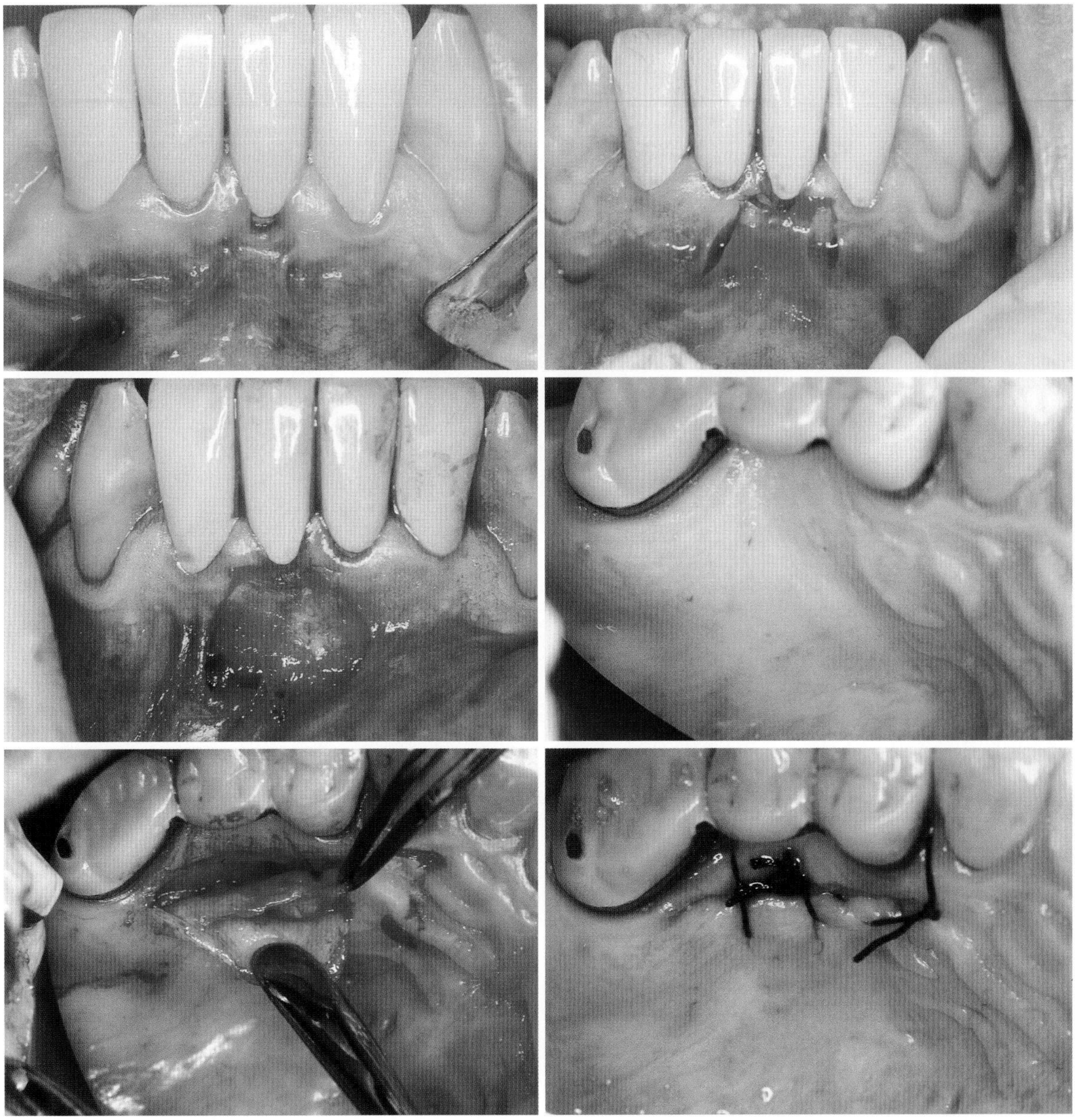

Figure 69-6 Free connective tissue graft. **A,** Lack of keratinized, attached gingiva buccal to central incisor. **B,** Vertical incisions to prepare recipient site. **C,** Recipient site prepared. **D,** Palate from which connective tissue will be removed for donor tissue. **E,** Removal of connective tissue. **F,** Donor site sutured.

Continued

flap, which is sutured back in primary closure; therefore, healing is by first intention. The patient has less discomfort postoperatively at the donor site. When resective flap surgery is planned for the palate, the connective tissue removed to thin the palatal flap can be used as the graft tissue to augment areas of recession.

Another advantage of the free connective tissue autograft is that better esthetics can be achieved because of a better color match of the grafted tissue to adjacent areas.

Apically Displaced Flap

This technique uses the apically positioned flap, either partial thickness or full thickness, to increase the zone of keratinized gingiva. Chapter 65 provides a step-by-step description of the surgical technique for apically displaced flaps, and Figure 69-7 illustrates the procedure.

ACCOMPLISHMENTS. The apically displaced flap technique increases the width of the keratinized gingiva but cannot predictability deepen the vestibule with attached gingiva. Adequate vestibular depth must be present before the surgery to allow apical positioning of the flap. The edge of the flap may be located in three positions in relation to the bone, as follows:

1. *Slightly coronal to the crest of the bone.* This location attempts to preserve the attachment of supracrestal fibers; it may also result in thick gingival margins

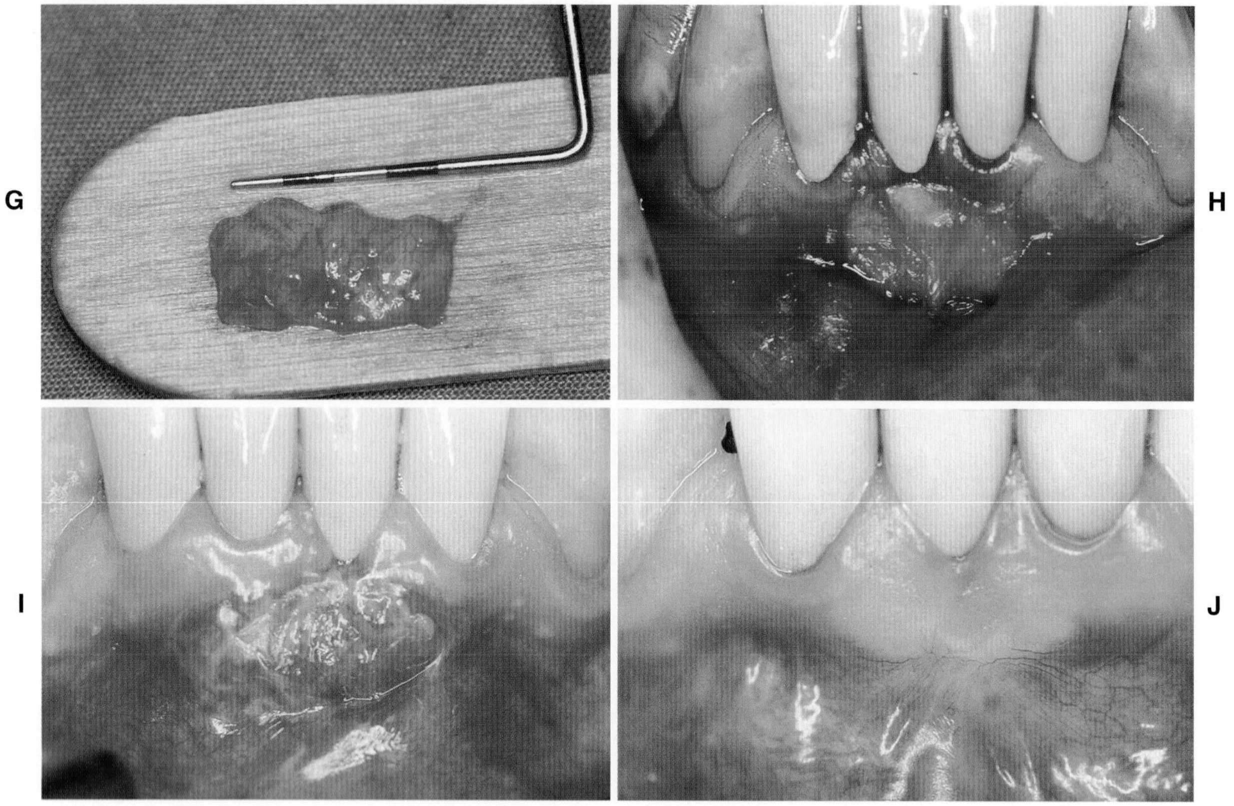

Figure 69-6, cont'd **G,** Connective tissue for graft. **H,** Free connective tissue placed at donor site. **I,** Postoperative healing at 10 days. **J,** Final healing at 3 months. Note wide, keratinized, attached gingiva.

and interdental papillae with deep sulci and may create the risk of recurrent pockets.

2. *At the level of the crest* (Figure 69-7, *C*). This results in a satisfactory gingival contour, provided that the flap is adequately thinned.
3. *Two millimeters short of the crest* (Figure 69-7, *D*). This position produces the most desirable gingival contour and the same posttreatment level of gingival attachment as obtained by placing the flap at the crest of the bone.[31] New tissue covers the crest of the bone to produce a firm, tapered gingival margin.

Placing the flap short of the crest increases the risk of a slight reduction in bone height,[21] but the advantages of a well-formed gingival margin compensate for this.

Other Techniques

The "vestibular extension technique," originally described by Edlan and Mejchar,[29] produced statistically significant widening of attached nonkeratinized tissue. This increase in width in the mandibular area reportedly persisted in patients observed for up to 5 years.[29,65,76] Currently, this technique is of historical interest only.

The *fenestration operation* was designed to widen the zone of attached gingiva with a minimum loss of bone height.[62,63] It has also been called *periosteal separation.*[19] It uses a partial-thickness flap, except in a rectangular area at the base of the operative field, where the periosteum is removed, exposing the bone. This is the area of fenestration. Its purpose is to create a scar that is firmly bound to the bone.[16] It prevents separation from the bone and postsurgical narrowing of the attached zone. Results obtained with this technique are not as predictable as with the free gingival graft; therefore, it is not widely performed except for small, isolated areas.

Gingival Augmentation Coronal to Recession (Root Coverage)

Understanding the different stages and condition of gingival recession is necessary for predictable root coverage. Several classifications of denuded roots have been proposed. In the 1960s, Sullivan and Atkins[71] classified gingival recession into four morphologic categories: (1) shallow-narrow, (2) shallow-wide, (3) deep-narrow, and (4) deep-wide.

This early classification was helpful to categorize the lesion better but did not enable the clinician to predict the outcome of therapy. The predictability of root coverage can be enhanced by the presurgical examination and the correlation of the recession by using the classification proposed by Miller,[51] as follows (Figure 69-8):

Class I. Marginal tissue recession does not extend to the mucogingival junction. There is no loss of bone or soft tissue in the interdental area. This type of recession can be narrow or wide.

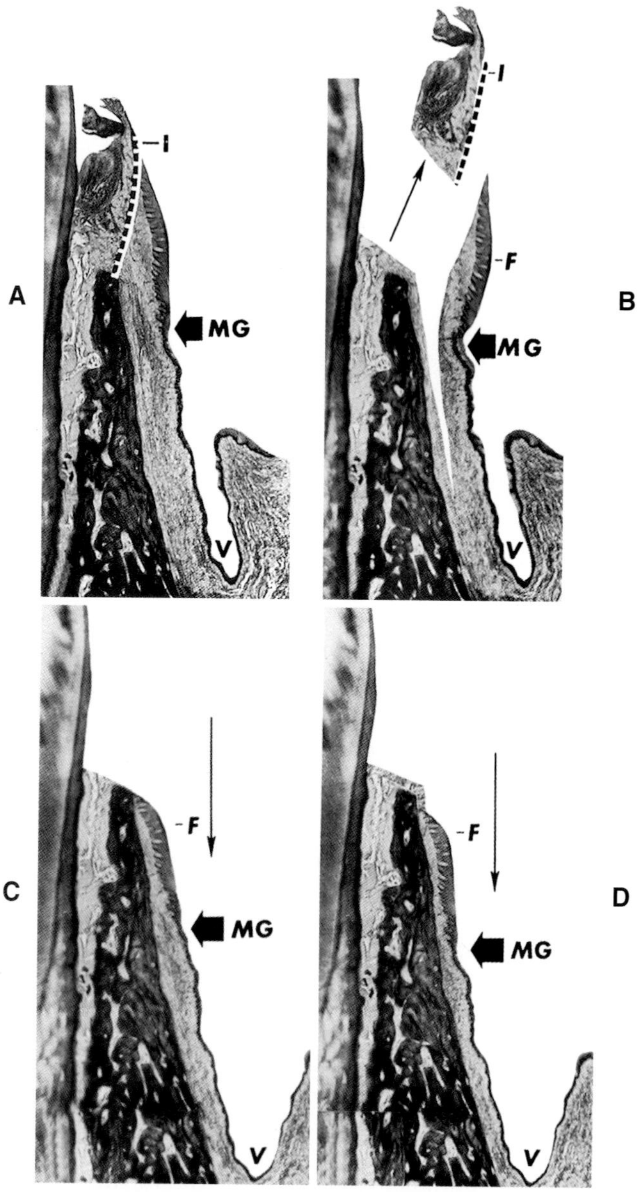

Figure 69-7 Apically displaced partial-thickness flap. **A,** Internal bevel incision *(I)* separates inner wall of periodontal pocket. *MG,* Mucogingival junction; *V,* vestibular fornix. **B,** Partial-thickness flap *(F)* separated, leaving periosteum and a layer of connective tissue on the bone. The inner wall of the periodontal pocket *(I)* is removed, and the tooth is scaled and planed. **C,** Partial-thickness flap *(F)* displaced apically, with edge of the flap at crest of the bone. Note that the vestibular fornix is also moved apically. **D,** Partial-thickness flap *(F)* displaced apically, with edge of the flap several millimeters below crest of the bone.

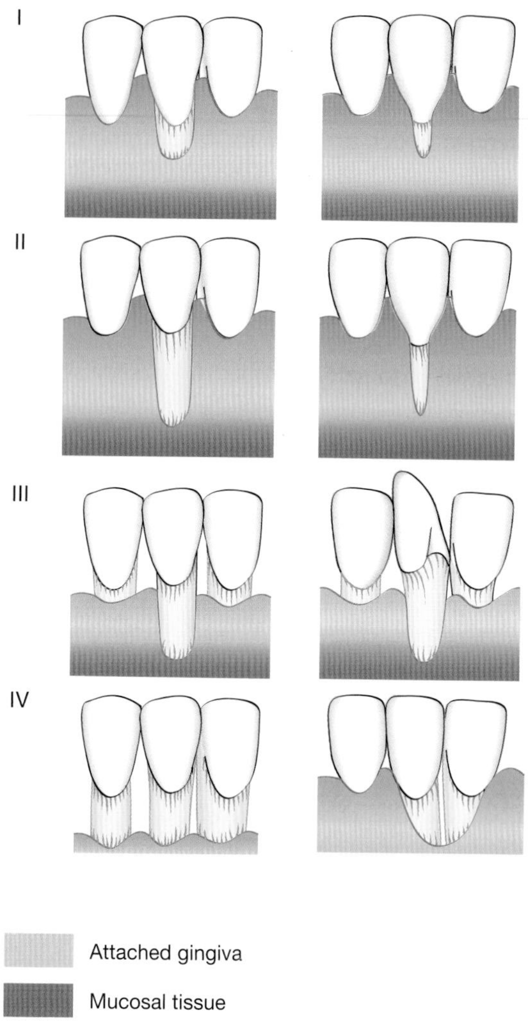

Figure 69-8 P.D. Miller's classification of denuded roots.

Class II. Marginal tissue recession extends to or beyond the mucogingival junction. There is no loss of bone or soft tissue in the interdental area. This type of recession can be subclassified into wide and narrow.

Class III. Marginal tissue recession extends to or beyond the mucogingival junction. There is bone and soft tissue loss interdentally or malpositioning of the tooth.

Class IV. Marginal tissue recession extends to or beyond the mucogingival junction. There is severe bone and soft tissue loss interdentally or severe tooth malposition.

In general, the prognosis for classes I and II is good to excellent; whereas for class III, only partial coverage can be expected. Class IV has a very poor prognosis with current techniques.

The following is a list of techniques used for gingival augmentation coronal to the recession (root coverage):

1. Free gingival autograft
2. Free connective tissue autograft
3. Pedicle autografts
   - Laterally (horizontally) positioned flap
   - Coronally positioned flap; includes semilunar pedicle (Tarnow)
4. Subepithelial connective tissue graft (Langer)
5. Guided tissue regeneration
6. Pouch and tunnel technique

Some of the techniques used for widening the attached gingiva apical to the area of recession can also be used for root coverage. Both the free gingival and the connective tissue autograft used for apical widening can be used for coronal augmentation by incorporating some modifications. In using the free grafts for root coverage, the recipient bed surrounding the denuded root surface must be extended wider to allow for better blood supply to the donor free graft, because a portion of the donor tissue overlies the root surface that has no blood supply.

Free Gingival Autograft

Successful and predictable root coverage has been reported using free gingival autografts.[50,52]

THE CLASSIC TECHNIQUE. Miller[52] applied the classic free gingival autograft described previously with a few modifications.

Step 1: Root Planing. Root planing is performed, with application of saturated citric acid for 5 minutes with a cotton pledget, burnishing it on the root. The advantage of citric acid application has not been confirmed by other studies.[40]

Step 2: Prepare the Recipient Site. Make a horizontal incision in the interdental papillae at right angles to create a margin against which the graft may have a butt joint with the incision. Vertical incisions are made at the proximal line angles of adjacent teeth, and the retracted tissue is excised. Maintain an intact periosteum in the apical area.

Steps 3 and 4. Refer to the step-by-step technique described for the classic gingival graft earlier in this chapter.

This technique results in predictable coverage of the denuded roots but may present esthetic color discrepancies with the adjacent gingiva because of a lighter color.

Free Connective Tissue Autograft

The free connective tissue technique was described by Levine in 1991.[46] The difference between this technique and the free gingival autograft is that the donor tissue is connective tissue (see Figure 69-6).

CONNECTIVE TISSUE TECHNIQUE

Step 1: Divergent Vertical Incisions. Divergent vertical incisions are made at the line angles of the tooth to be covered, creating a partial-thickness flap to at least 5 mm apical to the receded area.

Step 2: Suturing. Suture the apical mucosal border to the periosteum using gut suture.

Step 3: Scaling and Root Planing. Thoroughly scale and plane the root surface, reducing any prominence of the root surface.

Step 4: Obtain the Graft. From the palate, obtain a connective tissue graft. The donor site is sutured after the graft is removed.

Step 5: Transfer the Graft. Transfer the graft to the recipient site, and suture it to the periosteum with gut suture. Good stability of the graft must be attained with adequate sutures.

Step 6: Cover the Graft. Cover the grafted site with dry aluminum foil and periodontal dressing.

Pedicle Autograft

LATERALLY (HORIZONTALLY) DISPLACED FLAP. This technique, originally described by Grupe and Warren in 1956,[35] was the standard technique for many years and is still indicated in some cases. The laterally positioned flap can be used to cover isolated, denuded roots that have adequate donor tissue laterally and vestibular depth (Figures 66-9 and 69-10).

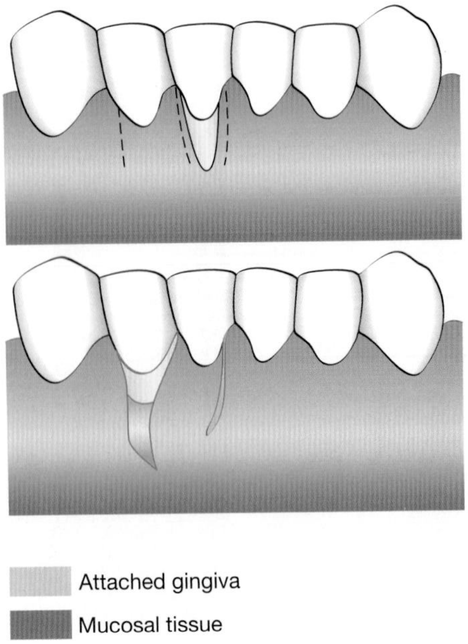

Figure 69-9 Laterally displaced flap for coverage of denuded root. *Top,* Incisions removing the gingival margin around the exposed root and outlining the flap. *Bottom,* After the gingiva around the exposed root is removed, the flap is separated, transferred, and sutured.

Step 1: Prepare the Recipient Site. Epithelium is removed around the denuded root surface. The exposed connective tissue will be the recipient site for the laterally displaced flap. The root surface will be thoroughly scaled and planed (Figure 69-10, *B*).

Step 2: Prepare the Flap. The periodontium of the donor site should have a satisfactory width of attached gingiva and minimal loss of bone, without dehiscence or fenestration. A full-thickness or partial-thickness flap may be used, but the latter is preferable because it offers the advantage of more rapid healing in the donor site and reduces the risk of loss of facial bone height, particularly if the bone is thin or a dehiscence or fenestration is suspected. However, if the gingiva is thin, partial thickness may not be sufficient for flap survival (Figure 69-10, *C*).

With a #15 blade, make a vertical incision from the gingival margin to outline a flap adjacent to the recipient site. Incise to the periosteum, and extend the incision into the oral mucosa to the level of the base of the recipient site. The flap should be sufficiently wider than the recipient site to cover the root and provide a broad margin for attachment to the connective tissue border around the root. The interdental papilla at the distal end of the flap, or a major portion of it, should be included to secure the flap in the interproximal space between the donor and the recipient teeth.

Make a vertical incision along the gingival margin and interdental papilla, and separate a flap consisting of

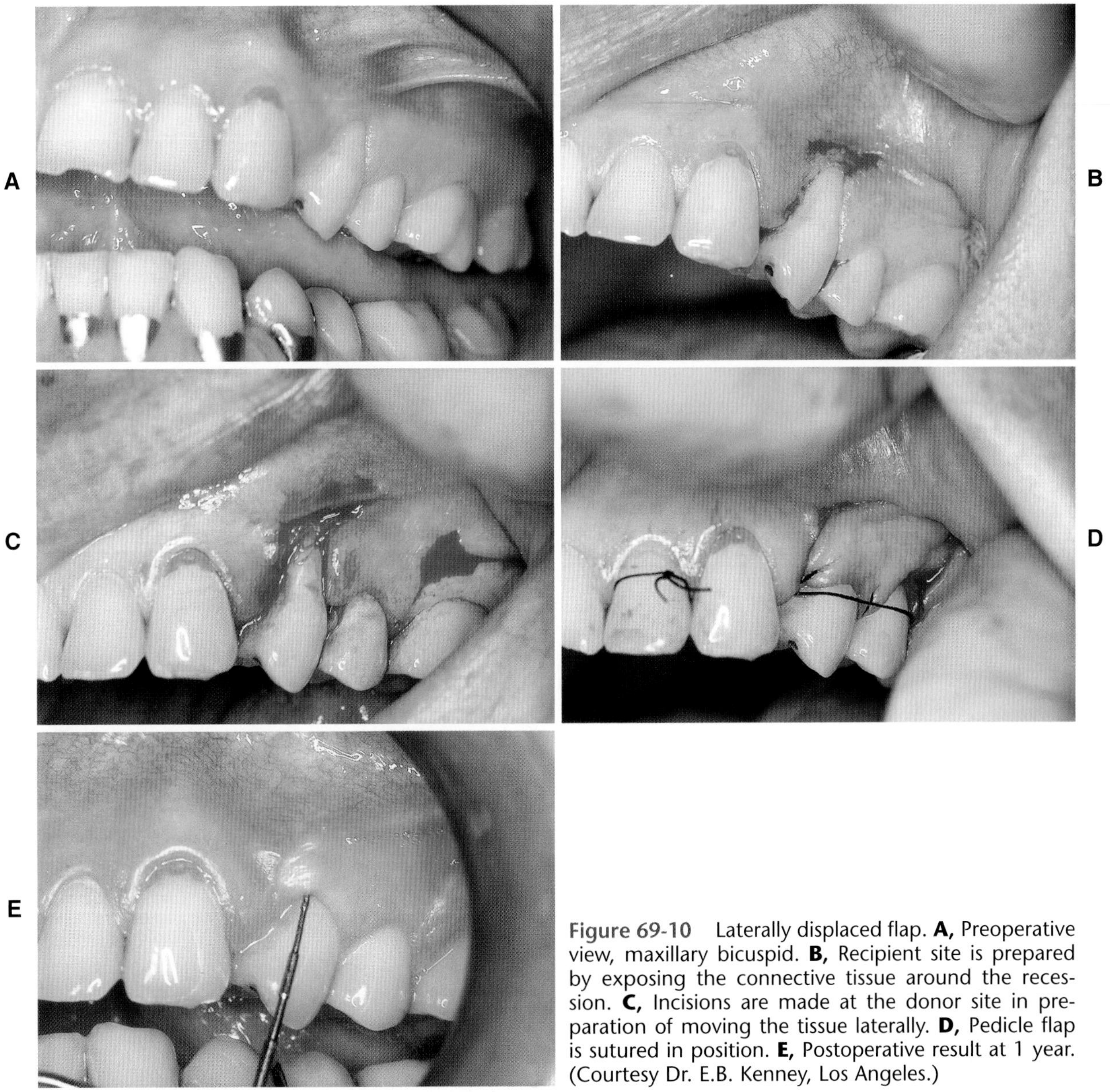

Figure 69-10 Laterally displaced flap. **A,** Preoperative view, maxillary bicuspid. **B,** Recipient site is prepared by exposing the connective tissue around the recession. **C,** Incisions are made at the donor site in preparation of moving the tissue laterally. **D,** Pedicle flap is sutured in position. **E,** Postoperative result at 1 year. (Courtesy Dr. E.B. Kenney, Los Angeles.)

epithelium and a thin layer of connective tissue, leaving the periosteum on the bone.

A releasing incision is sometimes needed to avoid tension on the base of the flap, which can impair the circulation when the flap is moved. To do this, make a short oblique incision into the alveolar mucosa at the distal corner of the flap, pointing in the direction of the recipient site.

Step 3: Transfer the Flap. Slide the flap laterally onto the adjacent root, making sure that it lies flat and firm without excess tension on the base. Fix the flap to the adjacent gingiva and alveolar mucosa with interrupted sutures (Figure 69-10, *D*). A suspensory suture may be made around the involved tooth to prevent the flap from slipping apically.

Step 4: Protect the Flap and Donor Site. Cover the operative field with aluminum foil and a soft periodontal pack, extending it interdentally and onto the lingual surface to secure it. Remove the pack and sutures after 1 week.

VARIANT TECHNIQUES. There are many variations in the incisions for the laterally displaced flap. A common alternative is the use of converging oblique incisions over the recipient site and a vertical or oblique incision at the distal end of the donor site so that the transposed flap is slightly wider at its base. In another modification, the marginal attachment at the donor site is preserved to reduce the likelihood of recession and marginal bone resorption, but this requires a donor site with a wider zone of attached gingiva.

Sliding partial-thickness grafts from neighboring edentulous areas (pedicle grafts)[34] can be used to restore attached gingiva on teeth adjacent to edentulous spaces with denuded roots and a small, vestibular fornix, often complicated by tension from a frenum. The "double-papilla flap" attempts to cover roots denuded by isolated gingival defects with a flap formed by joining the contiguous halves of the adjacent interdental papillae.[18,39] Results with this technique are often poor because blood supply is impaired by suturing the two flaps over the root surface.

ACCOMPLISHMENTS OF PEDICLE AUTOGRAFT. Coverage of the exposed root surface with the sliding-flap technique has been reported to be 60%,[32] 61%, and 72%.[61] Histologic studies in animals have reported 50% coverage.[17,79]

The extent to which the flap establishes a new attachment to the root with the formation of new cementum and the embedding of new connective tissue fibers has not been settled. New attachment on artificially denuded roots in experimental animals[79] and in some clinical studies in humans has been reported,[70,72] but it does not occur consistently enough to be predictable.

In the donor site, there is uneventful repair and restoration of gingival health and contours, with some loss of radicular bone (0.5 mm) and recession (1.5 mm) reported with full-thickness flaps.

CORONALLY DISPLACED FLAP. The purpose of the coronally displaced flap procedure is to create a split-thickness flap in the area apical to the denuded root and position it coronally to cover the root. Two techniques are available for this purpose.

First Technique

Step 1. With two vertical incisions, delineate the flap. These incisions should go beyond the mucogingival junction. Make an internal bevel incision from the gingival margin to the bottom of the pocket to eliminate the diseased pocket wall. Elevate a mucoperiosteal flap using careful sharp dissection.

Step 2. Scale and plane the root surface.

Step 3. Return the flap and suture it at a level coronal to the pretreatment position. Cover the area with a periodontal pack, which is removed along with the

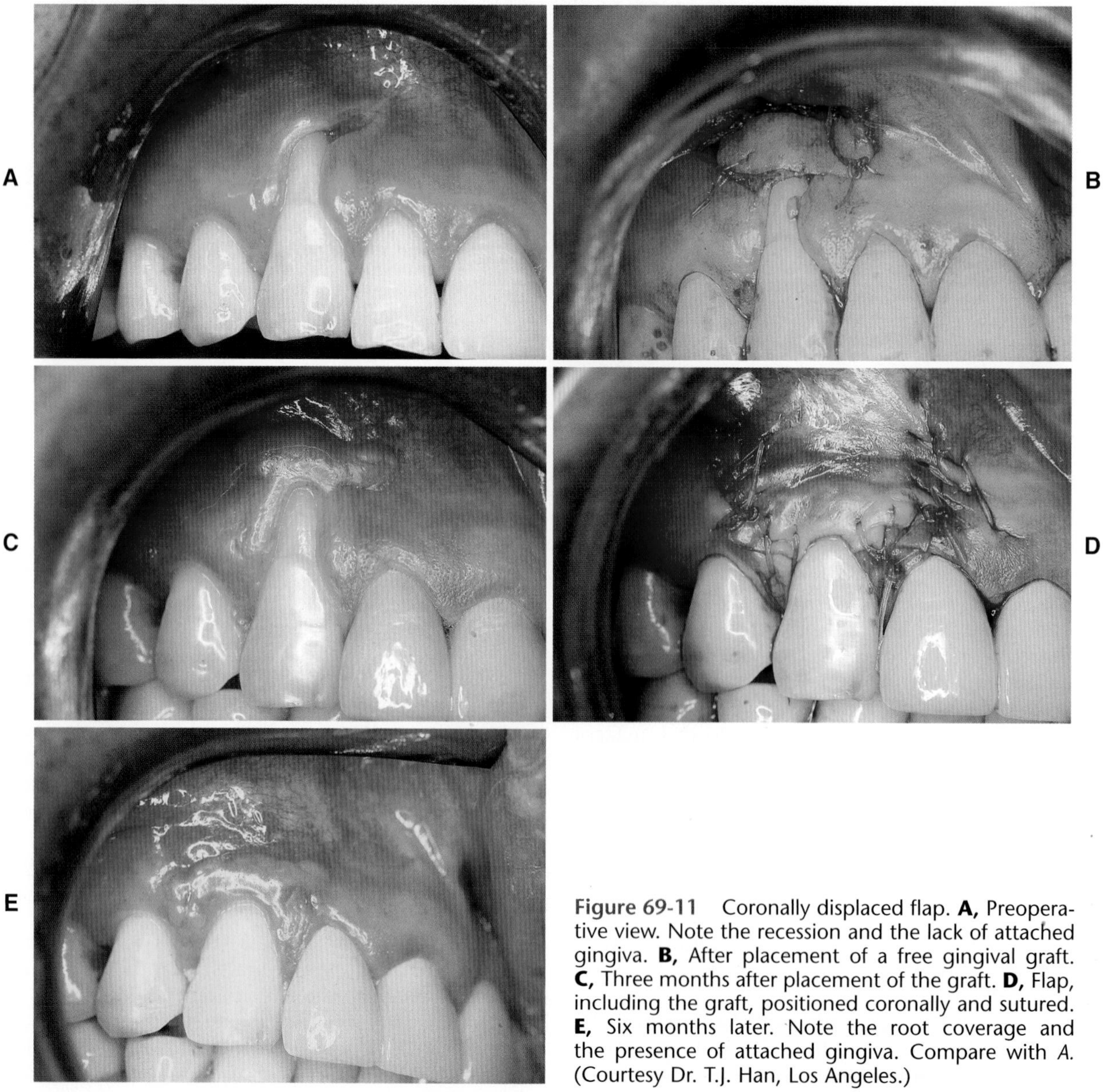

Figure 69-11 Coronally displaced flap. **A,** Preoperative view. Note the recession and the lack of attached gingiva. **B,** After placement of a free gingival graft. **C,** Three months after placement of the graft. **D,** Flap, including the graft, positioned coronally and sutured. **E,** Six months later. Note the root coverage and the presence of attached gingiva. Compare with *A.* (Courtesy Dr. T.J. Han, Los Angeles.)

sutures after 1 week. The pack is replaced for an additional week if necessary.

Variations to First Technique. Results with the coronally displaced flap technique are not often favorable[36] because of insufficient keratinized gingiva. To solve this and increase the chance of success, a gingival extension procedure with a free autogenous graft can be performed, as described earlier in this chapter. This creates several millimeters of attached keratinized gingiva apical to the denuded root (Figure 69-11).

Two months after this surgery, a second-stage procedure is performed, coronally positioning the flap that includes the free autogenous graft. The use of citric acid with a pH 1.0 for conditioning the root surface has been suggested.[47]

A significant degree of reduction in recession treated by this double-step procedure was reported after 2 years by Bernimoulin et al.[4] and confirmed by others.[11,48,49]

Second Technique. Tarnow has described the semilunar coronally repositioned flap to cover denuded root surfaces[73] (Figure 69-12).

Step 1. A semilunar incision is made following the curvature of the receded gingival margin and ending about 2 to 3 mm short of the tip of the papillae. This location is very important because the flap derives all its blood supply from the papillary areas. The incision may need to reach the alveolar mucosa if the attached gingiva is narrow.

Step 2. Perform a split-thickness dissection coronally from the incision, and connect it to an intrasulcular incision.

Step 3. The tissue will collapse coronally, covering the denuded root. It is then held in its new position for a few minutes with moist gauze; there is no need to suture or to pack.

This technique is very simple and predictably provides 2 to 3 mm of root coverage. It can be performed on several adjoining teeth, but even though the incision may be continuous, extreme care should be exercised not to dissect the blood supply. The Tarnow technique is successful for the maxilla, particularly in covering root left exposed by the gingival margin receding from a recently placed crown margin. It is not recommended for mandibular teeth.

Subepithelial Connective Tissue Graft (Langer)

The subepithelial connective tissue procedure is indicated for larger and multiple defects with good vestibular depth and gingival thickness to allow a split-thickness flap to be elevated. Adjacent to the denuded root surface, the donor connective tissue is sandwiched between the split flap (Figures 69-13 and 69-14). This technique was described by Langer and Langer in 1985.[45] Similar approaches had been previously reported by Perez-Fernandez[58] and Raetzke.[60]

Step 1. Raise a partial-thickness flap with a horizontal incision 2 mm away from the tip of the papilla and two vertical incisions 1 to 2 mm away from the gingival margin of the adjoining teeth. These incisions should extend at least half to one tooth wider mesiodistally than the area of gingival recession. Extend the flap to the mucobuccal fold

A B C

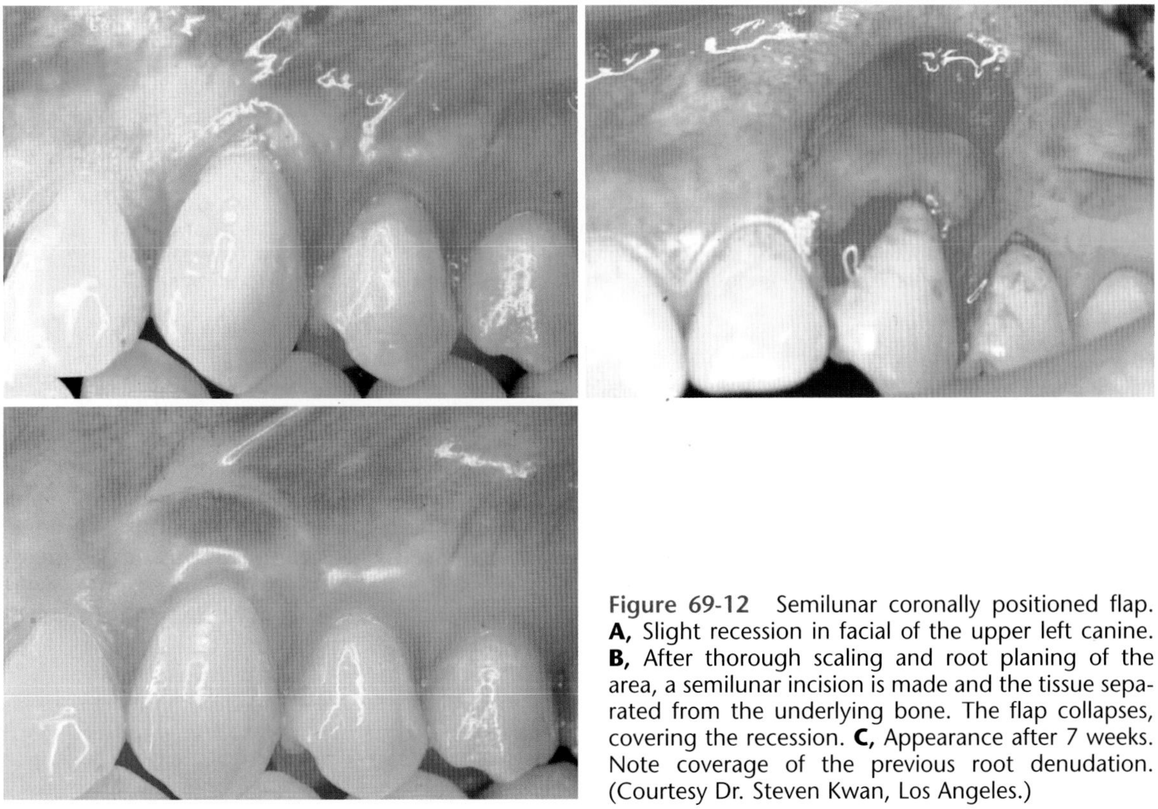

Figure 69-12 Semilunar coronally positioned flap. **A,** Slight recession in facial of the upper left canine. **B,** After thorough scaling and root planing of the area, a semilunar incision is made and the tissue separated from the underlying bone. The flap collapses, covering the recession. **C,** Appearance after 7 weeks. Note coverage of the previous root denudation. (Courtesy Dr. Steven Kwan, Los Angeles.)

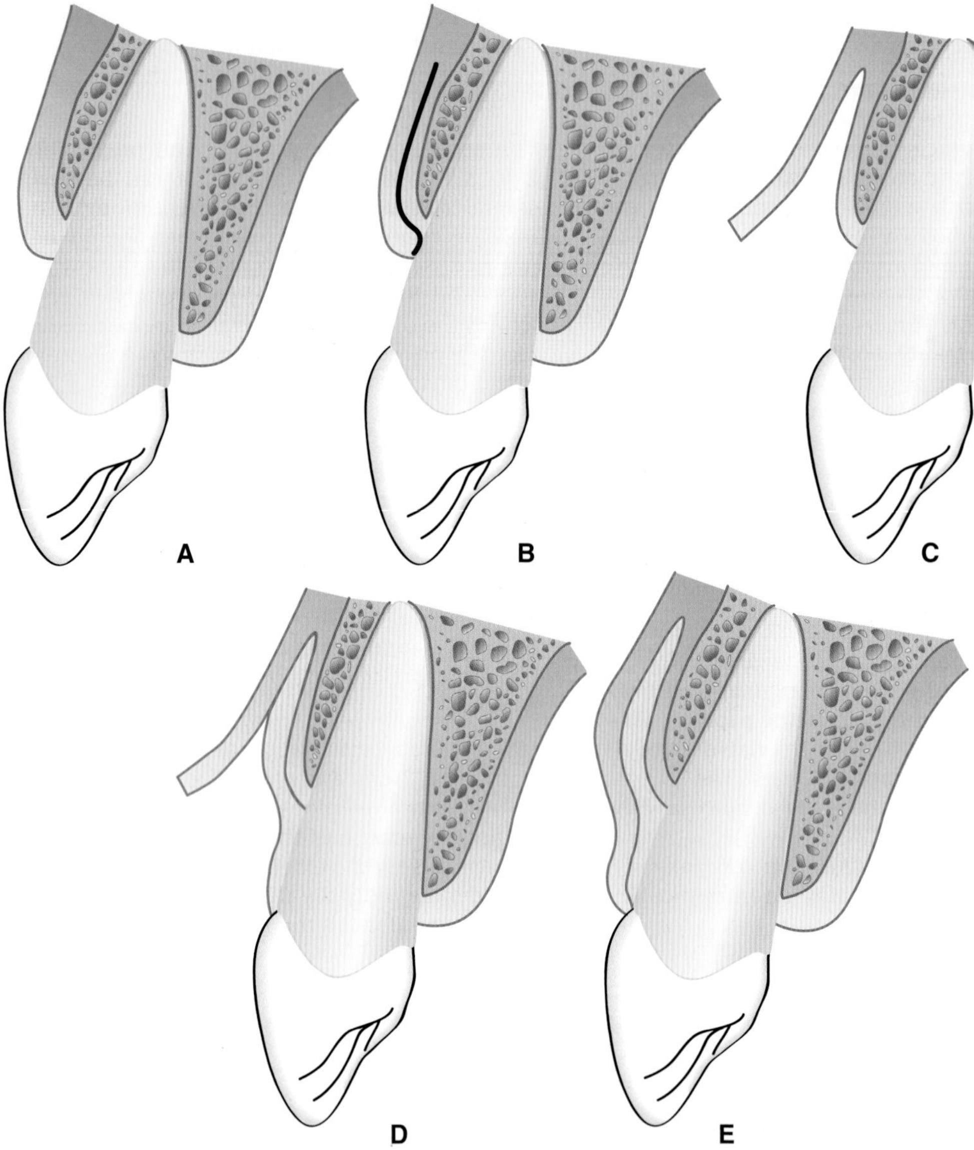

Figure 69-13 Subepithelial connective tissue graft for root coverage. **A** to **E,** Sagittal views. **A,** Preoperative view of facial recession on maxillary central incisor. **B,** Split-thickness incision for recipient site. **C,** Split-thickness flap reflected. **D,** Connective tissue placed over denuded root surface. Note that apical portion of the donor tissue is placed between the split flap. **E,** Recipient flap is closed. Subepithelial connective tissue graft for root coverage.

without perforations, which could affect the blood supply.

Step 2. Thoroughly plane the root, reducing its convexity.

Step 3. Obtain a connective tissue graft from the palate by means of a horizontal incision 5 to 6 mm from the gingival margin of molars and premolars. The connective tissue is carefully removed along with all adipose and glandular tissue. The palatal wound is sutured in a primary closure.

Step 4. Place the connective tissue on the denuded root(s). Suture it with resorbable sutures to the periosteum.

Step 5. Cover the graft with the outer portion of the partial-thickness flap and suture it interdentally. At least half to two thirds of the connective tissue graft must be covered by the flap for the exposed portion to survive over the denuded root.

Step 6. Cover the area with dry foil and surgical pack. After 7 days, the dressing and sutures are removed. The esthetics are favorable with this technique since the donor tissue is connective tissue (Figure 69-14, *E*). The donor site heals by primary intention, with considerably less discomfort than after a free gingival graft.

A variant of the subepithelial connective tissue graft, called a *subpedicle connective tissue graft,* was described by Nelson in 1987.[55] This technique uses a pedicle over the connective tissue that covers the denuded root surface.

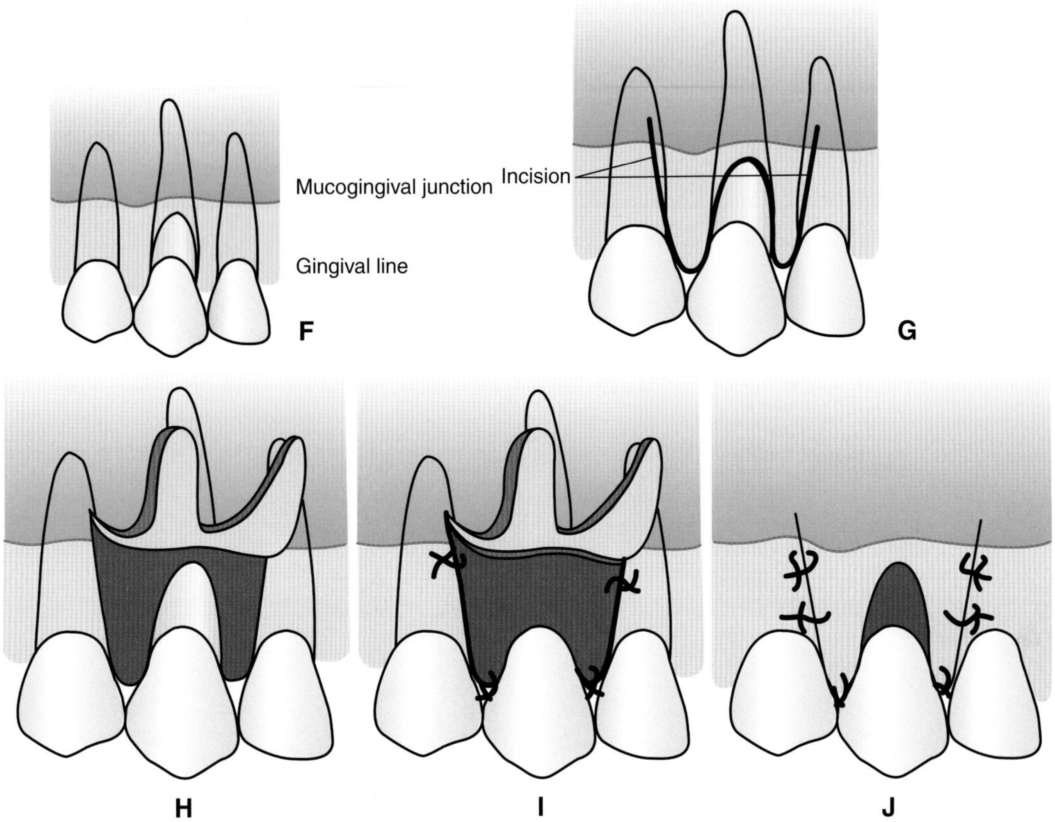

Figure 69-13, cont'd **F** to **J,** Facial views. **F,** Gingival recession. **G,** Vertical incisions to prepare recipient site. **H,** Split-thickness flap reflected. **I,** Connective tissue sutured over denuded root surface. **J,** Split-thickness flap sutured over donor connective tissue.

Therefore the blood supply is increased over the donor tissue.

Guided Tissue Regeneration Technique for Root Coverage

Pini-Prato et al.[59] described a technique based on the principle of guided tissue regeneration (GTR). Theoretically, GTR should result in reconstruction of the attachment apparatus, along with coverage of the denuded root surface (Figure 69-15).

Step 1. A full-thickness flap is reflected to the mucogingival junction, continuing as a partial-thickness flap 8 mm apical to the mucogingival junction.

Step 2. A microporous membrane is placed over the denuded root surface and the adjacent tissue. It is trimmed and adapted to the root surface and covers at least 2 mm of marginal periosteum.

Step 3. A suture is passed through the portion of the membrane that will cover the bone. This suture is knotted on the exterior and tied to bend the membrane, creating a space between the root and the membrane. This space allows for the growth of tissue beneath the membrane.

Step 4. The flap is then positioned coronally and sutured. Four weeks later a small envelope flap is performed, and the membrane is carefully removed. The flap is then again positioned coronally, to protect the growing tissue, and sutured. One week later these sutures are removed.

Tinti and Vincenzi[74] used titanium-reinforced membranes to create space beneath the membrane. Resorbable membranes have also been used to achieve root coverage. The inability to create space between the resorbable membrane and the denuded root, because of its softness, may present a problem, even though not needing a second surgery is an advantage.

Clinical studies comparing this technique with the coronally displaced flap have shown that the GTR technique is better when the recession is greater than 4.98 mm apico-coronally.[59] Histologically, one case reported 3.66 mm of new connective tissue attachment associated with 2.48 mm of new cementum and 1.84 mm of bone growth.[20]

Pouch and Tunnel Technique

To minimize incisions and reflection of flaps and to provide abundant blood supply to the donor tissue, the placement of subepithelial donor connective tissue into pouches beneath papillary tunnels allows for intimate contact of donor tissue to the recipient site.[81] After positioning the graft, the coronal placement of the recessed

A B C D E

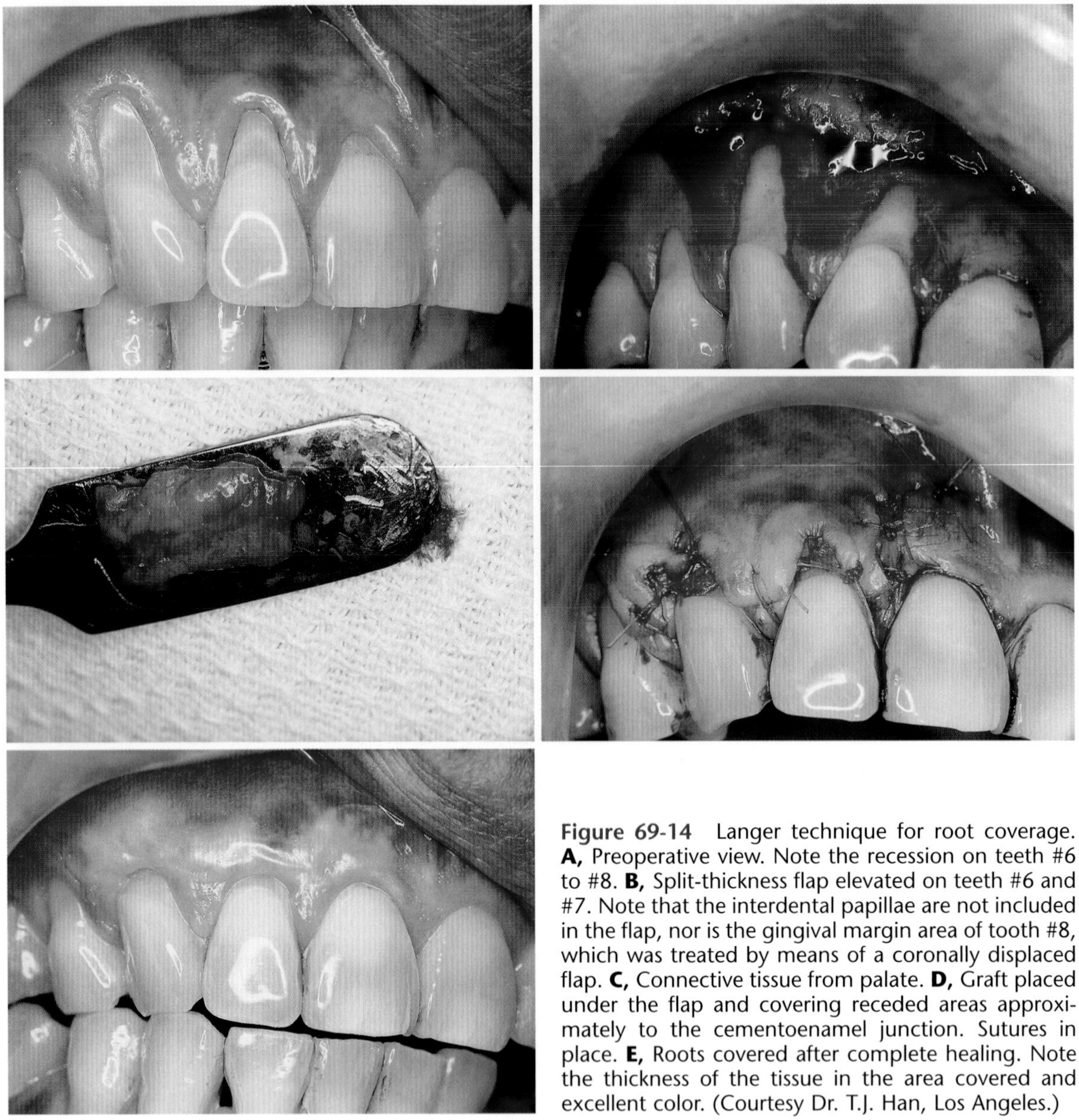

Figure 69-14 Langer technique for root coverage. **A,** Preoperative view. Note the recession on teeth #6 to #8. **B,** Split-thickness flap elevated on teeth #6 and #7. Note that the interdental papillae are not included in the flap, nor is the gingival margin area of tooth #8, which was treated by means of a coronally displaced flap. **C,** Connective tissue from palate. **D,** Graft placed under the flap and covering receded areas approximately to the cementoenamel junction. Sutures in place. **E,** Roots covered after complete healing. Note the thickness of the tissue in the area covered and excellent color. (Courtesy Dr. T.J. Han, Los Angeles.)

gingival margins completely covers the donor tissue. Therefore the esthetic result is excellent. This technique is especially effective for the anterior maxillary area, where vestibular depth is adequate and there is good gingival thickness (Figure 69-16).

One of the advantages to this technique is the thickening of the gingival margin after healing. The thicker gingival margin is more stable to allow for the possibility of "creeping reattachment" of the margin. The use of small, contoured blades enables the surgeon to incise and split the gingival tissues to create the recipient pouches and tunnels (Figure 69-17).

This technique consists of the following steps (see Figure 69-16):

Step 1. Using a #15C or #12D blade, a sulcular incision is made around the teeth adjacent to the recession. This incision separates the junctional epithelium and the connective tissue attachment from the root.

Step 2. Using either a curette or a small blade such as the #15C, a tunnel is created beneath the adjacent buccal papilla, into which the connective tissue is placed.

Step 3. A split-thickness pouch is created apical to the papilla, which has been tunneled, and the adjacent radicular surface. This pouch may extend 10 to 12 mm apical to the recessed gingival margin and papilla and 6 to 8 mm mesial and distal to the denuded root surface.

Step 4. The size of the pouch, which includes the area of the denuded root surface, is measured so that an equivalent size of donor connective tissue can be procured from the palate.

Step 5. Using sutures, curettes, and elevators, the connective tissue is placed under the pouch and

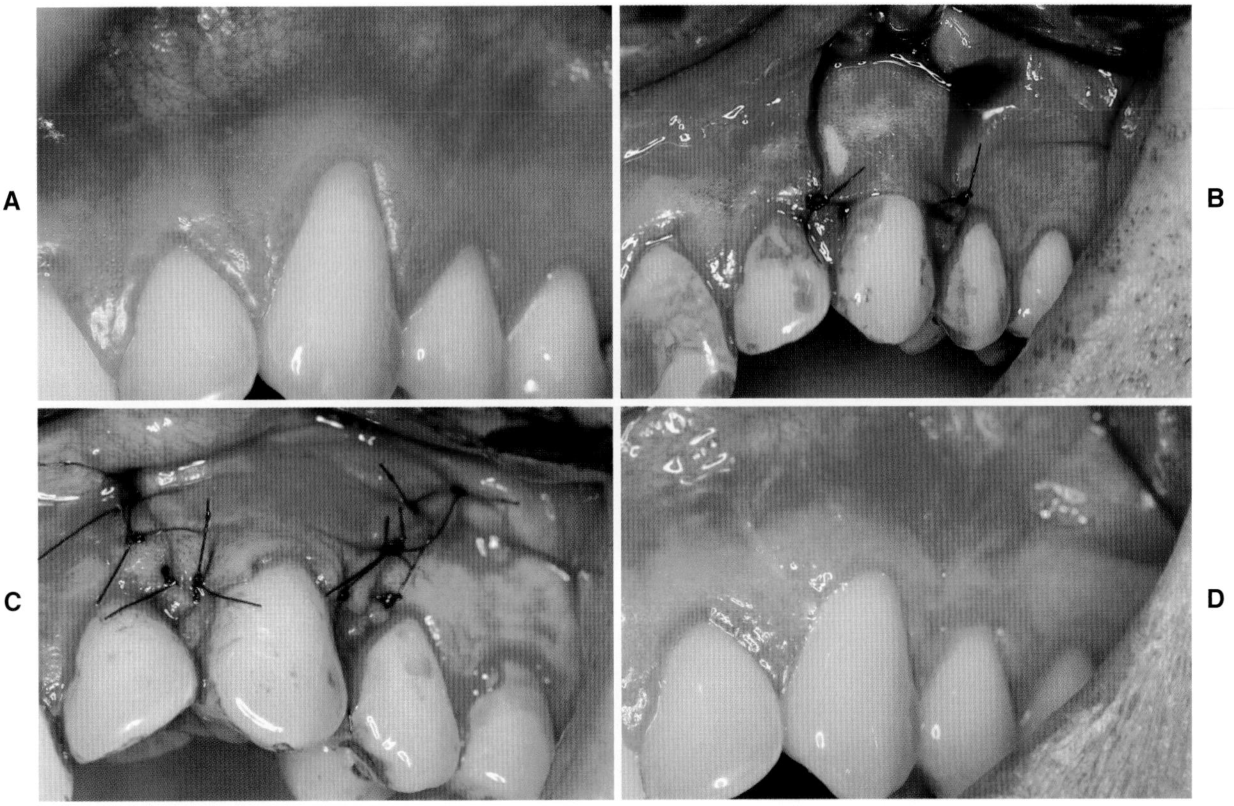

Figure 69-15 Guided tissue regeneration technique for root coverage. **A,** Marked recession of maxillary left cuspid. **B,** Vertical incisions made and membrane placed over recession. **C,** Flap sutured over the membrane. **D,** Postoperative result. Note complete coverage of recession. (Courtesy Dr. Zoran Aleksic.)

tunnel, with a portion covering the denuded root surface.

Step 6. The mesial and distal ends of the donor tissue are secured by gut sutures. The gingival margin of the flap is coronally placed and secured by horizontal mattress sutures that extend over the contact of the two adjacent teeth. If the teeth are not in contact, a small amount of composite material may be placed temporarily between the two teeth to allow the placement of the suture over the closed contact.

Step 7. Other holding sutures are placed through the overlying gingival tissue and donor tissue to the underlying periosteum to secure and stabilize the donor tissue beneath the gingiva.

Step 8. A periodontal dressing is used to cover the surgical site.

TECHNIQUES TO DEEPEN VESTIBULE

The presence of adequate vestibular depth is important for both oral hygiene and retention of prosthetic appliances. Numerous surgical techniques have been proposed to accomplish the objective of deepening the vestibule. The classic clinical studies in the early 1960s by Bohannan[7-9] indicated that deepening of the vestibule by non–free graft procedures were not successful when evaluated years later. Predictable deepening of the vestibule can only be accomplished by the use of free autogenous graft techniques and their variants, as covered in this chapter.

TECHNIQUES TO REMOVE FRENUM

A *frenum* is a fold of mucous membrane, usually with enclosed muscle fibers, that attaches the lips and cheeks to the alveolar mucosa and/or gingiva and underlying periosteum. A frenum becomes a problem if the attachment is too close to the marginal gingiva. Tension on the frenum may pull the gingival margin away from the tooth. This condition may be conducive to plaque accumulation and inhibit proper toothbrushing.

Frenectomy or Frenotomy

These terms refer to surgical procedures that differ in degree. *Frenectomy* is complete removal of the frenum, including its attachment to underlying bone, and may be required in the correction of an abnormal diastema between maxillary central incisors. *Frenotomy* is incision of the frenum. Both procedures are used, but frenotomy generally suffices for periodontal purposes, that is, relocating the frenal attachment so as to create a zone of attached gingiva between the gingival margin and the frenum.

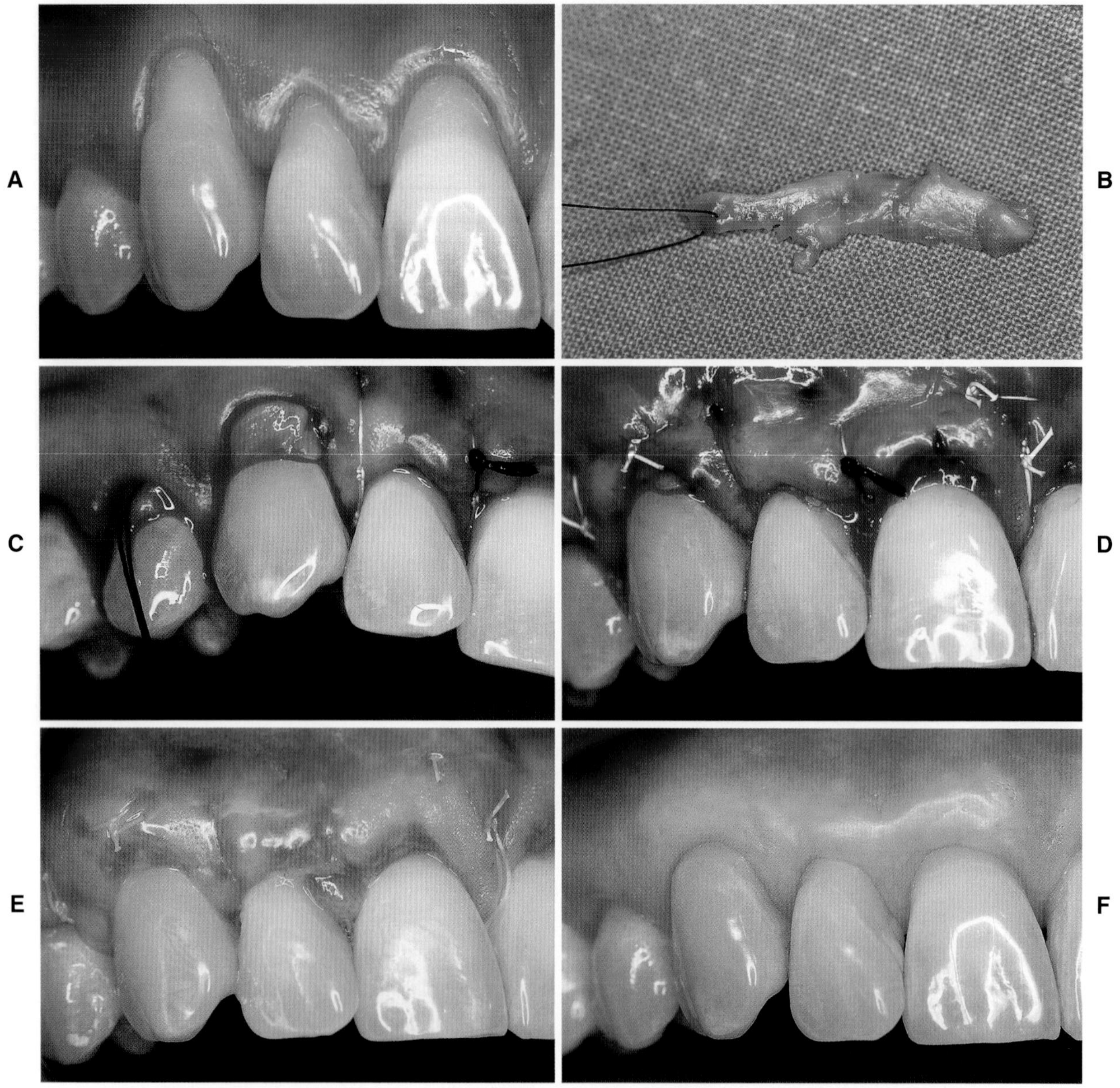

Figure 69-16 Pouch and tunnel technique for root coverage. **A,** Preoperative view. Note gingival recession. **B,** Donor connective tissue from palate. **C,** Donor tissue placed in pouch and tunnel. **D,** Facial gingiva is sutured coronally to cover donor tissue. **E,** Postoperative healing at 2 weeks. **F,** Final healing at 3 months. Note root coverage and thick marginal gingiva. (Courtesy Dr. Robert R. Azzi, Paris, France.)

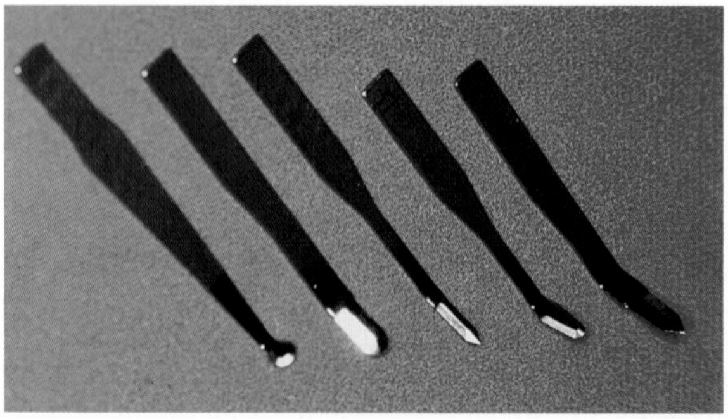

Figure 69-17 Small, contoured blades used for periodontal plastic surgery.

Frenectomy and frenotomy are usually performed in conjunction with other periodontal treatment procedures but occasionally are done as separate operations. Frenal problems occur most often on the facial surface between the maxillary and mandibular central incisors and in the canine and premolar areas[78] (see Figure 69-1, *D*). They occur less often on the lingual surface of the mandible.

Procedure

If the vestibule is deep enough, the procedure is confined to the frenum. It is often necessary to deepen the

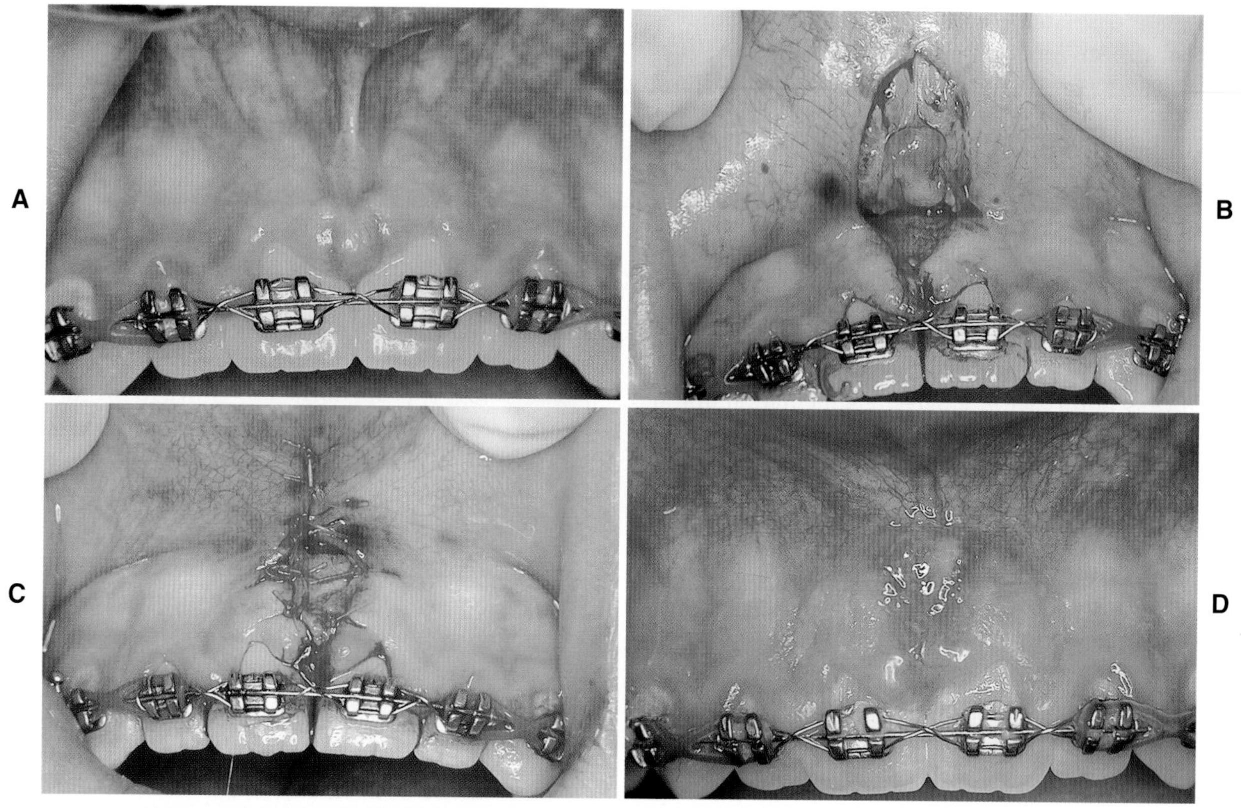

Figure 69-18 Removal of the frenum. **A,** Preoperative view of frenum between the two maxillary central incisors. **B,** Removal of the frenum from both the lip and gingiva. **C,** Site is sutured after it is placed over the wound. **D,** Postoperative view at 2 weeks.

vestibule to provide space for the repositioned frenum. This is accomplished as follows (Figure 69-18):

Step 1. After anesthetizing the area, engage the frenum with a hemostat inserted to the depth of the vestibule.
Step 2. Incise along the upper surface of the hemostat, extending beyond the tip.
Step 3. Make a similar incision along the undersurface of the hemostat.
Step 4. Remove the triangular resected portion of the frenum with the hemostat. This exposes the underlying brushlike fibrous attachment to the bone.
Step 5. Make a horizontal incision, separating the fibers, and bluntly dissect to the bone.
Step 6. If necessary, extend the incisions laterally and suture the labial mucosa to the apical periosteum. Sometimes the area is covered with a free gingival or connective tissue graft.
Step 7. Clean the surgical field and pack with gauze sponges until bleeding stops.
Step 8. Cover the area with dry aluminum foil and apply the periodontal pack.
Step 9. Remove the pack after 2 weeks and repack if necessary. One month is usually required for the formation of an intact mucosa with the frenum attached in its new position.

High frenal attachments on the lingual surface are uncommon. To correct these without involving the structures in the floor of the mouth, approximately 2 mm of the attachment is separated from the mucosa with a periodontal knife at weekly intervals until the desired level is reached. The area is covered with a periodontal pack in the intervals between treatments.

BOX 69-1

Criteria for Selection of Mucogingival Techniques

1. Surgical site free of plaque, calculus, and inflammation.
2. Adequate blood supply to the donor tissue.
3. Anatomy of the recipient and donor sites.
4. Stability of the grafted tissue to the recipient site.
5. Minimal trauma to the surgical site.

CRITERIA FOR SELECTION OF TECHNIQUES

Different techniques are presented for solving mucogingival problems outlined in this chapter. The proper selection of the numerous techniques must be based on the predictability of success, which in turn is based on the criteria described next (Box 69-1).

1. *Surgical site free of plaque, calculus, and inflammation.* Periodontal plastic surgical procedures should be

undertaken in a plaque-free and inflammation-free environment to enable the clinician to manage gingival tissue that is firm. Meticulous, precise incisions and flap reflection cannot be achieved when the tissue is inflamed and edematous. Thorough scaling and root planing as well as meticulous plaque removal by the patient must be accomplished before any surgical procedure.

2. *Adequate blood supply.* To obtain the maximum amount of blood supply to the donor tissue, gingival augmentation apical to the area of recession will provide a better blood supply than coronal augmentation, since the recipient site is entirely periosteal tissue. Root coverage procedures present a portion of the recipient site (denuded root surface) without blood supply. Therefore, if esthetics is not a factor, gingival augmentation apical to the recession may be more predictable. A pedicle-displaced flap has a better blood supply than a free graft, with the base of the flap intact. In root coverage, therefore, if the anatomy is favorable, the pedicle flap or any of its variants may be the best procedure.

The subepithelial connective tissue graft (Langer) and the pouch and tunnel techniques use a split flap with the connective tissue sandwiched between the flap. This flap design maximizes the blood supply to the donor tissue. If large areas require root coverage, these sandwich-type recipient sites provide the best flap design for blood supply.

3. *Anatomy of the recipient and donor sites.* The presence or absence of vestibular depth is an important anatomic criterion at the recipient site for gingival augmentation. If gingival augmentation is indicated apical to the area of recession, there must be adequate vestibular depth apical to the recessed gingival margin to provide space for either a free or a pedicle graft. If a vestibule is necessary, only a free graft can accomplish this objective apical to the recession.

Mucogingival techniques, such as free gingival grafts and free connective tissue grafts, can be used to create vestibular depth and widen the zone of attached gingiva. Other techniques require vestibular depth to be present before the surgery, including pedicle grafts (lateral and coronal), subepithelial connective tissue graft (Langer), and pouch and tunnel procedures.

The availability of donor tissue is another anatomic factor that must be considered. Pedicle displacement of tissue necessitates the presence of an adjacent donor site that presents gingival thickness and width. Palatal tissue thickness is also necessary for the connective tissue donor autograft. Gingival thickness is required at the recipient site for techniques using split-thickness, sandwich-type flap or the pouch and tunnel techniques.

4. *Stability of the grafted tissue to the recipient site.* Good communication of the blood vessels from the grafted donor tissue to the recipient site requires a stable environment. This necessitates sutures that stabilize the donor tissue firmly against the recipient site. The least amount of sutures and maximum stability should be achieved.

5. *Minimal trauma to the surgical site.* As with all surgical procedures, periodontal plastic surgery is based on the meticulous, delicate, and precise management of the oral tissues. Unnecessary tissue trauma caused by poor incisions, flap perforations, tears, or traumatic and excessive placement of sutures can lead to tissue necrosis. The selection of proper instruments, needles, and sutures is mandatory to minimize tissue trauma; sharp contoured blades (see Figure 69-17), smaller-diameter needles, and resorbable monofilament sutures all are important factors in achieving atraumatic surgery.

SCIENCE TRANSFER

As defined in this chapter, mucogingival surgery refers to soft tissue relationships and manipulations. *In all these procedures, blood supply is the most significant concern and must be the underlying issue for all decisions regarding the individual surgical procedure.* A major complicating factor is the avascular root surface, and many modifications to existing techniques are used to overcome this. Diffusion of fluids is short term and of limited benefit as tissue size increases. Thus the formation of a circulation through anastomosis and angiogenesis is crucial to the survival of these therapeutic procedures. The formation of vascularity is based on growth molecules, such as vascular endothelial growth factor (VEGF), and cellular migration, proliferation, and differentiation. As tissue-engineering techniques improve, the success and predictability of mucogingival surgery should dramatically increase. Undoubtedly, however, all advancements will have adequate circulation and blood supply as their basis.

Surgical techniques used solely to increase the width and thickness of the keratinized tissue are among the most predictable periodontal procedures. Periodontal plastic surgical procedures for root coverage have less predictability because of the absence of a foundation for blood supply over the root surface. The literature shows that the most predictable root coverage procedure is the use of connective tissue grafts in combination with split-thickness flaps. In cases where it is not possible to obtain a connective tissue graft because of the thinness of the palatal tissue, alternative procedures include coronally displaced flaps with membranes or Emdogain. In cases requiring root coverage where the gingival recession is 2 mm or less, a semilunar pedicle flap can be used. *Cigarette smoking is a contraindication for root coverage techniques because the compromised gingival blood supply results in many failures.*

CONCLUSION

New techniques are constantly being developed and are slowly being incorporated into periodontal practice. The practitioner should be aware that, at times, new methods are published without adequate clinical research to ensure the predictability of the results and the extent to which the techniques may benefit the patient. Critical analysis of newly presented techniques should guide our constant evolution toward better clinical methods.

REFERENCES

1. American Academy of Periodontology: Proceedings of the World Workshop in Clinical Periodontics. In *Annals of Periodontology,* Chicago, 1989, The Academy.
2. American Academy of Periodontology: Proceedings of the World Workshop in Periodontics. In *Annals of Periodontology,* Chicago, 1996, The Academy.
3. Becker NG: A free gingival graft utilizing a presuturing technique, *Periodontics* 5:194, 1967.
4. Bernimoulin JP, Loscher B, Muhlemann HR: Coronally repositioned periodontal flap, *J Clin Periodontol* 2:1, 1975.
5. Bjorn H: Free transplantation of gingiva propia, *Sveriges Tandlak T* 22:684, 1963.
6. Brackett RC, Gargiulo AW: Free gingival grafts in humans, *J Periodontol* 41:581, 1970.
7. Bohannan H: Studies in the alteration of vestibular depth. I. Complete denudation, *J Periodontol* 33:120, 1962.
8. Bohannan H: Studies in the alteration of vestibular depth. II. Periosteum retention, *J Periodontol* 33:120, 1962.
9. Bohannan H: Studies in the alteration of vestibular depth. III. Vestibular incision, *J Periodontol* 34:208, 1963.
10. Broome WC, Taggart EJ Jr: Free autogenous connective tissue grafting, *J Periodontol* 47:580, 1976.
11. Caffesse RG, Guinard E: Treatment of localized gingival recessions. II. Coronally repositioned flap with a free gingival graft, *J Periodontol* 49:358, 1978.
12. Caffesse RG, Albano E, Plot C: Injertos gingivalis libres en perros: analisis biometrico, *Rev Asoc Odontol Argent* 60:517, 1972.
13. Caffesse RG, Carraro JJ, Carranza FA Jr: Injertos givgivales libres en perros: estudio clinico e histologico, *Rev Asoc Odontol Argent* 60:465, 1972.
14. Caffesse RG, Burgett FG, Nasjleti CE, et al: Healing of free gingival grafts with and without periosteum. Part I. Histologic evaluation, *J Peridontol* 50:586, 1979.
15. Caffesse RG, Nasjleti CE, Burgett FG, et al: Healing of free gingival grafts with and without periosteum. II. Radioautographic evaluation, *J Periodontol* 50:595, 1979.
16. Carranza FA Jr, Carraro JJ, Dotto CA, et al: Effect of periosteal fenestration in gingival extension operations, *J Periodontol* 37:335, 1966.
17. Chacker FM, Cohen DW: Regeneration of gingival tissues in non-human primates, *J Dent Res* 39:743, 1960.
18. Cohen DW, Ross SE: The double papillae repositioned flap in periodontal therapy, *J Periodontol* 39:65, 1968.
19. Corn H: Periosteal separation: its clinical significance, *J Periodontol* 33:140, 1962.
20. Cortellini P, Clauser C, Pini-Prato GP: Histologic assessment of new attachment following the treatment of a human buccal recession by means of a guided tissue regeneration procedure, *J Periodontol* 64:387, 1993.
21. Costich ER, Ramfjord SP: Healing after partial denudation of the alveolar process, *J Periodontol* 39:127, 1968.
22. Donn BJ Jr: The free connective tissue autograft: a clinical and histologic wound healing study in humans, *J Periodontol* 49:253, 1978.
23. Donnenfeld OW, Glickman I: A biometric study of the effects of gingivectomy, *J Periodontol* 37:447, 1966.
24. Donnenfeld OW, Marks R, Glickman I: The apically repositioned flap: a clinical study, *J Periodontol* 35:381, 1964.
25. Dordick B, Coslet JG, Seibert JS: Clinical evaluation of free autogenous gingival grafts placed on alveolar bone. II. Coverage of non-pathologic dehiscences and fenestrations, *J Periodontol* 47:568, 1976.
26. Dorfman HS, Kennedy JE, Bird WC: Longitudinal evaluation of free autogenous gingival grafts: a four-year report, *J Periodontol* 1:185, 1974.
27. Dorfman HS, Kennedy JE, Bird WC: Longitudinal evaluation of free autogenous gingival grafts, *J Clin Periodontol* 7:316, 1980.
28. Edel A: Clinical evaluation of free connective tissue grafts used to increase the width of keratinized gingiva, *J Clin Periodontol* 1:185, 1974.
29. Edlan A, Mejchar B: Plastic surgery of the vestibulum in periodontal therapy, *Int Dent J* 13:593, 1963.
30. Friedman N: Mucogingival surgery, *Texas Dent J* 75:358, 1957.
31. Friedman N, Levine HL: Mucogingival surgery: current status, *J Periodontol* 35:5, 1964.
32. Gargiulo AW, Arrocha R: Histo-clinical evaluation of free gingival grafts, *Periodontics* 5:285, 1967.
33. Gordon HP, Sullivan HC, Atkins JH: Free autogenous gingival grafts. Part II. Supplemental findings: histology of the graft site, *Periodontics* 6:130, 1968.
34. Grupe HE: Modified technique for the sliding flap operation, *J Periodontol* 37:491, 1966.
35. Grupe HE, Warren RF Jr: Repair of gingival defects by a sliding flap operation, *J Periodontol* 27:92, 1956.
36. Hall WB: *Pure mucogingival problems: etiology, treatment and prevention,* Chicago, 1984, Quintessence.
37. Han TJ, Takei HH, Carranza FA Jr: The strip gingival autograft technique, *Int J Periodont Restor Dent* 13:181, 1993.
38. Hangorsky V, Bissada NF: Clinical assessment of free gingival graft effectiveness on the maintenance of periodontal health, *J Periodontol* 51:274, 1980.
39. Harvey PM: Management of advanced periodontitis. Part I. Preliminary report of a method of surgical reconstruction, *NZ Dent J* 61:180, 1965.
40. Ibbott CG, Oles RD, Laverty WH: Effects of citric acid treatment on autogenous free graft coverage of localized recession, *J Periodontol* 56:662, 1985.
41. James WC, McFall WT Jr: Placement of free gingival grafts on denuded alveolar bone. Part I. Clinical evaluations, *J Periodontol* 49:283, 1978.
42. James WC, McFall WT Jr, Burkes EJ: Placement of free gingival grafts on denuded alveolar bone. II. Microscopic observations, *J Periodontol* 49:291, 1978.
43. Janson WA, Ruben MP, Kraamer GM, et al: Development of the blood supply to split-thickness free gingival autografts, *J Periodontol* 40:707, 1969.
44. Karring T, Ostergaard E, Löe H: Conservation of tissue specificity after heterotopic transplantation of gingiva and alveolar mucosa, *J Periodontal Res* 6:282, 1971.
45. Langer B, Langer L: Subepithelial connective tissue graft technique for root coverage, *J Periodontol* 56:715, 1985.
46. Levine RA: Covering denuded root surface with the subepithelial connective tissue graft, *Compend Contin Educ Dent* 12:568, 1991.
47. Liu WWJ, Solt CW: A surgical procedure for the treatment of localized gingival recession in conjunction with root surface citric acid conditioning, *J Periodontol* 51:505, 1980.
48. Matter J: Free gingival graft and coronally repositioned flap: a 2-year follow-up report, *J Clin Periodontol* 6:437, 1979.
49. Matter J, Cimasoni G: Creeping attachment after free gingival grafts, *J Periodontol* 47:574, 1976.
50. Miller PD Jr: Root coverage using a free soft tissue autograft following citric acid application. Part I. Technique, *Int J Periodont Restor Dent* 2:65, 1982.
51. Miller PD Jr: A classification of marginal tissue recession, *Int J Periodont Restor Dent* 5:9, 1985.

52. Miller PD Jr: Root coverage using a free soft tissue autograft following citric acid application. III. A successful and predictable procedure in areas of deep wide recession, *Int J Periodont Restor Dent* 5:15, 1985.
53. Mormann W, Schaer F, Firestone AC: The relationship between success of free gingival grafts and transplant thickness, *J Periodontol* 52:74, 1981.
54. Nabers J: Free gingival grafts, *Periodontics* 4:243, 1966.
55. Nelson SW: The subpedicle connective tissue graft: a bilaminar reconstructive procedure for the coverage of denuded root surfaces, *J Periodontol* 58:95, 1987.
56. Oliver RC, Löe H, Karring T: Microscopic evaluation of the healing and revascularization of free gingival grafts, *J Periodontol* 3:84, 1968.
57. Pennel BM, Tabor JC, King KO, et al: Free masticatory mucosa graft, *J Periodontol* 40:162, 1969.
58. Perez-Fernandez A: Injerto submucoso libre de encia: una nueva perspectiva, *Bol Inform Dent* 42:63, 1982.
59. Pini-Prato G, Tinti C, Vincenzi G, et al: Guided tissue regeneration versus mucogingival surgery in the treatment of human buccal gingival recession, *J Periodontol* 63:919, 1992.
60. Raetzke PB: Covering localized areas of root exposure employing the "envelope" technique, *J Periodontol* 56:397, 1985.
61. Rateitschak KH, Rateitschak EM, Wolff HF, et al: *Color atlas of periodontology,* New York, 1985, Thieme.
62. Robinson RE: Periosteal fenestration in mucogingival surgery, *J West Soc Periodontol* 9:107, 1961.
63. Rosenberg MM: Vestibular alterations in periodontics, *J Periodontol* 31:231, 1960.
64. Rubenstein HS, Ruben MP, Levy C, et al: Evidence for successful acceptance of irradiated free gingival allografts in dogs, *J Periodontol* 46:195, 1975.
65. Schmid MO: The subperiosteal vestibule extension: literature review, rationale and technique, *J West Soc Periodontol* 24:89, 1976.
66. Schoo WH, Copes L: Use of palatal mucosa and lyophilized dura mater to create attached gingiva, *J Clin Periodontol* 3:166, 1976.
67. Staffileno H, Levy S, Gargiulo A: Histologic study of cellular mobilization and repair following a periosteal retention operation via split thickness mucogingival flap surgery, *J Periodontol* 40:311, 1969.
68. Stetler KJ, Bissada NF: Significance of the width of keratinized gingiva on the periodontal status of teeth with submarginal restorations, *J Periodontol* 58:696, 1987.
69. Strahan JD: The relation of the mucogingival junction to the alveolar bone margin, *Dent Pract Dent Rec* 14:72, 1963.
70. Sugarman EF: A clinical and histological study of the attachment of grafted tissue to bone and teeth, *J Periodontol* 40:381, 1969.
71. Sullivan HC, Atkins JC: Free autogenous gingival grafts. III. Utilization of grafts in the treatment of gingival recession, *Periodontics* 6:152, 1968.
72. Sullivan HC, Carman D, Dinner D: Histological evaluation of the laterally positioned flap, *IADR Abstr* 467:169, 1971.
73. Tarnow DP: Semilunar coronally repositioned flap, *J Clin Periodontol* 13:182, 1986.
74. Tinti C, Vincenzi GP: Expanded polytetrafluoroethylene titanium-reinforced membranes for regeneration of mucogingival recession defects: a 12-case report, *J Periodontol* 65:1088, 1994.
75. Trey E, Bernimoulin JP: Influence of free gingival grafts on the health of the marginal gingiva, *J Clin Periodontol* 7:381, 1980.
76. Wade AB: Vestibular deepening by the technique of Edlan and Meejchar, *J Periodontal Res* 4:300, 1969.
77. Ward VJ: A clinical assessment of the use of the free gingival graft for correcting localized recession associated with frenal pull, *J Periodontol* 45:78, 1974.
78. Whinston GJ: Frenotomy and mucobuccal fold resection used in periodontal therapy, *NY Dent J* 22:495, 1956.
79. Wilderman MN, Wentz FM: Repair of a dentogingival defect with a pedicle flap, *J Periodontol* 36:218, 1965.
80. Woofter C: The prevalence and etiology of gingival recession, *Periodont Abstr* 17:45, 1969.
81. Zabalegui I, Sicua A, Cambra J, et al: Treatment of multiple adjacent gingival recessions with the tunnel subepithelial connective tissue graft: a clinical report, *Int J Periodont Restor Dent* 19:199, 1999.

SUGGESTED READINGS

Albano EA, Caffesse RC, Carranza FA Jr: [A biometric analysis of laterally displaced pedicle flaps], *Rev Asoc Odontol Argent* 57:351, 1969.

American Academy of Periodontology: *Glossary of periodontal terms,* ed 3, Chicago, 1992, The Academy.

Ariaudo AA, Tyrrell HA: Elimination of pockets extending to or beyond mucogingival junction, *Dent Clin North Am* 4:67, 1960.

Becker BE, Becker W: Use of connective tissue autografts for treatment of mucogingival problems, *Int J Periodont Restor Dent* 6:89, 1986.

Bergenholtz A, Hugoson A: Vestibular sulcus extension surgery in cases with periodontal disease, *J Periodontal Res* 2:221, 1967.

Bhaskar SN, Cutright DE, Perez B, et al: Full and partial thickness pedicle grafts in miniature swine and man, *J Periodontol* 42:66, 1971.

Carranza FA Jr, Carraro JJ: Effect of removal of periosteum on postoperative result of mucogingival surgery, *J Periodontol* 34:223, 1963.

Carranza FA Jr, Carraro JJ: Mucogingival techniques in periodontal surgery, *J Periodontol* 41:294, 1970.

Carraro JJ, Carranza FA Jr, Albano EA, et al: Effect of bone denudation in mucogingival surgery in humans, *J Periodontol* 35:463, 1964.

Corn H: Edentulous area pedicle graft in mucogingival surgery, *Periodontics* 2:229, 1964.

Dordick B, Coslet JG, Siebert JS: Clinical evaluation of the free autogenous gingival grafts placed on alveolar bone. I. Clinical predictability, *J Periodontol* 47:559, 1976.

Friedman N: Mucogingival surgery: the apically repositioned flap, *J Periodontol* 35:5, 1964.

Grant DA: Experimental periodontal surgery: sequestration of alveolar bone, *J Periodontol* 38:409, 1967.

Guinard EA, Caffesse RG: Localized gingival recessions II. Treatment, *J West Soc Periodontol* 25:10, 1977.

Guinard EA, Caffesse RG: Treatment of localized gingival recessions. Part I. Lateral sliding flap, *J Periodontol* 49:351, 1978.

Hawley CE, Staffileno H: Clinical evaluation of free gingival grafts in periodontal surgery, *J Periodontol* 41:105, 1970.

Maynard JB: Coronal positioning of a previously placed autogenous gingival graft, *J Periodontol* 48:151, 1977.

Miller PD Jr: Root coverage with the free gingival graft: factors associated with incomplete coverage, *J Periodontol* 58:674, 1987.

Miller PD Jr: Regenerative and reconstructive periodontal plastic surgery, mucogingival surgery, *Dent Clin North Am* 32:287, 1988.

Miller PD Jr, Allen EP: The development of periodontal plastic surgery, *Periodontol 2000* 2:7, 1996.

Miyasato M, Crigger M, Egelberg J: Gingival conditions in areas of minimal and appreciable width of keratinized gingiva, *J Clin Periodontol* 4:200, 1977.

Nabers CL: Repositioning the attached gingiva, *J Periodontol* 25:38, 1954.

Nabers CL: When is gingival repositioning an indicated procedure? *J West Soc Periodontol* 5:4, 1957.

Neach K: The use of allogenic sclera and autogenous gingiva as free gingival grafts, University of California, Los Angeles, 1978 (thesis).

Pennel B, King KO, Higgason JD, et al: Retention of periosteum in mucogingival surgery, *J Periodontol* 36:39, 1965.

Pini-Prato G, Clauser C, Magnani C, et al: Resorbable membrane in the treatment of human buccal recession: a nine-case report, *Int J Periodont Restor Dent* 15:258, 1995.

Ramfjord SP, Costich ER: Healing after exposure of periosteum on the alveolar process, *J Periodontol* 39:199, 1968.

Rateitschak KH, Egli U, Fingeli G: Recession: a four-year longitudinal study after free gingival graft, *J Clin Periodontol* 6:158, 1979.

Redondo VF, Bustamante A, Carranza FA Jr: Evaluacion biometrica de la tecnica de extension gingival con fenestracion periostica, *Rev Asoc Odontol Argent* 56:346, 1968.

Robinson RE, Agnew RG: Periosteal fenestration at the mucogingival line, *J Periodontol* 34:503, 1963.

Roth H: Some speculations as to predictable fenestrations prior to mucogingival surgery, *Periodontics* 3:29, 1965.

Smith RM: A study of the intertransplantation of alveolar mucosa, *Oral Surg* 29:328, 1970.

Smith RM: A study of the intertransplantation of gingiva, *Oral Surg* 29:169, 1970.

Smukler H: Laterally positioned mucoperiosteal pedicle grafts in the treatment of denuded roots, *J Periodontol* 47:590, 1976.

Spengler DE, Hayward JR: Study of sulcus extension wound healing in dogs, *J Oral Surg* 22:413, 1964.

Staffileno H: Palatal flap surgery: mucosal flap (split thickness) and its advantages over the mucoperiosteal flap, *J Periodontol* 40:547, 1969.

Staffileno H, Levy S, Gargiulo A: Histologic study of cellular mobilization and repair following a periosteal retention operation via split thickness mucogingival flap surgery, *J Periodontol* 37:117, 1966.

Staffileno H, Wentz F, Orban B: Histologic study of healing of split-thickness flap surgery in dogs, *J Periodontol* 33:56, 1962.

Sullivan HC, Atkins JC: Free autogenous gingival grafts. Part I. Principles of successful grafting, *Periodontics* 6:5, 1968.

Sullivan HC, Atkins JC: The role of free gingival grafts in periodontal therapy, *Dent Clin North Am* 13:33, 1969.

Tavtigian R: The height of the facial radicular alveolar crest following apically positioned flap operations, *J Periodontol* 41:412, 1970.

Wennstrom J, Lindhe J, Nyman S: Role of keratinized gingiva for gingival health, *J Clin Periodontol* 8:311, 1981.

Wennstrom J, Lindhe J, Nyman S: The role of keratinized gingiva in plaque-associated gingivitis in dogs, *J Clin Periodontol* 9:75, 1982.

Wilderman MN: Exposure of bone in periodontal surgery, *Dent Clin North Am* 8:23, 1964.

Wood DL, Hoag PL, Donnenfeld OW, et al: Alveolar crest reduction following full and partial thickness flaps, *J Periodontol* 43:141, 1972.

Recent Advances in Surgical Technology

CHAPTER 70

CHAPTER OUTLINE

This chapter discusses surgical advances in the following two areas:

1. Recent developments in the use of magnification systems and especially periodontal microsurgery, part of a broad movement in medicine and dentistry toward minimally invasive approaches to replace procedures that previously required extensive surgical incisions.
2. Advances in the use of laser technology in periodontal surgery and other areas of periodontal therapy.

Both these techniques primarily are still in a developmental stage and are not fully recommended for clinical practice.

Microsurgery

Dennis A. Shanelec and Leonard S. Tibbetts

Microsurgery is defined as a refinement in surgical technique by which visual acuity is increased using a microscope at magnifications exceeding 10×. Although loupes improve normal vision, they do not increase visual acuity to the degree required for true microsurgery. Microsurgery is also an *ergonomic* methodology in which surgical manipulations are improved through better motor coordination. In addition to increasing clinical accuracy, the microscope is important for diagnostic and nonsurgical procedures in periodontics.[3,5,7,30,31]

MAGNIFICATION SYSTEMS

A variety of simple and complex magnification systems are available to dentists, ranging from simple loupes to prism telescopic loupes and surgical microscopes. Each magnification system has its specific advantages and limitations. Although magnification improves the accuracy of clinical and diagnostic skills, it requires an understanding of optical principles that govern all magnification systems. The assumption that "more magnification is better" must always be weighed against the decrease in field of view and depth of focus that can occur as magnification increases. This is a problem more common with dental loupes than with operating microscopes.

Magnifying Loupes

Dental loupes are the most common system of optical magnification used in periodontics. *Loupes* are fundamentally dual monocular telescopes with side-by-side lenses convergent to focus on the operative field. The magnified image formed has stereoscopic properties by virtue of their convergence. A convergent lens optical system is called a *Keplerian optical system.*

Although dental loupes are widely used, they have disadvantages compared with the microscope. The clinician's eyes must converge to view the operative field. This can result in eyestrain, fatigue, and even pathologic vision changes, especially after prolonged use.

Three types of Keplerian loupes are typically used in periodontics: simple or single-element loupes, compound loupes, and prism telescopic loupes. Each type may differ widely in optical sophistication and individual design.

Simple Loupes. Simple loupes consist of a pair of single meniscus lenses (Figure 70-1). Simple loupes are primitive magnifiers with limited capabilities. Each lens is limited to only two refracting surfaces. Their magnification can only increase by increasing lens diameter and thickness. Size and weight constraints make simple loupes impractical for magnification beyond 1.5×. Another disadvantage of simple loupes is that they are greatly affected by spherical and chromatic aberration. This distorts the image shape and color of objects being viewed.

Compound Loupes. Compound loupes use multi-element lenses with intervening air spaces to gain additional refracting surfaces (Figure 70-2). This allows increased magnification with more favorable working distance and depth of field. Magnification of compound loupes can be increased by lengthening the distance between lenses, thereby avoiding excessive size and weight.

In addition to offering improved optical performance, compound lenses can be *achromatic*. This is an optical feature that clinicians should always choose when selecting magnifying loupes. Achromatic lenses consist of two glass lenses, joined together with clear resin. The specific density of each lens counteracts the chromatic aberration of its paired lens to produce a color-correct image. However, multi-element compound loupes become optically inefficient at magnifications above 3×.

Prism Telescopic Loupes. The most advanced loupe optical magnification currently available is the prism telescopic loupe. Such loupes employ Schmidt or "rooftop" prisms to lengthen the light path through a series of switchback mirrors between the lenses. This arrangement folds the light so that the barrel of the loupes can be shortened. Prism loupes produce better magnification, wider depths of field, longer working distances, and larger fields of view than other types of loupes. The barrels of prism loupes are short enough to be mounted on either eyeglass frames (Figure 70-3) or headbands. However, increased weight of prism telescopic loupes with magnification above 4× makes headband mounting more comfortable and stable than eyeglass frame mounting. Recent innovations in prism telescopic loupes include coaxial fiberoptic lighting incorporated in the lens elements to improve illumination (Figure 70-4).

Magnification Range of Surgical Loupes. Dental loupes provide a limited range of magnification, 1.5× to 6×. Loupes delivering magnification of less than 3× are usually inadequate for the visual acuity necessary for clinical periodontics. Surgical loupes providing magnification of more than 4× are impractical because of their small field of view, shallow depth of focus, and excessive

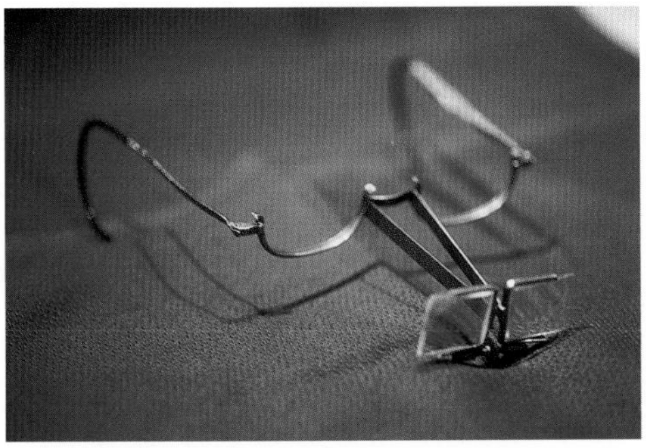

Figure 70-1 Simple loupes.

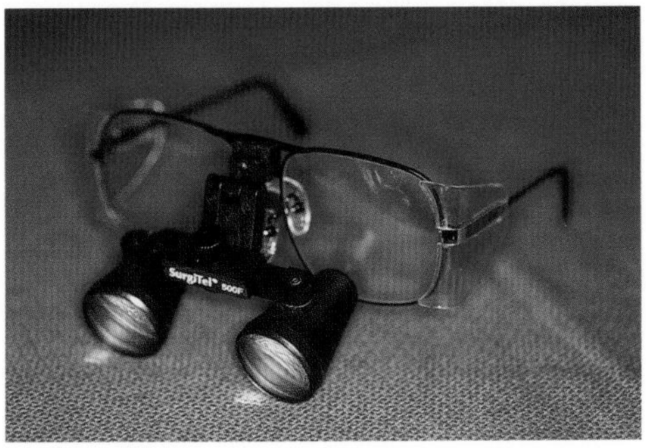

Figure 70-2 Compound loupes.

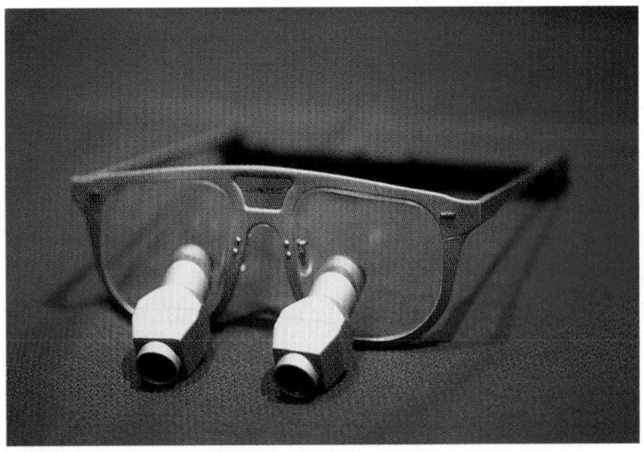

Figure 70-3 Eyeglass-mounted prism loupes.

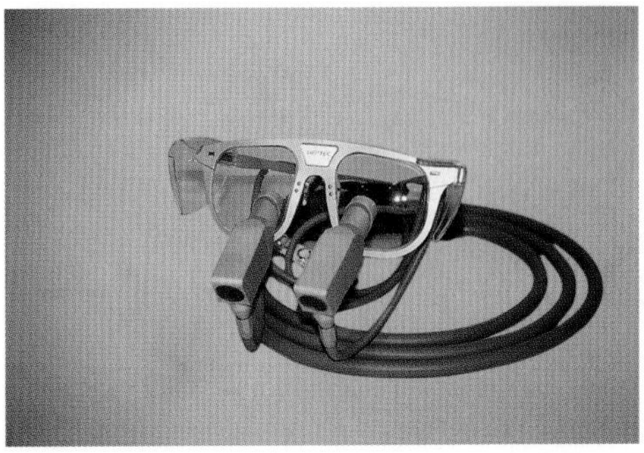

Figure 70-4 Coaxial lighted prism loupes.

weight. Excessively heavy loupes can make it difficult to maintain a stable visual field.

For some periodontal procedures, prism telescopic loupes with magnification of 4× provide an adequate combination of magnification, field of view, and depth of focus. However, the surgical microscope offers much higher magnification and superior optics compared with any of the loupe optical systems mentioned.

Surgical Microscope

The operating microscope provides higher magnification and superior optical performance compared with dental loupes (Figure 70-5). When one considers that a microscope lasts for a clinician's entire career, its expense is minimal. A microscope requires training and practice to gain proficiency but offers better performance and versatility than loupes. Surgical microscopes designed for dentistry employ Galilean optics with binocular eyepieces joined by offsetting prisms to establish parallel optical axes. Galilean optics permits stereoscopic vision without eye convergence. This aligns the eyes as if they were focused on infinity and permits a relaxed vision without eyestrain or fatigue. Operating microscopes incorporate coated optics with achromatic lenses to provide the best optical resolution and the most efficient illumination.

Perhaps the greatest advantage of the surgical microscope is that it allows the dentist to change working magnification easily to a value appropriate for the clinical task at hand.[12] Operating microscopes have a rotating variable-magnification element that changes magnification to match surgical needs. Some operating microscopes incorporate electronic foot-controlled focus and magnification for further convenience. Because the optical elements of surgical microscopes are more advanced than those found in loupes, depth-of-focus and field-of-view characteristics are enhanced.

The periodontal surgeon must establish adequate working distance between the surgical field and the objective microscope lens. This permits the surgical assistant to retract tissues and irrigate or evacuate the surgical site. Such assistant-aided control of surgical access is essential for microsurgical visibility. Assistant eyepiece attachments are available for surgical microscopes and can greatly aid the progress of microsurgical procedures. Surgical microscopes have objective lenses with various working distances. A useful range in dentistry is 250 to 350 mm. Because operating with indirect mirror vision adds 100 to 150 mm to the working distance, a ready means of changing working distances is valuable. Quick-change objective lenses are available for many surgical microscopes.

For practical use in periodontics, the surgical microscope must have both *maneuverability* and *stability*. Microscope mountings are available for ceiling, wall, or floor. Inclining eyepieces lend great postural flexibility to clinical use of the microscope in periodontics. Maneuverability must be sufficient to provide visual access to the posterior region of the mouth and to all anatomic structures addressed during periodontal treatment. The optical quality of various microscopes is comparable. Maneuverability, therefore, becomes more important than optics in choosing an appropriate microscope for periodontics.

Illumination of the microsurgical field is an important consideration. Periodontists are accustomed to lateral illumination from side-mounted dental lights. Clinicians who work with loupes often require a headlamp to compensate for the decreased illumination of dental loupes. Fiberoptic coaxial illumination is a major advantage of the operating microscope over surgical loupes. Coaxial lighting focuses the light parallel to the microscope's optical axis. With coaxial lighting, no shadows are produced. The surgeon can view perfectly the deepest reaches of the oral cavity, including into subgingival pockets and angular bony defects. Definitive visualization of root surface deposits and irregularities is only possible at magnification and resolution provided by a surgical microscope. Using the microscope, surgeons can view periodontal anatomy that previously could not be seen. Clinical decisions can be made based on certain knowledge of pathologic anatomy rather than decisions based on blind, educated guesses.

Documentation of periodontal procedures has become important for dental-legal reasons as well as for patient and professional education. The surgical microscope is ideal for documenting periodontal pathology and procedures of all types; digital or 35-mm images can be produced using a beam-splitter camera attachment (Figure 70-6). With a foot-operated shutter control, the surgeon can compose the photographic field as the procedure unfolds without interrupting surgery. In addition, the microphotographic image represents the surgical field

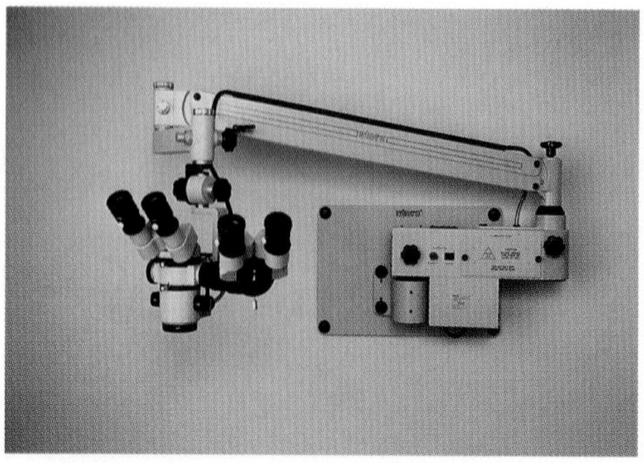

Figure 70-5 Surgical microscope.

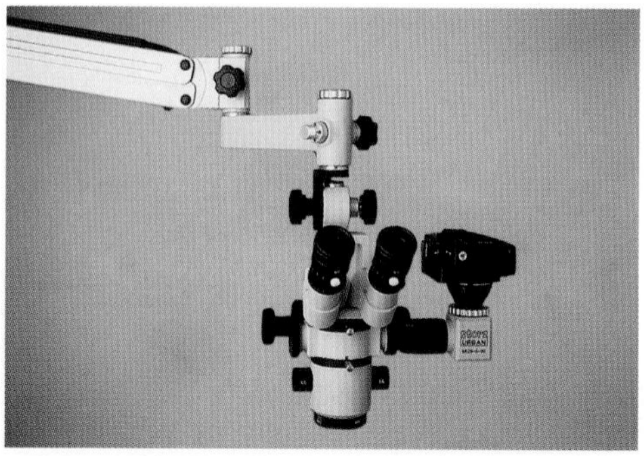

Figure 70-6 Microscope camera and beam splitter.

exactly as the surgeon sees it, as opposed to a camera view over the surgeon's shoulder. High-quality video documentation is also possible through the operating microscope using a video beam-splitter attachment. Digital cameras providing motion and still images are currently replacing 35-mm cameras for documentation in many microsurgical applications. Such high-resolution cameras bring new capabilities for live or recorded video of periodontal procedures for educational purposes.

PERIODONTAL MICROSURGERY

In recent years, periodontics has seen increasing application of procedures requiring progressively more intricate surgical skills. Regenerative and resective surgical procedures, periodontal plastic surgery, and dental implants all demand clinical performance levels that challenge the technical and motor skills of periodontal surgeons beyond a range possible with unassisted vision.

Periodontal microsurgery introduces the potential for a less invasive surgical approach in periodontics. This is exemplified by a decreased need for vertical releasing incisions and greater use of smaller surgical sites. Periodontal surgeons, as with other microsurgeons, continue to notice the extent to which reduced incision size and surgical retraction are directly related to decreased postoperative pain and rapid healing.[34]

Root Preparation

The importance of root debridement is recognized universally as an essential component of periodontal therapy.[11,18,23,27] Research in clinical dentistry has shown that microscope-enhanced vision more readily accomplishes the long-established clinical goals of endodontic and restorative dentistry. In periodontics, studies demonstrated that root debridement performed without magnification was incomplete. When debrided roots were examined with the aid of a microscope, substantial deposits remained. Even in the absence of clinical studies, it may be inferred that microscope-enhanced vision in periodontics permits more definitive root debridement.

The primary goals of periodontal surgery include visual access to the root surface for plaque and calculus removal and for removing pathologically altered tooth structure. Magnification greatly improves the surgeon's ability to create a clean, smooth root surface (Figure 70-7). The root surface represents one opposing edge of the periodontal wound. Root planing is therefore analogous to establishing a clean soft tissue incision. Magnification permits preparation of both hard and soft tissue wound surfaces so that they may be joined together according to the accepted microsurgical principle of butt-joint wound approximation. This encourages primary wound healing and enhanced periodontal reconstruction. Wound-healing studies show epithelial anastomosis of microsurgically joined surgical wounds in animals within 48 hours.[5,34]

Surgery under Magnification

Viewing periodontal surgery under magnification impresses the periodontal surgeon with the coarseness of conventional surgical manipulation. What appears to the unaided eye as gentle surgery is revealed under magnification to be gross crushing and tearing of delicate tissues. Periodontists have long advocated atraumatic surgery to achieve primary wound closure. However, the limits of normal vision made this goal impossible. Periodontal microsurgery is the natural transition from conventional surgical principles to a surgical ethic in which the microscope is employed to permit the most accurate and atraumatic handling of tissue to enhance wound healing.

Microsurgical Instruments

In addition to the use of magnification and reliance on atraumatic technique, microsurgery requires specially constructed instruments designed specifically to minimize trauma. An important characteristic of microsurgical instruments is their ability to create clean incisions that prepare wounds for healing by primary intention. Microsurgical incisions are established at a 90-degree angle to the surface using ophthalmic microsurgical scalpels (Figure 70-8). Microscopy permits easy identification of ragged wound edges for trimming and freshening. For primary wound closure, microsutures in the range of 6-0 to 9-0 are needed to approximate the wound edges accurately (Figure 70-9). Microsurgical wound apposition minimizes gaps or voids at the wound edges. This encourages rapid healing with less postoperative inflammation and with less pain.

Figures 70-10 and 70-11 illustrate periodontal surgery cases treated using microsurgical techniques.

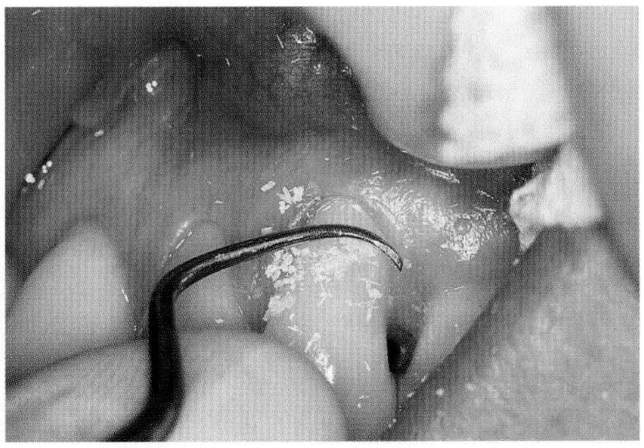

Figure 70-7 Magnified root planing.

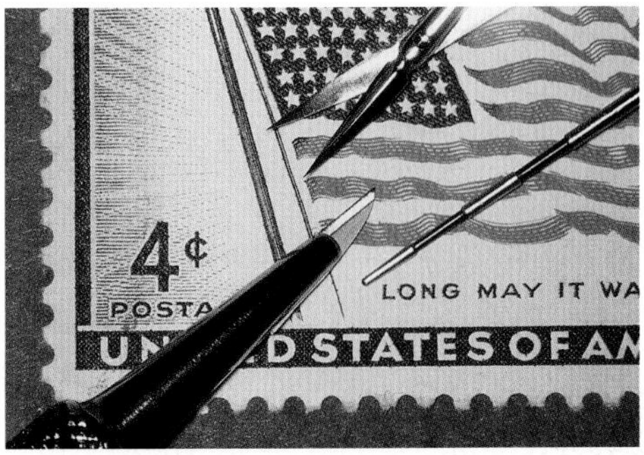

Figure 70-8 Castroviejo microsurgical scalpel.

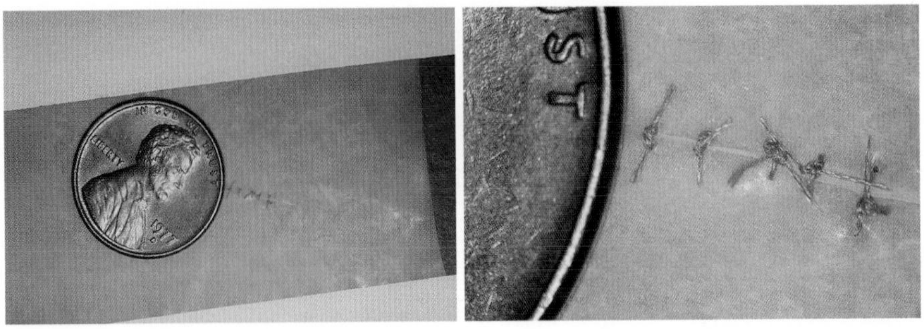

Figure 70-9 Microsurgical suturing.

A

B

C

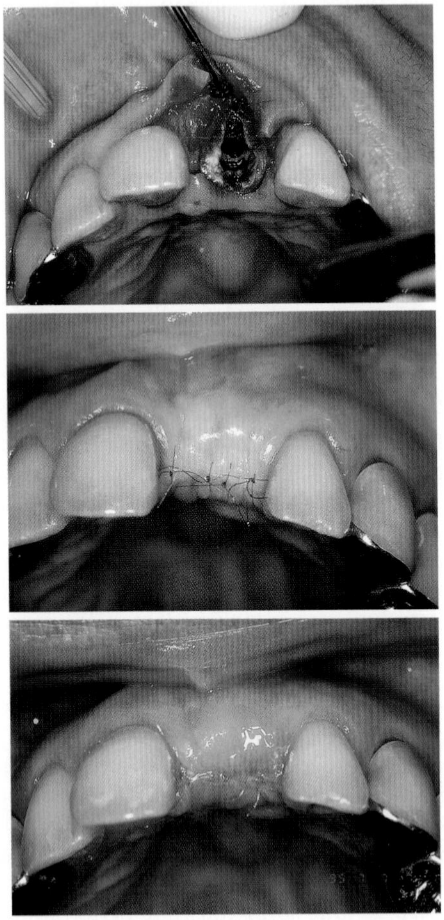

Figure 70-10 Microsurgical extraction. **A,** Before surgery. **B,** Microsurgical view. **C,** One week after surgery.

A

B

C

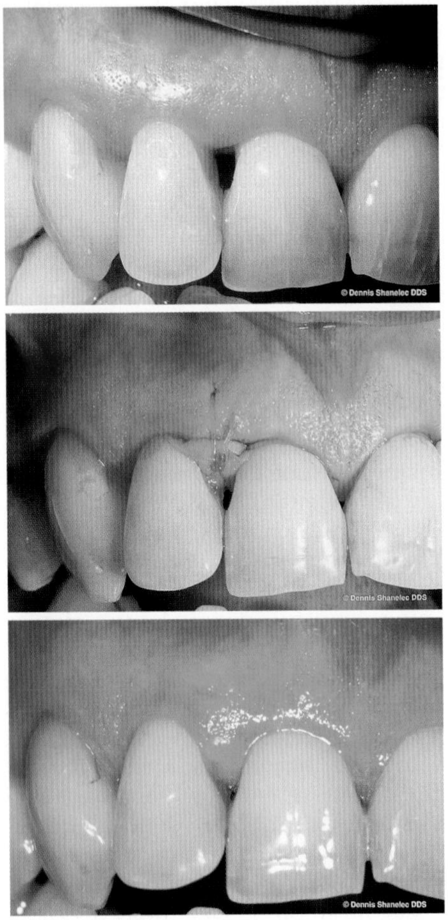

Figure 70-11 Papilla reconstruction. **A,** Before surgery. **B,** Microsurgical view. **C,** After surgery.

Ergonomics

The ergonomics of hand position and body posture are closely related to improved motor skills made possible by a microsurgical approach to therapy. Studies show that motor coordination is greatly improved when surgeons use microsurgical instruments specifically designed to employ a precision grip of the hand.

Microsurgical instruments are circular in cross section to permit precise rotational movements. They are manufactured of titanium because of its strength, lightness, and nonmagnetic characteristics. The various postural and ergonomic methods of reducing unwanted hand movements result in more precise surgeries. These methods also greatly reduce surgical fatigue as well as the spinal and occupational pathology common in periodontics. In the long term, the beneficial ergonomic aspects of microscopy may be the most influential factors in its adoption by the dental profession at large.

CONCLUSION

Microsurgery offers new opportunities for periodontal surgery that can enhance the therapeutic results for a

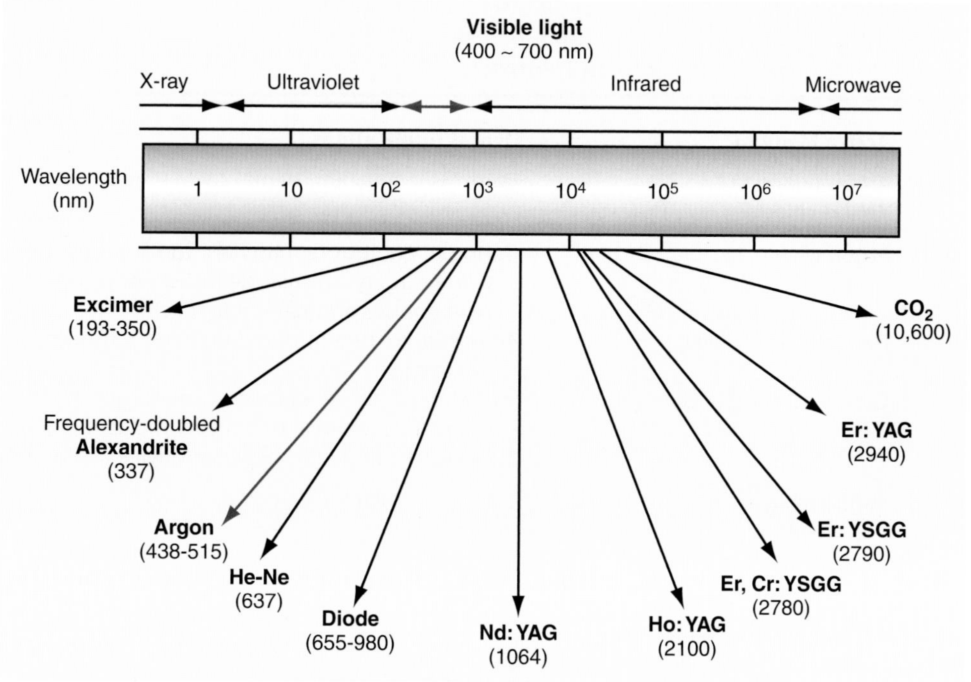

Figure 70-12 Wavelengths of various lasers.

variety of procedures. Its benefits include improved cosmetics, rapid healing, minimal discomfort, and enhanced patient acceptance. Periodontics of the future will see increasing use of magnification in all areas of practice, including implantology.

Lasers in Periodontics

Isao Ishikawa and Akira Aoki

Laser is an acronym for "*l*ight *a*mplification by *s*timulated *e*mission of *r*adiation." The stimulated emission of a photon by an excited atom, which triggers the release of a subsequent photon, is responsible for generation of a coherent, monochromatic, and collimated form of light, or laser. Lasers can concentrate light energy and exert a strong effect, targeting tissue at an energy level much lower than natural light. The wavelength of a laser determines its characteristics (Figure 70-12).

Maiman[19] invented the first laser device in 1960, based on theories derived by Einstein in the early 1900s. Since then, lasers have been used for various purposes in medicine and surgery. Once in contact with tissue, laser energy is reflected, scattered, absorbed, or transmitted to the neighboring tissues (Figure 70-13). The water molecules, proteins, pigments, and other macromolecules present in biologic tissue are responsible for absorption, but the absorption coefficient actually depends on the wavelength of the incoming laser irradiation.[22]

APPLICATION FOR PERIODONTAL THERAPY

The neodymium:yttrium-aluminum-garnet (Nd:YAG), carbon dioxide (CO_2), diode, erbium:YAG (Er:YAG), erbium, chromium:yttrium (Er,Cr:YSGG), and argon are the lasers most often used and studied in dentistry (Table 70-1). In dentistry, lasers were first used in the field of operative dentistry for caries removal and cavity preparation.[9] The effects of newer lasers (e.g., argon, CO_2, Nd:YAG, diode) on dental hard tissue and caries have been investigated[15,33] but reported to be unsuccessful because of thermal damage.

The use of lasers for periodontal treatment becomes more complex because the periodontium consists of both hard and soft tissues. Among the many lasers available, high-power lasers such as CO_2, Nd:YAG, and diode lasers can be used in periodontics. Because of their excellent soft tissue ablation and hemostatic characteristics, the use of these lasers has been approved for soft tissue

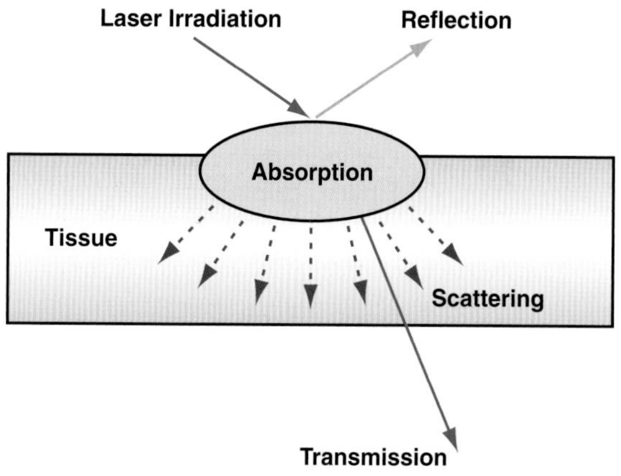

Figure 70-13 Interaction of human tissue and laser irradiation.

TABLE 70-1

Current and Potential Applications of Lasers in Dentistry

Type	Active Medium	Dental Applications
Excimer lasers	Argon-fluoride (ArF) Xenon-chloride (XeCl)	Hard tissue ablation, dental calculus removal
Gas lasers	Argon (Ar)	Curing of composite materials, tooth whitening, intraoral soft tissue surgery, sulcular debridement (subgingival curettage in periodontitis and periimplantitis)
	Helium-neon (HeNe)	Analgesia, treatment of dentin hypersensitivity, aphthous ulcer treatment
	Carbon dioxide (CO_2)	Intraoral soft tissue and soft tissue surgery, aphthous ulcer treatment, removal of gingival melanin pigmentation, treatment of dentin hypersensitivity, analgesia
Diode lasers	Indium-gallium-arsenide-phosphorus (InGaAsP)	Caries and calculus detection
	Galium-aluminum-arsenide (GaAlAs) Galium-arsenide (GaAs)	Intraoral general and implant soft tissue surgery, sulcular debridement (subgingival curettage in periodontitis and periimplantitis), analgesia, treatment of dentin hypersensitivity, pulpotomy, root canal disinfection, aphthous ulcer treatment, removal of gingival melanin pigmentation
Solid-state lasers	Frequency-doubled alexandrite	Selective ablation of dental plaque and calculus
	Neodymium:yttrium-aluminum-garnet (Nd:YAG)	Intraoral soft tissue surgery, sulcular debridement (subgingival curettage in periodontitis), analgesia, treatment of dentin hypersensitivity, pulpotomy, root canal disinfection, removal of enamel caries, aphthous ulcer treatment, removal of gingival melanin pigmentation
	Erbium group Erbium:YAG (Er:YAG) Erbium:yttrium (Er:YSGG) Erbium, chromium:YSGG (Er,Cr:YSGG)	Caries removal and cavity preparation, modification of enamel and dentin surfaces, intraoral general and implant soft tissue surgery, sulcular debridement (subgingival curettage in periodontitis and periimplantitis), scaling of root surfaces, osseous surgery, treatment of dentin hypersensitivity, analgesia, pulpotomy, root canal treatment and disinfection, aphthous ulcer treatment, removal of gingival melanin and metal-tattoo pigmentation

management in periodontal and oral surgery.[6,10,26,28] However, when applied to the root surface or alveolar bone, carbonization and major thermal damage have been reported on the target and adjacent tissues.[28] Therefore the use of these lasers is limited to gingivectomy, frenectomy, and similar soft tissue procedures,[6,10,26] including the removal of melanin pigmentation[4,32,38] and metal tattoos of the gingiva.[28]

The use of lasers also has been investigated for other indications in periodontal therapy, including subgingival debridement and curettage,[2] removal of granulation tissue during flap surgery,[36] and osseous recontouring,[21] as well as in implant surgery,[8] maintenance of implants, and management of periimplantitis.[16,20]

ADVANTAGES AND DISADVANTAGES

Advantages of laser treatment are greater hemostasis, bactericidal effect, and minimal wound contraction.[1,16,37] However, previous laser systems have strong thermal side effects, leading to melting, cracking, and carbonization of hard tissues.

Recently, Er:YAG and Er,Cr:YSGG lasers have been developed for dental applications. Of all dental lasers available, the absorption of the Er:YAG and Er,Cr:YSGG lasers in water is the highest. These lasers effectively ablate all biologic tissues that contain water molecules[1,16,37] and are applicable to both soft and hard tissues.[2,8,21] The erbium laser group has emerged as a promising laser system for periodontal indications.[2,14,29] Further research and development are needed, however, before they can be recommended for these purposes.[2,13,14]

The use of lasers also has disadvantages that require precautions to be taken during clinical application (Box 70-1).[6] Laser irradiation can interact with tissues even in the noncontact mode, which means that laser beams may reach the patient's eyes and other tissues surrounding the target in the oral cavity. Clinicians should be careful to prevent inadvertent irradiation to these tissues, especially to the eyes. Protective eyewear specific

BOX 70-1

Precautions and Risks Associated with Clinical Use of Lasers

Precautions before and during Irradiation

- Use glasses for eye protection (patient, operator, and assistants).
- Prevent inadvertent irradiation (action in noncontact mode).
- Protect the patient's eyes, throat, and oral tissues outside the target site.
- Use wet gauze packs to avoid reflection from shiny metal surfaces.
- Ensure adequate high-speed evacuation to capture the laser plume.

Potential Risks

- Excessive tissue destruction by direct ablation and thermal side effects.
- Destruction of the attachment apparatus at the bottom of pockets.
- Excessive ablation of root surface and gingival tissue within periodontal pockets.
- Thermal injury to the root surface, gingival tissue, pulp, and bone tissue.

for the wavelength of the laser in use must be worn by the patient, operator, and assistant.[6] Laser beams can be reflected by shiny surfaces of metal dental instruments, causing irradiation to other tissues, which should be avoided by using wet gauze packs over the area surrounding the target.[25]

During CO_2 or Nd:YAG irradiation for periodontal treatment, caution must be taken not to contact enamel surfaces because of the risk of melting. Improper irradiation in periodontal pockets could cause thermal damage to the root surface and pocket walls and destruction of the intact attachment apparatus at the base of the pocket, affecting the normal cell attachment during healing. Damage to the underlying bone and pulp tissue is another concern. Therefore, proper irradiation techniques and conditions need to be followed when using lasers.

SCIENCE TRANSFER

Challenges in dentistry include visualization of and access to the surgical site. Advances in lighting, magnification, and technology have greatly improved the clinician's ability to see and access the operative field. As with all advances, however, limitations exist, and therefore advantages must be balanced against disadvantages. Thus it is incumbent on the user of these newer technologies to learn all aspects of the technique and the required precautions. Ultimately, the question that must be answered is whether the outcome of the therapy is improved or unimproved. The use of all newer technologies, such as surgery with microscopes and with lasers, needs to be evaluated in prospective, randomized, masked clinical trials to determine if such advances provide an actual improvement in outcome.

Microsurgical approaches to periodontal therapy require the acquisition of precise surgical skills and the use of a surgical microscope. These approaches and skills result in more precise and less traumatic procedures. Microsurgery should expand the range of periodontal treatment by developing new surgical procedures rather than merely improving current techniques. Advances in magnification need to be followed by controlled human clinical trials that document their advantages and disadvantages in microsurgical periodontal procedures.

Lasers are being developed for a variety of uses in periodontal therapy. Much of the current viewpoint is based on the use of CO_2, Nd:YAG, and diode lasers. These high-power lasers are useful for soft tissue surgery such as gingivectomy and frenectomy, but when used on tooth surfaces or bone, they can produce unacceptable carbonization and major thermal damage. *The erbium laser group shows promise for use in periodontal surgical applications, and in the future, these lasers may be developed for other appropriate dental applications.*

REFERENCES

1. Ando Y, Aoki A, Watanabe H, Ishikawa I: Bactericidal effect of erbium YAG laser on periodontopathic bacteria, *Lasers Surg Med* 19:190, 1996.
2. Aoki A, Sasaki K, Watanabe H, Ishikawa I: Lasers in nonsurgical periodontal therapy, *Periodontol 2000* 36:59, 2004.
3. Apotheker H, Jako GJ: A microscope for use in dentistry, *J Microsurg* 3:7, 1981.
4. Atsawasuwan P, Greethong K, Nimmanon V: Treatment of gingival hyperpigmentation for esthetic purposes by Nd:YAG laser: report of 4 cases, *J Periodontol* 71:315, 2000.
5. Banowsky LH: Basic microvascular techniques and principles, *Urology* 23:495, 1984.
6. Cohen RE, Ammons WF: Lasers in periodontics. Report of Research, Science and Therapy Committee, American Academy of Periodontology (revised by LA Rossman), *J Periodontol* 73:1231, 2002.
7. Daniel RK: Microsurgery: through the looking glass, *N Engl J Med* 300:1251, 1979.
8. El-Montaser M, Devlin H, Dickinson MR, et al: Osseointegration of titanium metal implants in erbium-YAG laser–prepared bone, *Implant Dent* 8:79, 1999.
9. Goldman L, Hornby P, Meyer R, Goldman B: Impact of the laser on dental caries, *Nature* 25:417, 1964.
10. Gottsegen R, Ammons WF: Lasers in periodontics (position paper), Chicago, 1991, Research, Science and Therapy Committee, American Academy of Periodontology.
11. Hirchfeld L, Wasserman B: A long-term survey of tooth loss in 600 treated periodontal patients, *J Periodontol* 49:225, 1978.
12. Hoerenz P: The operating microscope. I. Optical principles, illumination systems and support systems, *J Microsurg* 1:367, 1980.

13. Ishikawa I: Re: Er:YAG laser scaling of diseased root surfaces (Frentzen M, Braun A, Aniol D: 73:524), *J Periodontol* 73:1227, 2002.
14. Ishikawa I, Aoki A, Takasaki AA: Potential applications of erbium:YAG laser in periodontics, *J Periodontal Res* 39:275, 2004.
15. Kinersly T, Jarabak JP, Phatak NM, DeMent J: Laser effects on tissue and materials related to dentistry, *J Am Dent Assoc* 70:593, 1965.
16. Kreisler M, Al Haj H, d'Hoedt B: Temperature changes at the implant-bone interface during simulated surface decontamination with an Er:YAG laser, *Int J Prosthodont* 15:582, 2002.
17. Kreisler P, Muller JH, Van Hattum AH: *Microsurgery and wound healing,* Amsterdam, 1979, Excerpta Medica.
18. Loos B, Nylund K, Claffey N, et al: Clinical effects of root debridement in molar and nonmolar teeth: a 2-year follow-up, *J Clin Periodontol* 16:498, 1989.
19. Maiman TH: Stimulated optical radiation in ruby, *Nature* 187:493, 1960.
20. Midda M, Renton-Harper P: Lasers in dentistry, *Br Dent J* 170:343, 1991.
21. Nelson JS, Orenstein A, Liaw LH, Berns MW: Mid-infrared erbium YAG laser ablation of bone: the effect of laser osteotomy on bone healing, *Lasers Surg Med* 9:362, 1989.
22. Niemz MH: *Laser-tissue interaction: fundamentals and applications,* Berlin, 1996, Springer-Verlag.
23. Nordland P, Garrett S, Kiger R, et al: The effect of plaque control and debridement in molar teeth, *J Clin Periodontol* 14:445, 1987.
24. Pecora G, Andreana S: Operating microscope in endodontic surgery, *Oral Surg Med Pathol* 75:751, 1993.
25. Pick RM, Pecaro BC, Silberman CJ: The laser gingivectomy: the use of the CO_2 laser for the removal of phenytoin hyperplasia, *J Periodontol* 56:492,1985.
26. Pick RM, Pecaro BC: Use of the CO_2 laser in soft tissue dental surgery, *Lasers Surg Med* 7:207, 1987.
27. Pihlstrom BL, Ortiz-Campos C, McHugh RB: A randomized 4-year study of periodontal therapy, *J Periodontol* 52:227, 1981.
28. Rossmann JA, Cobb CM: Lasers in periodontal therapy, *Periodontol 2000* 9:150, 1995.
29. Schwarz F, Sculean A, Georg T, Reich E: Periodontal treatment with an Er:YAG laser compared to scaling and root planing: a controlled clinical study, *J Periodontol* 72:361, 2001.
30. Serafin D: Microsurgery: past, present and future, *Plast Reconstr Surg* 66:781, 1979.
31. Shanelec DA: Optical principles of loupes, *Calif Dent Assoc J* 20:25, 1992.
32. Sharon E, Azaz B, Ulmansky M: Vaporization of melanin in oral tissues and skin with a carbon dioxide laser: a canine study, *J Oral Maxillofac Surg* 58:1387, 2000.
33. Stern RH, Vahl J, Sognnaes RF: Lased enamel: ultrastructural observations of pulsed carbon dioxide laser effects, *J Dent Res* 51:455, 1972.
34. Van Hattum A, James J, Klopper PJ: Epithelial migration in wound healing, *Virchows Arch B Cell Pathol* 30:221, 1979.
35. Way L: Changing therapy for gallstone disease, *N Engl J Med* 323:1273, 1990.
36. Williams TM, Cobb CM, Rapley JW, Killoy WJ: Histologic evaluation of alveolar bone following CO_2 laser removal of connective tissue from periodontal defects, *Int J Periodontol Restor Dent* 15:497, 1995.
37. Yamaguchi H, Kobayashi K, Osada R, et al: Effects of irradiation of an erbium:YAG laser on root surfaces, *J Periodontol* 68:1151, 1997.
38. Yousuf A, Hossain M, Nakamura Y, et al: Removal of gingival melanin pigmentation with the semiconductor diode laser: a case report, *J Clin Laser Med Surg* 18:263, 2000.

SECTION ▪ V ▪

Periodontal-Restorative Interrelationships

Henry H. Takei

Preparation of the Periodontium for Restorative Dentistry

Philip R. Melnick

71

CHAPTER

CHAPTER OUTLINE

Periodontal health is the "sine qua non," a prerequisite, of successful comprehensive dentistry.[23] To achieve the long-term therapeutic targets of comfort, good function, treatment predictability, longevity, and ease of restorative and maintenance care, active periodontal infection must be treated and controlled before the initiation of restorative, esthetic, and implant dentistry. In addition, the residual effects of periodontal disease or anatomic aberrations inconsistent with realizing and maintaining long-term stability must be addressed. More recently, this phase of treatment includes techniques performed in anticipation of esthetic or implant dentistry, such as clinical crown lengthening, covering denuded roots, alveolar ridge retention or augmentation, and implant site development.

RATIONALE FOR THERAPY

The many reasons for establishing periodontal health *before* performing restorative dentistry include the following[45]:

1. Periodontal treatment is undertaken to ensure the establishment of stable gingival margins before tooth preparation. Noninflamed, healthy tissues are less likely to change (e.g., shrink) as a result of subgingival restorative treatment or postrestoration periodontal care.[26,27] In addition, tissues that do not bleed during restorative manipulation allow for a more predictable restorative and esthetic result.[20,21]
2. Certain periodontal procedures are designed to provide for adequate tooth length for retention,

access for tooth preparation, impression making, tooth preparation, and finishing of restorative margins in anticipation of restorative dentistry.[20,41] Failure to complete these procedures before restorative care can add to the complexity of treatment and introduce unnecessary risk of failure.[20]

3. Periodontal therapy should antecede restorative care because the resolution of inflammation may result in the repositioning of teeth[40] or in soft tissue and mucosal changes. Failure to anticipate these changes may interfere with prosthetic designs planned or constructed before periodontal treatment.
4. Traumatic forces placed on teeth with ongoing periodontitis may increase tooth mobility, discomfort, and possibly the rate of attachment loss.[8] Restorations constructed on teeth free of periodontal inflammation, synchronous with a functionally appropriate occlusion, are more compatible with long-term periodontal stability and comfort (see Chapters 29 and 56).
5. Quality, quantity, and topography of the periodontium may play important roles as structural defense factors in maintaining periodontal health. Orthodontic tooth movement and restorations completed without the benefit of periodontal treatment designed for this purpose may be subject to negative changes that complicate construction and future maintenance.[47]
6. Successful esthetic and implant procedures may be difficult or impossible without the specialized periodontal procedures developed for this purpose.

SCIENCE TRANSFER

Periodontal disease involves an inflammatory reaction by the host. As in all inflammatory reactions in the body, the cardinal signs of inflammation are present. These include redness, swelling, and heat and therefore changes in the host tissues. Restorative dentistry generally involves margins between a material and the tooth or root structures. As such, these margins are placed in a specific relationship to the host tissues. If the host tissues are undergoing change, the dentist cannot predictably place margins in desired locations. Thus it is imperative that the host tissues are as stable (physiologic) as possible, meaning that they are free of change (pathology) or inflammation (periodontal disease). *Inflammation can therefore be considered the driving force for tissue change, and to ensure predictable restorative dentistry, this driving force should be eliminated. Thus, periodontal therapy to resolve inflammation should be completed before restorative dentistry.*

Clinicians need to combine periodontal and restorative procedures in a coordinated manner to optimize clinical outcomes. During Phase I therapy, periodontal tissues are treated to provide a stable, healthy foundation for restorative care. Orthodontic therapy may supplement this approach, and care must be taken to remove all subgingival deposits before tooth movement. This may involve performing flap procedures for access before orthodontic therapy. In Phase II therapy, periodontal surgical procedures, such as crown lengthening, mucogingival surgery, and surgical maintenance of alveolar ridges, are frequently performed and are necessary antecedents of restorative care.

SEQUENCE OF TREATMENT

Treatment sequencing should be based on logical and evidenced-based methodologies, taking into account not only the disease state encountered but also the psychologic and esthetic concerns of the patient. Because periodontal and restorative therapy is situational and specific to each patient, a plan must be adaptable to change depending on the variables encountered during the course of treatment. For example, teeth initially determined to be salvageable may be judged "hopeless," thus altering the established treatment scheme.

Generally, the preparation of the periodontium for restorative dentistry can be divided into two phases: (1) control of periodontal inflammation with nonsurgical and surgical approaches and (2) preprosthetic periodontal surgery (Box 71-1).

CONTROL OF ACTIVE DISEASE

Periodontal therapy is intended to control active disease (see Chapters 49-56). In addition to the removal of root surface accretions that are primary etiologic agents, secondary local factors such as plaque-retentive overhanging margins and untreated caries must be addressed.[13,18]

BOX 71-1

Sequence of Treatment in Preparing Periodontium for Restorative Dentistry

Control of Active Disease
Emergency treatment
Extraction of hopeless teeth
Oral hygiene instructions
Scaling and root planing
Reevaluation
Periodontal surgery
Adjunctive orthodontic therapy

Preprosthetic Surgery
Management of mucogingival problems
Preservation of ridge morphology after tooth extraction
Crown-lengthening procedures
Alveolar ridge reconstruction

Emergency Treatment

Emergency treatment is undertaken to alleviate symptoms and stabilize acute infection. This includes endodontic as well as periodontal conditions (see Chapters 48 and 58).

Extraction of Hopeless Teeth

Extraction of hopeless teeth is followed by provisionalization with fixed or removable prosthetics. Retention of hopeless teeth without periodontal treatment may result in bone loss on adjacent teeth.[30] Restorative margins are refined and provisional restorations refitted after the completion of active periodontal therapy.

Oral Hygiene Measures

Oral hygiene measures, when properly applied, have been shown to reduce plaque scores and gingival inflammation[28,44] (see Chapter 49). However, in patients with deep periodontal pockets (>5 mm), plaque control measures alone are insufficient in resolving subgingival infection and inflammation.[5,28]

Scaling and Root Planing

Scaling and root planing *combined* with oral hygiene measures have been demonstrated to significantly reduce gingival inflammation and the rate of progression of periodontitis[3,4,29] (see Chapter 51). This applies even to patients with deep periodontal pockets[5,14] (Figure 71-1).

Reevaluation

After 4 weeks the gingival tissues are evaluated to determine oral hygiene adequacy, soft tissue response, and pocket depth (see Chapter 59). This permits sufficient time for healing, reduction in inflammation and pocket depths, and gain in clinical attachment levels. In deeper pockets (>5 mm), however, plaque and calculus removal is often incomplete,[42,46] with risk of future breakdown[7] (Figure 71-2). As a result, periodontal surgery to access the root surfaces for instrumentation and to reduce periodontal pocket depths must be considered before restorative care may proceed.

Periodontal Surgery

Periodontal surgery may be required for some patients (see Chapters 59-70). This should be undertaken with future restorative and implant dentistry in mind. Some procedures are intended to treat active disease successfully,[11,34] and some are aimed at the preparation of the mouth for restorative or prosthetic care.[47]

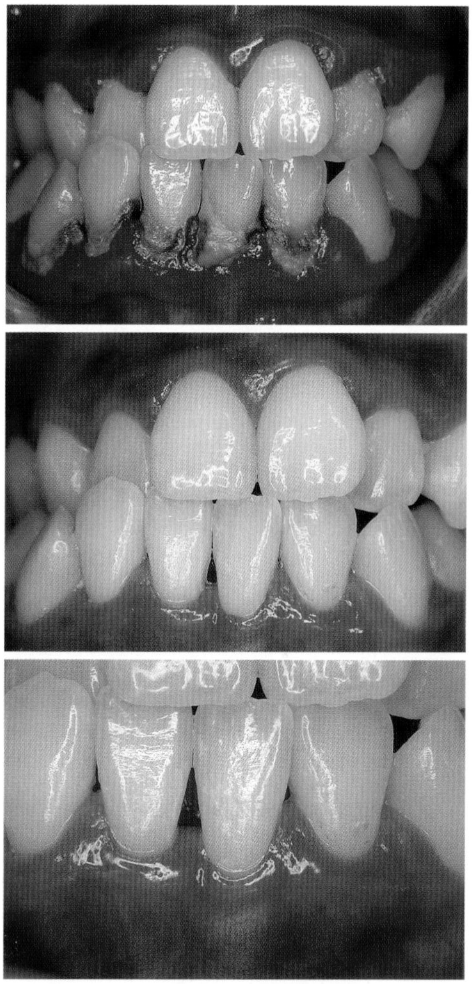

Figure 71-1 Root planing has resolved the gingival inflammation of this patient.

A 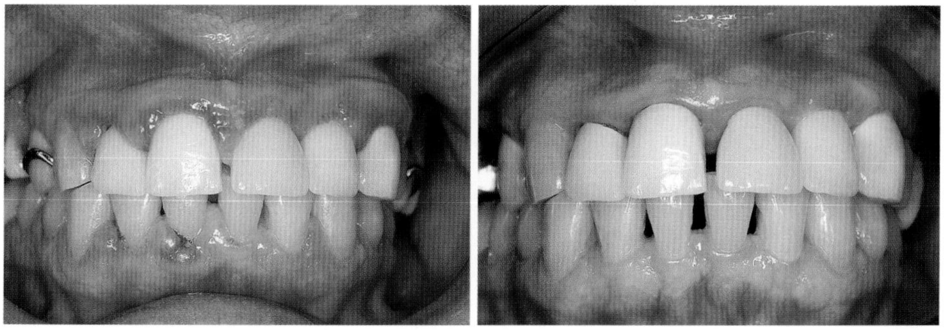 B

Figure 71-2 **A,** Before treatment. **B,** After 4 weeks, oral hygiene instructions and scaling and root planing have improved this patient's periodontal status. However, inflammation associated with pockets deeper than 5 mm suggests a need for periodontal surgery.

Adjunctive Orthodontic Therapy

Orthodontic treatment has been shown to be a useful adjunctive to periodontal therapy[6,16,17,22] (see Chapter 57). It should be undertaken only after active periodontal disease has been controlled. If nonsurgical treatment is sufficient, definitive periodontal pocket therapy may be postponed until after the completion of orthodontic tooth movement. This allows for the advantage of the positive bone changes that orthodontic therapy can provide. However, deep pockets and furcation invasions may require surgical access for root instrumentation in advance of orthodontic tooth movement. Failure to control active periodontitis can result in acute exacerbations and bone loss during tooth movement.[9] As long as they are periodontally healthy, teeth with preexisting bone loss may be moved orthodontically without incurring additional attachment loss.[36,37]

Soft tissue grafting procedures are often indicated in anticipation of orthodontic therapy to increase the dimension of attached tissue.[47]

PREPROSTHETIC SURGERY

Management of Mucogingival Problems

Periodontal plastic surgical procedures may be undertaken for a variety of reasons. The most common techniques include those that increase gingival dimensions and

A

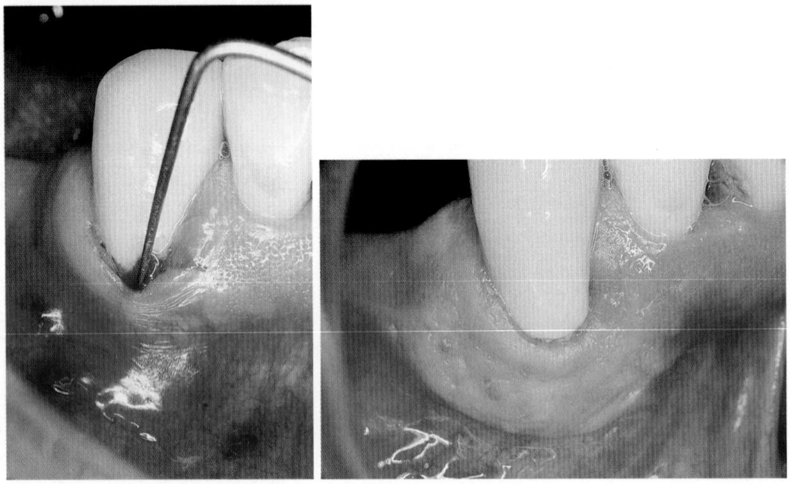

B

Figure 71-3 In preparation for a removable partial denture, this canine has received a gingival graft to increase attached gingiva and deepen the vestibule. **A,** Before therapy. Note minimal attached gingiva. **B,** After therapy, there is abundant attached gingiva and vestibular depth.

A B C D

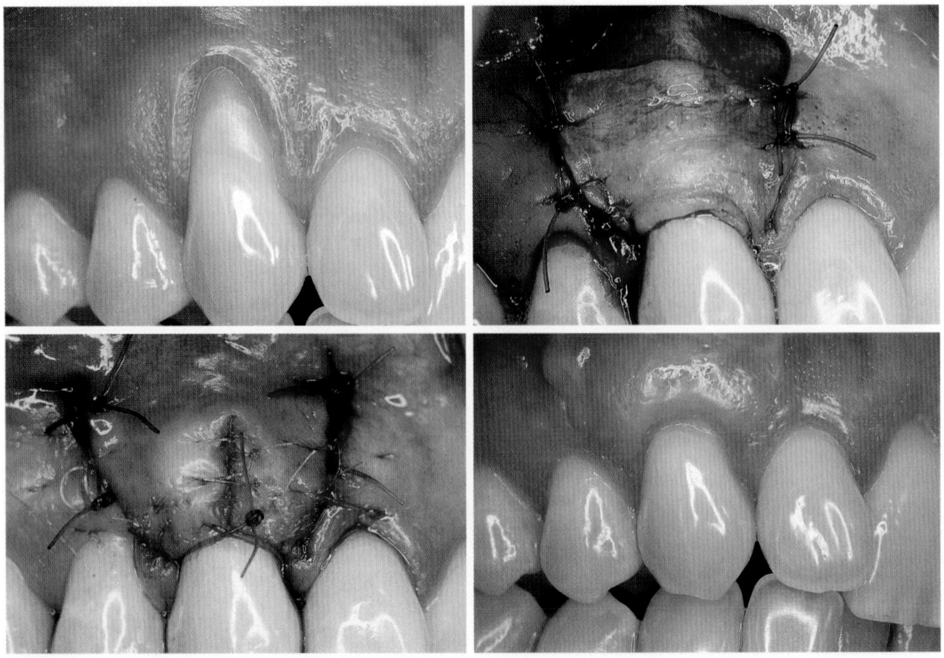

Figure 71-4 Connective tissue graft placed under a double-papilla flap has been used to provide root coverage for a maxillary right canine. **A,** Maxillary canine before therapy. **B,** Connective tissue graft placed over denuded root surface. **C,** Papilla placed over connective tissue. **D,** Final result.

achieve root coverage. These procedures are often indicated before restoration, for prosthetic reasons (Figure 71-3), and in conjunction with orthodontic tooth movement. Root coverage procedures may also be undertaken for purposes of comfort and esthetics (Figure 71-4).

At least 2 months of healing is recommended after soft tissue grafting procedures, before initiating restorative dentistry[47] (see Chapter 69).

Preservation of Ridge Morphology after Tooth Extraction

Alveolar ridge resorption is a common consequence of tooth loss.[1,2] Ridge preservation procedures have been shown to be useful in anticipation of the future placement of a dental implant or pontic, as well as in cases where unaided healing would result in an unesthetic deformity[15,24,25,31] (Figure 71-5).

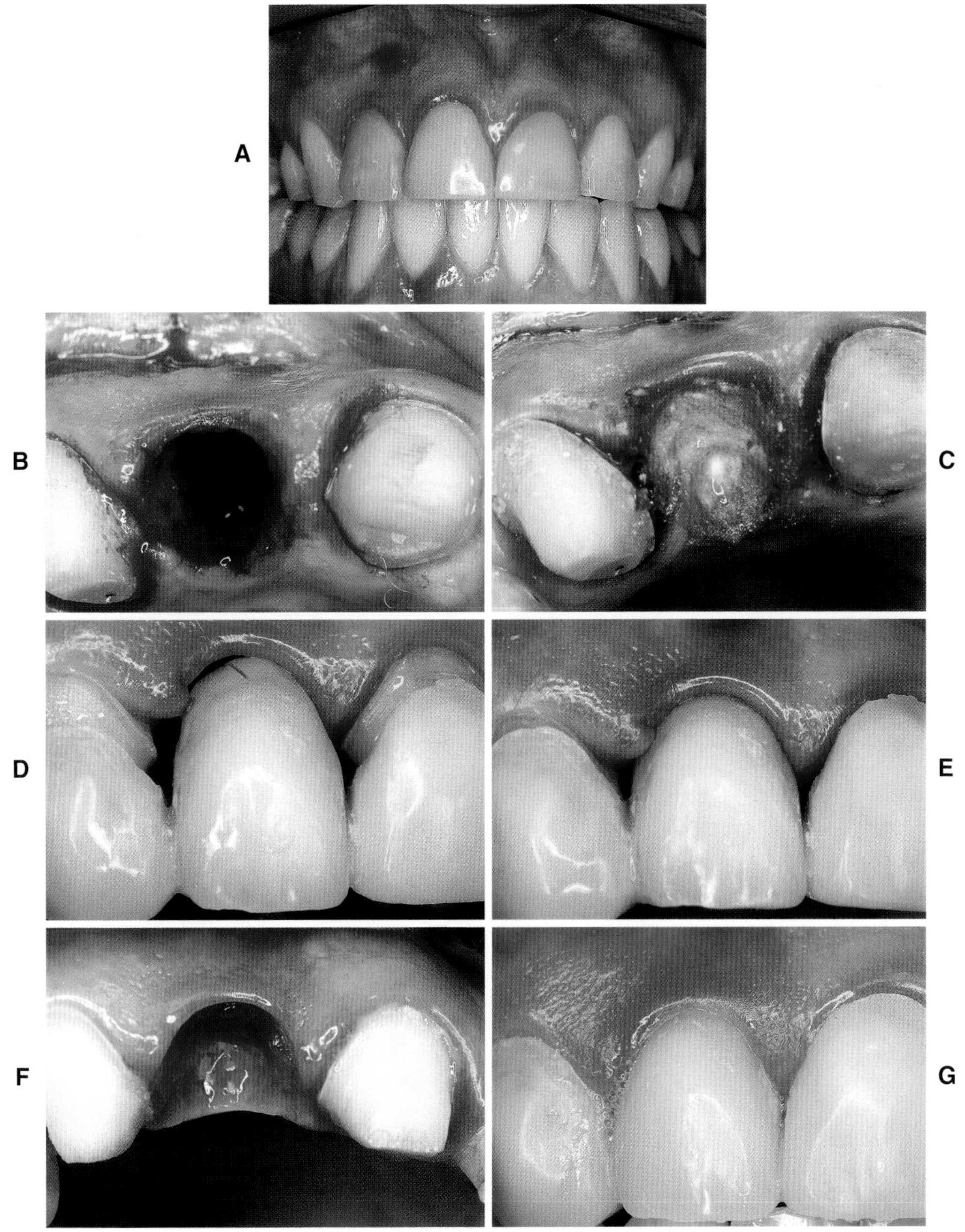

Figure 71-5 **A,** The maxillary right lateral incisor has failed endodontically, with a fistulous tract noted exiting from the attached gingiva. **B,** The tooth is atraumatically removed and the socket debrided while maintaining the surrounding anatomic integrity. **C,** In an effort to reduce ridge collapse, the socket is grafted with a combination of deproteinized bovine bone and calcium sulfate. **D,** Provisional fixed partial denture is placed, with an ovate pontic extending 2 mm into the socket and supporting the surrounding tissues. **E** and **F,** After 8 weeks the socket has healed, preserving the gingival and papillary architecture, in preparation for an esthetic final prosthesis. **G,** Final restoration.

Crown-Lengthening Procedures

Surgical crown-lengthening procedures are performed to provide retention form to allow for proper tooth preparation, impression procedures,[21] and placement of restorative margins (Figure 71-6)[21] and to adjust gingival levels for esthetics.[32,43] It is important that crown-lengthening surgery is done in such a manner that the biologic width is preserved. The *biologic width* is defined as the physiologic dimension of the junctional epithelium and connective tissue attachment (see Chapter 72). This measurement has been found to be relatively constant at approximately 2 mm (±30%).[10] The healthy gingival sulcus has shown an average depth of 0.69 mm (Figure 71-7).[19] It has been theorized that infringement on the biologic width by the placement of a restoration within its zone may result in gingival inflammation,[19]

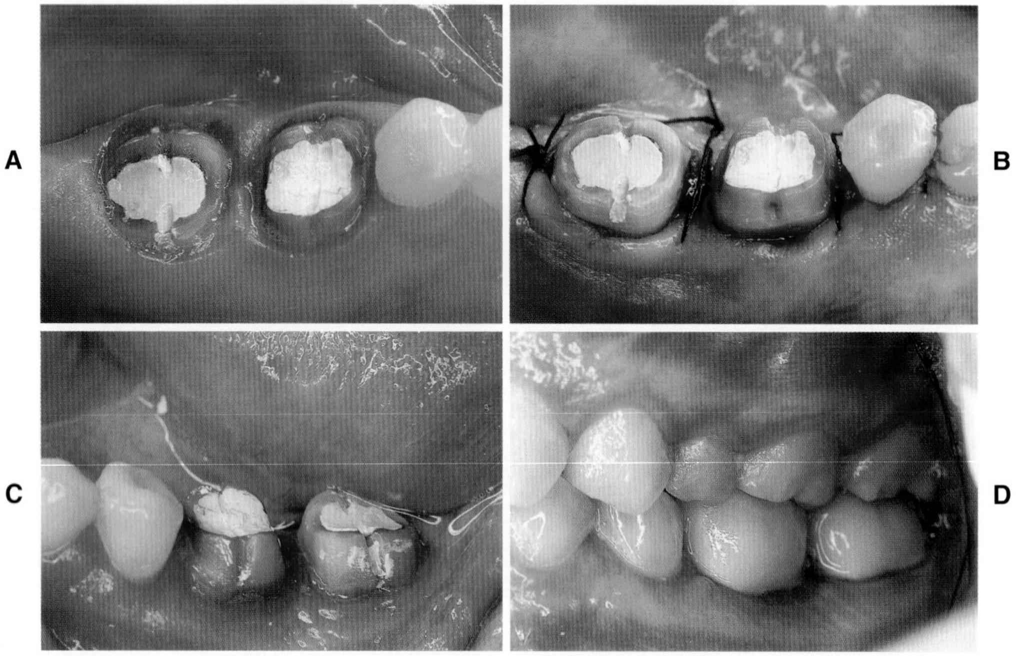

Figure 71-6 Surgical crown lengthening has provided these otherwise unrestorable mandibular molars with improved retention and restorative access for successful restorations. **A,** Before crown lengthening. **B,** Crown lengthening surgery completed. Note increased clinical crown. **C,** Buccal view after surgery. **D,** Final restorations.

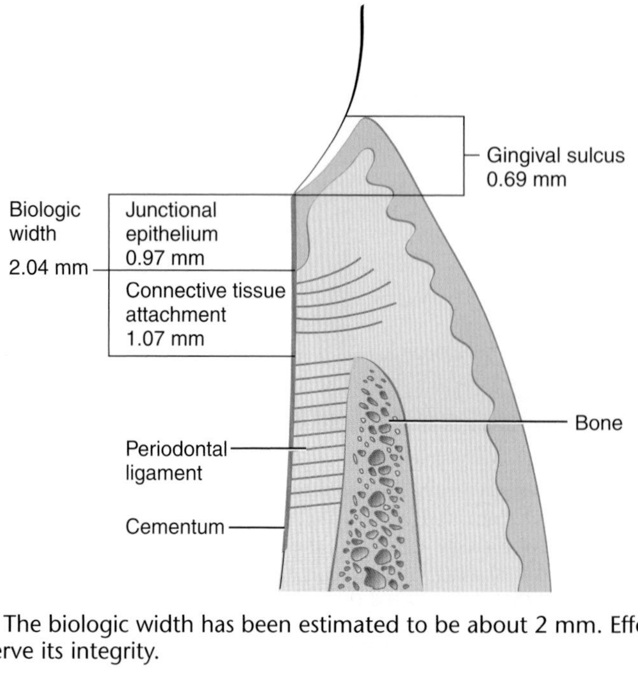

Figure 71-7 The biologic width has been estimated to be about 2 mm. Efforts should be made to preserve its integrity.

pocket formation, and alveolar bone loss[35] (Figure 71-8). Consequently, it is recommended that there be at least 3.0 mm between the gingival margin and bone crest.[12,38,39,41] This allows for adequate biologic width when the restoration is placed 0.5 mm within the gingival sulcus[39,41] (Figure 71-9).

Surgical crown lengthening may include the removal of soft tissue or both soft tissue and alveolar bone. Reduction of soft tissue alone is indicated if there is adequate attached gingiva and more than 3 mm of tissue coronal to the bone crest (Figure 71-10). This may be accomplished by either gingivectomy or flap technique (see Chapters 63-66). Inadequate attached gingiva and less than 3 mm of soft tissue require a flap procedure and bone recontouring (Figure 71-11). In the case of caries or tooth fracture, to ensure margin placement on sound tooth structure and retention form, the surgery should provide at least 4 mm from the apical extent of the caries or fracture to the bone crest (Figure 71-12).

With the advent of predictable implant dentistry, it is important to weigh carefully the value of crown lengthening for restorative ease as opposed to tooth removal and replacement with a dental implant (Box 71-2).

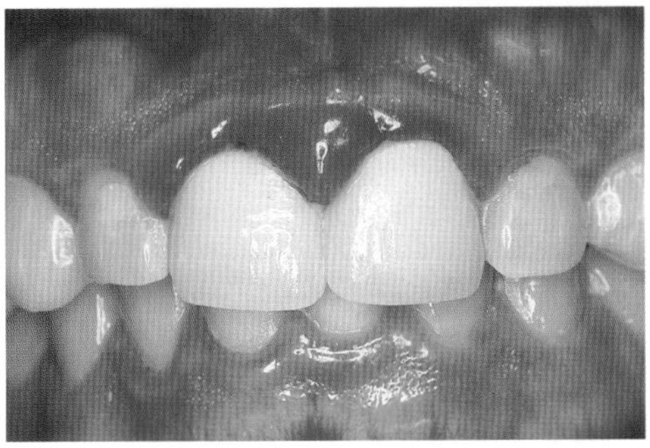

Figure 71-8 Although gingival inflammation around crowns may have a variety of causes, infringement of biologic width must be considered.

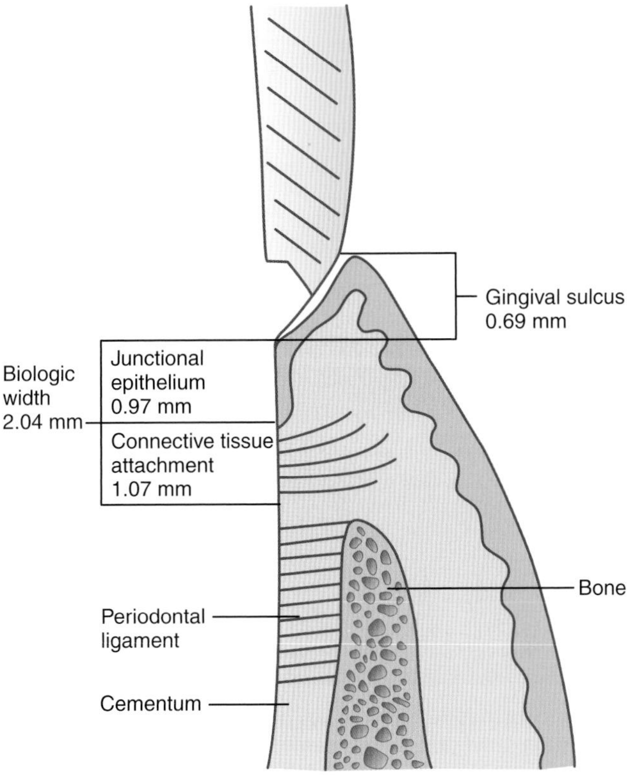

Figure 71-9 Placement of the restorative margin 0.5 mm into the sulcus allows for the maintenance of the biologic width.

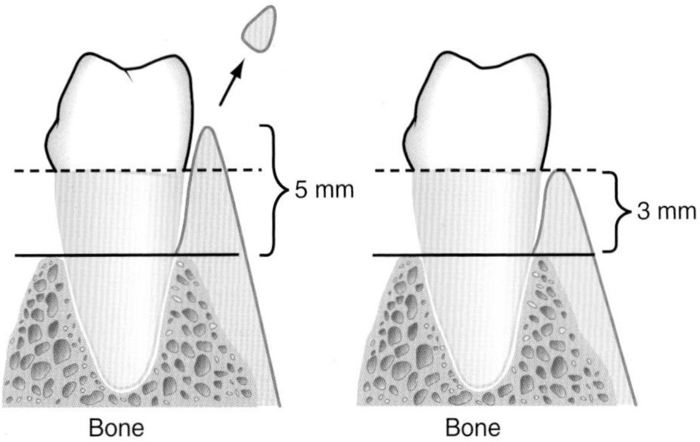

Figure 71-10 Greater than 3 mm of soft tissue between the bone and gingival margin, with adequate attached gingiva, allows crown lengthening by gingivectomy.

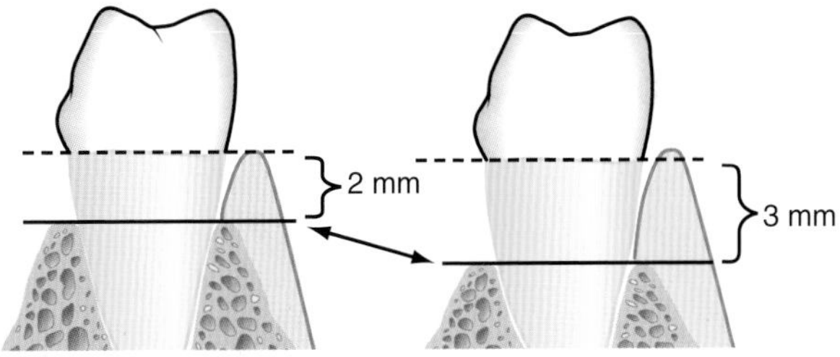

Figure 71-11 With less than 3 mm of soft tissue between the bone and gingival margin, or less-than-adequate attached gingiva, a flap procedure and osseous recontouring are required for crown lengthening.

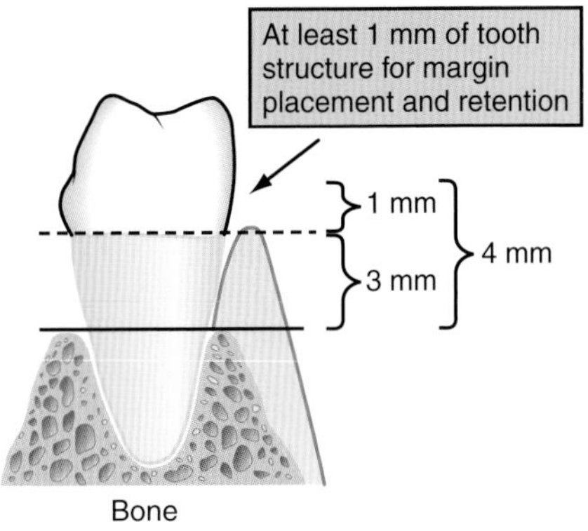

Figure 71-12 In the case of caries or fracture, at least 1 mm of sound tooth structure should be provided above the gingival margin for proper restoration.

BOX 71-2

Surgical Crown Lengthening

Indications	*Contraindications*
Subgingival caries or fracture	Surgery would create an unesthetic outcome.
Inadequate clinical crown length for retention	Deep caries or fracture would require excessive bone removal on contiguous teeth.
Unequal or unesthetic gingival heights	The tooth is a poor restorative risk.

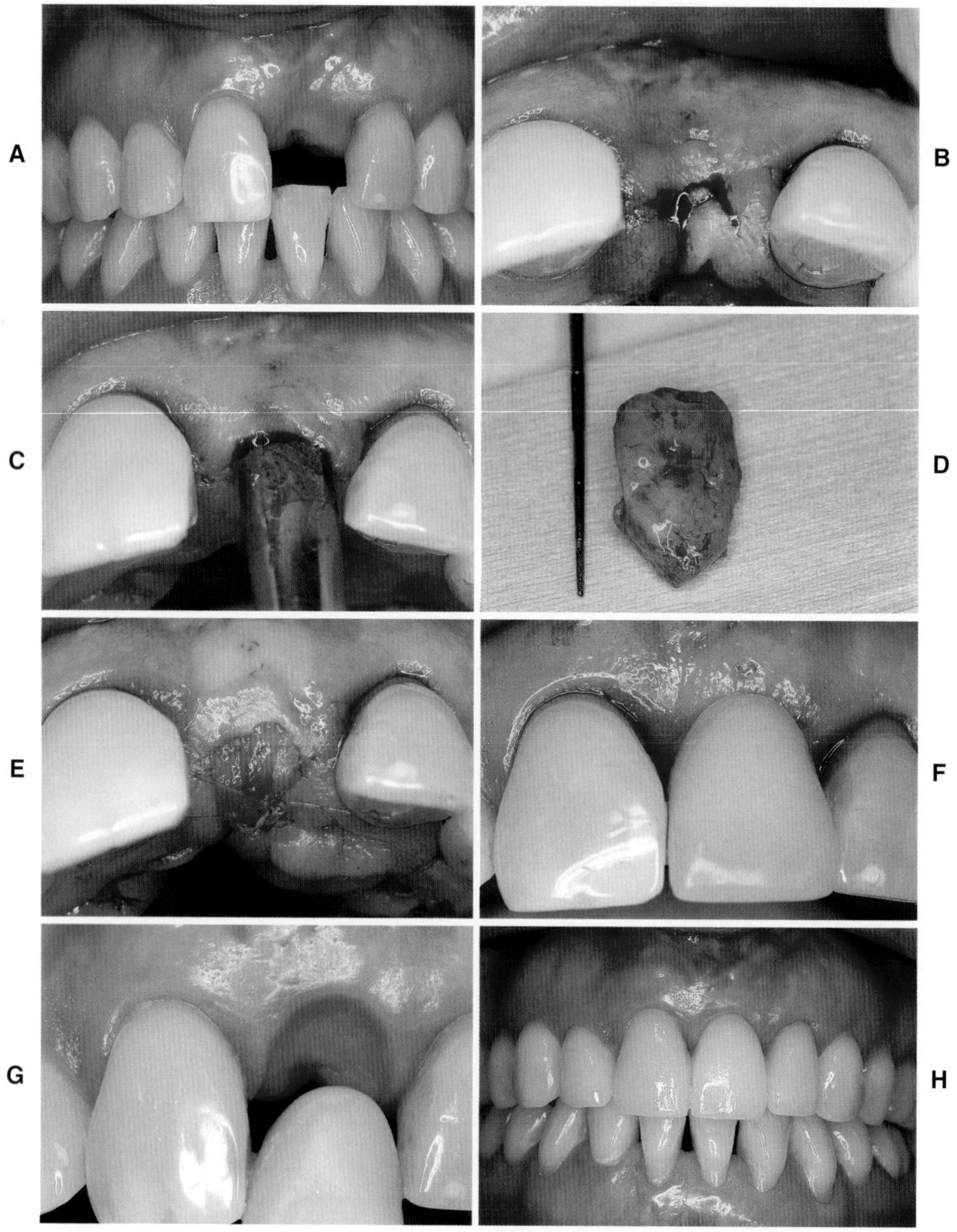

Figure 71-13 **A,** Loss of the maxillary left central incisor has resulted in an unesthetic alveolar ridge defect. **B** to **E,** An incision is made at ridge crest, a pouch is created, and a soft tissue graft harvested from the palate is placed into the pouch. **F** to **H,** A removable appliance with an ovate pontic is placed in light contact with the grafted site. Swelling around the pontic apex results in a tissue concavity from which the more natural-appearing final restoration emerges.

Alveolar Ridge Reconstruction

Patients are frequently seen after tooth loss and alveolar ridge resorption have occurred (see Chapter 77). To provide for adequate anatomic dimensions for the construction of an esthetic pontic (see Chapter 72) or the placement of dental implants (see Chapter 76), alveolar ridge reconstruction is undertaken. In the case of esthetic pontic construction, small defects may be treated with soft tissue ridge augmentation (Figure 71-13). For larger defects and in those sites receiving dental implants, hard tissue modalities are used (Figure 71-14).

CONCLUSION

As described in this and other sections of this textbook, the therapeutic goals of patient comfort, function,

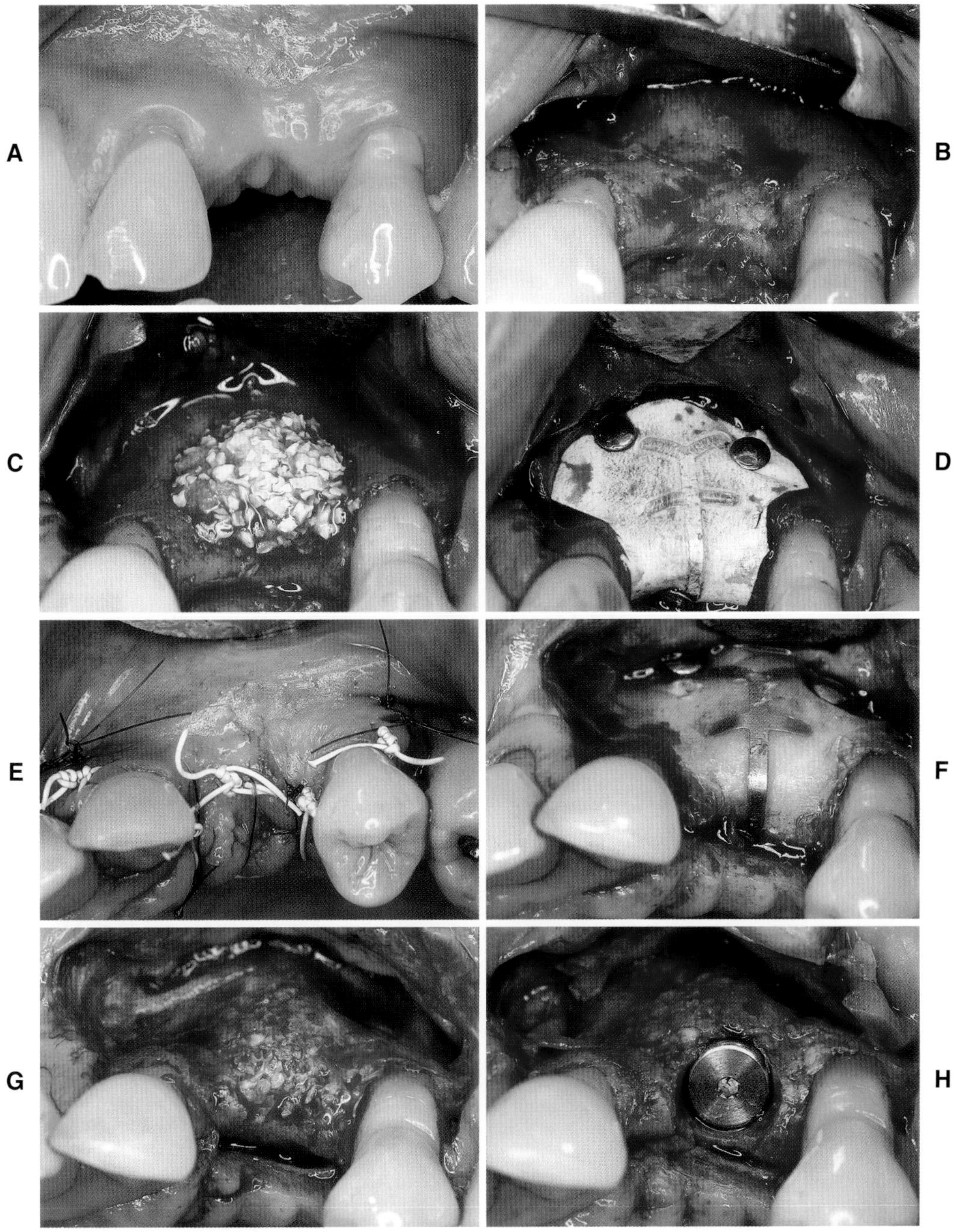

Figure 71-14 Postextraction ridge defect is grafted with a combination of autogenous and deproteinized bovine bone and contained by nonresorbable barrier membrane. After 8 months the site is reopened and the membrane removed. A comparison of *B* and *G* shows significant reconstitution of hard tissue, in this case used for the installation of a dental implant. **A,** Edentulous ridge before surgery. **B,** Flap reflection to visualize defect. **C,** Graft material placed over resorbed ridge. **D,** Nonresorbable titanium-reinforced membrane placed over graft material. **E,** Graft site sutured. **F,** Surgical site reopened 8 months after surgery. **G,** New bone over ridge. **H,** Implant placed into augmented ridge.

esthetics, predictability, longevity, and ease of restorative and maintenance care are attainable only by a carefully constructed interdisciplinary approach, with accurate diagnosis and comprehensive treatment planning serving as cornerstones. The complex interaction between periodontal therapy and successful restorative dentistry only serves to underscore this premise.

REFERENCES

1. Abrams H, Kopczyk RA, Kaplan AL: Incidence of anterior ridge deformities in partially edentulous patients, *J Prosthet Dent* 57:191, 1987.
2. Amler MH, Johnson PL, Salman I: Histological and histochemical investigation of human alveolar socket healing in undisturbed extraction wounds, *J Am Dent Assoc* 61:32, 1960.
3. Axelsson P, Lindhe J: Effect of controlled oral hygiene procedures on caries and periodontal disease in adults, *J Clin Periodontol* 5:133, 1978.
4. Axelsson P, Lindhe J: The significance of maintenance care in the treatment of periodontal disease, *J Clin Periodontol* 8:281, 1981.
5. Badersten A, Nilvens R, Egelberg J: Effect of nonsurgical periodontal therapy. II. Severely advanced periodontitis, *J Clin Periodontol* 11:63, 1984.
6. Brown SI: The effect of orthodontic therapy on certain types of periodontal defects. I. Clinical findings, *J Periodontol* 44:742, 1973.
7. Claffey N, Egelberg J: Clinical indicators of probing attachment loss following initial periodontal treatment in advanced periodontitis patients, *J Clin Periodontol* 22:690, 1995.
8. Ericsson I, Lindhe J: The effect of longstanding jiggling on experimental marginal periodontitis in the beagle dog, *J Clin Periodontol* 9:497, 1982.
9. Folio J, Rams TE, Keyes PH: Orthodontic therapy in patients with juvenile periodontitis: clinical and microbiological effects, *Am J Orthodont* 87:421, 1985.
10. Gargiulo AW: Dimensions and relations of the dentogingival junction in humans, *J Periodontol* 32:261, 1961.
11. Garret S: Periodontal regeneration around natural teeth, *Ann Periodontol* 1:621, 1996.
12. Herrero F, Scott JB, Maropis PS, Yukna RA: Clinical comparison of desired versus actual amount of surgical crown lengthening, *J Periodontol* 66:568, 1995.
13. Highfield JE, Powell RN: Effects of removal of posterior overhanging metallic margins of restoration upon the periodontal tissues, *J Clin Periodontol* 5:169, 1978.
14. Hirschfeld L, Wasserman B: A long-term survey of tooth loss in 600 treated periodontal patients, *J Periodontol* 5:225, 1978.
15. Iasella JM, Greenwell H, Miller RL, et al: Ridge preservation with freeze-dried bone allograft and a collagen membrane compared to extraction alone for implant site development: a clinical and histologic study in humans, *J Periodontol* 74:990, 2003.
16. Ingber JS: Forced eruption. Part I. A method of treating isolated one and two wall infrabony osseous defects: rationale and case report, *J Periodontol* 45:199, 1974.
17. Ingber JS: Forced eruption. Part II. A method of treating nonrestorable teeth: periodontal and restorative considerations, *J Periodontol* 47:203, 1976.
18. Jeffcoat MK, Howell TH: Alveolar bone destruction due to overhanging amalgam in periodontal disease, *J Periodontol* 51:599, 1980.
19. Kois JC: "The gingiva is red around my crowns," *Dent Economics,* April 1993, p 100.
20. Kois JC: The restorative-periodontal interface: biological parameters, *Periodontol 2000* 11:29, 1996.
21. Kois JC: Clinical techniques in prosthodontics: relationship of the periodontium to impression procedures, *Compend Contin Educ Dent* 21:684, 2000.
22. Kokich VG: Esthetics: the orthodontic-periodontic restorative connection, *Semin Orthodont* 2:21, 1996.
23. Kramer JM, Nevins M: *Int J Periodont Restor Dent* 1:4, 1981 (editorial).
24. Lekovic V, Camargo PM, Klokkevold PR, et al: Alterations of the position of the marginal soft tissue following periodontal surgery, *J Clin Periodontol* 7:525, 1980.
25. Lekovic V, Kenney EB, Weinlaender M, et al: A bone regenerative approach to alveolar ridge maintenance following tooth extraction: report of 10 cases, *J Periodontol* 68:563, 1997.
26. Lindhe J, Nyman S: Alterations of the position of the marginal soft tissue following periodontal surgery, *J Clin Periodontol* 7:525, 1980.
27. Lindhe J, Westfelt E, Nyman S, et al: Healing following surgical/non-surgical treatment of periodontal disease: a clinical study, *J Clin Periodontol* 9:115, 1982.
28. Listgarten MA, Lindhe J, Hellden L: Effect of tetracycline and/or scaling on human periodontal disease: clinical, microbiological and histological observations, *J Clin Periodontol* 5:246, 1978.
29. Lövdal A, Arno A, Schei O, Waerhaug J: Combined effect of subgingival scaling and controlled oral hygiene on the incidence of gingivitis, *Acta Odontol Scand* 19:537, 1961.
30. Machtei E, Zubrey YI, Ben Yahuda A, Soskolne W: Proximal bone loss adjacent to periodontally "hopeless" teeth with and without extraction, *J Periodontol* 60:512, 1989.
31. Melnick PR, Camargo PM: Preservation of alveolar ridge dimensions and interproximal papillae through periodontal procedures: long-term results, *Contemp Esthet Restor Pract,* November 2004, p 2.
32. Minsk L: Clinical techniques in periodontics: esthetic crown lengthening, *Compend Contin Educ Dent* 22:562, 2001.
33. Nedic M: Preservation of alveolar bone in extraction sockets using bioabsorbable membranes, *J Periodontol* 69:1044, 1998.
34. Palcanis KG: Surgical pocket therapy, *Ann Periodontol* 1:589, 1996.
35. Parma-Benfenati S, Fugazzotto PA, Ruben MP: The effect of restorative margins on the postsurgical development and nature of the periodontium. Part I, *Int J Periodont Restor Dent* 6:31, 1985.
36. Polson AM, Reed BE: Long-term effects of orthodontic treatment on crestal bone levels, *J Periodontol* 55:28, 1984.
37. Polson AM, Caton J, Polson A, et al: Periodontal response to tooth movement into intrabony defects, *J Periodontol* 55:197, 1984.
38. Pontoriero R, Carnevale G: Surgical crown lengthening: a 12-month clinical wound healing study, *J Periodontol* 72:841, 2001.
39. Rosenberg ES, Cho SC, Garber DA: Crown lengthening revisited, *Compend Contin Educ Dent* 20:527, 1999.
40. Sato S, Ujiie H, Ito K: Spontaneous correction of pathologic tooth migration and reduced infrabony pockets following nonsurgical periodontal therapy: a case report, *Int J Periodont Restor Dent* 24:456, 2004.
41. Smukler H, Chaibi M: Periodontal and dental considerations in clinical crown extension: a rational basis for treatment, *Int J Periodont Restor Dent* 17:465, 1997.
42. Stambaugh RV, Dragoo M, Smith DM, Carasali L: The limits of subgingival scaling, *Int J Periodont Restor Dent* 1:31, 1981.
43. Studer S, Zellweger U, Schärer P: The aesthetic guidelines of the mucogingival complex for fixed prosthodontics, *Pract Periodontics Aesthetic Dent* 4:333, 1996.

44. Tagge DL, O'Leary TJ, El-Kafrawy AH: The clinical and histological response of periodontal pockets to root planing and oral hygiene, *J Periodontol* 46:527, 1975.
45. Takei HH, Azzi RR, Han TJ: Preparation of the periodontium for restorative dentistry. In Newman MG, Takei HH, Carranza FA, editors: *Carranza's clinical periodontology,* ed 9, Philadelphia, 2002, Saunders.
46. Waerhaug J: The furcation problem: etiology, pathogenesis, diagnosis, therapy and prognosis, *J Clin Periodontol* 7:73, 1980.
47. Wennström JL: Mucogingival therapy. In Proceedings of the World Workshop on Periodontics, *Ann Periodontol* 1:671, 1996.

Restorative Interrelationships

Frank M. Spear and Joseph P. Cooney

72

CHAPTER

CHAPTER OUTLINE

The relationship between periodontal health and the restoration of teeth is intimate and inseparable. For restorations to survive long term, the periodontium must remain healthy so that the teeth are maintained. For the periodontium to remain healthy, restorations must be critically managed in several areas so that they are in harmony with their surrounding periodontal tissues. To maintain or enhance the patient's esthetic appearance, the tooth/tissue interface must present a healthy natural appearance, with gingival tissues framing the restored teeth in a harmonious manner. This chapter reviews the key areas of restorative management necessary to optimize periodontal health, with a focus on the esthetics and function of restorations.

BIOLOGIC CONSIDERATIONS

Margin Placement and Biologic Width

Restorative clinicians must understand the role of biologic width in preserving healthy gingival tissues and controlling the gingival form around restorations. They must also apply this information in the positioning of restoration margins, especially in the esthetic zone, where a primary treatment goal is to mask the junction of the margin with the tooth.

A clinician is presented with three options for margin placement: supragingival, equigingival (even with the tissue), and subgingival.[70] The *supragingival margin* will have the least impact on the periodontium. Classically, this margin location has been applied in unesthetic areas because of the marked contrast in color and opacity of traditional restorative materials against the tooth. With the advent of more translucent restorative materials, adhesive dentistry, and resin cements, the ability to place supragingival margins in esthetic areas is now a reality (Figures 72-1 and 72-2). Therefore, whenever possible, these restorations should be chosen, not only for their esthetic advantages, but for their favorable periodontal impact as well.

The use of *equigingival margins* traditionally was not desirable because they were thought to retain more plaque

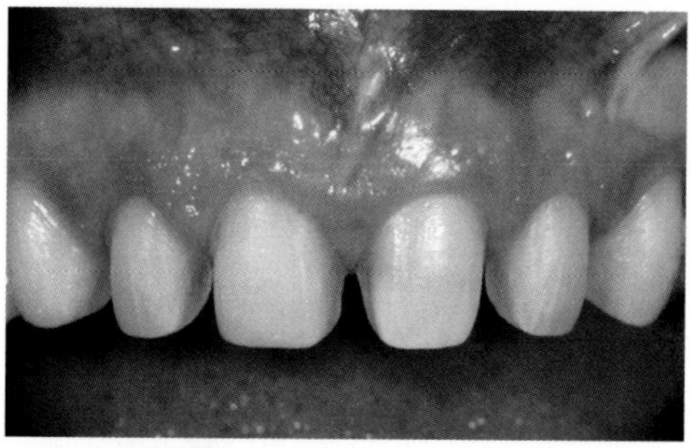

Figure 72-1 With the advent of adhesive dentistry and ultrathin ceramic veneers, it now is possible to prepare restorations *equigingival* without visible margins. The preparations for six porcelain veneers with the margins placed at the level of tissue are shown.

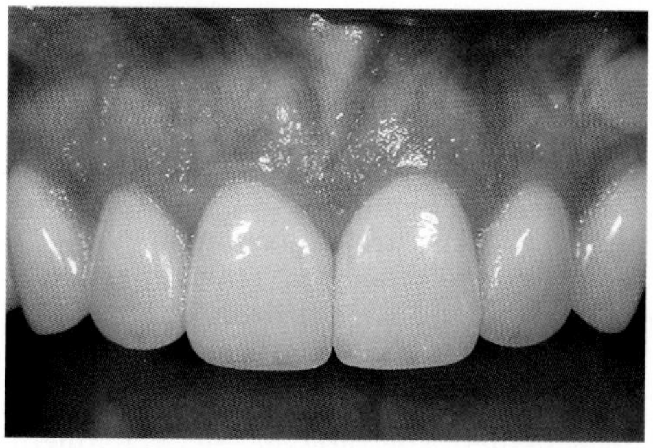

Figure 72-2 The completed veneers from Figure 72-1. Note the invisible gingival finish line, even though the margin has not been carried below tissue.

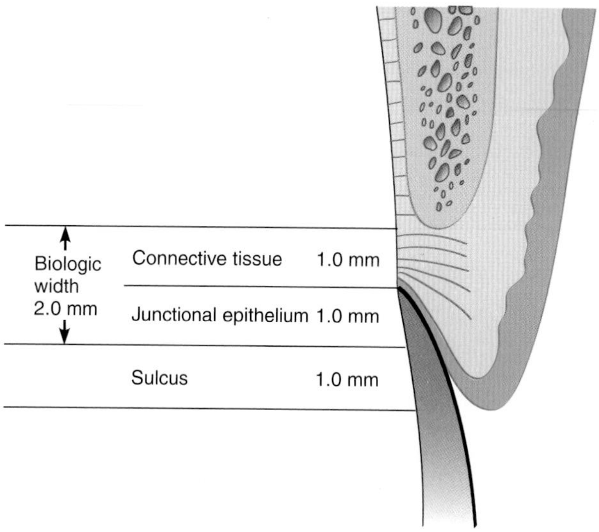

Figure 72-3 Average human biologic width: Connective tissue attachment 1 mm in height; junctional epithelial attachment 1 mm in height; sulcus depth of approximately 1 mm. The combined connective tissue attachment and junctional epithelial attachment, or biologic width, equals 2 mm.

than supragingival or subgingival margins and therefore result in greater gingival inflammation. There was also the concern that any minor gingival recession would create an unsightly margin display. These concerns are not valid today, not only because the restoration margins can be esthetically blended with the tooth, but also because restorations can be finished easily to provide a smooth, polished interface at the gingival margin. From a periodontal viewpoint, both supragingival and equigingival margins are well tolerated.

The greatest biologic risk occurs when placing *subgingival margins*.[44] These margins are not as accessible as supragingival or equigingival margins for finishing procedures. In addition, if the margin is placed too far below the gingival tissue crest, it will violate the gingival attachment apparatus.

The dimension of space that the healthy gingival tissues occupy above the alveolar bone is now identified as the *biologic width*. Most authors credit Gargiulo, Wentz, and Orban's study in 1961 on cadavers with the initial research establishing the dimensions of space required by the gingival tissues.[19] They found that, in the average human, the connective tissue attachment occupies 1.07 mm of space above the crest of the alveolar bone, and that the junctional epithelial attachment below the base of the gingival sulcus occupies another 0.97 mm of space above the connective tissue attachment. The combination of these two measurements constitutes the biologic width (Figure 72-3). Clinically, this information is applied to diagnose biologic width violations when the restoration margin is placed 2 mm or less away from the alveolar bone and the gingival tissues are inflamed with no other etiologic factors evident.

Restorative considerations will frequently dictate the placement of restoration margins beneath the gingival tissue crest. Restorations may need to be extended gingivally (1) to create adequate resistance and retentive form in the preparation, (2) to make significant contour alterations because of caries or other tooth deficiencies, or (3) to mask the tooth/restoration interface by locating it subgingivally. When the restoration margin is placed too far below the gingival tissue crest, it will impinge on the gingival attachment apparatus and create a violation of biologic width.[50] Two different responses can be observed from the involved gingival tissues (Figure 72-4).

One possibility is that bone loss of an unpredictable nature along with gingival tissue recession will occur as the body attempts to recreate room between the alveolar bone and the margin to allow space for tissue reattachment. This is more likely to occur in areas where the alveolar bone surrounding the tooth is very thin in width. Trauma from restorative procedures can play a major role in causing this fragile tissue to recede. Other factors that may impact the likelihood of recession include (1) whether the gingiva is thick and fibrotic or thin and fragile and (2) whether the periodontium is highly scalloped or flat in its gingival form. It has been found that highly scalloped, thin gingiva is more prone to recession than a flat periodontium with thick fibrous tissue.[48]

The more common finding with deep margin placement is that the bone level appears to remain unchanged, but gingival inflammation develops and persists. To

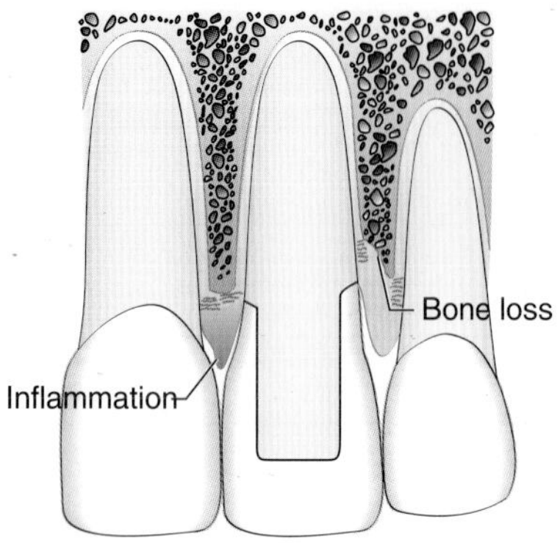

Figure 72-4 Ramifications of a biologic width violation if a restorative margin is placed within the zone of the attachment. On the mesial surface of the left central incisor, bone has not been lost, but gingival inflammation occurs. On the distal surface of the left central incisor, bone loss has occurred, and a normal biologic width has been reestablished.

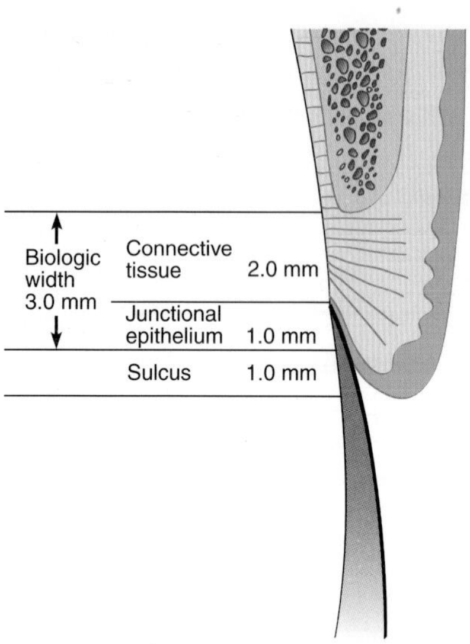

Figure 72-5 Possible variations exist in biologic width. Connective tissue attachments and junctional epithelial attachments may be variable. In this example the connective tissue attachment is 2 mm in height, the junctional epithelial attachment 1 mm in height, and the sulcus depth 1 mm, for a combined total tissue height above bone of 4 mm. However, the biologic width is 3 mm. This is just one variation that can occur from the average depicted in Figure 72-3.

restore gingival tissue health, it is necessary to establish space clinically between the alveolar bone and the margin. This can be accomplished either by surgery to alter the bone level or by orthodontic extrusion to move the restoration margin farther away from the bone level.

Biologic Width Evaluation

Radiographic interpretation can identify interproximal violations of biologic width. However, with the more common locations on the mesiofacial and distofacial line angles of teeth, radiographs are not diagnostic because of tooth superimposition. If a patient experiences tissue discomfort when the restoration margin levels are being assessed with a periodontal probe, it is a good indication that the margin extends into the attachment and that a biologic width violation has occurred.

A more positive assessment can be made clinically by measuring the distance between the bone and the restoration margin using a sterile periodontal probe. The probe is pushed through the anesthetized attachment tissues from the sulcus to the underlying bone. If this distance is less than 2 mm at one or more locations, a diagnosis of biologic width violation can be confirmed. This assessment is completed circumferentially around the tooth to evaluate the extent of the problem. However, biologic width violations can occur in some patients where the margins are located more than 2 mm above the alveolar bone level.[23] In 1994, Vacek et al.[71] also investigated the biologic width phenomenon. Although their average width finding of 2 mm was the same as that previously presented by Gargiulo et al.,[19] they also reported a range of different biologic widths that were patient specific. They reported biologic widths as narrow as 0.75 mm in some individuals, whereas others had biologic widths as tall as 4.3 mm (Figure 72-5).

This information dictates that specific biologic width assessment should be performed for each patient to determine if the patient needs additional biologic width, in excess of 2 mm, for restorations to be in harmony with the gingival tissues. The biologic, or attachment, width can be identified for the individual patient by probing to the bone level (referred to as "sounding to bone") and subtracting the sulcus depth from the resulting measurement. This measurement must be done on teeth with healthy gingival tissues and should be repeated on more than one tooth to ensure an accurate assessment. The technique allows the variations in sulcus depths found in individual patients to be assessed and factored into the diagnostic evaluation. The information obtained is then used for definitive diagnosis of biologic width violations, the extent of correction needed, and the parameters for placement of future restorations.

Correcting Biologic Width Violations

Biologic width violations can be corrected either by surgically removing bone away from proximity to the restoration margin or by orthodontically extruding the tooth and thus moving the margin away from the bone. Surgery is the more rapid of the two treatment options.[58] It is also preferred if the resulting crown lengthening will create a more pleasing tooth length. In these situations the bone should be moved away from the margin by the measured distance of the ideal biologic width for that patient, with an additional 0.5 mm of bone removed as a safety zone.

There is a potential risk of gingival recession after removal of bone.[7] If interproximal bone is removed, there is a high likelihood of papillary recession and the creation of an unesthetic triangle of space below the interproximal contacts. If the biologic width violation is on the interproximal side, or if the violation is across the facial surface and the gingival tissue level is correct,

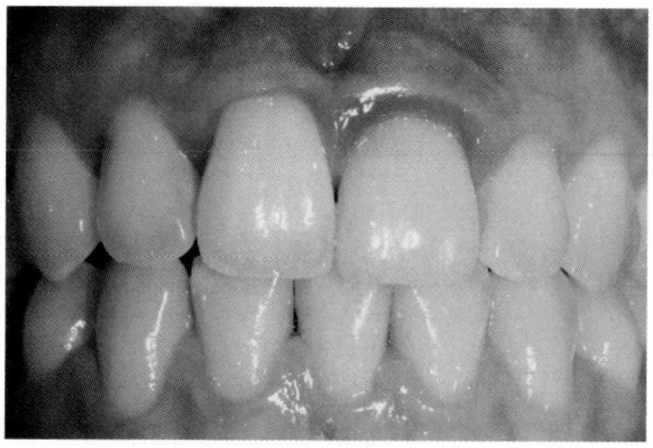

Figure 72-6 The left central incisor was fractured in an accident 12 months ago and restored at that time. The patient is unhappy with the appearance of the tissue surrounding the restoration. (See Figures 72-7, 72-8, and 72-9.)

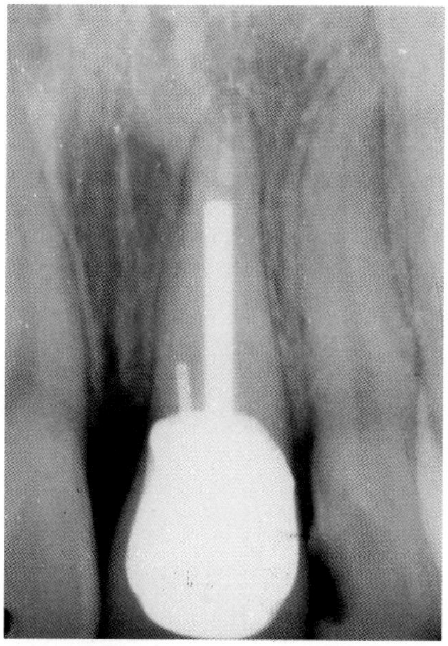

Figure 72-7 Radiograph reveals a biologic width violation on the mesial surface interproximally. Removal of interproximal bone would create an esthetic deformity. This patient is better treated with orthodontic extrusion. (See Figures 72-6 and 72-8.)

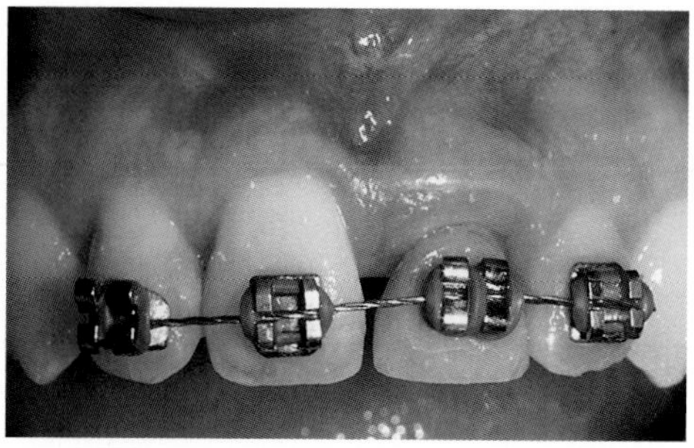

Figure 72-8 After orthodontic eruption. The tooth has been erupted 3 mm to move the bone and gingiva coronally 3 mm on the left central incisor. It is now possible to reposition the bone surgically to the correct level and position the gingiva to the correct level, reestablishing normal biologic width.

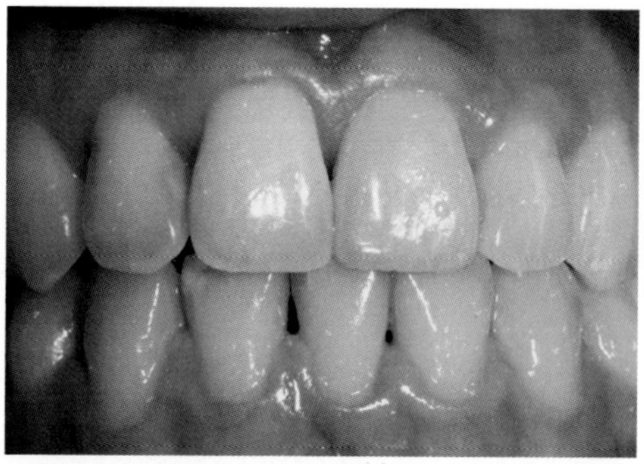

Figure 72-9 One-year recall photograph after orthodontic extrusion, osseous surgery, and placement of a new restoration for patient in Figure 72-6. Note the excellent tissue health after the reestablishment of biologic width.

orthodontic extrusion is indicated[28] (Figures 72-6 to 72-9). The extrusion can be performed in two ways. By applying low orthodontic extrusion force, the tooth will be erupted slowly, bringing the alveolar bone and gingival tissue with it. The tooth is extruded until the bone level has been carried coronal to the ideal level by the amount that will need to be removed surgically to correct the attachment violation. The tooth is stabilized in this new position and then is treated with surgery to correct the bone and gingival tissue levels. Another option is to perform rapid orthodontic extrusion where the tooth is erupted to the desired amount over several weeks.[32] During this period, a supercrestal fiberotomy is performed weekly in an effort to prevent the tissue and bone from following the tooth. The tooth is then stabilized for at least 12 weeks to confirm the position of the tissue and bone, and any coronal creep can be corrected surgically.

Margin Placement Guidelines

When determining where to place restorative margins relative to the periodontal attachment, it is recommended that the patient's existing sulcular depth be used as a guideline in assessing the biologic width requirement for that patient. The base of the sulcus can be viewed as the top of the attachment, and therefore the clinician accounts for variations in attachment height by ensuring that the margin is placed in the sulcus and not in the attachment.[4,37,38,57] The variations in sulcular probing depth are then used to predict how deep the margin can safely be placed below the gingival crest. With shallow probing depths (1.0-1.5 mm), extending the preparation more than 0.5 mm subgingivally will risk violating the attachment. This assumes that the periodontal probe will penetrate into the junctional epithelial attachment in healthy gingiva an average of 0.5 mm. With shallow probing depths, future recession is unlikely because the free gingival margin is located close to the top of the attachment. Deeper sulcular probing depths provide more freedom in locating restoration margins farther below the gingival crest. In most circumstances, however, the deeper the gingival sulcus, the greater is the risk of gingival recession.

The first step in using sulcus depth as a guide in margin placement is to manage gingival health. Once the tissue is healthy, the following three rules can be used to place intracrevicular margins:

Rule 1: If the sulcus probes 1.5 mm or less, place the restoration margin 0.5 mm below the gingival tissue crest. This is especially important on the facial aspect and will prevent a biologic width violation in a patient who is at high risk in that regard.

Rule 2: If the sulcus probes more than 1.5 mm, place the margin half the depth of the sulcus below the tissue crest. This places the margin far enough below tissue so that it will still be covered if the patient is at higher risk of recession.

Rule 3: If a sulcus greater than 2 mm is found, especially on the facial aspect of the tooth, evaluate to see if a gingivectomy could be performed to lengthen the teeth and create a 1.5-mm sulcus. Then the patient can be treated using Rule 1.

The rationale for Rule 3 is that deep margin placement is more difficult and the stability of the free gingival margin is less predictable when a deep sulcus exists. Reducing the sulcus depth will create a more predictable situation in which to place an intracrevicular margin. The clinician cannot be sure that the tissue will remain at the corrected level, however, because some gingival rebound can occur after gingevectomy. However, sulcular depth reduction ensures that the restorative margins will not be exposed and visible in the patient's mouth (Figures 72-10 to 72-14).

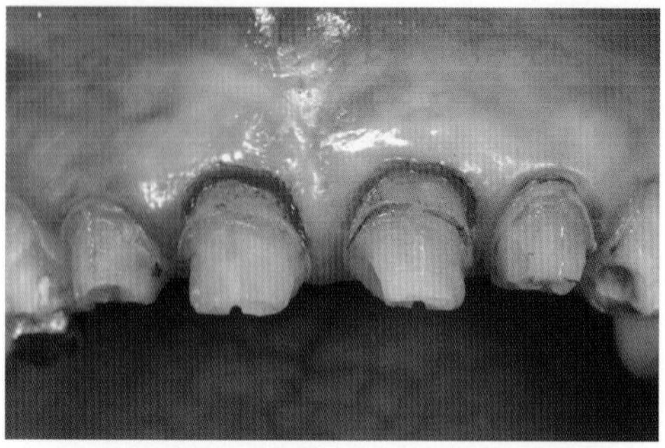

Figure 72-12 Two options were available to manage treatment appropriately: (1) place the original margins to half the depth of the sulcus, in which case the recession that occurred would not have exposed them, or (2) perform a gingivectomy, creating a 1-mm to 1.5-mm sulcus. The second option was chosen when the restorations were redone. The margins were then placed 0.5 mm below the tissue after the gingivectomy. (See Figures 72-11 and 72-13.)

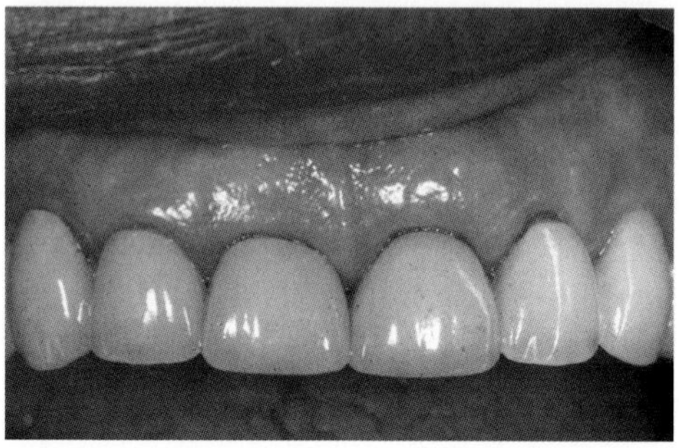

Figure 72-10 A 78-year-old woman presents with the maxillary anterior restorations placed 6 months earlier. She is unhappy with the exposed margins and notes that the margins were covered the day the restorations were placed. (See Figures 72-11 to 72-14.)

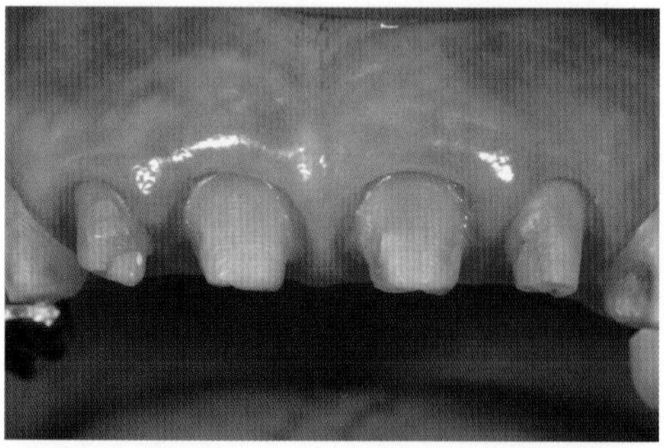

Figure 72-13 At 6 weeks after the gingivectomy and preparation of the teeth. Note the tissue level and that the tissue is rebounding coronally over the margins. This is a common finding when a pure gingivectomy is done.

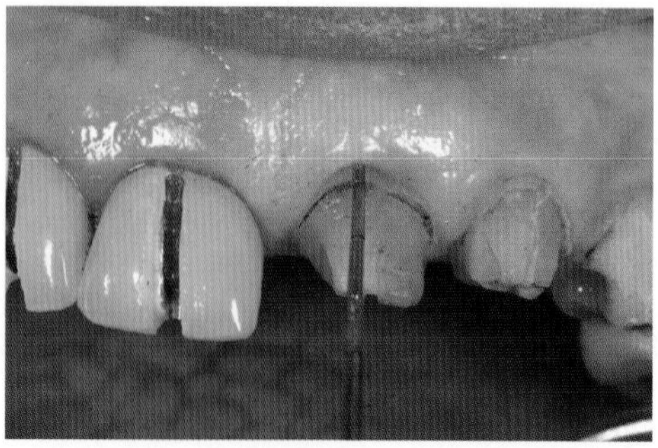

Figure 72-11 Depth from the attachment to the level of the preparation margin is greater than 3 mm. This patient in Figure 72-10 had an altered eruption pattern and a sulcus depth of more than 3 mm when these restorations were placed.

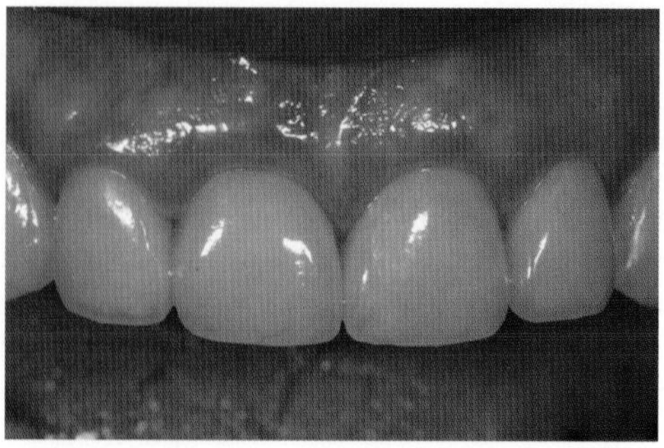

Figure 72-14 Four-year recall photograph after placement of the final restorations for patient in Figure 72-10. Note the tissue level has been maintained, with a sulcus depth of 2 mm on the facial surface.

Clinical Procedures in Margin Placement

The placement of supragingival or equigingival margins is simple because it requires no tissue manipulation. With regard to overall tooth preparation, the amount reduced incisally or occlusally, facially, lingually, and interproximally will be dictated by the choice of restorative materials. Before extending subgingivally, the preparation should be completed to the free gingival margin facially and interproximally. This allows the margin of the tooth preparation to be used as a reference for subgingival extension once the tissue is retracted (Figure 72-15).

Tissue Retraction

Once the supragingival portion of the preparation is completed, it is necessary to extend below the tissue.[6,24] The preparation margin must now be extended to the appropriate depth in the sulcus, applying the guidelines presented previously. In this process the tissue must be protected from abrasion, which will cause hemorrhage and can adversely affect the stability of the tissue level around the tooth. Access to the margin is also required for the final impression, with a clean, fluid-controlled environment. Tissue management is achieved with gingival retraction cords using the appropriate size to achieve the displacement required. Thin, fragile gingival tissues and shallow sulcus situations will usually dictate that smaller-diameter cords be chosen to achieve the desired tissue displacement.

For a Rule 1 margin, the cord should be placed so that the top of the cord will be located in the sulcus at the level where the final margin will be established, which will be 0.5 mm below the previously prepared margin (Figure 72-16). On the interproximal aspects of the tooth, the cord will usually be 1.0 to 1.5 mm below the tissue height, because the interproximal sulcus is often 2.5 to 3.0 mm in depth. With this initial cord in place, the preparation is extended to the top of the cord, with the bur angled to the tooth so that it will not abrade the tissue (Figure 72-17). This process protects the tissue, creates the correct axial reduction, and establishes the margin at the desired subgingival level. To create space and allow access for a final impression, it is now necessary to pack a second retraction cord. The second cord is pushed so that it displaces the first cord apically and sits between the margin and the tissue (Figure 72-18). For the final impression, only the top cord is removed, leaving the margins visible and accessible to be recorded with the impression material (Figure 72-19). The initial cord remains in place in the sulcus until the provisional restoration is completed.

As an alternative to additional retraction cords, electrosurgery can be used to remove any overlying tissue in the retraction process. A fine-wire electrode tip is held parallel to the tooth and against the margin in the sulcus and moved through the overhanging tissue, opening up the margin and the retraction cord to visual access (Figures 72-20 to 72-23). The electrosurgery tip sits on top of the retraction cord in place in the sulcus. This controls the vertical position of the tip and results in the removal of the least tissue needed for access.

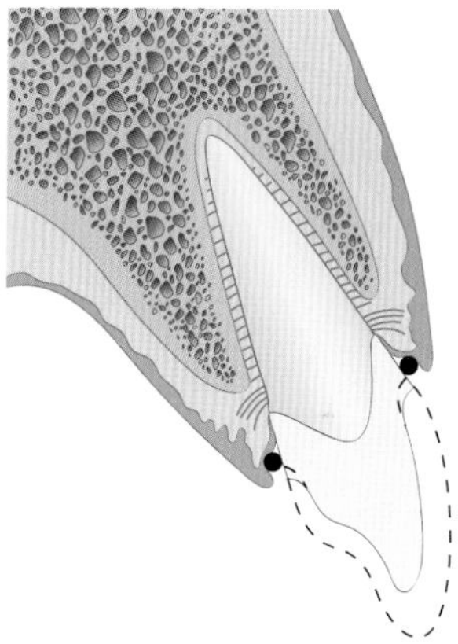

Figure 72-16 Second step in margin placement is to place a single layer of deflection cord below the previously prepared margin to the desired final margin level. Here, a single cord has been placed 0.5 mm below the previously prepared margin.

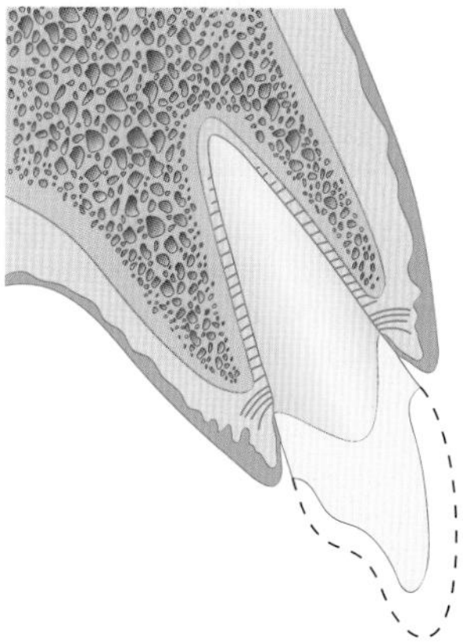

Figure 72-15 To provide a reference position for margin placement after tissue retraction, the margin of the tooth preparation is initially established level with the free gingival margin.

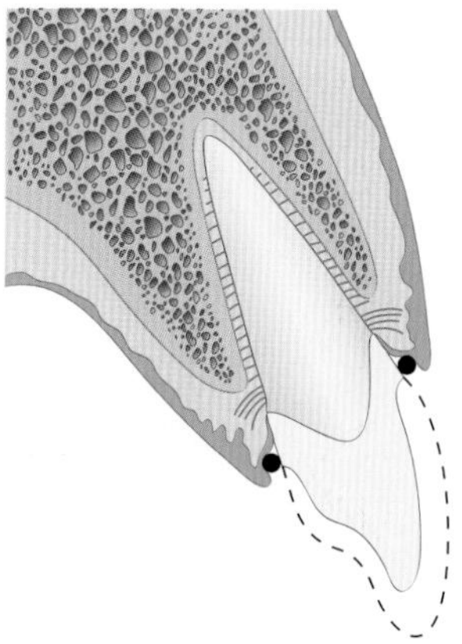

Figure 72-17 Margin of the preparation is now extended apically to the top of the retraction cord; this represents the correct placement of the margin below the previously nonreflected, free gingival margin.

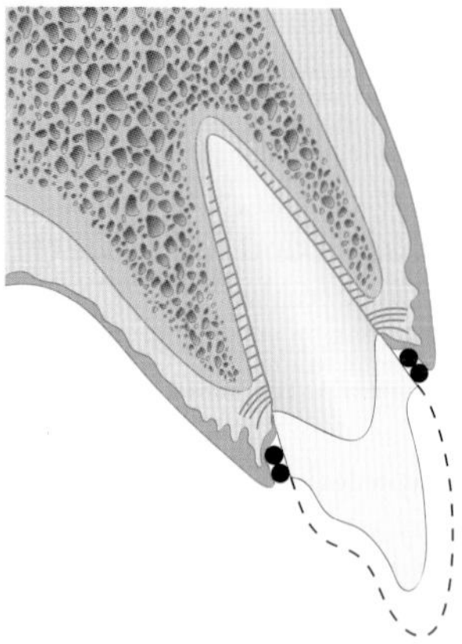

Figure 72-18 To provide space for impression material, a second impression cord is now placed on top of the first deflection cord. This impression cord is placed so that it is between the margin of the preparation and the gingiva to create adequate space for impression material after removal of the cord.

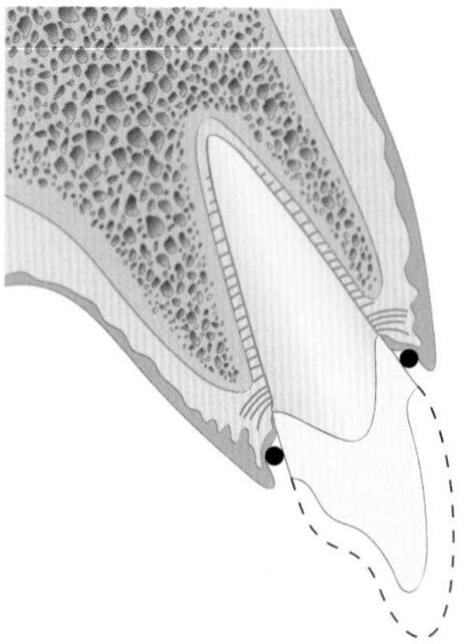

Figure 72-19 Ideal situation after removal of impression cord. The deflection cord is still in place maintaining the open sulcus but has been displaced apically another 0.5 mm by the placement of the impression cord, exposing tooth structure apical to the margin so that it can be captured in the impression.

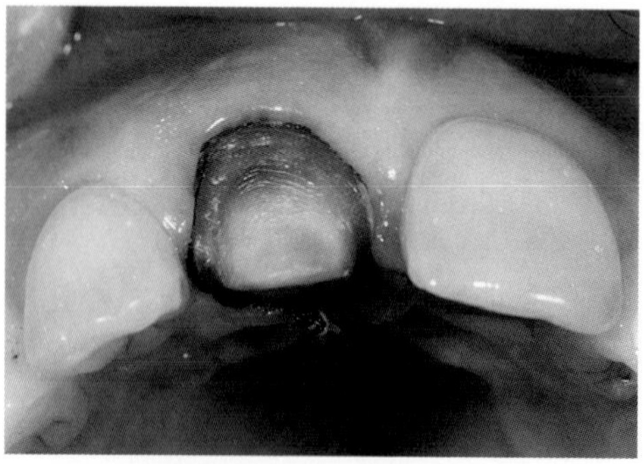

Figure 72-20 Deflection cord and impression cord are in place. The soft tissue is falling over the margins of the preparation. In this situation, if the impression cord were removed, the impression would not capture the margins in the areas where the tissue is overhanging.

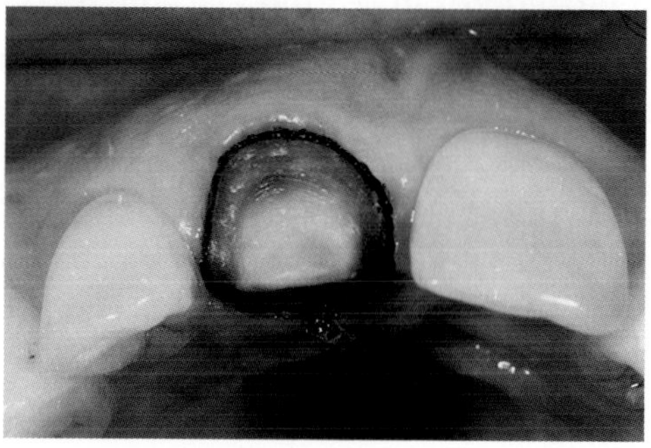

Figure 72-21 Overhanging tissue has been removed and space created for the impression material with electrosurgery. Note that the deflection cord and the impression cord are still in place. The impression cord is now visible completely around the tooth, allowing easy access for the impression material to the margin after removal of the impression cord.

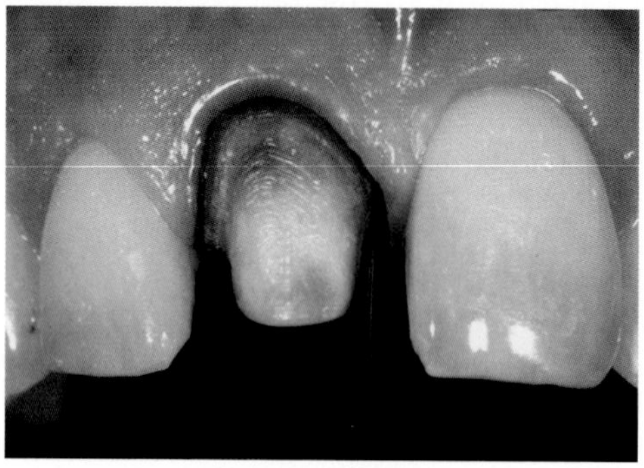

Figure 72-22 Using electrosurgery, the fine-wire electrode tip is held parallel to the tooth preparation and rests on the cord as the tip is moved around the tooth.

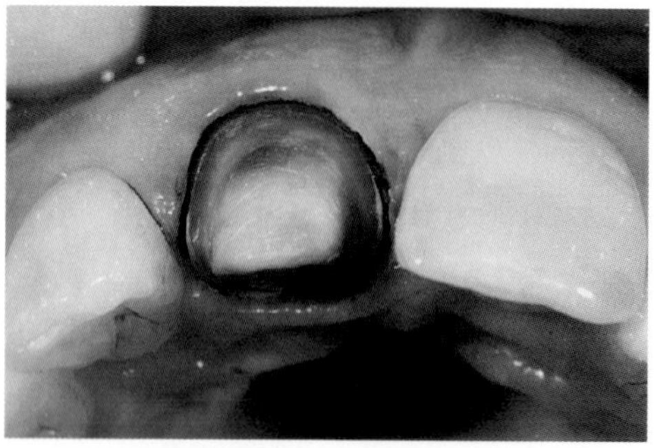

Figure 72-23 After removal of the impression cord, an adequate space is created for the impression material, with no soft tissue overhanging the margins to trap or tear the impression material. Note the first cord, or deflection cord, is still in place.

For Rule 2 situations where the sulcus is deeper, two larger-diameter cords are used to deflect the tissue before extending the margin apically (Figures 72-24 to 72-26). The top of the second cord is placed to identify the final margin location at the correct distance below the previously prepared margin, which was at the gingival

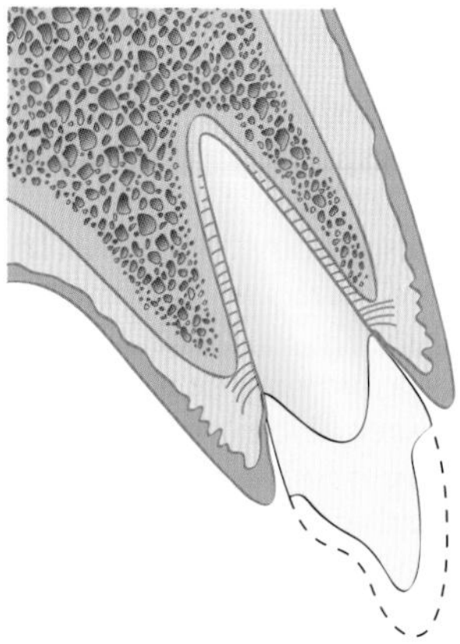

Figure 72-24 First step in margin placement for the patient with altered eruption or a deep sulcus is to prepare to the existing free gingival margin, as in the "Rule 1" patient (see text).

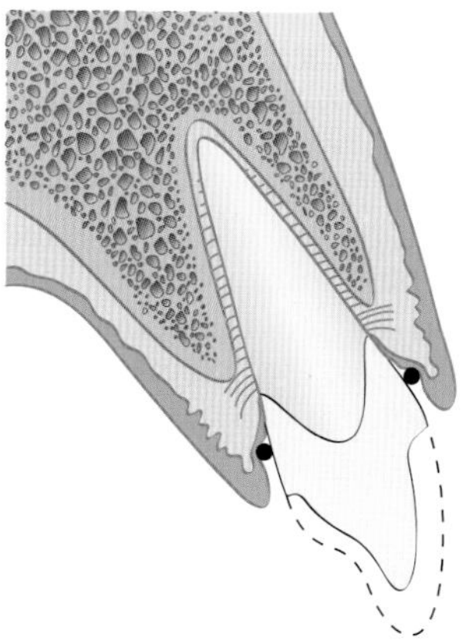

Figure 72-25 Second step for the patient with altered eruption is to place the deflection cord. Note that the placement of a single deflection cord does not provide adequate deflection of the tissue to allow the margin to be carried below tissue without abrading the gingiva with the bur.

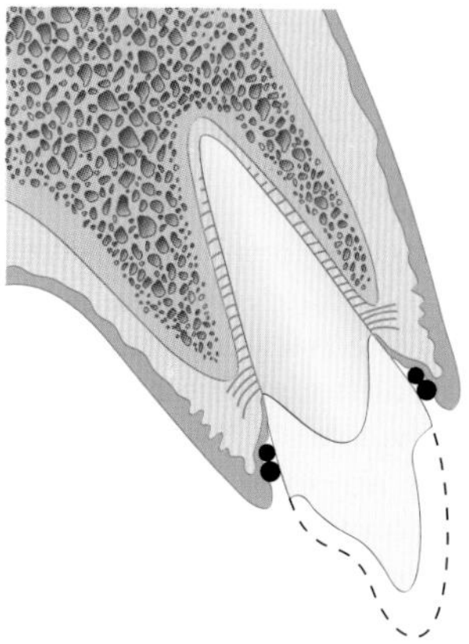

Figure 72-26 Third step for the patient with altered eruption and a deep sulcus is to place a second, larger-diameter deflection cord on top of the first deflection cord. Combined, these two cords allow adequate deflection to open up the sulcus so that the margin can be carried below tissue without abrading the gingiva.

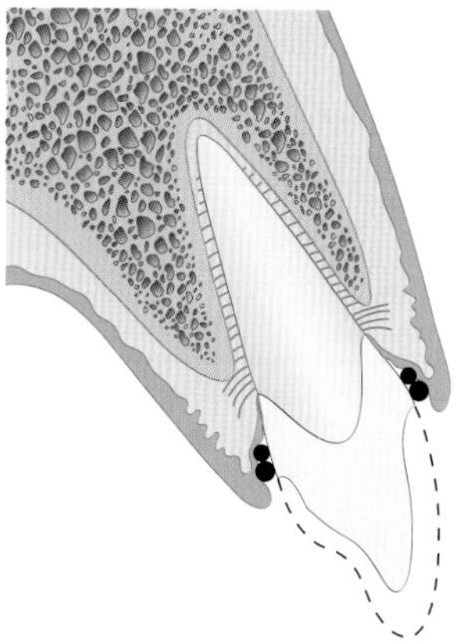

Figure 72-27 Preparation is now extended to the top of the second deflection cord, finalizing margin location.

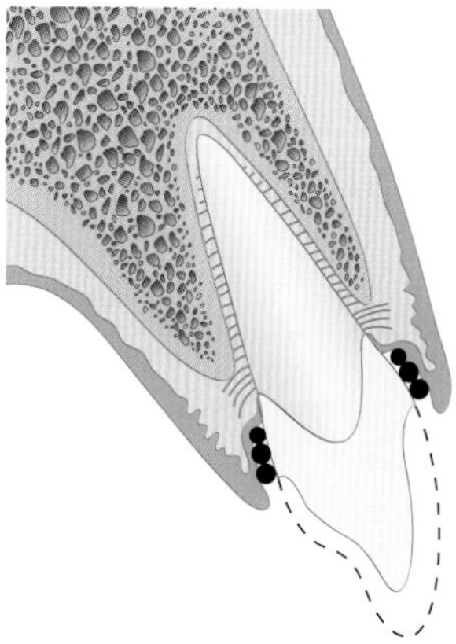

Figure 72-28 After extension of the margin to the top of the deflection cord, a third layer of cord is applied that will act as the impression cord. This impression cord should be placed so that it fits between the free gingival margin and the margin of the preparation. Its placement will also apically displace the two previously positioned deflection cords.

tissue crest level. The margin is lowered to the top of the second cord (Figure 72-27), then a third cord is placed in preparation for the impression (Figures 72-28 and 72-29). In the patient with a deep sulcus where the margin may be 1.5 to 2.0 mm below the tissue crest, electrosurgery is often required to remove overhanging tissue. To avoid altering the gingival tissue height, it is important to hold the electrosurgery tip parallel to the preparation (Figure 72-30).

Provisional Restorations

Three critical areas must be effectively managed to produce a favorable biologic response to provisional restorations.[3,75] The marginal fit, crown contour, and surface finish of the interim restorations must be appropriate to maintain the health and position of the gingival tissues during the interval until the final restorations are delivered. Provisional restorations that are poorly adapted at the margins, that are overcontoured or undercontoured,

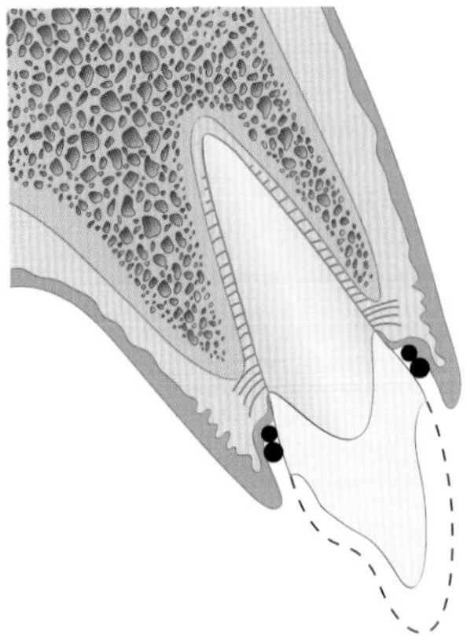

Figure 72-29 Removal of the impression cord creates an adequate space for the impression material to capture the margin and 0.5 mm of tooth structure below the margin where the impression cord had displaced the first two cords.

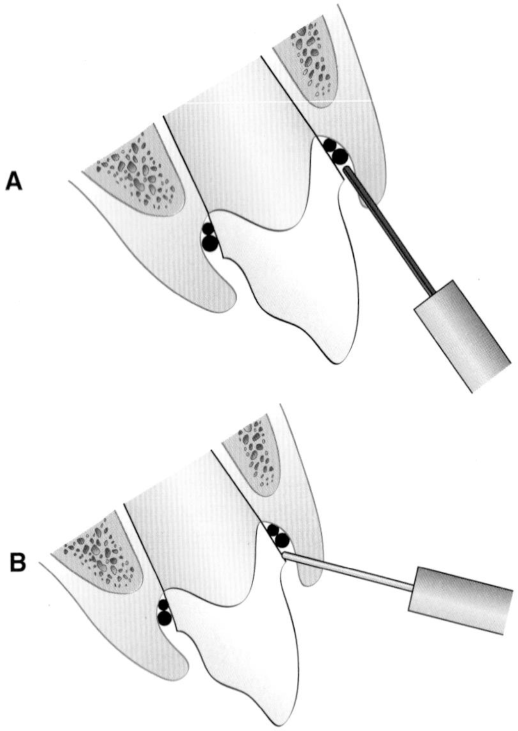

Figure 72-30 If it is necessary to use electrosurgery, either in the normal or altered-eruption patient, the correct inclination of the electrosurgery tip is important. **A,** Electrosurgery tip being held parallel to the preparation and resting on the previously placed retraction cord. This removes a minimal amount of tissue, and the presence of the retraction cord protects the attachment from the electrosurgery. **B,** Incorrect inclination of electrosurgery tip. The tip is leaning away from the preparation. This inclination results in excess tissue removal.

and that have rough or porous surfaces can cause inflammation, overgrowth, or recession of gingival tissues. The outcome can be unpredictable, and unfavorable changes in the tissue architecture can compromise the success of the final restoration.

Marginal Fit

Marginal fit has clearly been implicated in producing an inflammatory response in the periodontium. It has been shown that the level of gingival inflammation can increase corresponding with the level of marginal opening.[16] Margins that are significantly open (several tenths of a millimeter) are capable of harboring large numbers of bacteria and may be responsible for the inflammatory response seen. However, the quality of marginal finish and the margin location relative to the attachment are much more critical to the periodontium than the difference between a 20-μm fit and a 100-μm fit.[43,47,60]

Crown Contour

Restoration contour has been described as extremely important to the maintenance of periodontal health.[27,76] Ideal contour provides access for hygiene, has the fullness to create the desired gingival form, and has a pleasing visual tooth contour in esthetic areas. Evidence from human and animal studies clearly demonstrates a relationship between overcontouring and gingival inflammation, whereas undercontouring produces no adverse periodontal effect.[49,52] The most frequent cause of overcontoured restorations is inadequate tooth preparation by the dentist, which forces the technician to produce a bulky restoration to provide room for the restorative material. In areas of the mouth where esthetic considerations are not critical, a flatter contour is always acceptable.

Subgingival Debris

Leaving debris below the tissue during restorative procedures can create an adverse periodontal response. The cause can be retraction cord, impression material, provisional material, or either temporary or permanent cement.[56] The diagnosis of debris as the cause of gingival inflammation can be confirmed by examining the sulcus surrounding the restoration with an explorer, removing any foreign bodies, and then monitoring the tissue response. It may be necessary to provide tissue anesthesia for patient comfort during the procedure.

Hypersensitivity to Dental Materials

Inflammatory gingival responses have been reported related to the use of nonprecious alloys in dental restorations.[53] Typically, the responses have occurred to alloys containing nickel, although the frequency of these occurrences is controversial.[51] Hypersensitivity responses to precious alloys are extremely rare, and these alloys provide an easy solution to the problems encountered with the nonprecious alloys. More importantly, tissues respond more to the differences in surface roughness of the material rather than to the composition of the material.[1,67] The rougher the surface of the restoration subgingivally, the greater are the plaque accumulation and gingival inflammation. In clinical research, porcelain, highly polished gold, and highly polished resin all show similar plaque accumulation. Regardless of the restorative material selected, a smooth surface is essential on all materials subgingivally.

ESTHETIC TISSUE MANAGEMENT

Managing Interproximal Embrasures

The interproximal embrasure created by restorations and the form of the interdental papilla have a unique and intimate relationship.[62,63] The ideal interproximal embrasure should house the gingival papilla without impinging on it and should also extend the interproximal tooth contact to the top of the papilla so that no excess space exists to trap food or to be esthetically displeasing.

Papillary height is established by the level of the bone, the biologic width, and the form of the gingival embrasure. Changes in the shape of the embrasure can impact the height and form of the papilla. The tip of the papilla behaves differently than the free gingival margin on the facial aspect of the tooth. Whereas the free gingival margin averages 3 mm above the underlying facial bone, the tip of the papilla averages 4.5 to 5.0 mm above the interproximal bone (Figure 72-31). This means that if the papilla is farther above the bone than the facial tissue but has the same biologic width, the interproximal area will have a sulcus 1.0 to 1.5 mm deeper than that found on the facial surface.

Van der Veldon[73] completely removed healthy papillae to the bone level and found that they routinely regenerated 4.0 to 4.5 mm of total tissue above bone, with an average sulcus depth of 2.0 to 2.5 mm. The height above bone that the papilla strives to maintain was indirectly confirmed by Tarnow et al.,[68] who studied the relationship of the papilla between the interproximal contact and the underlying bone. When the gingival level of the interproximal tooth contacts measured 5 mm or less to the alveolar bone, the papilla always filled the space. When the contact was 6 mm from bone, only 56% of the papillae could fill the space. Finally, when the contact was 7 mm from bone, only 37% of the papillae could fill the spaces.

Knowing that there is individual variability to the required biologic width, this information relative to the papilla is applied by locating the lowest point of the interproximal contact in relation to the top of the epithelial attachment. The ideal contact should be 2 to 3 mm coronal to the attachment, which coincides with the depth of the average interproximal sulcus. As in assessing the facial tissues for margin location, this technique requires that the tissue is healthy to allow accurate probing. If the sulcus measures greater than 3 mm, there is some risk of papillary recession with restorative procedures.

The clinician most frequently confronts a normal or shallow sulcus with a papilla that appears too short rather than a tall papilla with a deep sulcus. Management of this situation is best approached by viewing the papilla as a balloon of a certain volume that sits on the attachment. This balloon of tissue has a form and height dictated by the gingival embrasure of the teeth. With an embrasure that is too wide, the balloon flattens out, assumes a blunted shape, and has a shallow sulcus (Figure 72-32). If the embrasure is the ideal width, the papilla assumes a pointed form, has a sulcus of 2.5 to 3.0 mm, and is healthy. If the embrasure is too narrow, the papilla may grow out to the facial and lingual, form a col, and become inflamed.

This information is applied when evaluating an individual papilla with an open embrasure. The papilla in question is compared to the adjacent papillae. If the papillae are all on the same level, and if the other areas do not have open embrasures, the problem is one of gingival embrasure form. If the papilla in the area of concern is apical to the adjacent papillae, however, the clinician should evaluate the interproximal bone levels. If the bone under that papilla is apical to the adjacent

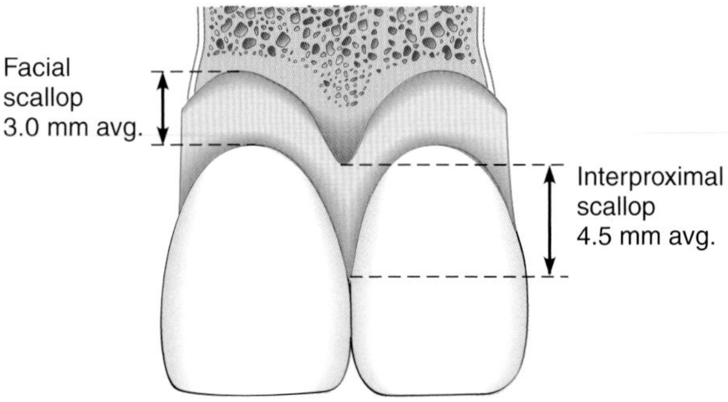

Figure 72-31 Comparison of the behavior of the interproximal papilla relative to bone and the free gingival margin relative to bone in the average human. There is a 3-mm scallop from the facial bone to the interproximal bone. However, on average, a 4.5- to 5.0-mm gingival scallop exists between the facial tissue height and the interproximal papilla height. This extra scallop of 1.5 to 2.0 mm of gingiva compared with bone is the result of the extra soft tissue height above the attachment interproximally.

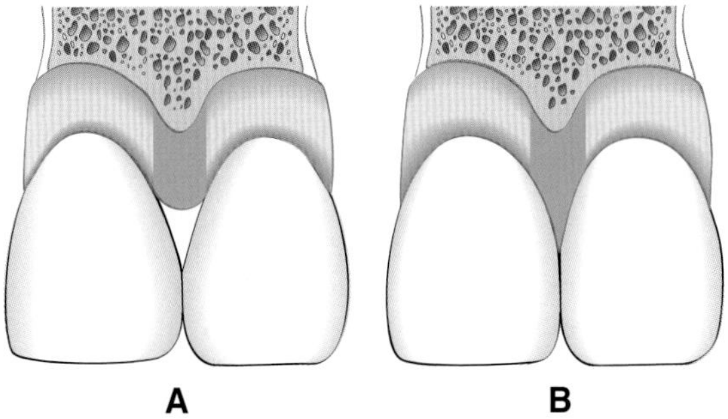

Figure 72-32 Relationship between gingival embrasure volume and papillary form. **A,** Gingival embrasure of the teeth is excessively large due to a tapered tooth form. Because of the large embrasure form, the volume of tissue sitting on top of the attachment is not molded to the shape of a normal papilla but rather has a blunted form and a shallower sulcus. **B,** Ideal tooth form where the same volume of tissue sits on top of the attachment as in *A*. Because of the more closed embrasure form from the teeth in *B,* however, the papilla completely fills the embrasure and has a deeper sulcus, averaging 2.5 to 3.0 mm. Note that the ideal contact position is 3 mm coronal to the attachment.

bone levels, the problem is caused by bone loss. If the bone is at the same level, the open embrasure is caused by the embrasure form of the teeth and not a periodontal problem with the papilla.

Correcting Open Gingival Embrasures Restoratively

There are two causes of open gingival embrasures: (1) the papilla is inadequate in height because of bone loss, or (2) the interproximal contact is located too high coronally. If a high contact has been diagnosed as the cause of the problem, there are two potential reasons. If the root angulation of the teeth diverges, the interproximal contact is moved coronally, resulting in the open embrasure. However, if the roots are parallel, the papilla form is normal, and an open embrasure exists, then the problem is probably related to tooth shape, specifically an excessively tapered form. Restorative dentistry can correct this problem by moving the contact point to the tip of the papilla. To accomplish this, the margins of the restoration must be carried subgingivally 1.0 to 1.5 mm, and the emergence profile of the restoration is designed to move the contact point toward the papilla while blending the contour into the tooth below the tissue (Figure 72-33). This can be accomplished easily with direct bonded restorations because the soft tissue can clearly be seen (Figures 72-34 to 72-36). For indirect restorations, the desired restoration contours and embrasure form should be established in the provisional restorations, and the gingival tissues are allowed to adapt for 4 to 6 weeks before the tissue contour information is relayed to the laboratory for use in the final restorations.

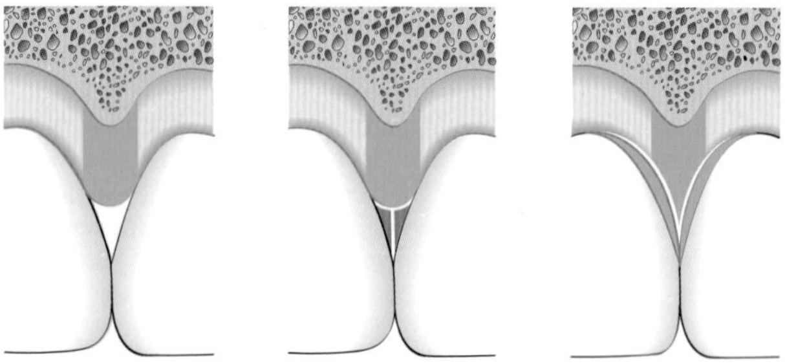

Figure 72-33 Methods of altering gingival embrasure form. **A,** Typical open gingival embrasure caused by excessively tapered tooth form. **B,** Common method employed by restorative dentists to correct the embrasure, in which material is added supragingivally. This closes the embrasure by moving the contact to the tip of the papilla but results in overhangs that cannot be cleaned using dental floss. Removing these overhangs restoratively reopens the embrasure. **C,** Correct method of closing the gingival embrasure, in which the margins of the restoration are carried 1.0 to 1.5 mm below the tip of the papilla. Note that this does not encroach on the attachment because the average interproximal sulcus probes 2.5 to 3.0 mm. This allows easy cleaning because of the convex profile. It also reshapes the papilla to a more pleasing profile esthetically.

Managing Gingival Embrasure Form for Patients with Gingival Recession

Management of the gingival embrasure form for patients who have experienced gingival recession will vary depending on whether the treatment is in the anterior or

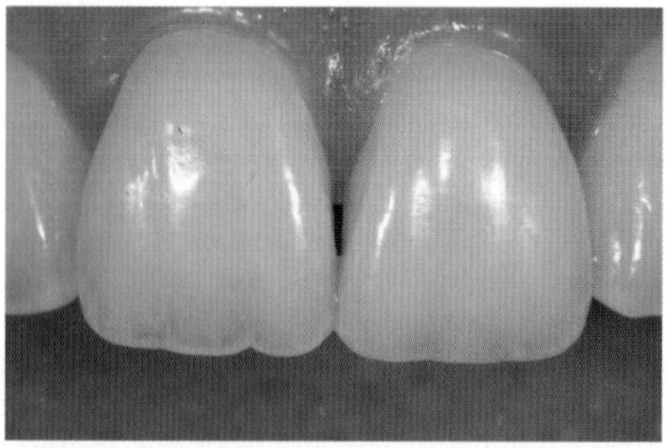

Figure 72-34 This patient has parallel roots, has recently completed orthodontic therapy, and is unhappy with the open gingival embrasure between her central incisors. An evaluation of papillary height reveals that all are at an equal level. This can only mean that the open embrasure is the result of an overly tapered tooth form. (See Figures 72-35 and 72-36.)

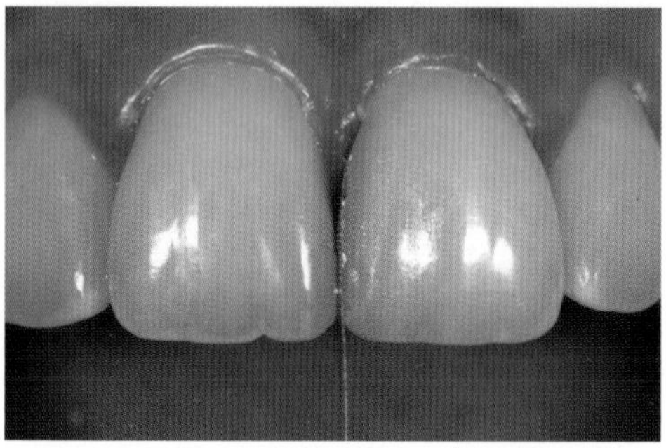

Figure 72-35 One method of correctly altering tooth form of patient in Figure 72-34. A metal matrix band has been shaped to the desired tooth form and placed 1.0 to 1.5 mm below the tip of the papilla. Restorative material then was added to the tooth against the matrix band, forming the new mesial surface of the left central incisor.

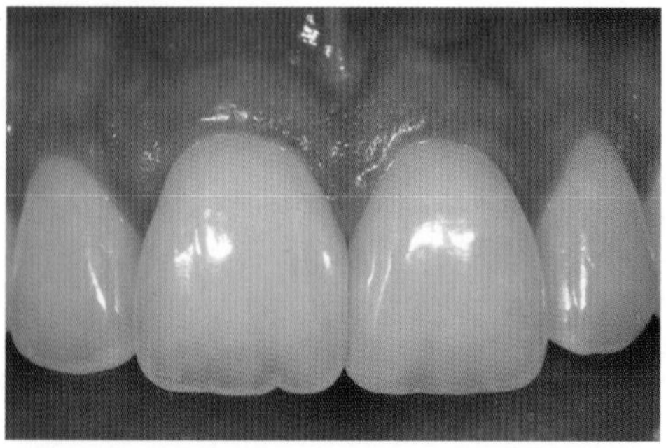

Figure 72-36 One-year recall photograph after restoring the mesial surfaces of the right and left central incisors, moving the proximal contact to the tip of the papilla and extending the restorations 1.0 to 1.5 mm below the papilla, blending them into the tooth and making an easily cleaned area. (See Figures 72-34 and 72-35.)

posterior regions of the mouth.[31] In esthetic areas, it is necessary to carry the interproximal contacts apically toward the papilla to eliminate the presence of large, open embrasures. With multiple-unit restorations, it is also possible with tissue-colored ceramics to bake porcelain papillae directly on the restoration. In the posterior areas where the interroot widths are significantly greater, it is often impossible to carry the proximal contacts to contact the tissue without creating large overhangs on the restorations. In these situations the contact should be moved far enough apically to minimize any large food traps while still leaving an embrasure of a convenient size to be accessed with an interdental brush for hygiene. It should be noted that developing excessively long interproximal contacts, whether on anterior or posterior teeth, will always create rectangular, somewhat unesthetic, tooth forms.

Pontic Design

Classically, there are four options to consider in evaluating pontic design: sanitary, ridge-lap, modified ridge-lap, and ovate designs (Figure 72-37). Regardless of design, the pontic should provide an occlusal surface that stabilizes the opposing teeth, allows for normal mastication, and does not overload the abutment teeth. The restorative material for all four designs can be glazed porcelain, polished gold, or polished resin. The biologic response of the tissue in contact with the restoration is no different in regard to of the material chosen, as long as it has a smooth surface finish.[26,54,64]

The key differences between the four pontic designs relate to the esthetics and access for hygiene procedures. The primary method for cleaning the undersurface of pontics is to draw dental floss mesiodistally along the undersurface. The shape of this undersurface determines the ease with which plaque and food debris can be removed in the process. The sanitary and ovate pontics have convex undersurfaces, which makes them easiest to clean. The ridge-lap and modified ridge-lap designs have concave surfaces, which are more difficult to access with the dental floss. Although the sanitary pontic design provides the easiest access for hygiene procedures, it is rarely used because of its unesthetic form and a variable acceptance of the open contour by patients.

The *ovate pontic* is the ideal pontic form.[62] It is created by forming a receptor site in the edentulous ridge with a diamond bur or by electrosurgery. The site is shaped to create either a flat or a concave contour so that when the pontic is created to adapt to the site, it will have a flat or convex outline. The depth of the receptor site depends on the esthetic requirements of the pontic. In highly esthetic areas such as the maxillary anterior region, it is necessary to create a receptor area that is 1.0 to 1.5 mm below the tissue on the facial aspect. This creates the appearance of a free gingival margin and produces optimal esthetics (Figure 72-38). This site can then be tapered to the height of the palatal tissue to facilitate hygiene access from the palatal side. In the posterior areas, a deep receptor site can complicate hygiene access. In these situations the ideal site has the facial portion of the pontic at the same level as the ridge, and then the site is created as a straight line to the lingual side of the pontic. This removes the convexity of the ridge and produces a flat, easily cleanable tissue surface on the pontic (Figure 72-39).

When the ridge is being surgically modified, it is important to know the thickness of soft tissue above the bone. This measurement is obtained by probing to the bone through the anesthetized tissue. If the tissue is removed to less than 2 mm in thickness, significant rebound in ridge height may occur. If it is necessary to reduce the tissue height to less than 2 mm above the bone to create the desired pontic form, some bone will need to be removed to achieve the desired result.

It is important when considering an ovate pontic to realize that certain soft tissue ridge parameters must exist to optimize the ovate pontic form. First, the ridge height needs to match the ideal height of the interproximal papillae where interproximal embrasures are planned,

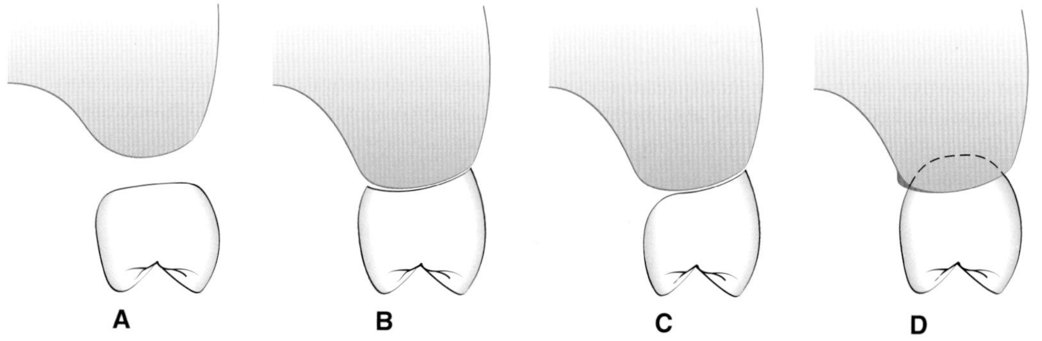

Figure 72-37 Four options to designing the shape of a pontic. **A,** *Sanitary pontic.* Tissue surface of the pontic is 3 mm from the underlying ridge. **B,** *Ridge-lap pontic.* Tissue surface of the pontic straddles the ridge in saddlelike fashion. The entire tissue surface of the ridge-lap pontic is convex and very difficult to clean. **C,** *Modified ridge-lap pontic.* Tissue surface on the facial is concave, following the ridge. However, the lingual saddle has been removed to allow access for oral hygiene. **D,** *Ovate pontic.* The pontic form fits into a receptor site within the ridge. This allows the tissue surface of the pontic to be convex and also optimizes esthetics.

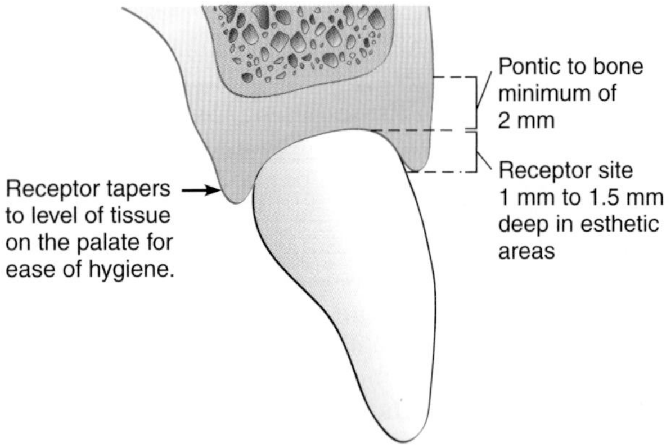

Figure 72-38 Ideal shape and form of an ovate pontic in the esthetic area. The receptor site has been created 1.0 to 1.5 mm apical to the free gingival margin on the facial aspect. This creates the illusion of the pontic erupting from the tissue. On the palatal side, the pontic is tapered so that the receptor site is not extended below tissue; this allows easier access for oral hygiene. Note that when the receptor site is created, the bone must be a minimum of 2 mm from the most apical portion of the pontic.

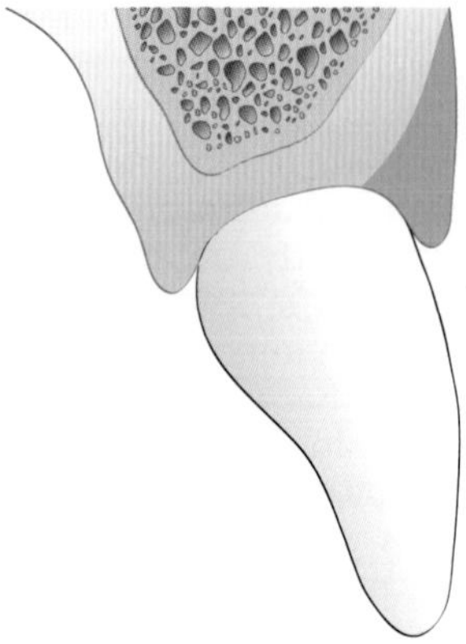

Figure 72-40 Ridge considerations when an ovate pontic is desired. For an ovate pontic to be properly created, the soft tissue ridge must be labial to the desired cervical portion of the pontic. When the pontic is facial to the ridge, it is not possible to create what appears to be a "free gingival margin" correctly. The shaded area represents the necessary amount of tissue that would be augmented to produce an ideal ovate pontic in this particular site.

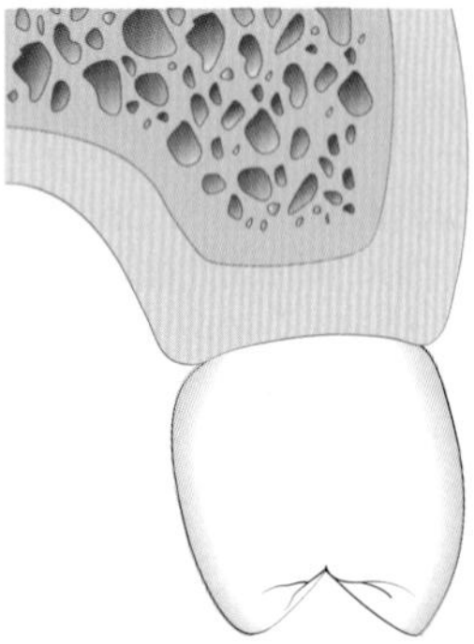

Figure 72-39 Option for creating an ovate pontic receptor site in less esthetic areas of the mouth. Rather than creating the receptor site so that the pontic extends into the ridge, it is possible to create a flattened receptor site where the pontic sits flush with the ridge. This facilitates oral hygiene.

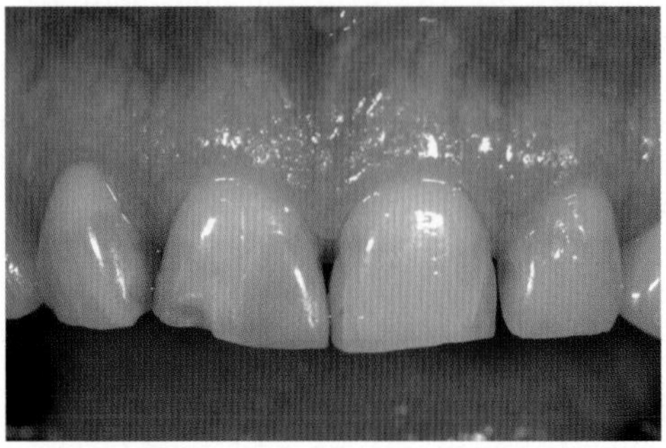

Figure 72-41 Patient who will have the right central incisor extracted because of periodontal disease. The patient is choosing to have a fixed partial denture rather than an implant as the method of replacement. An ovate pontic will be used to maintain the papillary form after the removal of this central incisor. (See Figures 72-42 to 72-48.)

either between pontics or next to abutment teeth. Second, the gingival margin height must also be at the ideal level, or the pontic will appear too long. Third, the ridge tissue must be facial to the ideal cervical facial form of the pontic so that the pontic can emerge from the tissue. If any of these three areas is inadequate, some form of ridge augmentation is needed to produce a ridge that can have an adequate receptor site created (Figure 72-40). Any ridge augmentation procedures should be completed before, or in conjunction with, fabricating an ovate pontic. When constructing the final restorations, the contours of the developed ovate pontic receptor site can be conveyed to the laboratory by capturing a soft tissue impression 4 to 6 weeks after the site has been created.

The ovate pontic can serve another important periodontal function by maintaining the interdental papilla next to abutment teeth after extraction.[62] When a tooth is removed, the gingival embrasure form is lost. The normal response of the papilla to this loss of embrasure form is to recede 1.5 to 2.0 mm, which corresponds to the additional soft tissue that exists above bone on the interproximal versus the facial aspect. However, this recession can be prevented. By inserting the correct pontic form 2.5 mm into the extraction site the day the tooth is removed, the gingival embrasure form and papilla can be maintained. At 4 weeks the 2.5-mm extension can be reduced to a 1.0- to 1.5-mm extension to facilitate hygiene. This procedure can maintain the papilla next to the abutment teeth as long as the bone on the abutment tooth is at a normal level (Figures 72-41 to 72-48).

The "full ridge-lap pontic" is an outdated design that straddles the convexity of the ridge buccolingually and

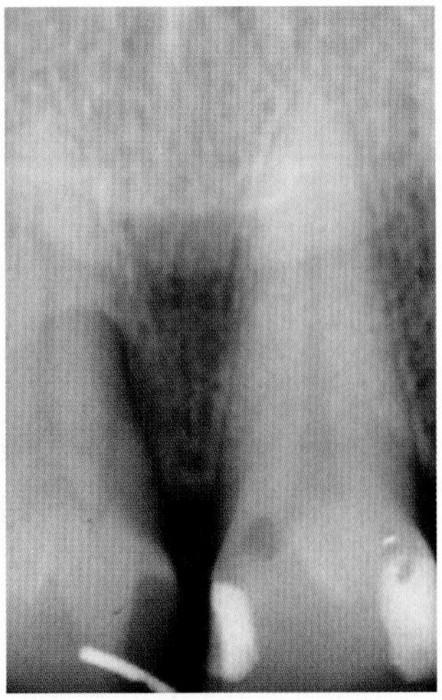

Figure 72-42 Note radiographic presence of a palatal well caused by a deep palatal groove on this right central incisor of patient in Figure 72-41. Two attempted periodontal surgeries have failed to correct this, and it still probes 10 mm with suppuration.

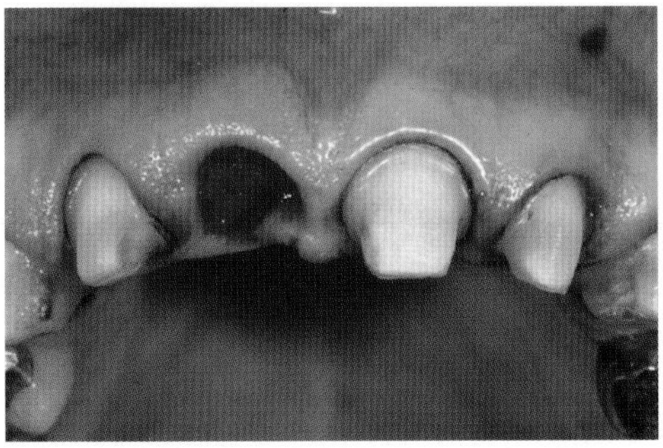

Figure 72-43 Because the patient in Figure 72-41 desired to alter the esthetics of her remaining anterior teeth, all the anterior teeth were prepared before removal of the right central incisor.

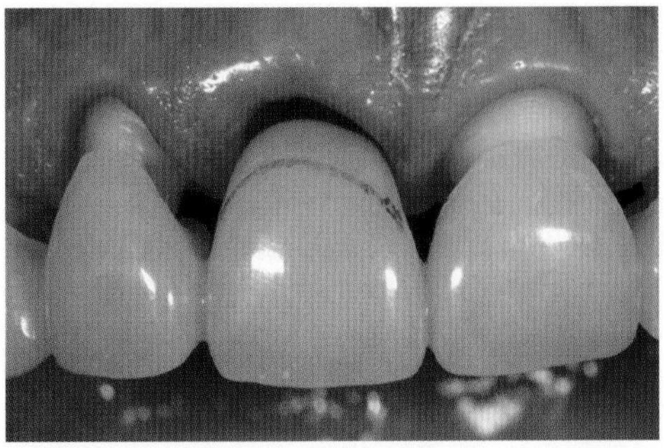

Figure 72-44 The key to maintenance of the interproximal papilla is that the ovate pontic extend 2.5 mm into the extraction site on the day of extraction. This will maintain gingival embrasure form and therefore maintain interproximal papillary height.

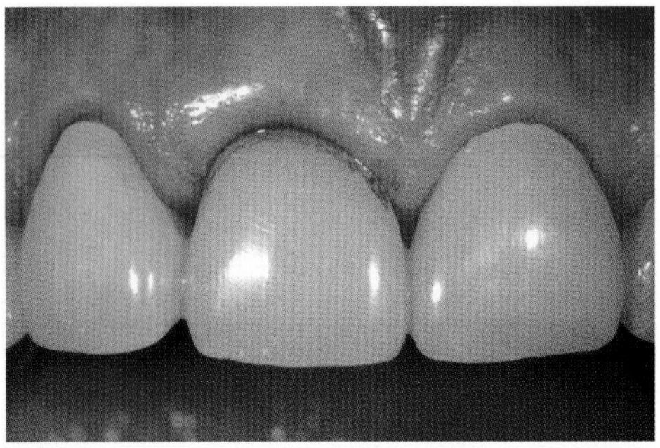

Figure 72-45 Note that when the provisional restoration is seated on the day of the extraction, 2.5 mm of the pontic extends upward into the extraction socket. Also note the open gingival embrasures present to allow space for the papillae to rebound coronally.

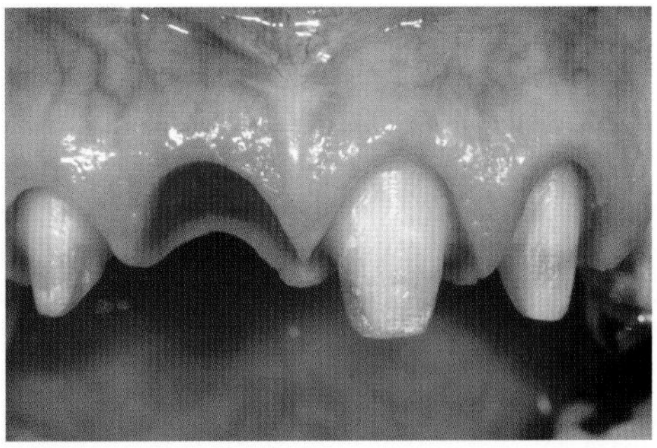

Figure 72-46 Nine months after placement of the provisional restoration. At 4 weeks after placement, the pontic was shortened to extend 1.5 mm into the extraction site to facilitate oral hygiene. Note maintenance of papillary form and free gingival margin height, predictable in this patient because she has excellent interproximal and facial bone.

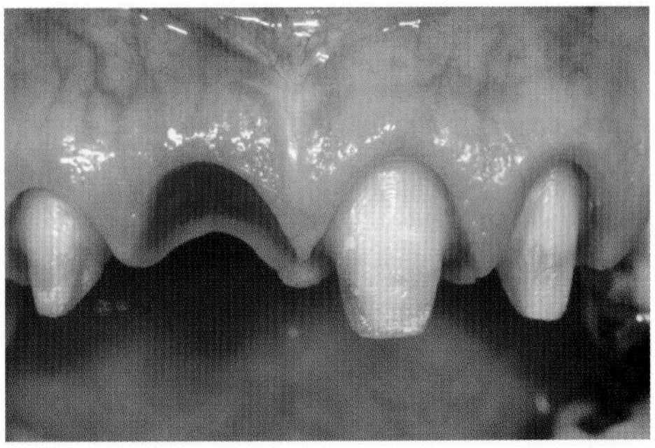

Figure 72-47 Ovate pontic site after removal of the provisional restoration and before final impressions. Note that the papillary form has been maintained because of the ovate pontic maintaining gingival embrasure volume.

creates an undersurface that is entirely concave and uncleanable. It is not recommended for use in any situations. However, a *modified ridge-lap pontic* can be an acceptable design if inadequate ridge exists to create an ovate pontic.

With the modified ridge-lap design, the pontic follows the convexity of the ridge on the facial aspect but stops on the lingual crest of the ridge without extending down the lingual side of the ridge. Although the facial aspect of the undersurface has a concave shape, the more open lingual form allows adequate access for oral hygiene.

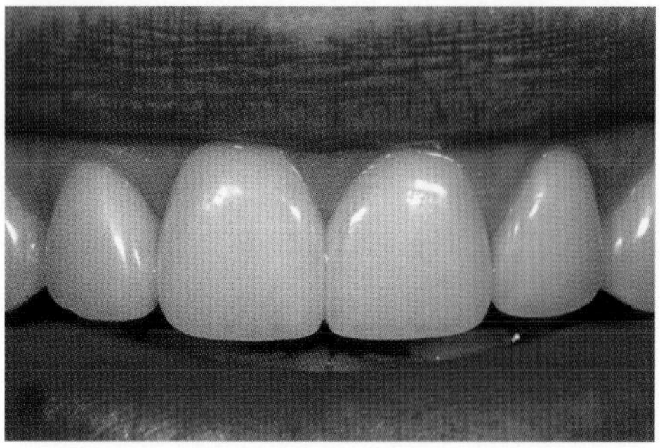

Figure 72-48 Two-year recall photograph of the final fixed prosthesis of patient in Figure 72-41. Note how the final ovate pontic also has maintained papillary form.

OCCLUSAL CONSIDERATIONS IN RESTORATIVE THERAPY

The importance of occlusion and its role in dentistry has been decreasing significantly over the past 20 years. Occlusal trauma as a factor in periodontal disease and its role in orofacial pain have been deemphasized in numerous papers.* However, the role that occlusion plays in restorative dentistry has been reemphasized. The increased use of dental implants and nonmetallic cosmetic restorations has resulted in greater concern over *force management.* These restorations are more sensitive to occlusal trauma, with subsequent structural failure, than are traditional restorations on teeth. Consequently, for the restorative dentist wanting a high degree of predictability in the final result, understanding occlusion is critical. The clinician must know how to create an occlusion, with the following guidelines as a goal:

1. There should be *even, simultaneous contacts* on all teeth during centric closure. This distributes the force of closure over all the teeth instead of the few teeth that may touch first.
2. When the mandible moves from centric closure, some form of *canine or anterior guidance* is desirable, with no posterior tooth contacts. This combination of anterior guidance and posterior disclusion reduces the ability of the elevator muscles to contract and distributes the force of the movement onto the anterior teeth, which receive less force because of the class III lever system being applied in this situation. It has been shown that, as a result of the class III lever action, the anterior teeth receive approximately one-ninth the force of a second molar.[25,61]
3. The anterior guidance needs to be in harmony with the patient's *neuromuscular envelope of function.* Harmony of this relationship is demonstrated by a lack of fremitus and mobility on the anterior teeth, by the ability of the patient to speak clearly and comfortably, and by the patient's general sense of comfort with the overbite, overjet, and guidance created during chewing and when holding the head upright.
4. The occlusion should be created at a *vertical dimension* that is stable for the patient. It is generally accepted that the patient's existing vertical dimension is at equilibrium between the eruptive forces of the teeth and the repetitive contracted length of the elevator muscles. It has been demonstrated that vertical dimension can be altered with no sense of pain from muscles and joints.[9,11,22,30] However, if this alteration lengthens the pterygomasseteric sling beyond its ability to adapt, the patient will not maintain the vertical change and will close the occlusal vertical dimension back down by intruding the teeth.[12,34,40-42]
5. When managing a pathologic occlusion or when restoring a complete occlusion, the clinician needs to work with a repeatable condylar reference position. *Centric relation,* defined as the most superior condylar position, provides such a starting point.[21] Centric relation has been shown to be reproducible over multiple appointments, allowing the clinician to create the occlusion indirectly on an articulator and return it to the same reference position in the mouth.[14,39,44,74] It is the only position that has been shown to shut off lateral pterygoid muscle contraction.[20] Because it is a border position, any mandibular movement will result in the condyle moving inferiorly. Therefore, centric relation is the only position from which an interference-free occlusion can be created.

To manage the occlusion as previously described, the clinician must be able to make accurate casts, use a facebow, and create centric relation records so that the information can be transferred to a suitable articulator. Although the details of these procedures are beyond the scope of this chapter, they are a routine part of any restorative treatment plan and must be mastered for the clinician to achieve predictable, long-term restorative success.

SPECIAL RESTORATIVE CONSIDERATIONS

Root-Resected Teeth

Although the availability of implant therapy has greatly reduced the frequency with which root-amputated teeth are saved, restoration of root-resected teeth is still a viable mode of treatment. Structural challenges are created in restoring these teeth because of the amount of tooth structure lost in the resection process (Figure 72-49). Conservative tooth preparation will maintain as much of the remaining tooth as possible, but the resulting supragingival or minimally prepared subgingival finish lines will require additional metal display in the final restoration. A cast post and core may be indicated to create an adequate foundation for the final restoration. Because the remaining roots are often very thin mesiodistally, it is difficult to cement premade posts and have adequate bulk to place a foundation core on the mesial and distal surfaces of the post. This problem is avoided with the one-piece cast post and core restoration.

*References 9, 15, 35, 36, 45, 46, 55, 66, 72.

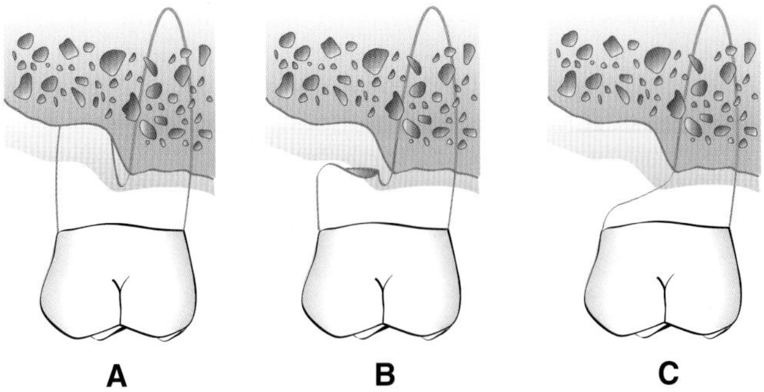

Figure 72-49 **A,** Maxillary molar with a class III furcation and bone loss surrounding the distal buccal root. **B,** Contour created when the distal buccal root is removed, but the coronal contour has not yet been reshaped. Note the overhang, which can trap food and plaque and create gingival inflammation. **C,** Correct contour after the restoration or reshaping of the tooth. Note this illustration is only of the facial portion of the tooth. The palatal portion of the crown and the palatal root do not appear. Note how the contour has been altered to allow easy access for an interdental brush to the gingival tissue and the tooth in the area where the root was removed.

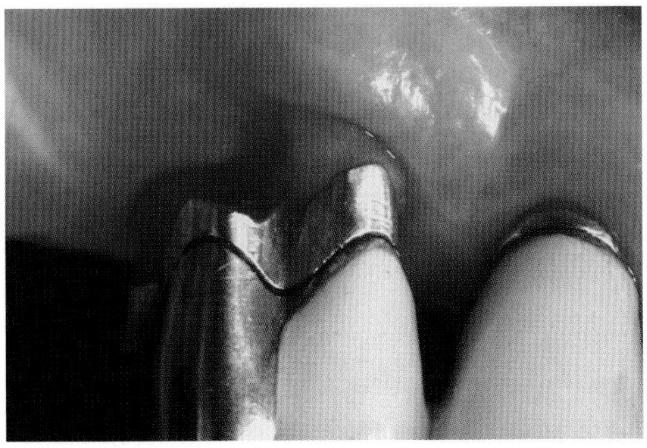

Figure 72-50 Photograph taken 6 weeks after the removal of the distal buccal root on this maxillary first molar. Note that the crown contour has not yet been altered. Also note the presence of a large overhang that easily traps debris.

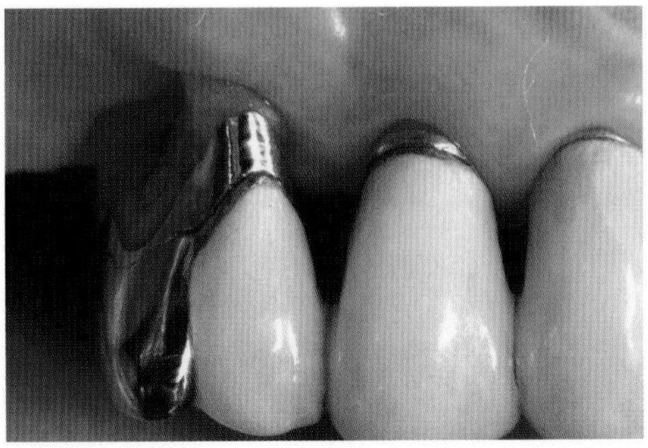

Figure 72-51 Correct modification of the crown form seen in Figure 72-50. The roof of the furcation of the remaining distal buccal root has been completely removed and the crown re-formed to allow easy access to the remaining roots and soft tissue.

Another area of concern when restoring root-resected teeth is the development of appropriate contours for hygiene access. The primary concern is to avoid any excessively heavy convexities of contour that would prevent access (Figures 72-50 and 72-51). Facially and lingually, the contours should be essentially a straight line from the margin coronally, while interproximally, the contour emerges from the margin as a straight line or is slightly convex as it slopes up to the contact point. The interproximal areas of root-amputated and hemisected teeth often present with surface concavities on the root trunk, and these areas cannot be adequately cleaned with floss because it will bridge across the concavity. The gingival embrasure form created in the restoration must be fluted into these areas so that the surfaces can be accessed with an interdental brush.

Esthetics is usually not a major concern unless the tooth in question is a maxillary molar with a mesiobuccal root amputation and the patient has a broad smile. The solution is to create an artificial mesiobuccal root with normal crown contour coronal to it and a furcation made of restorative material that is easily cleanable with an interdental brush.

Splinting

Splinting therapy may be applied with bonded external appliances, intracoronal appliances, or indirect cast restorations to connect multiple teeth, with the goal of improving tooth stability. Unstable teeth may be caused by a lack of periodontal support from bone loss, a lack of support from tooth loss, or the need to splint abutment teeth to support pontics. Indications for splinting are (1) mobility of teeth that is increasing or that impairs patient comfort, (2) migration of teeth, or (3) prosthetics where multiple abutments are necessary.

Before considering splinting, the clinician must identify the etiology of the instability.[2] Excessive occlusal forces from parafunction or deflective tooth contacts are frequent causes of excessive mobility. Whenever the occlusion is the cause, occlusal therapy is always performed first. The mobility is then evaluated over time to determine if it resolves before splinting is considered. In addition, any inflammation of the periodontal supporting apparatus must be controlled before making a decision on splinting, because inflammation can produce mobility in the presence of normal occlusal forces and normal periodontal support. When the teeth are splinted, all the teeth in the splint share the occlusal load to some extent.[17] The rigidity of the splint and the number of teeth utilized will determine how the forces are distributed.

The most common indication to splint mobile teeth is to improve patient comfort and to provide better control of the occlusion if the anterior teeth are mobile. Adequate crown length on the teeth being splinted is critical so that the interproximal connectors do not impinge on the interdental papilla. Also, adequate space must exist between the connector and the papilla for access with dental floss anteriorly and with an interproximal brush on posterior teeth.

Anterior Esthetic Surgery

The importance of gingiva in relation to anterior esthetics has been well documented.[10,29,59,65] Various methods for altering gingival levels have been described, including gingivectomy, apically positioned flaps with osseous recontouring, and the use of orthodontic therapy to position the gingival tissue level apically or coronally by intruding or extruding the teeth.[5,13,33,69]

Whenever an alteration in gingival levels is contemplated, the expected outcome must be communicated to the patient to determine if the planned surgery is acceptable. Computer imaging can be used to provide the patient with a visual plan for the final esthetic result.[18] However, the imaging process does not allow the dentist or patient to include the dynamics of lip movement in the evaluation of the proposed changes. Computer imaging will provide enough information to depict the final outcome accurately when the planned surgery will alter the gingiva on one or two teeth while leaving the gingival levels of adjacent teeth in their existing position.

However, when the surgery will involve many or all of the anterior teeth and will result in moving gingiva several millimeters, to the extent that a flap will be raised and bony levels altered, an additional guide is desirable before surgery. Constructing these guides directly on a stone cast is the easiest and least time-consuming method. Before constructing the guide, treatment planning is completed on the patient to determine the desired incisal edge position and the desired gingival level of the tissues. This will establish the amount of tooth display at rest and at full smile. The information is transferred to a stone cast of the patient's teeth, and the desired shape of the gingival margins for each tooth is drawn on the cast. The existing incisal edge position of each tooth is used as a reference in establishing the desired gingival level. A composite or acrylic resin veneer is then constructed on the cast, extending gingivally to the desired tissue position. The veneer guide can also be extended incisally to the desired incisal edge position so that this information can also be included in the veneer. The veneer is trimmed, polished, and tried in the patient's mouth.

When the patient approves the gingival levels established with the guide, the desired gingival correction can be completed using the veneer guide as a surgical template. In addition to locating the initial incisions at the correct level, the guide can also be employed after flap reflection to aid in the bony recontouring to ensure adequate biologic width and sulcus depth at the new gingival position. The surgeon will replace the flap at closure to the gingival level established with the guide. Employing an esthetic template in this manner optimizes the predictability of the surgical therapy and establishes the ideal tissue framework to complete the esthetic restorations (Figures 72-52 to 72-59).

SCIENCE TRANSFER

The biologic width is a physiologic phenomenon that occurs around the tooth and around implants. These implants, constructed as a solid piece of titanium emerging from the bone and soft tissues, were referred to as "nonsubmerged implants" and did not have an implant/abutment interface at the alveolar crest. Under both tooth and implant conditions, the body reacts physiologically and forms a constant linear dimension of junctional epithelium and connective tissue, the biologic width. As a physiologic structure, this occurs in all patients under healthy conditions; however, although the means are constant, there is a standard deviation to the mean. Therefore, patients can have different dimensions of biologic width (often varying more than 1 mm), but the mean of a large number of patients is constant. Margins of restorations and interfaces between implant components, however, are microbial niches and stimulate inflammation. *Because inflammation is the driving force for tissue change, the closer the margin or interface is to the soft or hard tissue, the more tissue change is expected.* Margins or interfaces close to the alveolar bone crest should be avoided because this situation would be expected to produce the greatest tissue change (bone loss).

Subgingival restorative dental margins can cause periodontal inflammation and bone loss if placed too far apically. Violations of biologic width predispose to these adverse effects when margins are placed closer than 2 mm to the alveolar bone crest. Overcontoured crowns also predispose patients to periodontal inflammation, and this chapter provides excellent guidelines for minimizing these changes. Ovate pontics are recommended, and the chapter also outlines the specific procedures for their design. Maintenance of healthy interdental tissues is also part of optimal restorative dentistry techniques. If the distance of the contact point to the crest of bone is greater than 5 mm, an unesthetic black triangular space is likely, so interdental bone maintenance is vital for interdental papillary esthetics.

A restorative occlusal scheme should provide for periodontal, neuromuscular, and joint stability. The use of centric relation gives a reproducible, stable position that reduces the risk of lateral pterygoid muscle hyperactivity, and any condylar movement will be in an inferior direction, thus lessening the risk of occlusal interferences in functional and parafunctional positions.

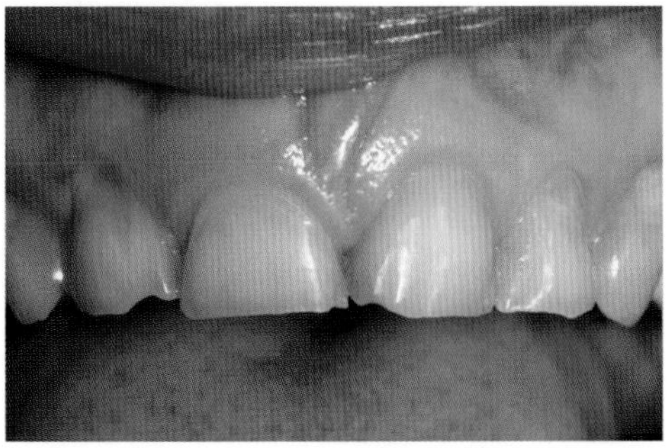

Figure 72-52 This patient is unhappy with the appearance of her maxillary teeth and the discrepancies of tissue height and tooth form. (See Figures 72-53 to 72-59.)

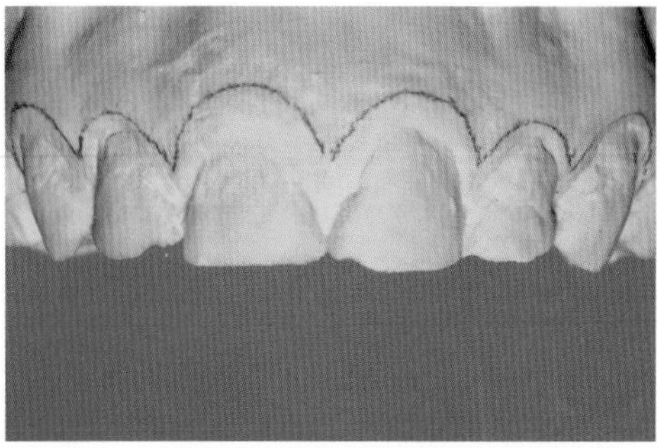

Figure 72-53 To create a surgical guide for patient in Figure 72-52, a stone cast is modified by drawing the desired soft tissue profile with a red wax pencil.

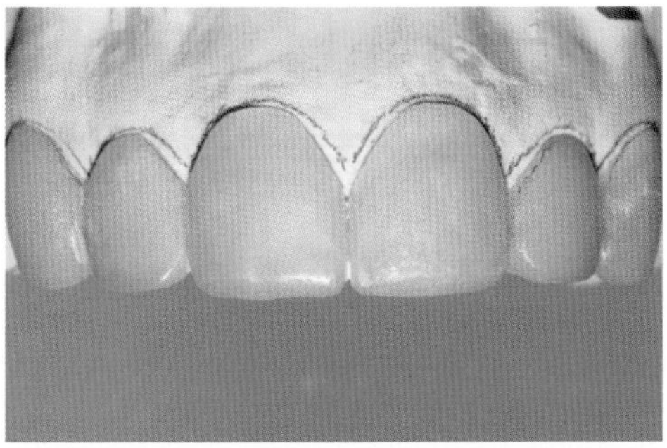

Figure 72-54 Composite-resin surgical guide is fabricated on this stone cast, extending to the line drawn. This guide can be taken to the mouth for try-in and verification by the patient (see Figure 72-52).

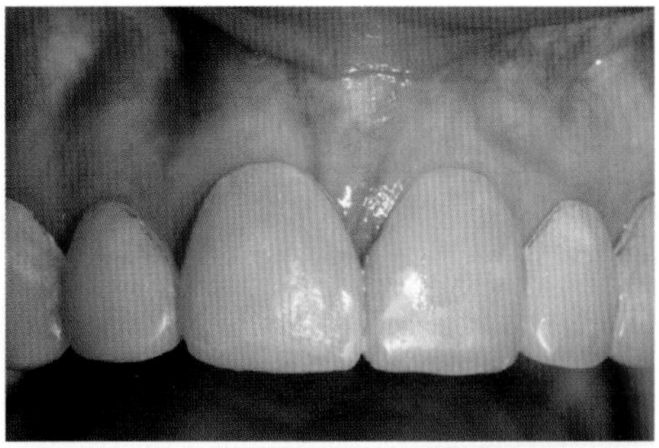

Figure 72-55 Photograph taken the day the surgical guide was tried-in. This patient in Figure 72-52 approved the new length of the maxillary anterior teeth and the form created by altering the soft tissue profile.

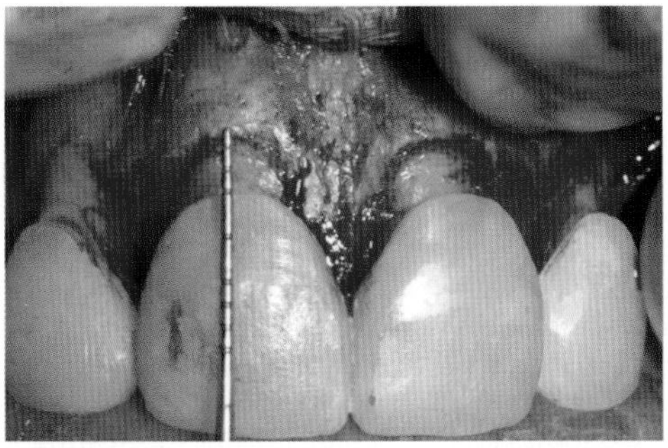

Figure 72-56 By placing the surgical guide during the surgery, it is possible to recognize where the bone needs to be placed. The surgical guide represents the desired final free gingival margin position and can be used as a reference for osseous recontouring. This patient had an average biologic width of 2 mm (see Figure 72-52). Allowing an additional 1 mm for sulcus depth, the desired distance between the bone and the free gingival margin will be 3 mm. With this knowledge, the periodontist can use the guide and remove bone until it is 3 mm from the position of the guide on each tooth.

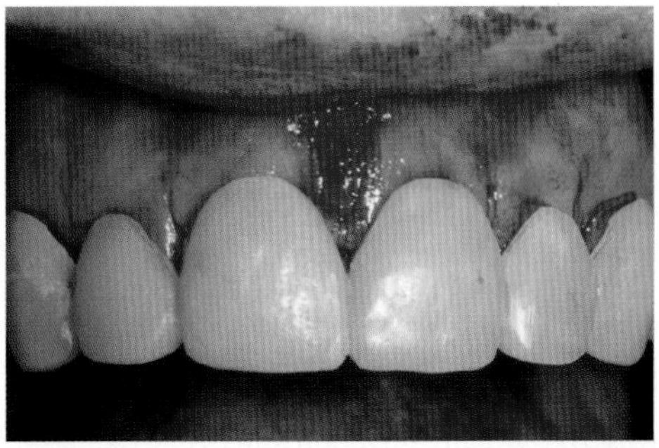

Figure 72-57 Surgical guide is also useful during suturing. Because the guide represents the desired free gingival margin position, it is possible to suture to the level of the guide, knowing that the surgery has now recreated biologic width and a 1-mm sulcus. This shortens the amount of time necessary for healing and eliminates the need to wait for tissue rebound before restorative dentistry.

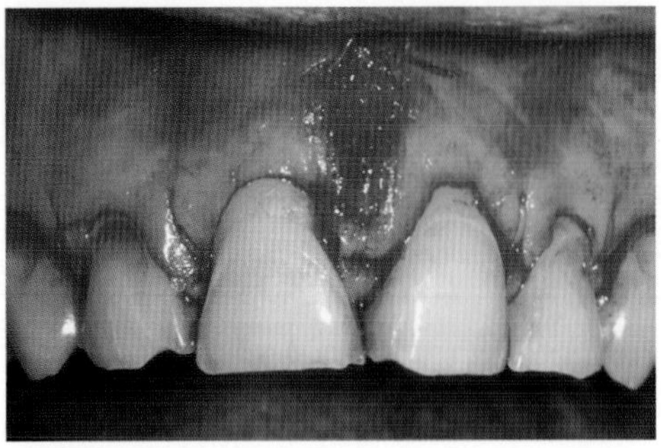

Figure 72-58 Soft tissue profile as seen the day of surgery with the guide removed. Note that in this patient, the interproximal papillae were not changed because the interproximal papillary form and height were deemed acceptable. (See Figures 72-52 to 72-57.)

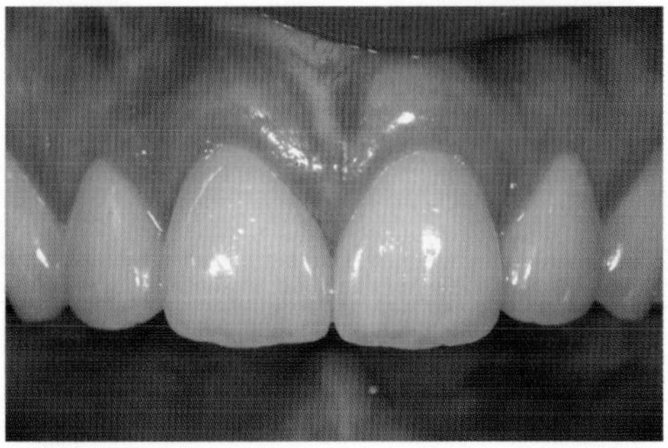

Figure 72-59 Photograph taken 4 years after placement of the final restoration of patient in Figure 72-52. Note the excellent soft tissue health and the attainment of the desired free gingival margin and papillary form.

REFERENCES

1. Adamczyk E, Speichowics E: Plaque accumulation on crowns made of various materials, *Int J Prosthodont* 3:285, 1990.
2. Amsterdam M: Periodontal prosthesis: twenty-five years in retrospect, *Alpha Omegan* 67:30, 1974.
3. Amsterdam M, Fox L: Provisional splinting: principles and techniques, *Dent Clin North Am* 4:73, 1959.
4. Armitage GC, Svanberg GK, Löe H: Microscopic evaluation of clinical measurements of connective tissue attachment levels, *J Clin Periodontol* 4:173, 1977.
5. Becker W, Ochsenbein C, Becker B: Crown lengthening: the periodontal-restorative connection, *Compend Contin Educ Dent* 19:239, 1998.
6. Benson BW, Bomberg TJ, Hatch RA, et al: Tissue displacement in fixed prosthodontics, *J Prosthet Dent* 55:175, 1986.
7. Bragger U, Laachenauer D, Lang NP: Surgical lengthening of the clinical crown, *J Clin Periodontol* 19:58, 1992.
8. Carlsson G, De Boever J: Epidemiology. In Zarb G, Carlsson G, Sessle B, et al, editors: *Epidemiology,* Copenhagen, 1994, Munksgaard.
9. Carlsson GE, Ingerval B, Kocak G: Effect of increasing vertical dimension on the masticatory system in subjects with natural teeth, *J Prosthet Dent* 41:284, 1979.
10. Chiche GJ, Pinault A: *Esthetics of anterior fixed prosthodontics,* Chicago, 1994, Quintessence.
11. Christensen J: Effect of occlusion-raising procedures on the chewing system, *Dent Pract Dent Rec* 20:233, 1970.
12. Dahl BL, Krogstad O: Long-term observations of an increased occlusal face height obtained by a combined orthodontic/prosthetic approach, *J Oral Rehabil* 12:173, 1985.
13. Dolt A, Robbins J: Altered passive eruption: an etiology of short clinical crowns, *Quintessence Int* 28:363, 1997.
14. Downs DH: An investigation into condylar position with leaf gauge and bimanual manipulation, *J Gnathol* 7:75, 1988.
15. Ericsson I, Lindhe J: Effect of longstanding jiggling on experimental periodontitis in the beagle dog, *J Clin Periodontol* 9:497, 1982.
16. Felton DA, Kanoy Be, Bayne SC, et al: Effect of in vivo crown margin discrepancies on periodontal health, *J Prosthet Dent* 65:357, 1991.
17. Foucher RR, Bryant RA: Bilateral fixed splints, *Int J Periodont Restor Dent* 5:9, 1983.
18. Ganz CH, Brisman SA, Tauro V: Computer video imaging: computerization, communication, and creation, *QDT Yearbook,* 1989, p 64.
19. Gargiulo AW, Wentz FM, Orban B: Dimension and relations of the dentogingival junction in humans, *J Periodontol* 32:262, 1961.
20. Gibb CH, Mahan PE, Wilkenson TM, et al: EMG activity of the superior belly of the lateral pterygoid muscle in relation to other jaw muscles, *J Prosthet Dent* 51:691, 1984.
21. *The glossary of prosthodontic terms,* ed 6, St Louis, 1994, Mosby.
22. Gross MD, Ormianer Z: A preliminary study on the effect of occlusal vertical dimension increases on mandibular postural rest position, *Int J Prosthodont* 7:216, 1994.
23. Günay H, Seeger A, Tschernitschek H, et al: Placement of the preparation line and periodontal health: a prospective 2-year clinical study, *Int J Periodont Restor Dent* 20:173, 2000.
24. Hansen PA, Tira DE, Barlow J: Current methods of finish line exposure by practicing prosthodontists, *J Prosthodont* 8:163, 1999.
25. Hatcher DC, Faulkner MG, Hay A: Development of mechanical and mathematic models to study temporomandibular joint loading, *J Prosthet Dent* 55:377, 1986.
26. Henry PJ, Johnson JF, Mitchell DF: Tissue changes beneath fixed partial dentures, *J Prosthet Dent* 16:937, 1966.
27. Hochman N, Yaffe A, Ehrlich J: Crown contour variation in gingival health, *Compend Contin Educ Dent* 4:360, 1983.
28. Ingber JS: Forced eruption. II. A method of treating nonrestorable teeth: periodontal and restorative considerations, *J Periodontol* 47:203, 1995.
29. Kay HB: Esthetic considerations in the definitive periodontal prosthetic management of the maxillary anterior segment, *Int J Periodont Restor Dent* 2(3):44, 1982.
30. Kohno S, Bando E: Die funcktionelle anpassung der kaumuskulatur bei starker beisshenbung [Functional adaptation of masticatory muscles as a result of large increases in the vertical dimension], *Dtsch Zahnartzl Z* 38:759, 1983.
31. Kois JC, Spear FM: Periodontal prosthesis: creating successful restorations, *J Am Dent Assoc* 123:108, 1992.
32. Kozlovsky A, Tal H, Lieberman M: Forced eruption combined with gingival fiberotomy: a technique for clinical crown lengthening, *J Clin Periodontol* 18:330, 1991.
33. Lie T: Periodontal surgery for the maxillary anterior area, *Int J Peridont Restor Dent* 12(1):73, 1992.
34. Lindauer SJ, Gay T, Rendell J: Effect of jaw opening on masticatory muscles: EMG-force characteristics, *J Dent Res* 72:51, 1993.
35. Lindhe J, Ericsson I: The influence of trauma from occlusion on progression of experimental periodontitis in dogs, *J Clin Periodontol* 53:562, 1982.
36. Lindhe J, Svanberg G: Influence of trauma from occlusion on progression of experimental periodontitis in the beagle dog, *J Clin Periodontol* 1:3, 1974.

37. Listgarten MA: Periodontal probing: what does it mean? *J Clin Periodontol* 7:165, 1980.
38. Listgarten MA, Mao R, Robinson PJ: Periodontal probing and the relationship of the probe tip to periodontal tissues, *J Periodontol* 47:511, 1976.
39. Long JH: Locating centric relation with a leaf gauge, *J Prosthet Dent* 29:608, 1973.
40. MacKenna BR, Türker KS: Jaw separation and maximum incising force, *J Prosthet Dent* 49:726, 1983.
41. Manns A, Mirallees R, Guerrs F: The changes in electrical activity of the postural muscles of the mandible upon varying the vertical dimension, *J Prosthet Dent* 45:438, 1981.
42. Manns A, Spreng M: EMG amplitude and frequency at different muscular elongations under constant masticatory force or EMG activity, *Acta Physiol Lat Am* 27:259, 1977.
43. Marcum JS: The effect of crown margin depth upon gingival tissue, *J Prosthet Dent* 17:479, 1967.
44. McKee JR: Comparing condylar position respectability for standardized versus nonstandardized methods of achieving centric relation, *J Prosthet Dent* 77:280, 1997.
45. Meitner S: Co-destructive factors of marginal periodontitis and repetitive mechanical injury, *J Dent Res* 54:78, 1975.
46. National Institutes of Health Technology: Management of temporomandibular disorders, Assessment conference statement, 1996, *Oral Surg Oral Med Oral Pathol Oral Radiol Endod* 83:177, 1997.
47. Newcomb GJ: The relationship between the location of subgingival crown margins and gingival inflammation, *J Periodontol* 45:151, 1974.
48. Olsson M, Lindhe S: Periodontol characteristics in individuals with varying forms of the upper central incisors, *J Clin Periodontol* 18:78, 1991.
49. Parkinson CF: Excessive crown contours facilitate endemic plaque niches, *J Prosthet Dent* 35:424, 1976.
50. Parma-Benfenati S, Fugazzoto PA, Ruben MP: The effect of restorative margins on the postsurgical development and nature of the periodontium. Part I, *Int J Periodont Restor Dent* 6:31, 1985.
51. Pelton L: Nickel sensibility in the general population, *Contact Derm* 5:27, 1979.
52. Perel ML: Axial crown contours, *J Prosthet Dent* 25:642, 1971.
53. Pierce LH, Goodkind RJ: A status report of possible risks in base metal alloys and their components, *J Prosthet Dent* 62:234, 1989.
54. Podshadley AG: Gingival response to pontics, *J Prosthet Dent* 19:51, 1968.
55. Polson AM, Meitner SW, Zander HA: Trauma and progression of marginal periodontitis in squirrel monkeys. III. Adaptation of interproximal alveolar bone to repetitive injury, *J Periodontal Res* 11:279, 1976.
56. Price C, Whitehead FJH: Impression material as foreign bodies, *Br Dent J* 133:9, 1972.
57. Robinson PJ, Vitek RM: The relationship between gingival inflammation and the probe resistance, *J Periodontal Res* 14:239, 1975.
58. Rosenburg ES, Garber DA, Evian CL: Tooth lengthening procedures, *Compend Contin Educ Dent* 1:161, 1980.
59. Rufenache CR: *Fundamentals of esthetics,* Chicago, 1990, Quintessence.
60. Sillness J: Treated with dental bridges. III. The relationship between the location of the crown margin and the periodontal condition, *J Periodontal Res* 5:225, 1970.
61. Smith DM, McLachlan KR, McCall WD Jr: A numerical model of temporomandibular joint loading, *J Dent Res* 65:1046, 1986.
62. Spear FM: Maintenance of the interdental papilla following anterior tooth removal, *Pract Periodont Aesthet Dent* 11:21, 1999.
63. Spear FM, Mathews DM, Kokich VG: Interdisciplinary treatment: integrating orthodontics with periodontics, endodontics, and restorative dentistry, *Semin Orthodont* 3(1), 1997.
64. Stein RS: Pontic-residual ridge relationship: a research report, *J Prosthet Dent* 16:251, 1966.
65. Studer S, Zellweger U, Scharer P: The esthetic guidelines of the mucogingival complex for fixed prosthodontics, *Pract Periodont Aesthet Dent* 8:333, 1996.
66. Suvinen T, Hanes K, Gerchman J, et al: Psychophysical subtypes of temporomandibular disorders, *J Orofac Pain* 11:200, 1997.
67. Swartz ML, Phillips RW: Comparison of bacterial accumulations on rough and smooth surfaces, *J Periodontol* 28:304, 1957.
68. Tarnow DP, Magner AW, Fletcher P: The effects of the distance from the contact point to the crest of bone on the presence or absence of the interproximal dental papilla, *J Periodontol* 63:995, 1992.
69. Townsend CL: Resective surgery: an esthetic application, *Quintessence Int* 24:535, 1993.
70. Tylman SD: *Theory and practice of crown and bridge prosthodontics,* ed 5, St Louis, 1965, Mosby.
71. Vacek JS, Gher ME, Assad DA, et al: The dimensions of the human dentogingival junction, *Int J Periodont Restor Dent* 14:155, 1994.
72. Vallon D: Studies of occlusion adjustment therapy in patients with craniomandibular disorders, Malmö, Lund University (thesis), *Swed Dent J,* suppl 124, 1997.
73. Van der Veldon U: Regeneration of the interdental soft tissue following denudation procedures, *J Clin Periodontol* 9:455, 1982.
74. Wood DP, Elliott RW: Reproducibility of the centric relation bite registration technique, *Angle Orthod* 64:211, 1994.
75. Yuodelis RA, Faucher R: Provisional restorations: an integrated approach to periodontics and restorative dentistry, *Dent Clin North Am* 24:285, 1980.
76. Yuodelis RA, Weaver JD, Sapko S: Facial and lingual contours of artificial complete crowns and their effect on the periodontium, *J Prosthet Dent* 29:61, 1973.

PART

8

Oral Implantology

Perry R. Klokkevold

The success and predictability of osseointegrated dental implants have forever changed the philosophy and practice of dentistry and, perhaps more than any other specialty, periodontics has changed dramatically. In the past two decades, there has been a paradigm shift in periodontics from the philosophy of saving teeth at all costs (albeit compromised) to one of extracting compromised teeth and replacing them with dental implants for a better and more predictable long-term outcome. All health care professionals, including but not limited to those who practice dentistry, dental specialties, and dental hygiene, today are compelled to become knowledgeable in all aspects of dental implant therapy and to continue their education as new information and evidence becomes available.

The chapters in Part 8 comprehensively present several important implant-related topics including biology, diagnosis, clinical evaluation, and surgical techniques. Biomechanics, treatment planning, prosthetics, and complications are covered as well. Readers are encouraged to consult the e-dition online version of *Carranza's Clinical Periodontology* for updates and additional learning modules.

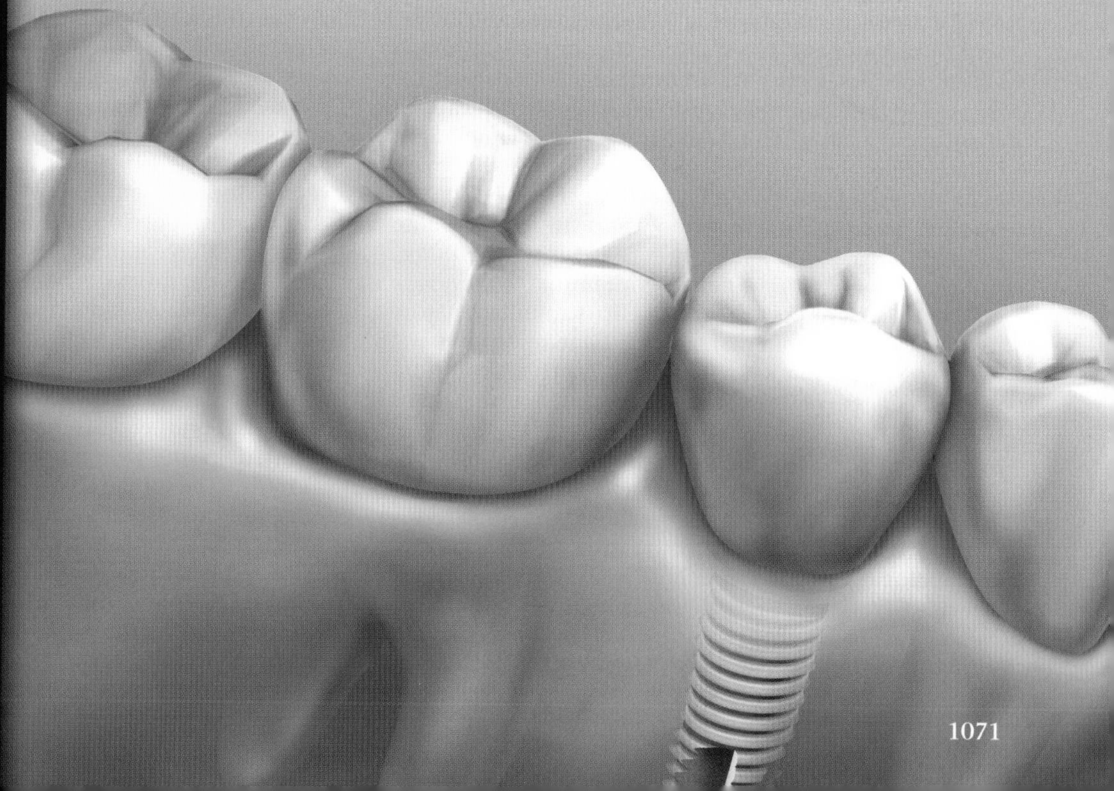

Biological Aspects of Oral Implants

Daniel van Steenberghe, Marina Maréchal, and Marc Quirynen

73

CHAPTER

Chapter Outline

The ability to rehabilitate an amputated limb or tooth by means of a bone-anchored substitute, or *prosthesis,* is a traditional endeavor. Although socket prostheses offer a comfortable solution both for amputated limbs and edentulism, many patients complain about soft tissue irritation and instability (Figure 73-1). Initial attempts at intraosseous anchorage failed because a soft tissue scar interposed between the bone and the implanted material allowed the downgrowth of epithelium (skin or mucosa), a phenomenon called *marsupialization.* Indigenous bacteria quickly contaminate the deep epithelial tracts or pockets, which elicits an inflammatory reaction with the potential to cause bone resorption and loosening of the implant (Figure 73-2). This gave (non-osseointegrated) endosseous implants (used intraorally) a bad reputation in medicine, dentistry, and the public at large. Indeed, the chronic infections and loss of jawbone often resulted in mutilations (Figure 73-3).

The lack of understanding about the underlying biology led many investigators to attempt new implant morphologies, which sometimes seemed "baroque art." The idea was that the complex retentive morphology would lead to a sufficient anchorage by bone growing into the convoluted spaces. Others believed that the quest for new biocompatible materials would offer the proper solution. By a trial-and-error approach on patients, titanium alloys, "precious" metals, ceramic materials, and carbons were used. Although the biocompatibility was definitely present, it did not lead to an intimate bone apposition on the implant surface. The quest continued.

In the late 1950s, Per-Ingvar Brånemark, a Swedish professor in anatomy studying blood circulation in bone and marrow, developed through a serendipitous finding a historical breakthrough in medicine: he predictably achieved an intimate bone-to-implant apposition that offered sufficient strength to cope with load transfer. He called the phenomenon "osseointegration."[15] The first patient was treated by means of this approach for a lower edentulous jaw in 1965.[16,46] A series of screw-shaped, commercially pure titanium implants were inserted in the symphysis and left covered for a few months. The gingival and mucosal tissues were then reopened, and titanium abutments were placed, on top of which a fixed prosthesis could be screwed. All implants appeared firmly anchored.

Since that time, millions of patients have been treated worldwide using this technique. The implants used sometimes had different geometries and surface characteristics.

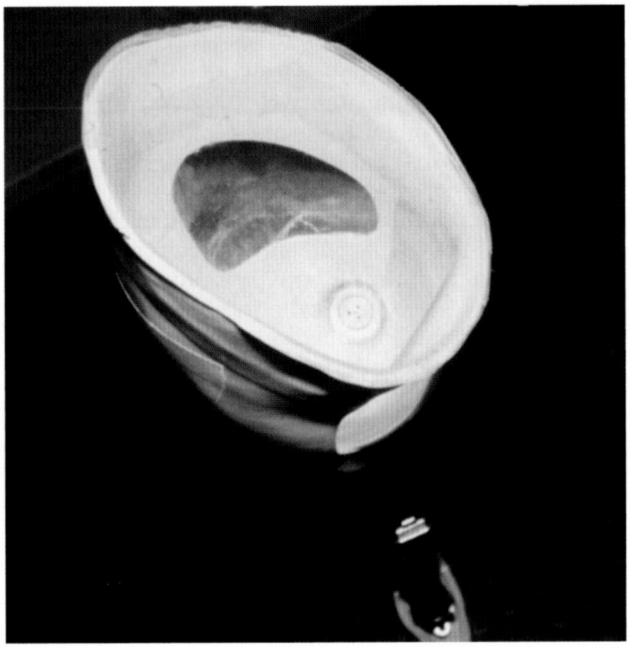

Figure 73-1 Socket prosthesis for a limb is similar to a complete denture in that it has a soft tissue interface, and a peripheral seal creates a vacuum for retention.

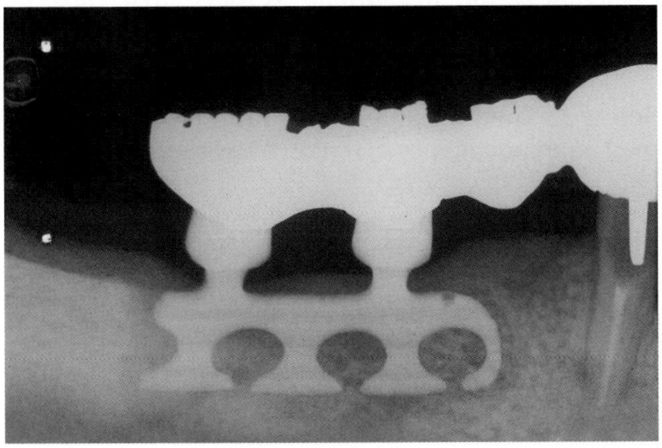

Figure 73-2 Blade implant shows a large radiolucency, indicating that the fibrous encapsulation has led to deep pocketing and subsequent bone loss. Neighboring teeth bear the load of the implant restoration.

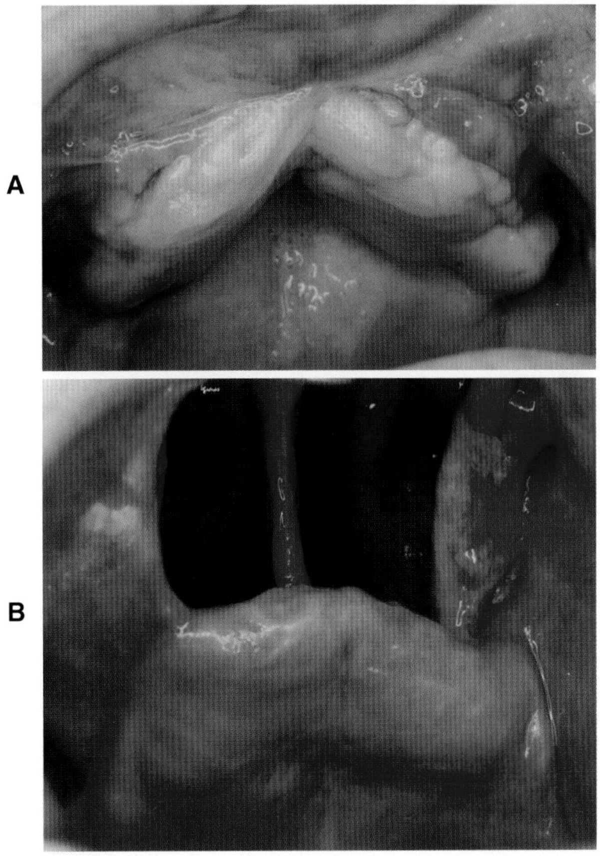

Figure 73-3 Clinical photographs of destruction caused by infection and removal of infected implants. The removal of non–root form, macroscopically retentive implants such as blades or subperiosteal implants can result in severe mutilation of the jawbone. **A,** Deformed maxilla resulting from an infected subperiosteal implant. **B,** Another patient lost a substantial portion of the anterior maxilla and nasal floor as a result of infections and removal of a subperiosteal implant. (Courtesy Dr. John Beumer, University of California, Los Angeles.)

Similar research followed, including that of André Schroeder in Switzerland in the mid-1970s. The serendipitous finding of Brånemark was that when a hole is prepared into bone without overheating or otherwise traumatizing the tissues, an inserted biocompatible implantable device would predictably achieve an intimate bone apposition as long as micromovements at the interface were prevented during the early healing period. The history of the research endeavors in Sweden provides a better understanding of the relevant biologic parameters involved.[46]

This chapter reviews the basic biology of the implant-tissue interface down to the cellular level, with a constant perspective on the clinical implications of the relationship. This discussion illustrates that biologic principles are common to all parts of the body, regardless of whether it is intraoral or extraoral.

IMPLANT GEOMETRY (MACRODESIGN)

The macroscopic configuration of implants has varied widely; the most common types are listed in Box 73-1. Currently, most endosseous implants have a cylindrical or tapered, screw-shaped, threaded design. The disastrous results with other implant configurations were largely responsible for the evolution toward the current popular designs.[5]

Endosseous Implants

Blade Implants. Blade implants, as associated with Linkow, were inserted into the jawbone after mucoperiosteal flap elevation. They were tapped in place in a

BOX 73-1

Implant Geometry (Macro design)

1. Endosseous implants
   - Bladelike
   - Pins
   - Cylindrical (hollow and full)
   - Disklike
   - Screw shaped
   - Tapered and screw shaped
2. Subperiosteal framelike implants
3. Transmandibular implants

narrow trench made with a rotary bur. One or several posts pierced through the mucoperiosteum after suturing of the flaps. After a few weeks of healing, a fixed prosthesis was fabricated by a classic method and cemented on top of it.

Because the high-speed drilling leads to ample bone necrosis at the histologic level, fibrous scar tissue formation occurs. This allows downgrowth of the epithelium, which leads to marsupialization of the blade implants (see Figure 73-2).[36] If a bacterial infection occurs, it can lead to an intractable periimplantitis with ample bone loss. More importantly, removal of such implants after complications implies sacrificing surrounding jawbone. Because of its retentive geometry, the blade implant cannot simply be extracted or removed by a trephine, as with a cylindrical or screw-shaped implant.

Pins. Although seldom used at present, in the classic technique, three diverging pins were inserted either transgingivally or after reflection of mucoperiosteal flaps in holes drilled by spiral drills. At the point of convergence, the pins were interconnected with cement to ensure the proper stability because of their divergence. On top of this arrangement, a single tooth could be installed. In edentulous jaws, several of these pin triads could be used to interconnect with a fixed prosthesis.

As with blade implants, the bone necrosis during drilling leads to fibrous encapsulation, marsupialization, and loss of the implants because of infections. A positive aspect, however, is that when such implants must be removed, removing the connection at the place of convergence is sufficient to allow easy extraction of each individual pin. Thus, bone loss from removal is minimal.

Cylindrical Implants. When discussing cylindrical implants, it is important to distinguish between *hollow* and *full* cylindrical implants. Straumann and co-workers introduced hollow cylinders in the mid-1970s with the ITI (International Team for Implantology) system.[67] The idea was that implant stability would benefit from the large bone-to-implant surface provided by means of the hollow geometry. It was also thought that the holes (vents) would favor the ingrowth of bone to offer additional fixation. The same concept was used in the Core-Vent system developed by Niznick.[50] Although it was not clarified whether the cause was geometry or the associated surface characteristics (titanium plasma–sprayed surface, titanium alloy), survival statistics were disappointing with the hollow cylinders.[73]

Full cylindrical implants were used by Kirsch and became available under the name *IMZ,* referring to the "internal mobile shock absorber."[40] Although early results were encouraging, especially in the symphyseal area, the long-term survival rates became unacceptable,[27] leading to the limited use of this implant type currently.

Even when an intimate bone apposition is achieved, extraction forces on such cylindrical implants lead to strong shear forces at the bone-to-implant interface. Only the microscopic surface irregularities offer some mechanical retention by interdigitation of bone growing onto the implant surface. With a screw-based geometry, forces acting parallel to the long axis of the implants are dispersed in many directions.[64]

Disk Implants. Disk implants are rarely used at present. The concept developed by Scortecci[62] is based on the lateral introduction into the jawbone of a pin with a disk on top. Once introduced into the bone volume, therefore, the implant has strong retention against extraction forces. Implants have been used with one, two, and even three disks. Unfortunately, as mentioned previously for blade implants, the cutting of the bone by means of high-speed drills leads to a fibrous scar tissue surrounding the implant, as revealed frequently by periimplant radiolucencies. Data on the clinical success of disk implants are mostly anecdotal.

Screw-Shaped (Tapered) Implants. Currently, the most common implant is the screw-shaped, threaded implant. Even systems that started with cylindrical geometries (hollow or not) progressively adopted screw-shaped implants, as discussed in detail in this chapter. Mostly on the basis of in vitro or finite element analysis studies, discussion is ongoing about the ideal thread profile, despite very good long-term (>15 years) clinical data available for a screw-shaped implant (Brånemark system).[45] For example, a decrease in interthread distance at the coronal end of the implant has been proposed to enhance the marginal bone level adaptation.[30]

Tapered implant forms have been used primarily because they require less space in the apical region, a relevant issue in some partially edentulous patients (i.e., between roots that approximate one another) and areas such as the anterior maxilla where apical concavities are common. No clinical data tend to support a superior success rate with tapered versus straight oral implants. In fact, some clinicians have experienced a higher incidence of non-integration with tapered implants. Presumably, the problems with a tapered implant result from a poor fit in the osteotomy site at the time of implant placement (e.g., implant too loose or too tight as a result of the vertical placement position being different than the vertical preparation of bone.)

Subperiosteal Implants

Subperiosteal implants are customized according to a plaster model derived from an impression of the exposed jawbone, prior to the surgery planned for implant insertion. Several posts, typically four or more for an edentulous jaw, are passed through the gingival tissues.[3] Subperiosteal implants are designed to retain an overdenture, although fixed prostheses have also been cemented onto the posts. As a result of epithelial migration, the framework of subperiosteal implants usually becomes surrounded by fibrous connective tissue (scar), including the space between the implant and the bone surface. The marsupialization, as described earlier, often leads to infectious complications, which often necessitates removal of the implant. Furthermore, while being loaded by jaw function, jawbone resorption occurs rapidly, resulting in a lack of adaptation of the frame to the bone surface. As a result of this type of outcome, subperiosteal implants are now rarely used.

Transmandibular Implants

Transmandibular implants were developed to retain dentures in the edentulous lower jaw. The implant was applied through a submandibular skin incision and required general anesthesia. Two models were available. The first, called the "Staple-Bone" implant, developed by Small, consisted of a splint adapted to the lower border of the mandible, to which it is fixed by stabilizing pins.[65] Two transmandibular screws were driven transgingivally into the mouth. The reported implant survival rate exceeded 90% after 15 years.[66] The other model, introduced by Bosker, has two metal splints, one below the lower border of the mandible and one intraorally to connect the four posts piercing through the soft tissues.[14] Despite the good long-term survival data reported for the Staple-Bone model, these transmandibular implants are rarely used at present. The Bosker implant seemed less reliable, achieving only 70% survival after 5 years in the symphyseal areas.[73]

IMPLANT SURFACE CHARACTERISTICS (MICRODESIGN)

A key element in the reaction of hard and soft tissues to an implant involves the implant's surface characteristics, that is, the chemical and physical properties. Some materials are not suitable for implantation because they have toxic cellular side effects. Some materials are biocompatible because they do not provoke an immune reaction and are "passive" toward the tissue-healing process (i.e., they do not cause adverse reactions, and they do not cause reactions that promote healing). On the other hand, some materials, as well as various surface characteristics, enhance bone apposition at the implant surface in an osteoconductive manner.

Before Brånemark clarified the proper surgical steps to be taken to obtain an intimate bone-to-implant contact, known as *osseointegration,* researchers focused on surface characteristics to obtain bone apposition. The quest was for biocompatible if not bioactive surfaces, achieved through additive or subtractive processes. Titanium, preferably commercially pure titanium, became the standard for endosseous implants both in orthopedics and in periodontology. Actually, titanium is a very reactive material that would not become integrated in tissues. However, its instantaneous surface oxidation creates a *passivation layer* of titanium oxides, which have ceramic-like properties, making it very compatible with tissues.

Additive Processes

The chemical nature of the implant surface can be modified dramatically by coating its surface. Calcium phosphates, especially *hydroxyapatite,* have been a popular coating material because of its resemblance to bone tissue. The content of this hydroxyapatite seems to be crucial; in vitro studies demonstrated that the cell response, exemplified by osteoblasts, varies according to the calcium-to-phosphate ratio and impurities.[11]

Another line of research used increased or modified *titanium oxide* (TiO_2) layers to enhance or accelerate the bone formation.[32] This is achieved by anodizing or chemical processing. The oxide content of the TiO_2 layer is essential for nucleation processes to form calcium phosphate precipitates, which lead to mineralized bone formation. Another line of research involves integrating fluoride in the TiO_2 layer. These ions can be displaced by oxygen originating from phosphates, thus achieving a covalent binding between bone and implant surface.[28] Fluoride release is also known to inhibit the adhesion of proteoglycans and glycoproteins on the hydroxyapatite surface, two macromolecules known to inhibit mineralization.[22] Besides this chemical change, surface additives primarily modify the microstructure of the implant surface, which influences adhesion of molecules and cells. The latter implant characteristics, with "micro-roughness" as a predominant aspect, are often the result of subtractive processes during manufacturing.

Subtractive Processes

The manufacturing processes to obtain a proper implant surface vary from machining (called "turned" for screw-shaped implants) to acid etching and blasting. Sometimes a combination of these processes is used. It is not known what degree of micro-roughness is ideal for bone adhesion; this depends greatly on the chemical nature of the implant.[21] Acid etching and blasting alter the micro-roughness of the implant surface. Their effect cannot be limited to this, however, because these processes can also modify the surface chemistry to a certain extent. Nevertheless, their impact on surface roughness predominates, which is why they are applied.

HARD TISSUE INTERFACE

Stages of Bone Healing and Osseointegration: Cell Kinetics and Tissue Remodeling

Any bone wounding leads to an inflammatory reaction with bone resorption and subsequently the activation of growth factors and attraction by chemotaxis of osteoprogenitor cells to the site of the lesion. The differentiation toward osteoblasts will lead to a reparative bone formation, which, in the case of a bone fracture, will lead

SCIENCE TRANSFER

The evaluation of implant design has ranged from the original flat, platelike designs such as blade implants to the cylindrical or tapered screw-shaped implants. The material that offers the best biologic attachment to bone and gingival tissue is titanium, which always has a layer of titanium oxide responsible for osseointegration. New surface technologies improve the early deposition of bone around implants primarily through an increase in the surface area by roughening the outer layers of the implant and an increase in the thickness of the titanium oxide layer. The next generation of implants will likely incorporate biologically active agents that stimulate osteoprogenitor cells to differentiate into osteoblasts and quickly lay down dense bone.

The ability of a titanium rod to integrate into bone tissue depends greatly on the host reaction to the surgical insult at the time of bone preparation and on the ability to stabilize the rod during the early wound-healing stage. A threshold appears to exist in which bone tissue repair is impossible. This is often attributed to irreparable bone cell necrosis but may involve other factors, including compromised blood supply and extracellular matrix modification resulting in fibrous tissue proliferation and blood clot stability, but these possible mechanisms are rarely mentioned. Similarly, a threshold may also exist in the amount of stability required of the implant in the early wound-healing process. Again, much attention is focused on the amount of movement allowed for bone healing, but the mechanisms to explain such results are rarely cited. Does the lack of stability only inhibit clot formation and stability, or does it also prevent angiogenesis and chemotaxis of cells or signals for such cellular activity? Future research should focus on such scientific principles rather than proprietary concerns.

to fusion of both ends. In the case of an implant insertion into a prepared hole, this will lead to bone apposition onto the implant surface if the latter is nontoxic. A "coupling" occurs between bone resorption and bone formation; the latter can occur only if an intercellular matrix is produced that favors apatite crystal integration in the collagen network. For example, osteocalcin, an extracellular matrix protein, modulates apatite crystal growth.[77]

The osseointegration process observed after implant insertion can be compared to bone fracture healing. Logically, a certain immobility of the implant surface toward the bone should be maintained. A mild inflammatory response, as triggered by movements or appropriate electrical stimuli, may enhance the bone-healing response, but above a certain threshold, this is detrimental.[2] It has been reported that when micromovements at the interface exceed 150 μm, differentiation to osteoblasts will not occur; rather, a fibrous scar tissue is laid down between the bone and implant surface.[74] Therefore, avoiding such forces as occlusal load during the early healing period seems to be a safe approach. If the neighboring bone has been overheated or crushed during drilling, however, the necrotic area will prevent ingrowth of stem cells, and a scar formation or sequestered formation will result. The critical temperature for bone cells is as low as 47° C at an exposure time of 1 minute. This corresponds to the denaturing temperature of alkaline phosphatase, the main bone cell enzyme.[23] Implant placement thus implies profuse cooling with intermittent moderate-speed drilling with sharp drills. Another complicating factor, well recognized from open wound fractures, is that microbial contamination jeopardizes the normal bone repair. Thus, when oral implants are placed, strict aseptic techniques should be maintained.

The limited damage to bone tissue must be cleared up by osteoclasts before the bone healing. These multinuclear cells, originating from the blood, can resorb bone at a pace of 50 to 100 μm per day. There is a coupling between bone apposition and bone resorption (Figures 73-4 and 73-5). The preosteoblasts, derived from the invading primary mesenchymal cells, depend on a favorable oxidation-reduction (redox) potential of the environment. Thus a proper vascular supply and oxygen tension are needed. This explains why, in the case of compromised oxygen supply, such as after local radiotherapy, hyperbaric oxygen therapy can be a key issue.[26] If the favorable conditions are not met because of one of the interfering factors previously cited, the primary stem cells may differentiate into fibroblasts, and the implant (or the bone fracture surfaces) will be facing scar tissue. Although this may be acceptable for endosseous implants, such as femoral implants, oral implants will eventually be connected to the outer environment with the potential for infection.

First, *woven bone* is quickly formed in the gap between the implant and the bone. Second, after several months, this is progressively replaced by *lamellar bone* under the load stimulation. Third, a steady state is reached after about 1½ years (Figure 73-6). Often, for oral implants,

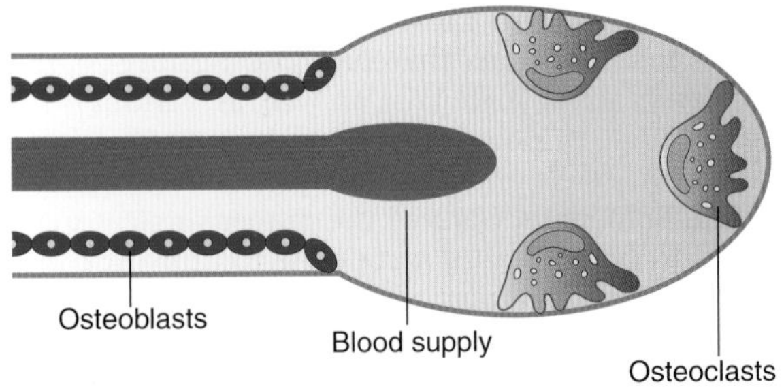

Figure 73-4 The basic multicellular unit is the basic remodeling process for bone renewal. Osteoclasts are imported by the vascular supply, and the resorption lacunae are soon filled by the lining osteoblasts.

occlusal load is allowed as soon as 2 to 3 months, while mostly woven bone is present.

Woven bone grows fast, up to 100 μm per day, and in all directions. It is characterized by a random orientation of its collagen fibrils, high cellularity, and limited degree of mineralization. Limited mineralization means that the bone's biomechanical capacity is poor, and thus occlusal load should be controlled. Woven bone can grow by apposition, originating from the bone lesion or by conduction, using the implant surface as a scaffold. The implant surface characteristics, such as material properties, surface free energy, and roughness profile, are determining factors that influence bone apposition. Altered implant surface topographies, such as those created by acid etching, blasting, combinations of acid etching and blasting, or increasing the titanium oxide layer appear to result in greater bone apposition to the implant surface as compared to a "turned" or machined surface.

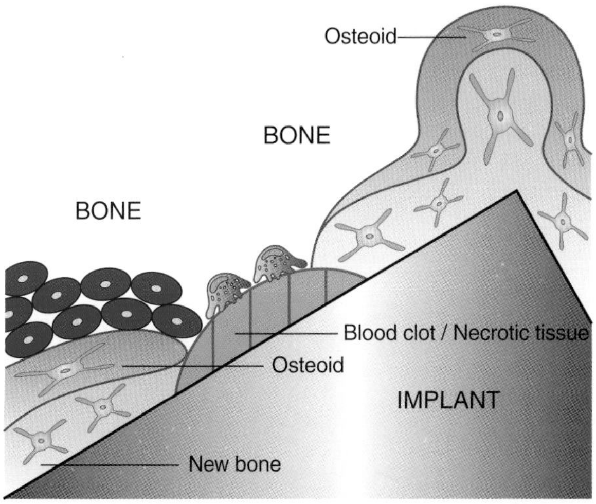

Figure 73-5 After insertion of an implant, slight tissue necrosis may result from surgical trauma. This tissue or the interposed blood clot is removed by the multinucleated osteoclasts and is replaced by osteoid (poorly mineralized) bone, which will then become woven and later lamellar bone.

After 1 to 2 months, under the effect of load, the woven bone surrounding the implant will slowly transform into lamellar bone. Parallel layers of collagen fibrils characterize the latter, each with their own orientation, which explains the typical polarized light aspect. Contrary to the fast growing woven bone, lamellar bone apposition occurs at a slow pace of a few microns per day.

An ongoing debate concerns the nature of the established bone-to-implant interface. At the light microscopic level, an intimate bone-to-implant contact has been reported extensively[60] (Figure 73-7). Depending on the bone type at the implantation site and on the type of implant surface, large variations exist in the percentage of the implant surface that actually contacts mineralized trabeculae. The remaining interface consists of vessels and bone marrow. Such analysis should also consider *time.* Thus, some implant surfaces may have an exponential bone apposition to stabilize after some time, whereas others may demonstrate a linear increase over months. Some eventually show a full coating of the implant surface by bone.

At the ultrastructural level, some doubt remains. Some claimed that only an ultrathin (about 10 nm) amorphous layer of proteoglycan exists between the implant surface and the structured bone, with no interposed fibrous tissue.[43] Others presented some evidence of interposition,

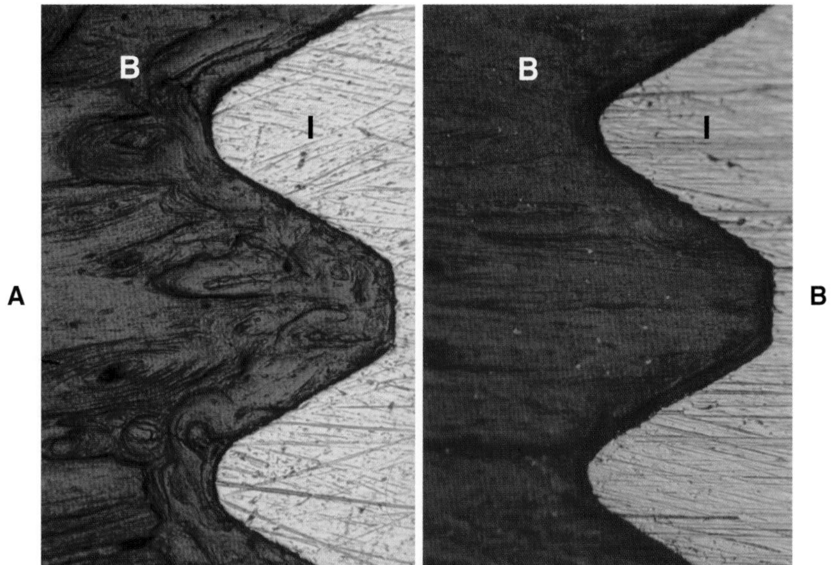

Figure 73-6 **A,** After initial healing, woven bone, as characterized by its irregular pattern, is laid down. **B,** After weeks or months, progressively a lamellar bone is laid down, with regular concentric lamellae. *B,* Bone; *I,* implant. (Courtesy Prof. T. Albrektsson, Gothenburg, Sweden.)

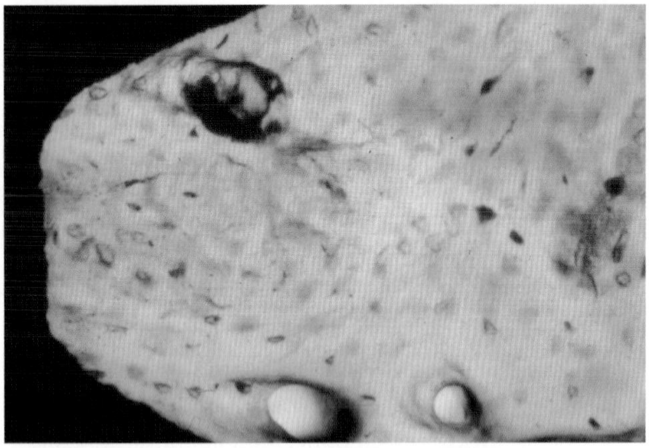

Figure 73-7 Once a steady state has been achieved at the bone-to-implant interface, an intimate contact can be observed, with some marrow spaces seen in between at the light microscopic level.

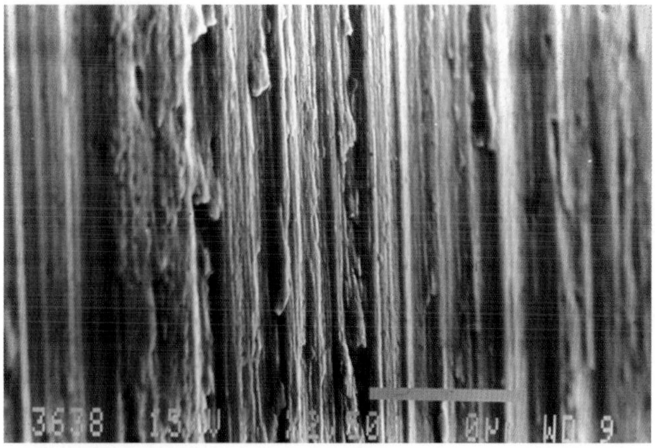

Figure 73-8 Even turned, or machined, implant surfaces are not "smooth." Scanning electron microscopic view of a Brånemark system implant. (Courtesy Nobel Biocare, Gothenburg, Sweden.)

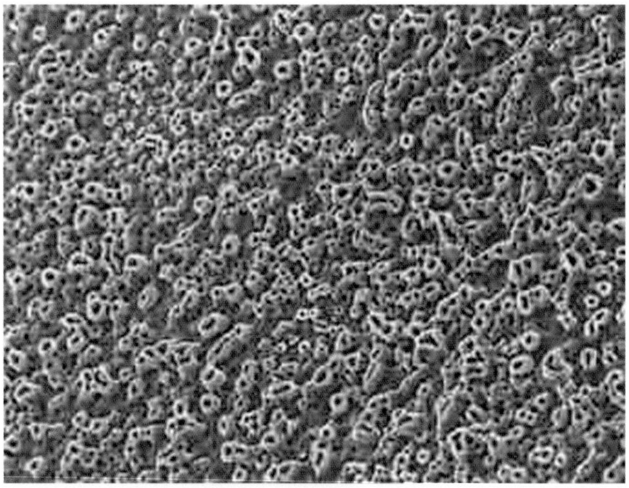

Figure 73-9 Roughened surfaces are achieved by plasma spraying, by acid etching, or as shown here, by oxidizing (TiUnite surface). (Courtesy Nobel Biocare, Gothenburg, Sweden.)

which may be caused by fracture artifacts.[68] The conflicting data were often presented at meetings, but were not published in peer-reviewed journals.

Once the bone-to-implant interface has reached a steady state, it can maintain itself over decades, as histologically ascertained from implants retrieved because of hardware fractures.[6]

Implant Surface Free Energy and Micro-Roughness

When an implant is brought into bodily tissues, in this case mostly bone, it faces a "bioliquid," an aqueous environment. Within milliseconds, water, ions, and small biomolecules are absorbed. One could imagine that this absorbed layer renders all surfaces equal. However, the large molecules and the cells that will subsequently adhere to this surface are influenced by the surface characteristics of this pellicle layer. The composition and structure of the initial layer are largely determined by the underlying surface.[59] Thus the three-dimensional shape of the molecules will be modified during their adherence to this pellicle layer and will unveil different radicals depending on this metamorphosis.

The *surface free energy,* often called "wettability," is an important parameter for these interactions. It can be assessed through the shape of a standardized drop of liquid put on the clean implant surface. The angle of this drop toward the underlying surface reveals that the cohesive forces between liquid molecules are stronger than the adhesive forces between the liquid and the surface. Thus a ball-shaped drop would reveal a low surface free energy.

Surface topography, at the cellular and molecular level, means microscopic roughness. A surface roughness can be measured with a *profilometer,* a stylus that follows the surface and measures the peak-to-valley dimensions (expressed as Ra values) or the spacing between irregularities (expressed as Scx values) (for review, see Wennerberg[76]). No implant surface is smooth, although several reports have incorrectly referred to the "turned" (machined) implant surface as "smooth" (Figure 73-8). Roughened implant surfaces speed up the bone apposition; as demonstrated in vitro, more prostaglandin E_2 (PGE_2) and transforming growth factor beta (TGF-β1) are produced on roughened than on smoother surfaces.[39] Roughened surfaces also show some disadvantages, such as increased ion leakage and increased adherence of macrophages and subsequent bone resorption[49] (Figure 73-9).

It was also reported that in vitro adsorption of fibronectin was higher on smooth than on roughened, commercially pure titanium surfaces.[24] Fibronectin is a glycoprotein quickly adhering on hard surfaces and known to determine subsequent cell adhesion.[53] Microtopography also influences the number and morphology of cell adhesion pseudopods and cell orientation.[31] Grooves in an implant surface will guide the cell migration

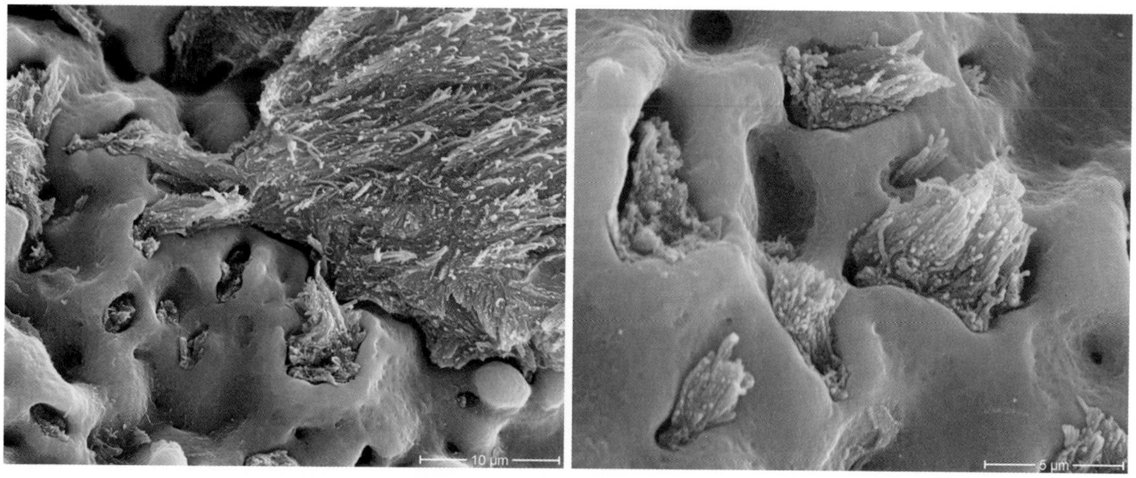

Figure 73-10 Even minute pores allow bone deposition. These scanning electron microscopic views show pore sizes of this TiUnite surface reach a few microns only. Apatite crystals deposition is evident in the oxide layer. (Courtesy Drs. Peter Schüpbach and Roland Glauser, University of Zurich, Zurich, Switzerland.)

along their direction. Bone growth can enter altered microtopographic features such as pits and porosities with internal dimensions that are only a few microns (Figure 73-10).

Implant Surface Chemical Composition

There have been unsuccessful trials with oral implants made of carbon or hydroxyapatite. Their lack of resistance, because of material properties, to the important occlusal forces led to frequent fractures. So-called noble metals or alloys, on the other hand, do not resist corrosion and have thus been abandoned. Because the vast majority of oral implants are made of commercially pure (c.p.) titanium, this type is the focus of this discussion.

Titanium is a very reactive metal that oxidizes within nanoseconds when exposed to air. Because of this passive oxide layer, the titanium then becomes very resistant to corrosion in its c.p. form. The alloys such as Ti6Al4V (for titanium-aluminum 6%, vanadium 4%) are known to provoke bone resorption because of leakage of some toxic components. The oxide layer of c.p. titanium reaches 10 nm of thickness. It grows over the years when facing a bioliquid. It consists mainly of titanium dioxide.

All titanium oxides have dielectric constants, which are higher than for most other metal oxides. This may be a crucial factor to explain titanium's tendency to adsorb biomolecules, as seen during surgery when the blood creeps up the implant surface while the implant is being inserted. The biomolecules normally appear as folded-up structures to hide their nonsoluble parts, while putting water-soluble radicals on their surface. Thus, they will adhere to the TiO_2 surface after displacing the original water molecules sitting on its surface. Although initially the weak van der Waals forces are acting, the high dielectric constant of titanium oxides and the polarizability of the molecules after adsorption will lead to high bond strengths, which are considered irreversible when they surpass 30 kcal/mol.[38] In fact, because of its propensity for being covered by an uninterrupted oxide layer, which has ceramic-like properties similar to other metal oxides (e.g., aluminum oxides), titanium makes the coating of implants superfluous. This should be stressed because many authors hope for even better osseointegration potential with calcium phosphate (CaP)–coated surfaces and strongly advocate their use. To date, clinical results with CaP-coated implants have not been encouraging in a long-term perspective.[12]

Thus the overall view of potential advantages for different implant surface characteristics is complex, and only clinical observations can determine their validity. For good-quality bone, after 15 years of follow-up, clinical success rates of 99% have been reported for implants with a turned surface.[45] Enhanced implant surface characteristics are likely to be most beneficial for the more challenging situations, such as poor-quality bone and early and immediate loading.

Rigidity and Strength of Established Bone-to-Implant Interface

Bone has a limited elasticity, with an elasticity modulus of about 10 gigapascals (GPa)/m^2 for the cortex and 1 to 5 GPa/m^2 for cancellous bone. The rigidity of a c.p. titanium screw-shaped implant, however, is about 100 GPa/m^2. These are only indicative values because large variations occur depending on the location and bone status of the subject. Thus, at the interface between implants and bone, even when a strong lamellar bone apposition has occurred, differences in elasticity are present.

Both the primary stability and the secondary stability of an implant determine its success and survival. *Primary stability* is that achieved at surgery. It depends on the bone quality and available volume, the relation between drill and implant diameter, and the implant geometry. The quantity of bone-to-implant contact area is a well-known parameter. Dense cortical bone, as often encountered in the symphyseal area, easily guarantees a rigid primary fixation, whereas this becomes questionable with an eggshell cortex in the maxillary tuberosity. This is reflected in the poorer clinical outcome observed for implants in the posterior maxilla.[7] In addition to the cortical bone, where a bicortical contact favors immobiliy,[72] the degree of mineralization of the trabecular bone should be considered. An established relationship exists between a low bone mineral density and implant rigidity. The role of compressive stresses at the implant-to-bone interface should not be neglected. By using an undersized drill in soft bone for preparation of the osteotomy site, the implant insertion, either by screwing or by "press-fit," achieves a slight local compression, which enhances the initial stability of the implant. This can result in hoop stresses, which, depending on their level, are either favoring bone apposition or leading to necrosis because of the compromised vascular supply and microfractures. At the bone-implant interface, once osseointegration has been achieved, both compressive and tensile stresses occur. Compact bone has a compressive strength of 100 to 200 megapascals (MPa), whereas for cancellous bone this reaches only 5 to 6 MPa.

Little is known about the fate of the bone-to-implant interface during the first days and weeks after surgery. Longitudinal biomechanical assessments seem to indicate that during the first weeks for one-stage implants, decreased rigidity can be observed.[25] Subsequently, rigidity increases and continues to increase for years.[69] This may reveal early bone resorption, which then questions the value of the initial biomechanical implant stability as previously described. Thus, when a prosthesis is installed immediately (in 1 day) or early (in 1-2 weeks), care must be taken to control against overload. Furthermore, it is established that the tactile sensation associated with endosseous implants is limited in the early stages.[34]

Overload, because of improper superstructure design or parafunctional habits, may cause microstrains and microfractures, which will lead to a bone loss of the bone at the interface to fibrous inflammatory tissue.[70] The threshold also depends on the bone mineral density. Several studies have indicated a higher failure rate after occlusal load is applied to implants in so-called poor-quality bone.[37]

Lack of load can also be detrimental and can lead to cortical bone resorption. This is well documented in orthopedics and termed "stress shielding."[33] This phenomenon has not been properly evaluated for oral implants where marginal bone resorption is thought to be associated with chronic inflammation of the overlying soft tissues.

The use of *finite element analysis* (FEA) has become popular but lacks value by itself; invalid assumptions, such as the isotropic nature of the bone (which it evidently is not), must be used in the modeling. The deviation of FEA data from in vivo data has been well documented.[47] FEA data should be considered "descriptive" models that require confirmation by biologic data.[20] However, as with photoelastic studies, FEA analyses do provide some insight on stress concentrations and their relation to implant geometry and rigidity and the prosthetic superstructures.

Assessment of implant biomechanics can easily be done at the clinical level by noninvasive devices such as the Periotest (Figure 73-11) and the Ostell (Figure 73-12). The Periotest (Gulden, Bensheim, Germany) projects a rod against the implant or abutment using a magnetic pulse at a certain speed. The apparatus measures the deceleration time needed before the rod comes to a standstill. This is transformed in an arbitrary unit, which reflects the rigidity of the bone-to-implant continuum.[51] Values should be below +7, the minimum, with the most rigid being −8. Osseointegrated implants are thought to demonstrate an increased rigidity over time.[71] The *resonance frequency analysis* (RFA) offers an alternative measurement.[48] With the Ostell device, a small transducer attached to the implant imposes a series of frequencies and measures the overall resonance frequency. Because the transducer and the structure are constant, any change in the resonance frequency reveals a change in the implant-bone interface, either in quality or in quantity. Primary stability measurements reveal a

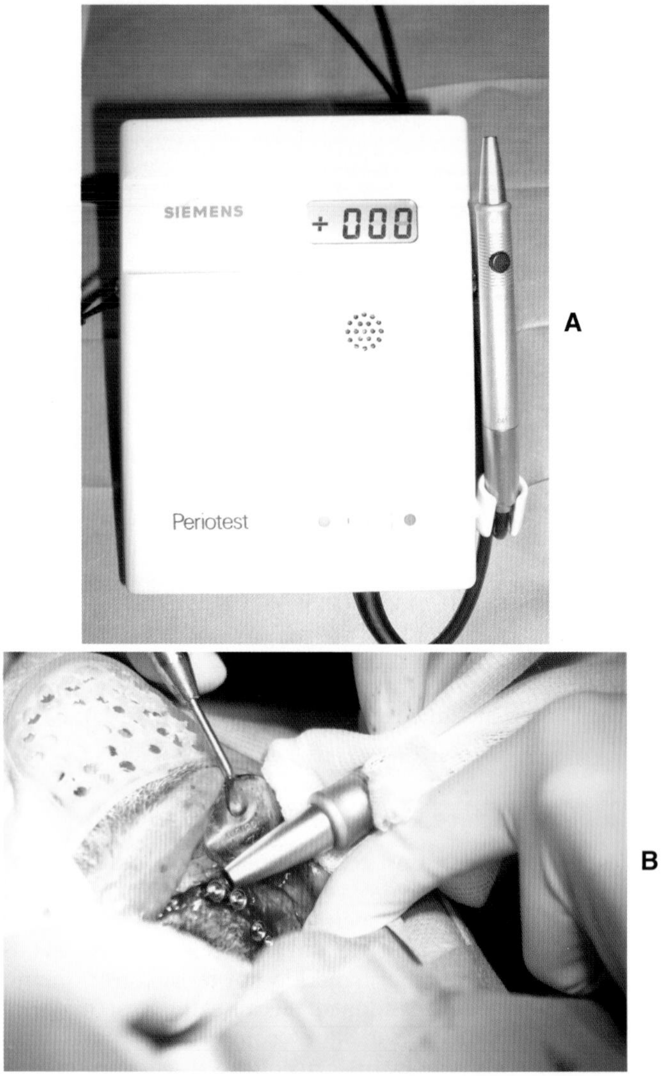

Figure 73-11 **A,** Periotest electronic apparatus (presently made by Gulden, Bensheim, Germany) provides objective means to measure endosseous implant rigidity. **B,** Periotest measurement performed at surgery to evaluate the increasing rigidity at future control visits.

A

B

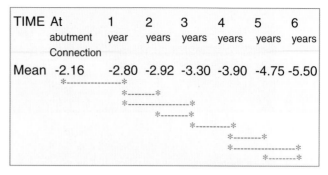

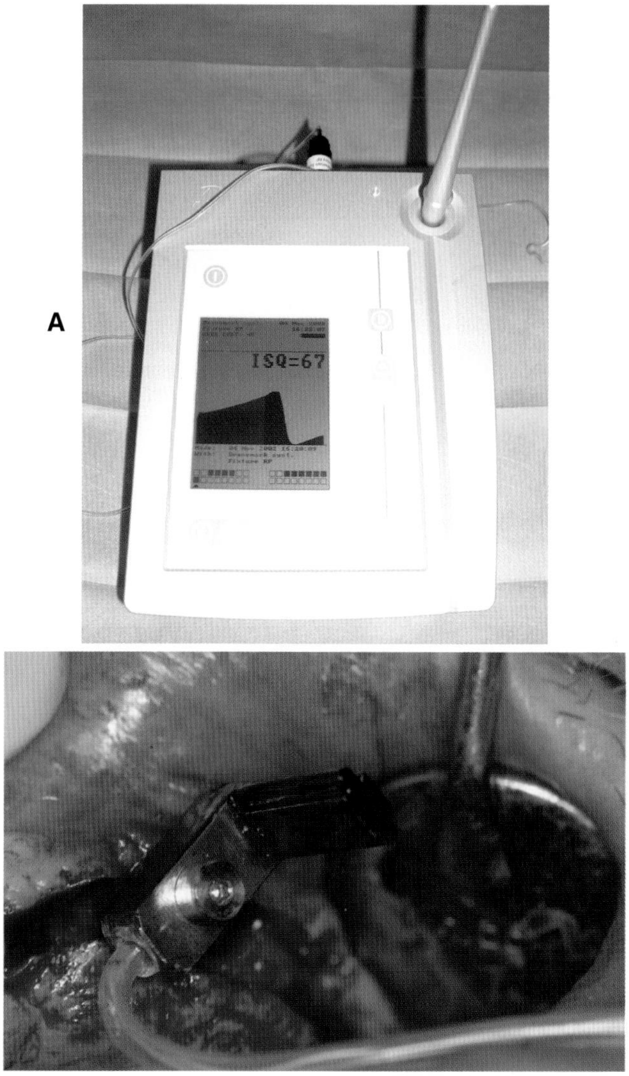

Figure 73-12 **A,** Ostell device measures changes in resonance frequency over time. **B,** Stimulator is fixed on the implant or abutment to transmit energy in a series of frequencies. Use of the Ostell allows measurement of the primary stability at surgery.

TIME	At abutment Connection	1 year	2 years	3 years	4 years	5 years	6 years
Mean	-2.16	-2.80	-2.92	-3.30	-3.90	-4.75	-5.50
	*	*					
		*	*				
		*	---	*			
			*	*			
				*	*		
					*	*	
					*	---	*
						*	*

Figure 73-13 Over time, Periotest values (*PTVs,* arbitrary units) indicate increasing rigidity, which parallels the increased bone density over time.

frequency range of 6 to 9 kHz, with higher values in the mandible. The measures are transformed into arbitrary values where measurements should exceed 56, which indicates a level of bone support that is consistent with osseointegration (Figure 73-13). These noninvasive tests reflect the *rigidity* of the bone-to-implant interface.

The *strength* of the bone-to-implant interface cannot be clinically assessed. Some investigators have measured the force needed to undo the tight adhesion of bone tissues. This has often been done by countertorque force measurements to determine the threshold at which loosening, or often fracturing, is observed. This methodology is questionable because it does not reveal the strength of the biologic interface as such, but rather the *congruency* of the implant surface irregularities with the surrounding bone.[18,29] Indeed, a very roughened surface, such as that achieved with a titanium plasma–sprayed implant, will demonstrate a higher torque resistance than a turned one, where the grooves are much smaller in scale and run parallel to the applied removal force. When the surface roughness is microscopic, such as that achieved with an acid-etched or blasted implant, the bone adaptation to the microtopography will increase the shear strength needed to fracture the bone from the surface to a level that is greater than a turned surface but less than a plasma-sprayed surface.[41]

Others have used pull-out tests of the implants as a whole in a coronal direction. For screw-shaped implants, which are very retentive in this axis because of the threads, this approach apparently cannot assess the biologic adhesion force. The real test should be a "pull-off" test in which a nonretentive surface is detached from the adhering bone. This is a difficult experimental model that is seldom used.[57]

SOFT TISSUE INTERFACES

Not surprisingly, for two decades, research and clinical interest focused on the bone-to-implant interface of osseointegrated implants, and the overlying tissues were largely unexplored. In the classic handbook by Brånemark et al.,[15] except for a few descriptive sentences, no data were presented. Because most patients were fully edentulous and Brånemark system implants had turned surfaces, the incidence of soft tissue inflammation was low,[1] as was the interest in the soft tissue seal around implants.

Because oral implants are used to support or anchor a dental prosthesis, the abutment and restoration must emerge through the connective tissue and epithelium. Thus, it is important to understand the anatomy and function of this soft tissue interface. It can be a keratinized mucosa, firmly anchored by collagen fibers to the underlying periosteum or a non-keratinized mucosa, which can be shifted over the underlying bone because of the presence of elastic fibers (i.e., non-keratinized mucosa is moveable). This soft tissue relationship around implants is comparable with teeth. The latter most often erupt in gingiva and therefore become surrounded by keratinzed tissue whereas implants placed in resorbed jaw often pierce non-kerratinized alveolar mucosa. In clinical studies, with half or more of the implant surfaces surrounded by non-keratinized mucosa, there does not seem to be a clinically significant difference in implant success.[42] On the other hand, mobility of soft tissues

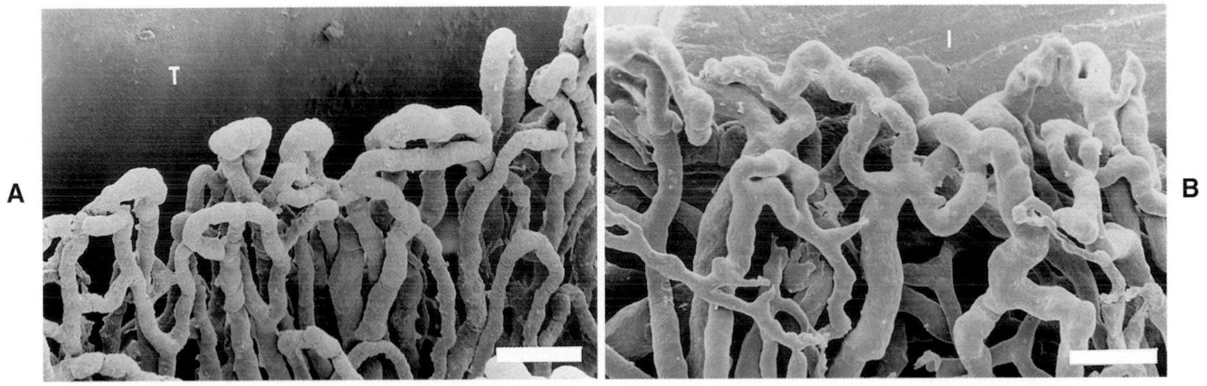

Figure 73-14 Microvascular topography surrounding a tooth **(A)** and an implant **(B)**. Bar = 5 μm. (Courtesy Drs. N. Selliseth and K. Selvig, Bergen, Norway.)

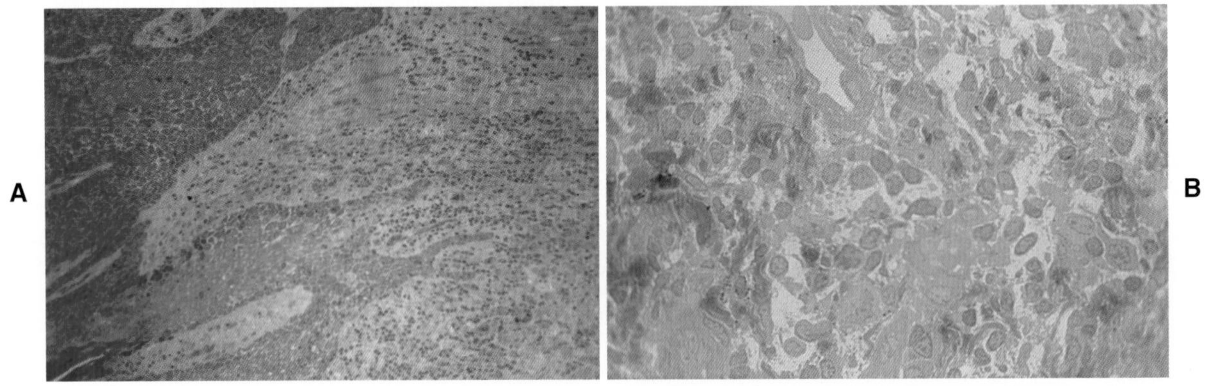

Figure 73-15 **A,** Histologic slide from healthy gingiva surrounding a well-functioning implant in human patient. No morphologic characteristics differentiate tissue around implant from that around teeth. **B,** When gingivitis occurs, a profuse migration of inflammatory cells through the pocket epithelium can be observed. (Courtesy Prof. Mariano Sanz, Madrid.)

surrounding extraoral implants, which pierce through the skin, seems to be associated with a higher incidence of implant failure.[4]

The interface between epithelial cells and the titanium surface is characterized by the presence of hemidesmosomes and a basal lamina. Histologically, studies indicate that these epithelial structures and the surrounding lamina propria cannot be distinguished from those structures around teeth.[17] Even capillary loops in the connective tissue under the junctional and sulcular epithelium around implants appear to be anatomically similar to those found in the normal periodontium (Figure 73-14).[63] In health, this sulcular epithelium has a thickness of about 0.5 mm, which shows transmigration of polymorphonuclear cells and more mononuclear cells (Figure 73-15).[58]

Between the epithelial attachment and the marginal bone is a dense connective tissue with a limited vascularity in the immediate vicinity of the implant surface. The total height of the "biologic width" is approximately 3 to 4 mm, where about 2 mm is the epithelial attachment and about 1 mm is the supracrestal connective tissue zone.[8] Clinically, the thickness of the periimplant soft tissues varies from 2 mm to several millimeters

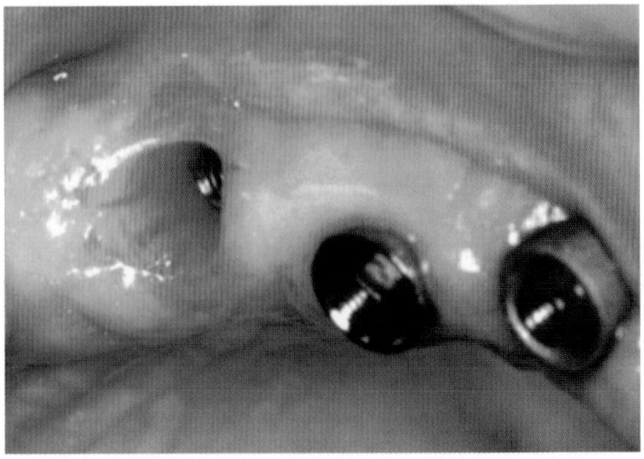

Figure 73-16 Clinical appearance of normal, healthy periimplant tissue with abutment removed. The tissue thickness varies, and the sulcular epithelium is very thin.

(Figure 73-16). Epithelial downgrowth does not occur in a healthy situation, indicating that factors other than collagen fiber bundles inserted in the root surface control this downgrowth. The apical edge of the epithelial attachment is about 1.5 to 2.0 mm of the bone margin.[56] This

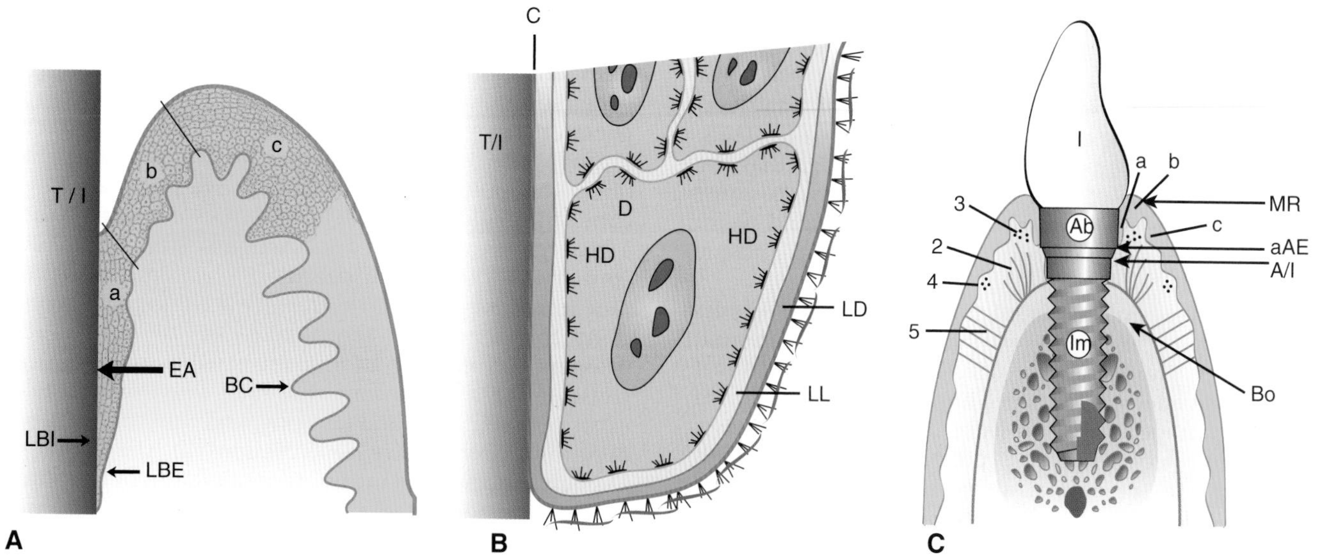

Figure 73-17 **A,** Histologic scheme of epithelial attachment *(EA)* (identical for tooth and implant). *T/I,* Titanium implant. *BC,* basal complex; *LBI,* lamina basalis interna; *LBE,* lamina basalis externa (only location where cell divisions occur); *a,* long junctional epithelial attachment zone; *b,* sulcular epithelial zone; *c,* oral epithelial zone. **B,** At electron microscopic level, basal complex at epithelial attachment (three most apical cells) and connection with stroma. *HD,* Hemidesmosomes; *D,* desmosome; *LL,* lamina lucida; *LD,* lamina densa; *C,* cuticle. **C,** Implant, abutment *(Ab),* and crown within alveolar bone and soft tissues. *Im,* Endosseous part of implant; *MR,* margin of gingiva/alveolar mucosa; *Bo,* marginal bone level; *1,* implant crown; *2,* vertical alveolar-gingival connective tissue fibers; *3,* circular gingival connective tissue fibers; *4,* circular gingival connective tissue fibers; *5,* periosteal-gingival connective tissue fibers; *a,* junctional epithelium; *b,* sulcular epithelium; *c,* oral epithelium; *A/I,* abutment/implant junction; *aAE,* apical (point) of attached epithelium.

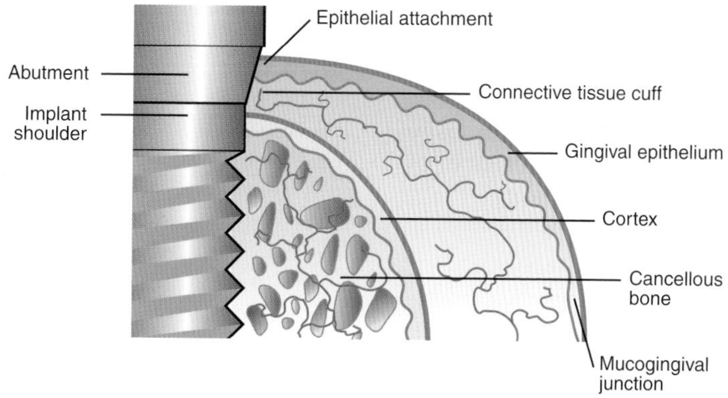

Figure 73-18 Blood supply of the connective tissue cuff surrounding the implant/abutment is scarcer than in the gingival complex around teeth because none originates from a periodontal ligament.

means that the attachment level measurement performed with a periodontal probe will be about 1.5 mm higher than the real bone level (Figure 73-17).

The average direction of the collagen fiber bundles of the gingiva is parallel with the implant or abutment surface. Even when the fiber bundles are oriented perpendicularly, which occurs more often in the gingiva than in the mucosa surrounding implants, the bundles apparently are never embedded in the implant surface, as occurs with dentogingival and dentoperiosteal fibers around teeth. The fiber bundles can also have a cufflike circular orientation. The role of these fibers remains unknown but it appears that there presence helps to create a soft-tissue "seal" around the implant.

At the biochemical level as well, there are no differences between the periimplant and the periodontal soft tissues, even if some higher amounts of collagen types V and VI were noticed.[19]

The vascular supply of the periimplant gingival or alveolar mucosa is more limited than that around teeth. Indeed, because of the lack of a periodontal ligament, this vascular supply is often reduced[9] (Figure 73-18).

Studies investigating the histology of healthy and inflamed tissues surrounding implants in humans have indicated that the reaction patterns toward plaque at both the light microscopic and the ultrastructural level are similar to those of tissues surrounding teeth.[58] Thus, one can derive from this emerging knowledge that the periimplant gingival or alveolar mucosa has the same morphology as the corresponding tissues around teeth. These soft tissues also react the same way to plaque accumulation.

As for the natural dentition, questions emerged decades ago on the need for a keratinized tissue to surround abutments. From many prospective and cross-sectional studies related to screw-shaped implants with a machined surface, it appears that presence or absence of gingiva, just as for teeth, is not a prerequisite for long-term stability.[61] In an animal study it was observed that ligature-induced periimplantitis occurs more frequently when alveolar mucosa surrounds the implant as compared to when keratinized mucosa surrounds the implant.[75]

Much attention has also been given to the microbial leakage originating from the abutment-to-implant connection in two-piece implants.[55] Although it has been shown in animals that this leakage results in an inflammatory reaction in the adjacent lamina propria,[44] no data indicate that this is clinically significant. A gingivitis lesion surrounding an endosseous implant can be a contained, non-progressing lesion. A periimplantitis lesion, on the other hand, is associated with a bacterial infection. Histologically, periimplantitis lesions demonstrate similarities with periodontitis lesions.[10] They can be progressive and lead to bone loss around the implant. Macroscopically rough implant surfaces, such as HA coated and TPS coated implants, seem to be associated with more significant periimplantitis problems due to the propensity of these surfaces to harbor bacteria and perpetuate the infection. Whereas the incidence of periimplantitis seems low with less rough (microscopically altered) implant surfaces even in the presence of periodontitis in the remaining natural dentition.[54]

COMPARISON OF TISSUES SURROUNDING NATURAL DENTITION AND OSSEOINTEGRATED ORAL IMPLANTS

Although the soft tissue–abutment/implant interface offers striking similarities with tissue surrounding the natural dentition, some differences should be considered. At the bone level, the lack of a periodontal ligament is the striking difference. The following discussion elaborates on the clinical perspectives of these similarities and differences.

In both cases the intimate adherence of soft tissues depends on the presence of a soft tissue free of inflammation. Air blowing does not provoke detachment of the lining tissues unless they are inflamed. Moving a probe just below the gingival margin will detach this and provoke bleeding, revealing the presence of an inflammatory reaction the same as around natural teeth.

When probing with a periodontal probe deep into the peri-implant sulcus or "pocket," the tip will penetrate nearly to the bone level. This occurs even when the tissues are healthy.[56] This probing depth can be explained by the lack of connective tissue fiber bundles embedded in the implant surface, which thus does not prevent the penetration of the tip. The depth of the pocket or probe penetration reveals the thickness of the mucoperiosteum through which the abutment/restoration is emerging rather than a loss of attachment. To assess the latter, the clinician should refer pocket depth measurements toward a fixed reference point and follow this over time.[56] Indeed, contrary to the natural dentition, the cementoenamel junction is not present as a reference point in the implant.

At the bone level the absence of the periodontal ligament surrounding an implant has important clinical consequences. This means that no resilient connection exists between teeth and jawbone, and thus any occlusal disharmony will have repercussions at the bone-to-implant interface. No intrusion or migration of teeth can compensate for the eventual presence of a premature contact. This can become even more challenging when osseointegrated, implant-supported fixed prostheses are present in both jaws.

The lack of a periodontal ligament also means that the clinician should be reluctant to use oral implants in growing individuals. The neighboring teeth and periodontal tissues will further erupt, leading to occlusal disharmonies.[52] Likewise, it may be problematic to place one or more implants in a location surrounded by teeth that are very mobile due to loss of periodontal support, because as the teeth move away from the occlusal forces, the implant(s) will bear the entire load.

Because the principal proprioception of the natural dentition comes from the periodontal ligament, its absence around implants reduces tactile sensitivity[35] and reflex function.[13] Even if a certain degree of tactile sensitivity by means of endosseous implants is present after a few months, a phenomenon called *osseoperception,* the clinician should instruct the patient about the necessary precautions with food intake during the early period. Interestingly, this phenomenon parallels the histologic observation in animals of increasing numbers of free nerve endings at the bone-to-implant interface. Considering the reduced tactile sensation with implants, especially during the first months, the restorative dentist should not rely on the patient's subjective perception when checking the occlusion.

CONCLUSION

The understanding of the osseointegration process is facilitated by a good knowledge of bone fracture healing. Many factors can interfere with the predictable establishment of a permanent rigid connection that is able to handle a load between an implant surface and the surrounding bone. Periodontists should familiarize themselves with the underlying molecular and cellular events, which will direct their surgical behavior and maintenance schemes.

The bone-to-implant interface and its rigidity are a predominant biomechanical aspect in coping with the time and intensity of loading. The osseoperception phenomenon deserves more attention from this perspective. The soft tissue–implant interface plays an important role in the long-term maintenance of a stable marginal bone level. Uncontrolled inflammatory reactions and subsequent epithelial downgrowth will jeopardize the implant's maintenance. The incidence of periimplantitis seems to depend on the implant surface characteristics.

REFERENCES

1. Adell R, Lekholm U, Rockler B, et al: Marginal tissue reactions at osseointegrated titanium fixtures. I. A 3-year longitudinal prospective study, *Int J Oral Maxillofac Surg* 15:39, 1986.
2. Albrektsson T: Bone tissue response. In Brånemark PI, Zarb GA, Albrektsson T, editors: *Tissue-integrated prostheses,* Chicago, 1985, Quintessence.
3. Albrektsson T, Sennerby L: State of the art in oral implants, *J Clin Periodontol* 18:474, 1991.
4. Albrektsson T, Brånemark PI, Jacobsson M, Tjellstrom A: Present clinical applications of osseointegrated percutaneous implants, *Plast Reconstr Surg* 79:721, 1987.
5. Albrektsson T, Zarb G, Worthington P, Eriksson AR: The long-term efficacy of currently used dental implants: a review and proposed criteria of success, *Int J Oral Maxillofac Implants* 1:11, 1986.
6. Albrektsson T, Eriksson AR, Friberg B, et al: Histologic investigations on 33 retrieved Nobelpharma implants, *Clin Mater* 12:1, 1993.
7. Bashi TJ, Wolfinger GJ: Management of the posterior maxilla in the compromised patient: historical, current, and future perspectives, *Periodontology 2000* 33:67, 2003.
8. Berglundh T, Lindhe J: Dimension of the peri-implant mucosa: biological width revisited, *J Clin Periodontol* 23:971, 1996.
9. Berglundh T, Lindhe J, Jonsson K, Ericsson I: The topography of the vascular systems in the periodontal and peri-implant tissues in the dog, *J Clin Periodontol* 21:189, 1994.
10. Berglundh T, Gislason Ö, Lekholm U, et al: Histopathological observations of human peri-implantitis lesions, *J Clin Periodontol* 31:341, 2004.
11. Best S, Sim B, Kayser M, Downes S: The dependence of osteoblastic response on variations in the chemical composition and physical properties of hydroxyapatite, *J Mater Sci Mater Med* 8:97, 1997.
12. Block MS, Kent JN: Long-term follow-up on hydroxylapatite-coated cylindrical dental implants: a comparison between developmental and recent periods, *J Oral Maxillofac Surg* 52:937, 1994.
13. Bonte B, van Steenberghe D: Masseteric post-stimulus EMG complex following mechanical stimulation of osseointegrated oral implants, *J Oral Rehabil* 18:221, 1991.
14. Bosker H, van Dijk L: The transmandibular implant: a 12-year follow-up study, *J Oral Maxillofac Surg* 47:442, 1989.
15. Brånemark PI, Zarb GA, Albrektsson T, editors: *Tissue-integrated prostheses,* Chicago, 1985, Quintessence.
16. Brånemark PI, Breine U, Adell B, et al: Intra-osseous anchorage of dental prostheses. 1. Experimental studies, *Scand J Plast Reconstr Surg* 3:81, 1969.
17. Buser D, Weber HP, Donath K, et al: Soft tissue reactions to non-submerged unloaded titanium implants in beagle dogs, *J Periodontol* 63:225, 1992.
18. Buser D, Nydegger T, Oxland T, et al: Interface shear strength of titanium implants with a sandblasted and acid-etched surface: a biomechanical study in the maxilla of miniature pigs, *J Biomed Mater Res* 45:75, 1999.
19. Chavrier C, Couble ML, Hartmann DJ: Qualitative study of collagenous and noncollagenous glycoproteins of the human healthy keratinized mucosa surrounding implants, *Clin Oral Implant Res* 5:117, 1994.
20. Currey J: The validation of algorithms used to explain remodeling in bone. In Odgaard A, Weinans H, editors: *Bone structure and remodeling,* Singapore, 1995, Worldscientific.
21. Ellingsen JE: Surface configurations of dental implants, *Periodontol 2000* 17:36, 1998.
22. Embery G, Rolla G: Interaction between sulphated macromolecules and hydroxyapatite studied by infrared spectroscopy, *Acta Odontol Scand* 38:105, 1980.
23. Eriksson AR, Albrektsson T: Temperature threshold levels for heat-induced bone tissue injury: a vital-microscopic study in the rabbit, *J Prosthet Dent* 50:101, 1983.
24. Francois P, Vaudaux P, Taborelli M, et al: Influence of surface treatments developed for oral implants on the physical and biological properties of titanium. II. Adsorption isotherms and biological activity of immobilized fibronectin, *Clin Oral Implant Res* 8:217, 1997.
25. Friberg B, Sennerby L, Linden B, et al: Stability measurements of one-stage Brånemark implants during healing in mandibles: a clinical resonance frequency analysis study, *Int J Oral Maxillofac Surg* 28:266, 1999.
26. Granström G: Radiotherapy, osseointegration and hyperbaric oxygen therapy, *Periodontol 2000* 33:145, 2003.
27. Haas R, Mensdorff-Pouilly N, Mailath G, Watzek G: Survival of 1920 IMZ implants followed for up to 100 months, *Int J Oral Maxillofac Implants* 11:581, 1996.
28. Hall R, Embery G, Waddington R, Gilmour A: The influence of fluoride on the adsorption of proteoglycans and glycosaminoglycans to hydroxyapatite, *Calcif Tissue Int* 56:236, 1995.
29. Han CH, Johansson CB, Wennerberg A, Albrektsson T: Quantitative and qualitative investigations of surface enlarged titanium and titanium alloy implants, *Clin Oral Implant Res* 9:1, 1998.
30. Hansson S, Werke M: The implant thread as a retention element in cortical bone: the effect of thread size and thread profile: a finite element study, *J Biomech* 36:1247, 2003.
31. Hong HL, Brunette DM: Effect of cell shape on proteinase secretion by epithelial cells, *J Cell Sci* 87:259, 1987.
32. Huang YH, Xiropaidis AV, Sorensen RG, et al: Bone formation at titanium porous oxide (TiUnite) oral implants in type IV bone, *Clin Oral Implant Res* 16:105, 2005.
33. Huiskes R, Weinans H, Dastra M: Adaptive bone remodeling and biomechanical design considerations for noncemented total hip arthroplasty, *Orthopedics* 12:1255, 1989.
34. Jacobs R: *Osseoperception,* Leuven, Belgium, 1998, Catholic University Leuven.
35. Jacobs R, van Steenberghe D: Role of periodontal ligament receptors in the tactile function of teeth: a review, *J Periodontal Res* 29:153, 1994.
36. James RA: Peri-implant considerations, *Dent Clin North Am* 24:415, 1980.
37. Jemt T: Failures and complications in 391 consecutively inserted fixed prostheses supported by Brånemark implants in edentulous jaws: a study of treatment from the time of prosthesis placement to the first annual check-up, *Int J Oral Maxillofac Implants* 6:270, 1991.
38. Kasemo B: Biocompatibility of titanium implants: surface science aspects, *J Prosthet Dent* 49:832, 1983.
39. Kieswetter K, Schwartz Z, Hummert TW, et al: Surface roughness modulates the local production of growth factors and cytokines by osteoblast-like MG-63 cells, *J Biomed Mater Res* 32:55, 1996.
40. Kirsch A: The two-phase implantation method using IMZ intramobile cylinder implants, *J Oral Implantol* 11:197, 1983.
41. Klokkevold PR, Johnson P, Dadgostari S, et al: Early endosseous integration enhanced by dual acid etching of titanium: a torque removal study in the rabbit, *Clin Oral Implants Res* 12:350, 2001.

42. Lekholm U, Ericsson I, Adell R, Slots J: The condition of the soft tissues at tooth and fixture abutments supporting fixed bridges: a microbiological and histological study, *J Clin Periodontol* 13:558, 1986.
43. Linder L, Albrektsson T, Brånemark PI, Hansson HA, et al: Electron microscopic analysis of the bone-titanium interface, *Acta Orthop Scand* 54:45, 1983.
44. Lindhe J, Berglundh T, Ericsson I, et al: Experimental breakdown of peri-implant and periodontal tissues: a study in the beagle dog, *Clin Oral Implant Res* 3:9, 1992.
45. Lindquist LW, Carlsson GE, Jemt T: A prospective 15-year follow-up study of mandibular fixed prostheses supported by osseointegrated implants: clinical results and marginal bone loss, *Clin Oral Implant Res* 7:329, 1996.
46. McClarence E: *Close to the edge: Brånemark and the development of osseointegration,* London, 2003, Quintessence.
47. Mellal A, Wiskott HW, Botsis J, et al: Stimulating effect of implant loading on surrounding bone: comparison of three numeral models and validation by in vivo data, *Clin Oral Implant Res* 15:239, 2004.
48. Meredith N, Alleyne D, Cawley P: Quantitative determination of the stability of the implant-tissue interface during resonance frequency analysis, *Clin Oral Implant Res* 7:261, 1996.
49. Murray DW, Rae T, Ruston N: The influence of the surface energy and roughness of implants on bone resorption, *J Bone Joint Surg* 71B:632, 1989.
50. Niznick GA: The Core-Vent implant system, *J Oral Implantol* 10:379, 1982.
51. Olivé J, Aparicio C: Periotest method as a measure of osseointegrated oral implant stability, *Int J Oral Maxillofac Implants* 5:390, 1990.
52. Op Heij DG, Opdebeeck H, van Steenberghe D, Quirynen M: Age as compromising factor for implant insertion, *Periodontology 2000* 33:172, 2003.
53. Pearson BS, Klebe RJ, Boyan BD, Moskowicz D: Comments on the clinical application of fibronectin in dentistry, *J Dent Res* 67:515, 1988.
54. Quirynen M, De Soete M, van Steenberghe D: Infectious risks for oral implants: a review of the literature, *Clin Oral Implant Res* 13:1, 2002.
55. Quirynen M, Bollen CML, Eyssen H, van Steenberghe D: Microbial penetration along the implant components of the Brånemark system: an *in vitro* study, *Clin Oral Implant Res* 5:239, 1994.
56. Quirynen M, van Steenberghe D, Jacobs R, et al: The reliability of pocket probing around screw-type implants, *Clin Oral Implant Res* 2:186, 1991.
57. Rupprecht S, Bloch A, Rosiwal S, et al: Examination of the bone-metal interface of titanium implants coated by the microwave plasma chemical vapor deposition method, *Int J Oral Maxillofac Implants* 17:778, 2002.
58. Sanz M, Alandez J, Lazaro P, et al: Histo-pathologic characteristics of peri-implant soft tissues in Brånemark implants with 2 distinct clinical & radiological patterns, *Clin Oral Implant Res* 2:128, 1991.
59. Schakenraad JM, Busscher HJ, Wildevuur CR, Arends J: The influence of substratum surface free energy on growth and spreading of human fibroblasts in the presence and absence of serum proteins, *J Biomed Mater Res* 20:773, 1986.
60. Schenk RK, Buser D: Osseointegration: a reality, *Periodontol 2000* 17:22, 1998.
61 Schou S, Holmstrup P, Hjorting-Hansen E, Lang NP: Plaque-induced marginal tissue reactions of osseointegrated oral implants: a review of the literature, *Clin Oral Implant Res* 3:149, 1992.
62. Scortecci G: Immediate function of cortically anchored disk-design implants without bone augmentation in moderately to severely resorbed completely edentulous maxillae, *J Oral Implantol* 25:70, 1999.
63. Selliseth NJ, Selvig KA: Microvascular adaptation to transmucosal implants: a scanning electron microscopic study in the rat, *Clin Oral Implant Res* 6:205, 1995.
64. Siegele D, Soltesz U: Numerical investigations of the influence of implant shape on stress distribution in the jawbone, *Int J Oral Maxillofac Implants* 4:333, 1989.
65. Small IA, Metz H, Kobernick S: The mandibular staple implant for the atrophic mandible, *J Biomed Mater Res* 8(4 Pt 2):365, 1974.
66. Small I, Misiek D: A sixteen-year evaluation of the mandibular staple bone plate, *J Oral Maxillofac Surg* 44:60, 1986.
67. Sutter F, Schroeder A, Straumann F: Engineering and design aspects of the I.T.I. hollow-basket implants, *J Oral Implantol* 10:535, 1983.
68. Thomsen P, Ericsson LE: Light and transmission electron microscopy used to study the tissue morphology close to implants, *Biomaterials* 6:421, 1985.
69. Tricio J, Laohapand PP, van Steenberghe D, et al: Mechanical state assessment of implant-bone continuum: a better understanding of the Periotest method, *Int J Oral Maxillofac Implants* 10:43, 1995.
70. Ueda M, Matsuki M, Jacobsson M, Tjellstrom A: Relationship between insertion torque and removal torque analysed in fresh temporal bone, *Int J Oral Maxillofac Implants* 6:442, 1991.
71. van Steenberghe D, Quirynen M: Reproducibility and detection threshold of peri-implant diagnostics, *Adv Dent Res* 7:191, 1993.
72. van Steenberghe D, Tricio J, Naert I, Nys M: Damping characteristics of bone-to-implant interfaces: a clinical study with the Periotest device, *Clin Oral Implant Res* 6:31, 1995.
73. Versteegh PA, van Beek GJ, Slagter AP, Ottervanger JP: Clinical evaluation of mandibular overdentures supported by multiple-bar fabrication: a follow-up study of two implant systems, *Int J Oral Maxillofac Implants* 10:595, 1995.
74. Von Recum AF, Shannon CE, Cannon CE, et al: Surface roughness, porosity and textures as modifiers of cellular adhesion, *Tissue Eng* 2:241, 1996.
75. Warrer K, Buser D, Lang NP, Karring T: Plaque-induced peri-implantitis in the presence or absence of keratinized mucosa, *Clin Oral Implant Res* 6:131, 1995.
76. Wennerberg A: On surface roughness and implant incorporation, Göteborg, Sweden, 1996, University of Göteborg (PhD thesis).
77. Xiao G, Cui Y, Ducy P, et al: Ascorbic acid–dependent activation of the osteocalcin promoter in MC3T3-E1 preosteoblasts: requirement for collagen matrix synthesis and the presence of an intact OSE2 sequence, *Mol Endocrinol* 11:1103, 1997.

Clinical Aspects and Evaluation of the Implant Patient

74

CHAPTER

Perry R. Klokkevold and David L. Cochran

CHAPTER OUTLINE

Endosseous dental implants and their retained prostheses have had great success over the past few decades following the landmark research and development of osseointegrated implants by Brånemark et al.[16-18] Initially, most prosthetic reconstructions with osseointegrated implants were limited to use in the edentulous patient, with many reports documenting excellent long-term success of implant-retained prostheses for edentulous patients.[1,2,30]

Following much success with implants in edentulous patients, the original implant treatment protocols were adapted for use in partially edentulous patients. Although some transitional problems were associated with the early use of dental implants in the partially edentulous patient, successes soon occurred for this population as well. Modifications in implant design, procedural techniques, and treatment planning greatly improved implant therapy for the partially edentulous patient. Currently, the long-term success of dental implants used to replace single and multiple missing teeth in the partially edentulous patient is very good.[35,48,49,57,64] Additionally, with the implementation of bone augmentation procedures, even patients with inadequate bone volume have a good opportunity to be successfully restored with implant-retained prostheses.[31,41,66] Virtually any patient with an edentulous space is a candidate for endosseous implants, and studies suggest that greater than 90% to 95% success rates can be expected in healthy patients with good bone and normal healing capacity.[27]

The ultimate goal of dental implant therapy is to satisfy the patient's desire to replace one or more missing teeth in an esthetic, secure, functional, and long-lasting manner. To achieve this goal, clinicians must accurately diagnose the current dentoalveolar condition as well as the overall mental and physical well-being of the patient to determine whether implant therapy is possible or practical and, perhaps most importantly, whether it is indicated for a particular patient. Local evaluation of potential jaw sites for implant placement (e.g., measuring available alveolar bone height, width, and spatial relationship) and prosthetic restorability is an essential part of determining whether an implant(s) is possible. However, determining whether the patient is a good candidate for implants is an equally important aspect of the evaluation process. This aspect of the patient evaluation includes identifying factors that might increase the risk of failure or complications as well as determining whether the patient's expectations are reasonable.

This chapter presents an overview of the clinical aspects of dental implant therapy, including an assessment of possible risk factors and contraindications. It also provides guidelines for the pretreatment evaluation of potential implant patients, posttreatment evaluation of patients with implants, and implant maintenance.

CASE TYPES AND INDICATIONS

Edentulous Patients

The patients who seem to benefit most from dental implants are those with fully edentulous arches. These patients can be effectively restored, both esthetically and functionally, with an implant-assisted removable prosthesis or an implant-supported fixed prosthesis.

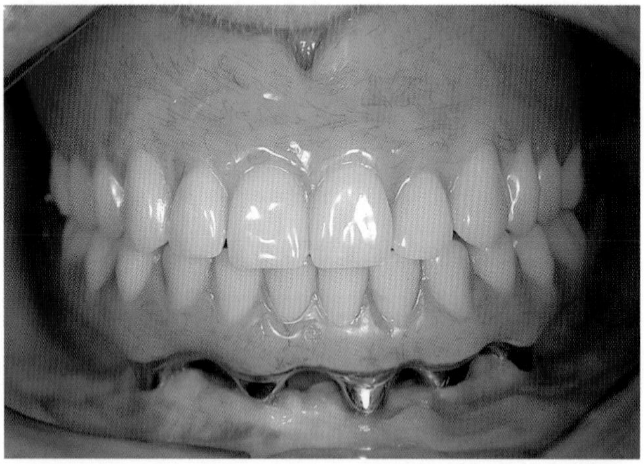

Figure 74-1 Clinical photograph of patient with a complete maxillary denture opposing a full-arch implant-supported fixed prosthesis in the mandibular arch.

The original design for the edentulous arch was a fixed-bone–anchored bridge that used five to six implants in the anterior area of the mandible or the maxilla to support a fixed, hybrid prosthesis. The design is a denturelike complete arch of teeth attached to a substructure (metal framework), which in turn is attached to the implants with cylindrical titanium abutments (Figure 74-1). The prosthesis is fabricated without flange extensions and does not rely on any soft tissue support. It is entirely implant supported (see Figure 80-11). Usually, the prosthesis includes bilateral distal cantilevers, which extend to replace posterior teeth (back to premolars or first molars).

Another implant-supported design used to restore an edentulous arch is the ceramic-metal fixed bridge (Figure 74-2). Some patients prefer this design because the ceramic restoration emerges directly from the gingival tissues in a manner similar to the appearance of natural teeth. One limitation of both hybrid and ceramometal implant-supported fixed prostheses is that they provide very little lip support and thus may not be indicated for patients who have lost significant alveolar dimension. This is often more problematic for maxillary reconstructions because lip support is more critical in the upper arch. For some patients, the lack of a complete seal (i.e., spaces under the framework) allows air to escape during speech, thus creating phonetic problems.

Depending on the volume of existing bone, the jaw relationship, the amount of lip support, and phonetics, some patients may not be able to be rehabilitated with an implant-supported fixed prosthesis. For these patients,

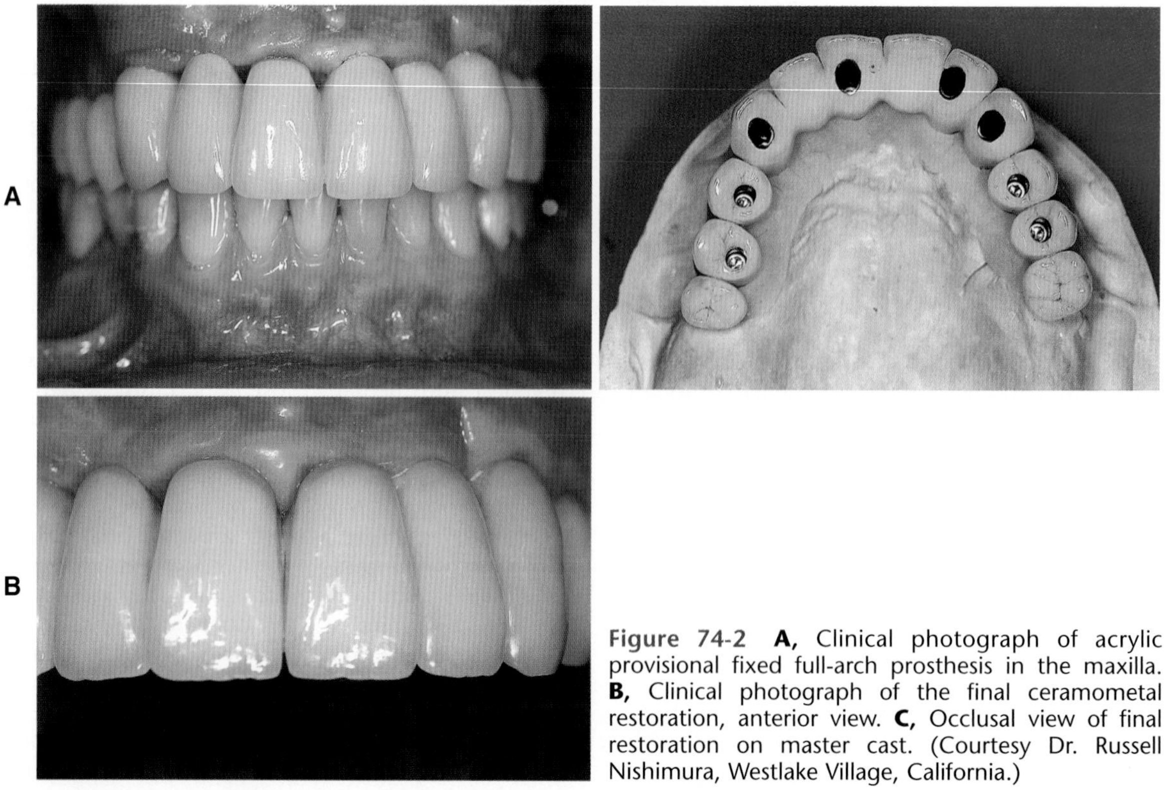

Figure 74-2 **A,** Clinical photograph of acrylic provisional fixed full-arch prosthesis in the maxilla. **B,** Clinical photograph of the final ceramometal restoration, anterior view. **C,** Occlusal view of final restoration on master cast. (Courtesy Dr. Russell Nishimura, Westlake Village, California.)

a removable, complete-denture type of prosthesis is a better choice because it provides a flange extension that can be adjusted and contoured to support the lip, and there are no spaces for unwanted air escape during speech. This type of prosthesis can be retained and stabilized by two or more implants placed in the anterior region of the maxilla or mandible. Methods used to secure the denture to the implants vary from separate attachments on each individual implant (see Figure 80-10) to clips or other attachments that connect to a bar, which splints the implants together (Figure 74-3). Advantages and disadvantages of these attachment designs are discussed in Chapter 80.

Although the stability of the implant-retained overdenture does not compare to the rigidly attached, implant-supported fixed prosthesis, the increased retention and stability over conventional complete dentures is an important advantage for denture wearers.[68] Additionally, implant-assisted and implant-supported prostheses are thought to protect alveolar bone from additional bone loss caused by long-term use of removable prostheses that are bearing directly on the alveolar ridges.

Partially Edentulous Patients

Multiple Teeth. Partially edentulous patients with multiple missing teeth represent another viable treatment population for osseointegrated implants, but the remaining natural dentition (occlusal schemes, periodontal health status, spatial relationships, and esthetics) introduces additional challenges for successful rehabilitation.[47] The juxtaposition of implants with natural teeth in the partially edentulous patient presents the clinician with challenges not encountered with implants in the edentulous patient. As a result of distinct differences in the biology and function of implants compared with natural teeth, clinicians must educate themselves and use a prescribed approach to the evaluation and treatment planning of implants for partially edentulous patients (see Chapter 80). In general, endosseous dental implants can support a freestanding fixed partial denture. Adjacent natural teeth are not necessary for support, but their close proximity requires special attention and planning.[10] The major advantage of implant-supported restorations in partially edentulous patients is that they are not invasive to adjacent teeth. Preparation of natural teeth becomes unnecessary, and larger edentulous spans can be restored with implant-supported fixed bridges.[59] Moreover, patients who previously did not have a fixed option, such as those with Kennedy Class I and II partially edentulous situations, can be restored with an implant-supported fixed restoration (Figure 74-4).

Early attempts to use endosseous implants to replace missing teeth in the partially edentulous patient were a challenge partly because the implants and armamentarium were designed for the edentulous patient and did not have much flexibility for adaptation and use in the partially edentulous patient (i.e., one standard-diameter

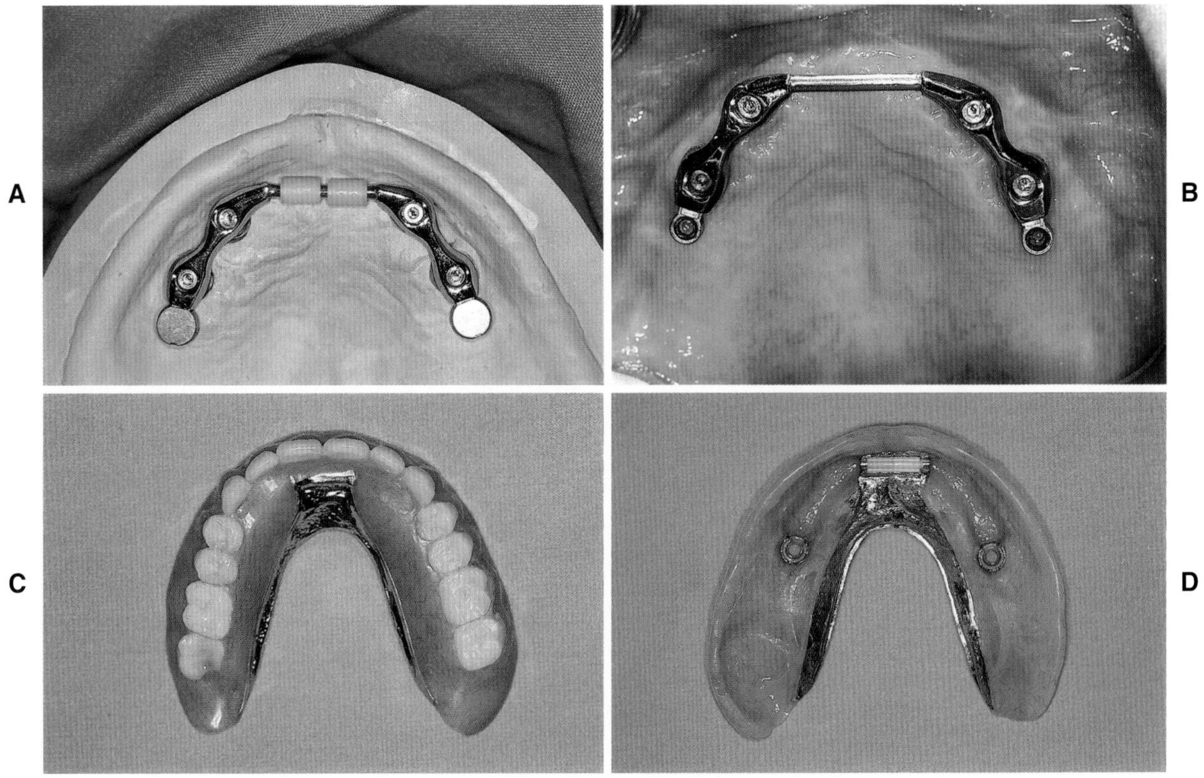

Figure 74-3 **A,** Laboratory view of maxillary overdenture bar attached to four implants with anterior clips and posterior extracoronal resilient attachments (ERAs). **B,** Clinical view of maxillary overdenture bar. **C,** Palateless maxillary complete overdenture. **D,** Tissue surface of same maxillary implant-assisted overdenture showing clips and ERAs.

A
B
C
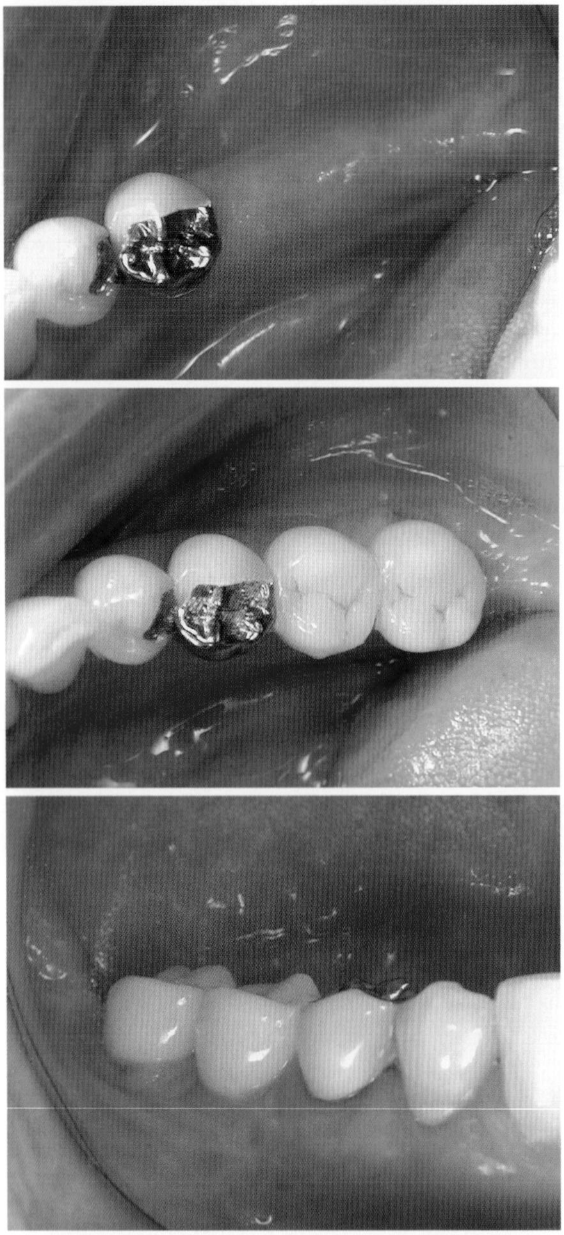

Figure 74-4 **A,** Clinical view of partially edentulous posterior mandible (Kennedy Class II distal extension). **B,** Occlusal view of same patient in *A* restored with implant-supported fixed restoration replacing teeth #18 and #19. Notice the dimensions of the crowns are smaller than typical mandibular molars (i.e., closer to bicuspid size). **C,** Buccal view of same restorations.

implant, one type of abutment, and one surgical kit with instrumentation that was difficult to use adjacent to teeth). As the demand for implants in the partially edentulous patient increased, implant manufacturers responded with the development of wide-diameter and narrow-diameter implants and a variety of abutment choices. They also developed instrumentation that was better suited for the placement of implants adjacent to natural teeth. Currently, clinicians have many choices in terms of implant length, diameter, and abutment connection to choose for the optimal replacement of any missing tooth, large or small (Figure 74-5).

Another difficulty with partially edentulous cases is an underestimation of the importance of treatment planning for implant-retained restorations with an adequate number of implants to withstand occlusal loads. For example, one problem that required correction was the misconception that two implants could be used to support a multiunit fixed bridge in the posterior area. Multiunit fixed restorations in the posterior jaw are more likely to experience complications or failures (mechanical or biologic) when they are inadequately supported either in terms of the number of implants, quality of bone, or strength of the implant material (see Chapter 80). The use of stronger implants and better treatment planning (more implants used to support more restorative units), particularly in areas of poor-quality bone, has solved many of these problems.

Single Tooth. Patients with a missing single tooth (anterior or posterior) represent another type of patient who benefits greatly from the success and predictability of endosseous dental implants. Replacement of a single missing tooth with an implant-supported crown is a much more conservative approach than preparing two adjacent teeth for the fabrication of a tooth-supported fixed partial denture. It is no longer necessary to "cut" healthy or minimally restored adjacent teeth to replace a missing tooth with a nonremovable prosthetic replacement (Figure 74-6). Reported success rates for single-tooth implants are excellent.[27]

Replacement of an individual missing posterior tooth with an implant-supported restoration has been successful as well. The greatest challenges to overcome with the single-tooth implant restorations were screw loosening and implant or component fracture. Because of increased potential to generate forces in the posterior area, the implants, components, and screws often failed. Both these problems have been addressed with the use of wider-diameter implants and internal fixation of components (Figure 74-7). Wide-diameter implants often have a wider platform (restorative interface) that resists tipping forces and thus reduces screw loosening. The wide-diameter implant also provides greater strength and resistance to fracture as a result of increased wall thickness (the thickness of the implant between the inner screw thread and the outer screw thread). Implants with an internal connection are inherently resistant to screw loosening and thus have an added advantage for single-tooth applications. Further, most dental implant manufacturers now sell implants with internal component fixation.

Esthetic Considerations. Anterior single-tooth implants present some of the same challenges as the single posterior tooth supported by an implant, but they also are an esthetic concern for patients. Some cases are more esthetically challenging than others because of the nature of each individual's smile and display of teeth. The prominence and occlusal relationship of existing teeth, the thickness and health of periodontal tissues, and the patient's own psychologic perception of esthetics all play

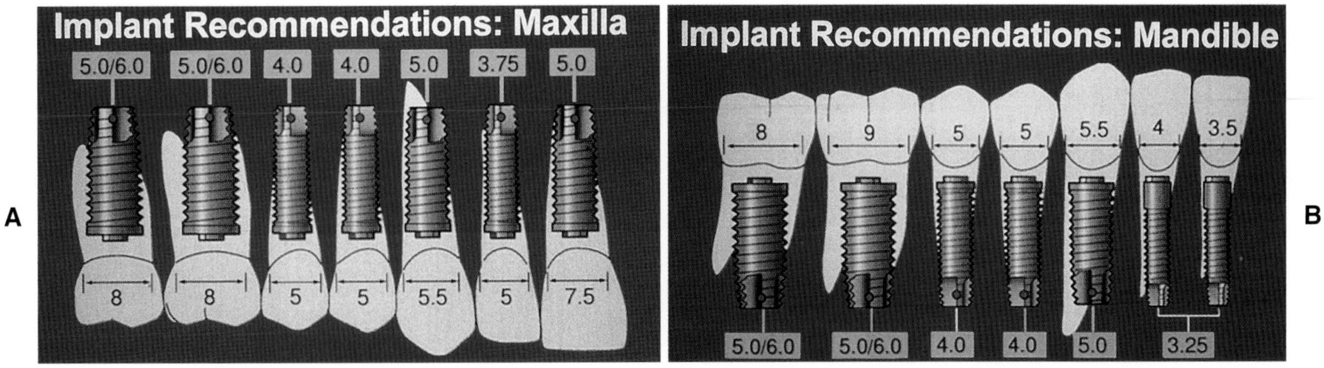

Figure 74-5 Diagram representing the use of wide-, narrow-, and standard-diameter implants superimposed over various teeth. **A,** Maxillary teeth. **B,** Mandibular teeth. (Courtesy 3i/Implant Innovations, Inc., Palm Beach Gardens, Fla.)

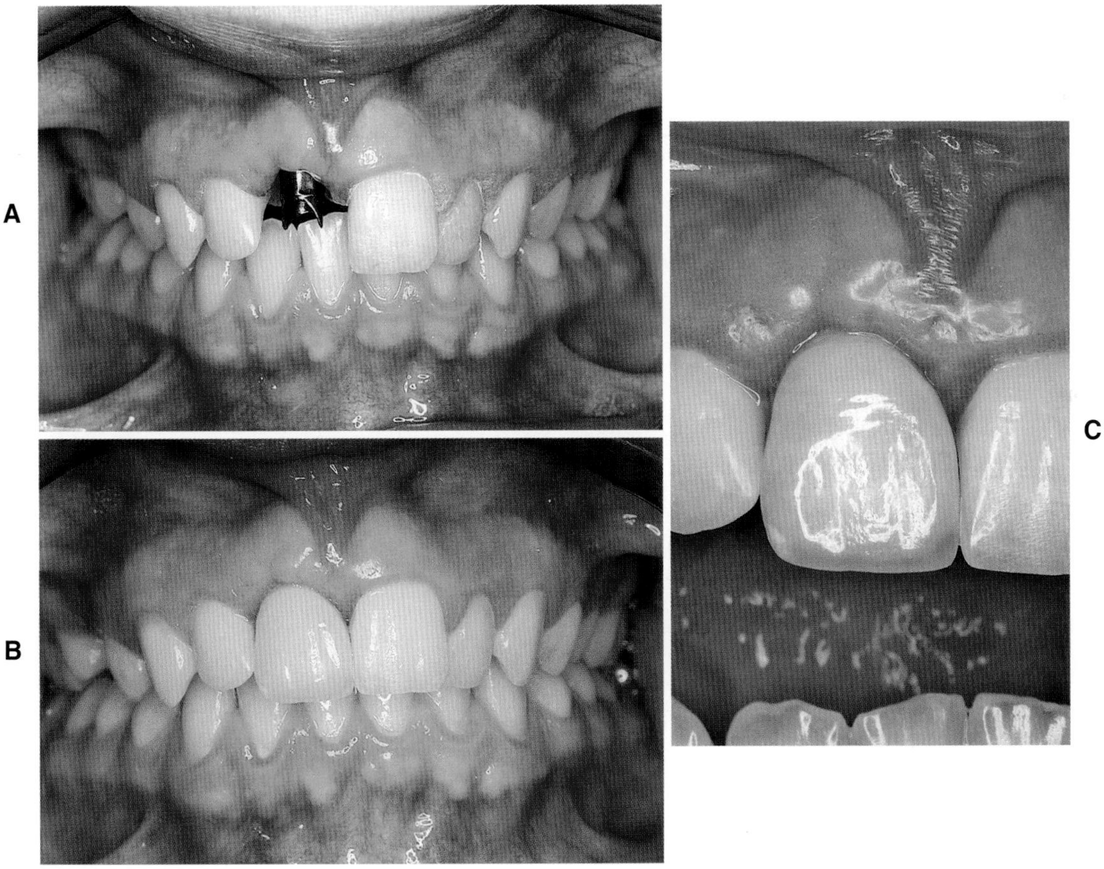

Figure 74-6 Single-tooth replacement. **A,** Implant in place. **B,** Metalloceramic crown. **C,** Close-up view.

a role in the esthetic challenge of the case. Cases with good bone volume, bone height, and tissue thickness can be predictable in terms of achieving satisfactory esthetic results (see Figure 74-6). However, achieving esthetic results for patients with less-than-ideal tissue qualities poses difficult challenges for the restorative and surgical team.[10] Replacing a single tooth with an implant-supported crown in a patient with a high smile line, compromised or thin periodontium, inadequate hard or soft tissues, and high expectations is probably one of the most difficult challenges in implant dentistry and should only be attempted by experienced clinicians.

SCIENCE TRANSFER

The goal of dental implant therapy is to replace missing teeth. The procedure is extremely effective in both edentulous and partially edentulous patients. The devices and technologies are well reported, but the important question is to determine *when endosseous dental therapy is indicated.* For example, in some patients, dental implant therapy may be contraindicated, or a higher risk of failure may exist. Therefore, all patients need to be carefully evaluated to determine the optional tooth replacement therapy for the individual patient. Dental implant therapy depends on the resorption and formation of hard connective tissue (bone); therefore the clinician must know the bone metabolic activity of the patient. As with all tooth placement therapy, the patient must be maintained and evaluated at periodic visits customized for the individual.

Cylindrical titanium implants with external hex abutment and 3.75-mm diameter were first used to treat edentulous patients. In these cases, four to six implants per arch may be used to support a fixed restoration, or two to four implants may be used for a removable overdenture prosthesis. Although the fixed type has advantages, in some fully edentulous patients the lip support, esthetics, and speech patterns are better controlled with an overdenture. Newer implant designs have been developed for replacement of single teeth, as well as for use in partially edentulous patients, with wider selection of platforms and the use of internal fixation systems for the prosthesis.

Diabetic patients, smokers, and patients with osteoporosis may have slightly lower success rates but can still be treated with implant therapy. In contrast, patients with a history of therapeutic radiation exposure exceeding 60 Gy and immunosuppressed patients are not usually treated with dental implants.

A

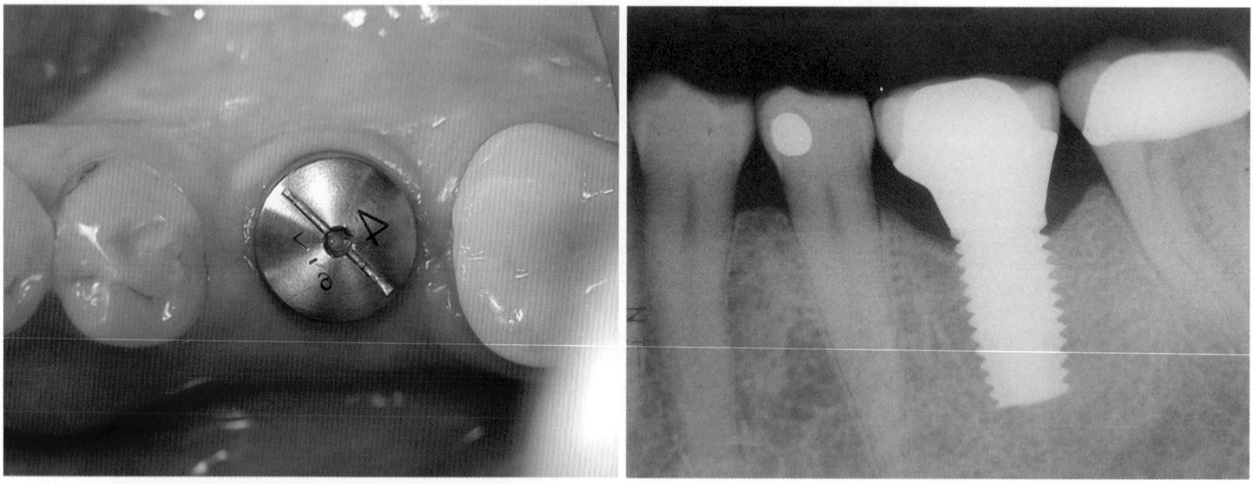

B

Figure 74-7 **A,** Occlusal view of healing abutment, which is attached to a wide-diameter implant used to replace a single missing molar. **B,** Radiograph of same patient depicted in *A,* showing the wide-diameter implant supporting the final restoration (molar replaced with a single-tooth implant-supported crown).

PRETREATMENT EVALUATION

A comprehensive evaluation is indicated for any patient who is being considered for dental implant therapy. The evaluation should assess all aspects of the patient's current health status, including a review the patient's past medical history, medications, and medical treatments. Patients should be questioned about parafunctional habits, such as clenching or grinding teeth, as well as any substance use or abuse, including tobacco, alcohol, and drugs. The assessment should also include an evaluation of the patient's motivations, level of understanding, compliance, and overall behavior. For most patients, this involves simply observing their demeanor and listening to their comments for an impression of their overall sensibility and coherence with other patient norms. For some individuals with questionable behavior, however, a professional psychologic assessment of their mental health status may be indicated.

An intraoral and radiographic examination must be done to determine whether it is possible to place implant(s) in the desired location(s). Properly mounted diagnostic study models and intraoral clinical photographs are a useful part of the clinical examination and treatment-planning process to aid in assessment of spatial and occlusal relationships. Once all the data collection is completed, the clinician will be able to determine whether implant therapy is possible, practical, and indicated for the patient.

Conducting an organized, systematic history and examination is essential to obtaining an accurate diagnosis and creating a treatment plan that is appropriate for the patient. Each treatment plan should be comprehensive and provide several treatment options for the patient, including periodontal and restorative therapies. Then, in consultation, the clinician can agree on the final treatment plan with the patient. Information gathered throughout the process will help the clinician's decision making and determination on whether a patient is a good candidate for dental implants. A thoughtful and well-executed evaluation will also reveal deficiencies and indicate what additional surgical procedures may be necessary to accomplish the desired goals of therapy (e.g., localized ridge augmentation, sinus bone augmentation). Each part of the pretreatment evaluation is briefly discussed here.

Chief Complaint

What is the problem or concern in the patient's own words? What is the patient's goal of treatment, and how realistic are the patient's expectations? The *patient's* chief concern, desires for treatment, and vision of the successful outcome must be taken into consideration. The patient will measure implant success according to personal criteria. The overall comfort and function of the implant restoration are often the most important factors, but satisfaction with the appearance of the final restoration will also influence the patient's perception of success. Furthermore, patient satisfaction may be influenced simply by the impact that the treatment has on the patient's perceived quality of life. Whether the clinician inquires about quality-of-life changes or not, the patient most likely will measure the success of treatment by comparison to the pretreatment condition. Patients will evaluate for themselves whether the treatment helped them to eat better, look better, or feel better about themselves.

The clinician could consider an implant(s) and the retained prosthesis a success using standard criteria of symptom-free implant function, implant stability, and lack of periimplant infection or bone loss. At the same time, however, the patient who does not like the esthetic result or does not think the condition has improved could consider the treatment a failure. Therefore it is critical to inquire, as specifically as possible, about the patient's expectations before initiating implant therapy and to appreciate the patient's desires and values. With this goal in mind, it is often helpful and advisable to invite patients to bring their spouse or a family member to the consultation and treatment-planning visits to add an independent "trusted" observer to the discussion of treatment options. Ultimately, it is the clinician's responsibility to determine if the patient has realistic expectations for the outcome of therapy and to educate the patient about realistic outcomes for each treatment option.

Medical History

A thorough medical history is required for any patient in need of dental treatment, regardless of whether implants are part of the plan. This history should be documented in writing by the patient's completion of a standard health history form and verbally through an interview with the treating clinician. The patient's health history should be reviewed for any condition that might put the patient at risk for adverse reactions or complications.

Patients must be in reasonably good health to undergo surgical therapy for the placement of dental implants. Any disorder that may impair the normal wound-healing process, especially as it relates to bone metabolism, should be carefully considered as a possible risk factor or contraindication to implant therapy (see later discussion).

A thorough physical examination is warranted if any questions arise about the health status of the patient.[17] Appropriate laboratory tests (e.g., coagulation tests for a patient receiving anticoagulant therapy) should be requested to evaluate further any conditions that may affect the patient's ability to undergo the planned surgical and restorative procedures safely and effectively. If any questions remain about the patient's health status, a medical clearance for surgery should be obtained from the patient's treating physician.

Dental History

A review of a patient's past dental experiences can be a valuable part of the overall evaluation. Does the patient report a history of recurrent or frequent abscesses, which may indicate a susceptibility to infections or diabetes? Does the patient have many restorations? How compliant has the patient been with previous dental recommendations? What are the patient's current oral hygiene practices?

The individual's previous experiences with surgery and prosthetics should be discussed. If a patient reports numerous problems and difficulties with past dental care, including a history of dissatisfaction with past treatment, the patient may have similar difficulties with implant therapy. It is essential to identify past problems and to elucidate any contributing factors. The clinician must also assess the patient's dental knowledge and understanding of the proposed treatment as well as the patient's attitude and motivation toward implants.

Intraoral Examination

The oral examination is performed to assess the current health and condition of existing teeth as well as to evaluate the condition of the oral hard and soft tissues. It is imperative that no pathologic conditions are present in any of the hard or soft tissues in the maxillofacial region. All oral lesions, especially infections, should be diagnosed and appropriately treated before implant therapy. Additional criteria to consider include the patient's habits, level of oral hygiene, overall dental and periodontal health, occlusion, jaw relationship, temporomandibular joint condition, and ability to open wide.

After a thorough intraoral examination, the clinician can evaluate potential implant sites. All sites should be

BOX 74-1

How Much Space Is Required for Placement of One or More Implants?*

Alveolar Bone
Assuming an implant that is 4 mm in diameter and 10 mm long, the minimal width of the jawbone needs to be 6 to 7 mm, and the minimal height should be 10 mm (minimum of 12 mm in the posterior mandible, where an additional margin of safety is required over the mandibular nerve). This dimension is desired to maintain at least 1.0 to 1.5 mm of bone around all surfaces of the implant after preparation and placement.

Interdental Space
Edentulous spaces need to be measured to determine whether enough space exists for the placement and restoration with one or more implant crowns. The minimal space requirements for the placement of one, two, or more implants are illustrated diagrammatically in Figures 74-9 and 74-10. The minimal mesial-distal space for an implant placed between two teeth is 7 mm. The minimal mesial-distal space required for the placement of two standard-diameter implants (4.0-mm diameter) between teeth is 14 mm. The required minimal dimensions for wide-diameter or narrow-diameter implants will increase or decrease incrementally according to the size of the implant. For example, the minimal space needed for the placement of an implant 6 mm in diameter is 9 mm (= 7 mm + 2 mm). Whenever the available space between teeth is greater than 7 mm and less than 14 mm, only one implant, such as placement of a wide-diameter implant, should be considered. The placement of a wide-diameter implant should be considered. Two narrow-diameter implants could be positioned in a space that is 12 mm. However, the smaller implant may be more vulnerable to implant fracture.

Interocclusal Space
The restoration consists of the abutment, the abutment screw, and the crown (it may also include a screw to secure the crown to the abutment if it is not cemented). This restorative "stack" is the total of all the components used to attach the crown to the implant. The dimensions of the restorative stack vary slightly depending on the type of abutment and the implant-restorative interface (i.e., internal or external connection). The minimum amount of interocclusal space required for the restorative "stack" on an external hex-type implant is 7 mm.

*All the minimal space requirements discussed here are generic averages. The actual space limitations for any particular implant system must be determined according to the manufacturer's specifications.

clinically evaluated to measure the available space in the bone for the placement of implants and in the dental space for prosthetic tooth replacement (Box 74-1). The mesial-distal and buccal-lingual dimensions of edentulous spaces can be approximated with a periodontal probe or other measuring instrument. The orientation or tilt of adjacent teeth and their roots should be noted as well. There may be enough space in the coronal area for the restoration but not enough space in the apical region for the implant if roots are directed into the area of interest (Figure 74-8). Conversely, there may be adequate space between roots, but the coronal aspects of the teeth may be too close for emergence and restoration of the implant. If either of these conditions is discovered, orthodontic tooth movement may be indicated. Ultimately, edentulous areas need to be precisely measured using diagnostic study models and imaging techniques to determine whether space is available and whether adequate bone volume exists to replace missing teeth with implants and implant restorations. Figure 74-9 diagrams the minimal space requirements for standard-, wide-, and narrow-diameter implants placed between natural teeth, and Figure 74-10 diagrams the minimal interocclusal space needed to restore implants.

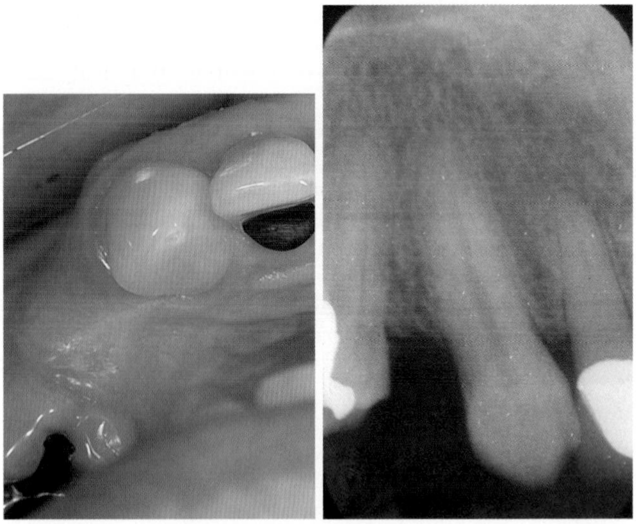

Figure 74-8 **A,** Clinical photograph of maxillary premolar space with apparently adequate space between the remaining teeth for an implant-supported crown. **B,** Radiograph clearly shows a lack of space between the roots of the adjacent teeth as a result of convergence into the space (same patient as in *A*).

Diagnostic Study Models. Mounted study models are an excellent means of assessing potential sites for dental implants. Properly articulated models with diagnostic wax-up of the proposed restorations allow the clinician to evaluate the available space and to determine potential limitations of the planned treatment (Figure 74-11). This is particularly useful when multiple teeth are to be replaced with implants or when a malocclusion is present.

Hard Tissue Evaluation. The amount of available bone is the next criterion to evaluate. Wide variations in jaw anatomy are encountered, and it is therefore important to analyze the anatomy of the dentoalveolar region of interest both clinically and radiographically. A visual examination can immediately identify deficient

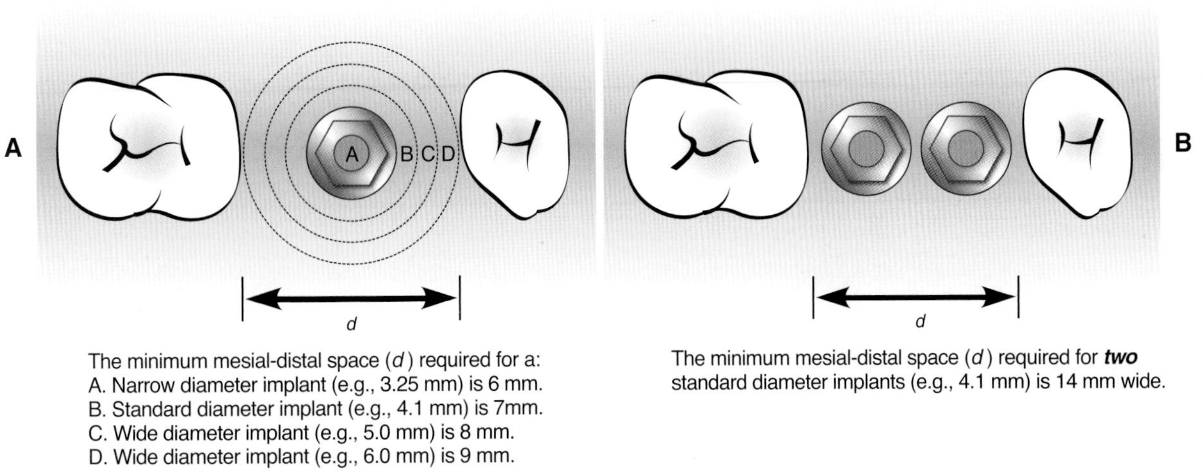

A
A
B
C
D
B
d
d
The minimum mesial-distal space (*d*) required for a:
A. Narrow diameter implant (e.g., 3.25 mm) is 6 mm.
B. Standard diameter implant (e.g., 4.1 mm) is 7mm.
C. Wide diameter implant (e.g., 5.0 mm) is 8 mm.
D. Wide diameter implant (e.g., 6.0 mm) is 9 mm.
The minimum mesial-distal space (*d*) required for ***two*** standard diameter implants (e.g., 4.1 mm) is 14 mm wide.

Figure 74-9 **A,** Minimum amount of mesial-distal space *(d)* required for placement of single-tooth implant between natural teeth: *A,* 6 mm for narrow-diameter implant (3.25 mm); *B,* 7 mm for standard-diameter implant (4.1 mm); *C* and *D,* 8 mm and 9 mm, respectively, for wide-diameter implants (5.0 mm and 6.0 mm). **B,** Minimum amount of mesial-distal space *(d)* required for placement of two standard-diameter (4.1-mm) implants between natural teeth is 14 mm. This allows approximately 2 mm between teeth/implants and between implant/implant.

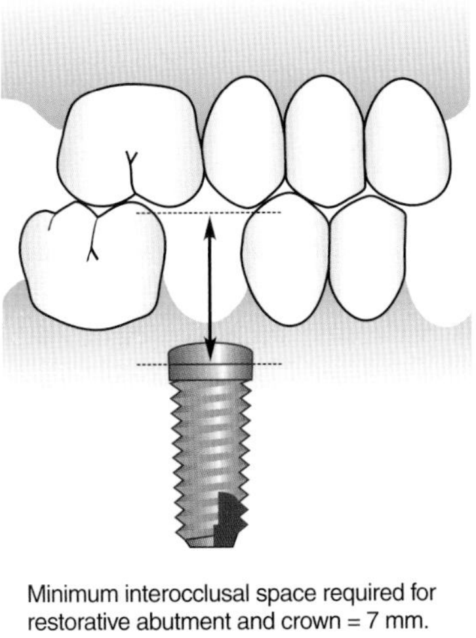

Minimum interocclusal space required for restorative abutment and crown = 7 mm.

Figure 74-10 Minimum amount of space required between implant/restoration interface and opposing occlusal surfaces for restoration of an implant. This dimension will vary depending on implant design and manufacturer component dimensions. The minimal dimension of 7 mm is based on an externally hexed implant and UCLA abutment.

areas (Figure 74-12), whereas other areas that appear to have good ridge width will require further evaluation (Figure 74-13). Clinical examination of the jawbone consists of palpation to feel for anatomic defects and variations in the jaw anatomy, such as concavities and undercuts. If desired, it is possible with local anesthesia to probe through the soft tissue (intraoral bone mapping) to assess the thickness of the soft tissues and measure the bone dimensions at the proposed surgical site.

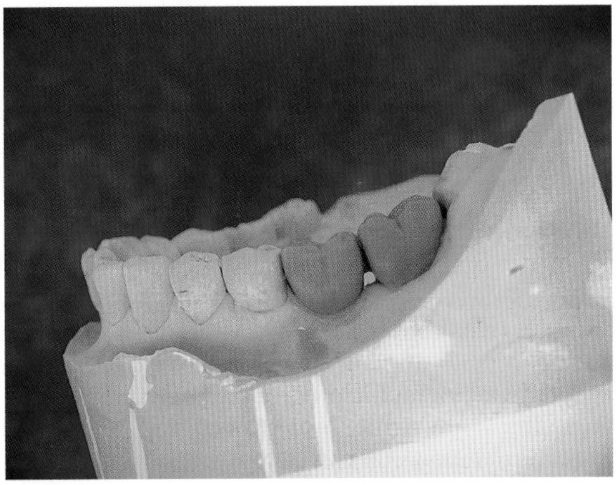

Figure 74-11 Photograph of a diagnostic model with proposed molar tooth replacement waxed to evaluate the amount of space and contours.

The spatial relationship of the bone must be evaluated in a three-dimensional view because the implant must be placed in the appropriate position relative to the prosthesis. It is possible that an adequate dimension of bone is available in the anticipated implant site (see Box 74-1), but that the bone and thus the implant placement might be located too lingual or too buccal for the desired prosthetic tooth replacement.[36] Bone augmentation procedures may be necessary to facilitate the placement of an implant in an acceptable prosthetic position despite the availability of an adequate quantity of bone (i.e., the bone is in the wrong location). Indications for the use of bone augmentation procedures are discussed in Chapter 77.

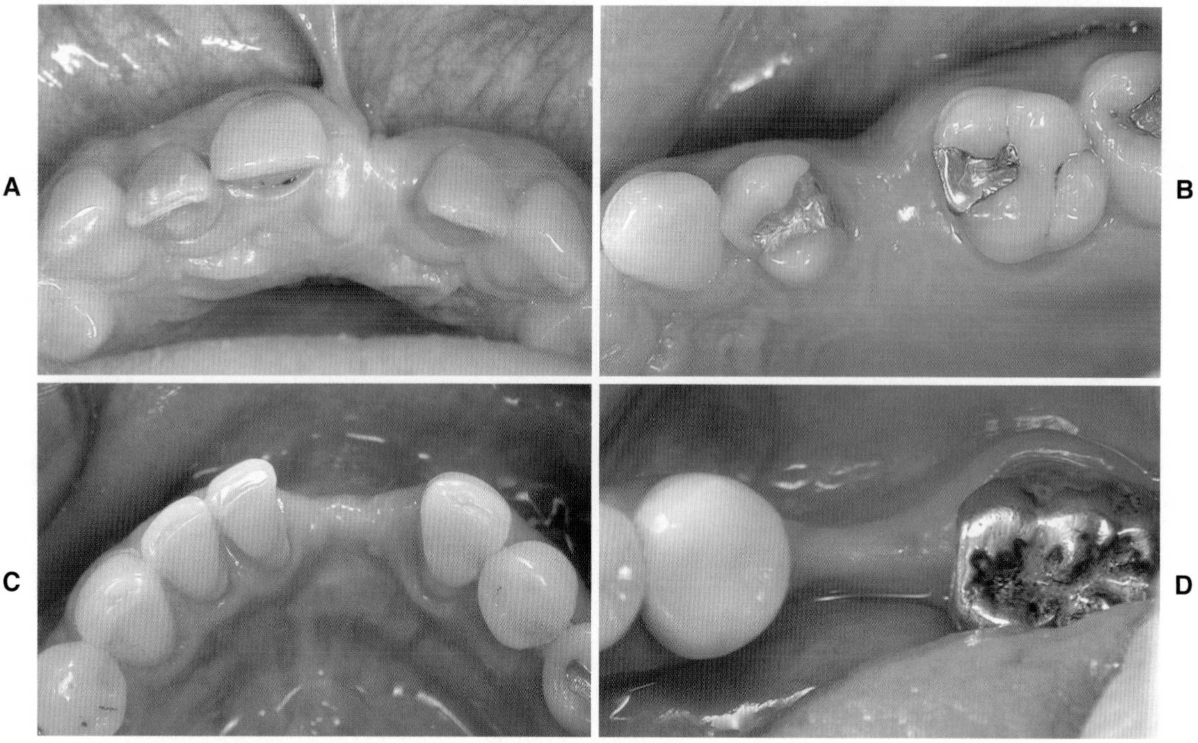

Figure 74-12 Clinical photographs of edentulous areas with obvious deficient areas of alveolar dimension noted on visual examination: **A,** anterior maxilla; **B,** posterior maxilla; **C,** anterior mandible; **D,** posterior mandible. These clinical images all represent buccolingual deficiencies in the alveolar dimensions.

Radiographic Examination. Radiographic assessment of the quantity, quality, and location of available alveolar bone in potential implant sites ultimately determines whether a patient is a candidate for implants and if a particular implant site needs bone augmentation. Appropriate radiographic procedures, including periapical radiographs, panoramic projections, and tomographic cross-sectional imaging, can help identify vital structures such as the floor of the nasal cavity, maxillary sinus, mandibular canal, and mental foramen (see Chapter 75). In addition to the absolute dimensional measurement of the alveolar bone, it is important to determine whether the volume of bone radiographically (as well as clinically) is located in a position to allow for the proper position of the implant to facilitate restoration of the tooth/teeth in proper esthetic and functional relationship with the adjacent and opposing dentition. The best way to evaluate the relationship of available bone to the dentition is to image the patient with a diagnostically accurate guide using radiopaque markers that accurately represent the proposed prosthetic contours (see Figure 75-5).

Soft Tissue Evaluation. Evaluation of the quality, quantity, and location of soft tissue present in the anticipated implant site helps to anticipate the type of tissue that will surround the implant(s) after treatment is completed (keratinized vs. nonkeratinized mucosa). For some cases, depending on the clinician's view of keratinized tissue, evaluation may reveal a need for soft tissue augmentation (Box 74-2). Areas with minimal or no existing keratinized mucosa may be augmented with gingival or connective tissue grafts. Additionally, any mucogingival concerns, such as frenum attachments or pulls, should be thoroughly evaluated.

RISK FACTORS AND CONTRAINDICATIONS

Clearly, there are numerous indications for the use of endosseous dental implants to replace missing teeth. Most patients who are missing one or more teeth can benefit from the application of an implant-retained prosthesis provided they meet the requirements for surgical and prosthetic rehabilitation. Edentulous patients who are unable to function with complete dentures and who have adequate bone for the placement of dental implants can be especially good dental implant candidates. More and more partially edentulous patients are also being treated with dental implant restorations. Many patients, whether they are missing one, several, or all of their teeth, can be predictably restored with implant-retained prostheses.

In this era of high implant success and predictability and thus possible complacency, it is imperative for clinicians to recognize risk factors and contraindications to implant therapy so that problems can be minimized and patients can be accurately informed about risks. As such, the clinician must be knowledgeable in this area and inform patients about risk factors and contraindications

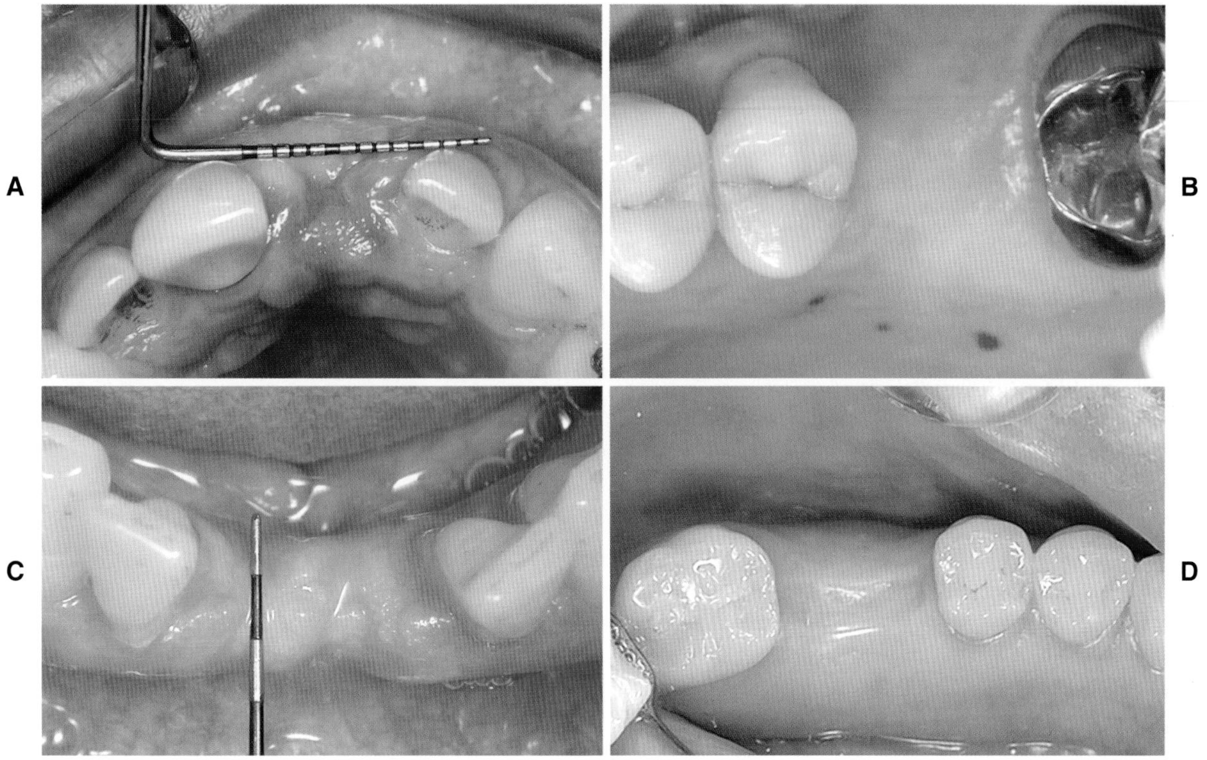

Figure 74-13 Clinical photograph of edentulous areas with apparent good alveolar dimension noted on visual examination: **A,** anterior maxilla; **B,** posterior maxilla; **C,** anterior mandible; **D,** posterior mandible. It is likely that these sites have adequate bone volume for implant placement. However, it is also possible to find alveolar deficiencies despite the appearance of wide ridges.

before initiating treatment. Contraindications for the use of dental implants, although relatively few and often not well defined, do exist. Some conditions are probably best described as "risk factors" rather than "contraindications" to treatment because implants can be successful in almost all patients; implants may be less *predictable* in some situations, and this distinction should be recognized. Ultimately, it is the clinician's responsibility with the patient to make decisions as to when implant therapy is not indicated.

Table 74-1 lists some conditions and factors that are thought to increase the risk for implant failure or otherwise deem the patient a poor candidate for implant therapy. Some of these conditions are briefly discussed here.

Medical and Systemic Health–Related Issues

Although few absolute medical contraindications to implant therapy exist, some relative contraindications are important to consider. The clinician must consider medical and health-related conditions that affect bone metabolism or any aspect of the patient's capacity to heal normally.[9] This category includes conditions such as diabetes, osteoporosis, and immune compromise and medical treatments such as chemotherapy and irradiation.

Diabetes Mellitus. Diabetes is a metabolic disease that can have significant effects on the patient's ability

BOX 74-2

How Much Keratinized Tissue Is Required for Health and Maintenance of Implants?

Debate continues about whether it is necessary to have a zone of keratinized tissue surrounding implants. Despite strong opinions and beliefs about the need for keratinized mucosa around implants versus this mucosa being unnecessary, neither argument has been proved.

Some studies have concluded that, in the presence of good oral hygiene, a lack of keratinized tissue does not impair the health or function of implants.[67] Others strongly believe that keratinized mucosa has better functional and esthetic results for implant restorations. Keratinized mucosa is typically thicker and denser than alveolar mucosa (nonkeratinized). It forms a strong seal around the implant with a cuff of circular (parallel) fibers around the implant, abutment, or restoration that is resistant to retracting with mastication forces and oral hygiene procedures. Implants with coated surfaces (i.e., HA or TPS coating) demonstrate greater peri-implant bone loss and failures in the absence of keratinized mucosa.[14,44]

TABLE 74-1

Risk Factors and Contraindications for Implant Therapy

	Risk Factor	Contraindication
Medical and Systemic Health–Related Issues		
Diabetes (poorly controlled)	?? -Possibly	Relative
Bone metabolic disease (e.g., osteoporosis)	?? -Probably	Relative
Radiation therapy (head and neck)	Yes	Relative/Absolute
Immunosuppressive medication	?? -Probably	Relative
Immunocompromising disease (e.g., HIV, AIDS)	?? -Possibly	Relative
Psychologic and Mental Conditions		
Psychiatric syndromes (e.g., schizophrenia, paranoia)	No	Absolute
Mental instability (e.g., neurotic, hysterical)	No	Absolute
Mentally impaired; uncooperative	No	Absolute
Irrational fears; phobias	No	Absolute
Unrealistic expectations	No	Absolute
Habits and Behavioral Considerations		
Smoking; tobacco use	Yes	Relative
Parafunctional habits	Yes	Relative
Substance abuse (e.g., alcohol, drugs)	?? -Possibly	Absolute
Intraoral Examination Findings		
Atrophic maxilla	Yes	Relative
Current infection (e.g., endodontic)	Yes	Relative
Periodontal disease	?? -Possibly	Relative

HIV, Human immunodeficiency virus; *AIDS*, acquired immunodeficiency syndrome.

to heal normally and resist infections. This is particularly true for diabetic patients who are not well controlled. Poorly controlled diabetics often have impaired wound healing and a predisposition to infections, whereas diabetic patients whose disease is well controlled experience few, if any, problems (see Chapter 17).

There is concern about the predictability of implants in patients with diabetes. Several studies have reported moderate failure rates in diabetic patients, with implant success ranging from 85.6% to 94.3%.[7,32,43] A prospective study demonstrated 2.2% early failures and 7.3% late failures in diabetic patients.[63] After 5 years the overall success rate for this group of diabetic patients was 90%.[56] None of these studies was able to correlate gender, age, smoking, diabetes type, or level of diabetic control with implant failure. In a meta-analytical review of implant failures in nondiabetic patients, the early implant failure rate was 3.2% and the late implant failure rate 5.2%.[26] The finding that diabetic patients experience slightly more late failures may be related to less tissue integrity caused by reduced tissue turnover and impaired tissue perfusion. These results suggest that diabetes may be a risk factor for implants, particularly for late failures. However, the risk does not appear to be particularly high.

Bone Metabolic Disease. Osteoporosis is a skeletal condition characterized by decreased mineral density. The two main classifications are primary (three types) and secondary (many types) osteoporosis. *Primary osteoporosis* has been attributed to menopausal changes (type I), age-related changes (type II), or idiopathic causes (type III). *Secondary osteoporosis* has been attributed to many different diseases and conditions, including diabetes, alcoholism, malnutrition, and smoking.[37]

All the various types of osteoporosis share the same fundamental problem of decreased bone mineral density, and the concern that this condition may impair the patient's ability to achieve and maintain implant osseointegration. The premise that implants will not perform as well in a patient with osteoporosis is reasonable given that osseointegration depends on bone formation adjacent to the implant surface and that success rates are highest in dense bone and lowest in poor-quality, loose trabecular bone. However, no clear evidence suggests that implants will not be successful in patients with osteoporosis, and the issue continues to be debated.[8,22] On the positive side, although the evidence is weak, case reports have demonstrated successful implant treatment in patients with osteoporosis.[36] Some investigators advocate the use of longer healing times for osseointegration to occur before loading the implants in patients with osteoporosis.[34] Conversely, evidence also suggests that implants placed in augmented bone in the maxillary sinus in patients with osteoporosis have significantly lower success rates.[13]

Interestingly, there is a trend in aging adults (men over 50 years and postmenopausal women) for bone mass to decrease progressively through bone demineralization at a rate of 1% to 2% per year and in some individuals as much as 5% to 8% per year throughout their later life.[24,42] If one considers this decline in bone mass with aging along with a continually increasing life expectancy in the population, the number of individuals with osteopenia or osteoporosis will continue to increase, and the concern about this condition's influence on implant success will become increasingly important for clinicians.

Immune Compromise and Immune Suppression. Individuals undergoing chemotherapy or taking medications that impair healing potential (e.g., steroids) are probably not good candidates for implant therapy because of the effects on normal healing. A lowered resistance to infection may also be problematic for these patients. Likewise, patients with an immunocompromising disease, such as human immunodeficiency virus (HIV) infection or acquired immunodeficiency syndrome (AIDS), are probably not good candidates for implants, especially when their immune system is seriously impaired. A past history of chemotherapy or immunosuppressive therapy may not be problematic if the patient has recovered from the side effects of treatment.

Radiation Therapy. Patients with a history of radiation treatment to the head and neck region may not heal well after surgery. Soft tissue dehiscence may follow surgical manipulation, which may lead to *osteoradionecrosis* (ORN), a serious condition of nonhealing exposure and infection of bone. This is especially problematic for patients who have received radiation dosages greater than 60 Gy. Surgical procedures, or any procedure that may initiate a wound, are generally avoided in patients with a history of radiation therapy. If deemed necessary, surgical procedures can be done in conjunction with hyperbaric oxygen (HBO) therapy to reduce the risk of ORN.

Several studies have documented poor success rates for implants in patients with a history of radiation therapy.[38,39,50] In a literature review, Sennerby and Roos[62] found irradiation to be associated with high failure rates, as did Esposito et al.[28] in their review. Beumer et al.[12] reported success rates as low as 60.4% in the irradiated maxilla. Granstrom et al.[38] reported a significant improvement in survival rates for implants in patients treated with HBO. However, in a systematic review, Coulthard et al.[21] concluded that the evidence is lacking to support the clinical effectiveness of HBO in irradiated patients receiving implants.

The application of implants in patients with a history of irradiation, with or without the use of HBO, is not resolved and continues to be debated. Clearly, irradiation is a risk factor for implant success and may be a contraindication.

Psychologic and Mental Conditions

In general, any type of psychologic abnormality can be considered a contraindication to dental implant treatment because of the patient's uncooperativeness, lack of understanding, or behavioral problems. Physiologically, there is no reason to suspect that implants could not become osseointegrated in these patients. However, the patient's ability to tolerate the number and type of treatment appointments required for implant placement, restoration, and maintenance could be problematic. All psychologic conditions have the potential to be absolute contraindications to implant treatment depending on the severity of the condition. The exception might be individuals who demonstrate good cooperative behavior with only mild psychologic or mental impairment. The clinician should take great care before accepting a mentally or psychologically impaired individual for treatment with implants.

Habits and Behavioral Considerations

Patients have a variety of habits and behaviors that may increase the risk of failure for implants. Smoking, clenching or grinding of teeth, and drug or alcohol abuse are among the most well-known habits that should be identified because of the increased risk for implant failure or complications.

Smoking and Tobacco Use. Moderate to heavy smoking has been documented to result in higher rates of early implant failure and adversely affect the long-term prognosis of dental implant restorations.[5,23,51] The mechanisms of action responsible for higher implant failures associated with smoking are not understood. Smoking is a known risk factor for osteoporosis and thus may adversely affect implant success through its effect on bone metabolism. Smoking cessation may improve the success rate of implants.[4] In a meta-analytical review, Bain et al.[6] found that implants with an altered surface microtopography (Osseotite, acid-etched surface) seemed to lessen significantly the adverse affects of smoking on implant success.

Parafunctional Habits. Parafunctional habits, such as clenching or grinding of teeth (consciously or unconsciously), has been associated with an increased rate of implant failure. Repeated lateral forces (i.e., parafunctional habits) applied to implants can be detrimental to the osseointegration process, especially during the early healing period. Patients with known parafunctional habits should be advised about an increased risk of complications or failures as a result of their clenching or grinding. Many consider bruxism to be a contraindication to implant treatment, especially in the case of a short-span, fixed partial denture or a single-tooth implant. If implants are planned for a patient with parafunctional habits, protective measures should be employed, such as creating a narrow occlusal table with flat cusp angles, protected occlusion, and the regular use of occlusal guards (see Chapter 80).

Substance Abuse. Drug and alcohol abuse should be considered a contraindication for implant therapy for reasons similar to the psychologic problems discussed earlier. Patients with drug or alcohol addictions can be irresponsible and noncompliant with treatment recommendations. Depending on the severity and duration of an individual's addiction, some patients may be malnourished or may even have impaired organ function and therefore may not be a good surgical candidate because of poor healing capacity. All elective treatments, including implant therapy, should be refused until addictions are treated and controlled.

POSTTREATMENT EVALUATION

Periodic examination of implants, the retained prosthesis, and the condition of the surrounding periimplant tissue is an important part of successful treatment. Aberrations and complications can often be treated if discovered early, but many problems will go unnoticed by the patient. Thus, periodic examination is essential to discovering problems early. Several parameters are available to evaluate the condition of the prosthesis, the stability of the implant(s), and the health of surrounding periimplant tissues after implant integration and prosthetic restoration. Many of these clinical measures are adaptations from dental and periodontal examination methods, such as clinical inspection, probing, and radiographic examination.

Clinical Examination

The clinical examination includes visual inspection and probing. Visual evaluation of the tissue color contour and consistency, periimplant probing, and radiographic images are some of the ways to evaluate implants in the posttreatment phase. Soft tissues can be visually inspected for signs of inflammation or swelling. They can also be palpated to detect areas of edema, tenderness, exudate, or suppuration. Periimplant probing can be used to assess the condition and level of hard and soft tissues surrounding implants.

Periimplant Probing. Periodontal probing around natural teeth is very useful to assess the health of periodontal tissues, the sulcus or pocket depth, and the level of attachment. However, using a periodontal probe around implants may not provide comparable results.[15] Clinicians should use caution when evaluating periimplant probing because these measures cannot be interpreted the same as probing depths around teeth. Because of distinct differences in the surrounding tissues that support teeth compared to those that support implants, the probe inserts and penetrates differently. Around teeth, the periodontal probe is resisted by the health of the periodontal tissues and, perhaps most importantly, by the insertion of supracrestal connective tissue fibers into the cementum of the root surface. These fibers, unique to teeth, are the primary source of resistance to the probe.[3] There is no equivalent fiber attachment around implants. Connective tissue fibers around implants generally run parallel to the implant or restorative surface and do not have perpendicular or inserting fibers (see Chapter 73). The primary source of resistance to the probe around an implant will differ depending on the conditions surrounding the implant.[25,46] At noninflamed sites, the probe will be resisted by the most coronal aspect of connective tissue adhesion to the implant. At inflamed sites, the probe tip consistently penetrates farther into the connective tissue until less inflamed connective tissue is encountered, which is often close to the level of bone.

The value of periimplant probing is different than periodontal probing and offers very limited information by comparison. Probing around implants can measure the level of the mucosal margin relative to a fixed position on the implant or restoration and can also measure the depth of tissue around the implant. The periimplant probing depth is often a measure of the thickness of the surrounding connective tissues and correlates most consistently with the level of surrounding bone. However, periimplant probing is affected by several conditions, including the size of the probe, the force and direction of insertion, the health and resistance of periimplant tissues, the level of bone support, and the features of the implant, abutment, and prosthesis design. In other words, the probe is not only a measure of tissue thickness, but also an indicator of access for the probe. In such situations, some areas will not be accurately measured as a result of the implant and prosthesis design. Furthermore, probing around implants is likely to be more variable than around teeth; studies have shown that a change in probing force around implants results in more dramatic changes than a similar change in probing force around teeth.[55]

The probing depth around implants presumed to be "healthy" (and without bleeding) has been documented to be about 3 mm around all surfaces.[1,19] The absence of bleeding on probing around teeth has been established as an indicator of health and a predictor of periodontal stability.[45] Studies comparing bleeding on probing around teeth and implants in the same patient have reported that bleeding around implants occurs more frequently. However, the ability to use bleeding as an indicator of assessing diseased versus healthy sites around implants has not been established. Microbiologic studies suggest that greater probing depth or "pockets" around implants harbor higher levels of pathogenic microorganisms.[54,60,61]

Microbial Testing. Studies in animals and humans have demonstrated the development of periimplant mucosal inflammation in response to the accumulation of bacterial plaque.[11,58] Studies have also documented similarities in the microbial composition of plaque in healthy periodontal sites compared with healthy periimplant sites.[53] Likewise, evidence indicates that the micobiota of inflamed periimplant sites (periimplantitis) harbors the same periodontal pathogenic microorganisms as those observed in diseased periodontal pockets.[53,61] However, there is no evidence to prove that periodontal pathogens cause periimplant disease, and the pathogenesis of inflammatory disease around implants has not been defined.[20] No convincing evidence indicates that laboratory tests for the identification of suspected periodontal pathogens are of any use in the evaluation of implants.[27] The usefulness of microbial testing may be limited to the evaluation of periimplant sites that are showing signs of infection and bone loss, so the clinician can prescribe appropriate antibiotics.

Stability Measures. The assessment of implant stability (or mobility) is an important measure for determining whether osseointegration is being maintained. Importantly, however, this measure has extremely low sensitivity but high specificity. That is, a large amount of bone loss can occur around an implant, but the implant remains stable (stability measure in this case has a low sensitivity for the detection of an implant that has lost much of its bone support). On the other hand, if significant mobility is detected, the implant has likely failed (mobility is highly specificity for the detection of implant failure). There is great interest in evaluating the stability of the bone-to-implant contact in a noninvasive manner. Two techniques that have been used as noninvasive ways of evaluating implant stability are impact resistance (e.g., Periotest) and resonance frequency analysis.

Originally designed to evaluate tooth mobility quantitatively, the Periotest (Gulden, Bensheim, Germany) is a noninvasive, electronic device that provides an objective measurement of the reaction of the periodontium to a defined impact load applied to the tooth crown. The Periotest value depends to some extent on tooth mobility but mainly on the damping characteristics of the periodontium.

Despite the dependence on the periodontium, the Periotest has been used to evaluate implant stability as well. However, unlike teeth, the movement of implants and the surrounding bone is minuscule, and therefore the Periotest values fall within a much smaller range compared to the range found with teeth. Detection of horizontal mobility may be a significant advantage for the use of the Periotest because it is much more sensitive to horizontal movement than similar detection by other means, such as manual assessment.[27] Additionally, many variables have been associated with the use of the Periotest related to positioning of the device.

Resonance frequency analysis (RFA) is another noninvasive method used to measure the stability of implants.[52] This method uses a transducer that is attached to the implant or abutment. A steady-state signal is applied to the implant through the transducer, and a response is measured. The RFA value is a function of the stiffness of the implant in the surrounding tissues. The stiffness is influenced by the implant, the interface between the implant and bone, and soft tissues as well as the surrounding bone. Additionally, the height of the implant or abutment above the bone will influence the RFA value. Unlike the Periotest, however, the RFA is not dependent on movement in only one direction. Thus the absolute RFA values will vary from one implant design to another and from one site to another, but there is high consistency for any one implant or location. The value of RFA is most appreciated with repeated measures of the same implant over time because it is very sensitive to changes in the bone-implant interface. Small changes in tissue support can be detected using RFA. An increase in RFA value indicates increased implant stability, whereas a decrease indicates loss of stability. However, it has not been determined whether RFA is capable of detecting impending failure before the implant actually fails.

Currently, much interest and research have focused on the use of noninvasive methods to evaluate implant stability. Mobility remains the cardinal sign of implant failure, and detecting mobility is therefore an important parameter.

Radiographic Examination

Intraoral radiographs should be taken at the time of placement (baseline), at the time of abutment connection (confirm seating and serve as another baseline), and subsequently to monitor marginal or periimplant bone changes. Periapical radiographs have excellent resolution and provide adequate details for evaluating bone support around implants if taken at a perpendicular direction. The limitation of periapical radiographs is that they are difficult to standardize, and great variability is inherent in the acquisition process. However, periapical films are relatively simple, inexpensive, and readily available in the dental office.

The objective of the radiographic examination is to measure the height of bone adjacent to the implant(s) and to evaluate the presence and quality of bone along the length of the implant. Finally, the periimplant areas are assessed for any radiolucent lesions around the implant. Although the predictive value of assessing implant stability with radiographs is low, films do offer a reasonable method to measure changes in bone levels.[65] The predictive value of detecting implant failure or loss of stability is good when radiolucent lesions are discovered with periapical radiographs. Radiographic identification of unstable implants is reliable when performed as part of annual examinations and when examining patients on a routine, long-term basis.[40]

The radiographic examination remains one of the primary tools for detection of failed implants in routine clinical evaluation, even though it is not as accurate as mobility tests. In one study designed to evaluate the accuracy and precision of radiographic diagnosis of mobility, the probability of predicting implant mobility in a population with a low prevalence of implant failures was found to be low.[65] Other studies, however, have demonstrated much higher predictive value for radiographic diagnosis of implant mobility.[33,40] The authors concluded that the most important factors for making an accurate radiographic diagnosis are the quality of the radiograph and the experience of the clinician.[40,65]

Oral Hygiene and Implant Maintenance

The long-term success of dental implants likely requires the maintenance of healthy periimplant tissues because the soft tissue "seal" around implants is best when the surrounding mucosa is not inflamed. For this reason, good oral hygiene and regular professional care are essential to maintaining implants. The importance of good oral hygiene should be stressed even before implants are placed, and oral hygiene instructions for plaque control should begin as early as possible. The patient's ability to maintain good oral hygiene should be monitored and reinforced at each visit, and the patient should be given instructions specific to individual needs. Interestingly, despite many years of experience with implants, a recent systematic review revealed that no well-designed studies with a high level of evidence (i.e., randomized controlled trials) have defined the most effective regimens for long-term implant maintenance.[29]

Professionally, several actions can be taken to enhance the patient's ability to perform good oral hygiene. For example, implant superstructures, frameworks, and restorations should be fabricated to accommodate and facilitate oral hygiene (e.g., embrasure spaces should be made to allow the passage of a proxybrush). Specific oral hygiene procedures with appropriate hygiene aids should be demonstrated for each implant area for every patient. Initially, for the first year after treatment is completed, recall maintenance visits should be scheduled at 3-month intervals and then adjusted to suit the patient's individual needs. Some patients, with good oral hygiene and minimal deposits, will require infrequent professional hygiene maintenance, whereas others, with poor oral hygiene and heavy deposits, will require more frequent follow-up care.

The use of plastic and gold-coated curettes has been advocated to protect the titanium implant surface and the titanium abutment from contamination by other metals. These curettes were also used to reduce the likelihood of scratching the surface. Unfortunately, plastic curettes do not work very well, and gold-coated curettes cannot be sharpened. Most current implant prostheses are made with gold alloys or ceramic materials, which are usually identical to the materials used in restorations for the natural dentition. Furthermore, the location of the connection between these restorative materials and the implant is typically below the mucosa and often near the crest of bone; most calculus removal will be above this level. Thus the fear of contaminating the titanium implant is unwarranted. The gold alloy or ceramic surfaces can be debrided with most scalers and curettes (plastic, gold coated, stainless steel) without damaging the surface. Rotary instruments (e.g., prophy cup) can be used to remove plaque or biofilms and polish surfaces. The use and sonic instruments (e.g., Cavitron) should be avoided because of irregularities that can easily be created in the surface, which can contribute to plaque and calculus accumulation.

Recall maintenance visits should include an evaluation of soft and hard tissue health, the patient's level of oral hygiene compliance and plaque control, prosthesis integrity and stability, and implant stability. Implant stability can be evaluated with a combination of mobility testing and radiographic assessment.

CONCLUSION

Dental clinicians can now predictably replace missing teeth with endosseous dental implants. Most patients, whether missing a single tooth, several teeth, or all their teeth, can be candidates for dental implant therapy. However, many factors influence the outcome; the clinician must consider the quantity, quality, and location of available bone; the patient's mental and physical health; and risk factors and contraindications. Patients should be advised about risk factors and provided treatment options both with and without dental implants. Periodic evaluation, good oral hygiene, and regular maintenance are important aspects of care for the long-term success and the prevention of complications with dental implants. Radiographic examination and mobility tests appear to be some of the most reliable parameters in the assessment of endosseous dental implants.

REFERENCES

1. Adell R, Lekholm U, Rockler B, et al: A 15-year study of osseointegrated implants in the treatment of the edentulous jaw, *Int J Oral Surg* 10:387, 1981.
2. Adell R, Eriksson B, Lekholm U, et al: A long-term follow-up study of osseointegrated implants in the treatment of totally edentulous jaws, *Int J Oral Maxillofac Implants* 5:347, 1990.
3. Armitage GC, Svanberg GK, Löe H: Microscopic evaluation of clinical measurements of connective tissue attachment levels, *J Clin Periodontol* 4:173, 1977.
4. Bain CA: Smoking and implant failure: benefits of a smoking cessation protocol, *Int J Oral Maxillofac Implants* 11:756, 1996.
5. Bain CA, Moy PK: The association between the failure of dental implants and cigarette smoking, *Int J Oral Maxillofac Implants* 8:609, 1993.
6. Bain CA, Weng D, Meltzer A, et al: A meta-analysis evaluating the risk for implant failure in patients who smoke, *Compend Contin Educ Dent* 23:695, 2002.
7. Balshi TJ, Wolfinger GJ: Dental implants in the diabetic patient: a retrospective study, *Implant Dent* 8:355, 1999.
8. Baxter JC, Fattore L: Osteoporosis and osseointegration of implants, *J Prosthodont* 2:120, 1993.
9. Beikler T, Flemmig, TF: Implants in the medically compromised patient, *Crit Rev Oral Biol Med* 14:305, 2003.
10. Belser UC, Buser D, Hess D, et al: Aesthetic implant restorations in partially edentulous patients: a critical appraisal, *Periodontol 2000* 17:132, 1998.
11. Berglundh T, Lindhe J, Marinello C, et al: Soft tissue reaction to de novo plaque formation on implants and teeth. an experimental study in the dog, *Clin Oral Implant Res* 3:1, 1992.
12. Beumer J III, Roumanas E, Nishimura R: Advances in osseointegrated implants for dental and facial rehabilitation following major head and neck surgery, *Semin Surg Oncol* 11:200, 1995.
13. Blomqvist JE, Alberius P, Isaksson S, et al: Factors in implant integration failure after bone grafting: an osteometric and endocrinologic matched analysis, *Int J Oral Maxillofac Surg* 25:63, 1996.
14. Block MS, Gardiner D, Kent JN, et al: Hydroxyapatite-coated cylindrical implants in the posterior mandible: 10-year observations, *Int J Oral Maxillofac Implants* 11:626, 1996.
15. Bragger U, Burgin WB, Hammerle CH, Lang NP: Associations between clinical parameters assessed around implants and teeth, *Clin Oral Implant Res* 8:412, 1997.
16. Brånemark PI: Osseointegration and its experimental background, *J Prosthet Dent* 50:399, 1983.
17. Brånemark PI, Zarb GA, Albrektsson T: *Tissue-integrated prostheses,* Chicago, 1985, Quintessence.
18. Brånemark PI, Breine U, Adell R, et al: Intraosseous anchorage of dental prostheses. I. Experimental studies, *Scand J Plast Reconstr Surg* 3:81, 1969.
19. Buser D, Weber HP, Bragger U: The treatment of partially edentulous patients with ITI hollow-screw implants: presurgical evaluation and surgical procedures, *Int J Oral Maxillofac Implants* 5:165, 1990.
20. Cooper L, Moriarty J: Prosthodontic and periodontal considerations for implant-supported dental restorations, *Curr Opin Periodontol* 4:119, 1997.

21. Coulthard P, Esposito M, Worthington HV, Jokstad A: Therapeutic use of hyperbaric oxygen for irradiated dental implant patients: a systematic review, *J Dent Educ* 67:64, 2003.
22. Dao TT, Anderson JD, Zarb GA: Is osteoporosis a risk factor for osseointegration of dental implants? *Int J Oral Maxillofac Implants* 8:137, 1993.
23. DeBruyn H, Collaert B: The effect of smoking on early implant failure, *Clin Oral Implant Res* 5:260, 1994.
24. Elders PJ, Netelenbos JC, Lips P, et al: Accelerated vertebral bone loss in relation to the menopause: a cross-sectional study on lumbar bone density in 286 women of 46 to 55 years of age, *Bone Miner* 5:11, 1988.
25. Ericsson I, Lindhe J: Probing depth at implants and teeth: an experimental study in the dog, *J Clin Periodontol* 20:623, 1993.
26. Esposito M, Hirsch JM, Lekholm U, Thomsen P: Failure patterns of four osseointegrated oral implant systems, *J Mater Sci Mater Med* 8:843, 1997.
27. Esposito M, Hirsch JM, Lekholm U, Thomsen P: Biological factors contributing to failures of osseointegrated oral implants. I. Success criteria and epidemiology, *Eur J Oral Sci* 106:527, 1998.
28. Esposito M, Hirsch JM, Lekholm U, Thomsen P: Biological factors contributing to failures of osseointegrated oral implants. II. Etiopathogenesis, *Eur J Oral Sci* 106:721, 1998.
29. Esposito M, Worthington HV, Thomsen P, Coulthard P: Interventions for replacing missing teeth: maintaining health around dental implants, *Cochrane Database Syst Rev* 3:CD003069, 2004.
30. Ferrigno N, Laureti M, Fanali S, Grippaudo G: A long-term follow-up study of non-submerged ITI implants in the treatment of totally edentulous jaws. Part I. Ten-year life table analysis of a prospective multicenter study with 1286 implants, *Clin Oral Implant Res* 13:260, 2002.
31. Fiorellini JP, Nevins ML: Localized ridge augmentation/preservation: a systematic review, *Ann Periodontol* 8:321, 2003.
32. Fiorellini JP, Chen PK, Nevins M, Nevins ML: A retrospective study of dental implants in diabetic patients, *Int J Periodont Restor Dent* 20:366, 2000.
33. Friberg B, Jemt T, Lekholm U: Early failures in 4,641 consecutively placed Brånemark dental implants: a study from stage 1 surgery to the connection of completed prostheses, *Int J Oral Maxillofac Implants* 6:142, 1991.
34. Friberg B, Ekestubbe A, Mellstrom D, Sennerby L: Brånemark implants and osteoporosis: a clinical exploratory study, *Clin Implant Dent Relat Res* 3:50, 2001.
35. Fugazzotto PA, Gulbransen HJ, Wheeler SL, Lindsay JA: The use of IMZ osseointegrated implants in partially and completely edentulous patients: success and failure rates of 2,023 implant cylinders up to 60+ months in function, *Int J Oral Maxillofac Implants* 8:617, 1993.
36. Fujimoto T, Niimi A, Nakai H, Ueda M: Osseointegrated implants in a patient with osteoporosis: a case report, *Int J Oral Maxillofac Implants* 11:539, 1996.
37. Glaser DL, Kaplan FS: Osteoporosis: definition and clinical presentation, *Spine* 22(24 suppl):12S, 1997.
38. Granstrom G, Tjellstrom A, Brånemark PI: Osseointegrated implants in irradiated bone: a case-controlled study using adjunctive hyperbaric oxygen therapy, *J Oral Maxillofac Surg* 57:493, 1999.
39. Granstrom G, Tjellstrom A, Brånemark PI, Fornander, J: Bone-anchored reconstruction of the irradiated head and neck cancer patient, *Otolaryngol Head Neck Surg* 108:334, 1993.
40. Grondahl K, Lekholm U: The predictive value of radiographic diagnosis of implant instability, *Int J Oral Maxillofac Implants* 12:59, 1997.
41. Hammerle CH, Jung RE, Feloutzis A: A systematic review of the survival of implants in bone sites augmented with barrier membranes (guided bone regeneration) in partially edentulous patients, *J Clin Periodontol* 29(suppl 3):226, 2002.
42. Hildebolt CF: Osteoporosis and oral bone loss, *Dentomaxillofac Radiol* 26:3, 1997.
43. Kapur KK, Garrett NR, Hamada MO, et al: A randomized clinical trial comparing the efficacy of mandibular implant-supported overdentures and conventional dentures in diabetic patients. Part I. Methodology and clinical outcomes, *J Prosthet Dent* 79:555, 1998.
44. Kirsch A, Ackermann KL: The IMZ osteointegrated implant system, *Dent Clin North Am* 33:733, 1989.
45. Lang NP, Adler R, Joss A, Nyman S: Absence of bleeding on probing: an indicator of periodontal stability, *J Clin Periodontol* 17:714, 1990.
46. Lang NP, Wetzel AC, Stich H, Caffesse RG: Histologic probe penetration in healthy and inflamed peri-implant tissues, *Clin Oral Implant Res* 5:191, 1994.
47. Lekholm U, van Steenberghe D, Herrmann I, et al: Osseointegrated implants in the treatment of partially edentulous jaws: a prospective 5-year multicenter study, *Int J Oral Maxillofac Implants* 9:627, 1994.
48. Lekholm U, Gunne J, Henry P, et al: Survival of the Brånemark implant in partially edentulous jaws: a 10-year prospective multicenter study, *Int J Oral Maxillofac Implants* 14:639, 1999.
49. Lindh T, Gunne J, Tillberg A, Molin M: A meta-analysis of implants in partial edentulism, *Clin Oral Implant Res* 9:80, 1998.
50. Lindquist LW, Rockler B, Carlsson GE: Bone resorption around fixtures in edentulous patients treated with mandibular fixed tissue-integrated prostheses, *J Prosthet Dent* 59:59, 1988.
51. Lindquist LW, Carlsson GE, Jemt T: Association between marginal bone loss around osseointegrated mandibular implants and smoking habits: a 10-year follow-up study, *J Dent Res* 76:1667, 1997.
52. Meredith N, Alleyne D, Cawley P: Quantitative determination of the stability of the implant-tissue interface using resonance frequency analysis, *Clin Oral Implant Res* 7:261, 1996.
53. Mombelli A: Microbiology and antimicrobial therapy of peri-implantitis, *Periodontol 2000* 28:177, 2002.
54. Mombelli A, van Oosten MA, Schurch E Jr, Lang NP: The microbiota associated with successful or failing osseointegrated titanium implants, *Oral Microbiol Immunol* 2:145, 1987.
55. Mombelli A, Muhle T, Bragger U, et al: Comparison of periodontal and peri-implant probing by depth-force pattern analysis, *Clin Oral Implant Res* 8:448, 1997.
56. Olson JW, Shernoff AF, Tarlow JL, et al: Dental endosseous implant assessments in a type 2 diabetic population: a prospective study, *Int J Oral Maxillofac Implants* 15:811, 2000.
57. Pjetursson BE, Tan K, Lang NP, et al: A systematic review of the survival and complication rates of fixed partial dentures (FPDs) after an observation period of at least 5 years, *Clin Oral Implant Res* 15:625, 2004.
58. Pontoriero R, Tonelli MP, Carnevale G, et al: Experimentally induced peri-implant mucositis. a clinical study in humans, *Clin Oral Implant Res* 5:254, 1994.
59. Pylant T, Triplett RG, Key MC, et al: A retrospective evaluation of endosseous titanium implants in the partially edentulous patient, *Int J Oral Maxillofac Implants* 7:195, 1992.
60. Rams TE, Link CC Jr: Microbiology of failing dental implants in humans: electron microscopic observations, *J Oral Implantol* 11:93, 1983.

61. Sanz M, Newman MG, Nachnani S, et al: Characterization of the subgingival microbial flora around endosteal sapphire dental implants in partially edentulous patients, *Int J Oral Maxillofac Implants* 5:247, 1990.
62. Sennerby L, Roos J: Surgical determinants of clinical success of osseointegrated oral implants: a review of the literature, *Int J Prosthodont* 11:408, 1998.
63. Shernoff AF, Colwell JA, Bingham SF: Implants for type II diabetic patients: interim report, VA Implants in Diabetes Study Group, *Implant Dent* 3:183, 1994.
64. Sullivan DY, Sherwood RL, Porter SS: Long-term performance of Osseotite implants: a 6-year clinical follow-up, *Compend Contin Educ Dent* 22:326, 2001.
65. Sunden S, Grondahl K, Grondahl HG: Accuracy and precision in the radiographic diagnosis of clinical instability in Brånemark dental implants, *Clin Oral Implant Res* 6:220, 1995.
66. Wallace SS, Froum SJ: Effect of maxillary sinus augmentation on the survival of endosseous dental implants. a systematic review, *Ann Periodontol* 8:328, 2003.
67. Wennstrom JL, Bengazi F, Lekholm U: The influence of the masticatory mucosa on the peri-implant soft tissue condition, *Clin Oral Implant Res* 5:1, 1994.
68. Zitzmann N, Marinello C: Treatment plan for restoring the edentulous maxilla with implant-supported restorations: removable overdenture versus fixed partial denture design, *J Prosthet Dent* 82:188, 1999.

Diagnostic Imaging for the Implant Patient

Sotirios Tetradis, Perry R. Klokkevold, and Robert C. Fazio

75

CHAPTER

CHAPTER OUTLINE

Several radiographic imaging options are available for diagnosis and treatment planning of patients receiving dental implants.[18,20] Options range from standard projections routinely available in the dental office to more complex radiographic techniques typically available only in radiology centers. Standard projections include intraoral (periapical, occlusal) and extraoral (panoramic, lateral cephalometric) radiographs. More complex imaging techniques include conventional x-ray tomography, computed tomography (CT), and cone-beam computed tomography (CBCT). The CT and CBCT image data files can be reformatted and viewed on a personal computer, using simulation software, making the diagnosis and treatment-planning process interactive and visually more meaningful. Often, combinations of various modalities are used because no single modality can provide all information pertinent to the radiographic evaluation of the implant patient. Familiarity with the benefits and limitations of various techniques and awareness of the specific clinical questions that need to be answered should guide the decision-making process and selection of radiographic examinations for individual patients.

Multiple factors influence the selection of radiographic technique(s) for a particular case, including cost, availability, radiation exposure, and case type. The decision is a balance between these factors and the desire to minimize risk of complications to the patient. Accurately identifying vital anatomic structures and being able to perform implant placement surgery without injury to these structures are critical to treatment success. Diagnostic imaging techniques must always be interpreted in conjunction with a good clinical examination.

This chapter discusses common imaging techniques used for evaluation of the implant patient. Indications for each technique are outlined, along with the advantages and limitations.

STANDARD PROJECTIONS

Standard diagnostic imaging modalities include periapical, panoramic, lateral cephalometric, and occlusal radiographs.

TABLE 75-1

Advantages and Disadvantages of Various Radiographic Projections

Modality	Advantages	Disadvantages
Periapical and occlusal radiography	High resolution and detail, easy acquisition, low exposure, inexpensive	Unpredictable magnification, small imaged area, 2D representation of anatomy
Panoramic radiography	Easy to acquire, images whole ridge, low exposure, inexpensive	Unpredictable magnification, 2D representation of anatomy, not detailed
Lateral cephalometric radiography	Easy to acquire, predictable magnification, low exposure, inexpensive	Limited use in area of midline, 2D representation of anatomy
Conventional tomography	3D representation, predictable magnification, sufficient detail, low exposure, images area of interest only	Requires special equipment; for evaluation of multiple sites, can be a lengthy procedure because patient must be repositioned for each site; blurring of image may occur depending on adjacent structures; expensive
Computed tomography (CT)	3D representation, predictable magnification, sufficient detail, digital format, images whole arch	Requires special equipment, expensive, high exposure dose, images whole arch
Cone-beam computed tomography (CBCT)	3D representation, predictable magnification, sufficient detail, digital format, images whole arch, low dose	Requires special equipment, expensive, images whole arch

2D, Two-dimensional; *3D,* three-dimensional.

The advantages and disadvantages of each modality are summarized in Table 75-1.

Periapical Radiographs

Periapical radiographs offer great advantages during the evaluation of the implant patient.[21,23] They provide an overall assessment of the quantity and quality of the edentulous alveolar ridge and the adjacent teeth. They are easy to obtain in the dental office, are inexpensive, and deliver low radiation to the patient (Table 75-2). Dentists are familiar with the depicted anatomy and possible pathology. Because these direct-exposure projections do not use intensifying screens, intraoral radiographs offer the highest detail and spatial resolution of all radiographic modalities (Figure 75-1). Thus, these films are the projection of choice when subtle pathology, such as a retained root tip, needs to be detected and evaluated.

Because of the ease of acquisition, periapical radiographs are very helpful during implant placement. Intraoperative radiographs can be taken during surgery to evaluate the proximity of adjacent teeth as well as other important anatomic structures. Sequential periapical films guide the clinician to visualize changes in direction and depth of the drilling procedure (Figure 75-2). Digital radiographs are particularly advantageous during intraoperative assessment of implant placement; images appear on the screen almost instantaneously and can be manipulated to extract the most pertinent diagnostic information (see Chapter 36).

The most significant disadvantage of periapical radiographs is their susceptibility to unpredictable magnification of anatomic structures, which does not allow reliable measurements.[17] Foreshortening or elongation can be minimized by the use of paralleling technique. However, distortion is particularly accentuated in edentulous areas, where missing teeth and resorption of the alveolus necessitate film placement at significant angulation in relation to the long axis of the teeth and alveolar bone. Additionally, periapical radiographs are two-dimensional representations of three-dimensional objects and do not provide any information of the buccal-lingual dimension of the alveolar ridge. Structures that are distinctly separated in the buccal-lingual dimension appear to be overlapping. Also, the periapical image is limited by the size of film being used. Often it is not possible to image the entire height of the remaining alveolar ridge, and

TABLE 75-2

Effective Dose of Ionizing Radiation Received from Common Projections during Evaluation of Implant Patient

Modality	Effective Dose (μSv)
Full-mouth x-ray series (FMX)	34-144
Panoramic radiography	5-30
Conventional tomography	26-187
Computed tomography (CT) of head	1202-3324
Cone-beam computed tomography (CBCT)	19.9-42.1

Data from Ludlow JB, Davies-Ludlow LE, Brooks SL: *Dentomaxillofac Radiol* 32:290, 2003; Scaf G, Lurie AG, Mosier KM, et al: *Oral Surg Oral Med Oral Pathol Oral Radiol Endod* 83:41, 1997; and White SC, Pharoah MJ: *Oral radiology: principles and interpretation,* ed 5, St Louis, 2004, Mosby.

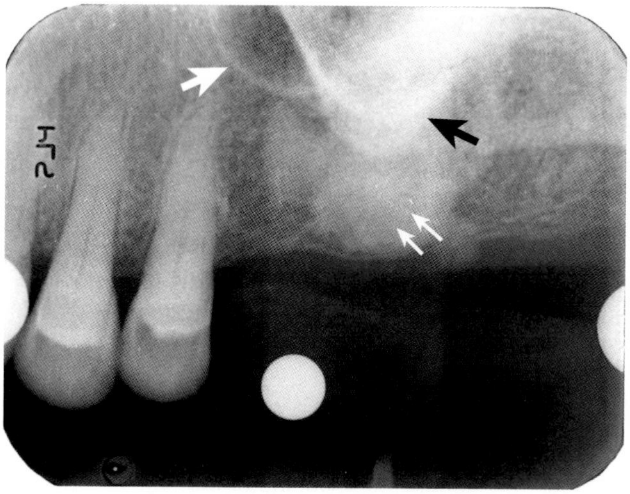

Figure 75-1 The periapical radiograph offers a high-resolution, detailed image of the edentulous area. Healing of the extraction socket with dense bone (socket sclerosis) can be seen *(small white arrows)*. Some anatomic structures, such as the maxillary sinus *(large white arrow)* and the zygomatic process of the maxilla *(black arrow)*, can also be visualized.

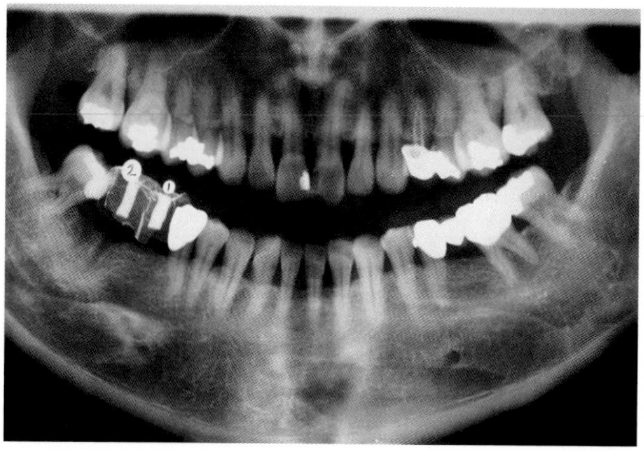

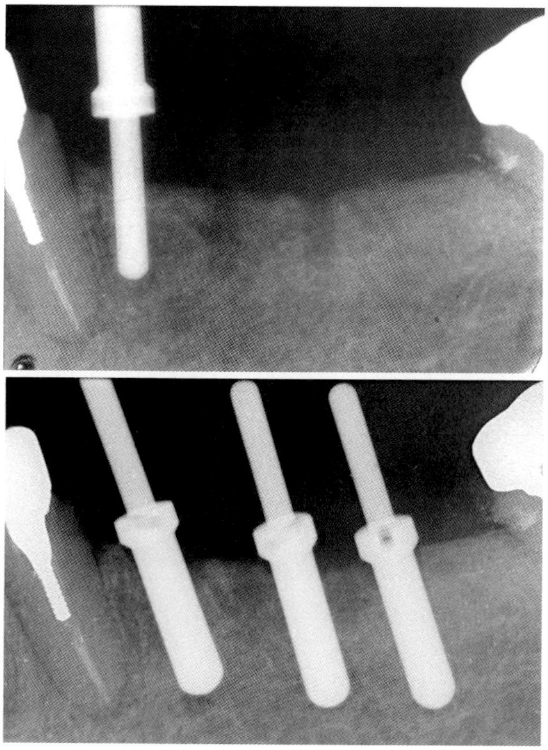

Figure 75-2 Intraoperative periapical radiographs are valuable in assessing the proximity of adjacent teeth. **A,** The 2-mm guide pin is used to determine direction of the osteotomy site and its proximity to the adjacent root. **B,** After angle correction, the osteotomy sites are completed to length with the final drill. Here the 3-mm guide pins confirm the correct angulation and spacing of the final osteotomy site preparation before implant placement.

Figure 75-3 Panoramic radiograph. Both jaws are visualized on the same film. An overall assessment of superoinferior and mesiodistal dimensions of the alveolar ridge can be formulated. Tooth and root positions relative to planned implant sites can be evaluated. Important anatomic structures, such as the maxillary sinus and mandibular canal, can be identified.

when extensive mesial-distal areas need to be evaluated, multiple periapical films are required.

In summary, periapical radiographs are useful screening images that offer a detailed view of a small area of the alveolar arch. Limitations that must be considered include the possibility of distortion and the two-dimensional representation of anatomic structures.

Occlusal Radiographs

Occlusal radiographs are intraoral projections that offer easy, economic, low-dose, and high-resolution images covering a larger area than periapical films.[23] Depending on film placement and the angulation of the x-ray tube, occlusal films can provide a cross-sectional image of the mandible or can depict an extended area of the edentulous ridge. Cross-sectional occlusal films allow the measurement of the buccal-lingual dimension of the mandible. This can be an important consideration when planning implants in the severely resorbed mandible. Occlusal films have the same limitations of distortion and overlapping anatomy as periapical films.

In summary, occlusal film projections are good screening images that can provide an overview of the mandibular width or can visualize larger areas of alveolar ridge compared with periapical film projections.

Panoramic Radiographs

Panoramic radiographs are often used in the evaluation of the implant patient because they offer several advantages over other modalities.[19] Panoramic films deliver low radiation (see Table 75-2) to provide a broad picture of both arches and thus allow assessment of extensive edentulous areas, angulation of existing teeth and occlusal plane, and important anatomy in implant treatment planning, such as the maxillary sinus, nasal cavity, mental foramen, and mandibular canal (Figure 75-3). Panoramic

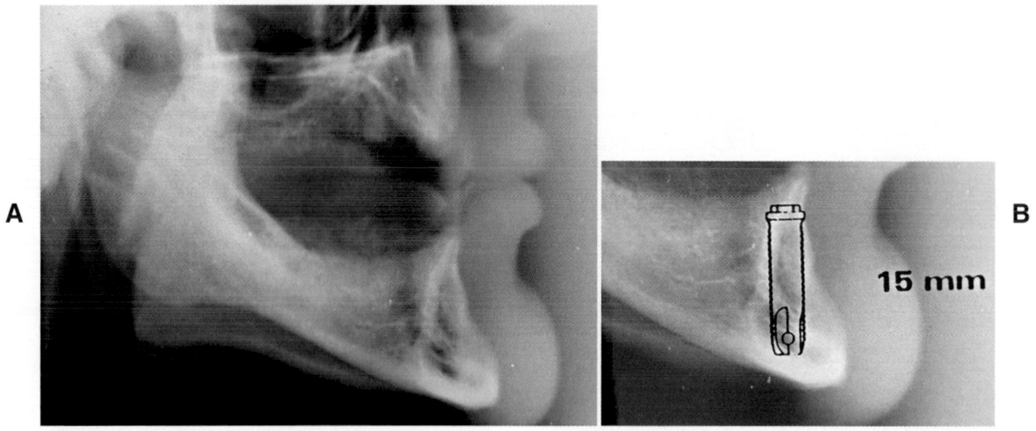

Figure 75-4 Lateral cephalometric radiograph can be used to evaluate cross-sectional dimensions of the alveolar ridge at the midline. **A,** Note the cortical bone outline of the anterior mandible and maxilla. **B,** Implant template with the same magnification is overlaid at the area of the midline to estimate available bone in mandible.

units are widely available and easy to operate, and dentists are familiar with the anatomy and pathology depicted by the images. Similar to intraoral projections, panoramic images are two-dimensional and thus do not offer diagnostic information for the buccolingual width of the alveolar arch.

Panoramic images appear intuitively familiar. However, they combine characteristic physical and radiographic principles that make them distinct from other intraoral and extraoral radiographs. Although outside the scope of this chapter, familiarity with the principles underlying panoramic radiography is central in understanding, and thus compensating for, the limitations and constraints of the images. The reader is referred to other textbooks for detailed discussion of this topic.[8,12] Briefly, the existence of ghost shadows, unpredictable horizontal and vertical magnification, distortion of structures outside the focal trough, projection geometry generated by the negative vertical angulation of the x-ray beam, and propensity to patient-positioning errors do not allow consistently detailed and accurate measurements to be generated. As a result, panoramic radiographs do not provide the highly detailed images that are generated by intraoral radiographs.

Measurement distortion is more prevalent and varies across the radiographic image. On average, panoramic radiographs are 25% magnifications of actual size. Implant manufacturers often provide transparency sheets with implant size outlines of 25% magnification. However, it is important to appreciate that the 25% magnification is an estimate. The actual magnification may range from 10% to 30% in different areas within the same film and depends greatly on patient positioning during panoramic radiography. For this reason, precise measurements on panoramic projections are not possible. Nonetheless, panoramic radiographs offer an overall view of the maxilla and mandible that can be used to estimate bone measurements and evaluate the approximate relationships between teeth and other anatomic structures. More precise diagnostic imaging should be used to measure proximity of critical anatomic structures, such as the maxillary sinus or the mandibular canal, to proposed implant positions.

In summary, panoramic projections are useful screening images of the jaws for approximations and relative special relationships. However, because of magnification and distortion errors, panoramic films should not be used for detailed measurements of proposed implant sites.

Lateral Cephalometric Radiographs

Lateral cephalometric radiographs are occasionally used to evaluate potential implant patients.[20] These films provide useful information for the cortical thickness, height, and width of the alveolar ridge at the midline, as well as the skeletal relationship between maxilla and mandible and facial profile. Lateral cephalometric radiographs are low in cost, readily available, and easy to interpret and have a predictable magnification of the depicted structures. However, their use for the implant patient is limited to structures at the midline, with minimal usefulness for other areas of the jaws (Figure 75-4).

In summary, lateral cephalometric radiographs have a limited use in implant treatment planning.

CROSS-SECTIONAL IMAGING

Cross-sectional diagnostic imaging modalities include conventional x-ray tomography, computer tomography, and cone-beam computer tomography.

Conventional X-Ray Tomography

In conventional tomography the x-ray source and the film are connected and rotate around a fixed point (fulcrum), usually performing simple (linear) or complex (elliptic or hypocycloidal) tomographic motions.[3] Structures that are in the plane (focal area) of rotation do not move in relation to the tube and the film and thus are depicted in sharp focus. Structures outside the plane of rotation are blurred progressively, depending on their distance from the focal plane. The resulting image is a true cross section

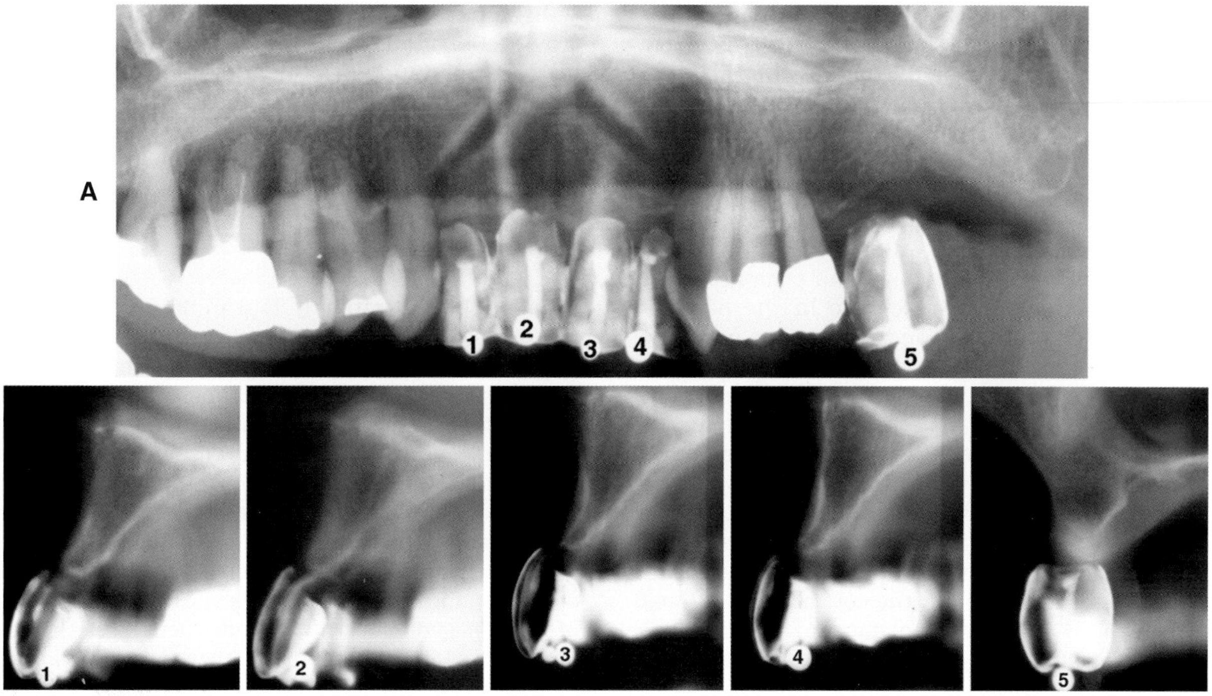

Figure 75-5 Panoramic radiograph **(A)** and conventional tomography **(B)** of five prospective implant sites in the anterior and posterior maxilla. Note the tooth-shaped markers used that allow the clinician to evaluate bone dimensions in the jaw relative to the planned prosthetic tooth position. The cortical outline of the alveolar ridge and the floor of the nasal cavity or maxillary sinus can be seen. Accurate measurements of the height and buccolingual width can be made. Although conventional x-ray tomographic images focus on a specific area, the image is often difficult to read because of the blurring of structures on either side of the plane.

of the structures within the imaged plane, which is perpendicular to the x-ray beam (Figures 75-5 and 75-6).

Proper patient positioning is essential to generate true cross sections of the jaws at the area of interest for planned implants.[4,6] The curvature of the alveolar ridge is usually evaluated from scout films, such as submentovertex (SMV) or occlusal projections, or from dental models. The thickness of the image and the appearance of the structures depend on the angle of rotation and the type of motion (simple vs. complex). The imaged structures are always magnified. However, the magnification is uniform, predictable, and specific to the equipment used for the acquisition of the image. Overlay templates with magnification values that match the magnification of the equipment can be used to measure dimensions on the film reliably.

Conventional x-ray tomography offers many advantages in evaluation of the implant patient.[9,10] With proper patient positioning, it can generate true cross sections of the alveolar ridge and provide diagnostic information of the cortical thickness, trabecular density, height and width of the alveolus, and location of vital anatomic structures. The generated images usually provide adequate resolution for the diagnostic task. The imaged structures are predictably magnified, so measurements made of the tomograms can be adjusted to provide accurate angular and linear assessments. Because during conventional tomography only a limited area of the jaws is imaged, the dose to the patient is limited (see Table 75-2).

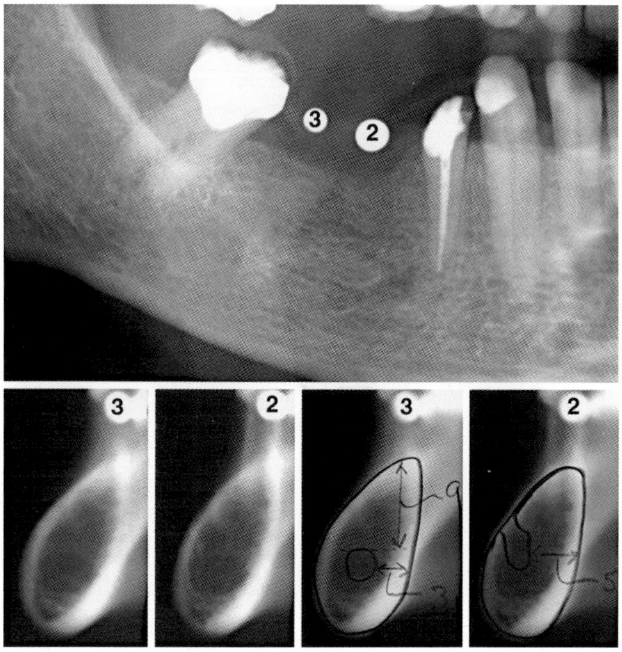

Figure 75-6 Panoramic radiograph **(A)** and conventional tomography **(B)** of two prospective implant sites in the posterior mandible. The cortical outline and trabecular architecture of the alveolar ridge can be seen. The last two tomograms are the same cross-sectional images shown with radiologist's overlay interpretation of bone height and position of mandibular canal and mental foramen.

The specialized equipment used for conventional x-ray tomography requires familiarity with the image acquisition. Interpretation of the images is sometimes challenging, especially when the anatomy of the jaws has been altered because of traumatic extractions, alveolar ridge resorption, or other conditions. Although images are true cross sections, the progressive blurring of structures outside the focal plane does not allow sharply defined tomographic slices, and prominent opaque structures can cast "ghost" shadows and complicate the images. This is especially problematic in the partially edentulous patient with teeth and restorations on either side of the area of interest. These problems can be reduced with the use of complex tomography and selection of various widths of tomographic sections. Conventional tomographic slices are generated one at a time, requiring the patient to be repositioned for each image area captured. This does not pose a problem if one or a few implant sites are being imaged. However, the procedure can be rather lengthy when evaluation of multiple edentulous areas is required. Finally, the cost of conventional x-ray tomography is higher than standard intraoral and extraoral radiographs.

In summary, conventional tomography offers true cross-sectional images of the alveolar ridge and is particularly useful during placement of single or few implants. Limitations of conventional tomography include blurring of images by structures on either side of the focal plane and the time required to reposition the patient for each image.

Computed Tomography

Computed tomography (CT) scanning is widely used in the evaluation of the implant patient.[2,7] The detailed physics behind image acquisition during CT scanning are beyond the scope of this chapter.[3] In general, a thin fan-beam of x-rays rotates around the patient to generate in one revolution a thin (0.5-1.0 mm wide) axial slice of the area of interest (Figure 75-7, *A*). Multiple overlapping axial slices are obtained by several revolutions of the x-ray beam until the whole area of interest is covered. These slices are then used to generate, with the help of a computer and sophisticated algorithms, a digital volume of the imaged object. The construction of this three-dimensional digital map of the jaws is the advantage of

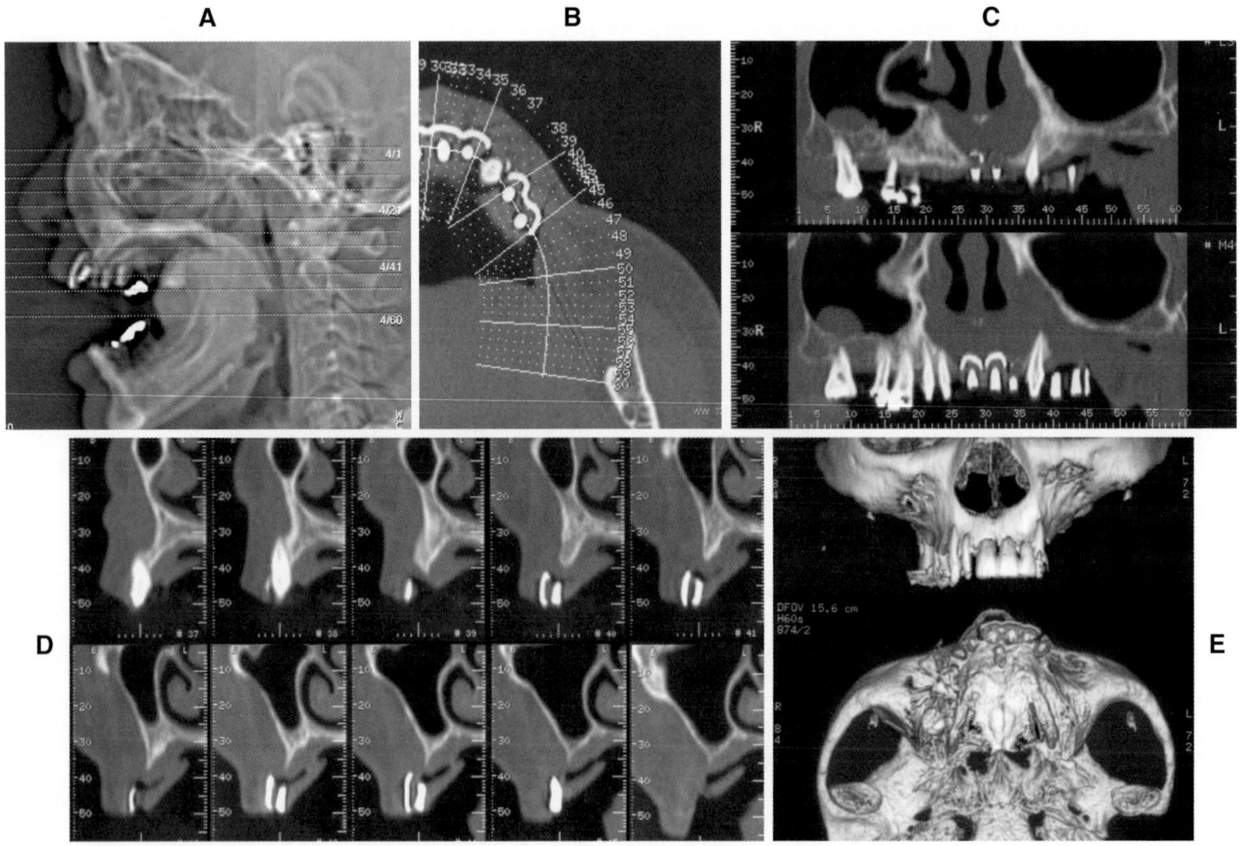

Figure 75-7 Computed tomography (CT) examination for evaluation of edentulous maxilla before implant placement. **A,** Scout view of the patient's head; axial sections through the area of interest are indicated. **B,** Axial slice through the markers is used to display the orientation of the panoramic and cross-sectional images through the alveolar ridge. **C,** Panoramic views through the alveolar ridge demonstrate the relation of the markers to adjacent teeth. **D,** Cross-sectional slices through the area of the markers reveal the height and buccolingual dimension of the alveolar ridge, as well as the relation of the markers to the ridge. **E,** Three-dimensional reconstructions provide an overall impression of the bone contours and shape of the alveolar ridge.

CT during evaluation of the implant patient. Specialized software can be used to generate appropriate views that best depict the dimensions of the jaws and the location of important anatomic structures.

Typical dental views obtained from a CT scan include axial (Figure 75-7, *B*), panoramic (Figure 75-7, *C*), and cross-sectional (Figure 75-7, *D*) views of the jaws. Appropriate axial slices through the alveolar ridge of interest are selected as scout views. The curvature of the maxillary or mandibular ridge is then drawn on the axial slices, and panoramic images along the drawn line are created. Finally, cross-sectional slices, every 1 to 2 mm and perpendicular to the drawn curvature, are created. In addition to these flat, two-dimensional views, complex, three-dimensional images with surface rendering can also be generated from the CT data (Figure 75-7, *E*). These images can provide useful information about the alveolar ridge defects that are easy to comprehend. Images can be printed on photographic paper or transparent film or can be displayed on the computer screen.

CT scans offer several advantages for evaluation of the implant patient. True cross sections offer a precise and detailed evaluation of the height and width of the alveolar ridge. The images can be adjusted and printed without magnification, facilitating measurements directly on the prints or films with standard rulers (i.e., not magnified). Vertical and horizontal rulers adjacent to each section allow the clinician to check for magnification and make direct measurements. The digital format allows for image enhancement tools, rapid communication between the radiologist and the surgeon, and generation of multiple copies of the images. Various anatomic structures can be visualized and analyzed at all three coordinate axes, such that their superoinferior, anteroposterior, and buccolingual location can be identified with precision. The process of CT scanning images the entire arch (usually one arch per scan), so several edentulous areas can be visualized with a single examination. The bone and soft tissue contrast and resolution are excellent for the diagnostic task.

CT scanning requires specialized equipment and setting. Radiologists and technicians need to be knowledgeable of the anatomy, anatomic variants, and pathology of the jaws, as well as considerations pertinent to implant treatment planning, so that optimal views will be provided. A CT scan delivers much higher radiation dose to the patient compared with the other modalities used during implant treatment planning[15] (see Table 75-2). Because a CT scan images the whole arch, radiation is delivered to the entire imaged area regardless of how many or few sites are actually needed. Metallic restorations can cause ring artifacts that impair the diagnostic quality of the images. This is particularly challenging in patients with heavily restored dentition. In general, the cost of CT is significantly higher than that of conventional tomography or the other standard intraoral and extraoral projections.

In summary, CT scanning offers many advantages during implant treatment planning, including accurate cross-sectional imaging and three-dimensional visualization of anatomic structures. High dose to the patient and ring artifacts caused by metallic restorations are concerns that should be considered.

Cone-Beam Computed Tomography

Cone-beam computed tomography (CBCT) is a new imaging modality that offers significant advantages for the evaluation of implant patients.[5,16] It was introduced to dentistry in the late 1990s.[1,14] Similar to CT scanners, the x-ray source and the detector are diametrically positioned and make a 360-degree rotation around the patient's head within the gantry. In contrast to the fan-beam generated by CT scanners, however, the CBCT scanner generates a cone-shaped x-ray beam, which images a larger area. Images are generated in 1-degree increments. Thus, at the end of a single complete rotation, 360 images of the area are generated. The computer uses these images to generate a digital, three-dimensional map of the face. Once this map is generated, multiplanar reconstructions as well as axial, coronal, sagittal, or oblique sections of various thicknesses can be reconstructed from the data (Figure 75-8), similar to the CT images.

In general, CBCT offers the same advantages and disadvantages as CT. However, the two modalities have a few basic differences that result from the different physical principles used during image acquisition. CT scan offers a greater *contrast resolution,* or the ability to distinguish two objects with small density differences. CBCT scans have a limited capacity to separate muscle from fat or connective tissue compared with CT scans. Fortunately, contrast resolution is not a significant concern in implant evaluation. Because bone has a much higher density than surrounding soft tissues, both CBCT and CT can clearly depict bone shape and architecture. One of the most significant advantages of CBCT scanning versus CT scanning is the reduced amount of radiation dose delivered to the patient[11] (see Table 75-2). CBCT delivers an effective dose approximately equal to a full-mouth x-ray series (FMX); this is 50 to 100 times less than the radiation dose delivered during a typical CT scan. The cost to patients for CT and CBCT scans is comparable.

In summary, CBCT scanning is a valuable imaging modality for three-dimensional and cross-sectional evaluation of the implant patient. It has similar advantages and disadvantages as CT scanning. The most significant difference is that CBCT imaging requires much less radiation exposure.

INTERACTIVE "SIMULATION" SOFTWARE PROGRAMS

In many challenging cases, implant treatment planning can be greatly enhanced by the use of specialized software. These programs utilize data from the CT or CBCT scans and allow the simulation of implant placement and restoration on the computer. The quantity and quality of bone can be evaluated. A database of popular implant (commercial size and design) images is usually available to use with the three-dimensional images. The length, width, angulation, and position of implants can be "simulated" in the desired positions. In cases of alveolar ridge deficiency or defects or when sinus bone augmentation is indicated, the additional bone volume needed can be evaluated and quantified. The restoration

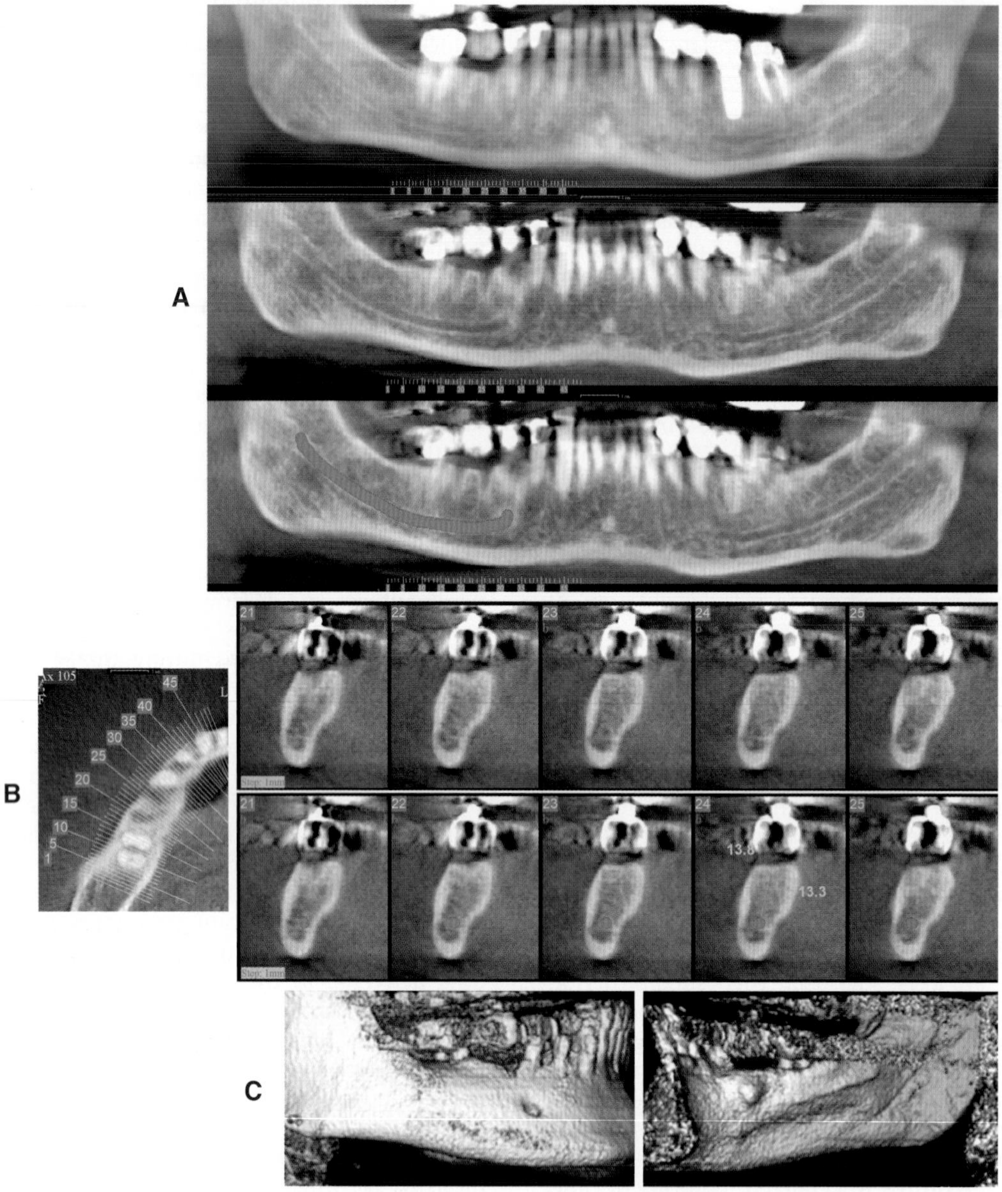

Figure 75-8 Cone-beam computed tomography images for the evaluation of the edentulous space at the area of missing tooth #30 before implant placement. Note the tooth-shaped marker used. **A,** Series of panoramic images through the alveolar ridge reveals the relationship of the marker to the adjacent teeth. The top panoramic view is 12 mm thick to depict most of the extent of the alveolar ridge and adjacent teeth. The middle panoramic image is 1 mm thick through the area of the mandibular canal. Note that adjacent teeth are out of the plane of the section and thus not depicted on the image. The bottom panoramic view is the same as the middle one, but the position of the mandibular canal has been depicted by the red line. **B,** Scout axial view and series of cross sections through the area of the marker. The bottom row shows the same axial slices as the top row. However, the position of the red line drawn on the panoramic view is also depicted to help localization of the mandibular canal. The height and width of the alveolar ridge have been measured in a selected section. **C,** Three-dimensional reconstructions provide an overall impression of the bone contours and shape of the alveolar ridge. Note the small exostosis on the lingual surface of the alveolar ridge.

of the implants can also be simulated and the distribution of mechanical forces onto the implant and adjacent bone predicted.

Software programs specialized in implant treatment planning, such as SIM/Plant (Materialise/Columbia Scientific, Glen Burnie, Md), can import CBCT or CT scan data. The clinician can use the reformatted images on a personal computer in an interactive manner to better appreciate relationships between planned implant positions and teeth or anatomic structures (Figure 75-9).

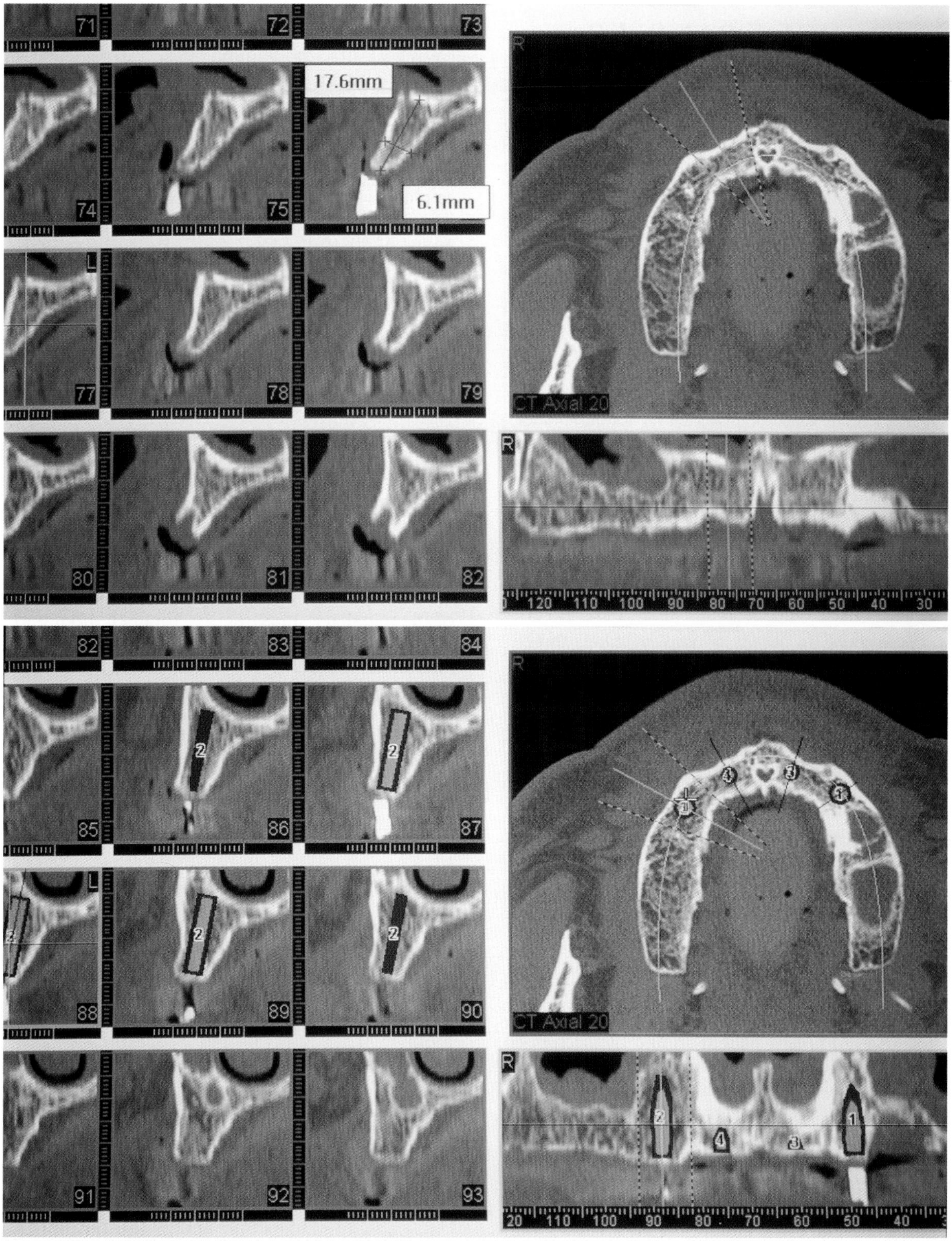

Figure 75-9 SIM/Plant images. The SIM/Plant software program allows clinicians to measure bone height, width, density, and volume on a personal computer. Scan data are reformatted for interactive evaluation and manipulation. Implant positions can be simulated on the patient's scan data before surgery, allowing the surgeon to anticipate areas of deficiency.

SCIENCE TRANSFER

Endosseous dental implant therapy, although highly efficient and predictable, cannot easily be performed for all patients. *The clinician must evaluate each potential candidate comprehensively.* The evaluation includes the exclusion of pathology, identification of anatomic structures, and evaluation of available bone tissue. Failure to evaluate accurately can lead to complications, including inability to place an implant. In other cases this information, obtained in large part through some form of diagnostic imaging, may lead to the need for bone augmentation. Thus, although diagnostic imaging is a critical evaluation tool, the implant must eventually be placed in a precise position that allows for functional and often esthetic tooth replacement. Knowledge of the options for diagnostic imaging, including advantages and disadvantages, is necessary to provide optimal dental treatment.

Two-dimensional radiographs, such as periapical and panoramic views, are valuable as screening modalities because they have high definition and result in low radiation exposure. In almost all implant cases, three-dimensional radiographs using a stent that localizes the ideal position of implants are necessary. Conventional tomography provides useful images while requiring only a radiation dose similar to a full-mouth periapical series. However, both computed tomography (CT) and the newer cone-beam tomography (CBCT) offer more complete data with the added benefit of software to manipulate images of implant placement and to fabricate CADCAM-generated, precise surgical guides.

PATIENT EVALUATION

Evaluation of the implant patient should be disciplined and objective. Specific questions that can affect implant placement and outcome should be considered and examined carefully and explicitly. The advantages and disadvantages of various radiographic projections should be considered and radiographic modalities chosen based on necessary information for the particular patient. The objectives for any radiographic evaluation, regardless of imaging technique used, should include an evaluation to (1) exclude pathology, (2) identify anatomic structures, and (3) measure the quantity, quality, and location of available bone.

Exclude Pathology

Healthy bone is prerequisite for successful osseointegration and long-term implant success. The first step in the radiographic evaluation of the implant site is to establish the health of the alveolar bone and other tissues imaged within a particular projection. Local and systemic diseases that affect bone homeostasis can preclude, modify, or alter placement of implants. Retained root fragments, residual periodontal disease, cysts, and tumors should be identified and resolved before implant placement. Systemic diseases, such as osteoporosis and hyperparathyroidism, alter bone metabolism and might affect implant osseointegration (Figure 75-10). Areas of poor bone quality should be identified and, if indicated, adjustments to the treatment plan incorporated. Maxillary sinusitis, polyps, or other sinus pathology should be diagnosed and treated when implants are considered in the posterior maxilla, especially if sinus bone augmentation procedures are planned (Figure 75-11).

Identify Anatomic Structures

Several important anatomic structures are found close to desired areas of implant placement in the maxilla and mandible (Box 75-1). Familiarity with the radiographic appearance of these structures is important during treatment planning and implant placement. Their exact localization is central to prevent unwanted complication and unnecessary morbidity. Important anatomic structures in the maxilla include the floor and anterior wall of the maxillary sinus, incisive foramen, floor and lateral wall of the nasal cavity, and canine fossa. Important anatomic structures in the mandible that should be recognized include the mandibular canal, anterior loop of the mandibular canal, mental foramen, anterior extension of the canal, and submandibular fossa. The existence of anatomic variants, such as incomplete healing of an extraction site, sinus loculation, double mandibular canal (Figure 75-12), or absence of a well-defined corticated canal, should also be recognized.

Assess Bone Quantity, Quality, and Volume

The primary goal of diagnostic imaging for potential implant patients is to evaluate the available bone volume

BOX 75-1

Anatomic Structures Pertinent to Treatment Planning of the Implant Patient

Maxilla
Maxillary sinus (floor and anterior wall)
Nasal cavity (floor and lateral wall)
Incisive foramen
Canine fossa

Mandible
Mandibular canal
Anterior loop of mandibular canal
Anterior extension of mandibular canal
Mental foramen
Submandibular fossa
Lingual inclination of alveolar ridge

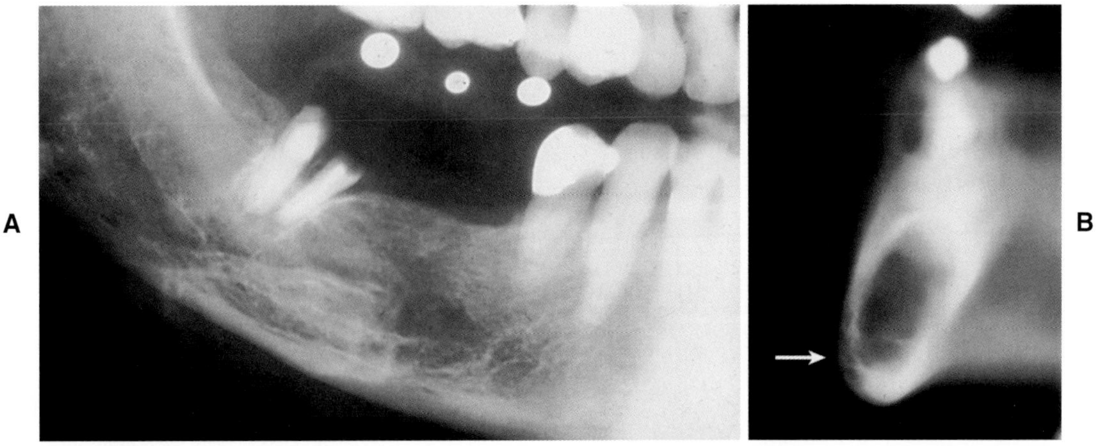

Figure 75-10 Panoramic film **(A)** and conventional tomography **(B)** of a postmenopausal patient. Note the large marrow spaces, thin trabeculae, and thin cortical outline of the inferior border of the alveolar ridge. **B,** Little if any trabeculation of the alveolar ridge is seen. The cortical outline shows areas of resorption *(white arrow)*. This patient has advanced osteoporosis, which has affected the mandible.

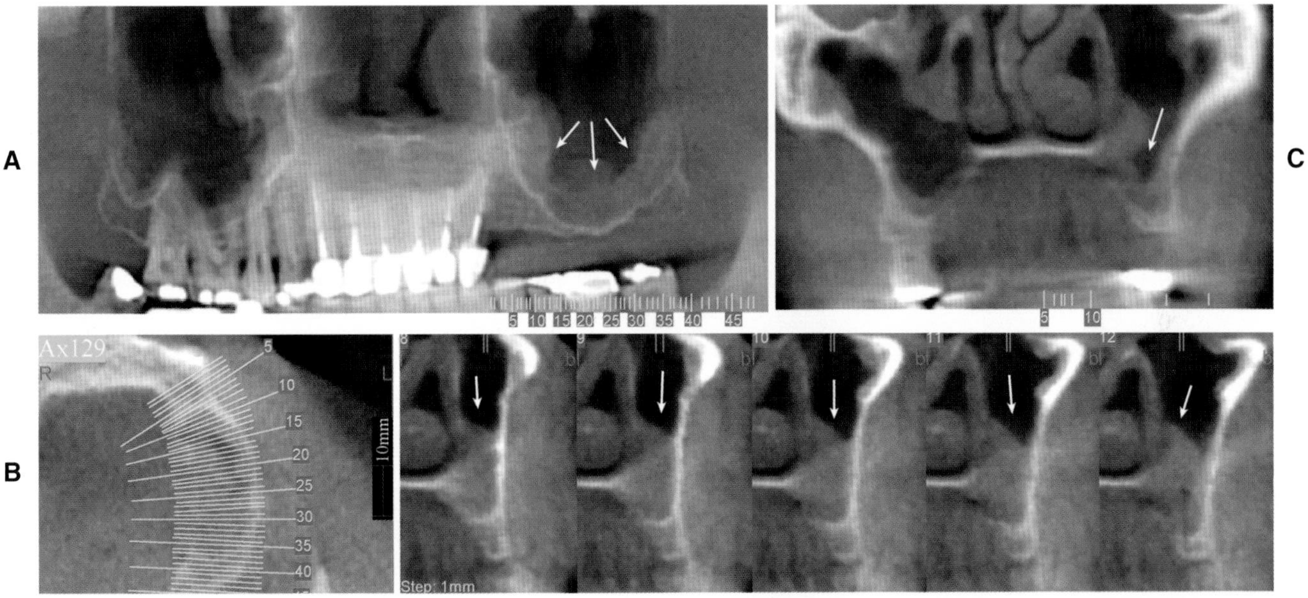

Figure 75-11 CBCT examination of the posterior left maxilla. Panoramic **(A),** coronal **(B),** axial and cross-sectional **(C)** views of the alveolar ridge. Note the thickened mucoperiosteal lining of the floor of the left maxillary sinus *(white arrow)*. The patient has chronic maxillary sinusitis.

for implant placement in desired anatomic locations. The clinician wants to estimate and verify exact adequate height, width, and density to the recipient bone while avoiding damage to critical anatomic structures. Failure to assess accurately the location of important anatomic structures can lead to unnecessary complications. For example, inadvertent penetration and damage to the inferior alveolar nerve can result in serious immediate-term (profuse bleeding), short-term, and long-term (nerve paresthesia/anesthesia) complications. The height and width of the alveolar bone should be accurately detailed. Depending on the technique, diagnostic imaging can estimate or measure the coronal-apical height, the buccal-lingual width, and the mesial-distal spacing available for implants that will be placed in proximity to teeth or relative to other planned implants.

This task can be simple in cases with good bone quality and sufficient bone volume in the desired implant location(s). However, in cases with moderate-severe bone resorption, alveolar defects, or recent extraction sites, obtaining a clear and accurate diagnostic image can be more challenging. The diagnostic imaging may reveal inadequate bone volume for the proposed implant(s) and indicate a need for bone augmentation or, depending on the severity of the deficiency, preclude the patient from the possibility of implant therapy (Figure 75-13).

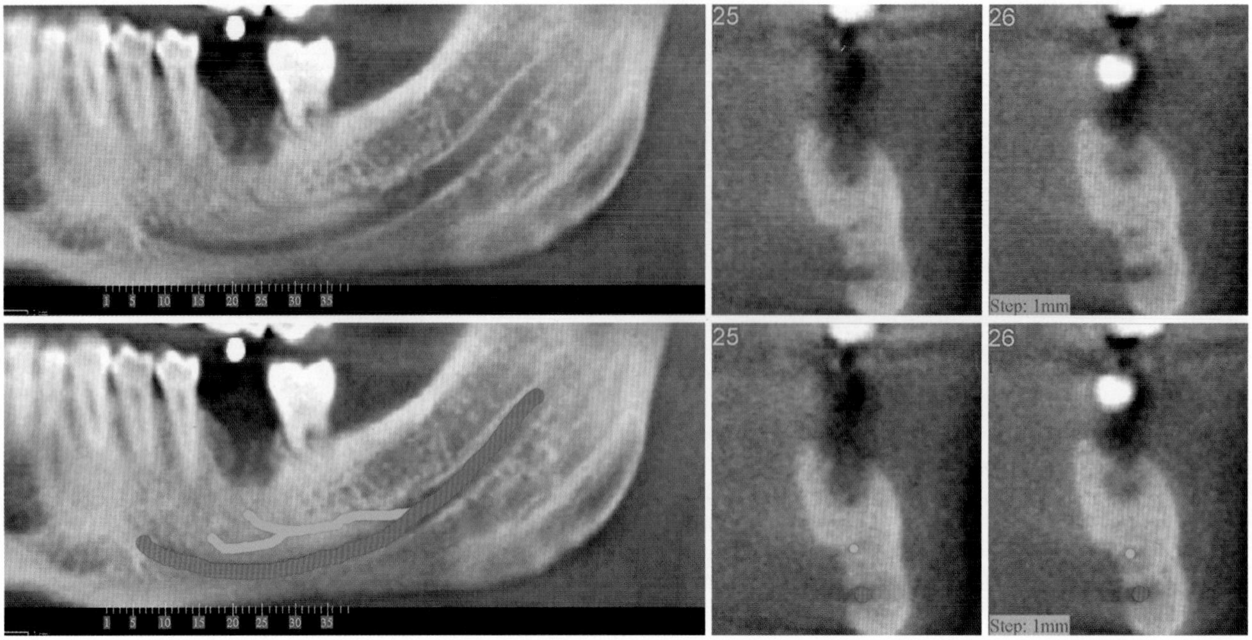

A B C D

Figure 75-12 CBCT examination of the area of missing tooth #19 before implant placement. **A,** Panoramic view of the area of interest depicts an accessory mandibular canal. **B,** Same panoramic view with the accessory mandibular canal colored blue and the main canal red. **C,** Cross-sectional views through the area of missing tooth #19. **D,** Same cross-sectional images depicting the blue and red markings. Note that the position of the markings coincides with the position of the accessory and main mandibular canals (compare *C* and *D*).

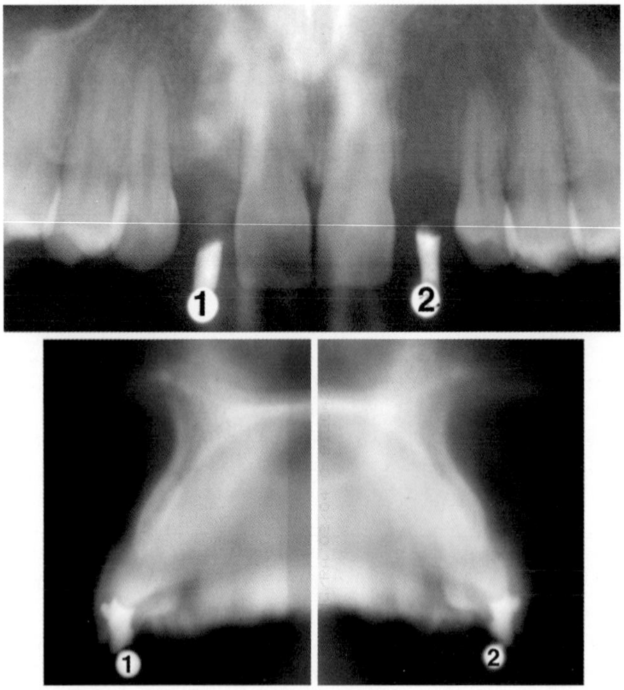

A B

Figure 75-13 Radiographic evaluation of a patient with congenitally missing maxillary lateral incisors before implant placement. **A,** Panoramic radiograph reveals sufficient height and mesiolateral width of the alveolar ridge. **B,** Cross-sectional conventional tomography of the edentulous areas reveals a narrow (<4 mm) buccolingual width of the alveolar ridge that needs to be addressed by modifications in the treatment planning, such as bone augmentation.

In addition to the amount, the *quality* of the available bone should also be evaluated. A uniform, continuous cortical outline and a lacy, well-defined trabecular core reflect the normal bone homeostasis necessary for appropriate bone response around the implant. Thin or discontinuous cortex, sparse trabeculation, large marrow spaces, and altered trabecular architecture should be noted because they might predict poor implant stabilization and less desirable response of the bone. Poor bone quality may necessitate modifications of the treatment planning, such as waiting longer for healing (osseointegration) to maximize bone-to-implant contact before loading.

Evaluate Relation of Alveolar Ridge with Existing Teeth and Desired Implant Position

Accurate placement (spatial position and angulation relative to adjacent teeth and occlusal plane) will greatly affect the restorative success and long-term prognosis of the implant (see Chapter 80). A significant variable during the preimplant evaluation is the relation of the desired implant position relative to the existing teeth, alveolar crest, and occlusal plane. Angled or custom abutments can accommodate slight variations in implant position and implant inclination. However, more significant deviations should be avoided.

Prolonged tooth loss is usually associated with atrophy of the alveolar ridge and, in the case of the maxilla, with pneumatization of the sinus floor toward the alveolar crest. Traumatic extractions can compromise the buccal or lingual cortex and alter the shape and buccolingual

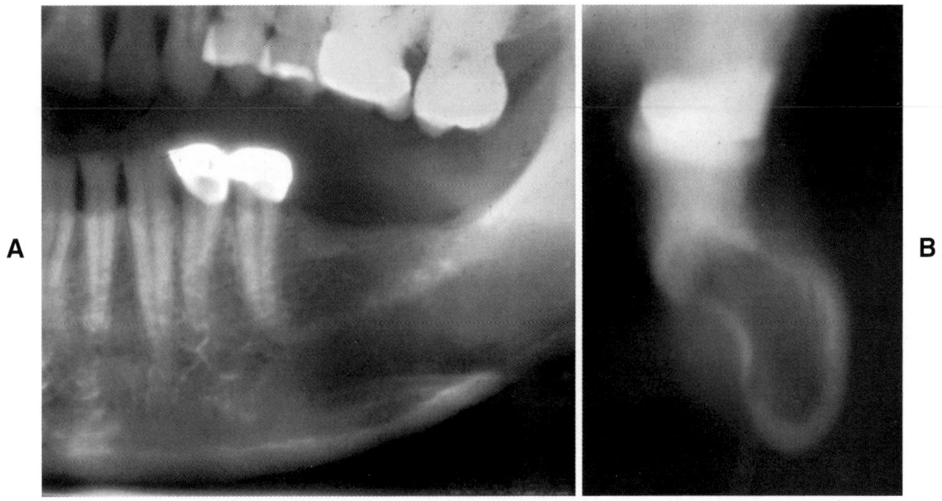

Figure 75-14 Radiographic evaluation of a patient with edentulous posterior left mandible before implant placement. **A,** Panoramic radiograph demonstrates sufficient height of the alveolar ridge with little or no resorption. **B,** Cross-sectional conventional tomography reveals significant lingual inclination of the alveolar ridge not depicted on the panoramic radiograph.

ridge dimension. Anatomic variants, such as lingual inclination of the alveolus or narrow ridges, should be considered during treatment planning of the implant patient (Figure 75-14).

An important part of diagnostic imaging must include an evaluation of the available bone relative to the "prosthetically driven" implant position. This aspect of the patient evaluation is best accomplished with diagnostic models, wax-up of planned tooth replacement, and radiographic markers in the desired tooth positions during imaging. Steel balls, brass tubes, and gutta percha have all been used to establish the proposed tooth positions relative to the existing alveolar bone. The use of these nonanatomic markers is helpful for evaluating bone height and width in specific anatomic locations. However, they do not accurately represent the tooth contours and do not allow the clinician to estimate variations in implant position and angulation relative to the position and emergence of the planned tooth replacement. Therefore, it is more desirable and beneficial to use radiopaque "tooth-shaped" markers so that the existing alveolar bone can be evaluated relative to the entire tooth position/contours (Figure 75-15; see also Figures 75-5 and 75-8). This is particularly important for anterior, esthetic implant cases. Patients should *always* be imaged with radiographic guides (markers).

CLINICAL SELECTION OF DIAGNOSTIC IMAGING

Radiography is an important diagnostic tool for the evaluation of the implant patient. However, radiographic imaging alone is not sufficient. It is important to correlate diagnostic information with a good clinical examination. Conversely, a clinical examination is insufficient to provide the information needed to plan implant treatment for a patient without some radiographic imaging.

Clinical Examination

Before taking any radiographs, a complete clinical examination of the implant patient is required. This should include the etiology and duration of tooth loss, any history of traumatic extraction, and a review of records and radiographs, if available. Clinical assessment of the edentulous area, covering mucosa, adjacent and opposing teeth, and occlusal plane should be performed. Temporomandibular function, mandibular maximal opening, and protrusive and lateral movements should be evaluated (see Chapter 74).

Screening Films

At this point, an overall assessment of the health of the jaws should be performed. Periapical films provide a high-resolution image of the alveolus and the surrounding structures, including adjacent teeth. For extended edentulous areas, panoramic, lateral cephalometric, and occlusal films can be used to estimate bone height and width. Any pathology of the bone at the prospective implant site, as well as of the surrounding structures, should be identified and treated as indicated.

Fabrication of Radiographic and Surgical Guides

Once the health of the soft and hard tissues is established, casts should be taken and detailed analysis performed. The clinician should decide on the number of implants and their desired location. Next, a radiographic guide should be fabricated, usually with clear acrylic. The position of the desired implants is indicated by the use of radiopaque objects such as metallic balls, cylinders, or rods; gutta percha; or composite resin. If CT imaging might be performed, the use of metallic markers should be avoided. The design of such a guide greatly enhances the diagnostic information provided by the radiographs

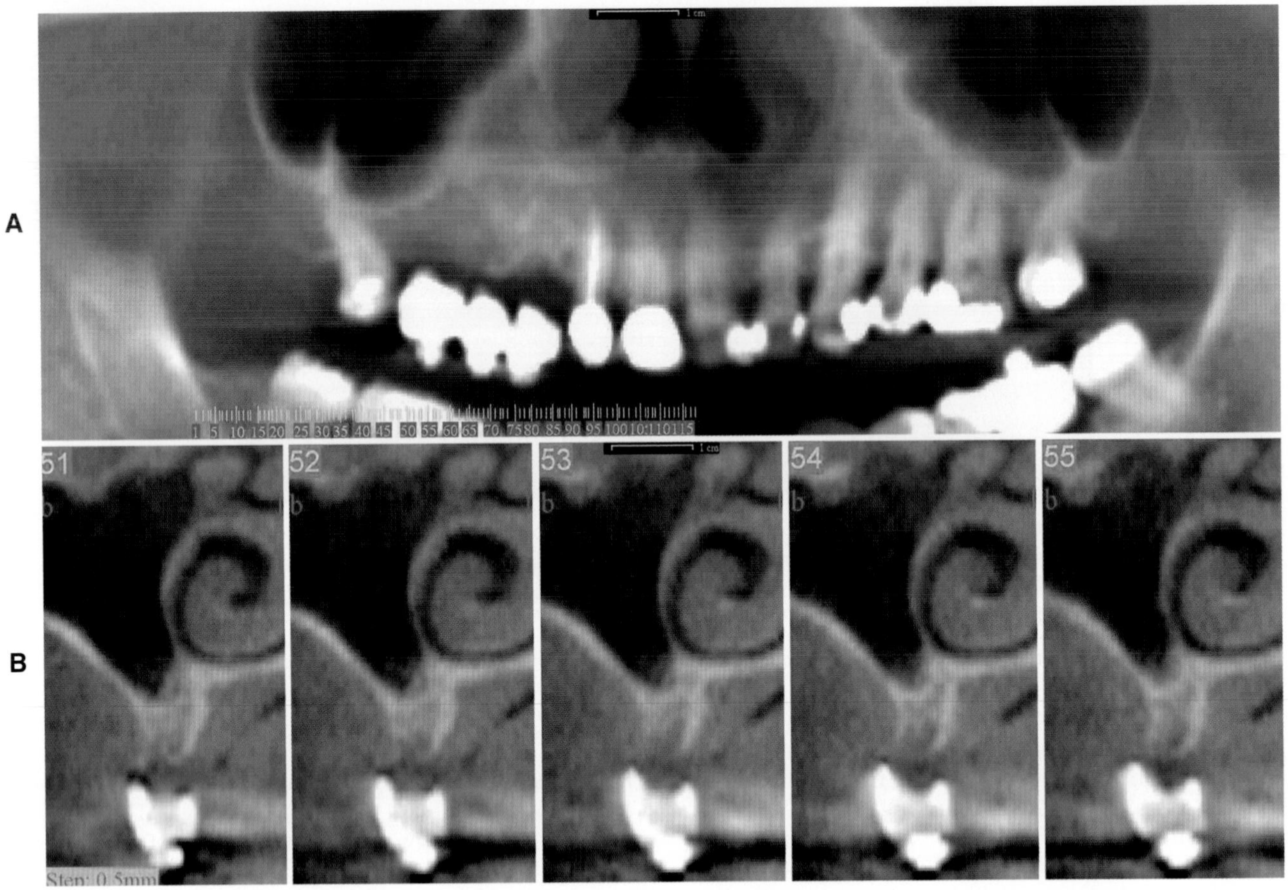

Figure 75-15 Panoramic **(A)** and cross-sectional **(B)** views from a CBCT examination before implant placement in the right maxilla. Markers in the shape and size of the missing teeth help evaluate the alveolar ridge relative to the prospective teeth positions and contours.

because it correlates the radiographic anatomy with the exact position of the proposed implant location.

Cross-Sectional Tomography

Some type of cross-sectional imaging, such as conventional tomography, CT, or CBCT, should be performed before implant placement in any site of the jaws.[20] Plain (two-dimensional) films might be sufficient in select implant cases. For example, a single anterior maxillary site with good interdental space and bone volume and no significant anatomic structures at risk might not require cross-sectional imaging. On the other hand, the potential morbidity of a compromised anatomic structure and the poor performance and potential failure of a misplaced implant, combined with the wide availability of tomographic facilities, favor the use of cross-sectional imaging in many cases of implant treatment planning. It is crucial that the cross sections are perpendicular to the curvature of the mandible and parallel to the planned implant. Improper patient positioning can lead to an overestimation of the height and width of the available bone. If the surgeon believes that sections were performed at the wrong angulation, new images should be requested. This might necessitate reexposure of the patient.

CONCLUSION

Many radiographic projections are available for the evaluation of implant placement, each with advantages and disadvantages. The clinician must follow sequential steps in patient evaluation, and radiography is an essential diagnostic tool for implant design and successful treatment of the implant patient. Selection of appropriate radiographic modalities will provide the maximum diagnostic information, help avoid unwanted complications, and maximize treatment outcomes while delivering "as low as reasonably achievable" (ALARA) radiation dose to the patient.[13]

REFERENCES

1. Arai Y, Tammisalo E, Iwai K, et al: Development of compact computed tomographic apparatus for dental use, *Dentomaxillofac Radiol* 28:245, 1999.
2. Cavalcanti MG, Yang J, Ruprecht A, Vannier MW: Validation of spiral computed tomography for dental implants, *Dentomaxillofac Radiol* 27:329, 1998.
3. Curry TS, Dowdey JE, Murry RC: *Christensen's physics of diagnostic radiology*, ed 4, Philadelphia, 1990, Lea & Febiger.
4. Ekkestubbe A, Grondahl K, Grondahl HG: The use of tomography for dental implant planning, *Dentomaxillofac Radiol* 26:206, 1997.

5. Hatcher DC, Dial C, Mayorga C: Cone beam CT for pre-surgical assessment of implant sites, *J Calif Dent Assoc* 31:824, 2003.
6. Kassebaum DK, Nummikoski PV, Triplett RG, Langlais RP: Cross-sectional radiography for implant site assessment, *Oral Surg Oral Med Oral Pathol* 70:674, 1990.
7. Kraut RA: Utilization of 3D/dental software for precise implant site selection: clinical reports, *Implant Dent* 1:134, 1992.
8. Langland OE, Langlais RP, Preece JW: Panoramic and special imaging techniques. In *Principles of dental imaging,* ed 2, Baltimore, 2002, Lippincott, Williams & Wilkins.
9. Lindh C, Petersson A: Radiologic examination for location of the mandibular canal: a comparison between panoramic radiography and conventional tomography, *Int J Oral Maxillofac Implants* 4:249, 1989.
10. Lindh C, Petersson A, Klinge B: Measurements of distances related to the mandibular canal in radiographs, *Clin Oral Implant Res* 6:96, 1995.
11. Ludlow JB, Davies-Ludlow LE, Brooks SL: Dosimetry of two extraoral direct digital imaging devices: NewTom cone beam CT and Orthophos Plus DS panoramic unit, *Dentomaxillofac Radiol* 32:290, 2003.
12. Lurie AG: Panoramic imaging in intraoral radiographic examinations. In White SC, Pharoah MJ: *Oral radiology: principles and interpretation,* ed 5, St Louis, 2004, Mosby.
13. Michel R, Zimmerman TL: Basic radiation protection considerations in dental practice, *Health Phys* 77:S81, 1999.
14. Mozzo P, Procacci C, Tacconi A, et al: A new volumetric CT machine for dental imaging based on the cone-beam technique: preliminary results, *Eur Radiol* 8:1558, 1998.
15. Scaf G, Lurie AG, Mosier KM, et al: Dosimetry and cost of imaging osseointegrated implants with film-based and computed tomography, *Oral Surg Oral Med Oral Pathol Oral Radiol Endod* 83:41, 1997.
16. Schulze D, Heiland M, Blake F, et al: Evaluation of quality of reformatted images from two cone-beam computed tomographic systems, *J Craniomaxillofac Surg* 33:19, 2005.
17. Sewerin IP: Errors in radiographic assessment of marginal bone height around osseointegrated implants, *Scand J Dent Res* 98:428, 1990.
18. Shetty V, Benson BW: Orofacial implants in intraoral radiographic examinations. In White SC, Pharoah MJ: *Oral radiology: principles and interpretation,* ed 5, St Louis, 2004, Mosby.
19. Truhlar RS, Morris HF, Ochi S: A review of panoramic radiography and its potential use in implant dentistry, *Implant Dent* 2:122, 1993.
20. Tyndall DA, Brooks SL: Selection criteria for dental implant site imaging: a position paper of the American Academy of Oral and Maxillofacial Radiology, *Oral Surg Oral Med Oral Pathol Oral Radiol Endod* 89:630, 2000.
21. Whaites E: Periapical radiography. In *Essentials of dental radiography and radiology,* ed 3, London, 2002, Churchill Livingstone.
22. White SC: Assessment of radiation risk from dental radiography, *Dentomaxillofac Radiol* 21:118, 1992.
23. White SC, Pharoah MJ: Intraoral radiographic examinations. In *Oral radiology: principles and interpretation,* ed 5, St Louis, 2004, Mosby.

Standard Implant Surgical Procedures

Thomas J. Han, Kwang Bum Park, and Perry R. Klokkevold

76

CHAPTER

■ ■ ■

CHAPTER OUTLINE

IMPLANT SELECTION AND DESIGN CONSIDERATIONS
 Implant Geometry (Macrodesign)
 Implant Surface Topography (Microdesign)
GENERAL PRINCIPLES OF IMPLANT SURGERY
 Patient Preparation
 Implant Site Preparation
 One-Stage versus Two-Stage Implant Surgeries
TWO-STAGE "SUBMERGED" IMPLANT PLACEMENT
 Flap Design, Incisions, and Elevation
 Implant Site Preparation

 Flap Closure and Suturing
 Postoperative Care
 Second-Stage Exposure Surgery
ONE-STAGE "NONSUBMERGED" IMPLANT PLACEMENT
 Flap Design, Incisions, and Elevation
 Implant Site Preparation
 Flap Closure and Suturing
 Postoperative Care
CONCLUSION

The surgical procedures for the placement of almost all endosseous dental implants currently used are based on the original work of Professor Per-Ingvar Brånemark and colleagues in Sweden approximately four decades ago. Their landmark research evaluated the biologic, physiologic, and mechanical aspects of the titanium screw-shaped implant subsequently known commercially as the Nobelpharma "Brånemark" implant system and currently manufactured by Nobel Biocare. The familiar Brånemark design is screw shaped and threaded with an external hex and a machined surface (Figure 76-1). Since Brånemark's original work, many different designs of root form implants have been developed and studied. At present, more than 50 implant manufacturers worldwide make implants with various shapes, dimensions, and surface characteristics. Regardless of which implant system is used, the same fundamental principles of atraumatic, precise implant site preparation apply. This involves gentle surgical techniques and progressive, incremental preparation of the bone for a precise fit of the implant.

This chapter presents general surgical considerations and outlines the standard surgical procedures for the placement of endosseous dental implants. The principles

apply to most of the common implant systems. Because the various implant systems have their own specific armamentarium and recommendations for use (e.g., drilling speeds), it is advisable to follow the detailed, step-by-step description usually found in the manufacturer's manual when using any particular implant system.

IMPLANT SELECTION AND DESIGN CONSIDERATIONS

Implant Geometry (Macrodesign)

Root form endosseous dental implants can be divided into two basic groups: (1) screw shaped with threads and (2) cylindrical and threadless (see Figure 76-1). The screw-shaped, threaded implants are rotated into the bone recipient site like a screw with a handpiece or handheld wrench after preparing an osteotomy site that is slightly smaller in diameter than the implant threads. Thus the threads engage the walls of the prepared osteotomy site and provide vertical stabilization. The cylinder-shaped, threadless implants are pushed or tapped into a recipient site that is prepared with a diameter and shape that is nearly identical to that of the implant. Thus the implant

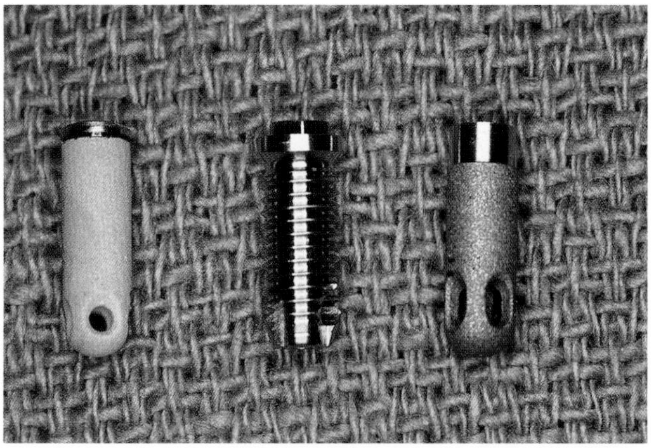

Figure 76-1 Two basic groups of the root form implants (macrodesign). *Center,* Brånemark screw-shaped, threaded design with external hex and machined surface. *Left* and *right,* Cylindrical, threadless design with hydroxyapatite-coated *(left)* and titanium plasma–sprayed *(right)* surfaces.

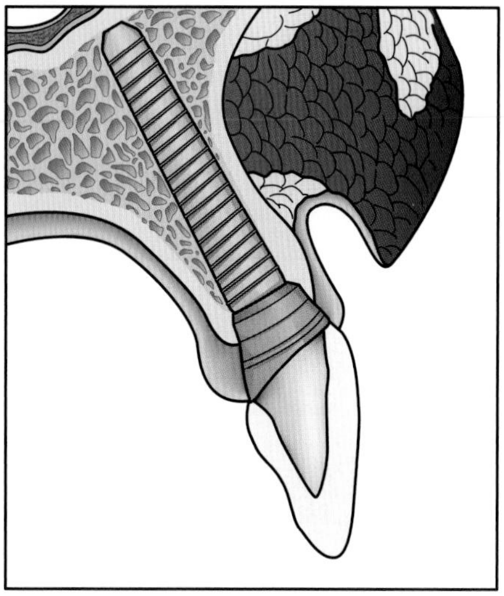

Figure 76-2 Conically shaped, threaded implant is helpful to minimize apical bone fenestration and also useful in placing implants into extraction sockets immediately. (Courtesy Nobel Biocare, Yorba Linda, Calif.)

achieves a tight "press-fit." Vertical stability comes from the apical end of the implant seating into the bottom of the osteotomy site.

The threaded implants are more widely used because they usually provide superior initial stability in bone, and vertical positioning of the implant during placement can be more precisely controlled. In dense bone, it may be necessary to "tap" the bone (i.e., create threads in the bone) for easier placement. Some screw-shaped, threaded implants are tapered to resemble the conical shape of a natural tooth root. Tapered implant designs help to minimize apical bone fenestration, allow for the placement of implants into narrower apical sites (between closely approximating roots), and are amenable to immediate placement into anterior extraction sockets (Figure 76-2).

Implant Surface Topography (Microdesign)

It is generally believed that the textured surfaces accelerate the initial healing phase and enhances bone formation at the implant surface.[9-11,13] Surface modifications can be additive or subtractive. Additive implant surfaces, such as titanium plasma–sprayed (TPS) and hydroxyapatite (HA)–coated surfaces, are considered highly textured because they have macroscopically visible surface "roughness" (Figure 76-3, *A* and *B*). Although these surfaces achieve secondary stability and integration earlier, progressive bone loss can occur if the rough surface of the implant becomes exposed to oral fluid and microorganisms. Therefore, when using implants with macroscopically rough surfaces, care must be taken to ensure complete submersion of the rough surface in bone with sufficient crestal bone thickness around the implant. Thinner areas of crestal bone have a greater risk of bone loss over time, which can expose the surface to contamination with oral bacteria, leading ultimately to infection and bone loss.

In contrast to the macroscopically rough TPS and HA-coated implant surfaces, machined implant surfaces are much more resistant to bacterial contamination and progressive bone loss. However, when compared to implants with "rough" surfaces, machined surfaces provide weaker secondary stability and consequently result in lower success rates in poor-quality or grafted bone[12] (Figure 76-3, *C*).

Over the past decade there has been great interest in implant surface modifications that alter the surface characteristics at the microscopic level (i.e., altered microtopography). Subtractive implant surface modifications such as blasting (e.g., RBM, Lifecore), acid etching (e.g., Osseotite®, Implant Innovations, Inc.), and a combination of both (e.g., SLA, Straumann) have gained favor because they are thought to enhance bone-to-implant contact through initial clot stabilization and osteoblast migration to the implant surface[10] (Figure 76-3, *D*). These implant surface modifications have been shown to enhance the bone-to-implant contact and strength of resistance compared with machined-surface implants.[8,13] Significantly, the altered microtopography appears to improve implant success in poor-quality bone sites.[16]

GENERAL PRINCIPLES OF IMPLANT SURGERY

Patient Preparation

Most implant surgical procedures can be done in the office using local anesthesia. For some patients, depending on individual preferences and complexity of the case, conscious sedation (oral or intravenous) may be indicated (see Chapter 60). The risks and benefits of implant surgery specific to the patient's needs should be thoroughly explained at an appointment before the day of surgery. Once the patient understands the proposed treatment and has questions answered, a written informed consent should be obtained for the procedure.

Implant Site Preparation

Some basic principles must be followed to achieve osseointegration with a high degree of predictability[4,6,7]

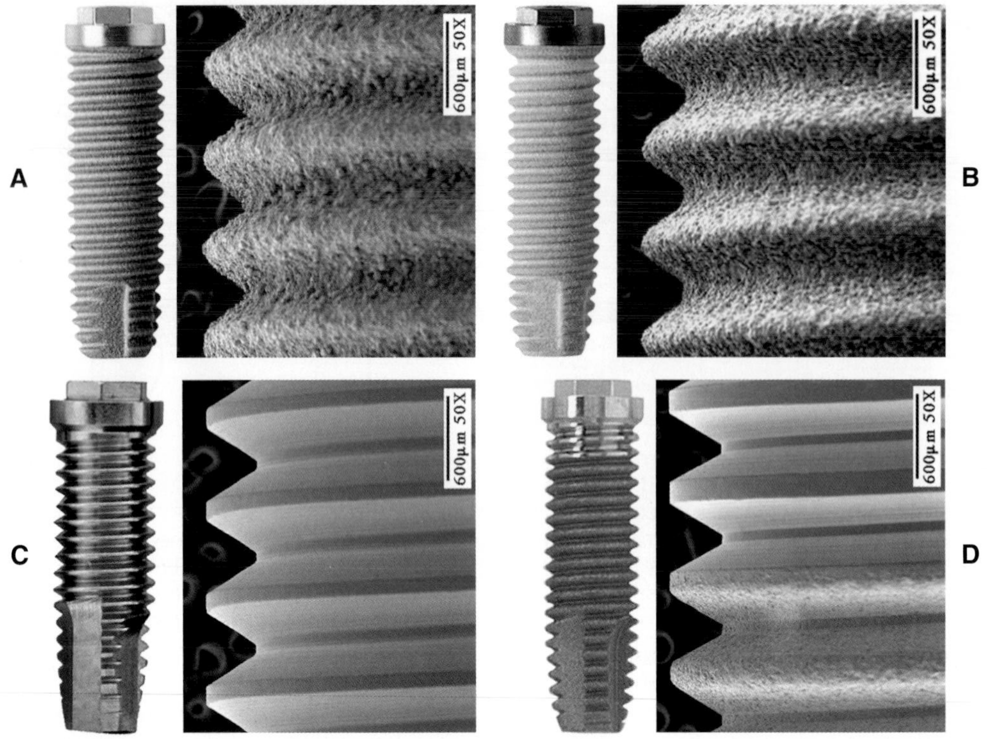

Figure 76-3 Surface topography of implant (microdesign). **A,** Highly textured implant with titanium plasma–sprayed surface. **B,** Highly textured implant with hydroxyapatite-coated surface. **C,** Implant with smooth, machined surface. **D,** Micro-textured implant with acid etched surface. (Courtesy 3i/Implant Innovations Inc., Palm Beach Gardens, Fla.)

BOX 76-1

Basic Principles of Implant Therapy to Achieve Osseointegration

1. Implants must be sterile and made of a biocompatible material (e.g., titanium).
2. Implant site preparation should be performed under sterile conditions.
3. Implant site preparation should be completed with an atraumatic surgical technique that avoids overheating of the bone during preparation of the recipient site.
4. Implants should be placed with good initial stability.
5. Implants should be allowed to heal without loading or micromovement (i.e., undisturbed healing period to allow for osseointegration) for 2 to 4 and 4 to 6 months in the mandible and maxilla, respectively.

(Box 76-1). The surgical site should be kept aseptic and the patient appropriately prepared and draped for an intraoral surgical procedure. It is recommended that the patient rinse with chlorhexidine gluconate for 30 seconds immediately before the procedure. Every effort should be made to maintain a sterile surgical field at all times and to avoid contamination of the implant surface. Implant sites should be prepared using gentle, atraumatic surgical techniques with a constant reminder to avoid overheating the bone. Finally, implants should be stable and allowed to heal without movement for a time.

When these clinical guidelines are followed, successful osseointegration occurs predictably for submerged[6] and nonsubmerged[15] dental implants. Well-controlled studies of patients with good plaque control and appropriate occlusal forces have demonstrated that root form, endosseous dental implants show little change in bone height around the implant.[1] After an initial remodeling in the first year that results in 1.0 to 1.5 mm of bone reduction (described as "normal remodeling around an externally hexed implant"),[1] the bone level around healthy functioning implants remains stable for many years, allowing implants to be a predictable means for tooth replacement. The annual bone loss after the first year in function is expected to be 0.1 mm or less.

Regardless of the type of surgical approach, the implant must be placed in healthy bone to achieve osseointegration, and an atraumatic technique must be followed to avoid damage to bone or vital structures. Bone quality at the recipient site influences the interface between bone and implant.[12] Compact bone offers a much greater surface area for mineralized tissue-to-implant contact than cancellous bone. Clinical studies have shown that areas of the jaw exhibiting thin layers of cortical bone and large cancellous spaces, such as the posterior maxilla, have significantly lower success rates than areas of denser bone structures.[12] The best results are obtained when contact between bone and implant is most intimate at implant placement.

SCIENCE TRANSFER

Successful implant placement requires stability by intimate bone-to-implant contact. This stability can be achieved by one of two ways. First, the implant can be stabilized if there is sufficient quantity and quality of bone. Second, the implant can be stabilized by rigidly connecting the coronal aspects intraorally and relying on the bone contact endosseously.

After the osteotomy has been prepared, areas of the native bone structure are left exposed. When the implant is placed into the preparation, some areas of the titanium rod make contact by "press-fit" to the exposed native bone; these areas are called *primary bone contact.* Because osseointegration is defined as bone-to-implant contact at the light microscopic level, primary bone contact results in instantaneous osseointegration. In areas between primary bone contact, bone formation begins to occur on the titanium surface and on the cut bone surfaces and trabeculae. At the same time, bone remodeling begins in the areas of primary bone contact, which also results in new bone formation along the implant surface. These areas of new bone formation are termed *secondary bone contact.*

The stability of the implant (vital to implant success) is a combination of primary bone–secondary bone contact areas.

As primary contact areas begin to remodel, the implant becomes slightly less stable overall until sufficient secondary bone contact is formed. Thus, there is a "dip" or decrease in the stability of the implant at an early stage of implant healing. This decrease or dip can be minimized by efforts to stimulate secondary bone contact.

Dental implants can be surgically placed with one-stage or two-stage procedures. In the one-stage procedure, a component of the implant is projected above the mucosa. With a two-stage approach, the implant is initially covered with mucosa, and later a second-stage surgery exposes the top of the implant, and an abutment is attached. The one-stage approach is valuable in many patients because of its simplicity and ability to provide support for adjacent gingival tissues. In complex cases with poor-quality bone or simultaneous bone grafting, the two-stage technique allows protection of the implant during the process of osseointegration.

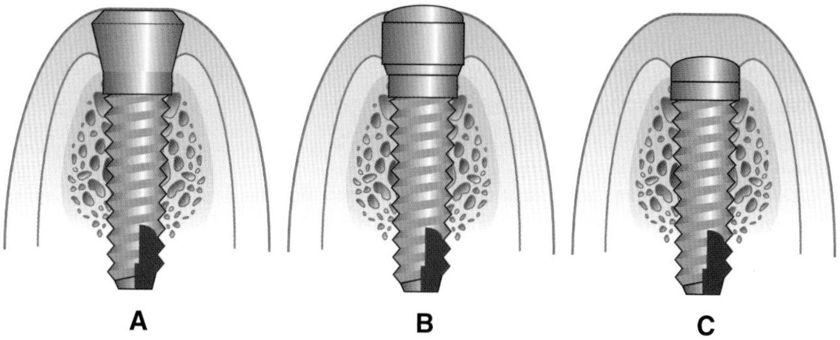

Figure 76-4 One-stage implant versus two-stage implant surgeries. **A,** One-stage surgery with the implant designed so that the coronal portion of the implant extends through the gingiva. **B,** One-stage surgery with implant designed to be used for two-stage surgery. A healing abutment is connected to the implant during the first-stage surgery. **C,** In the two-stage surgery, top of the implant is completely submerged under gingiva.

The surgical preparation of the tissues at the recipient site may also greatly affect healing. Drilling of the bone without proper cooling generates increased temperatures that can injure the bone and increase the risk of implant failure.[17]

One-Stage versus Two-Stage Implant Surgeries

Currently, most threaded endosseous implants can be placed using either a one-stage (nonsubmerged) or a two-stage (submerged) protocol. In the one-stage approach the implant or the abutment emerges through the mucoperiosteum at the time of implant placement, whereas in the two-stage approach the top of the implant and cover screw are completely covered with the flap closure (Figure 76-4). Implants are allowed to heal, without loading or micromovement, for a time. In two-stage implant surgery the implant must be surgically exposed following an undisturbed healing period. Some implants (e.g., ITI, Straumann; TG, Implant Innovations, Inc.) are specifically designed to have the coronal portion of the implant positioned above the crest of bone and extending through the gingival tissues during the healing period (Figure 76-4, *A*). Other systems require a healing abutment to be attached to the implant so that it can be used in a one-stage approach[8] (Figure 76-4, *B*).

The advantages of the one-stage surgical approach include easier mucogingival management around the implant in many cases. Patient management is simplified because a second-stage exposure surgery is not necessary.

The two-stage, submerged approach is advantageous for situations that require simultaneous bone augmentation procedures at the time of implant placement. This approach also prevents movement of the implant by the patient, who may inadvertently chew on it during the healing period. Fundamental differences in flap management for these two surgical techniques are described separately.

TWO-STAGE "SUBMERGED" IMPLANT PLACEMENT

In the two-stage implant surgical approach, the first-stage (placement) surgery ends by suturing the soft tissues over the implant cover screw so that it remains submerged and isolated from the oral cavity. In the mandible the implants are left undisturbed for 2 to 4 months, whereas in the maxilla they are allowed to heal for 4 to 6 months. Longer healing periods are indicated for implants placed in less dense bone (e.g., maxilla) or when there is less initial implant stability (i.e., slight looseness caused by limited bone-to-implant contact) regardless of jaw or specific site. Over time, osteoblasts migrate to the surface and form bone adjacent to the implant (osseointegration)[5] (see Chapter 73). Shorter healing periods are indicated for implants placed in good quality (dense) bone and for implants with an altered surface microtopography (e.g., acid etched, blasted or etched and blasted).

In the second-stage (exposure) surgery, the implant is uncovered and a healing abutment is connected to allow emergence of the implant/abutment through the soft tissues, thus facilitating access to the implant from the oral cavity. The restorative dentist then proceeds with the prosthodontic aspects of the implant therapy (impressions and fabrication of prosthesis).

The following paragraphs describe the steps for the first-stage implant placement surgery (Figures 76-5, 76-6, and 76-7).

Flap Design, Incisions, and Elevation

Flap management for implant surgery will vary slightly depending on the location and objective of the planned surgery. Two types of incisions, crestal or remote, can be used. The *remote* incision is made some distance from the planned osteotomy site. A periosteal elevator is then used to reflect a mucoperiosteal (full-thickness) flap. For the *crestal* design of flap, the incision is made along the crest of the ridge, bisecting the existing zone of keratinized mucosa (see Figures 76-5, *A,* and 76-7, *B*).

When extensive bone augmentation is planned, a remote incision with layer suturing technique is used to minimize the incidence of bone graft exposure. The crestal incision, however, is preferred in most cases because it is easier to manage and results in less bleeding, less edema, and faster healing.[14] Sutures placed over the implant generally do not interfere with healing.

A full-thickness flap is raised buccally and lingually to the level of the mucogingival junction, exposing the alveolar ridge of the implant surgical sites (Figures 76-5, *B,* and 76-7, *C*). Elevated flaps may be sutured to the buccal mucosa or the opposing teeth to keep the surgical site open during the surgery. The bone at the implant site(s) must be thoroughly debrided of all granulation tissue.

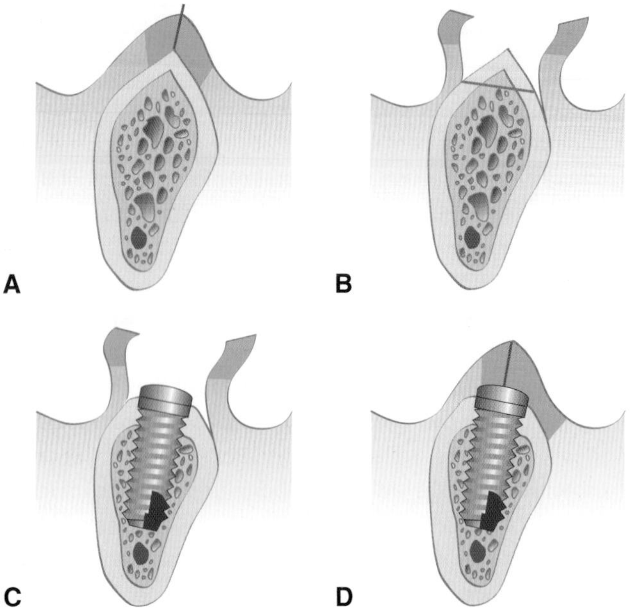

Figure 76-5 **A,** Crestal incision made along the crest of the ridge, bisecting the existing zone of keratinized mucosa. **B,** Full-thickness flap is raised buccally and lingually to the level of the mucogingival junction. A sharp ridge can be surgically contoured to provide a reasonably flat bed for the implant. **C,** Implant is placed in prepared osteotomy site. **D,** Crestal flap closure without tension.

For a "knife-edge" alveolar process with sufficient alveolar height and distance from vital structures (e.g., inferior alveolar nerve), a large round bur is used to recontour the bone to provide a reasonably flat bed for the implant site (Figure 76-5, *B*). However, if a site has less than 10 mm of remaining alveolar bone, the knife-edge alveolar bone should be preserved. Bone augmentation procedures can be used to increase the ridge width (see Chapter 77).

Implant Site Preparation

Once the flaps are reflected and the bone is prepared (i.e., all granulation tissue removed and knife-edge ridges flattened), the implant osteotomy site can be prepared. A series of drills are used to prepare the osteotomy site precisely and incrementally for an implant (Figure 76-8). A surgical guide or stent is inserted, checked for proper positioning, and used throughout the procedure to direct the proper implant placement (Figure 76-7, *E*).

Round Bur. A small round bur (or spiral drill) is used to mark the implant sites. The guide is removed, and the initial marks are checked for their appropriate buccal-lingual and mesial-distal location, as well as the positions relative to each other (see Figure 74-9). Slight modifications may be necessary to adjust spatial relationships and to avoid minor ridge defects. Any changes should

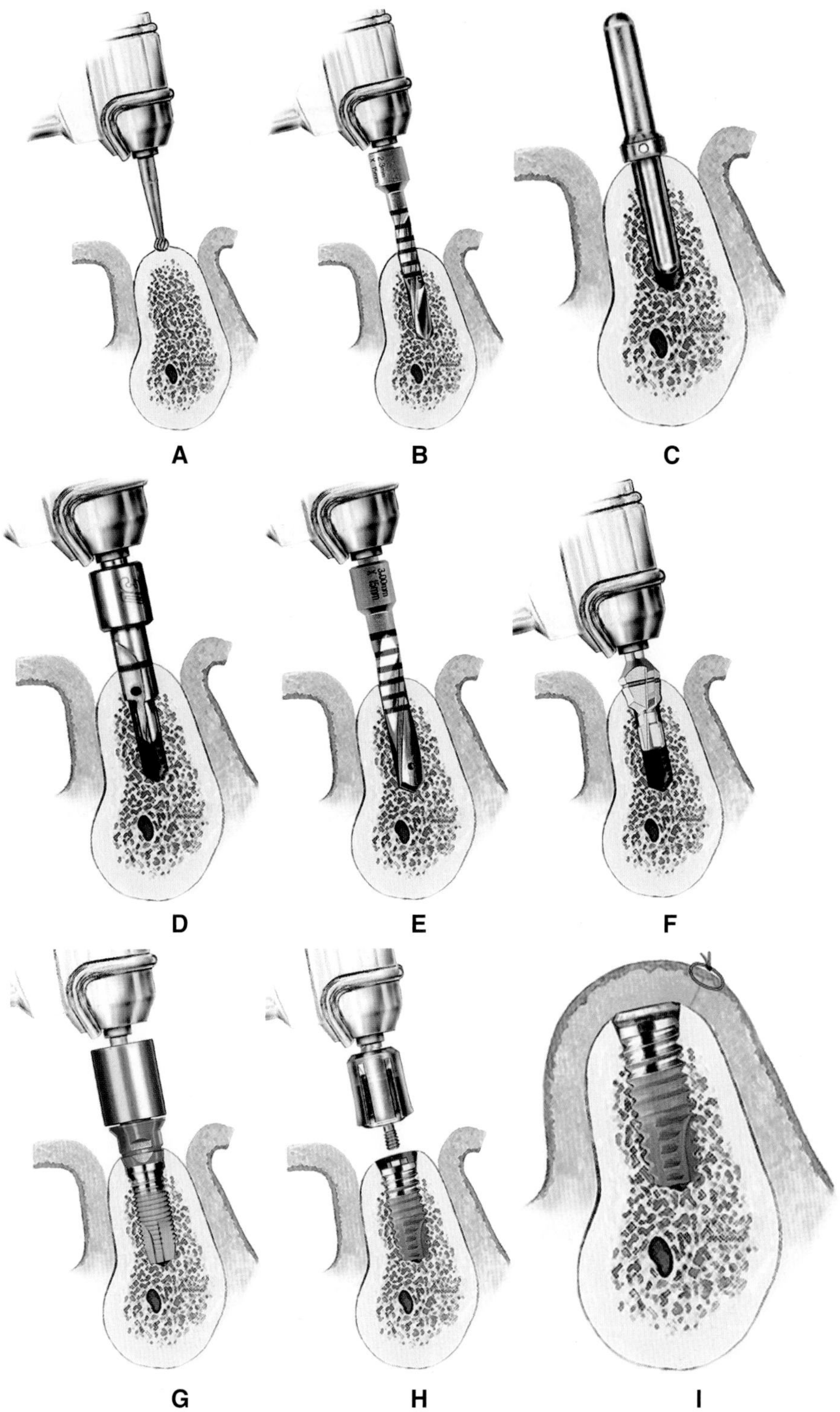

Figure 76-6 Implant site preparation (osteotomy) for a 4 × 10-mm screw-type, threaded (external hex) implant in a subcrestal position. **A,** Initial marking or preparation of the implant site with a round bur. **B,** Use of a 2-mm twist drill to establish depth and align the implant. **C,** Guide pin is placed in the osteotomy site to confirm position and angulation. **D,** Pilot drill is used to increase the coronal aspect of the osteotomy site. **E,** Final drill used is the 3-mm twist drill to finish preparation of the osteotomy site. **F,** Countersink drill is used to widen the entrance of the recipient site and allow for the subcrestal placement of the implant and coverscrew. NOTE: An optional tap (not shown) can be used at this point to create screw threads in areas of dense bone. **G,** Implant is inserted into the prepared osteotomy site. **H,** Implant mount is removed, and cover screw is placed. **I,** Soft tissues are closed and sutured. (Courtesy 3i/Implant Innovations, Inc., Palm Beach Gardens, Fla.)

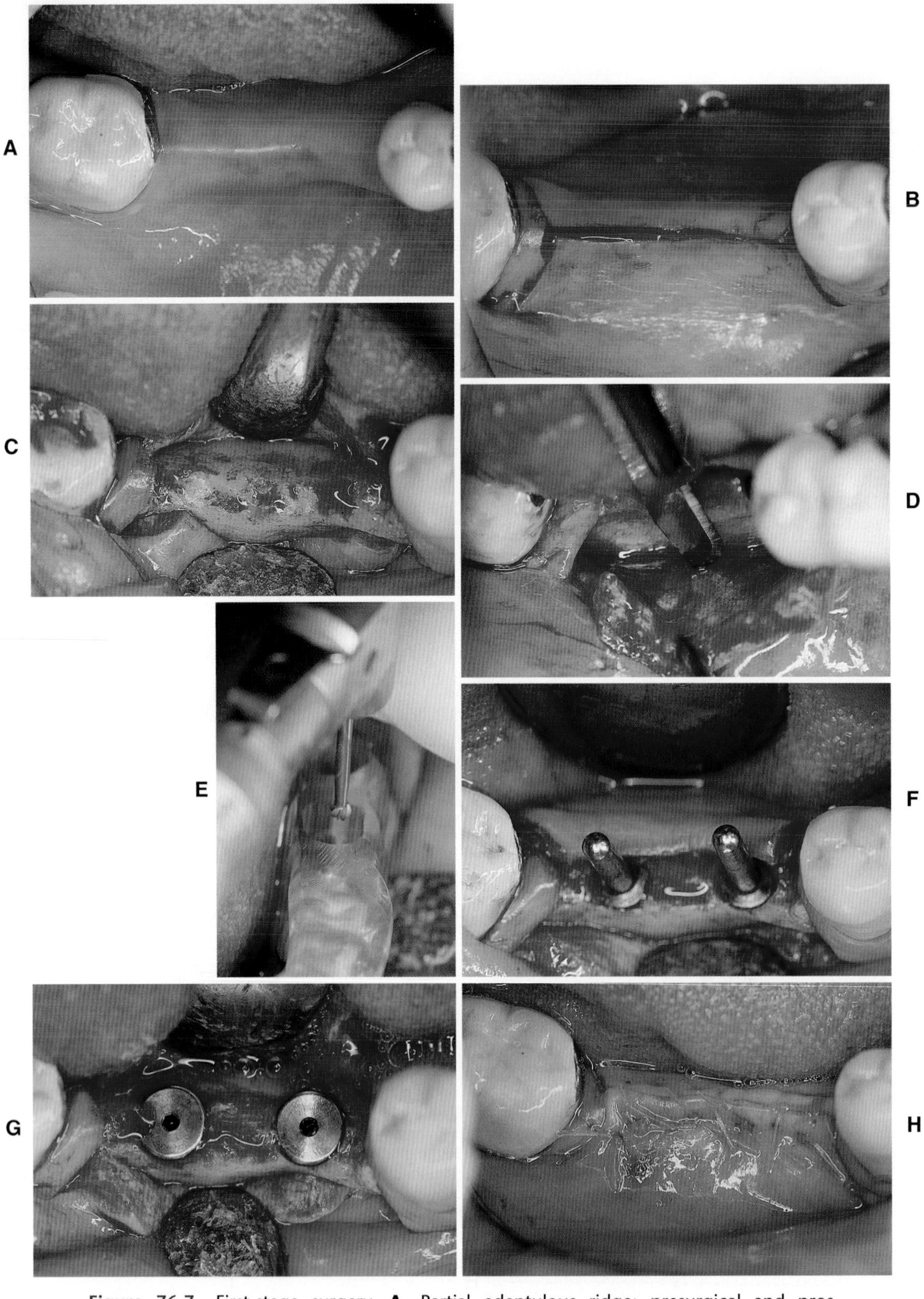

Figure 76-7 First-stage surgery. **A,** Partial edentulous ridge; presurgical and prosthodontic treatment has been completed. **B,** Mesial sulcular and distal vertical incisions are connected by a crestal incision. Notice that bands of gingival collars remain adjacent to the distal molar tooth. **C,** Minimal flap reflection is used to expose the alveolar bone. Sometimes a ridge modification is necessary to provide a flap recipient bed. **D,** Buccal flap is partially dissected at the apical portion to provide a flap extension. This is a critical step to ensure a tension-free closure of the flap after implant placement. **E,** It is important to use the surgical stent to determine the mesial-distal and buccal-lingual dimensions and proper angulation of the implant placement. **F,** Frequent use of the guide pins ensures parallelism of the implant placement. **G,** After placement of two Nobelpharma implants, the cover screws are placed. The cover screws should be flush with the rest of the ridge to minimize the chance of exposure. This is especially important if the patient will wear a partial denture during the healing phase. **H,** Suturing completed. Both regular interrupted and inverted mattress sutures are used intermittently to ensure tension-free, tight closure of the flaps.

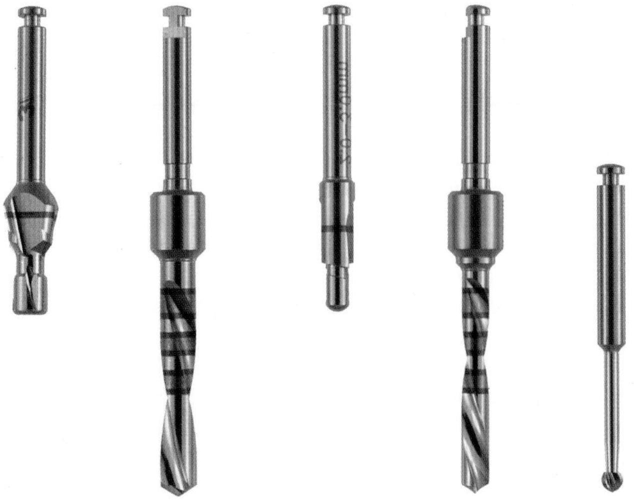

Figure 76-8 Sequence of drills used for standard-diameter (4.0-mm) implant site osteotomy preparation: round, 2-mm twist, pilot, 3-mm twist, and countersink. Bone tap (not shown here) is an optional drill that is sometimes used in dense bone before implant placement.

be compared to the surgical guide positions. Each marked site is then prepared to a depth of 1 to 2 mm with a round drill, breaking through the cortical bone and creating a starting point for the 2-mm twist drill (Figure 76-6, *A*).

The 2-mm Twist Drill. A small twist drill, usually 2 mm in diameter and marked to indicate various lengths (i.e., corresponding to the implant sizes), is used next to establish the depth and align the long axis of the implant recipient site (Figure 76-6, *B*). This drill may be externally or internally irrigated. In either case, the twist drill is used at a speed of approximately 800 to 1200 rpm, with copious irrigation to prevent overheating of the bone. Additionally, drills should be intermittently and repeatedly "pumped" or pulled out of the osteotomy sites while drilling to expose them to the water coolant and to facilitate clearing bone debris from the cutting surfaces. In other words, in an effort to reduce heat generation and the resistance of drills while in bone, clinicians should avoid preparing the bone with a unidirectional "push" of the drill in the apical direction only.

When multiple implants are being placed next to one another, a guide pin should be placed in the prepared sites to check alignment and parallelism throughout the preparation process. The relationship to neighboring vital structures can be determined by taking a periapical radiograph with a guide pin or radiographic marker in the osteotomy site(s) (see Figure 75-2). Implants should be positioned with approximately 3 mm between one another to ensure sufficient space for interimplant bone and soft tissue health and to facilitate oral hygiene procedures. Therefore the initial marks should be separated by at least 7 mm (center to center) for standard-diameter implants and more for wide-diameter implants (see Figure 74-9).

The 2-mm twist drill is used to establish the final depth of the osteotomy site for each planned implant. If the vertical height of the bone was reduced during the initial ridge preparation, this must be taken into account when preparing the site for a predetermined implant length.

The next step is to use a series of drills systematically to widen the size to accommodate the selected size of the implant. The shapes of the drills may differ slightly among different implant systems, but their general purpose is to prepare a recipient site with a precise diameter and depth for the selected implant without unduly traumatizing the surrounding bone. It is important to use copious irrigation for all drilling.

Pilot Drill. Following the 2-mm twist drill, a pilot drill with a noncutting 2-mm-diameter "guide" at the apical end and a cutting 3-mm-diameter (wider) midsection is used to enlarge the osteotomy site, thus facilitating the insertion of the subsequent drill in the sequence (Figure 76-6, *C*).

The 3-mm Twist Drill. The final drill in the preparation of a standard-diameter (4.0-mm) implant is the 3-mm twist drill. It is used to widen the site along the entire depth of the osteotomy from 2 to 3 mm. This final drill in the sequence will finish cutting the osteotomy site and will help the clinician determine whether the implant will be stable or not (Figure 76-6, *D*). Regardless of the system used, it is important that the final-diameter drilling be accomplished with a steady hand, without wobbling (Box 76-2).

Countersink Drill (Optional). When it is desirable to place the height of the cover screw slightly under the crestal bone to avoid a risk of premature exposure from the pressure of the temporary denture, countersink drilling is used to shape or flare the crestal aspect of the osteotomy site. This allows the coronal flare of the implant and cover screw to fit within the osteotomy site (Figure 76-6, *E*). As with all drills in the sequence, copious irrigation and gentle surgical techniques are used.

Bone Tap (Optional). Finally, for the placement of threaded implants, a tapping procedure may be necessary. With self-tapping implants becoming almost universal, there is less need for a tapping procedure. However, in dense cortical bone or when placing longer implants into moderately dense bone, it is prudent to tap the bone (create threads in the osteotomy site) before implant placement to facilitate implant insertion and to reduce the risk of implant binding (Figure 76-6, *F*).

Clinical comment: When faced with a very soft, poor-quality bone (e.g., loose trabecular bone in the posterior maxilla), tapping is not necessary or recommended (see Box 76-2).

Bone tapping and implant insertion are both done at very slow speeds (e.g., 25-30 rpm). All other drills in the sequence are used at higher speeds (800-1200 rpm).

It is important to create a recipient site that is very accurate in size and angulation. In partially edentulous cases, limited jaw opening may prevent appropriate positioning of the drills in posterior edentulous areas. In fact, implant therapy may be contraindicated in some patients because of a lack of interocclusal clearance or access for the instrumentation. Therefore a combination of longer drills and shorter drills, with or without extensions, may be necessary. Anticipating these needs before surgery facilitates the procedure and improves the results.

Note on wide-diameter implant site preparation: It is sometimes desirable to replace molars with wide-diameter implants because the larger diameter better approximates the size and the emergence profile of molar-sized teeth. When wide-diameter drills are used for implant site preparation, it is advisable to reduce the drilling speed (e.g., to 500-600 rpm), according to the manufacturer's guidelines, to prevent overheating the bone. Copious external irrigation is critical.

Implant Placement. Implants are inserted with a handpiece rotating at slow speeds (e.g., 25 rpm) or by hand with a wrench. Insertion of the implant must follow the same path or line as the osteotomy site. When multiple implants are being placed, it is helpful to use guide pins in the other sites to have a visual guide for the path of insertion.

BOX 76-2

Clinical Advice to Enhance Precision of Final Implant Site Preparation

Clinical Situation #1

If the final drill hits the bottom of the recipient site before reaching the desired depth, the added hand pressure necessary to achieve the proper depth often causes wobbling and funneling of the recipient site. This is especially true with "cannon" drills (used for cylindrical implants). To minimize this effect, the smaller-diameter drill should be used to prepare the site slightly deeper (e.g., 0.5 mm). This narrower drill does not affect the side walls and allows the desired depth to be reached with the final drill for a more precise osteotomy.

Clinical Situation #2

If the final drill is inserted at an inaccurate angle, the result is funneling of the coronal portion of the implant site. To minimize this potential problem, when drilling multiple implant sites, the operator should always keep a direction indicator in an adjacent site. For single-implant sites, the adjacent teeth and surgical guide should serve as direction indicators. When dealing with dense bone, a precise recipient site can be achieved more predictably if there is minimal diameter change from drill to drill. For example, switching from 3.0 to 5.0 mm is much more difficult than proceeding from 3.0 to 3.3 to 4.2 to 5.0 mm.

Clinical Situation #3

If the bone is "soft" (e.g., loose trabecular bone), it may be advantageous to underprepare the osteotomy site. A slightly underprepared site can be accomplished by using the final drill to a shallower depth than the previous drill (e.g., half the depth of the osteotomy site). This avoids removing too much bone and increases the implant stability or tightness at the time of placement.

Flap Closure and Suturing

Once the implants are inserted and the cover screws secured (Figures 76-6, *G*, and 76-7, *G*), the surgical sites should be thoroughly irrigated with sterile saline. Proper closure of the flap over the implant(s) is essential. One of the most important aspects of flap management is achieving good primary closure of the flap that is tension free. This is achieved by incising the periosteum (innermost layer of full-thickness flap), which is nonelastic. Once the periosteum is released, the flap becomes very elastic and is able to be stretched over the implant(s) without tension. One suturing technique that consistently provides the desired result is a combination of alternating horizontal mattress and interrupted sutures (Figure 76-7, *H*). Horizontal mattress sutures evert the wound edges and approximate the inner, connective tissue surfaces of the flap to facilitate wound healing. Interrupted sutures help to bring the wound edges together, counterbalancing the eversion caused by the horizontal mattress sutures.

The clinician should choose an appropriate suture for the given patient and procedure. For patient management, it is sometimes simpler to use a resorbable suture that does not require removal during the postoperative visit (e.g., 4.0 chromic gut suture). However, when moderate to severe postoperative swelling is anticipated, a nonresorbable suture is recommended to maintain a longer closure period (e.g., 4-0 monofilament suture). These sutures require removal at a postoperative visit.

Postoperative Care

Simple implant surgery in a healthy patient usually does not require antibiotic therapy. However, patients can be premedicated with antibiotics (e.g., amoxicillin, 500 mg tid) starting 1 hour before the surgery and continuing for 1 week postoperatively if the surgery is extensive, if it requires bone augmentation, or if the patient is medically compromised. Postoperative swelling is likely. As a preventive measure, patients should apply an ice pack to the area intermittently for 20 minutes (on and off) over the first 24 to 48 hours. Chlorhexidine gluconate oral rinses can also be prescribed to facilitate plaque control, especially in the days after surgery when oral hygiene is typically poorer. Adequate pain medication should be prescribed (e.g., ibuprofen, 600-800 mg tid).

Patients should be instructed to maintain a relatively soft diet for the first few days and then gradually return to a normal diet. If possible, patients should also refrain from tobacco and alcohol use for 1 to 2 weeks postoperatively. Provisional restorations, whether fixed or removable, should be checked and adjusted so that impingement on the surgical area is avoided.

Second-Stage Exposure Surgery

For implants placed using a two-stage "submerged" protocol, a second-stage exposure surgery is necessary after the prescribed healing period. Box 76-3 lists the objectives for second-stage, implant exposure surgery. Thin soft tissue with an adequate amount of keratinized attached gingiva, along with good oral hygiene, ensures healthier periimplant soft tissues and better clinical results. The need for keratinized tissue is somewhat controversial, depending on the type of implant prosthesis and location of the implant. However, one long-term study indicated that, at least in the posterior mandible and in partially edentulous patients, the presence of keratinized tissue is strongly correlated with soft and hard tissue health.[3]

BOX 76-3

Objectives of Second-Stage Implant Surgery

1. To expose the submerged implant without damaging the surrounding bone.
2. To control the thickness of the soft tissue surrounding the implant.
3. To preserve or create attached keratinized tissue around the implant.
4. To facilitate oral hygiene.
5. To ensure proper abutment seating.

Simple Circular "Punch" Incision. In areas with sufficient zones of keratinized tissue, the gingiva covering the head of the implant can be exposed with a circular or "punch" incision (Figure 76-9). Alternatively, a crestal incision through the middle of the keratinized tissue and full-thickness flap reflection can be used to expose implants.

Partial-Thickness Repositioned Flap. If inadequate keratinized tissue is available, a partial-thickness flap technique can be used to fulfill the objective of the second-stage surgery while increasing the width of keratinized tissue. The initial incision is made with approximately 2 mm of keratinized tissue. Vertical incisions are used on both the mesial and the distal end of the flap (Figure 76-10, *A* and *B*).

Clinical note: In esthetic anterior sites, the flap design should preserve the adjacent papilla.

A partial-thickness flap is then raised in such a manner that a relatively firm periosteum remains. The flap, containing a narrow band of keratinized tissue, is then repositioned to the facial side of the emerging head of the implant and sutured to the periosteum with a fine needle and suture (e.g., 5.0 gut suture) (Figure 76-11). If the initial amount of keratinized tissue is less than 2 mm, the flap may be started from the lingual part of the ridge, elevating a split-thickness flap and repositioning the keratinized band to the facial aspect. When a

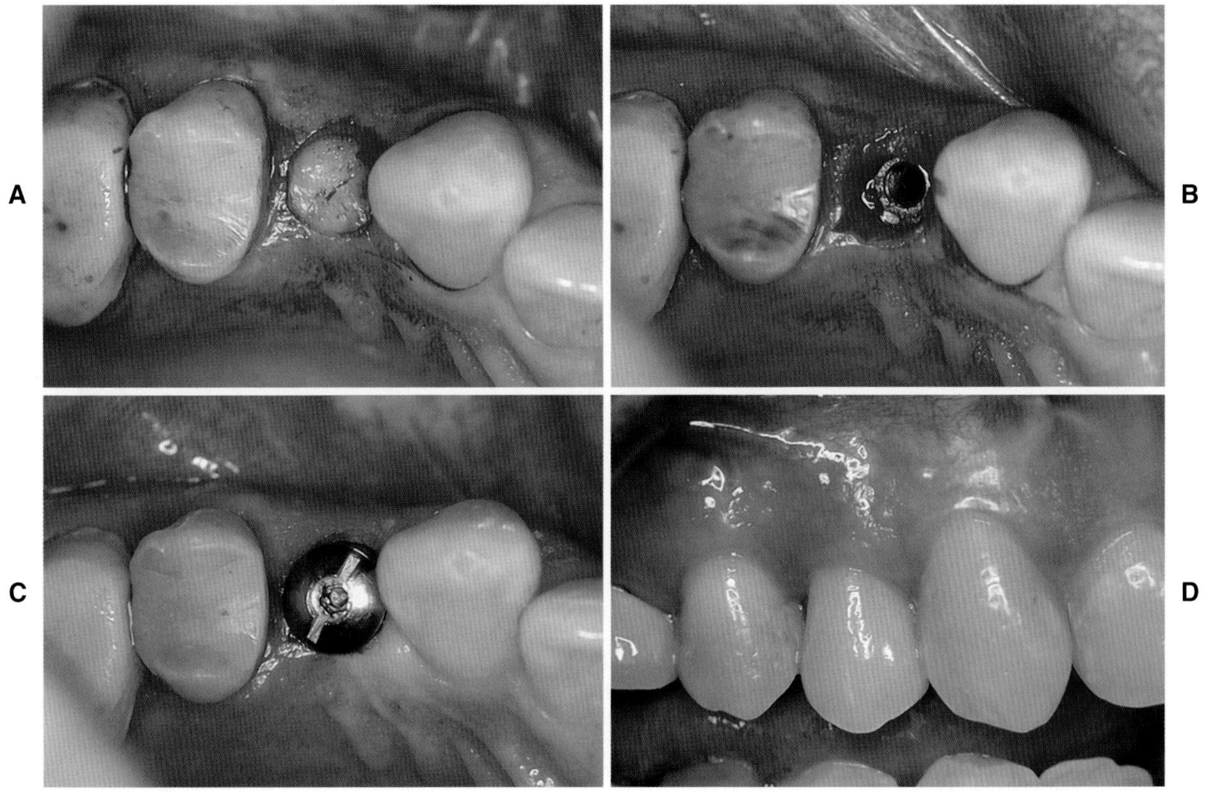

Figure 76-9 **A,** Simple circular "punch" incision used to expose implant when sufficient keratinized tissue is present around the implant(s). **B,** Implant exposed. **C,** Healing abutment attached. **D,** Final restoration in place, achieving an esthetic result with a good zone of keratinized tissue.

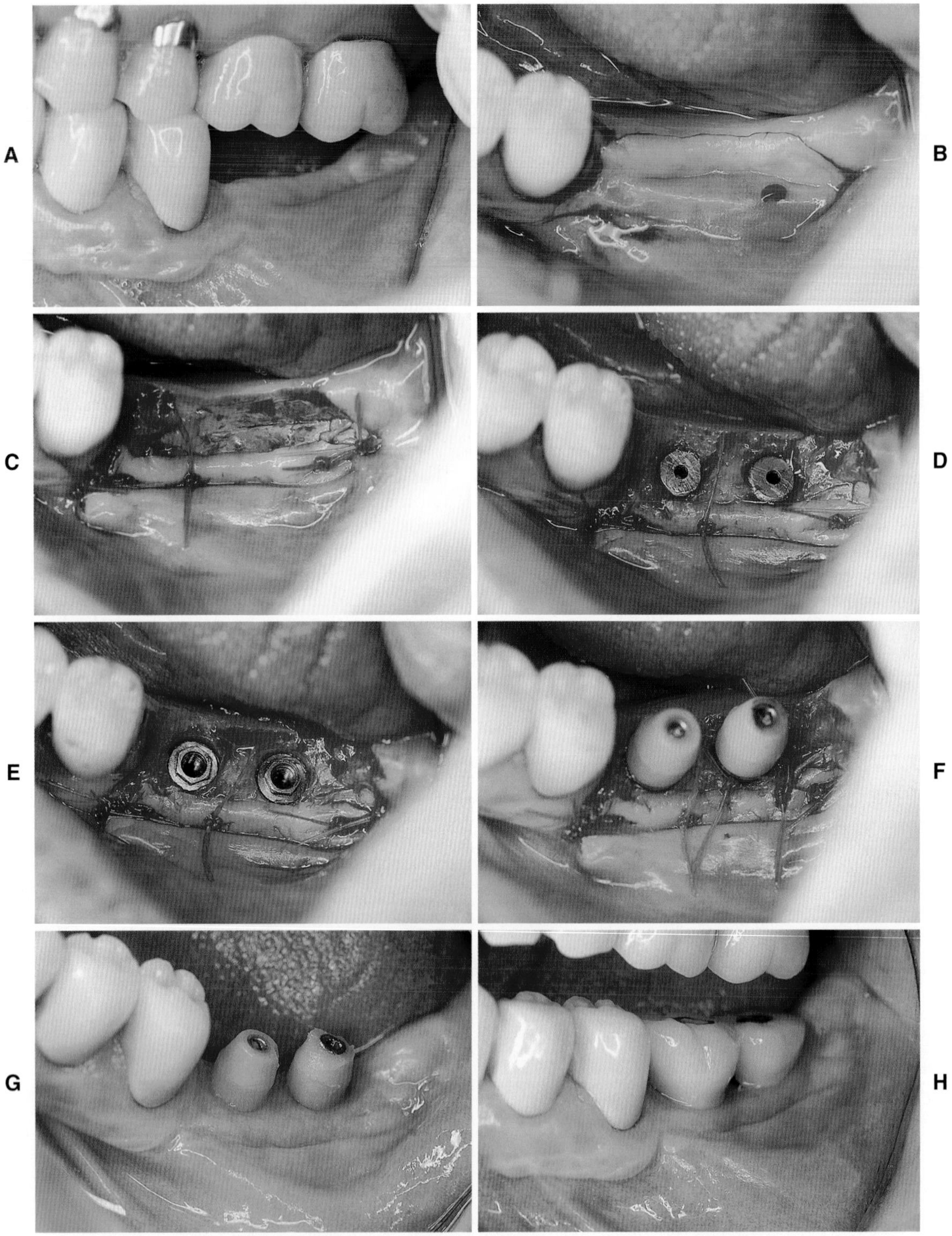

Figure 76-10 Second-stage surgery. **A,** Two endosseous implants were placed 4 months previously and are ready to be exposed. Note the narrow band of keratinized tissue. **B,** Two vertical incisions are connected by crestal incision. If facial keratinized tissue is insufficient, it is necessary to locate the crestal incision more lingually so that there is at least 2 to 3 mm of keratinized band. **C,** Buccal partial-thickness flap is sutured to the periosteum apical to the emerging implants. **D,** Gingival tissue coronal to the cover screws is excised using the gingivectomy technique. **E,** Cover screws are removed, and heads of the implants are cleared. **F,** Abutments are placed. Visual inspection ensures intimate contact between the abutments and the implants. **G,** Healing at 2 to 3 weeks after second-stage surgery. **H,** Four months after the final restoration. Note the healthy band of keratinized attached gingiva around the implants.

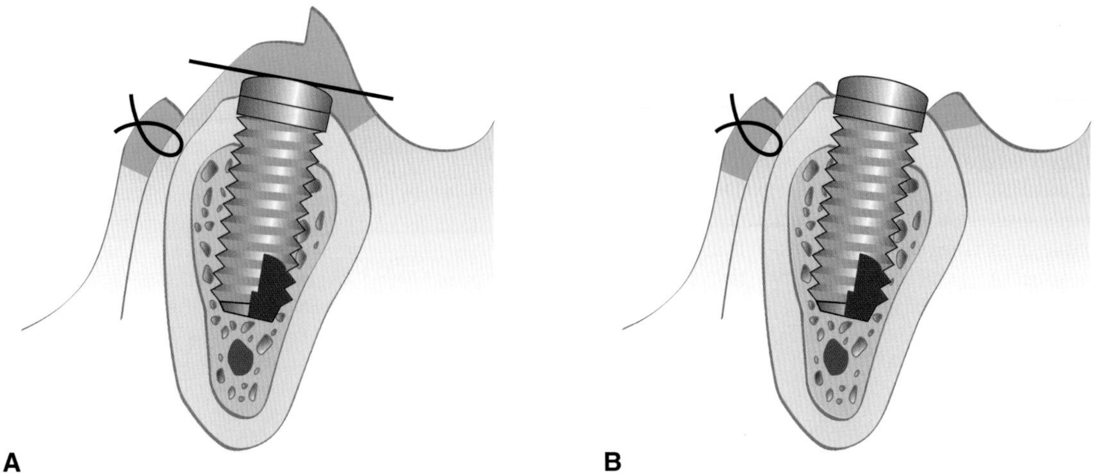

Figure 76-11 **A,** Partial-thickness flap is apically sutured to the periosteum, and excess connective tissue coronal to the cover screw is excised by gingivectomy. **B,** Sharp blade is used to eliminate all tissue coronal to the cover screw. (Care should be taken to avoid removing keratinized tissue from the lingual aspect of the implant.)

partial-thickness flap is apically displaced and sutured to the periosteum without exposing the alveolar bone, keratinized tissue will grow over the periosteum (i.e., connective tissue), and an increased zone of attached keratinized tissue will be created around the implants (Figure 76-10, *C*).

After the flap is repositioned and secured with periosteal sutures, the excess tissue coronal to the cover screw is excised, usually with a surgical blade (Figure 76-11, *B*). However, if removal of this tissue would jeopardize the amount of remaining keratinized tissue around the lingual aspect of the implant(s), a similar partial-thickness flap can be elevated and repositioned on the lingual side as well.

When the excess tissue over the cover screw is removed or displaced, the outline of the cover screw is visible. A sharp blade is used to eliminate all tissues coronal to the cover screw (Figure 76-10, *D*). The cover screw is then removed, the head of the implant is thoroughly cleaned of any soft or hard tissue overgrowth, and the healing abutments or standard abutments are placed on the implant (Figure 76-10, *E* and *F*). The fit of the implants to the healing abutments can often be visually evaluated. However, if it is not possible to visualize clearly the intimate connection between the implant and the abutment, an intraoral periapical x-ray film should be taken to confirm complete seating.

Postoperative Care. Once the implant is exposed, it is important to remind the patient of the need for good oral hygiene around the implant. A chlorhexidine rinse can be used to enhance oral hygiene for the initial 2 weeks while the tissues are healing. Any direct pressure to the soft tissue from dentures can delay healing. Fabrication of the suprastructure can begin in about 2 to 4 weeks. Figure 76-10, *G* and *H,* shows the postoperative results in a clinical case after 2 to 3 weeks and 4 months, respectively.

ONE-STAGE "NON-SUBMERGED" IMPLANT PLACEMENT

In the one-stage implant surgical approach, a second intervention is not needed because the implant is left exposed after the first surgery. Again, the implants are left unloaded and undisturbed for a period similar to that for the implants placed in the two-stage approach (2-4 months in mandible, 4-6 months in maxilla).

In the two-stage surgical approach, the implant is placed flush with the bone crest, and the soft tissue covering is purposely kept thick to minimize the risk of premature exposure of the cover screws. In the one-stage surgical approach, the implant or the healing abutment protrudes about 2 to 3 mm from the bone crest, and the flaps are adapted around the implant/abutment. In posterior areas of the mouth, the flap is thinned and sometimes sutured apically to periosteum to increase the zone of keratinized attached gingiva around the implant.

Flap Design, Incisions, and Elevation

The flap design for the one-stage surgical approach is always a crestal incision bisecting the existing keratinized tissue. Vertical incisions may be needed at one or both ends. Facial and lingual flaps in posterior areas should be carefully thinned before total reflection to minimize the soft tissue thickness. The soft tissue is not thinned in anterior or other esthetic areas of the mouth to prevent the metal collar from showing. Full-thickness flaps are elevated facially and lingually.

Implant Site Preparation

The implant site preparation for the one-stage approach is identical in principle to the two-stage implant surgical approach. The primary difference is that the implant or the healing abutment extension of the implant is placed in such way that the head of the implant protrudes about 2 to 3 mm from the bone crest.

Flap Closure and Suturing

The keratinized edges of the flap are sutured with single interrupted sutures around the implant. Depending on the clinician's preference, the wound may be sutured with resorbable or nonresorbable sutures. When keratinized tissue is abundant, scalloping around the implant(s) provides better flap adaptation.

Postoperative Care

The postoperative care for one-stage surgical approach is similar to that for the two-stage surgical approach except that the cover screw or healing abutment is exposed to the oral cavity. Patients are advised to avoid chewing in the area of the implant(s). Prosthetic appliances should not be used if direct chewing forces can be transmitted to the implant, particularly in the early healing period (first 4-8 weeks). Soft lining of denture is mandatory when a one stage, nonsubmerged surgical approach to implant placement is used.

CONCLUSION

It is essential to understand and follow basic guidelines to achieve osseointegration predictably. Fundamental protocols must be followed for implant placement (stage one) and implant exposure surgery (stage two). Additionally, specific protocols exist for a single-stage implant placement. These fundamentals apply to all implant systems.

REFERENCES

1. Adell R, Lekholm U, Rockler B, et al: A 15-year study of osseointegrated implants in the treatment of the edentulous jaw, *Int J Oral Surg* 10:387, 1981.
2. Adell R, Eriksson B, Lekholm U, et al: A long-term follow-up study of osseointegrated implants in the treatment of totally edentulous jaws, *Int J Oral Maxillofac Implants* 5:347, 1990.
3. Block MS, Kent JN: Factors associated with soft and hard tissue compromise of endosseous implants, *J Oral Maxillofac Implants* 48:1153, 1990.
4. Brånemark PI, Zarb GA, Albrektsson T: *Tissue-integrated prostheses,* Chicago, 1985, Quintessence.
5. Brånemark PI, Zarb G, Albrektsson T: Tissue-integrated prosthesis. In *Osseointegration in clinical dentistry,* Chicago, 1987, Quintessence.
6. Brånemark PI, Breine U, Adell R, et al: Intraosseous anchorage of dental prostheses. I. Experimental studies, *Scand J Plast Reconstr Surg* 3:81, 1969.
7. Brunski JB: Biomechanics of oral implants: future research directions, *J Dent Educ* 52:775, 1988.
8. Buser D, Weber HP, Bragger U: The treatment of partially edentulous patients with ITI hollow-screw implants: presurgical evaluation and surgical procedures, *Int J Oral Maxillofac Implants* 5:165, 1990.
9. Buser D, Nydegger T, Hirt HP, et al: Removal torque values of titanium implants in the maxilla of miniature pigs, *Int J Oral Maxillofac Implants* 13:611, 1998.
10. Davies JE: Understanding peri-implant endosseous healing, *J Dent Educ* 67:932, 2003.
11. Ericsson J, Johansson CB, Bystedt H, et al: A histomorphometric evaluation of bone-to-implant contact on machine-prepared and roughened titanium dental implants: a pilot study in dog, *Clin Oral Implant Res* 5:202, 1994.
12. Jaffin RA, Berman CI: The excessive loss of Brånemark implants in type IV bone: a 5-year analysis, *J Periodontol* 62:2 1991.
13. Klokkevold P, Nishimura T, Adachi M, et al: Osseointegration enhanced by chemical etching of the titanium surface, *Clin Oral Implant Res* 8:442, 1997.
14. Scharf DR, Tarnow DP: The effect of crestal versus mucobuccal incisions on the success rate of implant osseointegration, *Int J Oral Maxillofac Implants* 8:187, 1993.
15. Schroeder A, van der Zypen E, Stich H, et al: The reactions of bone, connective tissue, and epithelium to endosteal implants with titanium-sprayed surfaces, *J Maxillofac Surg* 9:15, 1981.
16. Sullivan DY, Sherwood RL, Porter SS: Long-term performance of Osseotite implants: a 6-year clinical follow-up, *Compend Contin Educ Dent* 22:326, 2001.
17. Watanabe F, Tawada Y, Komatsu S, et al: Heat distribution in bone during preparation of implant sites: heat analysis by real-time thermography, *Int J Oral Maxillofac Implants* 7:213, 1992.

Localized Bone Augmentation and Implant Site Development

Perry R. Klokkevold

77

CHAPTER

CHAPTER OUTLINE

The use of dental implants in the partially and fully edentulous patient with deficient jawbones creates a new demand for bone reconstruction before or during implant therapy, especially when natural esthetics is required. The most critical aspect of creating an implant restoration is the surgical placement of the implant in a "prosthetically driven" position to restore the natural position and to emulate the natural emergence of a tooth from the soft tissues. Implants placed without regard for prosthetic position often result in dental restorations that are functionally and esthetically compromised, and patients are left with a less-than-optimal reconstruction.

Periodontal bone loss, tooth extraction, and long-term use of removable appliances typically result in advanced alveolar bone loss that prevents the placement of implants in an optimal prosthetic position. Fortunately, continuous innovations in surgical techniques and advances in the biologic understanding of bone-regenerative techniques have led to advanced implant procedures and an increased predictability to reconstruct alveolar ridge defects.[26,38]

Conventional implant surgery, as described in Chapter 76, is based on adequate bone volume and quality in the desired implant location. The time-tested protocol allows for adequate remodeling and maturation of bone, with healing periods of 4 months and 6 months for the mandible and maxilla, respectively. Recent implant procedures often challenge these original conventions by placing implants in areas with inadequate bone volume, simultaneously augmenting bone and restoring or loading implants after shorter healing periods. This chapter presents an overview of implant surgical procedures currently used to prevent or overcome anatomic deficiencies for the optimal placement of dental implants.

GUIDED BONE REGENERATION

Much of what can be achieved with implant surgery and bone augmentation procedures is directly related to the achievements and understanding of guided bone regeneration. Historically, augmentation or "regeneration" of alveolar bone lost as a result of tooth extraction, resorption, or trauma presented a significant challenge for clinicians. Allowed to heal without the intervention of regenerative procedures, extraction site defects (especially those lacking a self-supporting bone structure) healed with fibrous connective tissue or scar formation and often did not fill with bone. The surrounding soft tissues collapsed, leaving an anatomic deficiency with respect to the natural tooth position. If a removable prosthetic appliance was used, the alveolar ridge resorbed even more.

Periodontal studies during the last several decades have led to new techniques and a new treatment approach referred to as *guided tissue regeneration* (GTR). Briefly, this concept is based on the principle that specific cells contribute to the formation of specific tissues. Exclusion of the faster-growing epithelium and connective tissue from a periodontal wound for 6 to 8 weeks allows the slower-growing tissues to occupy the space adjacent to the tooth. Osteoblasts, cementoblasts, and periodontal ligament cells are then afforded the opportunity to regenerate a new periodontal attachment (new bone and new connective tissue fibers inserted into newly formed cementum) on the previously diseased root surface. Chapter 67 discusses the concepts of GTR as related to periodontal regeneration.

The same basic principle of GTR has been applied to alveolar bone defects to regenerate new bone.[13] Using a canine model, Schenk et al.[47] demonstrated with histology that bone regeneration in membrane-protected defects healed in a sequence of steps that simulated bone formation after tooth extraction. They found that after blood clot formation, bone regeneration was initiated by the formation of woven bone initially along new blood vasculature at the periphery of the defect. The new vascular supply emanated from surgically created perforations in the cortical bone. The woven bone was subsequently replaced by lamellar bone, which resulted in mature bone anatomy. Ultimately, bone remodeling occurred with new, secondary osteons being formed. This concept employed the same principles of specific tissue exclusion but was not associated with teeth. Thus the term applied to this technique was *guided bone regeneration* (GBR). Because the objective of GBR is to regenerate a single tissue, namely bone, it is theoretically easier to accomplish than GTR, which strives to regenerate multiple tissues in a complex relationship.

Interestingly, long before the current concepts of GBR were introduced, Murray and Roschlau[40] demonstrated that when a cavity with a source of osteoblasts and a blood supply was isolated from adjacent soft tissues, it could fill with bone, whereas if the space were not protected, it would fill with fibrous connective tissue. In addition to this observation, they suggested that a bone graft placed in the space might interfere with bone formation because the graft would need to be resorbed before bone could occupy the space.

Bone is a unique tissue that has the capacity to regenerate itself completely. Because of its rigid calcified structure, however, bone has specific requirements that must be respected to achieve regeneration. Because the calcified structure of bone is not conducive to perfusion, new bone formation is critically dependent on establishing an adequate blood supply through new vasculature while maintaining rigid fixation or stabilization for bone formation. Any movement of the segments of bone relative to one another (even micromotion) during healing results in disruption of the blood supply and a change in the type of tissue formed in the site from bone to fibrous connective tissue. Table 77-1 lists the biologic requirements for bone regeneration along with the associated component of GBR surgical procedures needed to accomplish bone regeneration.

TABLE 77-1

Biologic Requirements for Bone Regeneration

Requirement	Surgical Procedure
Blood supply	Cortical perforations
Stabilization	Fixation screws, membrane tacks
Osteoblasts	Autogenous bone (graft or recipient site)
Confined space	Barrier membrane
Space maintenance	Tenting screws, bone graft materials
Wound coverage	Flap management, tension-free suturing

Barrier Membranes

Barrier membranes are biologically inert materials that serve to protect the blood clot and prevent soft tissue cells (epithelium and connective tissue) from migrating into the bone defect, allowing osteogenic cells to be established. Membranes have been manufactured from biocompatible materials that are both nonresorbable and resorbable. The ideal properties of a barrier membrane are (1) biocompatibility, (2) space maintenance, (3) cell occlusiveness, (4) good handling properties, and (5) resorbability. Advantages and disadvantages of the resorbable versus nonresorbable membranes are described here.

Nonresorbable Barrier Membranes

Various nonresorbable materials have been used as barrier membranes, including latex and Teflon. Teflon, an expanded polytetrafluoroethylene membrane (ePTFE, Gore-Tex Periodontal and Bone Regenerative Membranes, Gore and Associates, Flagstaff, Ariz), has been used extensively as a barrier membrane in both GTR and GBR procedures. A variety of shapes and sizes have been designed to custom-fit around teeth and osseous defects. These barrier membranes are nonresorbable and thus require a subsequent surgical procedure to remove them. The advantage of a nonresorbable barrier membrane is its ability to maintain separation of tissues over an extended time. Unless the barrier is exposed, it can remain in place for several months to years. Typically, GBR membranes are removed after 6 to 12 months.

The disadvantage of a nonresorbable barrier membrane is that if it becomes exposed, it will not heal spontaneously. Exposed membranes become contaminated with oral bacteria, which may lead to infection of the site and result in bone loss. Therefore, exposed membranes must be removed. Early removal may also result in less bone regeneration.

Space can be maintained under a barrier membrane with bone graft material or tenting screws, thereby facilitating the regeneration of increased bone volume.

Stiffer or titanium-reinforced (TR) membranes (Gore and Associates) with space-maintaining capabilities have been demonstrated to regenerate bone without bone grafts or tenting apparatus.[37,47] Stiffer membranes are able to promote significant amounts of new bone and maintain sufficient space without the addition of supportive devices. Ridge augmentation can be enhanced with a titanium-reinforced membrane in conjunction with implant placement in localized bone defects.[24]

Resorbable Barrier Membranes

The use of resorbable membranes continues to attract widespread interest. Copolymers of polylactide and polyglycolide (PLA/PGA) or collagen have been used to construct biodegradable membranes. The primary advantage of a resorbable membrane is the elimination of surgical reentry for membrane removal. In the case of subsequent implant placement procedure (or exposure surgery), this may not be a significant advantage.

A possible disadvantage is that most resorbable membranes degrade before bone formation is completed, and the degradation process is associated with varying degrees of inflammation.[61] Recent developments include cross-linking of collagen to increase resistance to biodegradation and thus increase longevity of the barrier function.[18] Fortunately, the mild inflammatory reaction caused by bioresorbable membranes does not seem to interfere with osteogenesis. Another disadvantage is that resorbable membranes are quite pliable. The lack in stiffness results in a collapse of the membrane into the defect area.[46] Thus, resorbable membranes are best suited for situations that allow the graft material or hardware (tenting screws, plates) or the adjacent alveolar bone to maintain the desired dimensions.

Human histology demonstrating the effectiveness of resorbable membranes is lacking, and further clinical research is needed before conclusions can be made about their use in bone regeneration. At present, it can be stated that biodegradable membranes have the potential to support bone formation if they are supported by bone graft material to resist collapse and if they are long-lasting enough to maintain their barrier function for extended periods in small to moderate bone defects.[28,29]

Bone Graft Materials

Unlike other tissues, as stated earlier, bone has the unique capacity to regenerate itself completely. The major limiting factor is maintenance of space for bone formation. Bone graft materials have been used to facilitate bone formation within a given space by occupying that space and allowing the subsequent bone growth (and graft replacement) to take place. The biologic mechanisms that support the use of bone graft materials are osteoconduction, osteoinduction, and osteogenesis.

Osteoconduction is the formation of bone by osteoblasts from the margins of the defect on the bone graft material. Materials that are osteoconductive serve as a scaffold for bone growth. They neither inhibit nor induce bone formation. They simply allow the normal formation of bone by osteoblasts into the grafted defect along the surface of the graft material. Osteoconductive bone graft materials facilitate bone formation by bridging the gap between the existing bone and a distant location that otherwise would not be occupied by bone.

TABLE 77-2

Biologic Properties of Various Bone Graft Materials

Source	Osteoconductive	Osteoinductive	Osteogenic
Alloplast	Yes	No	No
Xenograft	Yes	No	No
Allograft	Yes	Yes/No	No
Autograft	Yes	Yes	Yes

Osteoinduction involves new bone formation through stimulation of osteoprogenitors from the defect (or from the vasculature) to differentiate into osteoblasts and begin forming new bone. This induction of the bone-forming process by cells that would otherwise remain inactive occurs through cell mediators that "turn on" these bone-forming cells. The most widely studied of these mediators is the family of bone morphogenic proteins (BMPs). Chapter 78 discusses BMP use in bone augmentation.

Osteogenesis occurs when living osteoblasts are part of the bone graft, as in autogenous bone transplantation. Given an adequate blood supply and cellular viability, these transplanted osteoblasts form new centers of ossification within the graft. Thus, in addition to the bone formation from osteoblasts that already exist in the defect, osteoblasts added as part of the bone graft also form ossification centers and contribute to the total capacity for bone formation.

Numerous bone graft materials have been used to aid in the reconstruction of bone defects. These range from allografts (derived from the same species) to xenografts (derived from a different species) and alloplast or synthetic graft materials. At a minimum, bone graft materials should be *osteoconductive*. Bone graft materials that are *osteoinductive* are believed to be more advantageous than those that are only osteoconductive. Table 77-2 lists the properties of different classes of bone graft materials.

Decalcified, freeze-dried bone allograft (DFDBA) is thought to have osteoinductive effects because it retains some of the original BMPs within the donor tissue matrix.[58] In contrast to this view, more recent reports have suggested that bone augmentation with DFDBA is not osteoinductive because it does not contain the BMPs necessary to induce bone formation.[5,8] Schwartz et al.[48] reported that variations in the amount of bone formation induced by DFDBA may be related to the source and processing of the bone. In addition to processing variations, it has been demonstrated that young donor bone results in significantly greater quantities of BMPs retained in the bone allograft matrix compared with older donor bone.[49] Therefore the source of donor bone can greatly influence its osteoinductive capacity.

Bone graft materials help maintain space under a barrier membrane to facilitate the formation of bone within a confined space. Perhaps a more important requirement of bone graft materials is that they should facilitate the ingrowth of neovascularization and migration of osteoprogenitors. Because the size of the bone graft particles determines the resultant space available (between particles) for osseous formation, particle size has been carefully selected according to this concept. The typical size of bone graft particles ranges from 100 to 1000 µm, which is conducive to the ingrowth of bone. Bone forms in cones called *osteons* with a central blood supply. The dimension of these cones (100-µm radius) is determined by the distance that the central vasculature can supply nutrients to cells.

Harvesting Autogenous Bone

Compared with other bone graft materials, autogenous bone is thought to be the best bone graft because it is osteoinductive and osteogenic in addition to being osteoconductive. Furthermore, barring contamination, there is no risk of rejection or adverse reaction to the graft material when it is *autogenous* (harvested from same individual). Intraoral sources of autogenous bone include edentulous spaces, maxillary tuberosity, mandibular ramus, mandibular symphysis, and extraction sites. Bone from a recent extraction site (within 6-12 weeks) may have the advantage of increased osteogenic activity compared with other sites, which are more static and undergoing little or no osteogenesis. The maxillary tuberosity provides a more cellular source of autogenous bone compared with other sites. However, the trabecular nature of this site provides a lesser quantity of mineralized matrix, and the resultant total volume of bone available for grafting is often inadequate. For greater amounts of bone, it is more desirable to harvest bone from the mandibular ramus or symphysis. This bone, which is typically more cortical, can be harvested and used as a block graft or can be ground or shaved into small fragments and used as a particulate graft.

Although the mandibular ramus and symphysis offer good sources of bone for grafting, clinicians are sometimes reluctant to harvest bone from these sites because of an increased risk of morbidity from the surgical procedure. Risks of surgery in the mandibular symphysis region include postoperative bleeding, bruising, wound dehiscence, damage to lower incisors, disfigurement, and injury to nerves. Nerve injury may be the most significant concern because it can be a long-term, annoying alteration in sensation of the lower lip, chin, anterior teeth, and gingiva for the patient. A more serious risk is the alteration of facial appearance, particularly when the facial muscles are completely elevated from the bone beyond the inferior border of the mandible. A condition referred to as "witch's chin" can occur when the facial muscles and overlying skin of the chin fall, causing a disfiguring sag of facial tissues after surgery.

Hunt and Jovanovic[21] presented a retrospective analysis of 48 chin graft–harvesting procedures. They emphasized maintaining a 5-mm margin of safety between graft harvest sites and the lower incisors, the inferior border of the chin, and the mental foramen. Using both trephine and custom-block harvesting techniques, they reported minimal postoperative complications. In the 48 procedures, postoperative sequelae included bruising of lower face (48/48), bruising of upper neck (6/48), and paresthesia of lower lip and incisors (6/48). No patients experienced facial disfigurement or muscle prolapse (chin droop). Three of the six patients with paresthesia experienced transient symptoms and recovered completely within 2 months, whereas symptoms persisted longer than 6 months in the other three patients. Not surprisingly, the larger harvest defects (trephined six-ring sites) resulted in a higher incidence of paresthesia, which was longer lasting than that of the smaller defects (trephined four-ring sites). Harvesting bone in a custom-shaped "block" did not result in paresthesia, presumably because these harvest sites were smaller than the four-ring and six-ring trephine-harvested sites.

Observation of the following basic principles can minimize the risk of postoperative morbidity:

1. Carefully evaluate the harvest site for potential risks. A critical radiographic evaluation before surgery can identify individuals with inferior alveolar nerve branches that extend anterior beyond the mental foramen.
2. Use extreme care in making incisions laterally toward the mental nerve, and dissect the area with blunt instruments to locate the foramen.
3. Do not elevate and reflect muscle attachments beyond the inferior border of the mandible.
4. Limit bone cuts to an area at least 5 mm away from the tooth apices, the inferior border of the mandible, and the mental foramen. Do not extend cuts or harvest bone deeper than 6 mm, and do not include both labial and lingual cortical plates.
5. Suture the wound in layers (muscle and overlying mucosa separately) to prevent postoperative wound separation.

When harvesting autogenous bone, regardless of site or method used, it is important to use techniques that prevent overheating and maintain viability of the bone cells. Exceeding 47° C (116.6° F) is known to cause bone necrosis.[16] Thus, use of drills, trephines, or saws to cut bone should always be done with profuse irrigation to keep instruments and bone cooled.

LOCALIZED RIDGE AUGMENTATION

Patients often present for implant planning after tooth loss and alveolar ridge resorption. In these cases the clinician is obligated to perform advanced augmentation procedures to reconstruct lost bone and place implants in a prosthetically driven position.

Surgical reconstructive procedures for the preparation and placement of dental implants have become more numerous and complex. Depending on the size and morphology of the defect, various augmentation procedures can be used. These procedures have been categorized according to the deficient dimension: horizontal or vertical. Methods used to augment horizontal as well as vertical bone deficiencies include particulate bone grafts and monocortical block grafts. Barrier membranes can be used with bone grafts to reconstruct all types of alveolar bone defects. Chapter 78 discusses procedures used to achieve vertical augmentation.

All the proven principles of GBR and flap management must be followed to achieve good results. These include generating a blood supply; maintaining a stable, protected space for bone growth; and achieving tension-free flap closure.

Flap Management for Ridge Augmentation

Soft tissue management is a critical aspect of bone augmentation procedures. Incisions, reflection, and manipulation should be designed to optimize blood supply and wound closure. The design and management of mucoperiosteal flaps must consider the increased dimensions of the ridge after augmentation as well as esthetics and approximation of the wound margins. The surgical procedure needs to be executed with utmost care to preserve the maximum vascularity to the flap and to minimize tissue injury.[1]

Several flap techniques maintain a "submerged" position of bone grafts and barrier membranes during the entire healing process, including a remote or displaced incision.[9,25] The advantage of a remote incision is that the wound opening is positioned away from the graft. A conventional crestal incision can be used, even in large supracrestal defects, as long as a periosteal releasing incision and coronal advancement of the flap achieve the tension-free closure.[31] Most reports suggest removing sutures approximately 10 to 14 days after surgery. It is also suggested that no prosthesis be inserted for 2 to 3 weeks after surgery, to avoid pressure over the wound during the early healing period.

General concepts for flap management associated with ridge augmentation include the following:

1. Whenever possible, it is desirable to make incisions remote relative to the placement of barrier membranes (e.g., vertical releasing incisions at least one tooth away from the site to be grafted). In the anterior maxilla, keeping vertical incisions remote is also an esthetic advantage.
2. Full mucoperiosteal flap elevation at least 5 mm beyond the edge of the bone defect is desirable.
3. The use of vertical incisions, although often required for surgical access, should be minimized whenever possible.
4. Use of a periosteal releasing incision to give the flap elasticity and permit tension-free suturing is essential. This permits complete closure without stress on the wound margins.
5. Avoid postoperative trauma to the surgical site (i.e., no removable appliance should be inserted over the wound for 2 weeks or more).
6. Wound closure should incorporate a combination of mattress sutures to approximate connective tissues and interrupted sutures to adapt wound edges.

Horizontal Bone Augmentation

A deficiency in the horizontal dimension of bone may be minimal, such as a dehiscence or fenestration of an implant surface, or it may be more significant, such that the implant would have more than one axial surface exposed while having some bone along the entire vertical length. Dehiscence defects can usually be managed during implant placement because most of the implant is covered and stabilized by native bone. If the horizontal deficiency is large and the implant placement would result in significant exposure (i.e., implant body is significantly outside the alveolar bone), it may be better to reconstruct the bone before implant placement (staged implant placement).

Although reconstruction of deficient ridges with bone grafts alone (i.e., without barrier membrane) has proved to be effective, variable resorption of the grafted bone has been reported. Preliminary results in a 1- to 3-year study using autografts harvested from the maxillary tuberosity showed an increased ridge width, but resorption of 50% of the graft volume was also noted.[55]

Buser et al.[9] investigated the lateral ridge augmentation procedure using an autograft from the retromolar or symphysis area covered by a membrane in 40 consecutively treated patients and noted no clinical signs of resorption of the block graft. The researchers emphasized a remote incision technique, perforation of the cortex, stable placement of corticocancellous autografts, precise adaptation and stabilization (with miniscrews) of the ePTFE membranes, and a tension-free primary soft tissue closure. After 7 to 13 months, the sites were reopened for membrane removal and implant placement. Of the 40 patients, 38 exhibited excellent ridge augmentation, with two sites showing some soft tissue encapsulation of the grafted bone.

Nevins and Mellonig[42] and Doblin et al.[14] reported case results that the use of freeze-dried bone allografts with membranes increased the amount of new bone, even in the presence of a membrane exposure. The biopsies showed viable bone cells and visible osteocytes in lacunae, and a 9-month specimen showed no remaining allograft material. On the other hand, there are some contradictory results using DFDBA and membrane combinations.[2,7,8]

Particulate Bone Graft

Advantages of particulate bone grafts (or bone chips) are that the smaller pieces of bone demonstrate more rapid ingrowth of blood vessels (revascularization), larger osteoconduction surface, more exposure of osteoinductive growth factors, and easier biologic remodeling compared with a bone block. For reconstruction of large defects, however, particulate grafts often lack a rigid, supportive structure and are much more easily displaced than block grafts.

Autologous particulated bone grafts can be harvested from any edentulous jaw site, either in smaller particle sizes or in larger block size. If the bone has been harvested in block size, a bone mill is necessary to "particulate" the bone and prepare it for transplantation into the bone defect.

Particulate grafts are indicated (1) in defects with multiple osseous walls that will contain the graft or (2) in dehiscence or fenestration defects when implants are placed during the bone augmentation procedure. If a bone defect does not have sufficient osseous walls to contain the graft and if an implant is placed simultaneously, a barrier membrane is secured along the periphery with tacks or screws. This bone graft–implant–barrier membrane combination becomes an environment that is stable and supports bone formation.

Monocortical Block Graft

Horizontal alveolar deficiencies can easily be reconstructed with a monocortical block bone graft. The technique uses a cortical block of bone harvested from a remote site and used to increase the width of bone. The block graft taken from an intraoral (e.g., mandibular symphysis or ramus) or extraoral (e.g., iliac crest or tibia) site is fixated to the prepared recipient site with screws. The graft can be separated from overlying soft tissues with a barrier membrane or simply covered with the mucoperiosteal flap. Fixation hardware (screws and plates) should be removed after an adequate period of healing (approximately 6 months). The disadvantage of this technique is the biologic limitation of revascularizing large bone blocks. It therefore is crucial to have sufficient osteogenic cells in the residual surface of the surrounding bone and to limit this technique to horizontal augmentation and only minimal vertical defects.

Figure 77-1 shows the use of a monocortical block graft to reconstruct a horizontal deficiency in the posterior right mandible. The patient presented with a loss of the buccal cortical plate of bone after a traumatic extraction of endodontically treated tooth #29. The surgical extraction also resulted in a nonrestorable cut into the mesial root of tooth #30. Recommended treatment included extraction of tooth #30 with monocortical block graft to reconstruct the buccal defect of site #29. This case is discussed next.

Procedure. After local anesthesia, an incision was made in keratinized tissue along the crest and around the molar tooth (#30) with a vertical releasing incision mesial to the first bicuspid (#28). A full-thickness flap was elevated to expose the alveolar bone (Figure 77-1, *D*). All soft tissues were thoroughly removed from the recipient site before bone grafting. After simple forceps delivery of tooth #30, the defect to be grafted was measured to determine the size of block graft to harvest from the mandibular symphysis. Several bleeding points were created using a small round bur.

The autogenous monocortical block graft was harvested from the mandibular symphysis (see Autogenous Bone Harvesting). It was cut to an appropriate size and mortised to fit the recipient site (defect) intimately. Once properly positioned, the graft was fixated with two fixation screws (Leibinger, Kalamazoo, Mich) that passed through the graft and into the remaining native alveolar bone. A periosteal releasing incision was used to sever the periosteum from anterior to posterior and facilitate coronal advancement of the mucogingival flap.

After 6 months of healing, a full-thickness mucoperiosteal flap was elevated to expose the alveolar bone sites #29 and #30. Minimal resorption of the monocortical block graft is evident. Notice the position of the head of the fixation screws (especially the posterior screw), which are more protruded than the bone (Figure 77-1, *H* and *I*).

The fixation screws are removed and the sites are prepared in the usual manner for the placement of two

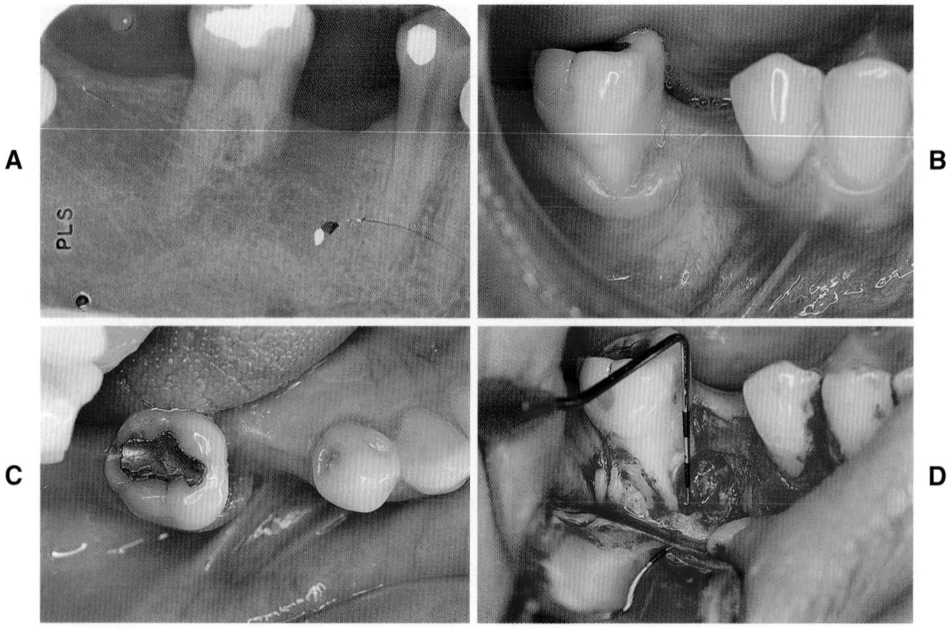

Figure 77-1 Use of a monocortical block graft to reconstruct a horizontal deficiency in the posterior right mandible. **A,** Periapical radiograph shows missing tooth #29 and severed mesial root #30. **B** and **C,** Labial and occlusal views, respectively, of site reveals deficient alveolar ridge on buccal side of #29. **D,** Full-thickness flap reflection reveals the extent of missing bone in the buccal aspect of site #29 as well as the periodontal defect and damaged mesial root #30.

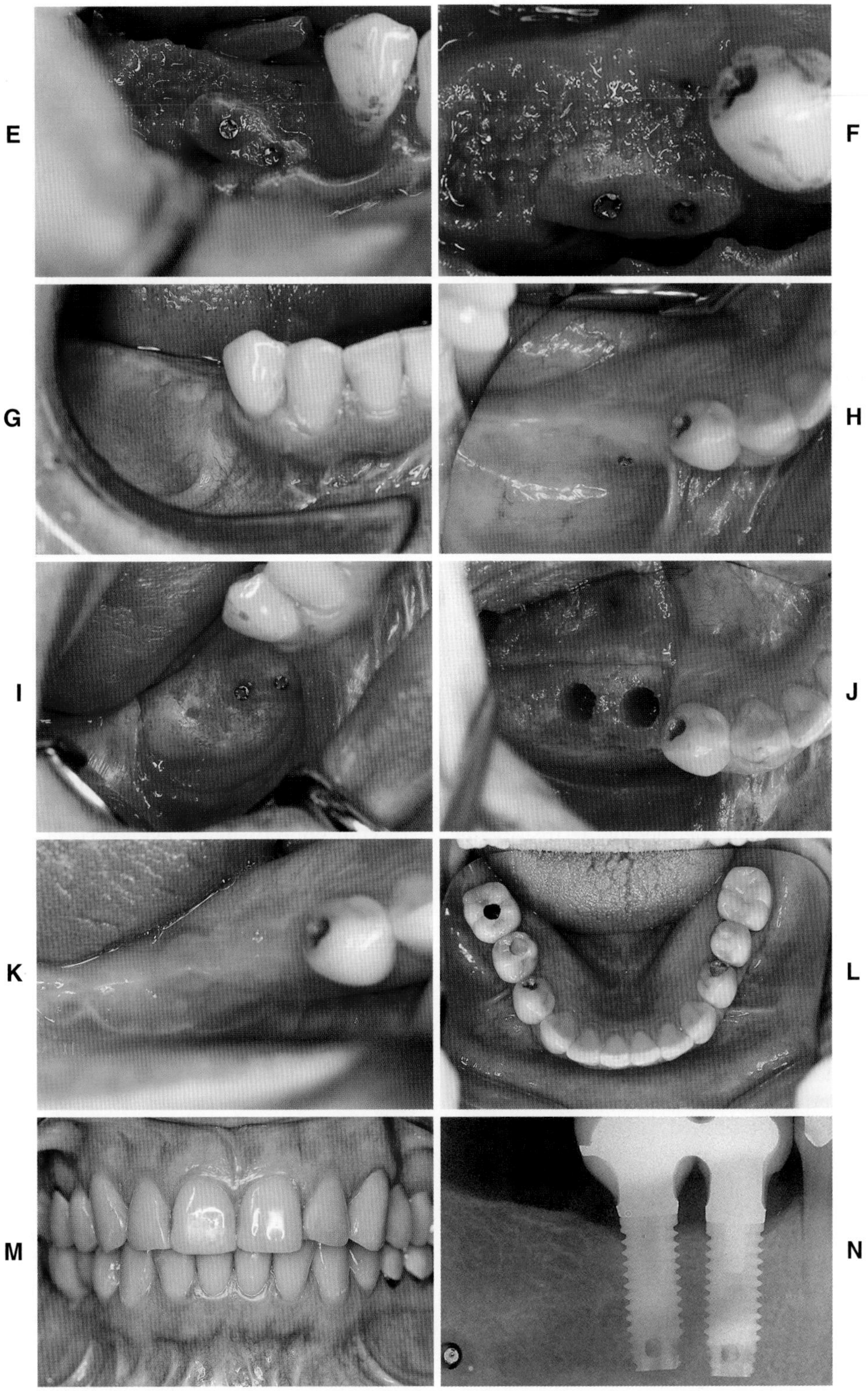

Figure 77-1, cont'd **E** and **F,** Autogenous monocortical bone block graft secured to native alveolar bone with fixation screws. **G,** Good tissue healing after block graft, with evidence of a widened alveolar ridge. **H,** After 6 months of healing, posterior fixation screw is observed protruding through the mucosa. **I,** Full-thickness flap reveals that bone resorption has resulted in exposure of part of the fixation screw. **J,** Osteotomy prepared for wide-diameter implants, taking care to avoid making the labial bone "graft" too thin. **K,** Complete closure and good healing of wound after implant placement. **L** and **M,** Clinical photographs of completed restorations. **N,** Final radiograph shows good restoration contours on wide-diameter implants.

screw-type, wide-diameter implants (Implant Innovations, Palm Beach Gardens, Fla). Care is taken to avoid preparing the grafted site too wide or too far labially because the grafted bone may be vulnerable to fracture or resorption (Figure 77-1, *J*).

Simultaneous Implant Placement and Guided Bone Regeneration

Large alveolar bone defects need to be augmented before implant placement and require a healing period of 6 months or longer. In selected cases, it is possible to perform a bone augmentation procedure simultaneously with the implant placement. It is essential to achieve good implant stability in the existing native bone so that endosseous integration can occur.

A very predictable osseous defect to manage with simultaneous implant placement is the implant dehiscence or fenestration defect. *Fenestration* defects are exposures of the implant's axial surface that do not include the coronal aspect of the implant. *Dehiscence* defects expose a part of the axial surface, including the coronal aspect of the implant, while maintaining sufficient bone volume around all remaining implant surfaces. In a dehiscence defect the implant remains within the confines of the existing bone.

Fenestration and dehiscence defects have been managed with barrier membranes or simply with flap closure. Bone grafts have also been used. The only controlled comparison studies between membrane treatment and periosteal flap coverage of exposed implant surfaces in humans demonstrated that the membrane treatment was far superior with regard to bone fill.[11] Another controlled study in humans showed better results in the membrane groups; four of six sites treated with a membrane resulted in 95% to 100% elimination of the dehiscence and total coverage of the threads. In the control sites, only two of six sites showed moderate to complete bone fill.[43] All other clinical studies are in the form of case reports.[38]

Figure 77-2, *M,* demonstrates coverage of an implant dehiscence using a barrier membrane. Admittedly, without a biopsy, it cannot be determined whether the tissue covering the implant is bone or firm connective tissue.[25,27]

A 1-year multicenter study evaluating 55 dehisced implants in 45 patients, treated by membrane alone, demonstrated an average bone fill of 82%.[12] The average initial defect size was 4.6 mm. The 1-year follow-up of these implants demonstrated a favorable response to loading. Of the 55 implants, a total of six failed, corresponding to a cumulative survival rate of 84.7% in the maxilla and 95% in the mandible, which is similar to previously published results.

A clinical report on the use of titanium-reinforced (TR) membranes demonstrated the biologic potential to fill a large protected space in four patients. The dehisced implant sites ranged from 5 to 12 mm (mean, 8.2 mm). They were covered with a TR membrane alone. Reentry after 7 to 8 months of submerged healing found complete bone coverage of the implants. Radiographic evaluation demonstrated the implants functioning with normal crestal bone support after 1 year.[24]

No clinical comparisons are available in the literature evaluating the placement of bone grafts with or without membranes on dehisced implant surfaces. Most evidence supports the use of graft materials in conjunction with membrane treatment, especially the use of freeze-dried bone allograft (FDBA) in conjunction with GBR. In a study with 40 patients, 110 implants were placed in conjunction with barrier membranes and FDBAs; a success rate of 96.8% was achieved with complete bone fill (defined as >90% fill of dehiscence). This study reported an exposure rate of 29% of the membranes, but little effect on the bone regeneration was noted.[45]

With respect to ridge preservation, Becker et al.[4] recently reported the effect of barrier membranes and autogenous bone grafts on the preservation of ridge width around implants. They evaluated the ridge width around 76 implants in 61 patients from a case series database. Comparison of 34 implants treated with barriers, 27 implants treated with autogenous bone grafts, and 15 implants placed without ridge preservation procedures (control group) revealed that the implant sites treated with barriers or autogenous grafts lost an average of 0.1 mm and 0.8 mm more ridge width, respectively, than the control group.

Another study evaluated the treatment of dehiscence bone defects associated with the placement of implants into fresh extraction sockets.[31] Augmentation procedures were conducted with demineralized (DFDBA) particles and ePTFE membranes. Complete flap closure resulted in complete bone regeneration. Histologic evaluation revealed remnants of the graft material and large areas of vital bone tissue, as evidenced by distinct osteocytes. Both woven bone and lamellar bone were observed in direct contact with graft particles. In a 1-year postgrafting biopsy, DFDBA particles were still present, and osteoblasts were observed engaged in bone formation. Figure 77-2, *L* and *M,* demonstrates a simultaneous GBR and implant placement in a dehiscence defect.

Complications of Localized Ridge Augmentation

Advanced procedures such as GBR and bone grafting to increase the bone volume in deficient alveolar ridges have been successful and have enabled the placement of implants into prosthetically driven positions.[51] Unfortunately, these advanced procedures carry an increased risk of morbidity and can require secondary surgeries to correct soft tissue changes resulting from the procedure.[60] For example, keratinized tissues that have been advanced to cover an increased volume of bone create unesthetic and non–load-bearing mucogingival discrepancies. The subsequent corrective surgeries required to correct mucogingival discrepancies add surgical time and complexity to the implant therapy.

Surgical complications are reported for a variety of bone reconstructive techniques.[15] With the use of bone grafts from the hip to rehabilitate extremely resorbed maxilla, exposure of bone transplants has been reported in up to 30% of cases.[57] The exposure rate usually correlates with an increased loss of transplanted tissue. Fenestration defects have the least risk and immediate extraction sites the highest risk for membrane exposure.

A review assessed the number and types of complications associated with bone reconstructive procedures for endosseous implants.[57] The review of literature (1976-1994) included 2315 implants in 733 autogenous block, particulate, and various other bone graft materials. Complications reported included bleeding, postoperative infection, bone fracture, nerve dysfunction, perforation of the mucosa, loss of a portion of the bone graft, pain, decubital ulcers, sinusitis, and wound dehiscence. Wound dehiscence seemed to have the most deleterious effect on implant survival. This finding emphasizes the importance of flap management, as discussed previously.

Typical findings include less bone fill with early exposure and membrane removal versus retaining the membrane without exposure for 6 to 8 months.[25,53] Buccolingual ridge deficiencies were treated in a prospective study involving 19 patients using ePTFE membranes and miniscrews as fixation and tenting devices.[33] The group of defects, which healed uneventfully, yielded on reentry a 90% to 100% bone regeneration compared with the maximal volume of the space defined by the membrane placement. In the exposed-membrane group, the percentage of regenerated bone ranged from 0% to 62%. When a late membrane removal was performed (3-5 months postsurgically), the regeneration varied between 42% and 62%. The authors concluded that the length of membrane healing and size of the defect played a significant role in the amount of new bone formation.[33]

Other authors have reported successful bone fill in situations where the membranes had to be removed because of an early exposure.[42,52] The use of a bone graft material under the membrane might account for the difference in results. This was confirmed in a clinical study evaluating 36 patients with 23 titanium plasma–sprayed (TPS) implants and 20 hydroxyapatite (HA)–coated implants placed in immediate extraction sites and treated with membrane alone or membrane in combination with DFDBA grafts.[20] When the effect of membrane exposure on bone gain was compared with membranes that remained covered, a significant difference was seen between the covered-membrane group and the exposed-membrane group, but no difference with the exposed-membrane/DFDBA group. A significantly greater fill of the osseous defects at the grafted sites was noted. The authors concluded that the regeneration of bone around the implants appeared most dependent on the anatomy of the bony defect at the time of implant placement.

Although the effect or amount of regenerated bone with regard to membrane exposure is somewhat contradictory, the goal should be to keep the membranes covered during the healing period so that the risk of infection and soft tissue and esthetic problems can be eliminated. Again, the importance of flap management for ridge augmentation procedures should be stressed.

It can be concluded that the selection of a localized ridge augmentation procedure depends on the size and dimension of the osseous defect. In cases of advanced bone resorption, ridge augmentation before implant placement may be a better choice. It seems reasonable to conclude that the predictability for bone formation is better in horizontal ridge augmentation procedures than in vertical ridge augmentation. This conclusion was also made for total maxillary and mandibular ridge reconstruction with calvarial bone grafts, because the implant survival rate was increased in cases with horizontal grafting versus vertical grafting techniques.[15]

Long-Term Results of Implants in Localized Bone-Augmented Sites

Long-term data (>3 years) on the outcome of the membrane technique are scarce; the few reports addressing the question of how regenerated bone behaves under functional loading with dental implants have shown a favorable result. A canine study showed that implants placed in regenerated bone have a normal interaction with the surrounding bone, resulting in direct bone-to-implant contact within 3 months. A loading period of 6 months demonstrated that the regenerated bone is capable of bearing functional load and reacts similarly to nonloaded regenerated bone sites. Regenerated bone sites that did not receive an implant demonstrated bone atrophy beneath the membrane.

One-year clinical follow-up data are available for implants placed in extraction sites with dehiscence or fenestration defects grafted with bone using a membrane technique. All were comparable to normal implant sites.[6,12] A multicenter study determining the predictability of implants placed in immediate extraction sockets and augmented by ePTFE membranes showed an implant survival rate of 93% after 1 year of loading.[6] Nonstandardized radiographs were evaluated for bone loss after an average loading of 7.5 months.

Dehiscence defects were analyzed in two separate studies.[12,25] Dahlin et al.[12] demonstrated in a multicenter study that implants with regenerated bone withstood loading for 1- to 2-year evaluation periods. The cumulative survival rate was 84.7% in the maxilla and 95% in the mandible, which is in line with previously published work with the Brånemark implant.

Jovanovic et al.[25] treated 19 dehisced implants with a membrane technique and demonstrated a 6- to 12-month loading result of 100% implant survival. Radiographic analysis showed an average of 1.73-mm mesiodistal bone loss. Differences between studies are related to the measurement method because the choice of a reference point can add or subtract 0.6 mm. If subtracted, a total crestal bone level of 1.13 mm remains, which is in line with other long-term studies of implant loading.

In a systematic review of survival rates of dental implants after ridge augmentation therapy, Fiorellini and Nevins[17] reported a high level of predictability for implants placed with GBR procedures. Thirteen studies (1741 patients) met the criteria for inclusion in the review. Survival rates for implants placed with GBR procedures were similar to implants placed in native bone.

MANAGEMENT OF EXTRACTIONS

Because tooth extraction (or tooth loss) often results in alveolar ridge resorption or collapse, preservation of bone volume at the time of extraction is a desirable goal. Most bone loss after extraction occurs in the first 6 to

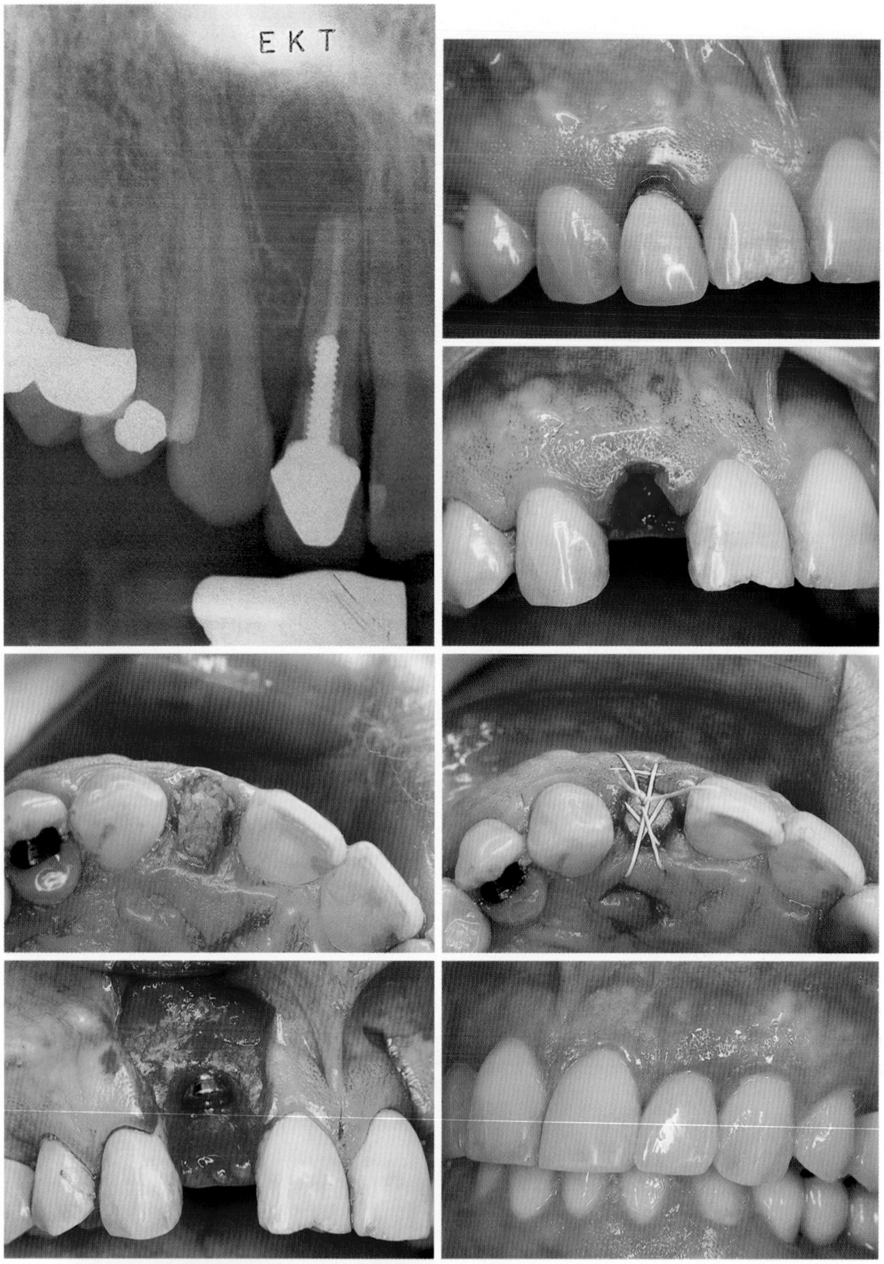

A B C D E F G

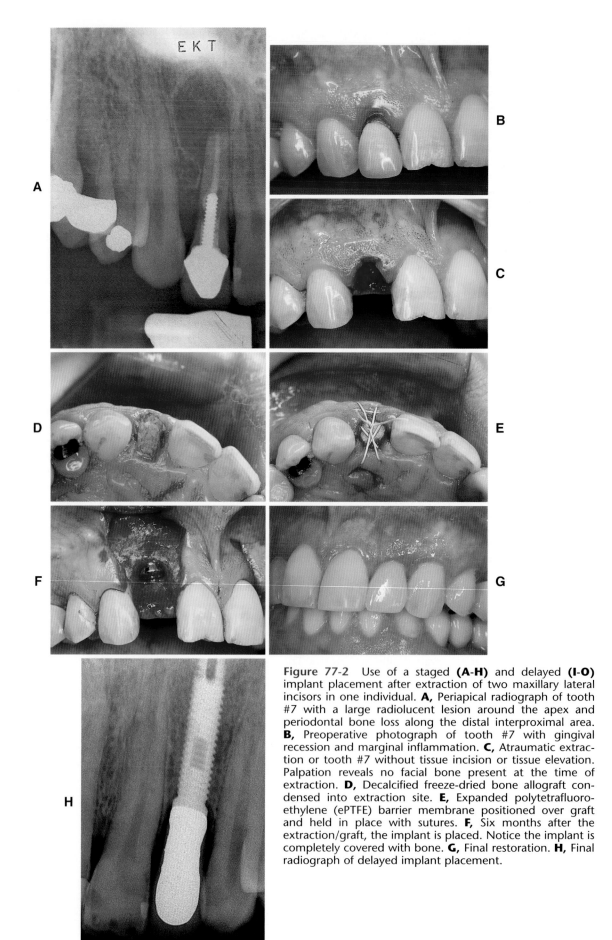

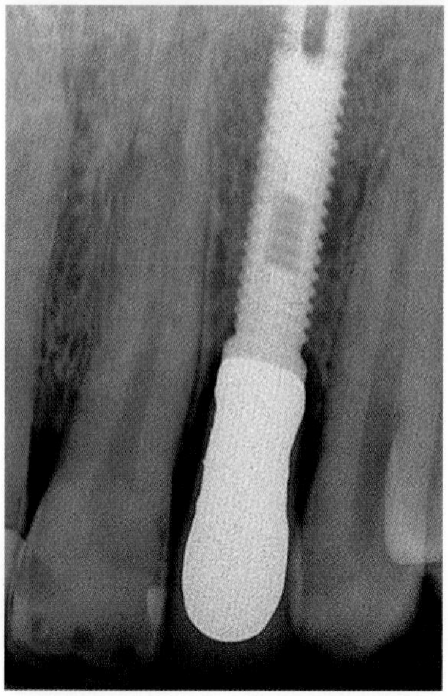

H

Figure 77-2 Use of a staged **(A-H)** and delayed **(I-O)** implant placement after extraction of two maxillary lateral incisors in one individual. **A,** Periapical radiograph of tooth #7 with a large radiolucent lesion around the apex and periodontal bone loss along the distal interproximal area. **B,** Preoperative photograph of tooth #7 with gingival recession and marginal inflammation. **C,** Atraumatic extraction or tooth #7 without tissue incision or tissue elevation. Palpation reveals no facial bone present at the time of extraction. **D,** Decalcified freeze-dried bone allograft condensed into extraction site. **E,** Expanded polytetrafluoroethylene (ePTFE) barrier membrane positioned over graft and held in place with sutures. **F,** Six months after the extraction/graft, the implant is placed. Notice the implant is completely covered with bone. **G,** Final restoration. **H,** Final radiograph of delayed implant placement.

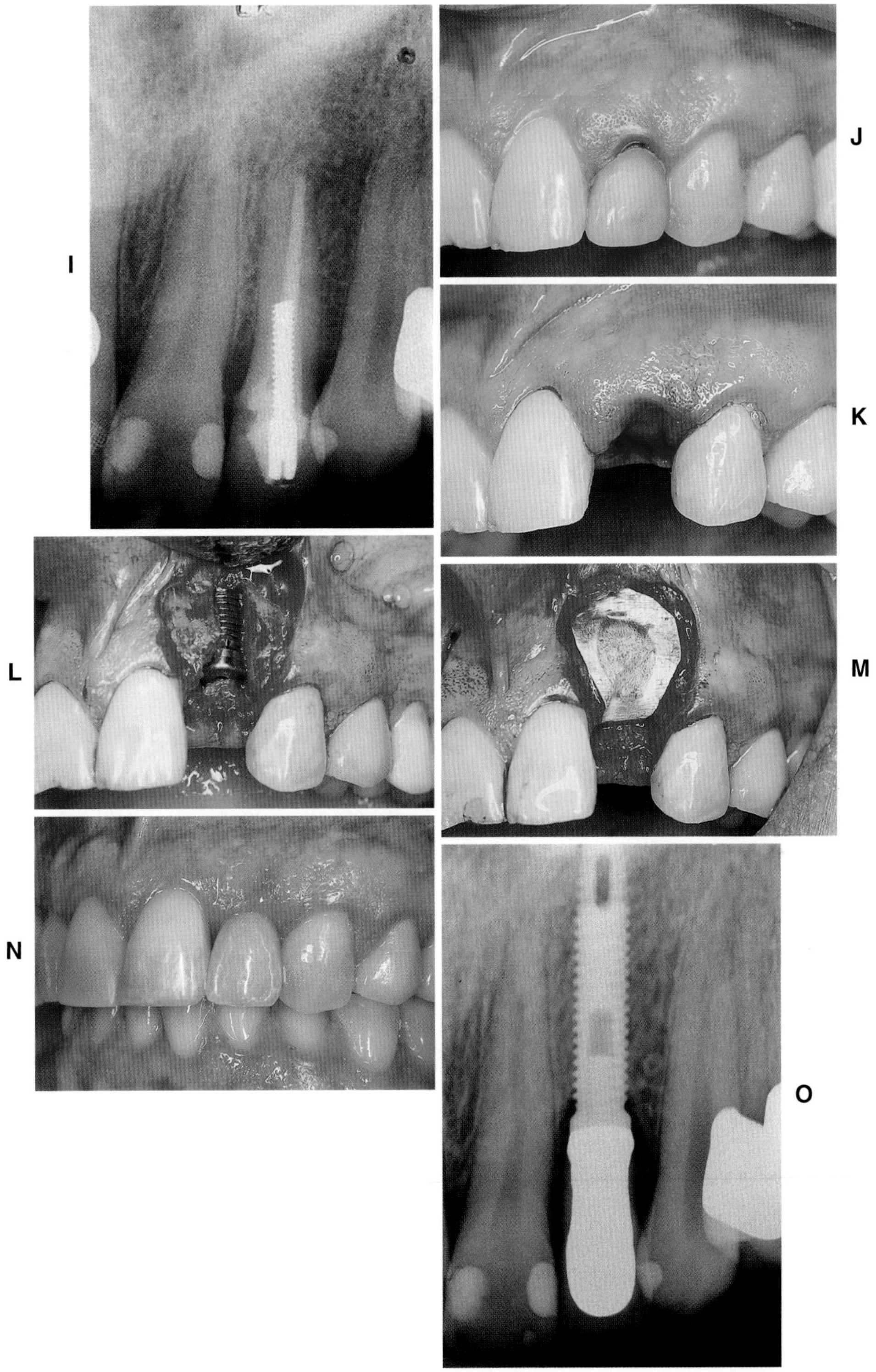

Figure 77-2, cont'd **I,** Periapical radiograph of tooth #10. **J,** Preoperative photograph of tooth #10 with exposed gingival margin. **K,** Atraumatic extraction #10 without tissue incision or tissue elevation. Palpation reveals no facial bone present, and dehiscence is expected. **L,** Two months after extraction, the implant is placed with dehiscence defect. **M,** Guided bone regeneration accomplished with ePTFE barrier membrane positioned over the dehiscence. **N,** Final restoration. **O,** Final radiograph. (**A, B, C, F, G, J, M, N,** and **O** from Klokkevold PR, Han TJ, Camargo PM: *Pract Periodont Aesthet Dent* 11:603, 1999.)

SCIENCE TRANSFER

Successful tooth replacement using dental implants requires stabilization of the implant in bone tissue in a specific location in the jaw. Under certain circumstances, inadequate bone tissue exists at the site for implant placement. In these cases, bone tissue can form using a number of different surgical approaches and techniques. Horizontal augmentation is now extremely predictable compared with vertical augmentation procedures. In any technique chosen for bone augmentation, however, the following principles must be observed:

1. The bone graft (if used) must be stable. This can be achieved by either protecting the graft material or by using fixation devices.
2. The area for bone formation must be protected from the ingrowth of the soft tissues. Also, to ensure optimal conditions, the barrier must be stabilized (fixed). In this way, soft tissues can shrink and swell without disturbing the bone healing.
3. The soft tissues should remain closed over the augmentation site to prevent bacterial contamination.

One significant question in regard to these augmentation procedures is how much time is required for graft stabilization and for barrier stabilization. These factors are critical in choosing materials for bone augmentation procedures because problems with either graft or barrier stability can compromise the outcome of the therapeutic procedure.

A variety of surgical procedures are available to promote bone formation around implants and implant sites. The use of guided bone regeneration (GBR) using membranes can be successful if postsurgical membrane exposure is avoided. Space-maintaining procedures are also widely used, including bone grafts and use of screws or titanium-reinforced Teflon membranes for a tentlike approach. Dehiscences and fenestrations can be successfully managed, and increased width of bone sites is also predictable. If no active infection is present and the implant can be stabilized by projection beyond the apex of the tooth socket, immediate placement into extraction sockets is generally successful with or without GBR.

24 months.[10] Therefore, when clinicians are afforded the opportunity to intervene at extraction, the preservation of alveolar bone should be initiated. A conservative approach to the management of extraction sites can eliminate or significantly reduce the necessity of advanced bone augmentation procedures.

When extracting a tooth and preparing for implant placement, alveolar bone resorption should be prevented. Experimental animal studies have shown that the use of a barrier membrane enhances the predictability of bone fill in the extraction site and therefore maintains original bone volume when compared with mucoperiosteal flap coverage alone.[7] Clinical studies have also demonstrated the benefits of a regenerative approach to tooth extraction.[35,36,41] These authors found that a nonresorbable barrier membrane resulted in minimal resorption of alveolar ridge size and shape.

Although earlier studies have proposed the concept of treating extraction sites without flap closure (i.e., an exposed membrane used to cover the graft), more recent studies concluded that complete wound closure over the physical barrier might be associated with greater bone fill.[6,53]

The timing of implant placement relative to the time of extraction has been widely debated. Depending on the quantity, quality, and support of existing bone, as well as the preferences of the clinician and patient, the placement of implants after tooth extraction can be immediate, delayed, or staged. By definition, *immediate* implant placement occurs at the time of extraction. *Delayed* implant placement is performed approximately 2 months after extraction to allow for soft tissue healing. *Staged* implant placement allows for substantial bone healing within the extraction site, which typically requires 4 to 6 months or longer.

Tooth extraction is managed with an atraumatic surgical technique that uses a narrow, flat instrument (e.g., Periotome, Hu-Friedy, Chicago) directed apically into the sulcus to sever the periodontal ligament and slightly expand the adjacent periodontal tissues. The tooth is elevated and removed with forceps using a gentle, rotational movement. Buccolingual forces are avoided to prevent damaging the integrity of the labial bone. No incisions are made, and care is taken to avoid soft tissue reflection. In this manner, soft tissues maintain their structural anatomy, and the periosteum (blood supply to the bone) remains intact. If the tooth has multiple roots, curved roots, or other anatomic features that make removal difficult, it may be necessary to cut the tooth using a high-speed drill and remove it in smaller pieces. It is important to cut only tooth structure and avoid cutting (overheating) bone when using high-speed drills. The bone within the extraction site is completely debrided of soft tissue with surgical curettes. After debridement, the extraction site is thoroughly irrigated with sterile saline. At this point, after evaluating bone level and support, the clinician decides whether to bone-graft the site and when to place the implant (immediate, delayed, or staged placement).

Immediate Implant Placement

The primary advantage of immediate implant placement is the reduction of the healing time.[34,39,50,59] Because the implant is placed at the time of extraction, the bone-to-implant healing begins immediately with extraction site healing. Another advantage is that the normal bone healing, which generally occurs within the extraction site, takes effect around the implant. This bone-forming activity may enhance the bone-to-implant contact compared with an implant placed in a less osteogenically active site.

Possible disadvantages of immediate implant placement include the need for subsequent mucogingival surgeries to correct tissues moved by repositioned flaps and the need for bone grafting to fill extraction site defects around the implant.

When a two-stage implant is placed at tooth extraction, the mucogingival flap is advanced, with releasing incisions, to cover the implant completely (exception: one-stage implants). It may also be necessary to graft bone into the extraction site in areas that do not contact the implant to avoid soft tissue invasion around the implant.[50] A 1-year study of 49 immediate extraction site implants treated by a membrane alone demonstrated a 93.6% bone fill. After 1 year (postloading), the implant success rate was 93.9%.[6]

The placement of 21 transmucosal implants in immediate extraction sites treated with a barrier membrane were tested for the implant success rate and the percentage of bone fill. Of 21 transmucosal implants, 20 yielded complete bone fill and coverage of the entire plasma-coated implant surface.[32] More clinical review is needed before the treatment of more advanced bone defects with transmucosal implants is recommended. Until then, submerging implants is preferred.[23]

A clinical report on the use of resorbable collagen membranes around extraction site implants demonstrated a variable degree of bone fill in nine patients.[44] More clinical review of the use of resorbable membranes for GBR is required because evidence is insufficient to evaluate the predictability.

If inadequate bone exists to stabilize the implant, immediate implant placement is not recommended. Also, preexisting infections associated with the tooth may impair healing and compromise implant success. Acute or subacute infection is a contraindication to immediate implant placement.

In a study of 30 patients, the use of autografts alone in 54 simultaneous extraction site implants was highly effective for implants placed completely within the envelope of bone. The study showed that extraction sites, including those with a buccal dehiscence, could be treated with autografts alone. Because ungrafted sites were not evaluated, the absolute need to graft small defects adjacent to implants was not ascertained by this study.[3] In another study, implants placed in extraction sockets were tested for their potential to regenerate bone with allograft alone, a membrane alone, and a combination treatment. Reentry confirmed 100% thread coverage in all but one implant in the "no-wall" group treated with DFDB alone.[19]

A clinical study of five patients evaluated different treatment modalities for extraction site implants together with bone graft combinations. It was demonstrated that "non–space-making defects" are best treated with a combination of barrier membrane and an autograft or allograft and achieve better results than a non-reinforced membrane without a graft.[54]

Delayed Implant Placement

Delayed implant placement shares some advantages of immediate implant placement, including extraction site preservation, and offers additional advantages. Unlike immediate implant placement, which is deficient of soft tissue for coverage, the delayed–implant placement technique allows time for soft tissue healing.[23] The delayed-placement technique still reduces the length of treatment by several months because it is not necessary to wait for complete bone healing. Furthermore, because bone formation is active within the first few months after tooth extraction, the delayed technique may facilitate more osteogenesis adjacent to the implant.

The primary advantage of delayed implant placement is that by allowing for soft tissue healing and closure of the extraction site, mucogingival flap advancement is not necessary. This alleviates the need for additional surgeries to correct mucogingival discrepancies. Delayed implant placement also allows time for resolution of infections that may have been present within the extraction site.

As with immediate implant placement, similar limitations of bone support and implant stability exist for delayed placement. The normal osseous healing that occurs within the first 2 months does not significantly affect the anatomy of the alveolar bone. Therefore, limitations in bone support after 2 months of healing are similar to those that exist at extraction.

Staged Implant Placement

Staged implant placement allows adequate time for osseous healing. This may be complete osseous healing of an extraction site without a bone graft (if circumferential bone support is good) or with a bone graft. Staged implant placement, by definition, allows for complete hard and soft tissue healing and permits the placement of implants into prosthetically driven positions with adequate coverage by hard and soft tissues.[51] This eliminates the necessity of mucogingival flap advancement, allows for the resolution of preexisting infections, and prevents soft tissue invasion. Furthermore, by using an extended healing period, the grafted bone also has the opportunity to become vascularized. Bone grafts performed simultaneously with implant placement do not share this advantage.

The primary disadvantage of staged implant placement is the length of time required for bone healing.

Delayed versus Staged Technique

Delayed and staged techniques for implant placement can be demonstrated in one individual using two extraction sites with similar bone morphologies in the anterior maxilla (see Figure 77-2). Both techniques facilitate the esthetic placement of implants into prosthetically driven positions. Delayed and staged approaches maintain alveolar bone volume, reduce the need for advanced bone augmentation, and eliminate the need for subsequent mucogingival surgery. The timing and management of delayed versus staged implant placement vary, as described next.

To decide which implant placement method to use, the quantity and location of bone surrounding the tooth should be assessed. Once the patient has been anesthetized, a periodontal probe can be used to "sound" for the level of bone support through the soft tissue. Using this method, the bone levels surrounding the tooth can be mapped. Bone support that surrounds the extraction site can also be evaluated and confirmed after tooth removal by palpation, probing, and direct (internal) visualization.

If the tooth to be extracted has sufficient bone support on all surfaces, the extraction site can be expected to fill with bone without additional augmentation procedures, except when the labial bone is very thin. A simple extraction followed by a healing period of 4 to 6 months would be sufficient for complete osseous healing. Subsequently, an implant could be placed in the usual manner without the need for bone augmentation. Conversely, if little or no bone exists on the labial surface, it should be anticipated that the site would require bone augmentation to facilitate placement of the implant. In this case, bone grafting at the time of extraction can be used to maintain the alveolar ridge dimensions occupied by the tooth.

CONCLUSION

Bone augmentation and simultaneous implant surgery procedures allow clinicians to reconstruct alveolar bone deficiencies, preserve alveolar dimensions, and replace missing teeth with dental implants in a prosthetically driven position with natural appearance and function. The predictable outcome of these procedures depends on several biologic principles that must be followed. Diagnosis, treatment planning, careful execution of the surgical treatment, postoperative follow-up, and appropriate implant loading are all important factors in achieving success.

REFERENCES

1. Bahat O, Handelsman M: Periodontal reconstructive flaps: classification and surgical considerations, *Int J Periodont Restor Dent* 11:481, 1991.
2. Becker W, Becker BE, Caffesse R: A comparison of demineralized freeze-dried bone and autologous bone to induce bone formation in human extraction sockets, *J Periodontol* 65:1128, 1994.
3. Becker W, Becker BE, Polizzi G: Autogenous bone grafting of bone defects adjacent to implants placed into immediate extraction sockets in patients: a prospective study, *Int J Oral Maxillofac Implants* 9:389, 1994.
4. Becker W, Hujoel P, Becker BE: Effect of barrier membranes and autogenous bone grafts on ridge width preservation around implants, *Clin Implant Dent Relat Res* 4:143, 2002.
5. Becker W, Clokie C, Sennerby L, et al: Histologic findings after implantation and evaluation of different grafting materials and titanium micro screws into extraction sockets: case reports, *J Periodontol* 69:414, 1998.
6. Becker W, Dahlin C, Becker BE, et al: The use of e-PTFE barrier membranes for bone promotion around titanium implants placed into extraction sockets: a prospective multicenter study, *Int J Oral Maxillofac Implants* 9:31, 1994.
7. Becker W, Schenk R, Higuchi K, et al: Variations in bone regeneration adjacent to implants augmented with barrier membranes alone or with demineralized freeze-dried bone or autologous grafts: a study in dogs, *Int J Oral Maxillofac Implants* 10:143, 1995.
8. Becker W, Urist MR, Tucker LM, et al: Human demineralized freeze-dried bone: inadequate induced bone formation in athymic mice—a preliminary report, *J Periodontol* 66:822, 1995.
9. Buser D, Dula K, Hirt HP, et al: Lateral ridge augmentation using autografts and barrier membranes: a clinical study with 40 partially edentulous patients, *J Oral Maxillofac Surg* 54:420, 1996.
10. Carlsson GE, Persson G: Morphologic changes of the mandible after extraction and wearing of dentures: a longitudinal, clinical and x-ray cephalometric study covering 5 years, *Odontol Rev* 18:27, 1967.
11. Dahlin C, Andersson L, Linde A: Bone augmentation at fenestrated implants by an osteopromotive membrane technique: a controlled clinical study, *Clin Oral Implant Res* 2:159, 1991.
12. Dahlin C, Lekholm U, Becker W, et al: Treatment of fenestration and dehiscence bone defects around oral implants using the guided tissue regeneration technique: a prospective multicenter study, *Int J Oral Maxillofac Implants* 10:312, 1995.
13. Dahlin C, Linde A, Gottlow J, et al: Healing of bone defects by guided tissue regeneration, *Plast Reconstr Surg* 81:672, 1988.
14. Doblin JM, Salkin LM, Mellado JR, et al: A histologic evaluation of localized ridge augmentation utilizing DFDBA in combination with e-PTFE membranes and stainless steel bone pins in humans, *Int J Periodont Restor Dent* 16:120, 1996.
15. Donovan MG, Dickerson NC, Hanson LJ: Maxillary and mandibular reconstruction using calvarial bone grafts and Branemark implants: a preliminary report, *Int J Oral Maxillofac Surg* 52:588, 1994.
16. Eriksson AR, Albrektsson T: Temperature threshold levels for heat-induced bone tissue injury: a vital-microscopic study in the rabbit, *J Prosthet Dent* 50:101, 1983.
17. Fiorellini JP, Nevins ML: Localized ridge augmentation/preservation: a systematic review, *Ann Periodontol* 8:321, 2003.
18. Friedmann A, Strietzel FP, Maretzki B, et al: Histological assessment of augmented jaw bone utilizing a new collagen barrier membrane compared to a standard barrier membrane to protect a granular bone substitute material, *Clin Oral Implant Res* 13:587, 2002.
19. Gelb DA: Immediate implant surgery: three-year retrospective evaluation of 50 consecutive cases, *Int J Oral Maxillofac Implants* 8:388, 1993.
20. Gher ME, Quintero G, Assad D: Bone grafting and guided bone regeneration for immediate dental implants in humans, *J Periodontol* 65:881, 1994.
21. Hunt D, Jovanovic S: Autogenous bone harvesting: a clinical graft technique for particulate and amniocortical bone blocks, *Int J Periodont Restor Dent* 19:165, 1999.
22. Jensen OT, Greer RO Jr, Johnson L, et al: Vertical guided bone-graft augmentation in a new canine mandibular model, *Int J Oral Maxillofac Implants* 10:335, 1995.
23. Jovanovic SA, Buser D: Guided bone regeneration in dehiscence defects and delayed extraction sockets. In Buser D, Dahlin C, Schenk RK: *Guided bone regeneration in implant dentistry,* Chicago, 1994, Quintessence.
24. Jovanovic SA, Nevins M: Bone formation utilizing titanium-reinforced barrier membranes, *Int J Periodont Restor Dent* 15:56, 1995.
25. Jovanovic SA, Spiekermann H, Richter EJ: Bone regeneration around titanium dental implants in dehisced defect sites: a clinical study, *Int J Oral Maxillofac Implants* 7:233, 1992.
26. Klokkevold PR, Newman MG: Current status of dental implants: a periodontal perspective, *Int J Oral Maxillofac Implants* 15:56, 2000.
27. Klokkevold PR, Han TJ, Camargo PM: Aesthetic management of extractions for implant site development: delayed

versus staged implant placement, *Pract Periodont Aesthet Dent* 11:603, 1999.
28. Kostopoulos L, Karring T: Guided bone regeneration in mandibular defects in rats using a bioresorbable polymer, *Clin Oral Implant Res* 5:66, 1994.
29. Kostopoulos L, Karring T: Augmentation of the rat mandible using guided tissue regeneration, *Clin Oral Implant Res* 5:75, 1994.
30. Landsberg CJ: The reversed crestal flap: a surgical modification in endosseous implant procedures, *Quintessence* 25:229, 1994.
31. Landsberg C, Grosskopf A, Weinreb M: Clinical and biological observations of demineralized freeze-dried bone allografts in augmentation procedures around dental implants, *Int J Oral Maxillofac Implants* 9:586, 1994.
32. Lang NP, Bragger U, Hammerle CH, et al: Immediate transmucosal implants using the principle of guided tissue regeneration. I. Rationale, clinical procedures and 30-month results, *Clin Oral Implant Res* 5:154, 1994.
33. Lang NP, Hammerle CH, Bragger U, et al: Guided tissue regeneration in jawbone defects prior to implant placement, *Clin Oral Implant Res* 5:92, 1994.
34. Lazzara RJ: Immediate implant placement into extraction sites: surgical and restorative advantages, *Int J Periodont Restor Dent* 9:332, 1989.
35. Lekovic V, Camargo P, Klokkevold P, et al: Preservation of alveolar bone in extraction sockets using bioabsorbable membranes, *J Periodontol* 69:1044, 1998.
36. Lekovic V, Kenney EB, Weinlaender M, et al: A bone regenerative approach to alveolar ridge maintenance following tooth extraction: report of 10 cases, *J Periodontol* 68:563, 1997.
37. Linde A, Thoren C, Dahlin C: Creation of new bone by an osteopromotive membrane technique, *Int J Oral Maxillofac Surg* 51:892, 1993.
38. Mellonig JT, Nevins M: Guided bone regeneration of bone defects associated with implants: an evidence-based outcome assessment, *Int J Periodont Restor Dent* 15:168, 1995.
39. Missika P, Abbou M, Rahal B: Osseous regeneration in immediate post-extraction implant placement: a literature review and clinical evaluation, *Pract Periodont Aesthet Dent* 9:165, 1997.
40. Murray G, Roschlau W: Experimental and clinical study of new growth of bone in a cavity, *Am J Surg* 93:385, 1957.
41. Nemcovsky CE, Serfaty V: Alveolar ridge preservation following extraction of maxillary anterior teeth: report on 23 consecutive cases, *J Periodontol* 67:390, 1996.
42. Nevins M, Mellonig JT: The advantages of localized ridge augmentation prior to implant placement: a staged event, *Int J Periodont Restor Dent* 14:96, 1994.
43. Palmer RM, Floyd PD, Palmer PJ: Healing implant dehiscence defects with and without expanded polytetrafluoroethylene membranes: a controlled clinical and histological study, *Clin Oral Implant Res* 5:98, 1994.
44. Parodi R, Santarelli G, Carusi G: Application of slow-resorbing collagen membrane to periodontal and peri-implant guided tissue regeneration, *Int J Periodont Restor Dent* 16:174, 1996.
45. Rominger JW, Triplett RG: The use of guided tissue regeneration to improve implant osseointegration [see comments], *J Oral Maxillofac Surg* 52:106, 1994.
46. Sandberg E, Dahlin C, Linde A: Bone regeneration by the osteopromotive technique using bioabsorbable membranes: an experimental study in rats, *Int J Oral Maxillofac Surg* 51:1106, 1993.
47. Schenk RK, Buser D, Hardwick WR: Healing pattern of bone regeneration in membrane-protected defects, *Int J Periodont Restor Dent* 9:13, 1994.
48. Schwartz Z, Mellonig JT, Carnes DL Jr, et al: Ability of commercial demineralized freeze-dried bone allograft to induce new bone formation, *J Periodontol* 67:918, 1996.
49. Schwartz Z, Somers A, Mellonig JT, et al: Ability of commercial demineralized freeze-dried bone allograft to induce new bone formation is dependent on donor age but not gender, *J Periodontol* 69:470, 1998.
50. Schwartz-Arad D, Chaushu G: Placement of implants into fresh extraction sites: 4 to 7 years retrospective evaluation of 95 immediate implants, *J Periodontol* 68:1110, 1997.
51. Shanaman RH: The use of guided tissue regeneration to facilitate ideal prosthetic placement of implants, *Int J Periodont Restor Dent* 12:257, 1992.
52. Shanaman RH: A retrospective study of 237 sites treated consecutively with guided tissue regeneration, *Int J Periodont Restor Dent* 14:292, 1994.
53. Simion M, Baldoni M, Rossi P, et al: A comparative study of the effectiveness of e-PTFE membranes with and without early exposure during the healing period, *Int J Periodont Restor Dent* 14:166, 1994.
54. Simion M, Dahlin C, Trisi P, et al: Qualitative and quantitative comparative study on different filling materials used in bone tissue regeneration: a controlled clinical study, *Int J Periodont Restor Dent* 14:198, 1994.
55. Ten Bruggenkate CM, Kraaijenhagen HA, van der Kwast WA: Autogenous maxillary bone grafts in conjunction with placement of I.T.I. endosseous implants: a preliminary report, *Int J Oral Maxillofac Surg* 21:81, 1992.
56. Tolman DE: Advanced residual ridge resorption: surgical management, *Int J Prosthodont* 6:118, 1993.
57. Tolman DE: Reconstructive procedures with endosseous implants in grafted bone: a review of literature, *Int J Oral Maxillofac Implants* 10:275, 1995.
58. Urist MR: Bone formation by autoinduction, *Science* 150:893, 1965.
59. Wilson TG Jr, Schenk R, Buser D, et al: Implants placed in immediate extraction sites: a report of histologic and histometric analyses of human biopsies, *Int J Oral Maxillofac Implants* 13:333, 1998.
60. Yildirim M, Hanisch O, Spiekermann H: Simultaneous hard and soft tissue augmentation for implant-supported single-tooth restorations [see comments], *Pract Periodont Aesthet Dent* 9:1023, 1997.
61. Zellin G, Gritli-Linde A, Linde A: Healing of mandibular defects with different biodegradable and non-biodegradable membranes: an experimental study in rats, *Biomaterials* 16:601, 1995.

Advanced Implant Surgical Procedures

78

CHAPTER

Perry R. Klokkevold

CHAPTER OUTLINE

The high predictability of endosseous dental implants has led to routine use and an expectation for success. However, the ultimate success for any patient or any particular implant relies on several factors, the most important of which is the *availability of bone*. The loss of teeth, whether caused by disease or trauma, can result in severe deficiency of the alveolar bone. Horizontal bone deficiencies are managed quite predictably with localized bone augmentation (see Chapter 77). However, vertical bone deficiency is a much more challenging problem. The edentulous posterior maxilla is particularly challenging because of a general lack of bone volume and the omnipresent poor bone quality of the area; that is, posterior maxillary bone is often sparse trabecular bone.

This chapter reviews advanced surgical procedures used to treat the most challenging patient-related factor, *a deficiency in vertical height of bone*. Maxillary sinus elevation and bone augmentation, vertical bone augmentation, and distraction osteogenesis are presented. The role of growth factors in bone augmentation procedures is also discussed.

MAXILLARY SINUS ELEVATION AND BONE AUGMENTATION

Rehabilitation of the edentulous posterior maxilla with endosseous dental implants often represents a clinical challenge because of the insufficient bone volume resulting from *pneumatization* of the maxillary sinus along with resorption or loss of alveolar crestal bone. Before the utilization of bone augmentation procedures, patients with deficient alveolar bone in the posterior maxilla were rehabilitated with removable prostheses, short implants, or cantilevered restorations (i.e., supported by adjacent teeth or implants). Unfortunately, implants placed in the posterior maxilla undergo significantly greater failures compared with all other intraoral anatomical locations.[9] Therefore, procedures are needed to increase the amount of vertical bone height in the posterior maxilla.

In 1980, Boyne and James[1] first described a procedure to graft the maxillary sinus floor with autogenous marrow and bone for placing an implant (blade type). Access to the maxillary sinus was gained through a "Caldwell-Luc" procedure (i.e., a superiorly located opening into the maxillary sinus). Since then, several other techniques have been described, including variations on the lateral window osteotomy and the use of osteotomes to elevate the floor of the sinus from an alveolar crest approach. Various bone graft materials have been used as well. The 1996 Consensus Conference on Maxillary Sinus Bone Grafting reviewed available data and concluded that allografts, alloplasts, and xenografts, alone or in combination with autogenous bone, can be effective as bone substitute graft materials for sinus bone augmentation.[10] More importantly, it was concluded that the sinus graft procedure with implant placement is a highly predictable and effective therapeutic modality for the rehabilitation of the posterior maxilla.

Sinus floor elevation with bone augmentation of the maxillary sinus is now a well-accepted procedure used to increase bone volume in the posterior maxilla. Numerous reports have validated the safety and efficacy of this procedure.[3,5,6] Success rates are equal to or better than that of implants placed in nongrafted maxillary bone (i.e., areas of the posterior maxilla with adequate height of existing native bone). Thus, in situations where the interocclusal dimension is normal or only moderately increased, bone augmentation of the maxillary sinus is indicated.

Indications and Contraindications

As with any therapeutic procedure, treatment success depends on appropriate patient selection, careful evaluation of the anatomy, identification and management of any pathology, sound surgical procedures, and appropriate postsurgical management. The primary indication for maxillary sinus elevation and bone augmentation, specific for the placement of endosseous dental implants, is an alveolar bone height in the posterior maxilla that is less than 10 mm. Other factors that must be considered include the health of the patient, the condition of the remaining dentition, and the likelihood of a beneficial outcome. A thorough evaluation of the patient and the judgment of the clinician will ultimately determine whether the procedure is indicated for any particular individual.

Contraindications to maxillary sinus elevation and bone augmentation are similar to contraindications for other surgical procedures, with the added consideration of the maxillary sinus (Box 78-1). Patients must be in good general health and free of diseases that affect the maxilla or maxillary sinus. Local factors that are considered contraindications to maxillary sinus elevation and bone augmentation include the presence of tumors, maxillary sinus infection, severe chronic sinusitis, scar or deformity of the sinus cavity from previous surgery, dental infection, severe allergic rhinitis, and chronic use of topical steroids. Systemic contraindications to treatment include radiation therapy, uncontrolled metabolic disease (e.g., diabetes), excessive tobacco use, drug or alcohol abuse, and psychologic or mental impairment.

BOX 78-1

Contraindications for Maxillary Sinus Elevation and Bone Augmentation

Local Factors

Tumors or pathologic growth in the sinus
Maxillary sinus infection
Severe chronic sinusitis
Surgical scar/deformity of sinus cavity
Dental infection involving or in proximity to sinus
Severe allergic rhinitis/sinusitis
Chronic topical steroid use

Systemic Factors

Radiation therapy involving the maxillary sinus
Metabolic disease (e.g., uncontrolled diabetes mellitus)
Excessive tobacco use
Drug/alcohol abuse
Psychologic/mental impairment

Anatomy and Physiology

The maxillary sinus is the largest of the paranasal sinuses. It is an air-filled cavity located in the posterior maxilla superior to the teeth. The lateral wall of the nasal cavity borders the sinus medially; it is bordered superiorly by the floor of the orbit and laterally by the lateral wall of the maxilla, the alveolar process, and the zygomatic arch (Figure 78-1). It is pyramidal in shape, with its apex is in the zygomatic arch and its base at the lateral wall of the nasal cavity. The size of the maxillary sinus varies from one individual to another (age and individual dependent), from very small and narrow to quite large and expansive.

The maxillary sinus is frequently subdivided (incompletely) into recesses by one or more *septa.* Maxillary sinus septa vary in size and location. Clinical and radiographic examinations suggest that septa are frequently present (up to 35.9% of sinuses).[12,25] Computed tomography (CT) scans are the preferred method for detecting septa because panoramic radiographs are not reliable (26.5% false diagnosis of the presence or absence of septa).[12,13] Septa are found in the anterior (24%), middle (41%), and posterior (35%) aspects of the maxillary sinus, with the most common location between the second premolar and the first molar.[11,25] The height of septa vary as well, ranging from 0 to 20.6 mm.[25] Only 0.5% of septa form complete separations.[14]

The entire maxillary sinus is lined with a thin mucosal membrane called the *schneiderian membrane.* The specialized structure of the respiratory mucous membrane, with its motile cilia and rich blood supply, is well adapted to purifying, moistening, and warming air to protect the

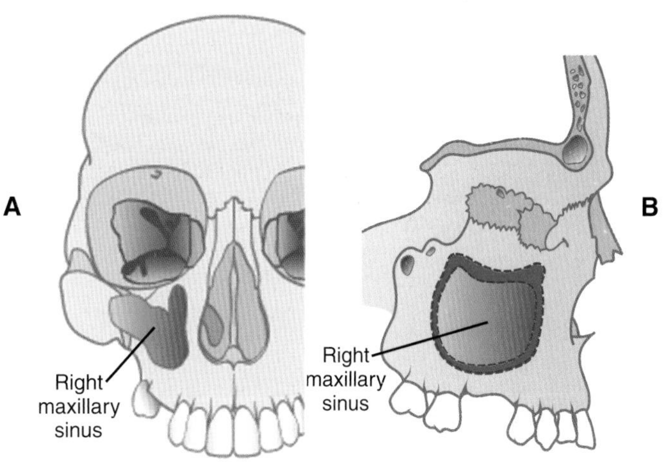

Figure 78-1 Location and anatomy of the maxillary sinus. **A,** Frontal view. **B,** Lateral view.

lungs. The entrance to the maxillary sinus, through the orifice or maxillary duct, is located at the superomedial aspect of the cavity. The orifice is relatively small, measuring only 3 to 6 mm in length and diameter. An accessory opening is occasionally found inferior and posterior to the main opening. The maxillary sinus drains into the middle meatus of the nasal cavity through the maxillary duct, which passes secretions medially to the semilunar hiatus. Normal amounts of secretion are moved from the sinus by the spiral pattern of beating cilia surrounding the orifice. If the maxillary sinus becomes infected or chronically inflamed, swelling of the mucosa around orifices impairs drainage.

The floor of the maxillary sinus extends down below the level of the nasal cavity into the alveolar process. The roots of the maxillary first and second molars are often close to the floor of the sinus. Less frequently, the roots of the premolars and third molars may protrude into the floor of the sinus. With increasing age the maxillary sinus expands, becoming more and more pneumatized down around the roots of the maxillary teeth, sometimes resulting in exposure of the roots through the bony floor into the sinus, with only the thin mucosal membrane covering the root surface.

Blood supply to the maxillary sinus arises from the superior alveolar (anterior, middle, and posterior) branches of the maxillary artery (Figure 78-2, *A*). Branches of the greater palatine artery contribute to a lesser extent. Venous blood drains via the pterygoid plexus. Much of the vasculature travels through channels in the bony walls of the maxillary sinus, with many branches anastomosing with the highly vascularized schneiderian membrane. Innervation of the maxillary sinus is supplied by the superior alveolar (anterior, middle, and posterior) nerve, branches of the maxillary nerve (Figure 78-2, *B*).

The goal of sinus elevation and bone augmentation procedure is to lift the schneiderian membrane (ideally without tearing or perforating) from the floor of the sinus, raising it up into the sinus cavity to create a new, more superiorly located sinus floor with a space above in relation to the deficient alveolar ridge. The newly created space can then be filled with bone (or a suitable bone substitute material) to increase the total vertical height of bone in the posterior maxilla for the placement of endosseous implants.

Surgical Procedures for Sinus Elevation

The maxillary sinus graft procedure was first described during the 1970s (unpublished oral presentations) and originally used as a preprosthetic surgical procedure for patients with large tuberosities and pneumatized sinuses. To reduce the size of the tuberosity without creating an oral-antral defect, bone was grafted into the sinus cavity. After healing, the bone-grafting procedure increased the volume of bone within the maxillary tuberosity, thus facilitating the ability to reduce surgically the tuberosity from the alveolar ridge crest. As stated earlier, Boyne and James[1] were the first to describe the use of the maxillary sinus bone-grafting procedure for placing an implant (blade type) to retain a prosthesis. Later, the success of root form, endosseous dental implants and the desire to replace missing posterior maxillary teeth with implant-retained restorations naturally led to greater use and further development of this procedure, with variations in the materials, techniques, and anatomic location of the *antrostomy* (i.e., surgically created opening into the maxillary sinus or antrum).

The techniques are primarily differentiated by the anatomic location of the osteotomy used to gain access to the maxillary sinus. Specifically, four different anatomic locations have been described: (1) the superior lateral wall, or "Caldwell-Luc," opening, which is located just anterior to the zygomatic arch; (2) the middle lateral wall opening, which is located midway between the alveolar ridge and the zygomatic arch; (3) the inferior lateral wall opening, which is located at the level of the alveolar ridge; and (4) the crestal approach with osteotomes

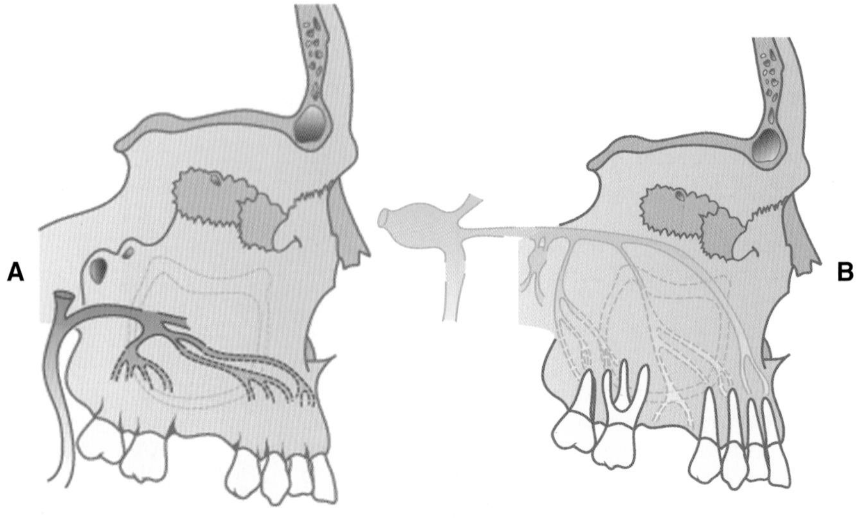

Figure 78-2 Blood supply and innervation of the maxillary sinus. **A,** Arterial blood supply. **B,** Innervation of the maxillary sinus.

through the alveolar bone crest superiorly to the floor of the sinus. At present, the most common procedures used for sinus elevation and bone augmentation are the lateral wall antrostomy (middle or inferior approach) and, to a lesser extent, the crestal approach.

Presurgical Evaluation of Maxillary Sinus

Presurgical evaluation of the maxillary sinus anatomy is primarily accomplished using radiographic examination techniques (Figure 78-3). Several observations can be made with a panoramic projection, but the internal anatomy is much better assessed with a three-dimensional scan, such as CT or cone-beam computed tomography (CBCT). The maxillary sinus should be evaluated for any pathology, masses, and the presence of septa. If three-dimensional scans are available, an investigation of the lateral wall for medium or large intraosseous vascular channels should be considered. Although rare, medium to large vessels occasionally traverse the lateral wall of the maxillary sinus, and identifying them would be helpful in avoiding a bleeding problem during surgery.

Simultaneous Implant Placement

Simultaneous implant placement is possible with sinus elevation and bone augmentation procedures as long as the implant can be stabilized in the desired location with the existing native bone (Figure 78-4). It has been suggested that a minimum of 5 mm of existing native bone in the alveolar crest is required for simultaneous implant placement. However, some clinicians claim that it is possible to place implants simultaneously with as little as 1 mm of remaining bone.[18,26] If inadequate native bone exists to place implants at the time of the bone augmentation procedure, they should be placed with a subsequent surgery after an appropriate healing period (e.g., 6 months) (Figure 78-5).

Bone Graft Materials

Autogenous bone is often considered the gold standard for bone augmentation because of its osteoconductive, osteoinductive, and osteogenic properties.[1] However, harvesting autogenous bone from other intraoral and extraoral sites creates a second surgical site with additional morbidity. Numerous studies have demonstrated clinical success using many variations of bone graft materials and combinations.[10]

Several recent clinical studies and reports have attempted to evaluate the maxillary sinus augmentation procedures using a variety of bone-grafting materials, including autogenous bone from the iliac crest or oral cavity and bone substitutes such as freeze-dried demineralized bone, resorbable and nonresorbable hydroxyapatite, and xenografts. However, only a few studies have critically evaluated the long-term clinical outcome of this procedure, and most have used a small study population. Short-term to long-term clinical studies of dental implants placed into grafted sinuses demonstrate a similar or even higher survival rate than reported in previous studies for implants placed in the maxilla without a sinus augmentation procedure.[10] The results of these studies support the clinical predictability of maxillary sinus augmentation procedures for the rehabilitation of the edentulous posterior maxilla with implant-supported prostheses.

The use of bone-substitute graft materials can reduce the morbidity introduced by a second surgical site while maintaining equally good implant success rates.[10] These materials form an osteoconductive scaffold for bone growth but do not have any osteoinductive properties. A possible exception is demineralized freeze-dried bone allograft (DFDBA). This material has demonstrated osteoinductive potential[24] but has not proved to be particularly advantageous in the maxillary sinus bone augmentation.[10]

Osteotome Technique

In cases demonstrating sufficient crestal bone height, a sinus elevation approach can be taken through the implant osteotomy (i.e., from a crestal approach). If the amount of available bone in the posterior maxilla is less than 10 mm and greater than 7 mm, the osteotome technique may be indicated. This procedure uses osteotomes (Figure 78-6) to compress bone (internally from the alveolar crest upward) against the floor of the sinus, ultimately leading to a controlled "inward fracture" of the sinus floor bone along with the schneiderian membrane, which should remain intact with the in-fractured bone.

Initially, an osteotomy site is prepared with a series of drills (implant preparation) to a depth that is approximately 2 to 3 mm from the floor of the maxillary sinus. Osteotomes are used to increase compressive forces gradually against the floor of the sinus by adding incremental quantities of graft material until the floor of the sinus fractures inward (Figure 78-7). After the controlled inward fracture of the maxillary sinus floor, bone graft materials continue to be slowly introduced, through the osteotomy site and into the maxillary sinus, which continues to elevate the membrane and thus allows a vertical expansion of the bone height in a localized area of the maxillary sinus. Once the sinus membrane is elevated with bone graft material to the desired height, the implant osteotomy can be completed, with a final drill used to finish preparation of the site (lateral walls), and an implant can be inserted. Multiple individual sites can be elevated and prepared simultaneously through separate osteotomy sites.

Published reports of this technique have demonstrated increased bone height from 2 to 7 mm (average, 3.8 mm).[23] Thus the crestal approach is a useful technique for increasing the vertical height of bone up to approximately 4 mm. If more vertical bone is needed, the lateral wall approach may be more advantageous.

In addition to the usual precautions and contraindications for sinus elevation and bone augmentation procedures, the osteotome technique may be contraindicated for sinuses that have an acutely sloped floor or septa in the location of the planned osteotomy. An acutely sloped sinus floor will tend to deflect the osteotome in an undesirable direction rather than allowing the osteotome to penetrate into the sinus space, and the presence of septa make it virtually impossible to fracture the sinus floor inward. Box 78-2 provides additional precautions and clinician comments on using the osteotome technique.

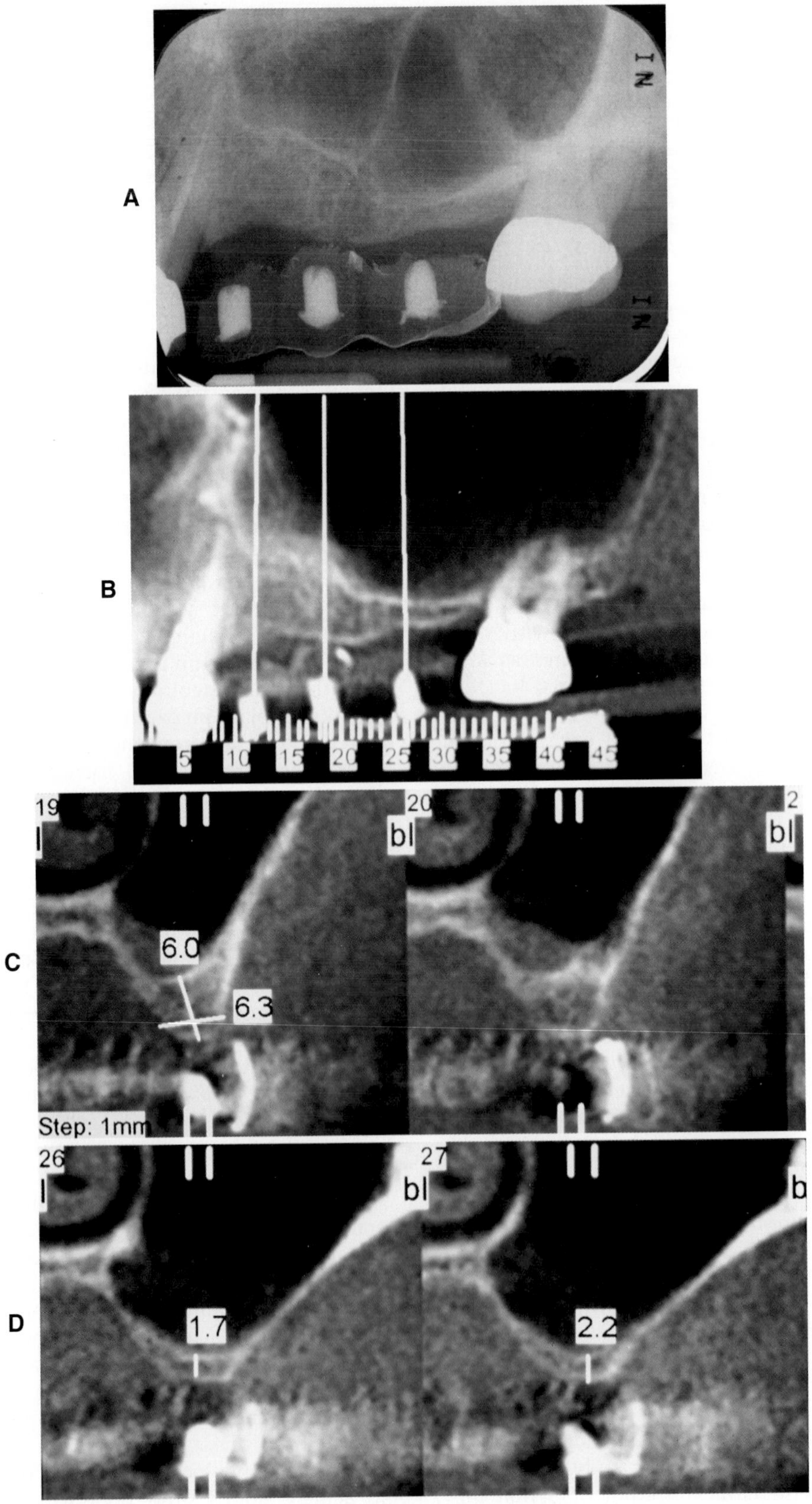

Figure 78-3 Presurgical evaluation of the maxillary sinus. **A,** Periapical radiograph. **B,** Panoramic projection from cone-beam scan. Notice the presence of maxillary septa in the premolar region. **C,** Cross-sectional image in premolar region showing about 6 mm of bone height and presence of maxillary septa. **D,** Cross-sectional image in molar region showing about 2 mm of bone height.

A

B

C

D

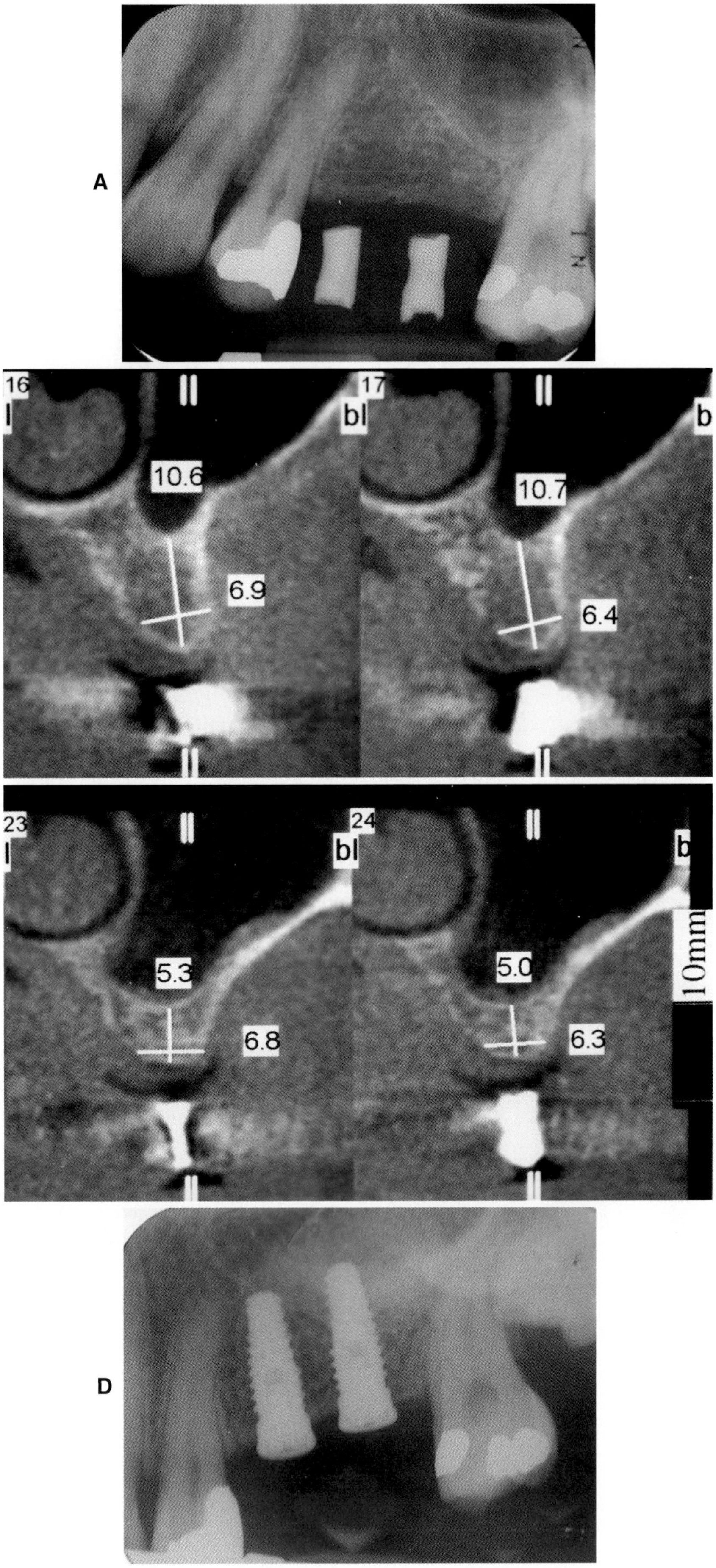

Figure 78-4 Simultaneous implant placement with maxillary sinus elevation and bone augmentation procedure. **A,** Preoperative periapical radiograph. **B,** Preoperative, cross-sectional image in premolar region demonstrating 10.6 mm of vertical bone height. **C,** Preoperative, cross-sectional image in molar region demonstrating 5.3 mm of vertical bone height. **D,** Postsurgical radiograph of graft and implants in place.

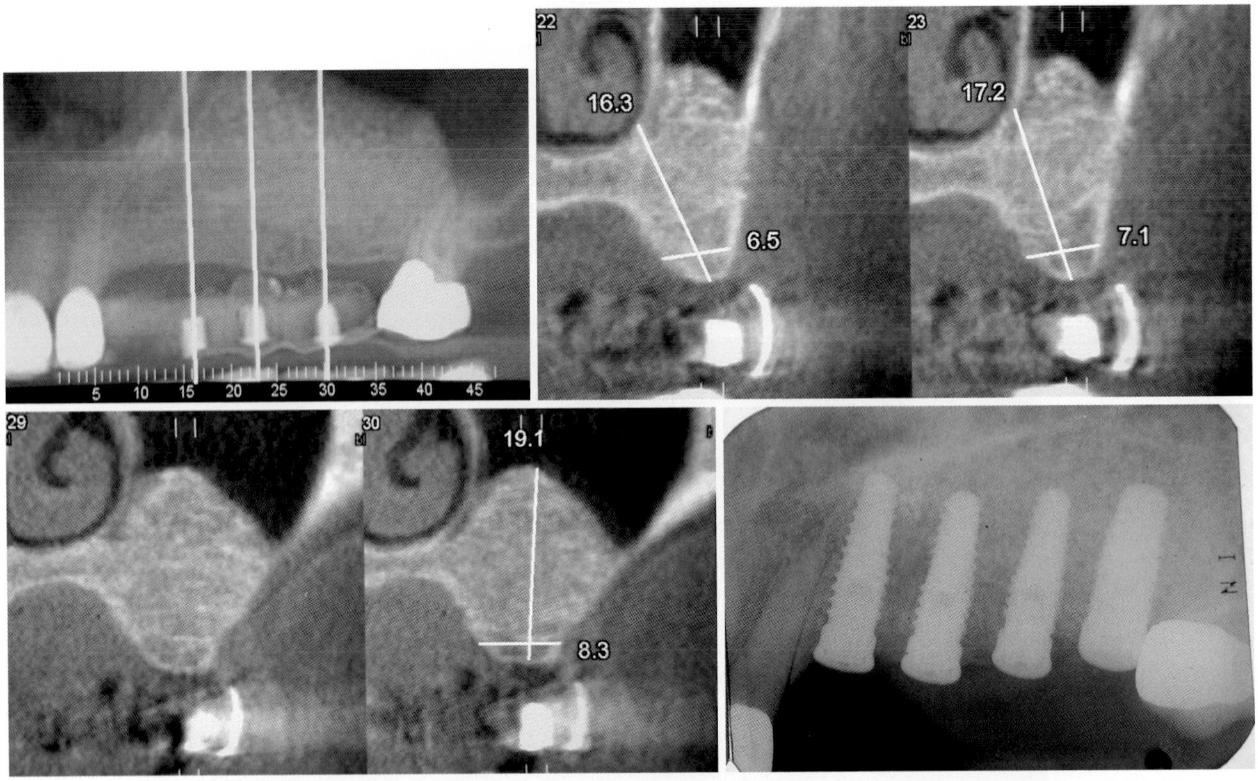

Figure 78-5 Staged implant placement after sinus elevation and bone augmentation procedure. Same patient as in Figure 78-3. See preoperative radiograph and preoperative cross-sectional images. **A,** Postsurgical panoramic view of bone-augmented maxillary sinus. The maxillary left cuspid has been extracted because of a vertical fracture. **B,** Postsurgical cross-sectional image in premolar region demonstrating more than 17-mm vertical bone height. **C,** Postsurgical cross-sectional image in molar region demonstrating 19.1-mm vertical bone height. **D,** Postsurgical radiograph of implants placed in the previously grafted maxillary sinus (and cuspid site).

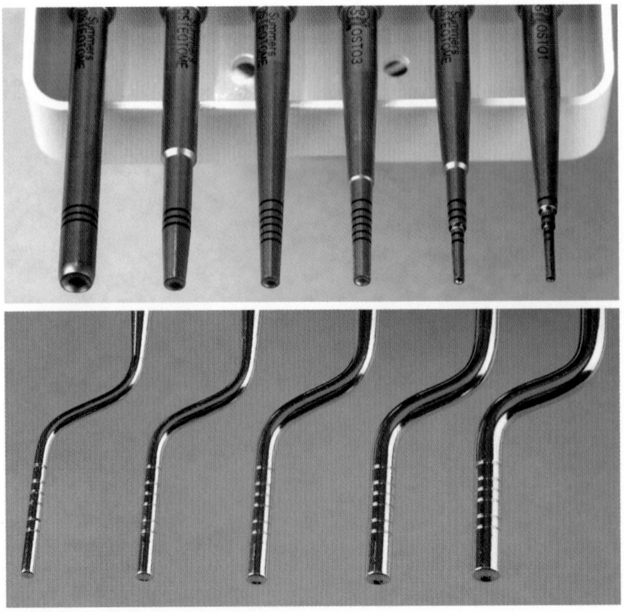

Figure 78-6 Osteotome instruments. **A,** Straight osteotomes. **B,** Offset osteotomes.

BOX 78-2

Clinician Comments on Use of Osteotome Technique

Clinical Perspective #1

The osteotome procedure involves repeated tapping of osteotomes with a mallet to create the necessary pressure to fracture the floor of the maxillary sinus. This tapping can be bothersome to some individuals, especially those patients who are not sedated for the procedure. The tapping procedure tends to be more bothersome for patients with dense cortical bone and for those with loose trabecular bone.

Clinical Perspective #2

The osteotome technique requires that the osteotome be properly aligned in the direction of the long axis of the planned implant. Thus, patients must be able to open wide enough to allow a direct insertion of the osteotome into the osteotomy site. Offset osteotomes are available that can facilitate the correct angulation (see Figure 78-6, *B*).

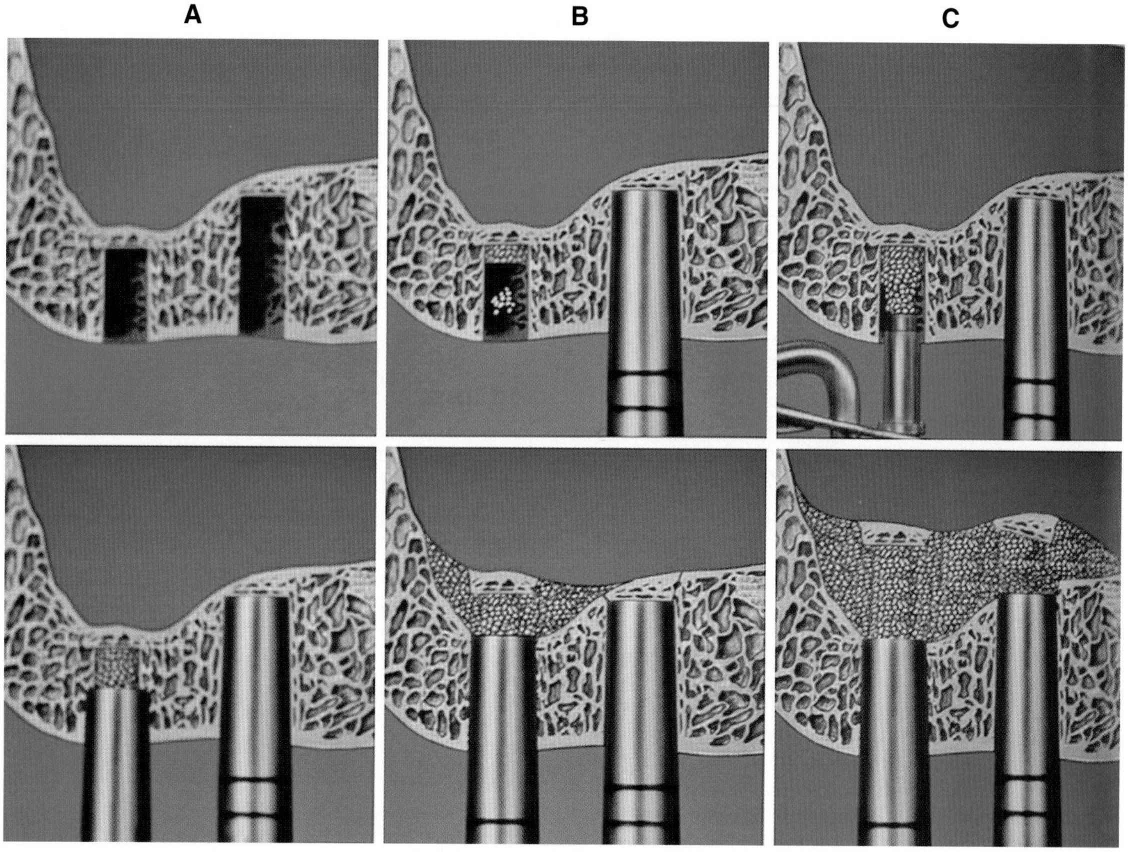

Figure 78-7 Osteotome technique. **A,** Osteotomy prepared with drills to a depth that is near the maxillary sinus floor. **B,** Graft material introduced into osteotomy and condensed with osteotome. **C,** Additional bone graft material is added to the osteotomy. **D,** Bone graft continues to be condensed by osteotomes. **E,** This process is continued until floor of sinus is lifted. **F,** Bone graft material continues to be added until sufficient height and volume are created in the maxillary sinus. (Courtesy Implant Innovations, Inc., Palm Beach Gardens, Fla.)

Lateral Window Technique

The lateral window technique is probably the most effective and efficient way to access the maxillary sinus and elevate the sinus floor. In this procedure, an opening into the maxillary sinus is created to elevate the schneiderian membrane and place bone graft in the space immediately above the existing alveolar bone. Some clinicians prefer to cut the lateral window (outline cut through to the mem-brane) and use the impacted bony wall as the superior wall of the space created for bone grafting (Figure 78-8, *A* and *B*). Others prefer to eliminate the bony window completely by using a bur to thin the bone down to a paper-thin layer, which is easily removed (Figure 78-8, *C* and *D*). With the former technique, it is important to create a window that is not too large, relative to the mediolateral width of the maxillary sinus, to allow the "window" to be pushed completely into the sinus cavity. If the window cannot be inserted completely, it must be carefully separated from the membrane and removed.

Elevation of the schneiderian membrane is accomplished with hand instruments that are inserted along the internal aspect of the bony walls of the sinus (Figure 78-9). Great care is taken to avoid perforation of the membrane. Small instruments are introduced along the inferior, anterior, posterior, and superior aspects of the prepared antrostomy window, gradually inserting further along the bone until the membrane begins to separate and lift away from the bone. Subsequently, larger instruments are gently introduced along the bone to continue lifting the membrane to the desired levels (height, width, and depth). Regardless of whether implants are being placed simultaneously, it is useful to estimate the dimensions of the augmentation needed by inserting a surgical guide with holes or markers indicating the ideal location for planned implants. Once elevated, the space can be grafted with bone (autogenous, bone substitute, or a combination). If implants are being simultaneously placed, the implant osteotomy sites should be prepared and implants placed after the medial, anterior, and posterior aspects are filled with bone (supporting the schneiderian membrane up and away from the drills and implants). After implant placement, the remaining lateral aspect is packed with bone graft. Finally, the antrostomy is covered with a barrier membrane (e.g., resorbable membrane).

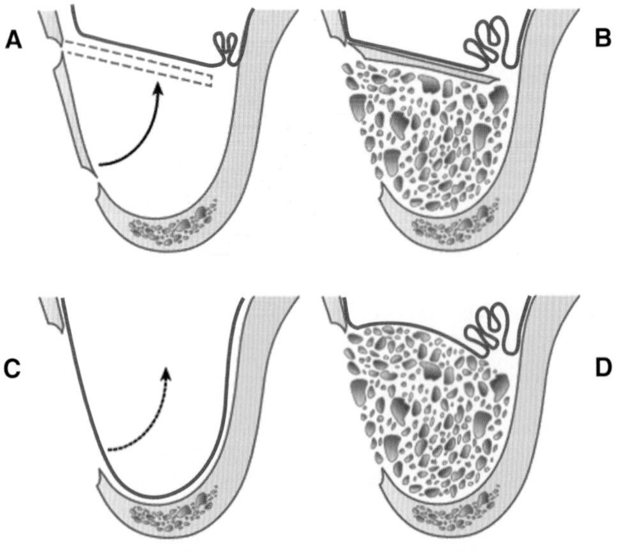

Figure 78-8 Illustrations showing two different techniques for the lateral window procedure to access the maxillary sinus for bone augmentation. **A,** Lateral window is cut at the periphery of the access window, leaving the lateral bony wall in the center of the window intact. **B,** The bony window is then pushed inward to become the superior wall of the grafted maxillary sinus space. **C,** Lateral window is cut completely away (including the bone at the center of the window). **D,** The schneiderian membrane is elevated inward and upward to become the superior containment of the grafted maxillary sinus space without a superior bony wall.

Risks and Complications

The maxillary sinus elevation and bone augmentation procedure is technique sensitive, requiring meticulous surgical skills. Risks and complications of the procedure include tearing or perforation of the schneiderian membrane, intraoperative or postoperative bleeding, postoperative infection, and loss of bone graft or implants.

The reported incidence of perforation or tearing of the schneiderian membrane varies greatly (up to 60%), which probably depends largely on the anatomy of the sinus and the skill and experience of the operator.[15,19,20] The presence of septa in the maxillary sinus increases the likelihood of membrane perforation. If the perforation is small, it often can be managed with a resorbable barrier membrane placed over the opening, followed by careful packing of the bone augmentation material. If a perforation or tear is extensive, it may be necessary to abort the procedure, close the wound, and attempt again at a later date.

Infections have been reported in a small (up to 10%) but significant number of cases following maxillary sinus elevation and bone augmentation procedures.[20] Prevention of infection is crucial for bone augmentation procedures. Surgery should always be performed using sterile technique. Patients should use a presurgical antimicrobial mouth rinse (e.g., chlorhexidine), and postoperative antibiotics (e.g., Augmentin) should be prescribed.

Opening a window through the lateral wall is accomplished by completely cutting through the bone of the lateral wall up to the schneiderian membrane. The membrane is highly vascularized and may bleed significantly. However, a more serious bleeding problem can arise if an intraosseous artery is severed in the process. Bone wax and topical hemostatic agents must be available to manage such an urgent surgical complication. If a medium to

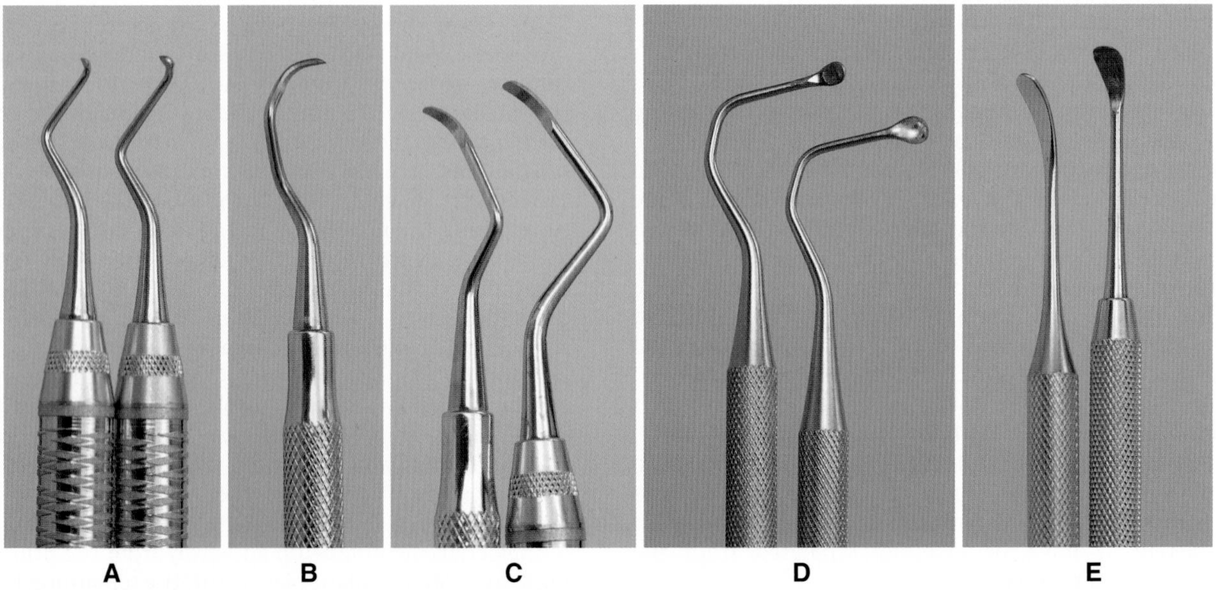

Figure 78-9 Instruments used to elevate the schneiderian membrane through lateral window antrostomy. **A,** DeMarco curettes. **B,** #13/14 Gracey curette. **C,** Universal curettes. **D,** Large spoon curettes. **E,** Medium-sized curved membrane elevators.

SCIENCE TRANSFER

Some implant placement procedures are extremely challenging because of the lack of vertical bone height and limiting anatomic structures. Some of these cases can be treated but require tedious surgical technique and different procedures than used in more common periodontal applications and routine implant placement. The maxillary sinus represents one such anatomic location that requires special techniques, largely because bone is not normally found in this sinus. Interestingly, even when large amounts of bone are grafted into the maxillary sinus and implants are extended into the bone, pneumatization occurs over time, and radiographically, a thin amount of bone is found only over the implant, similar to that found over root apices. Implant success continues, however, and patients can benefit for years. Why the bone remains around the apical area of the implant is not known but may relate to the stresses applied through the implant body.

Maxillary sinus bone augmentation allows implants to be placed in sites where there is limited bone height. If sufficient bone height is present to stabilize the implant, implants may be placed at the same time as the bone augmentation. Generally, a minimum of 5 mm of bone height is needed to stabilize implants, and implants 10 to 13 mm in length are positioned after elevating the sinus floor and placing bone graft material around the implant. A variety of bone graft materials are successful in sinus elevation procedures, and bovine-derived inorganic bone particles, alone or in combination with autogenous bone, have widespread application.

Augmentation of crestal bone height is more complex, and guided bone regeneration and bone distraction techniques are the procedures of choice.

large vascular channel is identified (with CT or CBCT scan) presurgically, it can usually be avoided.

SUPRACRESTAL/VERTICAL BONE AUGMENTATION

Supracrestal or vertical bone augmentation presents the greatest challenge in terms of regenerating bone for implant placement. Historical attempts to increase alveolar bone height vertically have failed. Such procedures as the onlay block graft and particulate hydroxyapatite grafts inserted after use of tissue expanders failed as a result of severe resorption and graft displacement. More recent attempts have used the principles of guided bone regeneration (GBR) to improve the outcomes for vertical bone augmentation.

Guided Bone Regeneration and Augmentation

The available evidence on GBR-associated and supracrestal implant placement is limited. Some published studies have evaluated the effect of space creation by a membrane alone or with an autogenous bone graft. Studies conducted in dogs have demonstrated the ability to gain about 2.7 mm (0.4-4.0 mm) of vertical bone height around implants placed simultaneously.[11] In one clinical study, five patients were treated with a supracrestal exposure of 3 to 7 mm (average of 4.67 mm) and showed a clinical bone gain of 0.5 to 4 mm (average of 2.97 mm) after 9 months.[22]

The incorporation of bone grafts covered by membranes demonstrated that graft sites without membranes around implants tended to be less well preserved than membrane-covered sites. The membrane treatment preserved the bone graft volume by 70% or greater. The membrane also helped increase bone-implant contact of the incorporated bone graft.[4] These studies suggest that supracrestal bone formation up to 3 mm is predictable using the GBR technique with a membrane–blood clot combination.

Simion et al.[21] and Jovanovic et al.[11] used a titanium-reinforced (TR) membrane for vertical bone regeneration around dental implants. No supportive bone substrates were used, except for a careful fill of space with a blood clot by perforating the bone surface or injecting it with venous blood. The variation in supracrestal bone regeneration achieved was 3.3 mm[21] and 1.82 mm.[11] Recent studies showed that supracrestal bone formation is more predictable using a TR membrane and bone graft filler material. Therefore, at present, an advanced surgical reconstruction technique for vertical bone gain is always combined with a bone graft (autogenous) and a nonresorbable TR membrane (Figure 78-10). A recent 1- to 5-year clinical follow-up clinical study has demonstrated that vertically augmented bone can be maintained with functionally loaded implants and that the periimplant bone structures are maintained similar to implants placed in native, nonregenerated bone.[22]

Distraction Osteogenesis

This surgical technique has been developed to increase vertical bone height in the deficient jaw site and contrasts with the more conventional method of bone grafting with or without membranes. Under the proper circumstances, most cells in bone can differentiate into osteogenic or chondrogenic cells needed for repair. Ilizarov[7,8] introduced the process of generating new bone by "stretching," referred to as *distraction osteogenesis.*

Based on experimental and clinical studies over 35 years, distraction osteogenesis can provide a surgeon with the ability to treat extremities, small bones in

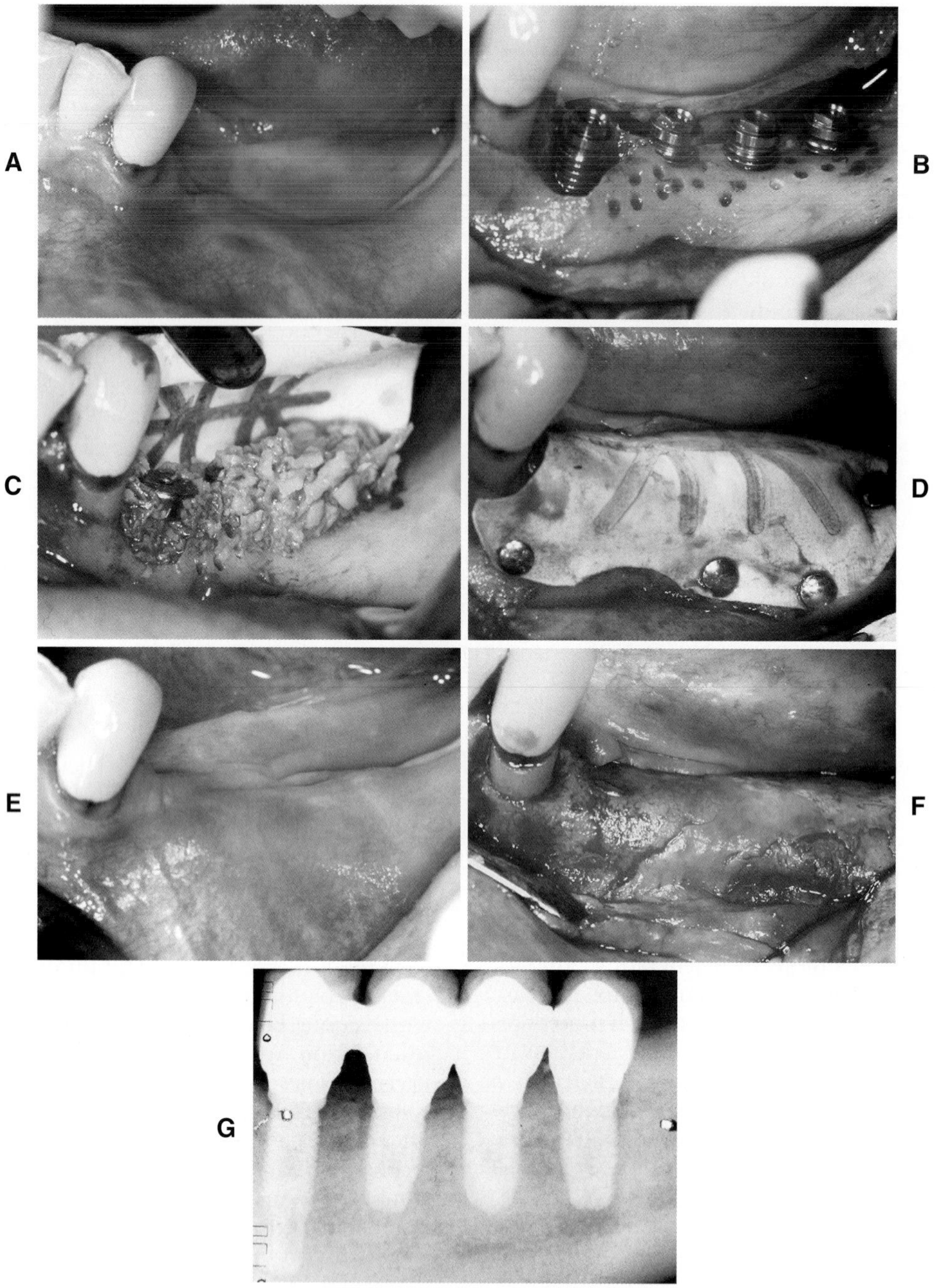

Figure 78-10 Vertical bone augmentation. **A,** Partially edentulous patient with a vertically resorbed posterior mandible, with 5 mm from the mandibular canal to the bone crest. Note the normal periodontal level around the anterior teeth. **B,** After full-thickness flap elevation and implant placement, a supracrestal position of 2 to 4 mm was achieved. The most anterior implant was 15 mm in length (mesial to the mental foramen), and the three posterior implants were 8.5 mm. Note the perforations in the cortical bone to open the marrow spaces and allow for blood supply. **C,** After an autogenous bone graft was harvested from the ramus and particulated, a nonresorbable, titanium-reinforced, expanded polytetrafluoroethylene membrane (TR-9Y) was trimmed and fixated with two pins on the lingual to act as an envelope for the bone graft. **D,** Membrane was closed on the buccal and fixated with four pins. Note the safety margin between the membrane and the tooth and mental foramen of at least 2 mm. **E,** Closure of the surgical site by periosteal release of the buccal and lingual flap. After advancement of the buccal flap and the lingual floor of the mouth, tension-free closure was achieved with horizontal mattress and interrupted sutures. During an uneventful healing of 7 months, no prosthesis was inserted. **F,** After full-thickness flap elevation and membrane removal, a vertical and horizontal bone gain of more than 5 mm was evident. Note that the vertical augmentation procedure with guided bone regeneration achieved vertical and horizontal bone reconstruction around the previously exposed implant surfaces. **G,** Radiograph after 1 year of loading shows normal maintenance of bone structures around the implants.

hands and feet, using external fixation devices. Recently, new intraoral devices for vertical bone growth of the alveolar process have been developed and successfully applied before dental implant placement. Other important advantages of distraction osteogenesis are that no second surgical site is needed to harvest bone, and the newly created bone has native bone at the crest, which are thought to withstand forces better than fully regenerated bone.

One of the most significant disadvantages of the distraction osteogenesis procedure for intraoral application is the unidirectional limitation of current devices. The application for vertical bone augmentation has shown a broad use in the preprosthetic surgical indication with good predictability, although limitations have been encountered in developing horizontal bone growth with this method. Secondary bone grafting is frequently needed for the extremely resorbed jaw.

GROWTH FACTORS IN BONE AUGMENTATION

Current research is exploring the use of various growth factors to induce bone formation.[2] These bone-inductive mediators are powerful modifiers of the healing process. Incorporation of osteoinductive mediators into bone graft material or other carriers can be applied to sites in conjunction with conventional bone augmentation procedures to enhance the outcome.

Bone Morphogenic Proteins

Perhaps the most studied of all the osteoinductive growth factors are the bone morphogenic proteins (BMPs), belonging to the transforming growth factor beta (TGF-β) superfamily. Of this family, *recombinant human bone morphogenic protein* (rhBMP-2) has shown significant signs of bone-enhancing potential.

Recently, studies have reported substantial preclinical data for rapid new bone formation using rhBMP-2 in critical-sized defects. The potential advantage of combining barrier membranes and rhBMP-2 for osteogenesis is evident. The inductive capacity of rhBMP-2 was demonstrated by impregnating a polymer carrier and placing the substrate in critical-sized rat mandibular defects with or without a barrier membrane.[16] The study evaluated 12- and 24-day healing times and showed a bony union of the defects for BMP-treated sites. The control site was not closed at the same intervals.

Autologous Platelet Concentration

In recent years, a new approach to enhance the vitality of bone grafts has been introduced by using platelet concentrate or platelet-rich plasma (PRP).[17] PRP is an autologous source of platelet-derived growth factors and transforming growth factors that is obtained by sequestering and concentrating platelets by centrifugation. The patient's own blood is withdrawn and separated into platelet-rich and platelet-poor components. The PRP is the important content, containing a high-level mixture of platelets and a concentration of growth factors. This PRP mixture is added to the autologous bone graft and has been shown to increase the quality of and reduce the time needed for bone regeneration. Clinical and experimental studies are scarce but suggest that this technique holds promise for large bone defects and bone defects with low osteogenic potential. Extrapolation to the possible effect of PRP on other bone-filler materials cannot be made at this time.

CONCLUSION

Bone augmentation and advanced implant surgery procedures allow clinicians to reconstruct vertical alveolar bone deficiencies and replace missing teeth with endosseous dental implants. As stated in Chapter 77, the predictable outcome of these procedures depends on several biologic principles that must be followed. Diagnosis, treatment planning, careful execution of the surgical treatment, postoperative follow-up, and appropriate implant loading are all important factors in achieving success.

REFERENCES

1. Boyne PJ, James RA: Grafting of the maxillary sinus floor with autogenous marrow and bone, *J Oral Surg* 38:613, 1980.
2. Boyne PJ, Marx RE, Nevins M, et al: A feasibility study evaluating rhBMP-2/absorbable collagen sponge for maxillary sinus floor augmentation, *Int J Periodont Restor Dent* 17:11, 1997.
3. Bruschi GB, Scipioni A, Calesini G, et al: Localized management of sinus floor with simultaneous implant placement: a clinical report, *Int J Oral Maxillofac Implants* 13:219, 1998.
4. Dahlin C, Andersson L, Linde A: Bone augmentation at fenestrated implants by an osteopromotive membrane technique: a controlled clinical study, *Clin Oral Implant Res* 2:159, 1991.
5. Del Fabbro M, Testori T, Francetti L, et al: Systematic review of survival rates for implants placed in the grafted maxillary sinus, *Int J Periodont Restor Dent* 24:565, 2004.
6. Geurs NC, Wang IC, Shulman LB, et al: Retrospective radiographic analysis of sinus graft and implant placement procedures from the Academy of Osseointegration Consensus Conference on Sinus Grafts, *Int J Periodont Restor Dent* 21:517, 2001.
7. Ilizarov GA: The tension-stress effect on the genesis and growth of tissues. Part 1. The influence of stability of fixation and soft tissue preservation, *Clin Orthop* 238:249, 1989.
8. Ilizarov GA: The tension-stress effect on the genesis and growth of tissues. Part 2. The influence of the rate and frequency of distraction, *Clin Orthop* 239:263, 1989.
9. Jaffin RA, Berman CL: The excessive loss of Brånemark fixtures in type IV bone: a 5-year analysis, *J Periodontol* 62:2, 1991.
10. Jensen OT, Shulman LB, Block MS, et al: Report of the Sinus Consensus Conference of 1996, *Int J Oral Maxillofac Implants* 13(suppl):11, 1998.
11. Jovanovic SA, Schenk RK, Orsini M: Supracrestal bone formation around dental implants: an experimental dog study, *Int J Oral Maxillofac Implants* 10:23, 1995.
12. Kasabah S, Slezak R, Simunek A, et al: Evaluation of the accuracy of panoramic radiograph in the definition of maxillary sinus septa, *Acta Medica (Hradec Kralove)* 45:173, 2002.
13. Krennmair G, Ulm C, Lugmayr H: Maxillary sinus septa: incidence, morphology and clinical implications, *J Craniomaxillofac Surg* 25:261, 1997.

14. Krennmair G, Ulm CW, Lugmayr H, et al: The incidence, location, and height of maxillary sinus septa in the edentulous and dentate maxilla, *J Oral Maxillofac Surg* 57:667, 1999.
15. Levin L, Herzberg R, Dolev E, et al: Smoking and complications of onlay bone grafts and sinus lift operations, *Int J Oral Maxillofac Implants* 19:369, 2004.
16. Linde A, Hedner E: Recombinant bone morphogenetic protein-2 enhances bone healing, guided by osteopromotive e-PTFE membranes: an experimental study in rats, *Calcif Tissue Int* 56:549, 1995.
17. Marx RE, Carlson ER, Eichstaedt RM, et al: Platelet rich plasma, *Oral Surg Oral Med Oral Pathol Oral Radiol Endod* 85:638, 1998.
18. Peleg M, Mazor Z, Chaushu G, et al: Sinus floor augmentation with simultaneous implant placement in the severely atrophic maxilla, *J Periodontol* 69:1397, 1998.
19. Raghoebar GM, Batenburg RH, Timmenga NM, et al: Morbidity and complications of bone grafting of the floor of the maxillary sinus for the placement of endosseous implants, *Mund Kiefer Gesichtschir* 3(suppl 1):S65, 1999.
20. Schwartz-Arad D, Herzberg R, Dolev E: The prevalence of surgical complications of the sinus graft procedure and their impact on implant survival, *J Periodontol* 75:511, 2004.
21. Simion M, Trisi P, Piattelli A: Vertical ridge augmentation using a membrane technique associated with osseointegrated implants, *Int J Periodont Restor Dent* 14:496, 1994.
22. Simion M, Jovanovic SA, Tinti C, et al: Long-term evaluation of osseointegrated implants inserted at the time or after vertical ridge augmentation, *Clin Oral Implant Res* 12:35, 2001.
23. Toffler M: Osteotome-mediated sinus floor elevation: a clinical report, *Int J Oral Maxillofac Implants* 19:266, 2004.
24. Urist MR: Bone formation by autoinduction, *Science* 150(698):893, 1965.
25. Velasquez-Plata D, Hovey LR, Peach CC, et al: Maxillary sinus septa: a 3-dimensional computerized tomographic scan analysis, *Int J Oral Maxillofac Implants* 17:854, 2002.
26. Winter AA, Pollack AS, Odrich RB: Placement of implants in the severely atrophic posterior maxilla using localized management of the sinus floor: a preliminary study, *Int J Oral Maxillofac Implants* 17:687, 2002.

Recent Advances in Implant Surgical Technology

Daniel H. Etienne, Raymond R. Derycke, Philippe C. Gault, and Perry R. Klokkevold

79

CHAPTER

CHAPTER OUTLINE

Implant surgical procedures have more or less remained the same since the introduction of osseointegrated dental implants. Briefly, implant placement surgery involves the use of a full-thickness flap elevation and a sequential series of drills with increasing diameters under profuse irrigation to create a precise osteotomy site in the bone for the placement of a dental implant (see Chapter 76). The site is prepared and the implant positioned to avoid important anatomic structures, such as the inferior alveolar nerve, sinus cavities, and natural teeth, and optimally support and emulate the planned prosthetic tooth replacement(s). Proper implant position is important for optimal function and esthetics.

Clinicians determine implant positions based on presurgical diagnostic imaging, study models, and the use of a diagnostic wax-up of the planned tooth replacement(s). The actual or final position of the implant(s) results from the surgeon's interpretation of diagnostic information and ability to translate that information to the patient at surgery. Most often the surgical "guide" between the diagnostic information and the patient is an acrylic stent, fabricated by a laboratory technician, that may or may not have precise guide channels for implant positioning. Therefore, inaccuracies in the stent fabrication and movement of the stent during surgery, as well as variations in the use of the stent during surgery, can lead to imprecise implant positioning.

Recent advances in implant surgical technology include use of the following:

- *Computer imaging software* to "simulate" preoperatively the implant position(s) into a virtual patient, that is, a three-dimensional (3D) computer image of the patient's jaw created from the computed tomography (CT) scan data.[20]
- *Computer-generated surgical guides* with drill holes based on the presurgical "virtual" implant positioning.[8,10,15]
- *Computer-assisted implant surgery* (CAIS) through simultaneous tracking and "guidance" of the implant instrumentation.[4]

CAIS is the most sophisticated and perhaps the most promising of these technologies because it has the greatest potential to reduce surgical time, minimize surgical invasiveness, and result in a more precise translation of implant planning to the actual surgical procedure.[19] Understandably, CAIS is also the technique that requires the greatest amount of preparation and coordination of the patient, image data, and surgical instrumentation. This chapter provides a conceptual overview of the techniques and terminology used in CAIS. Readers are referred to the *Carranza's Clinical Periodontology* electronic edition (e-dition) for a more detailed description and updates of this emerging technology.

COMPUTER-ASSISTED IMPLANT SURGERY

Uses and Requirements

Computerized navigation surgery evolved from early applications in neurosurgical procedures and continues to evolve with applications in several surgical specialties.[14,16] Clearly, the advantage of using a computer to assist surgery is the precision that it offers. As in medicine, 3D imaging can be used in dentistry to facilitate presurgical planning and guide the surgical placement of dental implants. This allows precise positioning while avoiding injury to important anatomic structures. Several different approaches to computers have been used in dental implant surgery, from the simple imaging software to visualize the implant positions in a 3D virtual patient to the more complex, simultaneous image monitoring and instrument navigation.[4]

The use of computer-assisted implant surgery requires precise and continuous coordination of the patient, the image data, and the surgical instrumentation. Therefore, CAIS requires an accurate alignment (identification and registration) of the patient with the patient's image data (3D CT scan data) and a system of tracking the precise movements of the surgical instrumentation (e.g., handpiece, drills) in relation to the actual patient. A variety of systems have been developed to acquire and register image data and to coordinate and track movements. These methods are generically described in the following sections.

Sequence of Steps

The clinical sequence of steps required for CAIS is as follows:

1. *Data acquisition.* The patient is scanned for image data acquisition (e.g., CT scan) with *fiducial* (artificial) radiographic markers (e.g., stent with markers or intentionally placed pins or screws into jaw) or *anatomic* (natural) markers such as teeth or bony landmarks. If fiducial markers are placed in a stent, the patient must have it in place when scanned.
2. *Identification.* The anatomic or fiducial markers will be identified with a probe tracked by the system. If markers were incorporated into a radiographic stent, the stent will again be placed in the mouth and the markers identified by hand with a probe tracked by the stereovision system.
3. *Registration.* After identification of the predetermined markers, the software will indicate the best localization or "match" on the arch between the image data and the patient. If registration is not validated, matching can be improved with additional points. A nonvalidated registration may be caused by an improper initialization or CT scan data.
4. *Navigation.* Ultimately, the operator will be able to visualize surgical instrument navigation (movement). The drilling instruments will be guided to a target point of impact with a 3D spatial orientation.
5. *Accuracy.* Sustained-accuracy procedures are critical during surgery and should prove reliability in regard to the system's overall accuracy. This sustained-accuracy procedure will be done through contact of the drill on the handpiece with selected teeth, by visualization of markers, which can be viewed by the stereovision system, or repositioning of the radiomarker stent.
6. *Feedback.* Variations from the ideal position can be restricted by the software through inactivation of the drill (stop-and-go action) or by an audible or visual cue.

Preoperative Data Acquisition

CT scans, and more recently cone-beam computed tomography (CBCT) scans, are widely used for 3D patient imaging (see Chapter 75). Factors that must be considered when deciding to use a CT scan include radiation exposure, limitations in accuracy, and the possibility of diffracted images as a result of metallic restorations. The evolution of scanner technology (spiral CT scan, CBCT scan) has made it possible to reduce the radiation dose to the level of a conventional panoramic radiograph while maintaining adequate diagnostic quality for preoperative implant planning.[6]

As for conventional diagnostic implant planning, radiographically identifiable markers are important for CAIS. However, unlike conventional planning, where orientation and simulation of implant positions are related to the planned prosthetic crown position (see Figures 75-5 and 75-7 through 75-9), CAIS markers must relate the image data to the actual patient anatomy. In other words, the position of the surgical instrumentation (and ultimately the implant) must be related to scan image data of the patient's jaw morphology. Thus, it is critically important to scan the patient with markers that will be identified in the scan and correlated to the patient at surgery. Markers can be anatomic markers, such as teeth or specific bony landmarks, or artificial markers (fiducial), such as small tacks or screws that are secured in the bone.

Identification and Registration

Following scan acquisition, the 3D image data of the patient's jaw(s) are interpreted by software as anatomic geometric elements. As previously stated, a sufficient number of markers (anatomic or fiducial) must be identified in the patient's mouth to correlate the image data with the patient anatomy. Several devices have been used to capture the actual patient anatomy for registration with the scan data, including a touch pointer and an ultrasound probe. The *touch pointer* allows the operator to touch specific anatomic points (or fiducial markers) while a tracking device "sees" the instrument and records each point of reference. This device is fairly accurate, but if the clinician is not careful, there is a tendency to define points that are not in contact to real surface, thus creating a false mapping. The *ultrasound probe* has a lower accuracy than the touch pointer but has the advantage of being able to capture continuous data of bone morphology through the mucosa or gingiva. Echo quality is subject to variations with the type of penetrated tissue.

Matching between the geometry of the image data with the patient anatomy is called *registration.* Five registration methods are used to compare anatomic points of the preoperative image data and the intraoperative patient anatomy: (1) point-based, (2) line-based or curve-based, (3) surface-based, (4) volume-based, and (5) projective methods. Point-based and line-based methods are described here to illustrate the requirements for an adequate registration.

In the *point-based method* a few particular points are identified in the preoperative image data and the patient anatomy. These can be natural (anatomic points) or artificial (fiducial) markers. In either case, points must be well defined and stable so that they can be precisely measured. The operator can manually click, with a tracking device, on the point in the patient corresponding to the image point. After several points are matched, the computer calculates a transformation equation that minimizes the mean distance between matched points to complete the registration. Three nonaligned points are necessary to obtain a nonambiguous result. The registration accuracy can be predicted, depending on the distribution of points (e.g., an equilateral tripod will give more accurate results than three co-linear points).[7,12]

The most intuitive algorithm may be the *Hough transformation,* in which the most simple geometric invariant, the distances between points, are computed, compared, and used to find a triangle in the preoperative set of points and a triangle in the intraoperative set of points that shares similar edge lengths. The triangle points are then registered using the best-fit algorithm. Once a first estimate of the transformation has been computed, the clinician can apply the transformation to the intraoperative points.

Line-based or curve-based methods are derived from point-based methods but require a few lines or curves to be measured and identified. Artificial lines can be extracted from the CT scan image data and measured intraoperatively by the operator with the tracking device. All lines and surfaces measured on image planning (after segmentation of anatomic structure of the jawbone in the CT scan), and the points taken on the patient anatomy by the tracking device are known as a *set* of points. These sets may be dense or sparse; a segmented bone surface may have hundreds or thousands of points. However, it is not practical to measure hundreds of points.

When the segmented surface is dense, one can assume that almost all points measured with the tracking device will be identified as points of the segmented surface. Thus, algorithms developed for the point-based registration, based on identification of matching between the preoperative and the intraoperative data, can be easily adapted. However, the number of possible errors in the identification process increases dramatically in line-based or curve-based methods.

Navigation and Positional Tracking

Numerous commercial products exist for navigation or positional tracking, but few meet the *computer-aided surgery* (CAS) requirements in terms of accuracy (about 1 mm in one cubic meter), reliability, and clinical usability.

SCIENCE TRANSFER

Successful tooth replacement with dental implants requires very precise placement and alignment of the implant in thee dimensions. Such placement allows for optimal restorative procedures. Intraoperatively, surgeons use their expertise and experience plus any presurgical aides to help with alignment and placement. Particularly useful is a second or third individual who can assist from different angulations during the surgery; for example, the surgeon watches placement from a buccal-lingual direction while an assistant provides guidance in a mesial-distal direction.

Recently, computer-aided implant surgical devices have become available. These devices integrate presurgical diagnostic information and hands-on surgical positioning information and allow for surgical placement by guidance from a computer and positioning/tracking devices. This equipment is becoming more affordable and more accurate and will be increasingly used in the future. Robot-assisted surgical placement of implants is a possible future application of computer-assisted implant surgery (CAIS). At present, however the limitations of accuracy, the complexity, the cost, and documentation of advantages over conventional techniques indicate that CAIS procedures require further development before they can have widespread application.

The "real-time" navigational technology is based on the global positioning system (GPS) technology.[17] Some of the technologies used in medical CAS to track movement include mechanical, magnetic, and optical tracking systems.

Mechanical tracking systems use a six-axis coding robot with a passive arm. The system is very reliable and highly accurate but has limitations when more than one instrument or patient marker needs to be located. Thus, mechanical tracking is less desirable for CAIS, which requires the use of several different instruments and multiple markers.

Magnetic tracking systems use a magnetic source and a field receiver.[13] The system loses accuracy in the presence of magnetic field interference. Relative inaccuracies result from changes in the magnetic field, which may be caused by any metallic mass that may be present, such as a drill motor (with or without activation).[2,3] Thus the obligatory presence of drill motors in the operatory during implant surgery make magnetic trackers impractical for CAIS.

Optical tracking systems are recognized for their dependability and accuracy. Positioning is made by intersecting the vision plane between two or three cameras to locate markers with stereovision. A *passive* system absorbs and processes ambient light, whereas an *active* system interprets reflected light.

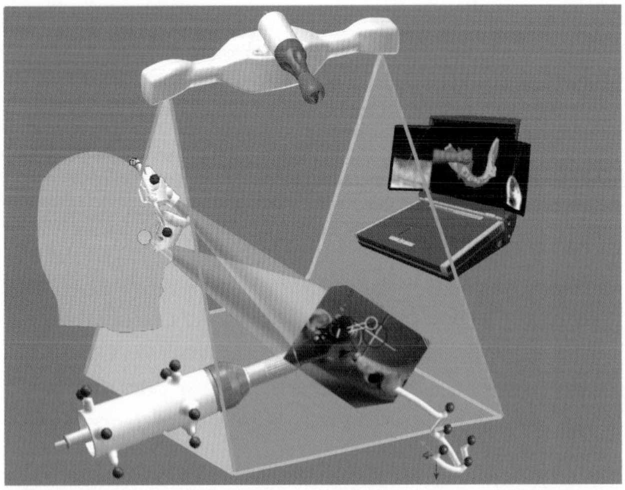

Figure 79-1 Global setup for surgical navigation. The basic setup for a navigation system consists of stereovision cameras (infrared or not) with several tools. Other technologies, such as electromagnetic or ultrasound tracking, are not available or have limited application in dentistry because of a lack of accuracy and dependability. The contra-angle probe, the ultrasound probe (if any), and the patient jig need to have markers, which are tracked by the cameras. The occlusal stent, with markers in the standard process and without markers in ultrasound registration, used during CT scan acquisition will be recognized in its three dimensions for prosthetic planning.

Active markers with infrared light–emitting diodes (IRED) have been widely used with superb accuracy but are sensitive to reflections and interference with the line of sight between the IRED markers and the cameras.[9,11] Although variations in optical localizers are adequate for medical applications,[1,5] they need to be improved for use in dental implant surgery. This is particularly problematic with the typical seating arrangement of surgeon and assistant (i.e., the direct line of sight to the cameras may be interrupted by the operators). A stereovision with natural-light cameras is a less expensive alternative compared with IRED. However, natural-light systems are more sensitive to surrounding light, background, and the shape of markers. In comparison, infrared cameras are less sensitive to these light variations.

With optical tracking devices, the surrounding light in the operatory is important, and a headset light is preferred with a camera sensitive to natural light. Patient motion will be tracked efficiently if the marker is stable during surgery. In case of loose teeth or unstable markers, cortical bone screws should be used.

External Viewer and Augmented Reality

Once registration between the data and the actual patient has been established, the instrumentation can be coordinated with the system and observed by the surgeon/operator (Figures 79-1 and 79-2). Visualization of the

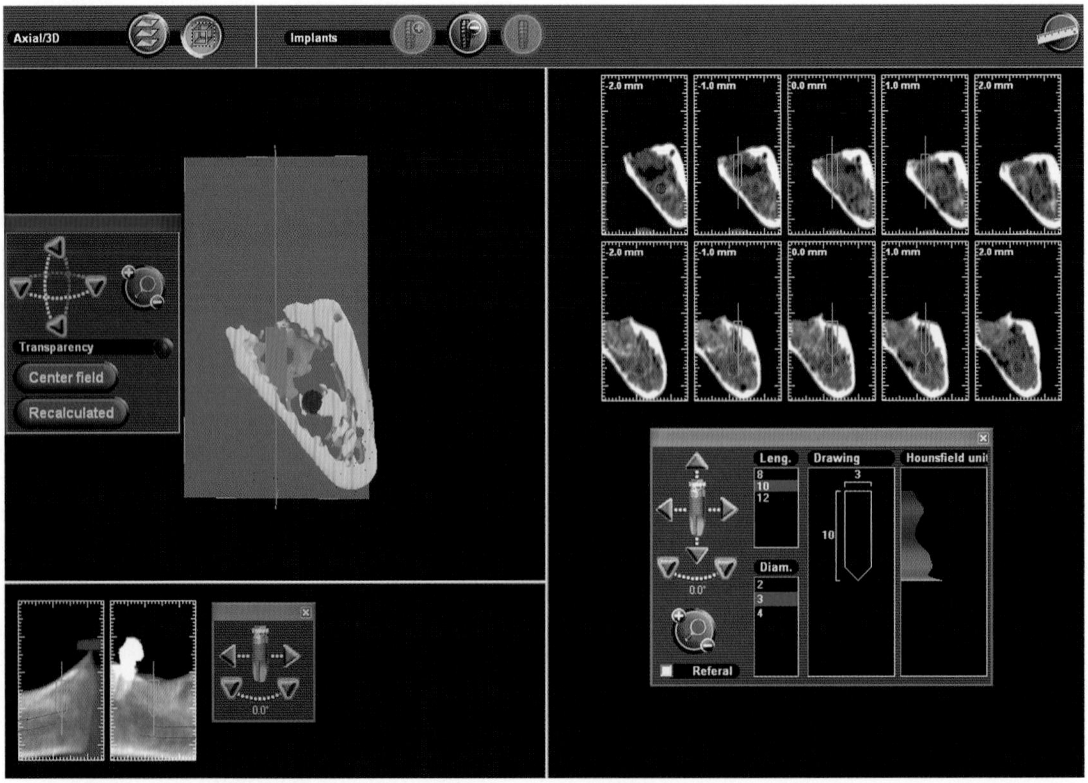

Figure 79-2 Images of computer screen and surgeon's view of CAIS navigation simulated with dry mandible. During navigation, the surgeon will concentrate visual cues seen on the eye viewer and not on the computer screen.

instrument movement relative to the image data (and through registration to the patient) may occur on an external monitor or may be visually projected in the surgeon's field of vision (resulting in a superimposed visual image seen over the surgical field) using a head-mounted projection system.[21] In this manner, the monitor or the projected image device will directly guide the surgeon to perform the planned procedure.

Side viewers display target data in two dimensions and require the surgeon to look away from the surgical field. However, see-through viewers display target data transparently in the surgeon's field of view and allow the operator to observe the surgical field continuously. An *augmented-reality viewer* allows the surgeon to see target data in three dimensions, superimposed over the surgical site through projected images in both eyes.[22] The augmented-reality method allows the operator to adapt to the system more naturally and therefore more rapidly, but there does not appear to be advantages over the use of a two-dimensional (2D) side-viewer devices in terms of accuracy.[18] Both systems allow simultaneous viewing of virtual information of the implant (axis and target) and a real vision of the surgical site. Augmented-reality devices are very sensitive to calibration before surgery and require care and monitoring intraoperatively to prevent misalignment during the surgery. The relative stability of a headset is critical to maintaining accuracy.

Advantages and Disadvantages

Benefits and advantages of computer-assisted implant surgery include the following:

1. CAIS results in improved accuracy and safety.
2. Surgeon validation and expertise are maintained.
3. Security features can stop the rotary instrument in proximity to important structures.
4. Simulation can be visualized before surgery.
5. Implant position can be planned before surgery.
6. Real-time information is provided to the surgeon.
7. Inexperienced surgeons will improve their skill with training.
8. Experienced surgeons can treat more challenging cases with greater comfort and confidence.
9. Surgical time is reduced using a surgical guide.
10. Noninvasive surgery is possible; some cases may be performed with minimal or no flap reflection.

Limitations and disadvantages of CAIS are as follows:

1. Initial cost of the system.
2. Increased installation time for surgery.
3. Training time is mandatory.
4. Accuracy depends on the various components of the system.
5. Inaccurate data (e.g., CT scan, displaced markers) can lead to difficulties in registration.
6. Three anatomic or fiducial markers must be visible.

CONCLUSION

The use of computer-assisted implant surgery with simultaneous tracking and "guidance" of the implant instrumentation facilitates the precise surgical placement of implants with "real-time" visual assessment of anatomic structures. The system is complex, and several steps must be coordinated for CAIS to be accurate and useful.

CAIS systems are expensive and therefore not readily available. Surgeons require training and experience to perform CAIS well. As a result, the more complex or difficult cases may be the most likely types of patients to benefit from the use of CAIS.[17]

REFERENCES

1. Armangué X., Salvi J: Overall view regarding fundamental matrix estimation, *Image Vision Comput* 1:205, 2003.
2. Birkfellner W, Watzinger F, Wanschitz F, et al: Calibration of tracking systems in a surgical environment, *IEEE Trans Med Imaging* 17:737, 1998.
3. Birkfellner W, Watzinger F, Wanschitz F, et al: Systematic distortions in magnetic position digitizers, *Med Phys* 25:2242, 1998.
4. Casap N, Tarazi E, Wexler A, et al: Intraoperative computerized navigation for flapless implant surgery and immediate loading in the edentulous mandible, *Int J Oral Maxillofac Implants* 20:92, 2005.
5. Chassat F, Lavallée S: Experimental protocol of accuracy evaluation of 6D localizers for computer integrated surgery: application for four optical localizers. In Dohi T, Kikinis R, editors: *Medical image computing and computer-assisted intervention,* Proceedings, Part II, MICCAI 2002, 5th International Conference, Tokyo, 2002.
6. Diederichs CG, Engelke WG, Richter B, et al: Must radiation dose for CT of the maxilla and mandible be higher than that for conventional radiography? *Am J Neuroradiol* 17:1758, 1996.
7. Fitzpatrick, West JB, Maurer CR Jr: Predicting error in rigid-body point-based registration, *IEEE Trans Med Imaging* 17:694, 1999.
8. Fortin T, Coudert JL, Champleboux G, et al: computer-assisted dental implant surgery using computed tomography, *J Image Guid Surg* 1:53, 1995.
9. Kai J, Shiomi H, Sasama T, et al: Optical high-precision three-dimensional position measurement system suitable for head motion tracking in frameless stereotactic radiosurgery, *Comput Aided Surg* 3:257, 1998.
10. Klein M, Abrams M: Computer-guided surgery utilizing a computer-milled surgical template, *Pract Proced Aesthet Dent* 13:165, 2001.
11. Malamas E, Petrakis E, et al: A survey of industrial vision systems: applications and tools, *Image Vision Comput* 21:171, 2003.
12. Pennec X, Thirion JP: A framework for uncertainty and validation of 3D registration methods based on points and frames, *Int J Comput Vision* 25:203, 1997.
13. Robert B, Richard B, et al: Accuracy of magnetic tracker for three-dimensional echography, *Innov Technol Biol Med* 20:9, 1999.
14. Roberts DW, Strohbehn JW, Hatch JF, et al: A frameless stereotaxic integration of computerized tomographic imaging and the operating microscope, *J Neurosurg* 65:545, 1986.
15. Sarment DP, Al-Shammari K, Kazor CE: Stereolithographic surgical templates for placement of dental implants in complex cases, *Int J Periodont Restor Dent* 23:287, 2003.
16. Satava RM: Emerging technologies for surgery in the 21st century, *Arch Surg* 134:1197, 1999.
17. Siessegger M: Use of an image-guided navigation system in dental implant surgery in anatomically complex operation sites, *J Craniomaxillofac Surg* 29:276, 2001.

18. Tian X, Ling KV: Magnetic tracker calibration for an augmented reality system for therapy, *Proc Inst Mech Eng* 215:51, 2001.
19. Verstreken K, van Cleynenbreugel J, Marchal G, et al: Computer-assisted planning of oral implant surgery: a three-dimensional approach, *Int J Oral Maxillofac Implants* 11:806, 1996.
20. Verstreken K, van Cleynenbreugel J, Martens K, et al: An image-guided planning system for endosseous oral implants, *IEEE Trans Med Imaging* 17:842, 1998.
21. Wanschitz F, Birkfellner W, Figl M, et al: Computer-enhanced stereoscopic vision in a head-mounted display for oral implant surgery, *Clin Oral Implant Res* 13:610, 2002.
22. Zamorano LJ, Nolte L, Kadi AM, et al: Interactive intra-operative localization using an infrared based system, *Neurol Res* 15:290, 1993.

CHAPTER 80

Biomechanics, Treatment Planning, and Prosthetic Considerations

Ting-Ling Chang, Eleni D. Roumanas, Perry R. Klokkevold, and John Beumer, III

CHAPTER OUTLINE

Clinical research has demonstrated excellent long-term success rates for implant-supported restorations in fully and partially edentulous patients. The predictability and longevity of these results have made dental implant restorations highly desirable and beneficial for patients. Tooth replacement with dental implants not only restores function and esthetics but also improves confidence and self-esteem, resulting in an enhanced quality of life. Appropriate case selection, good occlusal harmony, careful management of hard and soft tissues, and maintenance of good oral hygiene all contribute to the success and predictability of dental implants.

Although "mechanical" failures (implants, components, prosthesis) can be problematic, most of these issues have been resolved with improvements in materials and design of connecting components, as well as better biomechanical planning of cases. At present, the most critical remaining factor that requires consideration in the planning and success of implant-retained restorations is the "biologic" connection between the implants and the patient (i.e., the bone-to-implant contact). The quantity and quality of bone available to support implants in the desired anatomic locations and the ability to maintain the bone-to-implant contact and support under functional loading are essential for success.

After the first year of function, a relatively small amount of bone loss around the neck of (most) dental implants is expected. Subsequently, marginal bone levels stabilize, and very little additional bone loss occurs over years of function. However, if occlusal loads exceed the load-bearing capacity of the supporting alveolar bone, progressive bone loss can result. Ultimately, if bone loss continues to the point of implant failure (loss of osseointegration), the restoration may be lost as well. Thus, adverse or excessive occlusal loading not only can adversely affect the prognosis of individual implants, but also may result in loss of the prosthetic reconstructions. It is important to recognize that excessive occlusal loading is often the result of inadequate engineering (i.e., poor assessment and planning) rather than a sudden increase in occlusal loading. Clinical experience has demonstrated that the most predictable results are achieved when implant restorations are overengineered relative to the anticipated occlusal loads.

This chapter describes important biomechanical considerations and offers treatment-planning guidelines for the use of dental implants in edentulous, partially edentulous, and single-tooth applications. Additional prosthetic considerations that are addressed include connecting implants to teeth, immediate and early loading, and immediate provisionalization.

BIOMECHANICAL CONSIDERATIONS

Osseointegrated dental implants provide a predictable means of replacing missing teeth and restoring dental function. It is now clear that a thorough understanding of implant biomechanics is essential if implant-retained restorations are to be employed predictably. The load-bearing capacity of implants supporting the restoration must be greater than the anticipated loads during function. If the loads applied exceed load-bearing capacity of the implants, the prosthesis, or the supporting bone, implant overload may result in mechanical or biologic failure. In the case of *mechanical failure,* screws that secure the restoration may bend, loosen, or fracture. The most devastating type of mechanical failure is fracture of the implant. In the case of *biologic failure,* a resorption-remodeling response of the bone around the implant(s) is provoked, leading to progressive bone loss.[3,11] In some cases, bone loss around the implant progresses until the implant is no longer supported and osseointegration is lost.

The function and support of dental restorations by endosseous implants are quite different from similar restorations supported by the natural dentition. Teeth are suspended within the supporting alveolar bone by the periodontal ligament, which allows slight physiologic "movement" of teeth in function. If forces are excessive, teeth have the capacity to adjust or move in response to the applied forces. As long as inflammatory periodontal disease is controlled, teeth will adapt to these forces without appreciable bone loss. The controlled orthodontic movement of teeth through alveolar bone is an example of the capacity of teeth to adapt to excessive applied forces. As orthodontic forces move a tooth, new bone begins to form in its path as a result of tension applied to the bone by the "attached" periodontal ligament fibers.

Osseointegrated dental implants, by definition, are in direct contact with the alveolar bone without intervening soft tissues (i.e., there is no periodontal ligament).[2] Together, the implant(s) and prosthesis are rigidly connected with the jawbone, and no movement (relative to the jawbone) is possible. Any movement of a dental implant is indicative of failure or loss of osseointegration (e.g., fibrous encapsulation). As a result of this rigid relationship, the dental implant(s), the attached implant-retained restoration, and the surrounding bone are not forgiving or adaptive to adverse or excessive forces. If occlusal loads exceed the tolerance of the implant(s), the connecting component(s), the attached prosthesis, or the supporting bone to withstand the stress, then fatigue, fracture, or failure will ensue. Successful implant treatment planning requires a good understanding of the biomechanics, an appropriate assessment of the load-bearing capacity, and an adequate engineering plan to maintain osseointegration with resistance to the anticipated occlusal loads.

Load-Bearing Capacity

Several factors affect the load-bearing capacity of implant-retained prostheses, including the number, arrangement, size (length and width), and angulation (in relation to the plane of occlusion) of the implants used to support the restoration.[17] In addition to these "mechanical" issues, the quantity and quality of bone support around the dental implants will also influence their load-bearing capacity with respect to the "biologic" support and resistance to occlusal loading (Box 80-1).

The *bone appositional index* (percentage of bone-to-implant contact) may be the most important factor to consider when evaluating the load-bearing capacity. The lower the bone-to-implant contact and the lower the bone density surrounding the implants, the lower will be the support of the implants and the resistance to occlusal loading. As an example, consider the bone support of implants in the posterior maxilla; the bone quality is particularly poor compared with the anterior mandible. In the posterior maxilla the trabecular bone is less dense and the cortical bone layer is thin. As a result, the bone appositional index in the posterior maxilla is significantly less than what can be achieved in the anterior mandible, where the trabecular bone is typically denser with a thick cortical bone layer. The bone appositional index for implants in the posterior maxilla typically ranges from 30% to –60%, whereas the bone appositional index for implants placed in the anterior mandible typically ranges from 65% to 90%. Figure 80-1 illustrates the bone appositional index in poor-quality, trabecular bone of the posterior maxilla compared with better-quality, dense cortical bone of the anterior mandible.

BOX 80-1

Implant Biomechanics

Load-Bearing Capacity

Implant
- Number
- Length
- Arrangement
- Angulation

Quality of bone-implant interference

Anticipated Load (affected by)

Occlusal factors

Cusp angles

Width of occlusal table

Guidance type
- Anterior guidance
- Group function

Cantilever Forces

Connection to natural dentition

Size of occlusal table
- Buccal-lingual dimension
- Mesial-distal dimension

Cantilevered extensions

Parafunctional Habits

Chronic bruxism

Clenching habit

Grinding habit

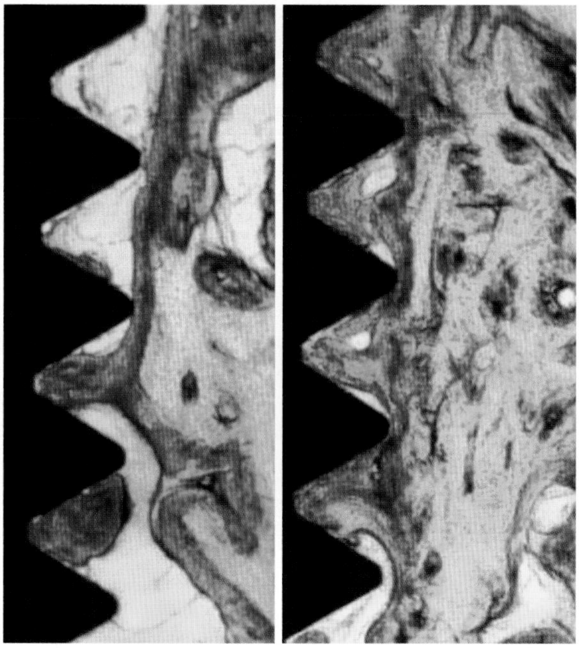

Figure 80-1 Bone quality influences the load-bearing capacity. In these histologic images obtained with light microscopy, note the difference in bone appositional index achieved in **A,** poor-quality bone, often found in the posterior maxilla, versus **B,** dense bone, typical of the anterior mandible.

Anatomic structures and a lack of bone height in the posterior mandible and maxilla limit the amount of available bone for placement of long implants and thus reduce the potential for bone-to-implant contact. In the lower jaw the inferior alveolar nerve and vessels travel through the body of the mandible until exiting the mental foramen in the premolar region. The location of the neurovascular bundle and resorption of the alveolar ridge limit the height of bone available for placement of long implants. Lateral nerve repositioning is possible but has a moderately high morbidity rate; therefore this technique is not advised. In the upper jaw, pneumatization of the maxillary sinus combined with loss of alveolar bone results in a decreased total height of available bone in the posterior maxilla, which limits the lengths of implants that can be used and thus reduces the bone appositional index and the load-carrying capacity of implants placed in this region. Sinus floor elevation and bone augmentation procedures have enabled clinicians to increase the height of bone available in the posterior maxilla, allowing for the placement of longer implants with improved success. Recent studies have suggested that implants with an altered microtopography (e.g., acid etched) can achieve a greater bone-to-implant contact in poor-quality bone (e.g., trabecular bone of posterior maxilla) than implants with a machined surface.[20,34]

The number of implants used obviously affects load-bearing capacity. In the 1980s and early 1990s, many posterior quadrants of the maxilla were restored with one or two implants, and in some patients, two implants were used to support restorations with three or four dental units. In many cases, soon after loading, a distinct pattern of bone loss was observed that led to loss of the implants in many patients (Figure 80-2). Additional implants significantly improve the biomechanics of these implant-supported fixed partial dentures. Currently, it is imperative to "engineer" the treatment of posterior segments with one implant for every missing tooth that will be restored. Furthermore, if space (and available bone) permits, it is desirable to use a minimum of three implants to replace missing posterior teeth in the maxilla. The same rule (one implant for every missing tooth being restored) applies to replacing teeth with implants in the posterior mandible. However, greater bone density (i.e., thickness of cortical bone) in the posterior mandible often permits the use of fewer implants.

Linear Configurations and Implant Overload

Both the angulation and the arrangement of implants used to retain and support prostheses can influence the load-bearing capacity of the system (implants, components, prosthesis, bone). When implants are arranged in a linear fashion, the biomechanics with respect to anticipated bone response are quite unfavorable compared with a configuration where the implants are arranged in a nonlinear (curvilinear or staggered) fashion. Arranging implants in a *nonlinear* manner creates a more stable base that is more resistant to the torquing forces created by off-center contacts and lateral loads (Figure 80-3). This is particularly true when loads are *not* applied along the long axis of the implant. In the 1980s, conventional dogma stated that once an implant became "osseointegrated," it did not matter whether occlusal loads were applied axially. However, as more clinical follow-up data and animal research data become available, it is increasingly apparent that in some clinical situations—namely, implant-supported fixed partial dentures restoring posterior quadrants—nonaxial loads can cause sufficient load magnification at the bone-to-implant interface, resulting in bone resorption and higher rates of implant failure. This concept is supported by numerous finite element analysis (FEA) studies, which clearly demonstrate that nonaxial forces significantly increase the stress concentration to the cortical bone around the neck of the implant[1,4,26,36] (Figure 80-4).

Nonaxial loads can lead to implant overload (through load magnification), which in turn precipitates a resorptive remodeling response of the bone around the neck of the implants. When loads persist, the bone loss progresses and can lead to implant failure. With regard to the biologic mechanisms initiated in bone when an implant is overloaded, Brunski et al.[3] proposed that excessive occlusal loads lead to microdamage (fractures, cracks, delamination) of the bone adjacent to the implant, which provokes a resorptive remodeling response. The bone remodeling at the implant surface results in less bone density adjacent to the implant (especially around the coronal aspect of the implant). Probably because of a lack of tension on the bone adjacent to the implants (no periodontal ligament fiber attachment), bone adjacent to the implant has a poor capacity for repair. Thus, a vicious cycle ensues in which continued excessive loading leads

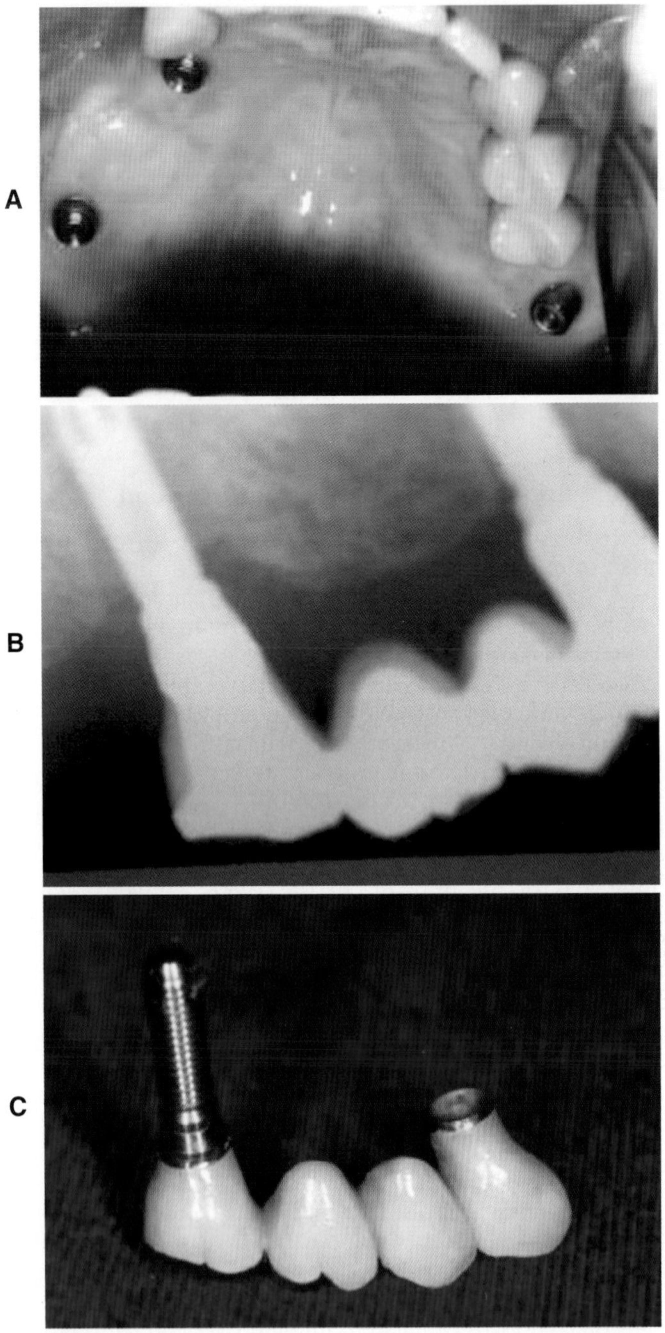

Figure 80-2 Four-unit fixed partial denture in the posterior maxilla supported by only two implants. **A,** Clinical photograph of implant abutments in posterior maxilla. Notice the long span between the two implants. **B,** Radiograph taken 30 months after restoration. Note bone loss around the distal implant. **C,** Failed distal implant attached to failed prosthesis. The biologic failure (distal implant) resulted in a long-span cantilever on the other (anterior) implant that ultimately led to its' mechanical failure (i.e., screw fracture).

to more microdamage and progressive bone loss until the implant fails (Box 80-2).

Linear implant configurations in the posterior mandible and posterior maxilla are particularly prone to bone loss when loads are not applied axially. Bone loss in posterior areas can be more damaging because implants

BOX 80-2

Implant Overload and Bone Resorption: Proposed Mechanisms of Implant Failure

- Excessive occlusal loads.
- Load resulting in microdamage: fractures, cracks, and delaminations.
- Resorption-remodeling response of bone.
- Loss of bone at the bone-to-implant interface as a result of remodeling.
- Vicious cycle of continued loading, additional microdamage, and bone loss progressing to implant failure.

Modified from Brunski J, Puelo D, Nanci A: *Int J Oral Maxillofac Implants* 15, 2000.

in these areas are primarily supported by the cortical bone around the most coronal aspect of the implant. This is particularly true for the posterior maxilla. The cortical bone is sometimes very thin, and unless the implant is positioned to engage the superior cortical bone (floor of maxillary sinus), the apical aspect of the implant is usually poorly supported by loose trabecular bone. Therefore the authors believe that every attempt should be made surgically to position posterior implants so that occlusal forces can be directed down the long axis of the implant (i.e., axial loads). When implants are perpendicular to the occlusal plane, occlusal forces can be directed down the long axis of the implant, which is tolerated better than nonaxial forces. In addition, the restoration is simpler and more cost effective to fabricate when angled or custom abutments are not required.

An extreme example of the damage that can result from nonaxial occlusal forces is observed in the posterior, implant-supported restoration with a cantilevered pontic. Before the use of sinus bone augmentation, implants were placed as far posterior as possible. The available bone, anterior to the maxillary sinus, frequently limited the position of the posterior implant to the bicuspid area. To restore first molar occlusion, a cantilevered pontic was added distal to the last implant. Subsequent occlusal forces directed to the pontic created torquing forces around the implant adjacent to the cantilever. As a result, load magnification caused bone loss around the neck of the implant closest to the cantilever (Figure 80-5). For this reason, cantilevered pontics (mesial or distal) are contraindicated for unilateral posterior, implant-supported restorations.

The *angulation* of implants in relation to the plane of occlusion and the direction of the occlusal load is also an important factor in optimizing the transfer of occlusal forces to implants used to restore posterior quadrants in partially edentulous patients. In the 1980s, before the use of the sinus floor elevation and bone augmentation procedures, many implants placed in the posterior maxilla exhibited excessive buccal angulations or resulted in restorations with buccal cantilevers. In addition, some implants placed in the posterior mandible presented with

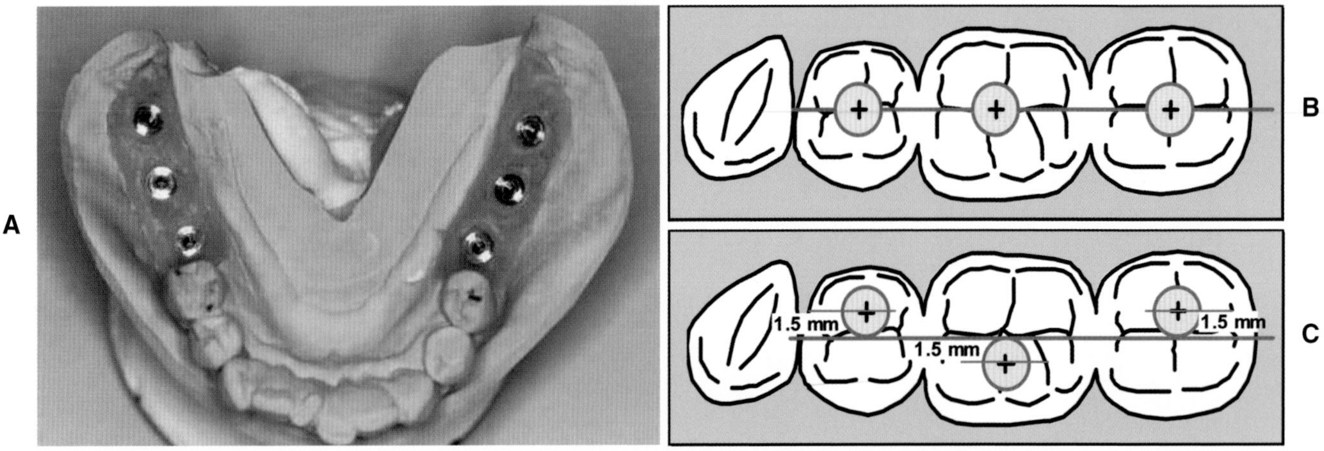

Figure 80-3 **A,** Study model and diagrams illustrating **B,** linear arrangement of posterior implants compared with **C,** a staggered arrangement. The nonlinear or staggered arrangement, if possible, provides better resistance to rotation with buccal-lingual forces.

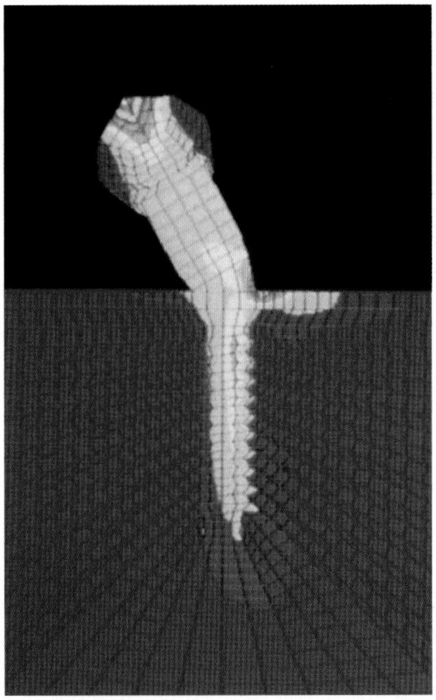

Figure 80-4 Nonaxial loads result in load magnification. Using finite element analysis, Cho and co-workers demonstrated that nonaxial loads concentrated stresses around the neck of the implant. (Courtesy Dr. In Ho Cho.)

excessive distal angulations. A high percentage of such implants exhibited signs of implant overload (i.e., progressive and irreversible bone loss around neck of implant adjacent to cantilever) after delivery of the prosthesis (Figure 80-6).

Minor discrepancies in angulation are probably not clinically significant, but if loads are at an angle of 20 degrees or more to the long axis of the implant, load magnification can result in some patients, provoking a resorptive remodeling response of the adjacent bone. The combination of short implants improperly positioned and angled in poor-quality bone makes implants prone to overload.

TREATMENT PLANNING WITH DENTAL IMPLANTS

The success of implant-retained restorations is measured not only by successful osseointegration but also by the lack of problems associated with the implants, components, prosthesis, and supporting bone. Implant complications (e.g., screw loosening, screw fracture) and implant failures (e.g., severe bone loss, loss of integration) have taught dental clinicians that the "engineering" of implant support for prosthetic appliances is essential for proper treatment planning and the key to the ultimate success of implant-retained restorations. Treatment planning with dental implants in the edentulous or partially edentulous patient must take these biomechanical issues into consideration to minimize failures and complications.

Edentulous Maxilla

Although a conventional denture is satisfactory for many patients with an edentulous maxilla, implants provide support and stability that may be desirable in some situations, including but not limited to the following:

1. There is poor ridge form, and the conventional maxillary denture is marginally stable. Two or four implants will provide greater stability and security of a maxillary denture in function when the maxillary ridge is severely resorbed and lacks resistance to lateral forces.
2. The patient has an intact mandibular anterior dentition but lacks posterior support. Implants in the maxilla can offset the potentially destructive effects on the premaxillary region when a mandible with natural anterior teeth and missing posterior teeth opposes an edentulous maxilla. In this situation the lack of posterior support leads to a condition often referred to as "combination syndrome," in which

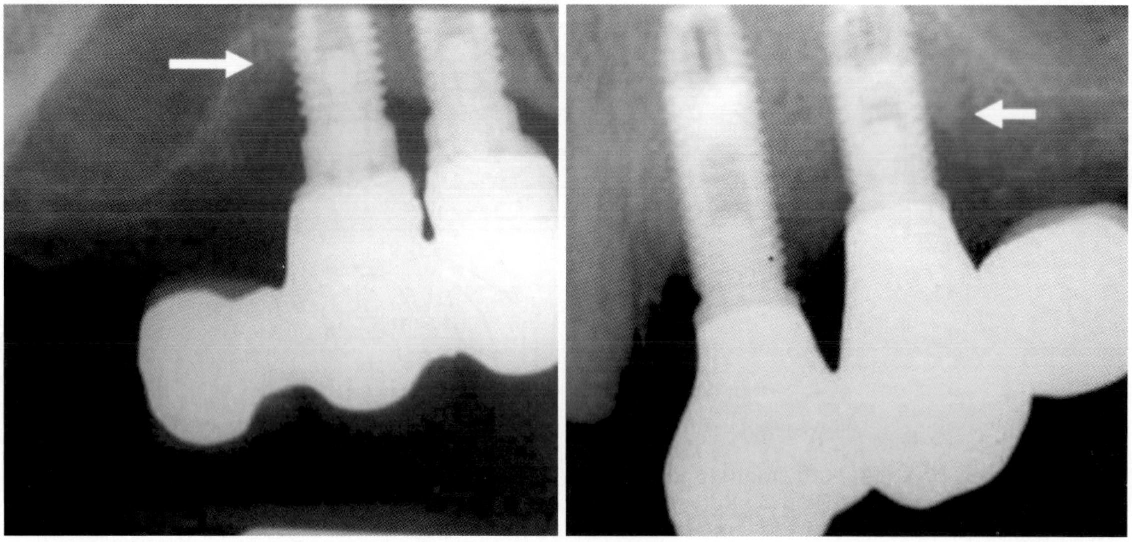

Figure 80-5 Cantilevers in posterior quadrants of partially edentulous patients should be avoided. These radiographs demonstrate two cases of bone loss *(arrows)* around the neck of short implants (closest to the cantilever) where load magnification occurs.

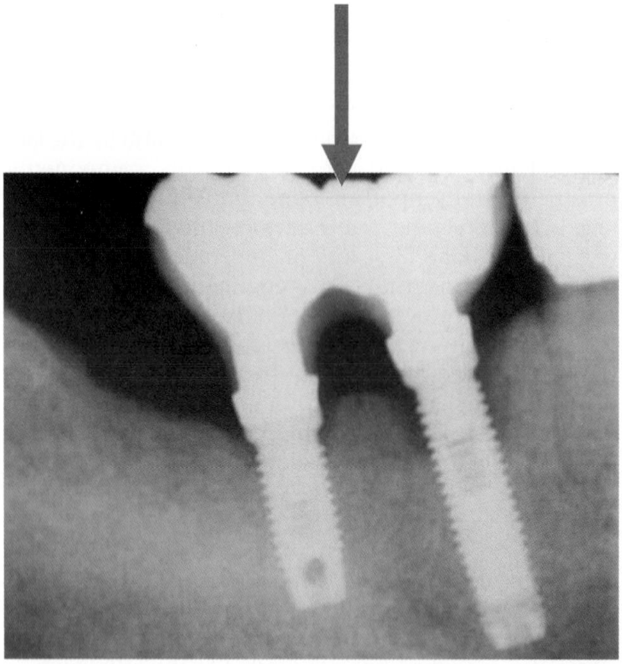

Figure 80-6 Because of the curve of Spee and the distal angulation of these implants (posterior mandible), the occlusal loads *(arrow)* are nonaxial. The nonaxial loading results in implant overload and bone loss around the neck of both implants.

overclosure of the anterior teeth causes destruction of the anterior maxilla.

3. The patient cannot tolerate palatal coverage. Some patients prefer a palateless denture, which may enhance their sensations of taste and texture or may simply provide a psychologic advantage. Some patients prefer a palateless denture because proximity of the denture with the soft palate induces a gag reflex. Patients with large palatal tori can also benefit from a palateless maxillary denture. A minimum of four implants with adequate *anterior-posterior* (A-P) *spread* allows the fabrication of an implant-assisted overdenture without palatal coverage.

The design of maxillary implant-retained prostheses is greatly influenced by the anatomic limitations of the maxilla. Most notably, the maxillary sinus limits the height of bone available for implant placement in the posterior region. As a result, the A-P spread achieved is often limited (Figure 80-7). If the A-P spread is inadequate to provide support, a full-palatal-coverage overlay denture is recommended.

The four-implant–assisted, palateless overlay denture ideally addresses the needs of most patients (Figure 80-8). Many patients who are edentulous in the maxilla have lost a significant amount of structure in the premaxillary region because of alveolar ridge resorption after tooth loss and prosthetic replacement. As a result, adequate support for the upper lip is lacking. Thus, in most patients, it is advisable to construct an implant-assisted maxillary overdenture (i.e., not an implant-supported fixed prosthesis) unless an unusual amount of alveolar bone is present. The usual resorption pattern of the alveolus places the gingival margin of a fixed restoration too far superiorly, too far palatally, or both. Even if the patient has a low smile line, a lack of lip support just beneath the nose can be unsightly with fixed prostheses. Most patients are best served with an implant-assisted overlay denture. Lower cost, improved hygiene access, and predictable speech articulation are additional benefits that favor the use of an overlay denture in the edentulous maxilla over an implant-supported fixed prosthesis.

Edentulous Mandible

A mandibular complete denture is more problematic for patients than a maxillary complete denture, especially for

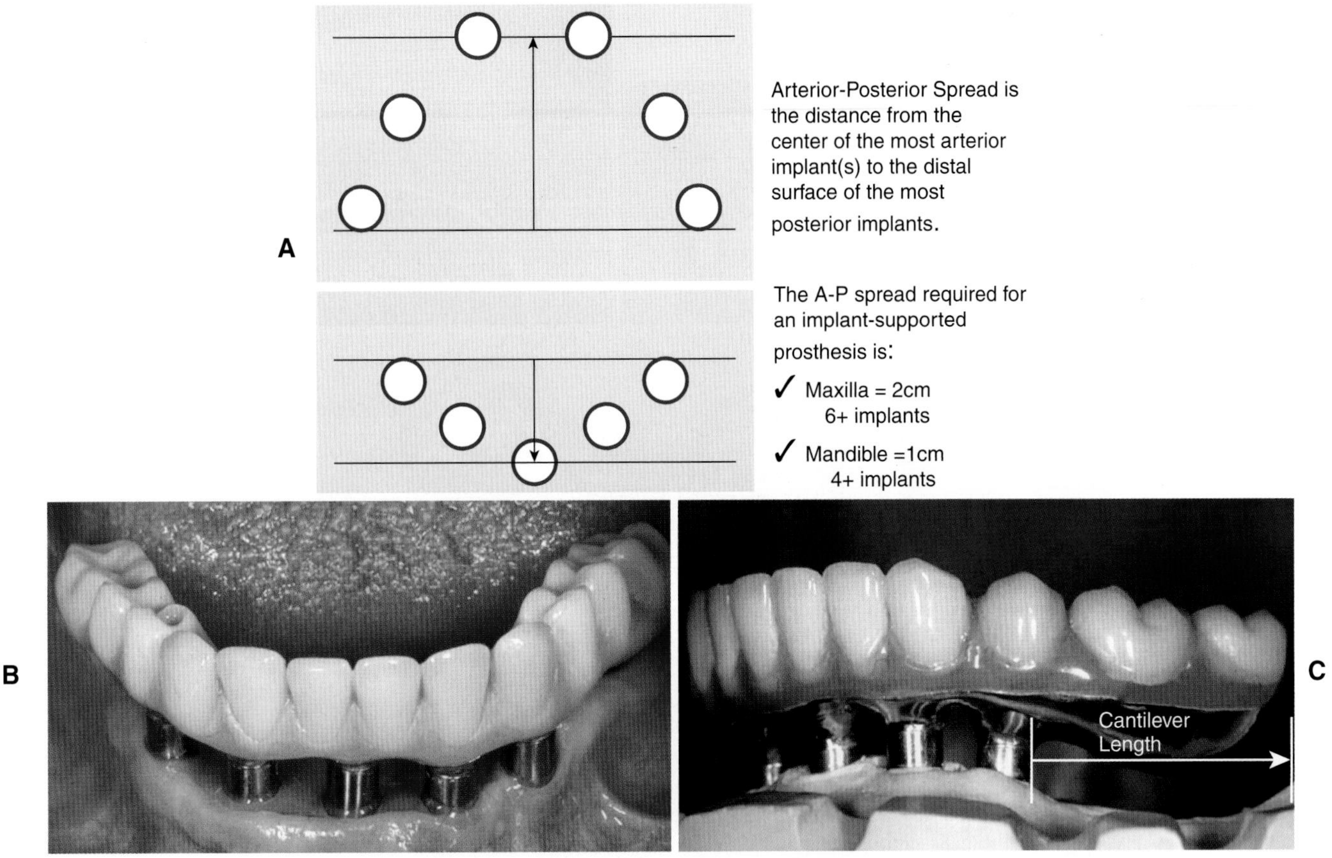

A
Arterior-Posterior Spread is the distance from the center of the most arterior implant(s) to the distal surface of the most posterior implants.
The A-P spread required for an implant-supported prosthesis is:
✓ Maxilla = 2cm
6+ implants
✓ Mandible =1cm
4+ implants
B
C
Cantilever Length

Figure 80-7 Anterior-posterior spread of implants. **A,** Diagram demonstrating anterior-posterior (A-P) implant spread (i.e., the distance from the middle of the anterior implant to the posterior edge of the most posterior implants). **B,** Clinical view of an implant-supported restoration replacing mandibular teeth. Notice that the restoration is supported by five implants in the anterior and has cantilever extensions in the posterior segments. **C,** Study model view of similar mandibular implant-supported restoration with posterior cantilever extensions. Cantilever length should not exceed twice the A-P spread.

SCIENCE TRANSFER

Restoration of missing teeth with dental implants involves consideration of the number of implants, their location, and their length and diameter. Much has been written about these topics, but little research has been performed. Consequently, many recommendations are empiric or based on operator experience. Also, experiences change as implant systems evolve. In the past, for example, single implants of the Brånemark design, when used to replace a mandibular molar, would occasionally break. This experience resulted in the recommendation to use two implants in these sites for better distribution of the occlusal load. Similarly, if three implants of the same design were placed in the posterior aspect in a straight line, clinicians observed screw, abutment, and implant complications. These experiences resulted in the placement of these implants using the phenomenon of "tripodization," or offsetting the middle implant. At present, however, the implant materials and connections have changed, with fewer complications, and such recommendations are less frequently made. More research is needed on the occlusal loading and tolerance of implant restorations.

Biomechanical considerations are the basis for determining the number of implants to be used, the size of each implant, the position of implants, and the optimal occlusal scheme. In general, it is wise to use at least three implants to replace missing posterior segments in the maxilla, with a guideline of one implant for each missing tooth. The more dense bone of the posterior mandible often permits the use of as few as two implants. It is advisable to use implants at least 10 mm long where possible and to position implants so they are loaded axially. Cantilevered pontics add to the biomechanical stress on the adjacent implant, so they are generally contraindicated for unilateral, posterior, implant-supported restorations. Connecting implant-supported prostheses to natural teeth should be avoided.

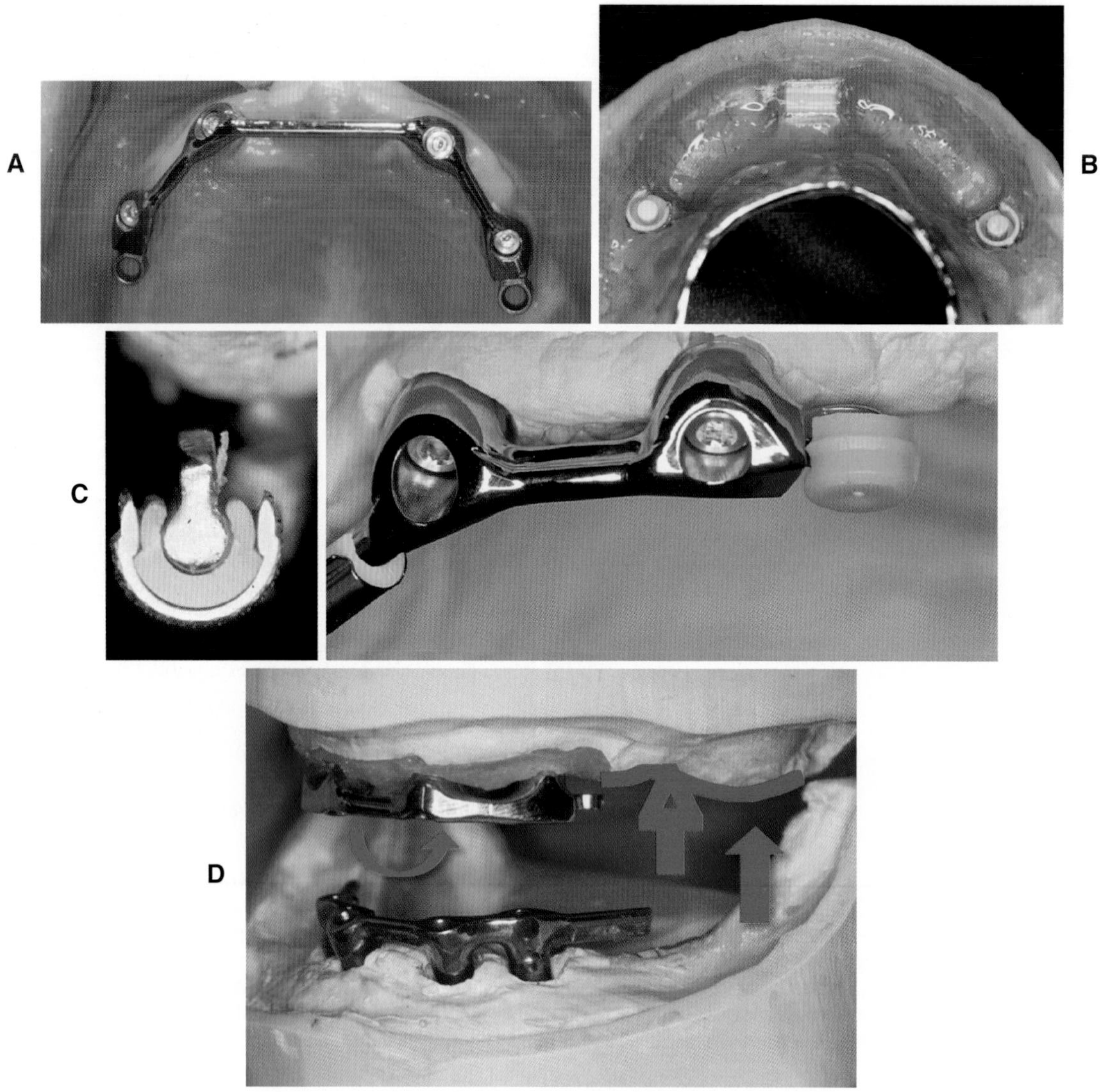

Figure 80-8 Implant-assisted overlay denture. **A,** Clinical photograph of four-implant bar in the maxilla designed to retain a palateless overlay denture. **B,** Photograph of clip and attachment design of palateless overlay denture. Anterior Hader clip attaches to anterior bar and posterior ERAs (Extra-coronal Resilient Attachment) attach to female connectors at posterior ends of the bar. **C,** Cross-section of Hader bar clip attached to anterior bar (inset). View of overdenture bar with Hader clip (left) and ERA (right) attached. These plastic components will be embedded in the overdenture as in (B). **D,** Axis of rotation and function of resilient attachment. When posterior occlusal forces *(solid vertical arrow)* are applied, the denture rotates around the bar clip anteriorly *(curved arrow)*, and resilient attachment *(arrow)* allows the denture to be compressed to primary denture-support areas posteriorly *(open arrow).*

patients with a severely resorbed (atrophic) mandibular ridge. The lack of stability and retention makes it very diffi-cult for patients to control the denture. In this situation, implants offer unprecedented stability and retention. The two-implant–assisted overdenture is now the treatment of choice for patients with an atrophic, edentulous mandible.

Implant-assisted dentures are designed so that most of the masticatory load is borne by the primary denture-support areas (retromolar pad, buccal shelf). The implants provide additional stability and retention while bearing little occlusal load. A common practice is to place two implants in the anterior mandible with a connecting bar. One or two clips retain the denture over the bar. When occlusal forces are applied, the denture rotates around the bar (anterior axis of rotation) and depresses slightly in the posterior aspect, directing the forces to the primary denture-bearing areas (Figure 80-9). Individual attachments secured to each implant offer a simple prosthetic solution (Figure 80-10). If this prosthodontic option is chosen, however, the implants must be parallel to one another to facilitate a proper path of insertion and to minimize stress during prosthetic seating and function.

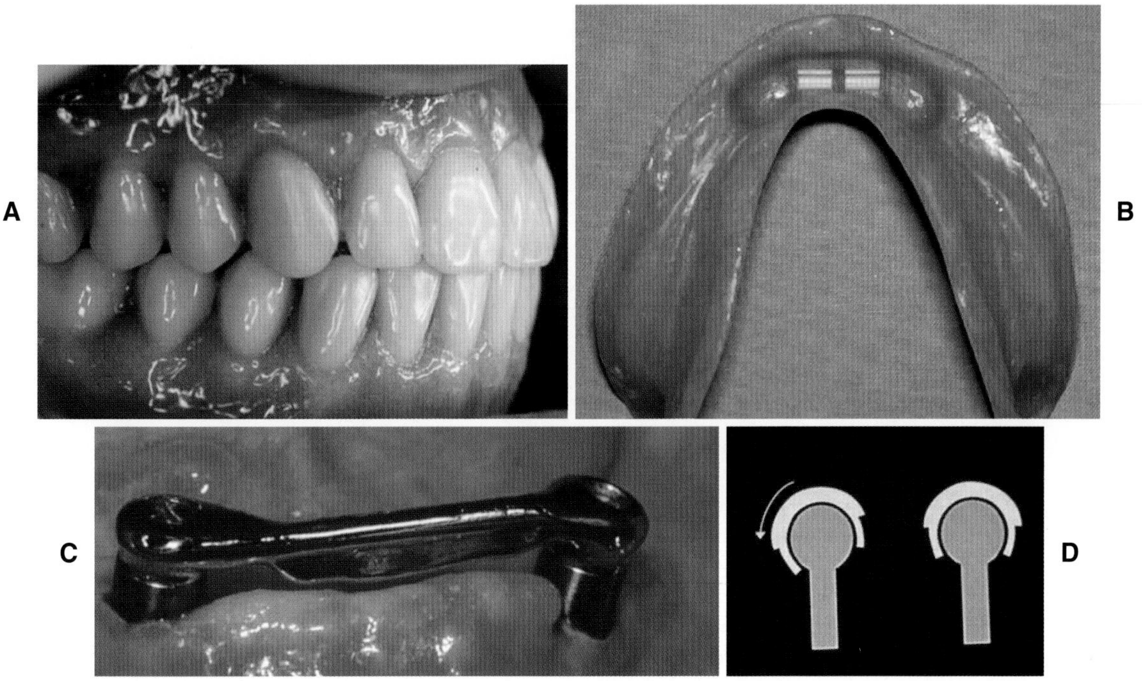

Figure 80-9 Implant-assisted overlay denture. **A,** Clinical view of overdenture in occlusion. **B,** Photograph of mandibular overlay denture (tissue-bearing surface) designed for an implant bar attached to two implants in the anterior mandible. Two Hader clips are embedded in the anterior acrylic. **C,** Clinical view of bar attached to two implants in the anterior mandible. **D,** Illustration demonstrating how axis of rotation allows denture to rotate around the bar. When the patient applies occlusal force posteriorly, the overlay denture rotates around the bar, and the load is absorbed by primary denture-bearing surfaces posteriorly.

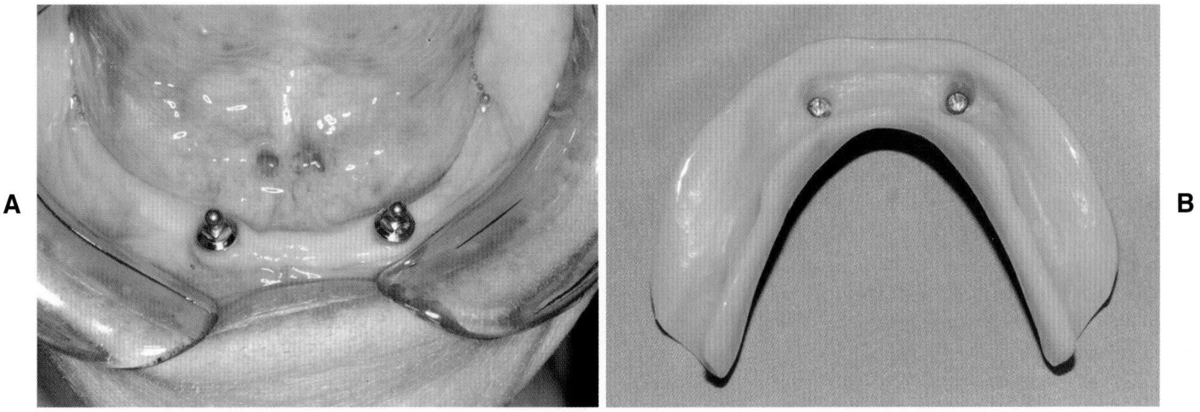

Figure 80-10 Individual attachments can be used on each implant to assist in retention of the mandibular overdenture. **A,** Clinical view of anterior mandible with individual ball attachments on two implants. **B,** Tissue-bearing surface of mandibular overdenture showing individual female attachments embedded in the denture. (Courtesy Dr. Sal Esposito, Beachwood, Ohio.)

Implant-assisted overlay dentures are most often employed to restore edentulous patients. Fixed, implant-supported prostheses require four, five, or six implants arranged in an appropriate arc of curvature with at least 1 cm of A-P spread. In this situation the fixed prosthesis can be fabricated with distal extension cantilevers up to half the A-P spread provided it does not exceed 10 mm (Figure 80-11). Many patients prefer this option for psychologic reasons, but the mastication efficiency provided by this prosthesis is only slightly better than that provided by an implant-assisted overlay denture. Evidence suggests that such fixed restorations tend to stop resorption of the body of the posterior mandible and in some cases enable regeneration of the bone in this region.[18]

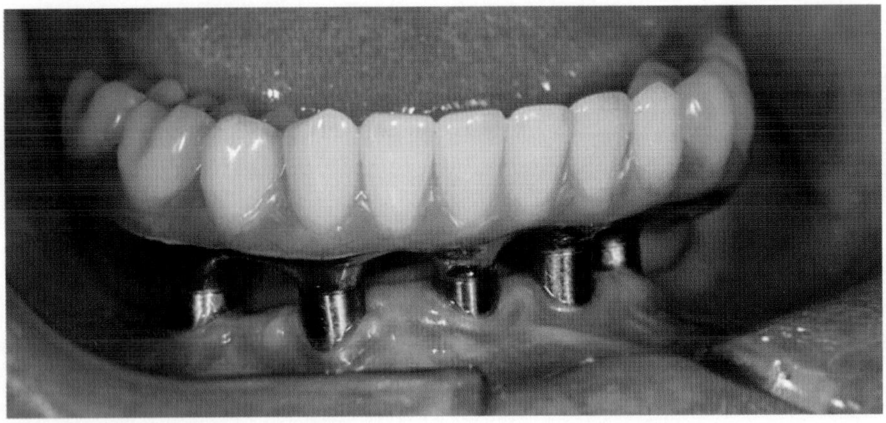

Figure 80-11 Implant-supported full-arch denture prosthesis fabricated from denture teeth and acrylic resin with a nonprecious metal support structure.

Partially Edentulous Patients

Multiunit Restorations in Posterior Quadrants

The lowest success rates for implants have consistently been reported for short-span (segmental) restorations in the posterior maxilla.[12] Anatomic limitations may prevent placement of implants of adequate length in the posterior quadrants. In the posterior quadrants of the maxilla, the maxillary sinus limits the lengths used, and in the mandible the inferior alveolar nerve limits the lengths of the implants used. Also in the posterior quadrants of the maxilla, the bone-implant interface or the bone anchorage for osseointegrated implants is compromised because the bone quality is poor. Primary anchorage for an implant placed in this region is provided by the implant engaging the cortical bone of the floor of the sinus and the cortical bone on the alveolar ridge. There is generally minimal bone-implant interface along the course of the implant. The use of implants with rougher surfaces may improve the bone anchorage in poor-quality bone but still may not provide all patients with sufficient anchorage to support unilateral, implant-supported, fixed partial dentures if the implants are too short (<10 mm in length).

The new, rough implant surfaces appear to have a significant effect on bone anchorage and therefore biomechanics.[17,19,22] The acid-etched surfaces, in particular, appear to achieve higher bone appositional indices than the machined surfaces initially introduced in the 1980s and appear to facilitate the biologic processes of bone formation, resulting in greater deposition of bone onto the surface of the implant (Figure 80-12). In addition, bone deposited on the surface of acid-etched implants appears to be harder and denser and may be more resistant to resorptive remodeling.[32]

Because many patients possess insufficient bone in the posterior maxilla to receive an implant of suitable length, bone augmentation of the alveolar ridge or maxillary sinus has been suggested.[24] Free bone grafts taken from intraoral (e.g., ramus, chin) or extraoral (e.g., iliac crest, fibula) sites, often mixed with bone substitutes, are now being used to supplement the existing bone at these sites.[33] Vertical augmentation of the alveolar ridge has not been predictable, but the "sinus lift and graft procedure" appears predictable and has achieved wide acceptance.[14,35]

In the posterior mandible the limiting factor with respect to implant placement is the presence of the inferior alveolar nerve. Based on clinical experience, the authors believe that the minimum length for implants used to restore posterior mandibular quadrants, regardless of implant width, is 10 mm. In general, the use of short implants (<10 mm) for posterior, implant-supported restorations is discouraged.

Single-Tooth Implants in Posterior Quadrants

Standard-diameter implants have been used to restore single-tooth defects in the posterior quadrants of the maxilla and mandible with mixed results. Solitary implants restoring maxillary molars have had unpredictable results, whereas single implants used to restore mandibular molars have had a better prognosis. In the 1980s, clinicians attempted to restore mandibular first molar sites with conventional implants 3.75 or 4.0 mm in diameter. Unfortunately, the results were quite disappointing. In some patients, occlusal overload led to loss of bone around the implant, and implant fixtures fractured in other patients; however, these occurrences were rare.

The most common problem observed, particularly when external hex-headed implants were used, was loosening of the screw retaining the restoration. This problem results because the diameter of the head of the implant is much smaller than the size of the occlusal surface. Tipping of the restoration during function eventually leads to stretching and loosening of the screw securing the crown to the implant fixture. The buccal-lingual width of the crown can be controlled, and this dimension should be kept to a minimum. However, clinicians do not have control over the mesial-distal dimension because this space must be filled. When the bolus of food becomes positioned on the mesial or distal side of the crown, tipping forces are generated that eventually lead to loosening of the screw retaining the crown. If hex-headed implants are used, the use of wide-diameter implants resolves the screw-loosening complication

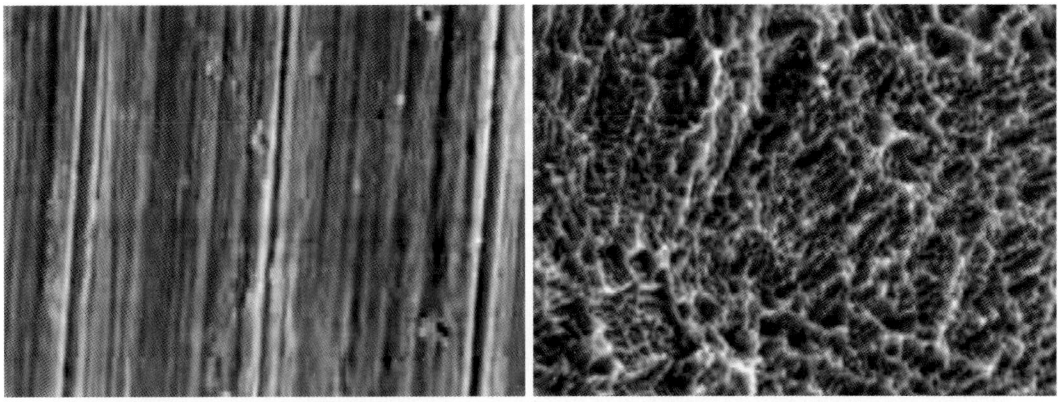

Figure 80-12 SEM comparison of machined and acid-etched surfaces. **A,** Machined surface has the characteristic grooved pattern. **B,** Acid-etched surface (Osseotite) has a characteristic porous pattern consisting of peaks and valleys. This surface appears to facilitate bone formation, leading to improved bone-to-implant contact. (Courtesy Implant Innovations, Inc., Palm Beach Gardens, Fla.)

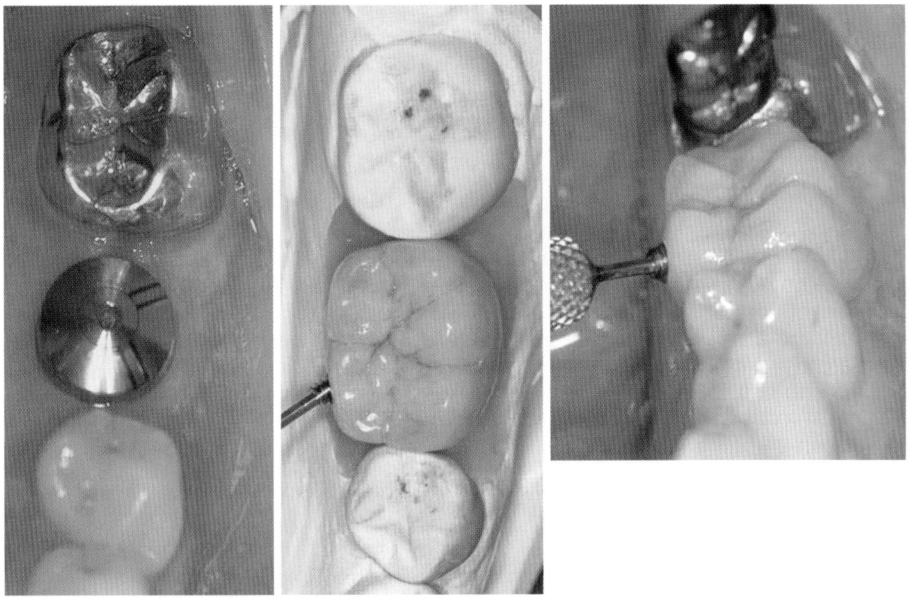

Figure 80-13 Single-tooth restoration in the posterior mandible supported by a wide diameter implant. **A,** Clinical photograph of healing abutment on wide-diameter implant. **B,** Photograph of laboratory model with single molar. **C,** Clinical photograph of molar crown supported by wide-diameter implant. The use of wide-diameter (external hex) implants eliminates the problem of screw loosening for single-tooth, posterior, implant-supported crowns. NOTE: This crown is secured to the abutment via a lingual set screw (small hex driver seen attaching set screw).

(Figure 80-13). The larger platform reduces the potential for tipping forces to stretch or break the screw.

If the first molar is lost and suitable abutments are present, a conventional three-unit, fixed partial denture is still a viable option, especially if the adjacent teeth already have large restorations. However, if adjacent teeth have small or no restorations, it is preferable and more conservative to replace the missing single tooth with an implant. This restoration is cost effective and predictable in compliant patients. In distal extension areas when restoring one molar tooth, the authors recommend that two conventionally sized implants be placed close together. This restoration is biomechanically sound and can be designed to allow adequate hygiene access (Figure 80-14).

Single implants can be used with a high rate of success in the premolar area. The bone-implant interface achieved in this area is good, and the size of the occlusal surface is generally small. Although similar considerations exist regarding screw loosening for single-implant restorations in the premolar region, these concerns are less because of a more anterior position (lesser forces) and typically better bone quantity and quality compared with more

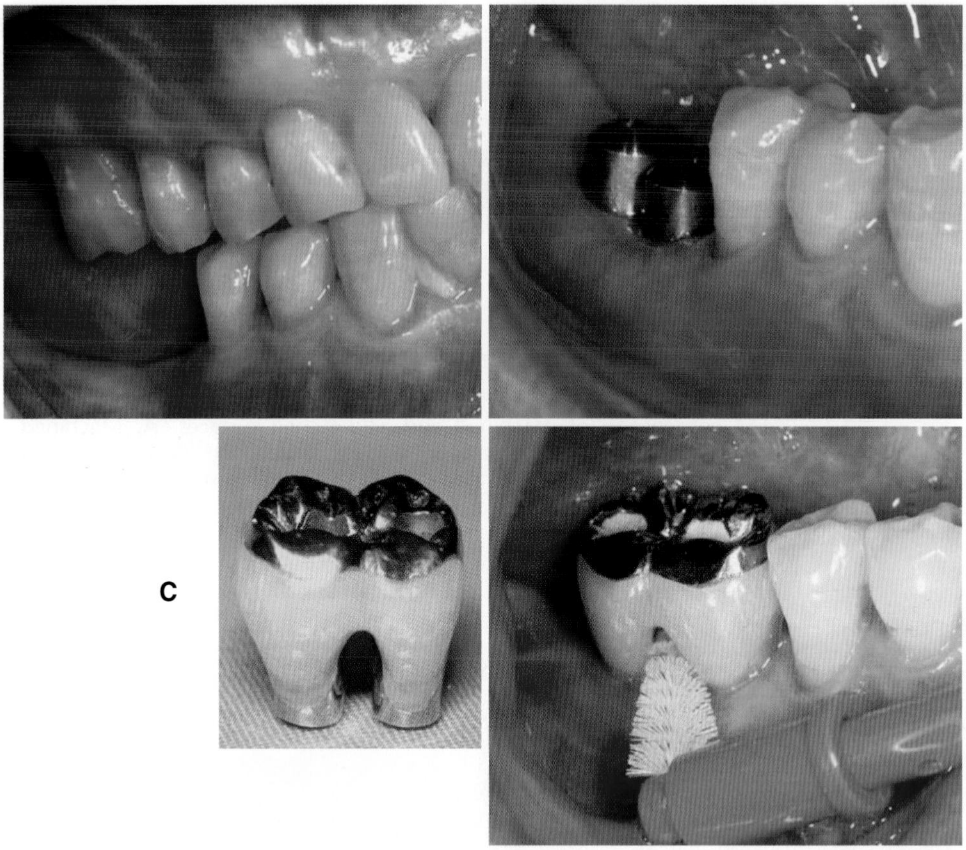

Figure 80-14 Single-tooth restoration in the posterior mandible in a distal extension defect supported by two implants. **A,** Clinical view of mandibular right edentulous area. **B,** Clinical view of healing abutments on two implants placed in right mandibular molar area. Two standard-diameter (4-mm) implants are used to replace the last mandibular tooth in the arch (first molar). **C,** Photograph of final restoration. Notice that restoration is designed similar to two splinted premolars with adequate space for cleaning between the implants. **D,** Clinical view of final restoration on implants. Access for a proxybrush is provided by open embrasure space between the two implants.

BOX 80-3

Strategies to Avoid Implant Overload*

1. Place implants perpendicular to the occlusal plane. (Note that the occlusal plane is not flat [i.e., curve of Wilson, curve of Spee].)
2. Place implants in tooth positions.
3. When in doubt, always add a third implant.
4. Avoid the use of cantilevers in linear configurations.
5. Avoid connecting implants to teeth.
6. If it is necessary to connect to the natural dentition, use a rigid attachment system.
7. Control occlusal factors (i.e., cusp angles and width of occlusal table).
8. Restore anterior guidance if possible.
9. Avoid the use of short implants (<10 mm).

*These strategies are used to avoid implant overload in the posterior quadrants of partially edentulous patients. When these conditions cannot be met, removable partial dentures are recommended.

posterior regions. The use of implants that are 10 mm or longer is still advised.

CLINICAL STRATEGIES TO AVOID IMPLANT OVERLOAD AND OTHER PROSTHETIC CONSIDERATIONS

Clinically, the risk of implant overload can also be minimized by limiting the width of the occlusal table of the implant-supported fixed partial denture, flattening the cusp angles, avoiding the use of cantilevered restorations, and restoring the anterior guidance provided by the residual anterior dentition. Box 80-3 lists strategies to avoid implant overload. Multiunit implant restorations should be splinted to maximize implant support (sharing the loads), and emergence profiles should be developed with open embrasure spaces to facilitate oral hygiene (Figure 80-15).

The use of cantilevered implant-supported restorations (i.e., unilateral, linear configurations) in posterior quadrants of the mandible or maxilla is strongly discouraged. Cantilever extensions result in load magnification and

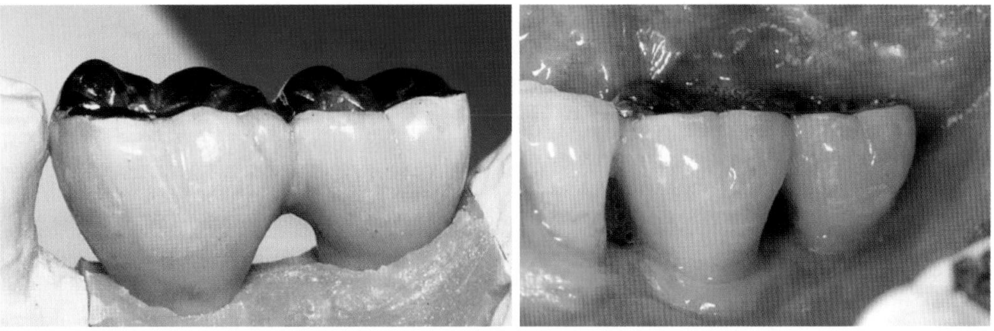

Figure 80-15 Guidelines for restoring posterior quadrants. Embrasures should be large enough for access with a proxybrush. The occlusal table must be narrow, cusp angles flattened, and proper emergence profiles developed. Anterior guidance should be restored with the natural dentition whenever possible. **A,** Laboratory model and **B,** clinical photograph of two-unit, fixed partial denture supported by two implants in the posterior mandible demonstrate these qualities.

can cause overloading of the implant next to the cantilever extension, which in turn may lead to bone loss and implant failure (see Figure 80-5).

Connecting Implants to Natural Dentition

In general, the authors advocate keeping implant-supported restorations separate from natural teeth (i.e., do not connect implant-supported restorations to teeth). As stated previously, implants and teeth function differently, and connecting them can lead to complications such as screw loosening and intrusion of natural dentition. Since teeth have the capacity to move under functional occlusal loads and implants do not, connecting implants to teeth with a fixed restoration results in a cantilever effect on the implant. In addition, designing the restoration so that it is independent of the natural dentition simplifies the biomechanics.

However, there are rare exceptions and situations that warrant connection of implants to teeth. In these cases, the authors recommend that implants be connected to the natural dentition in a rigid manner, either with screw-retained attachments or with copings secured by permanent cement. In making the case for such rigid connections, Gulbransen[10] showed that if implants are connected to the natural dentition with a rigid system of attachment, the implant failure and complication rates (e.g., screw loosening) were dramatically reduced. It appears that the intrusion problem (and other complications) is increased when implants and natural teeth are connected with "nonrigid" and "semirigid" attachments. In addition, the well-documented phenomenon of intrusion of the natural tooth abutment associated with the use of semiprecision attachments is prevented.

Immediate or Early Loading in Posterior Quadrants

Immediate or early loading may be feasible when implants are placed in good-quality bone (e.g., anterior mandible) and are used to retain implant-assisted overlay dentures. However, when implants are placed in posterior quadrants of partially edentulous patients where the bone sites are less dense and all the occlusal loads are borne by the implants, immediate or early loading is inadvisable.

BOX 80-4

Biologic Processes in Implant Anchorage*

- Blood clot
- Angiogenesis
- Osteoprogenitor cell migration
- Woven bone formation
- Deposition of lamellar bone
- Secondary remodeling of woven bone with lamellar bone

*These biologic processes need to be completed before an implant is firmly anchored in bone. This process takes about 4 months in humans.

Immediate or early loading of osseointegrated implants is generally not recommended when implants are used to restore posterior quadrant defects in partially edentulous patients. When an implant is placed into bone, the initial bone anchorage is not very good, and if it is loaded, the implant may become mobile and fail to osseointegrate. If an implant moves during the early stages of healing, a fibrous connective tissue capsule develops around the body of the implant. The initial biologic processes and bone remodeling needed to complete the first remodeling cycle of bone around an implant require an estimated 4 months in humans (Box 80-4). Some evidence suggests that implants with acid-etched surfaces resulting in a specific surface morphology may lead to the expression of specific genes that promote more rapid healing of the bone around implants.[24,25] However, these animal studies are yet to be confirmed by human follow-up studies.

CONCLUSION

In the early years (1980s) of treating patients with osseointegrated dental implants, we underestimated the importance of biomechanics and the limitations of the systems that we created (i.e., the bone-implant-connector-restoration). As in the natural dentition, we believed that multiunit fixed bridges could be supported by as few as two implants. Through clinical experience, research, and failures, we have learned to appreciate the importance of biomechanics and its role in the predictability and success of implant-retained prosthetics. A revised approach to treatment planning now must be applied when using dental implants because of the rigid nature of implant-retained restorations. Biomechanical considerations and the potential for implant overload must be assessed and factored into the decision-making process and treatment-planning guidelines for the use of dental implants in fully and partially edentulous patients.

If the clinician follows the strategies to avoid implant overload (see Box 80-3) and also places implants in tooth positions, (1) proper emergence profiles can be developed, (2) space is available in interproximal areas for hygienic access, (3) the clinician has better control over the occlusal anatomy (narrowed occlusal table and flat cusp angles), (4) occlusal loads are delivered axially, and (5) abutment selection is simplified.

REFERENCES

1. Akca K, Iplikcioglu H: Evaluation of the effect of the residual bone angulation on implant-supported fixed prosthesis in mandibular posterior edentulism. Part II. 3-D finite element stress analysis, *Implant Dent* 10:238, 2001.
2. Brånemark PI, Hansson BO, Adell R, et al: Osseointegrated implants in the treatment of the edentulous jaw: experience from a 10-year period, *Scand J Plast Reconstr Surg Suppl* 16:1, 1977.
3. Brunski J, Puelo D, Nanci A: Biomaterials and biomechanics of oral and maxillofacial implants: current status and future developments, *Int J Oral Maxillofac Implants* 15, 2000.
4. Canay S, Hersek N, Akpinar I, Asik Z: Comparison of stress distribution around vertical and angled implants with finite-element analysis, *Quintessence Int* 27:591, 1996.
5. Davis H: Neurologic complications in implant surgery. In American Association of Oral and Maxillofacial Surgeons: *1992 Clinical Congress: study guide,* 1992, p 42.
6. Davis H, Rydevik B, Lundborg S, et al: Mobilization of the inferior alveolar nerve to allow placement of osseointegrated fixtures. In Worthington P, Brånemark PI, editors: *Advanced osseointegration surgery applications in the maxillofacial region,* Chicago, 1992, Quintessence.
7. De Bruyn H, Collaert B: The effect of making an early implant failure, *Clin Oral Implant Res* 5:260, 1994.
8. Ehrenfeld N, Roser M, Altenmuller E: Transposition of the inferior alveolar nerve in pre-prosthetic surgery. In *Proceedings of the 6th International Congress of Pre-Prosthetic Surgery,* Palm Springs, Calif, 1995.
9. Garrett NR, Kapur KK, Hasse AL, Dent RJ: Veterans Administrations Cooperative Dental Implant Study. Comparisons between fixed partial dentures supported by blade vent implants and removable partial dentures. Part V. Comparisons of pretreatment and post-treatment dietary intakes, *J Prosthet Dent* 77:153, 1997.
10. Gulbransen H: Personal communication (unpublished data), 1995.
11. Hoshaw S, Brunski J, Cochran C: Mechanical loading of Brånemark implants affects interfacial bone modeling and remodeling, *Int J Oral Maxillofac Implants* 9:345, 1994.
12. Jemt T, Lekholm U, Adell R: Osseointegrated implants in the treatment of partially edentulous patients: a preliminary study of 876 consecutively placed fixtures, *Int J Oral Maxillofac Implants* 4:211, 1989.
13. Jensen O, Nock D: Inferior alveolar nerve repositioning in conjunction with placement of osseointegrated implants: a case report, *Oral Surg Oral Med Oral Path Oral Radiol* 63:263, 1987.
14. Jensen OT, Shulman LB, Block MS, Iacono VJ: Report of the Sinus Consensus Conference of 1996, *Int J Oral Maxillofac Implants* 13(suppl):11, 1998.
15. Kapur KK: Veterans Administrations Cooperative Dental Implant Study. Comparisons between fixed partial dentures supported by blade vent implants and removable partial dentures. Part III. Comparison of masticatory scores between two treatment modalities, *J Prosthet Dent* 65:272, 1991.
16. Kapur KK: Veterans Administrations Cooperative Dental Implant Study. Comparisons between fixed partial dentures supported by blade vent implants and removable partial dentures. Part IV. Comparisons of patient satisfaction between two treatment modalities, *J Prosthet Dent* 66:517, 1991.
17. Kinni ME, Hokama SN, Caputo AA: Force transfer by osseointegration implant devices, *Int J Oral Maxillofac Implants* 2:11, 1987.
18. Klokkevold PR, Nishimura RD, Adachi M, Caputo A: Osseointegration enhanced by chemical etching of the titanium surface: a torque removal study in the rabbit, *Clin Oral Implant Res* 8:442, 1997.
19. Klokkevold PR, Johnson P, Dadgostari S, et al: Early endosseous integration enhanced by dual acid etching of titanium: a torque removal study in the rabbit, *Clin Oral Implant Res* 12:350, 2001.
20. Lazzara RJ, Testori T, Trisi P, Porter SS, Weinstein RL: A human histologic analysis of osseotite and machined surfaces using implants with 2 opposing surfaces, *Int J Periodont Restor Dent* 19:117, 1999.
21. Lindquist LW, Rockler B, Carlsson GE: Bone resorption around fixtures in edentulous patients treated with mandibular fixed tissue-integrated prostheses, *J Prosthet Dent* 59:59, 1988.
22. Ogawa T, Nishimura I: Different bone integration profiles of turned and acid-etched implants associated with modulated expression of extracellular matrix genes, *Int J Oral Maxillofac Implants* 18:200, 2003.
23. Ogawa T, Sukotjo C, Nishimura I: Modulated bone matrix-related gene expression is associated with differences in interfacial strength of different implant surface roughness, *J Prosthodont* 11:241, 2002.
24. Ogawa T, Ozawa S, Shih JH, et al: Biomechanical evaluation of osseous implants having different surface topographies, *J Dent Res* 79:1857, 2000.
25. Ogawa T, Nishimura I: Different bone integration profiles of turned and acid-etched implants associated with modulated expression of extracellular matrix genes, *Int J Oral Maxillofac Implants* 18:200, 2003.
26. O'Mahony A, Bowles Q, Woolsey G, et al: Stress distribution in the single-unit osseointegrated dental implant: finite element analyses of axial and off-axial loading, *Implant Dent* 9:207, 2000.
27. Rangert B, Jemt T, Jorneus L: Forces and moments on Brånemark implants, *Int J Oral Maxillofac Implants* 4:241, 1989.
28. Rangert B, Sullivan R, Jemt T: Load factor control for implants in the posterior partially edentulous segment, *Int J Oral Maxillofac Implants* 12:360, 1997.
29. Rangert B, Krogh P, Langer B, et al: Bending overload and implant fracture: a retrospective clinical analysis, *Int J Oral Maxillofac Implants* 10:326, 1995.

30. Richter E: In vivo vertical forces on implant, *Int J Oral Maxillofac Implants* 10:99, 1995.
31. Simion M, Jovanovic SA, Trisi P, et al: Vertical ridge augmentation around dental implants using a membrane technique and bone auto or allografts in humans, *Int J Periodont Restor Dent* 18:9, 1998.
32. Takeuchi K, Saruwatari L, Nakamura HK, et al: Enhanced intrinsic biomechanical properties of osteoblastic mineralized tissue on roughened titanium surface, *J Biomed Mater Res A* 72:296, 2005..
33. Tolman D: Reconstructive procedures with endosseous implants in grafted bone: a review of the literature, *Int J Oral Maxillofac Implants* 10:275, 1995.
34. Trisi P, Lazzara R, Rebaudi A, et al: Bone-implant contact on machined and dual acid-etched surfaces after 2 months of healing in the human maxilla, *J Periodontol* 74:945, 2003.
35. Wallace SS, Froum SJ: Effect of maxillary sinus augmentation on the survival of endosseous dental implants: a systematic review, *Ann Periodontol* 8:328, 2003.
36. Watanabe F, Hata Y, Komatsu S, et al: Finite element analysis of the influence of implant inclination, loading position, and load direction on stress distribution, *Odontology* 91:31, 2003.

Implant-Related Complications and Failures

Perry R. Klokkevold

81

CHAPTER

CHAPTER OUTLINE

Patients have experienced much success with endosseous dental implants.[2,14,45] Despite the long-term predictability of implants, however, biologic, technical, and esthetic complications do occur in a percentage of cases.[1,3,12] Some complications are relatively minor and easy to correct, but others result in loss of implants and failure of prostheses.

Biologic complications and failures are those that involve the periimplant supporting hard and soft tissues. Changes in the periimplant soft tissues may be minor, such as inflammation and proliferation, or more significant, involving progressive bone loss. The ultimate biologic complication is implant loss or failure. Biologic loss of implants may be caused by a lack of osseointegration in the early stages before restoration or by a loss of osseointegration as a result of bone loss after the restoration is installed and functioning.

Technical complications and failures typically occur in the form of material failure, such as abutment and prosthetic screw loosening or fractures. The patient can recover from many of these mechanical problems if they are minor and recognized early. However, some technical complications are not salvageable, such as implant fractures.

Esthetic complications arise when patient expectations are not met. Patient satisfaction with the esthetic outcome of the implant prosthesis will vary from patient to patient depending on several factors. The risk for esthetic complications is increased for patients with high esthetic expectations and less-than-optimal patient-related factors (e.g., bone quantity and quality).

Finally, there are also risks involved in the surgical procedures used for implant site development, implant placement, and implant exposure. *Surgical* complications are those problems or adverse outcomes that result from surgery.

This chapter reviews several of the more common implant-related complications. A summary of findings from literature reviews on the subject is presented to offer some insight into the prevalence of technical and biologic complications. Implant failure is also discussed.

DEFINITION OF IMPLANT SUCCESS

Implant success (or failure) is reported in many ways. Case reports, case series, retrospective studies, controlled studies, and prospective studies all report levels of success and failure as related to the population being evaluated.

Each type of report or study has recognized limitations, but more importantly, tremendous variation exists in the way individual investigators measure and interpret success. At times, outcomes are measured simply by the presence or absence of the implant(s) at the time of the last examination. In contrast to this simplified assessment, some investigators use detailed criteria to measure success and failure, with variations of successful outcomes separated and defined by additional criteria. Criteria for success and failure have been defined over the years, but not all investigators use them. Sometimes these criteria are used as proposed, and at other times they are modified. Other investigators create new criteria. Thus, it is difficult to make comparisons between studies and often impossible to make absolute conclusions about any aspect of success or failure based on one or a few studies.

SCIENCE TRANSFER

Implant success rates are often reported in the high-90% range. This number reflects a very predictable procedure, but not a procedure that is always (100%) successful. *Thus, complications and failures do occur, and for the patient with the failure, the failure rate is 100%.* Complications and failures can become significant in terms of time, energy, and cost for both the patient and the dentist. Virtually all aspects of implant therapy have had reported problems, and many of these problems occurred more often in the past. New materials, designs, and techniques, as well as operator knowledge and experience, have contributed to the decrease in complications. As with all procedures, accurate and reasonable expectations are necessary for implant procedures, as is adequate informed consent. Thorough treatment planning, diagnosis, and evaluation, combined with excellent communication among the patient, surgeons, restorative dentist, and laboratory technicians, can be crucial to successful tooth replacement using endosseous dental implants.

Complications following fixed prosthetic implant therapy include fracture of veneers, loss of screw hole restoration, screw fractures, and less frequently, implant fracture. For single crowns the most common complication is screw loosening, with reports of recurrence ranging from 2% to 45%. Failures related to loss of osseointegration are more common in the posterior maxilla.

Neurosensory disturbances can be avoided by careful treatment planning and the use of accurate three-dimensional radiographs; damage to adjacent teeth can be similarly prevented. Placement of implants in the esthetic zone requires elaborate presurgical planning, precise surgical techniques using stents as guides, and appropriate soft tissue management.

If one considers "success" as the outcome without any adverse effects or problems, "implant success" should be defined as any implant-retained restoration in which (1) the original treatment plan is performed as intended without complications, (2) all implants that were placed remain stable and functioning without problems, (3) peri-implant hard and soft tissues are healthy, and (4) both the patient and the treating clinician(s) are pleased with the results. When these strict criteria are used, implant success (i.e., absence of complications) is projected to be only about 61%.[61]

"Implant survival," on the other hand, is simply defined as any implant that remains in place at the time of evaluation, regardless of any untoward signs, symptoms, or history of problems. Clearly, there is a difference between implants that are present and functioning under an implant-retained restoration and implants that are present but not connected to any restoration (not functioning). These latter implants are sometimes referred to as "sleepers" and should not be considered successful merely because they are present and remain osseointegrated. Rather, these sleeper implants should be included in the discussion as "surviving" but counted as "failures" because they failed to fulfill the originally intended treatment.

TYPES AND PREVALENCE OF IMPLANT COMPLICATIONS

The prevalence of implant-related complications has been reported in several reviews. In a systematic review of reports on the survival and complication rates of implant-supported fixed partial dentures (FPDs), Pjetursson et al.[61] found that the most common technical complication was fracture of veneers (13.2% after 5 years), followed by loss of the screw access hole restoration (8.2% after 5 years), abutment/occlusal screw loosening (5.8% after 5 years), and abutment/occlusal screw fracture (1.5% after 5 years; 2.5% after 10 years). Fracture of implants occurred infrequently (0.4% after 5 years; 1.8% after 10 years).

In a literature review that included all types of implant-retained prostheses, Goodacre et al.[22] found that the most common technical complications were loosening of the overdenture retentive mechanism (33%), resin veneer fracture with FPDs (22%), overdentures needing to be relined (19%), and overdenture clip/attachment fracture (16%). Their review, with the inclusion of edentulous patients having overdentures, seemed to indicate a significantly higher percentage of complications than Pjetursson's systematic review[61] of patients with implant-supported FPDs. Goodacre et al.[23] found it impossible to calculate an overall prosthesis complication rate because most studies included in their review did not report on several of the complication categories.

The most common complication reported for single crowns was abutment or prosthesis screw loosening. Abutment screw loosening varied dramatically from one study to another, ranging from 2% to 45%.[22] The highest rate of abutment screw loosening was associated with single crowns, followed by overdentures. The rate of prosthesis screw loosening was similar, ranging from 1% to 38% in various studies. A higher frequency was reported

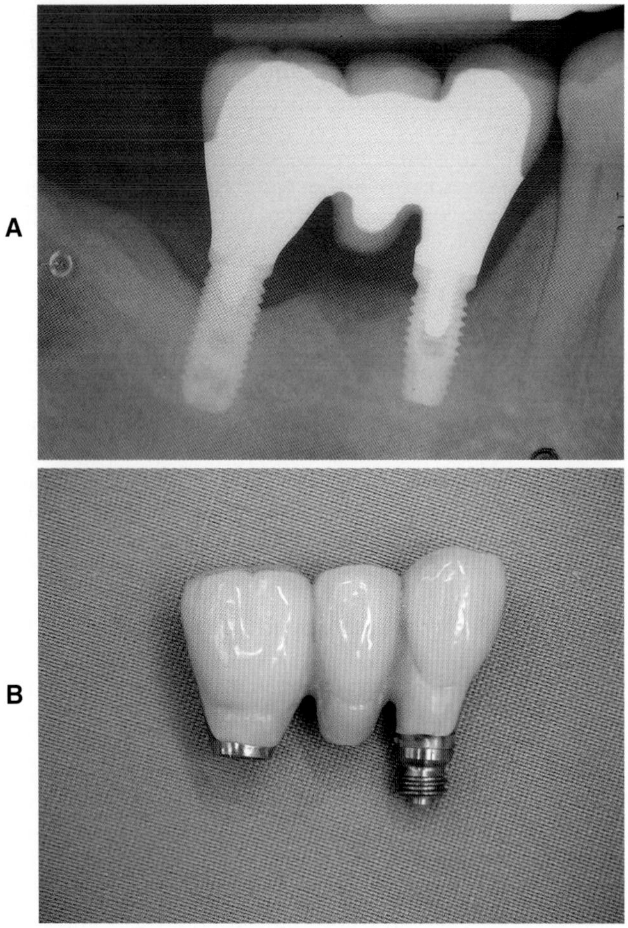

Figure 81-1 **A,** Radiograph of three-unit, posterior, fixed partial denture supported by two standard-diameter, screw-shaped threaded implants. Notice long crown height, relatively short implant length, and bone loss around posterior implant. **B,** Photograph of the ultimate implant-supported restoration failure. The anterior implant fractured between the second and third threads, which resulted in loss of the restoration.

for single crowns in the posterior areas (premolar and molar) than in the anterior region.

Implant fracture is an uncommon but significant complication. Goodacre et al.[23] reported a 1.5% incidence in their literature review.[3] The incidence of implant fracture was higher in FPDs supported by only two implants. Consistent with this finding, Rangert et al.[68] reported that most fractured implants occurred in single- and double-implant–supported restorations. They also indicated that most of these fractures were in posterior partially edentulous segments, where the generated occlusal forces can be greater, as opposed to anterior segments (Figure 81-1).

In a systematic review of prospective longitudinal studies (minimum of 5 years) reporting both biologic and technical complications associated with implant therapy (all restoration types included), Berglundh et al.[8] found that the incidence of technical complications was consistent with Pjetursson's findings, with implant fracture occurring in less than 1% (0.08%-0.74%) of cases. Interestingly, consistent with the findings in Goodacre's review, technical complications were higher for implants used in overdenture therapy than implants supporting fixed prostheses.

In Pjetursson's systematic review[61] of survival and complication rates for implant-supported FPDs, biologic complications such as periimplantitis and soft tissue lesions occurred in 8.6% of implant-supported FPDs after 5 years. A critical review of the literature by Esposito et al.[18] included 73 publications reporting early and late failures of Brånemark implants; biologically related implant failures were relatively low at 7.7%. The treatments involved all anatomic areas and all types of prosthetic design. The authors concluded that the predictability of implant treatment was especially good for partially edentulous patients compared with totally edentulous patients, with failures in the latter population twice as high as in the former. Also, the incidence of implant failure was three times higher for the edentulous maxilla than for the edentulous mandible, whereas failure rates for the partially edentulous maxilla were similar to those for the partially edentulous mandible.

SURGICAL COMPLICATIONS

As with any surgical procedure, there are risks involved with implant surgery. Proper precautions must be taken to prevent the risk of injury resulting from surgical procedures, including but not limited to (1) a thorough review of the patient's past medical history, (2) a comprehensive clinical and radiographic examination, and (3) good surgical techniques. Surgical complications include perilous bleeding, damage to adjacent teeth, injury to nerves, and iatrogenic jaw fracture. Additionally, postoperative complications may arise, such as hematoma or infection. Postoperative complications may be minor, transient, and easily managed or may be more serious or permanent and may require additional postoperative treatment.

Hemorrhage and Hematoma

Bleeding during surgery is expected and usually easily controlled. However, if a sizable vessel is incised or otherwise injured during surgery, the hemorrhage can be difficult to control. Smaller vessels will naturally constrict or retract to slow the hemorrhage. If bleeding continues, it may be necessary to apply pressure or to suture the hemorrhaging vessel. This can be especially difficult if there is a vascular injury to an artery that is inaccessible, such as the floor of the mouth or posterior maxilla. Serious bleeding from an inaccessible vessel can be life threatening, not by exsanguination but rather as a result of airway obstruction. This is most problematic when the point of bleeding is inaccessible and internal (within the connective tissues and soft tissue spaces).

Postoperative bleeding is an equally important problem to manage (Figure 81-2). Patients should be given postoperative instructions on normal expectations for bleeding and how to prevent and manage minor bleeding. They should also be advised to contact the treating practitioner if bleeding is excessive or persistent.

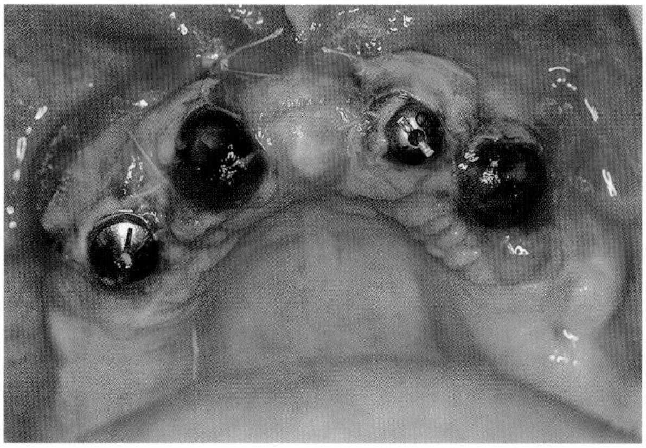

Figure 81-2 Clinical photograph of postoperative bleeding after second-stage implant exposure surgery.

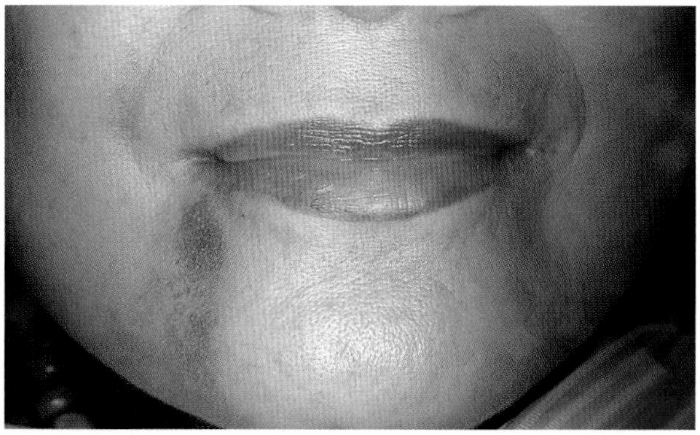

Figure 81-3 Clinical photograph of postoperative (extraoral) bruising indicative of subdermal bleeding into connective tissues spaces. This is a normal expectation that resolves within 7 to 14 days.

Submucosal or subdermal hemorrhage into the connective tissues and soft tissue spaces can result in hematoma formation. Postoperative bruising is a typical example of minor submucosal or subdermal bleeding into the connective tissues (Figure 81-3). Bruising and small hematomas typically resolve without special treatment or consequence. However, larger hematomas or those that occur in systemically compromised individuals are susceptible to infection as a result of the noncirculating blood that sits in the space. Thus, it is prudent to prescribe antibiotics for patients who develop a hematoma.

Although the incidence of a life-threatening hemorrhage from implant surgery is extremely low, the seriousness of the problem warrants the attention of everyone who participates in this type of surgery. Potentially fatal complications have been reported for implant surgical procedures in the mandible, particularly the anterior floor of the mouth.[20,27,59] Massive internal bleeding in the highly vascular region of the floor of the mouth can result from instrumentation that perforates the lingual cortical plate and severs or injures the arteries running along the lingual surface. Depending on the severity and location of the injury, bleeding may be apparent immediately or after some delay. In either case, the progressively increasing hematoma dissects and expands to displace the tongue and soft tissues of the floor of the mouth, ultimately leading to upper airway obstruction. Emergency treatment includes airway management (primary importance) and surgical intervention to isolate and stop bleeding. Clinicians must be aware of this risk and must be prepared to act quickly.

Neurosensory Disturbances

One of the more problematic surgical complications is an injury to nerves. Neurosensory alterations caused by damage to a nerve may be temporary or permanent. Neuropathy can be caused by a drilling injury (cut, tear, or puncture of the nerve) or by implant compression of the nerve. In either case, the injury produces neuroma formation, and two patterns of clinical neuropathy may follow. *Hypoesthesia* is a neuropathy defined by impaired sensory function that is sometimes associated with phantom pain. *Hyperesthesia* is a neuropathy defined by the presence of pain phenomena with minimal or no sensory impairment.[24] Some neuropathies will resolve, whereas other will persist. The type of neuropathy is not indicative of the potential for recovery.

It is likely that neurosensory disturbances occur more frequently after implant surgery than currently reported in the literature, for several reasons. First, many of these changes are transient in nature, and most patients recover completely or at least recover to a level that is below a threshold of annoyance or daily perception. Second, wide variation exists in the postoperative evaluation of patients by clinicians. Some clinicians do not examine or inquire about postsurgical neurosensory disturbances at all, thus allowing this complication to go unnoticed. Likewise, some patients may think that the altered sensation is part of the expected "side effect" of surgery and may never acknowledge or comment on its presence, especially if the disturbance is minor. Therefore, minor neuropathies likely are unreported.

Neurosensory disturbances reported in the literature are most prevalent and significant when they are more serious and occur more frequently, such as those associated with lateral transposition of the mandibular nerve.[30,38] This uncommon procedure is used to allow longer implants to be placed in the atrophic posterior mandible. Lateral nerve transposition procedures are associated with almost 100% incidence of neurosensory dysfunction immediately after surgery, and more than 50% of these neurosensory changes are permanent (30%–80%).[38]

Damage to Adjacent Teeth

Surgical procedures used to prepare osteotomy sites and place implants adjacent to teeth can injure the teeth either by directly cutting into the tooth structure or by damaging nearby supporting tissues and nerves. Instrumentation (e.g., drills) directed at or near the adjacent tooth may cause injury to the periodontal ligament, tooth structure, and nerve of the tooth. Depending on the extent of the injury, the tooth may require endodontic therapy or extraction.

Damage to adjacent teeth should be entirely preventable. Most often, damage results from a lack of appreciation of the local anatomy or disorientation in the direction of drilling with respect to the location and direction of the tooth root. Prevention is possible with diligent planning, familiarity with the local anatomy, and use of intraoperative periapical radiographs (see Figure 75-2).

The risks of surgery may always be present, but the complications can be minimized with an understanding of the etiologies.

BIOLOGIC COMPLICATIONS

Biologic complications involve pathology of the surrounding periimplant hard and soft tissues. Frequently, soft tissue problems are an inflammatory response to bacterial accumulation. The cause of bacterial accumulation around implants is key to understanding the problem. For example, bacteria may accumulate at the junction of an ill-fitting implant-abutment or abutment-crown connection. Some of the macroscopically rough implant surfaces (e.g., TPS or HA coated) may also perpetuate the accumulation of bacteria.

Inflammation and Proliferation

Inflammation in the periimplant soft tissues has been found to be similar to the inflammatory response in gingival and other periodontal tissues. Not surprisingly, the clinical appearance is similar as well. Inflamed periimplant tissues demonstrate the same erythema, edema, and swelling seen around teeth. Occasionally, however, the reaction of periimplant soft tissues to bacterial accumulation is profound, almost unusual, with a dramatic inflammatory proliferation (Figure 81-4). This type of lesion is somewhat characteristic around implants and is indicative of either a loose-fitting implant to abutment connection or trapped excess cement that remains buried within the soft tissue space or "pocket." The precipitating local factor ultimately becomes infected with bacterial pathogens, leading to mucosal hypertrophy or proliferation and possible abscess formation (Figure 81-5). Correction of the precipitating factor (e.g., loose connection, excess cement) quickly and effectively resolves the lesion. Another type of lesion resulting from a loose abutment connection is the fistula (Figure 81-6). Again, correcting the etiologic factor quickly resolves the fistula.

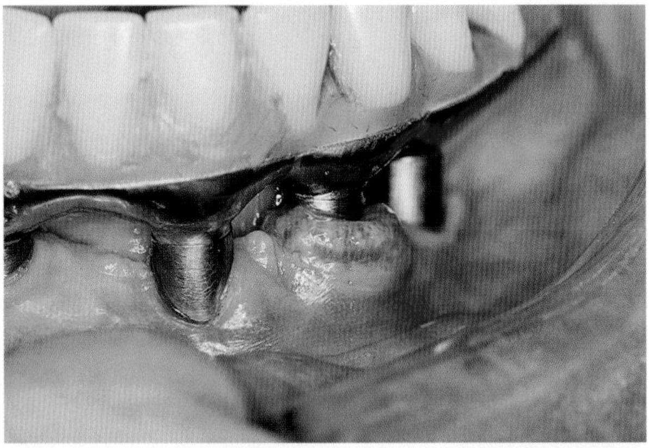

Figure 81-4 Inflammatory proliferation caused by a loose-fitting connection between the abutment and the implant.

A

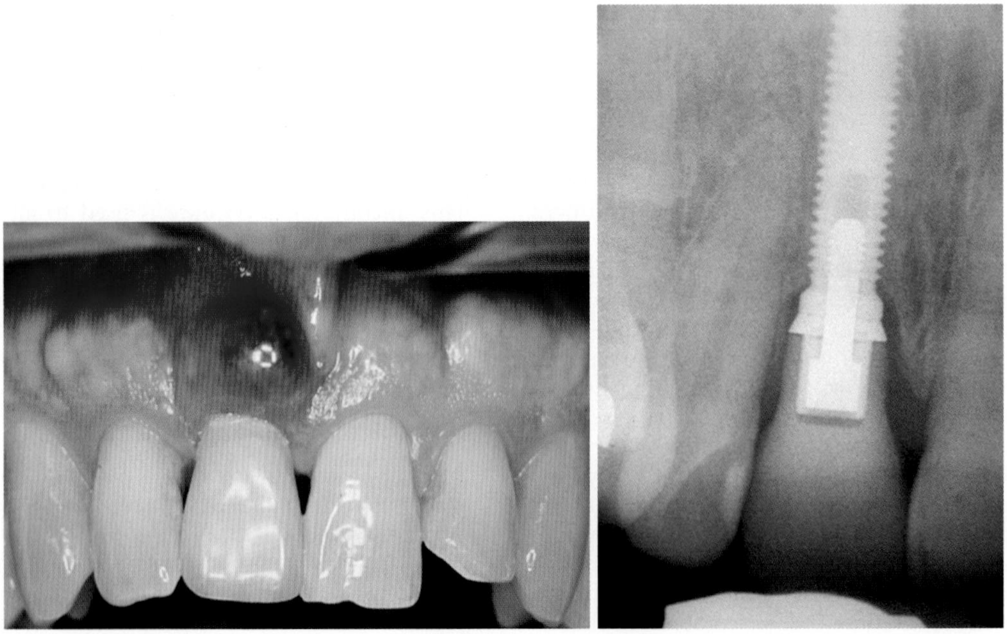

B

Figure 81-5 **A,** Clinical photograph of abscess caused by excess cement trapped within the soft tissues. **B,** Radiograph of implant with cemented crown (same patient as in A). Notice the subgingival depth of the crown-abutment (cement) junction, which is below the level of the adjacent interproximal bone and therefore impossible to adequately remove excess cement.

Dehiscence and Recession

Dehiscence or recession of the periimplant soft tissues occurs when support for those tissues is lacking or has been lost. Recession is a common finding after implant restoration and should be anticipated especially when soft tissues are thin and not well supported (Figure 81-7). The problem is particularly disconcerting in the anterior esthetic areas. Patients with a high smile line or high esthetic demands will consider such recession a failure.

The anatomy and soft tissue support around implants is different than that around teeth. Specifically, periodontal tissues have the distinct advantage of soft tissue support from circumferential and transeptal connective tissue fibers that insert into the cementum above the level of crestal bone. In the absence of inflammation, these fibers support periodontal soft tissues far above the level of crestal bone. As a result, gingival margins and interdental papillae are supported and maintained around teeth even when the periodontal tissues are very thin. Periimplant soft tissues, on the other hand, are entirely dependent on surrounding bone for support. Soft tissue thickness accounts for some soft tissue height, but there are no supracrestal inserting connective tissue fibers to aid in the soft tissue support around an implant. Therefore, soft tissue height around implants typically does not exceed about 3 to 4 mm, and bone loss around implants often leads to recession.

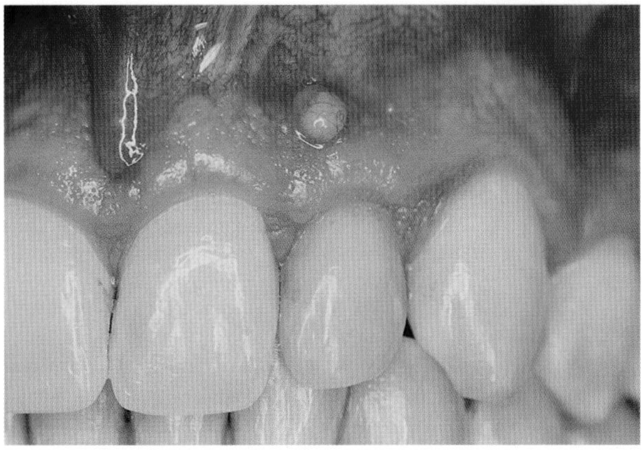

Figure 81-6 Fistula caused by loose implant-abutment connection (maxillary left lateral incisor).

Periimplantitis and Bone Loss

Periimplantitis is defined as an inflammatory process affecting the tissues around an osseointegrated implant in function, resulting in loss of supporting bone.[52] To diagnose a compromised implant site, soft tissue measurements using manual or automated probes have been suggested. Although some reports state that probing is contraindicated, careful monitoring of probing depth over time seems useful in detecting changes of the periimplant tissue.[15,67,77,78] Radiographic procedures to assess periimplant bone level have been shown to be useful. Standardized radiography, both with and without computerized analysis, has been well documented.[1,10,12,33,67] Together, periodic evaluation of tissue appearance, probing depth changes, and radiographic assessment are the best means of detecting changes in bone support. Clinicians should monitor the surrounding tissues for signs of periimplant disease by monitoring changes in probing depth and radiographic evidence of bone

A

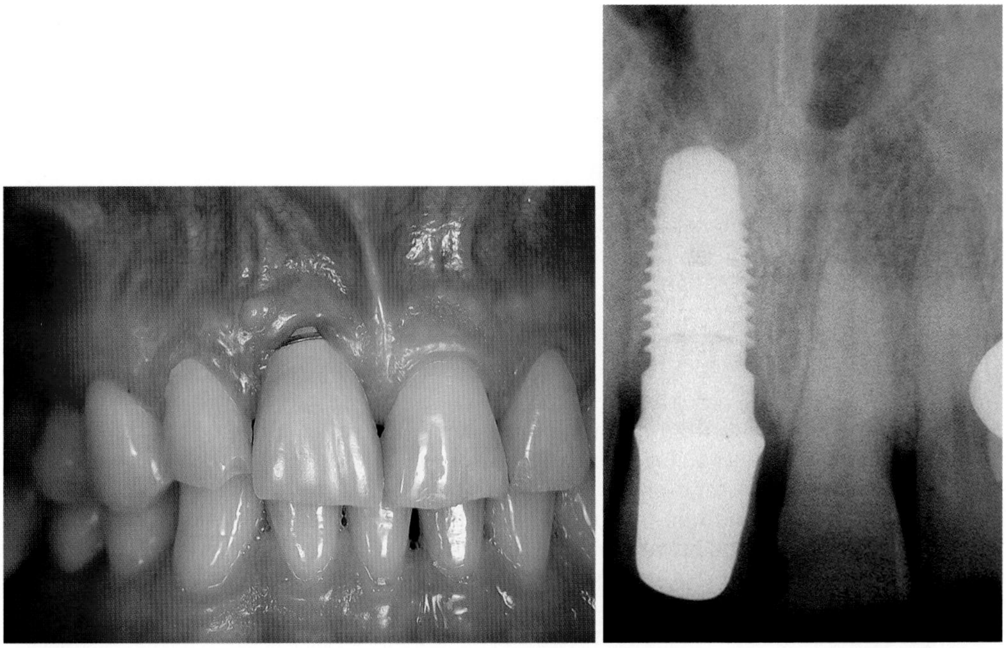

B

Figure 81-7 **A,** Clinical photograph of single-tooth implant crown (maxillary right central) with moderate recession that occurred 1 year after delivery of final restoration. Recession, in this case, most likely occurred because the labial bone around this wide-diameter implant was very thin or nonexistent. **B,** Radiograph of wide-diameter (6-mm) implant supporting maxillary central incisor crown (same patient as in *A*).

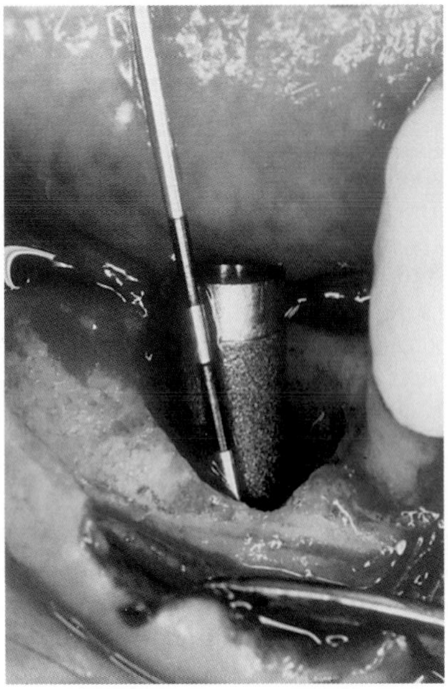

Figure 81-8 Advanced type IV bone loss around implant with titanium plasma–sprayed coating. Note the typical circumferential trough defect.

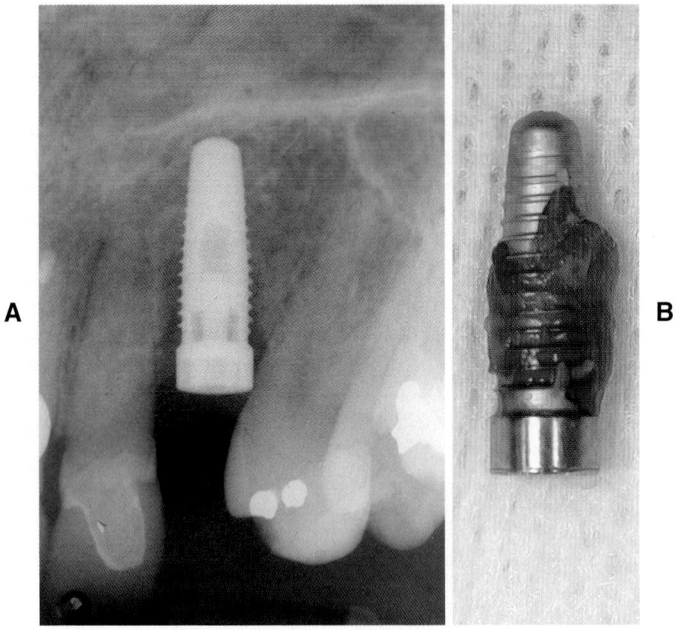

Figure 81-9 Implant loss (early failure or lack of osseointegration). **A,** Radiograph. **B,** Photograph of failed (non-integrated) implant removed with surrounding connective tissue.

destruction, suppuration, calculus buildup, swelling, color changes, and bleeding.[53,57]

Periimplantitis may be perpetuated by bacterial infection that has contaminated a rough (e.g., titanium plasma–sprayed, hydroxyapatite-coated) implant surface and by excessive biomechanical forces.[82,83] A classic trough-type defect is typically associated with peri-implantitis (Figure 81-8). The number of implants, the implant distribution, and the occlusion relationship influence the biomechanical forces on implants[66,69] (see Chapter 80).

In cases with severely reduced bone support extending into the apical half of the implant, or in cases demonstrating mobility, implant removal should be considered.[3,56] After the implants are removed, the ridge defects can be reconstructed using bone graft and membrane techniques. This treatment usually enables the clinician to place new implants in a previously compromised situation.

Implant Loss or Failure

Implant loss or failure is generally considered relative to the time of placement or restoration. Early implant failures occur before implant restoration. Late implant failures occur after the implant has been restored.

When an implant fails before restoration, it probably did not achieve osseointegration, or the integration was weak or jeopardized by infection, movement, or impaired wound healing (Figure 81-9). Late implant failures occur after delivery of the prosthesis for many reasons, including implant overload and infection.

Esposito et al.,[19] reviewing the literature to evaluate biologic causes for implant failure, found that infections, impaired healing, and overload were the most important contributing factors.

TECHNICAL OR MECHANICAL COMPLICATIONS

Technical or mechanical complications occur when the strength of materials is no longer able to resist the forces that are being applied. As materials fatigue, they begin to stretch and bend; ultimately, depending on the applied forces, they will fracture. Material failures, in turn, lead to prosthetic complications, such as loose, broken, and failed restorations.

Screw Loosening and Fracture

Screw loosening has been reported to occur quite frequently in screw-retained FPDs. Screw-retained single crowns attached to externally hexed implants (i.e., those with narrow- or standard-diameter restorative interface connection surfaces) are particularly prone to this type of technical complication. Reports have shown screw loosening in 6% to 49% of cases at the first annual checkup.[29,54] Screw loosening was a more prevalent problem with earlier designs. For example, abutment screws were previously made with titanium, which did not offer the clamping forces of current materials. Newer abutment designs and improved abutment screws allow for an increased clamping force to be achieved without excessive torque levels, which has helped to reduce the rate of screw loosening.

Abutment or prosthesis screw loosening is often corrected by retightening the screws. Over time, however, screws become fatigued and eventually fracture. This problem is evident to the patient with a loose single crown. In the patient with a prosthesis retained by multiple implants, however, the ability to detect a loose screw

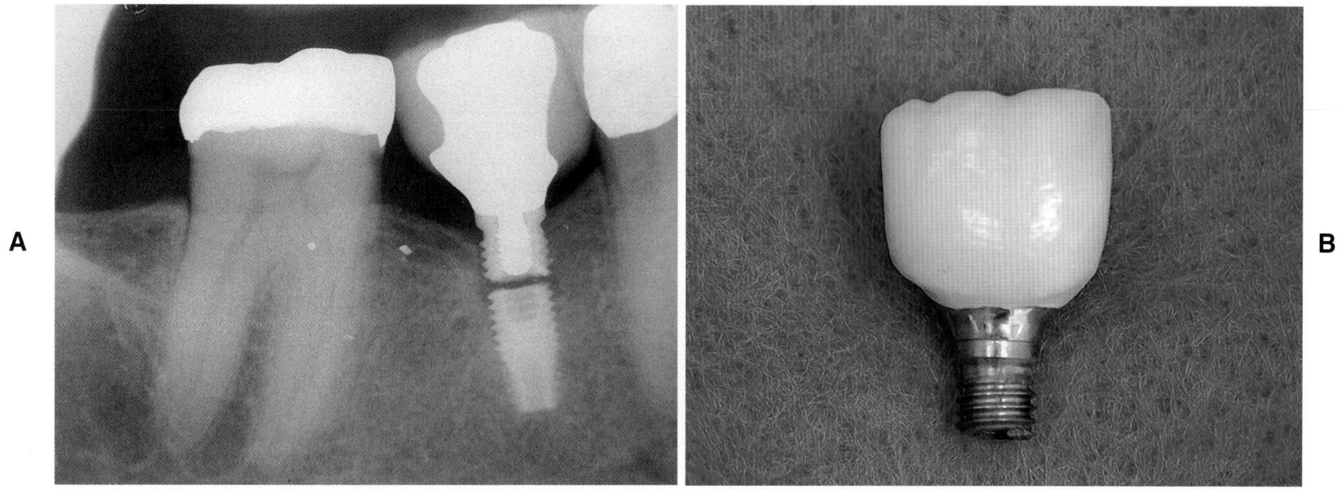

Figure 81-10 Fractured implant. **A,** Radiograph of fractured implant (standard diameter) used to support a molar-sized single crown in the posterior mandible. **B,** Crown and implant that fractured between the third and fourth threads.

is greatly diminished; the problem may go unnoticed until the other screws also fatigue and fracture. In either case, the biomechanical support (and resistance) for the restoration must be evaluated and, if possible, changed to prevent recurrence of the problem.

Implant Fracture

The ultimate mechanical failure is implant fracture because it results in loss of the implant and possibly the prosthesis (Figure 81-10). Furthermore, removal of a fractured implant will create a large osseous defect. Factors such as fatigue of implant materials and weakness in prosthetic design or dimension are the usual causes of implant fractures.[1,6] Balshi[6] listed three categories of causes that may explain implant fractures: (1) design and material, (2) nonpassive fit of the prosthetic framework, and (3) physiologic or biomechanical overload. Patients with bruxism seem to be at higher risk for such events and therefore need to be screened and informed accordingly.[5,6]

Fracture of Restorative Materials

Fracture or failure of materials used for implant-retained restorations can be a significant problem. This is particularly true for veneers (acrylic, composite, or ceramic) that are attached to superstructures.

ESTHETIC AND PHONETIC COMPLICATIONS

Esthetic Complications

Esthetic complications arise when patient expectations are not met. Patient satisfaction with the esthetic outcome of the implant prosthesis will vary from patient to patient depending on a number of factors. As mentioned earlier, the risk for esthetic complications is increased for patients with high esthetic expectations and less-than-optimal patient-related factors (e.g., bone quantity and quality). In addition to the actual appearance of the final restoration, individual perceptions and desires will be more or less accepting of the results. Esthetic complications result from poor implant placement and deficiencies in the existing anatomy of the edentulous sites that were reconstructed with implants.

Implant placement in the esthetic zone requires precise three-dimensional tissue reconstruction and ideal implant placement. This reconstructive procedure enables the restorative dentist to develop a natural emergence profile of the implant crown. If the amount of available bone does not allow for ideal implant placement, and if the implant is positioned too apical, buccal, or interproximal, a prosthetic profile will be developed with unesthetic dimensions (Figure 81-11). The same is true if a bone reconstruction procedure shows a compromised result and the implant is still placed, but in an inappropriate position.

If crown form, dimension, and shape and gingival harmony around the implants are not ideal, the patient may consider the implants or restorations as complications because the result does not represent a natural profile. If the patient is truly dissatisfied with the esthetic result and there is a problem with the position of the implants that can be corrected (i.e., the patient's expectations are reasonable), the implants could be removed; the case could be reevaluated and, if possible, retreated.

Appropriate treatment planning and implementation keep esthetic complications to a minimum, although anterior implant work is technique sensitive and time-consuming. Patients with a high smile line, high esthetic demands, thin periodontium, or lack of hard and soft tissue support in the anterior esthetic region are some of the most difficult cases to treat and should only be treated, after extensive planning, by experienced clinicians.

Phonetic Problems

Implant prostheses that are fabricated with unusual palatal contours (e.g., restricted or narrow palatal space)

A

B

C

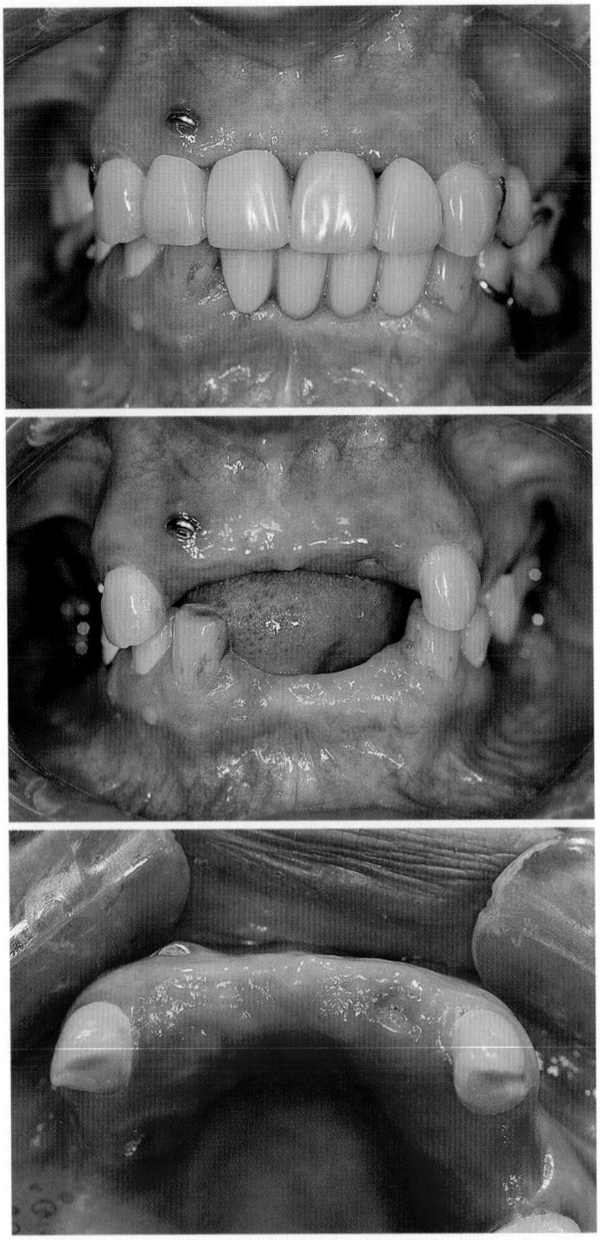

Figure 81-11 Poor implant position makes it impossible to restore with an esthetic restoration. **A,** Anterior view with removable partial dentures (RPDs). **B,** Anterior view without RPDs. Note the high exposure of the cover screw/head of implant in site #7 (right maxillary incisor). **C,** Occlusal view of same patient. Note the labial projection of implant in site #7 as well as the palatal position of the implant in premolar area. Any attempt to restore implant would not be esthetically acceptable.

or that have spaces under and around the superstructure can create phonetic problems for the patient. This is particularly problematic when full-arch, implant-supported, fixed restorations are fabricated for patients who have a severely atrophied maxilla. These patients are probably best served with an implant-assisted maxillary overdenture.

CONCLUSION

Endosseous dental implants are successful and predictable. Complications and failures appear to be a small but significant factor. Technical complications as well as some biologic complications can be effectively treated without loss of implants or prostheses. The key to minimizing implant-related complications is to understand the causes and plan cases so that known implant complications and failures associated with endosseous dental implants and the retained prosthetic appliances are avoided or minimized.

REFERENCES

1. Adell R, Lekholm U, Rockler B, et al: A 15-year study of osseointegrated implants in the treatment of the edentulous jaw, *Int J Oral Surg* 10:387, 1981.
2. Adell R, Eriksson B, Lekholm U, et al: Long-term follow-up study of osseointegrated implants in the treatment of totally edentulous jaws, *Int J Oral Maxillofac Implants* 5:347, 1990.
3. Albrektsson T, Zarb G, Worthington P, et al: The long-term efficacy of currently used dental implants: a review and prognosis criteria for success, *Int J Oral Maxillofac Implants* 1:11, 1986.
4. Apse P, Ellen RP, Overall CM, et al: Microbiota and crevicular fluid collagenase activity in the osseointegrated dental implant sulcus: a comparison of sites in edentulous and partially edentulous patients, *J Periodontal Res* 24:96, 1989.
5. Balshi TJ: Preventing and resolving complications with osseointegrated implants, *Dent Clin North Am* 33:821, 1989.
6. Balshi TJ: An analysis and management of fractured implants: a clinical report, *Int J Oral Maxillofac Implants* 11:660, 1996.
7. Becker W, Becker BE, Newman MG, et al: Clinical and microbiologic findings that may contribute to dental implant failure, *Int J Oral Maxillofac Implants* 5:31, 1980.
8. Berglundh T, Persson L, Klinge B: A systematic review of the incidence of biological and technical complications in implant dentistry reported in prospective longitudinal studies of at least 5 years, *J Clin Periodontol* 29(suppl 3):197, 2002.
9. Block M, Kent J: Factors associated with soft and hard tissue compromise of endosseous implants, *J Oral Maxillofac Surg* 48:1160, 1990.
10. Bragger U, Burgin W, Fourmousis J, et al: Image processing for the evaluations of dental implants, *Dentomaxillofac Radiol* 21:208, 1992.
11. Brown FH, Ogletree RC, Houston GD: Pneumoparotitis associated with the use of an air-power prophylaxis unit, *J Periodontol* 63:642, 1992.
12. Buser D, Weber HP, Bragger U, et al: Tissue integration of one stage ITI implants: 3-year results of a longitudinal study with hollow-cylinder and hollow-screw implants, *Int J Oral Maxillofac Implants* 6:405, 1991.
13. Buser D, Weber HP, Donath K, et al: Soft tissue reactions to non-submerged unloaded titanium implants in beagle dogs, *J Periodontol* 63:226, 1992.
14. Buser D, Mericske-Stern R, Bernard JP, et al: Long-term evaluation of non-submerged ITI implants. Part 1. 8-year life table analysis of a prospective multi-center study with 2359 implants, *Clin Oral Implant Res* 8:161, 1997.
15. Dahlin C, Sennerby L, Lekholm U, et al: Generation of new bone around titanium implants using a membrane technique: an experimental study in rabbits, *Int J Oral Maxillofac Implants* 4:19, 1989.
16. Dohm GJ, Stender E, Foitzik CH: Die Reinigung von Implantatoberflächen mit Strahl- und Zahnsteinentfernungsgeräten, *Dtsch Z Zahnärztl Implantol* 2:133, 1986.

17. Ericsson I, Persson LG, Glanz PO, et al: The effect of antimicrobial therapy on periimplantitis lesions: an experimental study in the dog, *Clin Oral Implant Res* 7:320, 1996.
18. Esposito M, Hirsch JM, Lekholm U, et al: Biological factors contributing to failures of osseointegrated oral implants. I. Success criteria and epidemiology, *Eur J Oral Sci* 106:527, 1998.
19. Esposito M, Hirsch J, Lekholm U, et al: Differential diagnosis and treatment strategies for biologic complications and failing oral implants: a review of the literature, *Int J Oral Maxillofac Implants* 14:473, 1999.
20. Flanagan D: Important arterial supply of the mandible, control of an arterial hemorrhage, and report of a hemorrhagic incident, *J Oral Implantol* 29:165, 2003.
21. Golec TS, Krauser JT: Long-term retrospective studies on hydroxyapatite-coated endosteal and subperiosteal implants, *Dent Clin North Am* 36:39, 1992.
22. Goodacre CJ, Kan JY, Rungcharassaeng K: Clinical complications of osseointegrated implants, *J Prosthet Dent* 81:537, 1999.
23. Goodacre CJ, Bernal G, Rungcharassaeng K, et al: Clinical complications with implants and implant prostheses, *J Prosthet Dent* 90:121, 2003.
24. Gregg JM: Neuropathic complications of mandibular implant surgery: review and case presentations, *Ann R Aust Coll Dent Surg* 15:176, 2000.
25. Hadeen G, Ismail Y, Garrana H, et al: Three-dimensional finite element stress analysis of Nobelpharma and Core-Vent implants and their supporting structures, *J Dent Res* 67:286, 1998 (abstract).
26. Hanisch O, Tatakis DN, Boskovic MM, et al: Bone formation and re-osseointegration in periimplantitis defects following surgical implantation of rhBMP-2, *Int J Oral Maxillofac Implants* 12:604, 1997.
27. Isaacson TJ: Sublingual hematoma formation during immediate placement of mandibular endosseous implants, *J Am Dent Assoc* 135:168, 2004.
28. James RA: Periodontal considerations in implant dentistry, *J Prosthet Dent* 30:202, 1973.
29. Jemt T: Fixed implant-supported prosthesis in the edentulous maxilla: a five-year follow-up report, *Clin Oral Implant Res* 5:142, 1994.
30. Jensen J, Reiche-Fischel O, Sindet-Pedersen S: Nerve transposition and implant placement in the atrophic posterior mandibular alveolar ridge, *J Oral Maxillofac Surg* 52:662, 1994.
31. Johnson B: HA-coated dental implants: long term consequences, *Calif Dent Assoc J* 20:33, 1992.
32. Jovanovic SA: The management of periimplant breakdown around functioning osseointegrated dental implants, *J Periodontol* 64:1176, 1993.
33. Jovanovic SA: Plaque-induced periimplant bone loss in mongrel dogs: a clinical, microbial, radiographic and histological study, University of California, Los Angeles, 1994 (master of science thesis).
34. Jovanovic SA, James RA, Lessard G: Bacterial morphotypes and PGE_2 levels from the pergingival site of dental implants with intact and compromised bone support, *J Dent Res* 67:28, 1988 (abstract).
35. Jovanovic SA, Spiekermann H, Richter EJ: Bone regeneration on titanium dental implants with dehisced defect sites: a clinical study, *Int J Oral Maxillofac Implants* 7:233, 1992.
36. Jovanovic SA, Spiekermann H, Richter EJ, et al: Guided tissue regeneration around titanium dental implants. In Laney WR, Tolmen DE, editors: *Tissue integration in oral, orthopedic and maxillofacial reconstruction,* Chicago, 1992, Quintessence.
37. Jovanovic SA, Kenney EB, Carranza FA, et al: The regenerative potential of plaque-induced periimplant bone defects treated by a submerged membrane technique: an experimental study, *Int J Oral Maxillofac Implants* 8:13, 1993.
38. Kan JY, Lozada JL, Goodacre CJ, et al: Endosseous implant placement in conjunction with inferior alveolar nerve transposition: an evaluation of neurosensory disturbance, *Int J Oral Maxillofac Implants* 12:463, 1997.
39. Koth DL, McKinney RV, Steflik DE: Microscopic study of hygiene effect on periimplant gingival tissues, *J Dent Res* 65:186, 1986.
40. Krauser J, Berthold P, Tamery I, et al: A SEM study of failed endosseous root formed dental implants, *J Dent Res* 70:274, 1991 (abstract).
41. Lang NP, Karring T: *Proceedings of the 1st European Workshop on Periodontology,* Chicago, 1994, Quintessence.
42. Lang NP, Bragger U, Walther D, et al: Ligature-induced periimplant infection in cynomolgus monkeys. I. Clinical and radiographic findings, *Clin Oral Implant Res* 4:2, 1993.
43. Lehmann B, Bragger U, Hammerle CH, et al: Treatment of an early failure according to the principles of guided tissue regeneration, *Clin Oral Implant Res* 3:43, 1992.
44. Lekholm U, Ericsson I, Adell R, et al: The condition of the soft tissues at tooth and fixture abutments supporting fixed bridges: a microbiological and histological study, *J Clin Periodontol* 13:558, 1986.
45. Lekholm U, Gunne J, Henry P, et al: Survival of the Branemark implant in partially edentulous jaws: a 10-year prospective multicenter study, *Int J Oral Maxillofac Implants* 14:639, 1999.
46. Lindhe J, Berglundh T, Ericsson I, et al: Experimental breakdown of periimplant and periodontal tissues: a study in the beagle dog, *Clin Oral Implant Res* 3:9, 1992.
47. Lindquist LW, Rockler B, Carlsson GE, et al: Bone resorption around fixtures in edentulous patients treated with mandibular fixed tissue-integrated prostheses, *J Prosthet Dent* 59:59, 1988.
48. Lozada J, James R, Boskovic M, et al: Surgical repair of periimplant defects, *J Oral Implant* 16:42, 1990.
49. Matarasso S, Quaremba G, Coraggio F, et al: Maintenance of implants: an in vitro study of titanium implant surface modifications subsequent to the application of different prophylaxis procedures, *Clin Oral Implant Res* 7:64, 1996.
50. Meffert RM: Treatment of the ailing, failing implants, *J Calif Dent Assoc* 20:42, 1992.
51. Mombelli A, Lang NP: Antimicrobial treatment of periimplant infections, *Clin Oral Implant Res* 3:162, 1992.
52. Mombelli A, Lang NP: The diagnosis and treatment of periimplantitis, *Periodontol 2000* 17:63, 1998.
53. Mombelli A, Marxer M, Gaberthuel T, et al: The microbiota of osseointegrated implants in patients with a history of periodontal disease, *J Clin Periodontol* 22:124, 1995.
54. Mombelli A, Van Oosten M, Schurch E, et al: The microbiota associated with successful or failing osseointegrated titanium implants, *Oral Microbiol Immunol* 2:145, 1987.
55. Naert I, Quirynen M, van Steenberghe D, et al: A study of 589 consecutive implants supporting complete fixed prosthesis. Part II. Prosthetic aspects, *J Prosthet Dent* 68:949, 1992.
56. Nakou M, Mikx FH, Oosterwaal PJ, et al: Early microbial colonization of perimucosal implants in edentulous patients, *J Dent Res* 66:1654, 1987.
57. Nevins M, Mellonig JT: Enhancement of the damaged edentulous ridge to receive dental implants: a combination of allograft and the Gore-Tex membrane, *Int J Periodont Rest Dent* 12:97, 1992.
58. Newman M, Flemmig T: Periodontal considerations of implants and implant associated microbiota, *J Dent Educ* 52:737, 1988.
59. Niamtu J 3rd: Near-fatal airway obstruction after routine implant placement, *Oral Surg Oral Med Oral Pathol Oral Radiol Endod* 92:597, 2001.

60. Philip L, Parham PL Jr, Charles M, et al: Effects of air-powder abrasive system on plasma-sprayed titanium implant surfaces: an in vitro evaluation, *J Oral Implant* 15:78, 1989.
61. Pjetursson BE, Tan K, Lang NP, et al: A systematic review of the survival and complication rates of fixed partial dentures (FPDs) after an observation period of at least 5 years, *Clin Oral Implant Res* 15:625, 2004.
62. Quirijnen M, Listgarten MA: The distribution of bacterial morphotypes around natural teeth and titanium implants ad modum Branemark, *Clin Implant Res* 1:8, 1990.
63. Quirijnen M, Naert I, van Steenberghe D: Fixture design and overload influence marginal bone loss and fixture success in the Branemark system, *Clin Oral Implant Res* 3:104, 1992.
64. Quirijnen M, Marechal M, Busscher HJ, et al: The influence of surface free energy and surface roughness on early plaque formation, *J Clin Periodontol* 17:138, 1990.
65. Quirijnen M, van Steenberghe D, Jacobs R, et al: The reliability of pocket probing around screw-type implants, *Clin Oral Implant Res* 2:186, 1991.
66. Rams TE, Link C: Microbiology of failing dental implants in humans: electron microscopic observations, *J Oral Implant* 11:93, 1983.
67. Rangert B, Jemt T, Jorneus L: Forces and moments on Branemark implants, *Int J Oral Maxillofac Implants* 4:241, 1989.
68. Rangert B, Krogh PH, Langer B, et al: Bending overload and implant fracture: a retrospective clinical analysis, *Int J Oral Maxillofac Implants* 10:326, 1995.
69. Richter EJ, Jansen V, Spiekermann H, et al: Langzeitergebnisse von IMZ-und TPS-Implantaten im interforaminalen Bereich des zahnlosen Unterkiefers, *Dtsch Zahnärztl Z* 47:449, 1992.
70. Roberts WE, Garetto LP, de Castro RA: Remodeling of devitalized bone threatens periosteal margin integrity of endosseous titanium implants with treated or smooth surfaces: indications for provisional loading and axillary directed occlusion, *J Indiana Dent Assoc* 68:19, 1989.
71. Sanz M, Newman M, Nachnani S, et al: Characterization of the subgingival microbial flora around endosteal dental implants in partially edentulous patie *Maxillofac Implants* 5:247, 1990.
72. Schou S, Holmstrup P, Stoltze K, et al: Ligature-induced marginal inflammation around osseointegrated implants and ankylosed teeth: clinical and radiographic observations in cynomolgus monkeys, *Clin Oral Implant Res* 4:12, 1993.
73. Simion M, Dahlin C, Trisi P, et al: Qualitative and quantitative comparative study on different filling materials used in bone regeneration, *Int J Periodont Restor Dent* 14:199, 1994.
74. Smedberg JI, Lothigius E, Bodin I, et al: A clinical and radiological two-year follow-up study of maxillary overdentures on osseointegrated implants, *Clin Oral Implant Res* 4:39, 1993.
75. Smithloff M, Fritz M: The use of blade implants in a population of partially edentulous adults: a 15-year report, *J Periodontol* 58:589, 1987.
76. Stefani LA: The care and maintenance of the dental implant patient, *J Dent Hyg* 62:447, 1988.
77. Strub JR: Langzeitprognose von enossalen oralen Implantaten unter spezieller Berücksichtigung von periimplantaren, materialkundlichen und okklusalen Gesichtspunkten. In *Habilitationsschriften der ZMK,* Berlin, 1986, Quintessenz Verlags.
78. Strub JR, Gaberthuel TW, Grunder U: The role of attached gingiva in the health of periimplant tissue in dogs. Part I. Clinical findings, *Int J Periodont Restor Dent* 11:317, 1991.
79. Thompson-Neal D, Evans G, Meffert R: Effects of various prophylactic treatments on titanium, sapphire, and hydroxyapatite-coated implants: an SEM study, *Int J Periodont Restor Dent* 9:301, 1989.
80. Tolman DE and Laney WR: Tissue-integrated prosthesis complications, *Int J Oral Maxillofac Implants* 7:477, 1992.
81. Weber HP, Buser D, Fiorellini JP, et al: Radiographic evaluation of crestal bone levels adjacent to nonsubmerged titanium implants, *Clin Oral Implant Res* 3:181, 1992.
82. Zablotsky M, Diedrich D, Meffert R: Detoxification of endotoxin-contaminated titanium and hydroxyapatite-coated surfaces utilizing various chemotherapeutic and mechanical modalities, *Implant Dent* 1:154, 1992.
83. Zablotsky M, Diedrich, D, Meffert R, et al: The ability of various chemotherapeutic agents to detoxify the endotoxin infected HA-coated implant surface, *Int J Oral Implant* 8:45, 1991.

PART

9

Periodontal Maintenance

Henry H. Takei

The successful management of periodontal disease requires a positive program directed at maintaining and improving the results of treatment as well as preventing the development of new disease. The gradual microbial recolonization of tooth surfaces begins soon after plaque is eliminated; therefore the measures to stop recolonization also must be a constant effort on the part of the patient, following the professional instructions and guidance and including periodic professional care visits. This part of the text also presents the overwhelming evidence that has been accumulated about the effectiveness of periodontal therapy.

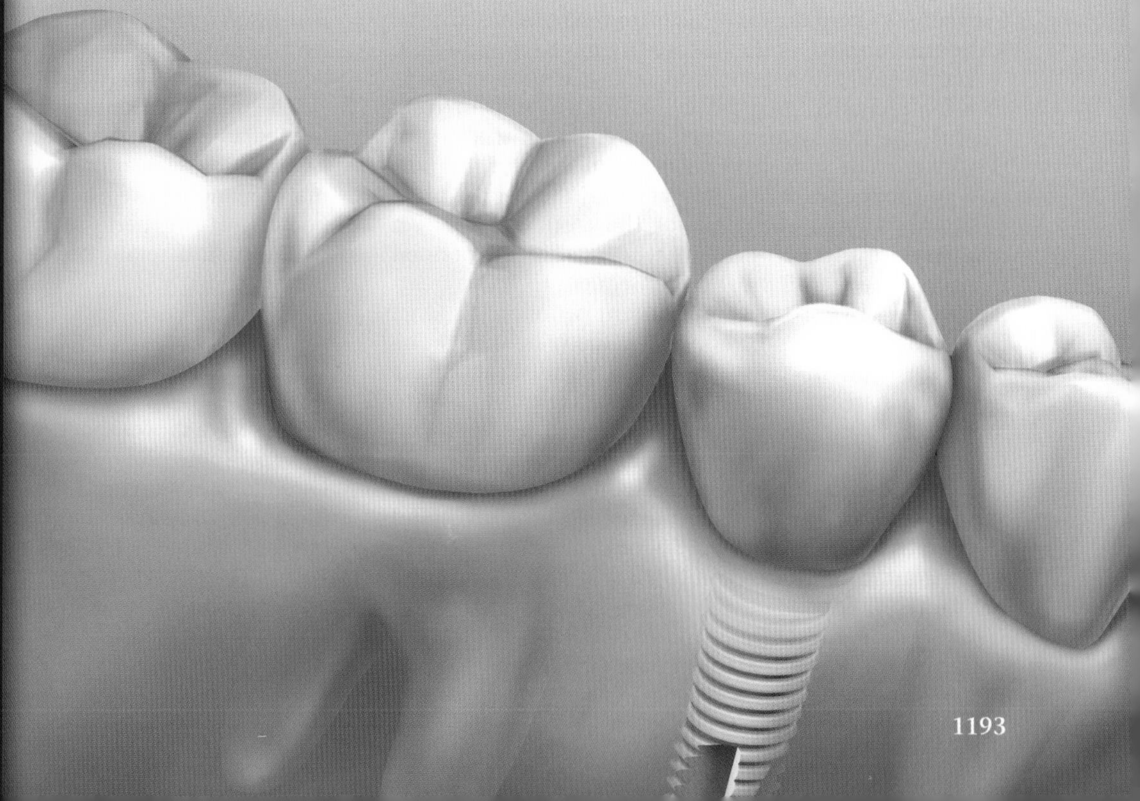

Supportive Periodontal Treatment

Robert L. Merin

82

CHAPTER

CHAPTER OUTLINE

Preservation of the periodontal health of the treated patient requires as positive a program as that required for the elimination of periodontal disease. After Phase I therapy is completed, patients are placed on a schedule of periodic recall visits for maintenance care to prevent recurrence of the disease (Figures 82-1 and 82-2).

Transfer of the patient from active treatment status to a maintenance program is a definitive step in total patient care that requires time and effort on the part of the dentist and staff. Patients must understand the purpose of the maintenance program, and the dentist must emphasize that preservation of the teeth depends on maintenance therapy. Patients who are not maintained in a supervised recall program subsequent to active treatment show obvious signs of recurrent periodontitis (e.g., increased pocket depth, bone loss, tooth loss).[5,8,14] The more often patients present for recommended supportive periodontal treatment (SPT), the less likely they are to lose teeth.[66] One study found that treated patients who do not return for regular recall are at 5.6 times greater risk for tooth loss than compliant patients.[14] Another study showed that patients with inadequate SPT after successful regenerative therapy have a 50-fold increase in risk of probing attachment loss compared with those who have regular recall visits.[16]

Motivational techniques and reinforcement of the importance of the maintenance phase of treatment should be considered before performing definitive periodontal surgery.[8] Studies have shown that few patients display complete compliance with recommended maintenance schedules* (Figure 82-3). *It is meaningless simply to inform patients that they are to return for periodic recall visits without clearly explaining the significance of these visits and describing what is expected of patients between visits.*

The maintenance phase of periodontal treatment starts immediately after the completion of Phase I therapy (see Figures 82-1 and 82-2). While the patient is in the maintenance phase, the necessary surgical and restorative procedures are performed. This ensures that all areas of the mouth retain the degree of health attained after Phase I therapy.

RATIONALE FOR SUPPORTIVE PERIODONTAL TREATMENT

Studies have shown that even with appropriate periodontal therapy, some progression of disease is possible.[21,24,40,45,59] One likely explanation for the recurrence of periodontal disease is *incomplete subgingival plaque removal.*[62] If subgingival plaque is left behind during scaling, it regrows within the pocket. The regrowth of subgingival plaque is a slow process compared with that of supragingival plaque.

*References 1, 36, 38, 39, 65, 67.

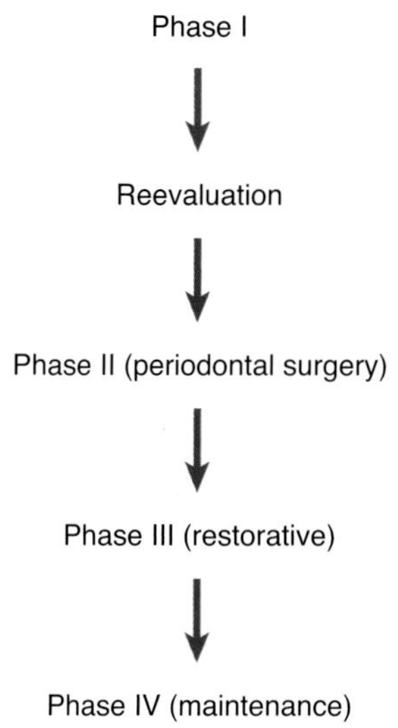

Figure 82-1 Incorrect sequence of periodontal treatment phases. Maintenance phase should be started immediately after the reevaluation of Phase I.

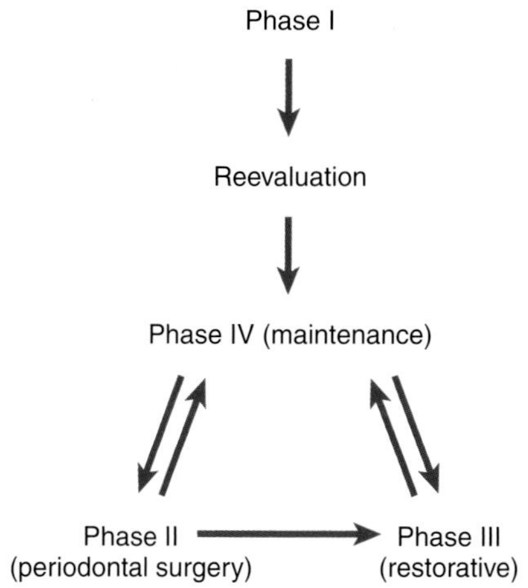

Figure 82-2 Correct sequence of periodontal treatment phases.

During this period (perhaps months), the subgingival plaque may not induce inflammatory reactions that can be discerned at the gingival margin. The clinical diagnosis may be further confused by the introduction of adequate supragingival plaque control, because the inflammatory reactions caused by the plaque in the soft tissue wall of the pocket are not likely to be manifested clinically as gingivitis. Thus, inadequate subgingival plaque control can lead to continued loss of attachment, even without the presence of clinical gingival inflammation.

Bacteria are present in the gingival tissues in chronic and aggressive periodontitis cases.[11,15,42,47] Eradication of intragingival microorganisms may be necessary for a stable periodontal result. Scaling, root planing, and even flap surgery may not eliminate intragingival bacteria in some areas.[16] These bacteria may recolonize the pocket and cause recurrent disease.

Bacteria associated with periodontitis can be transmitted between spouses and other family members.[2,60] Patients who

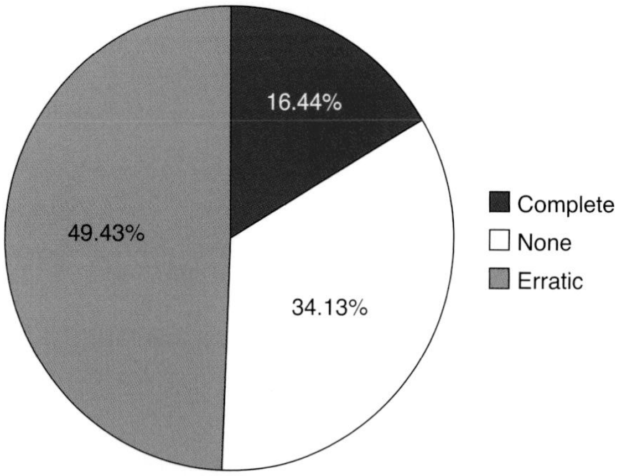

Figure 82-3 Compliance with maintenance therapy in 961 patients studied for 1 to 8 years. (Modified from Wilson TG Jr, Glover ME, Schoen J, et al: *J Periodontol* 55:468, 1984.)

appear to be successfully treated can become infected or reinfected with potential pathogens. This is especially likely in patients with remaining pockets.

Another possible explanation for the recurrence of periodontal disease is the microscopic nature of the dentogingival unit healing after periodontal treatment. Histologic studies have shown that after periodontal procedures, tissues usually do not heal by formation of new connective tissue attachment to root surfaces[12,53,54] but result in a long junctional epithelium. It has been speculated that this type of dentogingival unit may be weaker and that inflammation may rapidly separate the long junctional epithelium from the tooth. Thus, treated periodontal patients may be predisposed to recurrent pocket formation if maintenance care is not optimal.

Subgingival scaling alters the microflora of periodontal pockets.[37,44,51] In one study a single session of scaling and root planing in patients with chronic periodontitis resulted in significant changes in subgingival microflora.[37] Reported alterations included a decrease in the proportion of motile rods for 1 week, a marked elevation in the proportion of coccoid cells for 21 days, and a marked reduction in the proportion of spirochetes for 7 weeks.

Although pocket debridement suppresses components of the subgingival microflora associated with periodontitis, periodontal pathogens may return to baseline levels within days or months.[3,50] The return of pathogens to pretreatment levels generally occurs in approximately 9 to 11 weeks but can vary dramatically among patients.[3]

Both the mechanical debridement performed by the therapist and the motivational environment provided by the appointment seem to be necessary for good maintenance results. Patients tend to reduce their oral hygiene efforts between appointments.[5,67] Knowing that their hygiene will be evaluated motivates them to perform better oral hygiene in anticipation of the appointment.

In one study the proportion of spirochetes obtained in baseline samples of subgingival flora was highly correlated with clinical periodontal deterioration over 1 year.[29] However, subsequent reports in the same longitudinal study concluded that the arbitrary assignment of treated periodontitis patients to 3-month maintenance intervals appears to be as effective in preventing recurrences of periodontitis as assignment of recall intervals based on microscopic monitoring of the subgingival flora.[30,31] Microscopic monitoring was found not to be a reliable predictor of future periodontal destruction in patients on 3-month recall programs, presumably because of the alteration of subgingival flora produced by subgingival instrumentation.

In conclusion, *there is a sound scientific basis for recall maintenance because subgingival scaling alters the pocket microflora for variable but relatively long periods.*

MAINTENANCE PROGRAM

Periodic recall visits form the foundation of a meaningful long-term prevention program. The interval between visits is initially set at 3 months but may be varied according to the patient's needs.

Periodontal care at each recall visit comprises three parts (Box 82-1). The first part involves examination and evaluation of the patient's current oral health. The second part includes the necessary maintenance treatment and oral hygiene reinforcement. The third part involves scheduling the patient for the next recall appointment, additional periodontal treatment, or restorative dental procedures. The time required for a recall visit for patients with multiple teeth in both arches is approximately 1 hour,[48] which includes time for greeting the patient, setting up, and cleaning up.

BOX 82-1

Maintenance Recall Procedures

Part I: Examination
(Approximate time: 14 minutes)
Patient greeting
Medical history changes
Oral pathologic examination
Oral hygiene status
Gingival changes
Pocket depth changes
Mobility changes
Occlusal changes
Dental caries
Restorative, prosthetic, and implant status

Part II: Treatment
(Approximate time: 36 minutes)
Oral hygiene reinforcement
Scaling
Polishing
Chemical irrigation or site-specific antimicrobial placement

Part III: Report, Cleanup, and Scheduling
(Approximate time: 10 minutes)
Write report in chart.
Discuss report with patient.
Clean and disinfect operatory.
Schedule next recall visit.
Schedule further periodontal treatment.
Schedule or refer for restorative or prosthetic treatment.

Examination and Evaluation

The recall examination is similar to the initial evaluation of the patient (see Chapter 35). However, because the patient is not new to the office, the dentist primarily looks for changes that have occurred since the last evaluation. Analysis of the current oral hygiene status of the patient is essential. Updating of changes in the medical history and evaluation of restorations, caries, prostheses, occlusion, tooth mobility, gingival status, and periodontal and periimplant probing depths are important parts of the recall appointment. The oral mucosa should be carefully inspected for pathologic conditions (Figures 82-4 to 82-9).

Radiographic examination must be individualized,[32] depending on the initial severity of the case and the findings at the recall visit (Table 82-1). These are compared with findings on previous radiographs to check the bone height and look for repair of osseous defects, signs of trauma from occlusion, periapical pathologic changes, and caries.

Checking of Plaque Control

To assess the effectiveness of their plaque control, patients should perform their hygiene regimen immediately before the recall appointment. Plaque control must be reviewed and corrected until the patient demonstrates the necessary proficiency, even if additional instruction sessions are required. Patients instructed in plaque

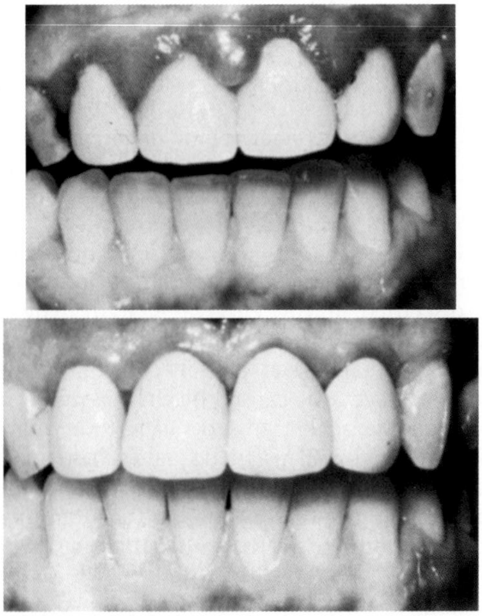

Figure 82-4 **A,** Hyperplastic gingivitis related to crown margins and plaque accumulation in a 27-year-old woman. **B,** Four months after treatment, there is significant improvement. However, some inflammation around crown margins still exists, which cannot be resolved without replacing the crowns.

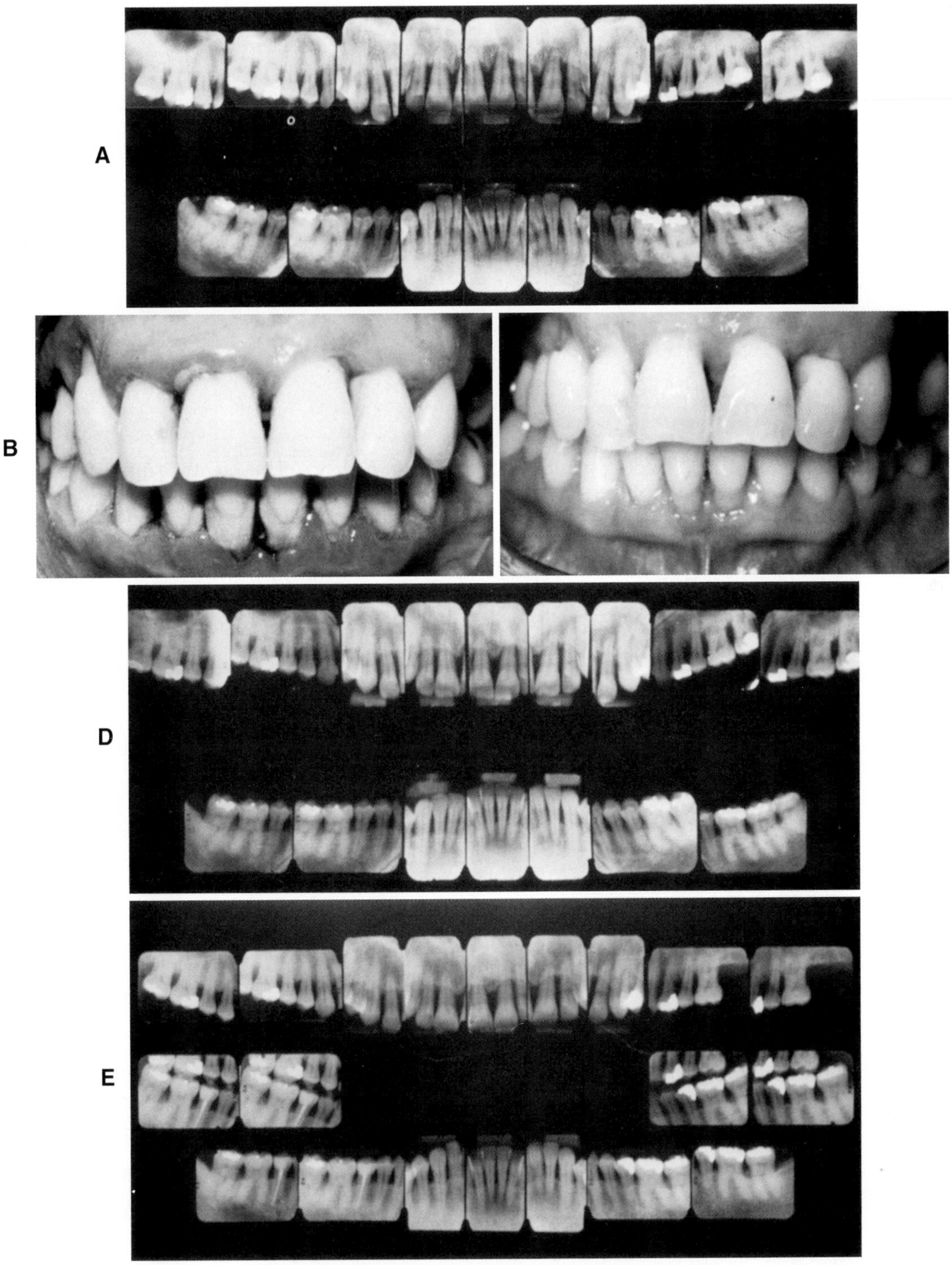

Figure 82-5 **A,** Patient was 38 years old when these original radiographs were taken and was treated with a combination of surgical and nonsurgical therapy. This individual is a classic class C maintenance patient. **B,** Pretreatment photographs. Note the inflammation and heavy calculus deposits. **C,** Photograph taken 10 years after treatment. **D,** Radiographs taken 5 years after treatment. **E,** Radiographs taken 10 years after treatment. The radiographic appearance is as good as can be expected in such a severe case. Teeth #15 and #17 were extracted 8 years after treatment.

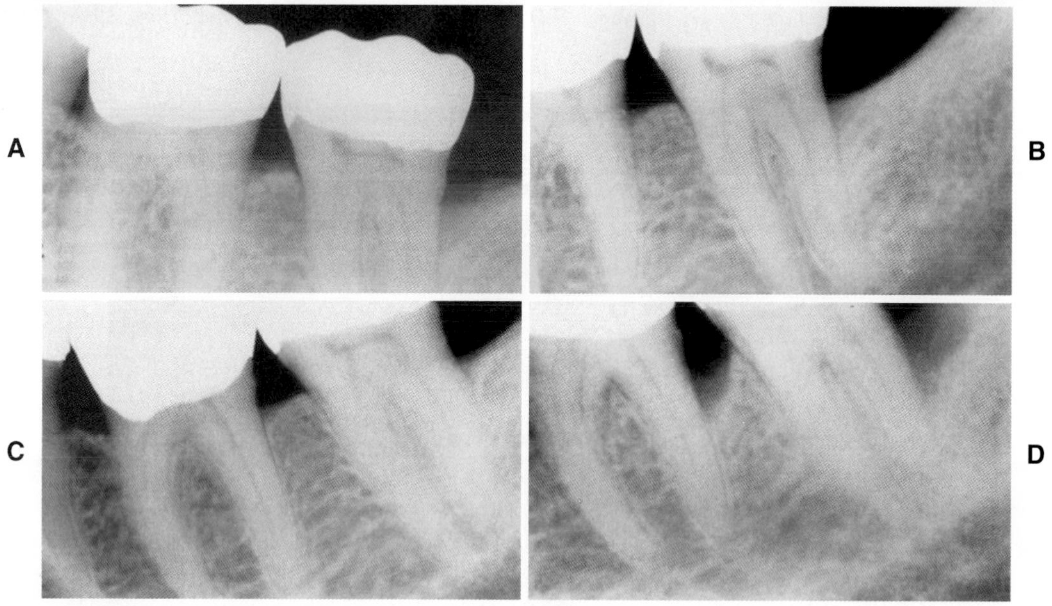

Figure 82-6 This series of radiographs clearly shows the importance of maintenance therapy. **A,** Original radiograph of a 58-year-old man. Note the deep distal bone loss on tooth #18 and the moderate distal lesion of tooth #19. Surgical treatment included osseous grafting. **B,** Radiograph 14 months after surgical therapy. The patient had recall maintenance performed every 3 to 4 months. **C,** Appearance 3 years after surgery, with regular recalls every 3 to 4 months. **D,** Appearance after 2 years without recalls (7 years after surgery). Note the progression of the disease on the distal surfaces of teeth #18 and #19.

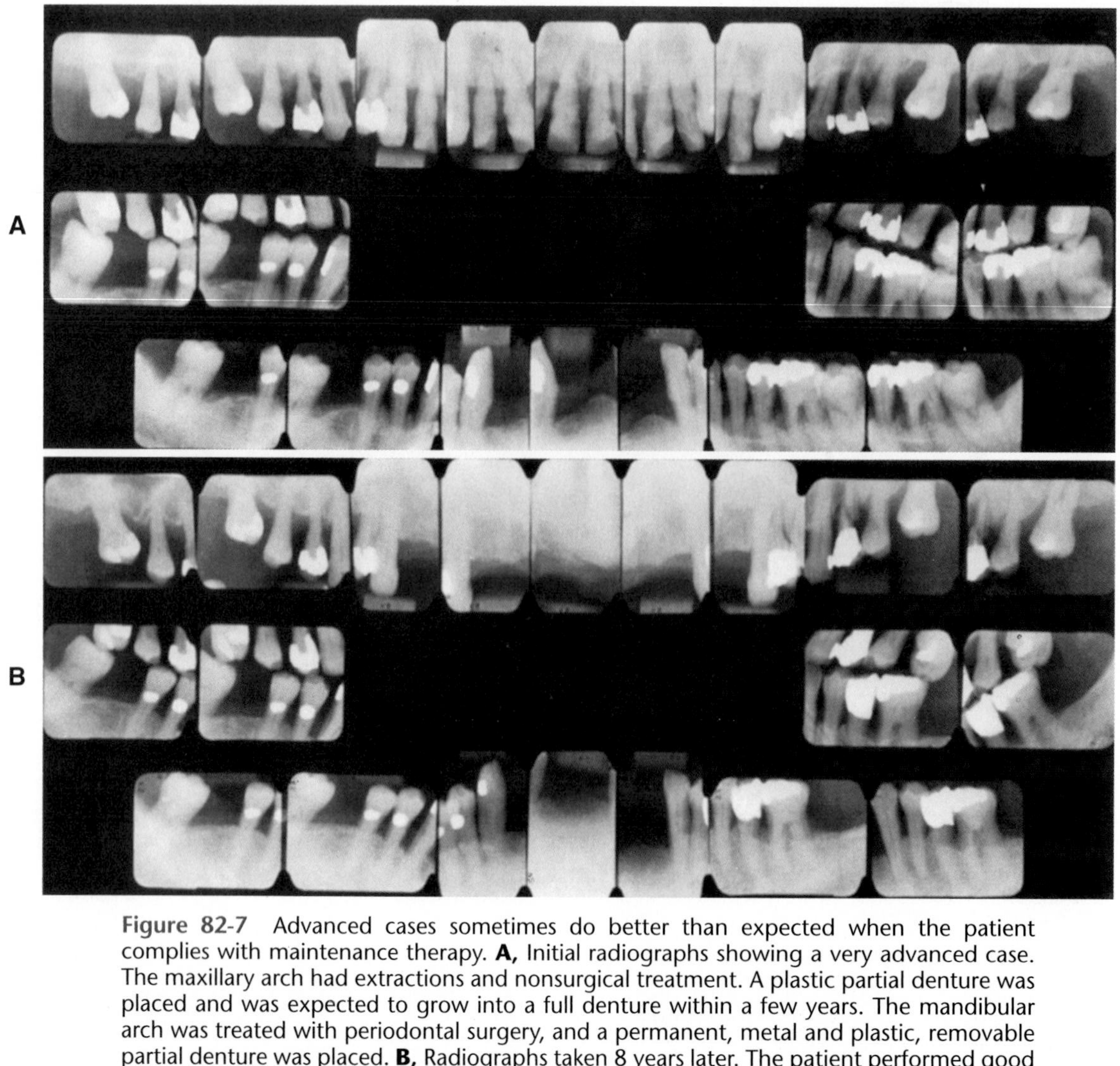

Figure 82-7 Advanced cases sometimes do better than expected when the patient complies with maintenance therapy. **A,** Initial radiographs showing a very advanced case. The maxillary arch had extractions and nonsurgical treatment. A plastic partial denture was placed and was expected to grow into a full denture within a few years. The mandibular arch was treated with periodontal surgery, and a permanent, metal and plastic, removable partial denture was placed. **B,** Radiographs taken 8 years later. The patient performed good oral hygiene and had 3-month recalls. Teeth #12 and #15 required extraction.

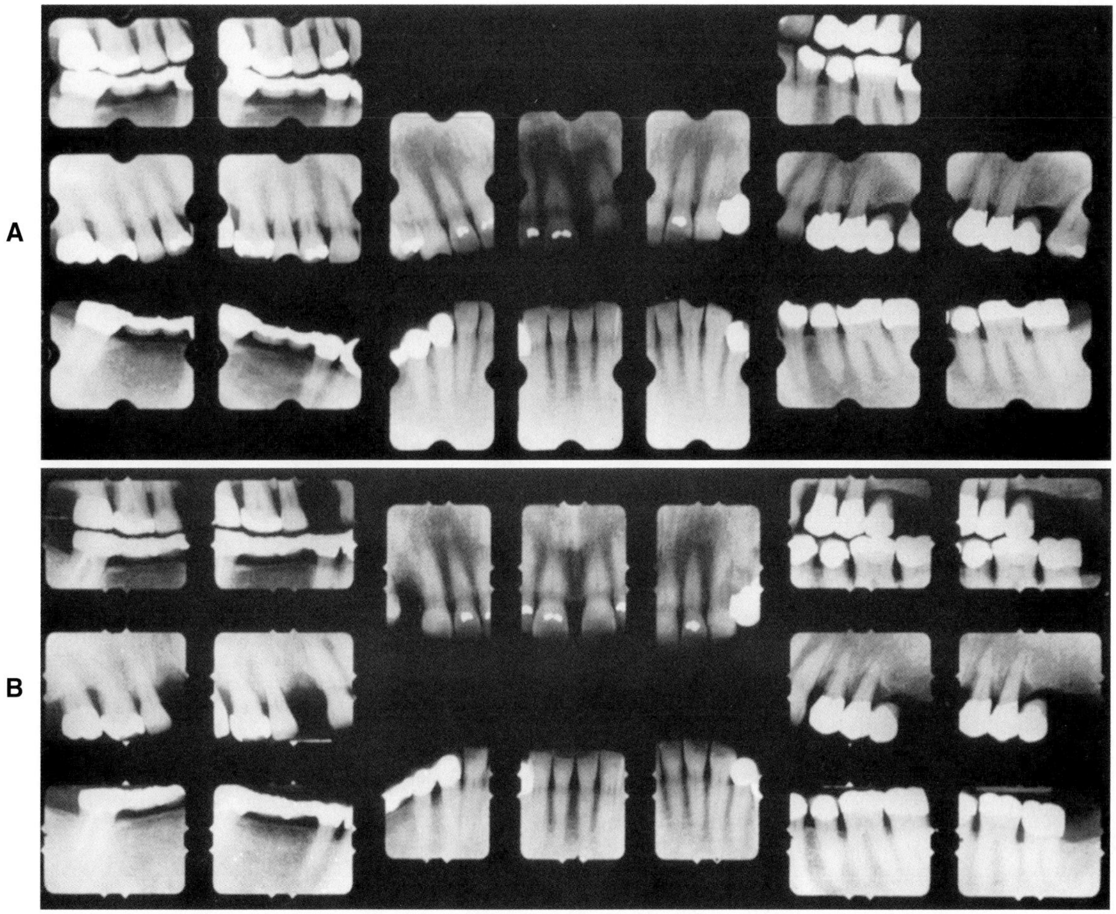

Figure 82-8 **A,** Initial radiographs. The patient was advised to have localized areas of periodontal surgery and periodontal recall every 3 months. However, the patient did not comply and only had dental cleanings once or twice yearly. **B,** Radiographs 4 years later. Note the loss of teeth #5 and #15 and the increased bone loss of several premolars and molars.

TABLE 82-1

Radiographic Examination of Recall Patients for Supportive Periodontal Treatment*

Patient Condition/Situation	Type of Examination
Clinical caries or high-risk factors for caries.	Posterior bite-wing examination at 12- to 18-month intervals.
Clinical caries and no high-risk factors for caries.	Posterior bite-wing examination at 24- to 36-month intervals.
Periodontal disease not under good control.	Periapical and/or vertical bite-wing radiographs of problem areas every 12 to 24 months; full-mouth series every 3 to 5 years.
History of periodontal treatment with disease under good control.	Bite-wing examination every 24 to 36 months; full-mouth series every 5 years.
Root form dental implants.	Periapical or vertical bite-wing radiographs at 6, 12, and 36 months after prosthetic placement, then every 36 months unless clinical problems arise.
Transfer of periodontal or implant maintenance patients.	Full-mouth series if a current set is not available. If full-mouth series has been taken within 24 months, radiographs of implants and periodontal problem areas should be taken.

Data from Matteson SR, Bottomley W, Finger H, et al: The selection of patients for x-ray examinations: dental radiographic examinations, DHHS Pub No FDA 88-8273, Washington, DC, 1987, US Department of Health and Human Services; and Wilson TG: *J Am Dent Assoc* 121:491, 1990.

*Radiographs should be taken when they are likely to affect diagnosis and patient treatment. The recommendations in this table are subject to clinical judgment and may not apply to every patient.

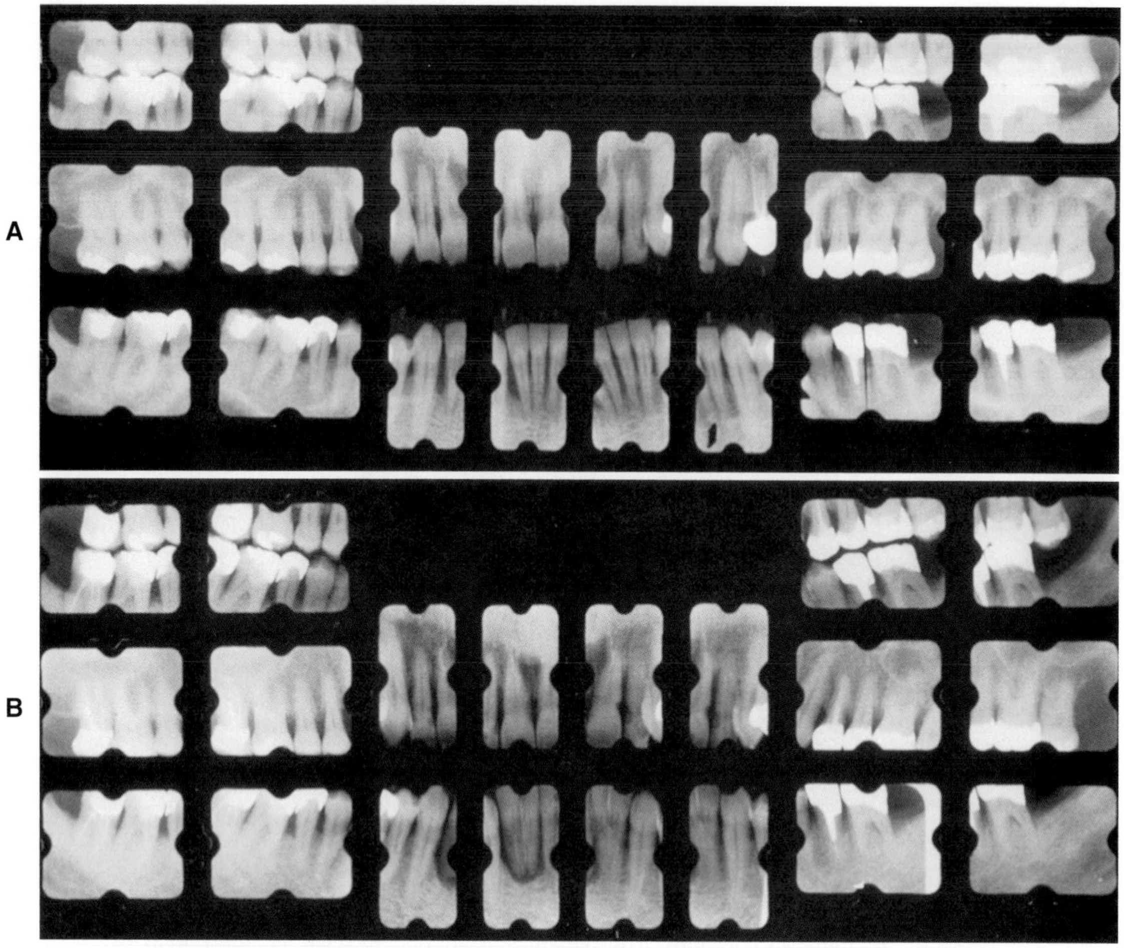

Figure 82-9 **A,** Initial radiographs. The patient was advised to have localized areas of periodontal surgery and periodontal recall every 3 months. However, the patient did not comply and had no treatment other than emergency care and occasional dental cleanings. **B,** Radiographs 7 years later. Note the advanced bone loss and caries on many teeth.

control have less plaque and gingivitis than uninstructed patients,[5,57,58] and the amount of supragingival plaque affects the number of subgingival anaerobic organisms.[17,52]

Treatment

The required scaling and root planing are performed, followed by an oral prophylaxis (see Chapter 51). Care must be taken not to instrument normal sites with shallow sulci (1-3 mm deep), because studies have shown that repeated subgingival scaling and root planing in initially normal periodontal sites result in significant loss of attachment.[27] Irrigation with antimicrobial agents or placement of site-specific antimicrobial devices is performed in maintenance patients with remaining pockets.[3,28,33,48]

Recurrence of Periodontal Disease

Occasionally, lesions may recur. This often can be traced to inadequate plaque control on the part of the patient or failure to comply with recommended SPT schedules. It should be understood, however, that it is the dentist's responsibility to teach, motivate, and control the patient's oral hygiene technique, and the patient's failure is the dentist's failure. Surgery should not be undertaken unless the patient has shown proficiency and willingness to cooperate by adequately performing his or her part of therapy.[8,55,66]

Other causes for recurrence include the following:

1. Inadequate or insufficient treatment that has failed to remove all the potential factors favoring plaque accumulation (see Figure 82-4). Incomplete calculus removal in areas of difficult access is a common source of problems.
2. Inadequate restorations placed after the periodontal treatment was completed.
3. Failure of the patient to return for periodic checkups (see Figure 82-6). This may be a result of the patient's conscious or unconscious decision not to continue treatment or the failure of the dentist and staff to emphasize the need for periodic examinations.
4. Presence of some systemic diseases that may affect host resistance to previously acceptable levels of plaque.

A failing case can be recognized by the following:

1. Recurring inflammation revealed by gingival changes and bleeding of the sulcus on probing.
2. Increasing depth of sulci, leading to the recurrence of pocket formation.
3. Gradual increases in bone loss, as determined by radiographs.
4. Gradual increases in tooth mobility, as ascertained by clinical examination.

Cases that do not respond to adequate therapy or recur for unknown reasons are referred to as *aggressive periodontitis* (see Chapters 33 and 46).

The decision to re-treat a periodontal patient should not be made at the preventive maintenance appointment but should be postponed for 1 to 2 weeks.[13] Often the mouth looks much better at that time because of the resolution of edema and the resulting improved tone of the gingiva. Table 82-2 summarizes the symptoms of recurrence of periodontal disease and their probable causes.

CLASSIFICATION OF POSTTREATMENT PATIENTS

The first year after periodontal therapy is important in terms of indoctrinating the patient in a recall pattern and reinforcing oral hygiene techniques. In addition, it may take several months to evaluate accurately the results of some periodontal surgical procedures. Consequently, some areas may have to be re-treated because the results may not be optimal. Furthermore, the first-year patient often has etiologic factors that may have been overlooked and may be more amenable to treatment at this early stage. For these reasons, *the recall interval for first-year patients should not be longer than 3 months.*

The patients who are on a periodontal recall schedule are a varied group. Table 82-3 lists several categories of maintenance patients and a suggested recall interval for each. Patients can improve or may relapse to a different classification, with a reduction in or exacerbation of periodontal disease. When one dental arch is more involved than the other, the patient's periodontal disease is classified by the arch with the worse condition.

In summary, maintenance care is a critical phase of therapy. *The long-term preservation of the dentition is closely associated with the frequency and quality of recall maintenance.*

REFERRAL OF PATIENTS TO THE PERIODONTIST

The majority of periodontal care belongs in the hands of the general dentist, because of (1) the overwhelming number of patients with periodontal disease and (2) the intimate relationship between periodontal disease and restorative dentistry.

For various reasons, an ever-greater number of periodontal maintenance patients are expected in future years. The number of caries per capita has dwindled since the mid-1970s by about 50%, and some evidence suggests that this decline will continue.[48] As more people retain their teeth throughout their lifetime and as the proportion

TABLE **82-2**	
Symptoms and Causes of Recurrence of Disease	
Symptom	**Possible Causes**
Increased mobility	Increased inflammation
	Poor oral hygiene
	Subgingival calculus
	Inadequate restorations
	Deteriorating or poorly designed prostheses
	Systemic disease modifying host response to plaque
Recession	Toothbrush abrasion
	Inadequate keratinized gingiva
	Frenum pull
	Orthodontic therapy
Increased mobility with no change in pocket depth and no radiographic change	Occlusal trauma caused by lateral occlusal interference
	Bruxism
	High restoration
	Poorly designed or worn-out prosthesis
	Poor crown-to-root ratio
Increased pocket depth with no radiographic change	Poor oral hygiene
	Infrequent recall visits
	Subgingival calculus
	Poorly fitting partial denture
	Mesial inclination into edentulous space
	Failure of new attachment surgery
	Cracked teeth
	Grooves in teeth
	New periodontal disease
	Gingival overgrowth caused by medication
Increased pocket depth with increased radiographic bone loss	Poor oral hygiene
	Subgingival calculus
	Infrequent recall visits
	Inadequate or deteriorating restorations
	Poorly designed prostheses
	Inadequate surgery
	Systemic disease modifying host response to plaque
	Cracked teeth
	Grooves in teeth
	New periodontal disease

of older people in the population increases, more teeth will be at risk of periodontal disease. Therefore the prevalence of patients requiring SPT is likely to increase in the future.

This expected increase in the number of periodontal patients will necessitate a greater understanding of periodontal problems and an increased level of expertise for the solution of such problems on the part of the general practitioner of dentistry. However, specialists always will be needed to treat particularly difficult cases, patients with systemic health problems, dental implant patients, and those with a complex prosthetic construction that requires reliable results.

The question of where to draw the line between the cases to be treated in the general dental office and those to be referred to a specialist varies for different practitioners and patients. The diagnosis indicates the type of periodontal treatment required. If periodontal destruction necessitates surgery on the distal surfaces of second molars, extensive osseous surgery, or complex regenerative procedures, the patient is usually best treated by a specialist. On the other hand, patients who require localized gingivectomy or flap curettage usually can be treated by the general dentist.

It is immediately obvious that some patients should be referred to a specialist, whereas most patients clearly have problems that can be treated by a general dentist. For a third group of patients, however, it will be difficult to decide whether treatment by a specialist is required. Any patient who does not clearly belong in the second of these categories should be considered a candidate for referral to a specialist.[41]

The decision to have the general practitioner treat a patient's periodontal problem should be guided by a consideration of the degree of risk that the patient will lose a tooth or teeth for periodontally related reasons.

The most important factors in the decision are the *extent and location of the periodontal deterioration.* Teeth with pockets of 5 mm or more, as measured from the cementoenamel junction, may have a prognosis of rapid decline. The location of the periodontal deterioration is also an important factor in determining the risk of tooth loss. Teeth with furcation lesions may be at risk even when more than 50% of bone support remains. Therefore, patients with strategically important teeth that fall into these categories are usually best treated by specialists.

An important question remains: *Should the maintenance phase of therapy be performed by the general practitioner or the specialist?* This should be determined by the amount of periodontal deterioration present. Class A recall patients should be maintained by the general dentist, whereas class C patients should be maintained by the specialist (see Table 82-3). Class B patients can alternate recall visits between the general practitioner and the specialist (Figure 82-10). The suggested rule is that the *patient's disease should dictate whether the general practitioner or the specialist should perform the maintenance therapy.*

TESTS FOR DISEASE ACTIVITY

Periodontal patients, even though they have received effective periodontal therapy, are at risk of disease recurrence for the rest of their lives.[23,24] In addition, many pockets in furcation areas may not have been eliminated by surgery. At present, the best way of determining areas that are losing attachment is to use a well-organized charting system.[46,64] Some computerized systems allow easy retrieval and comparison of past findings.

Comparison of sequential probing measurements gives the most accurate indication of the rate of loss of attachment.[4] A number of other clinical and laboratory variables have been correlated with disease activity (see Chapter 37). At present, no accurate method of predicting disease activity exists, and clinicians rely on the information provided by combining probing, bleeding on probing, and sequential attachment measurements.[26,30,64] Patients whose disease is clearly refractory are candidates for bacterial culturing and antibiotic therapy in conjunction with additional mechanical therapy.

New methods will undoubtedly be developed in the future to help predict disease activity.[3] The clinician must be able to interpret whether a test may be useful in determining disease activity and future loss of attachment.[9] Tests should be adopted only when they are based on research that includes a critical analysis of the sensitivity, specificity, disease incidence, and predictive value of the proposed test.

MAINTENANCE FOR DENTAL IMPLANT PATIENTS

Patients with implants are susceptible to a form of bone loss called *periimplantitis,* and evidence suggests that such patients may be more prone to plaque-induced inflammation with bone loss than those with natural teeth[7,49,61] (see Chapter 81).

The overall periodontal condition in partially edentulous implant patients can influence the clinical condition around implants.[10] The microflora of implants in partially edentulous patients differs from that in edentulous patients.[6] The implant microflora is similar to tooth microflora in the partially edentulous mouth. Periodontal and implant maintenance are linked because maintenance of a tooth microflora consistent with periodontal health is necessary to maintain implant microflora consistent with periimplant health.[6,56] Because periimplantitis is difficult to treat,[22] it is extremely important to treat periodontal disease before implant placement and to provide good supportive therapy with implant patients.

In general, procedures for maintenance of patients with implants are similar to those for patients with natural teeth,[3,19,25,35] with the following three differences:

1. Special instrumentation that will not scratch the implants are used for calculus removal on the implants.
2. Acidic fluoride prophylactic agents are avoided.
3. Nonabrasive prophy pastes are used.

During the phase after uncovering the implants, patients must use ultrasoft brushes, chemotherapeutic rinses, tartar control pastes, irrigation devices, and yarnlike materials to keep the implants and natural teeth clean. Patients often are reluctant to touch the implants but must be encouraged to keep the areas clean.

Special instruments should be used on the implants during recall appointments.[19,35] Metal hand instruments and ultrasonic and sonic tips should be avoided because they can alter the titanium surface.[20] Only plastic instruments or specially designed gold-plated curettes should be used for calculus removal because the implant surfaces

TABLE 82-3

Recall Intervals for Various Classes of Recall Patients

Merin Classification	Characteristics	Recall Interval
First year	First-year patient: routine therapy and uneventful healing.	3 months
	First-year patient: difficult case with complicated prosthesis, furcation involvement, poor crown-to-root ratios, or questionable patient cooperation.	1-2 months
Class A	Excellent results well maintained for 1 year or more. Patient displays good oral hygiene, minimal calculus, no occlusal problems, no complicated prostheses, no remaining pockets, and no teeth with less than 50% of alveolar bone remaining.	6 months to 1 year
Class B	Generally good results maintained reasonably well for 1 year or more, but patient displays some of the following factors: 1. Inconsistent or poor oral hygiene 2. Heavy calculus formation 3. Systemic disease that predisposes to periodontal breakdown 4. Some remaining pockets 5. Occlusal problems 6. Complicated prostheses 7. Ongoing orthodontic therapy 8. Recurrent dental caries 9. Some teeth with less than 50% of alveolar bone support 10. Smoking 11. Positive family history or genetic test 12. More than 20% of pockets bleed on probing	3-4 months (decide on recall interval based on number and severity of negative factors)
Class C	Generally poor results after periodontal therapy and/or several negative factors from the following list: 1. Inconsistent or poor oral hygiene 2. Heavy calculus formation 3. Systemic disease that predisposes to periodontal breakdown 4. Many remaining pockets 5. Occlusal problems 6. Complicated prostheses 7. Recurrent dental caries 8. Periodontal surgery indicated but not performed for medical, psychologic, or financial reasons 9. Many teeth with less than 50% of alveolar bone support 10. Condition too far advanced to be improved by periodontal surgery 11. Smoking 12. Positive family history or genetic test 13. More than 20% of pockets bleed on probing	1-3 months (decide on recall interval based on number and severity of negative factors; consider re-treating some areas or extracting severely involved teeth)

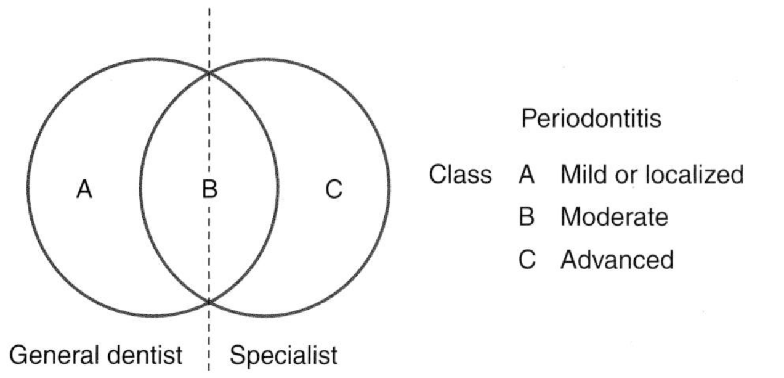

Figure 82-10 Scheme for determining which practitioner should perform periodontal maintenance in patients with different degrees of periodontitis.

can be easily scratched. The rubber cup with flour of pumice, tin oxide, or special implant-polishing pastes should be used on abutment surfaces with light, intermittent pressure.[34]

Although daily use of topically applied antimicrobials is advised,[35] acidic fluoride agents should not be used because they cause surface damage to titanium abutments.[43]

When prosthetics must be unscrewed and removed for maintenance, this is best done in the office responsible for placing the prosthetics. Each time the prosthetic appliances are reattached, a slight change in the occlusion occurs. Time must be allowed for occlusal corrections.

SCIENCE TRANSFER

All types of periodontal and implant therapy require continuous follow-up with periodic maintenance care because of the constant microbial challenge initiated by the formation of plaque. Thus the host must continually respond to this challenge, and this response must be effective to prevent further tissue damage. Maintenance therapy that has proved effective over time is periodic, professional recall visits.

The frequency of these recall visits depends on each patient. Some patients require frequent recall intervals to limit the inflammation around the teeth, whereas others may tolerate fewer recall visits. Most patients with periodontitis will need a long-term recall schedule, with visits for professional cleaning every 3 or 4 months and close supervision of their oral hygiene procedures. Monitoring of pocket depths and evaluation of other oral conditions will help detect problems early and allow treatment before extensive tissue loss. Ongoing work involves evaluating systems to determine the patient's risk for periodontal disease, and as these evolve, patient maintenance schedules can be better tailored to fit an individual's risk category.

REFERENCES

1. Ainamo J, Ainamo A: Risk assessment of recurrence of disease during supportive periodontal care, *J Clin Periodontol* 23:232, 1996.
2. Alaluusua S, Asikainen S, Lai CH: Intrafamilial transmission of *Actinobacillus actinomycetemcomitans, J Periodontol* 62:207, 1991.
3. American Academy of Periodontology: Position paper: Periodontal maintenance, *J Periodontol* 74:1395, 2003.
4. Armitage GC: Diagnosing periodontal diseases. In *Perspectives on oral antimicrobial therapeutics,* Littleton, Mass, 1987, PSG Publishing.
5. Axelson P, Lindhe J: The significance of maintenance care in the treatment of periodontal disease, *J Clin Periodontol* 8:281, 1981.
6. Bauman GR, Mills M, Rapley JW, et al: Plaque-induced inflammation around implants, *Int J Oral Maxillofac Implants* 7:330, 1992.
7. Bauman GR, Rapley JW, Hallmon WW, et al: The peri-implant sulcus, *Int J Oral Maxillofac Implants* 8:273, 1993.
8. Becker W, Becker BE, Berg LE: Periodontal treatment without maintenance: a retrospective study in 44 patients, *J Periodontol* 155:505, 1984.
9. Bennett WI: Screening for bowel cancer, *Harvard Med School Health Lett* 11:6, 1986.
10. Bragger U, Burgin WB, Hammerle CH, et al: Associations between clinical parameters assessed around implants and teeth, *Clin Oral Implant Res* 8:412, 1997.
11. Carranza FA Jr, Saglie FR, Newman MG, et al: Scanning and transmission electron microscope study of tissue invading microorganisms in localized juvenile periodontitis, *J Periodontol* 54:598, 1983.
12. Caton JG, Zander HA: The attachment between tooth and gingival tissues after periodic root planing and soft tissue curettage, *J Periodontol* 50:462, 1979.
13. Chace R: Retreatment in periodontal practice, *J Periodontol* 48:410, 1977.
14. Checchi L, Montevecchi M, Gatto MR, Trombelli L: Retrospective study of tooth loss in 92 periodontal patients, *J Clin Periodontol* 29:651, 2002.
15. Christersson LA, Albini B, Zambon JJ, et al: Tissue localization of *Actinobacillus actinomycetemcomitans* in human periodontitis. I. Light, immunofluorescence and electron microscopic studies, *J Periodontol* 58:529, 1987.
16. Cortellimi P, Pini-Prato G, Torretti M: Periodontal regeneration of human infrabony defects. V. Effects of oral hygiene on long-term stability, *J Clin Periodontol* 21:606, 1994.
17. Dahlen G, Lindhe J, Sato K, et al: The effect of supragingival plaque control on the subgingival microbiota in subjects with periodontal disease, *J Clin Periodontol* 19:802, 1992.
18. Egloff E, Saglie FR, Newman MG: Intragingival bacteria subsequent to scaling and root planing, *J Dent Res* 65:269, 1986 (abstract).
19. Eskow RN, Smith VS: Preventive periimplant protocol, *Compend Contin Educ Dent* 20:137, 1999.
20. Fox SC, Moriarty JD, Kusy RP: The effects of scaling a titanium implant surface with metal and plastic instruments: an in vitro study, *J Periodontol* 61:485, 1990.
21. Greenwell H, Bissada NB, Wittwer JW: Periodontics in general practice: perspectives on periodontal diagnosis, *J Am Dent Assoc* 119:537, 1989.
22. Grunder U, Hürzeler MB, Schüpbach P, et al: Treatment of ligature-induced peri-implantitis using guided tissue regeneration: a clinical and histologic study in the beagle dog, *Int J Oral Maxillofac Implants* 8:282, 1993.
23. Halazonetis TD, Smulow JB, Donnenfeld W, et al: Pocket formation 3 years after comprehensive periodontal therapy: a retrospective study, *J Periodontol* 56:515, 1985.
24. Hirschfeld L, Wasserman B: A long-term survey of tooth loss in 600 treated periodontal patients, *J Periodontol* 49:225, 1978.
25. Lang NP, Nyman SR: Supportive maintenance care for patients with implants and advanced restorative therapy, *Periodontol 2000* 4:119, 1994.
26. Lang NP, Joss A, Orsanic T, et al: Bleeding on probing, *J Clin Periodontol* 13:590, 1986.
27. Lindhe J, Nyman S, Karring T: Scaling and root planing in shallow pockets, *J Clin Periodontol* 9:415, 1982.
28. Lindhe J, Heijl L, Goodson JM, et al: Local tetracycline delivery using hollow fiber devices in periodontal therapy, *J Clin Periodontol* 6:141, 1979.
29. Listgarten MA, Hellden L: Relative distribution of bacteria at clinically healthy and periodontally diseased sites in humans, *J Clin Periodontol* 5:115, 1978.
30. Listgarten MA, Schifter CC, Sullivan P, et al: Failure of a microbiological assay to reliably predict disease recurrence in a treated periodontitis population receiving regularly scheduled prophylaxes, *J Clin Periodontol* 13:768, 1986.
31. Listgarten MA, Sullivan P, George C, et al: Comparative longitudinal study of 2 methods of scheduling maintenance visit: 4-year data, *J Clin Periodontol* 16:105, 1989.
32. Matteson SR, Bottomley W, Finger H, et al: The selection of patients for x-ray examinations: dental radiographic examinations, DHHS Pub No FDA 88-8273, Washington, DC, 1987, US Department of Health and Human Services.
33. Mazza JE, Newman MG, Sims TN: Clinical and antimicrobial effect of stannous fluoride on periodontitis, *J Clin Periodontol* 8:213, 1981.
34. McCollum J, O'Neal RB, Brennan WA, et al: The effect of titanium implant abutment surface irregularities on plaque accumulation in vivo, *J Periodontol* 63:802, 1992.

35. Meffert RM, Langer B, Fritz ME: Dental implants: a review, *J Periodontol* 63:859, 1992.
36. Mendoza AR, Newcomb GM, Nixon KC: Compliance with supportive periodontal therapy, *J Periodontol* 62:731, 1991.
37. Mousques T, Listgarten MA, Phillips RW: Effect of scaling and root planing on the composition of human subgingival microflora, *J Periodontal Res* 15:144, 1980.
38. Novaes AB Jr, Novaes AB: Compliance with supportive periodontal therapy. Part 1. Risk of non-compliance in the first 5-year period, *J Periodontol* 70:679, 1999.
39. Novaes AB Jr, Novaes AB: Compliance with supportive periodontal therapy. Part II, *Braz Dent J* 12:47, 2001.
40. Oliver RC: Tooth loss with and without periodontal therapy, *Periodont Abstracts* 17:8, 1969.
41. Parr RW, Pipe P, Watts T: *Periodontal maintenance therapy,* Berkeley, Calif, 1974, Praxis.
42. Pertuiset JH, Saglie FR, Lofthus J, et al: Recurrent periodontal disease and bacterial presence in the gingiva, *J Periodontol* 58:553, 1987.
43. Probster L, Lin W, Juttemann H: Effect of fluoride prophylactic agents on titanium surfaces, *Int J Oral Maxillofac Implants* 7:390, 1992.
44. Rosenberg ES, Evian CI, Listgarten MA: The composition of the subgingival microbiota after periodontal therapy, *J Periodontol* 52:435, 1981.
45. Ross IF, Thompson RH, Galdi M: The results of treatment: a long-term study of 180 patients, *Parodontologie* 25:125, 1971.
46. Ryan RJ: The accuracy of clinical parameters in detecting periodontal disease activity, *J Am Dent Assoc* 111:753, 1985.
47. Saglie FR, Newman MG, Carranza FA Jr, et al: Immunohistochemical localization of *Actinobacillus actinomycetemcomitans* in sections of gingival tissue in localized juvenile periodontitis, *Acta Odont Lat Am* 1:40, 1984.
48. Schallhorn RG, Snider LE: Periodontal maintenance therapy, *J Am Dent Assoc* 103:227, 1981.
49. Schou S, Holmstrup P, Reibel J, et al: Ligature-induced marginal inflammation around osseointegrated implants and ankylosed teeth: stereologic and histologic observations on cynomolgus monkeys, *J Periodontol* 64:529, 1993.
50. Shiloah J, Patters MR: Repopulation of periodontal pockets by microbial pathogens in the absence of supportive therapy, *J Periodontol* 67:130, 1996.
51. Slots J, Mashimo P, Levine MJ, et al: Periodontal therapy in humans. I. Microbiological and clinical effects of a single course of periodontal scaling and root planing, and of adjunctive tetracycline therapy, *J Periodontol* 50:495, 1979.
52. Smulow JB, Turesky SS, Hill RG: The effect of supragingival plaque removal on anaerobic bacteria in deep pockets, *J Am Dent Assoc* 107:737, 1983.
53. Stahl SS: Repair potential of the soft tissue-root interface, *J Periodontol* 48:545, 1977.
54. Stahl SS, Witkin GJ, Heller A, et al: Gingival healing. IV. The effects of home care on gingivectomy repair, *J Periodontol* 40:264, 1969.
55. Sternlich HC: Evaluating long-term periodontal therapy, *Texas Dent J* 92:4, 1974.
56. Sumida S, Ishihara K, Kishi M, Okuda K: Transmission of periodontal disease-associated bacteria from teeth to osseointegrated implant regions, *Int J Oral Maxillofac Implants* 17:696, 2002.
57. Suomi JD, Greene JC, Vermillion JR, et al: The effect of controlled oral hygiene procedures on the progression of periodontal disease in adults: results after the third and final year, *J Periodontol* 42:152, 1971.
58. Suomi JD, West JD, Chang JJ, et al: The effect of controlled oral hygiene procedures on the progression of periodontal disease in adults: radiographic findings, *J Periodontol* 42:562, 1971.
59. Tonetti MA, Muller-Campanile V, Lang NP: Changes in the prevalence of residual pockets and tooth loss in treated periodontal patients during a supportive maintenance care program, *J Clin Periodontol* 25:1008, 1998.
60. van Steenbergen TJ, Petit MD, van der Velden U, et al: Transmission of *Porphyromonas gingivalis* between spouses, *J Clin Periodontol* 20:340, 1993.
61. van Steenberghe D, Klinge B, Linden U, et al: Periodontal indices around natural and titanium abutments: a longitudinal multicenter study, *J Periodontol* 64:538, 1993.
62. Waerhaug J: Healing of the dentoepithelial junction following subgingival plaque control, *J Periodontol* 49:119, 1978.
63. Wilson TG: Maintaining periodontal treatment, *J Am Dent Assoc* 121:491, 1990.
64. Wilson TG, Kornman KS: Retreatment, *Periodontol 2000* 12:119, 1996.
65. Wilson TG Jr: Compliance: a review of the literature, *J Periodontol* 58:706, 1987.
66. Wilson TG Jr, Glover ME, Malik AK, et al: Tooth loss in maintenance patients in a private periodontal practice, *J Periodontol* 58:231, 1987.
67. Wilson TG Jr, Glover ME, Schoen J, et al: Compliance with maintenance therapy in a private periodontal practice, *J Periodontol* 55:468, 1984.

Results of Periodontal Treatment

Robert L. Merin

83

CHAPTER

CHAPTER OUTLINE

The prevalence of periodontal disease, the resulting high rate of tooth mortality, and the potential for multiple systemic health complications aggravated by chronic periodontitis raise an important question: Is periodontal treatment effective in preventing and controlling the chronic infection and progressive destruction of periodontal disease? Current concepts of evaluating health care require a scientific basis for treatment, referred to as **evidence-based therapy.** *Evidence is now overwhelming that periodontal therapy is effective in preventing periodontal disease, slowing the destruction of the periodontium, and reducing tooth loss.*

PREVENTION AND TREATMENT OF GINGIVITIS

For many years, the belief that good oral hygiene is necessary for the successful prevention and treatment of gingivitis has been widespread among periodontists. In addition, worldwide epidemiologic studies have confirmed a close relationship between the incidence of gingivitis and lack of oral hygiene.[5,6]

Löe and co-workers[16,35] provided conclusive evidence on the association between oral hygiene and gingivitis. After 9 to 21 days without performing oral hygiene measures, healthy dental students with previously excellent oral hygiene and healthy gingiva developed heavy accumulations of plaque and generalized mild gingivitis. When oral hygiene techniques were reinstituted, the plaque in most areas disappeared in 1 or 2 days, and gingival inflammation in these areas disappeared approximately 1 week after the plaque was removed. Thus, gingivitis is reversible and can be resolved by daily, effective plaque removal.

A number of long-term studies have shown that gingival health can be maintained by a combination of effective oral hygiene maintenance and scaling procedures.*

A 3-year study was conducted on 1248 General Telephone workers in California to determine whether progression of gingival inflammation is reduced in an oral environment in which high levels of hygiene are maintained.[33,34] Experimental and control groups were computer-matched based on periodontal and oral hygiene status, past caries experience, age, and gender. During the study period, several procedures were instituted to ensure that the oral hygiene status of the experimental group was maintained at a high level. Subjects were given a series of frequent oral prophylaxis treatments combined with oral hygiene instruction. Subjects in the control group received no attention from the study team except for annual examinations. They were advised to continue their usual daily practices and accustomed visits for

*References 1, 2, 8, 11, 12, 19, 33, 34.

professional care. After 3 years, the increase in plaque and debris in the control group was four times as great as that in the experimental group. Similarly, gingivitis scores were much higher in control subjects than in the matching experimental group. Therefore, *chronic marginal gingivitis can be controlled with good oral hygiene and dental prophylaxis.*

PREVENTION AND TREATMENT OF LOSS OF ATTACHMENT

Although periodontal therapy has been used for more than 100 years, it is only since the mid-1970s that a number of studies have been conducted to determine the effect of treatment on reducing the progressive loss of periodontal support for the natural dentition.

Prevention of Loss of Attachment

Löe et al.[17,18] conducted a longitudinal investigation to study the natural development and progression of periodontal disease. The first study group, established in Oslo, Norway, in 1969, consisted of 565 healthy male nondental students and academicians between 17 and 40 years of age. Oslo was selected mainly because this city had an ongoing preschool, school, and postschool dental program offering systematic preventive, restorative, endodontic, orthodontic, and surgical therapy on an annual recall basis for all children and adolescents, complete with a documented attendance record, for the previous 40 years. Members of the study population had experienced maximum exposure to conventional dental care throughout their lives. A second study group, established in Sri Lanka in 1970, consisted of 480 male tea laborers between 15 and 40 years of age. They were healthy and well built by local standards, and their nutritional condition was clinically fair. The workers had never been exposed to any programs relative to the prevention or treatment of dental diseases. Toothbrushing was unknown, and dental caries was virtually nonexistent.

The results of this study are interesting. The Norwegian group, as the members approached 40 years of age, had a mean individual loss of attachment of slightly above 1.5 mm, and the mean annual rate of attachment loss was 0.08 mm for interproximal surfaces and 0.10 mm for buccal surfaces. As the Sri Lankans approached 40 years of age, the mean individual loss of attachment was 4.50 mm, and the mean annual rate of progression of the lesion was 0.30 mm for interproximal surfaces and 0.20 mm for buccal surfaces. Figure 83-1 shows a graphic interpretation of the difference between the two groups. This study suggests that without interference, periodontal lesions progress continually and at a relatively even pace.

Further analysis of the Sri Lankan laborers showed that they were not all losing attachment at the same rate (Figures 83-2 and 83-3).[18] Virtually all gingival areas showed inflammation, but attachment loss varied tremendously. Based on interproximal loss of attachment and tooth mortality, three subpopulations were identified: individuals with "rapid progression" (RP) of periodontal disease (8%), individuals with moderate progression (MP) (81%), and individuals who exhibited "no progression" (NP) of periodontal disease beyond gingivitis (11%). At age 35, the mean loss of attachment in the RP group was 9 mm; in the MP group, 4 mm; and in the NP group, less than 1 mm. At the age of 45, the mean loss of attachment in the RP group was 13 mm and in the MP group, 7 mm. Therefore, under natural conditions and in the absence of therapy, 89% of the Sri Lankan laborers had severe periodontitis that progressed at much greater rates than in the Norwegian group.

In the previously discussed study of General Telephone workers in California, loss of attachment was measured clinically and alveolar bone loss measured radiographically.[33,34] After 3 years, the control group showed loss of attachment at a rate more than three times that of the matching experimental group during the same period (Figure 83-4). In addition, subjects who received frequent oral prophylaxis and were instructed in good oral hygiene practices showed less bone loss radiographically after 3 years than did control subjects. *It is clear that loss of attachment can be reduced by good oral hygiene and frequent dental prophylaxis.*

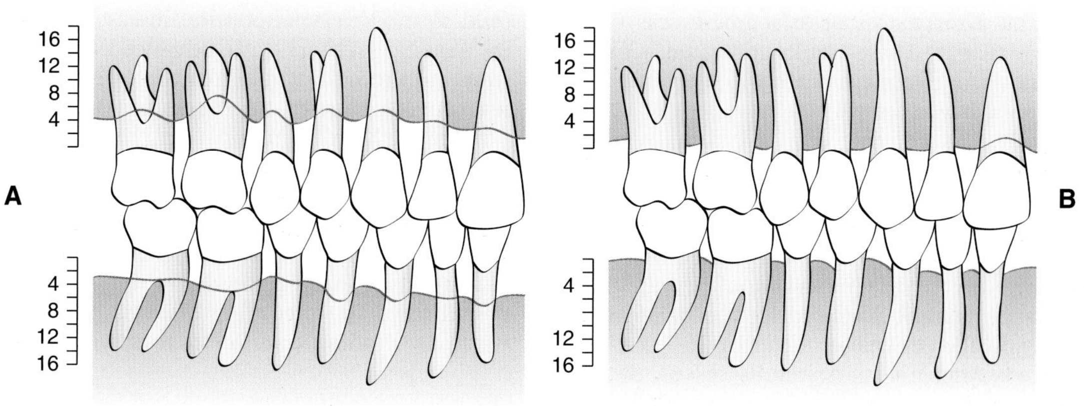

Figure 83-1 **A,** Mean periodontal support of teeth of Sri Lankan tea laborers at approximately 40 years of age. **B,** Mean periodontal support of teeth of Norwegian academicians at approximately 40 years of age. (From Löe H, Anerud A, Boysen H, et al: *J Periodontol* 49:607, 1978.)

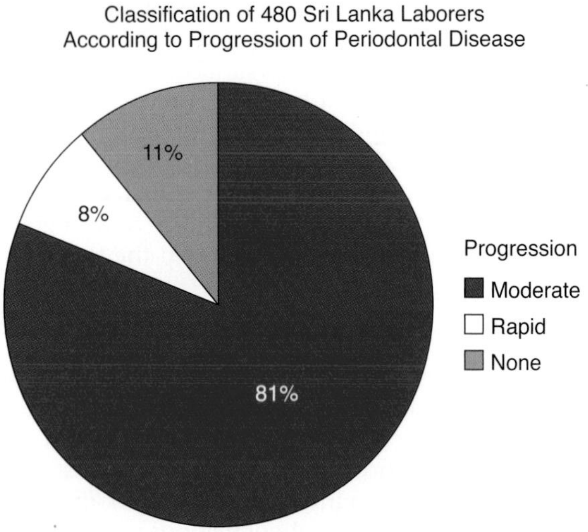

Figure 83-2 Progression of periodontal disease in an untreated population. (Data from Löe H, Anerud A, Boysen H, et al: *J Clin Periodontol* 13:431, 1986.)

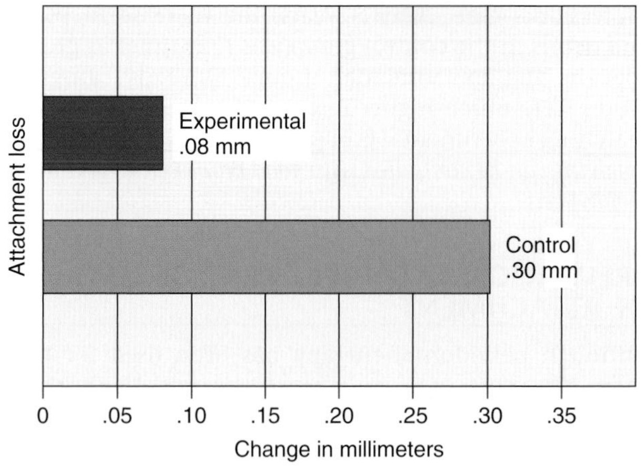

Figure 83-4 Change in mean attachment level from baseline to third-year examination for experimental and control groups. (From Suomi JD, West JD, Chang JJ, et al: *J Periodontol* 42:152, 1971.)

Mean Loss of Attachment at Various Ages (mm)

Age	Progression Group	
	Rapid	Moderate
35	9	4
45	13	7

Figure 83-3 Loss of attachment in untreated Sri Lankan laborers. (Data from Löe H, Anerud A, Boysen H, et al: *J Clin Periodontol* 13:431, 1986.)

Treatment of Loss of Attachment

A longitudinal study of patients with moderate to advanced periodontal disease conducted at the University of Michigan showed that the progression of periodontal disease can be stopped for 3 years postoperatively regardless of the modality of treatment.[25-28] With long-term observations, the average loss of attachment was only 0.3 mm over 7 years.[26] These results indicated a more favorable prognosis for treatment of advanced periodontal lesions than previously assumed.

Another study was conducted in 75 patients with advanced periodontal disease to determine the effect of plaque control and surgical pocket elimination on the establishment and maintenance of periodontal health.[14] This study showed that no further alveolar bone loss occurred during the 5-year observation period. The meticulous plaque control practiced by the patients in this study was considered a major factor in the excellent results produced. After 14 years, results for 61 of the initial 75 individuals were reported.[13] Repeated examinations demonstrated that treatment of advanced forms of periodontal disease resulted in clinically healthy periodontal conditions, and that this state of health was maintained in most patients and sites during the 14-year period. A more detailed analysis of the data, however, revealed that a small number of sites in a few patients lost a substantial amount of attachment. Approximately 43 surfaces in 15 different patients were exposed to recurrent periodontal disease of significant magnitude. The frequency of sites that lost more than 2 mm of attachment during the 14 years of maintenance was 0.8% to 0.1% per year.

Neither of these studies used a control group because failing to treat advanced periodontal patients cannot be justified for ethical reasons. However, in a study in private practice, an effort was made to find and evaluate patients with diagnosed moderate to advanced periodontitis who had not followed through with recommended periodontal therapy.[3] Thirty patients ranging in age from 25 to 71 years were evaluated after periods ranging from 18 to 115 months. All these untreated patients had progressive increases in pocket depth and radiographic evidence of progressive bone resorption.

In a study of the progression of periodontal disease in the absence of therapy, two different populations were monitored.[15] One group of 64 Swedish adults with mild to moderate periodontal disease and one group of 36 American adults with advanced destructive disease were monitored but not treated for 6 years and 1 year, respectively. During the course of 6 years, 11.6% of all sites in the Swedish population (1.9% per year) showed attachment loss of greater than 2 mm, and the corresponding figure for the American population was 3.2% per year. Thus the frequency of sites with disease progression was 20 to 30 times higher in untreated groups of patients than in the treated and well-maintained groups described in the preceding discussion.[15] *Thus, treatment is effective in reducing loss of attachment.*

TOOTH MORTALITY

The ultimate test for the effectiveness of periodontal treatment is whether the loss of teeth can be prevented. Sufficient studies from both private practice and research institutions are now available to document that loss of teeth is reduced or prevented by therapy.

The combined effect of subgingival scaling every 3 to 6 months and controlled oral hygiene was evaluated over a 5-year period in 1428 factory workers in Oslo.[19] Tooth loss was significantly reduced in all patients. This study showed that frequent subgingival scaling reduces tooth loss even when oral hygiene is "not good" (Table 83-1).

The previously mentioned longitudinal study conducted at the University of Michigan included 104 patients with a total of 2604 teeth.[25-28] After 1 to 7 years of treatment, 53 teeth were lost for various reasons (Table 83-2). Approximately 32 teeth were lost during the first and second years after initiation of treatment. The remaining 21 teeth were lost in a random pattern over the next 6 years. Therefore the loss of teeth caused by advanced periodontal disease after treatment was minimal (1.15%).

Another study was undertaken to test the effect of periodontal therapy in cases of advanced disease.[13,14] The subjects were 75 patients who had lost 50% or more of their periodontal support (Figure 83-5). Treatment consisted of oral hygiene measures, scaling procedures, extraction of untreatable teeth, periodontal surgery, and prosthetic therapy if indicated. After completion of periodontal treatment, no patient showed further loss of periodontal support for the next 5 years. No teeth were extracted in the 5-year posttreatment period. Patients in this study were selected because of their capacity to meet high requirements of plaque control after repeated instruction in oral hygiene techniques; this fact does not detract from the validity of the study but tends to show the etiologic importance of bacterial plaque. The results indicate that periodontal surgery coupled with a detailed plaque control program not only temporarily cures the disease but also reduces further progression of periodontal breakdown, even in patients with severely reduced periodontal support.

After 14 years, 61 of the original patients were still in the study.[14] Recurrence of destructive periodontal disease in isolated sites of the dentition resulted in loss of a certain number of teeth during the observation period (Figure 83-6). In the 6 to 10 years after active therapy, one tooth in each of three different patients was lost,

TABLE 83-1

Average Loss of Teeth during a 5-year Period Compared with Normal Loss of Teeth in 1428 Men and Women Ages 20 through 59

	GRADE OF ORAL HYGIENE		
	Good	**Fairly Good**	**Not Good**
"Normal" loss of teeth*	1.1	1.4	1.8
Actual loss of teeth during 5-year period	0.4	0.6	0.9

From Lovdal A, Arno A, Schei O, et al: *Acta Odontol Scand* 19:537, 1961.

*Estimate based on data recorded at initiation of study period.

TABLE 83-2

Tooth Mortality after Treatment of Advanced Periodontitis in 104 Patients with 2604 Teeth Treated over a 10-Year Period

Teeth Lost*	Reason
2	Pulpal disease
3	Accidents
4	Prosthetic considerations
14	Various reasons; for example, one patient wanted a maxillary denture for cosmetic reasons
30	Periodontal
53	All reasons

Data from Ramfjord SP, Knowles JW, Nissle RR, et al: *J Periodontol* 44:66, 1973.

*2% of the teeth were lost during the study period. *Note:* U.S. health surveys conducted in the 1960s indicated that an average of 4.3 teeth were lost after age 35 in the general population.[9]

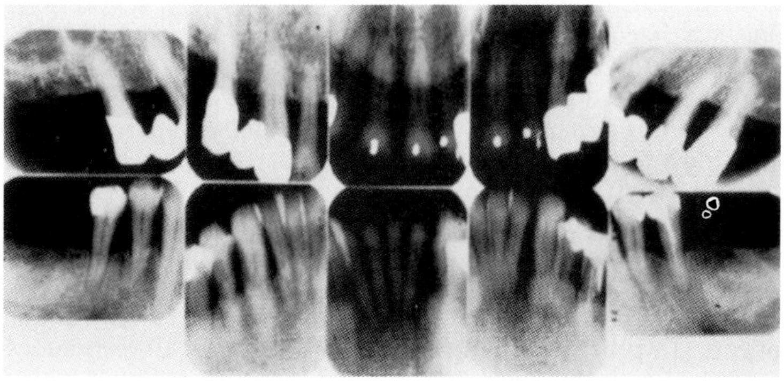

Figure 83-5 Radiographs taken 5 years after typical periodontal treatment. Note the advanced bone loss, despite the teeth retained in a healthy condition for the duration of the study. (From Lindhe J, Nyman S: *J Clin Periodontol* 2:67, 1975.)

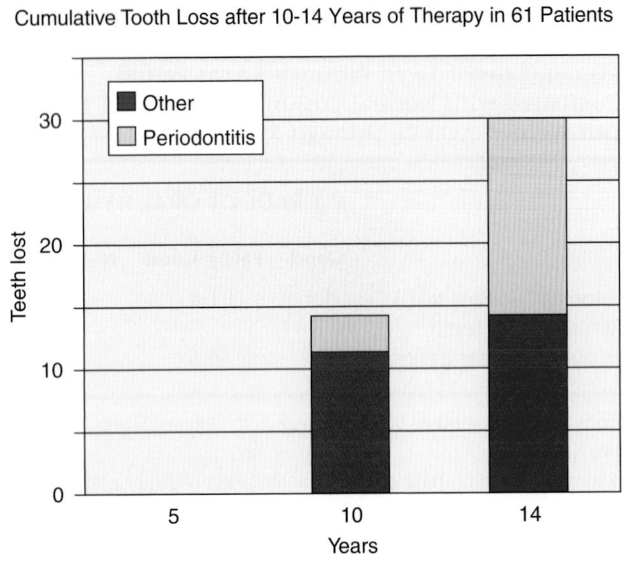

Figure 83-6 Tooth loss in treated patients with very advanced periodontal disease. (Data from Lindhe J, Nyman S: *J Clin Periodontol* 11:504, 1984.)

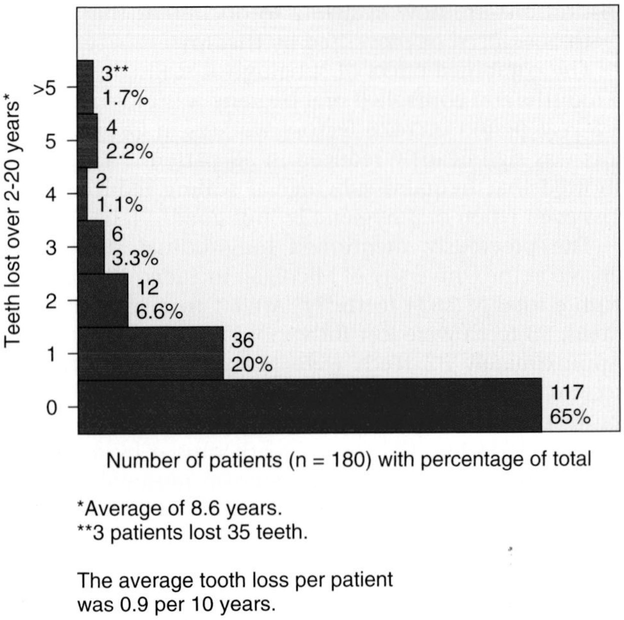

Figure 83-7 Tooth mortality. Average tooth loss per patient was 0.9 per 10 years. (Modified from Ross IF, Thompson RH, Galdi M: *Parodontologie* 25:125, 1971.)

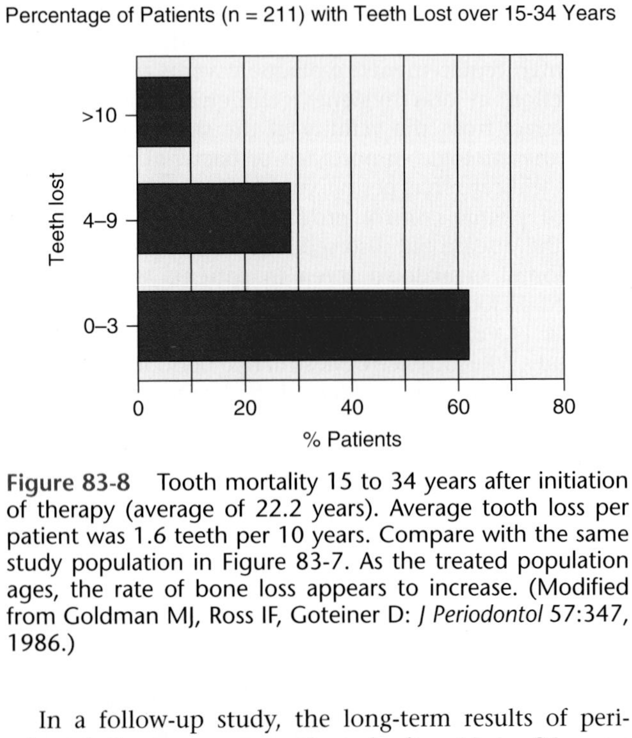

Figure 83-8 Tooth mortality 15 to 34 years after initiation of therapy (average of 22.2 years). Average tooth loss per patient was 1.6 teeth per 10 years. Compare with the same study population in Figure 83-7. As the treated population ages, the rate of bone loss appears to increase. (Modified from Goldman MJ, Ross IF, Goteiner D: *J Periodontol* 57:347, 1986.)

and during the final observation period (11 to 14 years), three teeth in one patient, two teeth in each of three patients, and one tooth in each of four patients had to be extracted because of recurrent periodontal disease. In addition, three teeth in each of three different patients and one tooth in each of five patients were extracted because of the development of extensive caries, periapical lesions, or other endodontic complications. During the entire course of the study, the total loss was 30 teeth (for all reasons) of 1330 teeth. The tooth mortality rate was therefore 2.3%.

Several studies in private practice have attempted to measure frequency of tooth loss after periodontal therapy. In one study, 180 patients who had been treated for chronic destructive periodontal disease were evaluated.[29,30] The average age of the patients before treatment was 43.7 years. A total of 141 teeth were lost. From the beginning of treatment to the time of the survey, the majority of patients lost no teeth (Figure 83-7). Three of 180 patients (1.7%) lost 35 teeth, approximately 25% of the teeth lost. Twelve additional patients lost 46 teeth, or 32.6% of the teeth lost. Many patients in the study had advanced alveolar bone loss, including extensive furcation involvements. However, only a relatively small number (141) of the teeth were lost in the study group of 180 patients between the beginning of periodontal treatment and the time of the study.

The teeth were lost for several reasons, including periodontal disease, caries, and other nonperiodontal causes. The length of time after treatment varied from 2 to 20 years, with an average of 8.6 years. Of considerable significance is the large number of teeth (81 teeth, or 57.5%) lost by a few patients (15 patients, or 8.4%). Even when this group is considered with the remaining 165 patients, the periodontal care helped to retain most teeth because the average tooth loss was slightly less than one tooth (0.9) over the 10 years after treatment.

In a follow-up study, the long-term results of periodontal therapy were evaluated after 15 to 34 years (average of 22.2 years).[4] The average tooth loss at this time was 1.6 teeth per 10 years. Patients were classified into three groups according to tooth loss. Approximately 62% had an average tooth loss of 0.45 per 10 years and were considered "well maintained"; 28% lost an average of 2.6 teeth per 10 years and were considered "downhill"; and 10% lost an average of 6.4 teeth per 10 years and were considered "extreme downhill" (Figure 83-8).

Another study included all patients in a practice who had been treated 5 or more years previously and

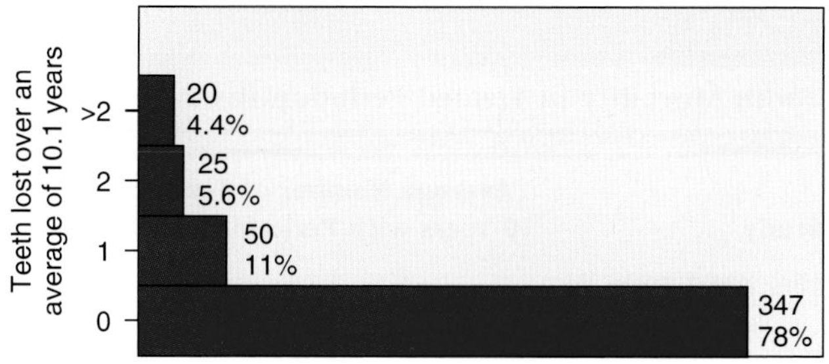

Figure 83-9 Tooth mortality in 442 periodontal patients treated over 10 years. (Courtesy Dr. R.C. Oliver, Rio Verde, Ariz.)

had received regular preventive periodontal care since that time.[24] The 442 patients had an average of 10.1 years since treatment. Two thirds of the patients were older than 40 at the time of treatment. These patients had been seen every 4.6 months, on average, for their preventive periodontal care, which consisted of oral hygiene instruction and prophylaxis (Figures 83-9 and 83-10).

The total tooth loss resulting from periodontal disease was 178 of more than 11,000 teeth available for treatment. More important, 78% of the patients did not lose a single tooth after periodontal therapy, and 11% lost only one tooth. Considering that more than 600 teeth had furcation involvements at the time of the original treatment and that well over 1000 teeth had less than half the alveolar bone support remaining, the tooth loss was low. During the same average 10-year period after periodontal therapy, only 45 teeth were lost through caries or pulpal involvement. Even more surprising are the statistics over an average 10-year period for teeth with a less-than-optimal prognosis. Only 85 (14%) of a total of 601 teeth with furcation involvement were lost, and 117 (11%) of 1039 teeth with half or less of the bone remaining were lost. Of the 1043 teeth listed as having a "guarded prognosis" for any reason by the clinician performing the initial examination, only 126 (12%) were lost over this 10-year average period. The average tooth mortality rate was 0.72 tooth lost per patient per 10 years.

In a third study in private practice, 600 patients were followed for 15 to 53 years after periodontal therapy (Figures 83-11 and 83-12).[7] The majority (76.5%) had advanced periodontal disease at the start of treatment. There were 15,666 teeth present, for an average of 26 teeth per patient. During the follow-up period (average of 22 years), a total of 1312 teeth were lost from all causes. Of this number, 1110 were lost for periodontal reasons. The average tooth mortality rate per patient was 2.2 teeth; when this is converted to a 10-year rate, an average of one tooth was lost per 10 years in each patient. During this period of observation, 666 teeth with a questionable prognosis were lost out of a total of 2141. This means that 31% of the teeth with a questionable prognosis were lost over 22 years of treatment. A total of 1464 teeth with furcation involvement were treated, and 31.6% were lost during the period of study. Approximately 83% of the patients lost fewer than three teeth over the 22-year average treatment period and were classified as "well maintained." The remaining 17% of the patients were

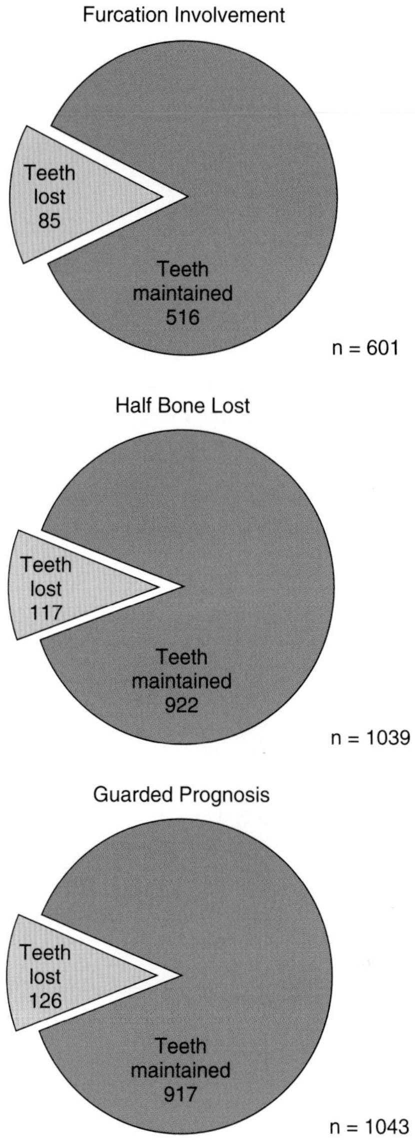

Figure 83-10 Loss of teeth with advanced periodontal disease over 10 years. (Courtesy Dr. R.C. Oliver, Rio Verde, Ariz.)

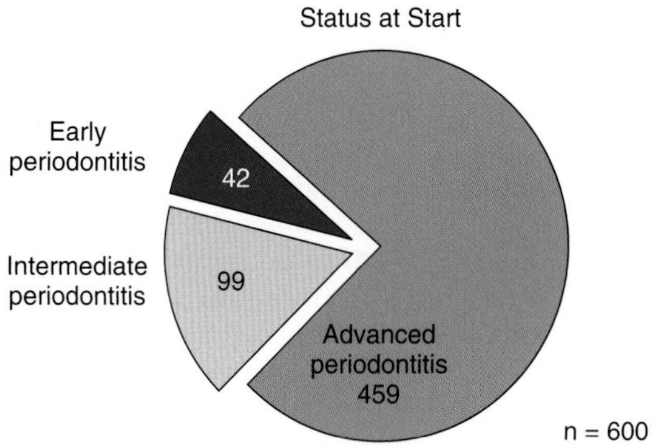

Figure 83-11 Status at the start of a study of 600 patients. (Data from Hirschfeld L, Wasserman B: *J Periodontol* 49:225, 1978.)

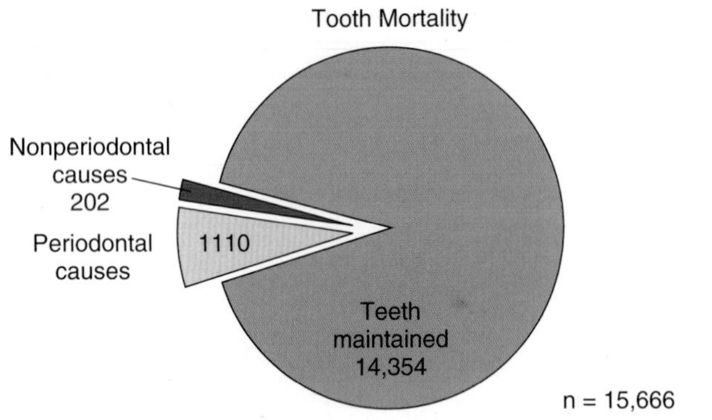

Figure 83-12 Loss of teeth in 600 patients over 15 to 53 years from nonperiodontal and periodontal causes. (Data from Hirschfeld L, Wasserman B: *J Periodontol* 49:225, 1978.)

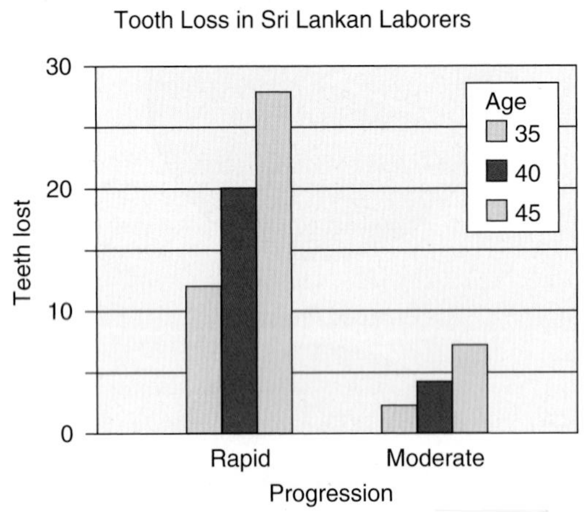

Figure 83-13 Tooth loss in a population with untreated periodontal disease. (Data from Löe H, Anerud A, Boysen H, et al: *J Clin Periodontol* 13:431, 1986.)

TABLE 83-3

Tooth Mortality in Treated Periodontitis Patients

Study	Average Number of Teeth Lost per 10 Years with Periodontal Treatment*
Hirschfeld and Wasserman[7]	1.0
Kocher et al[10]	1.6
McFall[20]	1.4
Oliver[24]	0.72
Ross et al[30]	0.9
Goldman et al[4]	1.6
McLeod et al[21]	1.5

*Tooth mortality adjusted to 10 years by chapter author.

TABLE 83-4

Tooth Mortality in Untreated Periodontitis Patients

Study	Average Number of Teeth Lost per 10 Years without Periodontal Treatment*
Becker et al[3]	6
Kocher et al[10]	5
Löe et al[18] (moderate progression)	5
Löe et al[18] (rapid progression)	16

*Tooth mortality adjusted to 10 years by chapter author.

divided into two groups: "downhill" (4-9 teeth lost) or "extreme downhill" (10-23 teeth lost). Thus, 17% of the patients studied accounted for 69% of the teeth lost from periodontal causes. This study also showed that relatively few teeth are lost after periodontal therapy. In addition, relatively few of the teeth with guarded prognosis, including those with furcation involvement, are lost, and a small percentage of patients lose most of the teeth.

Three studies give insight into tooth mortality in untreated patients. The studies of Löe et al.[18] in Sri Lankan laborers showed that after age 35, an average of 5 and 16 teeth were lost per 10 years in the "moderate progression" and "rapid progression" groups, respectively (Figure 83-13). In a previously discussed study in private practice,[3] an effort was made to find and evaluate patients with diagnosed moderate to advanced periodontitis who did not follow through with recommended periodontal therapy. Patients with untreated periodontal disease were losing teeth at a rate greater than 0.61 tooth per year (6.1 teeth per 10 years). A total of 83 teeth were lost in 30 patients, but the investigators excluded one patient who had lost 25 teeth. Including this patient would have increased the tooth loss in untreated patients to an even higher rate. In another study, reporting on patients with moderate to advanced periodontitis examined at the Department of Periodontology at the University of Kiel in Germany, Kocher et al.[10] found a marked increase in tooth loss in the untreated patients compared with the treated patients when they were examined after 7 years.

When Tables 83-3 and 83-4 are compared, it is obvious that tooth mortality is much greater in untreated groups.

SUMMARY

The prevalence of periodontal disease and the resulting high rate of tooth mortality have increased the need for effective treatment. Strong evidence now indicates that periodontal disease can contribute to numerous health problems, including pregnancy complications, heart disease, stroke, and diabetes.[22,23,31,32] Available treatment is effective in preventing periodontal disease and stopping the progression of bone destruction after periodontitis is present. In addition, overwhelming evidence suggests that periodontal therapy greatly reduces tooth mortality. Every dental practitioner should be familiar with the philosophy and techniques of periodontal therapy. Failure to diagnose and treat periodontal disease or to make periodontal treatment available to patients

SCIENCE TRANSFER

Untreated periodontal disease leads to loss of attachment, increased pocket depth, and eventually loss of teeth. There is abundant evidence that comprehensive periodontal therapy, followed by organized frequent recall visits, results in prevention of further significant attachment loss and maintains shallow pocket depths. Tooth mortality is also very low, ranging from less than 1% to 3%, when patients are followed for many years after treatment.

Thus, untreated periodontal disease results in tooth loss, and the treatment of periodontal disease significantly decreases tooth loss. Additionally, a small percentage of patients lose most of the teeth in studies. These data are particularly significant for two reasons.

First, because the host reacts to microbial plaque with an inflammatory and immune reaction, treatment to decrease the host's reaction is an effective way to inhibit tissue loss, including eventually tooth loss. This suggests, especially in certain individuals, that the host cannot tolerate a chronic infectious process and will eventually eliminate the infection by essentially exfoliating the source (the tooth and associated plaque and calculus).

Second, the data suggest that certain individuals have a more exaggerated host response to the infection (microbial plaque) than other patients. In other words, some patients are at a greater risk for periodontal disease than other patients. The questions then become, Why are some patients at greater risk? and can we determine who is at higher risk?

Future research will focus on these two questions. As the answers become more available, the treatment for periodontitis can become more directed to the patients who are at greater risk, and the therapy can be more focused on specific pathways of tissue loss in these individuals.

causes unnecessary dental problems and tooth loss and places the patient at risk for systemic health problems.

REFERENCES

1. Axelsson P, Lindhe J: Effect of controlled oral hygiene procedures on caries and periodontal disease in adults: results after 6 years, *J Clin Periodontol* 18:239, 1981.
2. Bay I, Moller IJ: The effect of a sodium monofluorophosphate dentifrice on the gingiva, *J Periodontal Res* 3:103, 1968.
3. Becker W, Berg L, Becker EB: Untreated periodontal disease: a longitudinal study, *J Periodontol* 50:234, 1979.
4. Goldman MJ, Ross IF, Goteiner D: Effect of periodontal therapy on patients maintained for 15 years or longer, *J Periodontol* 57:347, 1986.
5. Greene JC: Periodontal disease in India: report of an epidemiological study, *J Dent Res* 39:302, 1960.
6. Greville TN: United States life tables by dentulous or edentulous condition, 1971, and 1957–58, Pub No (HRA) 75-1338, Washington, DC, 1974, US Department of Health, Education, and Welfare.
7. Hirschfeld L, Wasserman B: A long-term survey of tooth loss in 600 treated periodontal patients, *J Periodontol* 49:225, 1978.
8. Hoover DR, Lefkowitz W: Reduction of gingivitis by toothbrushing, *J Periodontol* 36:193, 1955.
9. Kelly JE, Van Kirk LE Jr, Garst CC: Decayed, missing and filled teeth in adults: United States 1960–1962, PHS Pub No 1000, Series 11, No 23, Washington, DC, 1967, US Public Health Service.
10. Kocher T, Konig J, Dzierzon U, et al: Disease progression in periodontally treated and untreated patients: a retrospective study, *J Clin Periodontol* 27:866, 2000.
11. Ladavalya MR, Harris R: A study of the gingival and periodontal conditions of a group of people in Chieng Mai province, *J Periodontol* 30:219, 1959.
12. Lightner LM, O'Leary JT, Drake RB, et al: Preventive periodontic treatment procedures: results over 46 months, *J Periodontol* 42:555, 1971.
13. Lindhe J, Nyman S: The effect of plaque control and surgical pocket elimination on the establishment and maintenance of periodontal health: a longitudinal study of periodontal therapy in cases of advanced disease, *J Clin Periodontol* 2:67, 1975.
14. Lindhe J, Nyman S: Long-term maintenance of patients treated for advanced periodontal disease, *J Clin Periodontol* 11:504, 1984.
15. Lindhe J, Haffajee AD, Socransky SS: Progression of periodontal disease in adult subjects in the absence of periodontal therapy, *J Clin Periodontol* 10:433, 1983.
16. Löe H, Theilade E, Jensen SB: Experimental gingivitis in man, *J Periodontol* 36:177, 1965.
17. Löe H, Anerud A, Boysen H, et al: The natural history of periodontal disease in man, *J Periodontol* 49:607, 1978.
18. Löe H, Anerud A, Boysen H, et al: Natural history of periodontal disease in man, *J Clin Periodontol* 13:431, 1986.
19. Lovdal A, Arno A, Schei O, et al: Combined effect of subgingival scaling and controlled oral hygiene on the incidence of gingivitis, *Acta Odontol Scand* 19:537, 1961.
20. McFall WT Jr: Tooth loss with and without periodontal therapy, *Periodont Abstracts* 17:8, 1969.
21. McLeod DE, Lainson PA, Spivey JD: The effectiveness of periodontal treatment as measured by tooth loss, *J Am Dent Assoc* 128:316, 1997.
22. Meskin LH: Focal infection: back with a bang! *J Am Dent Assoc* 129:8, 1998.
23. Offenbacher S, Lieff S, Beck JD: Periodontitis-associated pregnancy complications, *Pregnancy Neonat Med* 3:82, 1988.
24. Oliver RC: Personal communication, 1977.
25. Ramfjord SP, Nissle RR: The modified Widman flap, *J Periodontol* 45:601, 1974.
26. Ramfjord SP, Knowles JW, Nissle RR, et al: Longitudinal study of periodontal therapy, *J Periodontol* 44:66, 1973.
27. Ramfjord SP, Knowles JW, Nissle RR, et al: Results following three modalities of periodontal therapy, *J Periodontol* 46:522, 1975.
28. Ramfjord SP, Nissle RR, Shick RA, et al: Subgingival curettage versus surgical elimination of periodontal pockets, *J Periodontol* 39:167, 1968.
29. Ross IF, Thompson RH: A long-term study of root retention in the treatment of maxillary molars with furcation involvement, *J Periodontol* 49:238, 1978.

30. Ross IF, Thompson RH, Galdi M: The results of treatment: a long-term study of one hundred and eighty patients, *Parodontologie* 25:125, 1971.
31. Slavkin HC: Does the mouth put the heart at risk? *J Am Dent Assoc* 130:109, 1999.
32. Stamm JW, editor: Proceedings of the Sunstar-Chapel Hill Symposium 1997 on Periodontal Diseases and Human Health: New directions in periodontal medicine, *Ann Periodontol* 3:1, 1998.
33. Suomi JD, Greene JC, Vermillion JR, et al: The effect of controlled oral hygiene on the progression of periodontal disease in adults: results after the third and final year, *J Periodontol* 42:152, 1971.
34. Suomi JD, West JD, Chang JJ, et al: The effect of controlled oral hygiene procedures on the progression of periodontal disease in adults: radiographic findings, *J Periodontol* 42:152, 1971.
35. Theilade E, Wright WH, Jensen SB, et al: Experimental gingivitis in man. II, *J Periodontal Res* 1:1, 1966.

Ethical, Legal, and Practical Issues in the Management of Periodontal Patients

Mark B. Lieberman

PART

10

As important as the biology of the periodontium is an understanding of patient management, dental ethics, and dental legal issues (jurisprudence). Educating patients so that informed consent can be obtained for treatment is an important prerequisite for successful periodontal care. Treating within the ethical guidelines of the profession allows for a satisfying outcome for both the practitioner and the patient. Learning to navigate managed care and associated insurance issues is also critical to a full comprehension of the subject.

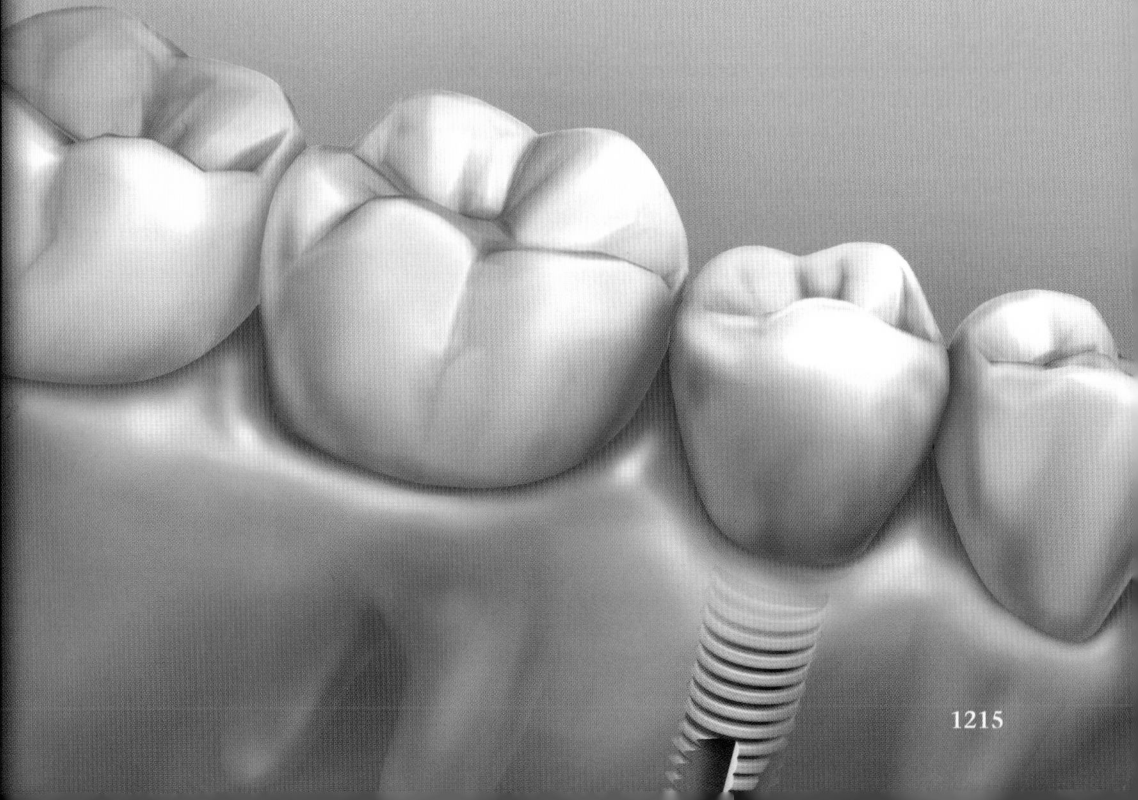

Dental Ethics

Mark B. Lieberman

84

CHAPTER

CHAPTER OUTLINE

To be professional means that the practitioner has the obligation to be mindful of the patient's physical and emotional well-being. These core values are entrusted to the dental professional, and they are critical to achieving successful outcomes.

Ethical behavior is not self-serving; rather, it is serving the larger community. Ethical obligations may, and often do, exceed legal duties. It is important that a dental practitioner have knowledge, skill, and technical competence; however, the traits of compassion, kindness, integrity, fairness, and charity will define the true professional.[9] *Whether it is local or international, ethical behavior depends on honesty and on protecting the patient.*

Ethical decisions can be difficult to make, and they may be subtle or encompassing. Ethics do not exist in a vacuum. They are relative to the culture where they are practiced. To define ethics is to determine how appropriate choices are made. The dentist's decisions must always be based on the best procedure available for each patient.

Organized dentistry mandates certain forms of ethical behavior beyond the primary activity of patient care. Community service is expected. Research and development performed in an evidence-based manner, along with patents and copyrights that do not restrict patient treatment, are needed to continually advance the level of care. All organizations must be self-governing to prevent discrimination, abuse, overtreatment or overbilling, and false or misleading advertising.

PROFESSIONAL ORGANIZATIONS

Dental Organizations and Dental Boards

Organized dentistry in the United States is composed of a tripartite system (Box 84-1):

1. Local dental societies are developed at the community level.
2. These local societies are under the auspices of the state dental associations.
3. The American Dental Association (ADA) is the largest national association. It governs in order to unite the systems and make policy at the national level.

Professional organizations such as the ADA issue guidelines to define and clarify how dentists can best carry out their duties.[9] It is also important to note that the ADA, while serving as the national "watchdog" on ethics, also

BOX 84-1

Tripartite Dental Governing System

- Local dental societies
- State dental associations
- National dental organizations such as the American Dental Association

BOX 84-2

Key Issues in American Dental Association (ADA) Code of Professional Conduct

Patient autonomy: Patient knowledge and participation.
Nonmaleficence: Do no harm to the patient.
Beneficence: Do only good for the patient.
Justice: Fairness.
Veracity: Truthfulness.

SCIENCE TRANSFER

The legal parameters of dental practice vary around the world, with licensing, continuing education requirements, and quality control of practicing dentists all governed by a variety of state, national, and international bodies. Ethics are universally important; one practical aspect of ethics is that clinicians should refer patients to specialists when the treatment requirements are outside their scope of competence.

Periodontists are professionals in the health care field who are specialists in a discipline of dentistry. As such, each individual is obligated to behave in specific ways in regard to other professionals, the public, and patients. One ethical obligation is to be truthful. Likewise, science reveals the truth, and the discipline of periodontics is based on science. Periodontology uses scientific methods, and as the truth guides the direction of the specialty, each specialist has the ethical obligation to practice truthfulness, among other attributes. This *veracity* involves all aspects of personal and professional life, including relationships with referring physicians, treatment planning with patients, and dealing with insurance and other companies and office staff. All dentists should be a role model in the community.

serves to protect the rights of organized dentistry through nationwide communication and by supporting local, state, and federal legislation (Box 84-2; see Chapter 85).

The ADA also serves as a major link to many international associations, allowing worldwide communication and interplay.[9] Within this framework, dentistry is connected to the legal, governing system through *state boards*. These boards issue licenses to practice dentistry. Most state boards are composed of dental and community individuals who are appointed by the state governor. They create, modify, and enforce the ethical and legal statutes of the state. These boards carry the full weight of the state law.[10] A number of states also have separate dental hygiene boards that are ancillary to the dental boards, allowing hygienists to work in concert with dentistry. Some states band together in socioeconomic, "symbiotic" regional boards that are more geographically encompassing, such as the Northeast Regional Boards and the Western Regional Boards.

Periodontal Specialty Organizations

The American Academy of Periodontology (AAP) is the national organization that governs the specialty of periodontics. Besides being one of the ethical arms of periodontology, the AAP strives to serve all of dentistry. It prescribes the requirements for advanced training and certifies specialty training programs. The American Board of Periodontology certifies individual members as *Diplomates* after they pass a series of competency and knowledge examinations. Also, general dentists can join the AAP as associate members. The AAP works to unite all phases of dentistry through education and communication.[15]

Various regional periodontal organizations are also formed to unite and promote the specialty of periodontics. For example, the Southeast Society of Periodontics and the Western Society of Periodontology serve their respective regions. Most states also have individual, local periodontal societies.

Internationally, periodontal organizations are well represented. The European Federation of Periodontology (EFP) comprises many national periodontal societies. The Pan Asian Society of Periodontology represents numerous Asian national societies. Independent periodontal societies in individual countries are also active. These organizations are somewhat analogous to the AAP, and their other functions include holding conferences, participating in continuing education, and publishing journals.

LICENSING

To practice dentistry in the United States, a state license is required; the candidate must take an examination. All the examinations are thorough and arduous, but the content and type of examination vary from state to state. The various basic subjects include periodontics, restorative dentistry, prosthetics, pathology, and ethics. The examination has written and practical sections. The chairman of the California Dental Board states, "The boards have an obligation to protect the dental health of the people of our state, and we believe that the current examination is a viable tool for that purpose."[11]

Other forms of licensure are currently being explored and employed by some states. Obtaining a license by "reciprocity" is available between certain states. Groups of states that are in geographic and socioeconomic proximity band together to administer regional boards. Other proposed forms of licensure include certification through graduation only, by residency, or by presentation of a portfolio of credentials. The ADA is currently exploring a national licensure examination that is relevant and can demonstrate clinical competency.[5] In contrast to the United States, Canada does not use human subjects for its examination, and dentists can move freely between provinces. In many countries in Europe, the European Union governs licensure. International students are accepted at American dental schools, and these dentists can enroll in intensive training programs at American dental schools to qualify to sit for the various boards.[12]

PRACTICAL CONSIDERATIONS IN ETHICAL PRACTICE OF DENTISTRY

The everyday practice of dentistry is typically filled with ethical decisions to be made by the dentist and dental hygienist. Ethics govern every phase of treatment, covering a wide range, as follows:

- Diagnosis and treatment planning.
- Patient education.
- Quality of work performed.
- Achieving satisfactory outcomes.
- Determining fees.
- Insurance company charges
- Communication with referring dentists.
- Accurate and honest record keeping.

Dentists who have recently graduated and who are building a practice face a confusing array of ethical choices. Most importantly, they must integrate their personal and monetary needs with the need to serve their community with quality work. "Value gaps" can arise. This concept states, "Patients' primary needs and wishes are that they be treated respectfully, ethically, and professionally."[8] The ethics of dentistry echo this goal, and dentists must not violate this principle by undertreating, overtreating, or overcharging.

Referral

A major issue facing all dentists is when to refer a patient. It is unethical to treat a patient beyond the practitioners' expertise. It is a good rule of thumb not to treat a patient if all the possible complications cannot be managed. A growing conundrum since the 1980s in periodontal treatment involves "practice management seminars which have been encouraging general practitioners to partake in soft tissue management protocols, and where nonsurgical treatment is looked upon as a much more important income center in the business model."[7] These "profit centers" should not supercede a patient's treatment needs. Clearly, the patient's best interest should determine treatment and referral patterns.

Evidence-Based Dentistry

Evidence-based dentistry is currently emerging as an ethical consideration in the clinical practice of dentistry. It entails the "integration of an individual practitioner's experience and expertise, with a critical appraisal of relevant best available external clinical evidence from systematic research, and with the consideration of the patient's needs and preferences."[6] This is a significant tool in aiding the dentist to determine the best treatment for their patients. (See Chapters 1 to 3.)

DENTAL BOARD DISCIPLINE

Negligence

Unfortunately, not all dentists are ethical throughout their careers. An important function of the dental boards and regulatory bodies involves investigating complaints from patients involving dental care. In some cases, boards will hold judicial hearings to determine whether a dentist was *negligent* in the treatment of the patient. The board is empowered to discipline the dentist. This ranges from public reprimands, to license suspension and probation, and even to license revocation.[11]

Insurance Fraud

Insurance fraud has become an important problem. Fraud involves the presentation of false information to an insurance administrator. This typically ranges from false diagnosis to false procedures and to overcharging. As third-party carriers (insurance companies) intrude further into the patient-dentist relationship, the temptation increases to use them as an improper financial source.

Using the insurance system to reap improper financial gain is a breach of this trust, and it is not only punishable by the board, but also through appropriate state and federals statutes. The national Healthcare Integrity and Protection Data Bank reports that the yearly losses sustained by all medical insurance fraud equals 3% to 10% of all health care expenditure, or $30 to $100 billion.[14]

Other Legal Issues

Other legal issues with ethical implications that dental boards must undertake encompass the following diverse areas:

- Aiding unlicensed practitioners.
- Improper billing issues.
- Improper use of auxiliary staff.
- Improper prescribing of controlled substances.
- Impaired practitioners who are addicted to drugs (substance abuse) are a great concern to the profession. It is important to note that confidential intervention programs are available through the boards.[11]
- Improper advertising has been a growing problem. As dentists compete for patients, unethical advertising has increased.[11]
- All aspects of the professional's conduct must be within the law. The boards can also investigate other transgressions, such as sexual abuse, or as they relate to the dentist's license.

Beyond civil matters, dentists are also liable in criminal cases when they break the law. In the United States, it is usually the individual state's attorney general's office that will prosecute criminal cases, assess fines, and pursue incarceration if necessary.[13]

CONTINUING EDUCATION

It is an ethical duty for all professionals to maintain, improve, and update their knowledge and skills. Continuing education (CE) has been an important and stimulating part of all dentists' practice life. Because of its importance, CE is now mandatory for maintaining licensure in most states. The type and amount of CE varies from state to state and is determined by their respective boards. For example, California requires 50 hours of study every 2 years. Half that amount must relate directly to clinical care; the other half can pertain to practical management issues, state law, federal regulations such as Occupational Safety and Health Administration (OSHA) and Health Insurance Portability and Accountability Act (HIPAA) guidelines, and cardiopulmonary resuscitation (CPR) certification.[12] Many CE courses are offered internationally. With the increasing use of the World Wide Web, many courses are offered online and are proving to be very valuable. UCLA School of Dentistry Section of Periodontics has pioneered the use of such a site, the *Periodontal Information Center,* which offers online tutorials and continuing education.[12] (See *Carranza's Clinical Periodontology Tenth Edition Online* [www.clinicalperiodontology.com] for other CE referrals.)

SCOPE OF PERIODONTAL SPECIALTY PRACTICE

In the United States, periodontics as a specialty involves the many areas of practice, education, research, public health, and industry. All these areas are aimed at preventing disease and restoring and maintaining the health of the periodontium. This involves nonsurgical as well as surgical procedures, maintenance care, and oral physiotherapy.[4,17] Another important area that falls under the large, important umbrella of oral medicine is diagnosing and treating systemic health as it relates to the periodontal process, as well as diagnosing and treating oral pathology (Figure 84-1).[1,19] A thorough knowledge of temporomandibular joint disorder and myofascial pain syndrome is also needed.

Periodontal plastic surgery is an important component in the scope of periodontics. These oral-surgical cosmetic procedures depend on partnership with the restorative dentist to achieve excellent esthetic results.[16]

Of great importance is patient comfort and safety. Periodontists in the United States have historically been trained in the use of intravenous, conscious sedation. To ensure complete patient safety, all postdoctoral periodontal training programs now train their residents for competency in use of conscious sedation.[3]

A crucial treatment modality in achieving and maintaining oral health and function is the surgical placement of implants. Periodontists have a thorough knowledge of the biology of soft tissue and bone and the necessary skills and training in the surgical techniques needed to place an implant. Further, periodontists have an excellent interrelationship with restorative dentists who restore the implants.[2] Implants have a great success rate when placed by periodontists (Figure 84-2). To this end, the periodontal programs train their residents to full competency in the application of implants.[18] The AAP's "2002 Vision" states, "Our specialty will be known for advancing oral health through expertise in dental implants, periodontal medicine, and oral plastic surgery."[15]

ETHICAL RESPONSIBILITIES OF GENERAL PRACTITIONERS IN TREATMENT OF PERIODONTAL DISEASE

Periodontal disease is a chronic disease process with far-reaching implications for oral health as well as the patient's systemic well-being. Therefore it is important for the dentist to diagnose and treat periodontal disease properly. Proactive and conservative care along with

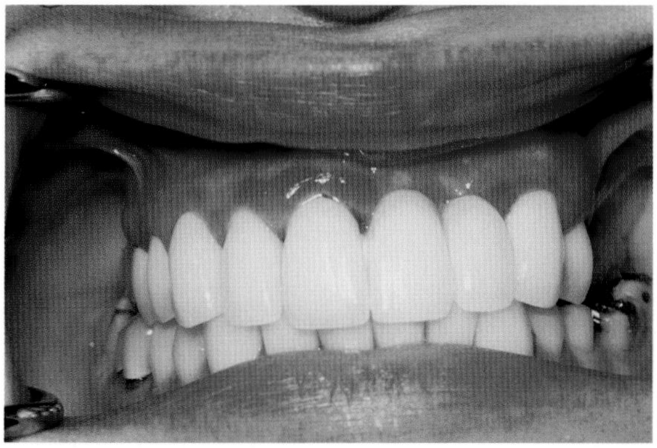

Figure 84-1 Oral medicine is an integral part of periodontal practice. Diagnosis of the patient's oral condition is essential.

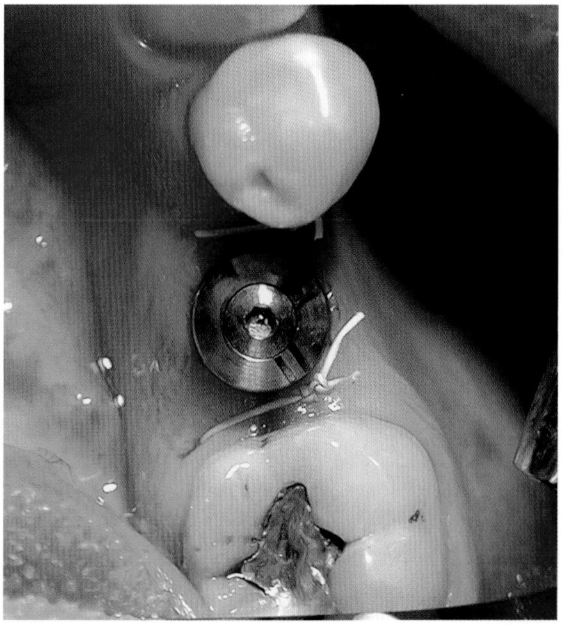

Figure 84-2 Surgical implant placement is an increasingly important aspect of periodontal practice.

long-term maintenance is critical. Patients with advanced disease who do not respond to initial treatment should be referred to the periodontist. One ethical quandary involves the patient who declines appropriate treatment or referral. Appropriate alternative treatment is acceptable, but it is improper as well as unethical to acquiesce to the patient's demands if the work rendered falls beneath the applicable standard of care (see Chapter 85).

SUMMARY

Periodontics and dentistry do not exist in a vacuum; they must function to serve the community. Ethical rules help guide dental professionals in their interactions with patients, other professionals, government agencies, and third-party payers. Professional organizations link, inform, speak collectively for, and promote their members. Dentistry and the specialty of periodontics have a strong mandate to treat with the highest level of ethical behavior.

REFERENCES

1. American Academy of Periodontology: Position paper: Periodontal disease as a potential risk factor for systemic disease, *J Periodontol* 69:841, 1998.
2. American Academy of Periodontology: Report: Dental implants in periodontal therapy, *J Periodontol* 71:1934, 2000.
3. American Academy of Periodontology: Report: The use of conscious sedation by periodontists, *J Periodontol* 72:1624, 2001.
4. American Academy of Periodontology: Position paper: Periodontal maintenance, *J Periodontol* 74:1395, 2003.
5. Ferris RT: A sea change in American dentistry: a national clinical licensure examination, or a residency-based pathway, *Journal of Evidence-Based Dental Practice* 6:136, 2006.
6. Kao R: CDA defines evidence-based dentistry, *Calif Dent Assoc J* 32:217, 2004.
7. McGuire M, Scheyer T: A referral based periodontics practice: yesterday-today-tomorrow, *J Periodontol* 74(10), 2003.
8. Newsome P, Wolfe I: Value gaps in dental practice, *J Am Dent Assoc* 134:1500, 2003.
9. www.ADA.org
10. www.CDA.org
11. www.dbc.ca.gov/
12. www.dent.ucla.edu/pic/
13. www.health-law.com/
14. www.npdb-hipdb.com/
15. www.perio.org
16. www.perio.org/consumer/smile.htm
17. www.perio.org/resources-products/pdf/41-maintenance.pdf
18. www.perio.org/resources-products/pdf/870.pdf
19. www.perio.org/resources-products/pdf/876.pdf

Legal Principles: Jurisprudence

Mark B. Lieberman and Brian Kamel

CHAPTER 85

CHAPTER OUTLINE

DEFINITIONS

Jurisprudence is the legal process in the United States. It addresses any damage, injury, or harm to a patient. This is termed a *tort,* and it becomes the cause to initiate legal action. All professionals, including dentists, are held to a higher standard when rendering care. When they fall below that standard, they become liable for a *malpractice* action. It is important to understand the principles and practice of the legal system to avoid its pitfalls.

Glossary of Legal Terms

Abandonment: Deliberate desertion of a patient.

Actual damages: Compensation for losses that can be proven to have occurred and for which the injured party has the right to recover an amount given for real loss or injury.

Allege: To make a contention in support or denial of a claim or accusation that has not yet been proven.

Battery: Unlawful and unwanted touching of one person by another with the intention of bringing about harmful contact.

Beneficence: Practice of doing good; an act to benefit the patient.

Compensatory damages: Compensation to replace the loss caused by the wrong or injury.

Demand letter: Correspondence from a lawyer on behalf of a client that requires payment or some other type of action; if such demand is not met, formal legal action will follow.

Deposition: Testimony that is made under oath, but not in open court, by a party or witness in response to oral examination and that is recorded by a court reporter.

Discovery: Methods used by parties to a civil or criminal action to obtain information or evidence held by the other party that is relevant to the action.

Expert witness: Professional who has knowledge not normally possessed by a layperson or other professionals regarding the topic that they are to testify about.

Informed consent: Agreement by a patient to undergo a medical or dental procedure after having an understanding of the relevant facts, benefits, and risks involved in the performance of that procedure.

Jurisprudence: The philosophy or science of the law; the knowledge of the laws, customs, and rights of men and women in a state or community.

Litigation: A legal action, including all proceedings; a contest in a court of law to determine and enforce legal rights.
Malpractice: Professional misconduct or breach of duty that results in injury or damage to an individual.
Mediator: Professional who intervenes between two parties in disagreement in an effort to reconcile them; a negotiator.
Negligence: Failure to use the degree of care considered reasonable under the circumstances, resulting in unintentional injury.
Plaintiff: The party who institutes or introduces a legal action or claim.
Punitive damages: Compensation in excess of actual and compensatory damage awarded in cases of malicious or willful misconduct, used to punish the defendant or set an example for similar wrongdoers; these damages are typically not covered by professional liability policies.
Standard of care: Degree of ability that is expected in a particular situation, specifically in the performance of medical, dental, and legal matters in the community. If the professional's conduct falls below this level, the person is responsible for any resulting damages or injuries.
Subpoena: Court order requiring an appearance at a certain time and place to give testimony regarding a certain matter or to produce records.
Tender: Presentation of proposed legal action to the plaintiff's malpractice insurance carrier initiating defense proceedings.
Tort: Damage, injury, or a wrongful act done deliberately, negligently, or in circumstance involving "strict liability" (e.g., hazardous, defective products causing injury).

COMMON PERIODONTAL MALPRACTICE ISSUES

Some malpractice problems are rare, but most periodontal missteps occur repeatedly. Recognizing these common problems will help to avoid them. When practicing periodontics, it is best for dentists to stay within their reasonable level of competency. Patients should be referred to the appropriate specialist when there is uncertainty or when problems first appear.

The most common periodontal malpractice issue involves the failure to diagnose, treat, or refer periodontal disease processes.

Most malpractice cases center on this issue. To avoid these pitfalls, it is critical to recognize and document the periodontal disease process, as follows:

- Scrupulous records, including charting and x-ray films, must be obtained.
- Appropriate treatment must be recommended and performed.
- Referral to a periodontal specialist should be given if careful, conservative treatment is unsuccessful.
- Monitoring patients receiving long-term maintenance therapy is especially important. With the aid of a conscientious, well-trained hygienist, these patients can be well treated. It is important to detect and remove any local irritants (e.g., plaque, calculus). Detailed home care instructions must be repeated, and any changes must be noted and followed carefully to allow for appropriate care.[3,9]

The other main cause of malpractice actions usually involves general dentists' attempt *to treat beyond their level of competence.* Although periodontal surgical procedures are taught in dental schools, it is important for dentists to be able to discriminate between surgical procedures they are qualified to perform and those they are not qualified to perform. Further, when unforeseen problems or consequences arise, the use of a specialist can save a case and prevent a subsequent malpractice lawsuit.

SCIENCE TRANSFER

The practice of periodontics demands that dentists adhere to certain laws, regulations, and standards of care. One of these is informed consent. Part of informed consent is the patient knowing the options for treatment. Similar to interpreting the results of scientific experimentation, several possibilities usually exist to explain the results (or treat the periodontal problem). Sometimes what may first appear to be the best explanation (or treatment) may not be correct for the experimental data (or might not be the choice of the patient). The scientist (and periodontist) must have an open mind and must be flexible. In the case of the scientist, new theories or discoveries might be revealed, and for the periodontist, the patient may be more satisfied and less prone to initiate legal action. Adherence to a standard of care, excellent documentation and record keeping, and informed consent can all help to avoid expensive legal processes. A major aspect can involve remembering, documenting, and treating the patient's chief complaint.

The need to provide periodontal therapy at a minimum to the standard of care means that clinicians must continually upgrade their clinical skills. The use of updated comprehensive textbooks, continuing education courses, and current studies in the scientific literature are all essential. Accurate patient records are the foundation for quality patient care. In particular, the measuring and recording of pocket depths on six locations for each tooth provide the minimal foundation necessary to document the clinician's legal responsibility for each patient. Pocket depth recordings should be done for every patient at the initial examination, on completion of treatment, and once or twice per year during maintenance care.

LEGAL ELEMENTS OF MALPRACTICE

The determination of whether malpractice has occurred depends on several legal elements. These factors act as signposts in the American legal system. To prevent lawsuits, it is critical to the practice of periodontics that these legal elements are followed and are not violated.

Standard of Care

Standard of care is the primary element in determining malpractice suits. Two major components must be considered, as follows:

- The care rendered to a patient must be given with the same skill, expertise, and comprehension as would be provided by a comparable practitioner in the dental community.
- The results of the treatment must be equivalent given the limitations of the case.

It is important to note that general practitioners are trained to perform many periodontal procedures, but their legal standard of care must also be equal to that of a periodontist.

The care given to patients being treated for periodontal disease encompasses many areas. First, an accurate diagnosis is essential, and then an appropriate treatment plan, including etiology and prognosis, must be formulated. Traditionally, treatment is divided into three phases: nonsurgical therapy, surgical therapy, and the maintenance phase. All must be performed satisfactorily and to the standard previously cited. It is common knowledge that dentistry is not a perfect science; therefore, outcomes of treatment do not need to be ideal to conform to the standard of care.[9] Treating beneath the standard of care is considered *negligence,* however, and it can become grounds for a malpractice action. It is incumbent on every dentist to make sure that every patient is treated with the skill and care that will ensure a satisfactory result (Figure 85-1).

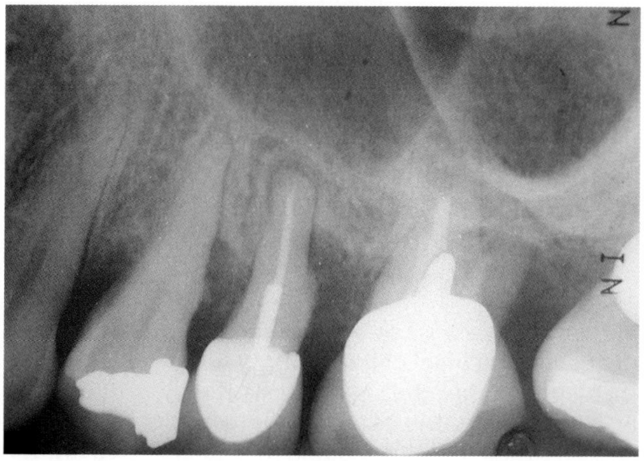

Figure 85-1 Patient was *not* diagnosed as having periodontitis. Radiograph shows bone loss, subgingival calculus, and furcation involvement. Failure to diagnose and treat periodontal disease falls below the standard of care.

Informed Consent

Informed consent is the other primary issue in any malpractice lawsuit. *Before patients can be treated, they must give consent.* The reason for obtaining consent involves the concept that patients are "active partners" with the clinician in their own care. They must feel comfortable and safe with their choice of treatment. To give consent, the patient needs to be given appropriate information by the dental office under the auspices of the dental practitioner. The consent has the following five areas:

1. There must be an understanding of the problem, that is, a diagnosis.
2. The proposed treatment and any alternative treatments must be fully explained.
3. No warranties or guarantees can be given.
4. Authorization must allow for a change in plan if unforeseen circumstances arise.
5. Discussion of all sequelae and side effects must be given.

The consent can be verbal or written, but it must be fully understood by the patient.[4] More recently, many practitioners are using videos to explain the informed consent to be sure the patient is fully informed. Lack of informed consent is a cause for malpractice action, and without it, *battery* (unlawful touching) can be alleged. In practical terms, this means physically or emotionally harming the patient. The dentist must never perform any procedure on a patient without first receiving permission from the patient (Figure 85-2).

Beneficence

Beneficence is the legal concept that refers to providing the patient with the best possible care. If the practitioner is unable to do this, the patient must be referred to a competent specialist for continuing or more advanced care. General dentists are currently treating more patients with mild to moderate periodontal disease, so they must ensure that treatment results or outcomes are at an acceptable level.

As of 2005, there were 4937 periodontists in the United States, and they currently perform the bulk of the

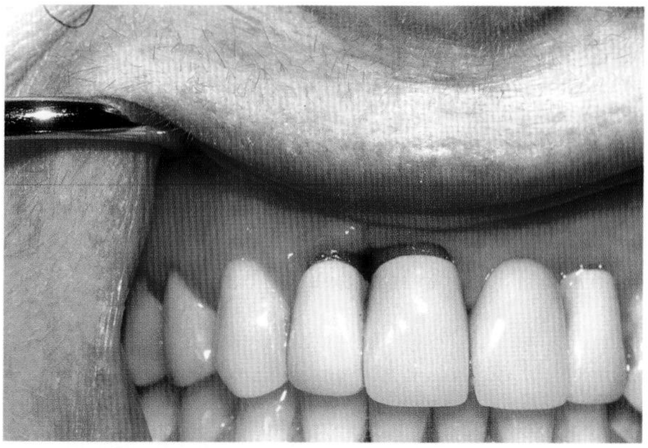

Figure 85-2 Patient must be informed of all possible cosmetic sequelae after periodontal treatment.

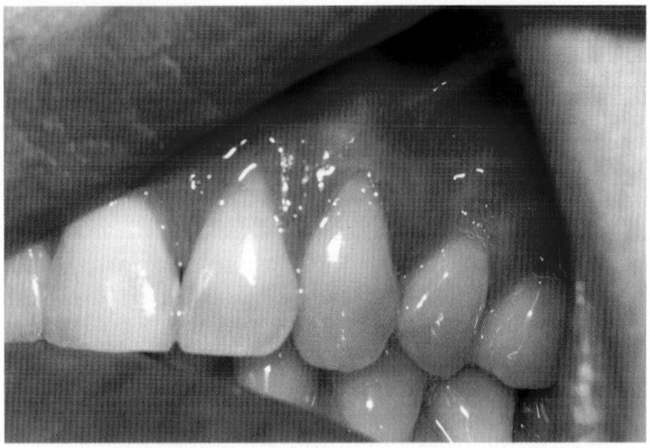

Figure 85-3 General dentists should refer complex surgical procedures, such as periodontal plastic surgery, to the appropriate specialist.

periodontal specialty procedures.[1] All cases where there is any question as to the degree of difficulty or outcome should be referred to the appropriate specialist. It appears that "the most significant roadblocks preventing appropriate treatment seem to be the patient's anxiety, fear, lack or education and lack of acceptance of being referred."[2] Regardless, dentists must use periodontists as treatment partners to avoid legal pitfalls (Figure 85-3).

Abandonment

Abandonment or "desertion" of a patient is a breach of the legal standard of care. Not all professional relationships are tenable. In some situations the dentist and patient cannot agree on treatment strategies or goals, but patients cannot be dismissed during the process of active treatment. Therefore, it is important to understand how legally to dismiss or stop treating a patient. Any discharge should be in writing and well documented and sent by registered mail, return receipt. Dismissal requires the following four elements:

1. The dentist must state a reasonable cause for the dismissal. In the United States the *Americans with Disabilities Act,* a federal statute enforced by the Department of Justice, prevents the dentist from discriminating against any disabled group.
2. The dentist must provide the patient with the names of competent new caregivers.
3. A time frame for dismissal is required (usually about 1 month). Also, the dentist must state that emergency treatment will be provided while the patient finds a new dentist.
4. The dentist must inform the patient that all records (or copies) will be forwarded to the new caregiver (nominal, clerical fees can be charged).

Record Keeping

Records are the most important factors needed to prevail in a lawsuit. Written records, including medical and dental history, chart notes, correspondence, informed consent, insurance request, and billing statements, as well as radiographs, photographs, and models, are the only available guidelines from which to deliberate in a malpractice lawsuit and must be meticulously kept (Box 85-1). All records must be contemporaneous, and they must be signed and dated. *Legally, a professional's written records carry more weight than a plaintiff's (patient's) recollections.*[10] If something is documented in the chart, it is deemed to have occurred. Conversely, if it is not documented, it is difficult to establish the event. The alteration of any records typically results in an adverse *verdict.* Also, punitive damages can be awarded to punish the dentist in these circumstances (see later discussion).

Radiographs are important records. Appropriate radiographs are needed to diagnose and document a case properly. Their number and timing depend on the severity and activity of the case. The U.S. Food and Drug Administration (FDA) issued guidelines advising full-mouth or panoramic x-ray surveys approximately every 5 years. Bite-wing films taken approximately every 12 to 18 months are sufficient to illustrate periodontal disease and its changes.

BOX 85-1

Essential Components of Record Keeping

- Medical and dental history
- Chart notes and results of examinations
- Professional correspondence
- Insurance requests
- Billing statements
- Informed consent
- HIPAA release
- Radiographs
- Model, photographs

PRACTICAL COMPONENTS IN LITIGATION

Once a malpractice lawsuit is filed against a dentist, a complex legal maze is opened. A dental practitioner needs the help of a competent attorney who specializes in dental malpractice *litigation.* The legal process moves slowly (often years) and can be very disconcerting; a calm, professional attitude is needed. Most lawsuits are won by the dentist, and those that are settled before a court trial can have their costs defrayed by appropriate dental malpractice insurance. *The best defense is avoiding the lawsuit in the first place.*

LEGAL PROCESS

The legal process starts when a patient perceives a poor treatment outcome and cannot obtain satisfaction from the dentist. A *plaintiff's* (patient's) *attorney* is hired, who first investigates the case. All the dentist's records will be *subpoenaed* (legally requested) and reviewed by the plaintiff's *expert dental witness,* who is usually a dental specialist. The review, along with the information from the dentist, determines if formal legal action is warranted. If warranted, a *letter of demand* will be sent to the dentist, requesting a substantial amount of money to repair the alleged damage and to compensate the patient for the pain and suffering allegedly endured.

At this point the dentist must *tender,* or report, the malpractice action to the malpractice insurance carrier.[10] The insurance company will start its own investigation to determine how best to defend the case. The dentist's input is needed, but dentists do not have the expertise to handle their own case. An important decision for the practitioner involves the right to demand that the case be defended all the way to a judicial or a courtroom verdict, rather than allowing the insurance company to settle the case for a reasonable amount.

Virtually every insurance policy contains a "consent clause." This means that a dentist must provide consent to the insurance company before a lawsuit can be settled. Generally, however, the policies also contain a "hammer clause," which gives the insurance carrier the authority to settle the case if the company thinks that the dentist is withholding consent unreasonably. Also, all awards are reported to the National Practitioner Data Bank.[6] Individual state data banks have thresholds below which awards are not reported. It is often crucial to the dentist that the award be below that amount, because a negative entry in the data bank can hinder applying for a new dental license or teaching position or receiving hospital privileges.

As the suit progresses, *discovery* occurs. This involves finding all other facts pertinent to the case. Records from other prior and subsequent treating dentists are obtained. Also, medical records can reveal other problems with the *allegedly* injured plaintiff. *Depositions,* or statements in front of a court reporter, are taken under oath. The plaintiff's attorney will meticulously question the defendant dentist regarding his or her qualifications, competence, and veracity and the accuracy of the dentist's records (see Box 85-1). The attorney may be adversarial. Depositions are also obtained from all the experts. The experts usually examine the patient and the records, and they testify to the standard of care being met or breached in the case.

When both sides have all the necessary information, the attorneys will attempt to reach a settlement, sometimes with the help of a court-appointed *mediator,* who will try to obtain a compromise from both sides. Another venue for resolution involves *binding arbitration.* This is a quasi–court trial process decided by a court-appointed arbitrator or judge. Insurance carriers and attorneys try to avoid this because it is rarely enforceable, and there are typically very few outright verdicts for the defense. This arbitration also lacks the right of appeal.

If no settlement is forthcoming, the case will go to trial. Interestingly, a legal defense before trial can cost up to $40,000. If a negative verdict is reached, the court will award monetary damages. The rule of thumb is to award *actual damages,* which are the cost of repair plus any future needed treatment. In addition, this amount is usually multiplied by a factor of three to arrive at an approximate amount for pain and suffering. Other *compensatory damage* amounts involve loss of plaintiff's earnings, loss of conjugal rights, and loss of enjoyment of life. Special damages can be awarded as well. These include *punitive damages,* and as the name implies, the court will award these damages to "punish" the defendant dentist. These are applicable only in onerous cases in which the dentist committed fraud, intentional injury was inflicted, or battery occurred. These awards are not covered by malpractice insurance, and there is no cap on the amount. Clearly, malpractice suits can be very expensive (Figure 85-4).

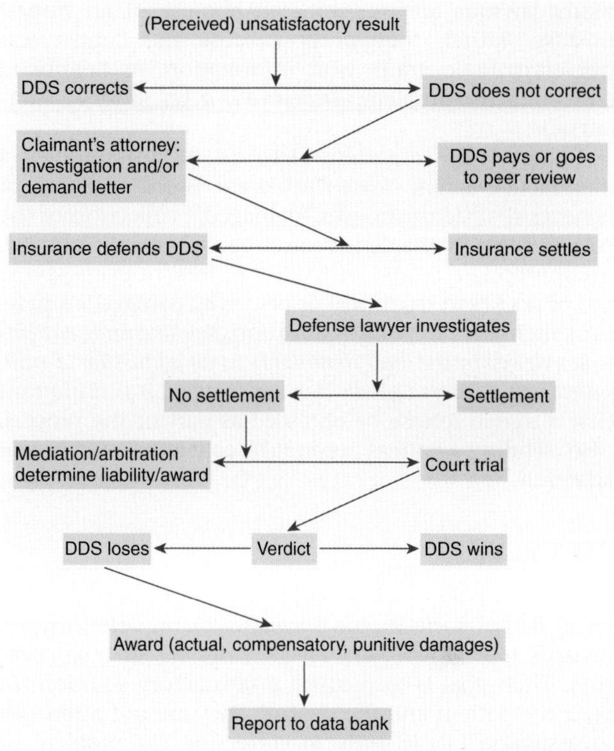

Figure 85-4 Anatomy of a malpractice claim.

MALPRACTICE INSURANCE

In the United States, malpractice insurance is essential for all practitioners. The cost of premiums spiralled out of control in the 1980s.[11] Organized dentistry has been instrumental in helping to enact legislation in order to contain costs. Many states now have a *MICRA law* (Medical Injury Compensation Reform Act), which places a monetary cap on noneconomic awards. In 2005 in California, the amount was $250,000. Insurance covers the costs of the defense as well as any awards to the plaintiff. It is important to use the insurance company's expertise very early in the process. The dentist should have no further contact with the patient once the lawsuit is initiated. The dentist also must start a separate file in communicating with the attorney because these patient records remain protected.

AVOIDANCE OF LAWSUITS

All lawsuits are detrimental to the practitioner and the profession. Not all treatment outcomes are satisfactory to the patient, so dentists must make every possible attempt to educate patients and make them comfortable.

Many lawsuits are not initiated because of an honest mistake; rather, they occur because the dentist was not empathetic, frank with information, or helpful in correcting the problem. *Arrogance is a key factor in many lawsuits.*

Money is an important factor in the initiation of a malpractice action. When a patient is truly injured or believes that he or she was "damaged," collection of the patient's fees by the dentist must be carefully scrutinized. An appropriate refund, reduction of fees, or even paying out of pocket to repair real or perceived damage is a practical alternative to years of litigation. *Remunerating patients is not viewed by the legal community as an admission of guilt; rather, it is a form of goodwill or compromise.* It is important that a signed release be obtained as part of the process. Also, sending a patient account to collections can trigger a lawsuit.

PEER REVIEW

Peer review is an excellent alternative to the legal process. Local dental societies have a panel of impartial, expert dentists (peers) who will review cases for member dentists. Their goal is to mediate a satisfactory solution for both the patient and the dentist. They are not interested in assigning blame, only in correcting the problem. If they decide that the dentist has improperly treated the patient, they award the amount of money needed to rectify the problem. This amount is not covered by insurance but may be well worth the cost.

FEDERAL LEGISLATION

Occupational Safety and Health Administration

The Occupational Safety and Health Administration (OSHA) enforces federal legislation designed to protect workers in all industries. Dentistry is of special concern because of the danger of infections. OSHA legislation covers the following four areas[8]:

- Universal precautions and blood-borne pathogens
- Hazard communication
- Waste management
- Illness and injury prevention

These regulations have a significant impact on the workplace and definitely make the dental office safer. The American Dental Association (ADA) has partnered with OSHA to ensure that dentists can follow the regulations in a practical manner. Violations can result in fines.

The Centers for Disease Control and Prevention (CDC) in Atlanta issued an update for office infection control in 2004.[7]

Health Insurance Portability and Accountability Act

The Health Insurance Portability and Accountability Act (HIPAA) is federal legislation designed to reduce health care administrative costs. With the increase of electronic data interchange, patients' protected health information must be in standardized form and carefully protected. HIPAA includes the following three standards:

- Electronic transaction standard
- Privacy standard
- Security standard

HIPAA is enforced by the Office of Civil Rights.[5] These regulations have a significant impact on the office workplace and are important in protecting patients' privacy. Again, violations can result in fines.

SUMMARY

Untoward or unsatisfactory outcomes can occur when treating dental or periodontal patients. Dental practitioners must be aware of the legal elements of malpractice, and they must strive to prevent their treatment from falling beneath the standard of care. The legal process is difficult and distressing to navigate, so it is best to avoid this when possible. A system of jurisprudence exists to determine liability and to award damages.

REFERENCES

1. Christensen G: What is the role of specialties in dentistry? *J Am Dent Assoc* 134:1517, 2003.
2. McGuire MK, Scheyer ET: A referral-based periodontal practice: yesterday, today, and tomorrow, *J Periodontol* 74:1542, 2003.
3. Position statement and guidelines for soft tissue management programs, 1996, www.perio.
4. Sfikas P: A duty to disclose, *J Am Dent Assoc* 134:1332, 2003.
5. www.aspe.hhs.gov.admnsimp/
6. www.bhpr.hrsa.gov/dqa/
7. www.cdc.gov/oralhealth
8. www.osha.gov
9. www.perio.org/resources-products/pdf/parameters.pdf
10. www.thedentists.com
11. www.Veatchfirm.com

Dental Insurance and Managed Care in Periodontal Practice

Maxwell H. Anderson and S. Jerome Zackin

86

CHAPTER

CHAPTER OUTLINE

HISTORY

Health Insurance

Health insurance emerged in the United States as the country was emerging from the Great Depression in the 1930s. Most of the original "insurance" programs were offered by hospital systems or groups of physicians and included diagnostic and radiographic services as well as "room and board" while patients were hospitalized. Insurance plans did not have great penetration in the United States until World War II.

World War II created a huge demand for labor in the United States. The labor force was significantly reduced by the Armed Forces as the United States fought the war. The posters of "Rosie the Riveter" were produced during this period as women moved into the wartime production economy to fulfill the needs for war materials in a depleted labor market. At the same time, the United States had frozen wartime wages and prices. This wage freeze was put in place to prevent individuals or groups from leveraging the shortage of goods and labor for personal gain, thereby hurting the wartime production efforts.

To compete for labor in these wage-restricted markets, employers began to offer "non-wage" compensation, and health insurance was a popular "total compensation" enticement to work for an employer. The effects of this "employment-based" health insurance system are still in place today, although its relevance to the current economy and health systems is increasingly debated.

Some progressive employers in World War II even opened their own clinics. This was seen as useful from a number of perspectives. In some cases, workers did not need to leave their workplace to receive medical services, thereby reducing the amount of time lost from production. The cost of the health system was also under the direct control of the employer. The Kaiser Health system of today is the evolutionary prodigy of Henry Kaiser's vision for the health care of the individuals employed in his shipyards.

Dental Insurance

Dental insurance has existed in one form or another for a substantial time. Figure 86-1 shows a proposal for a dental capitation plan from 1850.

Formally, dental insurance in the United States began in 1954 as a collaboration between the International Longshoreman and Warehouse Union (ILWU) and the three state dental associations on the West Coast. The ILWU suggested to the Washington State Dental Association that it help design a program for the ILWU's children

THE DAILY REPORTER

Baton Rouge, La., Tuesday Morning, March 5, 1850.

ADDRESS:

To the Heads of Families, Guardians, and the Superiors of Institutions

LONG AND PRACTICAL experience prompts us to believe that the teeth of man can be preserved to advanced age of life, provided he will give them that care and attention which their use and importance demands. It is our object then to reform the state and bad condition of the teeth and remove in a great measure the evils and sufferings of thousand, and more particularly the rising generation.

Our desire is to impress the young with a sense of the worth and usefulness of beautiful and sound teeth, and to accomplish this for the mutual good of all, we propose the following plan, viz:

To open a subscription book by which families can be served throughout the year, having all operation performed appertaining to Dentistry in the most skillful manner for the following prices, viz:

For adults......$15.00
For children from 10 to 16......10.00
For children from 5 to 10......5.00

In addition to the above allow us to mention some very important obversations which should be brought to your consideration. It is the various periods in the formation of the teeth which require the strictest observance and attention of some experienced and skillful dentist, and those periods in life are first, the infantile disease caused by inattention in teething and to facilitate matters at this critical time of life

Secondly, to the attention of the loss of the first denition and the proper arrangement and treatment of the second or permanent set, and thirdly, the treatment they may require in a more advanced time, for the importance of the teeth is such that they deserve our utmost care and attention as well with respect to the preservation of them when in their healthy state, as to the method of curing them when diseased. They required this attention. Not only for their preservation as organs useful to the body, but also on account of their intimate connection with other parts, for diseases of the teeth are apt to produce disease in the neighboring parts, frequently of very serious consequences, and there is no doubt but that disease in the mouth often severely affect the constitution, and are conducive to several diseases of the system, in fine many of you may be victims to these sad misfortunes and know too well the miseries of bad teeth, and the importance of an early and judicious attention to them, and such being the case many have been compelled to neglect them because they could not afford the means for relief, consequently to the advantage of all we now adopt this plan, and do most sincerely hope it will meet your approbation and gain your support.

Being permanently fixed at our office, where we have all the conveniences requisite, and where due attention will be given to all the different branches in dentistry in the shortest notice.

Our subscription book is now open, and all those desirous of subscribing and will engage their families, or single persons by the year will please call our office, corner of North Boulevard and Third Street.

A.L. PLOUGH & SON

Baton Rouge, La.

Figure 86-1 Newspaper advertisement from 1850.

or, following the World War II Kaiser example, the ILWU would open its own clinics.[2] At the time of this collaboration, dental care was considered uninsurable. Caries and periodontal diseases were pandemic, and edentulism was an expected outcome by the time individuals reached middle age[3] (Figures 86-2 and 86-3). Life expectancy at birth was 60 years.[5] Against this backdrop, three dental service corporations were formed in Washington, Oregon, and California within several months of each other.

There is some debate as to whether dental benefits coverage is insurance or prepaid health care. Typically, insurance covers large costs for events that occur infrequently (e.g., fire insurance, automobile insurance). However, dental needs across large populations are uniform, and the costs are relatively small compared with medical costs. The argument is actually one of perspective. For the purchaser of dental services from a third-party payer, this is prepaid health care. The carrier or the purchaser assumes the risk. The underwriting costs of dental care are very well known. In fact, an employer with more than about 1000 employees will probably be "self-insured." That is, the employer will pay the benefits costs while paying a third party to adjudicate the claims and manage the records. The employer assumes the risk, but actuaries have determined, with great precision, what their costs will be for the year. From the patient's perspective, dental coverage spreads the risk of incurring disease and its repair across a population and thus acts as insurance.

Given the high incidence and prevalence of dentistry's two primary diseases in the 1950s, dental insurance plans were written to treat the entire population. At present, neither dental caries nor periodontal diseases are pandemic, at least in populations covered by insurance. Using national data from both the NHANES II study[4] and dental insurance records[5] (Figure 86-4), it is clear that these diseases are sequestered in an increasingly smaller number

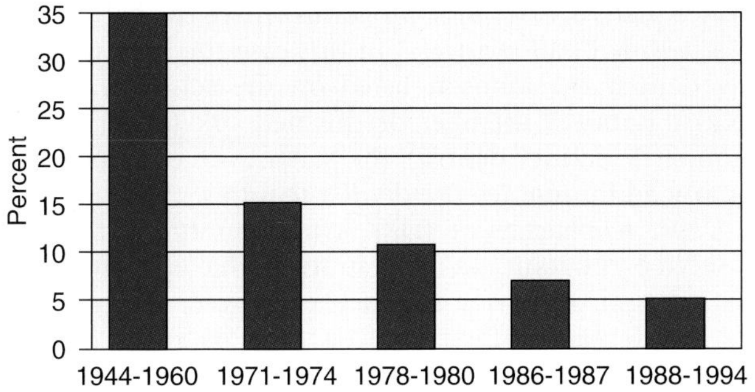

Figure 86-2 Decreasing incidence of caries in molar teeth. The probability that an erupting molar tooth would be restored in the year following eruption.

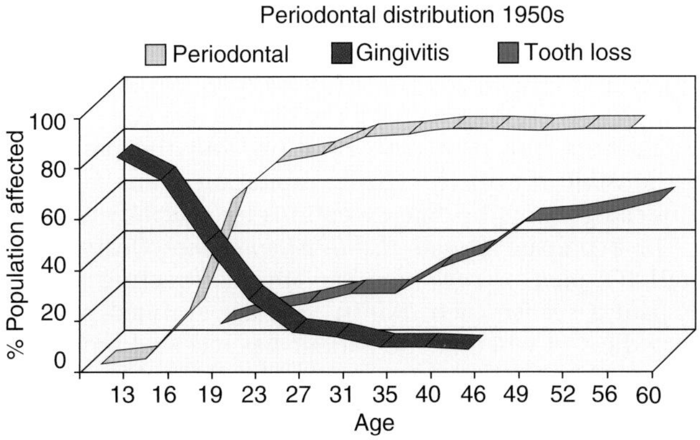

Figure 86-3 Penetration by age of gingivitis, periodontal disease, and tooth loss as recorded in 1950. (From Marshall-Day CD: *J Periodontal Res* 22:13, 1951.)

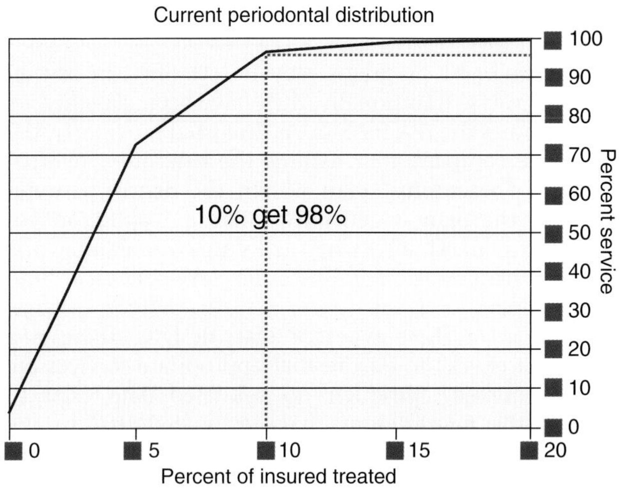

Figure 86-4 Penetration of periodontal services rendered to an insured population of approximately 2 million individuals. Treatments by general practitioners and specialists were examined and include all periodontal services, excluding implants.

of individuals. The penetration of both diseases has been declining for the past 50 years. This uneven distribution of disease makes dentistry much more like risk insurance than when everyone had dental diseases.

PRINCIPLES

In principle, there are only two major ways to provide dental benefits. In traditional *risk insurance* the dental insurance entity assumes the risk and potential gains or losses from revenue spent or not spent on treatment. This is the traditional view of "dental insurance." A less traditional type of "risk insurance" is capitation or prepaid care (DHMO), in which the dentist is paid a fixed amount per enrolled patient to provide a contractually specified level of treatment. Thus the dentist assumes the risk.

The second type of dental payment is aptly called an *administrative services contract* (ASC). Employers, generally with 1000 or more employees, are self-insured and pay third-party administrators, dental services corporations, or insurance companies to provide program management services. Employers have found that the administrative services contractor has more expertise in this domain and can perform these services better, faster, and cheaper than the purchaser can self-administer these functions. These services generally include all the record keeping (administration) and adjudicative practices (rules enforcement and professional determinations of the extent of benefits), but there is no potential for a gain or loss on the dental claims for the administrative company. For example, regardless of whether a specific claim for services is approved or denied by the ASC contractor, there is no impact on its revenues. It is paid a flat administrative rate to manage these activities for the self-insured business.

Within these two general insurance funding types, there are numerous administrative strategies. These include full-service programs in which the administrative entity provides all the services necessary to manage a dental plan. This involves suggesting and developing plan designs, writing the services contracts, receiving and keeping eligibility data, recruiting dentist networks, credentialing the dentists, and receiving, adjudicating, and paying claims for services. There are variations on this theme, with a "ratcheting back" of services until direct reimbursement is the remaining service. In the most basic form of direct reimbursement, the administrator manages only eligibility information, bookkeeping, and payment of submitted claims. No professional review services are rendered (see later discussion).

It should be noted that the purchasers of health care services make the final decisions about what they will and will not put in their benefits plans. Dental insurance companies advise purchasers about the costs of individual benefits, but ultimately this is the purchaser's decision. That decision may be determined by labor contracts because dental benefits are often negotiated benefits. In these cases the union(s) also has a voice in the benefits design. This is a complex process that is not simply a coverage choice for the insurance company, the purchaser, or the represented groups.

CLASSIFICATION OF PROGRAMS

Dental payment programs may be classified in several different ways. Traditionally, they have been classified by who assumes the risk for loss. As discussed previously, the insurance company may assume the risk, often referred to as an "indemnity" plan. When the dentist assumes the risk, the plan is generally called a "capitation" or "DHMO" plan. Finally, when the employer assumes the risk, the plan is an "administrative services" or a "self-insured" plan.

In most of these types of plan designs, there is a system of checks to ensure that appropriate services are being rendered. Although no validated data exist to support the figures, some have estimated that in the United States, approximately 7% to 10% of health care expenses are fraudulently claimed.[6] With a $1.7 trillion annual expenditure on health care, this means that at the high end, $170 billion would be fraudulently expended. With these staggering numbers, purchasers of health care services want external validation that services have been rendered and that the services rendered were consistent with the benefits they desire to provide. There is no evidence that the rate of fraud in dentistry is in this percentage range or that the incentives are equivalent. Most dental plans have annual maximums and patient co-insurance that do not permit extensive fraud. However, the dental industry is still part of the health care industry and is held to the same review principles.

Indemnity plans allow the patient to seek care from any general dentist or specialist of his or her choice. There is no contractual relation between the dentist and the third party. The plan provides benefits for covered services based on the plan's determination of some maximum plan allowance for a procedure or on a fee schedule ("table of allowances"). The patient is responsible for any balance beyond the benefit provided by the plan. Almost all these plans have a yearly or lifetime deductible and maximum payments for specific procedures and involve payment by the patient of a percentage (co-insurance) of the fee. That percentage varies with the type of treatment provided. For example, Class I treatment is generally diagnostic and preventive services and often has no required co-insurance contribution. Class II services (e.g., restorative, endodontics, periodontics, extractions) usually involve a patient payment of 20%. Fixed and removable prosthetics and major restorative procedures such as crowns typically are classified as Class III, with 50% co-insurance. Periodontal surgery, although most often considered a Class II expense, is categorized as type III by some plans.

Other plans offer a contractual relationship between the dentist and the plan. They many involve a *capitation* (prepaid) plan, *preferred provider organization* (PPO), *individual practice association* (IPA), service corporation, or discount plan. These plans may be further classified by access to dentists. In a *point-of-service plan* (POS), patients may see any dentist. The insurance plan may or may not pay a higher portion of the bill for a patient seeing dentists who have joined their network. If the plan pays more of the bill (and the patient less) when a patient sees a network dentist, the plan is called a *PPO*. Point-of-service plans also include programs where the patient has a "schedule of allowances." In this case the plan will pay any dentist the amount listed on the schedule. If the dentist is not a member of the network (also called a "nonparticipating" dentist), the patient will be responsible for any additional fee the dentist requires.

Direct reimbursement (DR) is another type of point-of-service program. In this strategy the employer sets aside a sum of money for each employee, and patients see the dentist of their choice, make payment directly to the dentist, and receive a statement demonstrating that payment. The plan then reimburses patients up to the limits of the plan. In this particular case there is no review of treatment for appropriateness or whether any particular service was actually rendered. This plan is attractive to many dentists and some employers. However, most major purchasers of health services desire external review.

When payment is restricted to only network dentists, the plan is termed an *exclusive provider organization* (EPO). If a patient chooses to see a dentist outside the network of dentists, the plan pays nothing, and the patient is responsible for all fees. Most capitation plans fall into this category, with some exceptions for specialty care.

In a prepaid *Dental Health Maintenance Organization (DHMO) plan* or *capitation plan* the contracting dentist is paid a set fee each month for each enrolled patient, regardless of whether the patient has received any treatment. The dentist agrees to provide all needed covered services with no patient payment except for specified co-payments for specified, usually more expensive, treatment, such as periodontal surgery and crowns and bridges. Although the contracting dentist usually is responsible for nonsurgical periodontal care, periodontal surgery typically is referred to a specialist, who is reimbursed according to a fee schedule. If the periodontist has contracted with the plan, the patient has no financial responsibility beyond a co-payment. If the specialist has not contracted with the plan, the patient is responsible for the difference between the plan payment and the dentist's fee. Payment for noncovered services also is the patient's responsibility. The dentist assumes the financial risk, so if the capitation fee, co-payments, and patient payment for services are not sufficient to cover the cost of treatment, the dentist, not the insurance company or the employer, is responsible for that difference. Conversely, if the patient uses fewer resources than the capitated amount, the dentist gains the difference.

There are different economic incentives and potential deterrents for dental offices to join panels, groups, or networks. With the PPO the reimbursement may be discounted from the dentist's usual fees. If there is a discount, the plan is referred to as a "fee-discounted PPO." The advantage of belonging to a PPO is the increased access to patients for the dental office. The increase in patients is driven by the listing of the dentist in a directory of dentists available to patients and by the patient's economic incentive to see a network dentist because the plan pays a greater portion of the bill. If a dentist needs additional patients in the practice, this may be an attractive program depending on the reimbursement offered or allowed by the insurance entity. However, the additional income generated by an increased patient load must be counterbalanced by the increased expenses incurred for supplies and materials (see later discussion on how to make this economic decision).

Participation in any dental program is a personal decision for each dentist, but before signing any contract, the dentist should obtain competent legal advice. The dentist also should read the contract carefully to be aware of the obligations he or she is incurring. It never is sufficient to look only at the fee schedule to determine if participation in a particular plan will be beneficial.

Government-funded programs in the United States such as Medicaid and Medicare provide limited coverage for dental care. *Medicaid* is a joint federal-state program. Benefits are determined by the states and vary greatly among them. In some cases, benefits may be limited to restorations and extractions for children. *Medicare* is the federally sponsored program under the Social Security Act and does not cover most routine dental services. In fact, it specifically excludes "services in conjunction with the care, treatment, filling, removal of teeth or structures directly supporting teeth." There are some limited benefits for treatment related to trauma or tumors.

SCIENCE TRANSFER

The wide variety of dental benefits programs available to both dentists and patients undergo changes over time. One reason for the changes is the distribution and penetration of periodontal disease (and other diseases). A significant aspect in all programs is a covered patient's risk of developing disease. Several lines of evidence clearly show that individual patients have different susceptibilities to periodontal disease, but presently it is difficult to identify these patients initially. Much ongoing work is attempting to define high-risk patients so that in the future, patients susceptible to periodontal disease can be easily identified, and dental benefit plans can focus efforts on these patients. This would permit more focused use of the dental benefits and money in the plan and could reduce overall costs for dental insurance.

Insurance coverage of dental care is provided through the following systems, in which the risk is borne by different sources:

- In government-sponsored insurance plans, taxpayers assume the risk.
- In an indemnity plan, the insurance company assumes the risk.
- In a capitation plan, the dentist assumes the risk.
- In an administrative services plan, the employer assumes the risk and uses an administrative group to provide supervision.
- In a direct reimbursement plan, the employer sets aside a specific sum of money for each employee, and the employee chooses how to spend these dental care funds.

The authors stress that, in all cases, it is important to remember that *dentists are treating the patient, not the insurance policy.*

BENEFITS DESIGN

Time Limits

Time limits are imposed on various procedures to control costs by holding the dentist responsible for his or her work for a finite period of time or in some cases to permit a reevaluation period. An example is the 2-year limitation on amalgam or resin restorations. Most plans will not pay for the replacement of a restoration placed within the preceding 24 months if the plan paid for the original restoration.

In periodontics, these limitations are imposed on surgical and nonsurgical services. Often a plan will not pay for a second surgery of the same type in the same site for 2 or 3 years. Some carriers interpret this so that benefits are provided for osseous surgery, but not for the bone grafts or guided tissue regeneration to repair or regenerate defects. Benefit frequencies for scaling and root planing are also limited in most plans. Many of these time limitations have not been based on scientific evidence or individual patient risk profiles in the past. Whether they will be based on such evidence in the future remains to be seen.

A separate example of time limitations is applicable to site-specific therapies in treating localized periodontal defects. Some carriers will not benefit the application of locally applied antibiotics, whereas others cover them with little or no restrictions. Others will provide a benefit only after a finite healing period has elapsed following scaling and root planing or periodontal surgery, and then the plan will only reimburse for application to residual pockets that show signs of active disease. The rationale is to allow a healing response to occur, thereby reducing the number of sites that need to be treated. This may or may not be appropriate, depending on the viewpoint of the dentist. This limitation is not validated by evidence because most studies for the current, locally delivered antibiotics have involved placement at the time of scaling and root planing and not after a healing period.

Balance Billing

Balance billing is a term used to describe how fee differences between a plan's allowance and a dentist's fees are handled. Depending on the dentist's relationship with the plan, the dentist may be unable to bill the patient for the fee difference.

Dentists who join a dental plan's group and who have their name listed in the directory and receive patients from among the plan's subscribers may be limited in their right to bill the patient for fee differences between their usual fees and those permitted by the plan. The dentist is trading this fee limitation for the additional patients received. This may or may not make economic sense. Determining whether it makes good business sense is quite simple but does require a careful analysis of treatment provided, the expenses incurred, and the remuneration received. Using the general equation provided below establishes whether this is an acceptable dental plan for any specific office.

First, an office needs to examine its mix of services. For a periodontal office, the mix of time spent in providing nonsurgical therapies, surgical services, and implant services needs to be calculated for a routine 3-month period. The results should be designed to show the percentage of time spent in each of the major areas of practice, and each area should include the associated case-planning and presentation times.

Using this percentage mix of services, the dentist should examine their fee schedule to determine the average hourly gross income for the office. Using the same percentages and the dental plan's schedule of maximum fees or its preapproved fee allowance, the office should calculate the cash flow that will be generated by the plan's subscribers.

It is important to measure these numbers as "dollars/hour of production" and not the total day's hours because unutilized chair time is costly to an office and may warrant participating in a plan to cover overhead, even with a reduced profit margin.

With the previous information, the following general equation applies:

Fees generated per hour at the plan's rates:

Office overhead + Additional expenses + Desired profit/hour

For the purposes of this chapter, "Office overhead" represents the fixed costs of running the office, including heat, lights, rent, computers, insurance, and staff salaries. "Additional expenses" are the variable costs associated with treating more patients and the mix of services they receive.

If this equation yields a number greater than 1, the plan's payments are at an acceptable level for the dentist.

If the number is less than 1, the dentist must determine whether to modify the desired profit. If the dentist has unwanted empty chair time, the calculation should be used to determine if the plan's allowable fees will cover the dentist's overhead and additional expenses.

More complex formulas exist to perform these calculations, but the underlying principles remain the same.

The dentist should do more than determine if the additional income is adequate. The contract itself must be analyzed to determine that all obligations imposed are acceptable to the dentist. Advice should be obtained from advisors who are familiar with dental benefits contracts.

Coordination of Benefits

When patients have access to more than one source of dental insurance, the insurance benefits are coordinated (generally by state law) to determine which plan pays first. Most states follow the lead of the National Association of Insurance Commissioners (NAIC) in setting up the rules for how the benefits are paid. It is important to know that in most cases, neither the insurance company nor the purchaser of the health care benefit controls these rules. It is also important to know what the rules are in your state.

In general, when the patient has dental coverage, his or her policy is *primary* (pays first). If the patient is covered as a dependent under two or more policies, the policyholder whose birthday is earlier in the year usually is considered primary. In most cases the *secondary* carrier will make a supplemental payment only to bring total benefits up the amount it would have paid had it been primary.

Lack of coordination of benefits information on a claim is the second most common claim problem encountered by dental insurance companies. If you know that there is only one form of coverage, make a note on the dental claim that there is no other coverage. Even if the patient is the policyholder, omitting this information may delay a claim because the insurance plan needs this information to determine the level of payment to make in a given situation.

There are a number of nuances in how plans will pay, within the state's rules for payment. It is important to know this information so that it can be discussed with the patient. An easy way to accomplish this with a new plan or when the situation is unclear is to submit an "estimate of benefits." This will allow both the dental office and the patient to review the insurance company's pre-estimates before financial commitments are made.

A caution regarding *pre-estimations* in general is that they are issued based on the claims that have been paid on the date of the pre-estimation. If other claims are being processed but have not been paid, or if additional treatment is received before the claim for actual services is processed, a plan's maximum may be exceeded by the time a claim for the pre-estimated treatment is actually submitted. The only rational solution to this dilemma is to work closely with patients to determine whether they have recently received or are planning to receive other services and, if so, the amount of those services. Pre-estimations also may not be valid if the insured individual no longer is covered because of job change or change in carrier.

As health care costs continue to escalate, an increasing number of purchasers choose variations on coordination of benefits. For example, when both members of a spousal pair are employed by the same employer, the employer may choose to provide coverage to only the employee and not provide secondary coverage from the other spouse's insurance. This is called "non-duplication" of benefits. Alternatively, an employer may choose to provide coverage for only the individual employee. Any additional coverage for a spouse or children is elective, and the employee will pay all or a portion of the additional costs. This listing is not all-inclusive and should be used only as a cautionary guide.

Alternate Benefits

When several treatments can be used to treat a given situation, plans may choose to pay for the least expensive, professionally acceptable treatment. Dentists and their patients are free to choose the therapy that they want, but the plan will limit payment to the lower-cost procedure. The dentist and the patient must then determine how to settle the cost difference between the two procedures.

A straightforward example is a plan paying for an amalgam restoration in a posterior tooth. If the dentist and patient choose to restore the tooth with a resin-based restorative material, the plan will pay for the equivalent amalgam restoration. Because posterior resin restorations are more labor and procedure intensive, the dentist will typically charge one-third to half more for an equivalent resin restoration. The payment of the additional fee is the patient's responsibility. Coverage for implants also may be affected by this contract provision. Although the dentist and patient may agree that replacement of a missing tooth with an implant is appropriate, the plan may determine that it could be replaced by a removable partial denture. In these cases the plan may provide a benefit to the restorative dentist equal to that for a removable partial denture, but no benefit for placement of the implant. In some cases, however, benefits will be provided only for the treatment provided, so the patient would not receive any reimbursement.

Exclusions

Purchasers of dental benefits may exclude certain procedures or classes of procedures as a mechanism for containing costs. For example, a purchaser may choose to exclude orthodontic treatment from its coverage or limit it to children under age 19 years. This represents a whole diagnostic category that is not covered by the plan.

Purchasers could also choose to limit how they will pay for the restoration of a bounded edentulous space. They may cover a three-unit bridge or a removable partial denture and not an implant. Alternatively, they may cover either the bridge or the implant but exclude preprosthetic procedures (e.g., sinus lift surgery).

Exclusions are generally considered totally outside the insurance plan and not limited by the plan. However, this statement requires a word of caution, particularly as it relates to implants. A number of plans will not pay for the placement of an implant (it is clearly excluded in the contract language), whereas the restoration of the implant may receive coverage at the standard rate for a crown. Although in this case the clinician placing the implant must be remunerated for those services outside the insurance plan, the patient should be advised to check with the plan to see if the prosthesis that will be placed on the implant is a covered benefit. Some contracts specify that payment for "non-covered" services (as distinct from excluded benefits) is determined by the carrier. This may occur even though that amount may not have been negotiated and, in some cases, is not made known to the patient or dentist before submission of a claim. In these cases, pre-estimation of benefits is in everyone's best interest.

Adjudication

Adjudication means "acting as a judge or referee." This is a function performed by a dental benefits carrier for the purchaser of health care services. The purchaser wants to ensure that needed and appropriate services for their employees are benefited and that the third-party payer has the expertise to provide this service. This can be an area of conflict between the periodontal office and the carrier in that differences of opinion can exist regarding whether a specific case meets the contract requirement for specific services. Most dental benefit plans "provide coverage for services and supplies that are determined [by the carrier] to be necessary for the diagnosis, care, or treatment of the condition involved." Because few, if any, dentists provide services they do not believe are necessary for the diagnosis, care, or treatment of the condition involved, there can be a difference of opinion between the dentist and the payer's dental consultant.

Differences of opinion occur for a number of reasons, but the most common reason is a lack of salient information being transferred between the dental office and the insurance entity. The key to obtaining coverage, within the scope of the purchased benefits, is providing the claims reviewer with enough information so that the person can make an informed decision. When information is lacking, the person adjudicating the claim is compelled to deny the service because the contract with the purchaser defines the reviewer's duties and responsibilities in this area. It would be a violation of the contract between the insurance entity and the purchaser to pay for services that do not meet the conditions of the contract. Carriers are audited regularly by plan purchasers and must refund moneys paid inappropriately.

To overcome this problem, the submitting dental office should provide enough information so that a person with similar training would be able to make the same treatment decision as the dental office. This can be in the form of a narrative or attachments. The narrative should be *clinically descriptive* rather than the expression of an opinion. The submitter should briefly describe the clinical condition in sufficient detail to allow a person who is not seeing the patient to make an informed decision about the service the clinician is performing or wants to perform. In most cases it is not necessary to describe the procedure in detail; dental consultants know what is done.

Attachments

Attachments such as periodontal charts, radiographs, and narratives are a useful way to augment the information on a claim. They can be submitted along with a paper claim or electronically. Electronic claims have limitations on the length of a narrative, so attachments can be provided either by mailing them to the insurance company or by providing them by electronic means. Some insurance companies are set up to receive electronic attachments directly; however, many do not have this capability.

To fill this electronic business need, a number of companies have entered the business of receiving electronic dental attachments and storing them for use by any insurance company or other professional. In general with these services, the dental office uses its direct digital images (e.g., digital radiographs, electronic periodontal charts) or converts existing documents (e.g., periodontal charts, radiographs) into a digital format. This format can usually be any of the standard formats that scanners or digital devices output. That digital information is transmitted via the Internet to the electronic attachment company using its software. In some cases these images have been integrated into electronic dental records so that only one data entry is required. When the electronic attachment company receives the image, it immediately transmits a randomized unique identification code for that image back to the dental office. The dental office then puts that unique code into the "Comments" box on the claim form and transmits it to the dental benefits company. Because the code is randomized and unique to the specific digital information transmitted from the dental office to the online storage facility, the carrier uses that code to view only that attachment. The images are available for a preset amount of time, often up to 3 years, so appeals and submissions for subsequent treatment or decision appeals do not require added transmissions.

The cost of these services varies slightly, but for periodontal offices they may represent a significant cost reduction mechanism. These stored images are available not only to the insurance company but also to the periodontal office and can be used to share patient information with a referring dentist, thereby saving time, handling, and other costs associated with moving information back and forth. It also eliminates the potential for lost records.

Health Insurance Portability and Accountability Act

The Health Insurance Portability and Accountability Act of 1996 (HIPAA) required the U.S. Department of Health and Human Services to adopt national standards for electronic submission of all electronic administrative and financial health care transactions. Dentists and all other health care providers who submit claims electronically either directly or through a billing service (clearinghouse) are considered covered entities and must comply with all HIPAA provisions. The law requires payers to accept and health care providers to submit all electronic claims in the standard format, but it does not require dentists to submit all (or any) claims electronically. Third parties still must accept paper claims. Because paper claims are substantially more expensive to manage for the benefits companies (as well as for dental offices), it is likely that they will charge a premium for them in the future. In other words, if the dental office chooses to submit paper claims, it will be charged for the increased transaction costs. It is unclear when this will occur, but it is being considered.

MOST COMMON ERRORS

The three most common submission errors that dental offices make when submitting claims to third-party payment systems are as follows:

1. Incorrect recording of the patient's birth date.
2. Providing no information about other potential insurance coverage.
3. Incorrect entering of Social Security numbers.

If these elements are double-checked by the office staff before submission, approximately 50% of all errors will be eliminated.

Third-party carriers also make errors, although electronic submission of claims lowers third-party error rates because the data entry function occurs in the dental office. The most common third-party errors are as follows:

1. Loss of submitted documentation, leading to repeated requests for the documentation and delay in adjudication of claims. This can be mitigated, as noted earlier, by electronically filing documentation.
2. Requests for unnecessary documentation, such as requesting radiographs for soft tissue grafts.
3. Failure to check patients' histories that document prior treatment.

CONCLUSION

Dental benefits are part of many patients' payment strategies for dental services. Therefore it is useful to understand the nature of dental insurance, why purchasers of benefits provide insurance for their employees, and how insurance is changing as the incidence, prevalence, and penetration of diseases change. These areas will continue to change as we learn more about treating the primary diseases of dentistry.

As in medicine, more individualized health plans, based on a patient's risk profile and the best currently available evidence will begin to emerge in dental plans. These risk calculations will take a number of forms and will evolve over time so that in the future, patients at higher risk for either caries or periodontal diseases will have increased access to proven preventive or interceptive techniques.

It is the responsibility of the treating dentist to provide the information on the best available therapies for patients regardless of the limitations of the patient's insurance. *It is important always to remember that the dentist is treating the patient, not the insurance policy.* Armed with this information, the patient and the dentist can reach an individual decision about treatment. It is also in the patient's best interest for a dental office to submit a preestimation of benefits for more expensive and nonroutine treatments. In this way, the office is helping the patient maximize the use of available benefits and is not making assumptions that may limit this opportunity.

REFERENCES

1. Anderson MH, del Augila M: Treatment distribution in an insured population, 1998 (Unpublished study of insurance data).
2. Goodman BF: Personal communication, 2000.
3. Marshall-Day CD: The epidemiology of periodontal disease, *J Periodontal Res* 22:13, 1951.
4. National Center for Health Statistics (NCHS): Second National Health and Nutrition Examination Survey (NHANES II), Hyattsville, Md, 1996, NCHS.
5. National Center for Health Statistics: Life expectancy at birth and at 65 years of age by sex and race, 1900-2000, http://www.cdc.gov/nchs/fastats/lifexpec.htm, 2005.
6. National Health Care Fraud Association: Health care fraud: a serious and costly reality for all Americans, http://www.nhcaa.org/pdf/all_about_hcf.pdf, 2005.

INDEX

Page numbers followed by f indicate figures; t, tables; b, boxes.

D

U